Morton Smith

# A Practice of Anaesthesia

WYLIE AND CHURCHILL-DAVIDSON'S

# A Practice of Anaesthesia

Edited by

H. C. CHURCHILL-DAVIDSON
M.A., M.D. (Cantab.), F.F.A.R.C.S.

*Consultant Anaesthetist, St. Thomas's Hospital and The Chelsea Hospital for Women*

*Fifth Edition*

1984

LLOYD-LUKE (MEDICAL BOOKS) LTD
49 NEWMAN STREET LONDON W1

| | |
|---|---|
| FIRST EDITION | 1960 |
| *Reprinted* | 1960 |
| *Reprinted* | 1962 |
| SECOND EDITION | 1966 |
| *Reprinted* | 1970 |
| THIRD EDITION | 1972 |
| FOURTH EDITION | 1978 |
| *Reprinted* | 1979 |
| FIFTH EDITION | 1984 |

(This work has also been translated into the Polish, Spanish, Italian and Portuguese languages)

FILMSET, PRINTED AND BOUND IN ENGLAND BY
HAZELL WATSON AND VINEY LTD
AYLESBURY, BUCKS
ISBN 0 85324 199 6

# Associate Editors

C. APS, M.B., B.S. (London), F.F.A.R.C.S.
*Consultant Anaesthetist, St. Thomas's Hospital, London*

T. H. S. BURNS, M.A., B.M., B.Ch. (Oxon), F.F.A.R.C.S.
*Consultant Anaesthetist, St. Thomas's Hospital and the Royal Northern Hospital, London*

A. J. CLEMENT, M.B., B.S. (London), F.F.A.R.C.S.
*Consultant Anaesthetist, St. Thomas's Hospital, London*

A. J. COLEMAN, M.B., B.S. (London), F.F.A.R.C.S.
*Consultant Anaesthetist, Northwick Park Hospital, London*

C. M. CONWAY, M.B., B.S. (London), F.F.A.R.C.S.
*Professor of Anaesthetics, Westminster Medical School, London*

G. J. DOBB, B.Sc., M.B., B.S. (London), M.R.C.P., F.F.A.R.C.S.
*Specialist in Intensive Care, Royal Perth Hospital, Perth, Western Australia*

S. A. FELDMAN, B.Sc. (London), M.B., B.S., F.F.A.R.C.S.
*Consultant Anaesthetist, Westminster Hospital, London*

J. W. W. GOTHARD, M.B., B.S. (London), F.F.A.R.C.S.
*Consultant Anaesthetist, Brompton Hospital, London*

I. C. GREGORY, M.D. (Cantab.), M.R.C.P., F.F.A.R.C.S.
*Consultant Anaesthetist, Charing Cross Hospital, London*

TESSA HUNT, M.B., B.S. (London), M.R.C.P., F.F.A.R.C.S.
*Consultant Anaesthetist, St. Thomas's Hospital, London*

D. M. JUSTINS, M.B., B.S. (Queensland), F.F.A.R.C.S.
*Consultant Anaesthetist, St. Thomas's Hospital, London*

R. A. F. LINTON, M.D. (London), F.F.A.R.C.S.
*Consultant Anaesthetist, St. Thomas's Hospital, London*

J. A. MATHIAS, M.B., B.S. (London), F.F.A.R.C.S.
*Consultant Anaesthetist, St. Thomas's Hospital, London*

FELICITY J. M. REYNOLDS, M.D. (London), F.F.A.R.C.S.
*Senior Lecturer, Department of Anaesthetics, St. Thomas's Hospital Medical School, London*

H. F. SEELEY, B.A., M.Sc. (Stanford), M.A., M.B., B.S. (London), F.F.A.R.C.S.
*Consultant Anaesthetist and Honorary Senior Lecturer, St. George's Hospital, London*

MARGARET J. SEMPLE, B.Sc., M.B., B.S. (London), M.R.C.P., M.R.C.Path.
*Lecturer in Haematology, St. Thomas's Hospital Medical School, London*

S. E. SMITH, M.A. (Oxon), Ph.D. (London), D.M. (Oxon), D.A.
*Professor of Applied Pharmacology and Therapeutics, St. Thomas's Hospital Medical School, London*

E. SUMNER, M.A., B.M., B.Ch. (Oxon), F.F.A.R.C.S.
*Consultant Anaesthetist, Hospital for Sick Children, London*

A. C. THURLOW, M.B., B.S. (London), F.F.A.R.C.S.
*Consultant Anaesthetist, St. George's Hospital, London*

D. J. WILKINSON, M.B., B.S. (London), F.F.A.R.C.S.
*Consultant Anaesthetist, St. Bartholomew's Hospital, London*

R. P. WISE, M.B., B.S. (London), F.F.A.R.C.S.
*Consultant Anaesthetist, St. Thomas's Hospital, London*

# Assistant Editors

M. LIM, B.Sc., M.B., B.S. (London), M.R.C.P., F.F.A.R.C.S.
*Senior Registrar, St. Thomas's Hospital, London*

D. J. LINTIN, M.B., B.S. (London), F.F.A.R.C.S.
*Lecturer, Department of Anaesthetics, St. Thomas's Hospital Medical School, London*

W. J. K. RICKFORD, M.B., B.S. (London), F.F.A.R.C.S.
*Senior Registrar, St. Thomas's Hospital, London*

# Preface to the Fifth Edition

First, the format has been radically changed in an attempt to make the whole more readable. For example, a double column lay-out has been introduced. At the beginning of every chapter there is a list of Contents which the reader can use both as a preliminary introduction, and for revision after perusal. Also, all figures have been acknowledged in the text. Finally, a modified version of the Vancouver system of references has been used; by removing names from the text, it was felt that it would lessen the disturbance for the first-time reader, whilst still providing the research worker with the vital information needed.

Many of the previous team of authors have volunteered to contribute to this new edition and to them, as always, I am extremely grateful. I would like to welcome some new members. Dr. Robert Linton, having played a major role in the production of the fourth edition, now has undertaken the revision of four chapters relating to Respiratory Physiology. Dr. Christopher Aps has joined with Dr. Tony Clement to produce four sparkling chapters on the Cardiovascular System. Dr. Hugh Seeley writing on Artificial Respiration and Dr. John Gothard on Thoracic Anaesthesia have produced two brilliant new chapters full of the latest information. The most important contribution to this fifth edition is the introduction of a new chapter on Intensive Therapy. Teaching in this subject is playing an increasingly important role in the training of anaesthetists. Dr. Geoffrey Dobb, with his anaesthetic background based on St. Thomas's Hospital, now works exclusively in the Intensive Therapy Unit at the Royal Perth Hospital in Australia. He brings his expertise to this subject as well as re-writing the chapter on Body Water, Electrolytes and Parenteral Fluid Therapy.

Their addition to the Board of Associate Editors and the excellent new chapters from Dr. Tessa Hunt with Dr. Margaret Semple of this hospital, writing on Blood Transfusion, Dr. Doug Justins' three chapters on Anaesthesia for Obstetrics and Gynaecology, Dr. Ted Sumner of Great Ormond Street Hospital on Paediatric Anaesthesia, Dr. Alex Thurlow of St. George's Hospital on Anaesthesia for Oral and Dental Surgery, and the concluding chapter by Dr. David Wilkinson of St. Bartholomew's Hospital on a Historical Perspective of Anaesthetic Equipment, have considerably strengthened the team and made the task of an Editor a pleasure. Finally, a new chapter has been produced by Dr. John Mathias on Anaesthesia for Special Situations. Without the help and enthusiasm of all these authors, this volume would never have reached fruition.

As in any large work of this kind, there are a number of people in the background who have played a leading role in its production. First and foremost is Mrs. Coral Feltham, who has borne the brunt of the typing and preparation of the manuscripts. I owe her a sincere debt of gratitude. Others I would like to mention are Professor Ian Phillips for his advice on sterilisation of anaesthetic equipment, Dr. Lucien Morris and Dr. Peter Horsey for their discussion on low flow anaesthesia, Dr. Cathy James for her help with Chapter 30, Mr. Tom Brandon and Mr. Alan Pache and their teams for all their photographic skills, Miss Valerie Martin for her artistic assistance with illustrations and diagrams and, finally, Drs. Morton Lim, Jeremy Rickford and David Lintin for their help with checking the manuscript. Dr. Rickford has also laboured long and hard on the compilation of the index.

In conclusion, I would like to thank our publisher—Douglas Luke—most sincerely for his unfailing courtesy, patience and skilful advice throughout the long period of the preparation of this book.

H. C. CHURCHILL-DAVIDSON

*January*, 1984

# Preface to the First Edition

Physiological and pharmacological principles now govern the choice of anaesthetic drugs and techniques; and, although many patients can be safely dealt with by routines born of experience, a sound understanding of the background of a particular patient enables the proper and best choice to be made.

In a sense anaesthesia is simply the application of a knowledge of the pharmacological action of drugs to known physiology and pathology, and for this reason the student of anaesthesia must be well-versed in the basic sciences and their application to anaesthesia. Moreover, he must be aware of the modern trends in the medical and surgical care of patients.

We have deliberately assumed that our readers are familiar with the elementary practice of anaesthesia, and practical methods are not always dealt with in great detail, unless they are either of special value though rarely performed, or likely to be required by only a small proportion of practitioners. By the addition of a little more than the bare requirements for competent anaesthesia in the operating theatre, and in some places by the description of a particular disease, pathological process or therapeutic measure, it is hoped to give the reader a broader view of the subject and a better foundation from which to assess the value of the specialty.

The preparation of a book of this nature has necessitated frequent reference to standard and specialised texts and papers in the world literature. These are acknowledged in the relevant parts of this work, but we wish to express our indebtedness to their authors since they have been the foundations upon which we have built, and to crave indulgence should any acknowledgement—through oversight—have been omitted.

A very special word of thanks must be made to Dr. M. D. Nosworthy, who first interested and instructed us in the art and science of anaesthesia. Not only has he read and corrected the greater part of the manuscript, and contributed a foreword to it, but he has never failed to give us helpful advice. We are very grateful to the contributors of special chapters, and to Dr. C. A. Foster for his continuous industry and unstinted aid during each stage of the preparation of the book.

It is a very great pleasure to acknowledge the help of Mr. Douglas Luke, our publisher, who, despite the many years that have passed during the preparation of this work, has never failed to understand the difficulties that beset medical authors.

Finally, without the expert secretarial care and continuous aid of Miss Jean Davenport and her assistants, it is very doubtful whether this book could ever have been completed.

W. D. WYLIE
H. C. CHURCHILL-DAVIDSON

*May*, 1959

# Contents

SECTION THREE *The Nervous System*



SECTION FOUR *The Metabolic, Digestive and Excretory Systems*



SECTION FIVE *The Endocrine System*



SECTION SIX *The Reproductive System*

## SECTION SEVEN *Special Situations*



## SECTION EIGHT *History*



## *Appendices*

# Abbreviations Used in the Book

| | |
|---|---|
| Å | Ångström |
| A-a | Alveolar-arterial |
| ACD | Acid citrate dextrose |
| ACE | Mixture of one part alcohol, 2 parts chloroform and 3 parts ether |
| ACh | Acetylcholine |
| ACTH | Adrenocorticotrophic hormone |
| ADH | Antidiuretic hormone |
| ADP | Adenosine diphosphate |
| AMP | Adenosine monophosphate |
| APUD | Amine percursor, uptake and decarboxylation |
| ARDS | Adult respiratory distress syndrome |
| ASA | American Society of Anesthesiologists |
| ATP | Adenosine triphosphate |
| AV | Atrioventricular |
| BART | Blood activated recalcification time |
| BBB | Bundle branch block |
| BUN | Blood urea nitrogen |
| BV | Blood volume |
| CAD | Coronary artery disease |
| $Cao_2$ | Oxygen content of arterial blood |
| CAS | Central anticholinergic syndrome |
| CAT | Computerised axial tomography |
| CBF | Coronary blood flow (sometimes Cerebral blood flow) |
| CC | Closing capacity |
| $Cc'o_2$ | Oxygen content of pulmonary end-capillary blood |
| CCU | Coronary Care Unit |
| CDP | Constant distending pressure |
| CFM | Cerebral function monitor |
| CK | Creatinine kinase |
| $CMRO_2$ | Cerebral oxygen consumption |
| CNS | Central nervous system |
| COP | Colloid osmotic or oncotic pressure |
| CPAP | Continuous positive airway pressure |
| CPD | Citrate phosphate dextrose |
| CPK | Creatinine phosphokinase |
| CPR | Cardiopulmonary resuscitation |
| CSF | Cerebrospinal fluid |
| CTZ | Chemoreceptor trigger zone |
| $C\bar{v}o_2$ | Oxygen content of mixed venous or pulmonary arterial blood |
| CVP | Central venous pressure |
| D and C | Dilatation and curettage |
| DC | Direct current |
| DIC | Disseminated intravascular coagulation |
| DNA | Deoxyribonucleic acid |
| DPG | Diphosphoglycerate |
| DPTI | Diastolic pressure time index |
| ECF | Extracellular fluid |
| ECF-A | Eosinophil chemotactic factor of anaphylaxis |
| ECG | Electrocardiograph |
| ECM | External cardiac massage |
| ECMO | Extracorporeal membrane oxygenation |
| ECT | Electroconvulsive therapy |
| $ED_{50}$ | Estimated dose to produce a 50% response |
| EEG | Electroencephalogram |
| EFP | Effective filtration pressure |
| EHBF | Estimated hepatic blood flow |

| | |
|---|---|
| EIP | End-inspiratory pause |
| e.m.f. | Electromotive force |
| EMG | Electromyograph |
| ER | Expiratory retard |
| ERPF | Effective renal plasma flow |
| ESR | Erythrocyte sedimentation rate |
| F.D.A. | Federal Drug Administration |
| FDP | Fibrin degradation products |
| $Fe^{++}$ | Ferrous iron |
| FEP | Fluoroethylenepropylene |
| $FEV_1$ | Forced expiratory volume in one second |
| FFP | Fresh frozen plasma |
| FGF | Fresh gas flow |
| FHR | Fetal heart rate |
| $F_{IO_2}$ | Inspired oxygen concentration |
| FRC | Functional residual capacity |
| FVC | Forced vital capacity |
| GABA | 5-gamma-aminobutyric acid |
| GFR | Glomerular filtration rate |
| GGT | Gamma-glutamyl transpeptidase |
| HAFOE | High air flow with oxygen enrichment |
| Hb.A | Normal adult haemoglobin |
| HBAg | Hepatitis B antigen |
| Hb.F | Fetal haemoglobin |
| Hb.S | Sickle-cell haemoglobin |
| HD | High density |
| HFJV | High-frequency jet ventilation |
| HFO | High-frequency oscillations |
| HFPPV | High-frequency positive-pressure ventilation |
| HFV | High-frequency ventilation |
| HLA | Human leucocyte antigen |
| HMD | Hyaline membrane disease |
| HT | High tension |
| HTIG | Human tetanus immunoglobulin |
| Hz | Hertz |
| IABP | Intra-aortic balloon pump |
| ICD | Isocitric dehydrogenase |
| ICF | Intracellular fluid |
| ICP | Intracranial pressure |
| ICU | Intensive Care Unit |
| I:E | Inspiratory : expiratory time ratio |
| IMV | Intermittent mandatory ventilation |
| INPV | Intermittent negative-pressure ventilation |
| IPPV | Intermittent positive-pressure ventilation |
| ISA | Intrinsic sympathomimetic activity |
| ISO | International Standards Organisation |
| IVC | Inferior vena cava |
| JVP | Jugular venous pressure |
| kPa | Kilopascal |
| LAHB | Left anterior hemiblock |
| LAP | Left atrial pressure |
| LD | Low density |
| LDH | Lactic dehydrogenase |
| LIS | Low ionic strength |
| LOS | Lower oesophageal sphincter |
| LPHB | Left posterior hemiblock |
| LSD | Lysergic acid diethylamide |
| LT | Low threshold |
| LVEDP | Left ventricular end-diastolic pressure |
| LVF | Left ventricular failure |
| MAC | Minimum alveolar anaesthetic concentration |
| MAST | Military anti-shock trousers |
| MAOI | Monoamine oxidase inhibitors |
| MBC | Maximum breathing capacity |
| MEPP | Miniature end-plate potential |
| MMV | Mandatory minute volume |
| MSH | Melanocyte stimulating hormone |
| NAD | Nicotinamide adenine dinucleotide |
| NADP | Nicotinamide adenosine diphosphate |
| NEEP | Negative end-expiratory pressure |
| NHS | National Health Service |
| $P_{50}$ | The oxygen tension at which haemoglobin is 50% saturated with oxygen |
| $Pa_{CO_2}$ | Arterial carbon dioxide tension |
| $P_{ACO_2}$ | Alveolar carbon dioxide tension |
| $Pa_{O_2}$ | Arterial oxygen tension |
| $P_{AO_2}$ | Alveolar oxygen tension |
| PAF | Platelet activating factor |
| PAH | Para-amino-hippuric acid |
| PAWP | Pulmonary artery wedge pressure |
| $P_{CO_2}$ | Carbon dioxide tension |
| PCV | Packed cell volume |
| PDA | Patent ductus arteriosus |
| $P\bar{E}_{CO_2}$ | Mixed expired carbon dioxide tension |
| PEEP | Positive end-expiratory pressure |
| PEFR | Peak expiratory flow rate |
| $P\bar{E}_{O_2}$ | Mixed expired oxygen tension |
| PET | Pre-eclamptic toxaemia |
| $PGE_1$, $PGE_2$ | Prostaglandin $E_1$, $E_2$ etc. |
| $P_{IO_2}$ | Inspired oxygen tension |
| PIVKA | Proteins induced by vitamin K absence or antagonists |
| pK′ | The negative logarithm of an apparent ionisation constant |
| $P_{O_2}$ | Oxygen tension |
| PPF | Plasma protein fraction |
| psi | Pounds per square inch |
| $P_{tc}CO_2$ | Transcutaneous $P_{CO_2}$ |
| $P_{tc}O_2$ | Transcutaneous $P_{O_2}$ |
| PT | Prothrombin time |

| | |
|---|---|
| PTR | Prothrombin time ratio |
| PTT | Partial thromboplastin time |
| PV | Plasma volume |
| PVC | Polyvinyl chloride |
| $P\bar{v}CO_2$ | Mixed venous carbon dioxide tension |
| $P\bar{v}O_2$ | Mixed venous blood oxygen tension |
| PVR | Peripheral vascular resistance |
| $\dot{Q}$ | Symbol denoting blood flow |
| $\dot{Q}_s$ | Blood flow through shunt |
| $\dot{Q}_s/\dot{Q}_T$ | Ratio of shunt flow to total flow or cardiac output |
| $\dot{Q}_T$ | Cardiac output |
| RBF | Renal blood flow |
| RCV | Red cell volume |
| REM | Rapid eye movement |
| RNA | Ribonucleic acid |
| RQ | Respiratory quotient |
| SA | Sino-atrial |
| SA | Sickle-cell trait |
| SβTHAL | Sickle-cell thalassaemia |
| SC | Sickle-cell Hb.C disease |
| SCUBA | Self-contained underwater breathing apparatus |
| SD | Standard deviation |
| SEM | Standard error of the mean |
| SGPT | Serum glutamic pyruvic transaminase |
| SPTI | Systolic pressure time index |
| SRS-A | Slow reacting substance of anaphylaxis |
| SS | Sickle-cell anaemia |
| SVC | Superior vena cava |
| SVR | Systemic vascular resistance |
| SWC | Submersible work chamber |
| TBH | Total body haematocrit |
| THA | Tetrahydroaminacrine |
| THAM | Tromethamine |
| TNS | Transcutaneous nerve stimulation |
| TSH | Thyroid stimulating hormone |
| TSS | Toxic shock syndrome |
| TT | Thrombin time |
| URTI | Upper respiratory tract infection |
| USP | United States Pharmacopeia |
| $\dot{V}A$ | Alveolar ventilation |
| $\dot{V}A/\dot{Q}$ | Alveolar ventilation/perfusion ratio |
| VC | Vital capacity |
| $V_D$ (anat) | Anatomical dead space |
| $V_D$ (phys) | Physiological dead space |
| VEB | Ventricular ectopic beat |
| VF | Ventricular fibrillation |
| VIC | Vaporisor inside circuit |
| VIP | Vasoactive intestinal polypeptide |
| VMA | Vanillylmandelic acid |
| Vmax | Maximum velocity of shortening (myocardial muscle) |
| VOC | Vaporisor outside circuit |
| VPG | Vessel poor group |
| $\dot{V}/\dot{Q}$ | Ventilation perfusion ratio |
| VRG | Vessel rich group |
| VSD | Ventricular septal defect |
| VT | Ventricular tachycardia |
| $V_T$ | Tidal volume |
| WBACT | Whole blood activated clotting time |
| WDR | Wide dynamic range |
| WFSA | World Federation of Societies of Anesthesiologists |

*Section One*

# THE RESPIRATORY SYSTEM

CHAPTER 1

# Structure and Function of the Respiratory Tract in Relation to Anaesthesia



## THE NOSE

### Functions

The nose has five important functions to perform:—

1. The adult patient breathes through his nose, unless there is some form of obstruction caused, for example, by nasal polypi or a severe catarrhal condition. In normal subjects the resistance created by breathing through the nose is 1½ times greater than mouth breathing. Deflection of the nasal septum may diminish the lumen of the respiratory airway and in some cases it is sufficiently severe to prevent the passage of all but the smallest of endotracheal tubes. Before attempting nasal intubation it is advisable to test the patency of each nostril in turn by listening for the sound that indicates a free flow of air. The side where the obstruction is greatest anteriorly (due to deflection of the nasal septum) often proves the easiest to intubate.

2. The stiff hairs in the anterior part of the nasal fossa together with the spongy mucous membrane and the ciliated epithelium comprise a powerful defence against the invasion of any organism. In reserve lie the flushing action of the watery secretions, the bactericidal properties of these secretions, and the extensive lymph drainage of the whole area.

3. Warming and humidifying the inspired air or gases is probably the most important work the nose performs. The enormity of the task can only be realised if it is recalled that 10,000 litres of air pass through every twenty-four hours. The great vascularity of the mucosa helps to maintain a constant temperature: inspired air at 17° C is heated to approximately 37° C during its passage through the nose and variations in external air temperature ranging from 25–0° C

produce less than 1° C change in the temperature of air reaching the laryngeal inlet.

The supply of moisture comes partly from transudations of fluid through the mucosal epithelium and to a lesser extent from secretions of glands and goblet cells in the nasal mucous membrane. The daily volume of nasal secretions is about 1 litre, of which about three-quarters is used in saturating the inspired air.

As a result of endotracheal intubation, or after tracheostomy, only relatively dry gases or air reach the lower part of the trachea, thus compelling the mucosa in this area to perform the duties of the nasal mucous membrane. Although in time the mucosa can adapt itself to the changed conditions, to begin with it becomes dry, and the absence of moisture, even for a few minutes, leads to a cessation of ciliary activity. When adaptation is slow there may be degeneration of the mucosal cells. Endotracheal anaesthesia is in fact frequently followed by a mild tracheitis; this incidence is accentuated when gases, which have had almost all their moisture removed before storage in cylinders, are used in an anaesthetic system that has a relatively low humidity.

4. Vocal resonance is influenced by the patency of the nasal passages.

5. The nose detects smells.

The blood supply to the nasal mucosa is controlled by an elaborate autonomic reflex which enables the mucosa to swell or shrink on demand. There is a dual nerve supply to this area. Parasympathetic fibres pass via the facial, greater superficial petrosal and vidian nerves to relay in the sphenopalatine ganglion. Sympathetic fibres reach the ganglion from the plexus surrounding the internal carotid artery, via the vidian nerve (nerve of the pterygoid canal).

The sensory nerve supply to the nasal mucosa is derived from the first and second divisions of the trigeminal nerve. The anterior third of both the septum and the lateral wall are supplied by the anterior ethmoidal branch of the nasociliary nerve (first division) and the posterior two-thirds by the nasopalatine nerves via the sphenopalatine ganglion (second division). For operations on the nasal septum local analgesia can be produced either by topical analgesia or by blocking the maxillary and anterior ethmoidal nerves on both sides.

In animals a notable reflex from this area is that known as the "Kratschmer" reflex in which stimulation of the anterior part of the nasal septum leads to constriction of the bronchioles. When a patient's nose is plugged with gauze after a nasal operation, intense restlessness often occurs during the recovery period even though the oral airway is adequate and there is no pain. This situation is frequently encountered in adolescents who have had a fractured nasal septum remodelled. It suggests a reflex from the nasal mucous membrane.

### Ciliary Activity

Throughout the respiratory tract the continuous activity of the cilia is probably the most important single factor in the prevention of the accumulation of secretions. In the nose the flow of material is swept towards the pharynx, whereas in the bronchial tree the flow is carried towards the entrance to the larynx.

Each cilium consists of a very fine hair-like structure approximately 7μm long and 0·3μm thick, in which the tip is always bent towards the direction of the flow of mucus (Fig. 1). The co-ordinated movement of numerous cilia is capable of moving large quantities of material but their activity is greatly assisted by their mucous covering, which consists of two layers: an outer layer of thick viscous mucus which is designed to entrap particulate matter such as dust, soot, or micro-organisms, and an inner layer of thin serous fluid designed to lubricate the action of the ciliary mechanism. The tips of the cilia come just in contact with the outer layer with each beat. Acting in unison, they set the outer mucous layer in motion and with gathering momentum this flows towards the pharynx and larynx.[1]

Ciliary movement consists of a rapid forward thrust followed by a slow recoil which occupies about four-fifths of the cycle. At 30° C the cilia of the nasal mucosa beat about 10–15 times per second. The streaming movement of the overlying mucus has been estimated at 0·25–1·0 centimetre per minute, the slowest speeds being in the bronchioles. The entire contents of the nose can thus be emptied into the pharynx every 20–30 minutes.

Human cilia have a similar structure to those found throughout the animal kingdom. As shown in Fig. 2, each cilium contains longitudinal fibrils—two single microtubules in the centre surrounded by nine double ones periph-

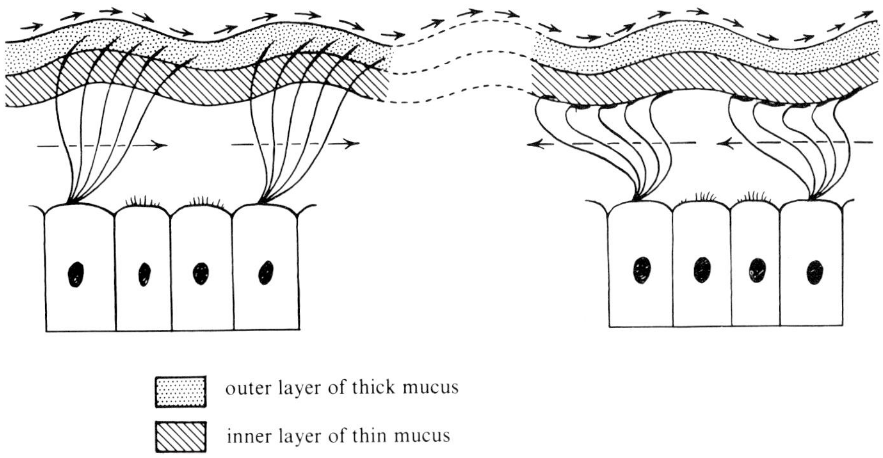


1/Fig. 1.—Ciliary movement.

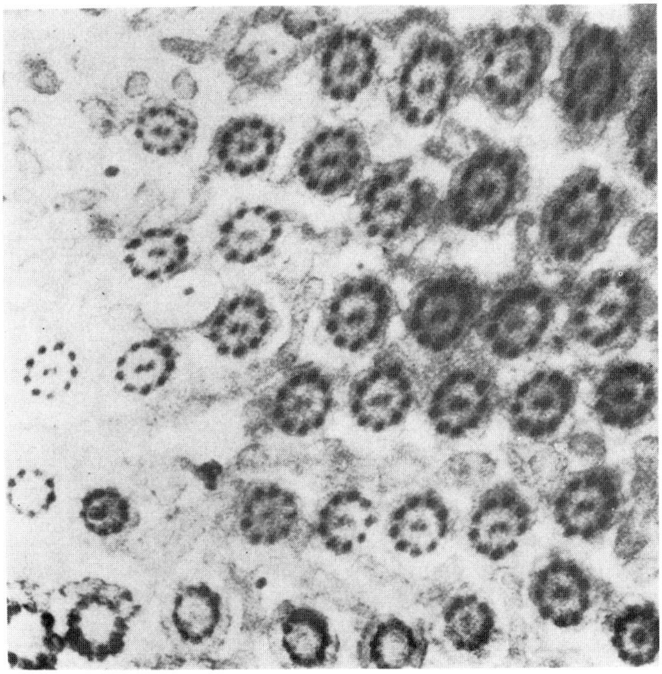

1/Fig. 2.—An electron micrograph of a transverse section of human bronchial cilia. Note the nine peripherally situated filaments (their paired structure cannot be seen) and the two central axial filaments. (Courtesy of Professor H. Spencer and Pergamon Press Ltd.[2])

erally. Ciliary function may be defective[3]; for example, in Kartagener's syndrome (situs inversus, chronic sinusitis and bronchiectasis) there is a genetic defect in the ultrastructure of the cilia due to the failure of synthesis of the protein dynein. Sperm tails have a similar structure to cilia, so that in this syndrome there is male infertility due to reduced sperm motility.

**Factors Influencing Ciliary Activity**

*Temperature*.—The optimum range of temperature for ciliary movement in excised human nasal mucosa is 28°–33° C, while the average nasal temperature is about 32° C. Ciliary activity ceases when the temperature of the mucosa falls to 7°–10° C and is depressed by temperatures rising above 35° C; however, only these extreme variations in temperature have much effect on ciliary action and any changes that do occur are largely caused by alterations in the amount of mucus secreted rather than by any direct influence on the ciliated epithelium.

*Mucus.*—Cilia cannot work without a blanket of mucus. The volatile general anaesthetics not only slow the propelling mechanism but also limit the production of suitable secretions. If a patient has an inadequate secretion of mucus after the use of atropine, or breathes dry gases for a long period, then evaporation will result in drying of the mucosa and ciliary activity will cease.

*Changes in pH.*—Cilia prefer a dilute alkaline solution and are readily paralysed by acid solutions with a pH of 6·4 or less. A rise of pH to 8·0 or more leads to swelling of the columnar cells bearing the cilia and thus to depression of their activity.

*Sleep.*—Natural sleep has little effect on ciliary activity and even several hours after death the cilia may still be found moving.

*Drugs.*—All volatile general anaesthetic agents in high concentrations depress ciliary activity[4,5] (Fig. 3). Nitrous oxide has no effect. The opiates have a direct depressant action, whereas atropine weakens ciliary activity only indirectly by altering the viscosity of the secreted mucus.

*Posture.*—Gravity appears to have no effect on ciliary action and the flow always continues in the same direction whatever the patient's position.

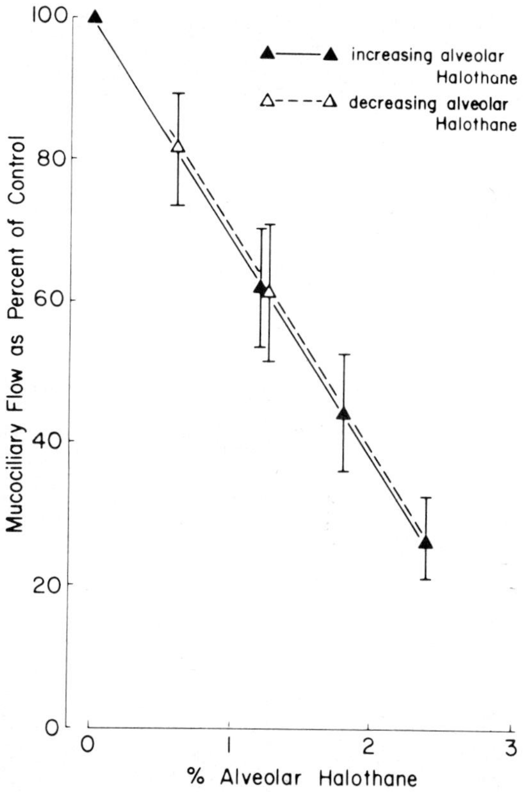


1/Fig. 3.—Effects of thiopentone and various concentrations of halothane on mucociliary flow in the dog trachea. Each value is a mean ± 1 SEM from six dogs, expressed as a percentage of the control (thiopentone) value. (Courtesy of Forbes (1976) and J. B. Lippincott Company.[4])

## Anaesthesia and Humidity

**Importance of humidity.**—The importance of humidifying the inspired gases is well-known to all those responsible for the management of patients on intermittent positive-pressure respiration. The anaesthetised patient undergoing a routine operation usually breathes virtually dry gases for long periods of time. With an artificial airway in position the gases tend to flow through the mouth so that the functions of the nose are largely short-circuited, while with an endotracheal tube, the whole role of providing adequate humidification falls on the lower respiratory tract. Proper humidification of the inspired gas of intubated patients reduces the incidence of pulmonary complications occurring after long operations.[6]

**Physical principles.**—The quantity of water needed to saturate air with water vapour increases with the temperature (Fig. 4).

At a room temperature of 17° C the air contains 2 volumes per cent of water when fully saturated. At a body temperature of 37° C the air in the trachea contains 6 volumes per cent of water vapour. The nose and respiratory tract, therefore, not only have the task of warming the inspired air but also of adding large quantities of water vapour. The value of this mechanism is appreciated to the full by anyone who runs rapidly on a cold, dry morning. The increased inhalation of air through the mouth leads to drying of the tracheal mucous membrane and an uncomfortable "soreness" in the chest.

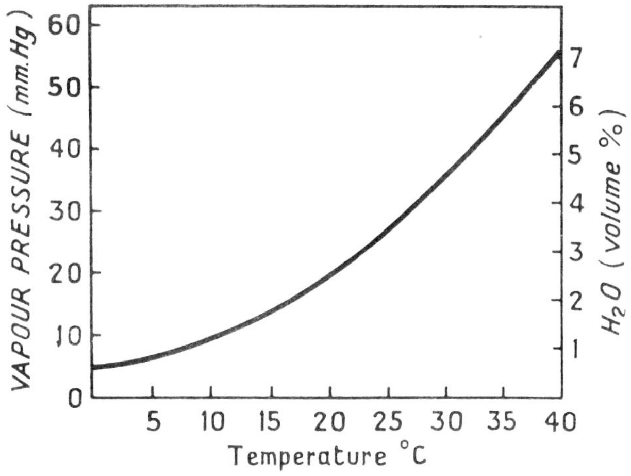


1/FIG. 4.—The relationship of water vapour tension in air to temperature. (Courtesy of Dr. J. D. K. Burton and the Editor of the *Lancet*[7])

**Anaesthetic Apparatus**

In most anaesthetic systems the temperature of the gases reaching the patient is approximately the same as the room temperature. This is because the gases are cooled or warmed during their passage through a long length of flexible rubber breathing tubing. The principal exception to this rule is in the to-and-fro' system where the temperature of the canister (near the patient's mouth) may rise to as high as 45° C and in which no time is available for the cooling of gases en route to the patient. This system, therefore, provides very efficient humidification but it has other disadvantages (see p. 80).

Two other principal types of anaesthetic system should be considered:

(*a*) *The non-rebreathing valve system* (Fig. 5).

The inspired air is always at room temperature (17° C) and therefore even if fully saturated it can only hold about 2 volumes per cent of water. Because there is no rebreathing the expired air (at 37° C and fully saturated) passes out through the valve and is lost to the atmosphere.

In this type of system anaesthetic gases are usually supplied direct from source without passing through a humidifier, and therefore are completely dry.

(*b*) *The circle absorption system.*

Here the inspired mixture consists not only of fresh dry gases but also of some expired gases containing water vapour at room temperature. The latter leave the patient at body temperature, but by the time they have traversed the apparatus they will have cooled to room temperature and so have lost the major part of their water content in the apparatus. Dry fresh gas is also added to the system.

Approximate values for the humidity of gases using various anaesthetic systems are shown in Table 1.

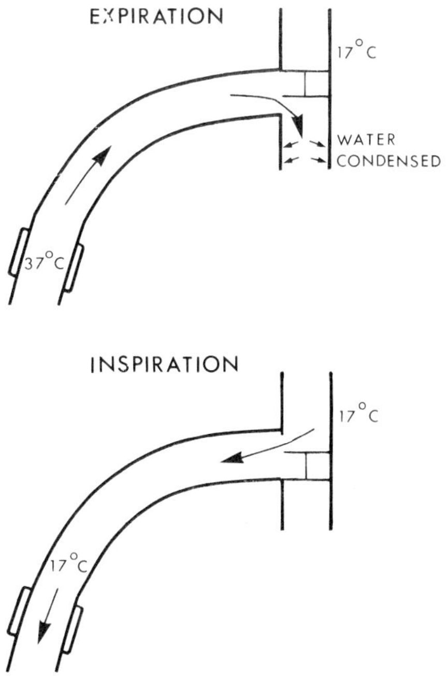


1/FIG. 5.—The non-rebreathing valve system. (Courtesy of Dr. J. D. K. Burton and the Editor of the *Lancet*[7])

1/TABLE 1
THE RELATIVE HUMIDITY OF GASES IN THE VARIOUS ANAESTHETIC SYSTEMS

| *Anaesthetic system* | *Percentage humidity of gases* |
|---|---|
| Non-rebreathing valve | 0 |
| T-piece | 0 |
| To and fro' | 40–100 |
| Closed circle | 40–60 |
| Human nose | 100 |

### Effect of Premedication, Intubation and Dry Gases

Burton[7] studied the effects of premedication, the endotracheal tube, and dry anaesthetic gases on ciliary activity by observing the movement of an ink marker placed at the carina of anaesthetised dogs. Under pentobarbitone anaesthesia alone the ink passed up the trachea and out through the vocal cords within 20–30 minutes.

After atropine premedication, the rate of movement of the ink was slowed to 10 cm in 30 minutes and normal movement was not resumed for some 4–5 hours. The endotracheal tube by itself had little untoward action if the gases were humidified, but the inflation of a cuff immediately produced a complete barrier to the passage of the marker ink. Dry anaesthetic gases, as delivered direct from a cylinder, produced gross reduction in ciliary movement. Thus, after 4½ hours anaesthesia using a Rubens non-rebreathing valve the maximal movement of the marker was only 2·5 cm in 30 minutes.

It is hardly surprising, therefore, that after a prolonged period of anaesthesia the mucosa of the trachea and lower respiratory tract shows evidence of dryness and an inflammatory reaction.

The whole process may be summarised as follows:

Atropine + Dry gas } → Dry mucosa →

Inflammatory reaction → Excessive mucus
↓ ↓
Tracheitis & Bronchitis — ? Pulmonary collapse

### Methods of Humidification

1. **Direct installation.**—Normal saline can be administered by direct instillation into an endotracheal tube or tracheostomy. Though not used much these days as a method of humidification, an extension of this practice is endobronchial lavage which is carried out to remove thick secretions or mucus plugs in the bronchi.

2. **Water-bath.**—The gas mixture is passed across the surface of a heated, thermostatically controlled, water-bath. This may be used in conjunction with an artificial ventilator, when the humidifier must be placed on the inspiratory side of the system, and the gases led to the patient by the shortest possible route. The tubing should be insulated to prevent heat loss, with consequent condensation. By raising the temperature in the humidifier slightly above body temperature it is possible to deliver gases to the patient which are at 37° C and completely saturated with water vapour. The exact temperature setting of the water-bath will depend on the surface area of water exposed to the gases, the flow rate of these gases and the amount of cooling and condensation taking place in the inspiratory tubing. Sterility of the water in the humidifier is greatly aided if the temperature is maintained at 60° C. It is important always to keep the humidifier at a low level to prevent water being blown into the patient.

This type of humidifier, when combined with a fan to blow air through it, can be used to humidify a tracheostomy. The attachment to the tracheostomy is of a T-piece design which allows the moistened air to flow freely across the opening. The weight of the tubing can be a serious disadvantage to the patient.

3. **Moisture exchanger.**—The heat and moisture exchanger offers a light and moderately efficient method of humidification for a patient breathing spontaneously through a tracheostomy or endotracheal tube. The modern version consists of a replaceable condenser that can be taken out and cleaned (Fig. 6). As it is at a lower temperature than the body, part of the water vapour of expiration is condensed on its inner surface where it is available to humidify the inspired air. It cannot, of course, achieve full saturation owing to the lower temperature. Nevertheless such a device can considerably

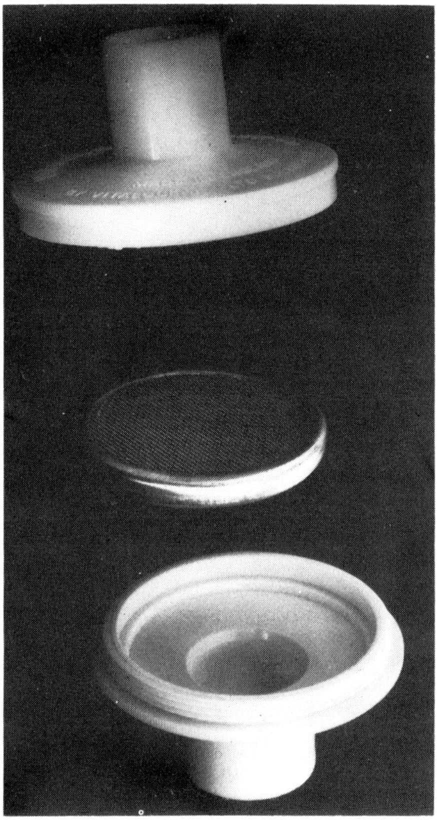

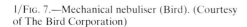

1/FIG. 6.—Artificial nose with replaceable heat and moisture exchanger. The central metal filter can be removed, sterilised and replaced.

improve the humidity of inspired air, especially if this already contains a little water vapour. Two problems are encountered with the use of an "artificial nose". First is colonisation by bacteria and the other is increasing airway resistance as the condenser becomes moisturised. These disadvantages can largely be overcome if the condenser unit is changeable and sterilisable.

4. **Mechanical nebuliser.**—This is a pneumatic device which breaks up a liquid into small particles. Water, when placed in the nebuliser, passes up a capillary tube at the summit of which it is nebulised by a jet of gas. The droplet leaving the capillary tube then crashes into the side of a ball where it is fractured into numerous small particles. Most particles of 5 microns and above cling to the ball, coalesce, and fall back into the reservoir. Those particles of 4 microns or less tend to float out and join the inspired gases. In this type of nebuliser 80 per cent of the particles are in the range 2–4 microns and the remainder are smaller. Most of these particles are deposited around the pharynx, and only a small percentage reach the bronchial level, but for many patients this is sufficient. Because it is compact this nebuliser can conveniently be placed in close proximity to the patient's airway (Fig. 7). It can also be used pre- or post-operatively with a face mask for the improve-

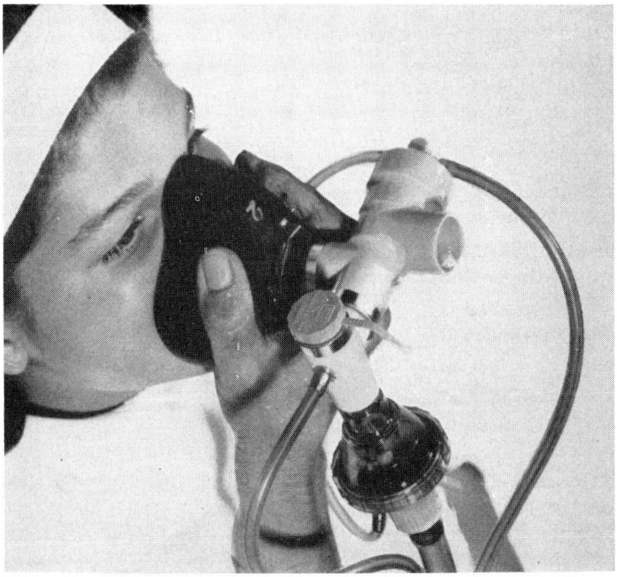

1/FIG. 7.—Mechanical nebuliser (Bird). (Courtesy of The Bird Corporation)

ment of lung function, or it can be attached directly to a tracheostomy tube.

5. **Ultrasonic nebuliser.**—In 1964 Herzog[8] and his colleagues introduced to clinical practice an ultrasonic nebuliser consisting of a plexiglass container to hold 150 ml of fluid and with a vibrating transducer head at its base. The transducer head is activated by a high-frequency (3 MHz) generator and is fed with drops of fluid by a capillary tube which passes through the top of the container. The nebuliser should be connected to the inspiratory side of a ventilator (Fig. 8).

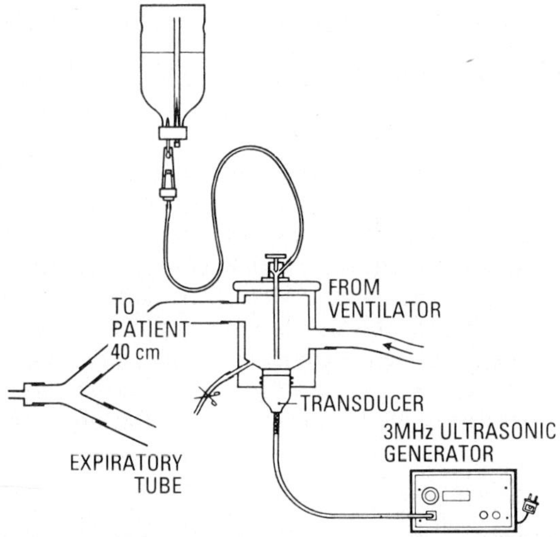


1/Fig. 8.—Diagram of an ultrasonic nebuliser. (Courtesy of Dr. P. Herzog, Dr. O. P. Norlander and Dr. C. G. Engstrom and the Editor of *Acta Anaesthesiologica Scandinavica*[8])

Each drop of fluid is completely nebulised to an aerosol in which 70 per cent of the particles have a size of 0·8 to 1 micron, the actual size being dependent on the frequency of vibration of the transducer head. Most particles of 1 micron or less are deposited in the lower airways and alveoli of the lungs. At the maximum rate of 12 drops per minute dripping on to the transducer head and with a ventilator delivering 10 litres of gas per minute, 72 mg of water are provided with each litre of gas. This corresponds to a relative humidity of 164 per cent at 37° C.

Ultrasonic nebulisers produce satisfactory humidification in patients who have very dry airways at the start of treatment (e.g. children with tracheobronchitis) and they can be used for the administration of water-soluble aerosol drugs, but they are not without dangers. Their extreme efficiency makes over-hydration possible, especially in children, and they are difficult to sterilise by conventional methods. Ringrose and his colleagues[9] have described how outbreaks of infection can follow inadequate cleaning of ultrasonic nebulisers. When used for a long time continuously on the same patient an ultrasonic nebuliser will increase the airway resistance,[10] and may cause pulmonary collapse.[11]

Variations on the design of Herzog's nebuliser are in production, their main difference being the frequency of vibration of the transducer head and hence an alteration in the size of the particles of fluid produced.

## PHARYNX

The pharynx extends from the posterior aspect of the nose at the base of the skull down to the level of the lower border of the cricoid cartilage where it becomes continuous with the oesophagus, and the respiratory tract through the larynx. The soft palate partially divides the pharynx into two—an upper nasopharyngeal portion and a lower orolaryngeal portion.

In the nasopharyngeal part a collection of lymphoid tissue—the nasopharyngeal tonsil or "adenoids"—lies embedded in the mucous membrane at the junction of the roof with the upper and posterior part of the pharynx. Lying close to the base of the nasopharyngeal tonsil is a small recess—the pharyngeal bursa. These structures often impede the passage of an endotracheal tube; if force is used the tube may penetrate the mucosa and create a false passage which can lead to trouble from sepsis and collection of secretions during the post-operative period.

The lymph drainage of the pharynx is often of clinical importance because enlargement of the lymphatic glands and swelling of the overlying mucosa may, in some instances, lead to partial obstruction of the airway. These lymph glands are numerous and are arranged in a circular fashion—the ring of Waldeyer (Fig. 9).

In essence the ring consists of the large palatine tonsils (P) lying between the pillars of

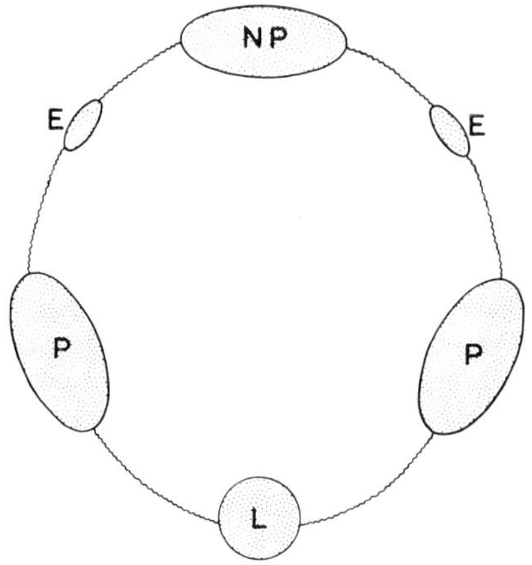


1/FIG. 9.—PHARYNGEAL AND TONSILLAR GLANDS (RING OF WALDEYER)
P = Palatine tonsil.
L = Lingual tonsil.
E = Eustachian tonsil.
NP = Nasopharyngeal tonsil or "adenoids".

the fauces; the smaller lingual tonsil (L) at the base of the tongue on each side of the midline and in front of the vallecula, the Eustachian tonsil (E) which is an accumulation of lymphoid follicles sometimes found on the posterior lip of the orifice of the Eustachian tube, and the nasopharyngeal tonsil (NP) which is a group of follicles united in one mass on the posterior wall of the nasopharynx. On the posterior wall of the pharynx at the level of the large palatine tonsils some small lymph nodes are often found. These are of particular importance when sepsis occurs in this neighbourhood because they swell up to form a retropharyngeal abscess. This may occur either in conjunction with sepsis tracking inwards from the spinal column or with a peritonsillar abscess ("quinsy"). The presence of a large retropharyngeal abscess makes nasal intubation extremely difficult and dangerous because the endotracheal tube may be deflected sharply forwards or it may impinge on and rupture the abscess.

**Pharyngeal obstruction and the airway.**—One of the principal duties of an anaesthetist is to learn the art of maintaining a completely unobstructed airway in an unconscious patient. Because intubation may lead to a sore throat, infection, or rarely, laryngeal lesions, it should only be used when indicated.

The principal difficulty in maintaining a perfect airway in an unconscious patient is the tendency of the tongue to fall backwards and obstruct the laryngeal opening. This occurs as soon as consciousness is lost and the muscles supporting the tongue start to relax. If the tongue is brought forward then the laryngeal opening once again is cleared.

Various manoeuvres may be used to achieve this.

1. The head should be extended (Fig. 10). In the supine unconscious subject flexion of the neck, such as occurs when the head is resting naturally on a pillow, is almost invariably associated with respiratory obstruction. The simple manoeuvre of extending the neck will

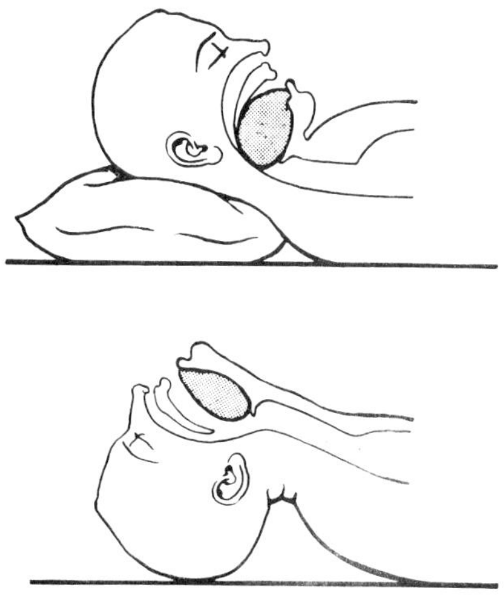

1/FIG. 10.—Maintenance of a clear airway.

clear the airway in about 75 per cent of cases by causing a forward movement of the mandible, to which the tongue is attached, and by stretching the anterior tissues of the neck, rather like straightening a washing line.

2. Extension of the neck causes the mouth to fall open due to the downward pull of the neck tissues. Simply closing the mouth will often improve the airway by straightening the tissues of the neck still further.

3. If the airway is still not perfect the mandible can be drawn forward by placing the fingers behind the angles of the jaw and exerting a forward pressure.

4. An oropharyngeal airway can be inserted. In neonates and infants a satisfactory airway is most often achieved if the mouth is allowed to fall open because the tongue is relatively large in this age group and closing the mouth tends to push the soft palate against the posterior wall of the nasopharynx and to obstruct the nasal airway.

An unconscious patient is safest in the lateral position. Unless there is a specific surgical contra-indication, an unconscious patient following anaesthesia should be nursed on his side. In this position the tongue tends to fall away from the posterior pharyngeal wall and foreign material is less likely to enter the larynx.

## LARYNX

The larynx lies at the levels of the 3rd–6th cervical vertebrae and comprises a number of articulated cartilages surrounding the upper end of the trachea (Fig. 11). The laryngeal cavity extends from the inlet at the top to the lower level of the cricoid cartilage below, where it becomes continuous with the trachea. The inlet is bounded anteriorly by the upper edge of the epiglottis, posteriorly by a sheath of mucous membrane stretched between the two arytenoid cartilages, and on each side by the free edge of a fold of mucous membrane—the aryepiglottic fold—which joins the apex of the arytenoid cartilage to the side of the epiglottis. When this fold is viewed down a laryngoscope the underlying cartilages protrude through the mucous membrane, making a ridge which appears to form the entrance to the larynx on each side. These projections are formed posteriorly by the arytenoid cartilages with the corniculate cartilages lying in close proximity; anteriorly the cuneiform cartilages can be seen.

The next structures in the laryngeal cavity are the vestibular folds which run on either side as narrow bands of fibrous tissue passing from the anterolateral surface of the arytenoid cartilages to the angle of the thyroid cartilage at the point

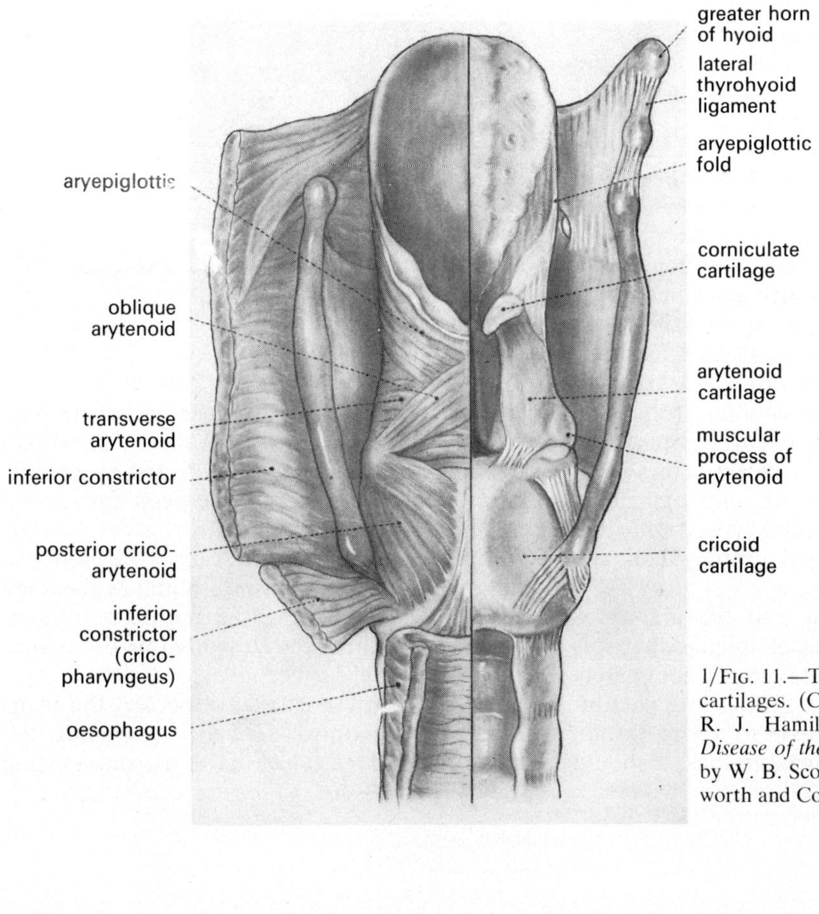


1/FIG. 11.—The larynx, showing muscles and cartilages. (Courtesy of W. J. Hampton and R. J. Hamilton, authors of a chapter in *Disease of the Ear, Nose and Throat*, Vol. 1, by W. B. Scott-Brown, published by Butterworth and Co.)

of attachment of the epiglottis. These folds are usually called the false vocal cords and are separated from the true vocal cords which lie below by the laryngeal sinus.

The vocal cords are two pearly-white folds of mucous membrane stretching from the angle of the thyroid cartilage to the vocal processes of the arytenoid cartilages. Beneath their outer lining of stratified squamous epithelium lies the tough fibrous vocal ligament. Since there is no true submucosa with the usual network of blood vessels, the vocal cords have a characteristic pale appearance.

In the adult, the narrowest part of the laryngeal cavity is the area between the vocal cords, whereas in children under about ten years of age it is just below the vocal cords at the cricoid ring. The clinical significance of this anatomical difference is to be found when small children are intubated, since an endotracheal tube which can pass between the vocal cords may yet be too large to pass beyond the cricoid ring.

### Movements of the Vocal Cords

It is not intended to give a detailed description of the actions of the intrinsic muscles but certain brief details of the laryngeal mechanism may be recalled. In each case the focal point of movement is the arytenoid cartilages which rotate and slide up and down on the sloping shoulders of the cricoid cartilage.

The muscles concerned are most conveniently thought of as pairs having opposing actions controlling three parts of the larynx:

First, the laryngeal inlet which is closed by the aryepiglottic and opened by the thyro-epiglottic muscles.

Secondly, the rima glottidis which is dilated by the posterior crico-arytenoid muscles assisted by the lateral crico-arytenoid muscle, and is closed by the inter-arytenoid muscles which approximate the arytenoids without rotation.

Thirdly, those acting on the vocal cords—the cricothyroid muscles which lengthen the vocal cords and the thyro-arytenoid muscles which shorten them.

The tension of the vocal cords is altered by the vocales, which are a part of the thyro-arytenoid muscles.

### Nerve Supply to the Larynx

The mucous membrane receives its nerve supply from both the superior and recurrent laryngeal nerves. The superior laryngeal nerve arises from the inferior ganglion of the vagus but receives a small branch from the superior cervical sympathetic ganglion. This nerve descends in the lateral wall of the pharynx, passing posteriorly to the internal carotid artery, and at the level of the greater horn of the hyoid divides into an internal and an external branch.

The internal laryngeal branch, which is entirely sensory apart from a few motor filaments to the arytenoid muscles, descends to the thyrohyoid membrane, pierces it above the superior laryngeal artery and then divides again into two branches. The upper branch supplies the mucous membrane of the lower part of the pharynx, epiglottis, vallecula and vestibule of the larynx. The lower branch passes medial to the pyriform fossa beneath the mucous membrane and supplies the aryepiglottic fold and the mucous membrane of the posterior part of the rima glottidis.

The external laryngeal branch carries motor fibres which innervate the cricothyroid muscle.

The recurrent laryngeal nerve accompanies the laryngeal branch of the inferior thyroid artery and travels upwards, deep to the lower border of the inferior constrictor muscle of the pharynx immediately behind the cricothyroid joint. Apart from sensory fibres which supply the mucous membrane of the larynx below the level of the vocal cords, this nerve innervates all the muscles of the larynx except the cricothyroid, and a small part of the arytenoid muscles.

### Cord Palsies

The cords can be visualised either indirectly by means of a mirror or—and this is the more familiar method for the anaesthetist—directly with a laryngoscope. This description of normal and abnormal cord movements is, therefore, written and illustrated from the point of view of direct laryngoscopy.

During phonation the vocal cords meet in the mid-line (Fig. 12*a*). On inspiration they abduct (Fig. 12*b*), returning to the mid-line on expiration, but leaving a small gap between them. The opening into the trachea between the vocal cords is maximal at the end of a deep inspiration. In order, therefore, to minimise the risk of any possible trauma to the cords, intubation and

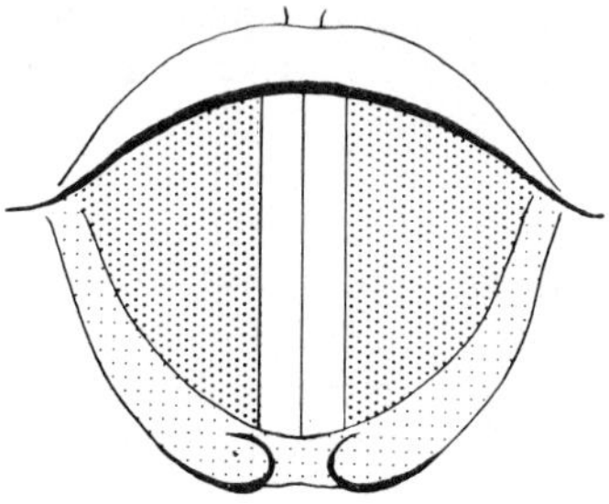

(*a*) Phonation

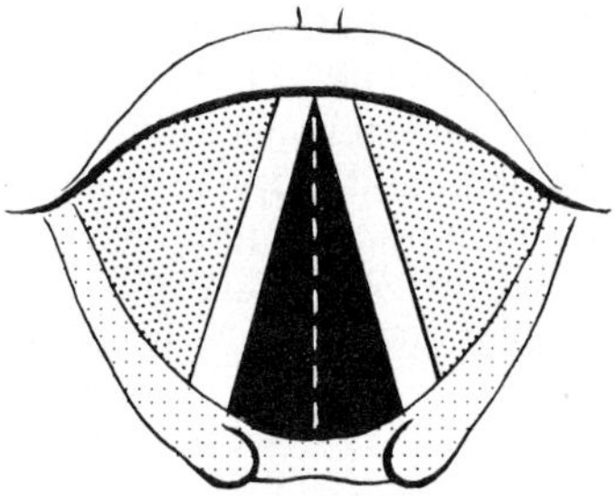

(*b*) Inspiration

1/FIG. 12.—The vocal cords.

extubation should be carried out during inspiration. When laryngeal spasm is present, both the false and the true cords are held tightly in apposition.

Topical analgesia of the throat and larynx blocks the sensory nerve endings of the superior and recurrent laryngeal nerves. Following this procedure, an occasional patient is unable to phonate clearly and develops a "gruff" voice—an effect which is probably due to some local analgesic solution reaching and blocking the external branch of the superior laryngeal nerve. This nerve carries motor fibres to the cricothyroid muscle, which is the principal tensor of the cords. Paralysis of the cricothyroid muscle produces visible alterations in the shape of the glottis and vocal cords—effects that must be remembered should they follow topical analgesia for diagnostic laryngoscopy. The superior laryngeal nerve itself may be traumatised during thyroidectomy when the superior thyroid artery is tied. Since the only motor fibres of the nerve are those that run on into its external branch, exactly similar effects to those just described will follow.

Damage to the recurrent laryngeal nerve may take the form of complete section or merely bruising. This nerve carries both the abductor and the adductor motor fibres of the vocal cords. The abductor fibres, however, are more vulnerable so that moderate trauma usually leads to a pure abductor paralysis. Severe trauma or section of the recurrent laryngeal nerve causes both abductor and adductor paralysis. A pure adductor paralysis does not occur as a clinical entity.

It is not always easy to differentiate between the various types of cord palsy but the main points are illustrated diagrammatically below. Unilateral lesions are assumed to exist on a patient's left side. The position of the cords during both phonation and inspiration is diagnostic.

**Pure abductor palsy—left.**—On phonation both cords meet in the mid-line because the adductor fibres on the left (damaged) side are still active. It will be noticed, however, that the right false cord tends to lie slightly anterior to that on the left (Fig. 13*a*). On inspiration the cord on the side of the injury remains in approximately the same position, but the cord on the unaffected side moves into full abduction (Fig. 13*b*).

**Abductor and adductor palsy–left.**—In this case both types of fibre are no longer functioning on the left, so that the cord tends to rest in a slightly more abducted position. On phonation, the right cord crosses the mid-line in an attempt to meet its opposite number (Fig. 14*a*). As it is forced to move in the arc of a circle, the right false cord appears to lie in front of the left. On inspiration, the unaffected cord moves back again into full abduction (Fig. 14*b*).

**Bilateral damage to the recurrent laryngeal nerves.**—This may occur during removal of the thyroid gland. The position of the vocal cords will depend upon the severity of the damage.

When the trauma is mild on both sides, then bilateral abductor paralysis may result. Severe trauma, or complete section, on both sides affects both abductor and adductor fibres. It is important to differentiate between these two conditions because they have differing effects on the laryngeal airway. After partial damage the vocal cords lie near the mid-line because the adductor fibres are still functioning, and the airway is reduced to a mere chink (Fig. 15*a*). A patient in this condition usually rapidly shows signs of severe respiratory obstruction, particularly when respiration is active due to fear or

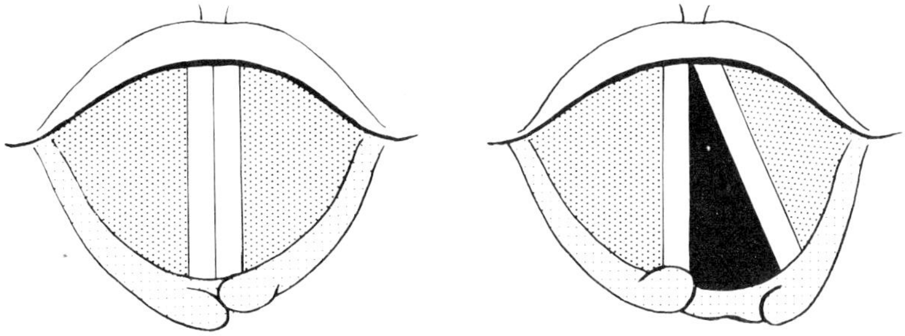

(*a*) Phonation (*b*) Inspiration

1/FIG. 13.—Pure abductor palsy—Left.

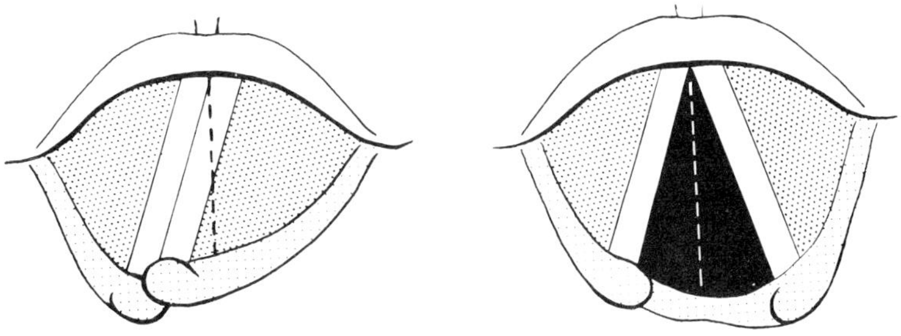

(*a*) Phonation (*b*) Inspiration

1/FIG. 14.—Abductor and adductor palsy—Left.

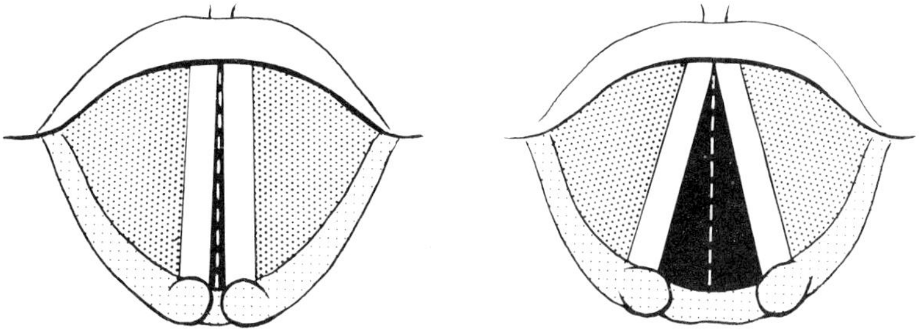

(*a*) Partial palsy (*b*) Total palsy

1/FIG. 15.—Bilateral damage to the recurrent laryngeal nerve.

other causes. When both nerves are severely damaged, or cut across, the vocal cords lie stationary in the mid position with a fair-sized lumen between them (Fig. 15*b*). Now, the airway is fairly adequate unless respiratory effort is very marked, when the cords tend to be sucked in with each inspiration.

**Bilateral palsy of the recurrent laryngeal nerves with palsy of the external branch of the superior laryngeal nerve.**—Total paralysis of the cords is now associated with paralysis of the cricothyroid muscles. The vocal cords are no longer tensed and the antero-posterior diameter of the glottis is reduced. This is the true cadaveric position. With complete relaxation, such as may be obtained by one of the muscle relaxants, exactly the same position is seen (Fig. 16).

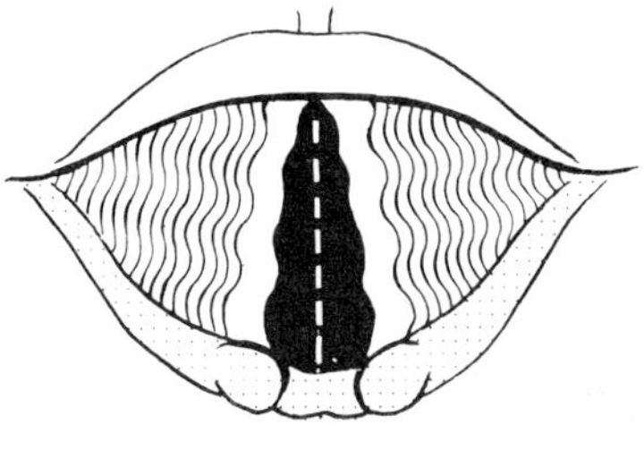

1/FIG. 16.—Bilateral palsy of the recurrent laryngeal nerves with palsy of the external branch of the superior laryngeal nerve.

### Laryngeal Trauma and Oedema

Trauma to the larynx during intubation of the trachea may lead to oedema (particularly in small children) and to a granuloma of the cords at a later date.

## TRACHEA AND BRONCHIAL TREE
(Figs. 20 and 21)

The trachea is a tube formed of rings of cartilage which are incomplete posteriorly. The cross-sectional shape shows considerable variation from subject to subject (Fig. 17) and this may be important from the point of view of the design of endotracheal tubes. It is about 10–11 cm long, extending downwards from the lower part of the larynx opposite the level of the 6th cervical vertebra to the point of its bifurcation into a right and left main bronchus at the carina, about the upper border of the 5th thoracic vertebra. It is lined by ciliated columnar epithelium.

The trachea moves with respiration and with alterations in the position of the head. Thus on deep inspiration the carina can descend as much as 2·5 cm. Extension of the head and neck—the ideal position in which to maintain an airway in an anaesthetised patient—can increase the length of the trachea by as much as 23 to 30 per cent. Clinically, if a patient is intubated with the head in a flexed position at the atlanto-occipital joint, and the endotracheal tube is so short that it just reaches beyond the vocal cords, the subsequent hyperextension of the head may withdraw the tube into the pharynx.

Bronchi divide dichotomously, eventually giving rise to several million terminal bronchioles which terminate in one or more respiratory bronchioles. Originating from each respiratory bronchiole are 2–11 alveolar ducts leading to the alveolar sacs which are extended as a group of alveoli. The total cross-sectional area of the tracheobronchial tree increases very rapidly as the peripheral parts of the lungs are reached (Fig. 18).

Bronchioles less than 1 mm in diameter do not have cartilage in their walls. Smooth muscle is found in the walls of all the airways down to the level of the alveolar ducts and is relatively most abundant in the terminal bronchioles.

### Right Bronchial Tree

The *right main bronchus* is wider and shorter than the left, being only 2·5 cm long. As it is more nearly vertical than the left main bronchus there is a much greater tendency for either endotracheal tubes or suction catheters to enter this lumen. In small children under the age of three years the angulation of the two main bronchi at the carina is equal on both sides (Fig.

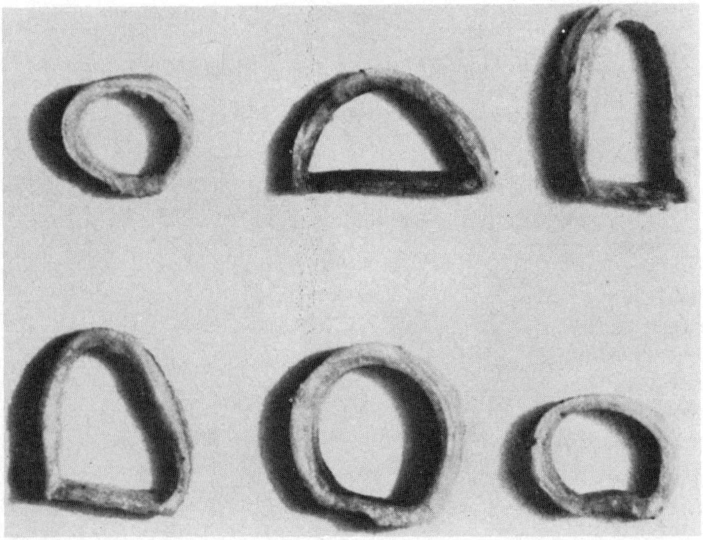

1/FIG. 17.—Examples of tracheal cross-sectional shapes at autopsy. (Courtesy of McKenzie *et al.* and the American Society of Anesthesiologists.[12])

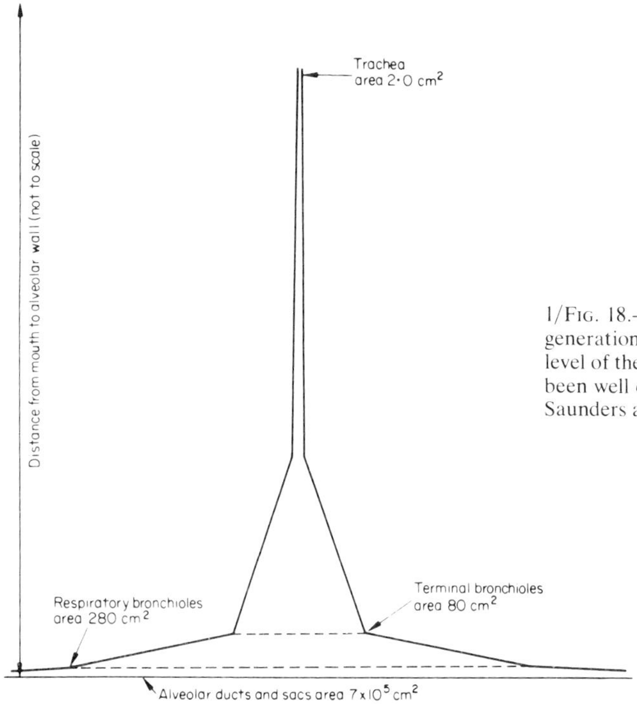

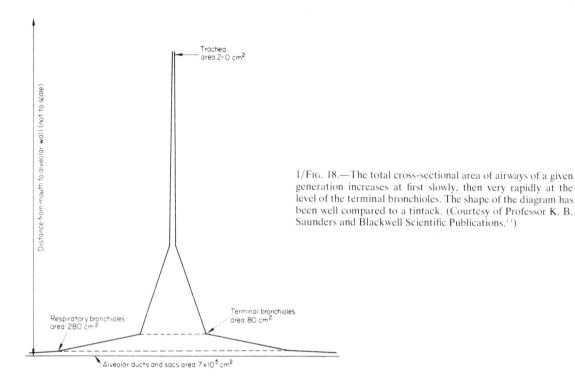

1/Fig. 18.—The total cross-sectional area of airways of a given generation increases at first slowly, then very rapidly at the level of the terminal bronchioles. The shape of the diagram has been well compared to a tintack. (Courtesy of Professor K. B. Saunders and Blackwell Scientific Publications.[13])

19). In the event of an endotracheal tube being inserted too far a further complication is that the bevelled end of the tube (as usually cut) may become blocked off by its lying against the mucosa on the medial wall of the main bronchus. The short length of this bronchus also makes the lumen difficult to occlude when this is required in thoracic anaesthesia.

The right main bronchus gives off branches to the upper and middle lobes before becoming continuous with the lower lobe bronchus.

The *right upper lobe bronchus* passes in an upward and lateral direction at 90° to the right main bronchus for 1 cm before dividing into its three main divisions.

The apical bronchus runs upwards with a lateral inclination and after about 1 cm usually gives off a lateral branch and then almost immediately divides into anterior and posterior branches.

The posterior bronchus runs in a backward, lateral, and slightly upward direction. After about 0·5–1·0 cm it gives off an important lateral branch and then ends by dividing into superior and inferior divisions.

The anterior bronchus runs in a downward, forward and slightly lateral direction. Soon after its origin it also gives off a lateral branch.

Each of these bronchi supplies a segment of the upper lobe. The posterior segment of the upper lobe, together with the apical segment of the lower lobe, is one of the common sites for the development of a lung abscess. When a patient is lying wholly or partly on his side, inhaled material tends to gravitate into the lateral portion of the posterior segment of the upper lobe—particularly on the right side (Fig. 22*a*). Alternatively, if the patient lies on his back the material accumulates in the apical segment of the lower lobe (Fig. 22*b*). The incidence of lung abscess is nearly twice as high in the upper lobes as in the lower ones. Surgery offers some of the most favourable conditions for aspiration of infected material, since if the anaesthetised patient is placed on his side either during or after operation then the upper lobe bronchus acts as the most dependent drain. The accumulation of secretions here, together with an inadequate cough reflex results in an area of pulmonary collapse which may later suppurate

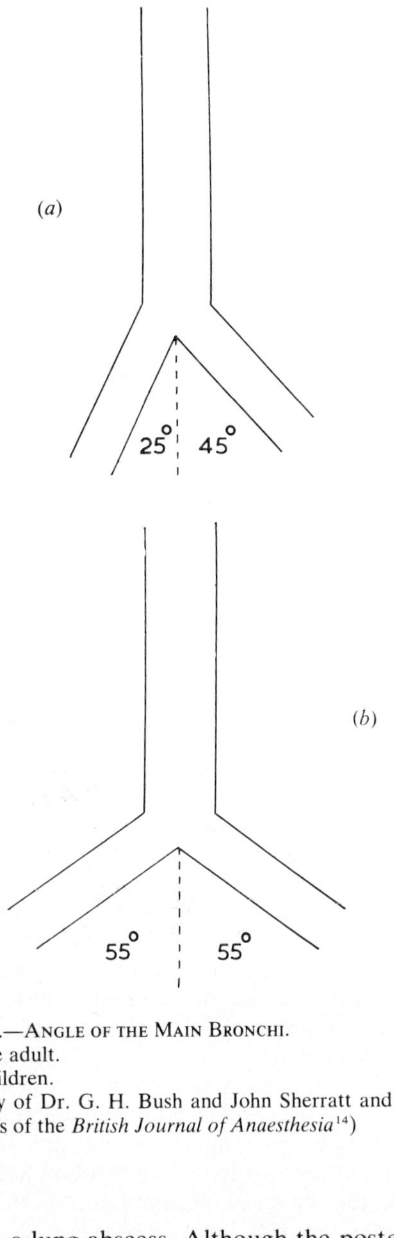


1/FIG. 19.—ANGLE OF THE MAIN BRONCHI.
(*a*) In the adult.
(*b*) In children.
(Courtesy of Dr. G. H. Bush and John Sherratt and Son, publishers of the *British Journal of Anaesthesia*[14])

to form a lung abscess. Although the posterior segment of the upper lobe is the commonest to be involved, it is the most difficult segment to examine radiographically or clinically, because being situated in the upper part of the axilla, it is almost completely hidden by the scapula.

The *right middle lobe bronchus* springs from the anterior aspect of the right bronchus about 3 cm from its origin. It arises just above the apical branch of the right lower lobe. After 1–1·5 cm the middle lobe bronchus divides into lateral and medial branches. The medial branch runs downwards and forwards with a convex curve following the contour of the right side of the heart. The patency of the middle lobe bronchus is particularly vulnerable to glandular swelling because it is closely related to the right tracheobronchial groups of glands.

The *right lower lobe bronchus* is the continuation of the right main bronchus and has five, or occasionally six, divisions. The apical branch comes off 0·5–1·0 cm below the origin of the middle lobe but slightly more laterally. About 1·5 cm below the apical bronchus the cardiac or medial basal branch arises from the medial side of the lower lobe stem and passes downwards for 2·5 cm before dividing into its two terminal branches—anterior and posterior. Sometimes there is a subapical branch which comes off the posterior wall of the main bronchus just below the cardiac branch. After giving off these branches the main stem divides into the basal bronchi—the anterior, lateral and posterior branches—to supply the appropriate segments.

The apical segment of either of the lower lobes is particularly vulnerable to inhaled material when the patient lies supine (Fig. 22*b*), and the right and left sides provide an approximately similar incidence of lung abscess. When a patient is propped up in bed in the post-operative period, secretions tend to gravitate to the lower lobes (Fig. 23).

### Left Bronchial Tree

The *left main bronchus* is narrower than the right and is nearly 5 cm long. It terminates at the origin of the upper lobe bronchus becoming the main stem to the lower lobe. It should be noted that this is in direct contrast to the right lung, where the branches to the upper lobe and middle lobes are offshoots of the parent main bronchus. The presence of 5 cm of bronchial lumen uninterrupted by any branching makes the left main bronchus particularly suitable for intubation and "blocking" during thoracic surgery.

The *left upper lobe bronchus* is unlike that of the right upper lobe, for it does not arise as an offshoot of the left main bronchus but as one part of the bifurcation of the main trunk. After its origin it begins to curve rapidly to the lateral side. The angle that it forms when visualised from within the main bronchial lumen often makes it possible to insert in it a very small

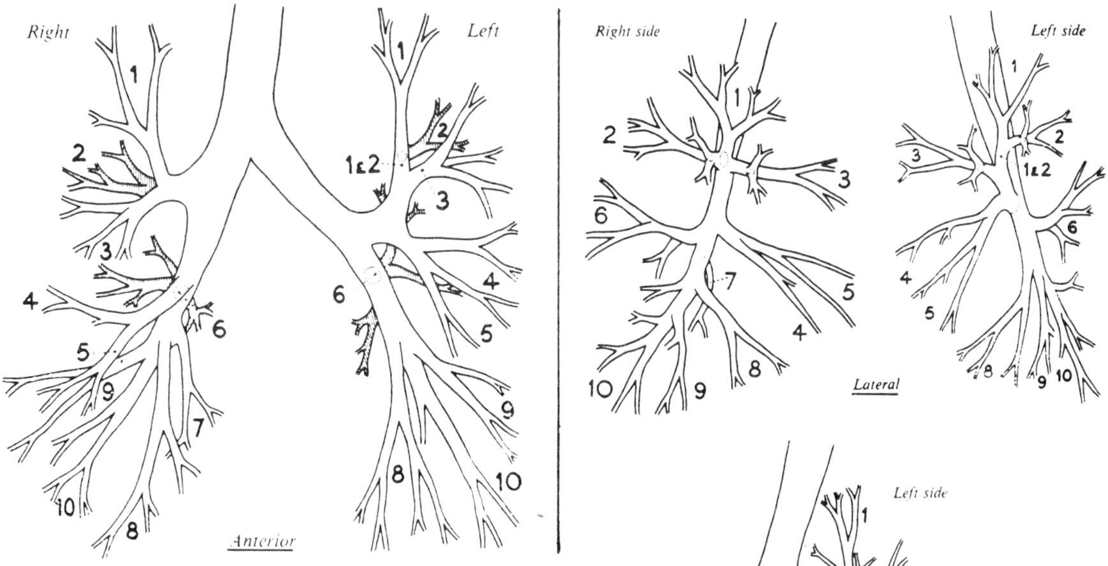


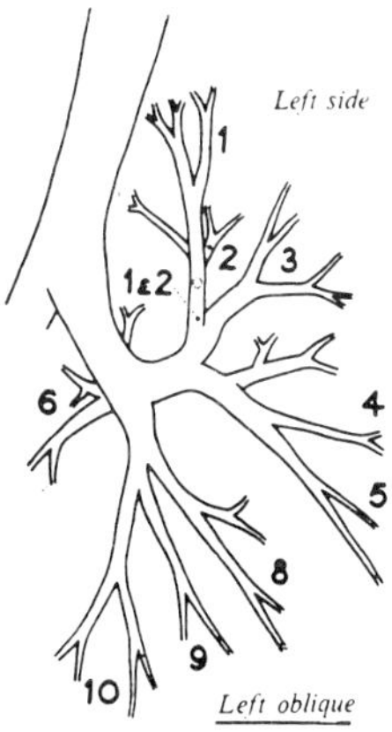

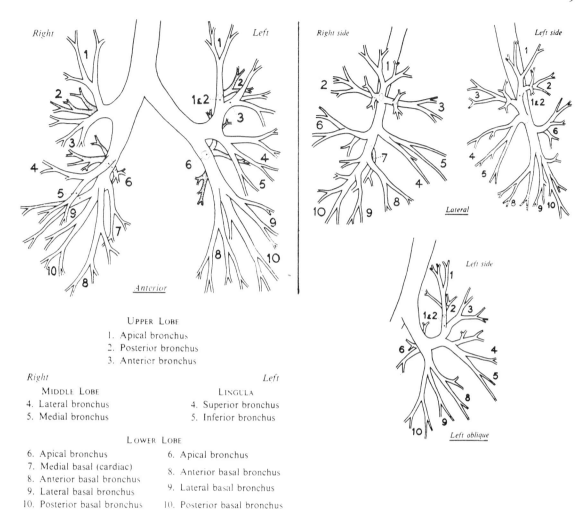

UPPER LOBE
1. Apical bronchus
2. Posterior bronchus
3. Anterior bronchus

| *Right* | *Left* |
| --- | --- |
| MIDDLE LOBE | LINGULA |
| 4. Lateral bronchus | 4. Superior bronchus |
| 5. Medial bronchus | 5. Inferior bronchus |

LOWER LOBE

| | |
| --- | --- |
| 6. Apical bronchus | 6. Apical bronchus |
| 7. Medial basal (cardiac) | |
| 8. Anterior basal bronchus | 8. Anterior basal bronchus |
| 9. Lateral basal bronchus | 9. Lateral basal bronchus |
| 10. Posterior basal bronchus | 10. Posterior basal bronchus |

1/FIG. 20.—Diagram illustrating the bronchopulmonary nomenclature approved by the Thoracic Society and reproduced by permission of the Editors of *Thorax*. (Figure courtesy of Drs. T. H. Sellors and J. L. Livingstone and the publishers Butterworth and Co.[15])

bronchial blocker. The upper lobe bronchus continues for 1–1·5 cm before bifurcating into an upper and a lower division. The upper division curves upwards in line with the main stem bronchus before dividing into apical, posterior and anterior branches. The lower division descends as the *lingular bronchus*.

The *left lower lobe bronchus* arises as a continuation of the left main bronchus and runs in a downward, backward and lateral direction. About 1 cm below its origin it gives off the apical branch from its posterior wall. This branch is important because, when the patient is lying on his back, inhaled material tends to flow through it into the apical segment of the lower lobe. The apical branch runs backwards as a short stem before dividing into three branches.

Sometimes, the left lower lobe bronchus gives off a subapical branch from its posterior wall about 1–1·5 cm below the origin of the apical branch before finally dividing into its main terminations—the basal bronchi. The anterior basal branch arises from the antero-lateral aspect of the lower lobe stem and runs downwards, forwards and slightly laterally. About 1 cm below its origin it may give off a small

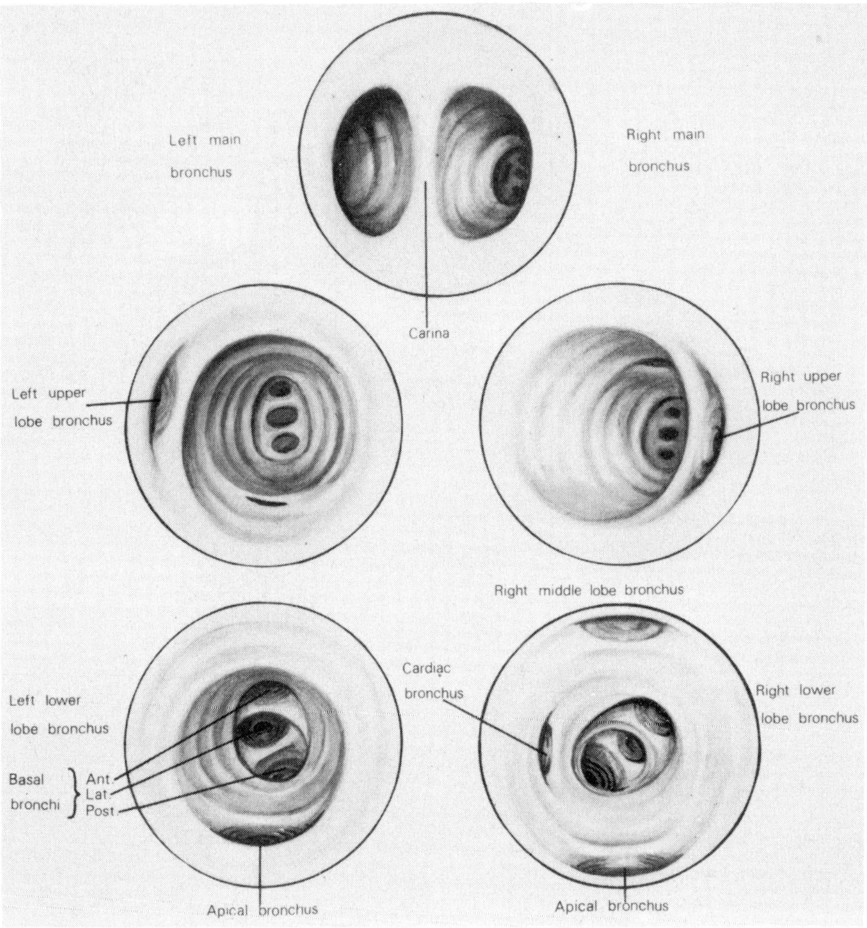


1/FIG. 21.—The normal bronchial tree as seen down a bronchoscope.

branch from its medial side which corresponds to the cardiac bronchus on the right side. The lateral basal bronchus runs in a downward and lateral direction. The posterior basal bronchus is the largest of three and sometimes appears as a continuation of the main stem running downwards, backwards and slightly laterally.

All three basal bronchi may give off lateral branches soon after their origin. These branches are often found to play an important part in the surgical anatomy of lung abscess.

**Bronchioles**

As a bronchiole is traced distally the cartilaginous rings gradually recede, forming irregular plates which occur sporadically until the diameter of the bronchiole is approximately 0·6 mm, when they disappear completely. Continuing the progress down the bronchial tree the tubular outline of the bronchiole wall changes and small projections in increasing numbers appear on all sides. This area is now termed a respiratory bronchiole and the small projections are alveolar ducts leading to the air sacs. The name "terminal bronchiole" has arisen in the English nomenclature and usually denotes that area of the bronchiole not containing cartilage which lies just before the origin of the respiratory bronchiole.

**The Bronchial and Bronchiolar Musculature**

The fundamental purpose of this muscle is to permit alterations in the length and width of the bronchial tube with the various phases of respiration. The particular arrangement of the muscle fibres is of great importance, for the

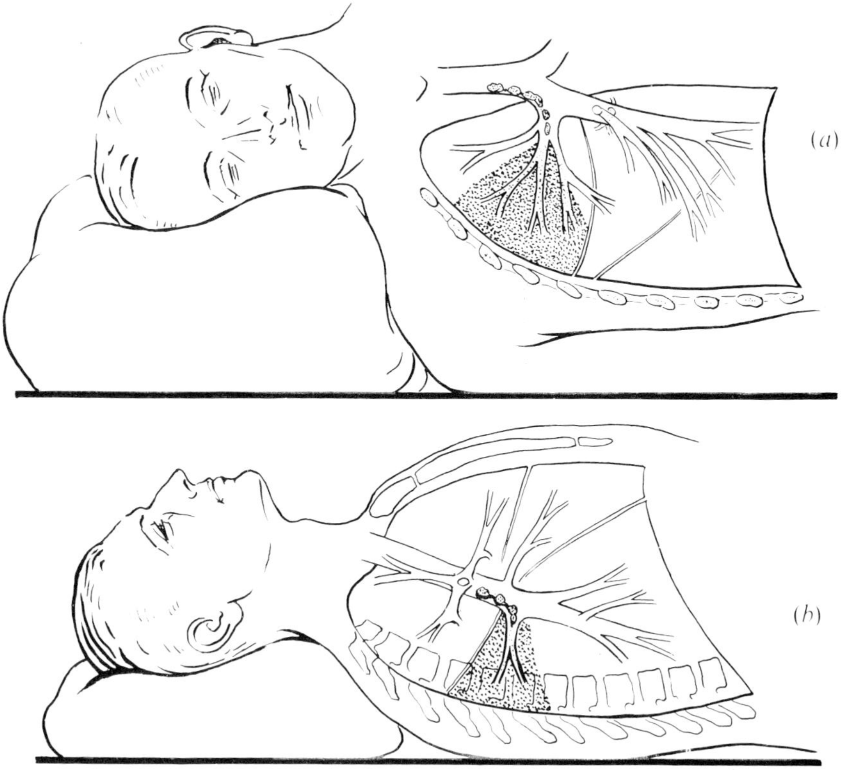


1/FIG. 22.—DIAGRAMS TO ILLUSTRATE THE RELATIONSHIP BETWEEN POSTURE AND THE FOCAL INCIDENCE OF LUNG ABSCESS
(*a*) Patient lying on side: inhaled material collects in posterior segment of right upper lobe.
(*b*) Patient lying on back: inhaled material collects in apical segment of right lower lobe.
(Courtesy of Lord Brock and the publishers, Oxford University Press, based on two figures in *The Anatomy of the Bronchial Tree*)

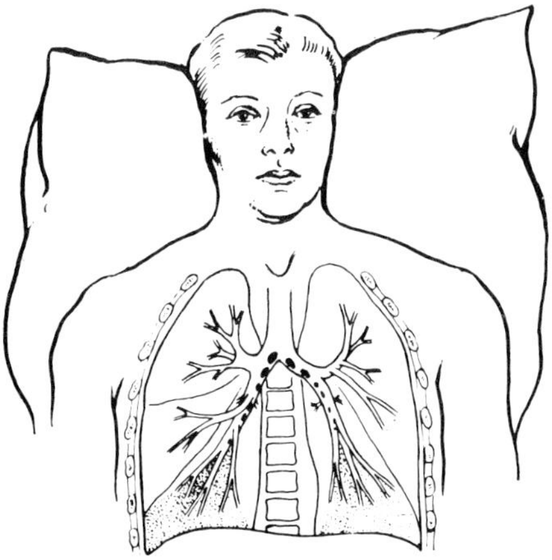

1/FIG. 23.—Figure to show the accumulation of secretions in the lower lobes of a patient in the sitting position.

muscle-pattern is best described as a "geodesic network" (a geodesic line on any curved surface is the one of shortest distance between two points, e.g. an arc of a great circle on a sphere). A geodesic pattern, therefore, is the ideal method of withstanding or producing pressures in a tubular structure without there being a tendency for the fibres to slip along the surface (Fig. 24).

As the muscle layer is followed down the bronchial tree so it becomes thinner, but the relative thickness of this layer in relation to that of the wall as a whole increases. Thus in a bronchiole of 1 mm diameter the muscle bands are relatively five times as strong as in a bronchus of 10 mm. The terminal bronchiole, which has the narrowest lumen, has therefore relatively the thickest muscle layer.

Elastic fibres run lengthwise between the mucosal and muscle layers. In general their course is longitudinal, but at the points where branching of the bronchioles occur the fibres swing over and encircle each branch as it leaves (Fig. 24). Since the smooth muscle fibres also undergo this arrangement the origin of each branch is reinforced by a series of interlacing fibres. So close is the admixture of elastic and muscle fibres that some authorities refer to this layer as a "myo-elastic layer".

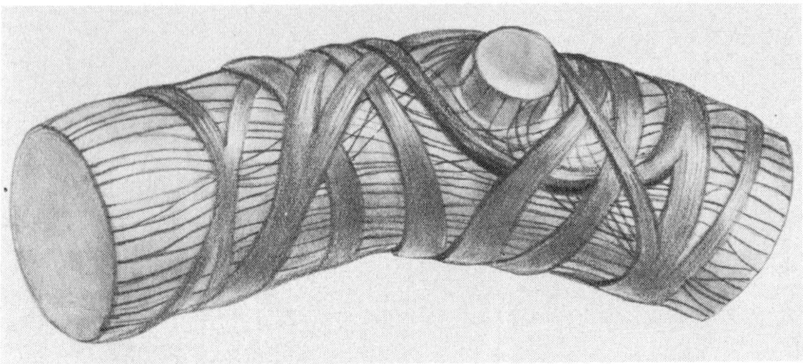

1/Fig. 24.—Diagram to show the geodesic arrangement of the musculature in a bronchiole. (Courtesy of Charles C. Thomas, publisher, based on reconstruction models from William Snow Miller's *The Lung*).

**Epithelium of the Tracheobronchial Tree** (Figs. 25 and 26)

The trachea down to the beginning of the respiratory bronchiole is lined by ciliated columnar epithelium freely interspersed with mucous or goblet cells lying on an intermediate layer of spindle-shaped cells; these are derived from the basal cells with round nuclei found in the deepest layer. In the lower part of the bronchial tree the ciliated cells far outnumber the other forms, but at the beginning of the respiratory bronchiole they give way to a cuboidal cell without any cilia.

**Bronchial Vessels**

The anatomy of the bronchial arteries is variable. Usually there are two left bronchial arteries arising from the thoracic aorta, and one right bronchial artery which arises either from an intercostal artery or the upper left bronchial artery. There may in addition be other smaller bronchial arteries.

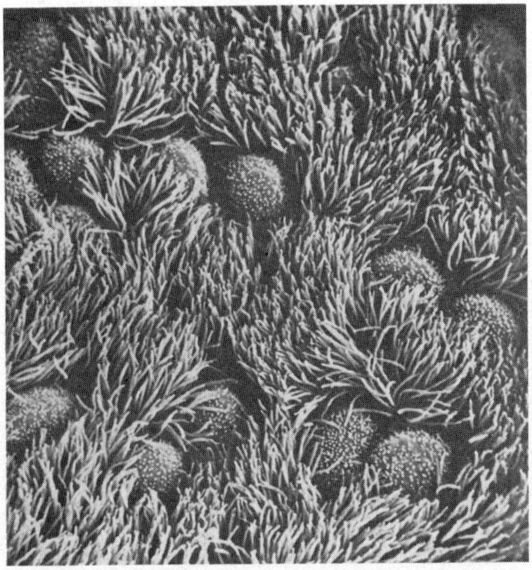

1/Fig. 25.—Scanning electron micrograph of epithelium of rat trachea. Groups of mucous cells are seen surrounded by ciliated cells. (Courtesy of Porter and Bonneville, 1973 and the publishers Lea and Febiger.[16])

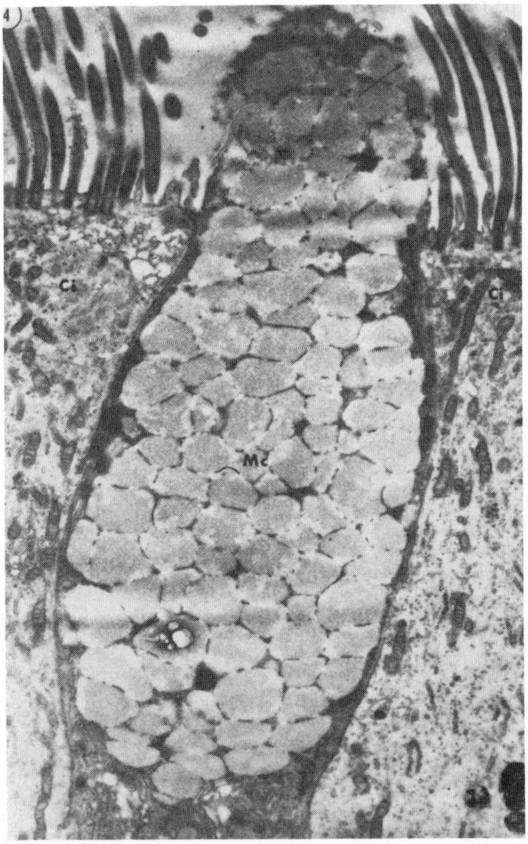


1/Fig. 26.—Section of human tracheal epithelium showing a mucous cell (Mc) surrounded by numerous ciliated cells (Ci). (Courtesy of Rhodin, 1966 and the *American Review of Respiratory Disease.*[17])

On entering the lung the bronchial arteries embed themselves in the layer of connective tissue surrounding the bronchus. Usually two or three branches of the bronchial artery run with the larger bronchi and bronchioli until finally each bronchial subdivision is accompanied by a corresponding division of the artery. In this manner the arteries continue until the distal end of the terminal bronchiole is reached.

Anastomotic branches from the bronchial artery pierce the outer fibrous coat of the bronchi and form an arterial plexus in the adventitia around the muscle layer. From this outer arterial plexus, branches pierce the muscle layer to enter the submucosa. The vessels run for a short distance parallel with the muscle fibres before splitting up into a fine capillary plexus which supplies the mucous membrane. From this capillary network venous radicles arise which in their turn pierce the muscle layer to reach a venous plexus in the outer adventitia. From this second plexus veins arise and form one of the sources of the pulmonary vein. It is evident, therefore, that an arterial and venous plexus lies on the outside of the muscle layers, whilst a capillary plexus lies on the inside. A point of great importance is that blood must pass through the muscle layer in its passage between the various plexuses.

Therefore, when the muscle layer contracts, it is probable that whilst the arterial plexus with its higher pressure can maintain a flow to the capillary plexus, the latter is unable to empty into the outer venous plexus. This must lead to swelling of the mucosa with a further narrowing of the lumen.

When the respiratory bronchiole is reached the bronchial arteries disappear as a distinct set of vessels. The internal capillary plexus, however, fuses with that of the pulmonary artery in the walls of the alveoli providing an example of normal "true shunt" (p. 98). It appears that the pulmonary artery supplies the respiratory bronchiole in a similar manner to the bronchial artery supplying the terminal bronchiole.

True bronchial veins are only seen at the hilum of the lung and do not play a significant part in the venous drainage of the bronchioles.

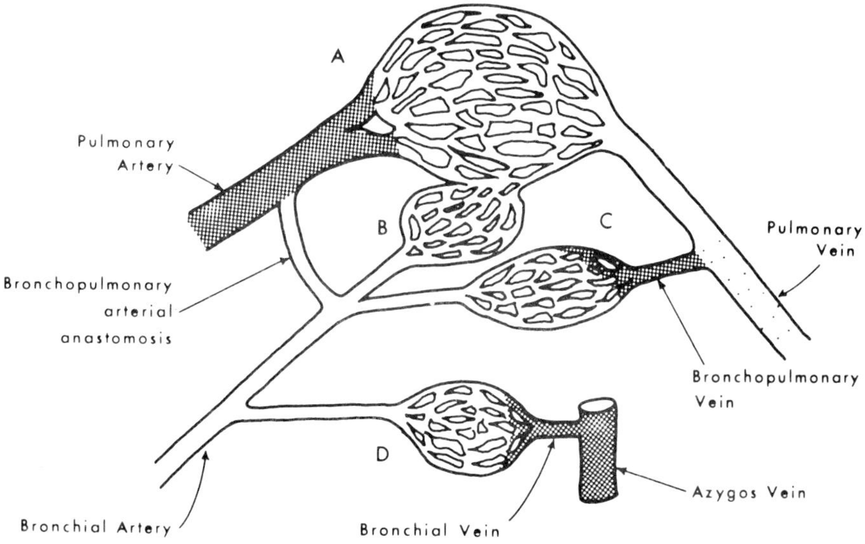


1/FIG. 27.—Schematic representation of the relationships between the bronchial pulmonary circulations. The pulmonary artery supplies the pulmonary capillary network A. The bronchial artery supplies capillary network B, C and D. Network B represents the bronchial capillary supply to bronchioles that anastomoses with pulmonary capillaries and drains through pulmonary veins. Network C represents the bronchial capillary supply to most bronchi; these vessels form bronchopulmonary veins that empty into pulmonary veins. Network D represents the bronchial capillary supply to lobar and segmental bronchi; these vessels form true bronchial veins that drain into the azygos, hemiazygos, or intercostal veins. (Courtesy of Murray (1976) and W. B. Saunders Company.[18])

They arise at the level of the first divisions of the main bronchial tree and usually drain into the azygos, hemi-azygos and intercostal veins. The pulmonary vein arises from the venous plexus in the terminal bronchiole wall, from that in the wall of the respiratory bronchiole down to and including the alveoli, and finally from the plexus underlying the pleura.

**Innervation of the Bronchial Tree**

The lung receives innervation from both sympathetic and parasympathetic sources. The sympathetic nerve fibres are derived from the 1st–5th thoracic ganglia along with branches from the inferior cervical ganglion, though some fibres may also be received from the middle cervical ganglion. The vagus nerve supplies the parasympathetic fibres, joining with the sympathetic fibres to form the posterior pulmonary plexus at the root of the lung. Fibres from this plexus pass round the root of the lung to form the anterior pulmonary plexus.

The posterior pulmonary plexus divides into a peri-arterial and peri-bronchial plexus. The latter again divides into an extrachondrial and intra-chondrial plexus in relation to cartilaginous plates in the bronchial wall. On reaching the non-cartilaginous parts of the lung the two plexuses again unite and continue distally as one. Ganglia are to be found at all levels of the bronchial tree so that short post-ganglionic fibres reach the bands of smooth muscle in which they break up into individual fibres. These fibres give off twigs to supply the smooth muscle fibres of the geodesic network.

In all probability the mucous glands are innervated solely by the vagus. As regards the nervous control of the vessel walls, recent evidence suggests that the vagus carries cholinergic dilator fibres whilst the thoraco-lumbar nerves carry predominantly adrenergic constrictor fibres to the bronchial arterial system.

**Control of Bronchial Calibre**

The bronchi dilate and retract passively with each phase of respiration. On inspiration the pressure in the air ducts is greater than that in the pleural cavity—consequently the bronchi are dilated by the pull of the negative intrapleural pressure. As the lung expands, therefore, the bronchial tree is dilated and lengthened, and as it diminishes in size the bronchi shorten and contract due to the retraction of the elastic tissue in their walls. In man, it is known that most sympathomimetic drugs produce bronchial relaxation whilst cholinergic drugs lead to constriction.

**Bronchomotor Tone**

Bronchomotor tone is a continuous and variable state of contraction of the bronchial musculature which is present during both phases of respiration. In the dog, section of the sympathetic nerves has no effect on bronchial calibre, while vagal section produces considerable alterations. In fact, bilateral vagal section results in the bronchi opening more widely during inspiration and narrowing to a greater degree than normal during expiration. These facts strongly suggest that it is predominantly the vagi that carry impulses influencing the diameter of the bronchial lumen and that they are responsible for normal bronchial muscle tone.

**Respiratory Tract Reflexes**

Because of the immense difficulties involved, most of the studies of respiratory reflexes have been made in animals rather than in man, yet these reflexes play a significant role in the control of the respiratory and the cardiovascular systems. This subject is well reviewed by Widdicombe.[19, 20]

**(a) Inflation.**—Hering and Breuer in 1868[21] showed that the inflation of the lungs inhibited the spontaneous contraction of the diaphragm in anaesthetised animals, and Adrian[22] concluded that the pulmonary stretch receptors were responsible for this inflation reflex. These receptors are unencapsulated, and are found in the airway smooth muscle without end-organs. They are generally believed to be responsible for signalling changes in the mechanical state of the lungs to the brain.

Barbiturate anaesthesia depresses the inflation reflex, but only abolishes it completely with very high doses.[23]

A weak inflation reflex has been demonstrated in man, but it may be absent in the anaesthetised subject.[24] It may be responsible for the apnoea produced on inflation of the newborn baby's lung, though this response only persists for the first few days of life.

**(b) Deflation.**—During expiration the tonic discharge of the stretch receptors diminishes so that soon inspiration can start again. Nevertheless, there is evidence that a deflation reflex exists in its own right; the receptors are sited differently in that they lie principally in the alveoli and terminal bronchioles. Sensitisation of these receptors leads to an increase in the rate and force of the inspiratory effort and its role may be designed primarily to protect the individual by increasing ventilation in the event of pulmonary collapse. Paintal[25] has shown that these receptors are stimulated by inhalational anaesthetics.

**(c) Paradoxical reflex.**—This reflex was described by Head in 1889 and can only be demonstrated when the vagus nerve is *partially* blocked. Inflation of the lungs under this condition leads to a strong diaphragmatic contraction. It does not occur if the vagus nerve is intact or completely blocked, and because it is the opposite response of the normal inflation reflex it has been termed "paradoxical". This reflex may account for the primitive gasp observed in newborn babies when the lungs are first inflated.[26]

**(d) Irritant receptors.**—Afferent nerve endings responding to both mechanical and chemical irritants have been described lying in the epithelium of the airways from the trachea to the respiratory bronchioles. They are concentrated mainly at the carina and at the points of branching of the bronchial tree. They are activated by (1) chemical irritants such as ether, ammonia, cigarette smoke; (2) mechanical irritants such as dust; (3) airway smooth muscle contraction; (4) airway distortion which may be caused for example by pneumothorax or atelectasis. Stimulation of these receptors results in hyperpnoea and laryngeal and bronchial constriction. Sometimes partial inflation of the lungs using positive pressure results in a deep breath. This is a vagal reflex probably involving irritant receptors.

Aspiration of fluid, whether it be fresh-water, sea-water, or vomit with a hydrochloric acid content, always leads to reflex closure of the glottis and bronchoconstriction. Animal experiments have demonstrated that even after both vagi have been sectioned atropine, neostigmine and isopropyl-noradrenaline are all capable of influencing the bronchial response.[27] This suggests that aspiration of fluid invokes a reflex response of the parasympathetic nervous system, but there is not only a central component acting via the vagus nerve, but also a peripheral fraction which is intrinsic within the bronchial wall.

**(e) J-receptors.**—J-receptors (or juxta-pulmonary capillary receptors) lie in the walls of the alveoli and possibly of the smaller airways. Like the other lung receptors their afferent pathway is vagal. They can respond to numerous different stimuli but they are chiefly stimulated by an increase in interstitial fluid between the capillary endothelium and alveolar epithelium, which may be caused by pulmonary oedema, micro-embolism, pneumonia or irritant gases such as chlorine. There is evidence to suggest that stimulation of J-receptors causes tachypnoea, bronchoconstriction and contraction of the adductor muscles of the larynx, but since the causes of their stimulation (above) often have other effects it is difficult to isolate those effects due to J-receptor stimulation alone.

### Bronchospasm

The term denotes spasm of the bronchi, but a better name would be bronchiolar spasm, as this is the area of the respiratory tree which is mainly involved. Stimulation can be initiated by chemical, mechanical or neurogenic factors. It is most commonly encountered in patients who have an "irritable" bronchial tree, i.e. chronic bronchitics and patients with a history of asthma. The constriction of the bronchiole is greater during expiration than inspiration. Inspiratory and expiratory wheezes can usually be heard on auscultation, although if the bronchospasm is very severe there may be insufficient air flow to make a noise. It is very important to be sure that the difficulty in ventilating the patient and high airway pressure are not due to mechanical obstruction of the tube. If there is any doubt about this the tube should be changed immediately. A tension pneumothorax can also simulate severe bronchospasm, as well as result from the high inflation pressures which may be required. Bronchospasm is a diagnosis that only should be made when all other causes of ventilatory difficulty have been excluded. The treatment of this condition is broadly the same as the treatment of an attack of asthma in an unanaesthetised patient.

1/TABLE 2
SUBSTANCES INFLUENCING BRONCHIAL SMOOTH MUSCLE TONE

| | |
|---|---|
| *Bronchodilatation* | |
| 1. $\beta_2$ Sympathomimetics. | Salbutamol, isoprenaline, adrenaline, ephedrine. |
| 2. Xanthine derivatives. | Aminophylline. |
| 3. Volatile anaesthetics. | Halothane, diethyl ether. |
| 4. Nitrites. | Amyl nitrite, glyceryl trinitrate. |
| 5. Prostaglandins $E_1$ and $E_2$. | Allergic response, infusion. |
| 6. Muscarinic cholinergic receptor blockers. | Atropine, hyoscine. |
| *Bronchoconstriction* | |
| 1. Muscarinic cholinomimetics. | |
| (a) Anticholinesterases. | Neostigmine, pyridostigmine, physostigmine, edrophonium. |
| (b) Choline esters and alkaloids. | Carbachol, pilocarpine. |
| 2. $\beta_2$ Adrenergic blockers. | Propranolol, etc. |
| 3. Autacoids. | Histamine, 5-hydroxytryptamine, kinins, prostaglandin $F_{2\alpha}$. (a) Histamine-releasing drugs: tubocurarine, morphine, thiopentone. (b) Allergic response. (c) Carcinoid tumours. (d) Prostaglandin infusion. |

The response to some of these agents may be minimal in the normal and enhanced in the presence of abnormal bronchial smooth muscle tone or in susceptible individuals, e.g. asthmatics.

## THE ALVEOLI

The respiratory bronchioles terminate in alveolar ducts from which the alveoli arise (Fig. 28). Gas exchange occurs not only at alveolar level but also in the respiratory bronchioles, alveolar ducts and air sacs, so that from the functional aspect the exact anatomical differences between these structures are not of great importance. The average diameter of an alveolus is about 0·2 mm at functional residual capacity, though the size obviously varies with the state of inflation of the lung. It is also affected by gravity, the alveolar diameter being smallest within the most dependent parts of the lung and largest in the uppermost parts. This is due to the weight of the lung tissue itself compressing the lowermost alveoli, and has important functional implications.

About 1500 miles of capillaries distribute blood to 300 million alveoli where blood and air are separated by a thin layer of tissue less than 2 μm thick and which is built up of four layers:

(1) **Alveolar lining fluid.**—This is a very thin fluid layer lining the alveoli. Its surface tension is reduced by surfactant (see below).

(2) **Alveolar epithelium.**—About 95 per cent of the alveolar epithelium is composed of epithelial type I cells which are also called agranular pneumocytes. They are large flat cells, only about 0·2 μm thick and joined to each other by tight junctions. Their main function is gas exchange, which they aid by providing a very thin layer through which diffusion of oxygen and carbon dioxide can take place. The granular pneumocytes or type II cells are interspersed in the alveolar epithelium and contain multilamellar bodies which are extruded into the alveolar space by a process of exocytosis (Figs. 29 and 30), and are probably the source of surfactant.

(3) **Interstitial layer.**—This is a thin layer separating the alveolar epithelium and the capillary endothelium. It contains two basement membranes as well as elastic fibres, collagen fibrils and a few fibroblasts in its thicker parts. It accounts for about half the thickness of the blood-gas barrier.

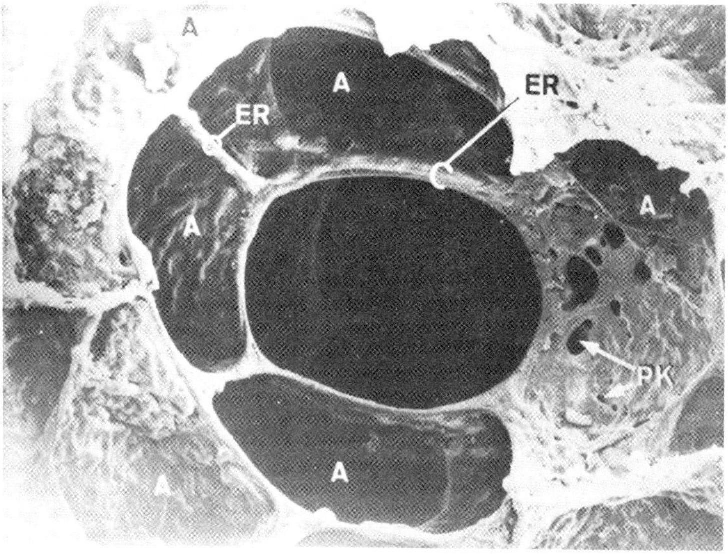


1/FIG. 28.—Scanning electron micrograph of alveolar duct leading to adjacent alveoli (A). The free edge of alveolar septa is reinforced by connective tissue which forms entrance rings (ER). Note the interalveolar pores of Kohn (PK) of varying size. (Courtesy of Gehr, Bachofen and Weibel (1978) and the North Holland Publishing Company.[28])

(4) **Capillary endothelium.**—The capillary endothelial cells are linked together by tight junctions and contain a large number of vesicles which are involved in bulk transport of fluid and macromolecules. Some of these vesicles are free in the cytoplasm, some are open to the blood side and some open to the tissue side. These cells are biochemically very active (see p. 29), and have access to the entire cardiac output.

**Alveolar Macrophages**

The alveolar surface area is about eighty times that of the skin and several defence mechanisms exist to protect it. Alveolar macrophages (Fig. 31) provide the last line of defence as they lurk within the alveoli armed with a variety of enzymes ready to ingest or destroy particles or organisms.

**Collateral Ventilation**

Pores of Kohn are holes 3–13 μm in diameter through alveolar walls (Figs. 28 and 31), allowing gas transfer between the two alveoli. Collateral ventilation can also occur at a more proximal level via canals of Lambert which connect bronchioles and possibly even some larger airways.

**Surfactant.**—It was originally believed that retraction of the lungs during passive expiration was due entirely to their elastic tissue. However, if the lungs are distended to peak capacity with air, the transpulmonary pressure is two to three times as great as when they are distended to the same volume with fluid. Because the only difference is the presence of an air-liquid interface in the air-filled lung, most of the lung recoil can be ascribed to surface forces. Mead and associates[30] also noted that the contribution of surface forces to the elastic recoil was less at low lung volumes. This was surprising in view of the formula of Laplace (an 18th century mathematician) which states that the pressure in a sphere is equal to twice the wall tension divided by the radius.

$$\text{Pressure} = \frac{2\ (\text{Wall Tension})}{\text{Radius}}$$

For the average alveolus, with its minute size, a very considerable pressure could thus be exerted by the fluid lining it; in fact, if pure water lined it, this pressure would equal 20 cm of water (2 kPa).

Laplace's formula implies that as the alveoli decrease in size during expiration, the pressure tending to collapse them increases and a vicious circle is established. In fact this does not happen because the alveoli are coated with surfactant, which causes a reduction in surface tension. As the alveoli deflate, the amount of surfactant per unit area of alveolar membrane increases and so surface tension is reduced even further. In

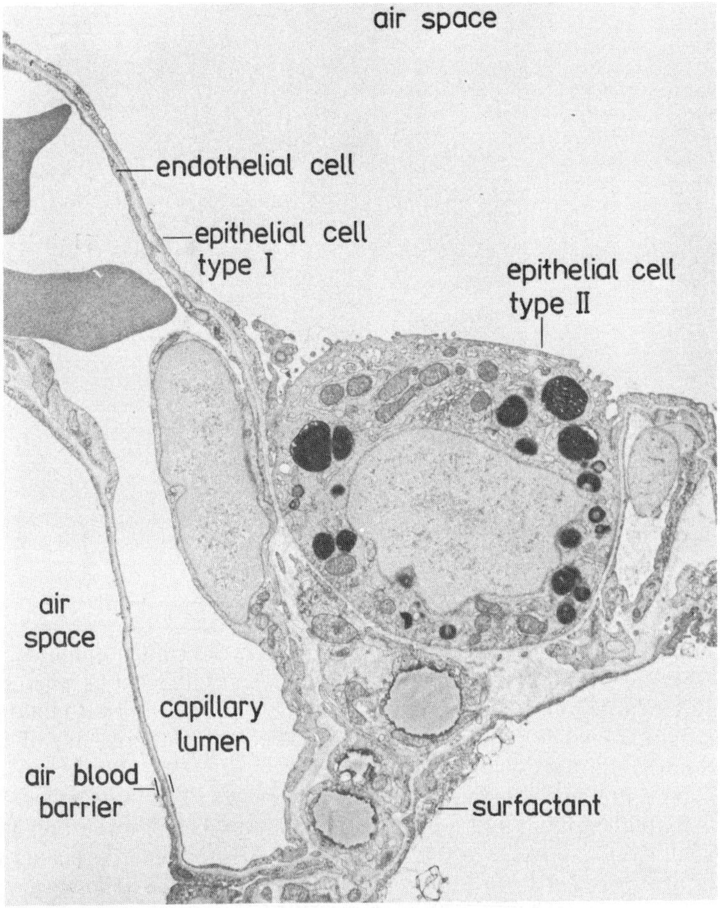


1/FIG. 29.—Cellular components of the alveolar-capillary unit of the rat lung. (Courtesy of Dr. M. Simionescu, and the Ciba Foundation Symposium, 1980.[29])

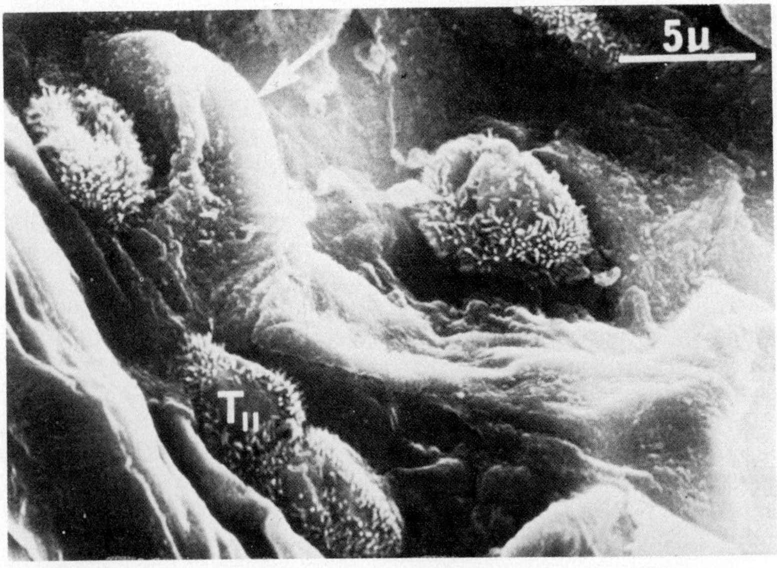


1/FIG. 30.—Scanning electron photomicrograph of the surface of a human alveolus showing several type II cells with characteristic microvilli; the rest of the surface is covered by the cytoplasmic extensions of type I cells. A red blood cell can be seen bulging in a pulmonary capillary (arrow). (Courtesy of Dr. N. S. Wang, the editor, J. F. Murray and the publishers W. B. Saunders Co.[18])

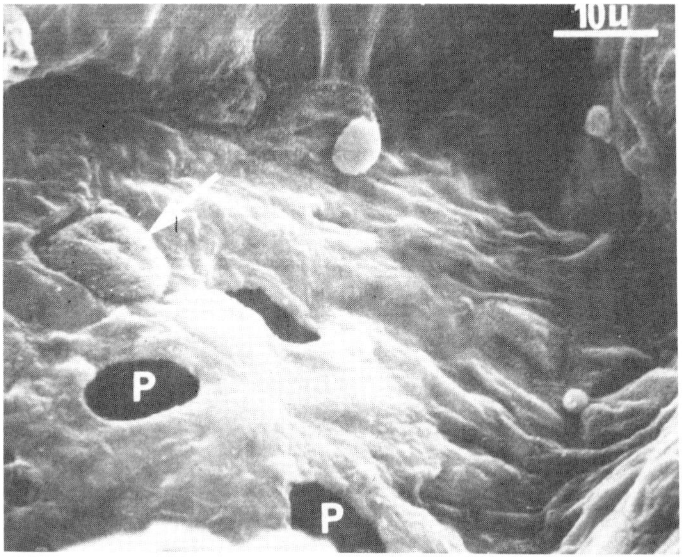


1/FIG. 31.—Scanning electron photomicrograph of the surface of a human alveolus showing pores of Kohn (P) and a macrophage (arrow). (Courtesy of Dr. N. S. Wang, and the editor J. F. Murray (1976) and the publishers W. B. Saunders Co.[18])

this way, the action of surfactant becomes more efficient as the alveoli decrease in size and therefore, contrary to what would be predicted just on the basis of Laplace's law, the smaller alveoli inflate more easily than the larger ones. If there was no surfactant the large alveoli would tend to inflate further at the expense of the smaller ones which would collapse. Non-wettability may be another important characteristic of surfactant.[31]

Surfactant is a mixture of phospholipids (mostly dipalmitoyl-phosphatidyl-choline) complexed with protein. It is secreted by type II epithelial cells (Fig. 32) and has a half-life of about 14 hours. In the foetal lung surfactant appears at about 6 months gestation, soon after lamellar bodies can be demonstrated in the type II cells.

**Clinical significance.**—Absence of this material in the infant at birth is believed to be one of the primary causes of the "respiratory distress syndrome" (see p. 1114). Attempts have been made to aerosolise one component of the surfactant (dipalmitoyl lecithin) into the airways of infants with the syndrome but these have not proved of value. Oxygen therapy may lead to a reduction in surfactant[32] and hence it should be used in the lowest possible concentration, and for the shortest time, necessary to achieve the desired effect, although if 100 per cent oxygen is needed to prevent arterial hypoxaemia then it should be used.[33]

Pulmonary collapse, whether occurring on its own or in association with a reduction in the pulmonary circulation—as from embolism or ligation—may well be associated with too little surfactant. Deficiency of it may also account for some of the respiratory difficulties that are encountered in patients after cardiopulmonary bypass.

### Metabolic Function of the Lungs

The enormous capillary surface area of the lungs makes them ideally suited for manipulating the chemistry of the blood. Gas exchange apart, it has only recently been appreciated how very active they are in this respect.[34]

The lungs are the major site of inactivation of 5-hydroxytryptamine; they also inactivate bradykinin and noradrenaline (about 30 per cent in one passage through the lungs) but not adrenaline. They are therefore chemically highly selective and, for example, more than 90 per cent of $PGE_1$*, $PGE_2$, or $PGF_2$ are removed in one passage through the lungs whereas $PGA_1$, $PGA_2$ and prostacyclin pass through unchanged.

Converting enzyme, present on the luminal surface of endothelial cells lining the pulmonary

* PG is the abbreviation for prostaglandin (see Chapter 38).

(a) (b) (c) (d)

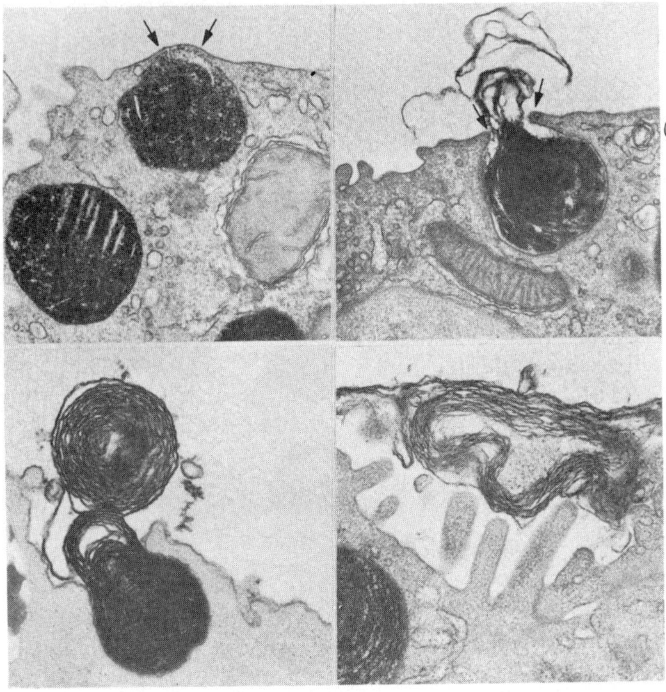

1/Fig. 32.—Multilamellar bodies of type II epithelial cells in different stages of their secretion into the alveolar space by exocytosis. (*a*) The body is found next to the apical plasmalemma (arrows); (*b*) the membrane surrounding the multilamellar body becomes continuous with the apical plasmalemma (arrows); (*c*) extrusion of a complex lamellar body; and (*d*) unravelling of the lamellae over the apical plasmalemma. (Courtesy of Dr. M. Simionescu, and the Ciba Foundation Symposium, 1980.[29])

blood vessels, catalyses the hydrolysis of angiotensin I to angiotensin II which is much more potent than the parent compound in causing smooth muscle contraction.

In addition to the processes of inactivation and conversion mentioned above, the lungs also secrete certain substances. During anaphylaxis, histamine and SRS-A (Slow Reacting Substances of Anaphylaxis) are released. Prostacyclin, which is a vasodilator and potent inhibitor of platelet aggregation is produced partly in the lungs. Its generation at this site is stimulated by angiotensin II and other peptides, and by hyperventilation probably as a result of simple stretching of lung tissue.

**Asthma**

Asthma is a condition characterised by attacks of bronchospasm often with a precipitating factor such as allergy (e.g. house dust, animal fur, etc.). Anxiety before surgery can often promote an attack so that it is vitally important for the anaesthetist to use pre-operative measures that calm, reassure and promote bronchodilatation. For example, disodium cromoglycate (Intal) is useful in the prevention of allergic attacks of asthma and the patient often gets great relief from the regular use of a salbutamol inhaler. Anxiolytic drugs (e.g. diazepam) and the antihistamines (e.g. promethazine) play an important role in the pre-operative preparation of the patient. For the severe asthmatic with a history of steroid therapy the administration of hydrocortisone with the premedication is essential.

During anaesthesia it is important to reduce irritation of the bronchial tree and intubation should be avoided if at all possible. Halothane, with its bronchodilating property, is particularly useful and all agents which are known to be liberators of histamine should be avoided. In the event of a severe attack of bronchospasm during anaesthesia, 250–500 mg of aminophylline (given intravenously over 5 minutes) will often improve ventilation. For the treatment of Status Asthmaticus the reader is referred to Chapter 9, page 281.

## REFERENCES


1. Camner, P. (1980). Clearance of particles from the human tracheobronchial tree. *Clinical Science and Molecular Medicine*, **59**, 79.
2. Spencer, H. (1977). *Pathology of the Lung*. Oxford: Pergamon Press Ltd.
3. Leading Article (1982). Pulmonary mucociliary clearance. *Lancet*, **1**, 203.
4. Forbes, A. R. (1976). Halothane depresses mucociliary flow in the trachea. *Anesthesiology*, **45**, 59.
5. Forbes, A. R. and Horrigan, R. W. (1977). Mucociliary flow in the trachea during anesthesia with enflurane, ether, nitrous oxide and morphine. *Anesthesiology*, **46**, 319.
6. Chalon, J., Patel, C., Ali, M., Ramanathan, S., Capan, L., Tang, C., Turndorf, H. (1979). Humidity and the anesthetized patient. *Anesthesiology*, **50**, 195.
7. Burton, J. D. K. (1962). Effects of dry anaesthetic gases on the respiratory mucous membrane. *Lancet*, **1**, 235.
8. Herzog, P., Norlander, O. P., and Engstrom, C. G. (1964). Ultrasonic generation of aerosol for the humidification of inspired gas during volume-controlled ventilation. *Acta anaesth. scand.*, **8**, 79.
9. Ringrose, R. E., McKown, B., Felton, F. G., Barclay, B. O., Muchmore, H. G., and Rhoades, E. R. (1968). A hospital outbreak of serratia marcescens associated with ultrasonic nebulizers. *Ann. intern. Med.*, **69**, 719.
10. Cheney, F. W., and Butler, J. (1968). The effects of ultrasonically produced aerosols on airway resistance in man. *Anesthesiology*, **29**, 1099.
11. Modell, J. H., Moya, F., Ruiz, B. C., Showers, A. V., and Newby, E. J. (1968). Blood, gas and electrolyte determinations during exposure to ultrasonic nebulised aerosols. *Brit. J. Anaesth.*, **40**, 20.
12. Mackenzie, C. F., McAslan, T. C., Shin, B., Schellinger, D., Helrich, M. (1978). The shape of the human adult trachea. *Anesthesiology*, **49**, 48.
13. Saunders, K. B. (1977). *Clinical Physiology of the Lung*. Oxford: Blackwell Scientific Publications.
14. Bush, G. H. (1963). Tracheo-bronchial suction in infants and children. *Brit. J. Anaesth.*, **35**, 322.
15. Sellors, T. H. and Livingstone, J. L. (1952). *Modern Practice in Tuberculosis*. London: Butterworth & Co.
16. Porter, K. R. and Bonneville, M. A. (1973). *Fine Structure of Cells and Tissues*. Philadelphia: Lea and Febiger.
17. Rhodin, J. A. G. (1966). Ultrastructure and function of the human tracheal mucosa. *American Review of Respiratory Diseases*—a Symposium on Structure, Function and Measurement of Respiratory Cilia. **93**, (3), 6.
18. Murray, J. F. (1976). *The Normal Lung*. Philadelphia: W. B. Saunders Co.
19. Widdicombe, J. G. (1974*a*). Reflex control of breathing. In: *International Review of Science, Respiratory Physiology*, pp. 273–301. Ed. by J. G. Widdicombe. London: Butterworth & Co.
20. Widdicombe, J. G. (1974*b*). Reflexes from the lungs in the control of breathing. In: *Recent Advances in Physiology*, No. 9, p. 239. Ed. by R. J. Linden. Edinburgh: Churchill Livingstone.
21. Hering, E., and Breuer, J. (1868). Die Selbsteuerung der Athmung durch den Nervus Vagus, *S.-B. Akad. Wiss. Wien*, **57**, 672.
22. Adrian, E. D. (1933). Afferent impulses in the vagus and their effects on respiration. *J. Physiol. (Lond.)*, **79**, 332.
23. May, A. J., and Widdicombe, J. G. (1954). Depression of the cough reflex by pentobarbitone and some opium derivatives. *Brit. J. Pharmacol.*, **9**, 338.
24. Widdicombe, J. G. (1961). Respiratory reflexes in man and other mammalian species. *Clin. Sci.*, **21**, 163.
25. Paintal, A. S. (1964). Effects of drugs on vertebrate mechano-receptors. *Pharmacol. Rev.*, **16**, 341.
26. Cross, K. W. (1961). Respiration in the new-born baby. *Brit. med. Bull.*, **17**, 163.
27. Colebatch, H. J. H., and Halmagyi, D. F. J. (1962). Reflex airway reaction to fluid aspiration. *J. appl. Physiol.*, **17**, 787.
28. Gehr, P., Bachofen, M. and Weibel, E. R. (1978). The normal human lung: ultrastructure and morphometric estimation of diffusion capacity. *Respiration Physiology*, **32**, 121.
29. Simionescu, M. (1980). *Metabolic Activities of the Lung* (Ciba Foundation Symposium). Amsterdam: Excerpta Medica.
30. Mead, J., Whittenberger, J. L., and Radford, E. P. (1957). Surface tension as a factor in pulmonary volume-pressure hysteresis, *J. appl. Physiol.*, **10**, 191.
31. Editorial. (1981). What is the true role of surfactant in the lung? *Thorax*, **36**, 1.
32. Norlander, O. P. (1968). The use of respirators in anaesthesia and surgery. *Acta anaesth. scand.*, (Suppl. 30), p. 35.
33. Gillbe, C. E., Salt, J. C. and Branthwaite, M. A. (1980). Pulmonary function after prolonged mechanical ventilation with high concentrations of oxygen. *Thorax*, **35**, 907.
34. Vane, J. R. (1980). Introduction. In: *Metabolic Activities of the Lung*. (Ciba Foundation Symposium, 78). Amsterdam: Excerpta Medica.

CHAPTER 2

# Pulmonary Ventilation



## CONTROL OF BREATHING

There are nerve cells in the brain stem which under normal circumstances generate the rhythm of breathing.[1] The exact localisation of these cells and their connections are not known, and although they do not form a discrete structure or even a collection of cells they are often referred to as the *respiratory centre*. Many of the early experiments involved study of respiratory activity before and after section of the brain and brain stem at various levels in animals. The relevance of these experiments to the control of breathing in Man is doubtful.

Classically, various respiratory centres have been described:

(1) *Inspiratory centre*. This lies in the dorsal part of the medulla on each side and is thought to generate the basic rhythm of respiration, although the existence of "inherent rhythmicity" has recently been questioned.

(2) *Pneumotaxic centre*. Situated in the pons, it transmits impulses to the inspiratory area limiting inspiration and so tending to produce a faster respiratory rate.

(3) *Apneustic centre*. This centre in the lower pons is normally overridden by the pneumotaxic centre. Transection of the pons just below the

pneumotaxic centre causes slow gasping breathing.

(4) *Expiratory centre.* This is situated ventrally on each side of the medulla and when stimulated causes expiratory muscle activity. Expiration is normally a passive process during quiet breathing but becomes active during exercise.

There is as much uncertainty concerning the origin of respiratory rhythmicity as there is concerning the respiratory centre. It is generally thought that there is an inherent rhythmicity in groups of neurons in the brain stem which is modified by their afferent input. Even this idea has been questioned recently[2] and it may be that there is no inherent rhythmicity, the respiratory centre merely transducing the afferent input into a rhythmic output, but in the absence of sufficient afferent input remaining silent. Further evidence in favour of this theory was produced by Phillipson and his associates,[3] who connected awake sheep to membrane oxygenators so that their venous blood could be oxygenated and $CO_2$ removed from it before it reached the lungs. If an amount of $CO_2$ equal to the sheep's $CO_2$ production was removed, the sheep remained apnoeic for up to an hour.

### The Stimulant Effect of Wakefulness on Respiration

Hyperventilation of the anaesthetised patient will lead to apnoea. This occurs at various levels of carbon dioxide tension in the blood and is partly dependent on the anaesthetic technique used. Fink[4] found that in *conscious* healthy volunteers the $Paco_2$ could be reduced to a mean of 22 mm Hg ± 4 (2·9 kPa ± 0·5) without apnoea developing at the end of the period of hyperventilation. On the contrary in the first minute of recovery, ventilation was usually greater than before the test. Subsequently the minute volume fell to about two-thirds of the control value. Thus wakeful subjects do not develop apnoea but continue to breathe rhythmically; this may be because, unlike the sheep described above, they think they ought to. It would appear from these observations that rhythmic respiration can be maintained by wakefulness in the presence of a reduced blood carbon dioxide, or by an increased carbon dioxide level in the blood in an anaesthetised patient, but not when both wakefulness and the carbon dioxide level of blood are below normal.

The stimulant effect of wakefulness on respiration can be ascribed tentatively to the brain stem reticular system. The depression of respiration at the onset of natural sleep may be due to lack of wakefulness.

### Other Centres Affecting the Respiratory Centre

Many of the higher centres exert some influence on respiration—for example, the acts of swallowing, speaking and coughing require a careful integration of the mechanical systems. These changes are due to impulses arising in the cerebral cortex. Similarly, impulses from the cortical and thalamic areas influence the respiratory pattern during crying and laughing.

### Effect of Anaesthetic Agents on the Respiratory Centres

Little is known of the effects which anaesthetic agents have on the respiratory centres, although it seems likely that their activity is depressed in common with that of other parts of the brain.

## THE CHEMICAL CONTROL OF BREATHING

Ventilation is normally controlled to:

(1) provide adequate oxygenation of blood passing through alveolar capillaries;

(2) excrete $CO_2$ so as to maintain brain pH within narrow limits.

One of the most obvious questions about this control system is: how does it regulate $Paco_2$ in the face of a widely varying $CO_2$ production? For example, during exercise $CO_2$ production is increased enormously and ventilation also increases by just the right amount so that $Paco_2$ remains constant (during severe exercise, $Paco_2$ falls due to the development of a metabolic acidosis). This is the fundamental question concerning chemical control of breathing but there is as yet no generally accepted answer, although recent evidence for a control system which matches ventilation to $CO_2$ production is presented below.

### Response to $CO_2$

The ventilatory response to $CO_2$ has been looked at in numerous different ways. Most of them can be criticised on the grounds of the old adage that "$CO_2$ is for breathing out not in". In awake subjects almost all measurements of breathing interfere to some extent with respiration, for example by making the subject aware that his breathing is being measured and by imposing added deadspace and resistance. Nevertheless, some of the classic ways in which respiratory control has been investigated will be presented.

### $CO_2$ Response Curve

The ventilatory response to $CO_2$ is usually measured using either the steady-state method or the rebreathing method.[5] In the steady-state method the subject inspires three different concentrations of $CO_2$ (e.g. 2 per cent, 4 per cent, 6 per cent) each for about 20 minutes or until ventilation is steady. Towards the end of each period the ventilation and end-tidal $CO_2$ concentrations are measured. Points relating ventilation to end-tidal $P_{CO_2}$ are derived and the line of best fit is obtained. This is called the carbon dioxide response curve, in spite of being a straight line. The slope of the line ($l\ min^{-1}\ kPa^{-1}$) is a measure of the subject's ventilatory sensitivity to $CO_2$. In the rebreathing method, the subject rebreathes for 4 minutes from a 6-litre bag which is filled initially with 7 per cent $CO_2$, 50 per cent $O_2$, 43 per cent $N_2$. During the first half-minute equilibration occurs between the $CO_2$ in the bag and the subject. During the next 3·5 minutes there is a linear increase in $P_{CO_2}$ and consequent increase in ventilation; a line relating ventilation to end-tidal $P_{CO_2}$ is derived from measurements made during this time. For comparable levels of $P_{O_2}$ the rebreathing and steady-state methods give similar results for the $CO_2$ sensitivity except during metabolic acidosis and alkalosis. The advantages of the rebreathing method are that it is rapid, less distressing to the subject and so can more readily be repeated.

The carbon dioxide response curve is a sensitive index of respiratory depression and as such has been used in the study of respiratory effects of narcotic drugs.[6]

### Factors Influencing the Carbon Dioxide Response Curve

Alterations in the $CO_2$ response curve may be of two types. (a) The *slope* may be increased or decreased, indicating an alteration in $CO_2$ sensitivity, or (b) the *curves* may be displaced either to the left or to the right. Both types may of course be seen together. Some of the factors which influence the $CO_2$ response are as follows:

(1) *Individual responses* vary widely from person to person, and in the same individual from time to time.

(2) *Hypoxia*. In the presence of hypoxia the $CO_2$ response curve becomes steeper. Hypoxia therefore reinforces the ventilatory response to $CO_2$.[7]

(3) *Metabolic acidosis and alkalosis*. With the steady-state method metabolic acidosis shifts the curve to the left and alkalosis shifts it to the right, although the slopes remain unchanged. When the ventilation is plotted as a function of CSF pH, however, no displacement occurs.[8] Figure 1 shows the effects of hypoxia and acidosis on the $CO_2$ response curve.

(4) *Chronic bronchitis*. In chronic bronchitis or other lung diseases causing chronic diffuse airway obstruction the slope of the curve is flattened, and is displaced to the right in the presence of $CO_2$ retention. If the increase in respiratory *work*, rather than the *ventilation*, is plotted against the $P_{CO_2}$, in some patients the increase in work when breathing $CO_2$ is close to normal, and in others it is reduced. It has been suggested that these different responses may characterise "blue bloaters" (reduced work response) and "pink puffers" (normal work response).[10]

(5) *Drugs*. Opiate analgesics depress the ventilatory response to $CO_2$. For example, morphine shifts the response curve to the right, but its slope is not usually affected. Pethidine depresses the slope as well as moving it to the right, although the dose of the drug which has been administered is probably important as regards its precise effect. In Table 1 are listed the doses of a number of analgesic drugs which depress the $CO_2$ response curve an equivalent amount to 10 mg of morphine.

(6) *Added airway resistance*. A dangerous increase in added airway resistance may occur if an anaesthetic circuit includes an inappropriate or malfunctioning component. Depression of the $CO_2$ response curve as shown in Fig. 2 will result, and this depression must be added to that caused by the anaesthetic agents and other drugs used.

(7) *Inhalation anaesthetics*. A number of studies into the effects of anaesthetic agents on the ventilatory response to inhaled $CO_2$ have

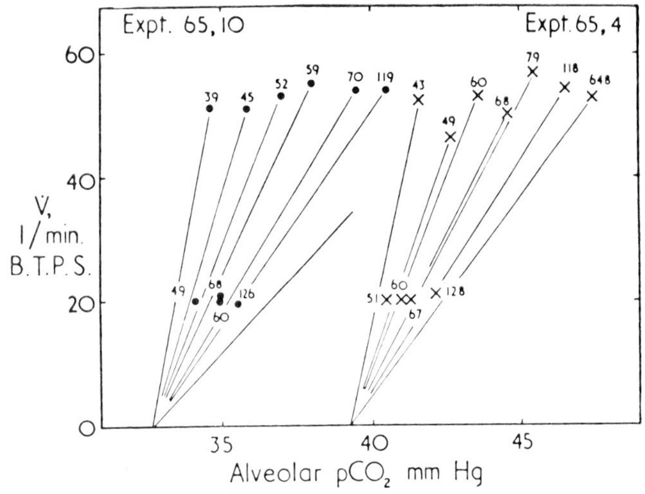


2/Fig. 1.—The effect of acidosis on the V̇, $P_{CO_2}$ relation. Crosses × – experiment before; closed circles • – experiment during acidosis. Number near points indicate $P_{O_2}$ (mm Hg). The fan of V̇ $P_{CO_2}$ lines is displaced 7 mm Hg $P_{CO_2}$ to the left during acidosis, but is otherwise similar. (Courtesy of Cunningham *et al.* (1961) and the *Quarterly Journal of Experimental Physiology*.[9])

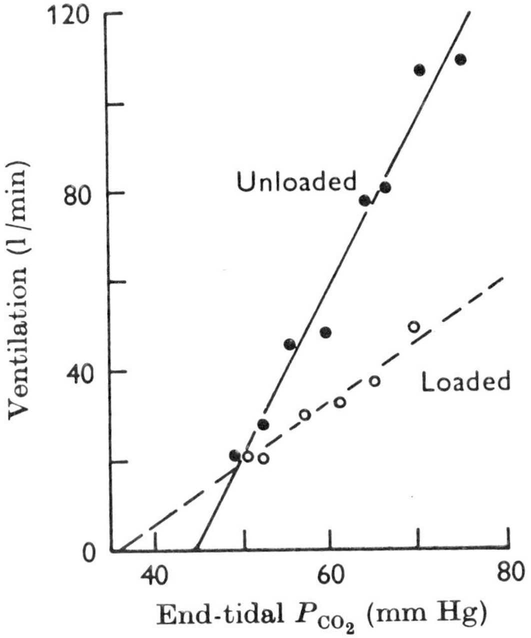


2/Fig. 2.—The effect of added resistance to breathing on the $CO_2$ response curve of a normal subject. (Courtesy of Clark and Godfrey, 1969, and the Cambridge University Press.[11])

2/Table 1

Doses of some Analgesic Drugs which have the Same Respiratory Depressant Effect as Morphine 10 mg. (Compiled from Various Sources)

| | |
|---|---|
| Pethidine | — 75 mg |
| Dihydrocodeine | — 60 mg |
| Codeine | — 100 to 120 mg |
| Methadone | — 10 mg |
| Oxymorphone | — 0·68 mg |
| Phenazocine | — 1·5 mg |
| Pentazocine | — 20 mg |
| Phenoperidine | — 2 mg |
| Fentanyl | — 0·1 mg |

appeared in the literature.[12, 13, 14] The use of the Minimum Alveolar Anaesthetic Concentration (MAC) to describe the depth of anaesthesia has enabled several different agents to be compared. Cyclopropane, halothane, fluroxene and methoxyflurane all cause a fall in ventilation and a rise in arterial $P_{CO_2}$, these changes increasing with the depth of anaesthesia (Fig. 3). The ventilatory response to inhaled $CO_2$ is also progressively reduced as anaesthesia becomes deeper with these agents, and eventually becomes almost flat.

**Inhalation of Carbon Dioxide**

A concentration of 5 per cent carbon dioxide, though unpleasant, can be inhaled for long periods without ill-effects. However, unconsciousness inevitably supervenes when the concentration is raised to 15 per cent or above. At this level, muscle rigidity and tremor may be observed. If 20–30 per cent carbon dioxide is inspired then generalised convulsions can be produced. Thus, the acidosis produced by a high $P_{CO_2}$ might play a part in deepening anaesthesia produced by other agents and may

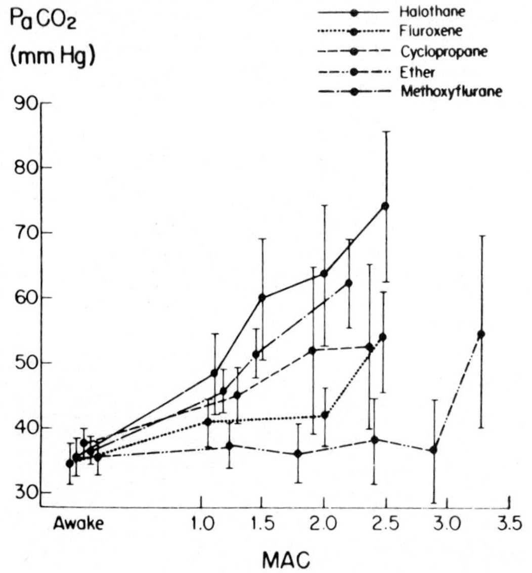

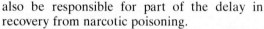

2/Fig. 3(*a*).—Alterations in $Pco_2$ with increasing depth of anaesthesia, the latter expressed as multiples of the Minimum Alveolar Anaesthetic Concentration (MAC). Note that with diethyl ether the $Pco_2$ remains around normal until deep levels of anaesthesia, and the wide variations in $Pco_2$ about the mean values. $Pco_2$ plotted as means ± one Standard Deviation. (Courtesy of Drs. C. P. Larson, Jr., E. I. Eger II, M. Muallem, D. R. Buechel, E. S. Munson and J. H. Eisele, and the Editors and publisher, J. B. Lippincott Company, of *Anesthesiology*[14])

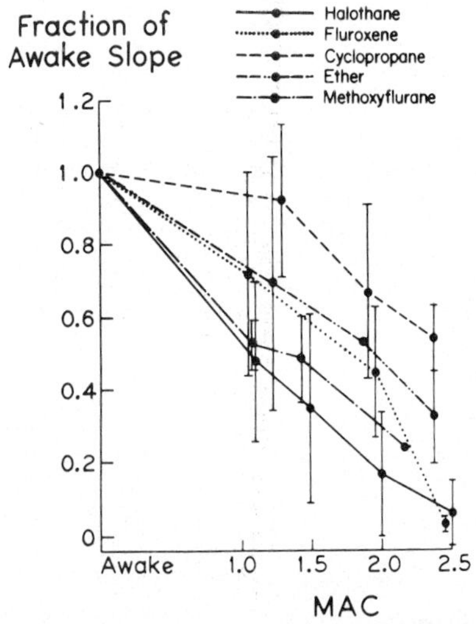


2/Fig. 3(*b*).—Alterations in the response to $CO_2$ inhalation with deepening anaesthesia. The slope of the ventilatory response to administering $CO_2$ in the inspired gases is plotted as a fraction of the slope obtained before the induction of anaesthesia. Note that as anaesthesia is deepened the response to $CO_2$ progressively falls and that, as in the conscious subject, there is a wide variation in the individual response. $CO_2$ response plotted as mean values ± one Standard Deviation. (Source: as for Fig. 3*a*)

also be responsible for part of the delay in recovery from narcotic poisoning.

About three-quarters of the ventilatory response to $CO_2$ is due to central chemoreceptor stimulation and the remainder is due to peripheral chemoreceptor activity. The peripheral chemoreceptor discharge is reduced by high levels of $Po_2$ and increased by low levels, providing the only drive to ventilation in response to hypoxia.

## The Central $H^+$ Chemoreceptor

The pioneer studies by Leusen first suggested the possible importance of the cerebrospinal fluid in the control of ventilation.[15, 16] Using anaesthetised animals he showed that perfusion of the ventriculo-cisternal system with mock CSF containing either a high $Pco_2$ or a low bicarbonate concentration (low pH) caused an increase in ventilation. In 1963 Mitchell and his colleagues[17] located a bilateral superficial chemoreceptor on the ventro-lateral surface of the medulla in the region of the origins of the IXth and Xth cranial nerves, extending towards the mid-line. These areas are termed the *Medullary $H^+$ Chemoreceptor*. The topical application to these sites of pledgets soaked in cerebrospinal fluid with a raised $H^+$ concentration leads to an almost immediate increase in ventilation which is proportional to the increase in $H^+$ concentration above normal. Furthermore, the application of a pledget containing a very low concentration of procaine causes apnoea even when the arterial $Pco_2$ is high. The area of the medullary respiratory centre below the floor of the IVth ventricle does not react to any of these manoeuvres.

In a series of most elegant experiments Pappenheimer and his colleagues[18] examined the responses mediated by the medullary chemoreceptor. They used normal unanaesthetised goats into which had been previously implanted nylon catheters leading to the lateral ventricles and the cisterna magna. The ventriculo-cisternal system could then be perfused with artificial

CSF of any desired composition. The goats were trained to tolerate masks for long periods, and samples of arterial blood could be withdrawn at will from carotid artery loops. The respiratory responses of the animals to various alterations in the $H^+$ concentration of both blood and CSF could then be studied. The main conclusions they reported were: (1) The sensitivity of the chemoreceptor in normal animals to changes in CSF pH was two to seven times that found when the animals were anaesthetised. (2) The $Pco_2$ in the outflow of CSF was constantly about 10 mm Hg (1·3 kPa) higher than that in the arterial blood, irrespective of the $Pco_2$ in the infused artificial CSF. The $Pco_2$ of the CSF is therefore controlled by the $Pco_2$ in the brain tissue adjacent to the walls of the ventricular cavities. (3) During the inhalation of $CO_2$ the difference between the $Pco_2$ in CSF and arterial blood decreased, and this effect was thought to be secondary to an increase in cerebral blood flow at this time. (4) $CO_2$ response curves were slightly more linear when referred to CSF $Pco_2$ than when referred to arterial blood $Pco_2$. (5) Ventilation was increased when the CSF $H^+$ concentration was raised by perfusing the cerebral ventricles with mock CSF containing a low bicarbonate concentration. This response to a "metabolic acidosis" within the CSF was much reduced if the increase in ventilation was allowed to cause a reduction in the $Pco_2$ of the CSF outflow. (6) During $CO_2$ inhalation it was estimated that about 40 per cent of the ventilatory response was due to the alteration of the CSF $H^+$ concentration, the remaining 60 per cent being the result of changes in $Pco_2$ or $H^+$ concentration elsewhere. Other estimates of the contribution of the medullary $H^+$ chemoreceptors to the response to the inhaled $CO_2$ vary from 30 per cent to over 80 per cent.

From these and other experiments there has emerged the concept of the medullary $H^+$ chemoreceptor and the factors which affect it. It is situated superficially near the surface of the medulla, and is sensitive to the $H^+$ concentration of the interstitial fluid bathing it. Because $CO_2$ combines with water to form $H^+$, it also reacts to changes in $Pco_2$ via this reaction. There is no convincing evidence that it is sensitive to changes in $Pco_2$ *per se*. The $H^+$ concentration of the all-important interstitial fluid is determined by its $Pco_2$ and bicarbonate concentration. These in turn are influenced by the $Pco_2$ of the CSF and the cerebral capillary blood and by the bicarbonate concentration of the CSF. The bicarbonate concentration in the blood has no immediate effect on the medullary $H^+$ chemoreceptor due to the diffusion barrier for bicarbonate ions which exists between blood and CSF and between blood and brain, although there appears to be free diffusion of bicarbonate between the CSF and the interstitial fluid bathing the receptor. Carbon dioxide, being rapidly diffusible throughout blood, tissues and CSF, provides the means whereby rapid changes in the $H^+$ concentration of the CSF and the fluid surrounding the receptor can be produced. Slower adjustments are mediated through alterations in the CSF bicarbonate concentration and the processes involved are probably more than diffusion alone. The evidence suggests that there is an active transport mechanism between blood and CSF which is capable of adjusting the CSF pH.

The normal values for the pH, $Pco_2$ and bicarbonate concentration in arterial plasma and cerebrospinal fluid in man are shown in Table 2.[19] Because the bicarbonate system is the only buffer in the cerebrospinal fluid, its chemical buffering power is small, and for a given rise in $Pco_2$ the CSF pH will, therefore, fall more than that of blood. Because of this the influence of the CSF on the activity of the medullary $H^+$ chemoreceptors is increased in response to changes in $CO_2$ in the body. In spite of this poor buffering capacity the CSF pH is kept remarkably constant in a wide variety of acid-base disturbances. Thus, it is normal or near normal in patients with chronic metabolic acidosis and alkalosis, moderate long-standing respiratory acidosis, and following acclimatisa-

2/TABLE 2

NORMAL VALUES FOR pH, $Pco_2$, AND $[HCO_3^-]$ IN ARTERIAL PLASMA AND CSF IN MAN. MEANS AND STANDARD DEVIATIONS

| | pH | $Pco_2$ mm Hg (kPa) | $[HCO_3^-]$ mmol/l |
|---|---|---|---|
| Arterial Plasma | 7·397 (0·022) | 41·1 (5·5) 3·6 (0·5) | 25·3 (1·8) |
| CSF | 7·307 (0·027) | 50·5 (6·7) 4·9 (0·7) | 23·3 (1·4) |

(Modified from Bradley and Semple[19])

tion to high altitude (respiratory alkalosis). Only in severe respiratory acidosis is the CSF pH below normal, and also during acute respiratory changes before compensation has had time to occur.

FACTORS REGULATING CSF pH

| | | |
|---|---|---|
| CSF pH | $P_{CO_2}$ | Arterial $P_{CO_2}$<br>Cerebral blood flow<br>Tissue metabolism |
| | $HCO_3^-$ | Bulk secretion of CSF<br>Active transport mechanisms<br>Slow passive diffusion |

If alterations in $P_{CO_2}$ in either direction are maintained beyond the acute stage, the CSF bicarbonate slowly alters so that the changes in CSF pH are minimised even though there is no further change in the blood bicarbonate. In contrast to the changes in $P_{CO_2}$ this change in bicarbonate is slow, and its time course can be measured in hours. McDowell and Harper[20] have reported on the changes occurring in the CSF during hyperventilation to an arterial $P_{CO_2}$ of 19–20 mm Hg (2·5–2·7 kPa) in baboons. They found that the CSF pH rose rapidly from an average value of 7·32 to 7·49 following the institution of hypocapnia. Over the next 3 hours the CSF pH fell slowly to an average value of 7·41, and during this time the CSF bicarbonate concentration fell from 21·4 mmol/l to 17·5 mmol/l. The CSF $P_{CO_2}$ remained stable at 29 ± 2 mm Hg (3·9 ± 0·3 kPa) during the whole period.

## Practical Implications

When a patient inspires a high concentration of carbon dioxide, the raised $P_{CO_2}$ of the blood reaching the brain causes a reduction in brain extracellular fluid pH and stimulates respiration. If this inhalation continues for a time, the $H^+$ ion concentration of the cerebrospinal fluid is decreased by a compensatory rise of $HCO_3^-$. A sudden withdrawal of the inhaled $CO_2$ will be accompanied by a diminution of ventilation below normal because the stimulus of a high $H^+$ ion content is no longer present in the cerebrospinal fluid.

## Effects of Anaesthetic Agents on the Medullary $H^+$ Chemoreceptor

Although the ventilatory response to inhaled $CO_2$ is depressed during general anaesthesia, the mechanism of this phenomenon is unknown. Experiments in which the central chemoreceptor have been stimulated by the application of pledgets to the medulla have shown that the ventilatory response to a given pH change is much less in anaesthetised animals than has been found in other experiments in conscious animals and man. This suggests that the chemoreceptor itself may be depressed by anaesthesia. The response of the central respiratory mechanisms to chemoreceptor activity may also be depressed. In total spinal analgesia the action of the local analgesic at this site may well explain the cessation of respiration which occurs.

## THE PERIPHERAL CHEMORECEPTORS

The peripheral chemoreceptors consist of the carotid and aortic bodies. Although the carotid body was first described in 1743 it was not until the 1920's that its more detailed anatomy was published. Also at this time Heymans and Heymans demonstrated that its stimulation by hypercapnia, hypoxia or increased acidity caused an increase in ventilation. The carotid bodies are about 5 mm in diameter and are situated at the bifurcations of the common carotid arteries. Although each carotid body is close to the respective carotid sinus, they are completely separate structures. They are innervated by the sinus nerves which are branches of the glossopharyngeal nerves. The most striking aspect of the anatomy of the carotid body is its vascularity. It has by far the highest blood flow of any organ of the body—2000 ml 100 $g^{-1}$ $min^{-1}$. It is generally accepted that stimulation by $CO_2$ is due to a pH change somewhere in the carotid body, which contains carbonic anhydrase, and the response to hypoxia is also probably mediated via its effect on pH.

Most of the work on peripheral chemoreceptors has centred on the carotid bodies, largely because of their greater accessibility. In most respects the aortic bodies, situated close to the arch of the aorta, are similar but they appear to be less important as chemoreceptors but may be important for their cardiovascular effect.

Central chemoreception is a relatively slow process so that the fast component of the respiratory response to $CO_2$ is due to peripheral chemoreceptor activity. In fact the peripheral chemoreceptor rate of response is fast enough to transduce respiratory oscillations in $Paco_2$ into an oscillating nerve discharge.

### Alveolar Gas Oscillations

At the beginning of the century, Haldane and Priestley sampled alveolar gas. By getting their subjects to exhale maximally at different points in the respiratory cycle they found that if an alveolar gas sample was collected at the end of inspiration the $Pco_2$ was lower than if the sample was collected at the end of expiration. In this way they demonstrated that tidal ventilation produces a corresponding fluctuation in alveolar $Pco_2$.

### Arterial pH/$Pco_2$ Oscillations

Continuous measurement of arterial pH has shown that these $Paco_2$ oscillations are transmitted to the arterial blood (Fig. 4). It is not possible to measure the $Paco_2$ oscillations directly because the response of a $Pco_2$ electrode is too slow, but the pH oscillations are due to corresponding fluctuations in $Pco_2$.

### Respiratory Oscillations in Chemoreceptor Discharge

Recordings of chemoreceptor activity made from single fibre preparations of the carotid sinus nerve have demonstrated that the oscillating $Paco_2$ is transduced into an oscillating chemoreceptor discharge (Fig. 5). This still occurs at rates of 70/min in cats although the stimuli at this frequency were outside the physiological range. Band and co-workers[23] made the important observation that when brief injections of saline equilibrated with $CO_2$ were made via an aortic root catheter, a respiratory response was obtained to pH changes whose amplitude was less than that of the naturally occurring arterial pH oscillations.

To summarise so far: Oscillations in alveolar $Pco_2$ are produced as a result of tidal breathing. These oscillations are transmitted to the arterial blood where the peripheral chemoreceptors are sufficiently sensitive and fast-responding to transduce them. The oscillating afferent chemoreceptor discharge so produced is transmitted to the medulla.

The mean level of this discharge reflects $Paco_2$/pH/$Pao_2$ but the amplitude of the discharge is proportional to the rate of rise of $Paco_2$ during a respiratory oscillation and this is closely related to $CO_2$ production. We therefore have a system whereby the brain receives information concerning $CO_2$ production. Is this information used in the control of breathing?

### Matching of Ventilation to $CO_2$ Production

The greatest increase in $CO_2$ production occurs during exercise. Ventilation increases by just the right amount to excrete this $CO_2$ load and maintain the mean $Paco_2$ constant.

Yamamoto and Edwards[24] used an extracor-

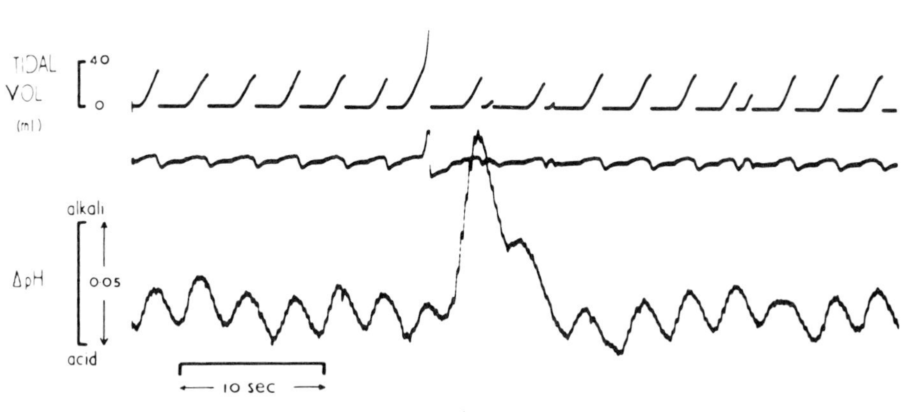


2/FIG. 4.—Arterial pH oscillations in an anaesthetised cat breathing spontaneously. The traces represent from the top downwards: tidal volume, tracheal air flow and arterial pH. Note the change in arterial pH following the gasp. (Courtesy of Dr. D. M. Band and co-workers, and the American Physiological Society.[21])

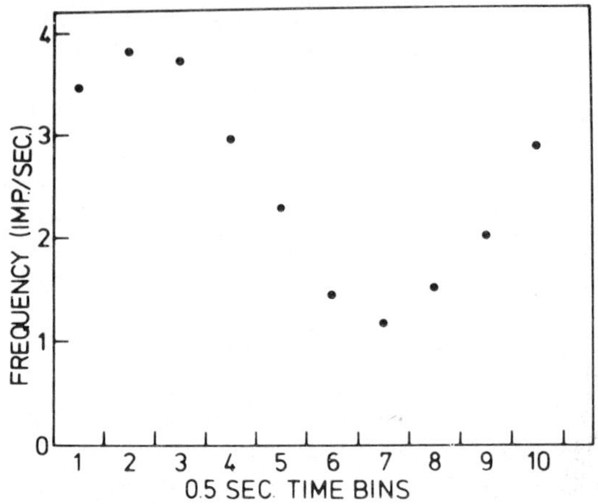


2/FIG. 5.—The respiratory cycle has been split up into 0·5 sec sections or 'bins'. The number of action potentials recorded from an afferent chemoreceptor fibre in each bin is added up for about thirty respiratory cycles. The summed counts are an estimate of the mean frequency of chemoreceptor firing for the portion of the cycle covered by any particular bin. This figure shows results obtained in a cat and indicates an oscillating chemoreceptor discharge. This oscillation has the same period as that of breathing and can be abolished if the carotid blood flow is passed through a mixing chamber (which removes the $Paco_2$ oscillations) before reaching the carotid bodies. (Courtesy of Dr. D. M. Band and colleagues and the American Physiological Society.[22])

poreal circuit to load the venous blood of rats with $CO_2$, so mimicking the increased $CO_2$ production of exercise in isolation from other changes due to exercise, e.g. joint and muscle movement, etc. They found that ventilation was linearly related to the $CO_2$ load up to amounts six times the normal resting metabolic $CO_2$ production and that $Paco_2$ remained constant. They suggested that the signal to breathing was related to $Paco_2$ oscillations. Phillipson and associates[3] used two membrane lungs in an extracorporeal circuit in awake sheep and measured ventilation during addition of $CO_2$ to venous blood and during removal of $CO_2$ from venous blood. As the rate of ventilation of the membrane lungs with 100 per cent oxygen was progressively increased, while maintaining a constant rate of blood flow, there was a progressive reduction in the depth and frequency of respiration until breathing stopped completely. This apnoea was maintained for periods up to 60 min and presumably could have been continued for longer. Figure 6 shows the one-to-one relationship between the $\dot{V}co_2$ of the membrane lungs and the $\dot{V}co_2$ of the sheep's lungs.

Results from one of the sheep are illustrated in Fig. 7 and show that up to a $\dot{V}co_2$ of 0·4 l/min (about twice the resting value) ventilation increases so as to maintain $Paco_2$ normal. With higher rates of $CO_2$ loading there is a small increase in $Paco_2$ implying that some other drive to breathing is also required at these levels in order to stimulate ventilation sufficiently to maintain $Paco_2$ constant.

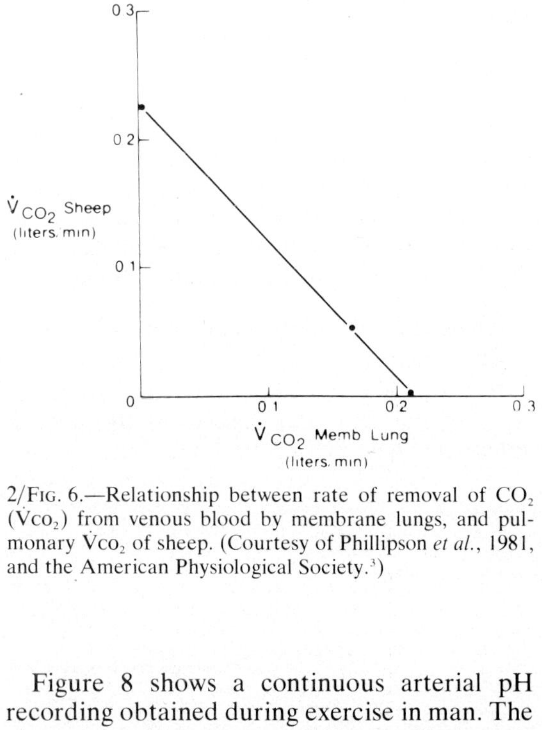


2/FIG. 6.—Relationship between rate of removal of $CO_2$ ($\dot{V}co_2$) from venous blood by membrane lungs, and pulmonary $\dot{V}co_2$ of sheep. (Courtesy of Phillipson *et al.*, 1981, and the American Physiological Society.[3])

Figure 8 shows a continuous arterial pH recording obtained during exercise in man. The change in the pattern of the oscillations is apparent within 10 seconds of the onset of exercise, so that the "humoral factor" may operate to drive breathing much earlier than previously supposed.

**Other Drives to Breathing During Exercise**

(1) *Temperature.*—A rise in body temperature results in an increase in ventilation and greatly exaggerates the respiratory response to

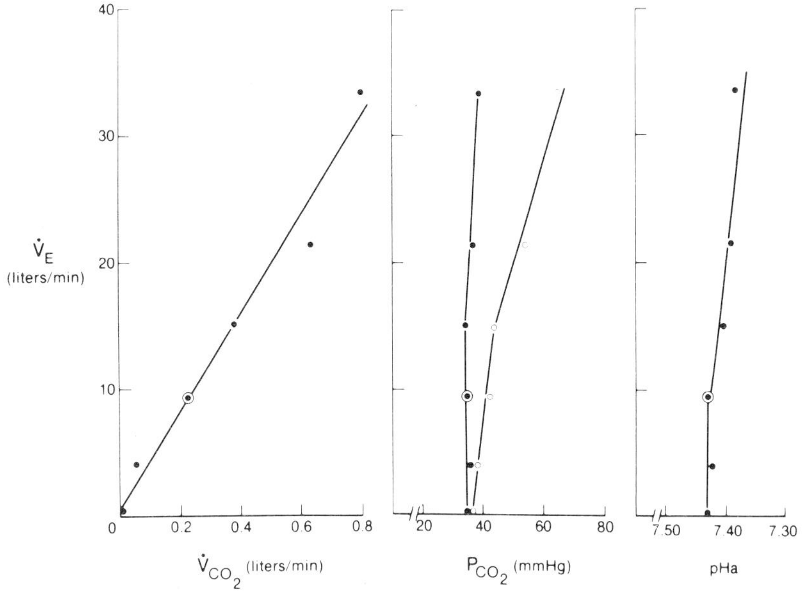


2/Fig. 7.—Effect of induced changes in rate of pulmonary $CO_2$ excretion ($\dot{V}co_2$) of a sheep on a minute volume of ventilation ($\dot{V}_E$), arterial $Pco_2$ (●), mixed venous (i.e. pulmonary arterial) $Pco_2$ (○) and arterial pH ($pH_a$). Circled data points represent control values. Decreases in $\dot{V}co_2$ below control value were achieved by removing $CO_2$ from venous blood through $CO_2$-membrane lung (CDML); Increases in $\dot{V}co_2$ above control value were achieved by adding $CO_2$ to venous blood through CDML. (Courtesy of Phillipson *et al*, 1981 and the American Physiological Society.[3])

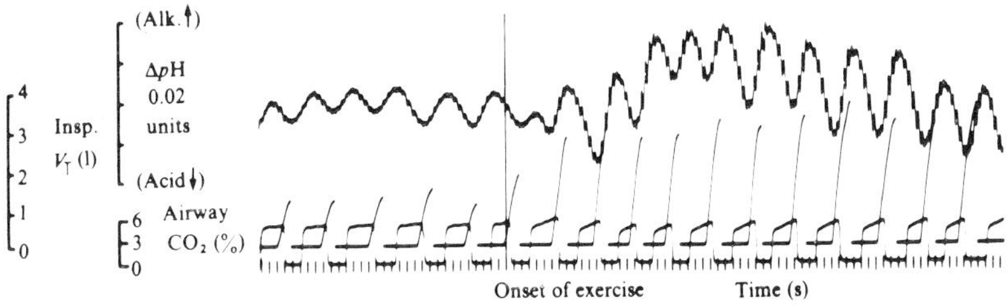


2/Fig. 8.—Arterial pH oscillations before and after the onset of exercise (40 W) in a healthy subject. The traces from above down are: arterial pH measured via the brachial artery, inspiratory tidal volume, airway $CO_2$ concentration and time. $CO_2$ production increased 2·7 times, from 304 to 827 ml/min, causing a corresponding increase in slopes of the arterial pH oscillations. (Courtesy of Band *et al*., 1980 and Macmillan Journals Ltd.[25])

$CO_2$. (Hypothermia causes a reduction in ventilation in excess of what would be expected on the basis of a reduced $CO_2$ production.)

(2) *Neural factors*.—Figure 9 shows that at the onset of exercise there is a rapid increase in ventilation, then a slower rise to a plateau. There is a rapid decrease in ventilation at the end of exercise followed by a slower return to the control value. The fast components are generally ascribed to neurogenic control on the basis that there has not been time for $CO_2$ production to increase (or decrease) within a few seconds. This neurogenic component may originate in mechanoreceptors in joints and muscle spindles; in addition there may be a central contribution from other areas of the brain. In fact, a very rapid increase in delivery of $CO_2$ to the lungs at the start of exercise can be achieved just by increasing cardiac output.

(3) *Humoral factors*.—Arterial pH and $Pco_2$.

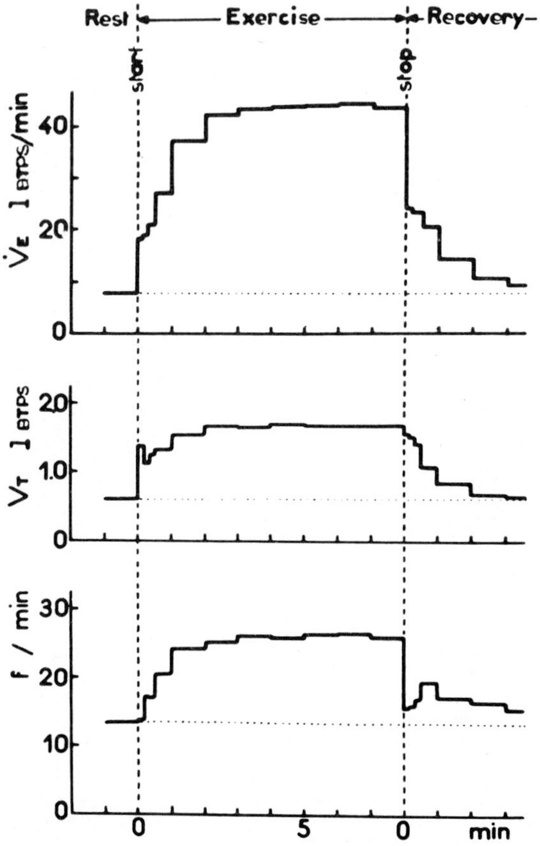


2/FIG. 9.—Expiratory minute volume $V_E$, tidal volume $V_T$, and respiratory frequency f in the course of a treadmill exercise (speed 4·6 km per hour; grade 15 per cent; $Vo_2$ 1·75 litres STPD per min) at sea level. At rest the subject was seated on a platform located at the side of the treadmill; at command "start" or "stop", the subject stepped on or off the running belt. (Courtesy of Dejours and the American Physiological Society.[26])

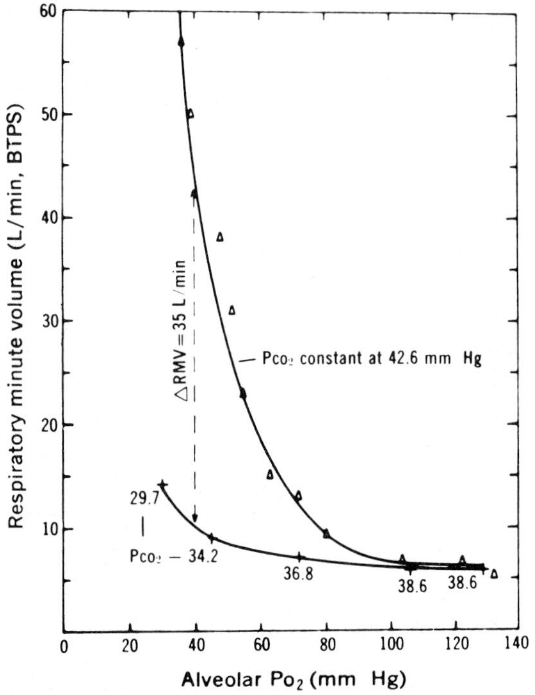


2/FIG. 10.—Interaction of $Po_2$ and $Pco_2$ in respiratory control. Influence of $Pco_2$ on respiratory response to $0_2$ lack. *Lower curve* shows that progressive lowering of alveolar $Po_2$ produces only slight respiratory stimulation, which, apparently by lowering alveolar and central $Pco_2$, tends to be self-limiting. Hypocapnia thus may mask anoxic drive. *Upper curve*, obtained over same range of hypoxia but while holding alveolar $Pco_2$ essentially constant, indicates true capacity of chemoreceptor influence on respiratory control system. Difference between curves, for example, 35 l/min at 40 mm Hg $Po_2$ represents loss of reactivity of centres resulting from effects of difference in alveolar $Pco_2$ of approximately 8 mm Hg. (Courtesy of C. J. Lambertsen and the editor, V. B. Mountcastle, and the publishers of *Medical Physiology*, C. V. Mosby Company.[27])

During heavy exercise a metabolic acidosis develops, which stimulates both central and peripheral chemoreceptors. Arterial $Po_2$ does not fall during exercise. Catecholamine levels are increased during exercise and it is known that they increase ventilation. Other chemical factors have also been postulated; the most important is potassium which is released from exercising muscle and causes peripheral chemoreceptor stimulation.

### The Ventilatory Response to Oxygen Lack

The respiratory response to hypoxia is mediated entirely via the peripheral chemoreceptors, the central effect of hypoxia being depressive. Acute hypoxia increases the respiratory sensitivity to $CO_2$, making the $CO_2$ response curve steeper; by measuring $CO_2$ responses at different oxygen tensions fans of lines can be obtained as in Fig. 1. Another way of looking at ventilatory response to hypoxia is to give the subject a progressively more hypoxic gas mixture to breathe and measure ventilation. Figure 10 shows this under two conditions; for the lower curve the $Pco_2$ has been allowed to fall and this of course will have tended to oppose the increase in ventilation; for the upper curve the response has been done under isocapnic conditions, $CO_2$ being added to the inspired gas so as to keep $Pa_{CO_2}$ constant; the ventilatory response to hypoxia is now much more impressive.

It used to be thought that the ventilatory response to hypoxia was a very rugged one, unaffected for example by anaesthetic drugs. This is now known to be wrong, and Knill and Gelb[28] have shown that halothane virtually abolishes the response at MAC 1·1 (Fig. 11).

Figure 12 shows two groups of subjects acclimatised to chronic hypoxia. One group is high altitude residents and the other is patients with chronic stable asthma living at sea level. As you can see there is no significant difference between the $P_{CO_2}/P_{O_2}$ relationships of the two groups. Figure 13 shows what happened when chronic stable asthmatics developed an acute attack—in all cases when they were first seen in hospital their $Pa_{CO_2}$ levels were *higher* than they should have been relative to their $Pa_{O_2}$ values. It is often said that in the early stages of status asthmaticus $Pa_{CO_2}$ is lower than normal; it may be less than 40 mm Hg (5·3 kPa), but it is none the less raised above the subject's usual level.

In response to chronic hypoxia, there is eventually a greater increase in ventilation than occurs in response to a similar degree of acute

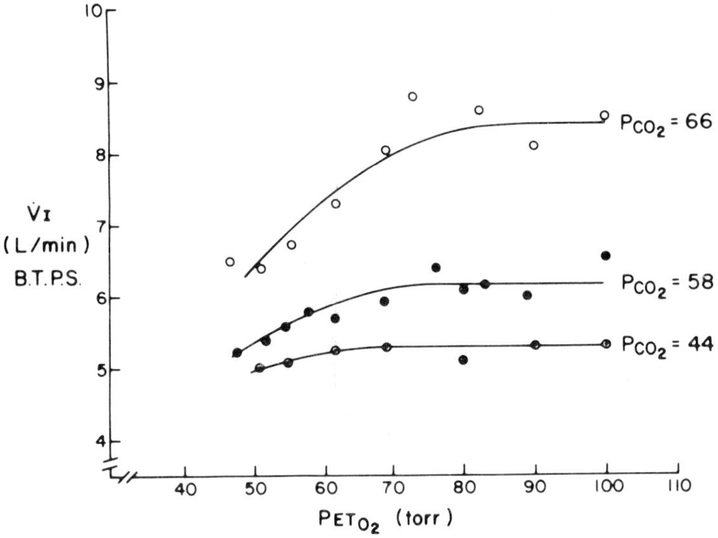


2/Fig. 11.—The relationship between inspiratory minute volume and end-tidal $P_{O_2}$ at 3 levels of $Pa_{CO_2}$ in a subject anaesthetised with halothane (1·1 MAC). Under these conditions hypoxia decreased the ventilatory response to $CO_2$. Note that hypoxia in the patient anaesthetised with halothane leads to *depression* of respiration. (Courtesy of Knill and Gelb, 1978 and the American Society of Anesthesiologists.[28])

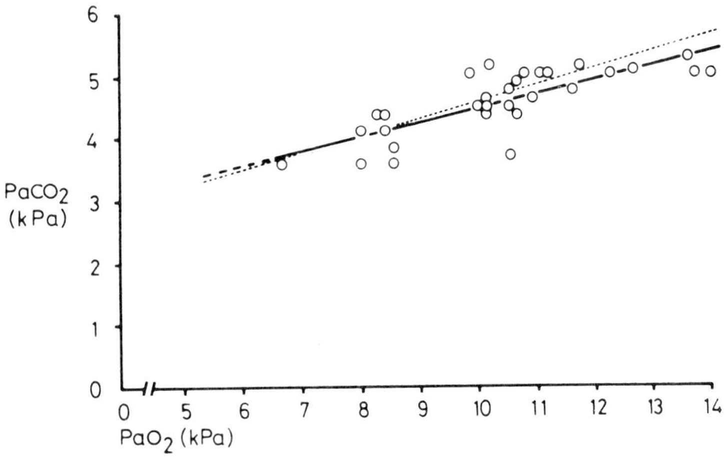


2/Fig. 12.—Relation between $Pa_{CO_2}$ and $Pa_{O_2}$ in 29 patients with chronic stable asthma. ——— least squares regression line. – – – Regression line extrapolated below 6·7 kPa (50 mm Hg), . . . . Relation between $Pa_{CO_2}$ and $Pa_{O_2}$ calculated by Wolff for normal subjects acclimatised to altitude hypoxia (1 kPa ≈ 7·5 mm Hg). (Courtesy of Cochrane, Prior and Wolff, 1980 and the Editor of the *British Medical Journal*.[29])

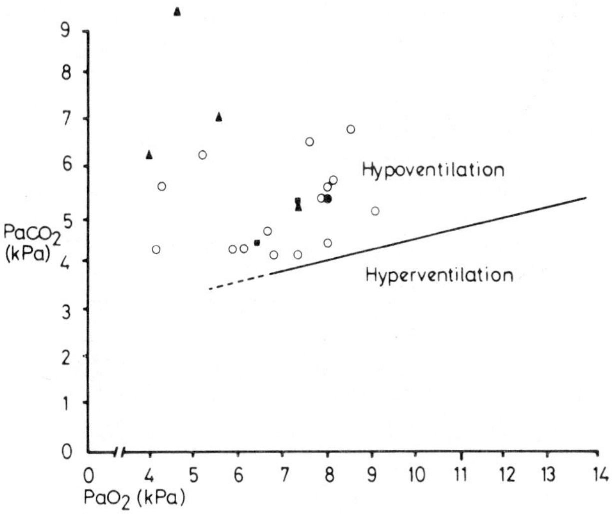


2/Fig. 13.—Relation of $Paco_2$ and $Pao_2$ in patients with status asthmaticus. The line is the least squares regression line in patients with chronic stable asthma. All the patients of Rees *et al.* had $Paco_2$ values above the line, reflecting hypoventilation in relation to the ventilation expected from the degree of hypoxia. ○ = patients with pH value 7·35–7·46. ■ = Patients with pH > 7·46. ▲ = patients with pH < 7·35. ⊙ = two patients at same point. (1 kPa ≈ 7·5 mm Hg). (Courtesy of Cochrane, Prior and Wolff, 1980 and the Editor of the *British Medical Journal*.[29])

hypoxia. The initial hyperventilation in response to hypoxia causes an increase in central chemoreceptor pH (due to a lowering of $Paco_2$) which opposes any further increase in ventilation. If the hypoxic stimulus is maintained, the CSF bicarbonate level falls bringing the central chemoreceptor pH back towards normal and so removing the inhibition to ventilation mentioned above; consequently ventilation increases further.

## PULMONARY REFLEXES

Widdicombe[30] studied the inflation and deflation reflexes in a number of mammalian species, including conscious and anaesthetised man, and concluded that in man the reflexes were relatively weak when compared with those of the other species he studied. In conscious man bilateral vagal blockade causes no change in the pattern of respiration, making man unique in this respect, but has been found to affect the sensation of breathlessness. In patients anaesthetised with nitrous oxide and halothane Guz and colleagues[31] found that (i) Bilateral vagal blockade caused no alteration in the respiratory pattern. (ii) Sudden lung inflation only caused a period of apnoea when large volumes (1 litre or more) were used. This effect was abolished by vagal block. (iii) Vagal stimulation, when intense, was capable of causing apnoea. They concluded that, although vagal afferent impulses were able to affect respiration in anaesthetised man, their influence was weak and probably of little physiological importance.

The cause of the tachypnoea which is so often seen under anaesthesia remains undecided, although many suggestions have been put forward. These include sensitisation of the pulmonary stretch receptors, irritation of the respiratory tract and stimulation of extrapulmonary receptors.

## THE RESPIRATORY MUSCLES

The diaphragm is the principal muscle of respiration, but many other muscles, including the intercostal, abdominal, scalene, sternomastoid and even some of the back muscles, have their part to play. All of these muscles have one thing in common—they are attached to the thoracic cage. Each group will now be considered in turn.

### The Diaphragm

#### Anatomy

The diaphragm (Fig. 14) consists of a central tendon which is arched on both sides to form a cupola. Muscle fibres radiate from each portion of the tendon and can be traced to their origin

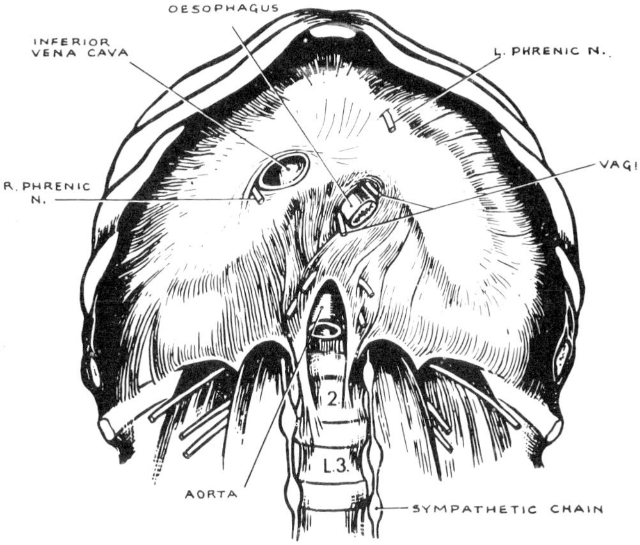


2/Fig. 14.—The diaphragm. (Courtesy of Professor H. Ellis and Miss McLarty and the publishers Blackwell Scientific Publications; based on a figure in *Anatomy for the Anaesthetist*.)

in three distant regions. First, the spinal or crural portion in which the fibres arise from the upper three or four lumbar vertebrae and from the arcuate ligaments. This division is inserted into the posterior margin of the central tendon. Secondly, the costal portion which arises by a series of digitations from the inner surface of the lower six ribs and cartilages. Finally there is a small contribution arising from the back of the ensiform process. The central or tendinous part of the diaphragm is domed upwards into the chest, partly due to the higher intra-abdominal pressure and partly due to the negative pressure pull exerted by the elastic recoil of the lung.

The motor innervation of the diaphragm is largely supplied by the phrenic nerves whose fibres are 90 per cent motor and 10 per cent sensory and autonomic. The two crura receive a motor supply from the 11th and 12th intercostal nerves. Peripheral parts of the diaphragm receive a sensory and autonomic innervation from the lower six intercostal nerves.

**Movements**

The diaphragm moves in a vertical plane and in quiet respiration is responsible for the major part of tidal exchange. As it descends, it increases intra-abdominal pressure, and by using the intra-abdominal contents as a fulcrum, it elevates and expands the lower rib cage. The exact extent to which it moves has been studied radiologically. Wade[32] gives it a range of about 1·5 cm upwards or downwards during quiet respiration, but this distance may be extended to 6–10 cm with deep breathing. Extension of the spine and lifting of the whole thoracic cage are associated with maximal respiratory effort and account for part of this extended movement. The details of diaphragmatic function are still controversial.[33]

Contrary to popular belief, the range of movement of the diaphragm does not alter with a change of posture from the standing to the supine position. The resting level, however, is higher when the subject is lying down.

In normal circumstances a movement of 1 cm downwards of the diaphragm causes about 350 ml of air to enter the lungs and thus the normal tidal exchange of 500 ml per breath is attained by a movement of about 1·5 cm.[32] This figure does not take into account the effects of any of the other muscles of respiration but it emphasises the fact that in quiet breathing the diaphragm produces the major contribution. During deep breathing the contraction of the diaphragm increases the volume of the thorax by an amount equal to 75 per cent of the volume of gas which is inhaled; the remaining 25 per cent is attributable to the movement of the ribs. Thus total paralysis of the diaphragm, as when both phrenic nerves are cut, greatly reduces the ability to ventilate the lungs, though adequate tidal exchange for rest and light acitivity can still be maintained. Unilateral phrenic crush produces little more than a 15–20 per cent reduction in Maximum Breathing Capacity (MBC) with a normal tidal exchange. The paralysed half of the diaphragm moves paradoxically by rising in the thorax during inspiration and falling during expiration, thus reflecting the differences in pressure between the thorax and the abdomen during the two phases of the respiratory cycle. Paralysis of the diaphragm may be diagnosed on X-ray screening of the chest by asking the patient to sniff.

It is interesting to reflect that morphologically all vertebrates except mammals use the principle of body-wall compression to provide an expiratory force. For them this is the fundamental act of breathing. In mammals, however, the demands for oxygen cannot be met by this type of respiration and a new principle of active inspiration is introduced and carried out by an entirely new structure—the muscular diaphragm—situated below the heart and lungs. The diaphragm thus provides mammals with a new and more efficient form of ventilation than that of other vertebrates.

## Intercostal Muscles

### Anatomy

The *external* intercostal muscle fibres, which are mostly in the posterior part of the intercostal space, run obliquely *downwards* and *forwards* from the lower and outer border of one rib to the upper and outer border of the rib below. Contraction of these fibres tends to draw the ribs closer together, but by virtue of their articulations the ribs move upwards and outwards. The result is that in the upper part of the chest the antero-posterior diameter and in the lower part the transverse diameter, is increased.

The *internal* intercostal muscle fibres, which are mostly in the anterior part of the intercostal space, run from the floor of the costal groove and corresponding costal cartilages *downwards* and *backwards* and are finally inserted into the upper and inner border of the rib below. It will be noted, therefore, that both types of intercostal muscles run downwards and their fibres cross obliquely in opposite directions, the one set going forwards and the other backwards.

Both groups of muscles are supplied by the intercostal nerves.

### Movements

Throughout the years the part played by the intercostal muscles in respiratory movement has been strongly debated.[34] Some believed that they were merely a relic of the past and did little more than regulate the tension in the intercostal spaces. Others felt that they had some part to play, but no general agreement on this could be reached. Campbell[35] has shown that the external intercostals, with the aid of those parts of the internal intercostals which run between the cartilaginous portions of the ribs, raise the ribs. They also contract during inspiration in both quiet and strenuous respiration. These muscles, therefore—particularly those lying in the fifth to ninth spaces—play an important part in inspiration. Campbell suggests that the external intercostals are second only in importance to the diaphragm as muscles of inspiration but found no evidence that they play any part in expiration.

Green and Howell[36] have made similar studies and are in agreement with these findings. In addition they note that although the external intercostal muscles in the fifth to ninth space contract during inspiration, this contraction persists into the first part of the expiration, especially during vigorous breathing: this has the effect of smoothing the transition between the two phases of the respiratory cycle. They found little evidence of activity in the other intercostal spaces.

The function of the internal intercostal muscles is in doubt. Campbell[37] believes that their action is determined by the incline of the structures to which they are attached. Thus those fibres which are parasternal lie between costal cartilages and slope upwards, paralleling therefore the external intercostal muscles in both direction and action during inspiration, while the fibres that lie between the ribs slope backwards as well as downwards and contract during expiration. These inter-osseous fibres also contract during speech.

## Abdominal Muscles

There are four principal groups of abdominal muscles that influence respiration—namely the

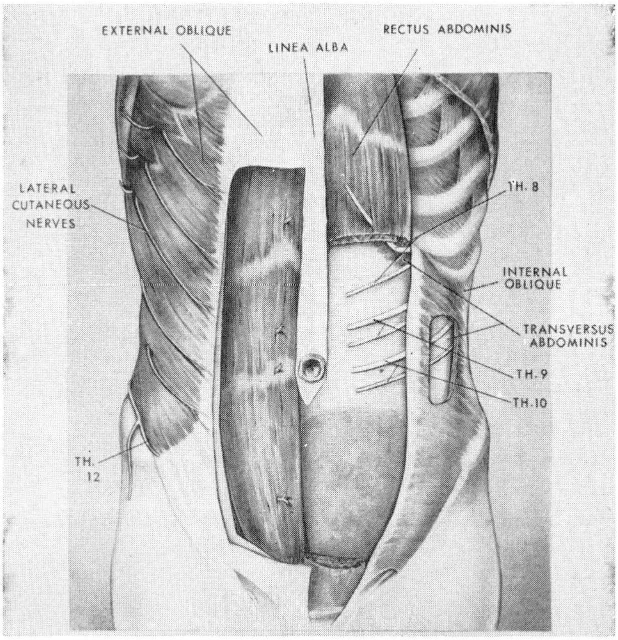


2/Fig. 15.—The muscles of the abdominal wall. (Based on anatomical dissections made available by Professor R. J. Last of the Royal College of Surgeons of England)

external and internal obliques, the transversi and the recti muscles (Fig. 15).

### Anatomy

The *external oblique* muscle arises from the outer surface of the lower eight ribs and the fibres pass downwards in a fan-shape to be inserted into the iliac crest posteriorly and into a fibrous aponeurosis blending with the rectus sheath anteriorly. The lower border of this aponeurosis forms the inguinal ligament.

In contrast, the *internal oblique* arises from the iliac crest, lumbar fascia and inguinal ligament, and the fibres pass vertically upwards to be inserted into the lower three ribs posteriorly and into the aponeurosis forming part of the rectus sheath anteriorly. The *transversus abdominis* muscle arises from the costal cartilages of the lower six ribs, the lumbar fascia, the iliac crest and a small portion of the inguinal ligament. The fibres run horizontally and are attached to the aponeurosis forming part of the rectus sheath. Finally, the *rectus abdominis* muscle arises from the pubic symphysis and crest and the fibres pass vertically upwards to become attached to the 5th, 6th and 7th costal cartilages. During their passage these fibres are enclosed in an aponeurosis or sheath which is closely related to the three abdominal muscles already mentioned.

### Movements in Conscious People

During quiet respiration, and any increase in ventilation up to 40 l/min (i.e. about five times the resting minute volume), the abdominal muscles remain inactive in the conscious subject when supine, and often even when the body is erect.[38] As the volume of respiration increases further so the abdominal muscles gradually start to take an active part (Fig. 16). By the time forceful abdominal contractions can be seen, ventilation will have risen to 90 l/min—the equivalent of strenuous exercise. These muscles also contract when a forced expiratory effort is made, and are the major muscles concerned in developing the enormously high expulsive pressures of defaecation and coughing.

### Movements in Anaesthetised Patients

Fink,[40] using an electromyographic technique, has studied the movements of both the abdominal muscles and the diaphragm during anaesthesia. Under all types of light anaesthesia some electrical activity can always be detected in the abdominal musculature (oblique-trans-

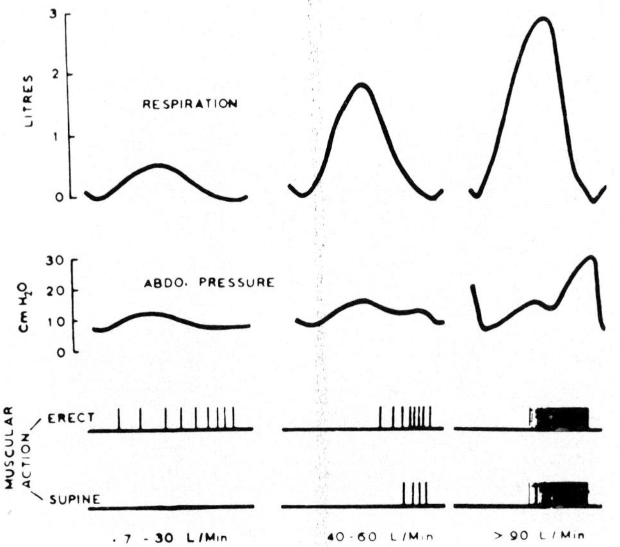


2/FIG. 16.—Schematic pattern of the activity of the muscles of the abdominal wall of the gastric pressure, and of the spirogram at different levels of ventilation. (Courtesy of Dr. E. J. M. Campbell and the publishers of the *Archives of the Middlesex Hospital*.[39])

verse group) during expiration. This can be abolished by the use of a muscle relaxant.

In anaesthetised patients under light anaesthesia the diaphragm contracts with inspiration and the abdominal muscles with expiration (see Fig. 17*a*). On the other hand, if the patient is now ventilated manually until spontaneous respiration is abolished, then activity ceases in the diaphragm during the period of apnoea but persists as continuous activity in the abdominal muscles (Fig. 17*b*). Fink favours the view that the diminished abdominal activity during a spontaneous inspiration is due to a direct inhibition of these muscles brought about by the respiratory centre. During apnoea this inhibition is removed, so that they enter a state of continuous activity.

## Other Accessory Muscles of Respiration

The *scalene muscles* contract during quiet inspiration and as such are almost entitled to be

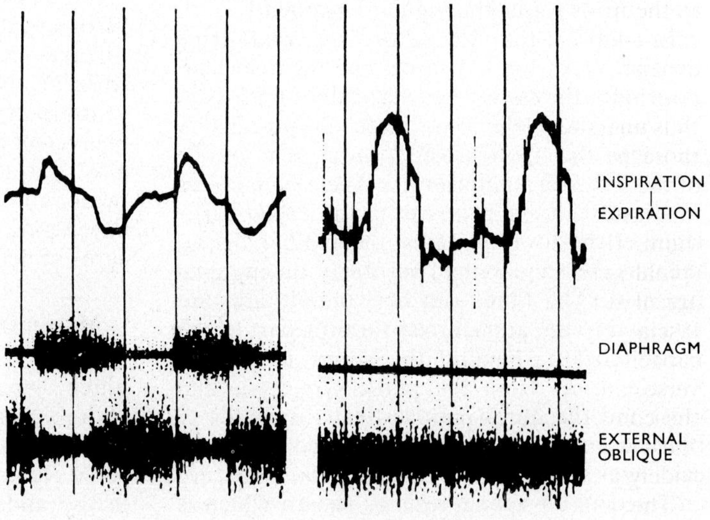


2/FIG. 17.—Electromyogram of diaphragmatic and abdominal muscle activity in an anaesthetised patient.

(*a*) Spontaneous respiration under halothane/nitrous oxide/oxygen anaesthesia.

(*b*) Controlled respiration (i.e. apnoea) under same anaesthesia.

(Courtesy of Dr. B. R. Fink and John Sherratt and Son, publishers of the *British Journal of Anaesthesia*[40]).

considered as a principal muscle of respiration. Their total contribution to the amount inspired, however, is not considered to be great. They also are believed to contract during violent expiratory motions such as coughing, presumably in an attempt to support the apex of the lung.

The *sternomastoid muscles*, on the other hand, are inactive during quiet breathing but become vigorous as ventilation increases. They then contract during inspiration and are regarded as important accessory muscles and their action can be seen well in patients with dyspnoea.

There are many other muscles attached to the thoracic cage which have, at one time or another, been considered as important accessory muscles of respiration. They do not play a significant part in respiration, although many of them contract during the act of coughing. The latissimus dorsi is important in this respect as it may become paralysed following section of its nerve supply at a radical amputation of the breast or division of the muscle fibres at a thoracotomy incision. As a result there is sometimes a serious limitation of the power to expel sputum. A posterior incision for thoracotomy alone may, by dividing the latissimus dorsi, cause a permanent reduction of lung function.

## NORMAL LUNG MOVEMENTS

Those parts of the lung lying in direct relation to the mobile or expansile parts of the thoracic cage—i.e. the ribs and diaphragm—are expanded in direct contact with their neighbouring wall. The peripheral parts of the lung thus undergo a greater degree of expansion than those nearer the hilum. There are three areas of the lung which are not expanded directly, the mediastinal surface in contact with the pericardium, the dorsal surface in contact with the spinal segments of the ribs, and the posterior apical surface lying close to the deep cervical fascia of Sibson. At each inspiration the capacity of the chest is increased in its transverse, antero-posterior and vertical diameters; the converse applies during expiration. As the chest wall expands, so the glottis opens more widely and air enters the lungs.

The movements of the lungs are best considered in relation to the change in position of the chest wall and diaphragm.

I. *The apex*.—The thoracic inlet, formed by the first two ribs, the vertebral column, and the manubrium sterni, moves upwards and forwards on inspiration to increase the antero-posterior diameter of the chest wall. In this manner the anterior part of the apex of the upper lobe is expanded directly. In later life (60 years and over) the manubrio-sternal junction becomes ankylosed and this part of the lung ceases to expand.

II. *The thoracic cage*.—This is best divided into two parts, the upper stretching from the second to the sixth ribs and the lower from the seventh to the tenth. The ribs move outwards and upwards on inspiration; in the upper portion it is the antero-posterior diameter of the thoracic cage that is chiefly increased, whereas in the lower portion the main enlargement lies in the transverse diameter.

III. *The diaphragm*.—The diaphragm has already been mentioned as the principal muscle of respiration. In quiet breathing it can account for the whole of the inspired air, whilst in a maximal inspiratory effort it can still claim over 60 per cent. It is hardly surprising, therefore, that the bases of the lung are the parts which undergo the greatest movement. Radiographically the position of the diaphragm can be seen to vary markedly with changes in posture. In the supine position the abdominal muscles are relaxed and the intestines push the diaphragm up to its highest level. In this position, therefore, the diaphragm possesses its greatest potential powers of contraction. In the erect posture, on the other hand, the weight of the intestines falls away and the level of the diaphragm descends. Frequently, however, the abdominal muscles are contracted, presumably in an attempt to maintain an even intra-abdominal pressure. A similar set of circumstances prevails in the sitting position because the cupola lies at a low level and the abdominal muscles may be contracting if the ventilation is large.

Patients with severe dyspnoea adopt the sitting posture for comfort. This is not due to any change in position of the diaphragm, which would tend to be detrimental rather than beneficial, but to a reduction in the pulmonary congestion and also an improved action of the accessory muscles of respiration. The most satisfying position is often found to be with the trunk bent forward and the head and arms fixed on a support.

IV. *Other factors.*—Vertical movements of the thoracic cage occur in some subjects, mainly at the end of deep inspiration, and are usually most marked in the standing position. These movements are caused by flexion and extension of the vertebral column, but they do not appear to play an important part in ventilating the lungs. They are especially marked during voluntary hyperventilation and thus may aid the contractions of the diaphragm.

## LUNG VOLUMES

The terminology used in this chapter to describe the lung volumes and capacities was introduced by a group of American physiologists in an attempt to simplify the subject, and has now gained general acceptance (Table 3 and Fig. 18).[41]

### Tidal Volume and Minute Volume

The tidal volume is the amount of air passing in and out of the lungs and respiratory passages

2/TABLE 3

NOMENCLATURE FOR LUNG VOLUMES AND CAPACITIES, with normal values in adults. Normal values have been taken from Needham *et al.*[42] The figures are mean values, with the standard deviation in brackets. 98 per cent of the population will lie within ± two standard deviations of the mean.

| *Terminology* | *Explanation* | *Normal Values* *M.* | *F.* |
|---|---|---|---|
| Tidal volume | Volume of air inspired or expired at each breath. | 660 (230) | 550 (160) |
| Inspiratory reserve volume | Maximum volume of air that can be inspired after a normal inspiration. | 2240 | 1480 |
| Expiratory reserve volume | Maximum volume of air that can be expired after a normal expiration. | 1240 (410) | 730 (300) |
| Residual volume | Volume of air remaining in the lungs after a maximum expiration. | 2100 (520) | 1570 (380) |
| Vital capacity | Maximum volume of air that can be expired after a maximum inspiration. | 4130 (750) | 2760 (540) |
| Total lung capacity | The total volume of air contained in the lungs at maximum inspiration. | 6230 (830) | 4330 (620) |
| Inspiratory capacity | The maximum volume of air that can be inspired after a normal expiration. | 2900 | 2030 |
| Functional residual capacity | The volume of gas remaining in the lungs after a normal expiration. | 3330 (680) | 2300 (490) |

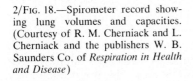

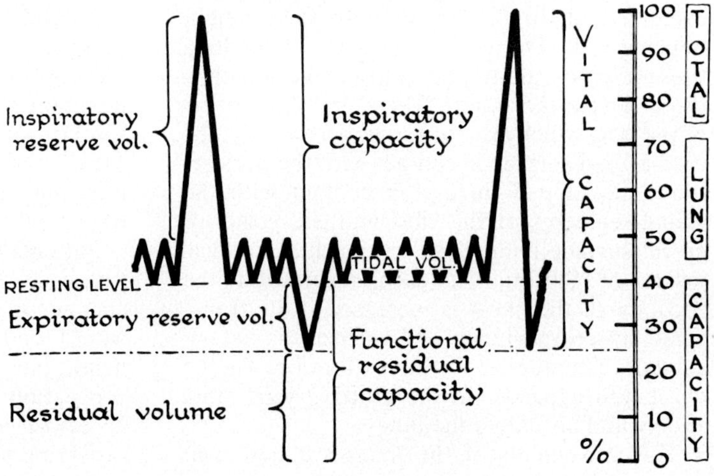


2/FIG. 18.—Spirometer record showing lung volumes and capacities. (Courtesy of R. M. Cherniack and L. Cherniack and the publishers W. B. Saunders Co. of *Respiration in Health and Disease*)

during each respiratory cycle. The quantity, therefore, varies with the size and age of the individual and the depth of respiration. It ranges from 19 ml in the average newborn infant (less in premature infants) to between 450 and 750 ml in resting adults. The tidal volume multiplied by the respiratory rate (breaths per minute) gives the minute volume.

**Measurement of tidal and minute volumes during anaesthesia.**—Of the various methods of measuring minute volume, the Wright respirometer has been found the most satisfactory (Fig. 19). After allowing the instrument to record for one minute, the minute volume can be read directly, and the tidal volume then calculated from this reading and the respiratory rate. A rough estimate of the tidal volume can also be made for each breath. The instrument is compact and light; it under-reads at low flow rates and over-reads at high flow rates, but in practice the respiratory waveform and the nature of the anaesthetic gases tend to minimise these errors. For clinical purposes the instrument offers an accurate assessment of the patient's minute volume (± 10 per cent) within the range of 3·7 to about 20 l/min.[43] A falsely high reading (+10 to 20 per cent) will be obtained if the instrument is connected directly to the catheter mount unless the baffled connecting piece provided by the manufacturers is also inserted into the circuit. This is done to avoid channelling of gases.

(*a*)

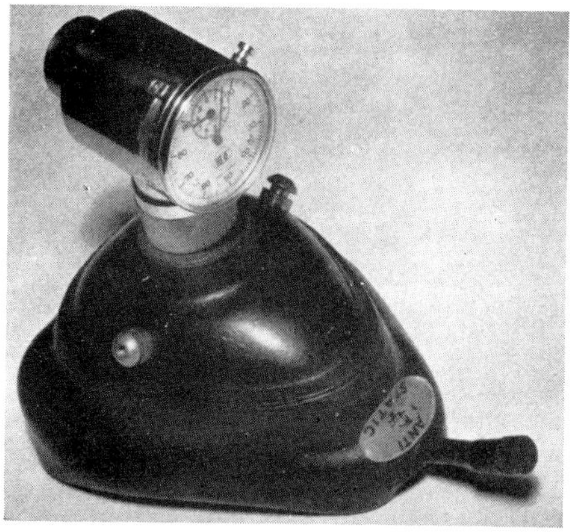

(*b*)

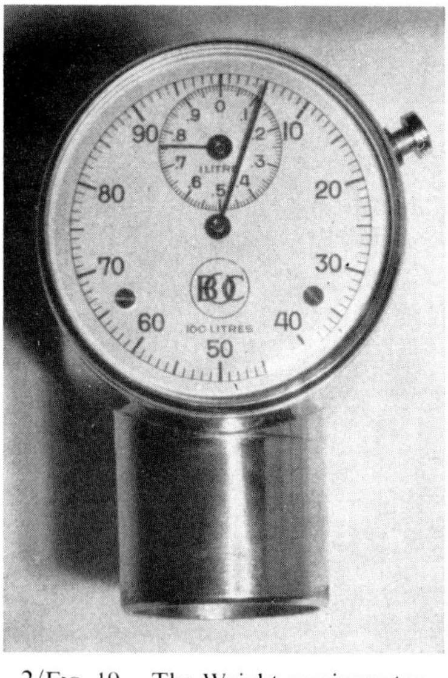


2/Fig. 19.—The Wright respirometer.

### Some Abnormalities of Ventilation

**Tachypnoea.**—Tachypnoea means an increase in the rate of respiration. The rate of respiration in any given situation is such, normally, that the work of breathing is at a minimum.

**Hyperpnoea.**—Hyperpnoea means an increase in ventilation which is in proportion to an increase in carbon dioxide production. The arterial $P_{CO_2}$ therefore remains near normal. The commonest example of this situation is the hyperpnoea which occurs on exercise. In hyperthyroid states the general body metabolism is raised, and the pulmonary ventilation may be increased by as much as 50–100 per cent.

**Hyperventilation.**—Hyperventilation is an increase in ventilation out of proportion to carbon dioxide production. It is a common occurrence during controlled ventilation. Another example is the hyperventilation which accompanies a metabolic acidosis, such as occurs in renal failure and especially in diabetic coma. It can also be due to psychological factors or it may follow brain damage.

**Hypoventilation.**—This means a decrease in ventilation so that the arterial $P_{CO_2}$ rises. Some degree of hypoventilation is the rule rather than the exception during anaesthesia with spontaneous respiration.

**Dyspnoea.**—Dyspnoea is a subjective sensation which is difficult to define. It is best described as an awareness of respiration which is unpleasant or distressing. This description does not include "breathlessness", which is not distressing, and may indeed be mildly pleasurable, such as is experienced after mild or moderate exercise.

The physiological mechanisms leading to dyspnoea are not well defined, and the most satisfying theory is that of Campbell and Howell,[44] who have suggested that the sensation arises when there is an inappropriate result (i.e. volume of inspiration) for a given muscular effort, or that a greater effort than expected is required to produce a given ventilation. They describe this as "length-tension inappropriateness", the normal situation being "learnt" by experience. The abnormal sensation of dyspnoea can then be recognised.

Dyspnoea is a common symptom of disease, and is the presenting symptom in many pulmonary and cardiac abnormalities. Its severity is very variable from person to person, so that in two patients with disease of apparently similar severity one may complain of crippling dyspnoea while it is of much less importance to the other.

In a normal subject, raising the $Pa_{CO_2}$ causes a progressively more severe sensation of "shortness of breath". This sensation appears to be related to the increased respiratory muscle activity which, in turn, is secondary to the increased drive to ventilation. The sensation is worse if this extra muscle activity does not produce the desired ventilation; for example, at the breakpoint of breath-holding, if the gas in the lungs is expired into a bag and then re-inspired, breath-holding can continue again for some time even though there has been no "improvement" in blood gas tensions. In a paralysed subject, there can be no respiratory muscle activity with the result that if the $Pa_{CO_2}$ is raised the normal feeling of shortness of breath does not occur.

Breath-holding time can be increased by prior hyperventilation to wash out $CO_2$. This is a dangerous manoeuvre, especially if carried out before diving, because the subject may become dangerously hypoxic. It can also be increased by breathing oxygen and by vagal or phrenic blockade. Neural blockade, up to a spinal segment of T1, does not affect breath-holding, but a patient with a C3 transection has no sensation of dyspnoea while breath-holding. It therefore appears that the normal "shortness of breath" occurring in response to a raised $Pa_{CO_2}$ and/or reduced $Pa_{O_2}$ is dependent on intact vagi and phrenic nerves.[45]

**Increased ventilation during anaesthesia.**—During anaesthesia with spontaneous respiration, an increase in ventilation is usually due to one of four causes; (1) Oxygen lack; (2) Carbon dioxide excess; (3) Irritation of the respiratory tract by an anaesthetic vapour or other stimulating procedure; (4) Reflex surgical stimulation.

*Carbon dioxide*, which acts mainly by central chemoreceptor stimulation but also to some extent by peripheral chemoreceptor stimulation brings about an increase mainly in the depth of respiration. In the past some anaesthetists deliberately added 5 per cent of carbon dioxide to produce a hyperpnoea when inducing with an agent such as ether. Provided this practice is only continued for a short time, and that once a physiological response has been obtained the concentration is gradually diminished, then little harm can follow in normal subjects. The danger, however, of the ill-advised use of carbon dioxide has led some people to dispense with it entirely.

Hyperventilation as a result of *reflex stimulation* from the operation site or stimulation of bronchial mucosa has already been discussed. Pulling on the mesentery, or dilating the anal sphincter under too light anaesthesia—in other words, inadequate reflex suppression—results in an increase in the depth of respiration. If the stimulus is even more severe or the depth of anaesthesia totally inadequate, then laryngeal spasm may result.

## DEAD SPACE

1. **Anatomical dead space** ($V_D$ anat) comprises the volume of the respiratory passages, extending from the nostrils and mouth down to (but not including) the respiratory bronchioles. The term "dead space" is used since in it there is no exchange of gases between blood and air. Its capacity varies with age and sex, the figure normally quoted being 150 ml, but in young women it may be as low as 100 ml, whereas in old men it can rise to as much as 200 ml. The position of the lower jaw can influence dead space. Depression of the jaw with flexion of the head (a common cause of respiratory obstruction in the anaesthetised patient) reduces dead space by 30 ml. On the other hand, protrusion of the jaw with extension of the head increases dead space by 40 ml[46]. Pneumonectomy or

tracheostomy clearly reduces the volume of dead space.

2. **Physiological dead space** ($V_D$ phys) is defined as that fraction of the tidal volume which is not available for gaseous exchange. It includes therefore not only the anatomical dead space, but also "alveolar dead space", which is the "wasted ventilation" occurring in zones of lung with high $\dot{V}/\dot{Q}$ ratios. In these zones, the extra ventilation beyond what would give a normal $\dot{V}/\dot{Q}$ ratio for that particular pulmonary capillary blood flow contributes to alveolar dead space. If there is no blood flow to a particular zone (infinite $\dot{V}/\dot{Q}$ ratio), for example due to a pulmonary embolus, then all the ventilation to that zone is "wasted". The relationships between ventilation and perfusion of alveoli are further discussed on page 95. In normal man, anatomical and physiological dead space are numerically almost equal, and amount to about one-third of the tidal volume. Because the relationship between physiological dead space ($V_D$ phys) and tidal volume ($V_T$) remains fairly constant when tidal volume is altered, the physiological dead space is often expressed as a fraction of the tidal volume ($V_D/V_T$ ratio; normal 0·25 to 0·4).

Physiological dead space is increased in old age, in the upright position when compared with supine subjects, with large tidal volumes or high respiratory rates, after the administration of atropine, when inspiratory time is reduced to 0·5 seconds or less during controlled ventilation, and in the presence of lung disease whenever ventilation-perfusion relationships are altered. For instance, in chronic bronchitis or asthma the physiological dead space may rise to 50–80 per cent of the tidal volume; it is also found to be high following pulmonary embolism. It is increased following haemorrhage[47] and during controlled hypotension, especially if the patient is tilted head up.[48]

The effect of anaesthesia on the physiological dead space appears to be very variable, but as a general rule it can be taken that both $V_D$ phys and $V_D/V_T$ are increased during anaesthesia, after taking into account any changes due to apparatus dead space. During intermittent positive pressure respiration, this increase in $V_D$ phys is approximately compensated for by intubation (which reduces dead space by about 70 ml); thus for ventilated, intubated and anaesthetised patients $V_D/V_T$ is found to be 0·3–0·45, but if the effect of intubation is corrected for, then $V_D/V_T$ appears to be in the 0·4–0·6 range. In one study the effects of intubation on total functional dead space during halothane anaesthesia during spontaneous ventilation has been studied.[49] These workers found that, using a mask and Frumin valve, the total dead space was increased considerably (mean $V_D/V_T = 0{\cdot}68$; SD $= 0{\cdot}062$), being reduced by intubation (mean $V_D/V_T = 0{\cdot}51$; SD $= 0{\cdot}073$), representing in absolute terms an average difference in total functional dead space of 82 ml between intubated patients and those anaesthetised with a mask. These subjects were able to compensate for changes in dead space by altering their tidal volumes.

As a general rule it may be said that the dead space is increased during anaesthesia, although the changes are very variable. Cooper[50] has suggested that the physiological dead space during anaesthesia with passive ventilation can be roughly estimated from the formula:

$$V_D/V_T = 33 + \frac{\text{Age}}{3} \text{ per cent}$$

*Measurement of physiological dead space.*— This is usually done by using Enghoff's modification of the Bohr equation which may be derived as follows:

$$(V_T - V_D)Pa_{CO_2} = V_T \times P\bar{E}_{CO_2}$$

This merely states that the volume of $CO_2$ in gas which has partaken in gas exchange (tidal volume $V_T$ – physiological dead space $V_D$) is the same as the volume of $CO_2$ in mixed expired gas, although it is now diluted to a larger volume, the tidal volume $V_T$.

Rearranging this equation:

$$V_D \text{ phys} = V_T \frac{(Pa_{CO_2} - P\bar{E}_{CO_2})}{Pa_{CO_2}}$$

The apparatus dead space should be subtracted from this amount. The assumption is made that $Pa_{CO_2}$ is equal to alveolar $P_{CO_2}$.

Measurement of physiological dead space requires the collection of a sample of mixed expired air into a Douglas bag over a known number of breaths, and measurement of its carbon dioxide content and total volume. The arterial $P_{CO_2}$ must also be measured in a blood sample taken during the period of gas collection. The values obtained for $Pa_{CO_2}$, $P\bar{E}_{CO_2}$ and $V_T$ are then substituted in the equation, and $V_D$

phys calculated. Allowance is then made for apparatus dead space.

3. **Apparatus dead space** consists of the volume of gas contained in any anaesthetic apparatus between the patient and that point in the system where rebreathing of exhaled carbon dioxide ceases to occur (e.g. the expiratory valve in a Magill system, or the side-arm in an Ayre's T-piece). The importance of apparatus dead space is so well known as hardly to need further emphasis, especially when anaesthetising small children. The interior volume of an adult face-piece and the connections up to the point of the expiratory valve in a Magill system may add as much as 125 ml of dead space to the patient. This problem is further discussed below.

### Alveolar Ventilation

Alveolar ventilation is defined as that part of the minute volume which takes part in gas exchange. The normal value for alveolar ventilations is 2·0 to 2·4 $l\ min^{-1}m^{-2}$ body surface area, or about 3·5 to 4·5 l/min in adults. Its importance lies in the fact that it is the pulmonary factor controlling the excretion of carbon dioxide by the lungs, and it is directly related to the tidal volume, physiological dead space and respiratory rate.

Alveolar Ventilation = (Tidal Volume − Physiological Dead Space) × Respiratory Rate.

$$\text{or } \dot{V}_A = (V_T - V_D\ \text{phys}) \times f$$

From this relationship it can be seen that a rise in physiological dead space or a fall in the respiratory rate will lead to a reduction in the alveolar ventilation provided the other factors remain fairly constant. So too will a fall in the tidal volume, although in normal man the physiological dead space also decreases, so that the effect on the alveolar ventilation is lessened.

For example, if we calculate the alveolar ventilation under various circumstances we find the following figures are obtained:

1. *Normal*
   $(V_T - V_D\ \text{phys}) \times f = V_A$
   $(450 - 150) \times 13 = 3{\cdot}9$ l/min ($P_{CO_2}$ normal)
2. *Tidal Volume Reduced*
   $(300 - 100) \times 13 = 2{\cdot}6$ l/min ($P_{CO_2}$ raised)
3. *Physiological Dead Space Increased by Anaesthetic Apparatus*
   $(450 - 225) \times 13 = 2{\cdot}7$ l/min ($P_{CO_2}$ raised)
4. *Respiratory Rate Decreased*
   $(450 - 150) \times 8 = 2{\cdot}4$ l/min ($P_{CO_2}$ raised)

These simple calculations, although useful as a guide, do not always represent the true state of affairs. For instance, the addition of apparatus dead space of 100 ml (measured by filling the relevant volume with water) may represent a rather smaller addition when in clinical use. This is due to patterns of gas flow and channelling of gases within the apparatus. For example, the central core of the gas stream moves rapidly whilst gas in the periphery moves relatively slowly. Thus the central element represents the major portion of the ventilation, so reducing the role of the dead space. It should also be noted that in practice physiological mechanisms react to any of these changes and tend to return the $P_{CO_2}$ towards normal values, so that the alterations in alveolar ventilation are not as great as those indicated above. However, under the influence of sedative or anaesthetic drugs these physiological responses may be depressed, so that any alteration in alveolar ventilation due to the addition of apparatus dead space may not be compensated fully. Deep anaesthesia and respiratory depressant drugs depress alveolar ventilation. The resulting rise in alveolar carbon dioxide tension will produce a fall in alveolar oxygen tension unless extra oxygen is added to the inspired air.

Because alveolar ventilation is almost invariably reduced by anaesthesia with spontaneous ventilation, and because other changes leading to arterial hypoxaemia occur in the lungs, it is always advisable to administer at least 33 per cent oxygen in all anaesthetic gas mixtures.

The clinical assessment of alveolar ventilation is one of the most important for the anaesthetist to make. Observation of the reservoir bag, the movements of the chest and abdomen, the rate of respiration, measurement of the minute volume using a respirometer, and the colour of the blood in the patient's capillary bed are all used in this assessment. In addition, the end-tidal $CO_2$ concentration, which gives a guide to the arterial $P_{CO_2}$, can be monitored. The dangers of hypoventilation during anaesthesia cannot be overstressed, Equally, it is not sufficient merely to oxygenate a patient by raising the inspired oxygen percentage if adequate steps are not being taken at the same time to remove the carbon dioxide. Many beginners fall into the trap of believing that all must be well if the patient has a good colour during anaesthesia.

### Vital Capacity

At the end of a normal expiration, a patient lying at rest and breathing quietly is capable of forcibly expiring a large quantity of air from his lungs—this is called the *expiratory reserve volume*. Similarly at the end of a normal inspiration, he is equally capable of taking in an even larger quantity of air—the *inspiratory reserve volume*. If the tidal volume is added to the sum of these two measurements, the patient's vital capacity will be known.

| | | *Approx. Figure* |
|---|---|---|
| Vital capacity = | Tidal volume | 500 ml |
| | Inspiratory reserve volume | 2500 ml |
| | Expiratory reserve volume | 1000 ml |
| | | 4000 ml |

The vital capacity can be simply measured with a spirometer. The patient is requested to take a maximum inspiration and then to expire completely into the spirometer. This test is not wholly reliable, as with a judicious use of the tongue some patients can give completely false readings. Modifications of it will be considered under the tests of lung function.

The vital capacity does not remain constant even in healthy adults, and is altered by such factors as age, physical training, changes in weight and an increase in height. For this reason it is often expressed in relation to the surface area of the body. Repeated examinations may lead, for no obvious reasons, to a steady improvement.

2/TABLE 4

NORMAL VALUES OF VITAL CAPACITY

| | *Athlete* | *Male* | *Female* |
|---|---|---|---|
| Average vital capacity in ml/m$^2$ of body surface area | 2800 | 2600 | 2100 |
| Average vital capacity in ml/m$^2$ of height | 2900 | 2500 | 2000 |

In view of the marked differences in values for normal people, a measurement of vital capacity cannot be considered abnormal unless it varies by more than 20 per cent from the above figures. A single reading is of little value, but repeated readings may be useful when undertaken on a comparative basis to study the progress of a patient's treatment.

The vital capacity may be reduced by many disease processes. Some of these are of particular interest to the anaesthetist.

1. **Alterations in muscle power.**—Clearly, any drug which depresses the activity of the ventilatory mechanisms, whether it be in the brain, nerve, or muscle fibre, must reduce the vital capacity. Similarly, lesions in the brain such as cerebral tumours, a raised intracranial pressure, lesions affecting the nerves, such as poliomyelitis and polyneuritis, or lesions of the neuromuscular mechanism such as occur in myasthenia gravis, will lead to a reduced vital capacity.

2. **Pulmonary disease.**—The commonest disease in this country in which a reduction in vital capacity is found is chronic bronchitis. Some other lung diseases which reduce the vital capacity are pulmonary fibrosis, lobar collapse, pneumonia, and asthma.

3. **Space-occupying lesion in the chest.**—Neurofibromata and other extra-pleural tumours, kyphoscoliosis, pericardial and pleural effusions, pneumothorax, and some diseases—such as carcinoma of the lung with infiltration or consolidation—will reduce the vital capacity.

4. **Abdominal tumours which impede the descent of the diaphragm.**—Abdominal distension may cause a reduction in vital capacity. Surprisingly, although the gravid uterus displaces the diaphragm upwards, the vital capacity of a pregnant woman is not decreased. On the contrary, it is increased on average 10 per cent over the normal, since the thoracic cage is enlarged transversely and antero-posteriorly and there is marked splaying of the subcostal angle.

5. **Abdominal pain.**—The pain experienced after an operation involving the abdominal musculature leads to a reduction in vital capacity of 70–75 per cent in upper abdominal and 50 per cent in lower abdominal operations.

These figures have been confirmed by Simpson and his associates[51], who advocated the use of a continuous thoracic epidural technique for the relief of post-operative pain. Using this method, they were able to produce not only complete freedom from pain, but also a very substantial improvement in the vital capacity (see Table 5). It is interesting to note, however, that in very few patients in their series was the vital capacity restored to the pre-operative level.

There seems to be little doubt that a continuous epidural technique provides the most effective form of pain relief in combination with the maximum ventilatory function. Nevertheless, such techniques are time-consuming and require a high degree of technical skill if the thoracic level is used. For these reasons this technique is best reserved for the special case.

6. **Abdominal splinting.**—Tight abdominal binders, strapping, or bandaging limit the range of respiratory movement. Elastic strapping applied in the vertical plane allows the greatest freedom of respiration in the post-operative period.

7. **Alterations in posture.**—Changes in posture in the conscious subject lead to considerable alterations in the vital capacity, and these are mainly related to positions which are calculated to alter the volume of blood in the lungs. Thus the capacity is greater when standing than when sitting or lying. It increases by as much as ¼–½ litre if there is an accumulation of blood in the legs.

The various positions in which an anaesthetised patient may be placed on the operating table have been shown to have a considerable effect on the vital capacity of the unanaesthetised subject. For example:

| | *Loss of Vital Capacity* |
|---|---|
| Trendelenburg position (20°) | 14·5 per cent |
| Lithotomy | 18·0 per cent |
| Left lateral | 10·0 per cent |
| Right lateral | 12·0 per cent |
| Bridge in dorsal position | 12·5 per cent |
| Prone position, unsupported | 10·0 per cent |

(Case and Stiles,[52])

**Significance during anaesthesia.**—Alterations in the vital capacity are of little significance during anaesthesia unless extremely pronounced. During spontaneous ventilation the patient can nearly always maintain a satisfactory $Paco_2$ and during artificial ventilation the only noticeable consequence is that the lungs feel "stiff". It is only when the vital capacity begins to fall below the required tidal volume that respiratory difficulties arise during anaesthesia. Examples of conditions in which this may occur are tension pneumothorax, a large haemothorax, diaphragmatic hernia, exomphalos in the newborn, neuromuscular diseases and upper respiratory obstruction. Reductions in vital capacity do, however, become important in the post-operative period when the expulsion of secretions may be seriously impeded. If the vital capacity falls below about three times the tidal volume artificial help may be needed to maintain the airways clear of excessive secretions.

### Residual Volume

Residual volume is the amount of air that still remains in the lungs after the patient has made

2/Table 5
Vital Capacity Readings Expressed as a % of the Pre-operative Value

| | *Before epidural (In pain)* | | | *1 hour after epidural (Pain-free)* | | | *24 hours after epidural (Pain-free)* | | |
|---|---|---|---|---|---|---|---|---|---|
| | *Range %* | *Mean %* | *No. of Cases* | *Range %* | *Mean %* | *No. of Cases* | *Range %* | *Mean %* | *No. of Cases* |
| Upper Abdominal | 20–56 | 35·2 | 54 | 44–139 | 69·0 | 54 | 61–139 | 83·2 | 50 |
| Lower Abdominal | 37–69 | 55·5 | 6 | 80–91 | 84·8 | 6 | 92–96 | 94·7 | 3 |

Vital capacity readings in 60 patients undergoing abdominal surgery (Simpson *et al.*[51]).

a maximal expiration. Normal average values range from 2,100 ml for males to 1,570 for females. Functional residual capacity is the amount of air remaining in the lungs after a normal expiration. Normal average values range from 3,300 ml for males to 2,300 ml for females.

Unfortunately neither of these two measurements can be made directly. There are, however, two indirect methods which use a known concentration of a relatively insoluble gas, i.e. one that does not readily traverse the alveolar membrane and become dissolved in the plasma.

**Nitrogen technique.**—The principle is to collect all the nitrogen that can be washed out of the patient's lungs. Following a maximal expiration (if residual volume is required) or a normal expiration (if functional residual capacity is required) the patient inspires oxygen from a special source and then expires into a spirometer which is known to be free of nitrogen. Over some minutes almost all the alveolar nitrogen is washed out of the lungs. In healthy adults this may be achieved after only two minutes, but in patients with severe emphysema as much as 20 minutes may be needed. At the beginning of the test all the nitrogen is in the lungs and at the end it has all passed to the spirometer. The concentration of nitrogen in the spirometer can now be measured. The total volume of gases in the spirometer is known so that the total volume of nitrogen in the mixture can be calculated. As air contains 80 per cent nitrogen a suitable correction will reveal the total alveolar gas volume at the moment the test began.

**Helium technique.**—In this case a spirometer with carbon dioxide absorption is used. This is filled with a mixture of 10 per cent helium and 90 per cent oxygen and the patient then breathes in and out of it. At first, there is no helium in the patient's lungs, but gradually mixing takes place until after a few minutes the concentration of helium in the patient's lungs and in the spirometer is the same. Again, the volume of gas in the alveoli can then be calculated.

**Significance.**—As the residual volume represents the amount of air remaining in the lungs at the end of a maximal expiration, any increase in it signifies that the lung is larger than usual and cannot empty adequately. Increases in residual volume are usually associated with air-trapping in the lungs, but may occur temporarily without any actual structural change. For example, obstruction to the airway, as in asthma or over-inflation of the lungs after a thoracic operation, may cause an increase. If there is a marked increase in residual air the act of respiration may be difficult, since by implication the patient is unable to reduce the volume even by forced expiration, and it is likely that respiration is carried out with the mechanical disadvantage of a thorax already larger than normal.

In severe emphysema some air is "trapped" completely in the alveoli and never comes in contact with the respired gases. In emphysematous patients it is impossible to obtain a true reading of the residual volume by either of the methods mentioned above. This can only be obtained in a specialised respiratory unit where a body plethysmograph is available. Such an instrument measures the thoracic gas volume whether it is in free communication with the airway or not.

### Functional Residual Capacity (FRC)

The functional residual capacity is the volume of gas held in the lungs at the normal relaxed end-expiratory point. It is increased in certain diseases (such as asthma and chronic bronchitis) and as a result of the application of a positive end-expiratory pressure (Fig. 20*a*). It is decreased as a result of the induction of anaesthesia (Fig. 20*b*) and post-operatively, especially following abdominal surgery. The FRC is especially important in relation to the Closing Capacity (see below) since if the latter rises above the FRC arterial hypoxaemia may occur.

### Closing Capacity (CC)

As the lungs become reduced in volume during expiration there comes a point at which some small airways begin to close and therefore prevent any further expulsion of gas from related alveoli, so that air-trapping occurs. The lung volume at which this phenomenon can first be detected is called the Closing Capacity (CC or the Closing Volume, CV). Measurements of this volume are made using a single breath nitrogen-washout technique. Whilst breathing air the subject slowly expires to residual volume, and then slowly takes a single breath of oxygen to maximum inhalation. The breath is held for a few seconds and then slowly and evenly expired. During this phase the instantaneous nitrogen concentration and volume of the expir-

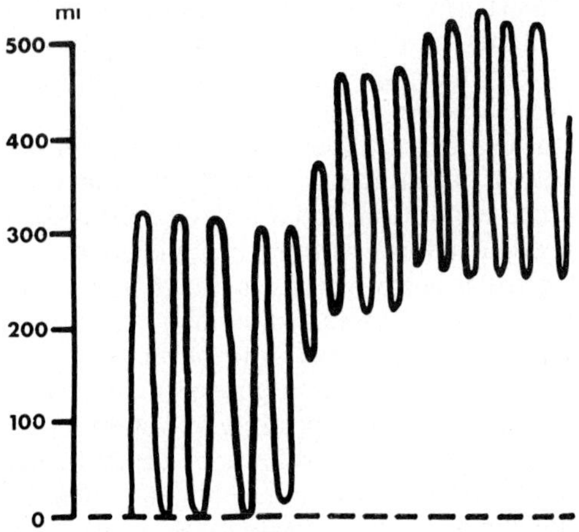


2/Fig. 20(*a*).—Spirometer tracing showing the effect of positive end-expiratory pressure (PEEP) on functional residual capacity (100 ml divisions).

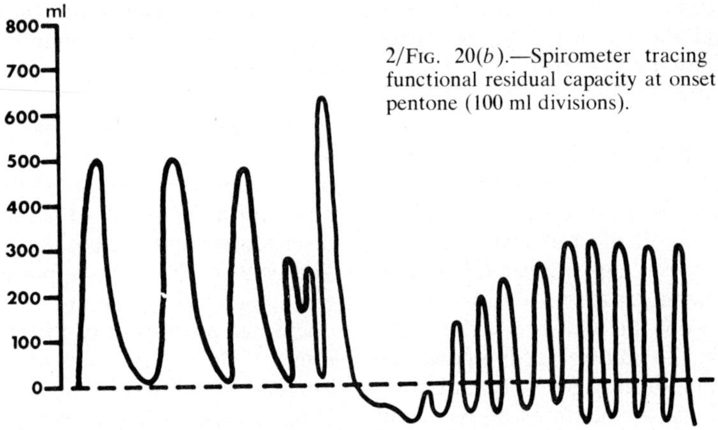


2/Fig. 20(*b*).—Spirometer tracing showing decrease in functional residual capacity at onset of anaesthesia—thiopentone (100 ml divisions).

ate are recorded, and a characteristic curve is obtained (Fig. 21). This curve has four phases: (I) Dead space gas; (II) Mixed dead space and alveolar gas; (III) Mixed alveolar gas from all alveoli; and (IV) A phase in which there is a sudden rising concentration of nitrogen. The CC is the volume at which phase IV begins. The reasoning behind this is as follows. During inhalation the oxygen is preferentially distributed to the smaller alveoli in the dependent parts of the lung due to the shape of the alveolar compliance curve which assures a larger change in volume in smaller alveoli than in larger ones. Therefore the nitrogen is more diluted in the smaller alveoli. During expiration the mixed alveolar nitrogen concentration from all alveoli is measured (Phase III) until the point at which airway closure begins. At this moment the nitrogen concentration increases because the expulsion of gases from the smaller airways ceases and exhalation continues from those areas of the lung where the nitrogen concentration is higher. Other tracer gases such as helium, argon and $^{133}$Xenon can be used in a similar fashion.

In subjects with normal lungs the normal value for CC is intimately related to the age and position of the subject. Normal regression lines for CC in supine subjects with respect to age are shown in Fig. 22. From this figure it can be seen that the lowest values for closing capacities are to be found in the late teens, and that below (down to the age of about 5 years) and above this age it is progressively increased.

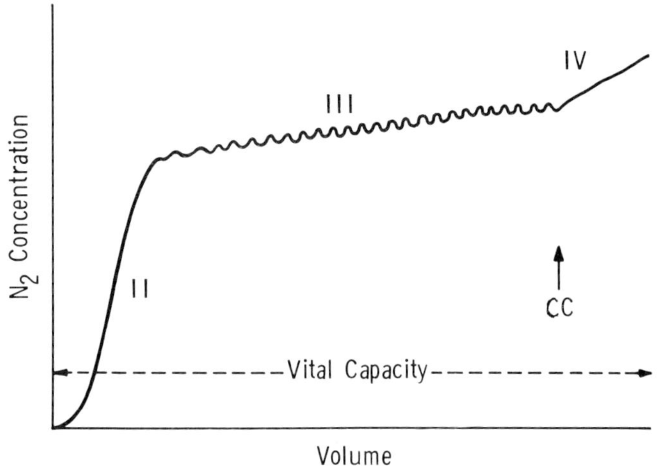


2/FIG. 21.—Measurement of closing capacity by nitrogen wash-out technique (full explanation in text).

The important point to note is the relationship of the CC to the FRC. If the CC rises above the FRC some airways will be closed during part, or later perhaps the whole, of the range of normal ventilation with the result that blood passing through the closed areas of lung will not be fully oxygenated, and the arterial $Po_2$ will fall. In subjects with normal lungs CC becomes equal to FRC in the 60's and in the 40's in supine subjects. After this the CC continues to rise as age increases, and the arterial $Po_2$ begins to fall. A rise in CC is seen in smokers, obesity, rapid intravenous transfusion, early chronic bronchitis, left ventricular failure and following myocardial infarction. It is almost certainly increased after surgery, and may be an important factor in the genesis of post-operative hypoxaemia.[53, 54] The use of a positive end-expiratory pressure probably raises the arterial $Po_2$ by increasing the FRC above the CC.

**Thoracic Gas Volume**

The principle of measuring the total volume of air contained in the thorax is based on a change of the air pressures inside and outside the thorax when the patient's airway is suddenly obstructed. First, the patient is enclosed in a body plethysmograph and permitted to breathe the air within the chamber. The airway pressure and the plethysmograph pressure are noted. At the desired moment (usually at the end of a normal expiration) the airway is suddenly occluded by an electrical shutter. The patient

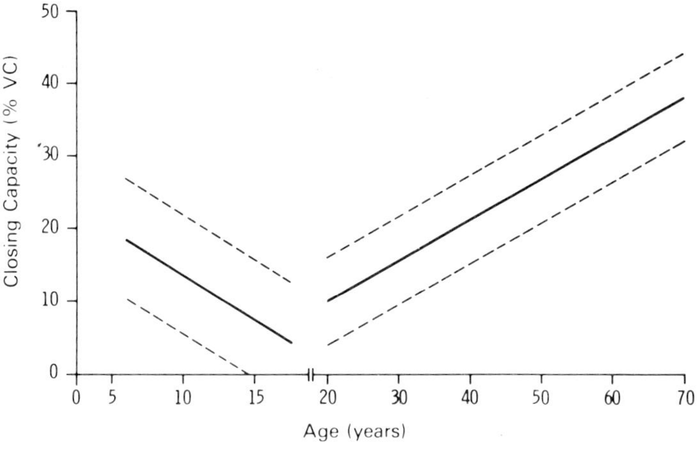


2/FIG. 22.—Relationship of age to closing capacity in normal subjects.

will then attempt to inspire against a total obstruction. The chest expands, the intrathoracic pressure falls whilst the pressure in the plethysmograph rises. Alveolar pressure is assumed to equal mouth pressure under these circumstances, so that the pressure differences now enable the original thoracic gas volume to be calculated.

This method is rapid and relatively simple. It is often used in combination with the dilution methods of nitrogen and helium for in this manner it is easy to determine the amount of "non-ventilated" areas of lung in a particular patient. In a patient with severe emphysema these tests may reveal that as much as 1–3 litres of air are trapped within the alveoli.

**Discussion.**—All these tests must be interpreted with caution because there is a wide margin for normal values even in the healthy adult. Nevertheless, an increase in functional residual capacity is usually assumed to denote structural emphysematous changes in the lung. In reality it represents hyperinflation of the lung during quiet breathing and though this is commonly caused by emphysema and partial obstruction of the airway, it could in rare cases be due to a deformity of the thorax.

### Minimal Air

Even after the pleural cavities have been opened and the lungs have collapsed, there still remains a very small, but nevertheless important, quantity of air entrapped in the lungs—the minimal air. In medico-legal circles the presence of air in the lungs of a newborn child suggests that it has breathed after birth, but this deduction does not hold if the lungs have been positively inflated during resuscitation. A piece of aerated lung when placed in water will float, whereas a piece of atelectatic lung (i.e. one which has not been aerated) will sink to the bottom.

### Dynamic Tests of Ventilation

The tests of ventilatory function so far discussed are more or less static in nature. However, ventilation is essentially a dynamic process, and other function tests have been devised which attempt to quantitate ventilatory function in terms of the *rate* at which ventilation can take place, rather than in terms of volumes.

1. **Maximum breathing capacity (MBC).**—This test is designed to measure the speed and efficiency of filling and emptying the lungs during increased respiratory effort, and is defined as the maximum volume of air that can be breathed per minute. It is usually measured for 15 seconds and the result expressed in litres per minute. It is therefore a dynamic test, as opposed to the static measurement of vital capacity. As age increases there is a large reduction in the maximum breathing capacity, but it is in patients with pulmonary emphysema that it shows the most impairment. It also falls in the presence of bronchospasm and bronchiolar obstruction. Average values for normal subjects range from 100–200 litres per minute depending upon the mode of measurement, but there is a big difference between these figures and those for abnormal subjects.

2. **Forced expiratory volume (FEV).**—The patient makes a maximal inspiration, expires as forcefully and rapidly as he can into a spirometer, and the total amount of air expelled over a given time is measured. The time intervals at which the total amount of air expelled is measured are 0·5, 1, 2 and 3 seconds. However, as there seems to be little advantage between the results taken at each of these intervals, it is customary to take only the volume expired at 1 second, called the $FEV_1$. This volume is expressed as a percentage of the forced vital capacity. In normal young subjects 83 per cent of the vital capacity should be expired during the first second. The lower limit of normal is usually taken as 70 per cent. In a patient with chronic bronchitis the $FEV_1$ may be only 50 per cent or less.

The dry spirometer is commonly used to measure the vital capacity and $FEV_1$. One such instrument is the Vitalograph (Fig. 23). Expiring into it causes a bellows to expand and results in the vertical deflection of a pen writing on a calibrated chart. The initial act of expiration activates a pressure switch, and the whole chart is then moved sideways at a constant speed by an electric motor. A graph is drawn out on the chart, in which the vertical axis is expressed in litres, and the horizontal axis as time in seconds (see Fig. 24). The result is a graphical analysis of the rate and volume of the patient's forced vital capacity, from which the $FEV_1$ can be calculated. One of the main advantages of this type of instrument is that the records are produced in a small flat sheet of paper which can be filed away for reference, and subsequent tests can then be compared with previous records. A rough estimate of the peak expiratory flow rate can be obtained by measuring the slope of the steepest part of the curve.

3. **Peak expiratory flow rate (PEFR).**—After a maximal inspiration, the patient expires as forcefully as he can, and the maximum flow rate of air is measured. The measurement can be made either into a pneumotachograph, or by a specially designed instrument, such as the Wright Peak Flow Meter. The normal limits for the PEFR are taken as 450–700 l/min in men, and 300–500 l/min in women, although like all tests of ventilatory function the normal value varies with the age and build of the subject.

*Discussion.*—The results from measurement of both the $FEV_1$ and the PEFR can be improved with a little practice on the patient's part. For this reason it is customary to perform the test five times, and then to take the average of the last three readings as the final result. Alternatively, the best of the five readings can be taken. It is of great importance to use apparatus with a low resistance to high gas flow rates.

Low values for the $FEV_1$ and PEFR usually

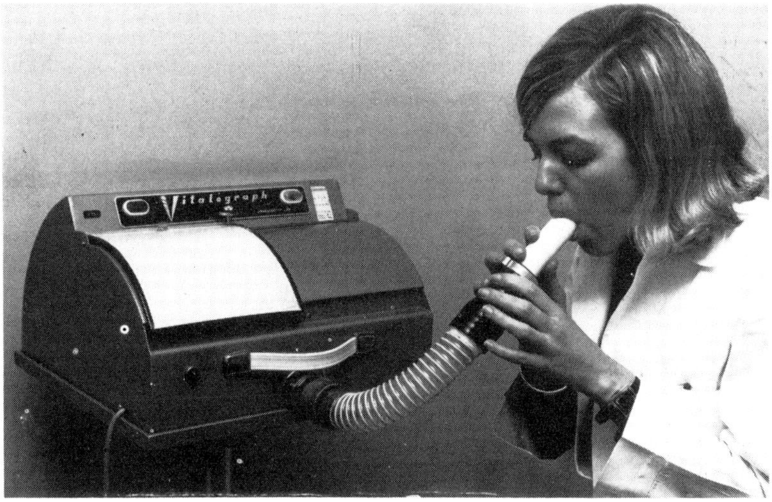


2/FIG. 23.—The "Vitalograph".

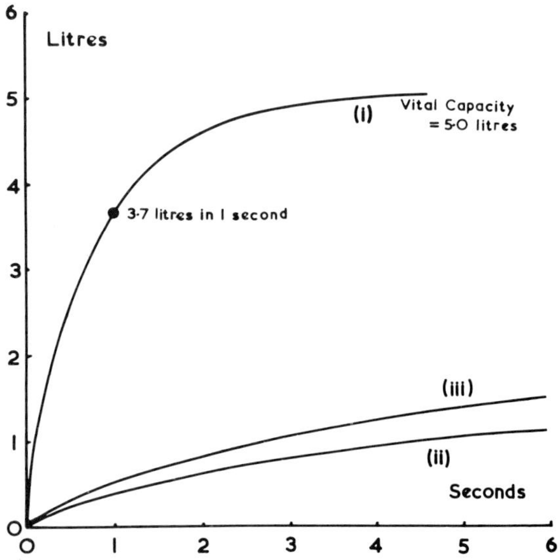


2/FIG. 24.—Examples of the time course of forced expiration taken with a "Vitalograph". Curve (i): normal male aged 40. $FEV_1 = 3{\cdot}7/5{\cdot}0 = 74$ per cent. Curve (ii): a patient with chronic bronchitis, showing both a restrictive and an obstructive lesion (see text). Curve (iii): the same patient after the inhalation of an isoprenaline aerosol, showing some improvement.

indicate a higher than normal resistance to gas flow within the conducting airways (i.e. a diffuse airways obstruction). This type of abnormality is termed "obstructive" and is found in such conditions as asthma, chronic bronchitis, bronchitis and bronchospasm. The response to the inhalation of a bronchodilator aerosol can readily be tested. If reversible bronchoconstriction is present, then both the PEFR and $FEV_1$, improve after aerosol inhalation (see Fig. 24). This gives a guide as to whether bronchodilator drugs will or will not be an effective form of treatment, for example in combination with physiotherapy during the pre-operative preparation of such a patient. Some patients are found to have a reduced vital capacity, although their PEFR and $FEV_1$ values are within normal limits. This type of ventilatory defect is described as "restrictive". Although this distinction between obstructive and restrictive abnormalities of ventilation has been made, it is usual to find that both the vital capacity and the tests of flow rate are reduced so that both types of abnormality are present. Such is the case in chronic bronchitis where, apart from diffuse airway obstruction, air trapping also contributes to abnormally low PEFR and $FEV_1$ values.

If no apparatus is available for estimating the severity of an obstructive lesion, this can be judged by a simple bedside test. The patient is asked to take a deep breath, and then to exhale as forcibly as possible through his mouth. Normally this forced expiration is virtually complete after three seconds. Prolongation beyond this time is abnormal, and the severity of the obstructive lesion can be roughly judged from the time it takes to complete the expiration.

## THE PLEURAL CAVITY

Each lung is invested with a thin serous covering on its outer surface (visceral pleura) and this is reflected on to the inner aspect of the chest wall and the upper surface of the diaphragm (parietal pleura). The potential space between these two layers is the pleural cavity and under normal conditions the two surfaces are in apposition save for a small quantity of lymph which acts as a lubricant. In disease, adhesions may form between the two surfaces, but if the underlying lung is not involved there is no appreciable change in respiratory function.

At the apex of the pleural cavity the outer surface is surrounded by loose areolar tissue (extrapleural or Sibson's fascia) in which small fibrous bands can sometimes be demonstrated coursing over the dome of the lung (bands of Sebalot).

### Intrapleural Pressure

Owing to the continual retractive force exerted by the elastic recoil of the lung, the intrapleural pressure under normal conditions is always negative. When the pleural cavity is opened the negative pressure returns to atmospheric, the lung collapses, and the mediastinum moves over towards the unaffected side.

The elastic recoil of the lung is made up of three factors:

1. The elastic tissue in the bronchial wall and also that coursing throughout the interstitial tissue of the lungs.
2. The arrangement of the muscle fibres of the bronchi and bronchioles in a "geodesic" network so that on contraction the bronchial tree not only becomes reduced in diameter but also shortened in length.
3. The surface tension of the fluid lining the alveolar walls.

In man the intrapleural pressure ranges from −5·6 mm Hg (−0·7 kPa) on inspiration to −2·6 mm Hg (−0·3 kPa) on expiration. It is less negative at the bottom than at the top of the lung. In normal circumstances the force required to separate the two pleural surfaces is prodigious unless air or fluid enters the pleural cavity. During a strong inspiratory effort with the glottis closed, pressures of −40 mm Hg (−5·3 kPa) have been recorded, whereas forced expiration under similar conditions may lead to pressures as high as +50 mm Hg (6·7 kPa). These variations in pressure have little bearing on the thoracic cage, but are reflected on the thin-walled surrounding structures, namely the heart and great vessels. A rise of intrathoracic pressure impedes the venous return and expels blood from the intrathoracic veins into the neck and abdomen.

### Intrapleural Pressure Changes in Pulmonary Collapse

With the pleura intact, collapse of lung can take place only if the surrounding soft tissue structures such as those at the apex of the lung, the diaphragm, and the mediastinum move inwards to fill the vacant space. In practice, as the lung collapses, so the pressure in the intrapleural space falls, causing a raised diaphragm on that side and the mediastinum to move across.

In cases of severe post-operative pulmonary collapse, negative intrapleural pressures four times greater than normal have been recorded.

### Pneumothorax

Air can enter the pleural cavity in a number of ways. If there is a free communication with the atmosphere, whether through a broncho-pleural fistula or a wound of the chest wall, the pneumothorax is described as *open*, whereas if there is no communication it is *closed*. A particularly dangerous type of pneumothorax is that in which air can enter but cannot escape (ball-valve), leading to a *tension* pneumothorax. Thus in an anaesthetised patient a pneumothorax may be found to be open, closed, or under tension.

It is important to remember in any discussion of the physiological changes occurring under these conditions that the pleural cavity in the experimental animal often differs profoundly from that in man. For example, the commonest animal to be used for such investigations is probably the dog, and in this animal the parietal and visceral pleura are of almost diaphanous texture, the mediastinum extremely mobile, and the two pleural cavities are often in direct communication. The extremely thin and lax pleural membranes permit pressure changes in one cavity to be rapidly transmitted to the other. In man, however, the pleural membrane is thicker and the mediastinum represents a fairly solid mass separating the two cavities, which have no communication. Thus a change of pressure in one cavity is only partially reflected in the other cavity.

Norris and his colleagues[55] have shown a correlation between the extent of a pneumothorax as judged from a radiograph and the size of the anatomical shunt producing arterial oxygen desaturation. When the ratio of lung to intrapleural space is greater than 75 per cent the shunt does not exceed the normal value of 2 per cent of the cardiac output. Below 65 per cent the shunt increases as the size of the lung decreases. When the air is removed from the pleural space a delay of several hours occurs before the ventilation-perfusion upset in the lung improves, and this despite an early increase in the size of the lung. This delay is probably due to the relatively greater pressure required to open a ventilatory unit which is completely closed as opposed to that needed for one that has remained at least partially open.

**Open pneumothorax.**—In the presence of an open pneumothorax the size of the opening in relation to the diameter of the trachea will determine how much air enters the lungs. Patients breathing quietly under local analgesia can tolerate large openings in their chest wall although there is no negative intrapleural pressure and the lung is partially collapsed. The reason for this is that in the resting state only a small tidal volume is required, and this is a small fraction of the vital capacity. If, however, the patient becomes alarmed and attempts deep respirations, more air is sucked into the pleural space, the lung collapses further, and dyspnoea and cyanosis result. It must be clear, therefore, that those patients with a reduced vital capacity tolerate a pneumothorax badly. Under anaesthesia the detrimental effects of a pneumothorax are countered by intermittent positive-pressure respiration when the opening is between the pleura and the chest wall. If the opening is via a broncho-pleural fistula this treatment may lead to a tension pneumothorax unless special precautions are taken.

The degree of collapse of lung with the chest open depends on a number of factors which are altered in both health and disease:

1. Size of opening in the pleura.
2. The elastic recoil of the lung.
3. Airways resistance and bronchiolar patency.

**Closed pneumothorax.**—This may occur spontaneously or result during the closure of a thoracotomy wound. Spontaneous pneumothorax may arise when an emphysematous bulla ruptures and partially fills the pleural space with air. As a thoracotomy wound is closed, a certain amount of air will remain entrapped in the pleural cavity. This volume can be considerably reduced if the anaesthetist ensures that the lung is fully distended just prior to complete closure of the wound. After such operations as lobectomy and pneumonectomy, a potential space is created which it is often impossible to fill with the surrounding soft tissues. In order to allow the remaining lung tissue to function adequately a negative intrapleural pressure must be re-established. Gases may be removed from this space in the following ways:

1. *Absorption.*—Any gas—including air—when introduced into the pleural cavity, is absorbed by the blood stream, because the visceral pleura is permeable to these gases. The rate of absorption of the contained gases depends largely on their respective partial pressures. Thus, air will be absorbed slowly, for the partial pressure of nitrogen is high in both the pleural space and the blood stream. Oxygen, however, is rapidly removed, and according to Dalton's Law this then raises the partial pressure of nitrogen so that it is now higher than that in the circulation; thus some nitrogen is absorbed. This process continues until all the air has been removed but, depending on the amount entrapped, may take up to three or four days to be completed.

2. *Aspiration.*—A pneumothorax apparatus may be used to take off small amounts of air in the operating theatre so that the patient returns to the ward with a normal negative intrapleural pressure.

3. *Water seal.*—This has two main functions—one to act as a drainage tube for any blood that may collect in the pleural cavity; the other to allow air to leave the cavity and to prevent its return. It is an efficient and simple type of unidirectional valve. A litre of sterile water is placed in a large glass bottle and the height of the water level is noted. A glass pipe starting just below the surface of the water is connected by a length of rubber tubing directly with the intrapleural space via a leak-proof circuit. On inspiration water is sucked up the glass pipe and falls again on expiration. If the patient coughs, or the lung is distended on expiration by increasing the respiratory resistance, then air is driven out of the chest and bubbles out into the bottle, which is in direct communication with the atmosphere. Using this method, provided there are no leaks either from the lung surface or bronchus, it is possible to re-establish a negative intrapleural pressure almost immediately after closure of the thoracic wound.

4. *Suction through a water seal.*—In order to be certain that all the air is removed from the pleural space suction may be applied to the air in the glass bottle. This will be transmitted via the drainage tube to the pleural cavity and thus rapidly establish a negative intrapleural pressure. It is an extremely useful method of treatment after segmental resection of lung, particularly where the remaining portion of lung continues to leak air into the pleural space. It must be remembered, however, that the indiscriminate use of suction may continue to keep open channels which might otherwise seal off.

**Tension Pneumothorax**

When air enters the intrapleural space but cannot leave it, a tension pneumothorax results. It may arise spontaneously or during anaesthesia, especially when intermittent positive pressure ventilation is used. In the earlier instance a bulla may rupture or a broncho-pleural fistula may be present. A quite normal lung may rupture if unduly high inflation pressures are allowed during anaesthesia.

Air enters the pleural space as if through a one-way valve and causes the pressure in the enclosed space to rise sometimes as high as +20 mm Hg (2·7 kPa)—thus displacing the mediastinum and compressing the great veins and heart.

Tension pneumothorax should be suspected during anaesthesia if inflation becomes increasingly difficult and the patient's condition steadily deteriorates. An unanaesthetised patient presents with cyanosis, hypotension and dyspnoea. Whether anaesthetised or not, tachycardia or bradycardia, depending on how far the condition has progressed, may be present. Pneumomediastinum and subcutaneous emphysema may or may not be present. In two recorded cases[56,57] the onset of marked respiratory wheezing led to the mistaken diagnosis of severe bronchospasm, and consequent ineffective treatment with bronchodilator drugs. Rarely a tension pneumothorax may occur due to the rupture of a bulla during an asthmatic attack when bronchospasm will also be present. It can be confirmed by the clinical findings of reduced chest movement on the side of the pneumothorax, deviation of the trachea to the other side, hyper-resonance to percussion and reduced breath sounds on the affected side. Often the patient's condition deteriorates rapidly so time must not be wasted waiting for X-ray confirmation. A large bore intravenous cannula is inserted in the second intercostal space in the mid-clavicular line. The needle is withdrawn leaving the cannula *in situ* so that the lung is not damaged as it expands. The patient's condition will rapidly improve as a result of this manoeuvre which converts the tension pneumothorax to an open pneumothorax. A chest drain can then be inserted in due course and connected to an underwater seal. Very occasionally, a tension pneumothorax may be bilateral[57] so that this possibility must always be borne in mind and the situation confirmed with a chest X-ray as soon as possible.

## ABNORMAL CHEST AND LUNG MOVEMENTS

When the stability of the thoracic cage is destroyed either by trauma or surgical intervention, then abnormal movements of both chest wall and the underlying lung may occur. There are three principal conditions that must be considered, paradoxical respiration, pendelluft and mediastinal flap.

### Paradoxical Respiration

In the presence of a crush injury of the chest wall or the deliberate surgical removal of part of the rib cage (as in a thoracoplasty), the affected part of the chest wall collapses inwards. On inspiration the unaffected side will expand in the normal fashion but the injured side will be sucked in. On expiration, the reverse takes place. This type of respiration—paradoxical respiration—is only seen in patients breathing spontaneously and is abolished by controlled ventilation. The presence of paradoxical respiration is usually an indication for artificial ventilation.

### Pendelluft

This signifies the pendulum-like movement of air that occurs from one lung to the other in the presence of an open pneumothorax in a patient breathing spontaneously. Thus, when the chest is opened the underlying lung partially deflates as the negative intrapleural pressure is lost. On inspiration, the lung on the normal side fills with air partly from the trachea and partly from the partially deflated lung on the affected side. On expiration, the converse takes place and some expired air from the normal lung passes over into the other side (Fig. 25). The physiological result of this pendulum-like flow of air is that there is rebreathing and the alveolar carbon dioxide tension rises.

In the presence of an open pneumothorax, pendelluft does not necessarily occur; much will

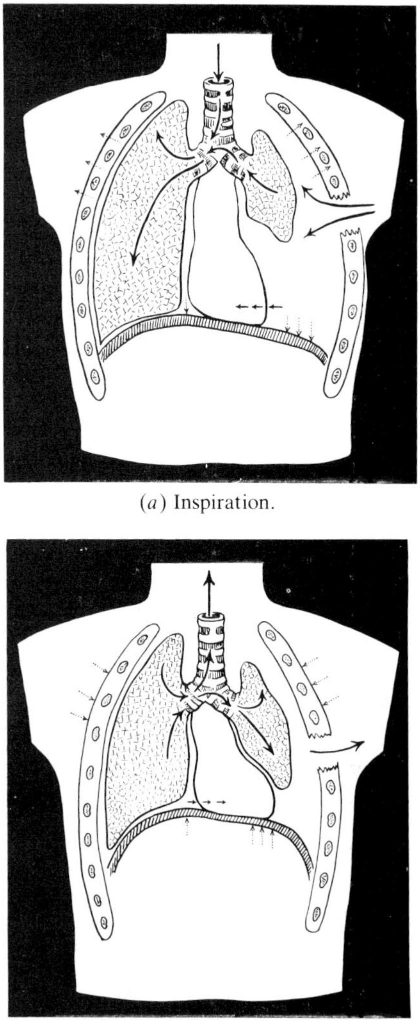

(*a*) Inspiration.

(*b*) Expiration.

2/FIG. 25.—PENDELLUFT

depend on the size of the opening in the chest wall and the volume of the ventilation. If the size of the hole in the chest wall is less than the diameter of the trachea, then it is easier for air to enter via the trachea, so very little air will be sucked into the affected side and both lungs will expand on inspiration. Similarly, a patient breathing spontaneously can often tolerate a large opening in his pleural cavity provided he is breathing quietly. The moment ventilation increases both paradoxical respiration and pendelluft may result.

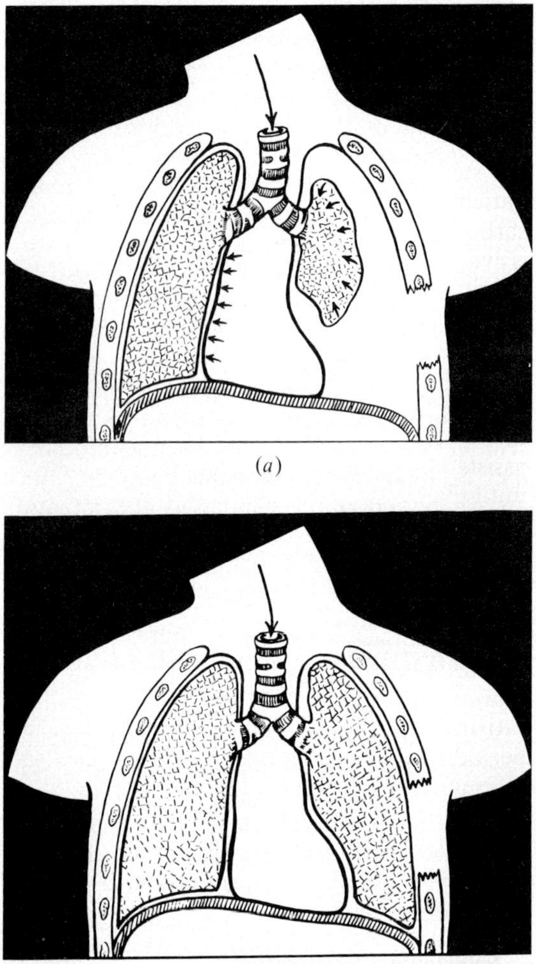

(*a*) (*b*)

2/Fig. 26.—Effect of Pneumothorax on Mediastinum (Inspiration)
(*a*) Mediastinal flap + weight of heart and great vessels (spontaneous respiration).
(*b*) These factors corrected by positive-pressure ventilation.

### Mediastinal Flap

In man the mediastinum can move freely with the different phases of respiration. It remains, however, approximately in the middle of the thorax because the negative pressures in the pleural cavities balance each other. When the pleural cavity is opened, so that the lung collapses and the pressure around it becomes atmospheric, the negative intrapleural pressure on the other side will pull the heart and great vessels in the mediastinum towards the sound lung. This negative pull reaches its maximum during inspiration and, therefore, the mediastinum comes furthest over at this time (Fig. 26*a*). On expiration the intrapleural pressure becomes less negative and the mediastinum passes back to its original position.

During quiet breathing, even in the presence of a large hole in the chest wall, the mediastinum merely moves with a slight to and fro' motion. As the volume of ventilation increases so the flapping movement becomes more obvious. Its presence tends to embarrass respiration because it impairs the filling of the lung on the normal side. The actual range of movement is greatest when the patient is in the supine position but it is more dangerous in the lateral position because, then, the whole weight of the mediastinal contents is compressing the dependent normal lung. In addition, mediastinal flap interferes with the filling of the great veins, leading to a fall in cardiac output.

**Treatment.**—Paradoxical respiration, pendelluft, mediastinal flap and the disturbances caused by the weight of the mediastinal viscera, can all be prevented by intermittent positive-pressure ventilation (Fig. 26*b*).

## ASSISTED AND CONTROLLED RESPIRATION

In a normal conscious subject breathing spontaneously, the carbon dioxide tension of the blood varies between 36 and 44 mm Hg (4·8–5·9 kPa), and only rarely can values outside this range be recorded. Under the conditions of anaesthesia, when spontaneous respiration is maintained, the effective tidal exchange can be impaired by anaesthetic, analgesic and relaxant drugs, so that the level of carbon dioxide in the body will consequently rise. Moreover the patient's efforts may be further impeded by the resistance of the anaesthetic system. As oxygen is usually added to anaesthetic mixtures the tidal volume may well be sufficient to ensure oxygenation of the patient, yet inadequate for normal excretion of carbon dioxide. If a suitable infrared analyser is available, end-tidal $CO_2$ concentration can be monitored or, alternatively, an arterial blood sample can be taken for blood gas estimation.

### Assisted Respiration

With this, the patient spontaneously commences inspiration and the anaesthetist then assists by providing a positive airway pressure until the lungs are sufficiently expanded. Expiration is then allowed to take place passively. Assisted respiration is useful when respiratory activity is temporarily depressed or hampered by such things as a small dose of central depressant like pethidine or a peripherally acting drug of the muscle relaxant type. It is, however, not easy to match spontaneous activity satisfactorily in this way, especially for long periods, and when it is possible to carry it out efficiently, apnoea tends to result as the carbon dioxide tension in the blood falls. Respiration is now said to be controlled. In other words efficient assisted respiration soon becomes controlled respiration.

### Controlled Respiration

Respiratory activity can be abolished in three different ways:

1. Paralysis of the muscles of respiration.
2. Depression of the respiratory centre.
3. Removal of the carbon dioxide stimulus to respiration.

In practice a combination of all three methods is often used. A reduction of arterial $Pco_2$ (hyperventilation) and a reduced activity of the respiratory centre (analgesics) can enable the total dose of relaxant to be reduced.

## DIFFUSION RESPIRATION

In a normal person the interchange of gases at the alveolar capillary membrane depends upon physical diffusion; at tidal volumes smaller than 1 litre the movement of gas molecules from the alveolar ducts to the alveoli is also almost entirely by diffusion. Some movement is caused by the contraction of the heart and by the ejection of blood from it leading to a pulsatile flow in the pulmonary vessels. If the nitrogen in the lungs is replaced by oxygen then these factors are sufficient to maintain an adequate uptake of oxygen in the blood in the absence of respiratory muscle activity. This process is known as diffusion respiration, but during it carbon dioxide is not removed from the blood. In fact the tension of carbon dioxide in the alveoli rises rapidly to equal that of the mixed venous blood (46 mm Hg—6·1 kPa) but thereafter more slowly, at approximately 3 mm Hg/min (0·4 kPa/min).

Diffusion respiration can be produced in an anaesthetised patient following the use of a muscle relaxant and the endotracheal administration of oxygen, and is sometimes used during bronchoscopy (see Chapter 11).

## Respiratory Movements in Anaesthesia

John Snow reported that inhalation of chloroform caused breathing "sometimes performed only by the diaphragm whilst the intercostal muscles are paralysed". During spontaneous ventilation under halothane anaesthesia it is common to see rib cage retraction during inspiration, but relative sparing of diaphragmatic activity. Using a technique which quantitatively partitions tidal volume into a contribution due to diaphragmatic descent and contribution due to rib cage expansion, Tusiewicz and associates[58] measured the ventilatory response to $CO_2$ of awake subjects and subjects anaesthetised with 0·8 per cent halothane. They plotted the results as:

(1) Ventilation due to diaphragmatic activity against $Pco_2$;

(2) Ventilation due to rib cage activity against $Pco_2$.

As shown for one subject in Fig. 27, halothane has an enormous effect on the rib cage contribution but little effect on the diaphragm. In their study, the total and compartmental minute ventilation (mean ± SEM) of 5 subjects at a $Pco_2$ of 60 mm Hg (8 kPa) were as follows:

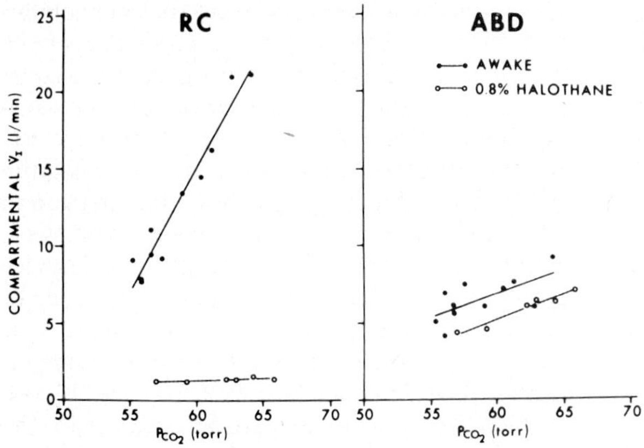


2/FIG. 27.—Compartmental minute ventilation during $CO_2$ rebreathing in subject, awake and anaesthetised. Rib cage response is on the left, diaphragmatic response on the right. (Courtesy of Tusiewica, Bryan and Froese (1977), and the J. B. Lippincott Co.[58])

| $\dot{V}_I$ (l/min) at a $Pco_2$ of 60 mm Hg (8 kPa) | | |
|---|---|---|
| | AWAKE | 0·8% HALOTHANE |
| Rib cage | 17·8 ± 3·4 | 1·7 ± 1·1 |
| Diaphragm | 13·5 ± 2·0 | 5·8 ± 0·5 |
| Total | 30·9 ± 3·4 | 7·5 ± 1·8 |

In awake subjects at a normal $Pco_2$, the rib cage contribution is usually less than 30 per cent of the total.[59]

### Tracheal Tug

In deep anaesthesia inspiration is associated with a tracheal tug. This is a sharp downward movement of the trachea on inspiration. The exact mechanism is obscure but there are two theories which deserve serious attention. Harris[60] believes it is associated with the dual origin of the muscle fibres of the diaphragm. In deep anaesthesia there is a general loss of muscle tone so that the sternocostal fibres of the diaphragm are no longer supported by a rigid costal margin when they contract on inspiration. In consequence, these costal fibres contract ineffectively leaving the crural fibres alone to appear to be functioning. The result is that a sharp contraction of the central part of the diaphragm on inspiration is transmitted to the whole mediastinum. The root of the lung and trachea is then pulled downwards with each inspiration. This explanation, however, does not account for the occurrence of this condition in respiratory failure.

Another approach has been made on the basis of the part played by the elevating muscles of the larynx. In rats, the sternothyroid and sternohyoid muscles contract during inspiration and are directly controlled by the respiratory centre. In man, these muscles may help to raise the sternum as accessory muscles of respiration but their size and mobility make it unlikely they play an important role. In normal breathing the larynx remains stationary in both phases of respiration. This is due to the pull of its stabilising muscles (mylohyoid, stylohyoid, styloglossus and the posterior belly of the digastric), all of which are elevators of the larynx. It has been suggested that tracheal tug is due to a failure of these stabilising muscles to stand up to the forceful traction of the diaphragm.[37]

Apart from deep anaesthesia, tracheal tug may be noticed in partially curarised patients and in the presence of respiratory obstruction. In most cases it can be cured by returning full power to the muscles of respiration or removing the cause of the respiratory obstruction. Tracheal tug at the end of anaesthesia— in the absence of muscular paralysis—may be an indication for endotracheal suction or bronchoscopy, as the cause is not infrequently inadequate ventilation of one lung due to an accumulation of mucus.

**Sigh.**—A deep sigh is occasionally seen in both conscious and anaesthetised subjects. In the latter it is commonly associated with deep anaesthesia. Its occurrence may be misinterpreted by the surgeon as denoting too light anaesthesia, but in practice it is unrelated to surgical stimuli, nor is its cause known. It must be distinguished from the inspiratory gasp or breath-holding which is clearly related to surgical stimulation in the presence of inadequate suppression of reflex activity.

Sighing in a conscious person is thought to be a mechanism by which during quiet respiration an occasional deep breath prevents underventilated alveoli from collapsing. However, Fletcher and Barber[61] investigated conscious subjects breathing spontaneously and found that sighing was not followed by any change in lung mechanics or in lung compliance. They were also unable to demonstrate any changes when sighing was almost completely abolished by intravenous morphine.

### Hiccup

Hiccup is an intermittent clonic spasm of the diaphragm, of reflex origin. With each contraction the bronchial lumen is constricted and, in unintubated patients, the glottis closed. In mild cases, unassociated with anaesthesia, the spasm is usually a unilateral contraction of the diaphragm which, if the condition persists, gradually spreads across the whole muscle.[62]. The left side is more often affected than the right.

Afferents can arise from almost any part of the body, including the central nervous system, but during anaesthesia are most frequently associated with visceral stimulation, usually in the upper abdomen, and probably transmitted through the vagus. Hiccup may also be caused by inflation of the stomach with anaesthetic gases, or from irritation below the diaphragm due to extraneous fluids, such as blood, pus or gastric juice. Persistent hiccups may be associated with uraemia.

Hiccup is not a common complication of deep anaesthesia but rather a product of modern methods when relaxation is produced by motor paralysis, and sensory reflex activity is by comparison relatively undepressed. It can be regarded as a reflex response of the partially anaesthetised respiratory centres and incompletely paralysed peripheral musculature to vagal stimulation.

**Treatment.**—Careful appraisal of the surgeon's technique will usually enable the anaesthetist to suppress reflex activity in advance of stimulation so that hiccup is prevented. A deeper level of anaesthesia than that previously maintained, or the addition of a further dose of relaxant just before a procedure which is known to be particularly stimulating, are often successful. Such preventive measures may be necessary even when the surgical conditions, in terms of relaxation, are satisfactory. Hiccups often occur "out of the blue" even in the presence of very adequate relaxation of the abdominal muscles.

Total paralysis will always prevent or stop hiccup, but the very large dose of muscle relaxant that this may entail in some patients is not always advisable, and may complicate the situation at the end of the operation. A large number of individual drugs, ranging from the administration of amyl nitrite to the addition of a sudden blast of ether vapour to the anaesthetic mixture, have been tried at one time or another. Salem[63] found that stimulation of the mid-pharynx behind the uvula, and opposite the second cervical vertebra, by gentle movement with the end of a catheter inserted through the nose stopped hiccups in 84 out of 85 patients. Such methods presumably act by reflex inhibition, and even though many of them stop the disturbance, they are usually only temporarily effective.

The best and most rational treatment for hiccup during anaesthesia is to block the reflex pathways concerned by a deeper level of anaesthesia (further supplementation with analgesic, hypnotic or more potent inhalational anaesthetic) or by incremental doses of a muscle relaxant.

In the post-operative period a cause for hiccup must be sought before special treatment is advised. Uraemia, subphrenic abscess and grossly distended bowels are some of the conditions which must be excluded, but in many patients no specific factor can be incriminated. Then, adequate sedation together with a phenothiazine should be tried. A method of treatment which often proves successful is initiation of the swallowing reflex with both nose and ears blocked. The patient sips repeatedly from a glass of water while his external auditory meatae and nose are obstructed. The success of this manoeuvre presumably depends on the afferent stimulus in the middle ear (from fluctuating pressure waves) being stronger than that which initiates the hiccup.

An oesophageal tube and suction are helpful to relieve distension. Carbon dioxide inhalation occasionally inhibits an attack. For prolonged and severe cases, after screening the patient to decide which side is affected, infiltration with local anaesthetic of a phrenic nerve in the neck should be considered.

## THE WORK OF BREATHING

As the term suggests, the work of breathing comprises all the energy required to ventilate the lungs. Unfortunately the task of the respiratory muscles is not simply the inflation of a passive balloon (the lungs). Certain forces which tend to prevent the lungs being inflated must be overcome. There are three essential components in this opposition: (*a*) the force needed to overcome the elastic resistance of the lung; (*b*) the force to move non-elastic tissues (structural resistance); and finally (*c*), the force to overcome resistance to the flow of air through the tracheo-bronchial tree.

The **elastic resistance** of the lung is defined as the force tending to return the lung to its original size after stretching. It should not be thought of as the force required to expand the lung, as this is also a measure of the rigidity of the lung which varies with pulmonary congestion. The *compliance of the lung* is a measure of its change in volume per unit of pressure change. In cardiac and pulmonary disease the congestion and fibrosis which are frequently present lead to a fall in the "compliance" of the lung.

The **structural resistance** is composed of the thoracic wall, the diaphragm and the abdominal contents. It is related to the speed of the flow of air so that when this is maximal so is the structural resistance.

The **air resistance** is important because it is dependent on the length and size of the lumen of the bronchial tree. The anaesthetist adds an extra air resistance when he inserts an endotracheal tube. This matter is of particular importance in the intubation of a young child for whom too small an endotracheal tube may increase the air resistance enormously.

The flow of air through the bronchial tree may be laminar (streamlined) or turbulent. In this latter condition the air pursues an erratic course with the creation of many eddy-currents. The air resistance in laminar flow can be lowered by reducing the *viscosity*, whereas in turbulent flow it is the *density* that must be lowered. Anaesthetists sometimes use a mixture of helium and oxygen (79 per cent: 21 per cent) in certain cases of upper respiratory obstruction with the object of improving the patient's oxygenation. As the viscosity of this mixture is slightly *greater* than air, the resistance to laminar flow will be increased. On the other hand, its density is less than that of air, so the resistance to turbulent flow is decreased. As partial upper respiratory obstruction sets up turbulence, this therapy produces a higher flow for a given pressure gradient.

### Compliance

The lungs and thoracic wall function as a single unit, and provided the tidal volume is in the normal range there is a linear relationship between the volume change and the pressure that produces it. If it is measured when the flow of air has ceased, as during breath-holding or during apnoea in anaesthesia, it is known as *static compliance*.

$$\text{Static compliance} = \frac{\text{Volume change in litres}}{\text{Pressure change in cm of } H_2O \text{ (kilopascals)}}$$

The compliance of the lungs and of the thoracic wall in a normal person are approximately the same, namely 0·2 litres/cm $H_2O$ (2·0 l/kPa). Thus a volume change of 0·2 litres in the thorax is obtained by a pressure of 1 cm of $H_2O$ ($9{\cdot}8 \times 10^{-2}$ kPa) exerted against the lungs in conjunction with a pressure of 1 cm of $H_2O$ ($9{\cdot}8 \times 10^{-2}$ kPa) against the thoracic wall, giving a total thoracic compliance of 0·1 litre/cm $H_2O$ (1·0 l/kPa)[64].

When the volume change of the thorax in relation to pressure changes is measured during respiration it is known as *dynamic compliance*.

**Measurement of total thoracic compliance.**—The pressure gradient to be measured is that between the airway and the atmosphere, but it is difficult to obtain a reliable result unless the patient is able to relax completely. Thus the measurement of total thoracic compliance is best made in a patient who is relaxed and ventilated, either with the aid of a tank ventilator (conscious patient) or an endotracheal tube (unconscious patient).

(a) *Tank ventilator*.—The conscious patient is placed in the ventilator so that the transthoracic pressure can be measured. The volume of air inspired at each level of subatmospheric pressure within the tank reveals the data for a pressure-volume curve.

(b) *Endotracheal method*.—In the anaesthetised patient an endotracheal tube is inserted and a relaxant used to abolish tone in the respiratory muscles. This tube is then occluded and the pressure within the system is measured. After this the tube is unclamped and the volume of air or gas expired is collected in a spirometer. Again, a pressure-volume curve is plotted.

**Measurement of lung compliance.**—The pressure gradient to be measured is that between the airway and the pleural space. Direct measurements by placing the tip of a sampling needle (connected to a manometer) within the pleural space are dangerous, so oesophageal pressure, which closely parallels intrapleural pressure, is measured instead using a balloon on the end of a catheter. Since this measurement is a static one, it is made with the patient holding his breath after having inspired a known volume of air from a spirometer. The procedure is then repeated many times with different volumes so that a pressure-volume curve can be constructed. This is usually linear provided large volumes are not used, and will give an average value for lung compliance.

**Measurement of thoracic wall compliance.**—This is obtained by subtraction of lung compliance from total thoracic compliance.

**Measurement of dynamic compliance.**—Dynamic compliance is measured during quiet breathing when lung volume (above FRC) is displayed on the vertical axis against intrapleural (oesophageal) pressure on the horizontal axis as shown in Fig. 28.

**Discussion**

Values for compliance should always be related to the predicted normal value for a person of the same sex, age, height, weight and lung volume, and are preferably related to the functional residual capacity (FRC). For example, a simple change in posture can alter the FRC and thus produce a change in compliance.

One of the principal factors causing the elastic recoil of the lungs is the presence of elastic fibres within the pulmonary tissue. The important role of the surface tension of the fluid lining the alveolar walls has also been emphasised (see p. 27). This tends to draw the opposing walls closer together and so collapse the alveoli. If this fluid were pure water it would exert the very considerable pull of about 70 dynes $cm^{-1}$ ($70 \times 10^{-3}$ $Nm^{-1}$), but fortunately it contains a "detergent-like" agent (surfactant) which reduces the surface tension to as little as 2–8 dynes $cm^{-1}$ ($2–8 \times 10^{-3}$ $Nm^{-1}$).

Much less pressure is required to inflate lungs filled with saline than those filled with air, the difference being due to abolition of the elastic pull of the surface tension exerted by the alveolar lining membrane. The detergent-like agent is believed to be absent in hyaline membrane disease of the newborn, and therefore to account for the very high inflationary pressures that are needed to expand the lungs in this condition.

Pulmonary oedema (altered surface tension with fluid in the alveoli), emphysema (destruc-

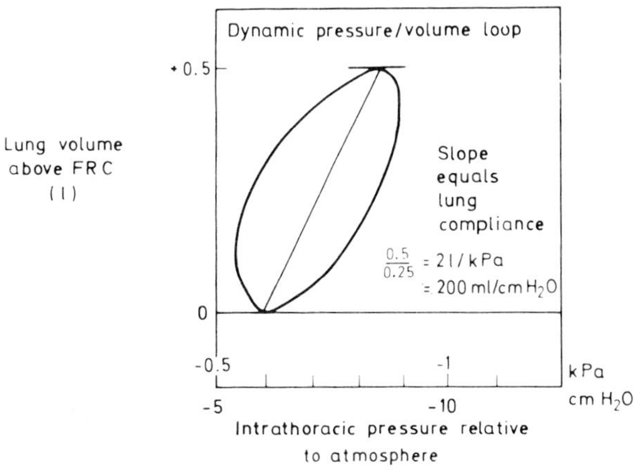


2/Fig. 28.—Measurement of dynamic compliance of lung by simultaneous measurement of tidal excursion (lung volume relative to FRC) and intrathoracic pressure (relative to atmosphere). These parameters are displayed as the Y and X co-ordinates on a two-dimensional plotting device, e.g. cathode ray oscillograph. Lung compliance is derived as lung volume change divided by transmural pressure gradient change. The transmural pressure gradient is indicated by the intrathoracic pressure (relative to atmosphere) when the lung volume is not changing. At these times the alveolar pressure must equal the atmospheric pressure because no gas is flowing. (Courtesy of Dr. J. F. Nunn and publishers Butterworth & Co.[65])

tion of elastic fibres) and mitral stenosis (increased pulmonary vascular congestion) are but some of the conditions that decrease the compliance of the lungs.

Under the conditions of anaesthesia so many factors are operating at the same time, and the situation changes so often, that it is frequently impossible to relate any change in compliance to a single agent or procedure. For example, a drug may affect the muscles of the thorax, the secretions in the respiratory tract, alter the cardiac output, constrict the bronchioles or dilate the pulmonary vessels.

However, very many investigations have been carried out and nearly all agree that induction of anaesthesia causes a fall in compliance.

**Breathing and Oxygen Consumption**

In a normal resting subject the work of breathing uses up approximately 0·5 ml oxygen for every litre of ventilation. Thus at average minute volume of 8 litres about 4 ml of oxygen are required, or about 1·5 per cent of the total oxygen consumption each minute. Increasing respiratory activity leads to a disproportionately high rate of oxygen consumption.

**Respiratory Work and Disease**

At a slow respiratory rate, the work done against elastic resistance tends to be increased, whereas at a faster rate work expended against flow resistance is increased. It is usually found that subjects breathe at a rate which overall results in the minimum respiratory work. In patients with mitral stenosis the severity of the dyspnoea is directly proportional to the degree of pulmonary rigidity, which is secondary to vascular congestion. Thus more work is required to inflate the lungs. It is this increase in respiratory work that makes the patient short of breath. The exact increase necessary to make the patient actually conscious of the respiratory effort varies from individual to individual.

Anaesthetists who commonly come in contact with cases of heart disease have often commented on the general improvement in the circulatory condition that frequently follows the induction of anaesthesia. This is particularly true when assisted or controlled respiration is used. The explanation may lie in the removal of this extra respiratory work by the mode of anaesthesia and the improved ventilation of the lungs.

In chest diseases, especially chronic ones, there is always an upset in respiratory mechanics with an increased work load. In pulmonary fibrosis the lung compliance is decreased, but to a small extent this is offset by a reduction in airway resistance which may occur because the traction exerted by the parenchymal tissue on the lung airways is increased. In diseases affecting the thoracic cage, such as ankylosing spondylitis or kyphoscoliosis, the chest wall compliance may be much reduced.

In obstructive lung conditions, such as severe asthma, chronic bronchitis, and emphysema there is an increased airway resistance and a reduced dynamic compliance. In emphysema marked changes take place in the structure of the lungs, associated with an increase in tissue rigidity leading to a complete loss of elasticity. This lack of elasticity markedly reduces the radial support of the peripheral airways and, combined with a possible intrinsic narrowing as well, means that during expiration the small bronchioles collapse before the alveoli distal to them have emptied completely, and air-trapping ensues. The lung-volume is increased, the intrathoracic pressure becomes less negative, and there is no lung-recoil when a pneumothorax is induced. The chest wall gradually becomes fixed in a position of inspiration. All these changes make the emphysematous patient work harder to ventilate his lungs, and, owing to the fixed chest wall, put the respiratory muscles at a mechanical disadvantage.

In the conscious state, the emphysematous patient can partially compensate for the loss of elastic tissue in the lung by actively contracting the abdominal muscles on expiration. It has already been pointed out that these muscles are the principal muscles of expiration. Anaesthesia, however, is frequently designed to relax them, so that while providing the surgeon with ideal conditions to explore the abdomen it deprives the emphysematous patient of his principal means for emptying the alveoli. In such circumstances, if spontaneous respiration is allowed, the level of carbon dioxide in the blood must rise. Therefore, on both theoretical and practical grounds, when marked abdominal relaxation is produced during general anaesthesia for an emphysematous patient, respiration should be controlled or assisted. Although intermittent positive-pressure respiration permits the anaesthetist to allow an adequate time for expiration to take place in these patients, it does not otherwise help to empty the alveoli.

## Resistance to Ventilation

Under normal conditions of breathing the respiratory resistance comprises the force required to drive air to and fro' along the bronchial tree from the mouth to the alveoli. The resistance to the flow of air in a tube is the pressure difference between the two ends at a given flow rate. If a subject breathes through an anaesthetic apparatus then the resistance of the extra breathing pathway must be taken into account, because the respiratory muscles will have to do more work. A simple test can be made by asking a conscious subject to breathe through a small endotracheal tube (Magill No. 4 or 6) held between his lips, when the extra effort required soon becomes apparent. Expiration is affected most, because there is a rise in intrapulmonary pressure with inadequate emptying of the alveoli. This leads to an increase in carbon dioxide and, therefore, an increase in the depth of respiration in an attempt to wash out more carbon dioxide. The abdominal muscles soon come into action during expiration in an endeavour to drive air out of the lungs.

Nearly every piece of anaesthetic apparatus increases in varying degree the respiratory resistance. One of the most important factors is the type of flow of the gases. This largely depends upon the diameter and shape of the breathing tubes and connection pieces, the number, style and setting of valves in the system, and the size and packing of the soda-lime canister.

**Gas flows.**—When the flow of gas along a tube is smooth and regular it is called laminar, but as the rate of flow increases a critical velocity is reached at which the flow becomes turbulent (Fig. 29). The flow of air in the respiratory tract of a normal patient is laminar, and the flow of gases during inspiration in anaesthetic practice does not reach sufficiently high rates to produce turbulent flow. The internal diameter of the tubes along which the gases flow and the presence of obstruction in them may, however, affect the critical velocity and hence produce turbulent flow. It is important, therefore, that the anaesthetist should use the largest sized tube that will pass easily through the glottic aperture, since in the adult this is the narrowest portion of the respiratory tract between the lips and the carina. In children the cricoid is the limiting factor. Furthermore, the endotracheal connections should be of a wide bore, and curved rather than sharply angled (Fig. 30).

**Valves.**—The number and the types of unidirectional valve used in the different pieces of anaesthetic apparatus vary, but the majority are of the disc type which is lifted by the flow of gases either against its own weight (simple disc type) or against the resistance of a spring (spring-loaded type). The disc should be as light as practicable and should have a lift approaching one quarter of the diameter of the duct. If a disc becomes wet from the moisture of the expired gases a slight increase in respiratory resistance will occur, not only from the greater weight of the disc but from the surface tension of the water between the disc edges and its seating. For paediatric anaesthesia not only is resistance of great importance but also the quantity of air contained in the valve, since this may markedly increase dead space in a small infant (see p. 1098 *et seq.*).

(*a*)

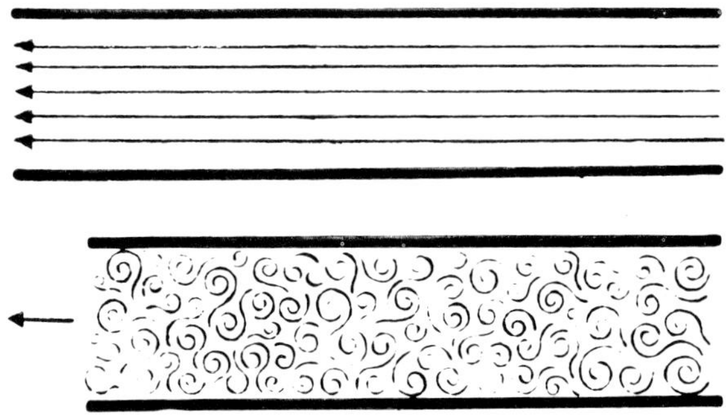

(*b*)

2/Fig. 29.—(*a*) Laminar flow. (*b*) Turbulent flow.

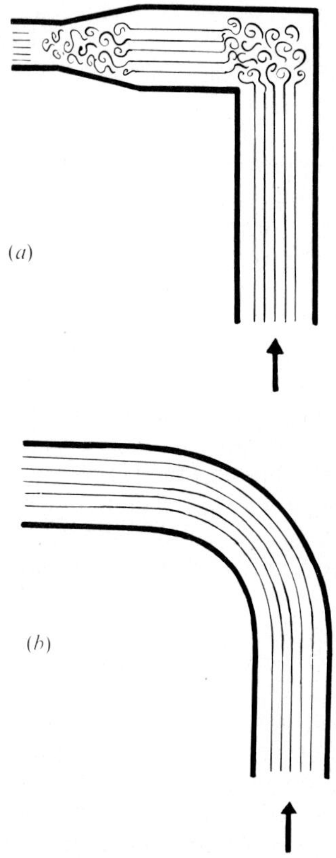


2/Fig. 30.—(*a*) Mixed laminar and turbulent flow. (*b*) Laminar flow in a curved tube. (These figures are adapted from illustrations in *Physics for the Anaesthetist*, courtesy of Sir Robert Macintosh, Professor W. W. Mushin and Dr. H. G. Epstein and published by Blackwell Scientific Publications[66])

**Soda-lime canister.**—The insertion of a soda-lime canister into a respiratory system is, in the mechanical sense, an obstruction. The difference between breathing in and out of a spirometer with or without a soda-lime container can be easily demonstrated. The resistance or obstruction to the flow of gases of a conventional soda-lime canister is very much larger than that of the average valve, except when using very small flow rates. The manner in which the granules are packed into the canister plays an important part, for vigorous compaction will increase the resistance for any given flow rate. It is clearly best, therefore, to select as large a granule as possible which is compatible with adequate absorption. For inhalational anaesthesia a blend of 4–8 mesh granules (see p. 79) has been found to offer optimum absorption efficiency with the minimum of resistance.

### Respiratory Effects of Resistance to Breathing

The diameter of the endotracheal tube, the pattern of the flow of gases along the flexible tubing, the valves, and the soda-lime canister are all capable of increasing resistance to respiration.

In a conscious patient a large rise in respiratory resistance produces a fall in ventilation and in the slope of the $CO_2$ response curve. More modest increases in resistance can be compensated for by an increased respiratory effort so that minute volume and $Paco_2$ remain normal. Nunn and Ezi-Ashi[67] found that anaesthetised patients had a remarkable ability to compensate in this way.

Another finding of interest was the difference in the effect of a 5-kilogram weight placed first on the chest and then on the epigastrium. The anaesthetised patient showed almost no change in ventilation following pressure on the chest, whereas there was a 20 per cent reduction in ventilation if the same weight was placed on the upper abdomen (Table 6).

The reason for this discrepancy is that the diaphragm is the principle muscle of respiration and any pressure in the epigastric region will seriously impede its function.

*The endotracheal tube* is always considered an important source of resistance to respiration. It is known that the resistance presented by a tube is proportional to the flow of gases and the diameter of the tube. Munson and his colleagues[68] have shown in a group of patients that whereas the mean peak flow rate in the conscious state was 21 $l\ min^{-1}$, it rose to 28–43 $l\ min^{-1}$ when anaesthesia was induced. A glance at Fig. 31 shows how the peak flow rate is high during light anaesthesia with most anaesthetic agents but drops down again when moderate or deep levels of anaesthesia are reached. With ether anaesthesia high peak flow rates are maintained at most levels of anaesthesia.

Interpretation of these flows in relation to the various sizes of endotracheal tube available reveals some interesting data. In adults, the difference in pressure gradients across a No. 10 and No. 7 Magill tube with a flow rate of

2/TABLE 6
EFFECT OF EXTERNAL INTERFERENCE WITH RESPIRATION ON VENTILATION

| | *Change in Lung volume* (*ml*) | *Change in tidal volume* (%) | *Change in respiratory rate* (%) | *Change in minute volume* (%) |
|---|---|---|---|---|
| 5 kg on sternum | −70 | −4·1 | +2·8 | −1·7 |
| 5 kg on epigastrium | −45 | −19·2 | +2·0 | −17·8 |

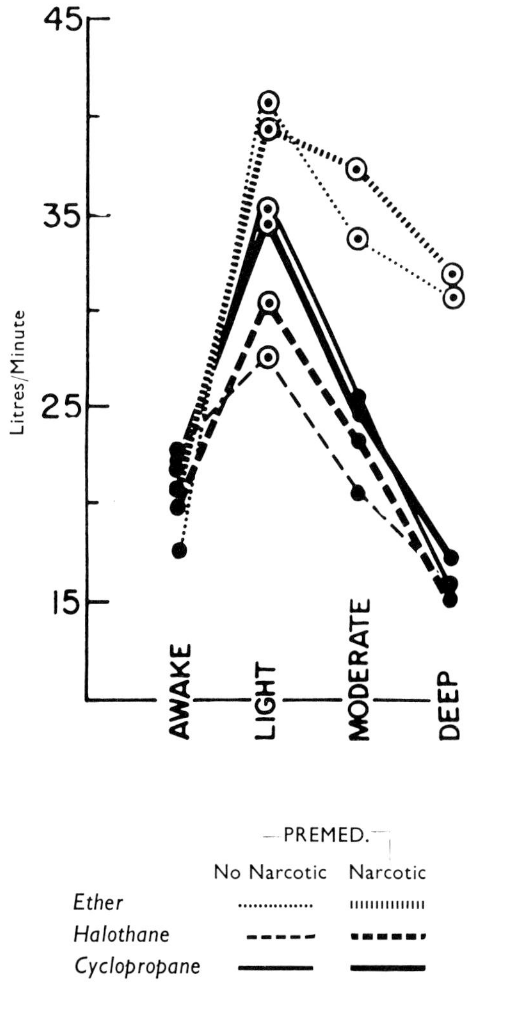


2/FIG. 31.—Peak inspiratory flow rate with various types of inhalational anaesthetic with and without narcotic premedication. (Courtesy of Dr. E. S. Munson and the Editors and publisher, J. B. Lippincott Company, of *Anesthesiology*[68]).

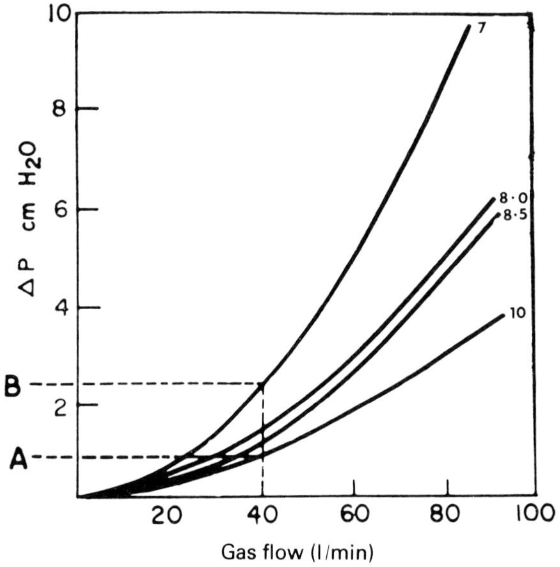


2/FIG. 32.—Resistance through endotracheal tubes. The Magill tube size is quoted. (Courtesy of Dr. E. S. Munson and the Editors and publisher, J. B. Lippincott Company, of *Anesthesiology*[68])

40 l/min is only 1 cm $H_2O$ (0·1 kPa) (Fig. 32). Thus at this flow rate there is a very small increase in resistance over a wide range of adult endotracheal tube sizes. This discrepancy may in part be due to the large bore of the trachea being required for fight or flight rather than the more tranquil event of anaesthesia where only relatively low flow rates are present.

By contrast, in children the size of the endotracheal tube is of much greater importance (Fig. 33).

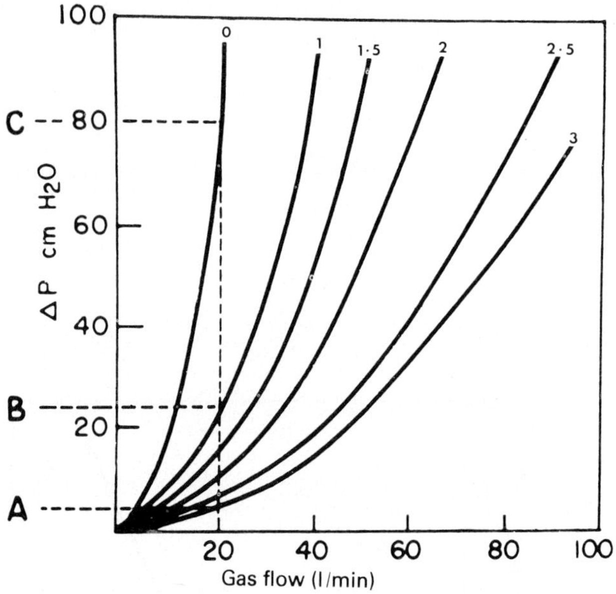


2/Fig. 33.—Resistance through endotracheal tubes. (Courtesy of Dr. E. S. Munson and the Editors and publisher, J. B. Lippincott Company, of *Anesthesiology*[68])

## ANAESTHETIC BREATHING SYSTEMS

A badly designed or improperly used anaesthetic breathing system adversely affects the respiratory function of the patient. At the extremes of age, and in ill patients, such a disturbance may have serious consequences. The principles of good practice must be recognised when selecting and administering anaesthesia with any particular system, and the advantages and disadvantages peculiar to it appreciated. None of the schemes to be described is perfect in itself, but some are of greater value for special types of case or anaesthesia than for routine use whatever the condition. When making a final choice, and after consideration of all the basic facts, the preference and experience of the anaesthetist concerned must be decisive.

The desirable features to be found in a good anaesthetic breathing system are:

1. Efficient elimination of exhaled $CO_2$.
2. The supply of an adequate inspired $O_2$ concentration.
3. Efficient exchange of anaesthetic gases.
4. A low apparatus dead space.
5. A low resistance to gas flow except in certain well-defined circumstances, such as the application of a positive end-expiratory pressure.
6. Safety.
7. Convenience in use.

Circuits can be classified as follows:

(*a*) Open-mask methods.
(*b*) Circuits relying on an adequate fresh gas flow for efficient performance.
(*c*) Circuits relying on soda-lime for the elimination of carbon dioxide, e.g. low flow systems.

### (A) Open-mask Methods

Volatile anaesthetic agents such as diethyl ether can be administered by a drop technique onto an open mask, though not much used today in developed countries. An example of such apparatus is the Schimmelbusch mask, in which a simple metal frame is covered with layers of gauze. The patient, breathes through the gauze so vaporising the volatile agent which is dropped onto the gauze from a dropper bottle. He therefore inhales an air-anaesthetic mixture which is at a low temperature and the respiratory tree is called upon to raise the temperature to 37° C and also to saturate it with water vapour. It has been estimated that there is a heat loss from the patient of about

300 calories per minute using diethyl ether as the anaesthetic agent. Oxygen can be added to the inspired gas mixture by delivering it through a narrow tube inserted under the edge of the mask. Examples of agents which have been administered by this method are diethyl ether, divinyl ether, ethyl chloride and halothane.

### (B) Circuits Requiring High Gas Flows

In this type of system $CO_2$ elimination is obtained by venting into the atmosphere, the volume of exhaled gas thus discarded depending on the amount of the fresh gas flow into the circuit. An expiratory valve or opening in the system allows the exhaled gases to pass into the atmosphere, and the position of the bag, the total flow of fresh gas and its site of entry into the circuit, and the position of the expiratory port, are all important to the efficiency of the circuit. Provided the apparatus dead space is low and that a sufficient fresh gas flow is available to ensure satisfactory $CO_2$ elimination, then an inspired concentration of oxygen equal to that in the fresh gas mixture and efficient exchange of anaesthetic gases are also assured. The total performance of these circuits can therefore be judged by examining the efficiency of $CO_2$ elimination. Various types of systems were classified and analysed by Mapleson,[69] and are depicted in Fig. 34. The fresh gas flows required to ensure $CO_2$ elimination are also shown and these flows are related to the minute volume of the patient, itself related to the $CO_2$ output and therefore the size and age of the patient.

**The Magill circuit (Mapleson "A").**—During anaesthesia with spontaneous ventilation the Magill attachment is still the best for an adult for economy in total gas flow with virtual elimination of rebreathing. The fresh gas flow into the Magill attachment has been investigated by Kain and Nunn.[70] These workers, measuring minute volume and end-tidal $CO_2$ while reducing the fresh gas flow in steps, found that significant rebreathing (as indicated by a rise in minute volume and end-tidal $CO_2$) did not occur until the gas inflow was reduced to between 2 and 4 l $min^{-1}$ or about equal to the patient's alveolar ventilation (Fig. 35). Previously it had been considered that a gas inflow equal to the patient's minute volume was necessary to prevent rebreathing. This state of affairs only holds when the patient is breathing spon-

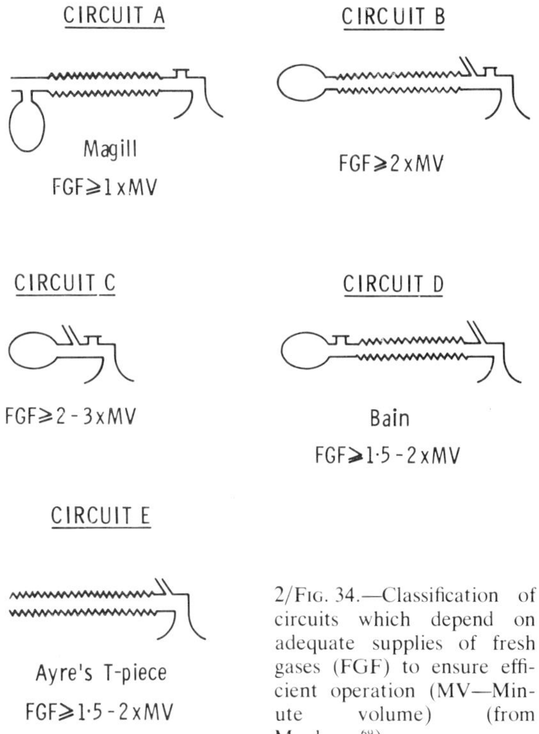


2/Fig. 34.—Classification of circuits which depend on adequate supplies of fresh gases (FGF) to ensure efficient operation (MV—Minute volume) (from Mapleson[69]).

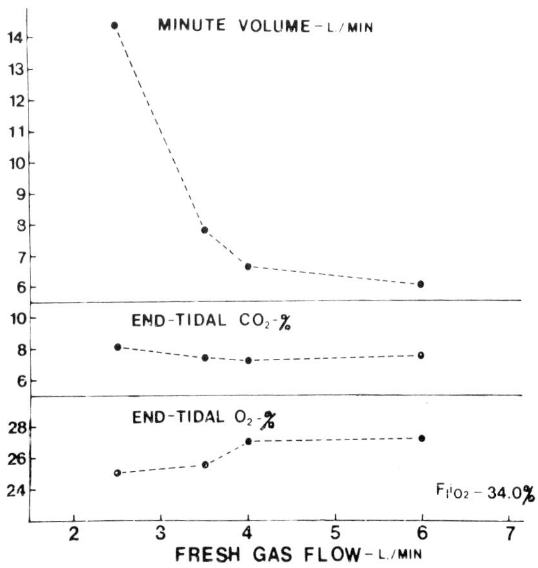


2/Fig. 35.—Diagram showing the changes in minute volume, end-tidal $CO_2$ and end-tidal $O_2$ with step-wise reductions in fresh gas flow into a Magill anaesthetic circuit. (Courtesy of Drs. M. L. Kain and J. F. Nunn and the Honorary Editors of the *Proceedings of the Royal Society of Medicine*[70]).

taneously, but not if such a system is used for intermittent positive-pressure respiration. Then a far greater flow of gases must be used to prevent carbon dioxide accumulation.

### Ayre's T Piece (Mapleson "E")

With a "T" piece the dead-space gases pass down the open end of the tube first, while the alveolar gases, leaving last, may be reinspired. A high flow of gases (one and a half to twice the respiratory minute volume of the patient) is needed to prevent rebreathing with a "T" piece if the capacity of the expiratory limb of the system is to be ignored. Rebreathing can be eliminated with a small expiratory limb provided that the volume of the gases that can be held in it is no greater than the volume of fresh gases that can enter it during an expiratory pause.[69] With a small expiratory limb some mixing with the atmospheric air may occur.

In paediatric anaesthesia an open-ended bag is usually attached to the open end of the expiratory limb converting the system to a Mapleson "D" type of circuit. With spontaneous ventilation the same fresh gas flow is required (1·5–2 times the minute volume) to prevent significant rebreathing depending on the length of the expiratory pause. With a short or absent pause twice the minute volume should be delivered, but if there is a significant pause then 1·5 times the minute volume is probably sufficient. When used to control the ventilation in adult patients the arterial $P_{CO_2}$ can be maintained at low or just below normal levels by a fresh gas flow of 70–100 ml $min^{-1}$ $kg^{-1}$ body weight.

### Coaxial Circuits

**Bain.**—This is a modification of the Mapleson "D" type of circuit in which the fresh gas flow is introduced through a narrow bore tube running inside a larger bore outer tube. For spontaneous ventilation a fresh gas flow of 1·5–2 times the minute volume is necessary to prevent significant rebreathing depending on the length of the expiratory pause. The characteristics of the circuit during controlled ventilation have been described by Henville and Adams.[71]

Using a tidal volume of 10 ml/kg and a respiratory rate of 10–15 breaths per minute the arterial $P_{CO_2}$ can be controlled by the supply of fresh gas. They found that at a fresh gas flow of 70 ml $kg^{-1}$ the mean arterial $P_{CO_2}$ was 40·8 mm Hg, S.D. = 4·3 (5·4±0·6 kPa) and with a flow of 100 ml $kg^{-1}$ the mean arterial $P_{CO_2}$ was 34·3 mm Hg, S.D. = 4·5 (4·6±0·6 kPa). The arterial $P_{CO_2}$ can therefore be fairly accurately controlled during anaesthesia. In patients weighing less than 40 kg the fresh gas flow should *not* be reduced below 3 l $min^{-1}$ or higher $P_{CO_2}$ values than predicted will result. This is a reflection of the higher metabolic rate of children and infants, and thus of a higher $CO_2$ output.

**Lack.**—In the Lack circuit, which has the Mapleson "A" configuration, expiration is via the inner tube and fresh gas flows down the outer tube. The circuit is suitable for spontaneous respiration and requires a lower fresh gas flow than the Magill[82].

**Humphrey (Mapleson A, D and E principle).**—This is a recently described sys-

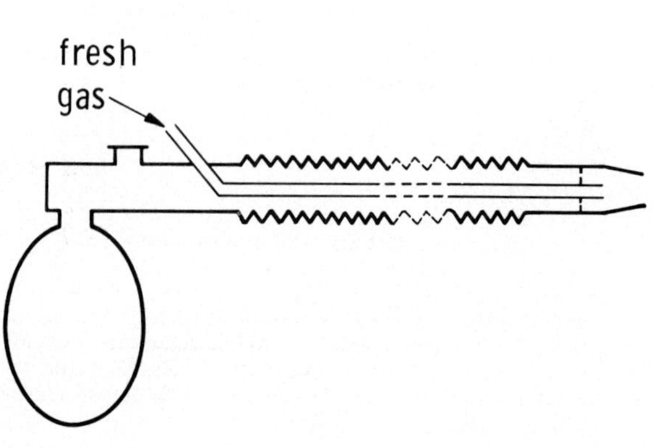


2/Fig. 36.—Bain circuit (Bain and Spoerel[72]).

tem[83] which is available in coaxial and non-coaxial forms. It is claimed that it functions with the efficiency of the Lack for spontaneous respiration and of the Bain for controlled ventilation. The non-coaxial form of the circuit overcomes the hazard of the inner tube kinking, obstructing or becoming disconnected but, of course, it is heavier and less convenient to use.

### Non-rebreathing Valves

The non-rebreathing valve may be considered as a modification of the semi-closed system. Designed primarily to prevent rebreathing by ensuring unidirectional flow of all expired gases, such valves have therefore the additional advantage of enabling the patient to inspire a constant proportion of gases from the anaesthetic machine, since there is no mixing of these with those which are expired. At any one moment the anaesthetist can tell the exact proportion of gases that the patient is inspiring. Non-rebreathing valves are also useful for intermittent positive-pressure ventilation, but unless specially designed, the exhalation part of the valve may need to be held closed when the pressure is applied. A further advantage is that the patient cannot be hyperventilated if the total flow of gases is set to match the required minute volume of the patient.

One valve of this type is the Frumin, which can be used for both spontaneous and controlled respiration.[73] It is so designed that a sudden rise in pressure (as produced by the anaesthetist's hand squeezing the reservoir bag) closes the expiratory leak so that all the gases pass to the patient. On release of the pressure at the end of inspiration the gases can then escape quietly again to the atmosphere. This valve can be used either with a face-mask or in a modified form to provide an "in-line" gas flow for use with an endotracheal tube. The resistance and dead space are minimal. The resistance to gas flow in the valve at either inspiration or expiration is 1·5 mm Hg at 60 l $min^{-1}$ (0·2 kPa $l^{-1}$ sec) flow rates.

Another valve of this type has been designed by Ruben[74] the exhalation part of which automatically closes during controlled or assisted respiration. One of its principal advantages is the small dead space—only 9 ml. Similarly, the resistance is low. It can, however, only be described as "noisy" in practice.

### (c) Circuits Relying on Soda-lime for the Elimination of Carbon Dioxide

Soda-lime consists mainly of calcium hydroxide, with small amounts of sodium hydroxide and potassium hydroxide added as activators. The ingredients are fused into sheets which are allowed to harden before being crushed. The granules so formed are graded according to size using wire mesh screens. A 4-mesh screen means that there are four quarter-inch square openings per inch (approximately four 6·2 mm square openings per 25 mm); an 8-mesh screen signifies eight eighth-inch openings per inch (approximately eight 3·1 mm openings per 25 mm), and so on. In general anaesthesia the granules should be in the 4–8 mesh range, as this size represents the optimum surface area of absorption with the minimum resistance.

Hardness is measured by placing the granules in a standard steel pan together with 15 steel balls of fixed diameter. The whole is then shaken for thirty minutes, after which the granules are placed on a 40-mesh sieve and again shaken for a further three minutes. The amount retained on the screen should be not less than 75 per cent of the original and is described as the hardness number.

2/Table 7
Specifications for Soda-lime

| | |
|---|---|
| *Content:* | Calcium hydroxide 90 per cent |
| | Sodium hydroxide 5 per cent |
| | Potassium hydroxide 1 per cent |
| | Silicate |
| *Moisture content:* | Not less than 14 per cent |
| | Not more than 19 per cent |
| *Granule size:* | 4–8 mesh |
| *Hardness number:* | 75 or more |

**Baralyme.**—This comprises 80 per cent calcium hydroxide and 20 per cent barium hydroxide. This mixture is sufficiently hard not to require the addition of silica. Barium hydroxide (like sodium hydroxide in soda-lime) plays the role of activator so that barium carbonate, calcium carbonate and water are formed. Heat is produced in a similar manner, but as both barium and calcium carbonate are insoluble, no interaction can take place. For this reason baralyme has no powers of regeneration like soda-lime, where any sodium carbonate (soluble) formed can combine with any unneutralised calcium hydroxide available, and so is less efficient than soda-lime.

**Indicators in soda-lime.**—Many dyes will

change colour as hydroxides are neutralised and converted to carbonates.

Ethyl violet is an example of a colourless base indicator which can be impregnated into soda-lime. The base of the indicator reacts with carbonic acid to form a soluble carbonate which is purple in colour. When all the sodium hydroxide is converted to sodium and calcium carbonate, a purple colour develops. Examples of other dyes are given in Table 8.

2/TABLE 8

| *Indicators* | *Soda-lime* | |
|---|---|---|
| | *Fresh* | *Exhausted* |
| Methyl orange | Orange | Yellow |
| Phenolphthalein | Colourless | Pink |
| Ethyl violet | Colourless | Purple |
| Clayton yellow | Pink | Yellow |

Too much reliance should never be placed on any indicator for soda-lime as hypercapnia can always develop before signs of soda-lime exhaustion are evident, especially if there is channelling of gases along the sides of a canister. Nevertheless, the presence of an indicator in soda-lime is a useful guide, particularly if a double canister system is being used, which allows one chamber to be replaced. The final proof of the efficacy of a particular soda-lime canister's contents can only lie in the periodic testing of the gases flowing through it for the possible presence of carbon dioxide.

**Mechanism of absorption.**—When the patient's expired gas is passed through the canister containing the soda-lime granules the carbon dioxide combines with the hydroxides to form carbonates and water. This chemical change requires the presence of some moisture, which is provided by the patient's expiration, and at the same time it produces heat. There is also an overall increase in the weight of the canister contents which amounts to about 33 per cent when they are worn out.

(1) $CO_2 + 2NaOH \rightarrow H_2O + Na_2CO_3 + \text{heat}$.
(2) $Na_2CO_3 + Ca(OH)_2 \rightarrow 2NaOH + CaCO_3$.

A small quantity is also absorbed thus:

$$CO_2 + Ca(OH)_2 \rightarrow H_2O + CaCO_3 + \text{heat}.$$

The heat produced is known as the *heat of neutralisation*. Temperatures up to 60° C have been recorded inside canisters, the production of some heat being a sign that the soda-lime is functioning efficiently. Modern soda-lime does not get as hot but even so it is recommended that trichloroethylene should not be used with $CO_2$ absorbers as hot alkaline conditions favour its decomposition to toxic substances such as phosgene which may cause cranial nerve palsies.

**Regeneration of soda-lime.**—In the old days, regeneration of soda-lime could be demonstrated. It was found that if "exhausted" soda-lime was taken out of the system and rested, after a few hours it was again able to absorb carbon dioxide efficiently. The explanation for this process was complex and probably related to the moisture content of the soda-lime and pores within the granules. With modern soda-lime in large canisters, regeneration does not occur to a significant extent.

**The to and fro'.**—The canister is placed between the breathing bag and mask or endotracheal tube. Fresh gases are introduced near the face-piece so that any alteration in the gas concentration is immediately transmitted to the patient. The presence of a warm canister so close to the patient's respiratory tract ensures that the heat and humidity loss is negligible, but the system has largely fallen into disfavour because of the inadequacy of the carbon dioxide absorption, the awkwardness of the apparatus so close to the patient's head, and the possibility of inhalation of dust particles.

A standard adult to-and-fro' canister is cylindrical and measures 8 by 13 cm. Ideally the air space should equal the patient's tidal volume. When filled with soda-lime the air capacity lies between 375 and 425 ml. As the patient breathes in and out of the canister, so the soda-lime nearest the mouth becomes exhausted. The respirations usually travel along the sides of the canister because in this region the flow of gases apparently encounters least resistance. With this system, as the soda-lime becomes exhausted, so the entrapped air around it becomes dead space because this air can now be rebreathed without first having the carbon dioxide removed. For the first 1½ hours the standard canister appears to be capable of absorbing almost all the carbon dioxide but after that there is a progressive rise up to 0·5 per cent after 5½ hours. It is seldom used nowadays, but may be useful for infected cases (e.g. tuberculosis) when the whole circuit can easily be sterilised afterwards.

**The circle.**—In this system the gases have to pass greater distances along flexible tubing so that the resistance to flow is higher than in a to and fro' apparatus. The presence of unidirectional valves also offers an increase in resistance, though if these are properly constructed with a wide surface area this is reduced to a minimum.

The capacity of the absorber should be at least equal to the patient's tidal volume; if the tidal volume is greater, then some of the expired gases will pass directly through the canister without coming to rest in the interior, thus impeding efficient absorption. The total air space normally available in an absorber lies between 40–60 per cent of the total volume of the unit, but this volume can be varied by changing the size of the granules and also the firmness of the packing. The ideal capacity has not yet been determined, but the greater this is the longer becomes the period of uninterrupted use before renewal is required. These units are often constructed of transparent plastic material so that a change in the colour of the indicator in the soda-lime can be seen. In some cases these large absorbers are made in two interchangeable sections so that one half can be replaced when exhausted.

## Low Flow and Closed Techniques of Anaesthesia

In recent years the use of truly "low flow" anaesthesia has not been widely practised; however, with the advent of new monitoring apparatus, a renewed interest has developed. The advantages must be weighed alongside the dangers. To help to understand the background to the debate, the reader is presented with two expert viewpoints—one from the U.S.A. and the other from the United Kingdom.

1. Dr. Lucien Morris (Toledo, U.S.A.) makes the following comment:

"The merits of the closed circuit absorption system are such that a redirection of our attention is warranted from both a practical and theoretical point of view. For a full appreciation of the merits of the closed absorption system, one needs to view it in some historic perspective. The closed system for absorption of carbon dioxide was introduced to avoid pollution, conserve agents and thereby gain economy and to reduce the effects of accumulations of carbon dioxide. It was early recognised that other benefits accrued in the form of retention of heat and improved humidity. All of these same concerns are among the valid reasons for our renewed interest in the clinical use of the closed circuit absorption system.

Closed absorption techniques became less common during the past twenty-five years as newer halogenated agents were introduced for which the clinical signs of deeper anaesthesia were less clearly defined and for which, coincidentally, the manufacturers provided specific direct reading vaporisers which purported to deliver appropriate inspired concentrations only when used with high flows. There were other factors which also mitigated against use of closed absorption techniques.

A. It is difficult for the neophyte to learn to maintain a truly closed leak-proof system of equipment.
B. It is difficult to stay within the narrow ranges of appropriate levels of inspired concentration for gases and vapours, including oxygen, when balancing the additions against the uptake of gas and vapour mass and the basal metabolic utilisation of oxygen while still maintaining appropriate partial pressures, particularly of oxygen.
C. It was thought easier to provide a known percentage of inspired vapour from a high flow of gases through a direct reading vaporiser than to counteract the general lack of understanding of the mysteries of uptake of agents.
D. Even the Copper Kettle, which was originally designed for incremental additions of vapour mass (of chloroform) to closed systems, has been more often taught for use with high flow systems. The reasons for this might be categorised as for comfort and convenience of the teachers.

The conflict of interest between profit motive and the avoidance of pollution seems to have been overlooked. The apparent success of commercial interests in modifying techniques of anaesthesia management which has resulted in greater sales of agents and possibly created a market for anti-pollution equipment seems to have been also overlooked by anaesthesiologists. We uncritically adopted wasteful habit patterns which have benefited commercial interests and in the process have lost not only the flexibility afforded by fine incremental changes in gases and vapours, but have also lost the opportunity to gain useful applicable information about the uptake requirements and metabolic alterations of individual patients.

Meantime, many of the small dissatisfactions identified by an older generation to be associated with the use of the closed absorption system have now been obviated. Indeed, new types of equipment are available which make a revival of interest in the closed system carbon dioxide technique completely logical.

A. The small size absorbers of the circle system have been replaced by larger ones which, with appropriate baffle design, are much more efficacious in the removal of carbon dioxide.
B. The valves of the circle system have been improved so that there is less resistance and more consistent closure.
C. Our concepts about the exponential reduction in uptake with elapsed time have improved to allow a more quantitative approach. The copper-kettle circuit by which a measured flow of carrier gas will pick up a known amount of vapour is a way of adding precise increments of vapour mass in accord with the need of demonstrated agent uptake.
D. The Revell circulator used with a divided chimney to provide a double entry to the mask effectively air-conditions the under-mask space and removes external dead space as well as resistance. In addition it mixes the respired gases and increases and stabilises a maximum appropriate inspiratory humidity.
E. There are monitors now available to measure the concentration of inspired gases. These include oxygen, carbon dioxide and anaesthetics.

One other important requisite for closed system anaesthesia is the fine flow measurement of all respired agents for discrete additions to the mixture. Unfortunately, many existing anaesthetic machines do not meet this requirement.

When one lists the advantages of using a closed circuit carbon dioxide absorption system with a Revell circulating flow it seems quite evident that the merits are such as to be worth the inconvenience of relearning all the nuances of the technique. In addition to the minimisation of pollution and the reduction of wastage a major advantage is the elimination of rebreathing in the dead space which is evident with all other anaesthetic systems and which has modified anaesthetic management away from spontaneous respiration in the past. With adequate removal of excess carbon dioxide the patients exhibit better relaxation and there is less apparent need for increasing anaesthetic depth. With the elimination of rebreathing there is also less chance for hypoxia or hypercarbia. The close attention required during use of the closed absorption system lends itself to a better titration of the anaesthetic depths in response to the clinical signs accompanying patient changes.

The current resurgence of interest in closed system techniques for carbon dioxide absorption is fully appropriate for all who consider themselves true specialists in anaesthesia. An opportunity is provided to demonstrate their art and understanding by regular use of the closed absorption technique."

Dr. Peter Horsey (Southampton, United Kingdom) writes as follows:

"Methods which make use of fresh gas flows of one to one-and-a-half litres per minute are called "low flow". They involve some quite different considerations from systems which are entirely closed and the term "closed" should be restricted to describe a circuit from which there is no intentional escape of gas. Both techniques introduce several concepts which can be ignored by proponents of conventional high flow methods and they provide fascination for those who master them. They demonstrate several aspects of respiratory and cardiovascular function which cannot be appreciated if high flows are used and they demand a degree of attention which does not encourage distraction or induce boredom. They are invaluable for teaching the physics and physiology of gas uptake and nitrogen elimination and of the use and behaviour of vaporisers outside (VOC) and inside (VIC) the breathing system. Their use demands meticulous attention to the elimination of leaks and there is no place for poorly maintained equipment if they are to be used effectively.

It is now possible to monitor accurately the oxygen concentration and the concentration of halothane or enflurane without abstracting any gas from the breathing system so that most of the earlier objections to the use of these techniques no longer apply. The methods are best learnt in the operating theatre by watching an experienced anaesthetist demonstrating them and using both oxygen and halogenated vapour analysers, although the descriptions which follow have been developed in order to make both techniques safe without the use of such devices.

Both methods necessitate the use of soda-lime for carbon dioxide absorption. This makes it possible to connect the patient to a breathing system which, as it were, acts as a buffer between the fresh gas inflow and the pulmonary circulation. Although the to-and-fro system can be used, the account which follows is based on the use of a circle absorber system with a large (1 kg) canister and a volume of about 4 litres, to which must be added the gas in the patient's lungs, amounting in all to some 6 or 7 litres. If a fresh gas inflow of one litre per minute is used, gases will leave the system at approximately equal rates into the pulmonary circulation and via the scavenging valve. When the system is closed, the only escape is into the patient. Although there are important differences between low flow and closed techniques, some characteristics are common to both and these will be dealt with first.

### Induction and Nitrogen Elimination

Whichever method is to be used, it is essential to replace the nitrogen in the lungs with the anaesthetic gases. For this reason, conventional high flows are used for the first three to five minutes, during which the total respiratory exchange should be 15 to 20 litres. This will reduce the nitrogen concentration in the lungs and breathing system to less than 5 per cent.* The fresh gas flow can then be reduced and only the nitrogen dissolved in the tissues can then diffuse into the alveolar gases. The volume of dissolved nitrogen is about 14 ml $kg^{-1}$ or one litre in an average adult and it takes about five hours for the entire nitrogen content of the body to be abstracted. With a low flow system there is sufficient escape of gas to prevent accumulation of nitrogen in the circuit, but if the system is closed, nitrogen will accumulate and may constitute as much as 15 per cent of the circuit gases after an hour.[75] This is of no consequence provided nitrous oxide is not given once the system is closed. With both methods it is essential to prevent the ingress of air as well as leaks of circuit gases. It is quite possible to achieve this without tracheal intubation. If air is inspired once flows have been reduced (for example when inserting an airway) it must be displaced by increasing the fresh gas flow and, if the circuit had been closed, opening the scavenging valve temporarily.

* Throughout this section, it is assumed average values for cardiac output and minute volume of ventilation obtain whenever gas uptake and output are mentioned.

### Flowmeters

Modern flowmeters are sufficiently accurate if either of the two techniques described below is followed. Before a machine is used, the preparatory check should ensure that the flowmeter bobbins are rotating and moving freely in the 0–1000 ml $min^{-1}$ range. The oxygen flowmeter should be set to deliver at least 2 l $min^{-1}$ and watched while the machine gas outlet is transiently occluded. Depression of the bobbin indicates that the rotameter tube and seatings are gas tight.

### Monitoring the Inspired Oxygen Concentration

If nitrous oxide is being used it is advisable to monitor the inspired oxygen concentration whenever fresh gas flow is reduced below 1·5 l $min^{-1}$. Apart from increasing the safety of any method, when low flows are used the oxygen meter will give a continuous indication of the rate of uptake of nitrous oxide. Earlier designs of oxygen monitor proved to be inaccurate when used in the presence of nitrous oxide.[76] Figure 37 shows a Ventronics Polarographic Oxygen Monitor with a digital display of oxygen concentration and a high and low setting oxygen alarm indicated by a flashing light and an audible signal. It is unaffected by nitrous oxide and has a means of indicating when the batteries need to be replaced. The sensor probe lasts about six months in normal use and is disposable. In the first few minutes of anaesthesia, nitrous oxide uptake is of the order of 500 ml $min^{-1}$, falling to about 200 ml $min^{-1}$ after half-an-hour and 100 ml $min^{-1}$ after about an hour, after which it tends to remain constant at 50–100 ml/hr due to inevitable losses through the skin and wound. Saturation of the tissues takes about five hours.[77] (Fig. 38).

At the end of a three-hour operation during

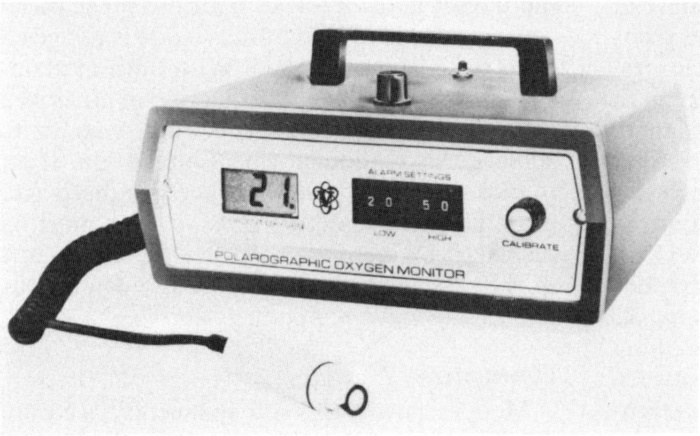


2/FIG. 37.—Polarographic oxygen monitor.

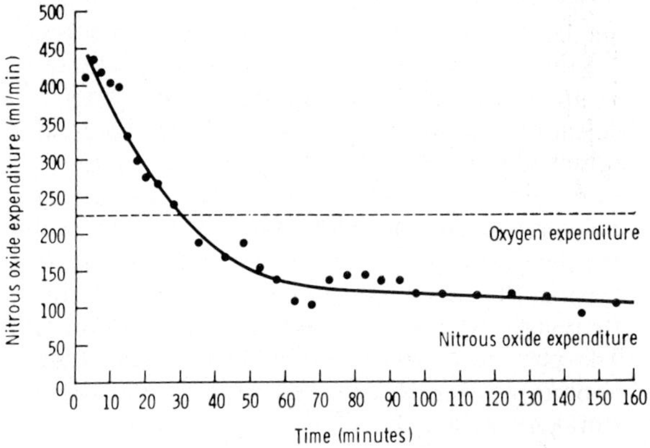


2/FIG. 38.—Expenditure of nitrous oxide in blocks of 2·5 to 25 min, 5 to 100 min and 10 min thereafter. Oxygen consumption did not change significantly with time and the mean value for all times is indicated by the broken line. All flows are given at ambient temperature and pressure (dry). (Courtesy of Dr. F. Barton and Dr. J. F. Nunn, 1975 and Macmillan Journals Ltd.[77])

which an inspired concentration of 70 per cent nitrous oxide has been maintained, the average adult will have 20 to 26 litres of the gas dissolved in his tissues. The fall in uptake of nitrous oxide from a circle system will be indicated by a gradual decrease in the inspired oxygen concentration which necessitates readjustment of the oxygen:nitrous oxide ratio.

For example, a setting of 500 ml $min^{-1}$ of oxygen and 1000 ml $min^{-1}$ of nitrous oxide will usually result in an $FIO_2$ of 0·3 in the early stages of an anaesthetic and after twenty minutes it may be necessary to reduce the flow of nitrous oxide to 800 ml $min^{-1}$ to achieve the same result.

Nitrous oxide should never be used in a closed system unless an oxygen analyser is in the circuit. If oxygen is used with isoflurane, enflurane or halothane without nitrous oxide, the system can be closed after the first few breaths and the oxygen inflow is set at 500 ml $min^{-1}$. There is then no necessity for a meter as the inspired oxygen concentration will be well above 30 per cent; most of the remaining alveolar gas will be nitrogen.

### Volatile Anaesthetics and Vaporisers

One of the main objections to both these techniques is that the anaesthetist does not know the inspired concentration of whatever volatile agent is in use. This is no longer so, now that accurate on-line crystal quartz meters are available. The Engström instrument can measure any halogenated vapour concentration with a rapid response time and it removes no gas from the circuit. With experience it becomes possible to assess the inspired concentration accurately whether the vaporiser is inside or outside the circuit and the use of a meter is not essential to safety.

**Vaporiser Outside the Circuit (VOC)**

The Mark 3 Fluotec and the Enfluratec are calibrated to deliver accurate concentrations from fresh gas flows of 250 ml $min^{-1}$ upwards. When high flows are used, the anaesthetist's only concern is with concentration of the vapour; as soon as the volume of fresh gas entering the circle falls below the patient's minute volume, the inspired concentration (due to dilution) will always be less than the concentration delivered from a vaporiser outside the path of the respired gases. This is because gases which have already been inhaled, and have therefore had halogenated anaesthetics abstracted from them, will form an increasing proportion of the inspired mixture as the fresh gas flow is reduced. For example, if the minute volume is five litres and the fresh gas flow one l $min^{-1}$, most of the inspired gases will have already had the volatile anaesthetic partially removed from them by the pulmonary circulation. It has been found that it is necessary to deliver approximately 15 ml of halothane vapour/minute to achieve an end-tidal concentration of one per cent halothane.[78] It will, therefore, be necessary to set the vaporiser at 1·5 per cent to deliver 15 ml of halothane vapour per minute and so achieve a one per cent end-tidal concentration. The uptake falls progressively with time and if a quartz crystal meter is used the vaporiser concentration can be adjusted to keep the inspired concentration constant.

A vaporiser designed to be used in the VOC mode can be used if the circuit is closed, but if the fresh gas flow is less than 500 ml $min^{-1}$ it may not be capable of delivering sufficient vapour. For example, if the fresh gas flow is 300 ml $min^{-1}$ of oxygen, it will be necessary to set the vaporiser to 5 per cent in order to deliver 15 ml $min^{-1}$ into the circuit and so maintain a one per cent end-tidal concentration. A copper kettle vaporiser is more appropriate for this purpose than any of the designs currently available in the U.K.

**Vaporiser in the Circuit (VIC)**

A simple method of ensuring that a sufficient mass of vapour is inspired in closed systems is to put the vaporiser in the path of the circulating gases. Any vaporiser can be used provided it offers minimal resistance to respiration and has a small vaporising chamber. It can be placed in either limb of the circle and although experience should be gained in its use with a meter for halogenated vapours, the closed circuit without a meter is a safe technique provided that nitrous oxide is not used.

**Low Flow Technique**

This method is suitable for spontaneous or mechanical ventilation. The ventilator may have its own circle absorber system, or a machine such as the Manley Servovent can be used with the circle system of the anaesthetic machine. Ventilators powered by the flow of fresh gases (minute volume dividers) cannot be used.

Anaesthesia is started in the usual way, using high fresh gas flows for at least three minutes, after which the flow is gradually reduced, keeping the $FIO_2$ at 0·33 throughout, until flows of 500 ml $min^{-1}$ of oxygen and 1000 ml $min^{-1}$ of nitrous oxide are set. If the operation lasts more than 20 minutes, the flow of nitrous oxide should be reduced to 800 ml $min^{-1}$.

As described above, it is for practical purposes always necessary to set the vaporiser concentration above the desired inspired concentration whenever a VOC method is used (except when reducing the depth of anaesthesia). A useful rough guide was provided by Mushin and Galloon[79] that with fresh gas flows of one litre per minute, the inspired concentration would be three-fifths of the vaporiser setting; thus a setting of 1·5 per cent would result in an inspired concentration of 0·9 per cent. As saturation of the tissues is approached, which takes many hours, this discrepancy will diminish. It will vary with minute volume, cardiac output and body mass and composition, but in practice these variables have surprisingly little effect.

If an oxygen meter is not being used, the method should be restricted to spontaneously breathing subjects and a volatile agent must be used to supplement anaesthesia. In this case a safe way to ensure that $FIO_2$ remains above 0·3 is to use a total flow of one litre per minute made up of equal volumes of oxygen and nitrous oxide.

**Closed Circuit Technique**

The development of accurate oxygen meters with high and low alarms and digital display of $FIO_2$ has brought closed circuit nitrous oxide/oxygen methods into the realms of clinical anaesthesia. If such a meter is not available, the only safe way is to maintain spontaneous respiration and not use nitrous oxide once the system is closed; isoflurane, enflurane or halothane must be used and the simplest way to do this is to use a vaporiser in the expiratory limb of the circuit.

This is the most popular method in the U.K. In America a method making use of a syringe to introduce small volumes of the anaesthetic into the expiratory limb at increasing intervals of time is more widely used.

The Goldman vaporiser, although not designed for the method, has been extensively used in the U.K. If halothane is vaporised, it is possible to achieve undesirable concentrations at the higher settings in certain circumstances—for example if the vaporiser is shaken. Enflurane is a much safer agent, being slightly less volatile and half as potent at any concentration. The interdiction prohibiting controlled ventilation when halothane is used in an in-circuit vaporiser need not be observed with enflurane once experience has been gained with a meter. Isoflurane has been extensively used in the closed circuit in America and proved very satisfactory, but it has yet to be used in the U.K.

Closed circuit enflurane or isoflurane is a safe technique for surgery which does not require profound muscular relaxation.

### Method

This will be described for enflurane, although with some modification it can be applied to any existing halogenated anaesthetic. Nitrous oxide and oxygen are used with conventional high flows for the first few minutes during which the vaporiser is turned fully "on". Once an airway has been inserted, the flows are reduced, as described above for the low-flow technique. Within five minutes it is possible to turn off the nitrous oxide, set the oxygen flowmeter to 500 ml $min^{-1}$ and close the system. The vaporiser is left fully "on" for 2–3 minutes during which time it will deliver approximately 2 to 2·5 MAC: it can then be set at the second notch which will result in a gradual fall of inspired enflurane towards 1 MAC. Meanwhile the $FIO_2$ will slowly increase from 0·3 to 0·5 during the next 20 minutes as nitrous oxide is absorbed from the system. It is usually possible to maintain anaesthesia for any operation not requiring abdominal muscle relaxation by varying the setting between the first and second notches. Even with the setting fully "on" it is unusual for the inspired concentration to exceed 4·5 per cent. If halothane is used, the second notch should be considered the maximum desirable setting once the system has been closed.

This technique takes advantage of the self-regulating characteristics of the in-circuit vaporiser. If anaesthesia is too light, the resulting increase in minute volume vaporises more of the agent, deepening the level of anaesthesia and so reducing the minute volume. Deepening anaesthesia has the reverse effect. This negative feedback system works extremely well in practice[80].

When it is desired to lighten the level of anaesthesia at the end of surgery, it is impossible to do this by simply switching off the vaporiser. It is also necessary to increase the fresh gas flow above 5 l $min^{-1}$ and open the scavenging valve to provide a gradient from pulmonary blood to the alveoli.

An excellent guide to the concepts one must master to use these methods has been produced by the Department of Anesthesiology of Yale University, by Stone and Greene.[81]"

## REFERENCES


1. Karczewski, W. A. (1974). *International Review of Science: Respiratory Physiology*, pp. 197–219. London: Butterworth & Co.
2. Sullivan, C. E., Kozar, L. F., Murphy, E., and Phillipson, E. A. (1978). Primary role of respiratory afferents in sustaining breathing rhythm. *J. Appl. Physiol.* **45**, 11.
3. Phillipson, E. A., Duffin, J. and Cooper, J. D. (1981). Critical dependence of respiratory rhythmicity on metabolic $CO_2$ load. *J. Appl. Physiol. Respirat. Environ. Exercise Physiology*. **50**, 45.
4. Fink, B. R. (1961). Influence of cerebral activity in wakefulness on regulation of breathing. *J. appl. Physiol.*, **16**, 15.
5. Read, D. J. (1967). A clinical method for assessing the ventilatory response to carbon dioxide. *Aust. Ann. Med.*, **16**, 20.
6. Bellville, J. W., and Seed, J. C. (1960). The effect of drugs on the respiratory response to carbon dioxide. *Anesthesiology*, **21**, 727.
7. Lloyd, B. B., Jukes, M. G. M., and Cunningham, D. J.

C. (1958). The relation between alveolar oxygen pressure and the respiratory response to carbon dioxide in man. *Quart. J. exp. Physiol.*, **43**, 214.
8. Fencl, V., Vale, J. R., and Broch, J. A. (1969). Respiration and cerebral blood flow in metabolic acidosis and alkalosis in humans, *J. appl. Physiol.*, **27**, 67.
9. Cunningham, D. J. C., Shaw, D. G., Lahiri, S. and Lloyd, B. B. (1961). The effect of maintained ammonium chloride acidosis on the relation between pulmonary ventilation and alveolar oxygen and carbon dioxide in man. *Quart. J. exp. Physiol.*, **46**, 323.
10. Lane, D. J. (1970). D. M. Thesis, University of Oxford.
11. Clark, T. J. H. and Godfrey, S. (1969). The effect of $CO_2$ on ventilation and breath-holding during exercise and while breathing through an added resistance. *J. Physiol.*, **201**, 55.
12. Munson, E. S., Larson, C. P., Jr., Babad, A. A., Regan, M. J., Buechel, D. R. and Eger, E. I., II (1966). The effects of halothane, fluroxene and cyclopropane on ventilation: a comparative study in man. *Anesthesiology*, **27**, 716.
13. Dunbar, B. S., Ovassapian, A., and Smith, T. C. (1967). The effects of methoxyflurane on ventilation in man. *Anesthesiology*, **28**, 1020.
14. Larson, C. P., Jr., Eger, E. I., II, Muallem, M., Buechel, D. R., Munson, E. S., and Eisele, J. H. (1969). Effects of diethylether and methoxyflurane on ventilation, II. A comparative study in man. *Anesthesiology*, **30**, 174.
15. Leusen, I. R. (1954). Chemosensitivity of the respiratory centre. Influence of $CO_2$ in the cerebral ventricles on respiration. *Amer. J. Physiol.*, **176**, 39.
16. Leusen, I. R. (1954). Chemosensitivity of the respiratory centre. Influence of changes on the $H^+$ and total buffer concentrations in the cerebral ventricles on respiration. *Amer. J. Physiol.*, **176**, 45.
17. Mitchell, R. A., Loeschcke, H. H., Massion, W. H., and Severinghaus, J. W. (1963). Respiratory responses mediated through superficial chemosensitive areas on the medulla. *J. appl. Physiol.*, **18**, 523.
18. Pappenheimer, J. R., Fencl, V., Heisey, S. R., and Held, D. (1965). Role of cerebral fluids in control of respiration as studied in unanesthetized goats. *Amer. J. Physiol.*, **208**, 436.
19. Bradley, R. D., and Semple, S. J. G. (1962). A comparison of certain acid-base characteristics of arterial blood, jugular venous blood and cerebrospinal fluid in man, and the effect on them of some acute and chronic acid-base disturbances. *J. Physiol. (Lond.)*, **169**, 381.
20. McDowall, D. G., and Harper, A. M. (1970). Cerebral blood flow and CSF pH during hyperventilation. In *Progress in Anaesthesiology. Proceedings of the Fourth World Congress of Anaesthesiologists*, p. 542. Amsterdam: Exerpta Medica Foundation.
21. Band, D. M., Cameron, I. R., and Semple, S. J. G. (1969). Oscillations in arterial pH with breathing in the cat. *J. Appl. Physiol*, **26**, 263.
22. Band, D. M., McLelland, M., Phillips, D. L., Saunders, K. B., and Wolff, C. B. (1978). Sensitivity of the carotid body to within-breath changes in arterial $PCO_2$. *J. Appl. Physiol. Respirat. Environ. Exercise Physiol.*, **45**, 768.
23. Band, D. M., Cameron, I. R., and Semple, S. J. G. (1970). The effects on respiration of abrupt changes in carotid artery pH and $PCO_2$ in the cat. *J. Physiol (Lond).*, **211**, 479.
24. Yamamoto, W. S. and Edwards, M. W. (1960). Homeostasis of carbon dioxide during intravenous infusion of carbon dioxide. *J. Appl. Physiol.*, **15**, 807.
25. Band, D. M., Cochrane, G. M., and Wolff, C. B. (1980). Respiratory oscillations in arterial carbon dioxide tension as a control signal in exercise. *Nature*, **283**, 84.
26. Dejours, P. (1964). Respiration in muscular exercise, In: *Handbook of Physiology—Respiration*, Chap. 25. Washington: American Physiological Society.
27. Lambertsen, C. J. (1980). Chemical control of respiration at rest. In: *Medical Physiology*, 14th edit. Mountcastle, V. B., ed. St. Louis: C.V. Mosby Co. (modified from Loeschcke, H. H., and Gertz, K. H. (1958) *Arch. Gesamte Physiol.* **267**, 460.)
28. Knill, R. L. and Gelb, A. W. (1978). Ventilatory responses to hypoxia and hypercapnia during halothane sedation and anaesthesia in man. *Anesthesiology*, **49**, 244.
29. Cochrane, G. M., Prior, J. G., and Wolff, C. B. (1980). Chronic stable asthma and the normal arterial pressure of carbon dioxide in hypoxia. *Brit. med. J.*, **281**, 706.
30. Widdicombe, J. G. (1961). Respiratory reflexes in man and other mammalian species. *Clin. Sci.*, **21**, 163.
31. Guz, A., Noble, M. I. M., Trenchard, D., Cochrane, H. L., and Makey, A. R. (1964). Studies on the vagus nerves in man: their role in respiratory and circulatory control. *Clin. Sci.*, **27**, 293.
32. Wade, O. L. (1954). Movements of the thoracic cage and diaphragm in respiration. *J. Physiol. (Lond.)*, **124**, 193.
33. Editorial (1981). Normal and abnormal function of the diaphragm. *Thorax*, **36**, 161.
34. Sharp, J. T. (1980). Respiratory muscles: a review of old and newer concepts. *Lung*, **157**, 185. (No. 4).
35. Campbell, E. J. M. (1955). An electromyographic examination of the role of the intercostal muscles in breathing in man. *J. Physiol. (Lond.)*, **129**, 12.
36. Green, J. H., and Howell, J. B. C. (1955). Correlation of respiratory airflow with intercostal muscle activity. *J. Physiol. (Lond.)*, **130**, 33P.
37. Campbell, E. J. M. (1958). *The Respiratory Muscles and the Mechanics of Breathing*. London: Lloyd-Luke (Medical Books).
38. Campbell, E. J. M., and Green, J. H. (1953). The variations in intra-abdominal pressure and the acitivity of the abdominal muscles during breathing: a study in man. *J. Physiol. (Lond.)*, **122**, 282.
39. Campbell, E. J. M. (1955). The functions of the abdominal muscles in relation to the intra-abdominal pressure and the respiration. *Arch. Middlx. Hosp.*, **5**, 87.
40. Fink B. R. (1961). Electromyography in general anaesthesia. *Brit. J. Anaesth.*, **33**, 555.
41. Pappenheimer, J. (1950). Standardisation of definitions and symbols in respiratory physiology. *Fed. Proc.*, **9**, 602.
42. Needham, C. D., Rogan, M. C., and McDonald, I. (1954). Normal standards for lung volumes, intrapulmonary gas mixing, and maximum breathing capacity. *Thorax*, **9**, 313.
43. Nunn, J. F., and Ezi-Ashi, T. I. (1962). The accuracy of the respirometer and ventigrator. *Brit. J. Anaesth.*, **34**, 422.
44. Campbell, E. J. M., and Howell, J. B. L. (1963). Sensation of breathlessness. *Brit. med. Bull.*, **19**, 36.
45. Noble, M. I. M., Eisele, J. H., Frankel, H. L., Else, W., and Guz, A. (1971). The role of the diaphragm in the sensation of holding the breath. *Clin. Sci.*, **41**, 275.
46. Nunn, J. F., Campbell, E. J. M., and Peckett, B. W.

(1959). Anatomical subdivisions of the volume of respiratory dead space and effect of position of the jaw. *J. appl. Physiol.*, **14**, 174.
47. Freeman, J., and Nunn, J. P. (1963). Ventilation-perfusion relationships after haemorrhage. *Clin. Sci.*, **24**, 135.
48. Askrog, V. F., Pender, J. W., and Eckenhoff, J. E. (1964). Changes in physiological deadspace during deliberate hypotension. *Anesthesiology*, **25**, 744.
49. Kain, M. L., Panday, J., and Nunn, J. F. (1969). The effect of intubation on the deadspace during halothane anaesthesia. *Brit. J. Anaesth.*, **41**, 94.
50. Cooper, E. A. (1967). Physiological deadspace in passive ventilation. *Anaesthesia*, **22**, 199.
51. Simpson, B. R., Parkhouse, J., Marshall, R., and Lambrechts, W. (1961). Extradural analgesia and the prevention of post-operative respiratory complications. *Brit. J. Anaesth.*, **33**, 628.
52. Case, E. H., and Stiles, J. A. (1946). The effect of various surgical positions on vital capacity. *Anesthesiology*, **7**, 29.
53. Alexander, J. I., Spence, A. A., Parikh, R. K., and Stuart, B. (1973). The role of airway closure in postoperative hypoxaemia. *Brit. J. Anaesth.*, **45**, 34.
54. Fibuch, E. E., Rehder, K., and Sessler, A. D. (1975). Preoperative CC/FRC ratio and postoperative hypoxemia. *Anesthesiology*, **43**, 481.
55. Norris, R. M., Jones, J. G., and Bishop, J. M. (1968). Respiratory gas exchange in patients with spontaneous pneumothorax. *Thorax*, **23**, 427.
56. Vance, J. P. (1968). Tension pneumothorax in labour. *Anaesthesia*, **23**, 94.
57. Rastogi, P. N., and Wright, J. E. (1969). Bilateral tension pneumothorax under anaesthesia. *Anaesthesia*, **24**, 249.
58. Tusiewicz, K., Bryan, A. C., and Froese (1977). Contributions of changing rib cage—diaphragm interactions to the ventilatory depression of halothane anaesthesia. *Anesthesiology*, **47**, 327.
59. Jones, J. G., Faithfull, D., Jordan, C., and Minty, B. (1979). Rib cage movement during halothane anaesthesia in man. *Brit. J. Anaesth.*, **51**, 399.
60. Harris, T. A. B. (1951). *The Mode of Action of Anaesthetics* Edinburgh: E. & S. Livingstone.
61. Fletcher, G., and Barber, J. L. (1966). Lung mechanics and physiologic shunt during spontaneous breathing in normal subjects. *Anesthesiology*, **27**, 638.
62. Samuels, L. (1952). Hiccup. A ten year review of anatomy, etiology and treatment. *Canad. med. Ass. J.*, **67**, 315.
63. Salem, M. R. (1967). An effective method for the treatment of hiccups during anesthesia. *Anesthesiology*, **28**, 463.
64. Comroe, J. H., Forster, R. E., Dubois, A. B., Briscoe, W. A., and Carlsen, E. (1962). *The Lung. Clinical Physiology and Pulmonary Function Tests*, 2nd edit. Chicago: Year Book Medical Publishers.
65. Nunn, J. F. (1977). *Applied Respiratory Physiology*. London: Butterworth & Co.
66. Macintosh, R. R., and Mushin, W. W. (1946). *Physics for the Anaesthetist.* Oxford: Blackwell Scientific Publications.
67. Nunn, J. F., and Ezi-Ashi, T. I. (1961). The respiratory effects of resistance to breathing in anesthetized man. *Anesthesiology*, **22**, 174.
68. Munson, E. S., Farnham, M., and Hamilton, W. H. (1963). Studies of respiratory gas flows: a comparison using different anesthetic agents. *Anesthesiology*, **24**, 61.
69. Mapleson, W. W. (1954). The elimination of rebreathing in various semi-closed anaesthetic systems. *Brit. J. Anaesth.*, **26**, 323.
70. Kain, M. L., and Nunn, J. F. (1967). Fresh gas flow and rebreathing in the Magill Circuit with spontaneous respiration. *Proc. roy. Soc. Med.*, **60**, 749.
71. Henville, J. D., and Adams, A. P. (1976). The Bain Anaesthetic System. An assessment during controlled ventilation. *Anaesthesia*, **31**, 247.
72. Bain, J. A., and Spoerel, W. E. (1972). A streamlined anesthetic system. *Canad. Anaesth. Soc. J.*, **20**, 426.
73. Frumin, M. J., Lee, A. S., and Papper, E. M. (1959). New valve for non-rebreathing systems. *Anesthesiology*, **20**, 383.
74. Ruben, H. (1955). A new non-rebreathing valve. *Anesthesiology*, **16**, 643.
75. Barton, F. and Nunn, J. F. (1975). Use of refractometry to determine nitrogen accumulation in closed circuits. *Brit. J. Anaesth.*, **47**, 346.
76. Orchard, C. H. and Sykes, M. K. (1980). Errors in oxygen concentration analysis: sensitivity of the IMI analyser to nitrous oxide. *Anaesthesia*, **35**, 1100.
77. Barton, F. and Nunn, J. F. (1975). Totally closed circuit nitrous oxide/oxygen anaesthesia. *Brit. J. Anaesth.*, **47**, 350.
78. Lin, C-Y., Mostert, J. W. and Benson, D. W. (1979). In: *Low Flow and Closed System Anaesthesia*. Ed. J. A. Aldrete, H. J. Lowe and R. W. Virtue. New York: Grune and Stratton.
79. Mushin, W. W. and Galloon, S. (1960). The concentration of anaesthetics in closed circuits with special reference to halothane. *Brit. J. Anaesth.*, **32**, 324.
80. Nunn, J. F. (1979). Control of vapor concentrations. In: *Low Flow and Closed System Anaesthesia*. Ed. J. A. Aldrete, H. J. Lowe and R. W. Virtue. New York: Grune and Stratton.
81. Stone, S. B. and Greene, N. M. (1981). Low-flow anaesthesia. *Curr. Rev. in Clin. Anesth.*, **1**, 114.
82. Humphrey, D. (1982). The Lack, Magill and Bain anaesthetic breathing system: a direct comparison in spontaneously breathing anaesthetised adults. *J. roy. Soc. Med.*, **75**, 513.
83. Humphrey D. (1983). A new anaesthetic breathing system combining Mapleson A, D and E principles. *Anaesthesia*, **38**, 361.

## FURTHER READING

The *Proceedings* of the First International Symposium on Low Flow and Closed System Anesthesia. Held at Denver in 1978.

CHAPTER 3

# Pulmonary Gas Exchange and Acid-Base Status



The function of the respiratory system is to provide an adequate supply of oxygen to the tissues and to regulate the excretion of carbon dioxide so as to help maintain a normal acid-base state. The lungs are one link in a complex chain of systems, and provide the mechanisms which allow the transfer of oxygen and carbon dioxide between blood and air. Three principal factors are concerned in their function, namely: ventilation, diffusion, and pulmonary blood flow. Ventilation must not only be sufficient to move an adequate volume of air, but its distribution throughout the lungs must be related to the distribution and quantity of pulmonary blood flow.

## VENTILATION

The subject of the overall ventilation of the lungs is dealt with in Chapter 2, and distribution of ventilation later in this Chapter.

## ALVEOLAR GAS TRANSFER

The exchange of gases within the lung occurs through a process of passive diffusion across the alveolar-capillary membrane. This membrane consists of the alveolar membrane, interstitial fluid, and the capillary endothelium. In the case of oxygen, the plasma, red cell membrane and intracellular fluid must also be considered, as the rate of reaction of oxygen with haemoglobin plays an important part in determining the rate of diffusion. For a given partial pressure gradient, $CO_2$ diffuses about twenty times more rapidly than $O_2$ across the alveolar-capillary membrane. This occurs in spite of its higher molecular weight and is due to the much greater water solubility of $CO_2$. In practice, roughly similar amounts of $CO_2$ and $O_2$ are exchanged between alveolar gas and alveolar capillary blood, with a gradient of 6 mm Hg (0·8 kPa) for $CO_2$ and 65 mm Hg (8·7 kPa) for $O_2$. Thus

| | *GRADIENT* |
|---|---|
| mixed venous $P_{CO_2}$ ($P_{\bar{v}CO_2}$) = 46 mm Hg (6·1 kPa); alveolar $P_{CO_2}$ ($P_{A}CO_2$) = 40 mm Hg (5·3 kPa) | 6 mm Hg (0·8 kPa) |
| mixed venous $P_{O_2}$ ($P_{\bar{v}O_2}$) = 40 mm Hg (5·3 kPa); alveolar $P_{O_2}$ ($P_{A}O_2$) = 105 mm Hg (14 kPa) | 65 mm Hg (8·7 kPa) |

The most important variable in considering the diffusion of oxygen is the partial pressure gradient across the capillary wall. As oxygen passes across the membrane, the $P_{O_2}$ of the blood rises, the rate of rise being determined by the rate of gas transfer and its rate of combination with haemoglobin, so that the pressure gradient driving the gas across the membrane falls. This process is shown in Fig. 1. From this diagram it can be seen that an average red blood corpuscle takes about 0·75 seconds to traverse a capillary, that the majority of the gas exchange occurs within the first third of this time, and that virtually complete equilibrium between blood and alveolus has been established at the venous end of the capillary. From this data it is evident that there is a great reserve capacity in the diffusion process. For example during exercise almost complete equilibration still occurs even though the time available for gas transfer may be reduced by two-thirds. A similar but opposite process occurs during diffusion of carbon dioxide.

The alveolar-capillary membrane can be seen to be thickened in certain diseases, such as sarcoidosis, asbestosis, pulmonary fibrosis, and infiltrating carcinoma, and this thickening can produce defects in the diffusion process. This state of affairs has been given the name "alveolar-capillary block", and is characterised clinically by dyspnoea and profound cyanosis, especially on exercise, associated with a low arterial $P_{CO_2}$. However, it has been shown that the diffusion defect in these conditions is not nearly so severe as was once supposed, and that most of the hypoxia is due to ventilation/perfusion abnormalities (see below). At present it is considered that impairment of diffusion does not play nearly such an important role in clinical practice as was at one time suspected.

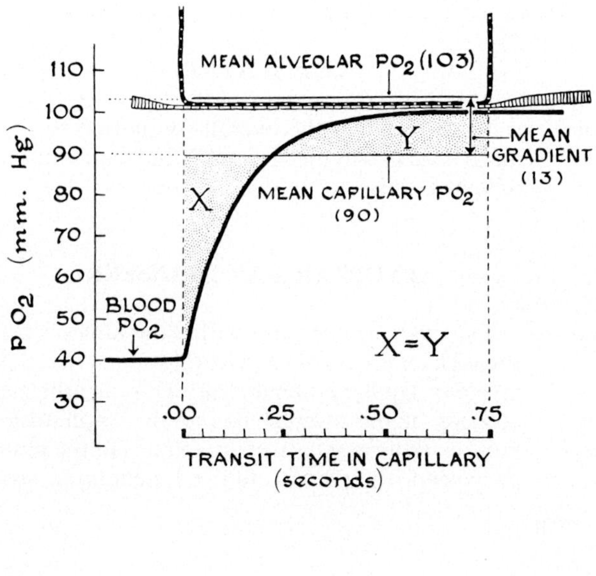


3/Fig. 1.—The change in oxygen tension of blood during its passage through a pulmonary capillary. (Courtesy of R. M. Cherniack and L. Cherniack, from *Respiration in Health and Disease*, published by W. B. Saunders Co.)

### Transfer Factor for Carbon Monoxide

An estimate of the efficiency of gas transfer from gas to blood can be made by measuring the Transfer Factor for carbon monoxide (CO). This is usually done by a single breath technique using a test gas mixture containing CO 0·3 per cent, helium 12 per cent and air. The subject exhales to residual volume, takes a single breath of the prepared gas mixture, holds it for 10 seconds and then exhales slowly and fully to residual volume. During exhalation a mid-expired sample is collected and analysed for CO and helium concentrations. The time for which the breath was held and the inspired volume are also noted. From these data the transfer factor can be calculated.[1]

The transfer of CO from inspired gas to blood depends on three factors.

(1) *Ventilation*. This is because the concentration of CO in the alveoli depends on the depth and the distribution of ventilation when inhaling the test gas, and is therefore influenced by airways obstruction. This distribution factor can to some extent be compensated for by an estimate of the volume of lung into which the test gas was distributed, hence the helium which is contained in the mixture.

(2) *Pulmonary capillary blood volume*, especially the volume of red cells which are available to take up the CO. Thus anaemic patients tend to have a low transfer factor and polycythaemic patients a high one.

(3) *Diffusion*. CO is so diffusible that it only leads to a reduction in gas transfer factor when a major diffusion defect is present, such as in severe pulmonary oedema.

Other factors affecting the transfer factor are less important. It increases during growth, is higher in men than in women and is low in the presence of a low cardiac output. During exercise it may be doubled. However, the most important single factor which lowers the transfer factor is ventilation-perfusion maldistribution.

Low values for transfer factor are found in bronchitis, emphysema, diffuse pulmonary infiltrations and loss of functioning lung tissue (e.g. pulmonary collapse, pulmonary embolus).

## THE PULMONARY CIRCULATION

The pulmonary circulation consists of the pulmonary artery and its branches, the pre-capillary vessels (which unlike those in the systemic circulation are thin-walled and easily distended), the pulmonary capillaries, and the pulmonary venous system. It is a low-pressure system, easily distensible, with a low resistance to blood flow, and accepts all the blood that leaves the right side of the heart. The normal pulmonary artery systolic pressure is 20–30 mm Hg (2·7–4·0 kPa), the diastolic pressure 8–12 mm Hg (1·1–1·6 kPa), with a mean pressure of 12–15 mm Hg (1·6–2·0 kPa) at rest. The normal mean left atrial pressure is about 8 mm Hg (1·1 kPa), with an upper limit of 15 mm Hg (2·0 kPa). The system is very flexible in adapting itself to changes in blood flow and blood volume, its adaptability being almost entirely passive in nature. Thus, immediately after blocking the pulmonary artery to one lung, the pressure in the other only rises by about 5 mm Hg (0·7 kPa). Also, the low pulse pressure in the pulmonary artery, compared with that in the aorta, is due to the high distensibility and low resistance of the system. The compliance of the entire pulmonary vascular tree resembles that of a large systemic vein in nature.

The pulmonary circulation normally contains about 10 per cent of the total blood volume, but this amount is easily altered by as much as 50 per cent. A rise in pulmonary blood volume is seen in negative-pressure breathing, the supine position when compared with the upright position, systemic vasoconstriction from any cause, over-transfusion, and left ventricular failure. A fall in pulmonary blood volume occurs during positive-pressure breathing, on assuming the upright posture, during Valsalva's manoeuvre, after haemorrhage, or as a result of systemic vasodilatation from any cause. Thus it is a simple matter to shift blood from the pulmonary circulation to the systemic circulation, and vice versa.

### Hypoxic Pulmonary Vasoconstriction

If alveolar hypoxia occurs for any reason, either generally or locally within the lung, the result is *vasoconstriction* and a reduction in blood flow in those vessels supplying the hypoxic area, so that the blood is diverted to oxygenated parts of the lung. For example, if pulmonary collapse occurs in a portion of the lung, ventilation will be reduced in the collapsed area, and oxygenation of the venous blood flowing to that area will be less effective. The blood is therefore diverted to parts of the lung where it can become adequately oxygenated, thus tending to maintain a normal arterial oxygen saturation. This response to hypoxia is the opposite to that which occurs in the systemic circulation. In man 50 per cent of the final shift in blood flow has occurred within 2 minutes of the onset of alveolar hypoxia, and it is complete after 7 minutes. The reflex is accentuated by a local rise in $H^+$ ion concentration.

The exact mechanism whereby the small pulmonary vessels constrict in response to alveolar hypoxia is obscure. Most of this response occurs locally and can be demonstrated in denervated animal lungs although there may be an autonomic contribution under some circumstances.[2] If hypoxic pulmonary vasoconstriction has occurred several drugs which cause a reduction in pulmonary vascular resistance may have an exaggerated effect[3]; the reported effects of halothane on hypoxic pulmonary vasoconstriction are conflicting. A list of some of the substances which affect pulmonary vascular resistance is given in Table 1.

3/TABLE 1
PULMONARY VASCULAR RESISTANCE

| *INCREASED* | *REDUCED* |
|---|---|
| hypoxia | α-blockers |
| α-sympathomimetics | β-sympathomimetics |
| β-blockers | prostaglandins $E_1$ and $E_2$ |
| protamine | acetylcholine |
| histamine | aminophylline |
| serotonin | alkalaemia |
| angiotensin 11 | sodium nitroprusside |
| prostaglandin $F_2\alpha$ | |
| acidaemia (respiratory or metabolic) | |
| cyclopropane | |
| diethyl ether | |

## Pulmonary Hypertension

Pulmonary hypertension is said to be present when the systolic pressure in the pulmonary artery rises above 30 mm Hg (4·0 kPa). It can be due either to an increase in flow, in pulmonary vascular resistance, or in left atrial pressure. An increase in pulmonary blood flow occurs when a left-to-right shunt is present, such as is found in atrial or ventricular defects or in the presence of a patent ductus arteriosus. In these conditions the blood flow through the lungs may be as much as three times the systemic cardiac output. If this state of affairs is allowed to persist, after some years the pulmonary vascular resistance begins to rise due to structural changes in the vessels and the pulmonary artery pressure rises even further. Eventually the pressure on the right side of the heart may exceed that on the left side, and a right-to-left shunt with central cyanosis then appears. The combination of a ventricular septal defect, pulmonary hypertension and a reversed shunt is called Eisenmenger's complex*.

A rise in left atrial and pulmonary venous pressures causes pulmonary arterial hypertension by back-pressure, and may be secondary to aortic or mitral valve disease, or to left ventricular failure from any cause. A rise in pulmonary vascular resistance occurs in such conditions as massive or multiple pulmonary emboli and in some lung diseases, notably advanced chronic bronchitis. Pulmonary hypertension in the latter condition is thought to be due to a combination of chronic hypoxia and obliteration of the pulmonary vascular bed by the disease process.

## Pulmonary Oedema

Normally the relationship between the pressure in the pulmonary capillaries, the colloid osmotic pressure of the plasma and the interstitial pressure of the lung tissue is such that only a small amount of fluid passes across the capillaries and this is returned to the circulation via the pulmonary lymphatics. If the amount of fluid passing across the capillary walls increases, due to a rise in pressure within the capillaries or an increase in their permeability, the capacity of the pulmonary lymphatics to drain this fluid may be exceeded in which case pulmonary oedema will result. This process will be accentuated if there is a low oncotic pressure due to hypoproteinaemia. For reviews of this subject see Snashall,[4] Noble[5] and Staub.[6]

## Measurement of Pulmonary Blood Flow

There are four principal methods: first, the use of radio-active gases, second, the direct Fick method requiring the measurement of the

* *Eisenmenger complex* is the condition which he originally described and comprises ventricular septal defect, a pulmonary resistance which is equal to or exceeds systemic vascular resistance, and right-to-left shunt.

*Eisenmenger syndrome* is any vascular connection between the left and right sides of the circulation at the atrial, ventricular or aortopulmonary level in which the pulmonary vascular resistance is equal to or exceeds systemic vascular resistance, causing a right-to-left shunt.

oxygen uptake per minute in the pulmonary circulation, third, the indicator-dilution method, and fourth, the body plethysmograph. The last method measures pulmonary capillary flow.

## DISTRIBUTION OF PULMONARY BLOOD FLOW

Many years ago it was suggested that in the erect posture the simple factor of the weight of a column of blood in the lung would cause the upper part of the lung to receive less blood than the lower part. Great advances have been made in the study of the amount and distribution of both air and blood in the lungs with the aid of radio-active techniques. The principle of the method of measurement is simple. The patient's chest is surrounded with multiple counters which can detect radio-activity in a particular area of the lung. The subject then takes a single breath of radio-active gas. The distribution of this gas in the lung will reveal the regional ventilation per unit of lung volume. Alternatively, if the value of the pulmonary blood flow is required, then the technique differs according to which gas is used. In the case of oxygen (or oxygen-labelled carbon dioxide) the patient takes a breath and then holds it: the rate of the removal of this gas from the different areas of the lung signifies the pulmonary blood flow. In contrast, xenon is a relatively insoluble gas and is injected into an arm vein as a solution in saline: the xenon passes to the pulmonary capillaries and out into the alveoli. The precise areas in which this takes place are revealed by the counters.

In the normal conscious subject, in the upright position, there is a nine-fold difference in the pulmonary blood flow between the first and fifth intercostal spaces, with almost no blood flow at the apex of the lung. From Fig. 2*a* it will be observed that in passing from the apex to the base of the lung, the volume of the organ at the relevant level only increases from 7 to 13 per cent, yet the blood flow alters from 0·07 l/min at the apex, to 1·29 l/min at the base. In the *supine* position the blood flow at the apex increases considerably, so that its distribution becomes uniform from apex to base, although now perfusion anteriorly is less than that posteriorly. It appears, therefore, that gravity plays a dominant role in determining the distribution of blood flow within the lungs. The mechanisms through which gravity controls the distribution of blood in the upright lung are shown in Fig.

| mm Hg | kPa |
|---|---|
| 132 | 17·6 |
| 28 | 3·7 |
| 89 | 11·9 |
| 42 | 5·6 |

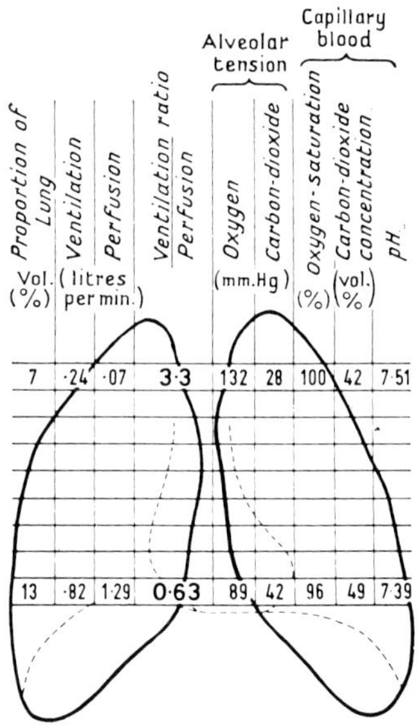


3/FIG. 2(*a*).—Differences in ventilation, blood flow and gas exchange in the normal upright lung. (Courtesy of Professor J. B. West and the Editor of the *Lancet*).

| mm Hg | kPa |
|---|---|
| 101 | 13·5 |
| 132 | 17·6 |
| 89 | 11·9 |
| 97 | 12·9 |
| 4 | 0·5 |

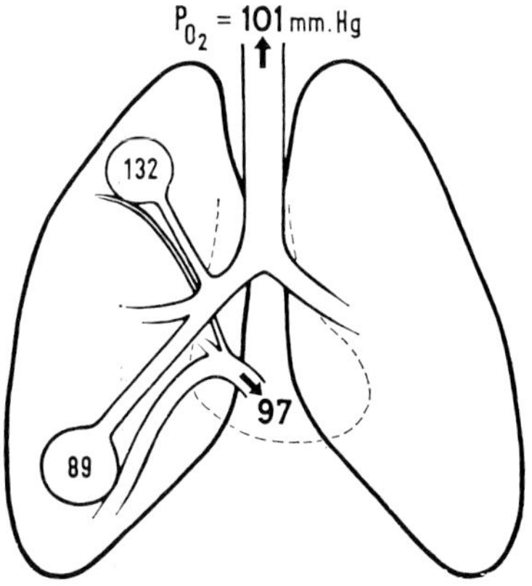

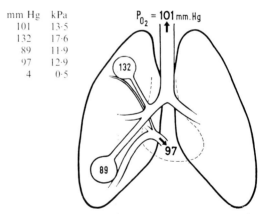

3/FIG. 2(*b*).—Diagram showing how the normal alveolar-arterial oxygen difference arises. The $Po_2$ values in alveoli at the top and bottom of the lungs, in the alveolar air (average value) and in mixed blood leaving the lungs are shown. Alveolar-arterial oxygen difference = 101 − 97 = 4 mm Hg (13·5 − 12·9 = 0·5 kPa). (Courtesy of Professor J. B. West and the Editor of the *Lancet*).

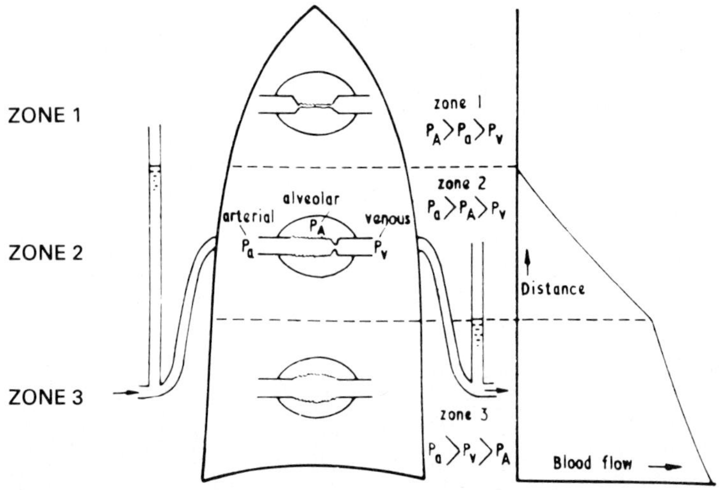


3/FIG. 2(*c*).—Diagram showing the distribution of blood flow in normal lung, and how this distribution arises. For a full explanation see text. (Courtesy of Professor J. B. West, Professor C. T. Dollery and Dr. A. Naimark, and the *Journal of Applied Physiology*[7]).

2*c*. The lung has been divided into three zones by considering the relationships between the alveolar pressure (PA), the pulmonary artery pressure (Pa) and the pulmonary venous pressure (Pv), and the effects these pressures have upon the collapsible pulmonary vessels. In zone 1, at the top of the lung, the alveolar pressure exceeds both the pulmonary artery and pulmonary venous pressures. The result is collapse of the local pulmonary vessels, and little or no blood flow. In zone 2 the pulmonary artery pressure exceeds the alveolar and pulmonary venous pressures. The pulmonary vessels are now held partly open, and blood flow begins to occur at the top of the zone, increasing rather rapidly down its length. In zone 3 the pulmonary artery pressure exceeds the pulmonary venous pressure, which itself is greater than the alveolar pressure. Blood flow continues to increase as we pass down zone 3, but at a slower rate than in zone 2. There is another important difference between zone 2 and zone 3. In zone 2, the blood flow depends mainly on the difference between the *alveolar* and *pulmonary artery* pressures, whereas in zone 3, it is the difference between the *pulmonary arterial* and *pulmonary venous* pressures which is important, the alveolar pressure having little influence.

The scheme outlined above satisfactorily explains most of the observed findings (e.g. the effect of lying supine). For instance, during exercise the perfusion of the lung becomes more evenly distributed, and this is probably due to the increase in pulmonary artery pressure which is observed under these conditions so that zone 1 becomes much smaller or disappears altogether.

In the normal lung at lung volumes below total lung capacity, the interstitial pressure at the lung base is raised because the lung parenchyma is less well expanded than at the lung apex. Perivascular oedema isolates the vessel from the normal expanding action of the lung parenchyma, with the result that the vessel closes by virtue of the inherent tension in its wall. A modification of the three zone model to take account of the reduction of blood flow in the most dependent regions of the lung has been proposed by Hughes and his colleagues.[8] Under pathological conditions, interstitial oedema may further raise the interstitial pressure, thus further reducing the basal blood flow.[7]

## DISTRIBUTION OF VENTILATION

In the normal upright lung the ventilation per unit lung volume is greater at the base than it is at the apex. The change in ventilation decreases approximately linearly with the distance up the lung, being about twice as great at the base than at the apex. These differences disappear in the supine position, the ventilation becoming almost even from apex to base. Also, the differences in regional ventilation become less during exercise, and are reversed in the inverted position. The mechanism by which ventilation is distributed within the normal lung has become clearer. In the upright position the lung tends to sag towards its most dependent part under the influence of gravity so that the alveoli are smaller at the base than they are at the apex. Small alveoli are more compliant than larger ones so that during inspiration a greater volume change occurs in the former and hence ventilation is preferentially distributed to the dependent parts of the lung, provided that the basal areas are not so compressed that airway closure has occurred (Fig. 3). The local tension of carbon dioxide may also play a part. Severinghaus and colleagues[10] found that a fall in alveolar $CO_2$ in one lung after occlusion of its pulmonary artery was accompanied by a fall in its ventilation of about 25 per cent.

In diseased lung the two main factors controlling the distribution of ventilation are the patency of the airways, and local changes in compliance within the lungs. Any factor which reduces the airway calibre, and therefore raises the resistance to airflow, will result in a fall in ventilation to the affected region. Similarly, any area in which the local compliance has decreased will be less well ventilated than the surrounding more expandable normal lung tissue.

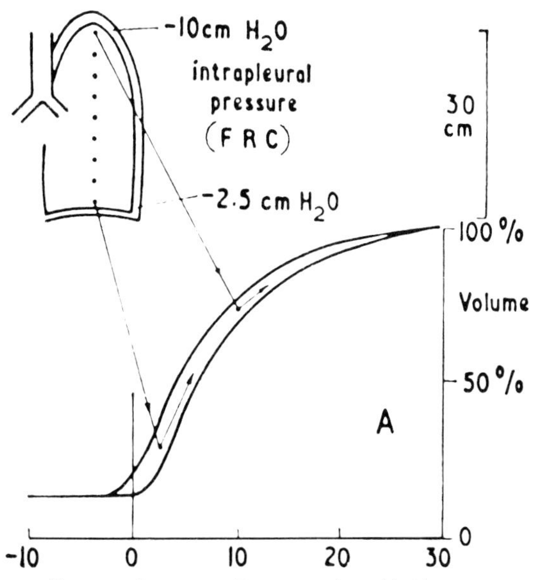


3/Fig. 3.—This figure shows an upright lung 30 cm from base to apex, at the end of a normal expiration—in other words at functional residual capacity (FRC). The apical and basal parts of the lung are operating on different segments of the pressure-volume curve with the result that the more compliant basal alveoli receive relatively more ventilation. (Courtesy of Dr. J. B. West and Blackwell Scientific Publications.[9])

## THE RELATIONSHIPS BETWEEN VENTILATION AND PERFUSION IN NORMAL AND ABNORMAL LUNGS

The normal alveolar ventilation ($\dot{V}_A$) in an adult is approximately 4 l/min, and the total perfusion ($\dot{Q}$) about 5 l/min. Therefore the proportion of ventilation to perfusion is $\frac{4}{5} = 0{\cdot}8$. This ratio is known as the VENTILATION/PERFUSION RATIO ($\dot{V}_A/\dot{Q}$). The ventilation/perfusion ratio for a whole lung is a composite of the ratios for each individual alveolus, and in an "ideal" lung the ratio for each alveolus should be the same as that for the whole lung (namely 0·8), so that ventilation and blood flow are distributed absolutely evenly to each individual alveolus. As is apparent from the foregoing discussions on the distribution of blood flow and ventilation within the normal lung, this is far from the case.

The differences in ventilation and perfusion at the top and bottom of the upright lung, together with their effects on gas exchange, are shown in Fig. 2*a*. At the bottom of the lung ventilation is exceeded by blood flow, so that $\dot{V}_A/\dot{Q}$ is low, namely 0·63. (In elderly people it is zero at the end of expiration because terminal airway closure results in zero ventilation of basal zones which are still being perfused; in these subjects the closing capacity exceeds functional residual capacity.) Because ventilation is proportionally low, the rate of supply of oxygen to these alveoli is less than the maximum rate at which it could be removed by the blood flow. This results in a low $P_{O_2}$ in these over-perfused alveoli (i.e. 89 mm Hg, 11·8 kPa), and therefore, a low $P_{O_2}$ in the blood leaving this portion of the lung. However, owing to the shape of the oxygen dissociation curve, a $P_{O_2}$ of 89 mm Hg (11·8 kPa), only results in a small fall in oxygen saturation (to 96 per cent), as the curve is nearly horizontal at this level of $P_{O_2}$. Similarly, the excretion of carbon dioxide is impaired, because the ventilation is not sufficient to wash out all the carbon dioxide passing into the alveoli from venous blood without a small rise in its alveolar concentration ($P_{ACO_2}$ = 42 mm Hg, 5·6 kPa). The result is that blood leaving the base of the lungs is slightly hypoxic and hypercapnic.

Passing up the lungs, both ventilation and perfusion decrease, but perfusion decreases at about three times the rate at which ventilation does. By the time the top of the lung is reached, perfusion is almost nil, so that ventilation at the apices is proportionally far greater than perfusion, and the ratio of the two becomes very high ($\dot{V}_A/\dot{Q}$ = 3·3). Therefore oxygen is supplied to the upper alveoli at a greater rate than it is removed, with the result that a new equilibrium is established, and the alveolar $Po_2$ is high ($P_{AO_2}$ = 132 mm Hg, 17·6 kPa). The blood leaving these areas has a similar $Po_2$ and the saturation rises to nearly 100 per cent. The alveolar carbon dioxide partial pressure is lower than at the bases ($P_{ACO_2}$ = 38 mm Hg, 5 kPa) owing to excessive washout. Thus blood leaving the apices is almost 100 per cent saturated with a slightly low carbon dioxide content. It is clear that at the top of the lung much of the ventilation is "wasted", as it does not have the opportunity to partake in gas exchange owing to the very low blood flow. This wasted ventilation, therefore, becomes part of the physiological dead space by definition. Any further increase in the proportion of alveoli which are over-ventilated (i.e. with a *high* $\dot{V}_A/\dot{Q}$ ratio) will result in an increase in physiological dead space. This may be secondary to either an increase in relative ventilation in parts of the lung, or to a reduction in relative perfusion, because in both instances a rise in $\dot{V}_A/\dot{Q}$ will occur.

The term $\dot{V}_A/\dot{Q}$ *mismatch* refers to the situation where alveoli are either over- or underperfused relative to their ventilation. Some degree of $\dot{V}_A/\dot{Q}$ mismatch is normal, as explained above, but this may be increased.

### $\dot{V}_A/\dot{Q}$ Mismatch and Carbon Dioxide Excretion

Variations in the relationship between ventilation and perfusion have a smaller effect on the excretion of carbon dioxide than on the uptake of oxygen. Because of the shape of the $CO_2$ dissociation curve (p. 108) blood passing through zones of lung with a high $\dot{V}_A/\dot{Q}$ ratio loses more $CO_2$ than normal and so can compensate for blood passing through zones of lungs with a low $\dot{V}_A/\dot{Q}$ ratio which will lose less $CO_2$ than normal. The same is not true for oxygen. Because of the shape of the haemoglobin-oxygen dissociation curve, blood passing through zones of lung with a high $\dot{V}_A/\dot{Q}$ ratio cannot pick up enough extra oxygen to compensate for blood passing through zones with a low $\dot{V}_A/\dot{Q}$ ratio. If blood from zones of high and low $\dot{V}_A/\dot{Q}$ ratios is mixed (Table 2) the $CO_2$ content and $Pco_2$ of the blood are close to normal whereas the oxygen content and $Po_2$ are reduced.

Blood leaving those parts of the lung with different $\dot{V}_A/\dot{Q}$ ratios will become mixed in the left atrium and left ventricle, so that the arterial tensions of oxygen and carbon dioxide will be somewhere in between the extreme values found at the top and bottom of the lungs.

### Alveolar-Arterial $Po_2$ Difference ($P_{AO_2}$ – $Pao_2$)

In normal young people the arterial $Po_2$ is about 97 mm Hg (12·9 kPa) and the $Pco_2$ about 40 mm Hg (5·3 kPa). As the normal average alveolar $Po_2$ is about 101 mm Hg (13·4 kPa) there is therefore a difference of about 4 mm Hg (0·5 kPa) between the alveolar and arterial $Po_2$ values. This difference is known as the

3/TABLE 2

| | *$O_2$ Content* | *$CO_2$ Content* |
|---|---|---|
| (1) $\dot{V}_A/\dot{Q}$ ratio low | Low | High |
| (2) $\dot{V}_A/\dot{Q}$ ratio high | Increase not great enough to compensate for (1) | Low |
| (1) & (2) arterial blood | Low | Normal |

*Alveolar-Arterial $PO_2$ Difference* ($P_{AO_2} - Pa_{O_2}$) (see Fig. 2*b*).

The normal value for $P_{AO_2} - Pa_{O_2}$ when breathing air ranges from 5–25 mm Hg (0·7–3·3 kPa), increasing with age[11]. The main factors responsible for an increase in this difference are shown below:

1. Increased partial pressure of oxygen in inspired gas ($P_{IO_2}\uparrow$)
2. Venous Admixture — LOW $\dot{V}_A/\dot{Q}$ / TRUE SHUNT
3. Reduced partial pressure of oxygen in mixed venous blood ($P\bar{v}O_2\downarrow$).

**Increased partial pressure of oxygen in inspired gas** ($P_{IO_2}$).—The higher the alveolar $Po_2$ the greater is the alveolar-arterial $Po_2$ difference. This is due to the shape of the haemoglobin-oxygen dissociation curve: a small difference in the oxygen content of blood at high levels of $Po_2$ is reflected by a large change in $Po_2$, whereas the same difference in the oxygen content of blood at low levels of $Po_2$ is reflected by a much smaller change in $Po_2$.

**Venous admixture.**—As a gross simplification, the blood returning to the left side of the heart can be considered to be made up of two fractions:

(*a*) Blood which has passed through "ideal" alveoli, that is alveoli with perfect ventilation and perfusion (i.e. no $\dot{V}_A/\dot{Q}$ mismatch).

(*b*) Mixed venous blood. The oxygen and carbon dioxide contents of venous blood vary according to which organ or part of the body the blood has come from. By the time the venous blood has reached the pulmonary artery mixing has occurred, so that a blood sample taken from the pulmonary artery consists of *mixed venous blood.*

The blood from "ideal" alveoli obviously has a $Po_2$ equal to "ideal" alveolar $Po_2$. In order to produce the observed alveolar-arterial $Po_2$ difference a certain quantity of mixed venous blood would have to be added. This quantity is termed *venous admixture* and can be defined as the *CALCULATED* amount of mixed venous blood which would be required to mix with blood draining "ideal" alveoli to produce the observed difference between "ideal" alveolar and arterial $Po_2$. This is an entirely theoretical concept since some of the blood contributing to the venous admixture effect has a $Po_2$ lower than $P\bar{v}O_2$, e.g. thebesian* venous blood from the myocardium; and some has a higher $Po_2$ than $P\bar{v}O_2$, e.g. blood which has picked up some oxygen in the lungs but is less than fully oxygenated. Venous admixture can be divided into

(*a*) blood which has passed from the right to the left side of the circulation and picked up *no* oxygen in the lungs—TRUE SHUNT;

(*b*) blood which has picked up *some* oxygen in the lungs but is still less than fully oxygenated, having passed through relatively overperfused or underventilated zones of lung—LOW $\dot{V}_A/\dot{Q}$ RATIO.

The causes of true shunt are summarised in Table 3. Other terms sometimes encountered are:

(i) *Anatomical shunt.* This is the same as "true shunt".

(ii) *Pathological shunt.* Those forms of anatomical shunt which are not present in the normal subject, e.g. congenital heart disease with right-to-left shunting.

(iii) *Physiological shunt.* This refers to the normal degree of venous admixture and comprises admixture due to normal true shunt (Table 3) and admixture due to blood which has passed through relatively overperfused or underventilated (low $\dot{V}_A/\dot{Q}$) zones of lung.

(iv) *Atelectatic shunt.* Blood which has passed through collapsed (unventilated) zones of lung.

Venous admixture causes an increase in arterial $CO_2$ *content* which is similar in magnitude to the reduction in arterial $O_2$ *content.* In the normal subject both quantities are very small, about 0·3 vols per cent. Because of the shapes of the $CO_2$ and $O_2$ dissociation curves this small increase in $CO_2$ content is reflected by only a small increase in $PaCO_2$ (less than 1 mm Hg, 0·1 kPa), whereas the small reduction in $O_2$ content is reflected by a large reduction in $PaO_2$ (15 mm Hg, 2·0 kPa). The arterial $Po_2$ is therefore the best indicator of venous admix-

*The thebesian veins, also called venae cordis minimae, are very small veins draining the myocardium and opening directly into the chambers of the heart. Those draining into the left atrium and ventricle fulfill the definition (above) of true shunt. Of course, by far the majority of the venous blood drains by large veins into the coronary sinus which, in turn, opens into the right atrium.

3/TABLE 3
CLASSIFICATION OF CAUSES OF "TRUE SHUNT"
(after Nunn[12])

| | *Normal* | *Abnormal* |
|---|---|---|
| Extrapulmonary | Thebesian veins | Congenital disease of the heart or great vessels with right-to-left shunting. |
| Intrapulmonary | Bronchial veins<br>Possibly some slight degree of atelectasis | Atelectasis<br>Pulmonary infection<br>Pulmonary arteriovenous shunts<br>Pulmonary neoplasm including haemangioma<br>Circulation through contused, damaged or oedematous lung. |

ture. Whether this is due to true shunt or to ventilation/perfusion mismatch can be determined by giving the subject 100 per cent $O_2$ to breathe. If there is only a relatively small increase in arterial $Po_2$, the hypoxaemia is likely to be due to true shunt. In the presence of a 50 per cent shunt, changes in inspired oxygen concentration have virtually no effect on arterial $Po_2$.

Venous admixture, which is normally up to 5 per cent of the cardiac output, may be calculated using the shunt equation and the alveolar air equation.

## SHUNT EQUATION AND ALVEOLAR AIR EQUATION

The "shunt" equation can be derived as follows:

Pulmonary capillary blood flow ($\dot{Q}c$)+blood flow through shunt ($\dot{Q}s$) = cardiac output ($\dot{Q}T$).

$$\dot{Q}c + \dot{Q}s = \dot{Q}T$$

This equation can be written in terms of oxygen content:

$$(Cc'O_2 \times \dot{Q}c) + (C\bar{v}O_2 \times \dot{Q}s) = (CaO_2 \times \dot{Q}T)$$

($Cc'O_2$ is the oxygen content of pulmonary end-capillary blood; $C\bar{v}O_2$ is the oxygen content of mixed venous or pulmonary arterial blood; $CaO_2$ is the oxygen content of arterial blood).

Since $\dot{Q}c = \dot{Q}T - \dot{Q}s$,

$$(Cc'O_2 \times \dot{Q}T) - (Cc'O_2 \times \dot{Q}s) + (C\bar{v}O_2 \times \dot{Q}s) = (CaO_2 \times \dot{Q}T)$$

Dividing both sides by $\dot{Q}T$,

$$Cc'O_2 - \left(Cc'O_2 \times \frac{\dot{Q}s}{\dot{Q}T}\right) + \left(C\bar{v}O_2 \times \frac{\dot{Q}s}{\dot{Q}T}\right) = CaO_2$$

$$Cc'O_2 - CaO_2 = (Cc'O_2 - C\bar{v}O_2)\frac{\dot{Q}s}{\dot{Q}T}$$

$$\text{Therefore } \frac{\dot{Q}s}{\dot{Q}T} = \frac{Cc'O_2 - CaO_2}{Cc'O_2 - C\bar{v}O_2}$$

Of the quantities on the right-hand side of the equation, $CaO_2$ and $C\bar{v}O_2$ can be obtained by analysis of arterial and pulmonary arterial blood samples respectively. $Cc'O_2$ refers to the oxygen content of blood in equilibrium with "ideal" alveolar gas, which cannot be sampled since it becomes contaminated with alveolar dead-space gas. "Ideal" alveolar $Po_2$ can be derived using the alveolar air equation.

Nunn[12] discusses different forms of the alveolar air equation, of which the following is the most satisfactory:

$$\text{ideal alveolar } Po_2 = P{\rm I}o_2 - Paco_2\left(\frac{P{\rm I}o_2 - P\bar{E}o_2}{P\bar{E}co_2}\right)$$

For the derivation of this equation the reader is referred to West[9] and Leigh and Tyrell[13].

If the patient is breathing 100 per cent oxygen, then since alveolar gas contains only oxygen and carbon dioxide,

$$\text{ideal alveolar } Po_2 = P{\rm I}o_2 - Paco_2$$

The error involved in assuming that $PaCO_2$ (which can be measured) is the same as the ideal alveolar $Pco_2$ (which cannot be measured) is small.

**Reduced partial pressure of oxygen in mixed venous blood ($P\bar{v}O_2$).**—The lower the $P\bar{v}O_2$ the greater will be the effect of a given amount of venous admixture on the $PAO_2$ – $PaO_2$ difference. The commonest cause of a reduced $P\bar{v}O_2$, apart from arterial hypoxia, is a low cardiac output.

Considering the magnitude of the variations in ventilation/perfusion relationships within the normal upright lung, it is remarkable how efficient the lungs are at oxygenating venous blood when compared with the "ideal" lung. As mentioned above, the normal alveolar-arterial oxygen difference is only about 4 mm Hg (0·5 kPa), with a venous admixture of less than 5 per cent of the cardiac output. This is due to the shape of the oxygen dissociation curve since, for blood leaving the over- or under-ventilated regions of normal lungs, only the flat upper portion of the curve is involved. In blood leaving the lung bases, therefore, a $Po_2$ of 89 mm Hg (11·9 kPa) corresponds to a saturation of 96 per cent, not far below full saturation. At the top of the lung the $Po_2$ in the blood is 132 mm Hg (17·6 kPa), corresponding to a saturation of nearly 100 per cent. The result is that when the two are mixed together the final $Po_2$ is 97 mm Hg (12·9 kPa) with a saturation of 97 per cent. However, arterial oxygenation is much less satisfactory when, for blood leaving the underventilated regions, the point of equilibration lies well down on the steep part of the dissociation curve. Under these circumstances significant desaturation occurs in the final blood mixture leaving the left ventricle. This situation occurs frequently in pathological states. For instance, if a region of atelectasis is present, in which no ventilation occurs, the blood leaving this part of the lung has an oxygen saturation equal to that in venous blood arriving at the lungs (i.e. $Po_2 = 40$ mm Hg (5·3 kPa); saturation = 75 per cent), as no oxygen has been added to the blood. Here we have a saturation which is considerably lower than that found in the under-ventilated areas of normal lung. The small rise in saturation in the overventilated regions is now unable to compensate for the low saturation in the blood which has passed through the atelectatic lung, and arterial desaturation inevitably follows. Clearly, compensation becomes even more difficult in the presence of a low cardiac output, when systemic venous saturation may fall to 50 per cent or less. The relation between cardiac output, venous admixture and arterial oxygenation is shown in Fig. 4. As can be seen, for a given venous admixture arterial oxygenation falls considerably at low cardiac outputs. This accounts for the very low arterial $Po_2$ values found in patients with cardiorespiratory failure.

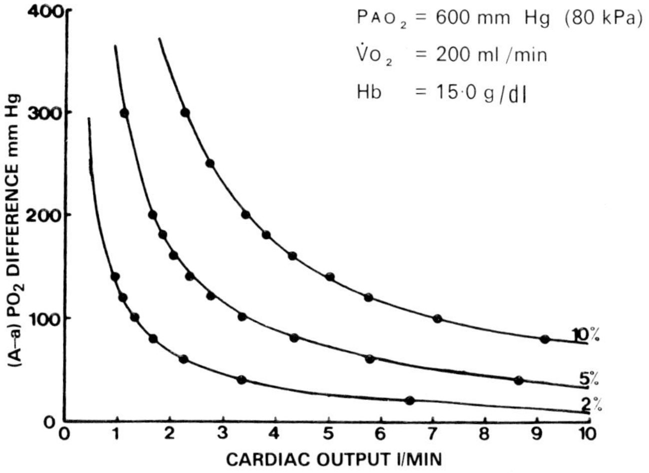


3/Fig.4.—Graph showing the effect of venous admixture and cardiac output on the alveolar-arterial oxygen difference while breathing oxygen. As can be seen, for a given venous admixture, the alveolar-arterial oxygen difference rises steeply at low cardiac outputs. Also, a change in venous admixture causes a greater change in alveolar-arterial oxygen difference when the cardiac output is low. (Courtesy of Dr. J. Panday and Dr. J. F. Nunn and the Editor of *Anaesthesia*.[14])

## SOME FACTORS AFFECTING PULMONARY FUNCTION
### with special reference to anaesthesia

**Advancing Age**

The results obtained from almost any lung function test must be interpreted with the subject's age in mind. For the tests of ventilation increasing age is associated with a fall in maximum breathing capacity, forced expiratory volume, peak expiratory flow rate, vital capacity and total lung capacity. A progressive rise is seen in the ratios functional residual capacity/total lung volume and residual volume/total lung capacity. The physiological dead space rises, but the arterial $P\mathrm{co}_2$ remains constant. The alveolar-arterial oxygen difference rises, and may be as high as 25 mm Hg (3·3 kPa) in old age. The arterial $P\mathrm{o}_2$ therefore falls progressively, and in an old person with clinically normal lungs may be as low as 75 mm Hg (10 kPa). A falling arterial $P\mathrm{o}_2$ with advancing age is almost certainly related to a rise in the closing capacity of the lungs (see p. 57). Once the closing capacity becomes greater than the functional residual capacity airway closure occurs and the arterial $P\mathrm{o}_2$ begins to fall.

**Posture**

Compared with the upright position, in a subject lying supine the distribution of both blood flow and ventilation becomes even from top to bottom of the lung. However, an anterior to posterior gradient now appears. In the inverted position ventilation is greater at the apex than at the base, the reverse of that found in the normal upright position.

In the lateral position, the blood flow is greater to the dependent lung. In the case of a normal conscious subject, the ventilation is also greater to the dependent lung so preventing a substantial fall in $\dot{V}/\dot{Q}$ ratio of this lung. The reason for this is that the lower diaphragm is pushed up high into the chest and so, on contraction, can produce a greater increase in volume of that hemithorax than can the upper one. In the *anaesthetised* subject breathing spontaneously, the ventilation is greater to the upper lung, so the $\dot{V}/\dot{Q}$ ratio of the lower lung falls. The same applies if the patient is paralysed and ventilated. This effect of anaesthesia may be related to the reduction in FRC which it produces,[15] and the greater ventilation of the upper lung can be prevented by PEEP, which of course increases FRC. If the chest is opened, the ventilation to the upper lung is now greatly increased—this causes a further increase in $\dot{V}/\dot{Q}$ mismatch and reduction in $PaO_2$.

**Effect of Artifical Ventilation**

It is now widely accepted that anaesthesia with artificial ventilation results in an increased physiological dead space, sometimes up to 50 per cent or more of the tidal volume. This means that parts of the lungs have become relatively overventilated. During positive pressure ventilation the alveolar pressure is increased. It is, therefore, possible to predict some of the effects of positive pressure ventilation on the distribution of blood flow. An increase in alveolar pressure will result in an enlargement of zone 1 (Fig. 2*c*), with the other two zones dropping down the lung. The amount of lung with a high $\dot{V}_A/\dot{Q}$ ratio is therefore greater, and an increased physiological dead space results.

**Effect of Duration of Inspiration**

During intermittent positive-pressure ventilation in a normal subject the duration of inspiration is usually set at 1·0–1·5 seconds. A long inspiratory time increases mean intrathoracic pressure so reducing venous return and cardiac output. A short inspiratory time causes poor distribution of the inspired gas due to the characteristics of "fast" and "slow" alveoli (see below). The following Table summarises the advantages and disadvantages of an inspiratory time which is longer or shorter than this.

| | | Venous Return Cardiac Output | Distribution of Inspired Gas |
|---|---|---|---|
| Inspiratory Time | More than 1·5 sec | Bad | Good |
| | Less than 1·0 sec | Good | Bad |

**"Fast" and "Slow" Alveoli**

Consider a balloon with a tube leading to it:

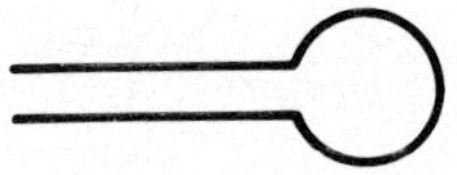

3/Fig. 5.

The inflation of the balloon in response to a given inflationary pressure is described by the exponential "wash-in" curve.

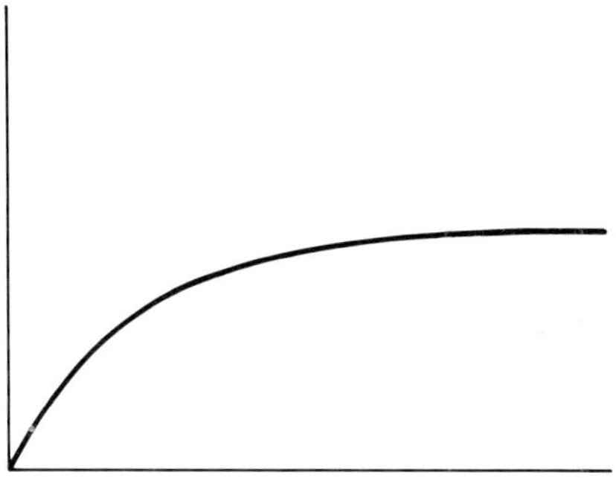


3/FIG. 6.

If the tube leading to the balloon is narrowed the balloon will still reach the same final volume when inflated at the same pressure, but it will take longer to do so (Fig. 7).

The compliance of the balloon wall is also of importance. If the wall has a low compliance (stiff) the balloon will reach a smaller final volume, when subjected to the same inflation pressure, and this volume will be reached after a shorter time (Fig. 8).

The exponential curve can be described in terms of its time constant ($\tau$) which is the time it would take for the balloon to reach its final volume if the initial gas flow rate was maintained throughout inflation ($\tau = 1{\cdot}44 \times$ the half-life). As we have seen, the time constant depends on the resistance and compliance of the system.

What has been said about the balloon can be applied to the lungs. Typical values for resistance (pulmonary and apparatus) and compliance for an anaesthetised patient are 10 cm $H_2O$ $l^{-1}$ sec (1·0 kPa $l^{-1}$ sec) and 50 ml/cm $H_2O$ (0·5 l/kPa) respectively; the two multiplied together give the time constant:

| RESISTANCE | × | COMPLIANCE | = | TIME CONSTANT |
|---|---|---|---|---|
| 10 | × | 0·05 | = | 0·5 |
| cm $H_2O$ $l^{-1}$ sec | | l/cm $H_2O$ | | sec |

An increase in resistance or compliance gives rise to a longer time constant. 95 per cent of the final volume will have been reached after 3 time constants. Different parts of the lungs may have different time constants and this scatter of time constants is exaggerated in some forms of res-

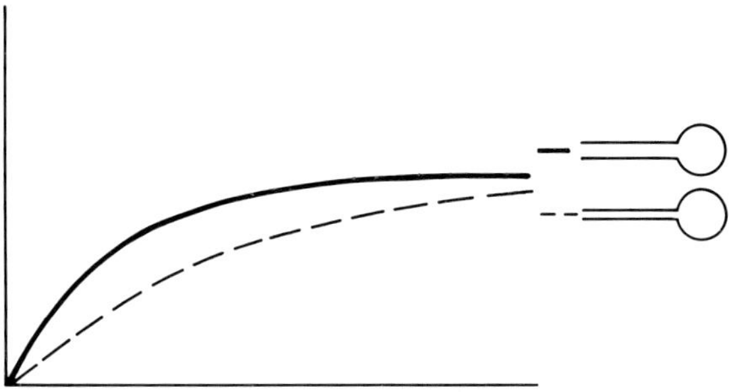


3/FIG. 7.

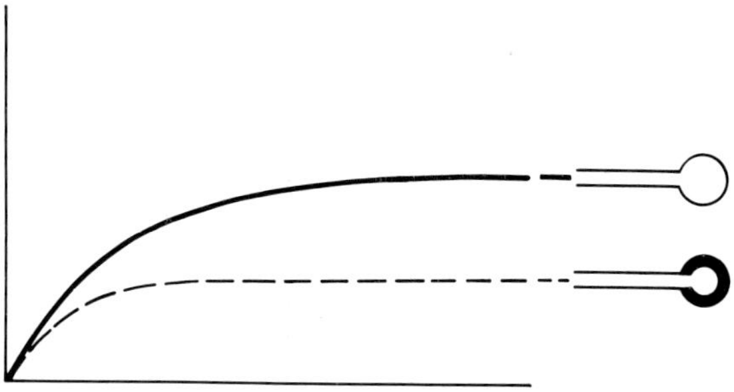


3/FIG. 8.

piratory disease such as asthma and emphysema. A short inspiratory time will result in poor ventilation of those zones of lung having a long time constant and there will be a resulting increase in $\dot{V}A/\dot{Q}$ mismatch.

**Effect of Total Blood Volume and its Distribution**

Freeman and Nunn[16] working with anaesthetised dogs, found an increase in physiological dead space in the presence of haemorrhage. In fact under these conditions it could be increased to nearly 80 per cent of the tidal volume. Askrog and associates[17] found similar changes during controlled hypotension in man, especially if the patient was tipped head up. Both experimental findings can be explained by a fall in pulmonary arterial and venous pressures, in one case secondary to a fall in total blood volume, in the other because of a shift of blood from the pulmonary to the systemic circulation. From Fig. 2*c* it can be seen that this will result in an increase in zone 1, with the other two zones dropping down the lung. Therefore, an increase in dead space results, the amount depending on the fall in pulmonary arterial and venous pressures.

**Premedication**

It has been suggested[18] that when arterial hypoxaemia is observed during and after general anaesthesia it may in part be due to the pulmonary effects of atropine. It was found that the mean oxygen saturation in a group of patients premedicated with atropine (93·4 per cent) was significantly lower than in a second unpremedicated group (96·0 per cent). In a second study there was a significant fall in arterial $Po_2$ following atropine given subcutaneously (from a mean of 95·4 mm Hg to 86·4 mm Hg, 12·7–11·5 kPa), and that postoperative hypoxaemia occurred in those patients premedicated with atropine but not in a group of unpremedicated patients. On the other hand, Nunn and Bergman,[19] in a study on conscious volunteers, observed that arterial oxygenation was unchanged in conscious subjects even after the administration of up to 2 mg of atropine intravenously. Conway[20] produced evidence that the route of administration may be important, hypoxaemia being most likely to appear after subcutaneous administration of the drug. Although the effect of atropine, if any, on arterial oxygenation has not yet finally been settled, there is general agreement that it increases both anatomical and physiological dead space. Nunn and Bergman[19] found an increase in $V_D/V_T$ ratio of 26·5 to 34·3 per cent. A similar increase in anatomical dead space has been reported by Smith and co-workers[21] after both atropine (+22 per cent) and hyoscine (+25 per cent). The precise mechanism of this effect is not known, but it is probably related either to an action on the bronchial musculature or to an action on the lining membrane.

Martinez and colleagues[22] investigated the pulmonary effects of various premedications in patients with pulmonary or cardiovascular disease, but who were well compensated at the time. They studied the effects of intramuscular morphine (1·3 mg/10 kg), pentobarbitone (15 mg/10 kg) and atropine (0·07 mg/10 kg), morphine and hyoscine (0·07 mg/10 kg), hyoscine alone and a placebo. Both arterial $Po_2$ and $Pco_2$ were unchanged in all groups after the drugs had been given, except for a small rise in $Pao_2$ after morphine alone and after pentobarbitone and atropine. The most significant finding was a fall in alveolar ventilation, ranging between 5·4 per cent and 12·7 per cent of control values, following each drug combination except the placebo. They considered that the arterial $Pco_2$ remained constant despite a fall in ventilation because this was accompanied by a reduction in $CO_2$ production. The study is remarkable for the lack of effects demonstrated. Gardiner and Palmer,[23] investigating healthy patients awaiting surgery, also found no change in arterial $Po_2$ or $Pco_2$ thirty minutes after premedication with either atropine alone or with papaveretum and hyoscine.

In spite of these studies it is well known that opiates, given in sufficient dosage, cause a reduction in alveolar ventilation and a rise in arterial $Pco_2$, and depress the ventilatory response to carbon dioxide.[21] They also cause systemic venodilatation, with a small shift of blood out of the pulmonary circulation (the likely mechanism through which they are effective in pulmonary oedema).

**Anaesthesia**

In most cases, anaesthesia causes an increase in the alveolar/arterial $Po_2$ difference. Several studies have demonstrated that venous admixture is increased, probably due to a combination of true shunt within the lungs and zones of very low $\dot{V}/\dot{Q}$ ratios. An increase in $P\bar{v}O_2$, which may result from a reduction in cardiac output will also increase venous admixture (page 97).

Induction of anaesthesia gives rise to an increased elastic recoil of the lungs and reduced compliance. These changes are associated with a marked reduction in FRC. When a conscious subject (say 1·7m tall) changes from the erect to the supine position FRC decreases from 3000 ml to 2200 ml (Fig. 9). A further reduction in FRC to about 1800 ml occurs after anaesthesia is induced. There is also an increase in airway resistance which correlates with the reduction in lung volume. The cause of the reduction in FRC is still not certain. Whether the patient is ventilated or breathes spontaneously seems to make little difference; there is no correlation between the magnitude of the reduction in FRC and the degree of expiratory muscle activity which is often observed under anaesthesia. There is no convincing evidence that the major cause of FRC reduction is impairment of surfactant activity, although this remains a theoretical possibility. The likeliest explanation is that the resting tone of the diaphragm is reduced as a result of induction of anaesthesia and that it is therefore pushed higher into the chest reducing the gas volume; there may also be an increase in central blood volume.

Closing capacity increases with age so that by 40–50 years it is equal to the FRC in the supine position. Any further reduction in FRC will then lead to the situation where closing capacity exceeds FRC with the result that at the end of expiration and beginning of inspiration there are zones of lung which are perfused but not ventilated. Although the FRC can be raised by the use of PEEP, the $PaO_2$ is still low. In view of the haemodynamic consequences of PEEP this is not very surprising.

It is clear that during general anaesthesia the transport of oxygen through the lungs is often impaired, and *that to ensure adequate arterial oxygenation during an anaesthetic at least 33 per cent oxygen should be administered in the inspired gas mixture.*

**The Ventilation/Perfusion Ratio and Carbon Dioxide Excretion**

As well as affecting oxygen transfer within the lungs, anaesthesia also impairs the efficiency of carbon dioxide excretion. The most important adverse effect is due to a reduction in alveolar ventilation, brought about by (1) direct depression of the respiratory centre; (2) decreased ventilatory response to a rise in arterial $Pco_2$; (3) the addition of apparatus dead space; and (4) an increase in physiological dead space. Another factor which has to be taken into account is that the alveolar-arterial $CO_2$

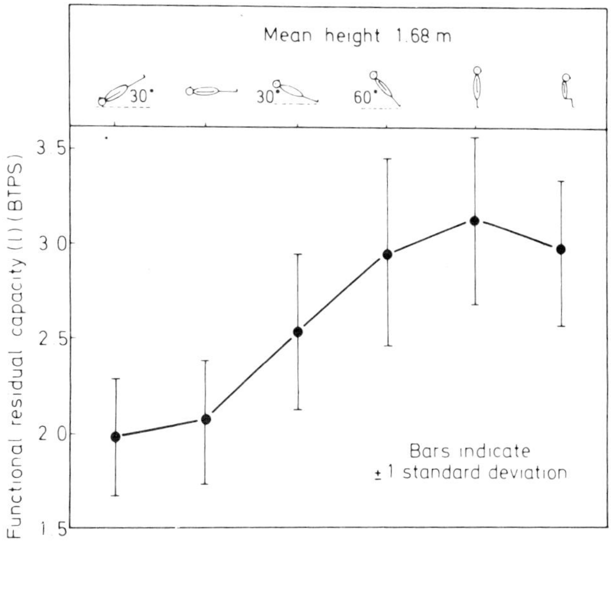


3/Fig. 9.—Studies of the functional residual capacity in various body positions. (Courtesy of Dr. J. F. Nunn and Butterworth and Co.[12])

difference (normal = less than 1 mm Hg, 0·1 kPa) rises during anaesthesia. Nunn and Hill[24] found an average value of 4·5 mm Hg (0·6 kPa) during spontaneous respiration, and 4·7 mm Hg (0·6 kPa) during controlled ventilation. It has been suggested that these findings might be secondary to a fall in pulmonary artery pressure.

### Post-operative Hypoxaemia

Although it has been known for many years that arterial hypoxaemia occurs after major thoracic and abdominal surgery, it has also been shown to be present after much simpler procedures. Nunn and Payne[25] reported a fall in arterial oxygen tension for as long as 12–24 hours following operation. The hypoxaemia is readily correctible by administering a modest concentration of oxygen.[26]

The mechanism of post-operative hypoxaemia may be the same as that during general anaesthesia, namely that the FRC falls below the closing volume of the lungs.

### Pre-operative Assessment and Lung Function

Milledge and Nunn[27] studied the criteria of fitness for anaesthesia in patients with chronic lung disease. They concluded that the forced expiratory volume in one second ($FEV_1$) was a useful pre-operative screening test. If the values of $FEV_1$ fell below 1 litre then it was advisable to supplement this information with blood gas studies. The combination of these results enabled an anaesthetist to predict the post-anaesthetic course. Thus:

Group I
  $FEV_1$ less than 1 litre
    + Normal $PaCO_2$ and $PaO_2$
      . . . normal post-operative course

Group II
  $FEV_1$ less than 1 litre
    + Normal $PaCO_2$ and low $PaO_2$
      . . . require prolonged use of oxygen therapy

Group III
  $FEV_1$ less than 1 litre
    + *high* $PaCO_2$ and *low* $PaO_2$
      . . . require ventilatory support

## THE TRANSPORT OF GASES IN THE BLOOD

### Oxygen

In alveolar air the tension of oxygen is 110 mm Hg (14·7 kPa), whereas it is only 40 mm Hg (5·3 kPa) in the venous blood entering the pulmonary capillaries. This pressure gradient is sufficient to induce oxygen to pass rapidly across the alveolar membrane. On reaching the blood stream the oxygen becomes dissolved in the plasma before finally uniting with haemoglobin for its carriage to the tissues.

**Simple solution of oxygen in the plasma.**—Only a very small proportion of the total oxygen carried in the arterial blood—namely, 0·3 ml per 100 ml of blood (0·3 volumes per cent) at a $PaO_2$ of 100 mm Hg (13·3 kPa)—is physically dissolved in the plasma. Nevertheless this small quantity is of vital importance for it alone reflects the tension of oxygen in the blood ($Po_2$) and also acts as a pathway for the supply of oxygen to haemoglobin. When the blood reaches the tissues it is this small quantity that is first transferred to the cells, while its place is rapidly taken by more oxygen liberated from haemoglobin.

**Haemoglobin.**—Haemoglobin consists of the protein "globin" joined with the pigment "haem", which is an iron-containing porphyrin.[28] The porphyrin nucleus consists of four pyrrol rings joined together by four methine bridges. The iron is in the ferrous ($Fe^{++}$) form and is attached to the N of each pyrrol ring and to the N of the imidazol group in the globin, thus creating a loose "bond" available for union with oxygen to form oxyhaemoglobin. The globin is made up of 4 amino acid chains. There are 2 $\alpha$ chains each containing 141 amino acids and 2 $\beta$ chains each containing 146 amino acids. Other chains having different amino acid sequences also occur.

| | | | |
|---|---|---|---|
| HbA | 2$\alpha$ | 2$\beta$— | adult haemoglobin |
| HbF | 2$\alpha$ | 2$\gamma$— | fetal haemoglobin |
| $HbA_2$ | 2$\alpha$ | 2$\gamma$— | accounts for 2 per cent of total haemoglobin in normal adults. |

In sickle-cell anaemia (p. 603) the $\beta$ chains are abnormal whereas in thalassaemia there is deficient production of either $\alpha$ or $\beta$ chains.

Methaemoglobin consists of haemoglobin in which the iron is present in the ferric ($Fe^{+++}$)

rather than ferrous ($Fe^{++}$) form, and is unable to combine with oxygen. Methaemoglobinaemia may occur

(*a*) because of inadequate conversion of methaemoglobin (which is normally present in small amounts) to haemoglobin—hereditary methaemoglobinaemia, or

(*b*) because of excessive production of methaemoglobin as occurs in poisoning by higher oxides of nitrogen—toxic or acquired methaemoglobinaemia. Conversion of methaemoglobin to haemoglobin can be hastened by reducing agents such as ascorbic acid or methylene blue.

### Oxyhaemoglobin

The reaction of haemoglobin with oxygen occurs in four stages; the rate at which the final stage takes place is much higher than the rate of the other stages and so counteracts the slowing down of the rate of reaction of haemoglobin with oxygen which would be expected, on the basis of the law of mass action, as saturation nears completion.[29]

$$Hb_4 + 0_2 \rightleftharpoons Hb_4 0_2$$
$$Hb_4 0_2 + 0_2 \rightleftharpoons Hb_4 0_4$$
$$Hb_4 0_4 + 0_2 \rightleftharpoons Hb_4 0_6$$
$$Hb_4 0_6 + 0_2 \rightleftharpoons Hb_4 0_8$$

In males the average haemoglobin content of blood is 15·8 g per 100 ml; in females it is 13·7 g. On a strictly molar basis 1 g of fully oxygenated haemoglobin would be expected to contain 1·39 ml oxygen. In practice it has been found that 1 g of oxyhaemoglobin carries 1·31 ml oxygen.[30] Confusion over this discrepancy has meant that several different figures for the oxygen carrying capacity of haemoglobin appear in different texts. At an arterial $Po_2$ of 100 mm Hg (13·3 kPa) haemoglobin is 97·5 per cent saturated. Thus the 15 g of haemoglobin present in 100 ml of blood can carry approximately 19 ml of oxygen. It will be seen, therefore, that every 100 ml of blood passing through the lungs takes up 5 ml of oxygen [19 ml (arterial) – 14 ml (venous) = 5 ml]. Equally, the tissues remove 5 ml per cent or about one-third to one quarter of the available total (Table 4).

### Oxygen Flux

The amount of oxygen leaving the left ventricle per minute in the arterial blood has been termed the "oxygen flux".[12] Ignoring the very small amount of oxygen in physical solution,

$$\text{Oxygen flux} = \begin{matrix}\text{cardiac}\\\text{output}\end{matrix} \times \begin{matrix}\text{arterial}\\\text{oxygen}\\\text{saturation}\end{matrix} \times \begin{matrix}\text{haemoglobin}\\\text{concentration}\end{matrix} \times 1{\cdot}31$$

$$= 5000 \text{ ml/min} \times \frac{98}{100} \times \frac{15{\cdot}6}{100} \text{ g/ml} \times 1{\cdot}31 \text{ ml/g}$$

$$= 1000 \text{ ml/min}$$

where 1·31 is the volume of oxygen (ml) which combines with 1g of haemoglobin. Normally about 250 ml of this oxygen is used up in cellular metabolism and the rest returns to the lungs in the mixed venous blood which is therefore about 75 per cent saturated with oxygen. Because the three variables in the equation (cardiac output, arterial oxygen saturation and haemoglobin concentration) are multiplied together, a relatively trivial reduction of each may result in a catastrophic reduction in oxygen

3/TABLE 4

| *Oxygen* | *Mixed Venous* | *Arterial* |
|---|---|---|
| 1. Amount in solution in plasma | 0·13 ml per cent | 0·3 ml per cent |
| 2. Tension . . . . . . . . | 40 mm Hg (5·3 kPa) | 100 mm Hg (13·3 kPa) |
| 3. Amount combined with haemoglobin (oxyhaemoglobin) | 14 ml per cent | 19 ml per cent |
| 4. Saturation . . . . . . | 75 per cent | 98 per cent |

flux; in addition the oxygen consumption may be increased above 250 ml/min for example in the post-operative patient suffering from "halothane shakes".

## Oxygen Dissociation Curve

The oxyhaemoglobin dissociation curve is shown in Fig. 10. At a pH of 7·4, the $Po_2$ at which the haemoglobin is 50 per cent saturated ($P_{50}$) is 27 mm Hg (3·6 kPa). A low $P_{50}$ implies that the curve is shifted to the left and vice versa. Note that at the upper flat part of the curve changes in $Po_2$ have relatively little effect on haemoglobin saturation and therefore blood oxygen content, whereas over the lower more vertical part of the curve changes in $Po_2$ have a very marked effect on percentage saturation, so facilitating the transfer of oxygen from haemoglobin to the tissues.

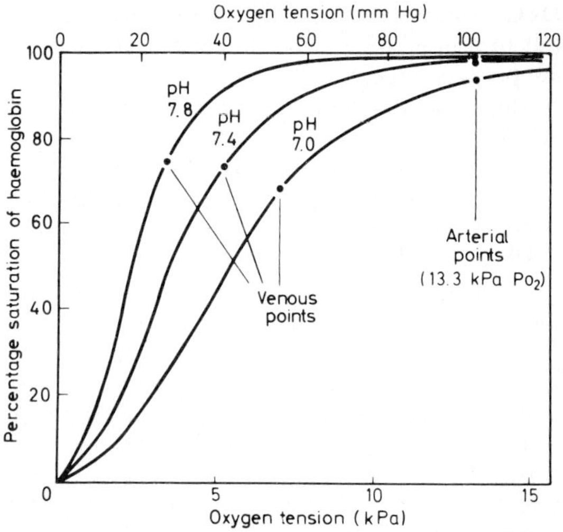


3/Fig. 10.—The oxyhaemoglobin dissociation curve at normal pH (7·4) and at high and low pH (Bohr effect). (Courtesy of Dr. J. F. Nunn and Butterworth and Co.[12])

| $Po_2$ mm Hg | $Po_2$ kPa | Hb saturation % | $O_2$ content of blood ml $O_2$/100 ml blood |
|---|---|---|---|
| 100 | 13·3 | 97·5 | 19·2 |
| ↓ 20* | ↓ 2·7* | ↓ 1·5 | ↓ 0·3 |
| 80 | 10·7 | 96·0 | 18·9 |
| 60 | 8·0 | 91 | 17·9 |
| ↓ 20* | ↓ 2·7* | ↓ 17 | ↓ 3·4 |
| 40 | 5·3 | 74 | 14·5 |

Similar reductions* (20 mm Hg, 2·7 kPa) in $Po_2$ over these two portions of the curve have very different effects. Reducing the $Po_2$ from 60 to 40 mm Hg (8·0 to 5·3 kPa) causes a roughly ten times greater fall in blood oxygen content than reducing the $Po_2$ from 100 to 80 mm Hg (13·3 to 10·7 kPa).

Other molecules as well as oxygen are carried by haemoglobin and these influence the exact position of the dissociation curve. The most important of these are carbon dioxide, hydrogen ions and 2,3 diphosphoglycerate (2,3 DPG), all associated with globin, and carbon monoxide which takes the place of oxygen on the haem radical. These molecules influence the position of the dissociation curve as follows.

(*a*) *pH* (*Bohr effect*).—A fall in pH shifts the curve to the right and a rise shifts it to the left, see Fig. 10. The pH change may be produced by either metabolic and/or respiratory disturbances. The higher carbon dioxide tensions in the tissues causes a shift to the right of the curve so that the haemoglobin more readily gives up its oxygen.

(*b*) *2,3 Diphosphoglycerate* (*2,3 DPG*).—Recently the importance of 2,3 DPG on oxygen uptake and release by haemoglobin has been highlighted.[31] The position of the dissociation curve is related to the concentration of 2,3 DPG within the red cell. This substance combines with globin and modifies oxygen access to the haem chain, a rise in 2,3 DPG being associated with a reduction in the affinity of haemoglobin for oxygen. Therefore a high concentration of 2,3 DPG shifts the curve to the right, and a low concentration shifts it to the left. The 2,3 DPG level is increased in anaemia.

(*c*) *Temperature*.—A fall in temperature shifts the curve to the left. There is no evidence, however, that the tissues suffer hypoxia because there is a coincidental fall in oxygen demand.

(*d*) *Storage of blood*.—In ACD blood there is a rapid fall-off in the concentration of 2,3 DPG in the red cells and the dissociation curve shifts to the left so that recently transfused blood is reluctant to give up oxygen to the tissues. This change becomes significant almost immediately the blood is taken and may take 2–3 days to recover after infusion. The use of citrate-phosphate-dextrose (CPD) as the anticoagulant in stored blood delays the fall in 2,3 DPG for about ten days, at which time the 2,3

DPG level is still near to normal in CPD blood, but in ACD blood has been reduced to about 30 per cent of normal. After two weeks of storage the 2,3 DPG level is virtually zero in ACD blood, and even in CPD blood falls off rapidly during the following week.

### Significance of Shifts in the Oxygen Dissociation Curve

Shifts in the dissociation curve of haemoglobin are usually presented as changes in the $P_{50}$ value, defined as the $Po_2$ at which haemoglobin is 50 per cent saturated. The normal value for the $P_{50}$ is 27 mm Hg (3·6 kPa). A shift to the left lowers the $P_{50}$ and a shift to the right raises it. Changes in $P_{50}$ have only a modest effect on the uptake of oxygen in the lungs, the main consequence of alterations being on the release of oxygen to the tissues. A low $P_{50}$ decreases oxygen availability to the tissues and may therefore lead to cellular hypoxia. The importance of these changes in clinical practice have yet to be determined, but they may be crucial to the survival of the patient following massive blood transfusion.

## Carbon Dioxide

The tissues produce carbon dioxide and this is then given up to the blood circulating through the capillaries. It rapidly enters the plasma and then passes into the red cells. On reaching the pulmonary capillaries the tension of carbon dioxide ($Pco_2$) in the venous blood is 46 mm Hg (6·1 kPa); in the alveoli the tension is 40 mm Hg (5·3 kPa). There is, therefore, a pressure gradient of 6 mm Hg (0·8 kPa) driving carbon dioxide across the alveolar membrane. In normal circumstances each 100 ml of arterial blood carries 48 ml of carbon dioxide.

Carbon dioxide is distributed in the blood in the following manner:

(*a*) *In solution in the plasma*.—Only a small yet very important proportion of the total carbon dioxide (i.e. 5 per cent) is carried in this manner. As with oxygen, this quantity is responsible for determining the tension of the gas in blood and also acts as the intermediary between the air in the alveoli and the inside of the red cell. The majority of the carbon dioxide is present in physical solution in the plasma, but a very small proportion is combined with water to form carbonic acid—$H_2CO_3$.

(*b*) *As bicarbonate* (90 per cent).—Except for the small proportion that is physically dissolved in the plasma, most of the carbon dioxide passes to the red cells where the enzyme *carbonic anhydrase* aids its rapid hydration to form carbonic acid ($H_2CO_3$) (Fig. 11). This enzyme is not found in the plasma. Normally carbon dioxide combines with water very slowly, but in the presence of carbonic anhydrase the whole process is greatly speeded up. Similarly, this enzyme accelerates the same process in the reverse direction when the pulmonary capillaries are reached since it reduces the time for the equilibrium of the reaction $CO_2+H_2O \rightleftharpoons H_2CO_3$ to be reached.

The role of carbonic anhydrase and haemoglobin is depicted in Fig. 11. The key to the whole process is the liberation of oxygen, thus:

$$Hb.O_2 \rightarrow Hb+O_2$$

Carbon dioxide diffuses into the red cell where in the presence of carbonic anhydrase it combines with water to form carbonic acid which dissociates into hydrogen ions and bicarbonate ions:

$$CO_2+H_2O \rightleftharpoons H_2CO_3 \rightleftharpoons H^+ + HCO_3^-$$

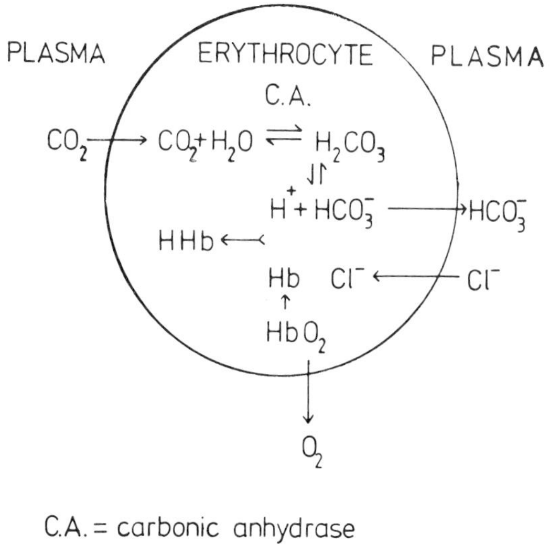


3/Fig. 11.—Chloride shift.

This formation of bicarbonate cannot take place to such an extent in the plasma due to the absence of carbonic anhydrase. Deoxygenated haemoglobin combines with the hydrogen ions

$$Hb + H^+ \rightarrow HHb$$

so favouring the formation of $HCO_3^-$ by displacing the equilibrium of the bicarbonate-forming equation (above) to the right according to the law of mass action. The bicarbonate diffuses out of the red cell into the plasma, and, so that ionic equilibrium is maintained, chloride ions ($Cl^-$) diffuse in the opposite direction from plasma into the red cells. This is called the chloride shift or Hamburger effect (Fig. 11).

When the blood reaches the capillaries of the lung there is a pressure difference of 46−40 = 6 mm Hg (6·1−5·3 = 0·8 kPa) of carbon dioxide on either side of the alveolar membrane, and as it diffuses across this barrier very rapidly this is quite sufficient to ensure an adequate interchange of gases. The process is the reverse of that already described for the uptake of carbon dioxide. First the small percentage physically dissolved in the plasma falls, then as the pressure gradient of dissolved carbon dioxide between the red cell and the plasma widens, so the carbon dioxide leaves the red cell and allows bicarbonate ions to enter, with an opposite movement of chloride ions. Following the formation of carbonic acid the enzyme carbonic anhydrase aids the breakdown to carbon dioxide and water so that finally carbon dioxide passes out into the plasma and from thence across the alveolar membrane.

Plasma bicarbonate, therefore, plays a very important role as the principal storehouse and carrier of carbon dioxide in the blood.

(*c*) *As a carbamino compound* (25 per cent).—Carbon dioxide can combine with the amino groupings of the haemoglobin to form carbamino-haemoglobin:

$$Hb.NH_2 + CO_2 \rightleftharpoons Hb.NH.COOH$$

A smaller amount combines in a similar manner with the plasma proteins. The combination takes place directly between the carbon dioxide and the haemoglobin or plasma protein, as no enzyme—such as carbonic anhydrase—is required. The amount formed is influenced mainly by the degree of oxygen saturation of the blood and not by the carbon dioxide tension.

**Carbon Dioxide Dissociation Curve**

The carbon dioxide dissociation curve relates the carbon dioxide content of blood to the $Pco_2$ to which it is exposed (Fig. 12). The position of this curve depends upon the degree of oxygenation of the blood. The more deoxygenated the blood becomes the more carbon dioxide it carries at a given $Pco_2$: this is called the *Haldane effect*. In Fig. 12 the upper curve is the $CO_2$ content/$Pco_2$ curve for fully deoxygenated blood and the lower curve is for fully oxygenated or arterial blood. Note that the arterial and

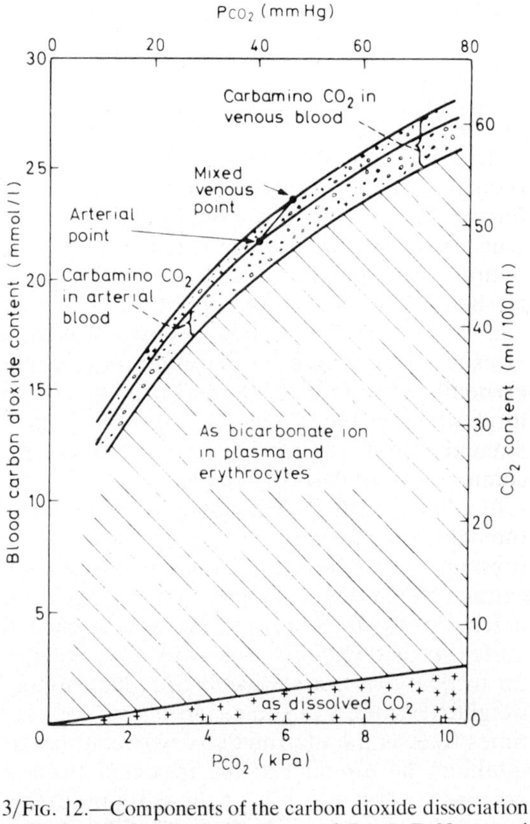


3/Fig. 12.—Components of the carbon dioxide dissociation curve for whole blood. (Courtesy of Dr. J. F. Nunn and Butterworth and Co.[12])

venous points, and that part of the curve for fully oxygenated blood below the arterial point, approximate to a straight line. It is for this reason that blood from zones of lung with high $\dot{V}A/\dot{Q}$ ratios can partly compensate for blood from zones with low $\dot{V}A/\dot{Q}$ ratios (p. 96). The major component of the Haldane effect is the increased carriage of $CO_2$ by reduced haemoglobin as carbamino haemoglobin. In addition, $CO_2$ carriage as bicarbonate is increased.

$$CO_2 + H_2O \rightleftharpoons H_2CO_3 \rightleftharpoons HCO_3^- + H^+$$

Reduced haemoglobin buffers the hydrogen ions, so displacing the equilibrium of this equation to the right and increasing the concentration of bicarbonate ($HCO_3^-$).

Due to the Haldane effect, the uptake of $CO_2$ by capillary blood is facilitated. When this blood reaches the lungs and becomes oxygenated elimination of $CO_2$ is facilitated.

## THE ACID-BASE STATUS OF THE BLOOD

Life is an acidogenic process and from birth until death the body is under a constant obligation to balance hydrogen ion output against hydrogen ion intake and production; the diet normally contains hydrogen ions, mostly in the form of sulphur-containing amino acids of proteins, and the urine is the sole channel of hydrogen ion excretion. The average intake is 50–80 mmol/day, much the same as sodium and potassium, but intermediate metabolism gives rise to enormous hydrogen ion loads: the carbon dioxide produced per day is equivalent to about 1500 mmol of hydrogen ions. Certain circumstances, of which tissue hypoxia is the commonest, give rise to acidosis because the rate of hydrogen ion production outstrips the rate of hydrogen ion neutralisation and excretion; the various buffer systems in the cells and extracellular fluid are the body's only means of defence against such accumulations. The acute buffer storage capacity is capable of absorbing up to 10 mmol of hydrogen ions per kg body weight, i.e. 500–700 in an adult, or nearly ten times the average daily intake. If hydrogen ion intake ceases, hydrogen ion production continues as is made evident by the gradually progressive acidosis which develops in anuric patients. It is of practical importance that hydrogen ion concentration does not reach lethal levels for 7–10 days or even longer. During this time the hydrogen ions produced by metabolism are absorbed by the various buffer systems in the cells and extracellular fluid. Renal control of hydrogen ion output is slow to develop and several days are needed for urinary excretion of hydrogen ions to increase from average to maximal amounts: the kidneys make no significant contribution to the control of sudden fluxes in hydrogen ion concentration. Tissue hypoxia, starvation and diminished ventilatory reserve are accompaniments of many surgical operations: all will tend to strain the buffer capacity of the body and it is therefore important that patients are brought to surgery with the least possible encroachment of their capacity to deal with acute rises in hydrogen ion concentration. For this among other reasons diabetes, heart failure and uraemia should all be brought under control as far as is practicable before operation. The contribution of haemoglobin to the buffer capacity of blood is considerable and tends to be overlooked on account of its more obvious importance in oxygen carriage.

### Terminology

The relationship between acids and bases can be described by the following equation:

$$\text{Acid} \rightleftharpoons H^+ + \text{Base}^-$$

*An acid* is a hydrogen ion donor. A strong acid, such as hydrochloric acid, is almost completely dissociated when in an aqueous solution, in other words, the equilibrium above is displaced far to the right. A weak acid is less completely dissociated. *A base* is a hydrogen ion acceptor. A strong base is one for which the above equilibrium is displaced almost completely to the left, and a weak base is one for which it is displaced only partly to the left. *Buffers* are substances which by their presence in solution increase the amount of acid or alkali which must be added to cause a unit shift in pH. The combination in solution of a weak acid and its strong base (as a salt) is called a *buffer pair.* The weak acid is the *buffer acid* and the strong base is the *buffer base.* A buffer system obeys the Law of Mass Action, so that

$$K\,[\text{Acid}] = [H^+] \times [\text{Base}^-]$$

where K is a constant. Rearranging this formula

$$[H^+] = K \frac{[Acid]}{[Base^-]}$$

and converting to negative logarithms to the base 10, this equation becomes:

$$pH = pK' + \log \frac{[Base^-]}{[Acid]}$$

For the bicarbonate buffer system the equation becomes:

$$pH = pK' + \log \frac{[HCO_3^-]}{[H_2CO_3]}$$

This is the Henderson-Hasselbalch equation. $[HCO_3^-]$ represents the plasma bicarbonate, and $[H_2CO_3]$ represents the sum of the dissolved carbon dioxide and carbonic acid, according to the equation

$$CO_2 + H_2O \rightleftharpoons H_2CO_3$$

For any given buffer system the pK is constant, so the pH will depend on the log of the ratio

$$\frac{[Base]}{[Acid]}$$

If acid or alkali is added the smallest change in this ratio and therefore in pH will result if initially [Base] = [Acid]. Under these circumstances pH = pK (since $\frac{[base]}{[acid]} = 1$, and log 1 = 0). So a buffer resists pH change best when it is operating at a pH close to its pK.

In the plasma, in the absence of carbonic anhydrase which is found inside the red cells the reaction

$$CO_2 + H_2O \rightleftharpoons H_2CO_3$$

is very slow and only about one-thousandth of the $CO_2$ dissolved in the plasma forms $H_2CO_3$, the vast majority being present in physical solution. (Remember that we are talking here about dissolved $CO_2$; most of the $CO_2$ formed by metabolism finds its way into red cells where its hydration to carbonic acid is sped up enormously by carbonic anhydrase. The carbonic acid then dissociates to give rise to $HCO_3^-$ which diffuses into plasma). The $H_2CO_3$ in the equation above for the bicarbonate buffering system can therefore be replaced by

$$\alpha \ Pco_2$$

where $\alpha$ is the solubility coefficient for $CO_2$, 0·03 mmol $l^{-1}$ mm $Hg^{-1}$ at 37° C (0·23 mmol $l^{-1}$ $kPa^{-1}$). The equation then becomes:

$$pH = pK + \log \frac{[HCO_3^-]}{\alpha \ Pco_2}$$

The value of pK is 6·1 at 37° C

At a $Pco_2$ of 40 mm Hg (5·3 kPa) the plasma bicarbonate concentration is about 25 mmol/l, therefore

$$pH = 6{\cdot}1 + \log \frac{25}{0{\cdot}03 \times 40} = 7{\cdot}4$$

Numerous graphic representations of the Henderson-Hasselbalch equation have been suggested, the best known being the pH-bicarbonate plot,[32] and the pH-log $Pco_2$ plot.[33]

The acidity of a solution depends on the concentration of hydrogen ions contained in it, and is most often expressed in pH units. pH is the negative logarithm of the molar hydrogen ion concentration (or, more correctly, the hydrogen ion activity).

The term pH (p stands for Potenz or Power) was introduced by Sorensen as a more convenient expression than molar hydrogen ion concentrations. The hydrogen ion concentration of pure water is $10^{-7}$ mol/l. Using the pH notation, the pH of pure water is 7·0, since $pH = \frac{1}{\log [H^+]} = -\log [H^+]$

The interconversion of $H^+$ and pH is best shown by two examples.

*Example 1.*

The normal pH of whole blood is 7·4. What is its hydrogen ion concentration?

We can say therefore that

$[H^+] = 10^{-7.4}$ mol/l or $10^{-7.4} \times 10^9$ nmol/l

(since $10^9$ nanomol = 1 mol)

$10^{-7.4} \times 10^9 = 10^{1.6} = 40$ nmol/l

(the antilog of 1·6 is 40)

*Example 2.*

If the hydrogen ion concentration is 80 nmol/l, what is the pH?

80 nmol/l = $80 \times 10^{-9}$ mol/l

The negative log of this quantity is the pH, so, the negative log of 80 = −1·9

the negative log of $10^{-9}$ = +9

Having taken logs we now add to effect multiplication −1·9+9 = 7·1

therefore pH = 7·1

You will notice from these two examples that a

pH reduction of 0·3 units represents a doubling of [$H^+$] and vice versa.

Table 5 shows equivalent values of $H^+$ and pH from the most acid level found in gastric acid, equivalent to decinormal (N/10) hydrochloric acid, to pancreatic secretion. The precise figures show considerable variation from subject to subject, so these are given only as a guide.

3/TABLE 5

| pH | $H^+$ (nmol/l) | |
|---|---|---|
| 1 | 100,000,000 ($10^8$) | gastric acid |
| 6·8 | 158 | |
| 7·0 | 100 | |
| 7·2 | 63 | |
| 7·4 | 40 | arterial blood |
| 7·6 | 25 | |
| 7·8 | 16 | |
| 8·0 | 10 | pancreatic secretion |

The *$P_{CO_2}$ of a liquid* is an extension of the concept of the $P_{CO_2}$ of gas mixtures. The $P_{CO_2}$ of a gas mixture saturated with water vapour at 37° C is given by the equation:

$$P_{CO_2} = F_{CO_2} \times (P_B - 47) \text{ mm Hg}$$
$$[F_{CO_2} \times (P_B - 6 \cdot 3) \text{ kPa}]$$

where $F_{CO_2}$ is the fractional concentration of carbon dioxide in the mixture, $P_B$ is the barometric pressure (760 mm Hg or 101 kPa), and 47 mm Hg (6·3 kPa) is the saturated vapour pressure of water at 37° C. The $P_{CO_2}$ of a solution of carbon dioxide in a liquid such as plasma is best understood by considering a gas-liquid system in equilibrium. The carbon dioxide tension of the liquid phase is equal to that in the gas phase when no net exchange of $CO_2$ occurs between the two phases. At any given equilibrium the carbon dioxide content of the liquid is a reflection of the $P_{CO_2}$ of the gas phase, and therefore the $CO_2$ content of the liquid can be described by stating the $P_{CO_2}$ of the gas phase. The $P_{CO_2}$ of blood is thus defined as that $P_{CO_2}$ in a gas mixture which, when in contact with the blood, results in no net exchange of $CO_2$ between the two phases.

An *acidosis* is said to be present when the hydrogen ion concentration in blood is higher than normal (low pH), or would be if no compensation had occurred. An *alkalosis* is present when the hydrogen ion concentration is lower than normal (high pH), or would be if compensation had not occurred. These definitions enable combinations of changes to be described, e.g. a respiratory acidosis and a metabolic alkalosis present at the same time, although the pH may lie within the normal range. A *respiratory acidosis* or *alkalosis* is a change, or potential change, in pH resulting from alterations in the $P_{CO_2}$. A *metabolic acidosis* or *alkalosis* is a change, or potential change, in pH resulting from alterations in the non-volatile acids in the blood, e.g. lactic acid.

It is not uncommon for there to be a mixed respiratory and metabolic acid/base disturbance. The 'base excess' measurement is one way of quantifying the metabolic component. Two examples will illustrate this term:

1. Initial measurements on an arterial blood sample (haemoglobin = 15 g/dl) are

   pH 7·50 $\quad$ $Pa_{CO_2}$ 52 mm Hg

   The blood sample is kept at 37° C and equilibrated with a $CO_2$ gas mixture which will make the $P_{CO_2}$ 40 and therefore remove the respiratory component of the pH abnormality. The pH is now 7·59.

   Next a strong acid, such as hydrochloric, is added to titrate the pH back to 7·4—the amount of acid required per litre of blood is found to be 15 mmol/l.

   The base excess of the original sample = 15 mmol/l.

2. Initial measurements on an arterial blood sample (haemoglobin = 15 g/dl) are

   pH 7·22 $\quad$ $Pa_{CO_2}$ 22 mm Hg

   Equilibrate the sample with a $CO_2$ gas mixture to make $Pa_{CO_2}$ 40 mm Hg:

   then pH = 7·1

   (this pH does not reflect the full extent of the acidosis as some hydrogen ions are bound to blood buffers).

   Titrate with strong alkali (NaOH) to bring pH to 7·40.

   Amount of alkali required = 18 mmol/l of blood

   Therefore

base excess = −18 mmol/l } both expressions
base deficit = 18 mmol/l } are commonly used

Obviously there should normally be neither a base excess nor deficit so the normal value for base excess is zero. Base excess is *defined* as the titratable base on titration to pH 7·40 at $P_{CO_2}$ 40 mm Hg (5·3 kPa) and temperature 37° C.

Nowadays, it is not necessary to perform this

time-consuming titration and in practice the base excess is derived from either

(*a*) nomograms, e.g. Figs. 13 and 14.
(*b*) acid-base slide rule (Severinghaus[36]).
(*c*) mathematically, as in many automatic blood gas analysers.

The base excess curve can be derived experimentally by diluting blood to different levels of haemoglobin, adding acid or alkali to give different levels of base excess and then equilibrating these samples with different $CO_2$ mixtures and plotting $P_{CO_2}$ against pH. Families of curves are produced (Fig. 15) and their points of intersection are plotted as the base excess curve. Unless the values of $P_{CO_2}$ and pH of a blood sample happen to give a point on the base excess curve, it is necessary to know the haemoglobin value in order to use the appropriate buffer slope to intersect the base excess curve; the higher the haemoglobin the better buffered the blood and so the steeper the buffer line as indicated in Fig. 15. The base excess measurement (unlike buffer base) is independent of the haemoglobin concentration—altering the haemoglobin concentration of a blood sample would result in a change in pH and $P_{CO_2}$ but *no* change in base excess.

*Buffer base* is the sum of the concentrations of all the buffer anions in the blood ($HCO_3^-$, phosphate, protein, haemoglobin, etc.). The

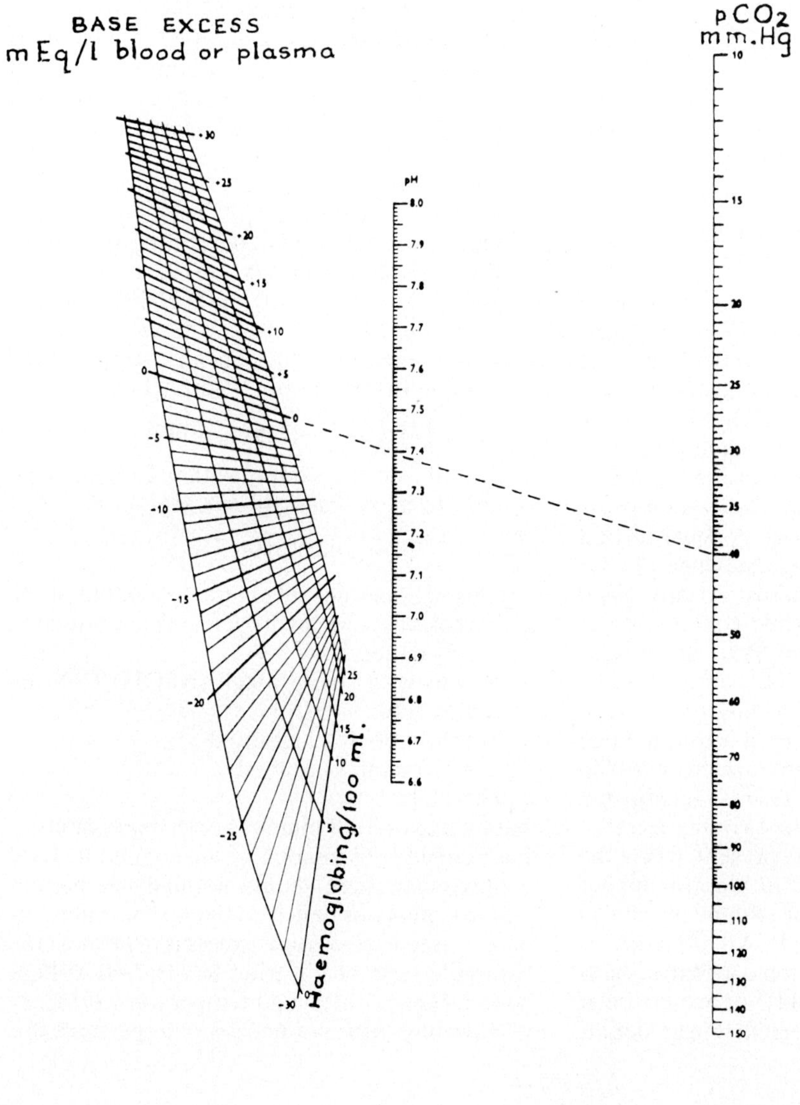


3/Fig. 13.—Nomogram for blood acid-base calculation. (Courtesy of O. Siggaard-Andersen and the Editor of the *Scandinavian Journal of Clinical and Laboratory Investigation*.[34])

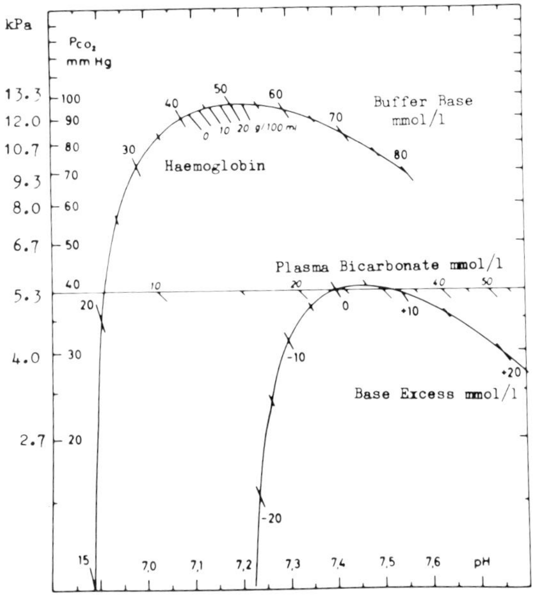


3/FIG. 14.—Nomogram for blood showing $P_{CO_2}$ plotted logarithmically against pH. (Courtesy of O. Sigaard-Andersen and the Editor of the *Scandinavian Journal of Clinical and Laboratory Investigation* and Radiometer A/S, Copenhagen.[34])

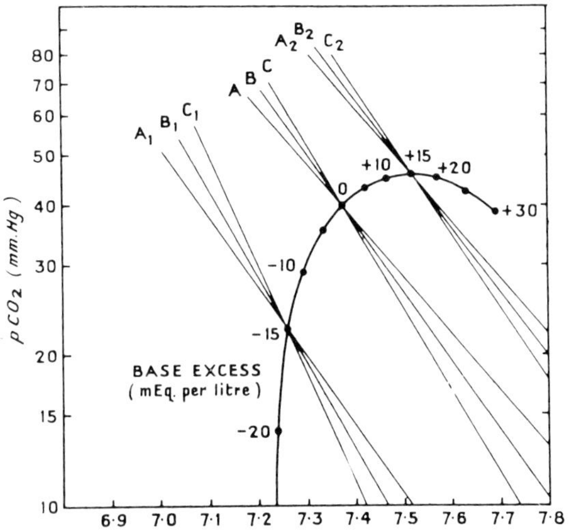


3/FIG. 15.—pH/log $P_{CO_2}$, lines for blood samples with different haemoglobin concentration and different content of base. A, B and C represent samples of normal blood with a haemoglobin concentration of 0, 10 and 20 g per 100 ml respectively. $A_1$, $B_1$ and $C_1$ show the displacement after addition of fixed acid (15mmol acetic acid per litre blood); and $A_2$, $B_2$ and $C_2$ after addition of base (15 mmol sodium carbonate per litre blood). The points of intersection of these lines form a curve (the base-excess curve) which indicates the amount of base excess (positive values) and base deficit (negative values) in any blood sample. (Courtesy of P. Astrup *et al.* and the Editor of the *Lancet*.[35])

normal value depends on the haemoglobin concentration and so is reduced in anaemia. Apart from changes in haemoglobin it is increased in metabolic alkalosis and decreased in metabolic acidosis. A rise in $P_{CO_2}$ does not affect it since although $[HCO_3^-]$ increases, the extra $[H^+]$ combine with $Hb^-$ so that the concentration of this ion is correspondingly reduced:

$$CO_2 + H_2O \rightleftharpoons H_2CO_3 \rightleftharpoons H^+ + HCO_3^-$$
$$\updownarrow$$
$$H^+ + Hb^- \rightleftharpoons HHb$$

*Standard bicarbonate* is the bicarbonate concentration (mmol/l) of plasma of fully oxygenated blood which has been equilibrated at 37° C with a gas mixture having a $P_{CO_2}$ of 40 mm Hg (5·3 kPa). The normal range is 22–26 mmol/l.

Of the three measurements—base excess, buffer base and standard bicarbonate—the first is the most widely used and the most useful, but like the others has the disadvantage that it depends on an assumed *in vitro* buffer line. In practice, the buffer line of the patient's blood *in vitro* may be different from the standard line. Furthermore, the *in vivo* buffering line is of greater significance although again the patient's *in vivo* buffering line may differ from the normal.

The normal values and changes found in the blood resulting from uncompensated alterations in acid-base status are shown in Table 6.

### Buffering Systems in the Body

About three-quarters of the chemical buffering power in the body lies within the cells, and is due to the high concentration of intracellular proteins, phosphate and other inorganic compounds. The remainder is due to the buffering power of the extracellular fluids. The buffering power of a system depends on the pH at which it is working and on the concentrations of the buffer elements.

**The bicarbonate buffer system.**—As previously explained this system consists of a mixture of $H_2CO_3$ (the weak acid) and $NaHCO_3$ (the strong base). The relationship between

3/TABLE 6
THE NORMAL VALUES AND CHANGES FOUND IN THE BLOOD RESULTING FROM UNCOMPENSATED CHANGES IN ACID-BASE STATUS

| | pH | $P_{CO_2}$ | *Plasma bicarbonate* | *Total buffer base* | *Base excess* | *Standard bicarbonate* |
|---|---|---|---|---|---|---|
| Normal values | 7·35–7·44 | 36–46 mm Hg (4·8–6·1 kPa) | 23–28 mmol/l | 44–48 mmol/l | 0 ± 3 mmol/l | 22–26 mmol/l |
| Respiratory acidosis | Low | High | High | Normal | Normal | Normal |
| Respiratory alkalosis | High | Low | Low | Normal | Normal | Normal |
| Metabolic acidosis | Low | Normal | Low | Low | Negative | Low |
| Metabolic alkalosis | High | Normal | High | High | Positive | High |

their concentrations and the pH is described by the Henderson-Hasselbalch equation:

$$pH = pK' + \log \frac{[HCO_3^-]}{[H_2CO_3]}$$

so that the pH is determined by the ratio $\frac{[HCO_3^-]}{[H_2CO_3]}$. In Fig. 16 the relation between the relative concentrations of the two and the pH is shown. This S-shaped curve is typical of many buffers. The following points should be noted: (1) The buffering power of the system is greatest when the slope of the curve is steepest so that, for the addition of a given amount of acid or base the smallest change in pH occurs around this part of the curve. (2) The buffer system is most efficient when the concentrations of $HCO_3^-$ and $H_2CO_3$ are equal, or when $pH = pK$ (under these conditions $\log \frac{[HCO_3^-]}{[H_2CO_3]} = O$). Once the relative concentrations of bicarbonate and carbonic acid exceed about 8:1 in either direction the buffering power of the system falls off rapidly. Normally the system functions at a pH of around 7·4, when the ratio of bicarbonate to carbonic acid is 20:1, well outside its optimal working range, but very well placed to combat acidosis.

From these considerations it is evident that the *chemical* buffering power of the bicarbonate system in the body is poor. However, its efficiency is vastly improved by the fact that both the carbonic acid and bicarbonate concentrations can be regulated by the body, the former by the lungs and the latter by the kidneys. Herein lies the importance of the bicarbonate buffer in the regulation of the acid-base state of the body. It is the only buffer which can be physiologically adjusted to maintain a normal pH. For instance, if a strong acid is added to the blood the following reactions occur:

$$HCl + NaHCO_3 = H_2CO_3 + NaCl$$

$$H_2CO_3 \rightleftarrows H_2O + \boxed{CO_2} \rightarrow$$

Excreted by the lungs

In the first instance the strong acid is "swapped" for a weak acid (chemical buffering). The carbonic acid dissociates into water and $CO_2$, and the latter is excreted by the lungs (physiological buffering).

**The phosphate buffering system.**—This works in exactly the same way as the bicarbonate system, except that the $NaH_2PO_4$ (sodium dihydrogen phosphate) is the weak acid and $Na_2HPO_4$ (disodium hydrogen phosphate) is

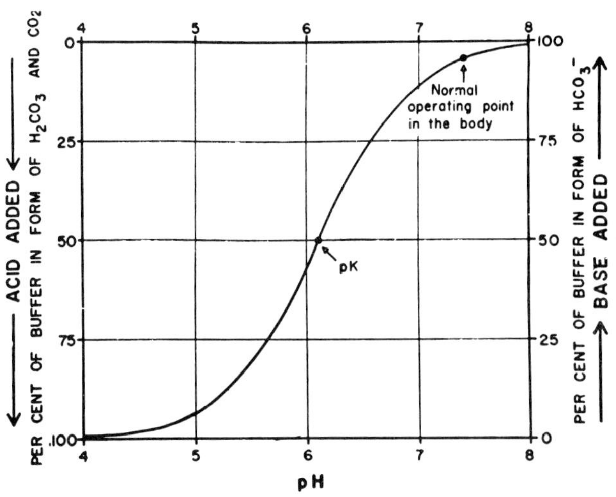


3/FIG. 16.—The reaction curve for the bicarbonate buffer system. (Courtesy of A. C. Guyton from *A Textbook of Medical Physiology*, published by W. B. Saunders Co.)

the strong base. The system is a chemical buffer. The pK of the system is 6·8, so that it is working fairly close to its optimal pH.

**Proteins as buffers.**—Proteins are quantitatively the most important buffers in the body. They contain acidic and basic groups, which make up "buffer pairs". An example of an acidic group is $-COOH$, which can dissociate into $-COO^- + H^+$, and an example of a basic group is $-NH_2$, which can accept a hydrogen ion to form $-NH_3^+$. The pKs of the different protein buffer systems vary, but many are around 7·4, so that in blood and extracellular fluid they are working at or near their most efficient ranges.

**Haemoglobin as a buffer.**—Haemoglobin is responsible for half the buffering power of the blood. It acts as a buffer both because it is a protein and, more important, because of the ability of the imidazole groups within the molecule to accept $H^+$ ions. The acidity of these groups is influenced by the oxygenation and reduction of haemoglobin, the point to remember being that haemoglobin is a weaker acid in the reduced form than when it is oxygenated (Fig. 17). When oxygenated haemoglobin gives up oxygen to the tissues it becomes reduced and is therefore more able to accept $H^+$ ions and $CO_2$. In the lungs the reverse effect occurs.

The buffers in the blood, in order of importance, are haemoglobin, bicarbonate and plasma proteins, and phosphate. In interstitial fluid the main buffers are bicarbonate, phosphate, and interstitial proteins. In the cells the main buffers are proteins, phosphate, and other inorganic substances.

### Carbon Dioxide Stores

A large amount of $CO_2$ is contained in the body, about 120 litres in all. Because of this great volume the total amount can only be altered rather slowly as a result of an inappropriate change in ventilation. The $CO_2$ stores can be considered to be contained in three compartments depending on the possible rate of exchange of the gas—fast, medium and slow. The fast compartment consists of the blood and high blood-flow organs such as the brain, heart and kidneys in which the tissues $Pco_2$ levels tend to follow the alveolar $Pco_2$ rather closely. The medium compartment consists mainly of resting skeletal muscle, and the slow compartment of bone and fatty tissue. The size of the three compartments is different, the slow compartment having the greatest capacity for storing $CO_2$, and the fast one the smallest.

From the above facts it follows that the final arterial $Pco_2$ changes resulting from a stepwise change in ventilation will be delayed, and it will take time for a new equilibrium to be attained. This time is faster for a stepwise increase in ventilation than it is for a decrease. Thus following a sudden increase in ventilation a new equilibrium is reached after about 20 minutes, the half-time for the change being 3–4 minutes. Following a sudden decrease in ventilation the

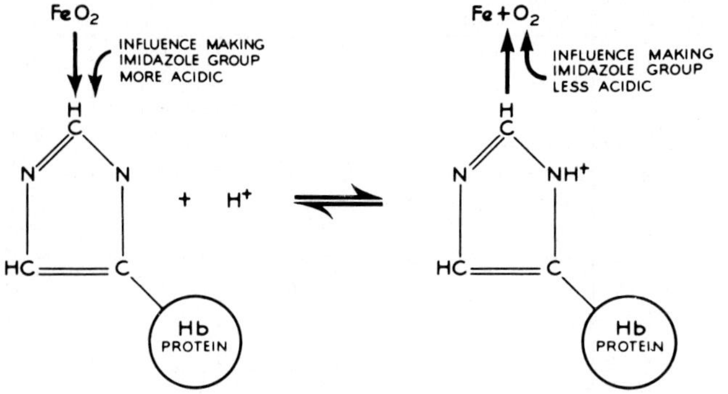


3/FIG. 17.—The effect of the oxygen saturation of haemoglobin upon the buffering power of the imidazole group. Reduced haemoglobin is a better buffer than oxygenated haemoglobin. (Courtesy of H. W. Davenport from *The ABC of Acid-Base Chemistry*, published by the University of Chicago Press.[32])

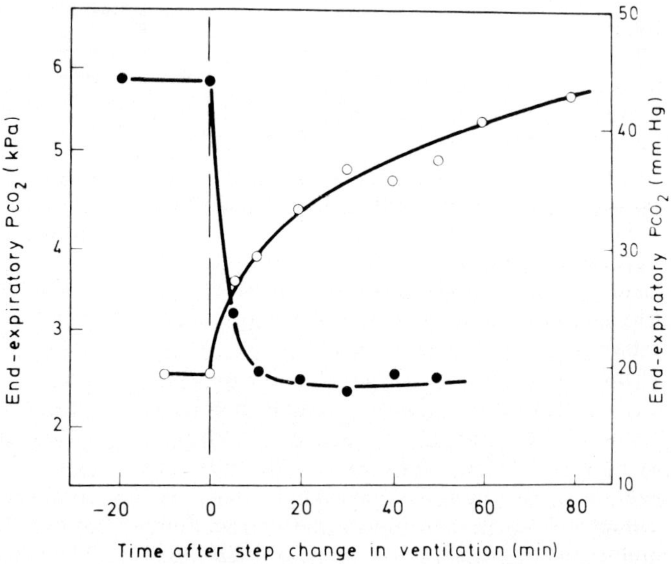


3/FIG. 18.—Changes in end-tidal $P_{CO_2}$ after a sudden increase (solid circles •) or decrease (open circles ○) in ventilation. (Courtesy of Dr. J. F. Nunn and Butterworth and Co.[12])

half-time is 15–20 minutes and new equilibrium may not have been reached after as long as one hour.

**Respiratory Acidosis** (Hypercapnia)

The normal arterial $P_{CO_2}$ (at normal $Pa_{O_2}$) is 35–45 mm Hg (4·7–6·0 kPa). The term "respiratory acidosis" means that the $Pa_{CO_2}$ is higher than normal. This can be produced by

1. $CO_2$ production constant; alveolar ventilation ($\dot{V}_A$) reduced
2. $CO_2$ production raised; $\dot{V}_A$ not raised sufficiently to excrete the extra $CO_2$

or 3. $F_{I}CO_2$ raised, e.g. rebreathing or breathing $CO_2$ gas mixture.

In addition to the rise in $Pa_{CO_2}$, there is an increase in bicarbonate and hydrogen ion concentrations (fall in pH):

$$CO_2 + H_2O \rightleftharpoons H_2CO_3 \rightleftharpoons H^+ + HCO_3^-$$

if $CO_2$ is increased, the equilibrium is displaced to the right.

The kidney compensates for acidosis by excreting $H^+$ ions and retaining bicarbonate. This secondary response is slow to develop, and it may take many days for full compensation to occur. The response to a chronic respiratory acidosis is therefore a metabolic alkalosis which tends to return the pH to normal, In the presence of acute hypercapnia, such as happens during general anaesthesia, there is no time for any appreciable renal compensation to occur.

During apnoea the arterial $P_{CO_2}$ rises about 3–6 mm Hg (0·4–0·8 kPa) per minute and $H^+$ ions accumulate at a rate of 10 mmol/min. This is some 20 times faster than the kidney can excrete them.

The systemic effects of hypercapnia are widespread. The central nervous effects include impairment of mental activity and loss of consciousness, a rise in cerebral blood flow and CSF pressure and the stimulation of respiration, followed by depression if the $P_{CO_2}$ rises further. 30 per cent carbon dioxide will produce anaesthesia but may cause convulsions. General sympathetic over-activity occurs. If a high inspired oxygen tension is not delivered to the patient hypoxaemia follows hypercapnia. Profound effects are seen in the circulation. The heart muscle is depressed, although this effect is offset by the increased sympathetic activity, and a rise in cardiac output follows, accompanied by peripheral, including cerebral, vasodilatation but pulmonary vasoconstriction.

High concentrations of carbon dioxide depress nervous conduction in the heart, particularly in the bundle of His, so that heart block and a slow ventricular rhythm are commonly observed with an increased myocardial irritability. A rise in the carbon dioxide level of the blood increases the secretion of catecholamines (principally noradrenaline) from the sympathetic nerve-endings within the myocardium, and there is also an increase in plasma adrenaline and noradrenaline due to secretion from the adrenal glands, although the sensitivity of target organs is reduced by a high $P_{CO_2}$. Thus, with most anaesthetic agents – principally cyclopropane and halothane – the higher the carbon dioxide level of the blood the greater is the chance of dysrhythmias. As both these agents are respiratory depressants, hypoventilation bears a close correlation with the onset of ventricular dysrhythmia. Furthermore, both these agents "sensitise" the myocardium to this increased catecholamine secretion so that both improving ventilation and reducing the depth of anaesthesia will help to restore normal rhythm.

Increased bleeding is seen in surgical wounds, the blood pressure rises, and the patient presents with a warm skin, dilated veins and a bounding pulse. Dysrhythmias occur, and are especially likely to happen during cyclopropane or halothane anaesthesia. There is a small rise in plasma potassium, and the oxyhaemoglobin dissociation curve is shifted to the right. It is important to remember that under anaesthesia many of the above signs may be masked.

Under anaesthesia hypercapnia may be caused by: (a) Badly chosen or malfunctioning apparatus, e.g. using adult apparatus on a child, incorrectly assembled apparatus or worn out soda-lime. (b) The accidental administration of carbon dioxide. (c) Hypoventilation due to such factors as central respiratory depression, the misuse of relaxants, airway obstruction and metabolic alkalosis.

**Hypoventilation during anaesthesia.**—Under anaesthesia the function of the lungs is often impeded. For example, most sedative and anaesthetic agents depress the activity of the respiratory centres. Thus, many patients breathing spontaneously through any anaesthetic system show a rise in the carbon dioxide tension of the blood. In some cases the degree of hypoventilation may be greater than realised and the $P_{CO_2}$ then rapidly reaches very high levels. It is, therefore, important to emphasise that during anaesthesia the anaesthetist (not the patient) is largely responsible for controlling the carbon dioxide tension at about the normal level. The principal difficulty for the anaesthetist is to recognise minor degrees of hypoventilation; the time-honoured custom of looking at the reservoir bag and thinking that ventilation is "adequate" is often grossly erroneous. Fluctuations in arterial $P_{CO_2}$ from 40–60 mm Hg (5·3–8·0 kPa) are probably of little consequence in the normal, healthy patient but values in excess of 80 mm Hg (10·7 kPa) denote severe and dangerous hypoventilation. When the level rises to 110 mm Hg (14·7 kPa), carbon dioxide narcosis occurs and the patient will not recover consciousness when the anaesthetic drugs are withdrawn. If, at this moment, the patient is allowed to breathe room air simply because the operation is finished, he will not only have to contend with the disadvantages of alveoli filled with anaesthetic gases escaping from the circulation (diffusion hypoxia) and the uneven ventilation-perfusion ratio which normally follows anaesthesia, but also with a reduced quantity of available oxygen from the lungs due to the high carbon dioxide tension. Hypoxia will occur, as shown in Table 7.

Fluctuations—both up and down—in the carbon dioxide content of the plasma are not

3/TABLE 7
PARTIAL PRESSURE OF GASES IN ALVEOLI, BREATHING AIR

| | *Normal ventilation (arterial* $P_{CO_2}$ *= 40 mm Hg or 5·3 kPA)* | *Hypoventilation (arterial* $P_{CO_2}$ *= 100 mm Hg or 13·3 kPa)* |
|---|---|---|
| Oxygen | 95 mm Hg (12·7 kPa) | 35 mm Hg (4·7 kPa) |
| Nitrogen | 578 mm Hg (77·1 kPa) | 578 mm Hg (77·1 kPa) |
| Carbon dioxide | 40 mm Hg (5·3 kPa) | 100 mm Hg (13·3 kPa) |
| Water vapour | 47 mm Hg (6·3 kPa) | 47 mm Hg (6·3 kPa) |
| Total | 760 mm Hg (101 kPa) | 760 mm Hg (101 kPa) |

always due to respiratory complications but may equally be the result of changes in tissue metabolism. Both respiratory acidosis and metabolic acidosis sometimes occur in a patient at the same time under conditions of anaesthesia.

**Respiratory Alkalosis** (Hypocapnia)

This state of affairs commonly occurs during controlled ventilation. Excessive ventilation leads to a reduction in the $P_{CO_2}$. The kidney compensates for a rise in pH by excreting more $HCO_3^-$ ions and reabsorbing more $H^+$ ions, thus producing an alkaline urine. The secondary response to a respiratory alkalosis is therefore a metabolic acidosis, but in an anaesthetised patient this secondary response is reduced by the fall in renal blood flow caused by the anaesthetic agents. However, it is not uncommon to find a mild metabolic acidosis in the anaesthetised and hyperventilated patient. An uncompensated respiratory alkalosis leads to the following changes in the blood: a low $P_{CO_2}$, a low plasma bicarbonate, a high pH and a normal base excess and standard bicarbonate.

Other features of alkalosis are hypokalaemia, increased neuromuscular excitability sometimes producing tetany, and a shift to the left of the haemoglobin-oxygen dissociation curve.

The principal theoretical danger of a respiratory alkalosis under anaesthesia is cerebral vasoconstriction, as it is known that the $P_{CO_2}$ of the blood reaching the brain largely controls the diameter of these vessels. Thus, a severe alkalosis may produce intense cerebral vasoconstriction. Cerebral effects of hyperventilation, such as euphoria and analgesia, have been demonstrated but whether they are due to cerebral vasoconstriction or to a direct action of a low $CO_2$ tension on the cells is not definitely known, although the latter seems to be much more likely. Satisfactory evidence that long periods of even severe respiratory alkalosis lead to cerebral damage is still lacking and most clinicians believe that a mild respiratory alkalosis is more beneficial for the patient than a mild respiratory acidosis. Furthermore, severe vasoconstriction is probably prevented by the reaction of the cerebral vessels to the change of oxygen tension, because a reduced oxygen tension leads to cerebral vasodilatation.

During anaesthesia with controlled ventilation a low $P_{CO_2}$ causes the cardiac output to fall. In fact one of the main determinants of the cardiac output during anaesthesia is the $P_{CO_2}$ level. As the $P_{CO_2}$ rises from low through normal to high values the cardiac output increases, at first due only to increases in the stroke volume, and then to increases in both stroke volume and in heart rate. These changes are accompanied by a rise in mean arterial pressure and in left ventricular stroke work, and by a fall in peripheral resistance. Other causes of respiratory alkalosis are hypoxia, pain and anxiety, pregnancy, metabolic acidosis and salicylate overdose.

**Metabolic Acidosis**

A metabolic acidosis follows the accumulation in the body of non-volatile acids, e.g. lactic acid, or aceto-acetic and $\alpha$-keto-glutaric acids in uncontrolled diabetes mellitus. Uncompensated, the changes seen in blood are as follows: a low pH, low plasma bicarbonate, normal $P_{CO_2}$, a negative base excess and a low standard bicarbonate. These changes are usually followed by a secondary hyperventilation with a fall in the $P_{CO_2}$, so that the pH tends to return towards normal.

The effects of a metabolic acidosis may be severe. The heart muscle is depressed and the cardiac output falls. Intense peripheral vasoconstriction may occur. These changes tend to perpetuate the acidosis so that a vicious circle is set up. The hydrogen ions will tend to displace potassium ions from the intracellular fluid with the result that hyperkalaemia can be produced, especially if renal function is poor. The cardiovascular responses to sympathetic activity and sympathomimetic drugs are reduced so that the natural protective mechanisms are interfered with. Metabolic acidosis stimulates the peripheral and central chemoreceptors. It must also be remembered that the haemoglobin-oxygen dissociation curve is moved to the right.

A mild metabolic acidosis sometimes occurs in patients undergoing general anaesthesia (see below). It is commonly observed after a period of extracorporeal perfusion, after circulatory arrest and hypothermia, and immediately following the temporary occlusion of a major vessel such as the aorta. Other causes are massive blood transfusion, renal failure, diabetic coma and salicylate poisoning, hypoxia, low cardiac output and lactic acidosis.

If the pH is very low (less than about 7·1) the acidosis itself is life-threatening because of its effect on the heart and, therefore, sodium bicarbonate should be given intravenously without delay. If the acidosis is less severe, management depends upon the diagnosis, associated disorders of electrolyte and fluid balance and whether the acidosis is still developing. So for example a patient with a diabetic ketoacidosis and base excess of −10 mmol/l will correct his own acidosis, given saline and insulin, and probably does not require bicarbonate. A patient with a base excess of −10 mmol/l during open heart surgery probably does require bicarbonate because they can ill-afford the depressant effect of the low pH on the myocardium. It is important not to give too much bicarbonate as this may have several undesirable effects:

1. Excessive sodium load, which is especially dangerous in patients with heart disease.
2. The rise in $Pa_{CO_2}$ due to the bicarbonate and due to the reduction in ventilation as the pH rises, may result in a further *fall* in CSF pH. This happens because the equilibration between $[HCO^-_3]$ in blood and CSF is slow, whereas that of $CO_2$ is fast.
3. The oxyhaemoglobin dissociation curve moves to the left, impairing oxygen delivery to the tissues.

The dose of bicarbonate can be calculated from the base excess, assuming that equilibration throughout the extracellular fluid will occur (about 20 per cent of the body weight).

$$\text{Dose (mmol)} = \frac{\text{Base deficit} \times \text{Body weight (kg)}}{3}$$

It is often recommended that half this dose be given and the blood gases then checked again. It is much better to undercorrect the acidosis than to overcorrect it. The results of administering the dose of bicarbonate as suggested above are not always predictable due to the possible development of further acidosis since the original blood sample was taken, because of altered equilibrium with the extracellular fluid in a deranged circulation, and because measuring the acid base state of the blood may give a very inaccurate index of the metabolic state of the body as a whole; measurement of intracellular pH as a clinical procedure is not yet possible. For these reasons it is essential to reassess the acid-base status of the arterial blood after the bicarbonate has been given, and to correct further if necessary. Sodium bicarbonate is a poor buffer in its own right, as explained previously, and acts mainly by combining with $H^+$ ions to form $CO_2$ and water:

$$H^+ + HCO_3^- \rightleftharpoons H_2CO_3 \rightleftharpoons CO_2 + H_2O$$

The administration of bicarbonate to correct a metabolic acidosis therefore presents a carbon dioxide load for the lungs to excrete, and efficient buffering of a metabolic acidosis depends on adequate pulmonary ventilation.

### Metabolic Alkalosis

Metabolic alkalosis may be caused by loss of acid, e.g. vomiting, ingestion or infusion of alkali or by potassium depletion. It usually does not require treatment although occasionally prolonged nasogastric drainage causes quite severe metabolic alkalosis which can easily be controlled with cimetidine which reduces the $[H^+]$ of gastric secretion.

3/TABLE 8

THE MECHANISMS BY WHICH PRIMARY ACID-BASE CHANGES ARE COMPENSATED. If the pH has been fully returned to normal the primary change is said to be FULLY COMPENSATED. If the pH has not been completely returned to normal the primary change is said to be PARTIALLY COMPENSATED.

| *Original acid-base change* | *Compensatory Mechanism* | *Compensating Organ* |
|---|---|---|
| Respiratory Acidosis | Metabolic alkalosis, with a further rise in plasma [$HCO_3^-$] | Kidney |
| Respiratory Alkalosis | Metabolic acidosis, with a further fall in plasma [$HCO_3^-$] | Kidney |
| Metabolic Acidosis | Respiratory alkalosis, with a further fall in plasma [$HCO_3^-$] | Lungs |
| Metabolic Alkalosis | Respiratory acidosis, with a further rise in plasma [$HCO_3^-$] | Lungs |

## MEASUREMENT OF BLOOD GASES AND ACID-BASE STATE

1. *pH electrode* (Fig. 19)

This electrode contains pH-sensitive glass which has the property that if each side of the glass is bathed in a solution of different pH, an e.m.f. is generated across it. This e.m.f. is directly and linearly proportional to the difference between the pH of the two solutions. If the pH on one side of the glass is stabilised, and a solution of unknown pH is introduced onto the other side of the glass, the e.m.f. thus generated gives an indication of the unknown pH. The e.m.f. across the pH sensitive glass can be measured by placing metal electrodes in the solutions on either side of it. But a problem arises here, because at any metal-electrolyte interface an e.m.f. is developed and this can obscure that across the glass. For this reason the electrodes on either side must be electrically very stable, so that little or no variation in potential occurs at their surfaces. If variations do occur it is impossible to separate these from alterations across the pH glass, which is what we are trying to measure. Suitably stable electrodes are (1) silver, coated with a layer of silver chloride, and immersed in a solution containing chloride ions; and (2) calomel coated mercury, in contact with saturated KCl. The general arrangement of a pH electrode is shown in Fig. 19. On one side of the glass is a solution of 0·1 M HCl (stable pH) into which is dipped a silver: silver chloride electrode. On the other side of the glass is the test solution. This is connected electrically via a liquid bridge to a saturated solution of KCl, which is itself in contact with a mercury: calomel electrode. A porous plug is inserted in the KCl to prevent contamination of the calomel electrode by the test solution. The e.m.f. across the whole assembly can now be measured by connecting the silver and calomel electrodes through a sensitive high resistance voltmeter. The instrument is calibrated by setting it up against solutions of known pH, and the pH of an unknown solution can then be measured by comparing the e.m.f. it generates with that produced by the solutions of known pH. Although for each measurement the potential across the whole apparatus is read, the stability of the system is such that changes in e.m.f. across the whole are due to changes across the pH sensitive glass.

2. *$PCO_2$ electrode* (Fig. 20)

A $CO_2$ electrode consists of a pH electrode separated from the blood sample by a nylon or cellophane spacer and teflon or latex rubber membrane. The nylon spacer allows the small gap between the membrane and the pH sensitive glass and this gap is filled with a bicarbonate solution. The membrane is permeable to $CO_2$ but not to hydrogen ions. When the blood

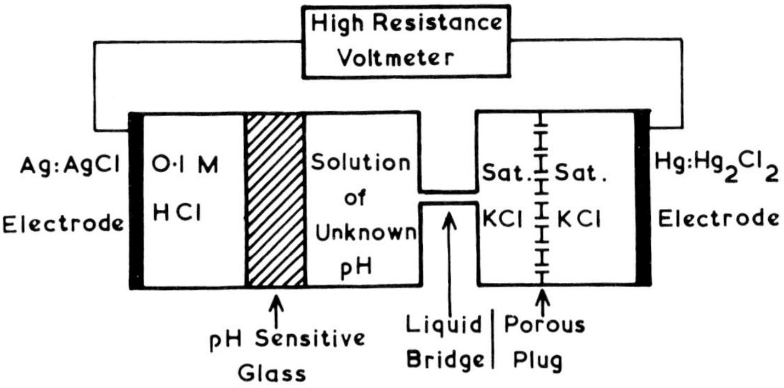


3/FIG. 19.—Schematic diagram of a pH electrode. See text for full details.

sample is introduced, $CO_2$ diffuses across the membrane into the bicarbonate layer where

$$CO_2 + H_2O \rightleftharpoons HCO_3 \rightleftharpoons HCO^-{}_3 + H^+$$

the change in $H^+$ and therefore pH causes a change in voltage across the glass which is measured via two silver/silver chloride reference electrodes, one in contact with the internal filling solution of the pH electrode and one in contact with the bicarbonate solution.

3. *$PO_2$ electrode* (Fig. 21)

The Clark polarographic electrode consists typically of a platinum cathode and a silver/silver chloride anode immersed in a buffered potassium hydroxide solution. The cathode, anode and electrolyte are separated from the blood by a plastic membrane which is permeable to oxygen but not to ions, water or protein. The cathode and anode are connected to a DC voltage source so that the cathode is 600 mV negative with respect to the anode. Oxygen molecules in the vicinity of the cathode become reduced

$$O_2 + 2\ H_2O + 4\ e \rightarrow 4\ OH^- \text{ overall reaction.}$$

The electrons drawn from the cathode cause a current to flow which is measured by an ammeter and is proportional to the $PO_2$ of the sample.

If blood and gas samples with identical $PO_2$ values are analysed a small difference will be found. This "blood-gas" difference is due to slower diffusion of oxygen from the blood sample to the cathode than from the gas sample. If very accurate results are needed, the electrode should be calibrated with blood tonometered with gases of known oxygen concentration.

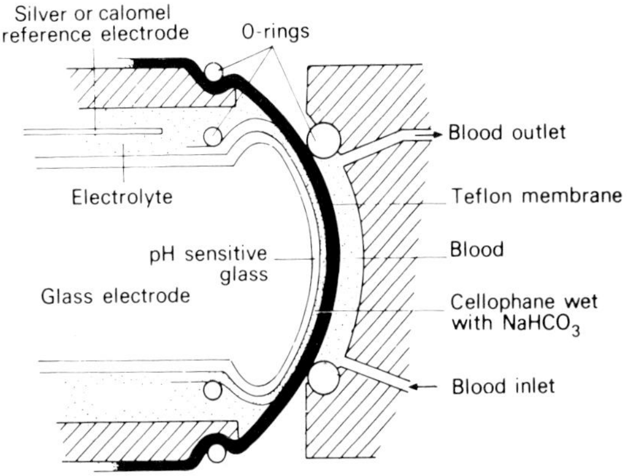


3/FIG. 20.—The $CO_2$ electrode and cuvette. (Courtesy of Professor M. K. Sykes, Dr. M. D. Vickers and Dr. C. J. Hull and Blackwell Scientific Publications.[37])

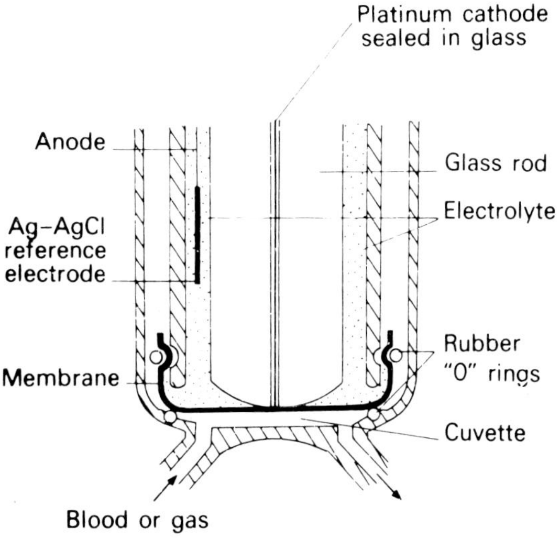


3/FIG. 21.—Time $0_2$ electrode and cuvette. (Courtesy of Professor M. K. Sykes, Dr. M. D. Vickers and Dr. C. J. Hull, and Blackwell Scientific Publications.[37])

### Arterial Blood-gas Samples

Arterial samples should be taken into a syringe whose dead space is filled with heparin (1000 units/ml). It is important to ensure that there are no air bubbles in the syringe and that the blood is well mixed with the heparin. Ideally the sample should be analysed straight away; alternatively it can be capped and stored in crushed ice. Storage at room temperature will result in a rise in $Pco_2$ and fall in pH and $Po_2$ due to the blood's metabolism. The temperature of the patient and the inspired oxygen concentration should be noted.

Capillary samples are often used in babies and are taken into special pre-heparinised glass capillary tubes. The $Pco_2$ and pH results on capillary blood are close to those of arterial blood taken at the same time. The $Po_2$ is less reliable.

### Interpretation of Blood-gas Analyses

It should be remembered that there is always more than a single explanation for any given set of blood-gas results, so it is not possible to make a diagnosis on the basis of these results alone, which must always be considered together with the patient's history, physical findings and other investigations.

1. $Paco_2$

Normal value 35–45 mm Hg (4·7–6·0 kPa).

A raised $Paco_2$ is synonymous with the term 'respiratory acidosis' irrespective of the pH.

A low $Paco_2$ is synonymous with the term "respiratory alkalosis" irrespective of the pH.

The $Paco_2$ reflects the relationship of alveolar ventilation ($\dot{V}_A$) to $CO_2$ production ($\dot{V}co_2$), thus an increase in $Paco_2$ may be due to a reduction in $\dot{V}_A$ or to an increase in $\dot{V}co_2$. During exercise $\dot{V}co_2$ increases considerably but $\dot{V}_A$ also increases appropriately so that $Paco_2$ remains constant.

The $Pao_2$ must be taken into account when assessing whether or not the $Paco_2$ is normal. For example, if an asthmatic with a $Pao_2$ of 60 mm Hg (8·0 kPa) has a $Paco_2$ of 40 mm Hg (5·3 kPa) this is higher than a normal subject would have at the same $Pao_2$ (see p. 43).

If the subject is hurt or frightened when the sample is taken, acute hyperventilation and an artificially low $Paco_2$ may result.

$Paco_2$ is relatively little affected by $\dot{V}/\dot{Q}$ mismatch (see p. 96).

2. pH

Normal value 7·35–7·45.

Abnormalities of pH may either be respiratory or metabolic in origin. If the pH is more acid than would be expected on the basis of the $Pco_2$ alone then a metabolic acidosis is present. If it is more alkaline than would be expected on the basis of the $Pco_2$ alone, then a metabolic alkalosis is present. The base excess (see above) is the index most commonly used to quantify the metabolic component.

3. $Pao_2$

Normal value 70–100 mm Hg (9·3–13·3 kPa), depending on age. The following relationship between age and $Pao_2$ has been found:

$$Pao_2 = 102 - 0{\cdot}33 \times \text{age in years (mm Hg)}$$
$$= 13{\cdot}6 - 0{\cdot}044 \times \text{age in years (kPa)}$$

the inspired oxygen concentration at the time thc blood sample is taken must be recorded. The $Pao_2$ is very sensitive to increases in $\dot{V}/\dot{Q}$ mismatch (see p. 96) but may be low for many reasons (see causes of hypoxic hypoxia, page 129).

*Examples*

1. pH = 7·18 $Paco_2 = 20$ $Pao_2 = 39$ (on air)

The $Paco_2$ is lower than normal so the patient has a *respiratory alkalosis*.
If there was no metabolic disturbance, this $Paco_2$ would give rise to a pH of nearly 7·6. The actual pH (7·18) is much more acid so the patient has a *metabolic acidosis*. If the haemoglobin is known, or measured with the blood gases as in some automatic blood gas analysers, the base excess can be derived:
if haemoglobin = 15 g/dl, base excess = −18 mmol/l, indicating a severe metabolic acidosis.
The $Pao_2$ indicates that the patient is *hypoxic*.

A common cause of the above findings (but NOT the only one) would be a major pulmonary embolus. The $Pao_2$ is low due to increased $\dot{V}/\dot{Q}$ mismatch. There is a low oxygen flux due to a reduced cardiac output of less than fully oxygenated blood which leads to tissue hypoxia, anaerobic metabolism and therefore metabolic acidosis. Hyperventilation due to the metabolic acidosis, hypoxia acting via the peripheral chemoreceptors and a local effect of the clot within the lungs cause a low $Pa_{CO_2}$; in addition the $\dot{V}_{CO_2}$ may be reduced because of insuffiicent oxygen for aerobic metabolism.

2. pH = 7·46 $Pa_{CO_2} = 51$ $Pa_{O_2} = 60$ (on air)

The $Pa_{CO_2}$ is higher than normal, so the patient has a *respiratory acidosis*. The pH is more alkaline than would be produced by the $Pa_{CO_2}$ alone, so the patient has a *metabolic alkalosis*. Assuming a haemoglobin of 15 g/dl, base excess = +10 mmol/l

The patient is *hypoxic*.

Several explanations are possible. The $Pa_{CO_2}$ and $Pa_{O_2}$ values would be typical of chronic bronchitis. The metabolic alkalosis could be partly compensatory (for the respiratory acidosis) and partly due to some other cause such as loss of gastric acid due to vomiting—a purely compensatory alkalosis would not over-correct the pH.

## REFERENCES


1. Cotes, J. E. (1975). *Lung Function*, 3rd edit. Oxford: Blackwell Scientific Publications.
2. Fishman, A. P. (1976). Hypoxia on the pulmonary circulation: how and where it acts. *Circulation Res.*, **28**, 221.
3. Editorial (1979). Hypoxic pulmonary vasoconstriction and infusion of sodium nitroprusside. *Anesthesiology*, **50**, 481.
4. Snashall, P. D. (1980). Pulmonary oedema. *Brit. J. Dis. Chest*, **74**, 2.
5. Noble, W. H. (1980). Pulmonary oedema: a review. *Canad. Anaesth. Soc. J.*, **27**, 286.
6. Staub, N. C. (1980). The pathogenesis of pulmonary oedema. *Progr. Cardiovasc. Dis.*, **23**, 53.
7. West, J. B., Dollery, C. T., and Heard, B. E. (1965). Increased pulmonary vascular resistance in the dependant zone of the isolated dog lung caused by perivascular oedema. *Circulat. Res.*, **12**, 301.
8. Hughes, J. M. B., Glazier, J. B., Maloney, J. E., and West, J. B. (1968). Effect of lung volume on the distribution of pulmonary blood flow in man. *Resp. Physiol.*, **4**, 58.
9. West, J. B. (1970). *Ventilation/Blood Flow and Gas Exchange*. Oxford: Blackwell Scientific Publications.
10. Severinghaus, J. W., Swenson, E. W., Finley, T. N., Lategola, M. T. and Williams, J. (1961). Unilateral hypoventilation produced in dogs by occluding one pulmonary artery. *J. appl. Physiol.*, **16**, 53.
11. Raine, J. M., and Bishop, J. M. (1963). A—a difference in $O_2$ tension and physiological deadspace in normal man. *J. appl. Physiol.*, **18**, 284.
12. Nunn, J. F. (1977). *Applied Respiratory Physiology*. London: Butterworth & Co.
13. Leigh, J. M., and Tyrrell, M. F. (1968). Respiratory gas equations: a geometric approach. *Brit. J. Anaesth.*, **40**, 430.
14. Panday, J., and Nunn, J. F. (1968). Failure to demonstrate progressive falls of arterial $P_{O_2}$ during anaesthesia. *Anaesthesia*, **23**, 38.
15. Rehder, K., and Sessler, A. D. (1973). Function of each lung in spontaneously breathing man anaesthetised with thiopental-meperidine. *Anesthesiology*, **38**, 320.
16. Freeman, J., and Nunn, J. P. (1963). Ventilation-perfusion relationships after haemorrhage. *Clin. Sci.*, **24**, 135.
17. Askrog, V. F., Pender, J. W. and Eckenhoff, J. E. (1964). Changes in physiological deadspace during deliberate hypotension. *Anesthesiology*, **25**, 744.
18. Tomlin, P. J., Conway, C. M., and Payne, J. P. (1964). Hypoxaemia due to atropine. *Lancet*, **1**, 14.
19. Nunn, J. F., and Bergman, N. A. (1964). The effect of atropine on pulmonary gas exchange. *Brit. J. Anaesth.*, **36**, 68.
20. Conway, C. M. (1964). Arterial oxygen tensions in surgical patients. In: *Oxygen Measurements in Blood and Tissue and their Significance*, p. 173. Eds. J. P. Payne & D. W. Hill. London: J. & A. Churchill.
21. Smith, T. C., Stephen, G. W., Zeiger, L., and Wollman, H. (1967). Effects of premedicant drugs on respiration and gas exchange in man. *Anesthesiology*, **28**, 883.
22. Martinez, L. R., von Euler, C., and Norlander, O. P. (1967). Ventilatory exchange and acid-base balance before and after preoperative medication. *Acta anaesth. scand.*, **11**, 139.
23. Gardiner, A. J. S., and Palmer, K. N. V. (1964). Effect of premedication and general anaesthesia on arterial blood gases. *Brit. med. J.*, **2**, 1433.
24. Nunn, J. F., and Hill, D. W. (1960). Respiratory deadspace and arterial to end-tidal $CO_2$ tension difference in anesthetized man. *J. appl. Physiol.*, **15**, 383.
25. Nunn, J. F., and Payne, J. P. (1962). Hypoxaemia after general anaesthesia. *Lancet*, **2**, 631.
26. Conway, C. M., and Payne, J. P. (1963). Post-operative hypoxaemia and oxygen therapy. *Brit. med. J.*, **1**, 844.
27. Milledge, J. S., and Nunn, J. F. (1975). Criteria for fitness for anaesthesia in patients with chronic obstructive lung disease. *Brit. med. J.*, **3**, 670.
28. Perutz, M. F. (1978). Hemoglobin structure and respiratory transport. *Scientific American*, December, 68.
29. Staub, N. C., Bishop, J. M., and Forster, R. E. (1961). Velocity of $O_2$ uptake by human red blood cells. *J. appl. Physiol.*, **16**, 511.
30. Gregory, I. C. (1974). The oxygen and carbon monoxide capacities of fetal and adult blood. *J. Physiol.* (*Lond.*), **236**, 625.
31. Thomas, H. M. (III), Lefrak, S. S., Irwin, R. S., Fritts,

H. W. jr., and Caldwell, P. R. B. (1974). The oxyhaemoglobin dissociation curve in health and disease. Role of 2, 3-diphosphoglycerate. *Amer. J. Med.*, **57**, 331.
32. Davenport, H. W. (1974). *The ABC of Acid-Base Chemistry*: Chicago: Univ. of Chicago Press.
33. Sigaard-Andersen, O. (1966). *The Acid-Base Status of the Blood*. Copenhagen: Munksgaard.
34. Sigaard-Andersen, O. (1963). The Acid-Base Status of the Blood. *Scand. J. Clin. Lab. Invest.*, **15**, Supp. 70.
35. Astrup, P., Siggaard-Andersen, O., Jørgensen, K., and Engel, K. (1960). The acid-base metabolism. A new approach. *Lancet*, **1**, 1037.
36. Severinghaus, J. W. (1966). Blood gas calculator. *J. Appl. Physiol.*, **21**, 1108.
37. Sykes, M. K., Vickers, M. D. and Hull, C. J. (1981). *Principles of Clinical Measurement*, 2nd edit. Oxford: Blackwell Scientific Publications.

## FURTHER READING

Adams, A. P. and Hahn, C. E. W. (1979). *Principles and Practice of Blood-gas Analysis*. London: Franklin Scientific Projects Ltd.
Cotes, J. E. (1975). *Lung Function*. Oxford: Blackwell Scientific Publications.
Davenport, H. W. (1974). *The ABC of Acid-Base Chemistry*. Chicago: Univ. of Chicago Press.
Nunn, J. F. (1977). *Applied Respiratory Physiology*. London: Butterworth & Co.
Siggaard-Andersen, O. (1966). *The Acid-Base Status of the Blood*. Copenhagen: Munksgaard.
West, J. B. (1970). *Ventilation/Blood Flow and Gas Exchange*. Oxford: Blackwell Scientific Publications.

CHAPTER 4

# Oxygen and Associated Gases



## OXYGEN ($O_2$)

### History

Although Stephen Hale prepared oxygen along with many other gases in 1727, the full credit for its discovery and the realisation of the importance of this gas as a normal constituent of air must go to Priestley (1777).[1] Following upon this discovery Lavoisier and his colleagues (1780 and 1789)[2,3] demonstrated that oxygen was absorbed by the lungs and, after metabolism in the body, eliminated as carbon dioxide and water. Since that time its value as a therapeutic agent has gradually increased with improved methods of administration.

### Properties

Oxygen is a tasteless, colourless, odourless gas which forms 20·95 per cent of the atmosphere (dry). It consists mainly of $O^{16}$, although small amounts of the $O^{17}$ and $O^{18}$ isotopes are also present. The boiling point at 1 atmosphere is −183° C; below this temperature it exists as a pale blue liquid, which on further cooling solidifies at −218° C. The critical temperature is −118° C, so at temperatures greater than this the oxygen exists as a gas rather than a vapour and cannot be liquefied by raising the pressure.

Oxygen is chemically very reactive and is the most plentiful element in and around Earth.

4/Table 1
Properties of Oxygen

| | | |
|---|---|---|
| Molecular weight | | 32·00 |
| Relative density (air = 1) | | 1·105 |
| Boiling point at 760 mm Hg | | −183° C |
| Melting point at 760 mm Hg | | −218° C |
| Critical temperature | | −118° C |
| Natural abundance: | | |
| Earth's crust, Hydrosphere, Atmosphere | together | 49·5% |
| Atmosphere alone | | 20·95 vol % |
| Human body | | 65% |
| Solubility in water (at 760 mm Hg) | at 0° C | 4·9 ml $O_2$/100 ml $H_2O$ |
| | at 37° C | 2·4 ml $O_2$/100 ml $H_2O$ |
| Solubility in blood at 37° C (not in combination with haemoglobin) | | 0·003 ml/100 ml blood per mm Hg $Po_2$ |

Although oxygen cannot be ignited, it aids combustion so that not only will substances burn far more vigorously or even explode in oxygen, but also the amount of energy needed to start combustion is much less. Explosions have occurred in this way due to grease on cylinder valves.

Due to the presence of unpaired electrons in the oxygen molecule the gas is attracted to regions of high flux in a magnetic field and is said to be paramagnetic. This property is exploited in some oxygen analysers.

## Preparation

Large scale commercial preparation of oxygen is by fractional distillation of liquid air. Electrolysis of water and many oxygen-producing chemical reactions are sometimes used to produce oxygen under special circumstances but will not be discussed further.

(i) *Liquefaction of air.*

When air is compressed it gets hot; if this heat is got rid of and then the air is allowed to expand, this expansion will result in a fall in temperature of the air (Joule-Thomson effect). By repeating this process of compression/expansion there is a progressive fall in the temperature of the air so that it starts to liquefy. In practice the process is rather more complicated than this in order to increase the efficiency, but the basic principle is the same.

(ii) *Distillation of liquid air.*

In the liquid air still, nitrogen and oxygen can be separated as the more volatile nitrogen (boiling point at 760 mm Hg = −196° C) is drawn off from the top of the still and the oxygen (boiling point = −183° C) from lower down. Other components of air can be separated as required, and the oxygen is usually liquefied for storage.

## Storage

Oxygen is either stored in liquid form in insulated tanks or as a gas at high pressure (102783·8 mm Hg, 13700 kPa, 2000 psig) in cylinders. For larger hospitals storage in the liquid form is much more economical. A tank with a capacity of up to 1500 kg of liquid oxygen and insulated by a high vacuum shell is used to maintain a temperature between −175 and −150° C.

With reference to Fig. 1, there is a continuous evaporation of liquid within the tank due to the

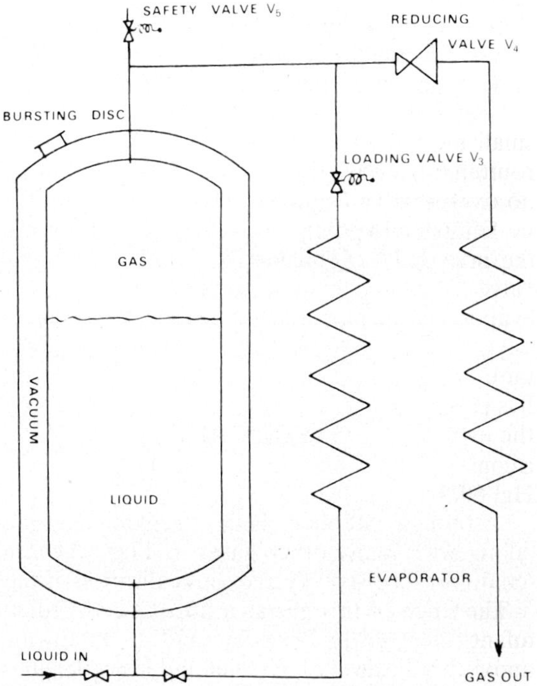


4/Fig. 1.—Diagram of a vacuum-insulated tank and evaporator. (Courtesy of Dr. W. J. Grant and HM & M Publishers Ltd.[4])

4/Fig. 2.—A liquid oxygen tank together with a bank of cylinders which provide a reserve supply in case of emergency. Liquid oxygen can be pumped into the tank from the supplier's road tanker and the tank weighed in order to measure the amount of liquid oxygen inside. For smaller consumers a bank of cylinders containing compressed gas can be used to feed a piped oxygen system. (Courtesy of Dr. W. J. Grant and HM & M Publishers Ltd.[4])

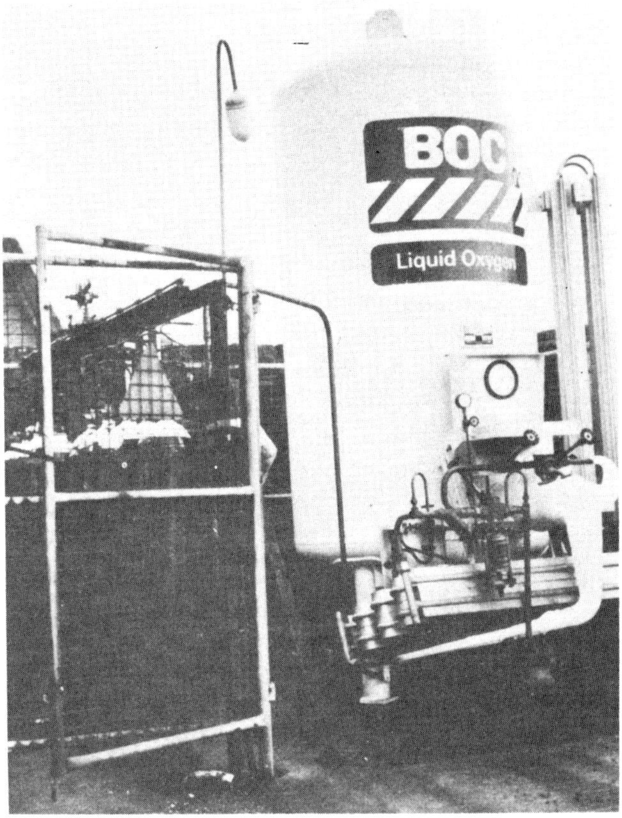


small amount of heat absorbed from the surroundings in spite of the vacuum insulation. If no oxygen is being drawn off then this gas will be vented to atmosphere through valve $V_5$. If the pressure in the tank falls below that set on valve $V_3$, more liquid oxygen will flow into the evaporator. So in response to demand, gaseous oxygen will be drawn off from the top of the tank and also will be derived from liquid which has passed from the bottom of the tank through the evaporator. A pressure regulator maintains a constant supply pressure of 400 kPa (3001 mm Hg, 60 psig) into the hospital pipe system.

## Oxygen Lack

The failure of the tissues to receive adequate quantities of oxygen is variously described as anoxia, hypoxia, or oxygen lack, but strictly interpreted anoxia means *total* lack of oxygen. The lack of oxygen represents a severe hazard to the tissues and has been aptly described by Haldane as causing "not only stoppage of the machine, but also total ruin of the supposed machinery." Under ordinary conditions the body has certain regulatory mechanisms which prevent the tissues from suffering oxygen deprivation, but during the course of anaesthesia oxygen lack may become a factor of prime importance.

We get the energy we need from the sun. Earth's atmosphere originally contained no oxygen and it was only when chemical evolution reached the stage of photosynthesis that plant-like organisms began to add oxygen to the atmosphere. 'Photosynthesis' implies that the energy for the reaction is derived from light

$$6\ CO_2 + 6\ H_2O \xrightarrow{\text{energy from sun}} C_6H_{12}O_6 + 6\ O_2$$

Within our cells this reaction is reversed so that the solar energy incorporated into the glucose molecule is released and made available for cell processes:

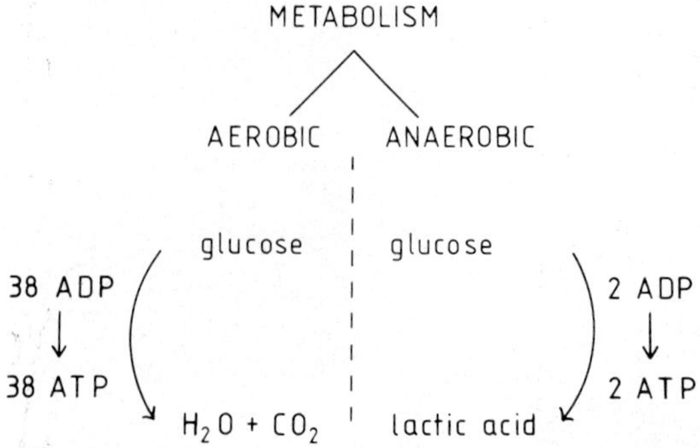


4/Fig. 3.—Synthesis of ATP by aerobic or anaerobic metabolism. The energy may of course be derived via other food substrates apart from glucose.

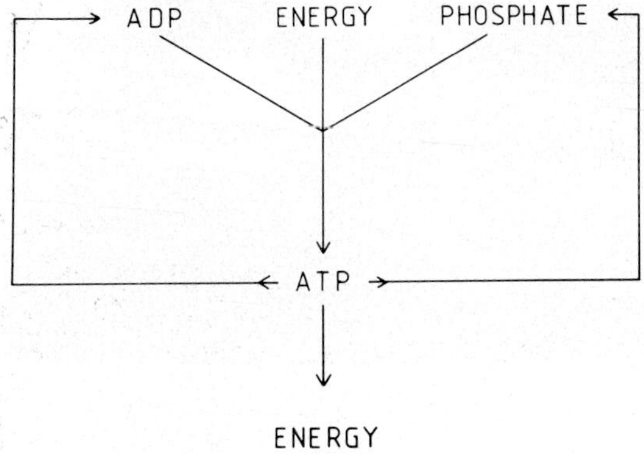


4/Fig. 4.—The transfer of energy by the synthesis and breakdown of ATP.

$$C_6H_{12}O_6 + 6\ O_2 \rightarrow 6H_2O + 6\ CO_2 + \text{energy}$$

Organisms such as ourselves are completely dependent on this process of oxidation in order to derive sufficient energy from food substrates to maintain life, but as can be seen from Fig. 3, some energy can be obtained from glucose in the absence of oxygen, although in terms of adenosine triphosphate (ATP) production anaerobic metabolism is only 1/19th as efficient as aerobic metabolism.

The energy is stored in the form of a high energy phosphate bond in the ATP molecule. When the energy is required, ATP is broken down to adenosine diphosphate (ADP) and phosphate. Lactic acid accumulation as a result of anaerobic metabolism will lead to a metabolic acidosis, although when oxygen becomes available the lactate can be metabolised to $CO_2$ and $H_2O$ with further energy release and ATP formation (Fig. 4).

Most of the oxygen is used in the mitochondria and if the level of $Po_2$ here falls below about 1–2 mm Hg (0·2 kPa), the so-called Pasteur point, then aerobic metabolism stops. The $Po_2$ drops in stages from 158 mm Hg (21 kPa) in dry air to the low levels in the mitochondria. The oxygen cascade (Fig. 5) shows these stages.

Alveolar $Po_2$ in fit young adults is about

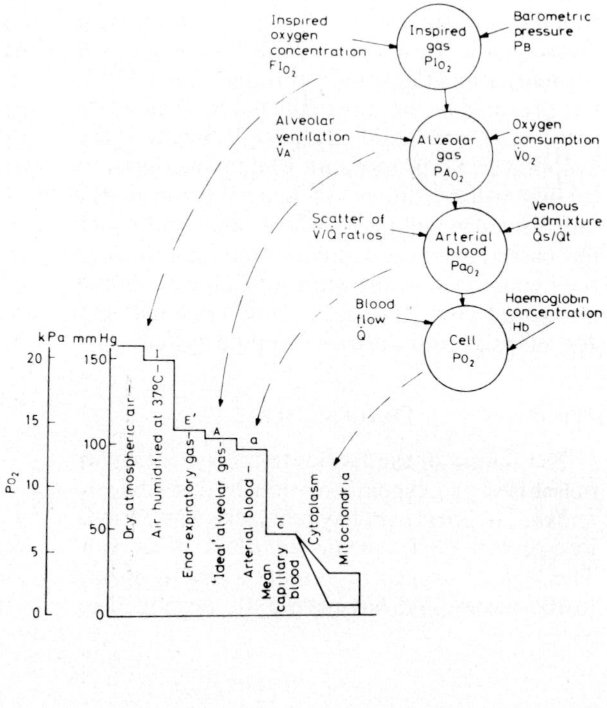


4/Fig. 5.—The oxygen cascade. The upper right-hand part of the figure shows factors influencing oxygenation at different levels in the cascade. (Courtesy of Dr. J. F. Nunn and Butterworth & Co.[5])

100 mm Hg (13 kPa). The drop from inspired to alveolar $Po_2$ depends mainly on alveolar ventilation and oxygen consumption and can be calculated using the alveolar air equation (see p. 98).

The first drop occurs as a result of humidification so that fully saturated air at 37° C has a $Po_2$ of 150 mm Hg (20 kPa), viz. (atmospheric pressure—saturated vapour pressure of water at body temperature) × fractional concentration of $O_2$ in air.

The difference between alveolar $Po_2$ and arterial $Po_2$, often referred to as the A–a gradient is normally of the order of a few mm Hg, but is increased if venous admixture is increased: that is to say, if there is a greater proportion of blood returning to the left atrium having passed through zones of lung with low $\dot{V}/\dot{Q}$ ratios or if there is an increase in true shunt (blood which has returned to the left side of the heart without picking up any oxygen in the lungs). For further discussion of venous admixture see page 97.

The $Po_2$ then falls progressively from the arterial to the venous ends of the capillaries and there will be variable $Po_2$ gradients from the capillary blood to the cells. The $Po_2$ is lowest in the mitochondria (see above). Venous $Po_2$ varies depending on the vascular bed concerned; for example the $Po_2$ in the coronary sinus blood draining from the myocardium is considerably less than that measured in the superior vena cava. Mixed venous $Po_2$ ($P\bar{v}o_2$) measured in blood sampled from the pulmonary artery is normally 40 mm Hg (5·3 kPa).

## 1. **Hypoxic Hypoxia**

This implies a reduction in $Pao_2$. The normal $Pao_2$ declines with age so that when breathing air

$$Pao_2\ (\text{mm Hg}) = 104 - 0{\cdot}24 \times \text{age} \qquad \text{S.D. } 7{\cdot}9$$

$$Pao_2\ (\text{kPa}) = (104 - 0{\cdot}24 \times \text{age}) \times 0{\cdot}133 \qquad \text{S.D. } 1{\cdot}1.$$

When assessing the significance of a value of $Pao_2$, the $F_{IO_2}$ and age of the patient must be borne in mind.

There are numerous causes of hypoxic hypoxia which will be considered in turn:

(a) *Reduced partial pressure of oxygen in inspired gas* ($P_{IO_2}\downarrow$).

This may be due either to a fall in the fractional concentration of oxygen in the inspired gas ($F_{IO_2}$), or to a fall in barometric pressure. The $F_{IO_2}$ will be low if the patient is rebreathing or if the fresh gas supplied is hypoxic. Barometric pressure decreases with altitude so that on top of Mount Everest at 8847 m (29028 ft) it is only about 236 mm Hg (31·5 kPa). Allowing for saturation of the inspired gas with water vapour, the $P_{IO_2}$ would be 40 mm Hg (5·3 kPa).

(b) *Fink effect or Diffusion hypoxia.*

Fink[6] described what he called "diffusion anoxia", occurring when nitrous oxide is withdrawn at the end of anaesthesia. While the patient is breathing nitrous oxide relatively large amounts of this gas replace the less soluble nitrogen present in the body fluids. When the anaesthetic is stopped, this nitrous oxide diffuses from body tissues via venous blood into the alveolar gas and nitrogen (now being breathed) diffuses from the alveolar gas back into the tissues. Because the solubility of nitrous oxide is much greater than that of nitrogen a relatively small amount of nitrogen passes from alveolar gas to restore the tissue $P_{N_2}$ but a much larger amount of $N_2O$ passes from the tissues to the alveoli, where it dilutes the alveolar gas and so reduces alveolar $Po_2$ (Fig. 6). The opposite occurs during induction and has a

4/Table 2
Classification of the Causes of Hypoxia

| | | | |
|---|---|---|---|
| HYPOXIC | | STAGNANT | |
| $P_{IO_2}\downarrow$ < $F_{IO_2}\downarrow$ / barometric pressure $\downarrow$ | Diffusing capacity $\downarrow$ | General—low cardiac output | Local |
| | $P\bar{v}O_2$ < $O_2$ consumption $\uparrow$ / $O_2$ flux $\downarrow$ | | |
| Fink effect | | HISTOTOXIC | |
| $\dot{V}_A\downarrow$ | Venous admixture $\uparrow$ < low $\dot{V}/\dot{Q}$ / true shunt | Cyanide poisoning | |
| ANAEMIC | | LOW $P_{50}$ | |
| Anaemia | Methaemoglobinaemia | pH $\uparrow$ | Hypothermia |
| CO poisoning | Sulphaemoglobinaemia | 2, 3 DPG $\downarrow$ | |

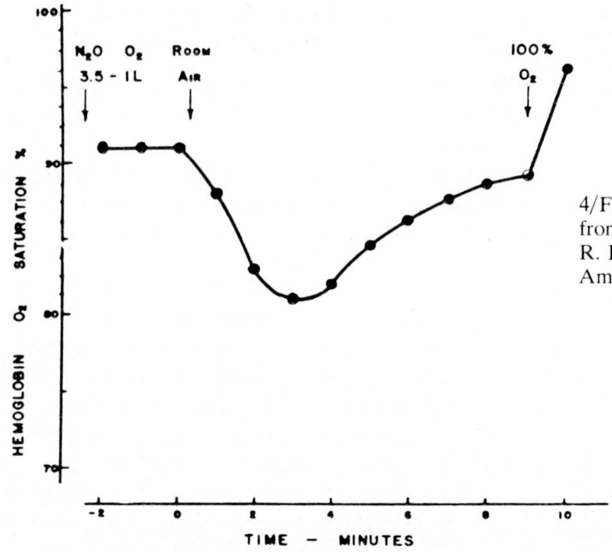


4/Fig. 6.—Arterial oxygenation saturation during recovery from nitrous oxide-oxygen anaesthesia. (Courtesy of Dr. B. R. Fink and J. B. Lippincott Company, publishers for the American Society of Anesthesiology.[6])

concentrating effect on the other gases including oxygen. Post-operative diffusion hypoxia is brief but may be important in the poor-risk patient. Figure 7 shows schematically the relative exchanges of nitrogen and nitrous oxide.

(c) *Reduced alveolar ventilation* ($\dot{V}A\downarrow$). Figure 8 shows the relationship between alveolar ventilation ($\dot{V}A$) and alveolar $Po_2$ ($PAO_2$)

The figure illustrates three important points:

(i) The $PAO_2$–$\dot{V}A$ relationship is hyperbolic. Because of this shape, if we look at the middle curve (21 per cent $O_2$), a reduction in ventilation of 2 l/min from 6 to 4 l/min has little effect on $PAO_2$ whereas a reduction from 4 to 2 l/min has a very marked effect on $PAO_2$.

(ii) Raising the inspired $Po_2$ by 64 mm Hg (8·5 kPa), achieved by increasing the $FIO_2$ from 0·21 to 0·3, results in a rise in $PAO_2$ of the same amount.

(iii) Raising the oxygen consumption shifts the relationship downwards and to the right so that what was previously a perfectly adequate alveolar ventilation may be grossly inadequate if the oxygen consumption increases. "Halothane shakes" is a common cause of increased $O_2$ consumption in the early post-operative period.

(d) *Reduced diffusing capacity*.
The term "alveolar/capillary block" has

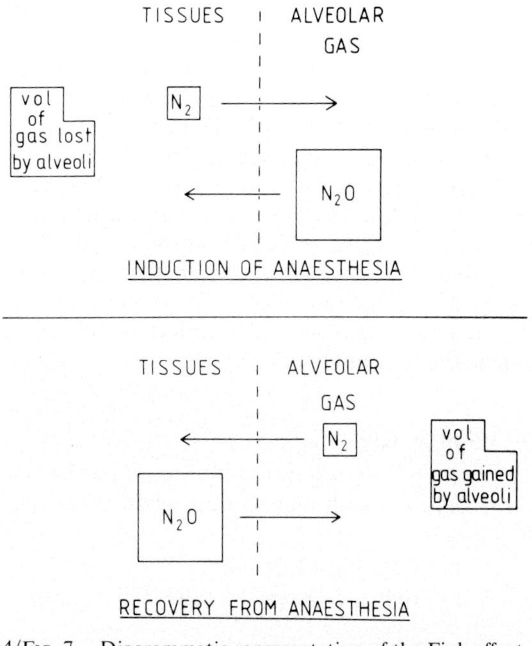


4/Fig. 7.—Diagrammatic representation of the Fink effect. During recovery from nitrous oxide/oxygen anaesthesia (lower half of diagram) a relatively large volume of the more soluble $N_2O$ diffuses from the tissues into the venous blood and thence to the alveoli and is replaced by a relatively small volume of $N_2$ which is less soluble. The alveolar gas therefore loses less $N_2$ than it gains $N_2O$, which dilutes the oxygen in the alveoli so causing the hypoxia illustrated in Fig. 6. The opposite of this process occurs during induction of anaesthesia as shown in the top half of the diagram.

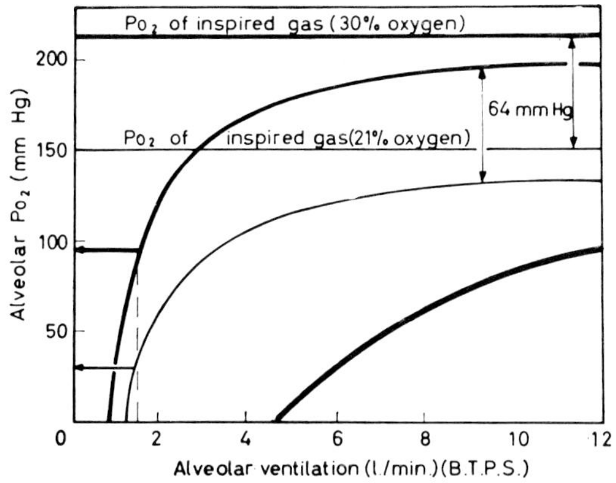


4/Fig. 8.—The relationship between alveolar $Po_2$ and alveolar ventilation.

Inspired $O_2$ concentration (%)

| *Top curve* | *Middle curve* | *Lower curve* |
|---|---|---|
| 30 | 21 | 21 |

$O_2$ consumption (ml/min)

| *Top curve* | *Middle curve* | *Lower curve* |
|---|---|---|
| 200 | 200 | 800 |

(Courtesy of Dr. J. F. Nunn and the publishers, Butterworths[5])

been used to describe impairment of oxygen diffusion from the alveolar gas across the alveolar membrane and pulmonary capillary wall into the pulmonary capillary blood as a result of thickening of the alveolar-capillary membrane. It is generally thought that this is a rare cause of hypoxia although such an abnormality is more likely to have a significant effect during exercise when the pulmonary capillary transit time is reduced.

(e) *Reduced mixed venous* $Po_2$ ($P\bar{v}o_2\downarrow$).
Mixing of venous blood from different vascular beds is not complete until the blood has reached the pulmonary artery, so it is from here that blood must be withdrawn to obtain a "mixed venous" sample. $P\bar{v}o_2$ may be reduced below the normal value of 40 mm Hg (5·3 kPa) either as a result of an increase in oxygen consumption or a reduction in oxygen flux. In the absence of any increase in alveolar ventilation or $P_{IO_2}$ a fall in $Pao_2$ will occur.

(f) *Venous admixture*.
This term refers to blood which has passed from the venous side of the circulation to the left side of the heart either having picked up no oxygen in the lungs (true shunt) or having passed through zones of lung with low $\dot{V}/\dot{Q}$ ratios so that it is less than fully oxygenated (low $\dot{V}/\dot{Q}$). Its role in producing post-operative hypoxia is mentioned on page 96.

## 2. Anaemic Hypoxia

In this form of hypoxia the oxygen content of arterial blood is reduced, although the arterial partial pressure of oxygen is normal (unless some form of hypoxic hypoxia coexists, which is not uncommon). If the total amount of haemoglobin is less than normal (anaemia) or if part of the haemoglobin is unavailable for oxygen transport (carbon monoxide poisoning, methaemoglobinaemia or sulphaemoglobinaemia) then anaemic hypoxia will result.

(a) *Anaemia*.
If we ignore the small amount of oxygen in physical solution in the blood, then halving the haemoglobin concentration will halve the oxygen content of the arterial blood. Anaemia causes an increase in 2, 3DPG synthesis and therefore a shift to the right of the oxyhaemoglobin dissociation curve, so favouring the unloading of oxygen from the blood to the tissues.

(b) *Carbon monoxide poisoning*.
Carbon monoxide causes anaemic hypoxia by combining with haemoglobin to form carboxyhaemoglobin, so that this fraction of the haemoglobin is unavailable for oxygen transport. A relatively low concentration of carbon monoxide will form a substantial amount of carboxyhaemoglobin because the affinity of haemoglobin for CO is about 250 times its affinity for oxygen. The other change produced by carbon monoxide is a shift to the left of the dissociation curve of the remaining oxyhaemoglobin. The significance of this (Fig. 9) is that in order to offload the same amount of oxygen to the tissues, the venous $Po_2$ is reduced to a much lower level. The venous points for the three curves shown in Fig. 9 are:

Normal curve (haemoglobin 14·4 g/dl) 40 mm Hg (5·3 kPa)
Anaemia curve (haemoglobin 7·2 g/dl) 27 mm Hg (3·6 kPa)
50% HbCO curve (total haemoglobin 14·4 g/dl) 14 mm Hg (1·9 kPa)

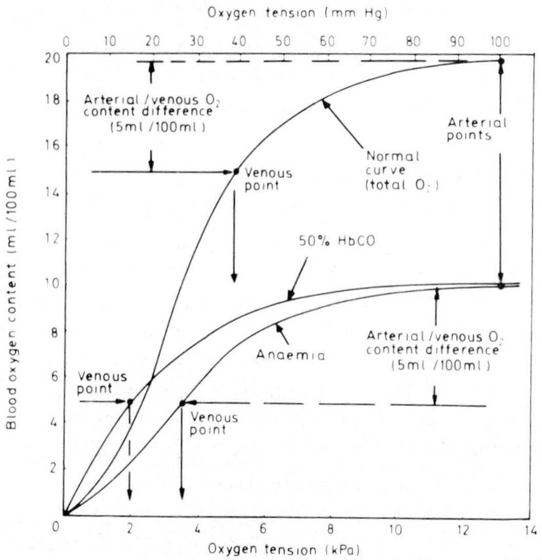


4/Fig. 9.—The relationship between blood oxygen content and oxygen tension in a normal subject (*top curve*) a subject with carbon monoxide poisoning (*middle curve*) and a subject with anaemia (*lower curve*). Note that the subject who has half his haemoglobin in combination with carbon monoxide is in a much worse state than the anaemic subject who just has half his haemoglobin absent (see text). (Courtesy of Dr. J. F. Nunn and Butterworth & Co.[5])

So although this shift of the oxyhaemoglobin dissociation curve has little effect on the arterial oxygen content, the effect on venous $Po_2$ is very significant—at a cerebral venous $Po_2$ of 14 mm Hg (1·9 kPa) the subject will be unconscious. Coal (or town) gas used to be a common cause of carbon monoxide poisoning as it contained 50 per cent hydrogen, about 25 per cent methane and about 10–15 per cent carbon monoxide. Now that coal gas has been replaced by natural gas (about 90 per cent methane, with only trace amounts of carbon monoxide), domestic gas is no longer a common cause of carbon monoxide poisoning. Cigarette smoking can produce levels of carboxyhaemoglobin of 10 per cent of the total haemoglobin. Car exhaust fumes and incomplete combustion during fires are other sources of the gas.

Commercial paint remover containing methylene chloride has caused severe carbon monoxide poisoning. In poorly ventilated surroundings the fumes are inhaled and metabolised to carbon monoxide.

Treatment consists of administration of oxygen (hyperbaric, if possible, for severe cases) with 5 per cent $CO_2$ in order to shift the dissociation curve of the remaining oxyhaemoglobin rightwards towards its normal position.

(c) *Methaemoglobinaemia and Sulphaemoglobinaemia*

Characteristically the cyanosis (due to the presence of either methaemoglobin or sulphaemoglobin in the blood) is unaccompanied by evidence of cardiac or respiratory abnormalities. In severe cases there may be symptoms and signs of hypoxaemia such as headache, tiredness, dizziness, dyspnoea, tachycardia and in chronic cases of polycythaemia. The condition can prove fatal.

Methaemoglobinaemia is the commonest of the two conditions and may be either *inherited* or *acquired*. The latter can be caused by a number of drugs and chemicals such as nitrites, nitrates (which are converted to nitrites in the gut) phenacetin, acetanilide, sulphanilamide and prilocaine (Citanest). Sulphaemoglobinaemia may be produced by most of the compounds that cause methaemoglobinaemia and the two conditions frequently coexist.

Methaemoglobin (Hb $Fe^{+++}$OH) is produced in small quantities by oxidation of the ferrous porphyrin complex, but, under normal circumstances, this ferric form is promptly reduced, thereby keeping the level of methaemoglobin in the blood at a low level. Coal-tar derivatives and other substances (mentioned above) interfere with this process and allow methaemoglobin to accumulate.

Methaemoglobinaemia gives a chocolate-brown appearance whereas sulphaemoglobinaemia produces a cyanotic tinge which is sometimes described as leaden-blue or mauve-lavender. The principal reason for attempting to distinguish between these two conditions is that methaemoglobinaemia can be treated whereas sulphaemoglobinaemia cannot. There are no known measures which will convert sulphaemoglobin to haemoglobin, though concentrations of sulphaemoglobin sufficient to endanger life do not seem to occur. The haemoglobin which is oxidised to methaemoglobin cannot transport oxygen; in addition, the dissociation curve of the remaining haemoglobin is shifted to the left, so impairing oxygen delivery to the tissues.

*Treatment of methaemoglobinaemia.*—The *inherited* form of methaemoglobinaemia can be successfully retarded by taking large doses of vitamin C (500 mg/day) or oral methylene blue. The *acquired* form requires removal of the causative agent and, if necessary, the intravenous administration of 1 per cent aqueous methylene blue (1–2 mg/kg body weight) over a period of 5 minutes.

### 3. Stagnant Hypoxia

This occurs as a result of reduced tissue perfusion which may be either general or local. General hypoperfusion is due to a low cardiac output, while local hypoperfusion may be due to arterial occlusion, for example by atheroma, embolism, trauma, vasoconstriction, or to venous occlusion.

### 4. Histotoxic Hypoxia

In the mitochondria food substrates are oxidized by nicotinamide adenine dinucleotide (NAD) which removes hydrogen. The hydrogen is passed down an enzyme chain containing several cytochromes and finally combines with oxygen to form water. Poisoning of this enzyme system means that the cells are unable to use the oxygen being delivered to them and aerobic metabolism therefore stops. A small amount of ATP can still be formed as a result of anaerobic metabolism. Reduced production of carbon dioxide and stimulation of ventilation produce a fall in arterial $Pco_2$; mixed venous $Po_2$ rises because the oxygen consumption has fallen.

Sodium nitroprusside contains a cyanide radical, so overdose of this drug can cause histotoxic hypoxia due to poisoning of intracellular enzymes.

### 5. Low $P_{50}$

This group is sometimes included under the heading "anaemic hypoxia" whose definition has to be appropriately altered. It is probably less confusing, albeit less tidy, to consider it separately.

The $P_{50}$ (see p. 106) is the partial pressure of oxygen at which haemoglobin is 50 per cent saturated, and normally has a value of 27 mm Hg (3·6 kPa). If the $P_{50}$ is reduced, this means that the haemoglobin dissociation curve is shifted to the left so that to offload a given amount of oxygen the $Po_2$ has to drop further. In this way a low $P_{50}$ can produce tissue hypoxia.

Causes of a shift to the left are alkalosis, reduced 2,3DPG and hypothermia.

### Cyanosis

This term refers to the bluish colour of skin or mucous membranes which occurs if there is more than 5·0 g of reduced haemoglobin in the blood passing through the capillaries. It follows that if a patient is very anaemic then even in the presence of gross hypoxia there may not be enough deoxygenated haemoglobin to produce cyanosis. Cyanosis may be central or peripheral. *Central* cyanosis, which is best detected by looking at the mucosa of the lips, implies arterial desaturation. *Peripheral* cyanosis may occur because there is central cyanosis, or it may occur alone due to poor peripheral blood flow. It is best detected by looking at the nail beds.* Detection of either form of cyanosis is prone to considerable observer error and of course patients are occasionally blue for other reasons, such as injection of dye to show up lymphatics prior to lymphangiography.

## Effects of Hypoxia

The effects of hypoxia are not always easy to predict. They depend on:

(i) whether one is considering the intact subject or an isolated preparation, for example the heart *in vivo* or *in vitro*;
(ii) the degree of hypoxia;
(iii) the duration of hypoxia;
(iv) the idiosyncrasy of the individual;
(v) other factors such as disease, drugs and temperature.

* If these are blue but the lips are not, then the cyanosis is peripheral.

1. **Cardiovascular System**

Systemic vasodilatation is a direct effect of hypoxia. The fall in blood pressure which this alone would produce is offset by an increase in cardiac output which is mainly due to an increase in sympathetic activity secondary to peripheral chemoreceptor stimulation by hypoxia. An animal which is peripherally chemodenervated will suffer profound hypotension in response to hypoxia. Of course, even in the intact subject, if the hypoxic insult is severe enough the cardiac output will no longer be able to compensate for the reduced systemic vascular resistance, the heart will fail and the blood pressure fall, the process culminating in hypoxic cardiac arrest. The prognosis for recovery following such a catastrophe is extremely poor because by the time the heart has stopped as a result of hypoxia there is nearly always irreversible brain damage.

Hypoxia increases the blood flow to most organs, especially to the brain, and causes a reduction in brain extracellular fluid pH which has a direct vasodilator effect on the cerebral vessels.

2. **Respiratory System**

Pulmonary arterioles constrict in response to hypoxia. This mechanism is of obvious benefit if part of the lung is more hypoxic than the rest, for example due to lobar consolidation, as it causes diversion of the blood flow to the better oxygenated regions. In patients with intracardiac shunts such as ventricular septal defect, hypoxia may cause an increase in right-sided pressure with a reversal of the shunt and consequent arterial desaturation. Chronic hypoxia can lead to an irreversible increase in pulmonary vascular resistance with pulmonary hypertension and cor pulmonale.

3. **Metabolism**

If there is insufficient oxygen for aerobic metabolism then a small amount of ATP can still be formed. The lactic acid produced accumulates and gives rise to a progressively more severe metabolic acidosis. The usual measure of blood pH gives little information concerning intracellular pH, which in the case of the brain may become so low as to cause structural damage.

4. **Organ Failure**

The brain and retina are very sensitive to oxygen lack. The sensitivity of the latter can be demonstrated by pressing gently on the side of one's eye to occlude the blood supply and within ten seconds observing a dark area advancing over the affected field. Cerebral function is a sensitive indicator of oxygen lack; changes of mood occur and performance gradually deteriorates leading to confusion and loss of consciousness. If the circulation is arrested the time taken for the brain to stop functioning to the extent of loss of consciousness is called its "survival time". The "revival time" is the time beyond which recovery of function is not possible. The brain cortex survival time is about 0·5 min whereas its revival time is about 5 min. As you would expect the spinal cord is also very sensitive to hypoxia and may be damaged as a result of clamping the aorta or of occlusion of the anterior spinal artery.

Hepatic cells, arranged in lobules with centrilobular (portal blood supply) and peripheral (systemic blood supply) distribution, show a characteristic pattern of disorder in hypoxic conditions. The centrilobular cells exhibit the first changes, being more remote from the systemic blood supply and therefore more hypoxic. In acute hypoxia centrilobular necrosis is seen while in more chronic hypoxic states a fibrosis develops. The kidney has a survival time of about ten minutes. More prolonged hypoxia produces acute tubular necrosis and then cortical necrosis. Chronic renal hypoxia increases synthesis of erythropoietin which stimulates marrow formation of erythrocytes, resulting in secondary polycythaemia. In a group of patients with polycythaemia secondary to hypoxic lung disease, although venesection which produced a fall in mean packed cell volume from 0·6 to 0·5 caused no increase in cerebral oxygen carriage, cerebral blood flow went up by 21 per cent and more importantly there was considerable symptomatic improvement.[7]

5. **Haemoglobin**

Reduced haemoglobin (Hb) is blue and if present in sufficient amount causes cyanosis (p. 133). It is a better buffer than oxyhaemoglobin ($HbO_2$) and so when $HbO_2$ gives up its oxygen (equation 1) Hb buffers the hydrogen ion (equation 2).

1. $HbO_2 \rightarrow Hb + O_2$
2. $Hb + H^+ \rightarrow HHb$

The increase in pH which this process tends to produce will partly offset the reduction in pH that occurs due to $CO_2$ production. The greater carriage of $CO_2$ by deoxygenated blood (Haldane effect) has been mentioned (p. 108).

The effect of hypoxia in reducing the solubility of haemoglobin S may have disastrous consequences (p. 604).

4/TABLE 3

EFFECTS OF HYPOXIA

| | |
|---|---|
| CVS | Systemic vascular resistance reduced<br>Cardiac output increased<br>Peripheral chemoreceptor stimulation→increase in sympathetic activity<br>Cerebral vasodilatation |
| RS | Ventilation increased<br>Pulmonary vascular resistance increased |
| METABOLISM | Aerobic metabolism reduced<br>Anaerobic metabolism→metabolic acidosis |
| ORGAN FAILURE | |
| Haemoglobin | Cyanosis<br>Reduced haemoglobin is a better buffer<br>Reduced solubility of haemoglobin S<br>Increased in chronic hypoxia |

## POSTOPERATIVE HYPOXIA

Nunn and Payne[8] showed that after general anaesthesia the arterial $P_{O_2}$ is lower than normal. There are several reasons for this which are considered briefly below. In addition to this hypoxic hypoxia, tissue oxygenation may also be reduced because of a low cardiac output (stagnant hypoxia) or because of anaemia (anaemic hypoxia). The important consideration is the oxygen flux, and this must match tissue oxygen requirement. The latter is commonly increased postoperatively as a result of shivering or pyrexia.

Factors contributing to hypoxic hypoxia in the post-anaesthetic period are:

1. Diffusion hypoxia or Fink effect.
2. Increased $\dot{V}/\dot{Q}$ mismatch.
   Anaesthesia produces a reduction in functional residual capacity (FRC) and the consequences of this are likely to be more serious in the elderly and patients who are fat or smoke. If the FRC decreases below the closing capacity there will be zones of lung perfused but not ventilated at the end of expiration and beginning of inspiration. Alexander[9] found that following upper abdominal surgery FRC was reduced by 30 per cent.
3. Reduced cardiac output.
   A reduced cardiac output will result in a reduced oxygen flux, which may be insufficient to meet the patient's oxygen demand especially if he is shivering. The fall in mixed venous $P_{O_2}$ will then produce a fall in arterial $P_{O_2}$, with further reduction in oxygen flux. This situation will be made worse if the patient is anaemic.
4. Hypoventilation
   (*a*) Drugs. Most anaesthetic drugs depress ventilation. If the dose has been judged correctly it is unlikely that dangerous hypoventilation will result from this alone, but even the so-called short-acting opiates such as fentanyl can cause respiratory depression lasting several hours. Relaxant drugs may not be fully reversed, although the degree of residual paralysis usually needs to be fairly gross for hypoventilation to result.
   (*b*) Obstruction. Partial respiratory obstruction in the postoperative period is often not recognised immediately.
   (*c*) Pain. In some patients, for example those who have had upper abdominal surgery, pain may be preventing them from breathing more deeply. Elevation of the diaphragm due to abdominal distension will also contribute to hypoventilation.
   (*d*) Intra-operative hyperventilation. Many patients are hyperventilated during operations. When spontaneous ventilation is restored there may be a considerable total body deficit of $CO_2$. Reduction of $CO_2$ excretion by hypoventilation during the early postoperative period allows this deficit to be made up.

Increasing the inspired oxygen concentration by using a 4 l/min flow of oxygen into a lightweight mask such as the Hudson or MC masks, will prevent hypoxia occurring in most patients.

Long operations, thoracic or upper abdominal incisions, old age, pre-existing lung disease, heart disease and sickle-cell disease place patients at special risk. The increase in pulmonary vascular resistance produced by hypoxia may initiate or increase a right-to-left shunt through a VSD. The protective effect of peripheral chemoreceptor stimulation by hypoxia and increased drive to ventilation may be reduced by halothane.

### Chronic Oxygen Lack

Chronic hypoxia may be due to disease or living at high altitude. As the altitude increases so the total atmospheric pressure is reduced and the partial pressure of oxygen declines proportionately. Thus:

Partial Pressure of $O_2$ in Air

| | | |
|---|---|---|
| At sea level | = | 159 mm Hg (21·2 kPa) |
| At 10,000 ft | = | 110 mm Hg (14·7 kPa) |
| At 20,000 ft | = | 73 mm Hg (9·7 kPa) |
| At 50,000 ft | = | 18 mm Hg (2·4 kPa) |

A normal person loses consciousness when the arterial oxygen saturation falls to about 50 per cent or below. Breathing air, this gives an upper ceiling of 23,000 feet (7010 metres), but if oxygen is substituted for air a height of 47,000 feet (14,326 metres) may be reached before unconsciousness ensues.

Studies of respiratory control in high altitude residents have shown that many of them produce no increase in ventilation in response to hypoxia. The question arises: is this absence of hypoxic sensitivity genetically determined or is it due to chronic hypoxia in early life? Children with Fallot's tetralogy have a blunted or absent ventilatory response to hypoxia and some have been shown to regain the response following corrective surgery. Adults who live at sea level and then move to an area at high altitude do not lose their ventilatory response to hypoxia (although it may decrease over many years), neither do adult residents at high altitudes who move to areas of low altitude regain it.

On ascent to high altitude the sequence of events is as follows. Acute hypoxia causes hyperventilation by stimulating the peripheral chemoreceptors. As $Paco_2$ falls, the pH in the CSF and in the region of the central chemoreceptor rises, so opposing to some extent the increase in ventilation. Over the next few days renal excretion of bicarbonate induces a compensatory metabolic acidosis and in addition CSF bicarbonate concentration falls, reducing the CSF pH almost to normal and so allowing the peripheral chemoreceptors to drive ventilation unopposed; ventilation reaches its maximum at four days. The mechanism of reduction in CSF bicarbonate concentration is not clear. If the subject remains at altitude there is a very slow reduction in ventilation extending over years. If he descends to sea level, $P_{AO_2}$ rises, peripheral chemoreceptor drive is reduced, $Paco_2$ rises and therefore brain $Pco_2$ rises. Because the pH of CSF and brain extracellular fluid is now lower than normal (since the bicarbonate concentration is still lower than normal) ventilation is driven by an increased central drive which declines as CSF bicarbonate reaccumulates bringing brain pH back to normal. Lenfant and Sullivan[10] have reviewed the physiology of high altitude adaptation.

Mountain sickness may occur in unacclimatised subjects who ascend rapidly to 3000 m or above. It can vary in severity from mild weakness, nausea and shortness of breath to fatal pulmonary and cerebral oedema. Prophylaxis is best achieved by slow ascent although acetazolamide has been shown to be worthwhile;[11] whether this drug, which is a carbonic anhydrase inhibitor, acts by stimulating breathing by the metabolic acidosis it produces is not known. If more than trivial symptoms are present, the subject must descend.[12]

**Oxygen Excess** (see also Chapter 5, p. 158)

"Oxygen remains a fascinating paradox. Essential to mammalian life within a narrow spectrum of partial pressures, it is lethal at pressures outside that range".[13]

A considerable weight of evidence is accumulating to substantiate this statement. It has long been known that fit adults breathing pure oxygen can suffer toxic effects.

#### Pulmonary Effects

Extensive investigation of American astronauts has revealed no lung damage as a result of breathing 100 per cent oxygen at one-third of an atmosphere pressure. It does not necessarily follow that a $P_{IO_2}$ of 238 mm Hg (32 kPa) is harmless in the presence of disease. Breathing 100 per cent oxygen at 1 atmosphere pressure can cause substernal discomfort and reduction in vital capacity after as little as 10 hours, and recovery of vital capacity may take several days after resumption of air breathing.

The lungs of animals which have died as a result of pulmonary oxygen toxicity show changes in the capillary endothelium with an increase in its permeability, allowing fluid to accumulate in the interstitial space and widen the diffusion pathway between alveolar gas and alveolar capillary blood. Other adverse effects of high oxygen concentrations on the lung include depression of mucociliary transport, inhibition of phagocytosis by alveolar macrophages and changes in surfactant activity and its production by the type 2 cells.

Although there is no doubt that high oxygen concentrations can cause lung damage, the highest safe concentration is not known and anyway it will vary depending on the individual, the pre-existing pulmonary pathology and duration of exposure. In intensive care it is customary to use the lowest level of $F_{IO_2}$ which produces an acceptable level of $Pa_{O_2}$, and patients should not be ventilated with high concentrations of oxygen for prolonged periods unless the alternative is dangerous hypoxia.

If there are high concentrations of oxygen in the alveolar gas of zones of lung with low $\dot{V}/\dot{Q}$ ratios, the oxygen passes into the pulmonary capillary blood and the alveoli collapse. This has been demonstrated in healthy volunteers by Nunn and co-workers.[14]

At sea level the normal subject has a small hypoxic drive to ventilation via the peripheral chemoreceptors. Some patients with chronic bronchitis and low $Pa_{O_2}$ rely heavily on their hypoxic drive and if this is removed by giving high concentrations of inspired oxygen, ventilation decreases, $P_{CO_2}$ rises and respiratory arrest soon to be followed by cardiac arrest may result. Such patients, if they do need oxygen, must be managed very carefully with repeated blood gas measurements and appropriate alteration of the inspired oxygen concentration.

**Circulatory system.**—In studies in volunteers breathing pure oxygen[15] it has been shown that there is a slight fall in both heart rate and cardiac output during the inhalation. The most striking feature was the generalised increase in peripheral resistance and systemic pressure. The effects of oxygen inhalation on the general circulation have been likened to the effects of administering a peripheral vasoconstrictor, for the blood pressure goes up and the heart rate goes down. On this basis it is suggested that the slowing of the heart rate may be a reflex action following upon stimulation of the baroreceptors rather than any direct action on the chemoreceptors.

**Elimination of nitrogen.**—The inhalation of 100 per cent oxygen leads to a rapid fall in the nitrogen content of the arterial circulation so that the blood is almost completely cleared in a few minutes, but the loss from other tissues is more gradual. The brain takes 15–20 minutes before it is largely free of nitrogen. The cerebrospinal fluid clears relatively slowly, only 50 per cent leaving in the first hour, while fat tissues—with their poor blood supply—may take many hours before denitrogenation is complete. Oxygen inhalation may be used to remove air from body cavities such as the gastro-intestinal tract and cerebral ventricles, as well as in the treatment of air embolism.

Typical arterial and mixed venous blood values for normal subjects breathing 100 per cent oxygen would be:

| | mm Hg | kPa | | mm Hg | kPa |
|---|---|---|---|---|---|
| $Pa_{O_2}$ | 600 | 80 | $P\bar{v}_{O_2}$ | 50 | 6·7 |
| $Pa_{CO_2}$ | 40 | 5·3 | $P\bar{v}_{CO_2}$ | 46 | 6·1 |
| $Pa_{N_2}$ | 0 | 0 | $P\bar{v}_{N_2}$ | 0 | 0 |

The reason the $P\bar{v}_{O_2}$ is only slightly higher than the normal value during air breathing (40 mm Hg, 5·3kPa) is because of the shape of the oxyhaemoglobin dissociation curve (p. 106). The top part of the curve is virtually horizontal, so since the amount of oxygen carried in physical solution is negligible compared with that in combination with haemoglobin, the oxygen *content* of arterial blood during oxygen breathing ($Pa_{O_2}$ = 600 mm Hg, 80 kPa) is only very slightly greater than that during air breathing ($Pa_{O_2}$ = 100 mm Hg, 13·3 kPa). There is therefore very little difference between the mixed venous oxygen content values; as we are now operating on the steep part of the curve this small content difference is reflected by only a small $P_{O_2}$ difference.

There is of course no need for the sum of the partial pressures of gases in the blood to approximate to atmospheric pressure (unlike alveolar gas) and because gases diffuse down partial pressure gradients, oxygen breathing will enormously increase elimination of nitrogen and other gases from a gas loculus within the body, for example a pneumothorax. If the loculus contains some gas other than nitrogen, then oxygen breathing removes the $P_{N_2}$ gradient favouring diffusion of nitrogen from the tissues into the loculus, and so again allows more rapid absorption of the gas.

### Other Effects of Oxygen Excess

Retrolental fibroplasia (see Chapter 42, p. 1116 in Treatment of Respiratory Distress Syndrome). Central nervous system effects of hyperbaric oxygen (see p. 162).

## METHODS OF OXYGEN THERAPY

**Spontaneously breathing patients.**—During inspiration gas flow starts from zero, reaches a peak which is usually about four times the minute volume and then declines to zero again. Since the peak inspiratory flow even at rest may be 30 l/min in an adult, unless the oxygen delivery device produces a flow in excess of this amount (high air flow with oxygen enrichment, HAFOE) or has a suitable reservoir the $F_{IO_2}$ will vary during inspiration, and different parts of the lungs will receive different oxygen concentrations.

**Oxygen masks.**—There are a great many different masks available, but only two representative ones will be mentioned.

The "MC" or Mary Catterall mask is illustrated in Fig. 10. It is very suitable for patients in recovery areas and is light, reasonably comfortable and cheap. At an oxygen flow rate of 5 l/min it provides very approximately 40 per cent inspired oxygen concentration, the oxygen being diluted by air drawn in through holes in the mask. The precise concentration will depend on the patient's size and therefore tidal volume, pattern of breathing and how well the mask fits their face. The mask adds a small volume to the patient's dead space.

"*Ventimask*" (Fig. 11).—This mask uses the venturi principle so that a low flow of oxygen can be used to draw in large quantities of air. The advantage of this principle is that it is not only economical with oxygen but it also permits accuracy in the concentration of oxygen delivered to the patient, even in the presence of a poorly fitting mask.

The mask is disposable and contains a single inlet tube. There are several types designed to give concentrations of 24, 28, 35, 40 or 60 per cent oxygen. They all produce at least 30 l/min of the desired mixture, but it is very important to ensure that the correct flow of oxygen (stated on the mask) is used. Other masks which have a reservoir arrangement have been produced but are not often used now.

**Nasal catheters.**—A nasal catheter or twin nasal cannula can be used to provide oxygen

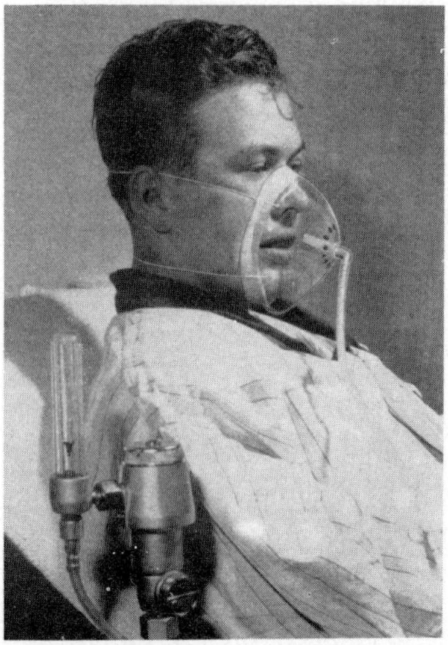

4/FIG. 10.—The "MC" mask. (Courtesy of Bakelite Xylonite Ltd.)

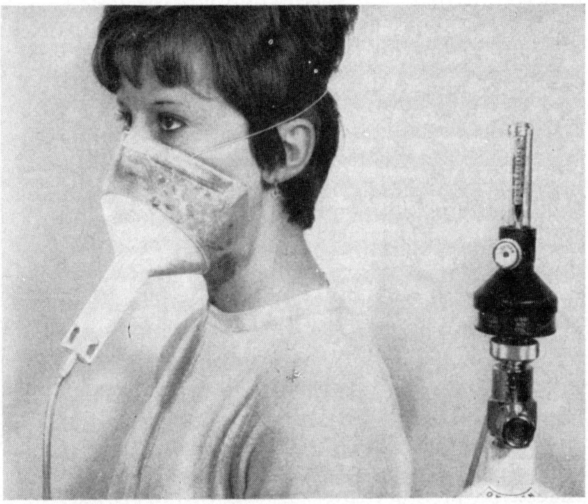

4/FIG. 11.—The "Ventimask". (Courtesy of Oxygenaire Ltd.)

enrichment of the inspired air. Flows up to 3 l/min are well tolerated, but the $FIO_2$ produced is unpredictable.

### Comment

The performance of these devices for oxygen therapy has been assessed on "patient-model" devices[17] and on patients.[18–20] The results emphasise the irregular performance of high-flow devices with regard to carbon dioxide accumulation, whilst the low-flow venturi devices provide inspired oxygen tensions close to the specification.

**Oxygen tents.**—A tent must be used when other methods of oxygen administration are impracticable. Such occasions arise when the patient is very young or incapable of tolerating a mask or catheter.

Hewer and Lee[21] have listed the essential characteristics of an oxygen tent:

1. Positive ventilation of the atmosphere in the tent must be secured.
2. The temperature and humidity of the atmosphere in the tent must be amenable to regulation.
3. Carbon dioxide must not be allowed to accumulate within the tent.
4. Adequate provision must be made for nursing, flushing the tent, and sampling the internal atmosphere.
5. The materials from which the tent is made must be non-inflammable.
6. It must be possible to sterilise the interior of the tent.

## CARBON DIOXIDE ($CO_2$)

### History

Carbon dioxide was first isolated by Black in 1757. Henry Hill Hickman (1800–1830) carried out experiments on animals with carbon dioxide, and he wrote a letter in 1824 on "Suspended Animation". A medal is awarded in commemoration of his work by the Royal Society of Medicine of London. The physiological significance of this gas was not fully appreciated until the work of Yandell Henderson in the United States[22] and J. S. Haldane in England.[23] It soon gained widespread popularity amongst anaesthetists as a stimulus to respiration, but in more recent years the emphasis has been on its elimination rather than its addition in view of the high figures for carbon dioxide tensions in the blood that have been recorded with certain anaesthetic systems and techniques.

### Properties

Carbon dioxide is a colourless gas, irritant to the mucosa when inhaled in high concentrations, and present in the atmosphere at a concentration of 0·03 vol per cent. If it is cooled to −78·5° C it solidifies without passing through the liquid state. Similarly if solid $CO_2$ ($CO_2$ snow or dry ice) is warmed it changes to the vapour state without liquefying. The liquid phase can only be achieved under conditions of increased pressure (greater than 517 kPa, 3878·8 mm Hg, 75 psig). Carbon dioxide for medical use is stored in grey cylinders at about 5000 kPa (37512·3 mm Hg, 750 psig) in liquid form. The physiological importance of $CO_2$ and the effects of hypercapnia and hypocapnia are discussed in Chapter 3.

4/TABLE 4
PROPERTIES OF CARBON DIOXIDE

| | |
|---|---|
| Molecular weight | 44·0 |
| Relative density (air = 1) | 1·53 |
| Sublimation point, 750 mm Hg (100 kPa) | −78·5° C |
| Critical temperature | 31·04° C |
| Solubility in plasma at 37° C | 0·03 mmol $l^{-1}$ mm $Hg^{-1}$ (0·23 mmol $l^{-1}$ $kPa^{-1}$) |
| Molar volume | 22·26 l* |

* $CO_2$ is a non-ideal gas. An ideal gas would have a molar volume of 22·41 l.

### Preparation

In Britain carbon dioxide is produced mainly as a by-product in the manufacture of hydrogen, and also as a by-product in the process of fermentation. For industrial chemical use, hydrogen is made by reacting a fuel such as petroleum or natural gas with steam. This results in a mixture of hydrogen and carbon monoxide which is reacted with more steam to produce carbon dioxide.

In the laboratory carbon dioxide can conveniently be made by adding any strong acid to a carbonate:

$$NaHCO_3 + HCl \rightarrow NaCl + H_2O + CO_2$$

### Use of Carbon Dioxide in Anaesthesia

It is important to remember that the patient's respiratory response to $CO_2$ may be grossly depressed or even absent as a result of drugs or disease, therefore failure-to-breathe of a non-paralysed patient may still occur in spite of a dangerously high $Paco_2$. 5 per cent $CO_2$ will raise the $Paco_2$ by about 35 mm Hg (4·7 kPa), for a given alveolar ventilation and $CO_2$ production, so care must be taken when using this mixture, while the use of higher concentrations is hazardous. Some anaesthetists consider that the provision of a $CO_2$ cylinder on an anaesthetic machine introduces an unacceptable hazard of accidental extreme hypercapnia. This must have happened on many occasions and has been reported.[24] Nevertheless it is useful to be able to raise the $FICO_2$ with exogenous (not produced by the patient) carbon dioxide in the following circumstances:

(i) to raise the $Paco_2$ when discontinuing IPPV so that spontaneous respiration is established more quickly. Patients ventilated during operations are frequently hypocapnic, so that the use of $CO_2$ under these circumstances is reasonable.

(ii) to stimulate respiration during induction of anaesthesia. If you intend a patient to breathe $N_2O/O_2$/halothane spontaneously, but he becomes apnoeic following the induction dose of thiopentone, you may decide just to wait for spontaneous respiration to be resumed. Sometimes, instead of starting to breathe quietly the patient coughs. If, during the apnoeic phase, the patient is gently ventilated with 5 per cent $CO_2$, $N_2O/O_2$/halothane, this problem is avoided. The ventilation must be gentle with a clear airway so that inflation of the stomach and regurgitation is avoided; 5 per cent $CO_2$ is used to prevent the hypocapnia which would otherwise result and which would lead to prolongation of apnoea and reduction in cerebral blood flow. $CO_2$ is sometimes used to stimulate respiration to facilitate blind nasal intubation.

## HELIUM (He)

### History

Helium was first noted by Lockyer and Eden in 1867 when examining the spectrum of the sun. It was isolated by Ramsay and Lockyer in 1895.[25]

### Preparation

The main source is from the abundant supplies of natural gas found in the United States, chiefly in Texas and Kansas. The other gases present are removed by absorption, liquefaction or scrubbing with water and sodium hydroxide. Helium has a very low boiling point (−269° C) so that when the temperature is lowered the other gases liquefy first and can be removed, leaving helium in the gaseous form.

### Physical Properties

Helium is an inert, colourless, odourless gas. It is one of the "rare gases", its concentration in air being 1 in 200 000 by volume, the others being radon, argon, xenon and krypton. Apart from hydrogen, helium is the lightest known gas, with a molecular weight of 4 and a relative density of 0·14 (air = 1). It diffuses through skin and rubber.

### Clinical Use

If there is a partial respiratory obstruction, for example tracheal stenosis, the speed of gas flow increases and may reach its critical velocity at which flow becomes fully turbulent. If gas flow is *laminar* the pressure gradient required to produce a given flow is proportional to the rate of flow and the *viscosity* of the gas. However, if gas flow is *turbulent* the pressure gradient required to produce a given flow is proportional to the *density* of the gas and to the square of the flow. Under these conditions a greater flow will occur with a mixture of 80 per cent helium and 20 per cent oxygen, having a relative density of 0·33, than with air (relative density = 1). In addition, because of the low density of helium, the critical velocity of this mixture is greater than that of air. It is important that the mixture be administered via a well-fitting face-mask because if it is diluted with air the advantage is lost.

Helium/oxygen mixtures are also used in deep-water diving to avoid nitrogen narcosis which occurs if air is breathed at high pressures (see p. 148).

## PRINCIPLES OF GAS ANALYSIS

In anaesthetic practice a knowledge of the concentration of a gas such as oxygen, carbon dioxide, or nitrous oxide is often required for the satisfactory management of the patient. This information can be obtained in a variety of ways depending on the apparatus available. In general the methods available can be classified in three groups—first, those based on *chemical* analysis; second, those requiring *physical* measurement; and third, the use of a *specific electrode*.

### Chemical Analysis

The principal methods require the absorption of a gas by a particular reagent and are especially applicable to the estimation of oxygen and carbon dioxide.

The Haldane apparatus, which over the years has been modified in various ways, is used for measurement of the $CO_2$ and $O_2$ concentrations of gas samples. Lloyd's[26] modification is shown in Fig. 12. The whole apparatus is enclosed in a water jacket which is kept stirred so as to minimise temperature fluctuations which would affect gas volume measurements. By raising and lowering the mercury reservoir (connected by tubing to the bottom of the apparatus) and turning the multiway tap to the appropriate position, the gas sample can be drawn into the central burette via I, then transferred to chamber K which contains potassium hydroxide. The KOH absorbs the $CO_2$, and by returning the

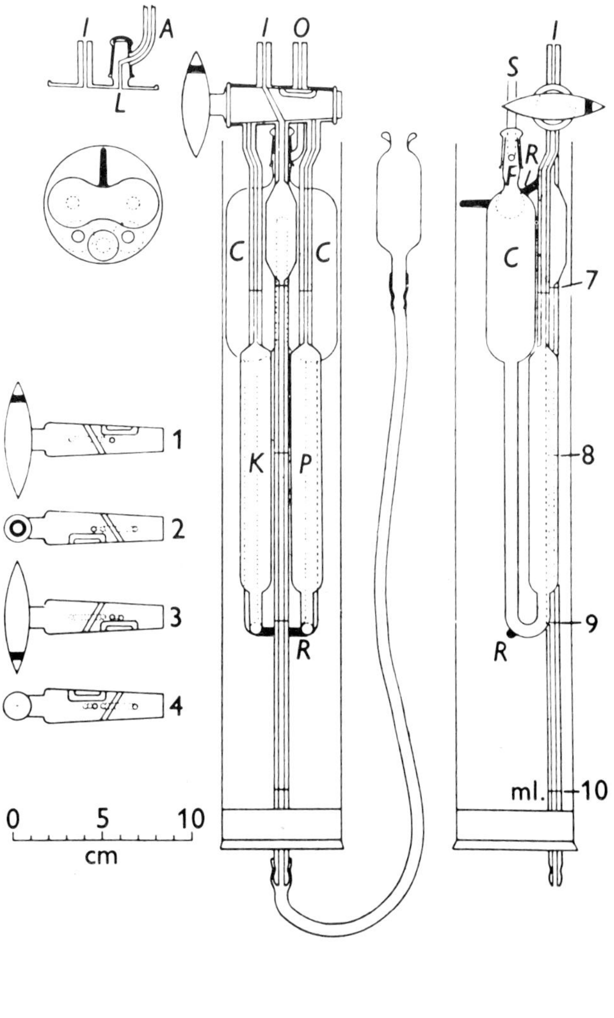


4/Fig. 12.—Haldane's gas analysis apparatus. (Courtesy of Dr. B. B. Lloyd and the publishers of the *Journal of Physiology*, the Cambridge University Press.[26])

remaining gas to the central burette its volume can be measured, then

$$\% \ CO_2 \text{ in gas sample} = \frac{\text{reduction in gas vol.}}{\text{original vol.}} \times 100$$

The gas can now be made to pass into chamber P where the oxygen is absorbed by pyrogallol. The remaining gas is then returned to the central burette, the change in volume measured and the oxygen concentration of the sample derived.

If $N_2O$ is present, inaccuracies will occur due to its absorption by KOH. Saturating the KOH with $N_2O$ before use is one method which has been used to overcome this problem. The $CO_2$ analysis must be done first since it will also be absorbed by pyrogallol. The accuracy of the Lloyd Haldane for $CO_2$ measurement is ±0·05 per cent.

The Van Slyke apparatus is used to measure the oxygen and carbon dioxide contents of blood. The blood sample is introduced into the apparatus where it is first of all mixed with acid-saponin to haemolyse it and drive off all the gases. Different solutions are then used to absorb $CO_2$ and $O_2$ and the blood content of these gases can be derived. The method is difficult and tedious.

A variation of this system is the manometric technique, where both the volume and the temperature are kept constant and variations in pressure can be measured by an apparatus such as that of Van Slyke and Niell. This type has the advantage of great accuracy and permits the determination of the pressure of gases in blood. Oxygen, for example, is absorbed by sodium hydrosulphite and carbon dioxide by sodium hydroxide. Nitrous oxide interferes with the estimation but allowance can be made for its presence.

**Physical Analysis**

The principal methods employed are:

**Magnetic.**—Unlike most gases, oxygen is paramagnetic and is therefore attracted into a magnetic field. A paramagnetic oxygen analyser exploits this property and consists of two glass spheres connected by a short bridge and suspended between the poles of a magnet. The spheres are filled with nitrogen which is weakly diamagnetic (moves away from a magnetic field), but are made to lie in the zone of high magnetic flux by means of the suspension. If oxygen is admitted to the cell it occupies the zone of greatest magnetic flux, displacing the nitrogen-containing spheres which rotate by an amount proportional to the concentration of oxygen present. This rotation is measured using a mirror and light source as shown in Fig. 13. Greater accuracy (to about 0·1 per cent) can be obtained by electrically offsetting this rotation and measuring the current needed to maintain the spheres in the 'zero' position.

**Infra-red analyser.**—Gases which contain two or more dissimilar atoms will absorb infra-red radiation, so $CO_2$ and $N_2O$ will absorb it but $O_2$ will not. In the usual type of infra-red $CO_2$ analyser the radiation from the source passes through a reference cell which is in parallel with the analyser cell. The radiation which emerges from the two cells passes into a detector unit. If one-half of this receives more infra-red radiation than the other, a pressure difference occurs across the diaphragm which separates the two halves. The infra-red radiation is "chopped" by a rotating shutter so that it switches on and off at 25–100 Hz, so prevent-

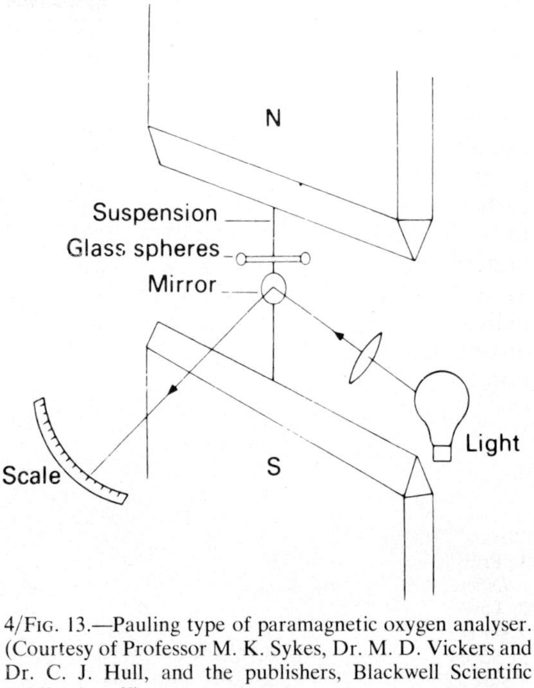


4/Fig. 13.—Pauling type of paramagnetic oxygen analyser. (Courtesy of Professor M. K. Sykes, Dr. M. D. Vickers and Dr. C. J. Hull, and the publishers, Blackwell Scientific Publications.[27])

ing excessive heating of the detector cells and producing an alternating output from the pressure transducer. The output is displayed as per cent $CO_2$ and is accurate to about ±0·1 per cent. Nitrous oxide has an absorption band very close to that of carbon dioxide and so will interfere with $CO_2$ measurement unless special precautions are taken.

**Oximeters.**—There are two types of oximeter—reflection and transmission. They are used to estimate the saturation of haemoglobin; light at certain wavelengths is shone on to the blood and the amount of light reflected or transmitted (depending on the type of oximeter) is measured. Transmission oximeters can be used on the ear lobe to provide a continuous non-invasive measurement.

**Fuel cell.**—Fuel cells can be used to measure oxygen concentration by converting energy from a chemical reaction into electrical energy. This reaction uses up the chemical components of the fuel cell, whose life therefore depends on the concentration of oxygen to which it is exposed and duration of exposure.

**Gas chromatography.**—The measurement of gases and vapours by the gas chromatograph has advanced considerably, but the basic technique remains the same in principle. Measurement of blood oxygen and carbon dioxide content may now be performed rapidly using this technique.[28]

A column consisting of crushed firebrick or Celite (or Kieselguhr, a diatomaceous earth) is usually heated to 70°–100° C. A carrier gas, being hydrogen, nitrogen, helium, argon or carbon dioxide, is used to carry the constituents to be distinguished. Each constituent then separates in the column and arrives at the detector as a separate entity and is revealed as an individual response. The various substances are distinguished by the time taken following injection for the response to appear. The record is usually displayed on a pen recorder and the amount of each constituent represented as a peak height. More exactly, it is proportional to the area under the peak, and the output of the detector may be fed directly to an integrating amplifier and the result obtained as a digital print out.

The detectors in gas chromatographs are of three main types:

1. Hot wire (katharometer) which detects changes in the thermal conductivity of the carrier gas.
2. Gas density.
3. Ionisation
   (i) Micro-argon using $Sr^{90}$ as a radioactive source of $\beta$ rays.
   (ii) Electron capture, using $Ni_{63}$ as a source of free electrons.
   (iii) Flame ionisation. A hydrogen flame is the means whereby ions are formed. This type of detector is extremely sensitive to organic compounds.

**Mass spectrometer.**—This device is able to analyse the concentrations of respirable gases. There are two types:

1. *The Magnetic Mass Spectrometer*

This analyser ionises the gas mixture as it is introduced into a high-vacuum chamber where it is subjected to a high magnetic field. The arc of ionic deflection is specific for each ion. Detectors distinguish the concentration of different ionised gases.

2. *Quadropole Mass Spectrometer*

The gas particles are again ionised in a vacuum chamber but subjected to an electrical field within 4 rods. The precise nature of this field may be altered, but at any given frequency only ions of a single mass will move along the axis. It, in effect, acts as an ion filter.

**Specific Electrodes** (see p. 120)

## REFERENCES

1. Priestley, J. (1777). *Experiments and Observations on Different Kinds of Air*. London.
2. Lavoisier, A. L., and de la Place, P. S. (1780). Mémoire sur la chaleur. *Mém. prés Acad. Sci. (Paris)*, **94**, 355.
3. Séguin, A., and Lavoisier, A. L. (1789). Premier mémoire sure la respiration des animaux. *Mém, prés. Acad. Sci. (Paris)*, **103**, 566.
4. Grant, W. J. (1978). *Medical Gases*, London: HM + M Publishers Ltd.
5. Nunn, J. F. (1977). *Applied Respiratory Physiology*, 2nd edit. London: Butterworths.
6. Fink, R. B. (1955). Diffusion anoxia. *Anesthesiology*, **16**, 511.
7. Wade, J. P. H., Pearson, T. C., Ross Russell, R. W. and

Wetherley-Mein, G. (1981). Cerebral blood flow and blood viscosity in patients with polycythaemia secondary to hypoxic lung disease. *Brit. med. J.*, **283**, 689.
8. Nunn, J. F., and Payne, J. P. (1962). Hypoxaemia after general anaesthesia. *Lancet*, **2**, 631.
9. Alexander, J. I., Spence, A. A., Parikh, R. K. and Stuart, B. (1973). The role of airway closure in postoperative hypoxaemia. *Brit. J. Anaesth.*, **45**, 34.
10. Lenfant, C. and Sullivan, K. (1971). Adaptation to high altitude. *New Eng. J. Med.*, **284**, 1298.
11. Greene, M. K., Kerr, A. M., McIntosh, I. B. and Prescott, R. J. (1981). Acetazolamide in prevention of acute mountain sickness: a double-blind controlled cross-over study. *Brit. med. J.*, **283**, 811.
12. Hackett, P. H., Rennie, D. and Levine, H. D. (1976). The incidence, importance and prophylaxis of acute mountain sickness. *Lancet*, **2**, 1149.
13. Smith, G. (1975). (Editorial) Oxygen and the lung. *Brit. J. Anaesth.*, **47**, 645.
14. Nunn, J. F., Coleman, A. J., Sachithanandan, T., Bergman, N. A. and Laws, J. W. (1965). Hypoxaemia and atelectasis produced by forced expiration. *Brit. J. Anaesth.*, **37**, 3.
15. Eggers, G. W. N., Jr., Paley, H. W., Leonard, J. J., and Warren, J. V. (1962). Haemodynamic responses to oxygen breathing in man. *J. appl. Physiol.*, **17**, 75.
16. Miller, W. F. (1962). Oxygen therapy catheter, mask, hood and tent. *Anesthesiology*, **23**, 445.
17. Bethune, D. W., and Collis, J. M. (1967). The evaluation of oxygen masks: a mechanical method. *Anaesthesia*, **22**, 43.
18. Leigh, J. M. (1970). Variation in performance of oxygen therapy devices. *Anaesthesia*, **25**, 210.
19. Leigh, J. M. (1974). Ideas and anomalies in the evolution of modern oxygen therapy. *Anaesthesia*, **29**, 335.
20. Leigh, J. M. (1974). The evolution of oxygen therapy apparatus. *Anaesthesia*, **29**, 462.
21. Hewer, C. L., and Lee, J. A. (1957). *Recent Advances in Anaesthesia and Analgesia*, 8th edit. London: J. & A. Churchill.
22. Henderson, Y. (1925). Physiological regulation of the acid-base balance of the blood and some related functions. *Physiol Rev.*, **5**, 131.
23. Haldane, J. S. (1926). Some bearings of the physiology of respiration on the administration of anaesthetics. *Proc. roy. Soc. Med.*, **19**, Sect. of Anaesth., p. 33.
24. Prys-Roberts, C., Smith, W. D. A. and Nunn, J. F. (1967). Accidental severe hypercapnia during anaesthesia. *Brit. J. Anaesth.*, **39**, 257.
25. Ramsay, —., and Lockyer, J. N. (1895). L'hélium, élément terrestre. (Abstr.) *Rev. Sci.*, **3**, 654.
26. Lloyd, B. B. (1958). A development of Haldane's gas analysis apparatus. *J. Physiol. (Lond).*, **143**, 5P.
27. Sykes, M. K., Vickers, M. D. and Hull, C. J. (1981). *Principles of Clinical Measurement*, 2nd edit. Oxford: Blackwell Scientific Publications.
28. Davies, D. D. (1970). A method of gas chromatography for quantitative analysis of blood gases. *Brit. J. Anaesth.*, **42**, 19.

## FURTHER READING

Drummond, G. B. (1975). Postoperative hypoxaemia and oxygen therapy. *Brit. J. Anaesth.*, **47**, 491.
Grant, W. J. (1978). *Medical Gases*. London: HM + M. Publishers Ltd.
Nunn, J. F. (1977). Oxygen. In: *Applied Respiratory Physiology*, 2nd edit. London: Butterworths.
Payne, J. P., and Hill, D. W. (1975). *Oxygen Measurements in Biology and Medicine*. London: Butterworths.
Sykes, M. K., Vickers, M. D. and Hull, C. J. (1981). *Principles of Clinical Measurement*, 2nd edit. Oxford: Blackwell Scientific Publications.

CHAPTER 5

# Hyperbaric Physiology and Medicine



INCREASE in environmental pressure however contrived, either by scuba diving, or within a specially constructed hyperbaric chamber, has medical implications: increase in oxygen levels may have certain therapeutic benefits, and increase in hydrostatic pressure may give rise to injuries. Increases in oxygen may be therapeutically useful in three general ways: in the management of certain forms of hypoxia, to treat certain anaerobic infections, or to render certain tumours more radio-sensitive. Increases in nitrogen confer no benefits but may depress cerebral function and give rise to embolic problems during decompression. Increase in hydrostatic pressure may give rise to injuries when pressure gradients occur between tissues. In this chapter the fundamental principles of hyperbaric physiology will be discussed, the dangers and complications of the hyperbaric environment described, details of the routines adopted in current deep water exploration will be given, the indications for hyperbaric oxygen will be enumerated, and the methods by which an anaesthetic may be given in a chamber will be considered.

**Definition.**—The scope of hyperbaric medicine embraces all those circumstances in which total environmental pressure increases and includes hyperbaric chambers at sea level, deep sea diving bells, and deep sea diving both with and without self-contained underwater breathing apparatus (SCUBA).

**Physics and physiology.**—At sea level the atmosphere exerts a pressure of 760 mm Hg (1 Atmosphere or 101·3 kPa). This pressure is referred to as one atmosphere absolute (1 AT.A). However, confusion arises because engineers tend to ignore the 760 mm Hg (101·3 kPa) pressure of our own atmosphere and set their gauges to read zero. Thus, when working with a hyperbaric chamber, if the gauge reads 760 mm Hg (101·3 kPa) the pressure in reality is 1 Atmosphere at sea level +1 Atmosphere (chamber pressure) i.e. 2 Atmospheres Absolute. As this terminology is so confusing throughout this chapter, the terms mm Hg and kPa pressures and Atmospheres Absolute will be used.

In physical terms, compression or decompression of a given amount of gas basically does three things: it changes volume, it changes density, and it changes the partial pressures of constituent gases. Physiological responses and problems due to exposure to a hyperbaric environment stem directly from these physical changes and may be categorised and differentiated into complications due to the direct *physical effects* of pressure, and *secondary complications* due to abnormally high volumes of respiratory gases dissolved in the blood and tissues. The first of these physical effects is due to hydrostatic pressure, which, when associated with injury, will be considered later under the broad heading of *Barotrauma*. The more elusive secondary reactions may be grouped together: a high inspired partial pressure of nitrogen is responsible for *Nitrogen Narcosis*, and *Decompression Sickness*; a high inspired partial pressure of oxygen has therapeutic applications and can in certain circumstances result in various forms of *Oxygen Toxicity*.

What happens then when man is placed in a compressed air environment? Both the soft tissues and the air cavities of the body must be considered. Soft tissues of the body behave as liquid and as such, are incompressible. The laws which apply to liquids can be applied to the tissues of the human body when subjected to an increase in environmental pressure as in a pressure chamber or with immersion in water. Gases in the cavities of the body obey the "gas laws", and of these Boyle's law is of fundamental importance. This law states that for a given quantity of gas whose temperature remains constant, the pressure varies inversely with volume. Put more simply this means that if the pressure of a given amount of gas is doubled, then it must be compressed to half its volume. These points are illustrated in Fig. 1 which represents the changes taking place in an inverted bucket or diving bell pushed under water. At sea level the bucket contains a given mass of air which occupies the volume of the bell and exerts a pressure equal to the environment of 1 AT.A (760 mm Hg, 101·3 kPa). If the

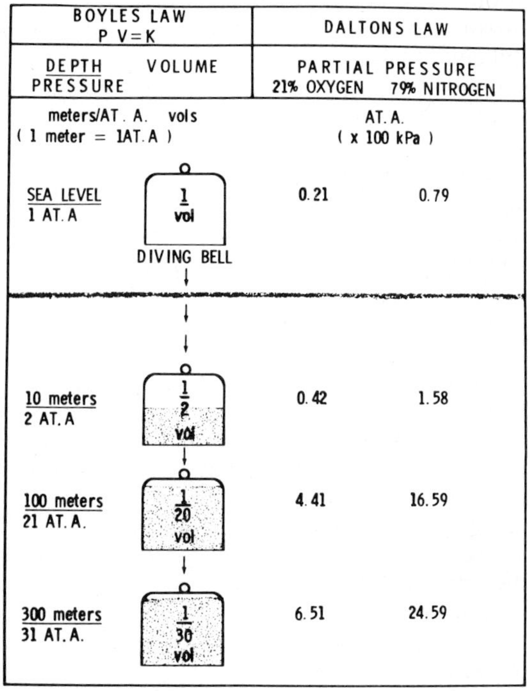


5/Fig. 1.—As the diving bell submerges, ambient pressure increases and water rises within the bell reducing the volume of trapped air (Boyle's law) and increasing the partial pressures of oxygen and nitrogen (Dalton's law).

bucket is now pushed down in water to a depth of 10 metres, the pressure inside the bucket is equal to that of the surrounding water which is 2 AT.A (1520 mm Hg, 203 kPa). The pressure has now been doubled and therefore the air within it must contract to half its volume. This is achieved by the water level rising halfway up inside the bucket. Similarly if the bucket is lowered to 30 metres, where the pressure is 4 AT.A (3040 mm Hg, 405 kPa), the air would be compressed to one-quarter of its original volume.

The air cavities of the body including respiratory passages, lungs, sinuses, middle ear and viscera are all subjected to changes in pressure as environmental pressure changes. As pressure increases either within the pressure chamber, or when submerged in water, the incompressible tissues take up the pressure of the environment but do not change their shape and are undistorted. This state, however, can only be upheld if the pressure within the air cavities of the body are also increased and equal to that of enclosing tissues. Within the pressure chamber, equalisation of pressure between gas cavities and surrounding tissue does not usually present difficulty; under water however, air must be supplied artificially by delivering compressed gas at a pressure equivalent to the water pressure at that depth. If this is not done two things may happen. If the surrounding tissues will allow it, the enclosing air may contract to meet the increasing pressure. Failing this, if the volume cannot be reduced the pressure will be unchanged and a pressure difference will build up between the air and the surrounding tissues. Barotrauma is the term used to describe tissue damage which may occur whenever pressure gradients exist between tissues.

Study of partial pressures of the gases within the inverted bucket will also serve to explain some of the *secondary complications* of increase in environmental pressure referred to above. These are also shown in Fig. 1. For example, in the inverted bucket at a depth of 30 metres, the partial pressure of oxygen has risen from 150 mm Hg (20 kPa) at sea level to 600 mm Hg (80 kPa). Pressure of nitrogen has increased from 600 mm Hg (80 kPa) at the surface to 2400 mm Hg (320 kPa) at 30 metres. Obviously, as a consequence of these greatly increased values of partial pressure, the amount of gas dissolved in body liquids will be proportionately increased.

### Deep Sea Diving Routines

Deep sea diving in the oil industry, currently on the Continental Shelf around the British Isles at depths of some 250 m, is a commercial enterprise and diving regimens are therefore designed to allow the maximum economic work load. Two diving techniques are in use; the "*bounce-dive*" and the "*saturation dive*". In the former, the scuba diver is rapidly compressed as he descends to his working depth, he carries out his allotted task and is then returned to the surface in a submersible work chamber (SWC) for a period of decompression. Decompression for a period of 15 minutes at a depth of 150 m is about 6 hours, and as long as 20 hours after one hour at pressure. Such long periods of inactivity for such a short work period are clearly uneconomical. In saturation diving, a team of divers live for periods of up to three weeks in a sea level habitat which is pressurised to the depth at which they are expected to work. Transfer of divers to their worksite is done in a submersible work chamber (SWC). Decompression after saturation dives is related solely to depth and not to its duration (Table 1).

5/TABLE 1
APPROXIMATE DECOMPRESSION TIMES FOLLOWING SATURATION DIVES

| Depth (meters) | 100 | 200 | 300 |
|---|---|---|---|
| Pressure (AT.A.) | 11 | 21 | 31 |
| Decompression Time (days) | 3 | 5 | 7 |

### Pulmonary Barotrauma

This condition is due to distortion of lung tissue which may occur during decompression either within a pressure chamber or during ascent in water. If during pressure reduction, there is any restriction or resistance to the release of air from the lungs, then as surrounding pressure falls, so the trapped air being unable to expand, will remain at a pressure above that of surrounding tissues. This excessive air-over-tissue pressure may expand the lungs and chest until the alveoli rupture and air escapes into the interstitial tissues, the pleural cavity, or into the circulation. Air may be trapped in this way in lung cysts, or by airway obstruction, bronchospasm, laryngospasm, or by breath holding. Sometimes air entering the pulmonary circulation through tears in lung tissue may pass to the left side of the heart to be distributed as arterial emboli.

Three clinical syndromes of pulmonary barotrauma, namely *pneumothorax*, *interstitial emphysema*, and *air embolism* can be recognised. Of these *air embolism* is by far the most serious. The clinical picture of air embolus depends on the final resting place of the offending bubble. The most serious sign is that of loss of consciousness immediately following decompression or soon after. Convulsions have occurred, and muscle paralysis and visual changes are also fairly common following air embolism. Any form of air embolism should respond to rapid recompression of the patient; the object being to reduce the volume of the embolism until it passes the point of obstruction or better, to redissolve the gas in the blood. Following resolution of symptoms, slow decompression is undertaken so that the bubbles will not form again. Schedules of treatment for these accidents have been published and are available in various forms as "Therapeutic Decompression Tables".

*Pneumothorax* or interstitial emphysema must be managed symptomatically. In the case of pneumothorax the air may be released by introducing a catheter into the pleural cavity and connecting it to some form of one-way valve, such as an underwater drain.

*Interstitial emphysema* is more difficult to manage by virtue of its position. Recompression will reduce the size of the trapped air but absorption of the gas from these sites is slow and sometimes other means for removal must be adopted. This may necessitate surgical intervention by direct cannulation of the air pockets.

### Aural Barotrauma

Normally the Eustachian tube serves to equalise pressures between nasopharynx and middle ear. In healthy individuals the Eustachian tube opens during swallowing and this is quite sufficient to maintain the necessary pressure adjustments without conscious awareness. When the Eustachian tube fails to open freely a pressure gradient develops across the tympanic membrane when environmental pressure increases; this results in inward bulging of the membrane with stretching, pain, haemorrhage and ultimately perforation. It is recommended that unconscious or anaesthetised patients should have a preliminary myringotomy to obviate this problem before being subjected to changes in environmental pressure. Sometimes underwater swimmers wear tight-fitting rubber hoods or caps which trap air in the external auditory meatus. As the water pressure rises so the hood is pressed firmly against the ear until the contained air volume can shrink no further. Meanwhile, as environmental pressure increases, the pressure in the respiratory tract also increases. If the Eustachian tube opens, this pressure may be passed to the middle ear resulting in the air pressure in the outer ear becoming relatively lower than the pressure in the middle ear. This results in outward bulging of the drum and the appearance of oedematous swelling of the linings of the external auditory meatus with blebs and large haemorrhagic blisters—a condition known as "reversed ear".

### Respiratory Sinuses

The air-filled sinuses of the skull are normally connected by foramina to the nasopharynx. This allows pressure equilibrium to be maintained between them and the rest of the respiratory system. When one of these channels becomes blocked, for example by catarrhal swelling, polypi, or deviated septa, air cannot pass freely in or out. Should environmental pressure be increased in these circumstances then the pressure of the surrounding tissue will exceed that within the sinus, its lining will swell and the space may fill with transudate and blood.

### Dental Problems

Small pockets of gas sometimes exist around the roots of teeth and are the result of fermentation. These being isolated, would, during compression, shrink and the space they occupy possibly fill with blood and transudate. On surfacing the bubble would expand resulting in an increase in pressure. The result is a severe toothache.

### Gas in the Intestinal Tract

Usually gas in abdominal viscera does not present any problems with changes in environmental pressure. However, on occasions fermentation continues in the gut and this can produce abdominal distension, discomfort and painful flatulence. Some people are air swallowers, particularly when anxious, and on occasions this can produce difficulties when swallowed air expands producing extreme discomfort and inconvenience.

### Pressure and Clothing

Pockets of compressed air trapped within clothing close to the skin of a patient or diver may produce a deep impression on the skin during exposure to high environmental pressure.

## Consequences of High Inspired Partial Pressure

### Nitrogen and Inert Gas Narcosis

It is now widely recognised that men and animals exposed to a hyperbaric environment of air will exhibit signs and symptoms of intoxication and narcosis. The occurrence of narcosis was first reported by Junod in 1835.[1] He noted that when breathing compressed air "the function of the brain was activated, imagination was lively, thoughts had a peculiar charm, and, in some persons, symptoms of intoxication". Since that time many workers have confirmed these observations. Cousteau in 1964,[2] referred to it in an apt and descriptive way as "l'ivresse des grands profondeurs" ("the raptures of the deep"). In Britain divers refer to it less romantically as "The Narks".

The narcosis observed when breathing compressed air is not an isolated phenomenon. The noble so called "rare gases" cause the same signs and symptoms but vary in the narcotic effect. The cause of inert gas narcosis is complex and cannot be related to any one factor. Many attempts have been made to correlate the narcotic effects of the inert gases: helium, neon, argon, krypton and xenon, to their various physical properties such as lipid solubility, partition coefficients, molecular weight, absorption coefficients, thermodynamic activity, and the formation of clathrates. However, the best correlation is afforded by lipid solubility (Table 2). Thus xenon is an anaesthetic at atmospheric pressure, and krypton causes dizziness. Helium is a very weak narcotic and it is mainly for this reason that it is used for deep diving or deep pressure chamber work beyond 10AT.A.

The narcosis observed when breathing compressed air is of particular relevance. Obviously medical personnel working in a hyperbaric chamber, compressed with air, would have their efficiency impaired if faced with some unusual or complicated clinical event. Also in deep-sea diving nitrogen narcosis is of considerable importance because it reduces the efficiency of the diver and can result in behaviour which is detrimental to safety. Sufficient is known about the responses of an average man to increasing inspired partial pressures of nitrogen, and it is possible to tabulate the sequence of events as follows: at a depth of 30–45 metres the atmospheric pressure is 4–5 AT.A and the inspired pressure of nitrogen will amount to 2500 mm Hg (333 kPa) with the result that euphoria, increasing self-confidence, and lightheadedness are noted. When depths of 60 to 75 metres are reached the atmospheric pressure is 8–9 AT.A, corresponding to an inspired nitrogen of about 5000 mm Hg (665 kPa). In this instance the power of concentration is considerably reduced and many mistakes are made in the performance of even simple tasks. There may be peripheral numbness and tingling. Personal safety tends to be disregarded. At even greater depths of 90–115 metres with an atmospheric pressure of 12–13 AT.A—corresponding to an inspired nitrogen pressure of 10,000 mm Hg (1330 kPa)—many individuals may be approaching unconsciousness, although it is possible that some of the signs and symptoms are due to oxygen poisoning. The first quantitative evidence of nitrogen narcosis reported by Shilling and Willgrube[3] perhaps serves to stress the dangers of compressed air narcosis in so far as operating room personnel and deep-sea divers are concerned.

### Decompression Sickness ("Bends", "Chokes", "Diver's Palsy" or "Caisson Disease")

At sea level body tissues are normally in equilibrium or saturated with the nitrogen in atmospheric air at atmospheric pressure. When ambient pressure is raised, as in a pressure chamber or during deep-sea diving, greater

5/TABLE 2

Correlation of narcotic potency of the inert gases with lipid solubility and other physical characteristics

| *Gas* | *Molecular weight* | *Sol. in lipid* | *Temp. °C* | *Oil–water sol. ratio* | *Relative narcotic potency* |
|---|---|---|---|---|---|
| | | | | | (least narcotic) |
| He | 4 | 0·015 | 37° | 1·7 | 4·26 |
| Ne | 20 | 0·019 | 37·6° | 2·07 | 3·58 |
| $H_2$ | 2 | 0·036 | 37° | 2·1 | 1·83 |
| $N_2$ | 28 | 0·067 | 37° | 5·2 | 1 |
| A | 40 | 0·14 | 37° | 5·3 | 0·43 |
| Kr | 83·7 | 0·43 | 37° | 9·6 | 0·14 |
| Xe | 131·3 | 1·7 | 37° | 20·0 | 0·039 |
| | | | | | (most narcotic) |

amounts of gas dissolve in the tissues until, after some time, tissue saturation is attained at the higher inspired pressures. When pressure is reduced gas dissolved in the tissues must be carried by the blood to the lungs to be eliminated. Should decompression be too rapid, bubble formation may occur with relatively insoluble nitrogen being the main constituent of the bubbles. The physiological basis of decompression sickness is the local release of nitrogen bubbles in the tissues and blood. The signs and symptoms will vary according to the extent and location of the bubbles. The term decompression sickness in practice refers only to those conditions which are the result of an excessively rapid reduction of environmental pressure and are caused by liberation of bubbles of gas from tissues and blood which have been supersaturated. This definition does not usually include those conditions which are caused mainly by the physical effect of gas expanding within a body cavity such as the lungs, and not actually dissolved in any tissue (barotrauma).

The early signs and symptoms of decompression sickness, the result of bubble formation, can be conveniently divided into two types.

*Type* 1.—This includes cases where pain is the only symptom, together with those showing cutaneous or lymphatic involvement either alone or with joint pain. Skin manifestations are usually preceded by intense itching localised in one or perhaps a number of areas asymmetrically distributed. Lymphatic occlusion may produce distal oedema for example in a painful limb. The skin distal to the obstruction may have the typical peau d'orange or orange peel appearance.

*Type* 2.—This category includes all cases of a more serious nature with central nervous and cardiopulmonary system involvement. The symptomatology may be multifocal and often unpredictable. The pulmonary manifestations sometimes known as the "Chokes" in traditional diving parlance, are probably the result of bubbles in pulmonary capillaries, and are usually evident at an early stage. Neurological upsets of many forms occur. Disturbances of cerebral function may account for almost any bizarre symptom or pattern of behaviour. Psychotic conditions have been simulated, but visual blurring, diplopia, scotomata, hemianopia, and migrainous headaches are commonly seen. Sometimes the clinical appearance suggests local involvement of the spinal cord with paralysis. Almost every possibility has been described. The effect on the legs, and consequently the gait, which may occur as a result of this condition, is referred to by divers as "The Staggers", and may be a disturbance of labyrinthine function with vertigo, nystagmus, nausea and vomiting.

### Delayed Decompression Sickness

Aseptic necrosis of bone is considered to be a form of decompression sickness which does not occur in the acute stages, but only after a delay of many months. It is suggested that this condition, like the other lesions of decompression sickness, is the result of bubbles of nitrogen producing infarcts in bones. This may, in time, cause joint deformity and arthritic changes. Common sites of aseptic necrosis are the head of the femur, proximal or distal ends of the humerus, and proximal end of the tibia.

### Prevention of Decompression Sickness

Decompression sickness can be almost completely avoided by the strict adherence to the rules which have been laid down to guide individuals working in a high pressure environment. The following factors are of importance:

1. **Limitation of pressure in the chamber.**—Since tissues can be moderately saturated with an inert gas without the formation of bubbles, it is possible to spend unlimited time in a chamber at 2 AT.A (1520 mm Hg, 203 kPa) without the need for slow decompression.

2. **Limitation of time.**—Experience with deep-sea diving has suggested that when the time spent at a given atmospheric pressure is limited, then no decompression is necessary. The longer the period spent in a compressed environment the greater the problems of decompression.

3. **Limitation of rate of decompression.**—It is apparently safe to be decompressed rapidly to half the original working pressure, but a suitable pause must be made at this new pressure before further decompression is undertaken.

4. **Use of helium and oxygen mixtures.**—Substitution of helium for nitrogen as the inert gas eliminates the dangers of narcosis and also reduces the problems of decompression sickness. Helium also reduces the time required for decompression because it is only about one-half

as soluble as nitrogen in the body, and in addition it diffuses out much more rapidly. Thus the amount of helium absorbed at a given time will be considerably less than nitrogen under the same conditions, and the rate of elimination will be faster.

5. **Oxygen decompression.**—It has already been stated that rapid decompression to half the original pressure can be achieved with safety. On reaching this stage, the time required at this new level can be shortened if the subject breathes oxygen. This ensures the maximum possible gradient between the nitrogen in the tissues and the zero level of nitrogen in the alveoli. This will speed the elimination of nitrogen and the decompression time will be shortened. In civil engineering practice involving tunnel work, workers may be frequently exposed to pressures in excess of 3 AT.A (2280 mm Hg, 304 kPa) for shift periods of up to 8 hours each. Here rigid adherence to decompression schedules is clearly of great importance.

## HYPERBARIC OXYGEN

**Physiology.**—Much of the recent interest and the benefits of hyperbaric therapy follow from its effects on the absorption and transport of oxygen. The higher the $Po_2$ of the inspired gas, the higher the arterial $Po_2$ in an almost linear relationship. The higher the arterial $Po_2$, the higher the actual amount of oxygen carried in physical solution in arterial blood. However it should be noted that a high arterial oxygen level does not necessarily mean that tissue levels will be elevated; these depend on a number of other factors including the properties of haemoglobin, the cardiac output, regional tissue perfusion, and upon the diffusion of oxygen from capillaries into tissues.

Fresh air contains 20·93 per cent oxygen, the remainder being mainly nitrogen. At the sea-level barometric pressure of 760 mm Hg (101·3 kPa) the partial pressure of oxygen in inspired air is thus 158 mm Hg (21 kPa), which is 20·93 per cent of 760 mm Hg (101·3 kPa). When air is inspired it rapidly becomes saturated with water vapour at body temperature, and on entering the lungs mixes with alveolar gas which contains carbon dioxide; the water vapour and the carbon dioxide accounts for 47 mm Hg (6·3 kPa) and about 40 mm Hg (5·3 kPa) respectively of the total alveolar pressure, leaving 673 mm Hg (90 kPa) for the combined pressures of nitrogen and oxygen. When oxygen alone is inspired, nitrogen is displaced from the alveoli, leaving only the oxygen water vapour and the carbon dioxide. The alveolar $Po_2$ then equals the total alveolar pressure minus the sum of the saturated water vapour pressure and the alveolar $Pco_2$. The alveolar oxygen pressures obtained when breathing oxygen at various ambient pressures can be readily calculated from the following formula:

$PAO_2 = PIO_2 - PH_2O - PACO_2$ where $PIO_2$ = inspired partial pressure of oxygen and $PACO_2$ = Alveolar partial pressure of $CO_2$ (usually 40 mm Hg or 5·3 kPa), $PH_2O$ = Alveolar pressure of water vapour (47 mm Hg or 6·3 kPa at 37° C).

Table 3 shows alveolar oxygen pressures calculated in this way for atmospheric pressures

5/TABLE 3

ALVEOLAR OXYGEN PRESSURES OBTAINABLE WITH OXYGEN ADMINISTRATION AT AMBIENT PRESSURES RANGING FROM 1–6 ATMOSPHERES (101·3–607·8 kPa)
(assuming body temperature 37° C and $PACO_2$ 40 mm Hg, 5·3 kPa)

| *Ambient pressure* | | *Alveolar* $Po_2$ | |
|---|---|---|---|
| AT.A | kPa | mm Hg | kPa |
| 1 | 101·3 | 673 | 90 |
| 2 | 202·6 | 1433 | 191 |
| 3 | 303·9 | 2193 | 292 |
| 4 | 405·2 | 2953 | 393 |
| 5 | 506·5 | 3713 | 494 |
| 6 | 607·8 | 4473 | 595 |

ranging from 1 to 6 atmospheres (101·3–609 kPa).

The alveolar $Po_2$ is the principal determinant of arterial $Po_2$, normally the difference between the two is small and is mainly due to venous admixture (see page 97).

Oxygen is carried in blood by chemical combination with haemoglobin, and in physical solution with plasma as dissolved oxygen (see page 104). One gram of haemoglobin combines with 1·34 ml of oxygen. Assuming a haemoglobin concentration of 14·6 grams per 100 ml of blood, the amount of oxygen which can be carried in the chemical combination with haemoglobin will be 19·6 ml per 100 ml of blood. When breathing air at atmospheric pressure, haemoglobin is only 97 per cent saturated with oxygen so only 19 ml of oxygen are carried per 100 ml of blood. In a healthy individual when 100 per cent oxygen is breathed at atmospheric pressure the haemoglobin becomes fully saturated.

The amount of physically dissolved oxygen is proportional to the partial pressure of oxygen in equilibrium with the blood no matter how high the oxygen pressure (Henry's Law) (i.e. 0·003 ml $O_2$/100 ml blood/mm Hg $Po_2$). When breathing room air at an alveolar $Po_2$ of 100 mm Hg (13·3 kPa) oxygen in physical solution mounts to 0·3 ml $O_2$ per 100 ml blood. If the $Po_2$ rose to 600 mm Hg (80 kPa) (because the patient breathed a high oxygen mixture) the dissolved oxygen would be 1·8 ml; if a subject breathed $O_2$ at 3 AT.A (2280 mm Hg, 304 kPa), and the arterial $Po_2$ was 2000 mm Hg (266 kPa), the dissolved oxygen would be 6 ml $O_2$/100 ml blood (Table 4 and Fig. 2). In the latter case dissolved oxygen would be sufficient to supply all the oxygen required by a resting man and venous blood would return to the lungs with the haemoglobin still fully saturated.

Thus at normal atmospheric pressure the oxygen content of arterial blood is largely dependent on the haemoglobin content. When hyperbaric oxygen is inhaled the haemoglobin cannot increase its oxygen load because it is already fully saturated, and, as the $Po_2$ rises, the oxygen content increases only by the carriage of additional oxygen as a simple solution in the plasma.

When an individual is breathing room air his oxygen stores are extremely limited and confined mainly to oxygen carried by haemoglobin and the small amount within the functional residual volume of the lungs. However oxygen stores are considerably increased when hyperbaric oxygen is given. At 3 AT.A (2280 mm Hg, 304 kPa) oxygen will be physically dissolved in body water to the extent of about 6 ml/100 ml. In a 70 kg adult with 50 litres body water this would create a potential oxygen reservoir of $6 \times 500 = 3000$ ml of oxygen. Such increases will theoretically allow tissues to survive temporary anoxia for much longer periods than are possible without hyperbaric oxygen.

It was stressed above that tissue oxygen levels depend not only on the arterial oxygen tension but also upon other factors which are responsible for oxygen delivery; these include haemoglobin, cardiac output and its distribution, and transfer factors. Hyperbaric oxygen may result in physiological adjustments which tend to offset increases in tissue oxygen levels. Cerebral blood vessels may constrict, for example, in response to changes in carbon dioxide transport thus limiting the increase in cerebral tissue oxygen tension.

### Indications for Hyperbaric Oxygen

The indications and current status of hyperbaric oxygen are difficult to define, and it would be perhaps prudent to regard it for the present, as experimental. On theoretical grounds hyperbaric oxygen has much to offer in certain disease processes; however the nub of the matter and the therapeutic objective, is the restoration or elevation of the tension of the gas in the probable area of maximum cellular activity—that is in the mitochondria. It should not be presumed that tissue oxygen is commensurate with the inhaled or arterial oxygen levels. A variety of haemodynamic adjustments are possible which may limit increases in the tissue oxygen levels.

Clinical applications of hyperbaric oxygen today are confined to relatively unusual disease processes and include: carbon monoxide poisoning, gas gangrene, congenital cardiac anomalies, peripheral vascular insufficiencies, disseminated sclerosis and cancer therapy. Such limited application makes comparative scientific evaluation of hyperbaric oxygen difficult, and a great deal of work needs to be done to establish the benefits of the technique in relation to the conventional therapeutic regimes. A

5/TABLE 4

OXYGEN LEVELS IN PLASMA OBTAINABLE WITH OXYGEN ADMINISTRATION AT AMBIENT PRESSURES RANGING FROM 1–6 ATMOSPHERES (101·3–607·8 kPa)
(Assuming body temperature of 37° C, a $PACO_2$ 40 mm Hg [5·3 kPa] and a physiological shunt of about 5 per cent cardiac output).

| | *Ambient pressure* | | *Approximate Arterial* $Po_2$ | | *Oxygen in simple solution* |
|---|---|---|---|---|---|
| AT.A | kPa | %$O_2$ | mm Hg | kPa | *ml/100 plasma* |
| 1 | 101·3 | 20·93 | 100 | 20 | 0·3 |
| 1 | 101·3 | 100 | 600 | 80 | 1·8 |
| 2 | 202·6 | 100 | 1400 | 186 | 4·2 |
| 3 | 303·9 | 100 | 2000 | 268 | 6·0 |
| 4 | 405·2 | 100 | 2850 | 372 | 8·5 |
| 5 | 506·5 | 100 | 3650 | 485 | 11·0 |
| 6 | 607·8 | 100 | 4350 | 579 | 13·1 |

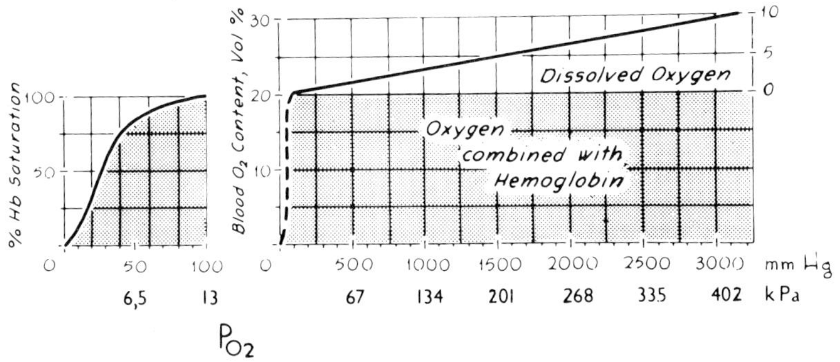


5/FIG. 2.—The oxygen content of blood when equilibrated with oxygen. From the standard oxygen dissociation curve on the left it can be seen that haemoglobin is almost fully saturated with oxygen when the $Po_2$ is 100 mm Hg (13·3 kPa). When the partial pressure is increased (right-hand graph) additional oxygen is carried in physical solution. At 3 atmospheres (2280 mm Hg, 304 kPa) oxygen, the pressure usually used in clinical hyperbaric chambers, an additional 6 ml oxygen/100 ml blood can be carried. From the graph it will be apparent that the amount of oxygen dissolved in plasma is very much less than that combined with haemoglobin, and that only a minor decrease in physically dissolved oxygen will reduce the $Po_2$ much more than a similar decrease in oxyhaemoglobin.

significant advance in hyperbaric oxygen would be the demonstration of its efficiency in the treatment of common diseases. Well controlled clinical trials of myocardial infarction or in the shock syndrome are currently being conducted in various centres throughout the world; their conclusions are awaited with interest.

The indications for hyperbaric oxygen may be classified in two groups according to their clinical application: current and possible.

## CURRENT APPLICATIONS OF HYPERBARIC OXYGEN

### Carbon Monoxide Poisoning

Carbon monoxide has considerably greater affinity for haemoglobin than oxygen; consequently exposure to even low concentrations of carbon monoxide rapidly leads to "anaemic hypoxaemia" because the gas interferes with the ability of haemoglobin to transport oxygen. Prompt institution of hyperbaric oxygen therapy has an important part to play in this condition. Oxygen at between 2 to 3 AT.A (1520–2280 mm Hg, 203–304 kPa) alleviates the situation in three ways: first, it provides enough dissolved oxygen in the plasma to keep the patient alive. Secondly it moves the oxygen-haemoglobin dissociation curve to the right, thus enabling the remaining oxyhaemoglobin to give up more oxygen. Thirdly, it accelerates the rate of dissociation of carboxyhaemoglobin to twice that achieved by conventional treatment with 5 per cent $CO_2$ in $O_2$. Treatment should be continued until carboxyhaemoglobin is no longer detectable in the blood, by which time consciousness will return provided there has been no brain damage. Clearance time seems to be related to the period of exposure to carbon monoxide rather than to the blood level of carboxyhaemoglobin or the clinical condition of the patient. Although few people doubt the efficacy of hyperbaric oxygen treatment in CO poisoning, there is little evidence to support the fact that such therapy saves many lives.

### Infections

It would seen reasonable to suspect that organisms such as *Clostridium welchii* and *Clostridium tetani*, which thrive under conditions of low oxygen level, might be adversely affected by hyperbaric oxygenation. In clostridial gas gangrene hyperbaric oxygen therapy appears to have an established place. Hyperbaric oxygen appears to inhibit the growth of the causative organisms, thus allowing normal body responses to deal with the bacteria, and stops the production of the clostridial alpha toxins. Van Zyl[4] analysed results from world-wide reports of other workers on the use of hyperbaric oxygen in the management of 170 patients with histotoxic clostridial infections. He compared these results with those obtained by conventional or traditional forms of therapy, including antibiotics, and concluded that high pressure oxygen eliminated the conventional requirements for urgent radical excision of infected tissue, and that after high pressure oxygen therapy subsequent tissue preservation was much greater than one would anticipate in patients who had been treated conservatively.

Although hyperbaric oxygen would seem to be logical in the treatment of tetanus, results have not been convincing. The total number of tetanus cases treated in which benefit has been claimed has been small, and in most the therapeutic effect of hyperbaric oxygen was masked by conventional therapy. Although hyperbaric oxygen therapy is unlikely to play a part in the treatment of established tetanus, it is possible it may find an adjunctive use in the early stages of the disease.

Certain aerobic organisms are known to be sensitive to hyperbaric oxygen; experimentally it is known to be effective against coagulase-positive staphlococci and *Pseudomonas pyocyaneus*. Clinically, the main benefit has been obtained in surface involvement, as in infected burns, leg ulcers, and areas of infected devitalised tissues such as pressure sores or amputation stumps.

### Cancer Therapy

Hyperbaric oxygen appears to have a useful part to play in potentiation of radiation therapy for inoperable cancer. The rationale for the use of hyperbaric oxygen in radiotherapy depends upon the fact that the radiosensitivity of a normal cell rendered hypoxic declines to about one-third of its original levels. On the other hand hyperoxygenation of a normal cell produces only a relatively small increase in sensitivity. Tumour cells are frequently hypoxic and treatment with hyperbaric oxygen raises their oxygen tension, restoring their sensitivity to radiation. Churchill-Davidson and colleagues[5] reported good results with this therapy, and Siegel and Morton[6] have commented favourably on its use with cytotoxic drugs.

### Arterial Insufficiency

Tissues deprived of their blood supply either by trauma, embolism or thrombosis can be supported during the critical period in an attempt to diminish the area of anoxaemia and permit the improvement of collateral flow. Hyperbaric oxygen has been used in plastic surgery for the treatment of ischaemic pedicle grafts.[7,8]

### Decompression Sickness and Air Embolism

It is customary to treat decompression sickness by recompression in air and the details of recompression procedures are well documented.[9] The purpose of recompression is to provide prompt and lasting relief of symptoms and signs in decompression sickness and air embolism. The recompression procedure is intended to reduce the size of the gas bubble rapidly and to ensure that no symptom-producing bubbles form upon subsequent decompression. The increase in pressure during recompression causes compression of bubbles according to Boyle's law. However, decrease in diameter of nitrogen bubbles with increasing pressure is disappointingly small (Fig. 3). Under normal conditions, any bubble containing normal atmospheric components tends to disappear by outward diffusion of gas. When tissues are super-saturated with gas this may no longer be true; the bubble may then grow by increasing diffusion of gas into it from surrounding tissues. To prevent this, the ambient pressure during treatment must at least equal the pressure of dissolved gas in the surroundings of the bubbles. The process of gas diffusion from bubbles may be slow and methods of speeding it up are desirable. Most effective is the administration of oxygen at increased pressure, preferably at about 3 AT.A (2280 mm Hg, 304 kPa).

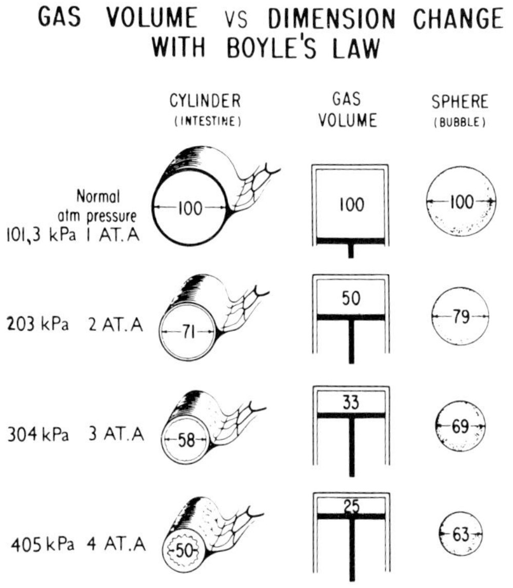


5/Fig. 3.—Change in diameter of gas bubbles of three different shapes with compression. The volume of each is progressively reduced as ambient pressure increases; however, reduction in diameter of cylindrical and spherical bubbles is disappointingly small, even negligible at higher pressures, and proportionately much less than the reduction in length of cylindrical bubbles. (Reproduced from *Advances in Surgery*, Vol. 1 courtesy of I. W. Brown *et al.*, Claude E. Welch (Ed.) and the publishers, Year Book Medical Publishers[10]).

### Possible Clinical Applications

The beneficial effect of hyperbaric oxygen therapy in hypoxia secondary to severe cardiac disease is obvious. During cardiac surgery hyperbaric oxygen will theoretically permit lower flows during cardiopulmonary bypass, will allow longer periods of circulatory arrest, and in addition will obviate the need for using red blood cells in the priming fluid of cardiopulmonary bypass pumps. Despite these theoretical benefits however, hyperbaric oxygen has not been adopted in current practice for this purpose.

The use of oxygen to correct arterial hypoxaemia due to increase in physiological shunt is well established. However it is important to realise that the increase in arterial oxygen tension for a given increase in alveolar oxygen tension decreases markedly as the shunt increases (Fig. 4). For high shunt fractions there is little increase in systemic oxygen as the fractional concentration of oxygen in inspired gas ($F_{IO_2}$) increases; on the other hand even a small reduction in shunt fraction is associated with a considerable increase in systemic oxygen.

## Methods of Administration of Hyperbaric Oxygen

Two types of hyperbaric chamber are in use for hyperbaric oxygen administration. One is a single-person chamber in which only the patient is subjected to compression, and the staff remain outside (Figs. 5 and 6). Here the patient alone is exposed to oxygen.

The other is a large operating room pressure chamber enclosing both the patient and medical attendants. Large pressure chambers can be used for surgery (Fig. 7). The chamber is compressed with air which is breathed by the medical attendants, while the patient breathes 100 per cent oxygen at the same ambient pressure either from a mask or cuffed endotracheal tube according to the state of consciousness. In the conscious patient, the efficacy of oxygen administration is dependent on the efficiency of the oxygen supply system; here the fit of the mask to the patient's face is of prime importance. Any leakage around the mask will lead to a fall in inspired oxygen tension. Best

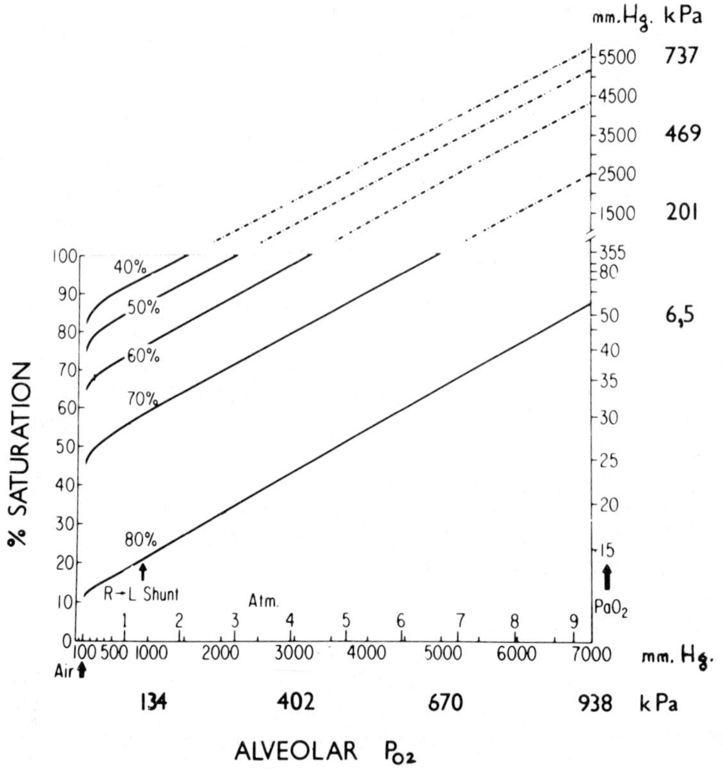


5/FIG. 4.—As physiological shunt increases ($Q_s/Q_t$) (diagonal lines), the effect of increasing the inspired oxygen tension (horizontal scale) upon the arterial oxygen tension or saturation (vertical scales) becomes less and less. At shunt fractions above 40 per cent the risk of oxygen toxicity must be carefully weighed against the small increase in $Pa_{O_2}$ as inspired oxygen is increased beyond 350 mm Hg (47 kPa). At a shunt of 80 per cent it is impossible to get a $Pa_{O_2}$ above 60 mm Hg (8 kPa) even with an alveolar $P_{O_2}$ of 7000 mm Hg (930 kPa).

(This graph was computed assuming a blood pH of 7·4; a body temperature of 37° C, and an A–V $O_2$ difference of 6 volumes per cent.) (Courtesy of Lanphier and Brown[9] and The National Academy of Sciences).

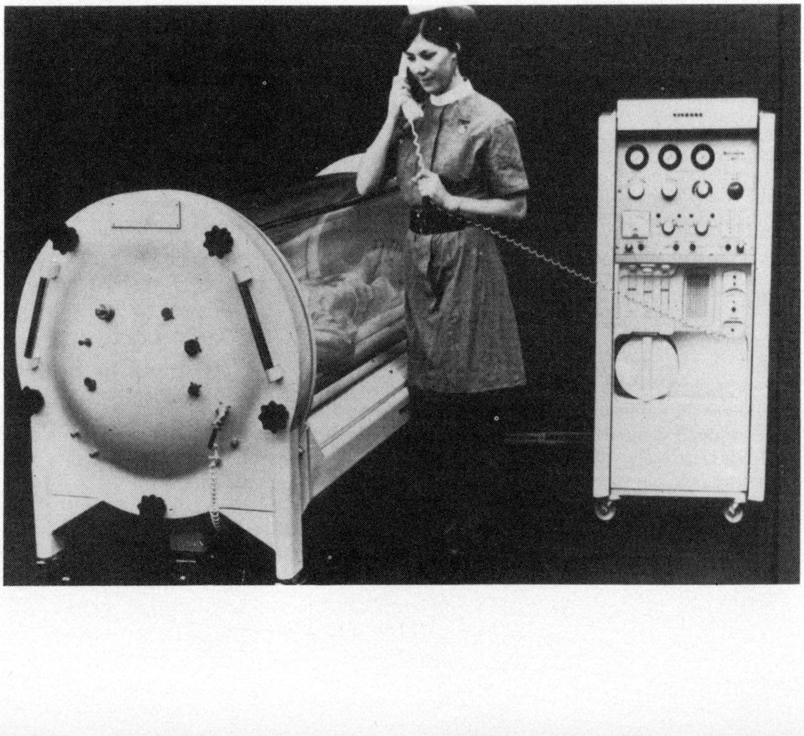

5/FIG. 5.—Single person transparent hyperbaric oxygen chamber (Vickers Ltd.). This general purpose model is designed to work at 3 atmospheres (2280 mm Hg, 304 kPa) pressure using recirculation with carbon dioxide absorption. (Courtesy of Vickers Ltd.)

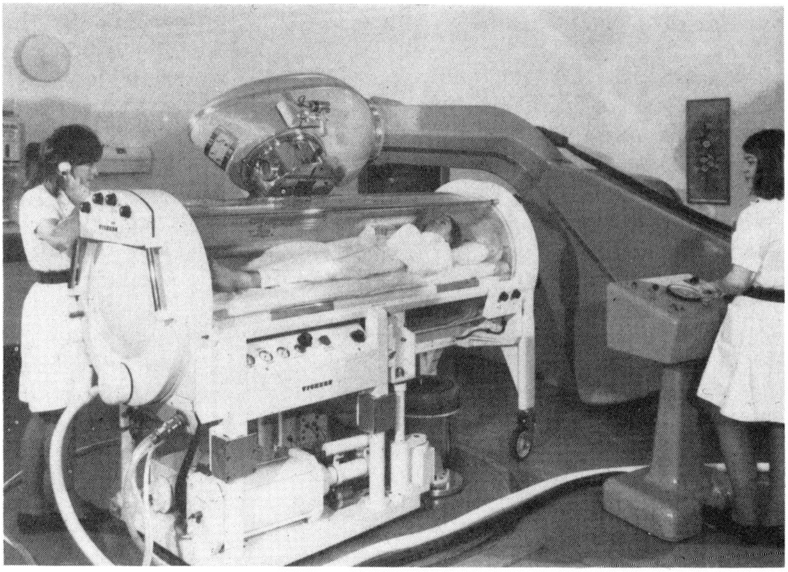

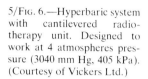

5/FIG. 6.—Hyperbaric system with cantilevered radiotherapy unit. Designed to work at 4 atmospheres pressure (3040 mm Hg, 405 kPa). (Courtesy of Vickers Ltd.)

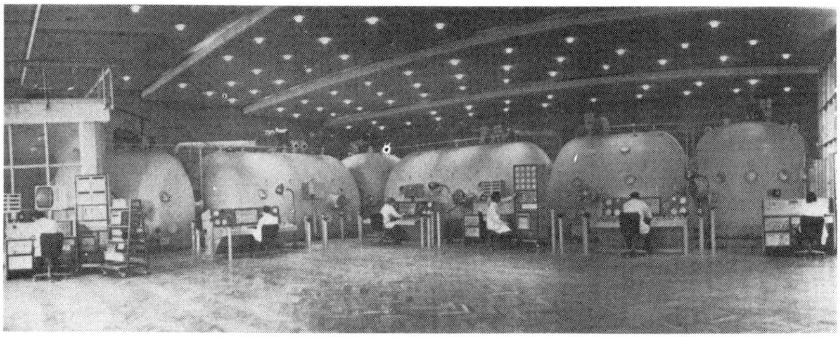

5/FIG. 7.—Hyperbaric facility at Research Institute of Clinical and Experimental Surgery in Moscow. This system consists of a series of interconnected hyperbaric chambers including entry locks, decompression chamber, group therapy chamber, operating theatre and experimental laboratory. Pressures range from 6–9 ats (4560–6840 mm Hg, 608–912 kPa). (Courtesy of Vickers Ltd.)

results are obtained by administering oxygen using a close-fitting pilot's type face mask connected to a low-pressure demand regulator.

### Basic Design Requirements of a Pressure Chamber

Five design features are important.

1. *Compressed air pump.*—Usually there are two. One pump is used for rapid compression, the other is used to maintain ventilation of the chamber once the requisite pressure has been reached. It is desirable that the compressors produce a steady rise of pressure within the chamber because this tends to reduce the incidence of painful effect of pressure changes on the middle ear and the skull sinuses. To avoid risk of explosion with high concentrations of oxygen the compressor pump must be oil-free.

2. *Climate control.*—There must be provision for heating, cooling and humidifying the air in the chamber.

3. *Electric equipment.*—All electric equipment within the chamber must be spark proof.

4. *Anaesthetic gases* and *oxygen* are best administered from cylinders stored within the chamber with facilities for spent gases to be vented.

5. *Sterile instruments.*—There must be some provision such as an air-lock for allowing instruments to be passed to and from the chamber.

## OXYGEN TOXICITY

Oxygen toxicity is a complex phenomenon which, in spite of much investigation over many years, remains an enigma. Although it is possible that high oxygen tensions could affect many, if not all, organ systems, it would appear that certain systems are more susceptible than others. These are:

1. *Pulmonary toxicity*, which is the most prominent manifestation of oxygen overdosage seen in clinical practice (Lorrain-Smith Effect[11]).
2. *Retrolental fibroplasia* in neonates.
3. *Hypoventilation*, seen in patients with chronic hypoxaemia and hypercarbia.
4. *Central nervous system oxygen toxicity* (Paul Bert Effect[12]).

### Pulmonary Oxygen Toxicity

The current clinical concept of oxygen toxicity has evolved from numerous observations in man and animals. With regard to pulmonary oxygen toxicity three clinically important generalisations may be justified from the many studies which have been done.

(*a*) There is at present no evidence that pulmonary oxygen toxicity develops in man at an inspired tension below about 0·5 atmospheres (382·6 mm Hg, 51 kPa) even with prolonged exposure.

(*b*) There is no reliable data to support the contention that measurable toxicity can develop in man breathing oxygen for 24 hours or less.

(*c*) There is no evidence that patients with pre-existing pulmonary disease are more sensitive to oxygen than normal volunteers.

A pathologist, Lorrain-Smith (1899),[11] was the first to carry out extensive investigations into the effects of increased oxygen tensions on the lungs of animals. He showed that oxygen was a lung irritant producing inflammation and congestion and that these effects occurred at a partial pressure of oxygen less than that required for the onset of convulsions. These findings, often referred to as the "Lorrain-Smith Effect", have been amplified by various workers in studies carried out usually within the range of 0·7 to 3·0 AT.A (525·2–2280·8 mm Hg, 70–304 kPa) oxygen; it is within this range that lung damage is the predominant sign of oxygen poisoning. At pressures less than 0·5 AT.A (382·6 mm Hg, 51 kPa) oxygen, the damage occurs very slowly if at all, as mentioned above, and at pressures greater than 3·0 AT.A (2280·8 mm Hg, 304 kPa) oxygen, the problem is overshadowed by the signs of central nervous system toxicity.

In man, despite the ethical difficulty in organising detailed studies, there is now sufficient data to demonstrate unequivocally that pulmonary oxygen toxicity is a real entity. The rate of development and degree of damage to the lungs appears to be proportional both to the dose of oxygen and to the duration of exposure. Because it is impossible to do detailed examinations of the lungs of normal volunteers to determine the rate of onset and course of toxicity, indirect measures have been adopted. Many have used "onset of symptoms" to describe tolerance curves. The earliest symptom is often described as substernal distress which begins as a mild irritation in the area of the carina and may be accompanied by occasional coughing. If exposure continues, pain becomes more intense, and is exacerbated by coughing or deep breathing. Time to onset of symptoms varies inversely with the partial pressure of oxygen (Fig. 8). Because of wide variability in the onset of symptoms, more objective critieria have been sought as indicators of the onset of oxygen toxicity. Among these, reduction in vital capacity is perhaps the most sensitive. It has been shown that vital capacity is progressively reduced during inhalation of between 0·5–1·0 AT.A (382·6–760 mm Hg, 51–101·3 kPa) oxygen, and at 2·0 AT.A (1520 mm Hg, 203 kPa).[13,14] As toxicity progresses, other changes become measurable. Minute ventilation, respiratory rate, compliance, and blood/gases all significantly deviate from normal as time passes.

Our understanding of the pathological changes of oxygen-poisoned lungs has been advanced considerably recently by application of histological techniques which enable quantification of lung damage, and in addition increasing application of electronmicroscopy has played a role. Although many of the changes described in detail refer to animal experiments, there is good reason to believe that the human lung behaves in a similar fashion when exposed

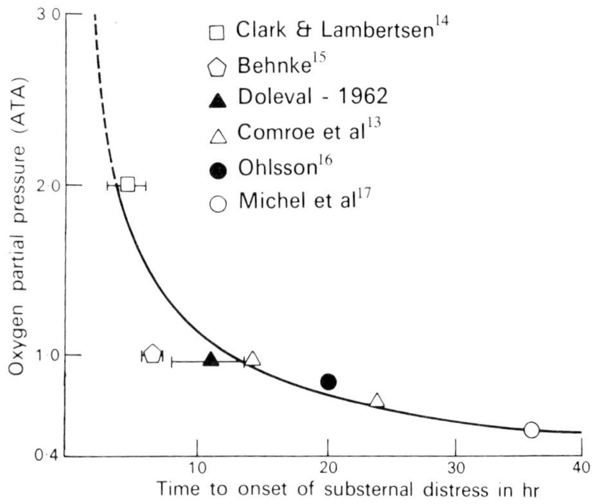


5/Fig. 8.—Time to onset of symptoms in normal volunteers[13–17]. (Courtesy of Bennett and Elliott and the publisher, Baillière Tindall[18].)

to high oxygen tensions for sufficient periods of time. When monkeys were exposed to concentrations of between 90 to 100 per cent oxygen at 1 AT.A (760 mm Hg, 101·3 kPa), the first change after a few days was slight swelling of endothelial cells, together with a small amount of interstitial oedema fluid. Following four days exposure, there was considerable destruction of alveolar cells, mainly of Type 1 (membranous pneumocytes). There was an increase in the thickness of the air-blood barrier, largely due to a 35 per cent increase in endothelial thickness and also an increase in the interstitial fluid volume (40 per cent of which was represented by an increase in oedematous tissues). After seven days, hyperplasia of Type 2 alveolar epithelial cells (granular pneumocytes) had led to a marked increase in alveolar thickness with almost complete destruction of Type 1 cells. The endothelium differed from region to region, with gross variations in thickness. At the end of twelve days, the proliferative changes seen in the granular pneumocytes were accentuated, which resulted in a further reduction in the alveolar spaces. The air-blood tissue barrier at the time was increased in thickness by approximately 370 per cent. During these experiments half of the animals died of acute toxicity within 7 days of commencing the experiment, some survived beyond that time apparently having become adapted. Two animals were weaned back to ambient air and then sacrificed 56 and 84 days after completion of the experiment. In both, considerable chronic change in lung structure had occurred. Although there are differences in the pathological changes seen in the lung of various species of animals exposed to high oxygen tensions, certain changes appeared consistently and are summarised in Fig. 9.

### Proposed Mechanisms of Oxygen Toxicity

Despite detailed documentation of the pathological effects induced by inhalation of oxygen, comparatively little progress has been made towards precise delineation of the mechanisms involved. A number of speculative hypotheses have been advanced regarding possible mechanisms, but supporting evidence is far from conclusive. These will be briefly discussed in turn.

### Absorption Collapse

It has been suggested that a major cause of oxygen-induced pulmonary damage is simple atelectasis resulting from a blockage of the small airways, with resultant absorption of gases trapped peripheral to the obstruction. However, this hypothesis has been challenged on the grounds that histologically the sequence of events in the course of the development of lung damage was capillary congestion progressing later to alveolar exudation and damage, and finally to secondary changes such as atelectasis.

While there is no doubt that collapse of lung is an important part of the clinical syndrome

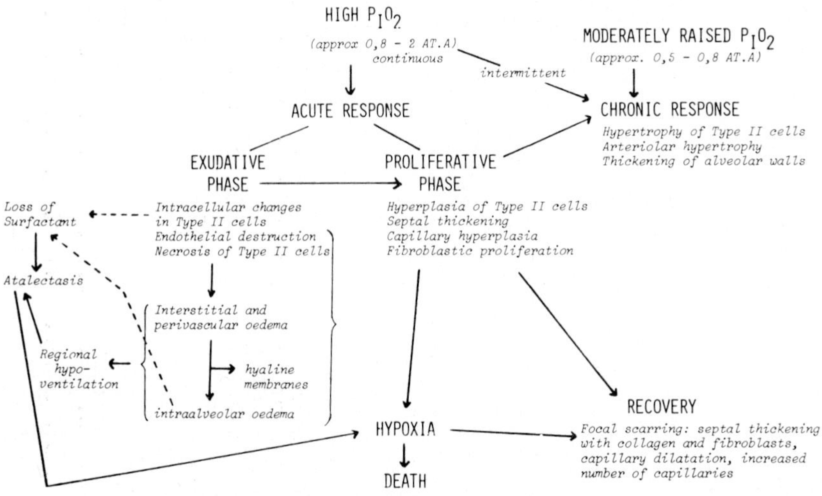


5/FIG. 9.—Diagrammatic representation of pathological responses of mammalian lung to oxygen. (Courtesy of Winter and Smith and the publisher, J. B. Lippincott Company.[19])

and sequelae of oxygen toxicity, it is not currently regarded as an initiating event. In clinical practice manoeuvres which ensure patency of the airways, such as physiotherapy of the chest, use of high tidal volumes, and techniques which increase the FRC by the use of positive end-expired pressures (PEEP) should receive particular attention.

### Lung Surfactant

Alveoli have a natural tendency to collapse because of mechanical properties of lung tissue; this collapse is prevented by a lining of lipoprotein material about 50 Å thick (surfactant), which lowers the surface tension of the lungs, thereby stabilising the alveoli.[20–23] The low surface tension also prevents transudation from capillaries which would otherwise occur. The surface-active properties of the lipoprotein material are believed to be due to phospholipid dipalmityl lecithin.[24] It follows from the above that if for any reason the amount of lung surfactant is decreased, the resultant rise in alveolar surface tension might be expected to bring about alveolar collapse and transudation. There have been many studies of the effect of oxygen at hyperbaric and atmospheric pressure on lung surfactant, some showing reduced surfactant activity, and others showing no effect. However, it is technically extremely difficult to obtain samples of lung extracts which give a true representation of the state of the surface tension of the fluid lining the alveoli. Although it seems certain that there are measurable changes in surface tension in the late stages of acute pulmonary oxygen toxicity, it is not clear whether these are the result of direct effects or indirect effects consequent upon mechanical changes induced by oxygen. Type 2 alveolar epithelial cells are thought to be the source of the surfactant.

In summary, the results obtained on the effects of oxygen on lung surfactant are inconclusive but sufficiently encouraging to warrant additional research on this subject with particular emphasis on improving experimental techniques.

### Metabolic Upset

The possibility that oxygen toxicity is brought about by inhibition of enzyme systems vital to the metabolism has received increasing attention. Although there is great variability in enzymatic resistance to high levels of oxygen, many reactions are very sensitive and easily inactivated. Those which have received much attention are those containing SH groups, the sulphydryl enzymes. Several mechanisms for the oxidation of SH groups have been proposed, and it is not known which pathways are involved. It is possible that the inactivation of sulphydryl groups is brought about either by oxidation or by the formation of free radicals produced under hyperbaric conditions. Inactivation of SH enzymes can have profound effects at many sites of action. Several such enzymes are involved in

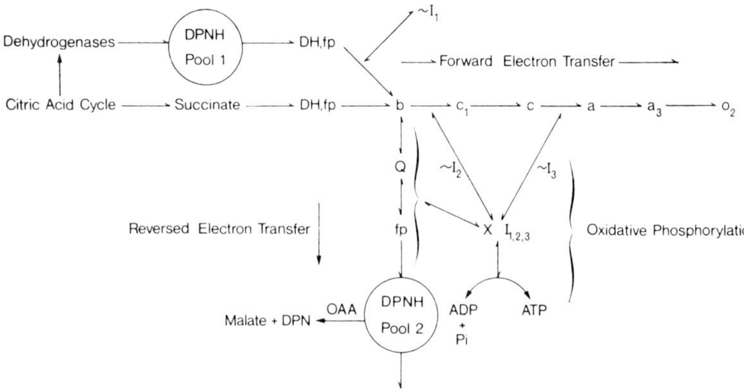


5/Fig. 10.—Schematic diagram of respiratory chain including reversed and forward pathways of electron transfer, with special emphasis on the possible site of action of hyperbaric oxygen. (Courtesy of Chance *et al.*, the editors, Brown and Cox and the National Academy of Sciences[26].)

the tricarboxylic acid cycle. An enzyme essential to glycolysis—glyceraldehyde phosphate dehydrogenase—is susceptible to oxygenation. In cellular respiration several flavo-proteins are particularly vulnerable, and Chance and associates[25,26] have demonstrated that oxygen interferes with chain electron transportation systems (Fig. 10). Other investigations have demonstrated altered metabolism of glutamate and *GABA*, which may be fundamental to central nervous system effects of high-pressure oxygen (Fig. 11).

### Myocardial Failure

Experiments *in vivo* have revealed that myocardial metabolism may be depressed by *high levels* of oxygen. This prompts the question that heart failure may be responsible for the pulmonary oedema of pulmonary oxygen toxicity. However, although evidence for this hypothesis is conflicting, it would appear to be unlikely that myocardial failure *per se* makes an important contribution to acute pulmonary oxygen toxicity.

### Role of the Endocrine System

The finding by Faulkner and Binger[28] that warm-blooded animals were more sensitive to oxygen than cold-blooded animals suggests that overall metabolic rate may exert an influence on the rate of development of pulmonary oxygen toxicity. Thus thyroxin or thyroid extract has been shown to hasten the onset of both convulsions and pulmonary oxygen damage in cats. Conversely, depression of metabolism by anaesthesia or hypothermia is associated with a reduction in susceptibility to oxygen. Part of the protective effects of hypophysectomy against pulmonary oxygen toxicity may be related to a reduction in TSH (Thyroid Secreting Hormone) secretions. Also it has been shown that the development of pulmonary damage is retarded by adrenalectomy, while conversely cortisone or similar adrenal corticoids increase the rate of development of pulmonary damage.

There is also considerable evidence that change in sympatho-adrenal medullary activity

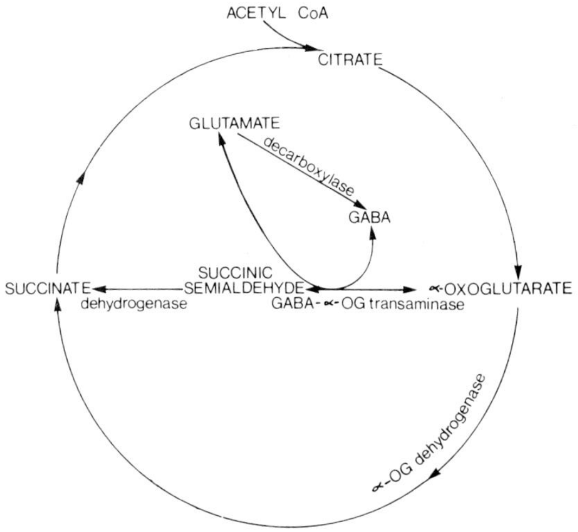


5/Fig. 11.—Metabolic reactions involving GABA and their relationship to the tricarboxylic acid cycle. Only the cycle intermediates relevant to the present discussion are shown. (Courtesy of Bennett and Elliott and the publisher, Baillière Tindall[27].)

may exert an influence on development of oxygen toxicity in animals; sympathomimetic agents augment the onset of the pulmonary oxygen damage, whilst sympatholytic agents delay development.

### Central Nervous System Toxicity

Paul Bert (1878)[12] noted convulsions in animals exposed to oxygen pressures in excess of 3 AT.A (2280 mm Hg, 304 kPa), which he was able to demonstrate were due to the partial pressure of oxygen and not the total environmental pressure. Man also is subject to the convulsive effects of hyperbaric oxygen. Bornstein and Stroink (1912)[29] reported muscle spasms in the legs with exercise after exposure for 50 minutes to oxygen at 3 AT.A (2280 mm Hg, 304 kPa).

These early findings have been amply confirmed and extended by others,[30–32] and our current understanding of the progressive nature of the clinical picture of oxygen poisoning is most aptly expressed by Lambertsen and colleagues[33] as follows:

"The convulsions are usually but not always preceded by the occurrence of localised muscular twitchings, especially about the eyes, mouth and forehead. Small muscles of the hand may be involved and inco-ordination of diaphragm activity in respiration may occur. These phenomena increase in severity over a period which may vary from a few minutes to nearly an hour with essentially clear consciousness being retained. Eventually an abrupt spread of excitation occurs and the rigid tonic phase of the convulsion begins. The tonic phase lasts for about 30 seconds and is accompanied by an abrupt loss of consciousness. Vigorous clonic contractions of the muscular groups of head and neck, trunk and limbs then occur, becoming progressively less violent over about one minute."

Our current knowledge on the toxic neurological effects of hyberbaric oxygen is derived from the extensive study of Donald.[34] In Donald's studies, the time to onset of symptoms was used as a quantitative measure of susceptibility. The symptom usually noted was lip twitching, but in a few instances it was nausea, vertigo or convulsions. In these studies an extremely large variation in susceptibility, not only between individuals, but also in any one person from day to day was noted. Also onset of symptoms occurred consistently sooner when studies were done during exercise, and in studies done under water rather than in a dry chamber. In view of this work and studies done at the U.S. Navy Experimental Diving Unit it is now current practice to limit the depth at which oxygen diving is done to about 10 metres; and Lanphier[35] has constructed an oxygen limit curve showing the underwater working limits (Fig. 12).

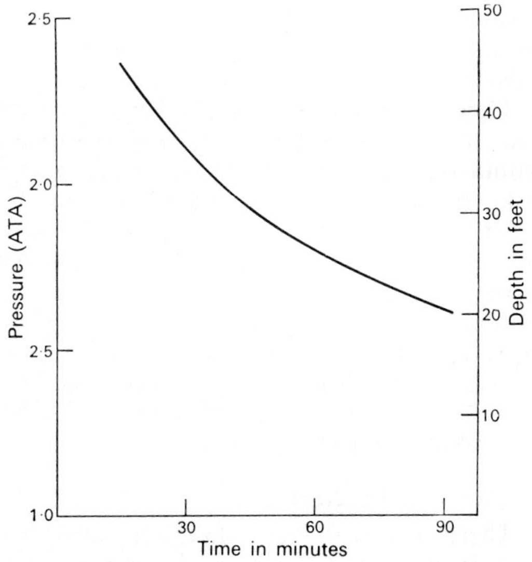


5/Fig. 12.—Oxygen limit curve for man. (Courtesy of Lanphier and the National Academy of Sciences.[35])

In dry conditions when no exercise is being undertaken, and when medical personnel are in attendance, a more lenient attitude can be tolerated. During radiotherapy for cancer Foster and Churchill-Davidson (1976 personal communications) reported only six cases of convulsions in 2965 exposures to 3 AT.A (2280 mm Hg, 304 kPa) oxygen for periods lasting 20 to 66 minutes.

**Diagnosis**

The suddenness of onset of convulsions make the detection of the pre-convulsive state difficult. However, the pattern of the electroencephalogram will reveal hyper-irritability prior to their onset and an electromyogram of the lip muscles has been used to detect the earliest signs of muscle twitching.

### Treatment

Provided the high pressure of oxygen is immediately withdrawn and the patient allowed to breathe air (either at atmospheric pressure or above) the convulsions will cease and no permanent cerebral damage will result. The danger of oxygen convulsions *per se* lies in the possible injury to the individual during a spasm in a small chamber.

However, if the patient is lying in a small single chamber then rapid decompression is not always advisable because in the conscious state laryngeal spasm may develop during the convulsions and close the glottis. In this case, a sudden drop of environmental pressure would lead to a dangerously high pressure trapped within the lungs thus increasing the possible risk of rupture. If the patient continues to breathe spontaneously (denoting an open glottis) or there is an endotracheal tube *in situ* (as in the anaesthetised subject), then the dangers of rapid decompression under hyperbaric oxygen are minimal.

## ANAESTHESIA IN A HYPERBARIC ENVIRONMENT

There is seldom need to provide anaesthesia in a single person chamber operating at 2–3 AT.A, as most patients tolerate this treatment with light sedation, but should full general anaesthesia be needed, the technique described below would suffice. Provision of an anaesthetic service for emergency surgery on deep sea divers operating at pressures of some 30–50 AT.A, constitutes a considerable challenge and will be considered in some detail. Large numbers of divers are currently employed in various commercial deep-sea enterprises, and most use a saturation diving programme which in practice has been found to be economically efficient. Thus divers live for periods of several weeks at a time in special habitats on the rigs or barges which are pressurised to depths of 300–400 metres, a pressure of 30–35 AT.A, only leaving for their work shifts on the ocean floor. Submersible capsules are used to lower the divers who, during the work period, remain tethered to their capsule by an umbilicus which conveys respiratory gases, heating water for the diver's suit, and communication cables. The work done by these men is very arduous and fraught with hazards, but even though divers are well trained and do their work with the utmost care, and are vetted to ensure physical and mental aptitude, the risks of injury and intercurrent illness are great. During a saturation programme urgent medical treatment demanding skilled attention would have to be done by doctors or rig medics actually within the pressurised facility; there can be no reduction of the decompression period (Table 1), which it should be noted was calculated for persons with normal circulations, and likely to be considerably prolonged after injury. First aid and initial treatment would have to be done by fellow divers possibly under radio-telephone instruction from a doctor. Generally habitats on oil rigs are unsuitable for medical treatment other than the most minor procedures, and patients would be far better moved from rig or barge to a shore base using a "transfer under pressure" (TUP) arrangement. At present there is no published information on a combination of helicopter and lightweight pressure chamber for this kind of transfer, but proposals have been made[36] for a TUP capsule to be available in Britain which will mate up with all rig chambers and with the International Underwater Contractors' saturation complex in Dundee, Scotland, where it will be possible to bring divers to medical attention with the advantage of the facilities of the NHS in the background. A similar facility is shortly to be available to the Royal Australian Navy which will work in conjunction with a "studio" at the diving school on HMSA *Penguin*, and with larger chambers in Fremantle and Sydney. Some of the problems encountered in providing medical services in a hyperbaric environment are enumerated in Table 5. Medical teams get access to the chamber via an air lock where they are compressed

5/TABLE 5
PROBLEMS OF ANAESTHESIA IN A HYPERBARIC CHAMBER

1. Problems due to compression of medical team
2. Problems of communication
3. Effect of pressure on clinical pharmacology of drugs
4. Risks of infection
5. Fire and explosion hazards
6. Effect of pressure on equipment

at a rate governed by the need to avoid aural barotrauma, high compression nervous syndrome, or excessive temperature rises.

Individual tolerance of medical team members participating in these programmes should be assessed by trial compressions. Once in the chamber communication may be a problem because speech is distorted by the altered density of the chamber's atmosphere (oxygen and helium, 0·4 AT.A & 46 AT.A). Special consideration needs to be given to medical apparatus. Space is at a premium so there is no room for bulky or cumbersome equipment. The ambient oxygen level increases fire risks; electric machines are therefore best avoided and should preferably be powered pneumatically. Drugs and transfusion solutions can be compressed, but if they are in rigid containers they should be vented to prevent implosion. Specimens for laboratory examination can be decompressed at about 3 metres/min, and analyses carried out at normal pressure. Blood gas and pH would not normally be available.

### Anaesthetic Technique

That high pressure can affect the intensity and duration of action of both intravenous and inhalation anaesthetic agents has been known for some time.[37] However, this factor is of little significance up to pressures of 50 AT.A and cannot, in practice, be differentiated from individual variation in responses to drugs given at sea-level pressure. (For example, some patients will sleep after as little as 50 mg i.v. thiopentone, whilst others require some 500 mg for the same effect.) Inhalation anaesthetic agents are not well suited to the pressure chamber: equipment needed is too cumbersome; some increase the fire risk; a high inspired oxygen level which may accompany inhalation anaesthesia is, as was noted above, potentially dangerous; and there is the problem of pollution in a chamber which usually relies on recirculating air conditioning; finally, nitrous oxide inhalation may aggravate decompression air emboli. For these reasons, some form of intravenous anaesthesia is recommended and may be the method of choice for intra-abdominal surgery. A suggested technique for major abdominal surgery (e.g. laparotomy for suspected peritonitis) would be as follows: induction of anaesthesia with an i.v. agent of short metabolic half-life, such as Althesin (70 μl/kg) or methohexitone (1 mg/kg) given by careful titration to its effect; muscle relaxation secured with pancuronium 100 μg/kg; intubation of the trachea using a cuffed tube inflated with sterile normal saline; hand controlled slight overventilation of the lungs with chamber gas using a non-rebreathing valve and self-inflating bag (Ambu bag or Laerdal Adult Resuscitator, or Hope Resuscitator in USA); maintenance of anaesthesia with increments of Althesin (about 10 μl/kg/min) or methohexitone (about 20 μg/kg/min); analgesia during surgery by i.v. pethidine (demerol) (15 mg/15 min) or morphine (0·2–0·3 mg/kg); at the end of surgery reversal of residual curarisation with an atropine/neostigmine mixture (atropine 17 μg/kg; neostigmine 50 μg/kg); continued ventilation of lungs until return of consciousness, muscle tone and reflexes. For short procedures, when muscle relaxation is not essential, Althesin or methohexitone may be used for induction and maintenance of anaesthesia in the same way as at sea level (1 AT.A[38], 31 AT.A[39]).

Regional anaesthesia can be used when indicated but there are a number of special problems peculiar to the hyperbaric environment; great care must be exercised to ensure that no air is injected, entrapped air could expand some 30 times on decompression; also it is important that bottles containing local drugs should be open prior to compression to prevent implosion and to allow at least some equilibration of dissolved gases in solution with the environment; it is of paramount importance to avoid risk of contamination of drugs because there are additional risks of sepsis in these conditions due to altered bacterial flora prevalent in the skin of divers as a result of long exposure to a hot, humid, compressed atmosphere. A suggested programme for handling anaesthetic drugs required for use in the pressure chamber is as follows: ampoules containing, for example, thiopentone, Althesin, atropine, neostigmine, Pavulon, adrenaline, calcium, lignocaine, Marcain, etc., should be placed in suitable stainless steel racks and autoclaved upright (134° C at 1658·1 mm Hg, 221 kPa for 3 min); drugs normally supplied in rubber-topped bottles can be handled in a similar manner. Prior to placing the drugs in the compression chamber, the autoclave drum should be opened under full aseptic surgical ritual and the tops of the ampoules should be removed and discarded, rubber caps should be perforated with a 21-gauge needle and the drum should then be closed and sealed with autoclavable tape. To allow pressure equalisation between the interior of the drum and the chamber during compression, several flexible plastic needles should be plunged through the tape into the drum and capped with bacterial filters (millipore filter, millex or 0·22 μm filter unit). The drum should be stored and handled upright at all times.

### Anaesthetic Equipment in the Hyperbaric Chamber at 2–4 AT.A

Cylinders containing the gases used in anaesthesia are usually at a pressure high enough to function normally in a hyperbaric environment. Reducing valves, similarly, work normally provided the supply pressure is sufficiently high; this means that any gas piped to them from outside the chamber must have a higher pressure than usual pipeline pressure of 60 lb per sq inch (32·3 mm Hg, 4·3 kPa).

Rotameters become inaccurate in the pressure chamber because of the gas density. At 2 AT.A (1520 mm Hg, 203 kPa) rotameters read about 30 per cent higher compared with readings from the same flows at 1 atmosphere (760 mm Hg, 101·3 kPa). Because of these discrepancies, flow meters should be individually calibrated using a spirometer at the pressure at which the flow meter is used. Vaporisers of the "Fluotec" type should deliver the set concentration because the partial pressure of vapour in equilibrium with its liquid is proportional to the absolute temperature, and is not affected by total ambient pressure. In practice, however, it has been shown that individual vaporisers exhibit variation in the partial pressure of halothane delivered, probably due to change in the ratio of gas passing through the bypass and vaporising chambers. They tend to be accurate when the concentration setting is 2 per cent or above, but below this, values tend to be high. Vaporisers, when not in use, should have their filler plug open during change in ambient pressure so as to avoid the danger of explosion. In some types of vaporiser liquid anaesthetic could be forced back up the inlet pipe during compression if appropriate precautions are not taken.

Changes in gas volume on compression or decompression necessitate a number of commonsense precautions. Cuffs on endotracheal tubes and intravenous and bladder catheters should be filled with water or saline to prevent large volume changes which would apply if they were filled with air. Similarly thoracotomy drainage tubes should be left open during decompression to avoid development of tension pneumothorax. Intragastric tubes should be left open. Intravenous transfusion may present problems because of expansion of air in the bottle; however, this may be prevented by the use of plastic infusion bottles. Multidose containers should have needles introduced through their tops to prevent pressure change of contents.

Electrically operated ventilators should not be used because of the potential fire hazard from sparking. Pressure-operated ventilators are satisfactory, but those powered by compressed air from outside the chamber will require an increase of pipeline pressure for efficient operation. Oil and grease must be excluded absolutely from those parts of the respirator exposed to high-pressure oxygen because of the fire hazard.

Suction apparatus taken from a direct suction pipeline outside the chamber tends to operate excessively when the chamber is functioning at high pressure because of the pressure differential. The recommended procedure is to have a pressure-reducing suction regulator within the chamber, thus making negative pressure of the sucker independent of the chamber pressure.

## REFERENCES


1. Junod, T. (1835). Recherches sur les effets physiologique et therapeutiques de la compression et des rarefaction de l'air taut sur le corps que les membres isoles. *Ann. gen. Med.*, **9**, 157.
2. Cousteau, J., (1964). At home under the sea. *Nat. Geograph.*, **125**, 465.
3. Shilling, C. W., and Willgrube, W. W. (1937). Quantitative study of mental and neuro-muscular reactions as influenced by increased air pressure. *U.S. nav. med. Bull.*, **35**, 373–380.
4. van Zyl, Jakobus J. W. (1967). Hyperbaric oxygenation in bacterial infections; with emphasis on those caused by the histotoxic clostridial organisms. From *Hyperbaric Oxygenation, a general review*. M.D. Thesis, University of Stellenbosch.
5. Churchill-Davidson, I., Sanger, C., and Thomlinson, R.

H. (1955). High pressure oxygen and radiotherapy. *Lancet*, **1**, 1091.
6. Siegel, B. V., and Morton, Jane I. (1967). Potentiation of the immunosuppressive effect of cytoxan by hyperbaric oxygen. *Experientia (Basel)*, **23**, 758.
7. Perrins, D. J. D. (1966). Hyperbaric oxygenation of ischaemic skin flaps and pedicles. *Proc. Third Internat. Conf. on Hyperbaric Medicine*. Ed. I. W. Brown, Jr. Washington, D.C.: Nat. Acad. Sci. Publication No. 1404, p. 613.
8. Perrins, D. J. D. (1967). Influence of hyperbaric oxygen on the survival of split skin grafts. *Lancet*, **1**, 868.
9. Lanphier, E. H., and Brown, I. W., Jr. (1966). The physiological basis of hyperbaric therapy. From *Fundamentals of Hyperbaric Medicine*. Publication No. 1298, p. 33. Washington, D.C.: Nat. Acad. Sci., Nat. Res. Council.
10. Brown, I. W. *et al.* (1965). Hyperbaric Oxygenation (Hybaroxia): Current Status, Possibilities and Limitations. *Advances in Surgery*, Vol 1. ed. Welch, C. E. Chicago: Year Book Medical Publishers.
11. Smith, J. Lorrain (1899). The pathological effects due to increase of oxygen tension in the air breathed. *J. Physiol.*, **24**, 19.
12. Bert, P. (1878). *La Pression Barometrique*. Eng. Trans. by Hitchcock, M. A. and Hitchcock, F. A., 1943. Columbus, Ohio: College Book Company.
13. Comroe, J. H., Dripps, R. D., Dumke, P. R., and Deming, M. (1945). Oxygen toxicity. The effect of inhalation of high concentrations of oxygen for twenty-four hours on normal men at sea level and at a simulated altitude of 18,000 feet. *J. Amer. med. Ass.*, **128**, 710.
14. Clark, J. M., and Lambertsen, C. J. (1966). Rate of devèlopment of pulmonary $O_2$ toxicity in normal men at 2 ATA ambient. *Fed. Proc.*, **25**, 566.
15. Behnke, A. R. Jr. (1940). High atmospheric pressure; physiological effects of increased and decreased pressure; application of these findings to clinical medicine. *Ann. Int. Med.*, **13**, 2217.
16. Ohlsson, W. T. L. (1947). Studies on oxygen toxicity at atmospheric pressure with special reference to the pathogenesis of pulmonary damage and clinical oxygen therapy. *Acta Med. Scand. Suppl.*, **190**, 1–19.
17. Michel, E. L., Langevin, R. W., and Gell, C. F. (1960). Effect of continuous human exposure to oxygen tensions of 418 mm Hg for 168 hours. *Aerospace Med.*, **31**, 138.
18. Bennett, P. B. and Elliott, D. H. (1975). *The Physiology and Medicine of Diving and Compressed Air Work*, 2nd edit. p. 167. London: Baillière Tindall.
19. Winter, P. M. and Smith, G. (1972). The toxicity of oxygen. *Anesthesiology*, **37**, 220.
20. Pattle, R. E. (1955). Properties, function and origin of the alveolar lining layer. *Nature (Lond.)*, **175**, 1125–1126.
21. Pattle, R. E., and Burgess, F., (1961). The lung lining film in some pathological conditions. *J. Path. Bact.*, **82**, 315–331.
22. Pattle, R. E., and Thomas, L. C. (1961). Lipoprotein composition of the film lining of the lung. *Nature (Lond.)*, **189**, 844.
23. Pattle, R. E. (1965). Surface lining of lung alveoli. *Physiol. Rev.*, **45**, 48–79.
24. Brown, E. S. (1964). Isolation and assay of dipalmityl lecithin in lung extracts. *Amer. J. Physiol.*, **207**, 402–406.
25. Chance, B., Jamieson, D., and Coles, H. (1965). Energy-linked pyridine nucleotide reduction: Inhibitory effects of hyperbaric oxygen *in vitro* and *in vivo. Nature (Lond.)*, **206**, 257–263.
26. Chance, B., Jamieson, D., and Williamson, J. R. (1966). Control of the oxidation-reduction state of reduced pyridine nucleotides *in vivo* and *in vitro* by hyperbaric oxygen. In *Proc. 3rd. Intern. Conference on Hyperbaric Medicine*. Ed. Brown, I. W., and Cox, B. G., pp. 15–41. Washington, D.C.: Nat. Acad. Sci., Nat. Res. Council.
27. Bennett, P. B. and Elliott, D. H. (1969). *The Physiology and Medicine of Diving and Compressed Air Work*, 1st edit. p. 130. London: Baillière Tindall.
28. Faulkner, J. M., Binger, C. A. L. (1927). Oxygen poisoning in cold blooded animals. *J. Exp. Med.*, **45**, 865–871.
29. Bornstein, A., and Stroink, M. (1912). Ueber Sauerstoffvergiftung. *Dtsch. med. Wschr.*, **38**, 1495–1497.
30. Behnke, A. R., Shaw, L. A., Shilling, C. W., Thomson, R. M. and Messer, A. C. (1934). Studies on the effects of high oxygen pressure. 1. Effect of high oxygen pressure upon the carbon dioxide and oxygen content, the acidity, and the carbon dioxide combining power of the blood. *Amer. J. Physiol.*, **107**, 13–28.
31. Behnke, A. R., Johnson, F. S., Poppen, J. R. and Motley, E. P. (1934–5). The effect of oxygen on man at pressures from 1 to 4 atmospheres. *Amer. J. Physiol.* **110**, 565–572.
32. Behnke, A. R., Forbes, H. S. and Motley, E. P. (1935–6). Circulatory and visual effects of oxygen at 3 atmospheres pressure. *Amer. J. Physiol.* **114**, 436–442.
33. Lambertsen, C. J., Kough, R. H., Cooper, D. Y., Emmel, G. L., Loeschcke, H. H., and Schmidt, C. F. (1953). Comparison of relationship of respiratory minute volume to $Pco_2$ and pH of arterial and internal jugular blood in normal man during hyperventilation produced by low concentrations of $CO_2$ at 1 atmosphere and by $O_2$ at 3·0 atmospheres. *J. appl. Physiol.*, **5**, 803–813.
34. Donald, K. W. (1947). Oxygen poisoning in man. *Brit. med. J.* **1**, 667–672.
35. Lanphier, E. H. (1955). Use of nitrogen oxygen mixtures in diving. From *Proceedings of the Underwater Physiology Symposium*, edited by L. G. Goff. Washington, D. C.: Nat. Acad. Sci., Nat. Res. Council.
36. Editorial (1975). High pressure medicine. *Brit. med. J.*, **4**, 541.
37. Johnson, F. H., Brown, D. E. S. and Marsland, D. A. (1942). Pressure reversal of the action of certain narcotics. *J. Cell. Comp. Physiol.*, **20**, 269.
38. Savege, T. M., Ramsay, M. A. E., Curran, J. P. J., Cotter, J., Walling, P. T. and Simpson, B. R. (1975). Intravenous anaesthesia by infusion. *Anaesthesia*, **30**, 757.
39. Dundas, C. R. (1979). Alphaxalone/Alphadolone in diving chamber anaesthesia. *Lancet*, **1**, 378.
40. Downing, J. W., Coleman, A. J., Meer, F. M. (1973). An intravenous method of anaesthesia for Caesarean section. *Brit. J. Anaesth.*, **45**, 381.

## FURTHER READING

Chew, H. E. R., Hanson, G. C., and Slack, W. K. (1969). Hyperbaric oxygenation. *Brit. J. Dis. Chest.*, **63**, 113.

Cox, J. and Robinson, D. J. (1980). Anaesthesia at depth. *Brit. J. Hosp. Med.*, **24**, 1.

Elliot, D. H., and Bennett, P. B. (1975). *The Physiology and Medicine of Diving*. London: Baillière Tindall.

CHAPTER 6

# Inhalational Anaesthetic Agents



THE continued dominance of inhalation methods of anaesthesia, over regional and intravenous techniques, is attributed to many factors but particularly to their inherent safety and almost universal applicability. Because of this, and the fact that new inhalational agents are in the process of development and introduction, it is proposed to state briefly the properties we should anticipate of the ideal inhalational agent; later certain aspects such as metabolism and potency standards which are common to all drugs in this group will be discussed. Finally each individual inhalational agent in current clinical use will be described in detail.

## PROPERTIES OF THE IDEAL INHALATIONAL ANAESTHETIC AGENT

New inhalational agents should allow a pleasant rapid induction, and rapid emergence. They should be non-inflammable and chemically stable during storage and while in contact with all materials used in construction of anaesthetic circuits. They should be biochemically stable and non-toxic to parenchymatous organs even with prolonged or repeated use; it would be a considerable advantage if the drug was excreted as given with virtually no biotransformation. The agent should be capable of inducing unconsciousness or sufficiently deep hypnosis to ensure amnesia, and sufficiently potent as an analgesic to prevent pain perception due to surgical stimuli; in addition it should produce some degree of skeletal muscle relaxation. Potency of the agent should be sufficient to allow high inspired oxygen levels which are occasionally required to compensate for increases in venous admixture during anaesthesia. It should have a high oil solubility which is usually indicative of anaesthetic potency, and rather low water solubility to ensure mobility. The ideal agent will have no deleterious affect upon the heart and will not be subject to serious interactions with drugs such as adrenaline or monoamine oxidase inhibitors.

## METABOLISM OF VOLATILE ANAESTHETIC AGENTS

Volatile anaesthetic agents were originally assumed to be unaffected by passage through the body and to be eliminated unchanged from the lungs. However, even though it was known that they may be liable to undergo biotransformation, in the case of chloroform since Zeller's report in 1883,[1] and in the case of trichloroethylene since the 1930s, these observations were considered to be esoteric unique features of two drugs and not applicable to other inhalational agents. These views had to be revised however in the early 1960s when Van Dyke and others[2] demonstrated in animals biodegradation of halothane, ether, chloroform, and methoxyflurane—observations which were soon to be amply confirmed by numerous investigators in man. Now it is known that all volatile agents are biotransformed, and in some it has been measured quantitatively: up to 10–20 per cent halothane,[3] or fluroxene,[4] and about 50 per cent methoxyflurane[5] taken up in man may be biodegraded rather than eliminated unchanged. Over the last 15 years anaesthetic metabolism has been the subject of many investigations which have in the main followed two general trends. Firstly, a number of studies have been biochemically orientated and have sought to demonstrate the chemical reactions involved, factors governing rate and extent of the reactions, and the fate of the resulting metabolites themselves. The second approach has had a clinical bias; of special interest has been the possibility that a relationship might exist between metabolism of anaesthetic agents and their toxicity. The three main aspects of toxicity which have received attention include: histotoxicity, abortifacient activity, and teratogenicity. A further clinical implication of anaesthetic metabolism has emerged from the reports of Tinker and colleagues[6] of plasma bromide levels after halothane, which clearly indicate a potential for prolonged sedation particularly after a long exposure to halothane. The close relationship between anaesthetic metabolism and histotoxicity can be demonstrated for both chloroform and methoxyflurane. Nephrotoxicity can readily be shown to be related to certain methoxyflurane metabolites, and hepatotoxicity is clearly directly and immediately related to chloroform metabolites. However, convincing evidence for hepatotoxicity following halothane has not been forthcoming despite considerable research, and the same may be said regarding the possibility that these metabolites might indirectly provoke damage by forming antigens capable of initiating sensitisation reactions involving the liver. Indeed, there is even doubt that the syndrome "halothane hepatitis" really exists (see Chapter 35).

The two other aspects of toxicity mentioned above: abortifacient activity and teratogenicity, mainly concern personnel and their associates working in or near operating units which are contaminated or polluted with anaesthetic gases and vapours. There appears to be some evidence that chronic exposure to traces of anaesthetic in the environment can be hazardous. A number of studies suggest that there is an increased incidence in operating-room workers of spontaneous abortion, congenital abnormalities in their offspring, cancer in female anaesthetists, liver disease, and renal disease in nurses.[7] Although a cause-effect relationship has not yet been established (and may indeed be impossible to prove conclusively) it would seem to be prudent to take all reasonable steps to monitor, and where feasible to reduce, ambient levels of anaesthetic gases and vapours within operating rooms, particularly as this may be effectively accomplished by relatively simple measures (see Chapter 8).

### Minimum Alveolar Concentration (MAC)

MAC is the minimum alveolar concentration of anaesthetic at 1 atmosphere that produces immobility in 50 per cent of those patients or animals exposed to a noxious stimulus. The term was first suggested in 1963 when Merkel and Eger[8] described a technique for the determination in dogs of the minimum alveolar concentration of anaesthetic (MAC) required to prevent gross muscular movement in response to a painful stimulus. Since then sufficient evidence has accumulated to lead us to accept MAC as a measure or index of anaesthetic potency (potency equals the reciprocal of the partial pressure of an agent to achieve a given anaesthetic effect), which would allow, for example, comparison of circulatory or respiratory effects of equipotent doses of two or more inhalational agents. The term MAC was chosen, and has gained wide acceptance, as an index of potency for three main reasons. Firstly MAC is perhaps the most readily measured index of partial pressure of drug at the anaesthetic site of action—the brain. Secondly MAC appears to be equally applicable to all inhalational agents; and does not rely on fickle physical signs or side-effects which vary from drug to drug. Finally MAC provides a useful number for the clinician in describing the dose of drug required to achieve the essential end point of anaesthesia: analgesia and amnesia.

## NITROUS OXIDE ($N_2O$)

Nitrous oxide was first prepared by Priestley in 1772,[9] and its anaesthetic properties were first demonstrated by Sir Humphry Davy in 1800.[10] It was not until 1844, however, that it came to be used in clinical practice. In that year Gardner Quincy Colton, a lecturer in chemistry, gave a demonstration of the effects of inhaling nitrous oxide at Hartford, Connecticut. Amongst his audience was Horace Wells, a local dentist, who was so impressed that he persuaded Colton to give him some nitrous oxide the following day for extraction of a tooth. The procedure was completely painless. Later that year Wells gave a demonstration of the technique to the Massachusetts General Hospital, Harvard Medical School, but the patient complained of pain and Wells was dubbed a fraud. The introduction of ether soon afterwards delayed a full appreciation of nitrous oxide until nearly twenty years later, when Colton reintroduced it for use in dental practice.

### Preparation

*In the laboratory*.—Small amounts may be prepared by allowing iron to react with nitric acid. Nitric oxide (NO) is first produced, but this is reduced to nitrous oxide by an excess of iron:

$$2NO + Fe \rightarrow FeO + N_2O$$

*Commercially*.—Nitrous oxide is produced by heating ammonium nitrate to between 245 and 270° C.

$$NH_4NO_3 \xrightarrow[245\text{–}270^\circ\,C]{\text{Heat}} N_2O + 2H_2O$$

The processes involved in drying and purifying the gas may vary but that used by the British Oxygen Company in the United Kingdom is briefly as follows.[11] A strong solution of ammonium nitrate when heated produces nitrous oxide with ammonia, nitric acid, nitrogen and traces of nitric oxide (NO) and nitrogen dioxide ($NO_2$). Cooling of the emerging gases results in reconstitution of the ammonia and nitric acid to ammonium nitrate and this is returned to the reactor. The gases are now passed through water scrubbers which remove any residual ammonia and nitric acid, and then through caustic permanganate scrubbers which remove the higher oxides of nitrogen to leave a residuum of 1 Vpm (volume per million) of nitric acid and nitrogen dioxide with the purified nitrous oxide and some nitrogen. Acid scrubbers now remove any final traces of ammonia and the gases are then compressed and dried in an aluminium drier. As the gases leave the drier continuous sampling takes place by passing a small stream of them through a visual bubbler. This consists of two solutions in series, the first containing acid potassium permanganate which converts any nitric oxide to nitrogen dioxide. The second consists of a colourless solution of Saltzman reagent in which any nitrogen dioxide present dissolves causing a chemical reaction which produces a magenta colour. The compressed and dried gases are now expanded into a liquefier with resultant liquefaction of the nitrous oxide and escape of the gaseous nitrogen. The pure nitrous oxide is now evaporated, compressed to a liquid, and passed through a second aluminium drier to the cylinder filling line. At this stage visual and electronic checks are carried out on samples leaving the drier to ensure that the nitrogen dioxide content does not exceed 1 Vpm.

About nine tenths of the contents of a full nitrous oxide cylinder are in liquid form. Great care is taken during manufacture to prevent moisture being included in the cylinder contents, since water vapour tends to freeze as it passes through a reducing valve and may lead to obstruction of gas flow.

When a nitrous oxide cylinder is turned on, the gas tension within is first reduced and then rapidly increases again as some of the liquid vaporises. In a discussion on the value of pressure gauges on nitrous oxide cylinders Jones[12] has pointed out that it is a misconception to believe that the pressure of the gas in the cylinder is maintained whilst liquid nitrous oxide is present. In fact, when flow rates of 10 litres/minute are used there is a sharp linear fall in pressure whereas only a small but never-

6/TABLE 1
PHYSICAL AND CHEMICAL CONSTANTS OF SOME INHALATIONAL AGENTS

| *Agents* | *Molecular Weight* | *Flammability* | *Vapour Pressure at 20° C* | *Solubilities* *Oil/Gas* | *Blood/Gas* | *$H_2O$/Gas* | *MAC* | *Maximum Safe Concentration (per cent)* |
|---|---|---|---|---|---|---|---|---|
| Nitrous Oxide $N_2O$ | 44 | no | 800 psi (5515 kPa) | 1·4 | 0·47 | 0·44 | 105 | 80 |
| Cyclopropane $C_3H_6$ | 42 | yes | 90 psi (620 kPa) | 11·2 | 0·42 | 0·20 | 9·2 | 30 |
| Xenon Xe | 131 | no | | 1·9 | 0·20 | 0·10 | 71 | 80 |
| Diethyl Ether $C_2H_5$—O—$C_2H_5$ | 74 | yes | 440 mm Hg (59 kPa) | 65 | 12·1 | 13·1 | 1·92 | 8 |
| Chloroform $CHCl_3$ | 119 | no | 170 mm Hg (23 kPa) | 265 | 8·4 | 3·8 | 0·7 | 1·0 |
| Trichloroethylene $CCl_2 = CHCl$ | 131 | no | 60 mm Hg (8 kPa) | 960 | 9·2 | 1·55 | | 1·5 |
| Halothane $CF_3CHClBr$ | 197·4 | 7·0 $N_2O$* 5·4 $O_2$ | 243 mm Hg (32 kPa) | 224 | 2·3 | 0·74 | 0·75 | 3 |
| Methoxyflurane $CH_3$—O—$CF_2CHCl_2$ | 165·0 | no | 22·5 mm Hg (3 kPa) | 825 | 13·0 | 4·5 | 0·16 | 1·5 |
| Enflurane $CHF_2$—O—$CF_2CHFCl$ | 184·5 | no | 184 mm Hg (24 kPa) | 98·5 | 1·8 | 0·82 | 1·68 | 5 |
| Isoflurane $CHF_2$—O—$CHClCF_3$ | 184·5 | no | 250 mm Hg (33 kPa) | 99 | 1·4 | 0·61 | 1·2 | 5 |

* Halothane is completely non-flammable even in oxygen at 2000 psi (13790 kPa)

theless progressive fall occurs with a flow rate of 2 litres/minute. However, he points out that even a short interruption in flow will rapidly allow the gas pressure to build up again as more liquid vaporises until finally no liquid remains. Then a pressure gauge would act in a similar manner to other gas cylinders. It is true, therefore, that pressure gauges on nitrous oxide cylinders will not indicate total contents until all the liquid is exhausted. Nevertheless they do warn against failure of flow. Most of the recent models of anaesthetic machines now incorporate them in their design.

Latent heat is required for the vaporisation of liquid nitrous oxide and this is obtained from the casing of the metal cylinder, which, as a result, rapidly cools. This in turn leads to freezing of the water vapour in the air immediately surrounding the cylinder, and to the formation of a layer of ice on the cylinder.

Nitrous oxide cylinders are marketed in various sizes, and coloured blue. In the United Kingdom 100 and 200 gallon cylinders are the most commonly used.*

*100 gallons of nitrous oxide weigh 30 oz: US gallon is 5/6th Imperial gallon.

**Physical Properties**

Nitrous oxide is non-irritating, sweet-smelling and colourless, and is the only inorganic gas in regular use today. The molecular weight is 44·01 and the specific gravity is 1·527 (air = 1). It is readily compressible under 50 atmospheres pressure at 28° C. to a clear and colourless fluid with a boiling point of −89° C. It is stable in the presence of soda-lime. The oil/water solubility ratio is 3·2. The blood/gas solubility coefficient is 0·47.

**Impurities**

The main impurities which may occur have already been mentioned, and to them carbon monoxide should be added. This may be produced from burning particles of the sacks in which ammonium nitrate is delivered. The consequences of inhaling higher oxides of nitrogen, especially nitrogen dioxide, in concentrations of over 50 Vpm are reflex inhibition of breathing with laryngospasm, and the rapid onset of intense cyanosis.[13] The last is due to both the formation of methaemoglobin and to altered pulmonary gas exchange. Pulmonary oedema may occur in the acute phase, but with concentrations lower than 50 Vpm it may not appear for some hours. If the patient does not die immediately, chronic chemical pneumonitis may follow, with resultant pulmonary fibrosis. Respiratory acidosis, from associated ventilatory failure, and metabolic acidosis, from production of nitric and nitrous oxide formed from solution of the gases in the body fluids, may occur. Hypotension may be marked and results from the effect of nitrate and nitrate ions on vascular smooth muscle. The cases of poisoning described by Clutton-Brock[14] illustrate vividly the clinical consequences.

The detection of higher oxides of nitrogen has been reviewed by Kain and associates.[15] In clinical practice the best method involves the use of a starch iodide paper. The moistened paper is placed in a 20 ml syringe and 15 ml of oxygen are drawn up, followed by 5 ml of the sample gas. Any nitric oxide will be oxidised by the oxygen to nitrogen dioxide, and the latter by oxidising iodide to iodine will turn the starch from a faint purple to a bright blue, depending on the amount of iodine present. The sensitivity of this test is 300 Vpm.

The principles of treatment of poisoning by the higher oxides of nitrogen have been discussed by Prys-Roberts.[16] He stresses that the advice he gives, although based on current concepts for the correction of the physiological disturbances that occur, is only a conjectural suggestion for those faced with the problem. Oxygen, either by spontaneous or assisted ventilation, and methylene blue, 2 mg/kg of body weight intravenously, will be required initially to overcome the intense cyanosis resulting from methaemoglobinaemia. Further increments of methylene blue may be required, but excessive amounts can result in the production of methaemoglobin and also haemolytic anaemia.

Bronchial lavage and suction, together with endobronchial and parenteral steroids, have been suggested for the treatment of the chemical pneumonitis. The use of fibre-optic endoscopic equipment will allow bronchial toilet to be done in a far more efficient and safe manner than has been hitherto possible using the standard bronchoscope. The acid-base and blood gas status of the patient should be regularly checked and appropriate measures taken to correct acidaemia, hypoxia, or hypercarbia. The cardiovascular status of the patient should be monitored at least by electrocardiograph, and occasionally measurement of central venous, pulmonary artery and pulmonary wedge pressures may be useful. The severe systemic hypotension from vasodilatation can be improved by intravenous fluid and minimal doses of a vasopressor. The use of dimercaprol is suggested for severe cases since it has a protective action against the higher oxides of nitrogen.

#### Inflammability

It is neither inflammable nor explosive but will support combustion of other agents, even in the absence of oxygen, because at temperatures above 450° C it does decompose to nitrogen and oxygen.

#### Pharmacological Actions

Nitrous oxide is rapidly absorbed from the alveoli and 100 ml of blood will carry 45 ml of nitrous oxide in its plasma. It does not combine with haemoglobin nor does it undergo any chemical combination within the body, so that elimination is as speedy as absorption.

**Anaesthetic action.**—Nitrous oxide is a weak anaesthetic, having a MAC of 105. At one time it was thought that any anaesthetic action that followed its use was produced solely by the exclusion of oxygen from the brain cells, since it is 15 times more soluble in plasma than nitrogen, and 100 times more so than oxygen.

At sea level, some patients lose consciousness when given 80 per cent nitrous oxide and 20 per cent oxygen—indeed a few subjects lose consciousness with mixtures containing equal parts of nitrous oxide and oxygen. If nitrogen is substituted for nitrous oxide in such a mixture anaesthesia rapidly ceases, and even if the oxygen is reduced to 10 per cent—with 90 per cent nitrogen—no anaesthesia occurs. Faulconer and associates[17] showed that a 50:50 mixture of nitrous oxide and oxygen at 2 atmospheres pressure rapidly produces surgical anaesthesia with complete oxygen saturation of the arterial blood, whereas the same concentration at atmospheric pressure in their patients did not produce loss of consciousness.

There is nowadays, therefore, no doubt that nitrous oxide is a weak anaesthetic agent, but the problem still remains as to how much of the anaesthesia produced (when it is used without supplement) is due to the potency of the gas and how much to the hypoxia which so frequently accompanies its use in these circumstances. The fact that these two features are intimately connected is emphasised by the following statement of Clement[18]: "... control of anaesthesia is synonymous with control of oxygen". In the past anoxic damage to the brain, or even death, has been reported following the use of nitrous oxide for a short period. Faulconer[17] showed that to produce in man surgical anaesthesia (stage III) with nitrous oxide, a partial pressure of 760 mm Hg (101·3 kPa) is required if full oxygenation is maintained. Since an 80 per cent mixture of nitrous oxide in oxygen at normal atmospheric pressure results in a partial pressure of nitrous oxide of only about 600 mm Hg (80 kPa), surgical anaesthesia cannot be achieved without some hypoxia. The use of a mixture of nitrous oxide and oxygen in the proportion 85:15 for induction causes a marked fall in arterial saturation in approximately two minutes, even when previous preoxygenation is carried out for three minutes. When nitrous oxide alone is used to induce anaesthesia, loss of consciousness is rapid enough—about 60 seconds—to suggest that this is primarily caused by displacement of oxygen from the brain rather than by saturation with nitrous oxide to a degree sufficient to cause anaesthesia without hypoxia.[19] In modern anaesthetic practice, nitrous oxide (even at sea level) is no longer used as an induction agent save in exceptional circumstances because of the danger of the accompanying hypoxia. However, when accompanied by at least 33⅓ per cent oxygen, it has proved an immensely valuable supplement to other anaesthetic agents.

### Circulatory Effects of Nitrous Oxide

Nitrous oxide has been long regarded as devoid of cardiovascular side-effects, a viewpoint supported both by considerable clinical experience extending over a period of more than a hundred years, and by a number of well-controlled haemodynamic trials. However the observations by Price and Helrich[20] that the drug possessed myocardial depressant properties was followed by isolated clinical reports in which it was blamed for the profound hypotension that occurred when the agent was given to patients anaesthetised with oxygen and halothane.[21,22] Interpretation of these observations is difficult because nitrous oxide was given against a background of other drugs with the possibility of complex interactions. In an attempt to resolve these difficulties two groups gave the drug on its own. Eisele and Smith[23] demonstrated that substitution of 40 per cent nitrogen by 40 per cent nitrous oxide in oxygen in trained healthy volunteers was associated with significant reductions in heart rate (6 to 9 per cent); there was no change in blood pressure and consequently derived peripheral vascular resistance increased significantly. Thornton and associates[24] confirmed these observations in a study on ten patients with heart disease during cardiac catheterisation.

In view of the widespread and expanding indications for nitrous oxide in the fields of post-operative, obstetric and coronary care analgesia, further studies were undertaken to determine the level at which nitrous oxide inhalation was associated with haemodynamic effects. Nitrous oxide was given in incremental steps of 10 per cent up to 50 per cent; 21 per cent oxygen and nitrogen formed the balance of the inspired mixtures. No change in heart rate, blood pressure or cardiac output was noted, suggesting that the high inspired oxygen level utilised in other studies was in some way responsible for the cardiovascular depression noted.[25]

In clinical practice therefore it would appear to be reasonable to ignore the possibility that nitrous oxide may be associated with cardiovascular depression.

Nitrous oxide does not sensitise the heart to adrenaline; the latter may therefore be infiltrated to produce ischaemia of the surgical field provided the concentration does not exceed about 1 in 200,000, the total dose 1 mg and the patient is moderately overventilated with arterial $Po_2$ of more than 100 mm Hg (13·3 kPa) and $Pco_2$ less than 35 mm Hg (4·6 kPa). Alternatively ornithine-8-vasopressin (POR 8) may be used.[26]

### Metabolism and Toxicity

Although nitrous oxide has no direct toxic activity, when given without physiological upsets such as hypoxia, there is evidence that its long-term use can indirectly produce haematological, neurological, and gestational defects.

(*a*) *Haematological*.—Pancytopaenia (aplastic anaemia) with a megaloblastic blood picture was first noted in 1956 by Lassen and colleagues[27] in patients given $N_2O$ (50%) for long periods as sedation in the respiratory management of tetanus; later Amess and colleagues[28] demonstrated in prospective studies that the severity of megaloblastic marrow depression was directly related to the duration of $N_2O$ inhalation (50%): mild depression after 6 hours became severe after 24 hours. The mechanism of these responses is probably due to $N_2O$ induced inactivation of vitamin $B_{12}$ which leads to impaired methionine and deoxythymidine synthesis and defects in folate metabolism, all essential factors in normal haemopoiesis. The cobalt in the corrin ring of $B_{12}$ is catalytic in a reaction in which $N_2O$ acts as a two-electron oxidising agent in a series of reactions which can be represented by:

$$Co^{I} + N_2O \rightarrow Co^{III} + N_2 + H_2O$$

This is followed by the rapid reaction of cob(III)alamin with cob(I)alamin:

$$Co^{III} + Co^{I} \rightarrow Co^{II}$$

Stoichiometry (the mathematics of chemistry) indicates that 2 moles of $B_{12}$ are oxidised by 1 mole of $N_2O$.

(*b*) *Neurological defects.*—These have been reported after long-term unintentional inhalation of $N_2O$ as an environmental contaminant by dentists and their assistants, and as a result of deliberate habitual abuse.[29–31] Neurological signs take the form of motor, sensory, co-ordination and reflex defects which appear to regress on discontinuation of $N_2O$. In monkey experiments, neurological lesions after long-term $N_2O$ inhalation appear to be the result of demyelinating lesions in posterior columns, lateral spinothalamic tracts and spinocerebellar tracts of the spinal cord. The mechanism of the neuropathy with $N_2O$ is probably similar to that described for the haematological defects and develops in response to vitamin $B_{12}$ lack. The failure to synthesise S-adenosylmethionine from methionine and ATP leads to failure of methylation of basic proteins in myelin sheaths, in particular there is impaired methylation of arginine-107 in the basic myelin protein.[32]

(*c*) *Gestational defects.*—The incidence of gestational defects appears to be increased in individuals associated with surgical operating theatres; studies on dental personnel exposed to trace amounts of $N_2O$ indicate an increased abortion rate among female assistants and among the wives of dentists.[33] The incidence of fetal death is increased in the incubated chick and in the rat by $N_2O$.[34,35] All fetuses born to $N_2O$ treated rats showed abnormalities of ribs and vertebrae, and some had visceral malformations.[36] Exposure of rats to a 1 in 200 concentration $N_2O$ in air resulted in a decreased incidence of pregnancy as well as an increased incidence of resorptions.[37–39] Thus there appears to be a sound experimental basis for the observation on the effect of $N_2O$ in producing abortion in man. The proposed mechanism of these effects, as with the haematological and neurological effects, is presumably through inactivation of $B_{12}$ and in turn the effect on folate metabolism. (See also Chapter 8, p. 250.)

What are the clinical implications of reports of toxic effects of $N_2O$? For routine use as a general anaesthethic, $N_2O$ may be regarded as non-toxic, and there need be no restriction on its use. When $N_2O$ is given for periods in excess of 6 hours, neurological and haematological defects may occur, which however are readily and rapidly reversible on discontinuation of inhalation. These problems are not sufficiently serious to restrict the use of $N_2O$, particularly in those instances in which opiates prove to be ineffective. The association between $N_2O$ and gestational defects is controversial, but it would seem sensible to avoid needless contamination of the operating-room environment by use of waste gas scavenging devices, provided these do not compromise clinical safety.

**Contra-indications to nitrous oxide anaesthesia.**—With the exception of the remarks above concerning duration of administration, there are no contra-indications to the use of nitrous oxide in combination with an adequate percentage of oxygen. It is always preferable either to precede the inhalation by an intravenous induction of anaesthesia or to supplement it with a more potent inhalational agent, thereby ensuring a satisfactory level of oxygenation in the inspired mixture at all times. Indeed, a minimum concentration of 30 per cent oxygen is recommended when nitrous oxide is used for anaesthetic purposes.

### Methods of Administration

Nitrous oxide can be administered by intermittent or continuous flow machines.

*Intermittent flow.*—This is an economical method as gas only flows during inspiration, and it is based upon two different techniques.

The first technique depends upon nitrous oxide and oxygen flowing into a mixing bag from which the patient inspires via corrugated tubing and a mask. As the bag empties, so it is refilled from the cylinders, and when it is full the flow of gases is automatically cut off until the next inspiratory effort starts the process once more (see Chapters 39 and 43). This type of apparatus is used almost entirely in midwifery and dental practice. The percentage of gas and oxygen in the mixture breathed can be readily adjusted by setting the dial to the required figure, and a simple device enables the intermittent flow to be replaced by a continuous flow at various pressures—a factor which may be particularly useful in dental anaesthesia. Many machines incorporate a small trichloroethylene or halothane inhaler and a reservoir bag between the patient and the machine.

The second technique makes use of a premixed cylinder of nitrous oxide and oxygen under pressure with a demand valve to allow a high flow of gas to the patient on inspiration. The premixing of these two gases in the same cylinder was first suggested by Barach and Rovenstine.[40] At room temperature and at a pressure of 2000 pounds per square inch certain proportions of nitrous oxide in oxygen exist as a single phase gas, due to the solvent action (Poynting effect) of the oxygen at this pressure. Tunstall[41] described this phenomenon, making the point that up to 75 per cent nitrous oxide-oxygen remains in the gas phase under these conditions. He also reported the clinical use of a mixture of 50 per cent nitrous oxide and 50 per cent oxygen contained in one cylinder for the relief of pain in childbirth. Cooling such a mixture produces liquid nitrous oxide at the bottom of the cylinder, and this remains even when the cylinder is rewarmed.[42] In these circumstances, if the cylinder is used it will first deliver a mixture with an oxygen content that is higher than intended, and then one that is lower. Delivery of a constant mixture from the cylinder can be assured either by preventing cooling or, should cooling occur, by briskly inverting the cylinder several times after rewarming.[42,43] The use of premixed nitrous oxide and oxygen (Entonox) for the relief of pain in labour is described in Chapter 39.

*Continuous flow*.—A continuous flow of gases is supplied from the anaesthetic machine, and a semi-closed system is most frequently used, with almost all the expired mixtures passing into the atmosphere through the expiratory valve. A completely closed system with absorption of carbon dioxide is not indicated when nitrous oxide is used, since it may be extremely difficult to ensure adequate oxygenation of the patient (see Chapter 2). Semi-closed anaesthesia is, however, frequently practised with a carbon dioxide absorber in place so that a more economical flow of gases can be used (see below).

### Clinical Uses of Nitrous Oxide

For the reasons already stated, there is no place for the use of nitrous oxide as the sole anaesthetic.

#### Nitrous Oxide Analgesia

The introduction of premixed cylinders of 50:50 nitrous oxide and oxygen has revolutionised the use of nitrous oxide for analgesia. Parbrook[44] has reviewed the possible indications, which include obstetric analgesia, the relief of pain in acute trauma and for cardiac ischaemia—particularly when a high oxygen content of the inspired gases is required—and other more traditional situations such as burns and painful dressings. Parbrook[45] has also outlined four zones of analgesia, which are essentially subdivisions of Stage I of anaesthesia, and he believes that the first of these is the most useful, because in it the patient remains in full contact with his surroundings. This zone is generally achieved with concentrations of 6–25 per cent of nitrous oxide.

#### Nitrous Oxide for Dental Anaesthesia (see Chapter 43)

#### Nitrous Oxide with Supplements

Though lacking in potency nitrous oxide is the least toxic of all the various anaesthetic agents available and has come to occupy an important role in anaesthetic technique. It is often used in conjunction with oxygen as the vehicle for delivering an anaesthetic vapour such as halothane or ether to the patient. In this respect, as a weak anaesthetic agent, it reduces the amount of the inhalational agent required for the same level of anaesthesia. It is also used extensively, with supplements of thiopentone and narcotic analgesic drugs in conjunction with the muscle relaxants in major surgery.

It is frequently administered in a ratio of 66⅔:33⅓ per cent nitrous oxide and oxygen. The 33⅓ per cent oxygen in the normal patient is sufficient to maintain adequate saturation of arterial blood; the increased inspired oxygen concentration is necessary to compensate for any alteration in the ventilation/perfusion ratio caused by anaesthesia as described in Chapter 3.

**Significance of uptake.**—The high cost of some inhalational anaesthetic agents has increased the interest in using a low-flow technique. As nitrous oxide is the principal carrier gas it is important to emphasise a few points in relation to its uptake by the blood. Nitrous oxide is relatively insoluble in blood, therefore the tension rises rapidly on induction and falls equally fast at the end of anaesthesia. The brain, an organ with a rich blood supply, has a similar solubility to that of blood so the brain tension also rises fast. Equilibrium between alveolar blood and brain concentrations is achieved in a few minutes, but this must not be interpreted as meaning that a state of complete saturation has been achieved. Other tissues such as muscle and fat with a relatively low blood supply will gradually extract nitrous oxide from the blood, so that even after many hours some gas is still leaving the circulation. For example, with a patient breathing 75:25 per cent nitrous oxide/oxygen the uptake by the body (mostly muscle and fat) is about 175 ml/minute at the end of one hour, and at two hours it is still around 100 ml/minute. After about thirty hours complete saturation could theoretically be achieved but this is thwarted by the constant loss of 5–10 ml/minute of nitrous oxide through the skin.

**Low-flow technique.**—The flow rate of nitrous oxide is important for two reasons. First, if it is the sole induction agent (in combination with oxygen) and it is used in a circle system (i.e. rebreathing allowed but carbon dioxide absorbed), then a 1 litre flow of 75:25 $N_2O/O_2$ will not render the patient unconscious even after 10 minutes of breathing this mixture. This is because the volume of air in the lungs and apparatus dead-space is too great and leads to dilution of inspired nitrous oxide to levels insufficient for narcosis. On the other hand, if an 8 litre flow of the same mixture is used then unconsciousness is lost within two minutes because the apparatus is rapidly flushed out.[46] Therefore, if a low-flow nitrous oxide technique is to be used it should always start with a high flow for a few minutes before reducing to smaller flows.

Once on a low-flow technique it must not be assumed that because the inspired concentration of oxygen is 25 per cent the alveolar concentration is at this level. Assuming for a moment that the input flow is 1·0 litre per minute and the oxygen consumption is 250 ml/minute and also that "complete saturation" with nitrous oxide has been achieved, then after one breath all the oxygen in the alveoli (i.e. 25 per cent of 1 litre = 250 ml) will be taken up by the blood and the alveoli will then contain pure nitrous oxide. This will remain to dilute the next breath containing the inspired concentration of 75:25 $N_2O/O_2$. Consequently the oxygen content in the alveoli is considerably below the 25 per cent in the inspired concentration. This example emphasises the paramount importance of using an oxygen analyser in the circle system when low flows of nitrous oxide are being administered. Provided the concentration of oxygen in the inspired mixture does not fall below 25 per cent and total minute volume is adequate then this technique can safely be used, but for reasons described in Chapter 2, it is best not to use an inspired mixture of less than 33 per cent oxygen.

Finally, it is interesting to consider the question of what happens to the patient with abdominal distension or a closed pneumothorax who also breathes a mixture of $N_2O/O_2$. Nitrous oxide, though relatively insoluble in blood, is still much more soluble than nitrogen. Therefore more molecules will present themselves at the cavity site and for every one molecule of nitrogen leaving, at least ten molecules of nitrous oxide will be available. On this basis the induction of nitrous oxide and oxygen anaesthesia might be predicted to increase distension of the gas bubble.

## ETHYLENE ($C_2H_4$)

There is a wide discrepancy in the anaesthetic literature as to the origin of the hydrocarbon, ethylene. In 1779 Priestley[47] gave the credit to Ingenhousz, but the exact date of preparation remains obscure. Other authorities claim that Becher, in 1669, was the first person to prepare the gas. In 1923 Brown,[48] whilst working in the Henderson Laboratory at Toronto, published some observations on the anaesthetic properties of this gas in animals. That same year Luckhardt and Carter[49] of Chicago reported their findings on the use of this drug in human subjects. The evidence available suggests that the credit for its introduction as an anaesthetic should go to Luckhardt, since he had observed its anaesthetic and analgesic properties in animals years before.

**Preparation**

*In the laboratory:* Ethyl bromide is reacted with alcoholic potassium hydroxide to form ethylene, potassium bromide, and water.

$$\underset{\text{Ethyl bromide}}{C_2H_5Br} + \underset{\substack{\text{potassium hydroxide}\\ \text{(alcoholic)}}}{KOH} \rightarrow$$

$$\underset{\text{Ethylene}}{C_2H_4} + \underset{\substack{\text{potassium}\\ \text{bromide}}}{KBr} + \underset{\text{water}}{H_2O}$$

*Commercially:* by dehydration of ethyl alcohol with either sulphuric ($H_2SO_4$) or phosphoric ($H_2PO_4$) acid.

$$\underset{\text{Ethyl alcohol}}{C_2H_5OH} + \underset{\text{Sulphuric acid}}{H_2SO_4} \xrightarrow{150^\circ\ C+}$$

$$\underset{\text{Ethylene}}{C_2H_4} + \underset{\text{Water}}{H_2O}$$

At temperatures below 150° C ethyl ether may be formed when sulphuric acid is used.

Natural gas can be used to produce ethylene by a process of breakdown or "cracking" with heat. Propane is formed as an intermediate process.

**Physical Properties**

Ethylene is a colourless, non-irritating gas with a slightly sweetish and unpleasant odour. It is lighter than air, having a specific gravity of 0·97 (air = 1). Molecular weight is 28·03. It liquefies at 10° C under 60 atmospheres pressure and the boiling point of this liquid is—104° C. It is the least soluble in blood of the commonly used anaesthetic agents having an Ostwald blood-gas solubility coefficient of 0·140 (*cf.* nitrous oxide = 0·468). The oil/gas coefficient is 1·28 and the solubility in blood and tissue (e.g. heart and brain) is about equal, i.e. 1·0 and 1·2 respectively.[50–52] It is not altered by soda-lime but diffuses through rubber.

**Impurities**

These are either contaminants from the manufacturing process or from decomposition. Alcohol, aldehydes, ether, oxides of sulphur or phosphorus, carbon dioxide, carbon monoxide, olefins or acetylenes may be present.

**Inflammability**

Ethylene is highly combustible, when mixed with oxygen or air, and exposed to sparks or flames. Thus in air 3·1–32·0 per cent ethylene is explosive, while in oxygen the range is from 3·0–80·0 per cent. The risk of explosion is increased on account of its low density which allows it to rise in the atmosphere.

The addition of nitrous oxide (40 per cent) to a mixture of ethylene (50 per cent) and oxygen (10 per cent) does not prevent an explosion, but helium and nitrogen, when used as diluents, reduce the explosive range.

**Pharmacological Actions**

Ethylene is rapidly absorbed from the alveoli and, when given in the maximum safe concentration of about 75 per cent, it brings about unconsciousness slightly more rapidly than nitrous oxide. Ethylene in mixtures of 20–40 per cent with oxygen is said to produce analgesia, but 80–90 per cent is required for anaesthesia. The main advantages over nitrous oxide are a more rapid induction, greater muscular relaxation, and the ability to use a slightly higher percentage of oxygen. Against these must be set the disadvantage of a highly explosive agent with an unpleasant odour.

In a report from the United States of nearly 200,000 cases of ethylene-oxygen anaesthesia, there were five deaths in the operating room and three in the post-operative period attributed to this agent. There were three non-fatal explosions in this series.

Ethylene is rapidly eliminated through the lungs, although a very small percentage may be excreted through the skin. The incidence of post-operative nausea and vomiting is greater than that with nitrous oxide.

### Method of Administration

This is similar to that already described for nitrous oxide.

## CYCLOPROPANE ($C_3H_6$)

Cyclopropane, or trimethylene, was first prepared by the chemist Freund in 1882.[53] Nearly fifty years later, in 1929, Lucas and Henderson[54,55] of Toronto noted that it possessed better anaesthetic properties than propylene, in which they were primarily interested. It was introduced into clinical anaesthesia in the 1930s by Waters and Schmidt, who developed a closed-circuit apparatus for its use since it was both expensive and highly explosive.

### Preparation

Cyclopropane can be prepared from the natural gas found in the United States, or from trimethylene glycol. This substance is produced during the fermentation of molasses to obtain glycol. In the first stage trimethylene glycol is reacted with hydrobromic acid to form trimethylene dibromide, and in the second stage this latter substance is treated with zinc which brings about the production of cyclopropane and zinc debromide.

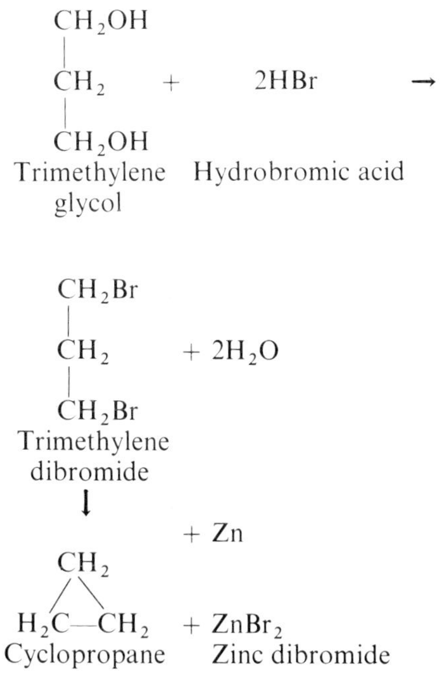


### Physical Properties

Cyclopropane is a pleasant, sweet-smelling gas, which is irritating to the respiratory tract when inhaled in concentrations over 40 per cent. The molecular weight is 42·08 and the vapour density 1·42 (air = 1), and because it is heavier than air it tends to gravitate towards the floor. When subjected to pressures of five atmospheres or more, it liquefies. It is stored as a liquid at a pressure of 75 lb per square inch in light metal cylinders which are coloured orange. Because of this relatively low pressure no reducing valves are required, the flow being regulated through a simple fine-adjustment pin. One ounce of the liquid gives 3·5 U.K. gallons or 4·29 U.S. gallons of gas. The boiling point is −33° C and freezing point −127° C. It has a solubility coefficient in blood of 0·415 (*cf.* nitrous oxide 0·468) and therefore it is relatively insoluble in blood. This accounts for the rapid induction and recovery that can be achieved with this agent. The solubility coefficient in human fat is 6·8 and the solubility in the tissues is about the same as in blood. Cyclopropane is not altered or decomposed by alkalis and so undergoes no change in the presence of soda-lime, but diffuses through rubber.

### Impurities

Propylene, allene, cyclohexane, carbon dioxide, various halides such as brom- or chlorpropane and, finally, nitrogen, are possible impurities. Concentrations of propylene above 3 per cent may prove dangerous.

### Inflammability

Cyclopropane, when mixed with air, oxygen or nitrous oxide, becomes explosive over a variable range. In air 2·4–10·4 per cent cyclopropane is explosive, in oxygen 2·5–60·0 per cent, and in nitrous oxide 3–30 per cent.

### Pharmacological Actions

*Uptake.*—Cyclopropane, when inhaled, is absorbed from the alveoli and carried in the circulation attached principally to the red cells by virtue of their high protein and lipoprotein content. Some is attached to the serum protein but as the water solubility of cyclopropane is relatively low (0·204 as opposed to 15·61 for ether) only a small portion is physically dissolved in the plasma.

*Elimination.*—Cyclopropane is excreted almost entirely by the lungs, although a small quantity is lost through the skin. Approximately 50 per cent of cyclopropane in the body is removed within ten minutes of discontinuing its administration.

*Concentration for anaesthesia.*—The amount of cyclopropane required for induction must necessarily be higher than that used for maintenance because of the dilution caused by the contents of the lungs and the anaesthetic apparatus. For a rapid induction of anaesthesia the reservoir bag of the apparatus should be filled with 50:50 cyclopropane and oxygen. The patient is asked to take five or six deep breaths of this mixture. Unconsciousness sets in within thirty seconds and this is rapidly followed by a period of apnoea in most cases. Sometimes unco-ordinated twitching movements may be observed throughout the body lasting for about half a minute.

Inhalation of a concentration of 4 per cent cyclopropane in oxygen produces analgesia, 6 per cent abolishes consciousness, 8 per cent light anaesthesia and 20–30 per cent deep anaesthesia. These figures, however, are of limited value since the concentration of cyclopropane inhaled and its effect vary widely, depending on the response of the patient and the duration of the inhalation.

**Action on the respiratory system.**—Cyclopropane given with oxygen to the unpremedicated patient produces a progressive decrease in alveolar ventilation as the depth of anaesthesia increases.[56] The depression of ventilation is due to a fall in tidal volume, for the respiratory rate increases as anaesthesia deepens. This increase in rate was at one time thought to result from a sensitisation by cyclopropane of the pulmonary stretch receptors in the respiratory tract, but there is strong evidence that anaesthetics abolish this reflex.[57] If morphine or pethidine are used as part of the premedication then there is a progressive decrease in tidal volume without any change in respiratory rate. This leads to profound hypoventilation at a much lighter level of anaesthesia than would be experienced in the unpremedicated patient. From a clinical standpoint heavy premedication with analgesics before cyclopropane anaesthesia invariably leads to apnoea long before a sufficient concentration is given for adequate muscular relaxation. Munson and his colleagues[58] suggest that at equipotent anaesthetic concentrations cyclopropane is less depressant to respiration than halothane.

In the experimental animal cyclopropane produces bronchial constriction and though such a response is not commonly seen in clinical practice, it should be remembered when considering this agent for anaesthesia for a patient liable to bronchospasm.

**Action on the circulatory system.**—*General reponse.* Much work has been done on the study of the effects of cyclopropane on the circulation.[59] In the past, most of the data concerning the effects of this anaesthetic have been based on studies involving premedication of the patient, intermittent positive-pressure ventilation, endotracheal intubation and the trauma of surgery. All of these are believed to influence the action of cyclopropane on the circulation and therefore the actions quoted below are those reported as being due solely to cyclopropane anaesthesia.

*Effect on the heart.*—Cyclopropane when administered to the heart-lung preparation causes a depression of cardiac contractility which is directly related to the concentration used. In direct contrast, in anaesthetised man cyclopropane brings about an increase in cardiac output with a rise in right ventricular stroke volume, stroke work and end-diastolic pressure. This increase in cardiac output is only seen under light anaesthesia, for the output falls to normal or below as depth is increased. The mechanism whereby cyclopropane can produce anaesthesia without causing a fall in arterial blood pressure or cardiac output has been a matter of debate for many years. Formerly these useful properties of cyclopropane were attributed to actions on the central sympathetic nervous system; Price and colleagues[293] proposed that the drug caused sympathetic excitation by direct effects on medullary vasomotor neurones; in low concentration, cyclopropane was stated to depress selectively the activity of the medullary vasomotor inhibitory neurones; while in higher concentration it directly stimulated the medullary excitatory pressor neurones.

However, these conclusions have been revised:— Sprague and Ngai[294] and Fukunaga and Epstein[60] have demonstrated that blood pressure is maintained during cyclopropane anaesthesia both by enhanced baroreceptor activity and by direct action on contractility of vascular smooth muscle. The regulatory mechanism controlling vascular smooth muscle is related to the level of cyclic 3′, 5′-adenosine monophospate (cyclic AMP). An increase in the intracellular concentration of cyclic AMP results in a decrease in tone and contractility (i.e. vasodilatation). Alternatively, a fall in the level will lead to vasoconstriction. Cyclopropane is now believed to maintain the peripheral vascular resistance and the arterial blood pressure by *decreasing* the formation of cyclic AMP.

*Effect on the heart rate.*—It is widely believed by all users of cyclopropane that this anaesthetic agent produces a slowing of the pulse rate. Yet, if the patient is not premedicated with a narcotic, the effect of cyclopropane on the heart rate is negligible. As the anaesthetic depth is increased no obvious change in pulse rate is observed. If, however, some premedication is given in the form of morphine, then a bradycardia may be observed with cyclopropane anaesthesia.[61]

In the absence of any premedicant drugs concentrations of cyclopropane as high as 14–18 vols per cent can be inspired without any observable change in pulse rate.[59] Furthermore, if a large dose of atropine (1·0–2·0 mg) is then given, a very dramatic increase in pulse rate takes place (i.e. an average increase of 70 beats/minute). This increase is far greater than that produced by the same dose of atropine without cyclopropane anaesthesia. The inference is made, therefore, that cyclopropane may increase vagal activity and this effects cardiac impulse generation, conduction and improved atrial contractility. At the time it increases vagal activity it also stimulates sympathetic activity within the heart. In the unpremedicated patient these two forces balance each other out and there is little change of pulse rate. When atropine is given not only is vagal activity blocked but sympathetic activity is allowed to proceed unheeded. Hence the dramatic tachycardia. However, atropine administration during cyclopropane anaesthesia leads to a high incidence of dysrhythmias, and might lead to ventricular fibrillation.[62]

*Dysrhythmias.*—An increase in the alveolar carbon dioxide tension precipitated the onset of dysrhythmias in every one of a series of twenty-eight patients anaesthetised with cyclopropane.[63] It is known that both hypercapnia and cyclopropane increase the rate of noradrenaline liberation from sympathetic nerves terminating in the myocardium. Catecholamines liberated from other areas of the body are relatively ineffective. It would appear, therefore, that the combination of a raised carbon dioxide tension of the blood and cyclopropane lead to an excessive noradrenaline excretion in the myocardium. Nevertheless, Price and colleagues[64] demonstrated that cyclopropane itself has a direct effect on the myocardium. Thus, during sympathetic nerve stimulation there is an increased chronotropic response and this is not directly related to the amount of transmitter substance released. Clinically, therefore dysrhythmias under cyclopropane anaesthesia can largely be prevented if particular attention is paid to the prevention of hypoventilation. In fact Price and his colleagues[65] concluded that "in persons anaesthetised with cyclopropane the most reliable circulatory indication of hypercarbia was the presence of cardiac dysrhythmias."

"*Cyclopropane shock.*"—This term became popular during the era of cyclopropane to explain the sudden cardiovascular collapse that was sometimes observed at the end of a long anaesthetic under deep cyclopropane. At first it was believed to be solely due to the accumulation of carbon dioxide brought about by the respiratory depression of the deep cyclopropane. Now it would seem that it is a combination of both cyclopropane and carbon dioxide causing a period of intense sympathetic nervous activity. The hypotension and collapse that occurs at the end of the anaesthesia is believed to be due to the sudden withdrawal of this activity.

**Action on various organs.**—*The kidney.* Cyclopropane produces a reduction of renal blood flow in direct proportion to the concentration. Thus under light anaesthetic there is about a 30 per cent fall in renal blood flow, whereas under deep anaesthesia this may fall to as low as 80 per cent of normal. This fall in renal blood flow with increasing concentrations of cyclopropane signifies that the agent produces a constriction of the renal vessels.[66] Deutsch and his co-workers,[67] studying normal unpremedicated human subjects, found that cyclopropane anaesthesia produced a dramatic reduction in both glomerular filtration and renal plasma flow (about 40 per cent). They concluded that their findings could be explained on the basis of increased sympathetic nervous system activity during cyclopropane anaesthesia. At the same time they observed that cyclopropane anaesthesia was associated with an antidiuresis which was probably brought about by increased production of antidiuretic hormone (ADH), and they also noted an increase in plasma renin levels. The latter finding is particularly interesting as the renin-angiotensin system has been considered to be responsible for the autoregulation of renal blood flow, so it is theoretically possible that cyclopropane may act on the renal blood flow through the mechanism of this system.

*The liver.*—Cyclopropane reduces liver blood flow in direct relation with the depth of anaesthesia.[68] This finding has been corroborated by the work of Price and his colleagues[69] who found that cyclopropane reduced splanchnic blood flow to both the gut and the liver. They concluded that this effect was brought about not only by increased sympathetic activity in the vasoconstrictor fibres to the liver and intestine but also by sensitisation of the vascular smooth muscle to the action of noradrenaline.

*The uterus.*—Cyclopropane depresses the contractions of the gravid uterus again in direct relation to the concentration used. It passes quickly through the placental barrier and equilibrium between maternal and fetal blood is rapidly established. For this reason high concentrations of cyclopropane are rarely used for Caesarean section or forceps delivery in obstetrical anaesthesia, though if cyclopropane is used as an induction agent only, the respiratory depression of the fetus is eliminated within a few minutes of the withdrawal of the agent.

*The lungs.*—Cyclopropane increases central venous pressure. This may be due to stimulating activity but it results in the right heart and great veins becoming firmer with increased tone. Thus, when the lungs are inflated with positive pressure the veins (and indirectly the cardiac output) are less susceptible to this compression. This may explain why the blood pressure does not usually fall under cyclopropane anaesthesia even in the seriously ill patient. Nevertheless, hypotension and diminished cardiac output do sometimes occur on induction with cyclopropane anaesthesia, particularly if a narcotic agent has been used. As time progresses this depression is usually offset and the blood pressure returns to normal, suggesting that some homeostatic mechanism is at work. This may be due to stimulation of baroreceptor reflex activity. Price and Widdicombe[70] have demonstrated in dogs and cats that cyclopropane anaesthesia acts by a direct stimulant effect on the baroreceptors in the carotid sinus. Another possible explanation, supported by some evidence in animal experiments, is that cyclopropane diminishes the sensitivity of the medullary vasomotor centre to afferent inhibitory impulses, causing an increase in the centre's efferent discharge and consequent vasoconstriction.

*Central nervous system.*—Price and his colleagues,[71] working with cats, have confirmed that cyclopropane increases sympathetic nervous activity and they conclude that this effect is brought about by a selective depression of certain neurones in the medulla oblongata. Thus, cyclopropane inhibited the "depressor" neurones whilst stimulating the "pressor" ones, although, as was noted above, an alternative explanation has been made for the haemodynamic effects of cyclopropane.[60] In common with other inhalational anaesthetic agents cyclopropane reduces cerebral oxygen consumption by 10–20 per cent. It has no effect on generation or utilisation of high energy compounds in the brain; no changes in the levels of ATP, creatine phosphate, NADH or NAD were found in the brains of animals anaesthetised with any popular volatile agent including cyclopropane.[72]

**Cyclopropane and adrenaline.**—Price and his co-workers[63] studied the different blood levels of adrenaline required to produce ventricular dysrhythmias with either a simple infusion technique or that produced by a raised carbon dioxide level of the blood. They found that hypercapnia was far more effective in producing dysrhythmias than adrenaline infusion. In fact, the catecholamine level under hypercapnia was only one-tenth as high as in the infusion series yet the incidence of dysrhythmias was high, suggesting that endogenous adrenaline is far more effective than the exogenous material.

Matteo and his associates,[73] however, found that the subcutaneous injection of a 1:60,000 solution of adrenaline during cyclopropane anaesthesia with adequate ventilation (i.e. normal $CO_2$ level) led to a 30 per cent incidence of ventricular dysrhythmias. From data available it would seem that the use of a subcutaneous infiltration with even a weak solution of adrenaline (i.e. 1:200,000) is contra-indicated during cyclopropane anaesthesia in man.

### Clinical Use

Owing to the risk of an explosion, the popularity of cyclopropane as an anaesthetic has gradually faded with the introduction of newer and non-inflammable anaesthetics. Cyclopropane may, however, be the agent of choice for the induction of anaesthesia when a rapid loss of consciousness is necessary, coupled with a high concentration of oxygen and maintenance of the systemic blood pressure. This type of induction is most commonly required in obstetric practice, but is also useful for those patients in whom any cardiovascular depression is dangerous. In such circumstances cyclopropane is best administered as a 50:50 mixture with oxygen.[19] The patient breathes from a six-litre bag filled with the mixture. Five to six breaths are sufficient to produce loss of consciousness. Some motor excitement (tonic or clonic contractions) may be observed at this point, and its onset is usually associated with a momentary period of breath-holding which lasts for a few seconds.

Its rapid onset of action has also made it a popular induction agent in paediatric anaesthesia.

### Metabolism of Cyclopropane

Cyclopropane does not appear to undergo biotransformation; Halsey and colleagues,[74] were unable to demonstrate that livers of miniature swines could metabolise cyclopropane, in contradistinction to halothane and methoxyflurane where considerable metabolism occurred. Absence of metabolism of cyclopropane was also noted by Sawyer and colleagues[75] at an inspired concentration of 0·9 vol per cent.

### Summary

Cyclopropane anaesthesia is particularly suitable as an anaesthetic agent for the seriously-ill patient because it is accompanied by a high oxygen concentration and a rise of cardiac output (under light anaesthesia only), peripheral vasoconstriction, and virtually no change in heart rate. The result is that the blood pressure is well maintained even when intermittent positive-pressure respiration is introduced. The latter procedure is often necessary because cyclopropane diminishes tidal volume. Most of the beneficial effects of cyclopropane on the myocardium are abolished if a narcotic is given as part of the premedication. Barbiturates, phenothiazine derivatives and atropine do not have this adverse effect. Morphine and pethidine also reduce ventilation in their own right so that when combined with cyclopropane there is a serious risk of hypoventilation; both the increased carbon dioxide level of the blood and cyclopropane combine to raise the amount of noradrenaline excreted in the myocardium so that the risk of dysrhythmias is increased. The presence of these dysrhythmias under cyclopropane anaesthesia should suggest inadequate ventilation or too deep anaesthesia; in either case it has often been observed that the inhalation of a low concentration of ether vapour will bring about a return of normal rhythm.

Disease, trauma and narcotic agents appear to influence both the sympathetic and the parasympathetic responses to cyclopropane. Atropine tends to remove the effect of increased vagal stimulation whereas ganglion-blocking drugs will remove the sympathetic response and may cause cyclopropane to produce a profound hypotension through direct myocardial depression.

## DIETHYL ETHER $(C_2H_5)_2O$

Ether was first described by Valerius Cordus in 1540. In 1841, Crawford Long used ether in his own home in Jefferson, Georgia, and, in the following year, he used it during three surgical operations. Unfortunately these events were not published until after William Morton's famous demonstration of the potentialities of ether as an anaesthetic at the Massachusetts General Hospital in 1846.[76] After this, ether became widely publicised and the news spread to London, where Drs. Boott and Squire soon used it on surgical cases at University College Hospital.

**Preparation.**—Dehydration of alcohol by sulphuric acid at a temperature below 140° C.

$$\underset{\text{Ethyl alcohol}}{C_2H_5OH} + \underset{\text{Sulphuric acid}}{H_2SO_4} \rightarrow C_2H_5HSO_4 + H_2O$$

$$C_2H_5HSO_4 + \underset{\text{Ethyl alcohol}}{C_2H_5OH} \rightarrow H_2SO_4 + \underset{\text{Diethyl ether}}{C_2H_5OC_2H_5}$$

**Physical properties.**—Ether is a colourless, volatile liquid (boiling point 36·5° C) with a characteristic pungent smell. At room temperature (20° C) it has a vapour pressure of approximately 425 mm Hg (57 kPa).

*Significance of vapour pressure.*—A knowledge of the vapour pressure of a volatile anaesthetic agent enables the anaesthetist quickly to calculate the inspired concentration being delivered to the patient by a "bubble-through" type of vaporiser e.g. copper kettle or "Vernitrol". It is of very little value if only a portion of the stream of gases are exposed to the liquid as in a "blow-over" type of vaporiser e.g. Boyle's bottle. Even when the latter type of vaporiser is converted to "bubbling" then the constantly changing temperature of the liquid makes a calculation difficult unless this temperature is known.

The principle of the copper kettle (Fig.1) is that the vaporiser is constructed of a highly conductive metal and when attached directly to an anaesthetic table-top of similar material it has a large heat reservoir available which will prevent the temperature in the vaporiser from falling. A known flow of oxygen is then bubbled through the liquid anaesthetic agent at room temperature.

Taking ether as an example, at a room temperature of 20° C the vapour pressure is 425 mm Hg (57 kPa). With flow rates of up to 500 ml of oxygen per minute passed through this instrument the temperature does not alter appreciably. Above this figure it falls in proportion to the flow rate. However, if the temperature of the liquid is known then the concentration of the ether vapour emitted can still be accurately predicted. For example, at a room temperature of 20° C the vapour pressure is 425 mm Hg (57 kPa) (Fig. 2) and the ether concentration is 52 vols per cent; if the temperature of the liquid dropped to −10° C (Fig.2) the same inflow would only meet ether at a vapour pressure of 120 mm Hg (16 kPa) giving a concentration of ether vapour of about 14 vols per cent.

The important part played by a changing temperature in vaporisation is well illustrated by studying the glass Boyle's bottle type of vaporiser during ether anaesthesia. When a liquid becomes a vapour, heat is required for

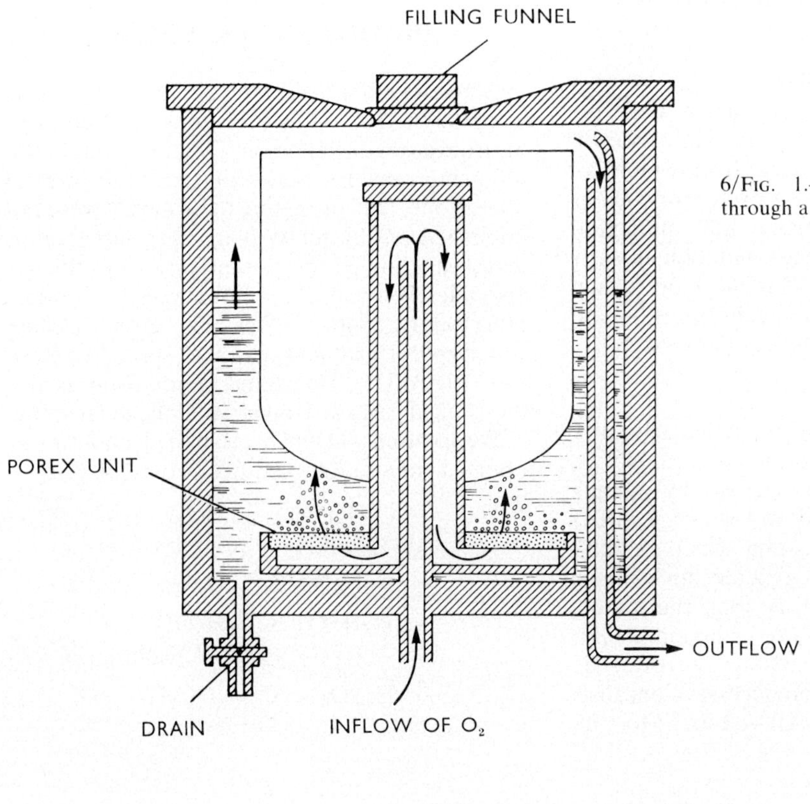


6/Fig. 1.—Diagram of flow of gases through a copper kettle. (After Morris.[77])

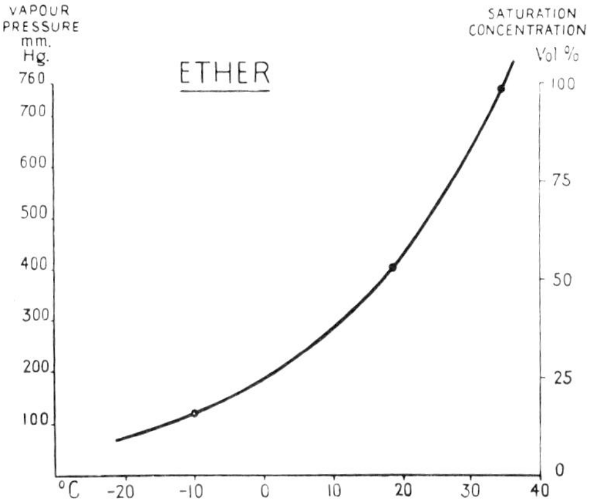


6/Fig. 2.—Influence of vapour pressure and temperature on ether concentration. (Courtesy of Sir Robert Macintosh, Professor W. W. Mushin and Dr. H. G. Epstein, published by Blackwell Scientific Publications.[296])

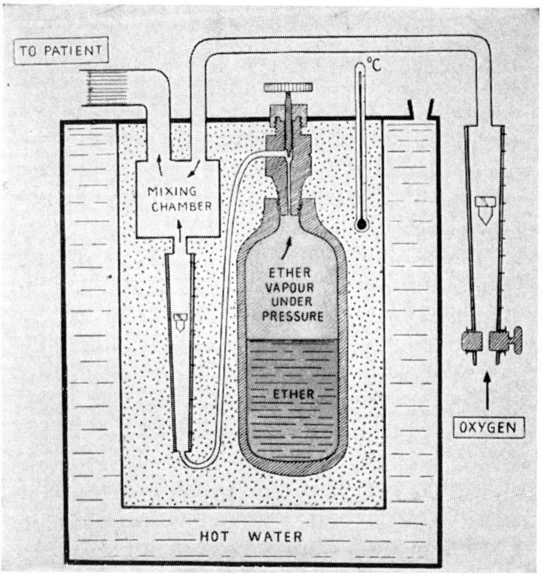


6/Fig. 3.—Oxford Vaporiser Mark II. (Courtesy of Sir Robert Macintosh, Professor W. W. Mushin and Dr. H. G. Epstein, published by Blackwell Scientific Publications.[296])

the process so the liquid cools (i.e. latent heat of vaporisation). A point is soon reached when the liquid is so cool that it freezes the moisture on the outside of the glass vaporiser and frost appears. This can be prevented by placing a jacket of warm water around the glass bottle. Alternatively, the ether can be kept constantly above its boiling point (36·5), so that it is under pressure trying to escape. This principle is used in the construction of the Oxford Vaporiser Mark II where the ether is surrounded by chemical crystals with a melting point above that of ether. Once these crystals have been melted by warm water then ether vapour will issue spontaneously (Fig. 3).

If a "bubble-through" vaporiser (copper kettle) is used at a room temperature of 20° C then a flow of 500 ml of oxygen through this instrument will give an output of 1000 ml of 50 per cent ether vapour. Except for the total volume involved it is easier to think of this as 500 ml of pure ether vapour. When this total is added to 4 litres of nitrous oxide and oxygen the patient will then receive a 10 per cent ether concentration, viz.

| | |
|---|---|
| 4 litres of $N_2O/O_2$ + 1 litre of 50 per cent ether vapour | 5 litres total gas flow including 500 ml of ether vapour |

= 5 litres of 10 per cent ether vapour in nitrous oxide/oxygen

**Inflammability.**—Ether is a highly inflammable liquid which ignites at a temperature of 154° C (the presence of peroxides may lower the ignition point to 100° C). Provided sufficient oxygen is present, low concentrations of ether burn with a clear blue flame, whereas high concentrations explode. In air, the range of inflammability of ether is 1·9–48·0 per cent, but with the addition of more oxygen this is increased to 2·0–82·0 per cent. Since ether vapour is two-and-a-half times heavier than air, the vapour collects like an invisible blanket over the floor. A spark from an electric motor or a switch can ignite this, causing a characteristic "cold blue" flame to spread slowly across the floor. In daylight this flame may be invisible. The chief danger is that it may reach a richer source of oxygen than the air, thus causing an explosion of devastating consequences. In practice, explosions with ether are extremely rare and can be prevented altogether by obvious and sensible precautions. The zone of flammability is confined to a relatively small area of about 25 cm around the exhalatory valve; and if diathermy is kept outside this area, and an efficient exhaust gas scavenging system is used, there should be little risk of explosion.

**Stability.**—The two important impurities

caused by decomposition of ether are acetic aldehyde and ether peroxide. The former can be detected by Nessler's solution (complex mercuric iodide solution), and the latter by potassium iodide solution—both of which are turned yellow. Decomposition is favoured by air, light and heat but prevented by copper and hydroquinone. Ether should, therefore, be kept in sealed, dark bottles in a cool cupboard.

Other impurities are alcohol, sulphuric acid, sulphur dioxide, mercaptans, and ethyl esters.

Some doubt has been expressed about the toxicity of these impurities of ether in man. An investigation in animals revealed that aldehyde (0·5 per cent) was without significant effect, whereas mercaptans (1·0 per cent) and peroxide (0·5 per cent) could cause gastric irritation but had no other obvious deleterious action. During anaesthesia the presence of mercaptans in the ether should be suspected if the patient's expirations have a peculiar "fishy" odour; in such cases tachycardia and an unexplained hypotension may also occur.

### Pharmacological Actions

*Uptake and distribution.*—Ether has a blood/gas solubility coefficient of 12·1.[78] This signifies that blood has a tremendous capacity for absorbing ether so that it is constantly being removed from the alveoli. Consequently it takes a long time for the alveolar tension to rise to the same height as the inspired tension. As alveolar tension is virtually synonymous with brain tension then induction of anaesthesia will be slow and equally recovery will be affected in the reverse manner. This combined with the fact that it is irritant to the respiratory tract means that it will take 15–25 minutes to achieve deep anaesthesia.

The solubility of ether in the various tissues is similar to that of blood (Table 2).

6/Table 2
The Tissue/Blood Coefficient for Ether

1·14 in Brain tissue
1·2 in Lung tissue
3·3 in Fat tissue
(Eger *et al.*, 1963[78])

*Significance of oil/gas solubility.*—The value for ether is 65; this signifies a relatively low lipid solubility when compared with other agents, e.g. 224 for halothane and 960 for trichloroethylene. The oil/gas solubility coefficient is another way of indicating anaesthetic potency. For example, to produce the 1st plane of surgical anaesthesia with ether an alveolar concentration of 2·5 vols per cent is required, whereas with trichloroethylene only 0·17 vols per cent is needed.

*Estimation of ether concentration.*—In the past the concentration of ether in the blood was measured by complex chemical analysis of the level in blood.[79] Newer methods such as gas chromatography or infra-red analysis are now available and these indicate the alveolar concentration of ether in vols per cent (Table 3).

*Excretion.*—Only a small quantity of ether undergoes biodegradation. The majority (85–90 per cent) is excreted unchanged through the lungs and the remainder is metabolised or eliminated via the skin, body secretions and urine.

**Action on the respiratory system.**—Ether, in

6/Table 3
Approximate Blood and Alveolar Levels of Ether in Relation to Depth of Anaesthesia

| | *Blood level in mg per cent* | *Alveolar concentration in vols per cent* |
|---|---|---|
| Stage I | 10–40 | 0·284–1·14 |
| Stage II | 40–80 | 1·14–2·27 |
| Stage III, Plane I | 80–110 | 2·27–3·12 |
| Plane II | 110–120 | 3·12–3·41 |
| Plane III | 120–130 | 3·41–3·69 |
| Plane IV | 130–140 | 3·69–3·98 |
| Stage IV | 140–180 | 3·98–5·11 |

anaesthetic concentrations, is an irritant to the mucosa of the respiratory tract. It increases the amount of bronchial secretions but at the same time it also increases the internal diameter of the bronchi and bronchioles. For this reason, it is an extremely useful anaesthetic agent for patients with asthma or bronchiolar spasm. Ether does not affect the action of surfactant in reducing surface tension in the alveoli.[80]

Ether is believed to stimulate the nerve endings in the bronchial tree and thus reflexly excite the respiratory centre. It may also sensitise the baroreceptors. The ultimate effect is to increase the *rate* of respiration. At a later stage, as the paralysant action of ether manifests itself in deep anaesthesia, the minute volume steadily declines until apnoea finally supervenes. Larson and his colleagues[81] have shown that in healthy unpremedicated patients, the resting preinduction arterial carbon dioxide tension does not rise until deep levels of ether anaesthesia (alveolar ether concentrations of 6 per cent) are reached. They doubt the need for controlled or assisted ventilation to maintain a satisfactory arterial carbon dioxide tension during anaesthesia.

**Action on the cardiovascular system.**—There is still a wide margin of discrepancy in the reported findings of the action of ether on the cardiovascular system in man. This is because countless studies have been made but each has varied the technique or the quantity or quality of premedicant and other drugs used. As most patients undergoing ether anaesthesia require premedication, it has been argued that studies made on patients without premedication are only academic, yet it is only through such studies that it is possible to determine the precise effect of ether anaesthesia in man.

If ether vapour is added to the circulation in a heart-lung preparation there is a dramatic depression of myocardial activity. Brewster and his colleagues[82] working with adrenalectomised dogs have convincingly shown that ether can depress the myocardium. Ether produces increased sympathetic nervous activity, mainly in the form of liberation of noradrenaline. The plasma level of noradrenaline rises with increasing depth of ether anaesthesia[83] (Fig. 4).

Ether anaesthesia produces remarkably small alterations in blood pressure and pulse rate. It rarely leads to cardiac irregularities and does not sensitise the myocardium (like cyclopropane) to the action of noradrenaline and adrenaline. In fact, in the past, small concentrations of ether were often given to stop irregularities produced by cyclopropane anaesthesia. The evidence of tachycardia when ether is given without atropine premedication is taken as an indication of the parasympathetic blocking action of ether. To summarise, ether appears to increase sympathetic nervous activity and block parasympathetic activity in normal man.[59] The increase in noradrenaline liberation under ether anaesthesia partially offsets the direct myocardial depressant action of ether seen in the isolated heart preparation. Deep ether anaesthesia, therefore, should be used with caution in those patients with reduced catecholamine secretion or in the presence of ganglion blockade. β-blocking agents, such as propranolol, may be dangerous during ether anaesthesia.[84]

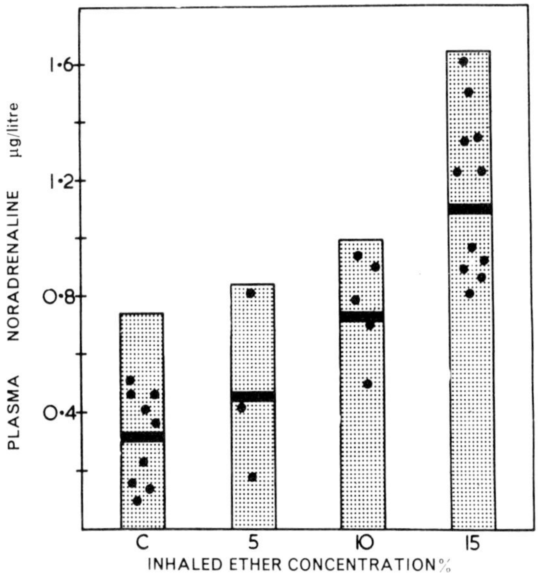


6/Fig. 4.—Plasma noradrenaline levels in relation to increasing concentration of inhaled ether. The horizontal black lines indicate mean values. (Courtesy of Dr. G. W. Black, Dr. L. McArdle, Dr. H. McCullough and Dr. V. K. N. Unni and the Editor of *Anaesthesia*[83]).

**Action on the peripheral circulation.**—McArdle and his colleagues[85] have measured the effects on forearm blood flow and conclude that increasing the concentration leads to a reduction in flow. There is no change in flow with inspired concentrations of 5 per cent ether, a slight fall with 10 per cent and a significant reduction with 15 per cent. When the sympathetic nerve supply to one forearm is blocked by local analgesia, the reduction in blood flow to that side still equals the fall on the unblocked side as increasing concentrations of ether are inspired, thus suggesting that the vasoconstriction is not nervously mediated. Black and associates[83] suggest that there is a close relationship between the increase in vascular resistance and a rising plasma noradrenaline concentration.

**Action on skeletal muscle.**—Ether causes skeletal muscle relaxation by depressing the central nervous system,[86] and by affecting the nerve, the motor end-plate and the muscle itself. Concentrations used in clinical practice cause a block at the motor end-plate,[87] and there is some evidence that the post-junctional membrane is affected.[88] The mode of action is probably similar (but not identical) to that of tubocurarine,[89] so that when these two drugs are used in the same patient an additive effect results from their synergism. The effect of ether at the motor end-plate can be reversed by neostigmine.[90]

**Action on other organs.**—Ether provokes sickness in two ways. First, it is absorbed in saliva and passed to the stomach where it irritates the mucosa. Secondly, it stimulates the vomiting centre in the medulla.

The smooth muscle of the intestines is depressed by ether in direct relation to the concentration of the anaesthetic in the blood.

Prolonged administration of ether, particularly in the presence of hypoxia, may lead to damage of liver cells. Since ether stimulates the autonomic nervous system and leads to the release of adrenaline, glycogen is mobilised from both the liver and muscle tissue and a marked rise in blood sugar follows.

Renal blood flow is depressed, and albuminuria from tubular irritation, occurs in a proportion of patients.

Ether reduces the tone of the gravid uterus even in slight concentrations. High concentrations lead to complete relaxation. It rapidly passes from the maternal placental circulation into that of the fetus, so that equilibrium between the two is soon achieved.

### Metabolism and Toxicity of Ether

The American National Halothane study[91] found that ether was associated with the lowest death rate and incidence of liver damage. About 4 per cent of ether is metabolised in the liver to acetaldehyde and ethanol. Transient alterations in liver function occur as with most inhalation agents, but the most marked effect is endogenous catecholamine-induced glycolysis. Ether is, like phenobarbitone, a powerful inducer of hepatic microsomal enzymes, and may after prolonged inhalation result in increased rate of metabolism of other drugs. There is no evidence of serious toxic effects on other organs with ether.

### Clinical Use

The objective in the administration of any anaesthetic is not only to produce unconsciousness but also to suppress the reflex activity of the patient to just a sufficient degree to enable the surgeon to perform a particular operation. Modern anaesthetic techniques often go far beyond this maxim, but ether still remains the safest and most effective means of gradually producing reflex suppression.

In the conscious state, if the skin of a patient's hand is incised with a knife, the hand is rapidly withdrawn unless the patient deliberately brings other muscles into force which overcome this withdrawal reflex. The moment unconsciousness is produced, the central controlling force is removed, and the patient responds to stimuli in a reflex manner. Now, if the skin is cut, not only is the limb withdrawn but, owing to "facilitation" produced by the reflex, there is a spread to many other pathways, so that the larynx may close, the abdominal muscles may contract, and the other limbs move across in an unco-ordinated effort to ward off the stimulus. As the depth of anaesthesia increases so, one by one, the reflex pathways become blocked, until finally all are suppressed. The exact position in which the reflex arc is broken differs with the various anaesthetic agents. Ether not only has a direct suppressant action on the central nervous system but also raises the excitation threshold of the motor end-plate, in a similar manner to tubocurarine chloride, thus producing a neuromuscular block.

Even in minimal concentrations ether irritates the bronchial tree, stimulating the vagal afferent fibres leading to an increase in depth and rate of respiration together with an outpouring of mucous secretions. The latter reflex is successfully depressed by adequate doses of atropine or hyoscine. As the depth of anaesthesia increases the respiratory pattern changes, more reflexes become suppressed, and characteristic changes in the size of the pupil can be seen. This slow progression of change has made it possible to divide up the various alterations in reflex activity into stages of ether anaesthesia. First described by Guedel[92] after an exhaustive study of open ether anaesthetics, these stages remain today amongst the basic requirements for the student of anaesthesia. They are given in Table 4.

The pre-operative use of even small doses of the opiates prevents the correct interpretation of the pupil signs. The changes are best seen in children premedicated with barbiturates. During rapid lightening of ether anaesthesia the changes in pupillary diameter (together with all the other reflexes) tend to lag behind the more accurate respiratory-pattern changes. Sometimes even the respiratory patterns of deep anaesthesia may persist until the patient is practically awake.

**Guedel's classification refashioned.**—Many authors have attempted to refashion Guedel's classification to embrace the changes seen with such anaesthetic drugs as halothane or the muscle relaxants. With ether, a relatively slow process of events underlines the stages and enhances the intrinsic safety of the drug. Newer agents do not respect such an orderly sequence; amongst others, the capacity of the intravenous thiobarbiturates to depress respiration in light anaesthesia, and of muscle relaxants to simulate most of the signs of anaesthesia yet produce no

6/TABLE 4
THE STAGES AND SIGNS OF ETHER ANAESTHESIA

| | *Respiration* | | | *Pupils* | | *Reflex Depression* |
|---|---|---|---|---|---|---|
| | *Rhythm* | *Volume* | *Pattern* | *Size* | *Position* | |
| *Stage I* (Analgesia)<br>Analgesia to loss of consciousness | Irregular | Small | 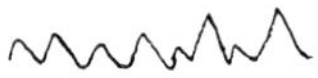 | Small | Divergent | Nil |
| *Stage II* (Excitement)<br>Loss of consciousness to rhythmical respiration | Irregular | Large | 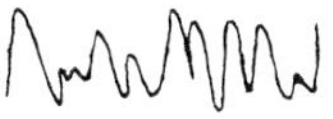 | Large | Divergent | Eyelash<br>Eyelid |
| *Stage III* (Surgicalanaesthesia)<br>*Plane I*<br>Rhythmical respiration to cessation of eye movement | Regular | Large | 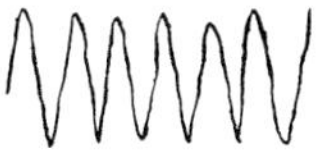 | Small | Divergent | Skin<br>Vomiting<br>Conjunctival<br>Pharyngeal<br>Stretch from limb muscles |
| *Plane II*<br>Cessation of eye movement to start of respiratory muscle paresis (excl. diaphragm) | Regular | Medium | * 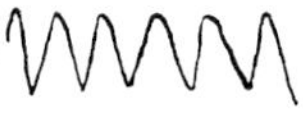 | ½ dilated | Fixed centrally | Corneal |
| *Plane III*<br>Respiratory muscle paresis to paralysis | Regular<br>Pause after expiration | Small | 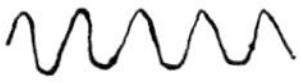 | ¾ dilated | Fixed centrally | Laryngeal<br>Peritoneal |
| *Plane IV*<br>Diaphragmatic paresis to paralysis | Jerky<br>Irregular<br>Quick inspiration<br>Prolonged expiration, i.e. "see-saw" | Small | 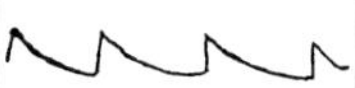 | Fully dilated | Fixed centrally | Anal sphincter<br>Carinal |
| *Stage IV*<br>Apnoea | | | | | | |

* If the respiration rate is slow, an expiratory pause may be seen in Plane II.

anaesthesia at all, are well known. The idea of anaesthetic depth is outmoded when combinations of drugs are used, but the need for a guide to the assessment of anaesthesia remains. Mushin[93] and Laycock[94] have restated the orthodox stages in modern terms. Analgesia, characterised by consciousness and disorientation, is an essential feature of the first stage, and merges into the second, when unconsciousness supervenes, often with marked reflex activity. Both these stages may be lost, however, when the induction of anaesthesia is rapid. It is in the third stage that surgery is performed when the reflexes are depressed. The fourth stage represents overdosage.

Each or all of these stages of general anaesthesia can usually be assessed from the specific and objective signs that surgical stimuli produce. Thus modern polypharmacy in anaesthesia is devised to select a combination of drugs, each with a more or less distinct action, and to avoid the unnecessary depression of other parts of the body that must occur occasionally when a single agent is used. Gray[95] has summarised this type of technique in the single word "control". Others have termed it "balanced anaesthesia", but this idea of utilising more than one agent to offset the disadvantages of a single one, was suggested long before anaesthesia reached its present state[96].

The anaesthetist chooses a drug or mixture of drugs that best fits the anticipated needs of the operation, and as Laycock[94] has written, reflexes are his essential guides in this matter. He must understand them, look out for them, nurse them, leave them alone, depress or abolish them.

### Methods of Administration

A patient can be anaesthetised with ether by any one of the three standard methods, namely open, semi-closed and closed with carbon dioxide absorption.

For an open technique the Schimmelbusch mask is commonly used. This consists of a wire frame covered with a layer or two of gauze or a single layer of lint. The ether is dropped on to it from a suitable bottle, the aim being to supply the maximum concentration that the patient will tolerate without coughing or breath-holding. The mask should be kept moist over its whole surface since this will provide the maximum vapour concentration, bearing in mind that the liquid vaporises very rapidly. It is helpful during open ether administration to allow a slow trickle of oxygen under the margin of the mask, and during the induction of anaesthesia to add a little carbon dioxide to increase the depth of respiration. An alternative to the addition of carbon dioxide is to allow some of this gas to accumulate from the patient's exhalations by covering the mask with gamgee gauze so that the system becomes semi-open. Such an arrangement also helps to contain the ether vapour.

The chief disadvantage of these techniques is the unpleasant induction, but this can be mitigated by the use of ethyl chloride prior to ether. Very high vapour concentrations are seldom achieved—indeed the concentration may be insufficient for some adults. Under experimental conditions, using an external method of warming, concentrations of 40 per cent or more have been obtained, but in clinical practice the rapid evaporation of ether results in a corresponding fall in temperature and therefore in the volume concentration of the inspired vapour.

In the semi-closed method the ether is vaporised in a glass container by a flow of anaesthetic gases and oxygen. One of the factors adding to the safety of ether as an anaesthetic agent, when used in this way, is that as vaporisation increases, so the temperature of the liquid ether falls which in turn slows the rate of vaporisation. If, therefore, the control is set to deliver a strong concentration of ether vapour, the depth of anaesthesia increases, but after a time, with the control still in the same position, there is a reduction in the vapour concentration. It is inadvisable to warm the outside of the glass container unless a strong concentration is required during the induction of anaesthesia. Even then this practice is generally considered too dangerous and it is safer to surround the bottle with cold water to prevent icing.

The vaporisation of ether in a closed system depends upon the particular type of apparatus. When it is to and fro', vaporisation is exactly as in a semi-closed system, but owing to the small basal flow of gases, only slight concentrations of ether can be obtained. In a circular system the whole volume of ventilation can be passed through an ether bottle, so that high concentrations of ether can be relatively quickly built up. Moreover, vaporisation is assisted both by heat from the patient and by heat produced in the canister.

**The E.M.O. inhaler.**—This "draw-over" inhaler was designed by Epstein and Macintosh[97] to deliver a required concentration of anaesthetic vapour irrespective of variations in the temperature of the liquid anaesthetic throughout the range likely to be met in clinical practice. The apparatus incorporates a water bath which surrounds the vaporising chamber and, by acting as a heat buffer, prevents sudden, marked changes in the temperature of the liquid anaesthetic. A bellows type thermostat automatically ensures that a constant vapour concentration of anaesthetic leaves the inhaler. The E.M.O. inhaler must be calibrated to suit the particular volatile anaesthetic used in it.

**Convulsions occurring during ether anaesthesia** (see Chapter 29).

## DIVINYL ETHER $(C_2H_3)_2O$

In 1887 Semmler described a substance which he believed to be divinyl ether. The anaesthetic properties of divinyl ether were first described by Leake and Chen in 1930,[98] and three years later Gelfan and Bell[99] published the first report on its use in clinical anaesthesia.

**Preparation.**—This is a complicated and costly process. Ether is first chlorinated to prepare $\beta\beta$-dichlor-ether which is then fused with molten potassium hydroxide to produce divinyl ether, potassium chloride and water.

$$(C_2H_4Cl)_2O + 2KOH \rightarrow$$
$\beta\beta$-dichlor-ether + Potassium hydroxide →

$$(C_2H_3)_2O + 2KCl + 2H_2O$$
Divinyl ether + Potassium chloride + Water

**Physical properties.**—Divinyl ether is a colourless, non-irritating liquid with a sweet odour. The molecular weight is 70, the specific gravity of the liquid is 0·77 and of the vapour 2·2 (air = 1). The boiling point is 28·3° C. Divinyl ether is believed to be less soluble in water than ethyl ether, but the oil/water solubility ratio is a matter of disagreement. Adriani[100] claims it is 41·3, whereas Kochmann[101] states it is similar to that of diethyl ether, or 3·2. The very rapid recovery from anaesthesia with this agent favours Adriani's figure.

**Stability.**—Divinyl ether has a relatively low stability, which is made worse by acids and improved by alkalis. When it is chemically pure it is so volatile that moisture tends to freeze on the anaesthetic face-piece. For this reason 3·5 per cent absolute alcohol is added to diminish volatility. A non-volatile organic base—phenyl-alpha-naphthylamine—in a concentration of 0·01 per cent is also added to improve the stability. The commercial product is known as "Vinesthene" in the United Kingdom. The liquid decomposes on exposure to air, light and heat to form formaldehyde, acetaldehyde, formic and acetic acid. It is, therefore, best kept in dark, well-stoppered bottles in a cool place. The manufacturers do not recommend use two years after production and it is inadvisable to use the contents of a bottle that has been opened for more than two weeks. It is not affected by soda-lime even when the heat in the canister reaches temperatures as high as 70° C.

**Inflammability.**—Divinyl ether is explosive when mixed with air in concentrations between 1·7 and 27·0 per cent, and with oxygen between 1·8 and 85·0 per cent.

### Pharmacological Actions

Divinyl ether is absorbed and eliminated almost entirely through the lungs, but a small percentage is excreted through the skin. A vapour, with a concentration of 4 per cent, will give a light plane of anaesthesia with a blood concentration of 20–30 mg per cent, whereas a vapour with 10 per cent divinyl ether may lead to a blood level of 70 mg per cent and respiratory arrest. Induction is more rapid and pleasant than with ether owing to the increased potency and the absence of irritation of the bronchial tree. Recovery is also more rapid than after ether.

**Action on the cardiovascular system.**—Divinyl ether has similar effects to diethyl ether. The pacemaker may be displaced, leading to auricular extrasystoles, but the adrenergic stimulation leads to improvement in myocardial contraction.

**Action on the respiratory system.**—Bronchial dilatation is produced, and in light anaesthesia respiration is increased in rate. An overdose leads to failure of the respiratory centre before the heart finally stops beating.

**Action on the alimentary system.**—Divinyl ether can cause toxic damage to the liver if used in high concentrations for prolonged periods. Central lobular necrosis is produced, and though this complication is rare it is inadvisable to use the agent for more than 30 minutes at one administration. As with chloroform, the incidence of this complication can be greatly reduced by pre-operative treatment with glucose, protein and amino acids in order to protect the liver, and also by a high percentage of oxygen with a low carbon dioxide tension during anaesthesia.

**Other actions.**—Salivation is apt to be produced by divinyl ether, particularly if premedication has been omitted. It has few side-effects and causes little or no nausea and vomiting after short administrations. It depresses uterine tone in labour and quickly crosses the placenta into the fetus.

### Clinical Use

Divinyl ether is both volatile and expensive, so that its clinical use is restricted; although it has some value for the induction of anaesthesia, divinyl ether alone is generally used in a special closed inhaler as a single dose method. A quantity of the agent is evaporated in the bag of an inhaler which has previously been filled with oxygen. About 3–5 ml of divinyl ether will produce anaesthesia in about six breaths and give approximately 2–3 minutes of unconsciousness, depending upon the size of the patient. The method is particularly suitable for guillotine tonsillectomy, and sometimes for dental extractions, in children.

A mixture of 75 per cent diethyl ether and 25 per cent divinyl ether marketed under the trade name of "Vinesthene Anaesthetic Mixture" (V.A.M.) has a wider application, however, since it gives a rapid induction of anaesthesia with less irritation of the bronchial tract than does diethyl ether alone. V.A.M. may be vaporised by any of the methods described for ether.

## ETHYL CHLORIDE ($C_2H_5Cl$)

Ethyl chloride was first prepared by Basil Valentine during the early part of the seventeenth century. Flourens in 1847[102, 103] and Heyfelder in 1848[104] described its general anaesthetic properties, but it continued to be used solely for local refrigeration analgesia until in 1894 Carlson inadvertently produced unconsciousness in a patient whilst spraying the gum for a dental extraction. In the past it has been used extensively in anaesthesia.

**Preparation.**—There are two common methods of preparation:

(a) By reacting ethylene with hydrochloric acid:

$$C_2H_4 + HCl \rightarrow C_2H_5Cl.$$

(b) By treating ethyl alcohol with hydrochloric acid:

$$C_2H_5OH + HCl \rightarrow C_2H_5Cl + H_2O.$$

**Physical properties.**—Ethyl chloride is a clear fluid with an ethereal odour which is not irritating to the respiratory tract. Frequently this is masked by the addition of eau-de-Cologne. The molecular weight is 64·5. The specific gravity of the liquid is 0·921 at 20° C and of the vapour 2·28 (air = 1). The boiling point is 12·5° C, so that at ordinary room temperatures it is a vapour. Nevertheless, it is easily compressed to form a highly volatile liquid which can be stored in glass or metal tubes. It has a high lipoid solubility, for at 38° C five volumes of vapour dissolves in one volume of blood.

**Impurities.**—It may contain traces of alcohol, aldehydes, chlorides or polyhalogenated ethanes.

**Inflammability.**—The vapour is heavier than air and is capable of explosion when mixed with air in concentrations between 3·8–15·4 per cent and with oxygen between 4·0 and 67·0 per cent.

### Pharmacological Actions

Ethyl chloride is non-irritant to the respiratory mucosa. Concentrations of 3–4·5 per cent in the inspired air produce anaesthesia and a blood concentration of 20–30 mg per cent leads to the signs of surgical anaesthesia. Forty mg per cent leads to respiratory arrest.

**Action on the cardiovascular system.**—There is very little evidence that ethyl chloride produces an irritable myocardium, and dysrhythmias are rare during induction. The pulse rate may be slowed from stimulation of the vagal centre and there is widespread vasodilatation due to vasomotor depression. As anaesthesia progresses the heart dilates slightly, owing to the effect on the myocardium. Although both the cardiac output and peripheral vascular tone are depressed in deep anaesthesia, there is no evidence that myocardial failure will occur before respiratory arrest—most cases of sudden circulatory failure during the induction of anaesthesia can be traced to relative overdosage at the time rather than to peculiar side-effects. Overdosage easily and quickly results on account of the physical properties of the drug.

**Other actions.**—Ethyl chloride anaesthesia is frequently followed by headache, nausea and vomiting. It depresses uterine tone in labour and quickly crosses the placenta into the fetus.

### Clinical Use

**Local analgesia.**—A fine spray is allowed to fall on the operation area. The liquid vaporises and the skin cools to $-20°$ C, and the surrounding water vapour freezes and deposits fine snowy crystals over the wound. The incision is painless but as the thaw sets in the pain may become excruciating.

**General anaesthesia.**—Ethyl chloride is an extremely potent and simple anaesthetic to administer—so much so that the greatest possible care should be exercised in its use. It is particularly suitable for induction in children, but once a rhythmical respiratory exchange has commenced it should be abandoned: if necessary, the anaesthesia can be maintained by the much safer agent—diethyl ether.

It is inadvisable to spray more than 5 ml of the ethyl chloride on to an open mask for the induction of anaesthesia; subsequent doses should be much smaller. Great care should be taken to prevent a child holding its breath for a prolonged period and then taking a large inspiration of a highly-concentrated vapour, which can lead to circulatory collapse.

Ethyl chloride may be used with oxygen in a closed inhaler in a manner similar to that described for divinyl ether. A dose of 3–5 ml is sufficient for a single administration.

## TRICHLOROETHYLENE ($CCl_2CHCl$)

Originally described by E. Fischer, a German chemist, in 1864,[105] it was first used as an anaesthetic agent in animals by Lehmann in 1911[106] whilst working at Würzburg University.

The finding that trichloroethylene was a powerful grease solvent led to its wide application in industry for the removal of grease from metal and machinery. This led to toxic symptoms in some of the factory workers, however, and in 1915 Plessner[107] described the syndrome of acute trichloroethylene poisoning—one of the main features of which is sensory paralysis of the fifth cranial nerve. Such symptoms were almost certainly due to the impurities associated with trichloroethylene. In the same year Oppenheim[108] described twelve cases of trigeminal neuralgia that were successfully treated by inhalations of trichloroethylene vapour.

In 1934, Dennis Jackson[109] of Cincinnati University redescribed its anaesthetic properties and one year later, at the same University, Striker and his colleagues[110] published the first report of the successful administration of trichloroethylene to 304 patients for dental extractions or minor operative procedures. Hewer and Hadfield[111] popularised it in the United Kingdom.

**Preparation.**—Acetylene when treated with chlorine forms tetrachlorethane; this is reacted with calcium hydroxide in a "lime slurry" to form trichloroethylene, which is purified by distillation.

$$\underset{\text{Acetylene}}{C_2H_2} + \underset{\text{Chlorine}}{2Cl_2} \rightarrow \underset{\text{Tetrachlorethane}}{C_2H_2Cl_4}$$

$$\underset{\text{Tetrachlorethane}}{2C_2H_2Cl_4} + \underset{\text{Calcium hydroxide}}{Ca(OH)_2} \rightarrow$$

$$\underset{\text{Trichloroethylene}}{2C_2HCl_3} + \underset{\text{Calcium chloride}}{CaCl_2} + \underset{\text{Water}}{2H_2O}$$

**Physical properties.**—Trichloroethylene is a heavy colourless liquid with a low volatility (boiling point 87·5° C) and has a smell similar to that of chloroform but not so sweet. The vapour pressure at 20° C is about 57 mm Hg (7·6 kPa). Thus with a high boiling point and low vapour pressure it is relatively difficult to vaporise high concentrations.

However, it has an oil/gas solubility coefficient of 960; on this basis it is the most potent of all known anaesthetic agents and it is calculated that a concentration as low as 0·17 vols per cent will achieve the 1st plane of surgical anaesthesia (or minimal anaesthetic concentration).

Trilene, the trade name for the preparation which is used in anaesthesia in Great Britain, consists of purified trichloroethylene, thymol (stabilising agent) 1:10,000 and waxoline blue (dye) 1:200,000. The dye is added to distinguish it from chloroform.

In the United States the trade name is Trimar. It consists of 99–99·5 per cent purified trichloroethylene with the remainder alcohol. Ammonium carbonate is added as a preservative.

**Stability.**—Trichloroethylene is decomposed by strong light or by contact with hot surfaces into phosgene and hydrochloric acid. It is, therefore, best kept in metal containers.

It is contra-indicated in the presence of soda-lime for two reasons—first, it decomposes to phosgene and hydrochloric acid when in contact with a hot surface. Secondly, in the presence of an alkali and heat it may be broken down to hydrochloric acid and dichloracetylene, a substance which is both inflammable and toxic. Dichloracetylene may itself decompose to phosgene and carbon monoxide. Thus:

1. $$CHCl{=}CCl_2 \xrightarrow{NaOH} CCl{\equiv}CCl + HCl \text{ (absorbed by NaOH)}$$
Trichloroethylene + Heat → Dichloracetylene + Hydrochloric acid

2. $$CCl{\equiv}CCl + O_2 \longrightarrow COCl_2 + CO$$
Dichloracetylene + Oxygen → Phosgene + Carbon monoxide

The rate of decomposition of trichloroethylene in the presence of soda-lime depends largely on the temperature. At 15° C it is slow, but over 60° C the rate rises sharply (Fig. 5). It has been suggested that decomposition can be inhibited by the addition of 10 per cent silica.

Some of the early cases of cranial nerve palsy following the use of trichloroethylene in the presence of soda-lime are believed to have been due to the high percentage of sodium hydroxide present in the absorbents used. Soda-lime of this type was five times more hygroscopic and also generated more heat than that available today. It has also been shown that the temperature of modern soda-lime rarely rises above 40° C during clinical anaesthesia, nevertheless at this temperature small amounts of dichloracetylene can be formed.

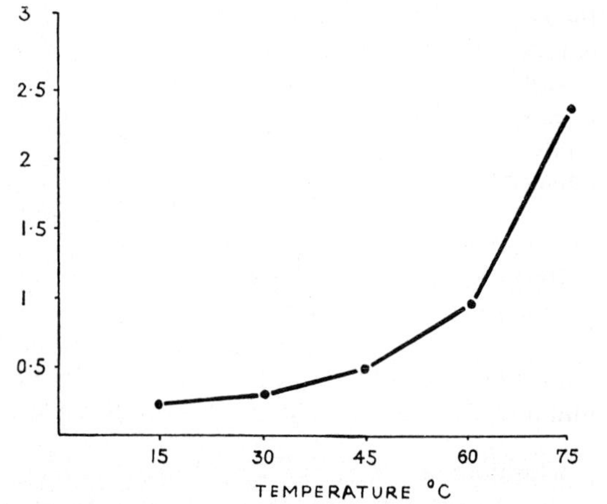


6/Fig. 5.—Chart to show how the rate of decomposition of trichloroethylene to dichloracetylene rises rapidly with temperature. (Reproduced from *Trichloroethylene Anaesthesia*, courtesy of Gordon Ostlere and E. & S. Livingstone Ltd.[297])

It is inadvisable to use cautery or diathermy in the immediate presence of trichloroethylene vapour, such as during an oral operation, because at temperatures above 125° C phosgene and hydrochloric acid may be rapidly formed, particularly if a high percentage of oxygen is present.[112,113]

**Toxicity.**—Cranial nerve lesions are amongst the commonest toxic manifestations of impure trichloroethylene or its degradation products, such as dichloracetylene. The fifth nerve is the most commonly involved but lesions of all the nerves except the first, ninth and eleventh have been reported.

The onset of toxic symptoms and signs is usually characterised by a complaint of numbness or coldness around the lips starting about twenty-four to forty-eight hours after the anaesthetic ceased. During the next few days the area of sensory loss spreads to involve the whole field supplied by the trigeminal nerve. There is no motor involvement. Recovery usually begins between the fifth and tenth days and may be complete in a fortnight.

**Inflammability.**—Trichloroethylene vapour is non-inflammable and non-explosive in the concentrations used in anaesthesia (see also Chapter 8).

### Pharmacological Actions

*Uptake and distribution.*—Trichloroethylene has a blood/gas solubility coefficient of 9·15, which indicates that it is relatively soluble in blood. In other words blood has a great capacity for taking up trichloroethylene. A long time will elapse, therefore, before alveolar tension reaches equilibrium with the inspired concentration. Clayton and Parkhouse[114] found that the administration of a 1 per cent v/v trichloroethylene concentration resulted in an arterial concentration in the blood of 12·17 mg/100 ml. Furthermore, in slim subjects the concentration in venous blood approximated to that of arterial blood after about 30 minutes, whereas in fat subjects it took twice as long. This is because trichloroethylene is extremely soluble in human fat due to its high oil/gas solubility; in fact, it is probably 100 times more soluble in fat than in muscle.

To summarise, this agent has a low volatility and a high blood solubility. The slow induction is partially offset by the high degree of potency due to the remarkable oil/gas solubility. Recovery, however, is prolonged.

Trichloroethylene is partly excreted unchanged by the lungs and partly metabolised. Depending upon the duration of time for which the vapour is inhaled, the percentage recovery of trichloroethylene in expired gases varies from 67 to 83 per cent.[115] Metabolic degradation is slow, and the metabolic products are found in the urine from 10 to 18 days following a single period of trichloroethylene administration. Assuming that approximately 20 per cent of inspired trichloroethylene is metabolised, then 10 per cent of trichloroethanol and 10 per cent of trichloracetic acid will result.[116]

**Action on the cardiovascular system.**—Almost every known form of cardiac dysrhythmia has been reported during trichloroethylene anaesthesia, but always in association with high concentrations of the inhaled vapour. Sinus tachycardia and bradycardia, nodal rhythm and partial heart block are usually associated with light anaesthesia, whereas ventricular extrasystoles may occur in deep anaesthesia.

The incidence of cardiac dysrhythmias is likely to be increased if adrenaline is used during anaesthesia. Opinion is divided on the incidence of primary cardiac failure due to trichloroethylene, though it appears that this condition may very rarely occur.[117]

Trichloroethylene produces no significant alteration in forearm blood flow, heart rate or mean arterial blood pressure.[118]

**Action on the respiratory system.**—Trichloroethylene in moderate concentrations (1–3 per cent) is non-irritant to the respiratory tract; in high concentrations, however, it may cause tachypnoea. The increased respiratory rate leads to a diminished tidal volume and in severe cases this may be so reduced that hypoxia occurs.

**Other actions.**—Post-operative vomiting and headache occasionally follow trichloroethylene anaesthesia, while circumoral herpes has been reported.

Trichloroethylene causes a rise in intracranial pressure. Jennett and his associates[119] report that such an increase occurs even when the arterial carbon dioxide is low, and that it is associated with cerebral vasodilatation and an increased cerebral blood flow.

Trichloroethylene will depress the contractions of the uterus during labour. Analgesic concentrations—0·5 per cent v/v in air or less—have little effect on uterine muscle unless inhaled for periods approaching 4 hours, when accumulation of the drug in the body occurs. At this stage both the rate and tone of uterine contraction may be decreased. Trichloroethylene rapidly crosses the placenta into the fetal circulation, and animal experiments (sheep) show that within sixteen minutes the fetal concentration is higher than that in the maternal circulation.[120]

The effect of trichloroethylene on the liver has been studied by determining concentrations of glutamic acid, pyruvic acid, transaminase and lactic dehydrogenase in the blood of patients undergoing anaesthesia. Elevated values were not found in any case.[121]

### Clinical Use

The fact that trichloroethylene is non-inflammable, relatively non-irritant and with minimum post-operative side-effects, has made it popular as a supplement in the sequence thiopentone, nitrous oxide and oxygen for the maintenance of light anaesthesia. The chief disadvantage in general surgery is that it is unsuitable for the production of muscle relaxation, because when this is attempted tachypnoea and cardiac dysrhythmias are soon encountered. Nevertheless within the safe limits of its application it is a useful agent. It was once widely used for the production of analgesia in obstetrics and dentistry, and it also appeared to have a place for post-operative and physiotherapeutic analgesia.[122,123] However, at present, the use of trichloroethylene in the U.K. has declined to the point that the makers ("Trilene"), I.C.I., announced in 1979 that they intended to discontinue manufacture; a decision soon withdrawn following protests from clinical anaesthetists. In the United States, trichloroethylene is no longer in use having been banned by the FDA as a health hazard in the workplace due to possible carcinogenic activity in mice.

Those anaesthetists supporting the retention of trichloroethylene suggest that it still has an important part to play in current practice: as an alternative to halothane, if, when during spontaneous breathing, unacceptable hypotension occurs; in obstetrics, to allow up to 60 per cent oxygen in inhaled mixtures, without risk of awareness, and without risk to fetus; as a keystone analgesic in balanced anaesthesia with muscle relaxants, without cardiovascular depression; in situations when nitrous oxide is contra-indicated, to limit increase-by-diffusion volume of a pneumothorax or embolism at cardiopulmonary bypass surgery.[124–126]

## CHLOROFORM ($CHCl_3$)

Chloroform was independently discovered by Soubeiran, Liebig and Guthrie in 1831. Its chemical and physical properties were first described by Alexandre Dumas in 1835, and twelve years later, in 1847, Flourens reported on its anaesthetic properties.[102,103] That same year James Simpson,[127] acting on a suggestion from a Liverpool chemist David Waldie, experimented upon himself and his colleagues, and finally gave it to patients with great success. Soon after its introduction into clinical practice chloroform largely replaced ether in popularity, but since then its popularity has gradually waned.

**Preparation.**—Chloroform may be prepared in a number of ways, but those most commonly encountered are:

*In the laboratory:* acetone or ethyl alcohol is heated with bleaching powder and the mixture is then submitted to steam distillation.

$$\underset{\text{Acetone}}{2CH_3.CO.CH_3} + \underset{\text{Bleaching powder}}{Ca(OCl)_2} \rightarrow$$

$$\underset{\text{Trichlor-acetone}}{CH_3COCCl_3} + \underset{\text{Chloroform}}{CHCl_3} + \underset{\text{Calcium acetate}}{Ca(CH_3.COO)_2}$$

*Commercially:* carbon tetrachloride and hydrogen are allowed to react in the presence of iron.

$$\underset{\text{Carbon tetrachloride}}{CCl_4} + \underset{\text{Hydrogen}}{2H} \xrightarrow[\text{Iron}]{Fe} \underset{\text{Chloroform}}{CHCl_3} + \underset{\text{Hydrochloric acid}}{HCl}$$

**Physical properties.**—Chloroform is a colourless transparent fluid with a sweet-smelling odour. The boiling point is 61° C and the vapour pressure at 20° C is 150 mm Hg (20 kPa).

The oil/gas solubility coefficient is 265 (*cf.* 960 for trichloroethylene and 11·2 for cyclopropane) denoting considerable solubility in lipoid tissues and also anaesthetic potency. In fact, an alveolar concentration of only 0·62 vols per cent is required for 1st plane surgical anaesthesia.

**Stability.**—Prolonged exposure to light or heat results in the breakdown of chloroform, the most serious oxidation product being phosgene, which is highly irritant to the respiratory tract. For this reason it should be stored in dark bottles in a cool place. Stability is increased by the addition of 1 per cent ethyl alcohol, an agent which would also convert any phosgene present to diethyl carbonate.

Chloroform can be used with soda-lime without danger of undue decomposition. In theory several reactions may take place when chloroform comes into contact with an alkali.[128]

1. Decomposition of chloroform into sodium formate

$$\underset{\text{Chloroform}}{CHCl_3} + \underset{\text{Sodium hydroxide}}{4NaOH} \rightarrow$$

$$\underset{\text{Sodium chloride}}{3NaCl} + \underset{\text{Sodium formate}}{H.COONa} + \underset{\text{Water}}{2H_2O}$$

2. Decomposition of chloroform into sodium chloride and carbon monoxide

$$\underset{\text{Chloroform}}{CHCl_3} + \underset{\text{Sodium hydroxide}}{3NaOH} \rightarrow$$

$$\underset{\text{Sodium chloride}}{3NaCl} + \underset{\text{Carbon monoxide}}{CO} + \underset{\text{Water}}{2H_2O}$$

3. Decomposition of chloroform into sodium chloride and phosgene

$$\underset{\text{Chloroform}}{CHCl_3} + \underset{\text{Sodium hydroxide}}{NaOH} + \underset{\text{Oxygen}}{O} \rightarrow$$

$$\underset{\text{Sodium chloride}}{NaCl} + \underset{\text{Phosgene}}{COCl_2} + \underset{\text{Water}}{H_2O}$$

There seems little doubt that under the conditions of anaesthesia little, if any, decomposition takes place, particularly if fresh soda-lime is used, and that the courses represented in equations 1 and 2 are the most likely, while the production of phosgene is extremely improbable. Bassett[128] was able to show in soda-lime used clinically with chloroform that only very slight decomposition had taken place. Even if all the chloroform destroyed in his cases had been converted to carbon monoxide, only about 16 ml of the gas would have been produced throughout the anaesthetic. Other products which may be present are hydrochloric acid, acetone, free halogens, organic halides, ethyl chloride, aldehydes and peroxides.

**Inflammability.**—Chloroform is non-inflammable.

### Pharmacological Actions

*Uptake and distribution.*—The blood/gas solubility coefficient of chloroform is 10·3 denoting that the blood is capable of taking up large quantities. Induction, therefore, is slow but this is partially offset by the high degree of anaesthetic potency of this agent. Recovery is slow.

The greater part of the chloroform inhaled is not altered in the body but is excreted unchanged by the lungs, nearly all of it leaving the circulation within sixty minutes of the end of anaesthesia. That which remains may not be eliminated for many hours and a small part is broken down in the body to hydrochloric acid and a residual hydrocarbon. Animal studies suggest that about 4 per cent of inhaled chloroform is metabolised.[129]

Chloroform has a direct depressant action on the myocardium, the respiratory centre, the vasomotor centre, and tissue cells in general, so that all of the four types of anoxia—anaemic, anoxic, stagnant and histotoxic—are possible in some degree when it is used.

**Action on the cardiovascular system.**—Chloroform depresses cardiac muscle and conducting tissue and also the smooth muscle of the peripheral vessels, with a resulting general depression of the circulation. These are direct effects, but both heart and circulation are also depressed reflexly from an action on the vagal and vasomotor centres. The situation is aggravated by anoxaemia resulting from respiratory depression and a reduction of the oxygen-carrying capacity of the blood.

Vagal inhibition of the heart may occur during induction. Since Levy's classical work in 1912 on ventricular fibrillation during chloroform anaesthesia[130] there has been a tendency to discountenance the view that irritant concentrations of chloroform reaching vagal receptors in the respiratory tract can induce cardiac arrest. Although this complication may be rare it seems very likely that it can occur, and not only with chloroform but with trichloroethylene and even agents such as ether, provided sufficiently irritant concentrations reach the vagal receptors in the lower air passages.[131] It is particularly likely to happen when any one of these volatile agents is given to a patient who has had some muscle relaxant. During the period of paralysis abnormally high concentrations may be blown into the patient's lungs, creating a situation which would be impossible were the volatile anaesthetic agent alone used.

In spite of the possibility of vagal inhibition of the heart, death during the induction with chloroform in man is probably most commonly due to ventricular fibrillation. This was first suggested by Levy working with cats; he demonstrated that chloroform sensitises the myocardium to the stimulating effects of injected adrenaline. In man during chloroform induction the pulse rate is slowed, partly due to vagal stimulation in the medulla, and partly due to direct depression of conducting tissue in the heart. Moreover, the efficiency of the myocardium is decreased by a reduction in its refractory period. All in all, the heart is sensitised to the effects of sympathetic stimulation, which are frequently met during the induction of anaesthesia. It is believed, too, that chloroform may stimulate the afferent endings of the vagus nerve in the upper respiratory tract, causing a reflex excitation of the cardiac sympathetic nerves. Cardiac irregularities are also accentuated by carbon dioxide retention and hypoxia, both of which are likely concomitants of chloroform anaesthesia.

The pre-operative use of atropine, by reducing vagal tone, will decrease the incidence of cardiac irregularities, but not by any means prevent them all from occurring. Indeed electrocardiographic monitoring during chloroform anaesthesia has shown that irregularities of all types, but particularly multifocal ventricular extrasystoles—the precursors of ventricular fibrillation—occur more frequently than not.[132] Waters[133] studied fifty-two patients, and in this small series noted four cases of temporary cardiac arrest, and only seven cases in which no cardiac irregularities occurred. In all induction deaths with chloroform the heart stops before respiration ceases.

During the inhalation of moderate concentrations of chloroform (1·5–2 per cent) the cardiac output and peripheral resistance are progressively decreased, together with a continuous fall in blood pressure. It is incorrect to assume, however, that maintenance of light anaesthesia with low constant concentrations of chloroform leads to a steady fall in blood pressure. In fact perfectly reasonable pressures can be maintained.

**Action on the respiratory system.**—Chloroform depresses respiration both by a direct effect on the respiratory centre and by the production of progressive depression of the respiratory muscles.

**Action on the liver.**—It is generally accepted that central hepatic necrosis occurs in some degree after chloroform anaesthesia or analgesia irrespective of the concentration used or the length of administration. But Rollason[134] using serum glutamic pyruvic transaminase (SGPT) activity in patients with good nutrition could find no evidence of liver damage following chloroform anaesthesia, provided the concentration did not exceed 2·25 per cent in an oxygen-rich mixture and there was no carbon dioxide retention. Repeated short administrations may sensitise the liver, and certainly increase the risk of a bad attack. In severe cases, leading to death, section of the liver will show necrosis with fatty degeneration of the cells surrounding the vein in the centre of the lobule. Signs and symptoms of poisoning are produced only by severe necrosis. The first symptoms may occur as early as six hours after the operation, although more commonly they present themselves twenty-four to forty-eight hours later. Nausea and vomiting start early and progressively increase in severity. The diagnosis becomes certain with the development of jaundice, and death, preceded by coma, may occur at any time during the first ten days. Delayed chloroform poisoning is not restricted in its symptomatology to the liver, the heart and kidneys also being affected. Fatty degeneration of the heart and necrosis of the tubular epithelium of the kidneys take place and result in incipient cardiac and renal failure.

A poor nutritional state increases the risk of this complication, whereas the pre-operative use of carbohydrates, proteins and amino acids helps to protect the liver. Moreover, the avoidance of hypoxia and carbon dioxide retention is of practical help. Waters[133] has shown that if chloroform is given in the presence of a high percentage of oxygen, and if steps are taken to avoid carbon dioxide accumulation, hepatic and renal function tests in a group of patients show no significant difference from those of controls.

The treatment of delayed chloroform poisoning consists primarily of the administration of intravenous fluids, together with carbohydrates, protein and amino acids. Of the various amino acids methionine is the most useful because it plays an important part in building up the reserves of glycogen in the liver.

**Action on the kidneys.**—The toxic effects of chloroform are mainly on the renal tubules, which at microscopy can be seen to be swollen with the lumina filled with fat globules and coagulated serum. After chloroform anaesthesia transient albuminuria is a common occurrence, while prolonged administration often leads to glycosuria. In cases of delayed poisoning as described above ketonuria also occurs.

**Other actions.**—Toxic effects may be found in other organs. In severe cases fatty degeneration occurs in the pancreas and spleen, while nausea and vomiting in some degree usually follow all but the briefest anaesthetic. Chloroform depresses uterine contractions during labour and quickly crosses the placenta to reach the fetus.

### Clinical Use

The main advantages of chloroform are a sweet-smelling, non-irritant vapour, portability, potency, and non-inflammability. It permits a rapid, smooth induction, while the decreased bleeding which results from circulatory depression was the forerunner of the "hypotensive" technique. Low volatility and a high potency make it particularly valuable in hot and humid countries, while the fact that an experienced administrator can produce such excellent conditions for surgery from a small bottle and simple mask has undoubtedly done much to recommend it in the past. It is interesting to recall in this respect that John Snow is believed to have given 4000 chloroform anaesthetics without any mortality.

Nevertheless, despite all these advantages, chloroform is not nowadays commonly used. The reason for its elimination from major anaesthetic practice is to be found in the toxic effects it produces on the various parts of the body, and the fact that most, if not all, of its advantages can be obtained with a combination of other agents and with less risk to the patient. Only on an occasion where there is no suitable alternative, such as may occur for instance in certain circumstances in domiciliary midwifery, should chloroform now be used.

### Administration

Chloroform may be dropped on to an open mask. One drop weighing 20 mg, if vaporised in 500 ml of air, forms a 1 per cent concentration of the vapour. At the start of induction 20 drops a minute is adequate, increasing later to 30 drops a minute. Great care should be taken to prevent the sudden inspiration of a high concentration, which is most likely with a struggling patient, and to avoid liquid chloroform reaching the skin, since it may cause a burn. Sometimes patients breathe shallowly during induction and then suddenly take a deep inspiration just before the second stage is reached. It can be avoided by adding a little carbon dioxide to the inspired mixture so that the depth of respiration could be regulated from the onset of unconsciousness. Once rhythmical and regular respiration has become established it is advisable to change over to ether or a chloroform-ether mixture (1 part chloroform to 4 parts diethyl ether). The safety of chloroform is at all times increased by the addition of oxygen to the inhaled mixture.

Administration in a semi-closed system has the advantage that it can be combined with an adequate oxygen flow and a more accurate increase in vapour concentration, but both in this type of system, and particularly in a closed system, the danger of accumulation cannot be over-emphasised.

## THE FLUORINATED HYDROCARBONS

The introduction of halothane into clinical practice provides one of the great landmarks in the development of anaesthesia. In an attempt to find an agent that was basically as "safe" as ether yet non-inflammable, Suckling[135] examined a number of fluorinated hydrocarbons. This group was known to be highly stable, volatile and non-inflammable (under clinical conditions).

In these compounds the fluorine atoms have a strong chemical bond with the carbon atoms. The result is that the fluorine atom is quite unreactive, particularly when the compound contains a $CF_2$ or $CF_3$ grouping. Such agents would be unlikely to interfere with body metabolism because of their high chemical stability, and therefore would tend to have a low toxicity.[136]

Robbins[137] in a study of many fluorinated hydrocarbons found that those with low boiling points produced convulsive movements; that the potency increased as the boiling point rose, yet recovery time became more prolonged, and that substitution of a bromine atom in the fluorohydrocarbon not only increased potency but also appeared to improve the safety margin.

The inclusion of several halogen atoms in a compound confers inflammability in the clinical range. If the halogen selected is a fluorine atom then there is no decrease in volatility, but the presence of at least one hydrogen atom is necessary for anaesthetic potency.

A large number of fluorinated hydrocarbons have been synthesised but only a few have to date received extensive clinical trials. Early amongst these were halothane, methoxyflurane and fluroxene:

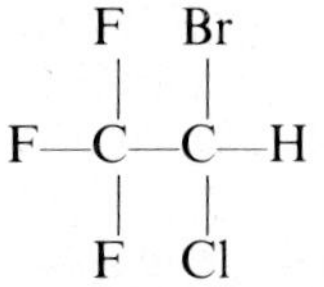

Halothane
(B.P. 50·2° C)

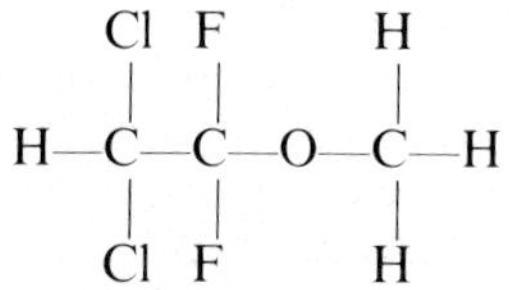

Methoxyflurane
(B.P. 104·65° C)

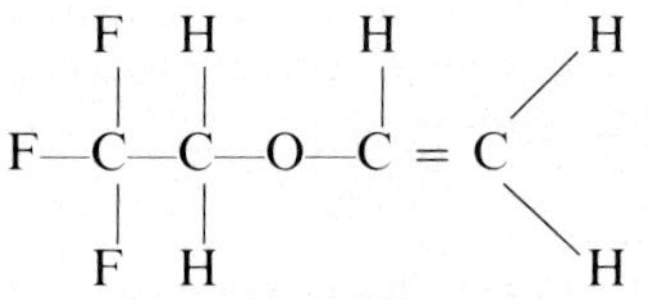

Fluroxene
(B.P. 43·2° C)

Later came enflurane and isoflurane:

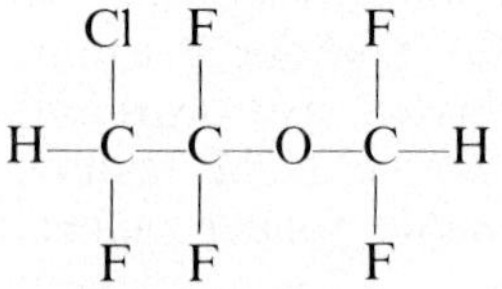

Enflurane (Ethrane)

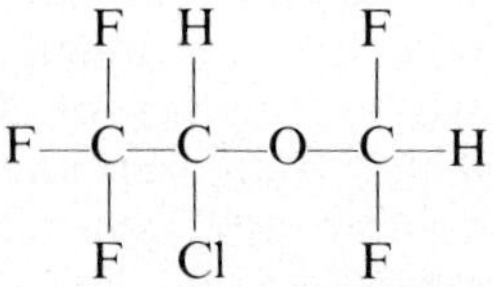

Isoflurane (Forane)

Of these compounds halothane has received the widest clinical acclaim. One of the principal features of these fluorohydrocarbons is that they have relatively low boiling points (with the exception of methoxyflurane) when compared with similar agents containing only chlorine or bromine. For example, if all of the five halogens in halothane were chlorine then the boiling point would be 162° C. In fact, the boiling point of halothane is 50·2° C at atmospheric pressure.

## Halothane (Fluothane)

Halothane was prepared and examined by Raventós.[138] It was introduced into clinical anaesthesia by Johnstone[139] and Bryce-Smith and O'Brien.[140]

**Physical properties.**—Halothane is a heavy, colourless liquid with a sweet smell somewhat resembling chloroform. It contains 0·01 per cent of thymol for stability. The formula is:

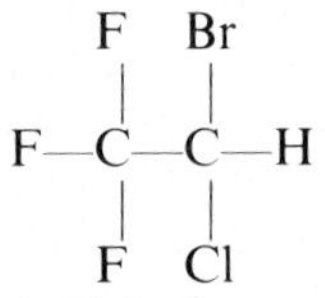

Halothane

It has a molecular weight of 197·39 and a boiling point of 50·2° C (at 760 mm Hg, 101·1 kPa). It does not react with soda-lime. One of the contaminants is betene in a concentration of 0·001 per cent. When exposed to light for several days it will decompose to various halide acids such as HCl, HBr, free chlorine, bromine radicles and phosgene. The presence of thymol helps to prevent the liberation of free bromine.

The vapour pressure of halothane is 241 mm Hg (32 kPa) at 20° C. It is, therefore, very suitable for vaporisation in a bubble-through (e.g. copper kettle) or temperature and flow-controlled vaporiser (e.g. "Fluotec"). If a flow of 100 ml of oxygen is passed through the copper kettle (or "Vernitrol") vaporiser then as the vapour pressure is $\frac{240}{760}$ mm Hg or approximately ⅓ of an atmosphere 100 ml of oxygen will pick up 50 ml of halothane (i.e. a total of 150 ml of 33⅓ per cent halothane or 50 ml of pure halothane vapour). If this quantity (i.e. 50 ml of halothane vapour) is added to 5 litres of nitrous oxide and oxygen then the patient will receive an inspired concentration of 1 per cent halothane. Similarly, if 200 ml is put through the vaporiser and this is again added to

5 litres of nitrous oxide and oxygen the patient will receive a 2 per cent halothane vapour.

In the absence of water vapour halothane does not attack most metals. However, if water vapour is present it will attack aluminium, brass and lead. Copper and fault-free chromium are not attacked.

Halothane is readily soluble in rubber (coefficient 121·1 at 760 mm and 24° C) and less so in polyethylene (coefficient 26·3). This significant rubber solubility together with the large amount of this material used in an anaesthetic system means that the uptake of halothane by rubber could be significant if a low-flow circle absorption technique is used. High flows eliminate this problem.[141]

**Analysis.**—Halothane can be estimated by gas chromatography[142] or by infra-red[143] or ultra-violet light analysis.

### Pharmacology

**Minimum alveolar concentration (MAC).**—The MAC for halothane is about 0·8 but is reduced to about 0·3 when, as in common practice, $N_2O$ 70 per cent is added as a carrier gas (approximately 1 per cent reduction in halothane MAC for every 1 per cent increase in alveolar $N_2O$). Premedicant drugs will also reduce halothane requirements.

*Uptake and distribution.*—Halothane has a blood solubility coefficient of 2·3 (*cf.* nitrous oxide 0·46 and ether 12·1) and might be described as being in the medium range of solubility. Because it is relatively insoluble in blood it is not taken up very rapidly from the alveoli. This means that the alveolar concentration or tension can soon approach the inspired concentration. Now alveolar *tension* is virtually synonymous with brain *tension*, so a high tension is rapidly achieved in the brain. This means induction of anaesthesia is relatively rapid. On withdrawal of the anaesthetic the same process is reversed so that recovery is rapid.

Mapleson[144] has shown that though the rate of uptake is high at the start, after twenty minutes, for every 1 per cent of halothane vapour in the inspired mixture, the patient has an uptake of 10 ml of halothane vapour per minute. This first goes to the organs with a rich blood supply such as the heart and brain. Resting muscle and fat have a much poorer blood supply so that they receive their quota of halothane long after the tension in the alveoli and brain have reached equilibrium. Thus, in the first few minutes of halothane anaesthesia most goes to the heart, brain, liver and kidneys. After ten or twenty minutes the muscles are tending to remove their quota from the circulation so that 10 ml of halothane vapour is removed from the lungs every minute. In time even the poorly perfused fat receives its share. In this manner the body continues almost indefinitely to keep removing halothane vapour from the lungs. If, therefore, a 1 per cent inspired concentration is given to a patient it is estimated that it will take 5 days or more for the concentration in the alveoli to rise to this level. In fact, equilibrium between inspired and alveolar concentrations is probably never reached because a small amount is lost through the skin.

One of the principal reasons for the prolonged uptake of halothane by the body is the remarkable capacity of human fat to absorb it. So great is this affinity—the solubility coefficient of halothane in fat is 60·0 (*cf.* nitrous oxide = 1·0)—that it is capable of removing almost all the halothane it receives in the circulation. Other tissues also show a slightly greater affinity for halothane than blood.

6/TABLE 5
TISSUE/BLOOD SOLUBILITY COEFFICIENT OF HALOTHANE

| |
|---|
| 2·6 in Brain |
| 2·6 in Lung |
| 1·6 in Kidney |
| 3·5 in Muscle |
| 60 in Fat |

*Metabolism.*—Isotope labelling techniques have now established that about 12 per cent of inspired halothane is metabolised by the liver microsomes and the resulting products are excreted in the urine.[145] Halothane undergoes both oxidation and dehalogenation to form trifluoracetic acid, as well as bromide and chloride radicals.[3] This metabolism may be stimulated by barbiturates and also by further doses of halothane itself.[146]

Work with mice has shown that the metabolites of halothane may persist in the liver for as long as twelve days after administration[147] Chronic exposure to halothane can impair liver cell function in small mammals and this may be due to the accumulation of metabolites. A matter of some concern to all anaesthetists, as well as those working in operating theatres, is whether such small concentrations of expired halothane from patients could have any harmful effects on the attendant staff.

**Action on respiration.**—Halothane is a respiratory depressant. This is more marked in the presence of narcotic premedication. Increasing the inspired concentration of halothane leads to a progressive diminution of volume rather than rate of respiration. In fact, surgical stimulation under light anaesthesia decreases basal metabolism in direct proportion to the depth of anaesthesia; in surgical anaesthesia the oxygen consumption is reduced about 20 per cent.[148, 149]

In view of the respiratory depressant action of halothane it is advisable occasionally to assist the ventilation whenever spontaneous respiration is present. At least 30 per cent oxygen should always be present in the inspired mixture.

The action of surfactant in the lungs is not affected by halothane anaesthesia.[80]

Halothane may be accidentally injected intravenously, in which case severe pulmonary lesions may occur, leading to death. Sandison and his colleagues,[150] in an experimental study of intravenous halothane in dogs, found that the predominant lesions produced in the lungs were generalised oedema and patchy alveolar haemorrhages, and that pathological changes occurred in other organs and in the blood. They note that in the dog, a dose equivalent to 3–5 ml for an adult human can cause severe lung damage.

**Action on the heart.**—One of the principal problems in the study of the action of halothane on the cardiovascular system is the wealth of contradictory evidence. This appears to be largely due to the multiplicity of premedicant and intravenous drugs used in the study. Price,[151] however, administered halothane and oxygen alone to a group of unpremedicated patients and observed the results. The cardiac contractile force was diminished; stroke volume and cardiac output were reduced despite an increased venous pressure. The heart rate and arterial pressure were also reduced, but the total systemic peripheral resistance was only slightly affected. Atropine reversed the bradycardia but failed to correct the arterial hypotension or to improve the cardiac output.

There appears to be unanimity of opinion amongst authors that myocardial depression is directly related to the depth of halothane anaesthesia,[148, 152, 153, 154] and animal experiments suggest that this is due to inhibition of enzyme activity in the muscle.[155] Nevertheless, an overall picture of the action of halothane is more complex. For example, the ability of atropine to reverse the bradycardia suggests that halothane has a parasympathetic stimulant action as well as producing myocardial depression.

An interesting hypothesis that might explain most of the actions of halothane throughout the body is that in increasing concentration it gradually blocks the action of noradrenaline at the effector sites in the heart, central nervous system and peripheral tissues.[151] Two important findings support this suggestion. First, unlike most other anaesthetic agents, halothane does not produce an increase in the plasma catecholamine level of blood. Secondly, halothane partially blocks the constrictor action of noradrenaline on the skin vessels.[156] On this basis the effect of halothane on the heart would be to reduce the secretion and activity of noradrenaline at the sympathetic nerve endings in the myocardium and at the same time to sensitise the parasympathetic nerve endings leading to bradycardia. There is experimental evidence from dogs to show that halothane can inhibit and, in adequate concentration, completely block stellate ganglion transmission.[157]

Dysrhythmias occurring during halothane anaesthesia bear a direct relationship to hypercapnia from respiratory depression. Adrenaline can be safely used in the presence of halothane provided the concentration and total dose are within acceptable limits and the patient is neither hypercapnic nor hypoxic. Katz and Katz[158] suggest concentrations of 1 in 100,000 to 1 in 200,000 and a total dose of the former of not more than 10 ml in any one ten-minute period. Whenever an infiltration of adrenaline is used during anaesthesia it is important to remember that the adrenaline itself is the most dangerous factor, and that this danger is enhanced when the injection is made in a vascular part of the body. The prophylactic administration of propranolol intravenously before infiltrating with adrenaline has been recommended,[159] but there are inherent dangers in using propranolol during general anaesthesia, particularly with halothane, and these may well be greater than those of the controlled use of adrenaline.

**Action on the peripheral circulation.**—

Despite a wealth of studies on the action of halothane on the myocardium, there are singularly few available on the action of this drug on the peripheral circulation. Black and McArdle[156] investigated a group of unpremedicated patients inhaling 1–4 per cent halothane (with thiopentone induction and nitrous oxide/oxygen maintenance). They found a persistent vasodilatation of the skin and muscle vessels along with a fall in both the arterial pressure and the vascular resistance.

In an attempt to explain the mechanism of the vasodilatation produced by halothane they infused a solution of noradrenaline into the brachial artery of a series of patients. In the absence of halothane anaesthesia, noradrenaline promptly produced severe vasoconstriction, but when halothane was inhaled this constrictor action of noradrenaline was partially blocked.

In another study they found that if a nerve block was produced in one arm then halothane anaesthesia had no effect on the blood flow through this arm, yet it produced an increase in the normal arm.

These results suggest that halothane does not have a direct action on the vessel wall itself but acts rather by blocking the action of noradrenaline. This concept fits well with the possible action of halothane on the myocardium mentioned above.

**Action on kidney and liver.**—Halothane causes a decrease in renal flow probably related to a fall in glomerular filtration rate and a reduction in ADH release.[160] It also leads to a fall in hepatic blood flow.[161] The possible association of halothane and liver damage is considered below.

**Action on uterus.**—Halothane anaesthesia relaxes uterine muscle in direct relation to the depth of anaesthesia and *in vitro* studies suggest that this may be due to stimulation of the adrenergic $\beta$-receptors in the uterus.[162] For this reason it has been expressly recommended in anaesthesia for external version, manual removal or contraction ring.[163] Vasicka and Kretchmer,[164] from experimental studies in women, found that uterine contractions recurred twice as quickly after halothane as compared with ether, when these anaesthetics were given in concentrations that produced comparable levels of clinical anaesthesia.

This last observation suggests that halothane may not be so liable to produce postpartum haemorrhage as has been stated. Some authors have stressed the possible dangers of increased bleeding from the uterus after the use of halothane. Like most other inhalational anaesthetic agents it readily crosses the placental barrier.

**Action on gastro-intestinal tract.**—In anaesthetic concentrations halothane depresses the motility of the jejunum, colon and stomach in dogs; activity promptly returns on withdrawal of the agent. It is also capable of antagonising the contractions produced by the parenteral administration of neostigmine.[165]

**Action on skeletal muscles.**—Halothane has minimal neuromuscular blocking action but potentiates the action of the non-depolarising agents, whilst antagonising the effect of drugs which act by depolarisation.[166–168]

**Action on the cerebral blood flow and intracranial contents.**—Cerebral blood flow is increased and cerebral vascular resistance decreased during halothane anaesthesia. These changes occur when the arterial carbon dioxide tension is maintained within normal limits and provided there is not a considerable fall in mean arterial blood pressure.[169,170] At normal arterial carbon dioxide tension halothane causes a rise in cerebrospinal fluid pressure, but this can be prevented if the patient is hyperventilated before the addition of halothane to the anaesthetic gases.[171] Intracranial pressure rises during halothane anaesthesia, especially so in those patients who have space-occupying intracranial lesions.[119] Headache may follow halothane anaesthesia.[172]

**Shivering.**—Intense muscle spasms are occasionally observed in the early part of the post-operative period. These movements are sometimes jocularly referred to as the "halothane shakes". Moir and Doyle[173] studied a large group of patients and found that the body temperature in those who "shivered" after operation was 0·5° C lower than those who did not shiver, and Jones and McLaren[174] noted a close relationship between falls in central body temperature and shivering following halothane anaesthesia. Bay and his colleagues[175] studied arterial oxygen and carbon dioxide tensions and cardiac output during post-operative shivering. They found that both ventilation and cardiac output were adequate for the increased demands imposed by shivering, but that there is a potential danger of hypoxaemia in patients who have ventilatory embarrassment or a fixed low cardiac output. The high incidence of shivering after halothane anaesthesia is probably related to the vasodilatory action of the drug and the environmental temperature.

**Action on cells.**—Experimental work by Nunn and associates[176] has shown that halothane interferes with mitosis in cells.

### Clinical Use

There is little doubt that halothane has proved one of the most useful agents in the whole history of clinical anaesthesia. It is non-inflammable, potent and non-irritating to the respiratory tract in anaesthetic concentrations. Furthermore, it has a low post-operative incidence of nausea and vomiting. In abdominal surgery it is often combined with a muscle relaxant in order to achieve good relaxation without resorting to high concentrations of halothane that would depress the systemic pressure. It is widely used in anaesthesia for all types of surgery including neurosurgery, ear, nose and throat, orthopaedic and paediatric cases. A reduction in blood pressure, which at one time was regarded as an undesirable side-effect, is now often used to advantage in major surgery to reduce the blood loss.

*Methods of vaporisation.*—Halothane can be vaporised in a number of ways but its high cost demands that reasonable economy be used. For this reason it is unsuitable for open-mask application. When placed in a bubble-through vaporiser (copper kettle, see Fig. 1),[77] a flow rate of 100 ml of oxygen through the apparatus (at room temperature) when added to 5 litres of nitrous oxide and oxygen will give an inspired concentration of 1 per cent. Similarly 200 ml of oxygen will give a concentration of 2 per cent.

On the other hand, the "Fluotec" vaporiser (Fig. 6*a*) receives all the inspired gas en route to the patient and adds a predicted amount of halothane to the mixture of gases. This apparatus is both temperature- and flow-controlled (Fig. 6*b*) and it is a satisfactory vaporiser for routine clinical use.[177]

*Vaporiser inside or outside circle system.*—Various authorities have argued for and against the policy of whether the vaporiser should be always placed outside the circle system or whether it is safe to incorporate it inside the system to permit rebreathing and thereby exercise economy.

Halothane with a relatively high vapour pressure, low boiling point and low blood solubility can be regarded as a potent anaesthetic in which low concentrations (i.e. 0·4 per cent with nitrous oxide/oxygen) are capable of maintaining unconsciousness. The only justification, therefore, for using a vaporiser within the circle system is on the grounds of economy.

*Vaporiser inside the circle system.*—One of the principal fears of using a halothane vaporiser within the circle system has been the possibility that the concentration of halothane would rapidly rise to a fatal level; in fact this does not occur if the patient is breathing spontaneously because not only does the patient continue to remove halothane from the system but as soon as the anaesthetic concentration rises the respiratory minute volume becomes depressed. In this manner the patient will then vaporise less halothane and this acts to prevent a rapid build up of halothane within the system. The patient, at this point, will show all the clinical signs of deep halothane anaesthesia, i.e. depressed ventilation, slow pulse rate and hypotension. Provided the anaesthetist uses these signs and reduces (or turns off) the concentration delivered by the vaporiser then this method can be used. However, to achieve a satisfactory level of anaesthesia, in some cases it is necessary to depress ventilation below normal. If the anaesthetist then institutes assisted or controlled respiration without modifying the vaporiser setting a rapid and fatal concentration of halothane may develop. In short, the vaporiser should only be used within the circle system in the presence of spontaneous respiration. If assisted respiration is required then great care must be exercised to see that the concentration of halothane does not rise unexpectedly.

*Vaporiser outside the circuit.*—If the vaporiser is placed outside the circle system then the concentration within the system cannot rise above that entering it. In fact, due to the constant uptake of halothane by the body it takes many hours or even days for the alveolar concentration to reach equilibrium with the inspired concentration. A vaporiser outside the circle system, therefore, is relatively safe provided an excessive concentration is not used and the patient is carefully observed for the signs of increasing depth of anaesthesia.

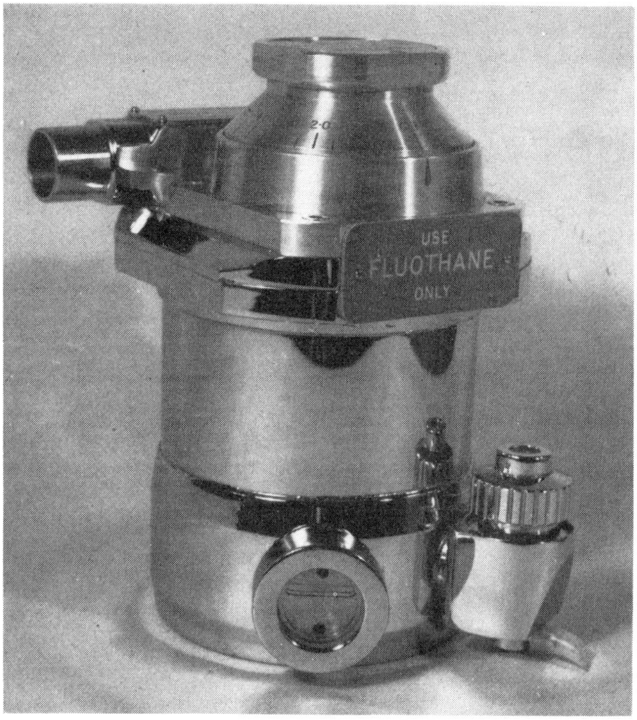


6/FIG. 6(*a*).—The "Fluotec" Mark III vaporiser. (Courtesy of Cyprane Ltd.)

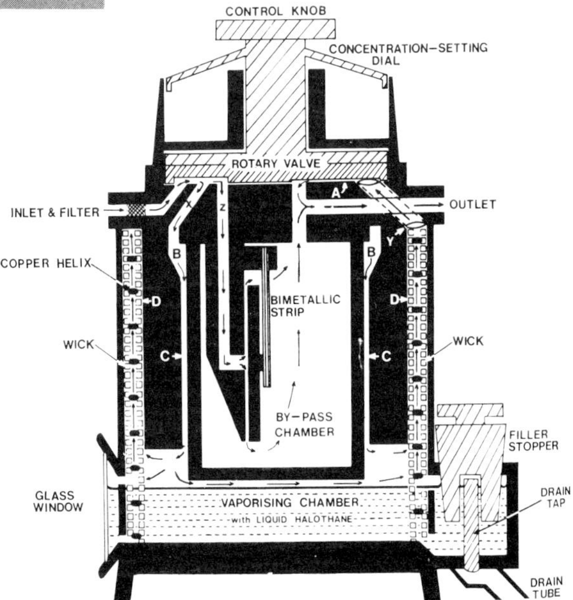


6/FIG. 6(*b*).—Diagram to illustrate the interior of the "Fluotec" Mark III showing direction of flow of gases. The rotary valve controls the amount of the gas passing to the vaporising chamber. The remainder of the gas flows into the by-pass chamber and then to the outlet. (Courtesy of Drs. J. A. and S. E. Dorsch and Williams & Wilkins Co.[295])

It is often not fully realised that even though the vaporiser is placed outside the circle system, fluctuations in concentration can occur when assisted or controlled respiration is used.[178] On squeezing the bag the back-pressure in the anaesthetic apparatus rises to 15–20 cm of water. This forces more gases into the interior of the vaporiser and this increased volume of gases collects additional vapour. The exact increase in the vapour concentration delivered

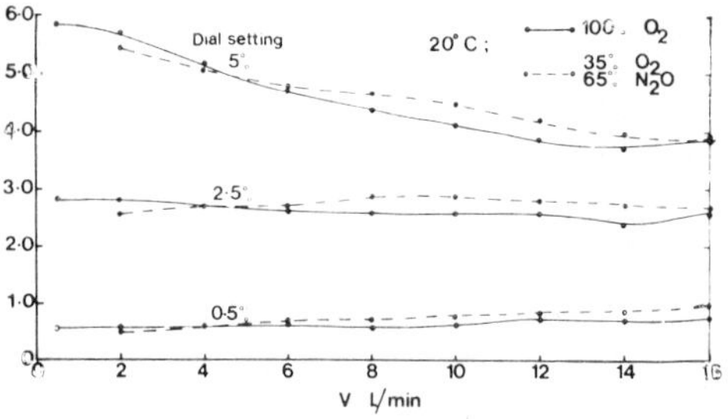


6/FIG. 7.—The effects of varying flow rates on halothane concentration ("Fluotec" Mark III). (Courtesy of Dr. G. M. Paterson, Dr. G. H. Hulands and Professor J. F. Nunn and John Sherratt and Son, publishers of the *British Journal of Anaesthesia*[177]).

to the patient will depend on the flow of gases used. If a high flow of gases is used then the extra 50 ml or so that can be compressed into the vaporiser does not pick up enough vapour to seriously increase the concentration. On the other hand, if a low flow is used then it is possible the concentration received by the patient may actually be double that indicated by the vaporiser. For this reason a flow of gases of at least 4 litres/minute is recommended for use on the circle system even when the vaporiser is outside the circuit. Some vaporisers contain a special device to prevent this back-flow of anaesthetic gases during controlled respiration.

A small, convenient and inexpensive vaporiser that will only develop a maximum concentration of halothane of not more than 2·3 vols per cent is illustrated in Fig. 8.

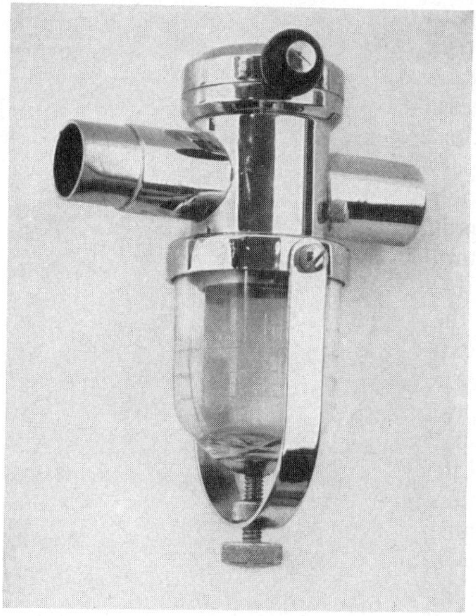

6/FIG. 8.—The Goldman vaporiser.

### Halogenated Hydrocarbons and Hepatotoxicity

When a patient becomes jaundiced after a general anaesthetic there is a tendency, in the absence of obvious diagnostic clues to the contrary, to blame the inhalational agent; this is a natural tendency perhaps, and stems from the chloroform legacy; an authentic story of hepatotoxicity. But because 80 per cent of general anaesthetics in the United Kingdom include halothane, it is the drug which has earned the sobriquet "halothane hepatitis", a conclusion which, in many studies, often lacks true objectivity; is based on circumstantial evidence; and gives only cursory attention to other possible contributory factors. Indeed the term "halothane hepatitis" has been used as a convenient dumping ground into which patients developing jaundice after surgery have been grouped—an intellectually deceitful approach when based on inadequate or non-existent control data, and apparently ignoring the incidence of jaundice after nonhalothane anaesthesia, or when no anaesthetic is given.

Halothane has served a long and meritorious apprenticeship and has been subjected to thorough, competent scrutiny in countless studies, and no toxicity has been found; indeed one authority has aptly noted that many workers appear to be in pursuit of the non-existent; "Obviously, when what you are searching for doesn't exist, you'll have trouble finding it even with an infinite number of experiments. Although halothane (or enflurane or diazepam . . .) may not be toxic, you cannot construct a study that will conclusively document non-toxicity."[179] All halogenated anaesthetics have at some time been blamed for rare and unpredictable incidence of hepatic necrosis, and because new agents such as enflurane and isoflurane are of this genre, the stigma is unlikely to disappear spontaneously. In this section the problem is reviewed, and halothane has been selected for special attention because more research studies and clinical experience has accumulated on this drug than with any other anaesthetic agent in contemporary use.

Soon after the introduction of halothane into clinical practice, anecdotal case reports of jaundice after routine and uncomplicated anaesthesia appeared, and with it the label "halothane hepatitis".[180,181] These, and the continuing flurry of anecdotal reports, led to the American National Halothane Study;[91] a randomised retrospective study in which co-operating institutions pooled data on the incidence of massive hepatic necrosis after surgery in some 1 million patients. This study found that the incidence of massive hepatic necrosis was 1·02 in 10,000 administrations, similar to the overall frequency of the entity, and therefore inconclusive. Later, in the 1960s several investigators noted that unexplained hepatitis after halothane (UHFH) was more prevalent after second and multiple exposures, and thus the concept "Halothane Hepatitis" arose.

Little[182] reported that 49 per cent of the patients in his series had received two or more halothane anaesthetics before developing jaundice, and Klatskin[183] noted that 68 per cent in his series had been given halothane more than once. In the U.K. the Committee on Safety of Medicines produced two analyses of reports of jaundice submitted to them.[184,185] The 1974 paper discussed 130 cases of jaundice occurring after anaesthetic with halothane, and showed "a significant relationship between the number of exposures to this anaesthetic and the rapidity with which jaundice develops after exposure." They considered that "this provided strong evidence of a cause-effect relationship between the use of halothane and jaundice". Of the 114 patients with complete anaesthetic histories, 82 per cent had been exposed more than once; of those exposed, 80 per cent had been anaesthetised with halothane more than once within 28 days. These reports led to a conviction mainly expressed by hepatologists and pathologists that repeated exposure to halothane may lead in some patients to a sensitivity reaction to the drug. This concept was reinforced by the following evidence: Paronetta and Popper[186] found that lymphocytes harvested from patients with suspected halothane hepatitis had increased thymidine uptake in the presence of halothane, the so-called positive lymphocyte stimulation test, which they suggested was a sign of an antigen-antibody interaction; secondly, a number of susceptible individuals had positive "challenge tests" to inhalation of sub-anaesthetic concentrations of halothane, and developed fever and increased transaminase levels;[187] and recently, circulating antibodies which react specifically with the cell membrane of hepatocytes isolated from halothane-anaesthetised rabbits have been detected in 9 of 11 patients who had fulminant hepatic failure after halothane.[188] However, there are a number of points counter to the allergy theory: all attempts to confirm the lymphocyte stimulation test have failed;[189] attempts to sensitise animals to halothane fail consistently;[190] infants and children readily develop drug allergies but do not appear prone to halothane-associated jaundice; some patients are jaundiced on their first encounter with halothane; a positive halothane challenge is not necessarily a sign of sensitivity to the drug, or mechanistically due to an antigen-antibody reaction; the diagnosis of hepatitis is frequently one of exclusion, and cases attributed to halothane not infrequently are proven to be due to viral hepatitis; finally there are some patients who have had jaundice after a second halothane anaesthetic who have received the drug on a third occasion without incident. Such discrepancies have led investigators to seek other mechanisms for the syndrome of hepatitis following halogenated anaesthetics, and of these the "Metabolic Activation Theory" has persuasive merits. It has been appreciated for a long time that classic hepatotoxins like carbon tetrachloride are not injurious *per se*, but depend on biotransformation to reactive intermediates to produce cell damage. In common with many drugs, carbon tetrachloride is metabolised by the mixed function oxidase cytochrome P-450 enzyme system of hepatic microsomes, and in the resultant chain of by-products, a toxic intermediate substance is produced which possesses a reactive unpaired covalent electron. This ephemeral reactive species may damage the liver by a number of mechanisms. Fatty acids and esters are broken down by a process of lipoperoxidation with eventual aldehyde formation. In a second mechanism liver glutathione level is reduced and structural lipid of hepatocytes are deprived of a valuable free radical scavenger. And finally, hepatic protein and lipoprotein lose their functional intregrity when firm covalent attachments are formed with reactive intermediates. So much for the hepatotoxicity of carbon tetrachloride; is there a way that halothane can fit into this scheme? Halothane is preferentially metabolised oxidatively in the hepatic mixed oxidase enzyme system to relatively innocuous trifluoroacetic acid with the release of chloride and bromide ions; and even if this pathway is enhanced by enzyme induction, there is no danger of toxicity. However, anaerobic "reductive type biotransformation" of halothane is possible, and may in certain circumstances lead to the formation of considerable reactive intermediates. Although these metabolites are found in man after incident-free routine anaesthesia with halothane, their concentration is too low to be a threat. On the other hand it has been speculated that the reductive pathway may be enhanced to toxic proportions by a subtle combination of events: genetic influence with increase in P-450 reductase activity, coupled with environmental events triggering further reductase activity through enzyme induction and, augmented by an episode of hepatic hypoxia from reduced splanchnic blood flow (Fig. 9). These events can be reproduced in animal models; Maclain, Sipes and Brown[191] have shown the potential role of tissue hypoxia, from reduced hepatic blood flow, coupled with microsomal enzyme induction, directing halothane along a reductive and hepatotoxic pathway.

In the present state of knowledge it is impossible to state whether human halothane hepatitis is a real entity, and if so, is due to "halothane hypersensitivity" or "metabolic activation". Against the allergy theory are cases with hepatitis after first exposure to halothane; the absence of animal models, and the apparent insusceptibility of children. Counter to bioactivation is the increased incidence of hepatitis with multiple exposures to halothane, and although an animal model exists, the disease is short-lived compared with the human disease.

However, despite the disparate views on the origin of post-operative hepatitis, it is possible to reach a compromise explanation which is compatible with both the allergic and the metabolic activation theory. Perhaps mild and transient cases of jaundice, including cases of non-icteric enzyme upsets, are due to reactive intermediates generated by bioactivation of halothane through the reductive pathway in susceptible individuals. On the other hand, delayed onset, fulminant severe hepatitis may well be due to an allergic sensitisation episode produced by a halothane metabolite to the hepatocyte; antibody formation and continued reaction could produce a chronic hepatitis in man.

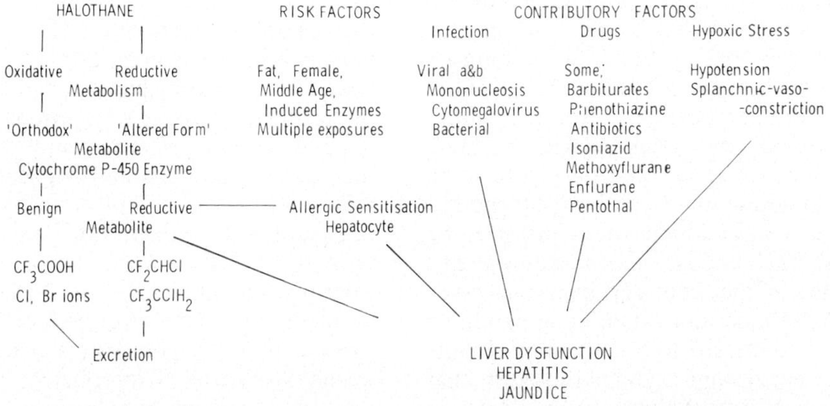


6/FIG. 9.—Some patients are more susceptible than others to liver dysfunction after surgery. This is, in most instances, due to infection, drugs or hypoxic stress to the liver; halothane has been implicated as a cause of liver dysfunction, but convincing proof is lacking.

It is unfortunate that it is still impossible to predict the individual for whom surgical intervention constitutes a hepatic risk; whether for halothane or any other form of anaesthesia. From epidemiological data (Swedish Adverse Drug Reaction Committee, 1966–1973[192]) and the evidence of prospective surveys[193, 194] it has been suggested that post-operative liver dysfunction is related to repeated exposure to halothane. However, none of the studies referred to above gives data on the response of the liver to non-halothane anaesthesia. All patient groups were highly selected and it is not possible to estimate the incidence of hepatitis after halothane, or to make comparisons with non-halothane anaesthesia. Indeed some studies report hepatitis after repeat methoxflurane[195] and $N_2O$ oxide anaesthesia.[196]

What then should be the anaesthetist's attitude to halothane anaesthesia? It was the conclusion of the working party set up by the British Medical Research Council[197] "That unexplained jaundice may occur in rare instances after multiple halothane anaesthesia, especially within 28 days. However there is insufficient evidence to indicate whether repeated exposure to halothane carries greater overall risk to the patient than substitution of other general anaesthetics after the first use of halothane; nor is there sufficient comparable information on the risks associated with repeated exposure to anaesthetics other than halothane."

A conservative, prudent and even defensive approach to the provision of anaesthesia for multiple surgical procedures, would perhaps dictate that attempts be made in pre-operative evaluation to acknowledge liver dysfunction risk factors: obesity; female middle-age; hypoxaemia; history of enzyme inducing medications; unexplained hepatitis after previous exposure; conditions requiring multiple anaesthesia. In such patients halothane should be avoided if an alternative satisfactory agent is available. In addition it would seem to be prudent, in "high-risk hepatitis" patients to adopt a prophylactic regimen: oxygen should be continued for longer periods into the post-operative period; and nutritional aspects should be evaluated by giving amino acid and glucose infusions during operation as well as time-honoured balanced salt. For a further commentary, see Chapter 35.

## METHOXYFLURANE ($CHCl_2$ $CF_2OCH_3$)

Methoxyflurane (Penthrane) is 2·2 dichlorofluroethyl methyl ether. It was first studied by Van Poznak and Artusio;[198] the formula is as follows:

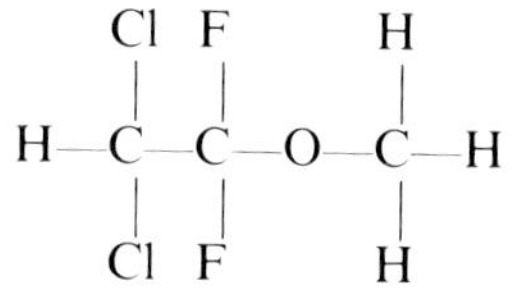

Methoxyflurane

**Physical properties.**—It is a clear colourless liquid with a characteristic fruity odour. The boiling point is just greater than that of the water i.e. 104·65° C at atmospheric pressure (760 mm Hg—101·3 kPa). The vapour pressure of methoxyflurane at room temperature (20° C) is approximately 23 mm Hg (3·1 kPa); in other words at this temperature the maximum concentration of vapour that can be obtained with a bubble-through vaporiser (e.g. copper kettle) is $\frac{23}{760} \times 100 = 3$ per cent.

Methoxyflurane is extremely soluble in rubber. This solubility is so great that 25–35 per cent of all the methoxyflurane introduced into the anaesthetic circuit can be absorbed by the rubber, and even after one hour as much as 20 per cent may still continue to be removed by the rubber.[199]

**Inflammability.**—Methoxyflurane is not flammable except at abnormally high vapour concentrations and temperatures. Up to 4 per cent in concentration and below a temperature of 75° C it will not ignite. Thus, under conditions of clinical anaesthesia it can be considered as a non-inflammable agent unless some unusual method of vaporisation (involving heat) is used. Under hyperbaric conditions methoxyflurane shows evidence of becoming flammable though not explosive, in the presence of a sustained high voltage spark.[200]

### Pharmacology

*Uptake and distribution.*—The blood/gas solubility coefficient of methoxyflurane is 13·0 (*cf.* nitrous oxide 0·46). This signifies it is very soluble in blood. The high blood solubility together with the high solubility in rubber means that it takes a long time for the inspired concentration to equal alveolar concentration.

Thus, about one-third of the output of the vaporiser is lost to rubber and that which reaches the alveoli is rapidly absorbed into the circulation. As tension of the vapour in the alveoli is virtually the same as brain tension, the build-up of tension in alveoli and brain is slow.

Methoxyflurane, however, has one very unusual physical attribute, namely a very high lipid solubility; the oil/gas coefficient is 825 (*cf.* ether = 65). A high lipid solubility signifies good anaesthetic potency, and this is borne out in practice. A steady alveolar concentration of only 0·30 vols per cent is required to maintain the 1st plane of surgical anaesthesia. This high anaesthetic potency, together with the absence of irritation of the respiratory tract, helps to reduce the time taken for induction of anaesthesia.

With the exception of the fatty tissue, methoxyflurane is only a little more soluble in other tissues than it is in blood (Table 6).

6/TABLE 6
TISSUE/BLOOD SOLUBILITY COEFFICIENT OF METHOXYFLURANE

| | |
|---|---|
| 2·34 | Brain tissue/White matter |
| 1·70 | Brain tissue/Grey matter |
| 1·34 | Muscle |
| 38·5 | Fat |

**Action on the respiratory system.**—Methoxyflurane depresses respiration in direct relationship with the depth of anaesthesia. The tidal volume is affected more than the rate of respiration. This agent does not appear to stimulate salivation or bronchial secretions and is relatively free from irritant effects on the respiratory mucosa.

**Action on the cardiovascular system.**—Walker and his colleagues[201] have measured the effects of methoxyflurane in unpremedicated patients. They observed a decrease in cardiac output, systemic vascular resistance and stroke volume. There was an increase in heart rate. The cardiovascular effects of methoxyflurane resembled halothane rather than ether, and they concluded that the hypotension produced by methoxyflurane was primarily due to a fall in cardiac output. Bagwell and Woods[202] working with dogs found that methoxyflurane produced a progressive depression of ventricular contractile force, aortic pressure and total aortic flow with increasing concentration of the anaesthetic agent. Miller and Morris[203] demonstrated that methoxyflurane does not increase the concentration of plasma catecholamines in the dog.

**Action on skeletal muscle.**—The basis for the profound muscular relaxation during methoxyflurane anaesthesia has been studied in man.[204] It was found that even when anaesthesia was deepened to a stage where electromyographic activity in the diaphragm was abolished, the twitch reponse to ulnar nerve stimulation remained unaffeced. This suggests that the principle cause of muscle paralysis in methoxyflurane anaesthesia is an action on the central nervous system (probably the spinal cord).

**Action on the kidney.**—Cousins and Mazze[205] have conclusively demonstrated that there is a relationship between the total amount of methoxyflurane administered and the incidence of renal damage. High concentrations over a long period of time may lead to nephrotoxicity. A metabolite (an inorganic fluoride) is believed to be responsible. For this reason, methoxyflurane should only be used (if necessary) for short periods of time and in low concentrations. It is contra-indicated in the presence of nephrotoxic drugs or renal insufficiency.

**Action on other organs.**—As with all the halogenated hydrocarbon anaesthetic agents there is no positive evidence definitely proving that these drugs produce toxic reactions in the liver. Such damage, however, has been reported in patients who have received these agents, yet there is no evidence at present definitely connecting the two events. Moricca and his coworkers[206] studied liver function in normal dogs and found a consistant modification of cellular function after methoxyflurane anaesthesia.

### Clinical use

Methoxyflurane can be used as the principal anaesthetic agent for most surgical procedures.[207–209] It has a relatively slow induction time[210] and some patients may complain about the unpleasant odour. In abdominal surgery the relaxation obtained is not as profound as that with a muscle relaxant.[211] Deep anaesthesia leads to respiratory depression and hypotension. If high concentrations are used for a long period of time then recovery time is delayed and the patient may undergo a prolonged period of somnolence.[212]

## Enflurane (Ethrane)

Enflurane ($CHF_2$—O—$F_2CHFCl$) is, like its isomer isoflurane, a methyl ethyl ether. It was first synthesised in 1963 by Terrell at Ohio Medical Products, and introduced into clinical practice in 1966 by Virtue and his colleagues.[213]

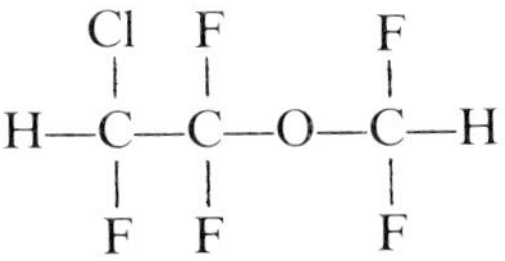

Enflurane (Ethrane)

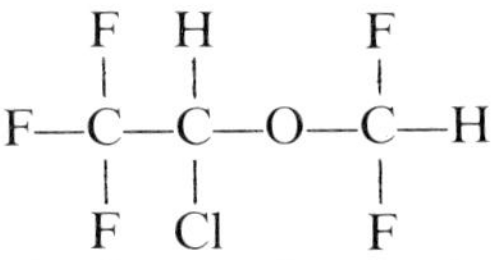

Isoflurane (Forane)

Enflurane has now outstripped the popularity of halothane in the United States, and has been employed in more than 20 million cases up to 1981.[214] In Britain enflurane has been available for 5 years, and now accounts for some 5 per cent of the inhalation anaesthetic market.

### Physical Properties

Enflurane is a clear, colourless, non-inflammable liquid with a specific gravity 1·52 at 25° C. It boils at 56·5° C and has a vapour pressure of 184 mm Hg (24·5 kPa) at room temperature of 20° C. Both enflurane and halothane vapour are inflammable under certain unusual circumstances,[215] but these are unlikely to be reproduced in everyday clinical practice. Enflurane contains no chemical stabiliser, is non-corrosive, does not attack materials used in the construction of anaesthetic apparatus, and may be stored in clear glass. Enflurane has a pleasant ethereal smell, is entirely compatible with soda-lime, and as suggested by its physico chemical properties, behaves like halothane in clinical practice. The relatively low blood/gas solubility coefficient of 1·91 at 37° C indicates the possibility of rapid change in alveolar and brain tensions, and explains the swift induction and emergence from anaesthesia with enflurane—features of particular value in the growing field of out-patient anaesthesia.[216]

The greater chemical stability of enflurane is reflected in lesser metabolism by body tissues, which may in turn reduce the likelihood of toxicity due to metabolites. The rate of metabolism of enflurane is about one-fifth that of halothane:[74] more than 80 per cent is excreted unchanged in exhaled gases,[217] and 2·4 per cent as non-volatile fluorinated metabolite in the urine.

### Pharmacology

**Minimum alveolar concentration (MAC).**—The MAC for enflurane is about 1·68 in young adults, (about twice that of halothane 0·8 per cent), and decreases to 0·6 per cent when 70 per cent nitrous oxide is used as carrier gas. Premedicant drugs will also reduce enflurane requirements.

*Uptake and distribution.*—The blood/gas solubility coefficient of enflurane is 1·8 (*cf.* nitrous oxide 0·46). This signifies that it is relatively insoluble in blood. Under these circumstances a relatively rapid induction and recovery from anaesthesia could be anticipated. In clinical practice, induction does not appear to be as rapid as with halothane given in equipotent concentrations. Recovery, on the other hand, would appear to be more rapid than with halothane and this may be explained on the basis of the lower solubility of enflurane in blood and the demonstrably more rapid rate of elimination.[218] A 25–35 per cent lower solubility in fatty tissues for enflurane as compared with halothane was also found (Table 7), but this poorly perfused area is hardly likely to influence recovery time.

6/Table 7
Tissue/Blood Solubility Coefficient of Enflurane

| | |
|---|---|
| 1·45 | Brain Tissue |
| 2·1 | Liver |
| 1·7 | Muscle |
| 36·2 | Fat (Halothane 60) |

**Action on respiratory system.**—Enflurane is non-irritant to the respiratory tract with no excessive salivation, but in high concentrations it can cause breath-holding, coughing and even laryngospasm. All general anaesthetics depress ventilation and ventilatory responses to carbon dioxide; and enflurane has the highest "apnoea index" (ratio of apnoeic dose to anaesthetic dose) compared to other agents as follows: enflurane > halothane > methoxyflurane > isoflurane.[219] It also depresses the ventilatory responses to hypoxia in dogs: enflurane at 1 MAC is more depressant than 1 MAC isoflurane; however, at 1·5 MAC, enflurane, isoflurane and halothane are equally depressant.[220] All volatile anaesthetic agents tend to produce bronchodilatation, and halothane[221] and enflurane[222] have both been recommended as particularly suitable for anaesthetising patients with obstructive airways disease. Two factors may influence airway calibre in an anaesthetised patient: change in bronchomotor tone, and change in lung volume; when these are taken into account, both halothane and enflurane diminish airflow resistance by "substantial reduction in bronchomotor tone".[223] Enflurane has been shown to have no effect on the regional pulmonary hypoxic vasoconstrictor responses in intact dogs.[224]

**Action on cardiovascular system.**—In common with other volatile agents, enflurane at 1 MAC will reduce cardiac output, arterial pressure, systemic vascular resistance, and rate of rise of pressure in the aorta.[225, 226] At 1·5 MAC, further reductions in stroke volume and rate of pressure rise occurred, but no further drops in cardiac output or blood pressure were noted. At 2·0 MAC substantial hypotension precluded further detailed observations. With long-term anaesthesia with enflurane at 1 MAC some recovery from cardiovascular depression occurs. Enflurane has been found to potentiate the hypotensive effects of sodium nitroprusside,[227] and fentanyl (e.g. 200 μg).[228, 229] Enflurane does not stimulate the sympatho-adrenal axis;[230] its use therefore in hypovolaemia (e.g. due to blood loss) in the presence of beta-adrenoceptor blockade would, without initial circulatory volume correction, result in severe haemodynamic depression.

In common with other volatile agents, enflurane depresses the mechanics and contractility of cardiac muscle; at equivalent MAC values it appears to be the most depressant; enflurane > halothane > methoxyflurane > cyclopropane > diethyl ether.[231] The probable mechanism of depression is due to inhibition of uptake of calcium ions by the sarcoplasmic reticulum of cardiac muscle.[232]

Myocardial work and oxygen demands are reduced during enflurane anaesthesia, and, unless myocardial perfusion is critically pressure-dependent as in ischaemic heart disease, oxygen needs are fulfilled by proportional reductions in oxygen extraction and myocardial blood flow.

Enflurane has no adverse effects on autonomic rhythmicity of the heart,[233] and the incidence of serious dysrhythmias is very low, and certainly no greater than with other anaesthetic agents in general use. Increases in both endogenous and exogenous catecholamines appear to be well tolerated during enflurane anaesthesia.[234, 235] Enflurane and halothane prolong conduction time at the A-V node in dogs, but enflurane, unlike halothane, has a sparing effect on His-Purkinje and ventricular conduction, and may by this mechanism result in relatively fewer ventricular dysrythmias.[236]

**Action on the central nervous system.**—Change in the electro-encephalograph pattern is seen with increasing depth of anaesthesia characterised by high voltage, high frequency spike and dome activity alternating with periods of silence or frank "seizure" activity. These observations are aggravated by hypocapnia and may be terminated by reduction of the enflurane level.[237] In a few instances abnormal neuromuscular activity is seen taking the form of twitching, clonus, or stiffness of the extremities: movements like those seen after bolus injections of some intravenous induction agents. The number of halogen atoms in the drug molecule is an important determinant for convulsive activities; with progressive halogenation, methyl ethyl ethers follow the stages of other ethers: anaesthesia → anaesthesia with convulsions → convulsions. With enflurane a fine balance has been achieved with sufficient halogenation to ensure non-flammability, anaesthetic potency, but minimum convulsive potential.[238] On rare occasions enflurane has been associated with convulsions in the immediate post-operative period,[239] or about 1 week later.[240] However, long-term follow-up studies show less abnormal EEG activity with enflurane than with halothane;[241] and no intellectual or personality defects can be demonstrated.[242] Enflurane may be useful as a tool to demonstrate epileptogenic foci in the surgery of epilepsy.[243]

In man, cerebral blood flow is unchanged or reduced by enflurane anaesthesia;[244, 245] cerebral oxygen consumption ($CMRo_2$) decreases markedly with low-dose enflurane anaesthesia (< 1MAC), but with increasing depths (> 1MAC) reductions are less marked.[246]

**Enflurane in obstetrics.**—Although there is no evidence that enflurane anaesthesia is associated with teratogenetic effects, its safety in pregnancy has not yet been established. Low dose enflurane (0·5–1·0 per cent) has been used to supplement anaesthesia in obstetric surgery; there was no awareness or factual recall, clinical conditions were good for the mothers, Apgar scores of infants compared well with other anaesthetic agents, and blood loss was not excessive relative to other techniques.[247, 248] Enflurane, isoflurane and halothane depress contractions and tone of gravid and non-gravid human myometrium *in vitro*, but resting tension is little altered by 0·5 MAC values[249], thus confirming clinical impression that blood loss does not appear to be excessive when low dose enflurane or halothane is used to supplement anaesthesia in obstetrics.

**Action on skeletal muscle.**—All volatile anaesthetic agents have intrinsic muscle relaxant properties by depression of post-synaptic responses to acetylcholine, thus inhibiting end-plate depolarisation. Isoflurane, enflurane, and di-ethyl ether, will, by this mechanism, provide a quality of skeletal muscle relaxation sufficient for laryngoscopy or manipulation, at a depth of anaesthesia equivalent to 1 MAC. Halothane and methoxyflurane, however, are relatively poor muscle relaxants. All patients anaesthetised with volatile anaesthetics require less muscle relaxant drug to block neuromuscular transmission; this potentiation is more marked with enflurane than with halothane. The enhancement by enflurane of the muscle paralysis produced by tubocurarine, pancuronium and suxamethonium was demonstrated in man by Fogdall and Miller.[250] They studied the effects of 1·25 MAC in oxygen on 50 per cent depression of twitch height ($ED_{50}$) produced by these drugs and found that 3·1, 1·7 and 1·0 times less amounts of tubocurarine, pancuronium and suxamethonium were required during enflurane than during halothane anaesthesia. The depression of twitch response was directly related to the alveolar concentration of enflurane. Such reductions in dose requirements of muscle relaxant drugs during anaesthesia with volatile agents is believed to be due to a change in the chemosensitivity of the end-plate region.[251] During enflurane anaesthesia there is a time-dependent increase in the sensitivity of neuromuscular junction to tubocurarine which becomes stable after 2–3 hours.[252]

### Toxicity

It is now generally accepted that volatile anaesthetic agents must undergo biological activation before the onset of toxicity. Enflurane, on this basis, is less likely to cause harmful effects on the liver and kidneys than others in

6/Table 8

Site of action of volatile anaesthetic agents and muscle relaxant drugs at the neuromuscular junction. Volatile anaesthetic agents do not appear to alter the affinity of the acetylcholine receptor to muscle relaxant drugs (the dissociation constant of tubocurarine, for example, is unchanged); thus volatile agents appear to exert their effect at a stage subsequent to the receptor

ACETYLCHOLINE
+
RECEPTOR

Muscle relaxant drug→ ↓
ACETYL CHOLINE RECEPTOR COMPLEX — END PLATE REGION
Volatile anaesthetic→ ↓
DEPOLARISATION
↓
MUSCLE CONTRACTION

common use, by virtue of inherent physicochemical characteristics: high degree of fluorination, chemical stability, and relative insolubility in blood and tissues. Most of the enflurane given during anaesthesia is excreted unchanged; 82·7 per cent can be recovered from the exhaled air; 2·4 per cent can be recovered in urine as non-volatile fluorinated metabolites; the remaining 15 per cent is lost through skin, sweat, and faeces, but some is lost unaccountably in expired air. Kidney injury occurs from inorganic fluoride but this is dose-related and unlikely to occur unless serum inorganic fluorides are in excess of 50 $\mu$mol $l^{-1}$ [253] or a "nephrotoxic threshold" of 2500 $\mu$mol/day is attained.[254] It is now generally accepted that there is greater potential for metabolite formation from prolonged exposure to low anaesthetic concentrations than from brief exposure to high concentrations. In studies of several sub-anaesthetic doses of enflurane in man, a dose-response relationship between the dose of enflurane and the amount of fluoride in both the urine and serum has been established.[255, 256] The mean peak enflurane level after the largest dose of enflurane (2 MAC-hour) was 23·6 $\mu$mol $l^{-1}$ and the "nephrotoxic" level 50 $\mu$mol $l^{-1}$ was never reached. Long-term exposure to low concentrations of anaesthetic is a prominent source of metabolite; and drugs emerging from fat stores in the recovery period are important factors. An important determinant of alterations in the biotransformation of enflurane is obesity rather than total body weight. The blood/gas partition coefficient of enflurane is lower in obese patients by some 30 per cent compared to non-obese patients; obese patients therefore absorb enflurane more rapidly and partition it in poorly perfused fat depots. Such patients generally have higher peak serum fluoride levels than controls. However, there was no evidence of nephrotoxicity.[257]

Uptake of fluoride ion from serum into bone is as important as excretion in urine, and accounts for almost half the fluoride load. This mechanism is important in renal dysfunction because greater amounts of fluoride enter bone thus protecting the kidney from prolonged exposure.

Second administrations of enflurane one week after a previous exposure do not cause increase in fluoride excretion.[254] Chronic exposure to enflurane does not have adverse effects on reproductive physiology.[258] Sub-clinical liver damage and jaundice after enflurane has not been proven; a number of cases of "hepatitis" have been reported but the picture was confused by coincidental administration of halothane[259–261] or prolonged use of chlorpheniramine,[262] or chlorpromazine.[263]

**Ophthalmology.**—Enflurane (1·0 per cent), halothane (0·5 per cent), or trichloroethylene (0·4 per cent) with controlled ventilation with $N_2O$ and $O_2$, and normocapnia will lower intraocular pressure by 10 to 40 per cent. This drop is mirrored by an almost identical decline in arterial blood pressure, which possibly explains its mechanism.

## Isoflurane (Forane; Aerrane)

Isoflurane $CHF_2$—O—CHCl—$CF_3$ is like its isomer enflurane, a methyl ethyl ether. It was discovered in 1965, by R. C. Terrell at Ohio Medical Products, and, following early difficulties with synthesis and purification, introduced into clinical practice by W. C. Stevens and colleagues at the University of California in 1971.[264]

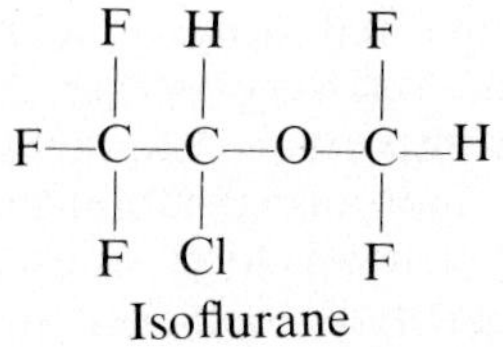

Isoflurane

Broad clinical studies were delayed by the Federal Drug Administration (F.D.A.) in the U.S. until evidence was produced that enflurane was without carcinogenic potential. In 1976 Corbett[265] reported a pilot study in which isoflurane administered to mice during gestation and early life produced hepatic neoplasias; but in 1978 these experiments were disproved by Eger and colleagues[266] in studies which, in addition to clearing isoflurane, provided negative evidence for the carcinogenic potential of $N_2O$, enflurane, halothane, and methoxyflurane.

### Physical Properties

Isoflurane is a clear, colourless, non-inflammable liquid with a specific gravity 1·52 at 25° C. It boils at 48·5° C, and has a vapour pressure of 250 mm Hg (33·3 kPa) at 20° C. Isoflurane contains no chemical stabilizer, is non-corrosive, does not attack materials used in the construction of anaesthetic apparatus, and may be stored in clear glass. It is stable in warm soda-lime. Isoflurane has a slightly pungent ethereal smell which limits the rate at which the inspired concentration may be increased and thus the induction of anaesthesia. Isoflurane, as suggested by its physicochemical properties, behaves like enflurane and halothane in clinical practice. The relatively low blood/gas solubility coefficient of 1·4 at 37° C, suggests the possibility of swift induction of anaesthesia, and emergence from anaesthesia with isoflurane.

The greater chemical stability of isoflurane is reflected in lesser metabolism in body tissues, which may in turn reduce the likelihood of toxicity due to metabolites. Animal studies suggest that isoflurane undergoes minimal or no metabolism,[74] and fluoride levels in bone are not increased.[267] The rate of metabolism of isoflurane is considerably less than that of enflurane: as much as 95 per cent is excreted unchanged in exhaled air; and less than 0·2 per cent as fluoride in urine.[268]

### Pharmacology

**Minimum alveolar concentration (MAC).**—The MAC for isoflurane is about 1·3 per cent in young adults, and decreases to about 1·0 per cent in the elderly; addition of 70 per cent $N_2O$ as carrier gas decreases MAC to about 0·6 per cent in the young, and to about 0·4 per cent in elderly patients.[269] Premedicant drugs will also reduce isoflurane requirements.

*Uptake and distribution.*—The blood/gas partition coefficient of this drug (1·4) is lower than that of halothane (2·3), and it is therefore predictably faster acting. However, the oil/gas partition coefficient is 98, and much lower than halothane (244), thus making isoflurane a weaker anaesthetic. Its vapour pressure of 250 mm Hg (33·3 kPa) makes it possible to deliver whatever concentration is required from the same vaporisers usually used for halothane. Thus it may be possible to recondition surplus halothane vaporisers by replacing wicks and labels. Awakening from isoflurane is predictably rapid.

As mentioned above, the pungent odour of isoflurane may, through breath-holding and coughing, limit speed of induction of anaesthesia; this limitation may be overcome by premedicant and intravenous induction drugs, and step-by-step increases in inspired concentration of 0·5 per cent every 5 breaths or so to a maximum of 4·0 per cent. Isoflurane is only slightly soluble in materials used for construction of anaesthetic circuits, and consequently will not affect ingress or egress of the agent.

**Action on the respiratory system.**—Isoflurane is a potent respiratory depressant. At 1 MAC isoflurane, spontaneous ventilation in unstimulated man is reduced so that $Paco_2$ is 50 mm Hg (6·37 kPa), at 1·5 MAC it is 65 mm Hg (8·7 kPa); and ventilatory responses to imposed increases in $Paco_2$ progressively and linearly approach zero at about 2·0 MAC.[270] This depression limits delivery of the anaesthetic to the lungs during spontaneous ventilation, limiting the alveolar concentration to about 3 per cent regardless of the inspired level. Surgical stimulation produces substantial increases in ventilation and reductions in $Paco_2$ of between 5 and 15 mm Hg (0·66–1·98 kPa).

Ventilatory reponses to hypoxia are markedly reduced by isoflurane at 0·1 MAC, and virtually disappear at 1 MAC.[271] Reduction of ventilatory responses to hypercarbia and hypoxia may lead to grossly impaired gas exchange in patients with impediments to breathing such as airway obstruction or partial curarisation.

Isoflurane produces a small drop in total lung compliance and functional residual volume.[272]

**Actions on the cardiovascular system.**—Studies in animals on isolated cardiac tissue, suggest that isoflurane is a direct myocardial depressant; and dose related decrease in maximum velocity of shortening (Vmax), and mean maximum developed force (Fm) of 36 per cent and 40 per cent of control values have been reported.[273] In contrast, studies in man suggest that isoflurane produces substantially less depression; 1 to 2 MAC does not extend the pre-ejection period, mean rate of ventricular ejection, ejection time, or the IJ wave of the ballistocardiogram.[264]

Arterial blood pressure and total peripheral vascular resistance are reduced in a dose-related manner by isoflurane; and reach 50 per cent of awake control values at 2 MAC. Cardiac output and right atrial pressure, however, are maintained at close to control levels.[274] The decrease in arterial blood pressure is due to vasodilatation; possibly a result of direct relaxation of vascular smooth muscle, by enhanced formation of cyclic adenosine-5-monophosphate, in regional circulations of skin, muscle, brain, splanchnic, and heart. Blood flow to muscle is particularly enhanced 2 or 3 fold, despite the drop in perfusion pressure, by general vasodilatation. In dogs, isoflurane decreases myocardial oxygen consumption, but because coronary blood flow is unaltered, coronary venous oxygen levels increase.[275]

There appears to be a wide margin of cardiovascular safety with isoflurane; the cardiac index (ratio of dose producing circulatory arrest versus MAC) is 5·7 and significantly larger than that for enflurane (3·3), or halothane (3·0).[219]

There is no evidence of tissue hypoperfusion with isoflurane; central venous oxygen saturation increases and base excess changes are minimal.[264]

Isoflurane does not affect heart rhythm,[274] and dysrhythmias following injection of adrenaline are less likely than with halothane.[235]

Isoflurane does not slow impulse conduction through the His-Purkinje system—a factor which promotes rhythm stability.[276] Vasopressors and ouabain are comparatively well tolerated.[277, 278]

In summary, isoflurane sustains myocardial contractility, does not sensitise the heart to adrenaline or vasopressors, maintains central venous pressure, and assures a relatively high margin of safety. Blood pressure falls due to decrease in vascular resistance in nearly all tissues, but heart rate is increased, and peripheral flow well maintained. Ventricular work and oxygen consumption are decreased. Pulmonary vasoconstrictor responses to hypoxia may be depressed, but pulmonary artery and wedge pressures are normal, and physiological shunt and dead space ventilation are no worse with isoflurane than with other potent inhalational agents.

**Effect on central nervous system.**—Isoflurane causes a dose-related depression, substantial changes occur between 0·25 and 0·5 MAC, and amnesia at 0·25.[279]

Isoflurane, unlike enflurane, does not promote convulsive activity,[280] or impair intellectual functions.[281]

Isoflurane does not increase cerebral blood flow at 0·6 to 1·1 MAC, but it doubles at 1·6 MAC.[282] Cerebral metabolism is decreased which may lead to a decrease in blood flow, a factor which may be useful in conditions of elevated intracranial pressure.[283]

**Neuromuscular effects.**—Isoflurane can produce adequate muscle relaxation for most surgical manoeuvres,[284] but for abdominal procedures it is desirable to use muscle relaxant drugs to avoid undesirable effects of prolonged inhalation of concentrations in excess of 1·0 MAC. Isoflurane enhances the action of non-depolarising muscle relaxants to the same extent as enflurane.[285] Isoflurane enhances the action of suxamethonium; possibly due to improved delivery by augmented muscle blood flow,[250] and reduction in time-dependent degradation by pseudocholinesterases.

These features may be of particular value in patients with limited neuromuscular reserves as in myasthenia gravis, or patients with excretory impairment through liver or kidney disease.

### Metabolism and Toxicity

Isoflurane is physicochemically very stable and this is reflected in its resistance to biodegradation. 95 per cent is excreted unchanged in exhaled air; and less than 0·2 per cent as urinary metabolite,[268] inorganic fluoride and trifluoroacetic acid.

The importance of anaesthetic metabolism lies in possible production of metabolites toxic to the kidney and liver; however, the near absence of metabolism of isoflurane implies that the possibility of such toxic effects is remote.

Repeated or prolonged isoflurane does not produce hepatorenal injury in animals;[286, 287] and no hepatic necrosis occurred in enzyme-induced hypoxic rats at 1 MAC isoflurane and enflurane, although necrosis was seen with 1 MAC halothane.[288]

### Mutagenicity, Teratogenicity and Carcinogenicity

Tests in mice have failed to reveal evidence of carcinogenicity with isoflurane;[266] and the Ames test,[289] widely accepted as a test of mutagenicity and carcinogenicity of both test drug and its metabolites, is negative for isoflurane, enflurane, methoxyflurane, and nitrous oxide; but positive for halothane metabolites.[290]

Reproductive physiology appears unimpaired by isoflurane.[271]

**Use of isoflurane in obstetrics.**—All potent inhalational agents relax the uterus in a dose-related manner, and because it may increase bleeding, isoflurane is not recommended as an anaesthetic for termination of pregnancy.[291] There are no studies to establish the place of isoflurane in obstetric anaesthesia, although animal studies suggest that 2·0 MAC isoflurane or halothane introduce an element of fetal asphyxia.[292]

## REFERENCES

1. Zeller, A. (1883). Ueber die schicksale des iodoforms und chloroforms im organismus. *Z. Physiol. Chem.*, **8**, 70.
2. Van Dyke, R. A., Chenoweth, M. B. and Van Poznak, A. (1964). Metabolism of volatile anaesthetics. I. Conversion *in vivo* of several anaesthetics to 14CO-2 and chloride. *Biochem. Pharmacol.*, **13**, 1239.
3. Rehder, K., Forbes, J., Alter, H., Hessler, O. and Stier, A. (1967). Biotransformation in man; a quantitive study. *Anesthesiology*, **31**, 560.
4. Blake, D. A. and Cascorbi, H. F., (1970). A note on the biotransformation of fluroxene in two volunteers. *Anesthesiology*, **32**, 560.
5. Holaday, D. A., Rudofsky, S. F. and Treuhaft, P. S. (1970). The metabolic degradation of methoxyflurane in man. *Anesthesiology*, **33**, 579.
6. Tinker, J. H., Gandolfi, A. J. and Van Dyke, R. A. (1976). Elevation of plasma bromide levels in patients following halothane anesthesia. Time correlation with total halothane dosage. *Anesthesiology*, **44**, 194.
7. Cohen, E. N. (Chairman) *et al.* (1974). Occupational disease among operating-room personnel: a national

study. (Report of an ad hoc Committee on the effect of trace anesthetics on the health of operating-room personnel, American Society of Anesthesiologists, 1974). *Anesthesiology*, **41**, 321.
8. Merkel, G. and Eger, E. I., (II) (1963). A comparative study of halothane and halopropane anesthesia—including a method for determining equipotency. *Anesthesiology*, **24**, 346.
9. Priestley, J. (1774). *Experiments and observations on different kinds of Air*. London.
10. Davy, H. (1800). *Researches, Chemical and Philosophical, chiefly concerning Nitrous Oxide*. London.
11. British Oxygen Co. Ltd. (1967). Current methods of commercial production of nitrous oxide. *Brit. J. Anaesth.*, **39**, 440.
12. Jones, P. L. (1974). Some observations on nitrous oxide cylinders during emptying. *Brit. J. Anaesth.*, **46**, 534.
13. Greenbaum, R., Bay, J., Hargreaves, M. D., Kain, M. L., Kalman, G. R., Nunn, J. F., Prys-Roberts, C. and Siebold, K. (1967). Effects of higher oxides of nitrogen on the anaesthetized dog. *Brit. J. Anaesth.*, **39**, 393.
14. Clutton-Brock, J. (1967). Two cases of poisoning by contamination of nitrous oxide with higher oxides of nitrogen during anaesthesia. *Brit. J. Anaesth.*, **39**, 388.
15. Kain, M. L., Commins, B. T., Dixon-Lewis, G. and Nunn, J. F. (1967). Detection and determination of higher oxides of nitrogen. *Brit. J. Anaesth.*, **39**, 425.
16. Prys-Roberts, C. (1967). Principles of treatment of poisoning by higher oxides of nitrogen. *Brit. J. Anaesth.*, **39**, 432.
17. Faulconer, A., Pender, J. W. and Bickford, R. G. (1949). The influence of partial pressure of nitrous oxide on the depth of anesthesia and the electro-encephalogram in man. *Anesthesiology*, **10**, 601.
18. Clement. F. W. (1951). *Nitrous Oxide-Oxygen Anesthesia*, 3rd edit. Philadelphia: Lea & Febiger.
19. Bourne, J. G. (1954). General anaesthesia for out-patients with special reference to dental extraction. *Proc. roy. Soc. Med.* **47**, 416.
20. Price, H. L. and Helrich, M. (1955). The effect of cyclopropane and diethyl ether, nitrous oxide, thiopentone and hydrogen ion concentration on myocardial function in the dog. *J. Pharmacol. exp. Ther.*, **115**, 206.
21. Johnstone, M. (1959). Collapse after halothane. *Anaesthesia*, **14**, 410.
22. Bloch, M. (1963). Some systemic effects of nitrous oxide. *Brit. J. Anaesth.*, **35**, 631.
23. Eisele, J. H. and Smith, N. Ty. (1972). Cardiovascular effects of 40 per cent nitrous oxide in man. *Anesth. Analg. Curr. Res.*, **51**, 956.
24. Thornton, J. A., Fleming, J. S., Goldberg, A. D. and Baird, D. (1973). Cardiovascular effects of 50% nitrous oxide and 50% oxygen mixture. *Anaesthesia*, **28**, 484.
25. Kaul, S. U. and Coleman, A. J., (1975). Unpublished observations of the effects of nitrous oxide, oxygen, nitrogen mixtures.
26. Coleman, A. J. and Baker, L. W. (1973). Some cardiovascular effects of ornithine-8-vasopressin. *Brit. J. Anaesth.*, **45**, 511.
27. Lassen, H. C. A., Henriksen, E., Neukirch, F. and Kristensen, H. S. (1956). Treatment of tetanus. Severe bone-marrow depression after prolonged nitrous-oxide anaesthesia. *Lancet*, **1**, 527.
28. Amess, J. A. L., Burman, J. F., Rees, G. M., Nancekievill, D. G. and Mollin, D. L. (1978). Megaloblastic haemopoiesis in patients receiving nitrous oxide. *Lancet*, **2**, 339.
29. Sahenk, Z., Mendel, J. R., Couri, D. and Nachtman, J. (1978). Polyneuropathy from inhalation of $N_2O$ cartridges through a whipped-cream dispenser. *Neurology*, **28**, 485.
30. Layzer, R. B., Fishman, R. A. and Schafer, J. A. (1978). Neuropathy following abuse of nitrous oxide. *Neurology*, **28**, 504.
31. Layzer, R. B. (1978). Myeloneuropathy after prolonged exposure to nitrous oxide. *Lancet*, **2**, 1227.
32. Small, D. H., Carnegie, P. R. and Anderson, R. McD. (1980). Inhibition of protein methylation in myelin mimics lesions due to vitamin $B_{12}$ deficiency. *Proc. Aust. Biochem. Soc.*, **13**, 113.
33. Cohen, E. N., Brown, B. W. Wu, M. L., Whitcher, C. E., Brodsky, J. B., Gift, H. C., Greenfield, W., Jones, T. W. and Driscoll, E. J. (1980). Occupational disease in dentistry and exposure to anesthetic gases. *J. Amer. Dent. Assoc.*, **101**, 21.
34. Rector, G. H. and Eastwood, D. W. (1964). The effects of an atmosphere of nitrous oxide and oxygen on the incubating chick. *Anesthesiology*, **25**, 109.
35. Fink, B. R., Shepard, T. H. and Blandau, R. J. (1967). Teratogenic activity of nitrous oxide. *Nature*, **214**, 146.
36. Pope, W. D. B., Halsey, M. J., Lansdown, A. B. G., Simmonds, A. and Bateman, P. E. (1978). Fetotoxicity in rats following chronic exposure to halothane, nitrous oxide, or methoxyflurane. *Anesthesiology*, **48**, 11.
37. Lane, G. A., Nahrwold, M. L., Tait, A. R., Taylor-Busch, M., Cohen, P. J. and Beaudoin, A. R. (1980). Anesthetics as teratogens: nitrous oxide is fetotoxic, xenon is not. *Science*, **210**, 899.
38. Ramazzotto, L., Carlin, R. and Warchalowski, G. (1980). Effects of chronic exposure to nitrous oxide on gestation in the rat. *Fed. Proc.*, **39**, 506.
39. Viera, E. (1979). Effect of the chronic administration of nitrous oxide 0·5% to gravid rats. *Brit. J. Anaesth.*, **51**, 283.
40. Barach, A. L. and Rovenstine, E. A. (1945). The hazards of anoxia during nitrous oxide anesthesia. *Anesthesiology*, **6**, 449.
41. Tunstall, M. E. (1961). Obstetric analgesia. The use of fixed nitrous oxide and oxygen mixture from one cylinder. *Lancet*, **2**, 964.
42. Cole, P. V. (1964). Nitrous oxide and oxygen from a single cylinder. *Anaesthesia*, **19**, 3.
43. Tunstall, M. E. (1963). Effect of cooling on premixed gas mixtures for obstetric analgesia. *Brit. med. J.*, **2**, 915.
44. Parbrook, G. D. (1968). Therapeutic uses of nitrous oxide. *Brit. J. Anaesth.*, **40**, 365.
45. Parbrook, G. D. (1967). The levels of nitrous oxide analgesia. *Brit. J. Anaesth.*, **39**, 974.
46. Eger, E. I. (II) (1960). Factors affecting the rapidity of alteration of nitrous oxide concentration in a circle system. *Anesthesiology*, **21**, 348–358.
47. Priestley, J. (1779). *Experiments in Natural Philosophy, with continuation of the Observations on Air*. Vol. I.
48. Brown, W. E. (1923). Preliminary report on experiments with ethylene as a general anaesthetic. *Canad. med. Ass. J.*, **13**, 210.
49. Luckhardt, A. B. and Carter, J. B. (1923). Ethylene as a gas anesthetic: preliminary communication. Clinical experience in 106 surgical operations. *J. Amer. med. Ass.*, **80**, 1440.
50. Marshall, E. K. and Grollman, A. (1928). Method for

determination of the circulatory minute volume in man. *Amer. J. Physiol.*, **86**, 117.

51. Meyer, K. H. and Hopff, H. (1923). Theorieder Narkose durch Inhalationoanesthetika. *Hoppe-Seylers Z. physiol. Chem.*, **126**, 281.
52. Kety, S. S. (1951). Theory and application of exchange of inert gas at the lungs and tissues. *Pharmacol. Rev.*, **3**, 1.
53. Freund, A. (1882). Über Trimethylene. *Mschr. Chemie.*, **3**, 625.
54. Lucas, G. H. W. and Henderson, V. E. (1929). A new anaesthetic gas: cyclopropane. A preliminary report. *Canad. med. Ass. J.*, **21**, 173.
55. Henderson, V. E. and Lucas, G. H. W. (1930). Cyclopropane: a new anesthetic. *Curr. Res. Anesth.*, **9**, 1.
56. Jones, R. E., Guldmann, N., Linde, H. W., Dripps, R. D. and Price, H. L. (1960). Cyclopropane Anesthesia III. Effects of cyclopropane on respiration and circulation in normal man. *Anesthesiology*, **21**, 380.
57. Paskin, S., Skovsted, P. and Smith, T. C. (1968). Failure of the Hering-Breuer reflex to account for tachypnea in anesthetized man. *Anesthesiology*, **29**, 550.
58. Munson, E. S., Larson, C. P., Jr., Babad, A. A., Regan, M. J., Buechel, D. R. and Eger, E. I. (II) (1966). The effects of halothane, fluroxene and cyclopropane on ventilation. A comparative study in man. *Anesthesiology*, **27**, 716.
59. Price, H. L. (1961). Circulatory actions of general anesthetic agents. *Clin. Pharmacol. Ther.*, **2**, 163.
60. Fukunaga, A. F. and Epstein, R. M. (1974). Effects of cyclopropane on the sympathetic nervous system and on neural regulation of circulation in the cat. *Anesthesiology*, **40**, 323.
61. Li, T. H. and Etsten, B. (1957). Effect of cyclopropane anesthesia on cardiac output and related hemodynamics in man. *Anesthesiology*, **18**, 15.
62. Eger, E. I. (II) (1962). Atropine, scopolamine, and related compounds. *Anesthesiology*, **23**, 365.
63. Price. H. L., Lurie, A. A., Jones, F. E., Price, M. L. and Linde, H. W. (1958). Cyclopropane anesthesia. *Anesthesiology*, **19**, 619.
64. Price, H. L., Warden, J. C., Cooperman, L. H. and Price, Mary L. (1968). Enhancement by cyclopropane and halothane of heart rate responses to sympathetic stimulation. *Anesthesiology*, **29**, 478.
65. Price, H. L., Lurie, A. A., Black, G. W., Sechzer, P. H., Linde, H. W. and Price, M. L. (1960). Modifications by general anesthetics (cyclopropane and halothane) of circulatory and sympathoadrenal responses to respiratory acidosis. *Ann. Surg.*, **152**, 1071.
66. Miles, B. E., de Wardener, H. E., Churchill-Davidson, H. C. and Wylie, W. D. (1952). The effect of the renal circulation of pentamethonium bromide during anaesthesia. *Clin. Sci.*, **11**, 73.
67. Deutsch, S., Pierce, E. C. and Vandam, L. D. (1967). Cyclopropane effects on renal function in normal man. *Anesthesiology*, **28**, 547.
68. Shackman, R., Graber, I. G. and Melrose, D. G. (1953). Liver blood flow and general anaesthesia. *Clin. Sci.*, **12**, 307.
69. Price, H. L., Deutsch, S., Cooperman, L. H., Clement, A. J. and Epstein, R. M. (1965). Splanchnic circulation during cyclopropane anesthesia in normal man. *Anesthesiology*, **26**, 312.
70. Price, H. L. and Widdicombe, J. (1962). Actions of cyclopropane on carotid sinus baroreceptors and carotid body chemoreceptors. *J. Pharmacol. exp. Ther.*, **135**, 233.
71. Price, H. L., Warden, J. C., Cooperman, L. H. and Millar, R. A. (1969). Central sympathetic excitation caused by cyclopropane. *Anesthesiology*, **30**, 426.
72. Biebuyck, J. F., Dedrick, D. F. and Scherer, V. D. (1975). In: *Molecular Mechanisms of Anesthesia.* New York: Raven Press.
73. Matteo, R. S., Katz, R. L. and Papper, E. M. (1963). The injection of epinephrine during general anesthesia with halogenated hydrocarbons and cyclopropane in man. *Anesthesiology*, **24**, 327.
74. Halsey, M. J., Sawyer, D. C., Eger, E. I. (II), Bahlman, S. H. and Impelman, D. J. K. (1971). Hepatic metabolism of halothane, methoxyflurane, cyclopropane, ethrane and forane in miniature swine. *Anesthesiology*, **35**, 43.
75. Sawyer, D. C., Eger, E. I. and Bahman, S. H. C. (1971). *Metabolism of inhalation anesthetics.* Conference on Cellular Toxicity of Anaesthetics, Seattle, 1970.
76. Morton, W. T. G. (1847). *A memoir to the Academy of Sciences at Paris on a new use of sulphuric ether.* Reprinted by Henry Schuman, New York, 1946.
77. Morris, L. E. (1952). A new vaporiser for liquid anesthetics. *Anesthesiology*, **13**, 586.
78. Eger, E. I. (II), Shargel, R. and Merkel, G. (1963). Solubility of diethyl ether in water, blood and oil. *Anesthesiology*, **24**, 676.
79. Andrews, E., Potter, R. M., Friedman, J. E. and Livingstone, H. M. (1940). Determination of ethyl ether in blood. *J. Lab. clin. Med.*, **25**, 966.
80. Miller, R. N. and Thomas, P. A. (1967). Determination from lung extracts of patients receiving diethyl ether or halothane. *Anesthesiology*, **28**, 1089.
81. Larson, C. B., Jr., Eger, E. I. (II), Muallem, M., Buechel, D. R., Munson, E. S. and Eisele, J. H. (1969). The effects of diethyl ether and methoxyflurane on ventilation: II. A comparative study in man. *Anesthesiology*, **30**, 174.
82. Brewster, W. R., Jr., Isaacs, J. P. and Wainø-Andersen, T. (1953). Depressant effect of ether on myocardium of the dog and its modification by reflex release of epinephrine and nor-epinephrine. *Amer. J. Physiol.*, **75**, 399.
83. Black, G. W., McArdle, L., McCullough, H. and Unni, V. K. N. (1969). Circulatory catecholamines and some cardiovascular, respiratory, metabolic and pupillary responses during diethyl ether anaesthesia. *Anaesthesia*, **24**, 168.
84. Jorfeldt, K., Löfström, B., Möller, J. and Rosen, A. (1967). Propranolol in ether anesthesia. Cardiovascular studies in man. *Acta anaesth. scand.*, **11**, 159.
85. McArdle, L., Black, G. W. and Unni, V. K. N. (1968). Peripheral vascular changes during diethyl ether anaesthesia. *Anaesthesia*, **23**, 203.
86. Ngai, S. H., Hanks, E. C. and Farhie, S. E. (1965). Effects of anesthetics on neuromuscular transmission and somatic reflexes. *Anesthesiology*, **26**, 162.
87. Secher, O. (1951). The peripheral action of ether estimated on isolated nerve-muscle preparation. (IV.) Measurement of action potentials in nerve. *Acta pharmacol. (Kbh.)*, **7**, 119.
88. Karis, J. H., Gissen, A. J. and Nastuk, W. L. (1966). Mode of action of diethyl ether in blocking neuromuscular transmission. *Anesthesiology*, **27**, 42.
89. Secher, O. (1951). The peripheral action of ether estimated on isolated nerve-muscle preparation. (III.)

Antagonistic and synergistic action of ether and neostigmine. *Acta pharmacol. (Kbh.)*, **7**, 103.

90. Gross, E. G. and Cullen, S. C. (1943). The effect of anesthetic agents on muscular contraction. *J. Pharmacol. exp. Ther.*, **78**, 358.
91. Bunker, J. P., Forrest, W. H., Mosteller, F. and Vandam, L. D. (1969). The National Halothane Study, Washington D.C.: U.S. Government Printing Office.
92. Guedel. A. E. (1951). *Inhalation Anesthesia*, 2nd edit. New York: The Macmillan Co.
93. Mushin, W. W. (1948). The signs of anaesthesia. *Anaesthesia*, **3**, 154.
94. Laycock, J. D. (1953). Signs and stages of anaesthesia. A restatement. *Anaesthesia*, **8**, 15.
95. Gray, T. C. (1957). Reflections on circulatory control. *Lancet*, **1**, 383.
96. Lundy, J. S. (1926). Balanced anesthesia. *Minn. Med.*, **9**, 399.
97. Epstein, H. G. and Macintosh, Sir R. (1956). An anaesthetic inhaler with automatic thermo-compensation. *Anaesthesia*,**11**, 83.
98. Leake, C. D. and Chen, M. Y. (1930). Anesthetic properties of certain unsaturated ethers. *Proc. Soc. exp. Biol. (N.Y.)*, **28**, 151.
99. Gelfan, S. and Bell, I. R. (1933). The anesthetic action of divinyl oxide on humans. *J. Pharmacol. exp. Ther.*, **47**, 1.
100. Adriani, J. (1952). *The Pharmacology of Anaesthetic Drugs*, 3rd edit. Springfield, Ill.: Charles C. Thomas.
101. Kochmann, M. (1936). Narkotica der Fettreihe. *In* Heffter's *Handbuch der experimentellen Pharmakologie*. Berlin: Ergünzungswerk, Vol. 2.
102. Flourens, M. J. P. (1847). Note touchant l'action de l'éther sur les centres nerveux. *C. R. Acad. Sci. (Paris)*, **24**, 340.
103. Flourens, M. J. P. (1847). Note touchant l'action de l'éther injecte dans les artères. *C. R. Acad. Sci. (Paris)*, **24**, 482.
104. Heyfelder, F. (1848). *Die Versuche mit dem Schwefeläther, Salzäther und Chloroform, und die daraus gewonnenen Resultate in der chirurgischen Klinik zu Erlangen*. Erlangen.
105. Fischer, E. (1864). Ueber die Einwirkung von Wasserstoff aus Einfach-Chlorkohlenstoff. *Jena Z. Med. Naturw.*, **1**, 123.
106. Lehmann, K. B. (1911). Experimentelle Studien über den Einfluss technisch and hygienisch wichtiger Gase und Dämpfe auf den Organismus. Die gechlorten Kohlenwasserstoffe der Fettreihe nebst Betrachtungen über die einphasische und zweiphasische Giftigkeit ötherischer Körper. *Arch. Hyg. (Berl.)*, **74**, 1.
107. Plessner, W. (1915). Uber Trigeminuserkrankung infolge von Trichloräthylenvergiftung. *Neurol. Zbl.*, **34**, 916.
108. Oppenheim, H. (1915). Über Trigeminuserkrankung infolge von Trichloräthylenvergiftung (Discussion), *Neurol. Zbl.*, **34**, 918.
109. Jackson, D. E. (1934). A study of analgesia and anesthesia with special reference to such substances as trichlorethylene and vinesthene (divinyl ether), together with apparatus for their administration. *Curr. Res. Anesth.*, **13**, 198.
110. Striker, C., Goldblatt, S., Warm, I. S. and Jackson, D. E. (1935). Clinical experiences with the use of trichloroethylene in the production of over 300 analgesias and anesthesias. *Curr. Res. Anesth.*, **14**, 68.
111. Hewer, C. L. and Hadfield, C. F. (1941). Trichlorethylene as an inhalation anaesthetic. *Brit. med. J.*, **1**, 924.
112. Carney, T. P. and Gillespie, N. A. (1945). (Letter) *Brit. J. Anaesth.*, **19**, 39.
113. Firth, J. B. and Stuckey, R. E. (1945). Decomposition of Trilene in closed circuit anaesthesia. *Lancet*, **1**, 814.
114. Clayton, J. I. and Parkhouse, J. (1962). Blood trichloroethylene concentrations during anaesthesia under controlled conditions. *Brit. J. Anaesth.*, **34**, 141.
115. Malchy, H. and Parkhouse, J. (1969). Respiratory studies with trichloroethylene. *Canad. Anaesth. Soc. J.*, **16**, 119.
116. Greene, N. M. (1968). The metabolism of drugs employed in anesthesia. Part II. *Anesthesiology*, **29**, 327.
117. Edwards, G., Morton, H. J. V., Pask, E. A. and Wylie, W. D. (1956). Deaths associated with anaesthesia. A report on 1,000 cases. *Anaesthesia*, **11**, 194.
118. McArdle, L., Unni, V. K. N. and Black, G. W. (1968). The effects of trichloroethylene on limb blood flow in man. *Brit. J. Anaesth.*, **40**, 767.
119. Jennett, W. B., Barker, J., Fitch, W. and McDowall, D. G. (1969). Effect of anaesthesia on intracranial pressure in patients with space occupying lesions. *Lancet*, **1**, 61.
120. Helliwell, P. J. and Hutton, A. M. (1950). Trichlorethylene anaesthesia. *Anaesthesia*, **5**, 4.
121. Blønda1, B. and Fagerlund, B. (1963). Trichloroethylene anaesthesia and hepatic function. *Acta anaesth. scand.*, **7**, 147.
122. Ellis, M. W. and Bryce-Smith, R. (1965). Use of trichloroethylene inhalation during physiotherapy. *Brit. med. J.*, **2**, 1412.
123. Hovell, B. C., Masson, A. H. B. and Wilson, J. (1967). Trichloroethylene for post-operative analgesia. *Anaesthesia*, **22**, 284.
124. Atkinson, R. S., Beynon, D. G., Birt, R. C., Cameron, A., Alfred Lee, J., Rushman, G. B., Thorne, T. C. and Watt, M. J. (1979). Trichloroethylene: a most valuable agent. *Anaesthesia*, **34**, 903.
125. Prior, F. N. (1972). Trichloroethylene in air with muscle relaxants. *Anaesthesia*, **27**, 66.
126. Crawford, J. S. (1978). *Principles and Practice of Obstetric Anaesthesia*, 4th edit., p. 259. Oxford: Blackwell.
127. Simpson, J. Y. (1847). *Account of a new anaesthetic agent as a substitute for sulphuric ether in surgery and midwifery*. Edinburgh.
128. Bassett, H. L. (1949). Action of soda-lime on chloroform. *Lancet*, **2**, 561.
129. Cohen, E. N. and Hood, N. (1969). Application of low-temperature autoradiography to studies of the uptake and metabolism of volatile anesthetics in the mouse. I. Chloroform. *Anesthesiology*, **30**, 306.
130. Levy, A. G. (1913). The exciting causes of ventricular fibrillation in animals under chloroform anaesthesia. *Heart*, **4**, 319.
131. Johnstone, M. (1955). Some mechanisms of cardiac arrest during anaesthesia. *Brit. J. Anaesth.*, **27**, 566.
132. Hill, I. G. W. (1932). The human heart in anaesthesia. An electrocardiographic study. *Edinb. med. J.*, **39**, 533.
133. Waters, R. M. (1951). *Chloroform. A Study after 100 years*. Madison: Univ. Wisconsin Press.

134. Rollason, W. N. (1964). Chloroform, halothane, and hepatotoxicity. *Proc. roy. Soc. Med.*, **57**, 307.
135. Suckling, C. W. (1957). Some chemical and physical features in the development of Fluothane. *Brit. J. Anaesth.*, **29**, 466.
136. Sadove, M. S. and Wallace, V. E. (1962). *Halothane*. Philadelphia: F. A. Davis Co.
137. Robbins, B. H. (1946). Preliminary studies of the anaesthetic activity of fluorinated hydrocarbons, *J. Pharmacol. exp. Ther.*, **86**, 197.
138. Raventos, J. (1956). The action of Fluothane—a new volatile anaesthetic. *Brit. J. Pharmacol.*, **11**, 394.
139. Johnstone, M. (1956). The human cardiovascular response to Fluothane anaesthesia. *Brit. J. Anaesth.*, **28**, 392.
140. Bryce-Smith, R. and O'Brien, H. D. (1956). Fluothane. A non-explosive anaesthetic agent. *Brit. med. J.*, **2**, 969.
141. Eger, E. I. (II), Larson, P. and Severinghaus, J. (1962). The solubility of halothane in rubber, soda lime and various plastics. *Anesthesiology*, **23**, 356.
142. Dyjverman, A. and Sjövall, J. (1962). Estimation of Fluothane by gas chromotography. *Acta anaesth, scand.*, **6**, 171.
143. Robson, G., Gillies, D. M., Cullen, W. G. and Griffith, H. R. (1959). Fluothane (Halothane) in closed circuit anesthesia. *Anesthesiology*, **20**, 251.
144. Mapleson, W. W. (1962). The rate of uptake of halothane vapour in man. *Brit. J. Anaesth.* **34**, 11.
145. Van Dyke, R. A. and Chenoweth, M. B. (1965). Metabolism of volatile anaesthetics II. *Biochem. Pharmacol.*, **14**, 603.
146. Cascorbi, H. F., Blake, D. A. and Helrich, M. (1970). Differences in the biotransformation of halothane in man. *Anesthesiology*, **32**, 119.
147. Cohen, E. N. (1969). Halothane-$2^{14}C$ metabolism in the mouse. *Anesthesiology*, **31**, 560.
148. Severinghaus, J. and Cullen, S. C. (1958). Depression of myocardium and body oxygen consumption with Fluothane in man. *Anesthesiology*, **19**, 165.
149. Nunn, J. F. and Matthews, R. L. (1959). Gaseous exchange during halothane anaesthesia: the steady respiratory state. *Brit. J. Anaesth.*, **31**, 330.
150. Sandison, J. W., Sivapragasam, S., Hayes, J. A. and Woo-Ming, M. O. (1970). An experimental study of pulmonary damage associated with intravenous injection of halothane in dogs. *Brit. J. Anaesth.*, **42**, 419.
151. Price, H. L. (1960). General anaesthesia and circulatory homeostasis. *Physiol. Rev.*, **40**, 187.
152. Mahaffey, J. E., Aldinger, E. E., Sprouse, J. H., Darby, T. D. and Thrower, W. B. (1961). The cardiovascular effects of halothane. *Anesthesiology*, **22**, 982.
153. Morrow, D. H. and Morrow, A. G. (1961). The effects of halothane on myocardial contractile force and vascular resistance. *Anesthesiology*, **22**, 537.
154. Wenthe, F. M., Patrick, R. T. and Wood, E. H. (1962). Effects of anesthesia with halothane on the human circulation. *Anesth. Analg. Curr. Res.*, **41**, 381.
155. Brodkin, W. E., Goldberg, A. H. and Kayne, H. L. (1967). Depression of myofibrillar A.T.Pase activity of halothane. *Acta anaesth. scand.*, **11**, 97.
156. Black, G. W. and McArdle, L. (1962). The effects of halothane on the peripheral circulation in man. *Brit. J. Anaesth.*, **34**, 2.
157. Price, H. L. and Price, M. L. (1967). Relative ganglionic blocking potencies of cyclopropane, halothane, nitrous oxide and the interaction of nitrous oxide with halothane. *Anesthesiology*, **28**, 349.
158. Katz, R. L. and Katz, G. J. (1966). Surgical infiltration of pressor drugs and their interaction with volatile anaesthetics. *Brit. J. Anaesth.*, **38**, 712.
159. Ikezono, E., Yasudo, K. and Hattori, Y. (1969). Effects of propanolol on epinephrine-induced arrhythmias during halothane anesthesia in man and cats. *Anesth. Analg. Curr. Res.*, **48**, 598.
160. Deutsch, S., Goldberg, M., Stephen, G. W. and Wen-Hsien, W. U. (1966). Effect of halothane on renal function in normal man. *Anesthesiology*, **27**, 793.
161. Epstein, R. M., Deutsch, S., Cooperman, L. H., Clement, A. J. and Price. H. L. (1966). Splanchnic circulation during halothane anaesthesia and hypercapnia in normal man. *Anesthesiology*, **27**, 654.
162. Klide, A. M., Penna, M. and Aviado, D. M. (1969). Stimulation of adrenergic beta receptors by halothane and its antagonism by two new drugs. *Anesth. Analg. Curr. Res.*, **48**, 58.
163. Crawford, J. S. (1962). The place of halothane in obstetrics. *Brit. J. Anaesth.*, **34**, 386.
164. Vasicka, A. and Kretchmer, H. (1961). Effect of conduction and inhalation anesthesia on uterine contraction. *Amer. J. Obstet. Gynec.*, **82**, 600.
165. Marshall, F. N., Pittinger, C. B. and Long, J. P. (1961). Effects of halothane on gastro-intestinal motility. *Anesthesiology*, **22**, 363.
166. Graham, J. D. P. (1958). The myoneural blocking action of anaesthetic drugs. *Brit. med. Bull.*, **14**, 15.
167. Hanquet, M. (1961). The action of halothane on inhibitors of neuromuscular transmission (observations carried out in humans). *Anesth. et Analg.*, **18**, 461.
168. Katz, R. L. and Gissen, A. J. (1967). Neuromuscular and electromyographic effects of halothane and its interaction with *d*-tubocurarine in man. *Anesthesiology*, **28**, 564.
169. McDowall, D. G. (1967). Effects of clinical concentrations of halothane on the blood flow and oxygen uptake of the cerebral cortex. *Brit. J. Anaesth.*, **39**, 186.
170. Christensen, M.Stig., Høedt-Rasmussen, K. and Lassen, N. A. (1967). Cerebral vasodilatation by halothane anaesthesia in man and its potentiation by hypotension and hypercapnia. *Brit. J. Anaesth.*, **39**, 927.
171. McDowall, D. G., Barker, J. and Jennett, W. B. (1966). Cerebrospinal fluid pressure measurements during anaesthesia. *Anaesthesia*, **21**, 189.
172. Tyrell, M. F. and Feldman, S. (1968). Headache following halothane anaesthesia. *Brit. J. Anaesth.*, **40**, 99.
173. Moir, D. D. and Doyle, P. M. (1963). Halothane and post-operative shivering. *Anesth. Analg. Curr. Res.*, **42**, 423.
174. Jones, H. D. and McLaren, A. B. (1965). Postoperative shivering and hypoxaemia after halothane, nitrous oxide, oxygen anaesthesia. *Brit. J. Anaesth.*, **37**, 35.
175. Bay, J., Nunn, J. F. and Prys-Roberts, C. (1968). Factors influencing arterial $Po_2$ during recovery from anaesthesia. *Brit. J. Anaesth.*, **40**, 398.
176. Nunn, J. F., Dixon, K. L. and Louis, J. D. (1969). Effects of halothane on mitosis. *Anesthesiology*, **30**, 348.
177. Paterson, G. M., Hulands, G. H. and Nunn, J. F. (1969). Evaluation of a new halothane vaporiser. The Cyprane Fluotec Mark 3. *Brit. J. Anaesth.*, **41**, 109.
178. Hill, D. W. and Lowe, H. J., (1962). Comparison of

concentration of halothane in closed and semiclosed circuits during controlled ventilation. *Anesthesiology*, **23**, 291.
179. Eger, E. I. (1979). Editorial Views: Dragons and other scientific hazards. *Anesthesiology*, **50**, 1.
180. Brody, G. L. and Sweet, R. B. (1963). Halothane anesthesia as a possible cause of massive hepatic necrosis. *Anesthesiology*, **24**, 29.
181. Lindenbaum, J. and Leifer, E. (1963). Hepatic necrosis associated with halothane anesthesia. *New Engl. J. Med.*, **268**, 525.
182. Little, D. M. (1968). *Halothane*. Edited by Green, N. M. Philadelphia: F. A. Davis.
183. Klatskin, G. (1968). *Toxicity of Anesthetics*. ed. Fink, B. R. Baltimore: Williams and Wilkins.
184. Inman, W. H. W. and Mushin, W. W. (1974). Jaundice after repeated exposure to halothane: an analysis of reports to the Committee of Safety of Medicines. *Brit. med. J.*, **1**, 5.
185. Inman, W. H. W. and Mushin, W. W. (1978). Jaundice after repeated exposure to halothane: a further analysis of reports to the Committee of Safety of Medicines. *Brit. med. J.*, **2**, 1455.
186. Paronetto, F. and Popper, H. (1970). Lymphocyte stimulation induced by halothane in patients with hepatitis following exposure to halothane. *New Eng. Med. J.*, **283**, 277.
187. Klatskin, G. and Kimberg, D. V. (1969). Recurrent hepatitis attributable to halothane sensitization in an anesthetist. *New Engl. J. Med.*, **280**, 515.
188. Vergani, D., Tsantoulas, D., Eddleston, A. L. W. F., Davis, M. and Williams, R. (1978). Sensitisation to halothane altered liver components in severe hepatic necrosis after halothane anaesthesia. *Lancet*, **2**, 801.
189. Moult, P. J. A., Ajduckiewicz, A., Gaylarde, P. M., Sarkany, I. and Sherlock, S. (1975). Lymphocyte transformation in halothane related hepatitis. *Brit. med. J.*, **2**, 69.
190. Reeves, J. G. and McCracken, L. E. (1976). Failure to induce hepatic necrosis in animals sensitised to halothane and subsequently given halothane. *Anesth. Analg. Curr. Res.*, **55**, 235.
191. McLain, G. E., Sipes, I. G. and Brown, B. R. (1979). An animal model of halothane hepatotoxicity: role of enzyme induction and hypoxia. *Anesthesiology*, **51**, 321.
192. Bottinger, L. E., Dalen, E. and Hallen, B. (1976). Halothane induced liver damage: an analysis of material reported to the Swedish Adverse Drug Reaction Committee, 1973–1976. *Acta anaesth. scand.*, **20**, 40.
193. Trowell, J., Peto, R. and Crampton-Smith, A. (1975). Controlled trial of repeated halothane anaesthetics in patients with carcinoma of the uterine cervix treated with radium. *Lancet*, **1**, 821.
194. Wright, R., Chisholm, M., Lloyd, B., Edwards, J. C., Eade, D., Hawksley, L., Moles, T. M. and Gardner, M. J. (1975). Controlled prospective study of the effects on liver function of multiple exposure to halothane. *Lancet*, **1**, 821.
195. Joshi, P. H. and Conn, H. O. (1974). The syndrome of methoxyflurane associated hepatitis. *Ann. Int. Med.*, **80**, 395.
196. McEwan, J. (1976). Liver function tests following anaesthetics. *Brit. J. Anaesth.*, **48**, 1065.
197. Statement by the Medical Research Council (1976). Conclusions of a Working Party on the effects of repeated exposure to anaesthetics. *Brit. J. Anaesth.*, **48**, 1037.
198. Van Poznak, A. and Artusio, J. F. (1960). Anaesthetic properties of a series of fluorinated compounds. *Toxicol. appl. Pharmacol.*, **2**, 374.
199. Eger, E. I. (II), and Brandstater, B. (1963). Solubility of methoxyflurane in rubber. *Anesthesiology*, **24**, 679.
200. Gottlieb, S. F., Fegan, F. J. and Tieslink, J. (1966). Flammability of halothane, methoxyflurane and fluroxene under hyperbaric conditions. *Anesthesiology*, **27**, 195.
201. Walker, J. A., Eggers, G. W. N. and Allen, C. R. (1962). Cardiovascular effects of methoxyflurane anesthesia in man. *Anesthesiology*, **23**, 639.
202. Bagwell, E. E. and Woods, E. F. 1962). Cardiovascular effects of methoxyflurane. *Anesthesiology*, **23**, 51.
203. Miller, R. A. and Morris, M. E. (1961). A study of methoxyflurane anaesthesia. *Canad. Anaesth. Soc. J.*, **8**, 210.
204. Ngai, S. H., Hanks, E. C. and Brody, D. C. (1962). Effect of methoxyflurane on electromyogram, neuromuscular transmission and spinal reflexes. *Anesthesiology*, **23**, 158.
205. Cousins, M. J. and Mazze, R. I. (1973). Methoxyflurane toxicity. A study of dose response in man. *J. Amer. med. Ass.*, **255**, 1611.
206. Morrica, G., Cavaliere, R., Manni, C. and Massoni, P. (1962). Effects of methoxyflurane on the liver. *Gazz. int. Med. Chir.*, **67**, 1293.
207. Boisvert, M. and Hudon, F. (1962). Clinical evaluation of methoxyflurane in obstetrical anaesthesia: a report on 500 cases. *Canad. Anaesth. Soc. J.*, **9**, 325.
208. Denton, M. V. H. and Torda, T. A. G. (1963). Methoxyflurane: clinical experience in fifty orthopaedic cases. *Anaesthesia*, **18**, 279.
209. McCaffrey, F. W. and Mate, M. J. (1963). Methoxyflurane. A report of 1,200 cases. *Canad. Anaesth. Soc. J.*, **10**, 103.
210. Thomason, R., Light, G. and Holaday, D. A. (1962). Methoxyflurane anesthesia. *Anesth. Analg. Curr. Res.*, **41**, 225.
211. Jarman, R. and Edghill, H. B. (1963). Methoxyflurane (Penthrane): a clinical investigation. *Anaesthesia*, **18**, 265.
212. Campbell, M. W., Hvolboll, A. P. and Brechner, V. L. (1962). Penthrane. A clinical evaluation in fifty cases. *Anesth. Analg. Curr. Res.*, **41**, 134.
213. Virtue, R. W., Lund, L. O., Phelps, M., Jr., Vogel, J. H. K., Beckwitt, H. and Heron, M. (1966). Difluoromethyl 1,1,2-trifluoro-2-chloroethyl ether as an anaesthetic agent: results with dogs and a preliminary note on observations with man. *Canad. Anaesth. Soc. J.*, **13**, 233.
214. Brown, B. R. (1981). Halogenated analgesics and hepato-toxicity. *S. Afr. Med. J.*, **59**, 422.
215. Leonard, P. F. (1975). The lower limits of flammability of halothane, enflurane, and isoflurane. *Anesthesiology*, **54**, 238.
216. Stanford, B. J., Plantevin, O. M. and Gilbert, J. R. (1979). Morbidity after day-case gynaecological surgery. Comparison of enflurane with halothane. *Brit. J. Anaesth.*, **51**, 1143.
217. Chase, R. E., Holaday, D. A., Fiserova-Bergerova, V., Saidman, L. J. and Mack. F. E. (1971). The biotransformation of ethrane in man. *Anesthesiology*, **35**, 262.
218. Torri, G., Damia, G., Fabiani, M. L. and Frova, G. (1972). Uptake and elimination of enflurane in man. *Brit. J. Anaesth.*, **44**, 789.

219. Wolfson, B., Hetrick, W. D., Lake, C. L. and Siker, E. S. (1978). Anesthetic indices—further data. *Anesthesiology*, **48**, 187.
220. Hirshman, C. A., McCullough, R. E., Cohen, P. J. and Weil, J. V. (1977). Depression of hypoxic ventilatory response by halothane, enflurane and isoflurane in dogs. *Brit. J. Anaesth.*, **49**, 957.
221. Gold, M. I. (1970). Anesthesia for the asthmatic patient. *Anesth. Analg. (Cleve.)*, **49**, 881.
222. Rodriguez, R. and Gold, M. I. (1976). Enflurane as a primary anesthetic agent for patients with chronic obstructive pulmonary disease. *Anesth. Analg. Curr. Res.*, **55**, 806.
223. Lehane, J. R., Jordan, C. and Jones, J. G. (1980). Influence of halothane and enflurane on respiratory airflow resistance and specific conductance in anaesthetised man. *Brit. J. Anaesth.*, **52**, 773.
224. Mathers, J., Benumof, J. L. and Waahrenbrock, E. A. (1977). General anesthetics and regional hypoxic pulmonary vasoconstriction. *Anesthesiology*, **46**, 1.
225. Calverley, R. K., Smith, N. T., Jones, C. W., Prys-Roberts, C. and Eger, E. I. (1978). Ventilatory and cardiovascular effects of enflurane anaesthesia during spontaneous ventilation in man. *Anesth. Analg. (Cleve.)*, **57**, 610.
226. Calverley, R. K., Smith, N. T., Prys-Roberts, C., Eger, E. I. and Jones, C. W. (1978). Cardiovascular effects of enflurane anaesthesia during controlled ventilation in man. *Anesth. Analg. (Cleve.)*, **57**, 619.
227. Bedford, R. F. (1979). Sodium nitroprusside: haemodynamic dose-response during enflurane and morphine anaesthesia. *Anesth. Analg. (Cleve.)*, **58**, 174.
228. Karliczek, G., Hampelmann, G., Piepenbrock, S. and Büter, F. (1974). Die beeinflussung der hämodynamik durch enflurane bei myokardial vorgeschädigten patienten. *Anaesthesist*, **23**, 457.
229. Bennett, G. M. and Stanley, T. H. (1979). Cardiovascular effects of fentanyl during enflurane anaesthesia in man. *Anesth. Analg. (Cleve)*, **58**, 179.
230. Li, T. H., Shaul, M. S. and Etsten, B. E. (1968). Decreased adrenal venous catecholamine concentrations during methoxyflurane anesthesia. *Anesthesiology*, **29**, 1145.
231. Brown, B. R., jr. and Crout, R. J. (1971). A comparative study of the effects of general anesthetics on myocardial contractility. *Anesthesiology*, **34**, 236.
232. Su, J. Y. and Kerrick, W. G. L. (1980). Effects of enflurane on functionally skinned myocardial fibres from rabbits. *Anesthesiology*, **52**, 385.
233. Marshall, B. E., Cohen, P. J., Klingenmaier, C. H., Neigh, J. L. and Pender, J. W. (1971). Some pulmonary and cardiovascular effects of enflurane (Ethrane) anaesthesia with varying $Paco_2$ in man. *Brit. J. Anaesth.*, **43**, 996.
234. Reisner, L. S. and Lippmann, M. (1975). Ventricular arrhythmias after epinephrine injection in enflurane and in halothane anesthesia. *Anesth. Analg.* (*Cleve.*), **54**, 468.
235. Johnston, R. R., Eger, E. I. and Wilson, C. (1976). A comparative interaction of epinephrine with enflurane, isoflurane, and halothane in man. *Anesth. Analg. (Cleve.)*, **55**, 709.
236. Atlee, J. L. and Alexander, S. C. (1977). Halothane effects of conductivity of the AV node and His Purkinje system in the dog. *Anesth. Analg. Curr. Res.*, **56**, 378.
237. Neigh, J. L., Garman, J. K. and Harp, J. R. (1971). The electroencephalographic pattern during anesthesia with Ethrane: effects of depth of anesthesia, $Paco_2$ and nitrous oxide. *Anesthesiology*, **35**, 482.
238. Rudo, F. B., Krantz, J. C., Jr (1974). Anaesthetic molecules. *Brit. J. Anaesth.*, **46**, 181.
239. Kruczek, M., Albin, M. S., Wolf, S. and Bertoni, J. M. (1980). Postoperative seizure activity following enflurane anaesthesia. *Anesthesiology*, **53**, 175.
240. Ohm, W. W., Cullen, B., Amory, D. W. and Kennedy, R. D. (1975). Delayed seizure activity following enflurane anaesthesia. *Anesthesiology*, **42**, 367.
241. Burchiel, K. J., Stockard, J. J., Calverley, R. K. and Smith, N. T. (1977). Relationship of pre- and post-anesthetic EEG abnormalities to enflurane-induced seizure activity. *Anesth. Analg. (Cleve.)*, **56**, 509.
242. Stark, A. H., Storms, L. H., Calverley, R. K. and Smith, N. T. (1975). The effect of enflurane on psychological functioning. American Society of Anesthesiologists, 1975 Annual Meeting, *Abstracts*, p. 229.
243. Flemming, D. C., Fitzpatrick, J., Fariello, R. G., Duff, T., Hellman, D. and Hoff, B. H. (1980). Diagnostic activation of epileptogenic foci by enflurane. *Anesthesiology*, **52**, 431.
244. Wollman, H., Smith, A. L. and Hoffman, J. C. (1969). Cerebral blood flow and oxygen consumption in man during electroencephalographic seizure patterns induced by anesthesia with Ethrane. *Fed. Proc.*, **28**, 356.
245. Reinhold, H., de Rood, M., Capon, A., Mouawade, E., Fruling, J. and Verbist, A. (1974). The action of Ethrane (enflurane) on cerebral blood flow. *Acta Anaesth. Belg.*, **25**, 257.
246. Stullken, G. H., Milde, J. H., Michenfelder, J. D. and Tinker, J. H. (1977). The non-linear responses of cerebral metabolism to low concentrations of halothane, enflurane, isoflurane and thiopental. *Anesthesiology*, **46**, 28.
247. Coleman, A. J. and Downing, J. W. (1975). Enflurane anesthesia for cesarean section. *Anesthesiology*, **43**, 354.
248. Abboud, T., Henriksen, E., Kim, S. H., Chen, T. C., Levinson, G. and Shnider, S. K. (1979). Enflurane and halothane effects of placental transfer. *Anesthesiology*, **51**, (Suppl. S306).
249. Munson, E. S. and Embro, W. J. (1977). Enflurane, isoflurane and halothane and isolated human uterine muscle. *Anesthesiology*, **46**, 11.
250. Fogdall, R. P. and Miller, R. D. (1975). Neuromuscular effects of enflurane, alone and combined with d-tubocurarine, pancuronium and succinylcholine in man. *Anesthesiology*, **42**, 173.
251. Waud, B. E. (1979). Decrease in dose-requirement of d-tubocurarine by volatile anesthetics. *Anesthesiology*, **51**, 289.
252. Stanski, D. R., Ham, J., Miller, R. D. and Sheinter, L. B., (1979). Time-dependant increase in sensitivity to dTC during enflurane anesthesia. Abstracts of Scientific Papers, Annual Meeting of Society of Anesthesiologists, Paper No. 5269. *Anesthesiology*, **51**, (Suppl.), S3.
253. Cousins, M. J., Greenstein, L. R., Hitt, B. A. and Mazze, R. I. (1976). Metabolism and renal effects of enflurane in man. *Anesthesiology*, **44**, 44.
254. Norgate, C. E., Sharp, J. H. and Cousins, M. J. (1976). Metabolism of enflurane in man following a second exposure. *Anaesth. Intens. Care*, **4**, 186.
255. Carter, R., Heerdt, M. and Acchiardo, S. (1976). Fluoride kinetics after enflurane anaesthesia in healthy

and anephric patients and in patients with poor renal function. *Clin. Pharmacol. Ther.*, **20**, 565.
256. Lowry, C. J., Sharp, J. H., Shumacher, J. E. and Cousins, M. J. (1977). A dose-response study in man of the metabolism of enflurane used as a supplement. *Anaesth. Intens. Care*, **5**, 198.
257. Bentley, J. B., Vaughn, R. W., Miller, M. S. Calkins, J. M. and Gandolfi, A. J. (1979). Serum inorganic fluoride levels in obese patients during and after enflurane anaesthesia. *Anesth. Analg. (Cleve.)*, **58**, 409.
258. Wharton, R. S. and Mazze, R. I. (1979). Reproductive safety of enflurane in female mice. Abstracts of Scientific Papers, 1979. Annual Meeting. American Society of Anesthesiologists, paper No. S 261. *Anesthesiology*, **51** (Suppl.), S3.
259. Denlinger, J. K., Lecky, J. H. and Nahrwold, M. L. (1974). Hepatocellular dysfunction without jaundice after enflurane anaesthesia. *Anesthesiology*, **41**, 86.
260. Sadove, M. S. and Kim, S. I. (1974). Hepatitis after the use of different fluorinated anesthetic agents. *Anesth. Analg. (Cleve.)*, **53**, 336.
261. Danilewitz, M. D., Brande, B. M., Bloch, H. M., Botha, J. and Kew, M. C. (1980). Acute hepatitis following enflurane anaesthesia. *Brit. J. Anaesth.*, **52**, 1151.
262. Ona, F. V., Patanella, H. and Ayub, A. (1980). Hepatitis associated with enflurane anaesthesia. *Anesth. Analg. (Cleve.)*, **59**, 146.
263. Van der Reis, L., Skin, S. J., Frecker, G. N. and Fitzgerald, W. J. (1974). Hepatic necrosis after enflurane anesthesia. *J. Amer. med. Ass.*, **227**, 76.
264. Stevens, W. C., Cromwell, T. H., Halsey, M. J., Eger, E. I., Shakespeare, T. F. and Bahlman, S. (1971). The cardiovascular effects of a new inhalation anaesthetic in human volunteers. *Anesthesiology*, **35**, 8.
265. Corbett, T. H. (1976). Cancer and congenital anomalies associated with anesthetics. *Ann. N.Y. Acad. Sci.*, **271**, 58.
266. Eger, E. I., White, A. E., Brown, C. L., Biava, C. G., Corbett, T. A. and Stevens, W. C. (1978). A test of the carcinogenicity of enflurane, isoflurane, halothane, methoxyflurane, and nitrous oxide in mice. *Anesth. Analg. (Cleve.)*, **57**, 678.
267. Fiserova-Bergerova, V. (1973). Changes in fluoride content in bone. *Anesthesiology* **38**, 345.
268. Holaday, D. A., Fiserova-Bergerova, V., Latto, I. P. (1975). Resistance of isoflurane to biotransformation in man. *Anesthesiology*, **43**, 325.
269. Stevens, W. C., Dolan, W. M., Gibbons, R. T., White, A., Eger, E. I., Miller, R. D., De Jong, R. H. and Elashoff, R. M. (1975). Minimum alveolar concentrations (MAC), of isoflurane with and without nitrous oxide in patients of various ages. *Anesthesiology*, **42**, 197.
270. Fourcade, H. E., Stevens, W. C., Larson, C. P., Cromwell, T. H., Bahlman, S. H., Hickey, R. F., Halsey, M. J. and Eger, E. I. (1971). The ventilatory effects of Forane, a new inhaled anesthetic. *Anesthesiology*, **35**, 26.
271. Eger, E. I. (1981). Isoflurane: A review. *Anesthesiology*, **55**, 559.
272. Rehder, K., Mallow, J. D., Fibuch, E. E., Krabill, D. R. and Sessler, A. A. (1974). Effects of isoflurane anesthesia and muscle paralysis on respiratory mechanics in normal man. *Anesthesiology*, **41**, 477.
273. Kemotsu, O., Hasimoto, Y., Shimosato, S. (1973). Inotropic effects of isoflurane on mechanics of contraction in isolated cat papillary muscles from normal and failing hearts. *Anesthesiology*, **39**, 470.
274. Eger, E. I. (1981). Isoflurane (Forane): A compendium and reference. Madison, Wisconsin: Ohio Medical Products.
275. Tarnow, J., Bruckner, J. B., Eberlein, H. J., Hess, W. and Patschke, D. (1976). Haemodynamics and myocardial oxygen consumption during isoflurane (Forane) anesthesia in geriatric patients. *Brit. J. Anaesth.*, **48**, 669.
276. Blitt, C. D., Raessler, K. L., Wightman, M. A., Groves, B. M., Wall, C. L., Geha, D. G. (1979). Atrioventricular conduction in dogs during anesthesia with isoflurane. *Anesthesiology*, **50**, 210.
277. Tucker, W. K., Rackstein, A. D. and Munson, E. S. (1974). Comparison of arrhythmic doses of adrenaline, metaraminol, ephedrine and phenylephrine during isoflurane and halothane anesthesia in dogs. *Brit. J. Anaesth.*, **46**, 392.
278. Ivankovich, A. D., Miletich, D. J. and Grossman, R. K. (1976). The effect of enflurane, isoflurane, fluroxene, methoxyflurane and diethyl ether anesthesia on ouabain tolerance in the dog. *Anesth. Analg. (Cleve.)*, **55**, 360.
279. Adam, N. (1973). Effects of general anesthetics on memory functions in man. *J. Comp. Physiol. Psychol.*, **83**, 294.
280. Clark, D. L., Hosick, E. C., Adam, N., Castro, A. D., Rosner, B. S. and Neigh, J. L. (1973). Neural effects of isoflurane (Forane) in man. *Anesthesiology*, **39**, 261.
281. Davidson, L. A., Steinhelber, J. C., Eger, E. I., II, and Stevens, W. C. (1975). Psychological effects of halothane and isoflurane anesthesia. *Anesthesiology*, **43**, 313.
282. Murphy, F. L., Nelson, T. E. and Stroben, G. E. (1973). A comparison of halothane, isoflurane, enflurane, and fluroxene in triggering malignant hyperthermia in susceptible swine. *Abstracts of Scientific Papers*, Annual Meeting of American Society of Anesthesiologists, p. 181.
283. Adams, R. W., Cucchiara, R. F., Gronert, G. A., Messick, J. M. and Michenfelder, M. D. (1981). Isoflurane and cerebrospinal fluid pressure in neurosurgical patients. *Anesthesiology*, **54**, 97.
284. Raj, P. P., Tod, M. J. and Jenkins, M. T. (1976). Clinical comparison of isoflurane and halothane anaesthetics. *South Med. J.*, **69**, 1128.
285. Miller, R. D., Way, W. L., Dolan, W. M., Stevens, W. C. and Eger, E. I. (1971). Comparative neuromuscular effects of pancuronium, gallamine, and succinylcholine during Forane and halothane anesthesia in man. *Anesthesiology*, **35**, 509.
286. Byles, P. H., Dobkin, A. B., Ferguson, J. H. and Levy, A. A. (1971). Forane (Compound 469): 2. Biochemical effects of repeated administration to animals, reponse to bleeding, and compatability with epinephrine. *Canad. Anaesth. Soc. J.*, **18**, 387.
287. Steffey, E. P., Zinkl, J., Howland, J. L. (1979). Minimal changes in blood cell counts and biochemical values associated with prolonged isoflurane anesthesia of horses. *Am. J. Vet. Res.*, **40**, 1646.
288. Harper, M. H., Johnson, B. H. and Collins, P. (1980). Hepatic injury following halothane, enflurane, and isoflurane anesthesia in rats. *Anesthesiology*, **53**, S242.
289. Ames, B. N., McCann, J., Yamasaki, E. (1975). Methods for detecting carcinogens and mutagens with the Salmonella/mammalian microsome mutagenicity test. *Mutat. Res.*, **31**, 347.

290. Baden, J. M., Kelley, M., Wharton, R. S., Hitt, B. A., Simon, V. F. and Mazze, R. I. (1977). Mutagenicity of halogenated ether anesthetics. *Anesthesiology*, **46**, 346.
291. Dolan. W. M., Eger, E. I., II, and Margolis, A. J. (1972). Forane increases bleeding in therapeutic suction abortion. *Anesthesiology*, **36**, 96.
292. Palahniuk, R. J. and Shnider, S. M. (1974). Maternal and fetal cardiovascular and acid base changes during halothane and isoflurane anesthesia in the pregnant ewe. *Anesthesiology*, **41**, 462.
293. Price, H. L., Cook, W. A., Deutsch, S. (1963). Hemodynamic and central nervous actions of cyclopropane in the dog. *Anesthesiology*, **24**, 1.
294. Sprague, D. H., Ngai, S. H. (1974). Effects of cyclopropane on contractility and the cyclic 3′, 5′-adenosine monophosphate system in the rat aorta. *Anesthesiology*, **40**, 336.
295. Dorsch, J. A. and Dorsch, S. E. (1974). *Understanding Anaesthesia Equipment*. Baltimore: Williams & Wilkins Co.
296. Macintosh, R. R., Mushin, W. W. and Epstein, H. G. (1963). *Physics for the Anaesthetist*, 3rd edit. Oxford: Blackwell Scientific Publications
297. Ostlere, G. (1953). *Trichlorethylene Anaesthesia*. Edinburgh: E. & S. Livingstone.

CHAPTER 7

# Uptake and Distribution of Inhalational Anaesthetic Agents



Surgical anaesthesia continues to rely today mainly on drugs given by inhalation, but although the principles governing uptake and distribution of inhaled anaesthetics are often overlooked, an understanding of the fundamentals involved reveals valuable and diverse information on speed of induction, maintenance procedure, safety, and rate of recovery from a particular agent. It is possible to master techniques of inhalation anaesthesia by empiric methods, learning slowly by trial and error and adopting rules of thumb; but this approach is time consuming and potentially hazardous. The proper and rational way to learn is to base practical experience on a sound background knowledge of the principles involved. This chapter considers these principles in detail.

The goal in inhalational anaesthesia is the development of a critical tension of anaesthetic agent within the brain; depth of anaesthesia and its side-effects correlate closely with brain tension. The factors controlling brain levels are consequently of fundamental importance in applying techniques of inhalational anaesthesia. These can be considered in a logical sequence of four interrelated steps: firstly, the production and delivery of a suitable concentration of anaesthetic drug for inhalation; secondly, the factors influencing distribution of the agent to the lungs; thirdly, uptake therefrom, and finally, the delivery of anaesthetic agent from circulation to brain (Fig. 1).

## Form and Functions of Anaesthetic Systems

An anaesthetic system is a device for presenting a suitable anaesthetic mixture to the

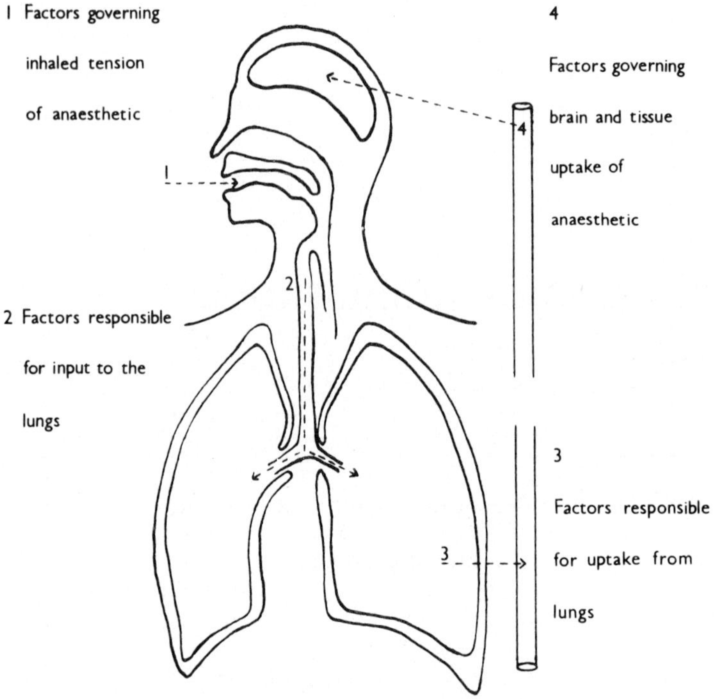


7/FIG. 1.—Diagrammatic illustration of the four factors influencing the brain tension of volatile anaesthetic agents and gases.

patient. Many different systems are available, and although the performance of each may be scrutinised and judged according to the criteria itemised in Table 1, we need here to consider only the factors affecting the inspired level of anaesthetic agent. The anaesthetic circuit and the manner in which it is used exert considerable influence because it is difficult to give a well-controlled anaesthetic without accurate knowledge of the inspired level of anaesthetic agent, and there are often considerable differences between the level of anaesthetic agent set by the anaesthetist on the machine, and the level actually inspired by the patient (see also Chapter 2).

7/TABLE 1
FUNCTION OF ANAESTHETIC SYSTEM

*Principal criteria*
1. PREDICTABLE INSPIRED ANAESTHETIC CONCENTRATION.
2. ELIMINATION OF CARBON DIOXIDE.
3. PREDICTABLE INSPIRED OXYGEN LEVEL.
4. ABILITY TO MONITOR OR CONTROL VENTILATION OF LUNGS.

*Secondary criteria*
5. ECONOMY OF EQUIPMENT AND DRUGS.
6. EASE OF CLEANING AND STERILISATION.
7. SIMPLICITY IN CLINICAL USE.
8. POLLUTION OF THEATRE ENVIRONMENT. (Noise and gases).

### Open Systems

Circuits which have no reservoir and do not permit rebreathing such as an open-drop mask, the insufflation method, and the Ayre's T-piece may be described as open systems. These systems are inexpensive, and simple in construction, but make prediction of inspired anaesthetic gas and oxygen levels difficult. Dilution of anaesthetic with ambient air may occur with high patient inspiratory flow rates, therefore it is difficult to maintain a steady level of inhalational anaesthetic agent.

### Semi-open Systems

Semi-open circuits such as the Magill (Mapleson-A), the Magill with non-rebreathing valve, the Jackson Rees modification of the Ayre's T-piece (Mapleson-E) all have a reservoir, and when properly used prevent rebreathing. Prediction of the inspired level of anaesthetic with these circuits presents no difficulty, it is the same as that set by the anaesthetist. These circuits do not suffer the defects of the open system, an increase in minute ventilation cannot dilute inspired anaesthetic gas concentration.

### Closed Systems

In addition to reducing theatre pollution, absorption of carbon dioxide gives a closed system great economic advantages over open and semi-open systems, but they are more cumbersome. If proper adjustments are made, they allow reduction of inspired anaesthetic gas levels to take any rebreathing into account.

### Vaporisers

Some vaporisers are more efficient than others. The familiar glass Boyle's bottle will deliver varying concentrations depending on such factors as temperature of the liquid, the vapour pressure, and the surface area exposed to vaporisation. Other vaporisers such as "the copper kettle" and "Fluotec" are more accurate because they can compensate for changes in temperature due to latent heat of vaporisation. The output of most modern vaporisers is not affected by the flow rate of fresh gas passing through them; however it should be noted that the efficiency of certain of the older types of vaporiser is reduced by either very low or very high fresh gas flow rates. When a vaporiser is used in conjunction with a closed circuit, it may be either placed within the circle sytem (vaporiser in circle, V.I.C.), or outside (vaporiser outside circle V.O.C.). In these circumstances inspired concentrations of anaesthetic may differ substantially from that set on the vaporiser controls, and depend upon a number of facts including the minute ventilation, and the fresh carrier gas flow rate.

## Delivery of Anaesthetic Agent to the Lungs and Alveolar Levels

For an understanding of the many factors involved in the uptake and distribution of anaesthetic agents the author acknowledges with gratitude the contribution and help of Dr. Eger and the publishers Williams & Wilkins Co.[1]

The tension of anaesthetic agent achieved within the lungs is of paramount importance because it is mirrored closely by levels within the brain; thus depth and some of the side-effects of anaesthesia correlate closely with the alveolar level. The alveolar level of an anaesthetic is the resultant of two entities: factors which promote delivery to the lungs on the one hand, and the factors which are responsible for uptake from the lungs on the other.

Delivery depends upon two factors: the inspired concentration, and the level of the alveolar ventilation.

### Effect of Inspired Concentration

The inspired concentration is of obvious importance, the rate of rise of anaesthetic drug within the lungs must bear some direct relationship to the concentration inspired. The "concentration effect" rules that the higher the inspired concentration, the more rapid the rise in alveolar concentration. Two elements are responsible for this: the first is a *concentrating* effect which is illustrated as follows:

Consider a mythical lung filled with 100 per cent of an anaesthetic agent. Under these conditions no matter how much or how little gas is removed by the circulation, the concentration in the lungs must remain at 100 per cent even though the lung gets smaller. If, however, this lung is filled with only 80 per cent anaesthetic agent, and the remaining 20 per cent is an insoluble diluent gas, then as the anaesthetic agent is absorbed, so the proportion must be altered as the amount of diluent gas remains the same. In other words, the diluent gas comes to represent a greater proportion of the whole and the concentration of anaesthetic gas must fall. Rate and degree of fall depends largely on the solubility of the particular anaesthetic agent in blood (Fig. 2).

The second element of the concentration effect is an increase in the input or inspired ventilation. When appreciable volumes of anaesthetic are taken up rapidly, the lungs do not collapse; instead subatmospheric pressure created by anaesthetic uptake causes passive inspiration of an additional volume of gas to replace that lost by uptake.

The concentration effect modifies the influence of uptake from the lung on rate of rise of alveolar concentration towards the concentration inspired. At low inspired concentration, the alveolar concentration results from a balance between ventilatory input and circulatory uptake: if the latter removes half the anaesthetic

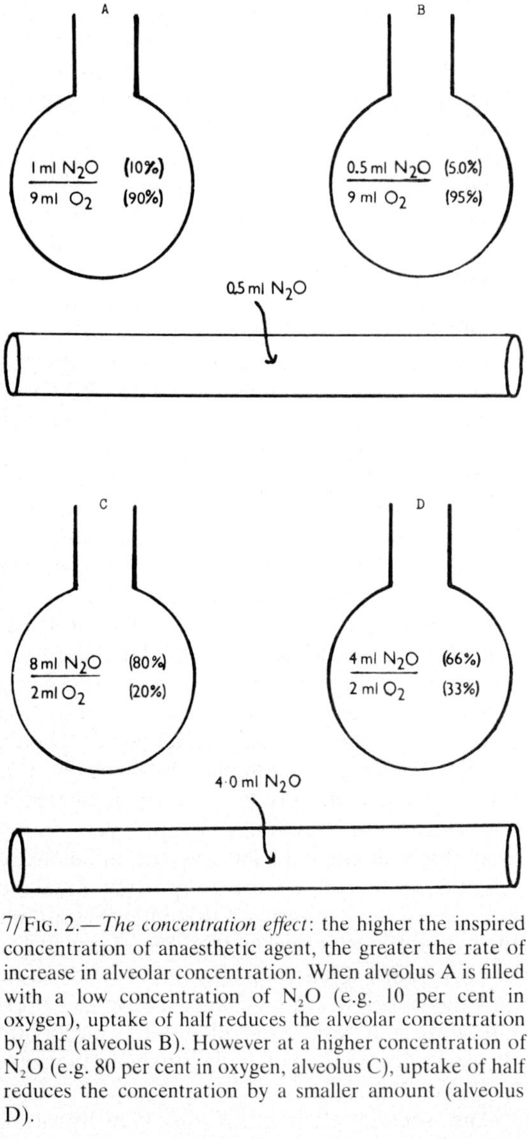


7/Fig. 2.—*The concentration effect*: the higher the inspired concentration of anaesthetic agent, the greater the rate of increase in alveolar concentration. When alveolus A is filled with a low concentration of $N_2O$ (e.g. 10 per cent in oxygen), uptake of half reduces the alveolar concentration by half (alveolus B). However at a higher concentration of $N_2O$ (e.g. 80 per cent in oxygen, alveolus C), uptake of half reduces the concentration by a smaller amount (alveolus D).

introduced by ventilation, then the alveolar concentration is half that inspired. The influence of uptake diminishes as inspired concentration increases. At 100 per cent inspired concentration, uptake ceases to influence the alveolar concentration, and the relationship of ventilation to functional residual capacity alone determines the rate of rise in concentration of anaesthetic within the alveoli (Figs. 3 and 4).

**Second Gas Effect**

Passive increase in inspired ventilation, due to rapid uptake of large volumes of anaesthetic (e.g. $N_2O$), may have secondary consequences when a second gas is given concomitantly (e.g. halothane). This increase in alveolar ventilation accelerates the rate of rise of the second gas regardless of its inspired concentration (Fig. 5).

**Effect of Ventilation**

The second factor governing the delivery of anaesthetic agent to the lungs is the level of alveolar ventilation. The greater the ventilation the more rapid the approach of the alveolar gas level to that which is inspired. This effect is limited only by lung volume; the larger the functional residual volume (FRC), the slower the wash-in of new gas. If uptake is ignored for the present, ventilation in the early moments of induction of anaesthesia produces a rapid increase in alveolar level of anaesthetic. Imagine a hypothetical lung with an FRC of 2 litres during induction of anaesthesia with 100 per cent nitrous oxide. Allow each breath to amount to 500 ml and alveolar ventilation to be 4 litres per minute. At the end of the first breath the alveolar concentration of nitrous oxide would be 20 per cent (500 ml $N_2O$+2000 ml FRC); at the end of the second breath 36 per cent (500 ml $N_2O$ introduced by ventilation plus 400 ml $N_2O$ already within FRC making 900 ml in a total of 2500 ml). By application of simple but tedious arithmetic, calculation of the concentration of $N_2O$ at the end of the first minute would be approximately 86 per cent. A quicker way of determining the rate of wash-in of a new gas would be to determine the *time constant*: in this context, the time constant is the time required for the flow (ventilation) through a container to equal the capacity of the container (Lung volume FRC). It is also the time required for 63 per cent wash-in of a new gas into the lungs. The time constant in the example above is half a minute, because it took half a minute for a 4-litre flow (4 l/min alveolar ventilation) to equal the 2-litre capacity of the container (FRC = 2 litres). In this example the concentration of $N_2O$ in the lungs after half a minute was 63 per cent; doubling this period to one minute allows the $N_2O$ concentration to increase to 86 per cent (63 per cent of difference between 63 per cent and 100 per cent) (Fig. 6).

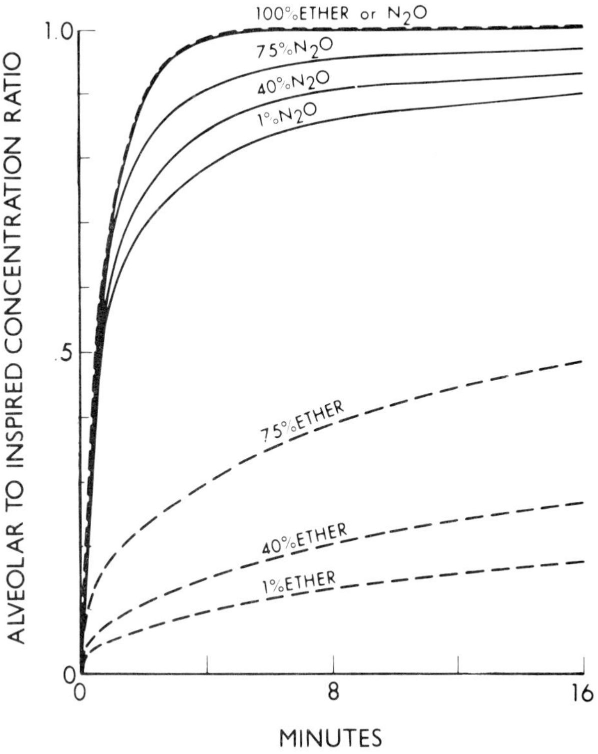


7/Fig. 3.—Increase in the inspired concentration of nitrous oxide and ether from 1 to 40 per cent and to 75 per cent increases the rate of increase of alveolar concentration. At 100 per cent inspired concentration, the rate of nitrous oxide and ether is identical and depends on rate of wash-in. (Courtesy of Dr. E. I. Eger and Williams & Wilkins Co.)[1]

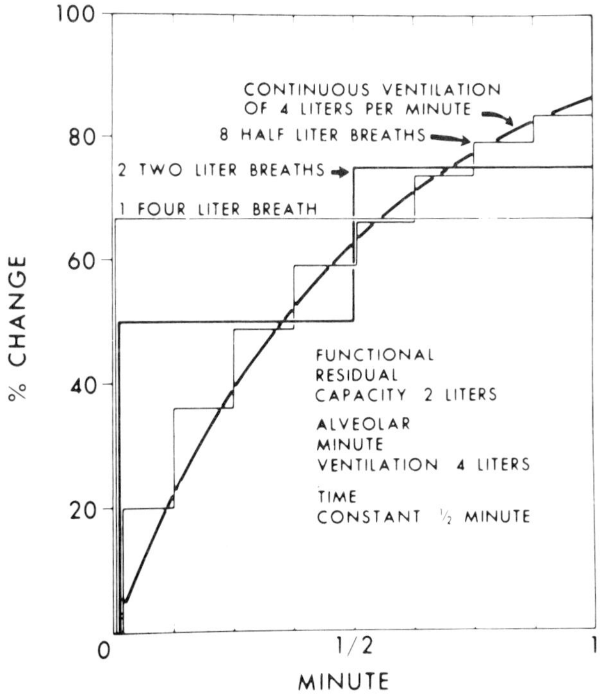


7/Fig. 4.—Rate of increase in alveolar concentration of an insoluble gas, expressed as a percentage of the inspired concentration, depends on the ratio of alveolar ventilation to functional residual volume. The larger the ratio, the greater the rate of rise of alveolar concentration. Size of tidal volume is relatively unimportant, two 2-litre breaths produce almost the same increase as 8 half-litre breaths. (Courtesy of Dr. E. I. Eger and Williams & Wilkins Co.)[1]

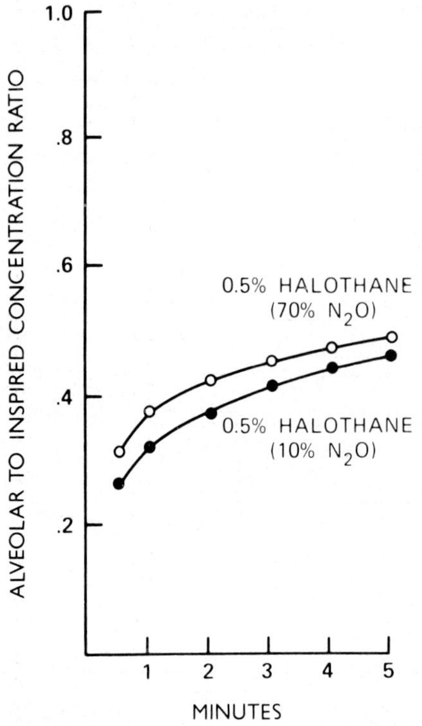


7/FIG. 5.—The second gas effect. The rate of increase in alveolar concentration of halothane is more rapid when it is administered together with 70 per cent compared with 10 per cent nitrous oxide. (Courtesy of Dr. E. I. Eger and Williams & Wilkins Co.)[1]

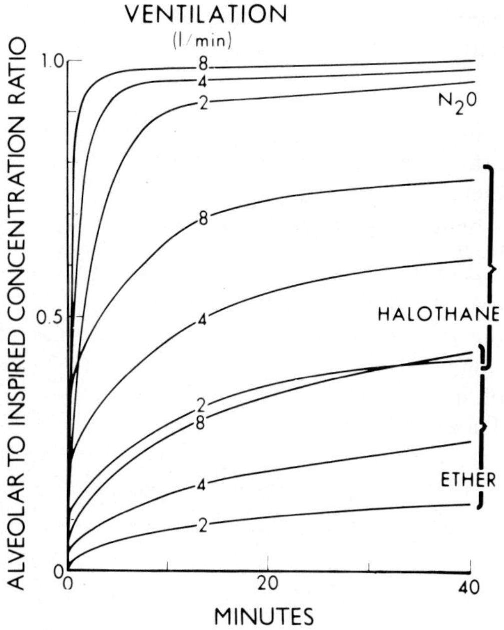


7/FIG. 6.—Influence of ventilation on alveolar level of anaesthetic agent. If uptake (cardiac output) is held constant, then rate of increase of alveolar concentration will be accelerated by increases in ventilation. This effect is greater with soluble anaesthetics. (Courtesy of Dr. E. I. Eger and Williams & Wilkins Co.)[1]

## Uptake of Anaesthetics from the Lung

As mentioned above, alveolar levels of anaesthetic are the result of rate of delivery on the one hand, versus rate of uptake on the other. Uptake from the lungs is the product of three factors: solubility of anaesthetic in blood, the cardiac output, and the difference between the level of agent in venous blood and the level in the alveolar gas. An increase in any of these factors will increase anaesthetic uptake and consequently will slow the rate of rise of alveolar tension.

### Solubility

There are a number of ways of expressing or describing the extent to which an anaesthetic will dissolve in blood and tissues. "Solubility" is the term used to describe how a gas or vapour is distributed between two media, for example between blood and gas or between tissue and blood. Figure 7 illustrates the derivation of the

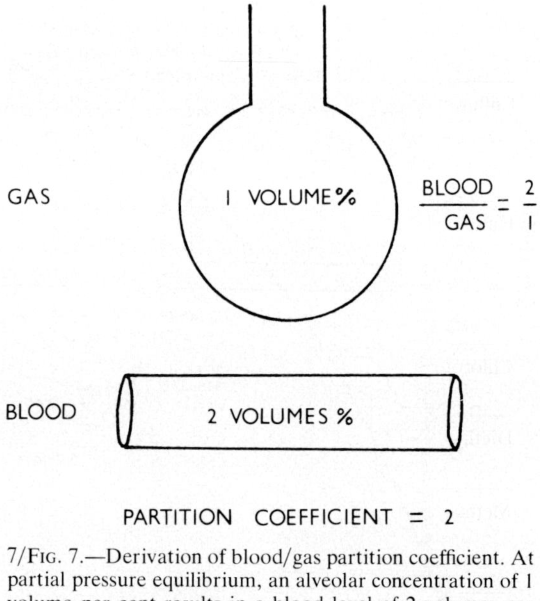


7/FIG. 7.—Derivation of blood/gas partition coefficient. At partial pressure equilibrium, an alveolar concentration of 1 volume per cent results in a blood level of 2 volumes per cent; the blood/gas partition coefficient is therefore 2.

blood/gas partition coefficient. At equilibrium, that is when the partial pressure of anaesthetic in the two phases is equal, concentration of anaesthetic in the blood was two volumes per cent, and in the alveoli was one volume per cent. The blood/gas solubility coefficient is therefore 2. Partition coefficients of some inhalational anaesthetics in common use are illustrated in Table 2. If other things are equal, the greater the blood/gas partition coefficient, the greater the uptake of anaesthetic, and the slower the rate of increase in the alveolar concentration. Table 2 also lists the anaesthetics in order of increasing blood gas partition coefficients. Those at the top of the list achieve their effects rapidly compared with those at the bottom, or higher coefficients result in slow inductions. This impediment to rapid induction may be partly or completely overcome by raising the inspired concentrations to levels well in excess of that required for maintenance of anaesthesia (overpressure). The importance of solubility on the behaviour of the drug in clinical practice is illustrated in the following examples: if an anaesthetic is totally insoluble in blood (i.e. blood/gas partition coefficient = 0), then none of it will be taken into the circulation; consequently the alveolar concentration will rise at a rate determined solely by ventilation and the functional residual volume and will soon equal the inspired concentration (Fig. 8). On the other hand, if an anaesthetic has a low blood solubility, then only small quantities can be carried by the blood stream, and both alveolar concentration and tension will consequently rise rapidly. As concentration determines the tension of the anaesthetic in the arterial circulation, the tension in the blood will also rise rapidly even though only a very small amount is present in the circulation. As this blood passes round the various tissues in the body, it gives up some of the anaesthetic molecules, so venous blood returning to the lungs has a reduced tension. Nevertheless, the fact that the venous blood contains some of the anaesthetic agent means that the tension gradient between it and the alveoli is necessarily reduced. Nitrous oxide and cyclopropane are examples of inhalational anaesthetics with low blood solubilities. When fixed concentrations of such gases are given, diffusion across alveolar capillary membranes is rapid. Because of the low blood solubility only a small quantity is absorbed, the alveolar concentration therefore rises rapidly so that the tension of the gas is also rapidly increased (Fig. 9).

If the gas or vapour has a high solubility, then large amounts can be absorbed just as though the blood were like a piece of blotting paper, so that it is difficult for the alveolar concentration to rise rapidly (Fig. 10). As concentration in the alveolus remains low, the tension in the blood is also low, so that induction of anaesthesia is slow.

Figure 11 illustrates this point further; the approach of alveolar concentration to the concentration inspired varies inversely with solubility. It is slow with a very soluble agent such

7/Table 2
Partition Coefficients of Some Inhalational Anaesthetics
at 37° C±0·5° C

| *Agent* | *Blood/Gas* | *Tissue/Blood* |
|---|---|---|
| Cyclopropane | 0·42 | 1·34 (brain)<br>0·81 (muscle) |
| Nitrous oxide | 0·47 | 1·0 (lung)<br>1·06 (brain)<br>1·13 (heart) |
| Fluroxene | 1·37 | 1·44 (brain) |
| Isoflurane | 1·41 | 2·6 (brain)<br>2·5 (liver)<br>4·0 (muscle)<br>45·0 (fat) |
| Enflurane | 1·78 | 1·45 (brain)<br>2·1 (liver)<br>1·7 (muscle)<br>36·2 (fat) |
| Halothane | 2·36 | 1·6 (kidney)<br>2·6 (brain)<br>2·6 (liver)<br>3·5 (muscle)<br>60·0 (fat) |
| Chloroform | 10·3 | 1·0 (heart)<br>1·0 (brain) |
| Diethyl ether | 12·1 | 1·2 (lung)<br>1·14 (brain) |
| Methoxyflurane | 13·0 | 1·34 (muscle)<br>1·70 (brain—grey)<br>2·34 (brain—white) |

(After Eger and Larsen)[2]

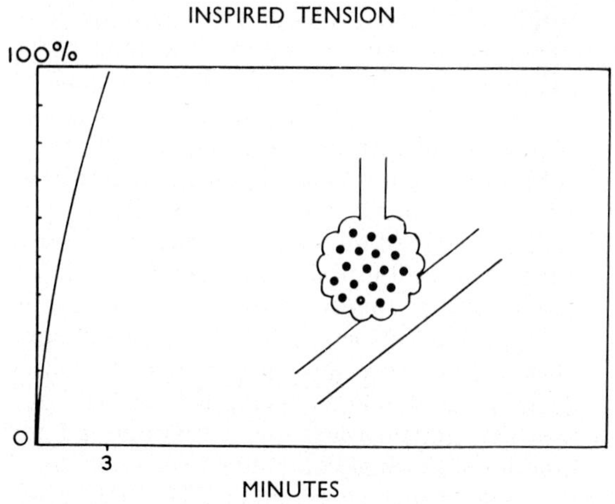


7/Fig. 8.—Rate of increase in alveolar tension of a gas which is totally insoluble in blood.

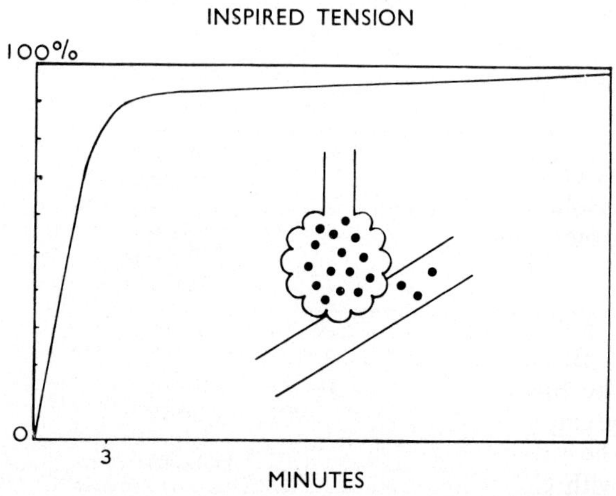


7/Fig. 9.—Rate of increase in alveolar tension of a gas which is poorly soluble in blood (e.g. $N_2O$).

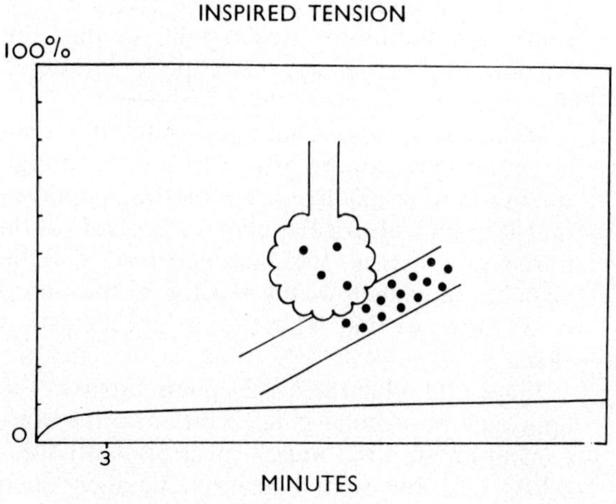


7/Fig. 10.—Rate of increase in alveolar tension of a gas which is highly soluble in blood (e.g. ether).

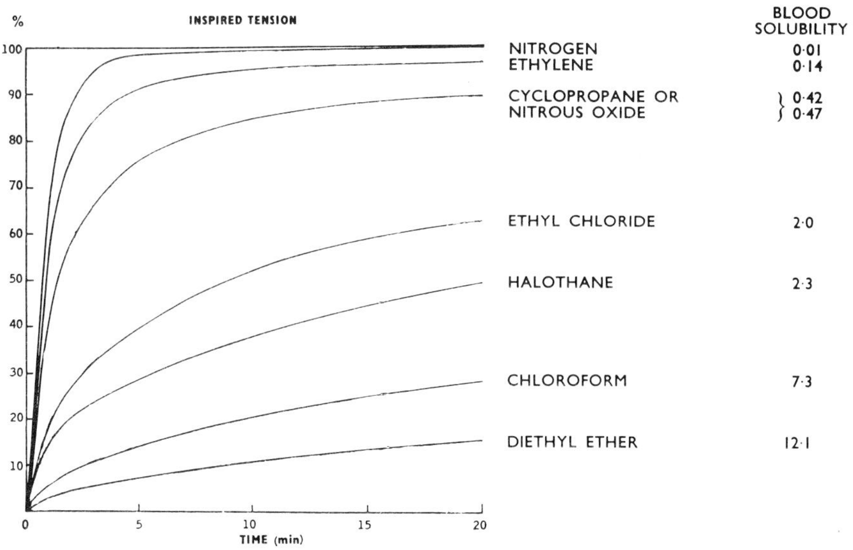


7/Fig. 11.—The influence of solubility of an anaesthetic agent on alveolar concentration. (After Bourne[3])

as ether, but quickly nears 100 per cent with insoluble agents like nitrous oxide or cyclopropane.

### Cardiac Output

Because blood carries anaesthetic away from the lungs, the greater the cardiac output, the greater the uptake, and consequently the slower the rate of rise of alveolar level (Fig. 12). As with changes in ventilation, the magnitude of this effect is related to solubility: the most soluble agents are affected more than the least soluble. This effect is more readily visualised at extremes of solubility. There is no uptake of a totally insoluble agent, and therefore changes in cardiac output do not affect the alveolar concentration. If an agent is highly soluble, then most of the anaesthetic molecules that reach the alveoli are taken up by the blood. Doubling the cardiac output cannot appreciably increase the extraction of an agent from the lungs because most of the molecules will have been absorbed anyway. This is illustrated in Fig. 12. Thus induction of anaesthesia in a patient with a high cardiac output, as for example an extremely nervous or thyrotoxic patient, will take longer than usual when a soluble agent such as ether is used. On the other hand if there is a low cardiac output (for example due to haemor-

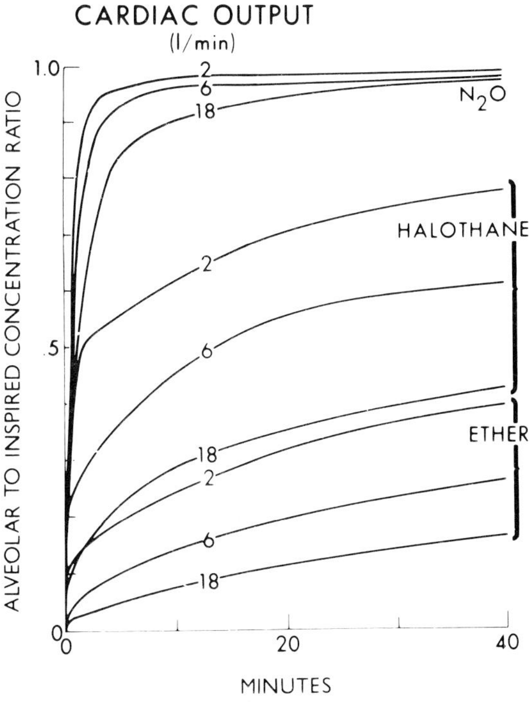


7/Fig. 12.—Influence of cardiac output on alveolar level of anaesthetic agent. If delivery (ventilation and inspired concentration) is held constant, then rate of increase of alveolar concentration will be retarded by increases in cardiac output. This effect is greater with soluble anaesthetics. (Courtesy of Dr. E. I. Eger and Williams & Wilkins Co.)[1]

rhage or heart disease) then the rate of induction of anaesthesia will be greatly increased.

**Influence of Alveolar to Venous Anaesthetic Difference**

The difference between the alveolar anaesthetic partial pressure and partial pressure in the returning venous blood is the third determinant of uptake. During induction the tissues remove nearly all the anaesthetic brought to them. This lowers the venous anaesthetic partial pressure far below that of arterial blood. The result is a large alveolar to venous anaesthetic partial pressure difference which causes the maximum anaesthetic uptake. As time passes, the increasing tissue anaesthetic concentrations reduce the rate of uptake and the anaesthetic concentration in venous blood rises. The resulting rise in venous anaesthetic partial pressure narrows the alveolar to venous difference and thereby reduces uptake.

### Delivery of Anaesthetic to Tissues

The uptake of anaesthetic from the lungs is equal to the sum of uptakes by the individual tissues. If the tissues were not removing the anaesthetic, then the blood would return to the lungs with as much anaesthetic as it carried away. The alveolar to venous difference would be zero, there would be no uptake, and the alveolar concentration would quickly approach the concentration inspired.

The uptake by the tissues is governed by the same considerations that determined uptake from the lungs; firstly the solubility of anaesthetic drug in the tissues, secondly tissue blood flow, and finally the anaesthetic partial pressure difference between arterial blood and tissue. An increase in any of these factors will increase uptake and vice versa. Similarly these factors may limit uptake; if a factor approaches zero then uptake must approach zero regardless of the magnitude of the remaining factors. Thus as tissues become saturated uptake must approach zero.

The capacity of the tissues to hold anaesthetic depends on the size of the tissue and on the affinity or the solubility of the anaesthetic in the tissue under consideration. Therefore the capacity of a tissue to absorb anaesthetic drugs equals the product of tissue solubility (tissue-blood partition coefficient) and tissue volume. The greater the solubility or the tissue volume, the greater the capacity of that tissue for the anaesthetic. In a tissue which has a large capacity and a small blood flow, the rate of rise of anaesthetic level is slow, permitting the tissue to continue to extract the anaesthetic for a long time. Conversely the rate of rise usually is rapid in highly perfused tissue, and uptake by such a tissue soon ceases.

Tissue-blood partition coefficients vary far less than blood/gas partition coefficients (ignoring fat which is relatively avascular). The lowest tissue-blood/gas partition coefficient is about 1 (nitrous oxide), and the highest about 4 (halothane). This means that the rate at which tissue anaesthetic partial pressure approaches the arterial level is fairly uniform for all anaesthetics, and depends on the blood supply to the tissue. It is possible on the basis of blood flow to tissues, and their volume, to assign each body tissue to a group, and in this way to get an idea of the contribution each group makes to overall uptake and to the mixed venous anaesthetic partial pressure of anaesthetic agent. In this way the tissues may be divided into four groups. There are tissues with an extremely good blood supply—the vessel rich group (VRG); a group made up of body muscle and skin which has a moderately good blood supply (MG); a group comprising skeleton, ligaments and cartilages with a negligible blood supply (VPG); and finally body fat which has a relatively poor blood supply, but by virtue of high solubility, relatively far greater capacity for absorbing anaesthetic drugs (FG). The VRG includes highly perfused tissues such as brain, heart, kidneys, splanchnic bed (including liver) and endocrine glands. Although these tissues make up only about 10 per cent of the total body mass, they receive about three-quarters of the cardiac output. The high flow per unit volume of such tissue results in a small time constant, and rapid equilibration to the arterial anaesthetic partial pressure. These organs cease to remove appreciable volumes of anaesthetic from the lungs within 5 to 15 minutes of induction of anaesthesia. The relationship between tissue blood supply and organ size is illustrated in Table 3. The importance of blood supply may be illustrated by considering uptake of a relatively insoluble agent such as nitrous oxide (Fig. 13). The initial uptake of nitrous oxide is undertaken by those organs with a large

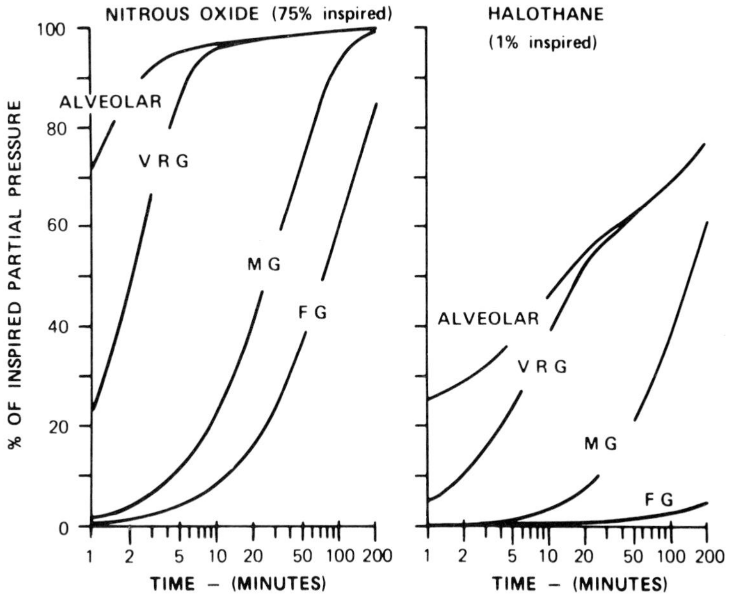


7/FIG. 13.—Influence of tissue uptake on alveolar level of anaesthetic agent. Tissue groups with relatively good blood supply (VRG) equilibrate to the alveolar tension more rapidly than the regions with relatively poor perfusion (MG and FG). Uptake into VRG tissues virtually ceases after 15 minutes for both nitrous oxide and halothane. Thereafter the muscle group dominates uptake. (Courtesy of Dr. E. I. Eger and Williams & Wilkins Co.)[1]

7/TABLE 3

| *Group* | *Region* | *Mass in kg* | *Per cent Cardiac output* |
|---|---|---|---|
| Vessel-rich | Brain | 1·4 | 14 |
| | Liver (splanchnic) | 2·6 | 28 |
| | Heart | 0·3 | 5 |
| | Kidney | 0·3 | 23 |
| Intermediate | Muscle | 31·0 | 16 |
| | Skin | 3·6 | 8 |
| Fat | Adipose tissue | 12·5 | 6 |
| Vessel-poor | Residual tissue | 11·3 | Nil |
| Total | — | 63·0 | 100 |

(After Bard)[4]

blood supply (e.g. brain), and equilibrium is established in about ten minutes. After this period, the importance of the intermediate group (e.g. muscle) becomes obvious, and these structures are responsible for a large proportion of the total anaesthetic uptake in succeeding minutes. In time, even these organs achieve equilibrium with the alveolar concentration and the task of further uptake finally falls upon fatty tissues. Fat depots, having a large lipoid content with special affinity for anaesthetic agents, continue to remove the drugs from the circulation for many hours.

The effect of tissue uptake on rate of alveolar rise of ether, halothane, cyclopropane and nitrous oxide is illustrated in Fig. 14. Dissimilarities in uptake caused by differences in solubility determine the position of each curve; the greater the solubility, the lower the alveolar concentration. Although the curves vary in position they have a common shape; the alveolar concentration initially rises rapidly regardless of solubility. Even the start of the ether curve shows this rapid upswing. The reason for this is that at the start of anaesthesia, the alveolar concentration is zero and remains low during the first few breaths. The alveolar to mixed venous anaesthetic partial pressure difference at this time is too small, and there is little uptake of anaesthetic. Without uptake, alveolar ventilation produces a rapid and unopposed increase in alveolar concentration. After a few minutes, however, a significant partial pressure difference develops and uptake increases in proportion with this difference. When uptake of anaesthetic from alveoli equals input by ventilation, a balance is achieved and the rapid rise in alveolar concentration slows consider-

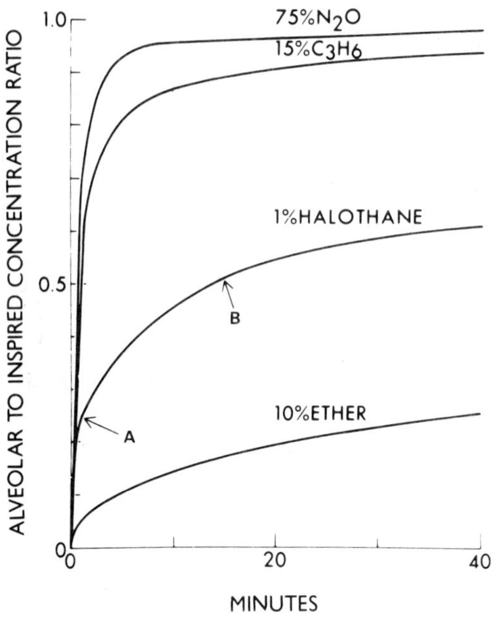


7/FIG. 14.—Influence of solubility of anaesthetic agent on shape and position of the alveolar concentration curves. The curves for nitrous oxide, cyclopropane, halothane and ether have different heights according to solubility, but are similar in shape. The rapid upswing to point A (halothane curve) is due to unopposed ventilation, whilst a slower continuing upswing to point B is due to uptake by VRG (vessel-rich group). The line continues with a slower uptake by MG (muscle) and FG (fat). (Courtesy of Dr. E. I. Eger and Williams & Wilkins Co.)[1]

ably. This results in the first bend or knee in the curves corresponding to point A on Fig. 14. If uptake were to continue at the same rate as at induction of anaesthesia, then the alveolar curves would plateau. However, because of the progressive and rapid saturation of the VRG, initial uptake is not maintained. As the vessel-rich group reaches saturation, 75 per cent of the blood returning to the lungs contains anaesthetic at the same partial pressure as when it left. This reduction in the tension difference between alveolar and mixed venous blood thereby reduces uptake, and continued ventilation of the lungs permits the alveolar concentration to rise. Thus equilibration of the VRG to the arterial anaesthetic tension is nearly complete within 5 to 15 minutes. A second bend or knee is then seen corresponding to point B in Fig. 14. Uptake now is into the MG and FG. Were uptake to these groups to continue indefinitely, there would be no further rise in the curves. It should be noted, however, that equilibration of muscle and fat has little influence on the alveolar partial pressure during the first hour of anaesthesia. The VRG saturation is of overwhelming importance during this time.

### The Effect of Abnormalities of Cardiopulmonary Function on Uptake of Anaesthetic Agents

Thus far uptake of anaesthetic agents has been considered against a background of ventilation, cardiac output and regional perfusion within the normal range. When disease or drugs adversely affect respiratory or circulatory function obviously there must be some change in anaesthetic uptake. The effect of certain changes in ventilation and cardiac output have been considered above. Here the effects of hyperventilation, ventilation-perfusion inequalities, reduced cardiac output, and changes in cerebral blood flow will be considered.

#### Hyperventilation and Cerebral Blood Flow

Although hyperventilation increases the rate at which an anaesthetic agent is delivered to the lungs, it also lowers the arterial carbon dioxide level which in turn reduces cerebral blood flow. Thus increasing ventilation twofold may halve both the arterial $CO_2$ and the cerebral blood flow. This reduction in cerebral perfusion delays the rate of rise of anaesthetic in the brain and thus opposes the tendency for the more rapid rise in alveolar anaesthetic concentration to hasten induction. The balance between these effects differs according to the solubilities of different anaesthetics. The effect of a modest increase in alveolar concentration of a poorly soluble agent such as cyclopropane or nitrous oxide produced by hyperventilation is more than offset by the reduction of cerebral blood flow, with the result that induction of anaesthesia is delayed. On the other hand the considerable rise in alveolar concentration induced by hyperventilation with a very soluble agent cannot be offset by reduced cerebral blood flow. Thus, induction of anaesthesia with methoxyflurane or ether is accelerated by hyperventilation. The intermediate solubility of halothane permits an almost perfect balancing of the increased alveolar anaesthetic rate of rise and reduced brain perfusion.

### Reduction of Cardiac Output and Cerebral Blood Flow

Uptake of anaesthetic from the lungs is reduced by low cardiac output thus increasing the rate of rise in alveolar partial pressure. However, when low cardiac output is associated with low cerebral blood flow, then the rate of transfer of anaesthetic agent from lung to brain is diminished. With soluble agents the increased rate of rise of anaesthetic agent within the lungs is sufficient to balance the effect of reduced cerebral perfusion. The initial rise in the brain, therefore, is normal; eventually however, the higher alveolar partial pressure resulting from a reduced cardiac output is associated with a higher brain level regardless of difference in solubility.

### The Effect of Venous Admixture

Some degree of venous admixture (physiological shunt) is normal, and is due to venous blood entering the left ventricle both from pleural, bronchial and thebesian veins, and from ventilation-perfusion mismatch, which together amounts to about 5 per cent of cardiac output. However, in many cardiopulmonary diseases and during anaesthesia venous admixture may be greatly increased (see Chapter 3). Referring to Fig. 15, all the anaesthetic agent is now being delivered to lung B. If the agent is soluble, the blood flow to that lung will take up an increased amount of the agent and so compensate to some extent for the blood flow from lung A which has taken up none of the agent. If the anaesthetic agent is insoluble, then partial pressure equilibration occurs rapidly between alveolar gas and alveolar capillary blood, limiting further uptake of the agent. The amount of the agent in the blood coming from lung B is therefore only slightly increased and cannot compensate for the absent uptake by blood passing through lung A.

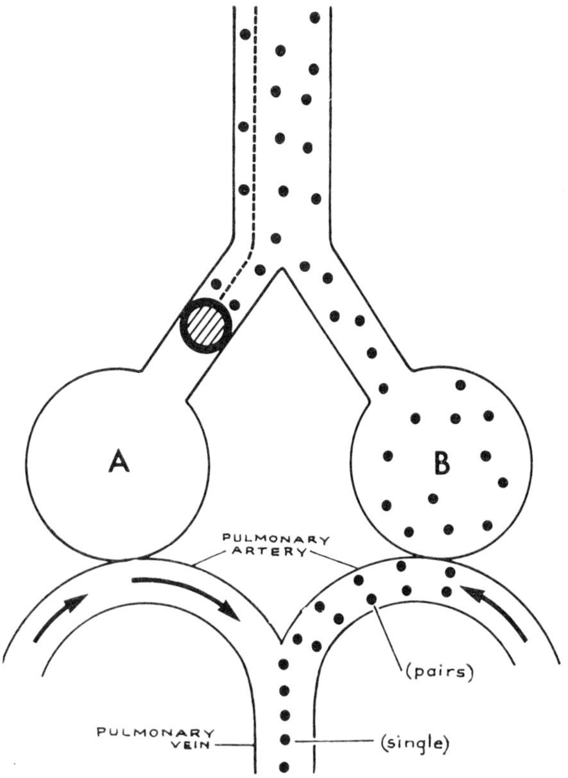


7/FIG. 15.—Effect of ventilation-perfusion inequality on uptake of anaesthetic agent. The dots represent molecules of anaesthetic agent.

### The Effect of Anaesthetic Agents on Air and Gases in Closed Body Cavities

Under normal circumstances, with the exception of the lungs, middle ear, sinuses, and intestines, there is no air in the various body cavities. However, during a pneumo-encephalogram, air is introduced into the ventricles of the brain; in a pneumothorax it is found in the pleural cavity, and in acute intestinal obstruction it accumulates in the lumen of the intestines. If such patients are anaesthetised with nitrous oxide and oxygen (70 per cent and 30 per cent), the anaesthetic gas will rapidly enter the enclosed space and the volume will increase. The reason for this is that nitrous oxide is 34 times more soluble than nitrogen in blood, but because of partial pressure difference between $N_2O$ in the blood and the air in the body cavity, a larger quantity of nitrous oxide will enter the gas cavity than nitrogen will diffuse out. When the wall of the cavity is elastic, as in the case of intestines, distention occurs, but when it is rigid there is an increase in pressure. Eger and Saidman[5] using 70–75 per cent nitrous oxide with oxygen for pneumo-encephalography in dogs, and in man, have shown that there is a dramatic rise in cerebral fluid pressure. Their finding suggested that this form of anaesthesia could cause a considerable increase in the cerebrospinal fluid pressure if used when air is present or injected into the ventricles; and that this rise in pressure might be clinically harmful in the presence of an already increased intracranial pressure. When the nitrous oxide is turned off, the cerebrospinal fluid pressure returns to its original value in about 10 minutes. Clinically, therefore, on the basis of this evidence, it would appear to be potentially harmful to use nitrous oxide/oxygen for a pneumo-encephalogram if air is to be used as a filling medium. However, this risk would be removed if either nitrous oxide or oxygen were used to outline the ventricles. Similar problems occur when a pneumothorax, pneumoperitoneum, or pneumopericardium are present or when air is trapped either in the middle ear, intestine or respiratory tract (Fig. 16).

### Recovery from Anaesthesia

When an inhalation anaesthetic is withdrawn at the end of surgery, the factors which affect elimination of the anaesthetic agent and recovery from anaesthesia are identical to those which were present during induction of anaesthesia. The effect of pulmonary ventilation to lower alveolar concentration is opposed by the same three factors which controlled uptake of drug from alveoli to blood. These are solubility of the anaesthetic agents in blood, cardiac output, and the venous to alveolar anaesthetic partial pressure difference. An increase in any one of these three factors will oppose the effect of ventilation, limit the fall in alveolar level, and

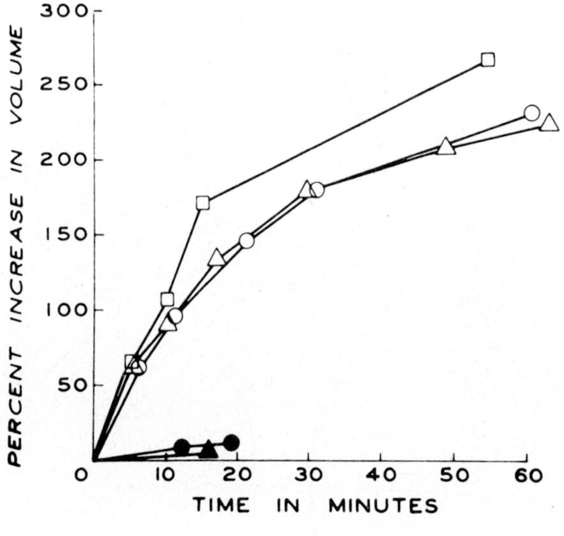


7/Fig. 16.—Intrapleural gas volume increases rapidly in the presence of 75 per cent nitrous oxide with halothane and oxygen (open circles, squares and triangles) but show little change when only halothane and oxygen is inspired (filled triangle and circles). (Courtesy of Dr. E. I. Eger and Williams & Wilkins Co.)[1]

thus prolong the time period for recovery from anaesthesia. The concentration effect which during uptake operated to increase uptake proportional to the inspired concentration has no effect on the output of the anaesthetic agent. However, there is a concentrating effect on non-anaesthetic gases; the outpouring of nitrous oxide at the end of anaesthesia may dilute the alveolar oxygen, thereby producing "diffusion hypoxia".

### Diffusion Hypoxia

At the end of an anaesthetic when the mask is withdrawn the patient breathes room air. The alveoli will soon become filled with a mixture of nitrogen, oxygen, carbon dioxide and water vapour. Nevertheless, there is still an appreciable quantity of nitrous oxide dissolved in the circulation and tissues because although nitrous oxide is always referred to as an insoluble anaesthetic agent, it is some 34 times more soluble than nitrogen. This means that blood can carry that much more nitrous oxide than nitrogen. Thus during the first few minutes of breathing air large quantities of nitrous oxide leave the body. Following an anaesthetic with a 75:25 per cent mixture of nitrous oxide and oxygen, as much as 1500 ml of nitrous oxide may be expired in the first minute, 1200 ml in the second and 1000 ml during the third. The net result of this exodus is that temporarily the volume of expiration exceeds that of inspiration, so that an increased volume of carbon dioxide is removed from the alveoli. This lowers the arterial carbon dioxide tension and thus reduces ventilatory drive, even producing apnoea.

The other and even more important effect of this mass movement of nitrous oxide into the alveoli is the dilution of alveolar oxygen tension. Normally in the alveoli there is approximately 14 per cent oxygen, but under these conditions the concentration may drop to as low as 10 per cent. This results in a degree of hypoxia which may be extremely dangerous in the elderly and critically ill (Fig. 17).

Clinically, diffusion hypoxia is only significant when nitrous oxide is employed, because this is the only anaesthetic agent that is commonly used in high concentrations. The effect is only likely to persist in a rapidly diminishing manner, for about ten minutes at the end of a nitrous oxide anaesthetic. After anaesthesia, in the presence of normal ventilation, diffusion hypoxia is of little significance in healthy patients; however when ventilation is depressed it becomes increasingly important. The adverse effects of diffusion hypoxia can be prevented by giving the patient oxygen for about five minutes after discontinuation of nitrous oxide, and the concomitant drop in alveolar carbon dioxide may be prevented by judicious addition of 5 per

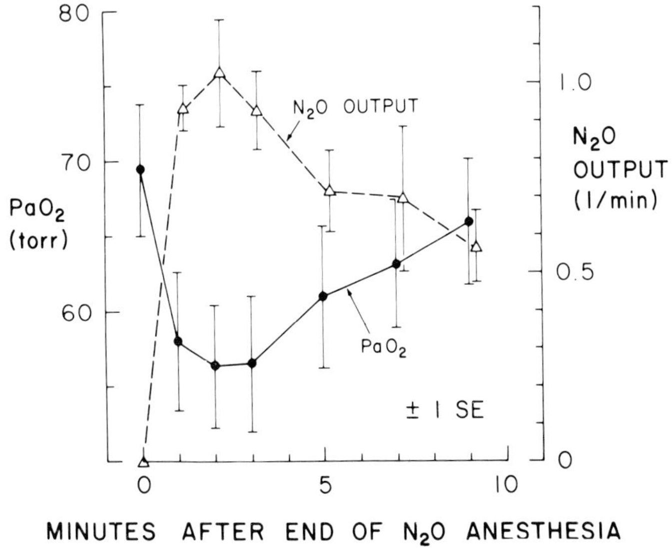


7/FIG. 17.—Diffusion hypoxia. A change in inspired gases from 21 per cent oxygen and 79 per cent $N_2O$ to 21 per cent oxygen and 79 per cent nitrogen causes a fall in arterial oxygen tension which at its nadir coincides with the period of maximum nitrous oxide excretion. (Courtesy of Dr. E. I. Eger (1974) and Williams and Wilkins Co.)[1]

cent carbon dioxide to the oxygen. This may be particularly important after controlled hyperventilation anaesthesia in which body stores of carbon dioxide are much depleted.

A reduced cardiac output or increased ventilation permits a more rapid fall in the alveolar anaesthetic concentrations. These changes may hasten recovery following anaesthesia with more soluble agents but the concomitant delay in tissue wash-out may retard recovery with poorly soluble agents. Concomitant increases in ventilation and circulation will accelerate recovery unless the increased perfusion is directed mainly to tissues of normally low perfusion, such as muscle or fat.

Finally, it should be noted that if a patient continues to breathe from an anaesthetic circuit at termination of anaesthesia, recovery may be delayed both by rebreathing and by the presence of anaesthetic vapour emerging from tubes and other components of the anaesthetic apparatus.

The point at which the patient is said to have recovered from anaesthesia is difficult to define. Safety aspects suggest a suitable endpoint to be the stage at which reflexes have recovered sufficiently for a patient to tolerate cardiopulmonary stresses. A patient cannot be regarded as recovered, for example, unless he can maintain a safe airway in all eventualities, and can tolerate postural changes without clinical signs of a drop in cardiac output. The anaesthetic level corresponding to this stage is unknown, but Eger[1] suggests that at "MAC awake" (the level at which a patient will obey a command), airways can be maintained without assistance. "MAC awake" appears to be about 0·6 of the MAC value of the particular anaesthetic.

**REFERENCES**

1. Eger, E. I. (II) (1974). *Anaesthetic Uptake and Action*. Baltimore: Williams and Wilkins Co.
2. Eger, E. I. (II) and Larson, C. P., Jr. (1964). Anaesthetic solubility in blood and tissues: values and significance. *Brit. J. Anaesth.*, **36**, 140.
3. Bourne, J. G. (1964). Uptake, elimination and potency of the inhalational anaesthetics. *Anaesthesia*, **19**, 12.
4. Bard, P. (1961). *Medical Physiology*, 11th edit., p. 240, St. Louis: C. V. Mosby Co.
5. Eger, E. I. (II) and Saidman, L. J. (1965). Hazards of nitrous oxide anesthesia in bowel obstruction and pneumothorax. *Anesthesiology*, **26**, 61.

FURTHER READING

Chenoweth, M. B., Ed. (1972). *Modern Inhalation Anaesthetics*. Berlin: Springer-Verlag.

Eger, E. I. (II) (1974). *Anaesthetic Uptake and Action*. Baltimore: Williams & Wilkins Co.

Papper, E. M., and Kitz, R. J., Eds. (1962). *Uptake and Distribution of Anesthetic Agents*. New York: McGraw-Hill.

Symposium and Pharmacokinetics of Inhalation Anaesthetic Agents (1964). *Brit. J. Anaesth.* (No. 3), **36**.

CHAPTER 8

# Environmental Hazards in the Operating Room



RISKS are involved whenever an anaesthetic is administered, because anaesthesia requires the depression of many of a patient's protective reflexes, in order to allow access to a given part by a surgeon. Other chapters describe how this access may be achieved with minimal risk to the patient from drugs and apparatus used to administer them. This chapter is concerned with acute risks to the patient and operating room staff which the reaction of anaesthetic techniques with the environment may produce, and risks to staff from prolonged exposure to unusual conditions.

## FIRES, EXPLOSIONS AND DETONATIONS

The first of such acute risks to be described was the explosion which could occur because of the flammable nature of some anaesthetics. These anaesthetics as well as some other agents, such as fluids used for skin or instrument cleaning, could also be involved in fires.

There is no essential difference between a fire and an explosion. A *fire* becomes an *explosion* if the combustion is sufficiently rapid to cause pressure changes which result in the production of sound waves. For example, paraffin poured on to a red coal fire will increase the rate of combustion sufficiently to make it "roar". Ether vapour and oxygen, in certain proportions, will, if ignited in a confined space, cause an explosion. In certain circumstances, the speed of combustion may be so high that a pressure wave is produced which ignites adjacent gas mixtures by compression rather than by the speed of a flame. Such combustion is extremely violent and is known as *detonation*. This phenomenon is similar to the compression ignition which occurs in diesel engines. Ether will detonate in certain circumstances in oxygen, but not in air.

The risk of an anaesthetic explosion in the United Kingdom has never been high. Even before the Report of the Working Party on Anaesthetic Explosions by the Ministry of Health[1] the risk of death from explosion of a flammable anaesthetic was less than one in three million. After the introduction of antistatic precautions which followed the publication of the Report of the Working Party and the introduction of halothane in the same year, the number of fires and explosions associated with anaesthesia fell to almost insignificant proportions in England and Wales. In 1966 and 1967 no explosion was reported. In 1968 there was one. Since 1968, no anaesthetic explosion had been reported in England and Wales until, in 1979, in an effort to avoid another risk—that of "pollution"—there was an explosion with ether. This was being scavenged by a passive system and was ignited by the blowlamp of a workman sealing bitumen close to the outlet. The ether bottle shattered, injuring three nurses with flying glass and a small fire developed near the patient, who, fortunately, appeared to be completely uninjured. The anaesthetist and operating department assistant were shocked and deafened for some time afterwards (Smith, 1981, Personal communication). This is a salutary reminder that steps to reduce one risk in the operating theatre may actually increase other risks. The last time a death was reported following an anaesthetic explosion was in 1964.

It is still necessary to discuss these risks, because ether and cyclopropane have their uses, and more detailed investigations into the flammability of newer compounds such as halothane, enflurane and isoflurane have shown that these and other drugs are not "non-flammable" in an absolute sense. Indeed some workers[2] have been able to make even nitrous oxide burn, given an ignition source of enormous energy (200 watts for 0·5–1·0 second), and others,[3] using 900 joules per second, have produced some combustion with halothane, enflurane and isoflurane in the presence of nitrous oxide, but no reliable combustion with pure oxygen. Such freak conditions would never be encountered in clinical anaesthetic practice, but whenever a new technique or apparatus is introduced into the operating room, its effect as an ignition source must be considered. At present, even the cautery has an energy of only approximately 20 watts and the energy produced by the carbon dioxide laser is of about the same order. It must be remembered that the laser beam gives off no energy until it hits something, so it will not ignite gases as it passes through them. However, the theoretical risk of flammability should not necessarily rule out the use of new volatile drugs which may have outstanding pharmacological advantages. For example, hexafluorobenzene[4] is a drug with interesting anaesthetic properties. It has been shown to support blood pressure and respiration and to be safe when adrenaline is used.[5] It has also been shown[6] to double cardiac output in ponies under deep anaesthesia. Although it is non-flammable in air, 6 per cent can be made to burn in oxygen, and about 4 per cent is needed to produce anaesthesia. This might be an acceptable risk in some circumstances.

### Flammable Anaesthetic Vapours

The essential conditions for an explosion are the presence, close enough together, of an *explosive mixture* and a spark of sufficient *energy*, or a surface hot enough to cause *ignition*. Whenever ether, cyclopropane, ethyl chloride or ethylene is used in anaesthetic concentrations, an *explosive mixture* is present, and even the low energy spark provided by static electricity (about 0·05 joules) is sufficient to cause *ignition*. Flammability limits of other drugs shown in Table 1 are either outside the anaesthetic concentrations or cannot be obtained in unheated vaporisers at room temperature (18–22° C). This table shows the flammability limits of inhalational anaesthetic drugs in air, oxygen and nitrous oxide. Nitrous oxide lowers the *lower* limit of flammability for each drug.

It is interesting and not always recognised that all inhalational anaesthetics in use today are more flammable in nitrous oxide than in oxygen. This is illustrated graphically in Fig. 1 where the flammability of halothane in oxygen/nitrous oxide mixtures at 20° C is shown. The experimental data, supplied by the manufacturers of Fluothane (halothane) only covered concentrations up to 20 per cent v/v. Extrapolation of this data to include all concentrations up to saturation at 20° C has been made. The concentrations of oxygen and nitrous oxide are given on the X-axis. 100 per cent oxygen is shown on the left; 100 per cent nitrous oxide on the right. The halothane concentration is given on the Y-axis and increases from 0–32 per cent v/v, the saturated vapour pressure concentration at 20° C. If atmospheric pressure is increased, the saturation vapour pressure of halothane is reduced. The two intermediate horizontal lines show the greatest concentration of halothane possible at 2 and 4 atmospheres pressure. The figures were obtained using a

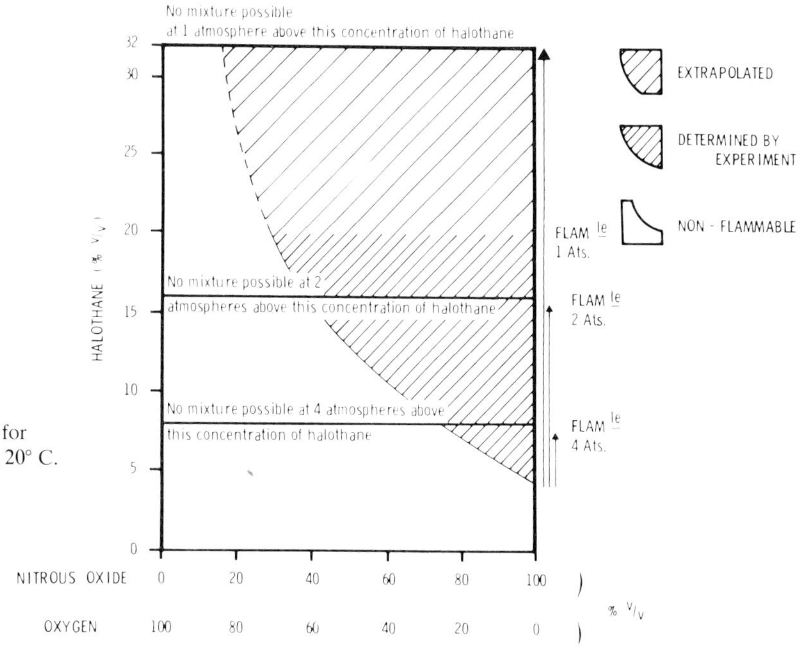


8/FIG. 1.—Flammability diagram for halothane in $O_2/N_2O$ mixtures at 20° C.

cerium-magnesium fusehead ignition source which can be regarded as having a total flash energy in the region of 80–120 joules. This is more powerful than any ignition source likely to be found in an operating theatre.

The figure also shows that 70 per cent nitrous oxide and 30 per cent oxygen would be safely non-flammable with up to 7 per cent halothane. If the cautery or laser is to be used in the patient's airway, it is just possible that the nitrous oxide concentration might rise and the halothane concentration reach 5 or 6 per cent and a fire might occur. To be absolutely safe, it would appear wise not to use nitrous oxide when using halothane for operations which involve the burning of tissue in the airway. The same remarks appear to apply to enflurane (Ethrane) and isoflurane (Forane), because 2·5 per cent enflurane and 4 per cent isoflurane have been made to burn in a 10 per cent oxygen/90 per cent nitrous oxide mixture, when an enormous energy source (900 watts) was used,[3] and the mixtures became progressively less flammable as the nitrous oxide concentration was reduced.

The addition of a non-combustible material, such as water vapour, to flammable mixtures of any kind will reduce their flammability. This led Miller and Dornette[7] to recommend the use of fluroxene in closed circuits even when the cautery is used. They claim that the water vapour present from the patient's expired gases raises the lower limit of flammability of fluroxene to 7·5 per cent.

A fully closed circuit, using proper antistatic equipment, makes it reasonable to use ether or cyclopropane when the lungs are not exposed if the anaesthetist feels that the pharmacological properties of these drugs are in the best interests of a patient.[8]

As well as flammable anaesthetic vapours in use on a patient, other combustible substances must be considered.

**Residual gases.**—Bracken and Wilton-Davies[13] showed that 29 ml of cyclopropane gas could be dissolved in 1 ml of liquid trichloroethylene at 20° C. If cyclopropane is run through a trichloroethylene vaporiser, an explosive mixture could be delivered during subsequent use. The risk would last for about three minutes, if a gas flow of eight litres per minute were used.

Cyclopropane and ether are adsorbed on to rubber, and a rubber hose recently used with these flammable gases will pass them into a subsequent gas mixture. It is wise to flush out

8/TABLE 1

| *Drug* | *Flammability limits in air per cent v/v* | | *Flammability limits in oxygen per cent v/v* | | *Flammability limits in 100% nitrous oxide per cent v/v* | |
|---|---|---|---|---|---|---|
| | lower | higher | lower | higher | lower | higher |
| Diethyl ether 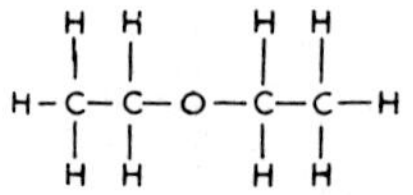 | 1·9 | 48·0 | 2·0 | 82·0 | 1·5 | 24·0 |
| Divinyl ether 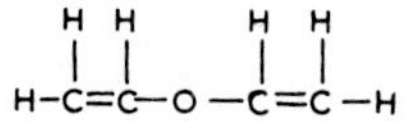 | 1·7 | 27·0 | 1·8 | 85·0 | 1·4 | 25·0 |
| Cyclopropane 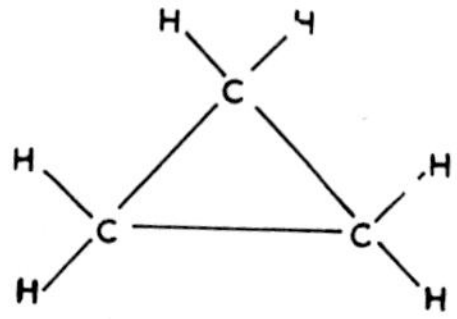 | 2·4 | 10·4 | 2·5 | 60·0 | — | — |
| Ethyl chloride 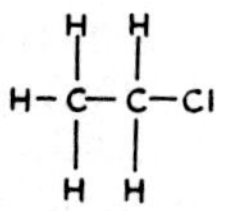 | 3·8 | 15·4 | 4·0 | 67·0 | 2·0 | 33·0 |
| Trifluoro-ethyl-vinyl-ether, fluroxene (Fluoromar) 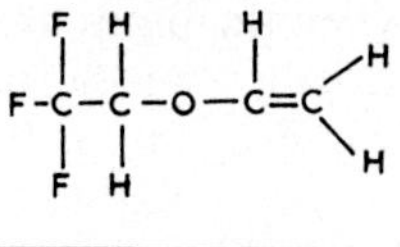 | 3·0 (Krantz *et al.*, 1953[9]) | — | 4·5 (Miller and Dornette, 1961[7]) | 80·0 | — | — |
| Ethylene 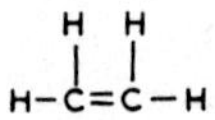 | 3·1 | 32·0 | 3·0 | 80·0 | 1·9 | 40·0 |
| Trichloroethylene (Trilene) 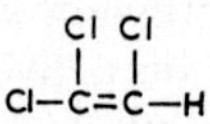 | non-flammable | | 10·0 | 65·0 | 2·0/2·5* | |

These values are taken from the U.S. Bureau of Mines Bulletin 503, Washington 1952, except for those marked (*) which are manufacturers' figures and those for the last four compounds, where other references are given. Although figures are given for lower limits of flammability in oxygen for trichloroethylene and in air and oxygen for methoxyflurane, it should be remembered that these concentrations cannot be obtained in unheated vaporisers at normal operating theatre temperatures (18–22° C).

8/TABLE 1 (*continued*)

| *Drug* | LOWER FLAMMABILITY LIMITS IN: | | |
|---|---|---|---|
| | *air per cent v/v* | *oxygen per cent v/v* | *70 per cent nitrous oxide with 30 per cent oxygen per cent v/v* |
| Halothane (Fluothane) 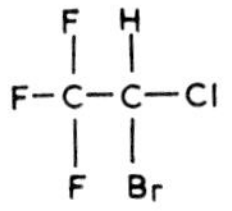 | non-flammable* | non-flammable* | 8·5 |
| Methoxyflurane (Penthrane) 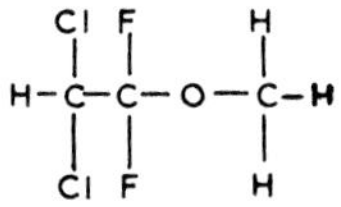 | 9·0* | 5·2* | 4·0* |
| Enflurane (Ethrane) 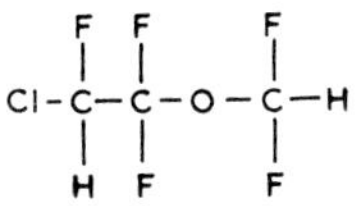 | non-flammable† | 9·75† | 5·75† |
| Isoflurane (Forane) 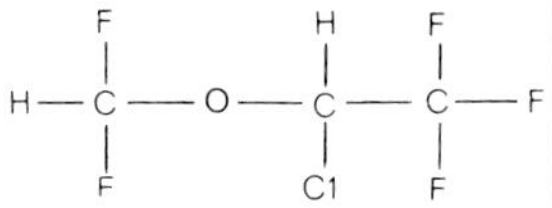 | non-flammable† | 8·75† | 7·0† |
| Halopropane 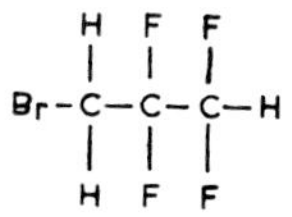 | non-flammable (Fabian *et al.*[12]) | | |
| Teflurane 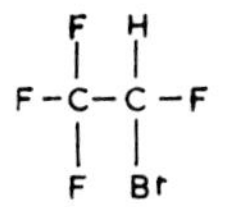 | "non-flammable" (Artusio, 1963[10]) | | |

†Leonard, 1975.[11]

**Anaesthesia at hyperbaric pressures.**—The manufacturers of Fluothane (halothane) give the following recommendation for this drug when it is used with oxygen in hyperbaric conditions up to 4 atmospheres pressure and at ordinary temperatures: "In small volumes, such as closed circuit anaesthetic equipment, the concentration of Fluothane should not exceed 2 per cent v/v; in large volumes, any concentration up to that given by its saturated vapour pressure may by used." They do not recommend the use of oxygen/nitrous oxide mixtures with halothane at hyperbaric pressures.

rubber hoses and breathing bags with oxygen before use.

**Persistence of flammable exhalation.**—Vickers,[14] and Nicholson and Crehan[15] have shown that even after long periods of cylopropane or ether administration the exhaled flammable agent is present in the patient's breath at concentrations well below those which are flammable, once the patient has breathed a non-flammable mixture for five minutes.

**Body gases.**—Carroll[16] describes an incident when a patient with a distended stomach had it opened with diathermy. The gases which escaped were ignited, and burned for some ten seconds with an intense blue flame. A loud explosion was heard outside the operating room. Gases present in the alimentary tract include hydrogen and methane, both of which are flammable. Woodward[17] proposed a scheme for clearing the bowel, and introducing carbon dioxide. In the absence of such precautions, some would question whether diathermy should be used for opening the stomach or large intestine.

### Other Flammable Substances

(*a*) Drapes which cover expiratory valves emitting oxygen or nitrous oxide and oxygen have been known to catch fire and have caused damage to patients when the cautery has been used. It is recommended that a closed gas system be employed if drapes are put near the head and neck, or the gases be vented well away from the material.[18]

(*b*) Some skin-cleaning solutions are flammable, and the diathermy can ignite their vapour if a pool of the liquid is allowed to remain when the diathermy is used.

## Prevention

Fires in operating theatres may be prevented in three main ways—the use of non-flammable gas mixtures, the elimination of every sort of spark or flame of sufficient energy to ignite any flammable mixture which might be present, or the separation at a safe distance of flammable gases from ignition sources.

### Non-flammable Gas Mixtures

There is no doubt that from a physical point of view the soundest method of preventing explosions is to use drugs which cannot be made to burn in any circumstances in the operating room; but the prevention of explosions is by no means the only problem for the anaesthetist. Many regard ether or cyclopropane, or both, as indispensable to the production of good anaesthesia in certain cases, and there are occasions when the physiological risk to the patient of a non-explosive anaesthetic is greater than the risk of an explosion. Vapours with highly desirable pharmacological properties, but capable of ignition, may be discovered. In such cases, if the diathermy can be dispensed with, or its spark kept at a safe distance, without increasing the risk to the patient, a flammable agent may be the drug of choice. In such a case, both the surgeon and anaesthetist must be prepared to understand the other's problems. The removal of a foreign body from the lungs of an infant may call for the use of ether, and cyclopropane is a very safe and pleasant induction agent for many children, as well as being preferred by some anaesthetists for poor-risk patients.

**A non-flammable theatre.**—It has been suggested that if a group of anaesthetists agreed to use only non-flammable drugs, their operating rooms need not be designed to eliminate sources of ignition. But such a suggestion is not without risk. A visiting anaesthetist, in the habit of using ether or cyclopropane, might well come to work in such theatres and not be in agreement with the view that flammable gases are unnecessary, or he might forget the limitations of the theatres. Furthermore, if a new drug were introduced, having extremely desirable pharmacological properties but ignitable in some extreme conditions, the existence of such theatres might stand in the way of progress in clinical anaesthesia.

**Existing non-flammable drugs.**—Although the introduction into clinical use of halothane and other fluorinated anaesthetics has greatly simplified the problem, it has not completely solved it. The pharmacological properties of drugs available are sometimes considered to be unsuitable for certain patients.

**New drugs.**—The most promising method of removing all flammable mixtures from the operating room is the discovery of new drugs. Shortly after the end of the Second World War, the introduction of tubocurare into clinical use made it possible to provide good operating conditions for the surgeon with analgesia and safety for the patient. The only gases involved were nitrous oxide and oxygen, which are completely non-flammable in clinical use.

During the war, fluorinated hydrocarbons were studied in an effort to produce non-flammable lubricants and refrigerants. When it was realised that the substitution of fluorine for hydrogen did not significantly alter the properties of the compounds, apart from making them less "reactive", the possibility of producing a non-flammable ether was investigated. Go Lu and colleagues[19] were among the first to demonstrate the anaesthetic properties of fluorinated hydrocarbons. The most promising of those he investigated was trifluoroethyl vinyl ether (fluroxene—Fluoromar) which contains three fluorine atoms in place of three hydrogen atoms. Its formula is given in Table 1. Presumably because of its five remaining hydrogen atoms, this drug is still flammable, but less so than diethyl ether. Its lower ignition limit in air is given as 3 per cent,[9] although Miller and Dornette[7] give the lower limit as 7·5 per cent in the moist conditions of the closed circuit. Substitution of more hydrogen atoms by fluorine was found to reduce anaesthetic potency greatly. It is interesting that more recent work suggests that diethyl ether, with seven of its hydrogen atoms replaced by fluorine, has anaesthetic properties.[20]

Halothane was the first truly non-flammable fluorinated drug to be introduced into anaesthesia[21] and has many useful properties besides that of non-flammability. It may be used with soda-lime in a closed system, is a potent anaesthetic with a relatively low solubility in blood, and shares with ether the ability to minimise expiratory spasm in asthmatic patients.

Other fluorine compounds which have reached clinical practice since the introduction of halothane and fluroxene are teflurane,[22] which may be regarded as halothane with the chlorine replaced by fluorine, enflurane (Ethrane) which is an ethyl methyl ether of similar structure to methoxyflurane, and isoflurane (Forane)[23] which is an isomer of enflurane.

**Inert diluents added to otherwise flammable drugs.**—In theory, volatile drugs such as ether and cyclopropane could be made effectively non-flammable by the addition of an inert diluent. This could work either by (a) absorbing the *thermal energy* of an incipient explosion or (b) absorbing *free radicals*. These free radicals result from the absorption of thermal energy by a molecule of an explosive gas, and, if they are not deactivated, will combine with oxygen and initiate a chain reaction, which results in an explosion.[24,25]

**(a) Energy absorbing diluents.**—Nitrogen is a member of this group. As it is added to a mixture of oxygen and trichloroethylene the upper limit of flammability is lowered until, at about 75 per cent nitrogen, it is the same as the lower limit. With concentrations above 75 per cent nitrogen, trichloroethylene is completely non-flammable.

Figure 2 is a "triple graph", showing the flammability limits for trichloroethylene/oxygen/nitrogen mixtures.[26]

"Air" is shown as a line joining pure air, on

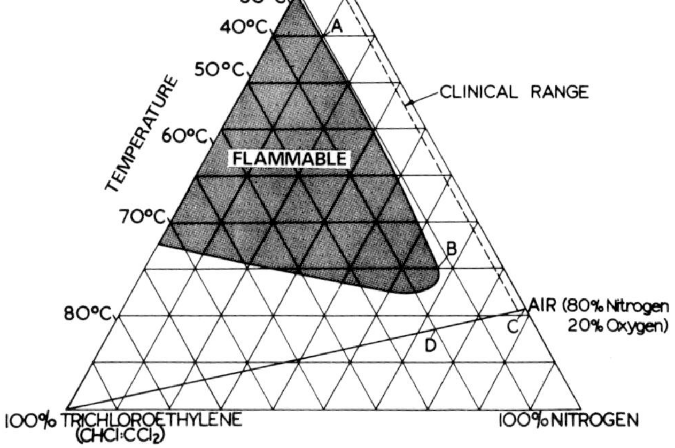


8/Fig. 2.—The flammability limits for trichloroethylene/oxygen/nitrogen mixtures.

the right side of the graph, at 79 per cent nitrogen and 21 per cent oxygen, with 100 per cent trichloroethylene at the bottom left corner. This line shows that no mixture of trichloroethylene in air passes through the flammable area. It may also be seen from the parallel line next to and to the left of the line joining "100 per cent oxygen" and "100 per cent nitrogen" (the "10 per cent trichloroethylene line") that less than 10 per cent trichloroethylene will never burn, in any mixtures of oxygen and nitrogen. The temperatures down the left side of the graph show that 10 per cent trichloroethylene cannot exist below 20° C, and so it is almost impossible to produce a flammable mixture of trichloroethylene in air or oxygen at room temperature. It is regarded as non-flammable in such mixtures, because the concentration needed for anaesthesia is only about 1 per cent. However, if nitrous oxide and oxygen are used, instead of air, flammable mixtures are produced with about 5 per cent trichloroethylene (see Table 1).

The lack of effect of increasing concentrations of nitrogen on the *lower limit* of flammability of gas is a fairly constant phenomenon.[27] The upper limit is affected to a much greater extent. Hence the range of flammability is always greater in oxygen than in air, although the *lower limit* is not significantly different.

**(b) "Free-radical" absorbers.**—The value of a free radical absorbing diluent has been investigated by Coleman[28] who has shown that only about 4 per cent of some bromine containing fluorocarbons is necessary to inhibit the combustion of n-hexane in air. This is a readily ignitable substance, often used in the testing of fire extinguishers. It is thus possible that a chemical could be found which would render a flammable gas non-flammable and yet leave it clinically useful. It has been shown that 7 per cent halothane will prevent the ignition of cyclopropane/oxygen mixtures (Bracken, personal communication) but as this is more than enough halothane to produce deep anaesthesia itself, the discovery is not of practical use.

## Ignition Sources and their Separation from Flammable Gases

The *energy* required to ignite gases varies according to the nature of the gases and how nearly their concentration approaches the stoichiometric, at which ignition is most easy. The *stoichiometric* mixture of any fuel is that at which, theoretically, combustion can be complete and all the fuel and oxygen molecules in the mixture react to form the products of combustion. The main sources of ignition in the operating theatre are static electricity, diathermy and other energy-producing apparatus.

### Static Electricity

It is almost impossible to ensure that a dangerous accumulation of static electricity will never occur in an operating room. Nevertheless most explosions due to static can be traced to a failure to observe fairly simple precautions. It is now believed that the danger from static is confined to a space even smaller than the area of 25 cm round the anaesthetic equipment outlined by Vickers.[8] The most important precaution for the anaesthetist to take against a dangerous accumulation of static electricity is to make sure that all breathing tubes and masks and apparatus locally associated with them are anti-static. In England and Wales equipment which is not anti-static is now allowed in parts of the operating room which are more than 25 cm from anaesthetic equipment. For the same reason, switches and electrical apparatus at a greater distance than 25 cm from anaesthetic apparatus need not be sparkproof.

Anti-static precautions in operating rooms are aimed at removing all non-essential articles which readily acquire static charges and at providing a limited path to earth from all personnel and equipment close to anaesthetic circuits. In this way any static charges that develop are dissipated as quickly as possible, without significantly increasing the risk of electrocution. In general terms it involves ensuring that there is a resistance of not more than 100 megohms* and not less than 50,000 ohms between each such person or article in the operating room and earth.

Static charges may be produced by *movement, friction* and *induction*. Trolleys when *moved* about the theatre can acquire dangerous static charges. This risk may be minimised by using wheels fitted with conducting rubber tyres.

Charges may be produced by *friction* in woollen blankets when these are quickly shaken or drawn across a trolley, and may be *induced* on equipment by the presence of certain types of electrical apparatus in the theatre. In such

*1 megohm = 1 million ohms.

cases there is no contact between the source of the current and the article on which the charge is induced.

*Materials*.—Certain materials, such as Perspex and nylon, are inherently dangerous, since they readily acquire static charges. It is usually possible to find suitable alternative materials which are not so troublesome, but where this is not possible the offending materials can be treated with an anti-static wax.

*Personnel*.—Theatre staff should not wear clothing which readily acquires a static charge. Plastic aprons and woollen garments should therefore not be worn unless they have been rendered anti-static.

Conducting footwear should be worn by everyone in the operating room involved in anaesthesia. Anti-static shoes or boots are most satisfactory, but light canvas shoes with anti-static rubber soles can also be worn with safety. People who enter the operating room for only a short time are no longer required to wear anti-static footwear (in Great Britain) unless they are concerned with anaesthesia.

Woollen blankets should not be brought into the theatre. They should be replaced by cotton blankets, a towel, or some other anti-static fabric. Closely fitting woollen stockings worn by patients are not a serious static risk since they become moist, and provided they are not removed or roughly handled in the theatre, are not likely to acquire a charge of static electricity. Furthermore, they are usually more than 25 cm from anaesthetic equipment.

It is sometimes suggested that nurses and others should not wear nylon stockings in the theatre, as this material might insulate the wearers. Quinton[29] has shown that this does not occur. No significant difference in resistance between the thigh and the outside of the sole of the shoe was found in a volunteer nurse who wore different types of stockings. Apparently the skin of the foot makes contact with the inside of the shoe through the mesh of the stocking.

*Floors*.—It is obviously essential that the floor in an operating theatre should have a conductivity of the same order as the items resting on it. The most satisfactory types of flooring in use at present are terrazzo or concrete with a resistance of from 0·1 to 10 megohms. To replace all unsatisfactory floors would be a most expensive undertaking, but it is now possible to lay conductive rubber or plastic on top of an existing floor and so render it satisfactory. Where an anaesthetic is only occasionally given, and the floor is unsuitable, it is sufficient to stand the anaesthetic trolley on a moistened sheet large enough to prevent anyone from touching the trolley without himself also making contact with the sheet.

*Relative humidity*.—The generation of static electricity is most difficult in a damp atmosphere, while moisture on the surface of an article renders it more conductive. It is good practice, therefore, to wet rubber breathing tubes before use if their anti-static properties are in doubt. A 1 per cent solution of a wetting agent is more effective than plain water.

A high relative humidity reduces the risk of a static explosion, but cannot entirely remove the hazard. It must also be remembered that articles have to be exposed to a humid atmosphere for about ten minutes before any significant amount of moisture collects on their surfaces.

No exact figure can be given for an optimum relative humidity, and different authorities recommend from 50–65 per cent. It is, however, very difficult to raise the humidity in a theatre; washing down the floor with hot water barely raises it by 8 per cent—and even if it were possible, there are few theatres in which the temperature could be kept low enough to make it comfortable to work in a high humidity. Where full air conditioning exists, a relative humidity of over 70 per cent is quite comfortable provided the temperature is not allowed to rise above 20–21° C (68–70°F).

*Rubber equipment*.—Only anti-static rubber should be used in association with anaesthetic equipment. This rubber is made by the addition of carbon to the rubber "mix". It owes its conductivity to the proximity of the carbon particles and it is thus possible for ordinary wear and tear to reduce its conducting properties. For complete safety, therefore, all anti-static rubber should be tested about once every year.

From the practical point of view, when there is any doubt about the anti-static properties of rubber equipment, it should be kept moist. If an anti-static article does not retain all the desirable properties of its non-conductive equivalent, an ordinary rubber one may be used, provided it is kept moist. The only anti-static item which is really markedly unsatisfactory in practice is the endotracheal tube. It is reasonable to use endotracheal tubes made of ordinary rubber or plastic, since they are kept moist when in position in the patient.

The instrument most commonly used for testing the conductivity of a material is a 500-volt D.C. insulation tester. The two leads of the apparatus are applied to different areas of the object to be tested, and the handle of the instrument is turned. A direct reading of the conductivity between the two test points is then given on a scale.

### Ignition from Electrical Apparatus

The spark from the *diathermy* can ignite flammable anaesthetic mixtures but Vickers[8] has shown that as close as 10 cm from an expiratory valve delivering 15 per cent ether in eight litres of air per minute, the highest concentration of ether detectable was only 0·85 per cent of the lower limit of flammability. He concluded that, "as far as the mixtures escaping in clinical anaesthesia are concerned, there seems no likelihood of explosive concentrations occurring at a distance greater than 25 cm from the expiratory valve". If closed circuit anaesthesia is used with full anti-static precautions, it appears safe to use flammable anaesthetic gases with diathermy, provided the chest is not opened.

The energy of a spark within 25 cm of an anaesthetic circuit has become more interesting recently, with the introduction of new equipment into the operating room. Tests for flammability of anaesthetic gases have, in the past, been carried out with ignition sources of around 9 joules per second. Hazards Research Corporation[3] have shown from tests using an ignition source of 900 joules per second that 9·75 per cent enflurane will burn in pure oxygen, although it is regarded as non-flammable in clinical use. When the same authors used 9 joules per second, no mixture of enflurane would burn.

At present, the main danger to be considered is the use of the *carbon dioxide laser* in the airway where energy, of the order of 20 watts, or 20 joules per second, is available in intimate contact with anaesthetic gases. The manufacturers of Fluothane (halothane) have managed to make about 4 per cent halothane burn in three parts of nitrous oxide and one part of oxygen, with this sort of ignition energy. Such a concentration of gases might exist at the beginning of anaesthesia for laryngoscopy, and so it would appear wise to wait for halothane levels to fall below 4 per cent, or to avoid the use of nitrous oxide as a carrier gas. When oxygen was the only carrier gas, the lower limit of flammability for halothane was 20 per cent, as opposed to 4 per cent in the nitrous oxide/oxygen mixture.

Gas mixtures themselves will not absorb a laser beam and therefore cannot be heated, ignited, decomposed or exploded, unless some solid object first absorbs the beam. Tissues in the larynx which are treated with laser beams will, of course, absorb energy and produce heat of about the same strength as an electric cautery. Any object which interferes with the path of the beam will absorb heat, including an endotracheal tube, which may burn. It has been suggested that tubes should be wrapped in foil, until a completely non-flammable plastic tube has been marketed.[30] A prototype of such a tube is shown in Fig. 3. There is, of course, a risk that a laser beam could be deflected by foil and cause a burn in a part of the larynx not intended for treatment.

## OTHER ELECTRICAL HAZARDS

The second group of hazards is concerned with the side-effects of electricity, other than the ignition of flammable gases and materials. According to Dobbie[31] *surgical diathermy* is responsible for the greatest number of accidents in this group. The commonest trouble is failure of the earth lead. If this is not intact, current will return to earth by the shortest possible route, and if this is via some other lead which is small, such as that of an ECG, a burn may occur where the small electrode makes contact with the skin. If part of the patient's skin is touching a piece of metal which is connected to earth, current may take this course, and a burn occur at the point of contact.

To minimise these and other risks of damage from the diathermy, the following precautions may be taken:

1. Use a "ground-free" diathermy set.
2. Use a monitored plate lead on the patient. This lead should sound an alarm when broken, and the alarm should be tested regularly.
3. Use a large area with good blood supply for application of the plate and place it

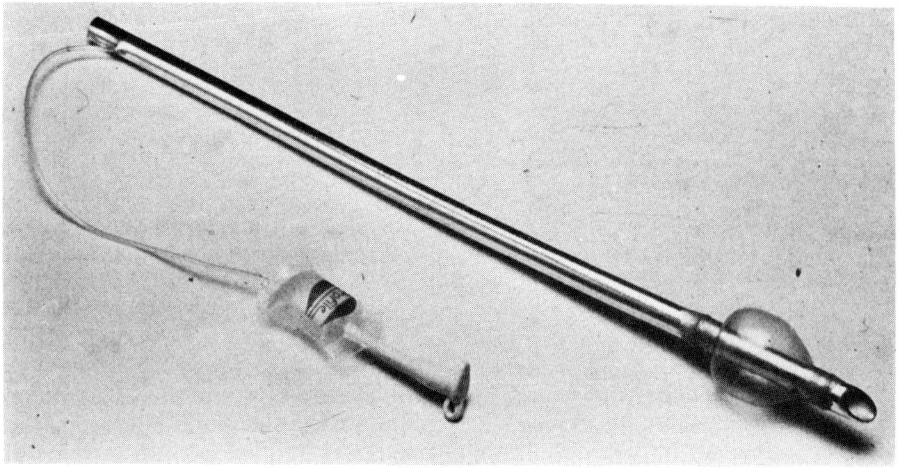

8/FIG. 3.—Prototype of Wainwright's non-flammable plastic tube. (Courtesy of Wainwright, and Blackwell Scientific Publications.[30])

as near to the surgical site as possible, remembering that the knee joint is a poor conductor of electricity.

4. Place ECG and other monitoring electrodes as far away as possible from the operation site. They should be at least one square centimetre in area. As far as possible, fully isolated equipment should be used and *all ECG leads should have a 10,000 ohms resister moulded into them.*
5. Encourage the operating surgeon to use the foot pedal himself. This should have an audible warning when the current is flowing, and as little current as possible should be used.
6. Encourage the return of the active electrode to its quiver, whenever not in use, and beware of pushing the foot pedal under the operating table.
7. The diathermy should be used with extra care in the neighbourhood of plastic drapes, if they are close to the outlet of anaesthetic gases. There is a risk that certain mixtures of nitrous oxide and oxygen could cause the ignition of such drapes by the diathermy.[18]
8. Use of the diathermy presents real problems if the patient has an artificial cardiac pace-maker. In most cases, the safest thing for such a patient is to avoid diathermy.
9. Grounded electric blankets should not be used on patients who are being treated with a diathermy machine.[32]
10. Ensure regular servicing of apparatus.
11. Train staff in the *reasons* for the precautions.

*Mains electricity* can be dangerous if the "live" lead in a grounded system makes contact with a grounded person. This can produce "macroshock", which can be prevented by the use of properly designed and maintained equipment. Such equipment should be enclosed in grounded metal cases, which should be regularly checked. Some countries favour the use of non-grounded mains supplies for the operating rooms. If the power supply is isolated from the ground, no lethal current can pass to ground through a victim. This isolation is achieved by the use of a 1:1 transformer in which the secondary winding is not grounded (Fig. 4). Contact between any *one* wire and ground will not result in a current flow. But if one wire of such a system is accidentally grounded, the system is just as dangerous as a normal grounded one. Isolated systems therefore require expensive monitors and power transfer is limited.

Very much smaller currents can be dangerous if they flow to a contact in, or very close to, the myocardium, and so bypass the protective impedance of skin and other tissue. Such contacts can be provided by cardiac pace-makers

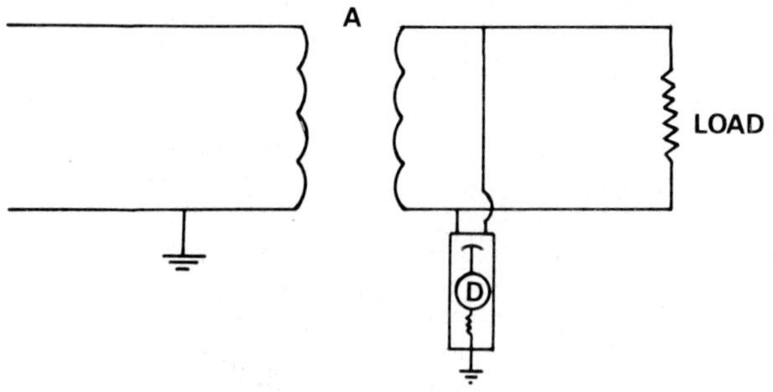


8/FIG. 4.—Isolation transformer (A) and its associated line-isolation monitor (D). The secondary circuit is not connected to ground except through the high impedance of the line-isolation monitor, which alternately connects both sides of the secondary circuit to ground for brief intervals. If another ground connection occurs inadvertently, a circuit will be completed through the line-isolation monitor and an alarm will be activated. (Courtesy of Dr. Kerr and Dr. Malhotra, 1981, and Little Brown and Co.[32])

or catheters which may be filled with conductive fluids. In order to prevent such "*microshock*", Hull[33] recommends that all intracardiac leads and catheters should be *totally isolated* from earth, including circuitry and transducers which may be attached to them.

Although more and more monitoring devices are being used on anaesthetised patients to increase their safety, it must be remembered that even monitors carry risks, such as giving a false alarm, electrocution or a burn. An artificial monitoring device should only be connected to a patient if the anaesthetist in charge of the case believes that he will be able to give a better anaesthetic with it than without it. False alarms such as the malfunctioning of one or more monitoring devices, can distract an anaesthetist from clinical observation, and more serious failure of monitoring devices can cause burns or even death. The anaesthetist should not hesitate to disconnect completely from a patient any piece of equipment whose functioning is worrying him. He should leave the safe repair and maintenance of sophisticated electrical life support, monitoring and surgical equipment to those with specialised knowledge.

## POLLUTION

It is now possible to measure volumes per million (vpm) of gases by portable and fairly simple physical methods such as gas chromatography and mass spectrometry. With the growing interest in general environmental conditions, such instruments have been used to measure small amounts of anaesthetic vapours present in operating rooms and other areas involved in anaesthesia. Whitcher and associates[34] measured halothane concentrations within a three-foot radius of anaesthesia equipment, and found about nine vpm when a semi-open (10 l/min) circuit was used in an operating room with about ten air changes per hour without recirculation. The writer (1974) has measured halothane concentrations of 45 vpm in semi-open systems, 3 vpm in closed systems with a small leak and less than 1 vpm with fully closed systems at two feet (60 cm) from anaesthesia equipment in an operating room with twelve air changes per hour without recirculation. The figures for nitrous oxide in similar systems were semi-open 4400 vpm, semi-closed 200 vpm, and closed—nil.

Nothing is known about the effects on general health of breathing such concentrations of anaesthetic vapours for long periods intermittently over many years, but a retrospective national study of disease among operating room personnel was published in *Anesthesiology.*[35] The authors believed that their results showed that female workers in the exposed group were subject to increased risk of spontaneous abortion, congenital abnormalities in their children, cancer and hepatic and renal disease, but their title was biased in that they described their report as being on "The effect of *trace anaesthetics* on the health of operating room personnel". The investigation could only be described fairly as being on the *effects of employment in a certain type of work*. Others[36] criticised the logic used by the authors of the national study. They believe that the data on spontaneous abortion, for example, would lead to the conclusion that "any increase in its rate amongst operating room personnel is LESS likely to be due to inhalation of trace anesthetic vapours, than to result from other environmental factors". They show from the Study's figures that "the tendency towards spontaneous abortion is not dose

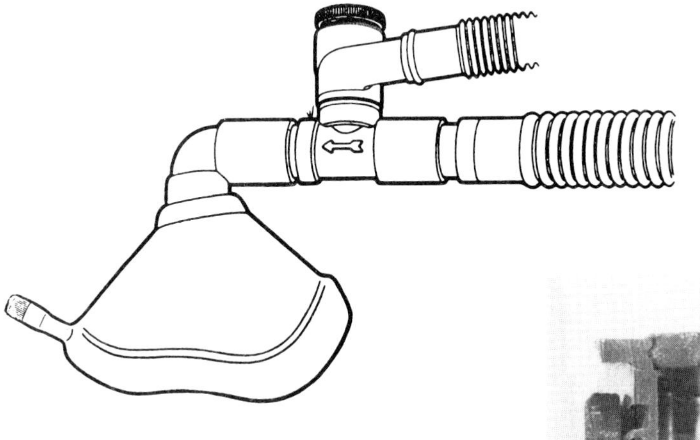

8/FIG. 5(*a*).—Shows one take-off arrangement for waste gases via a modified expiratory valve.

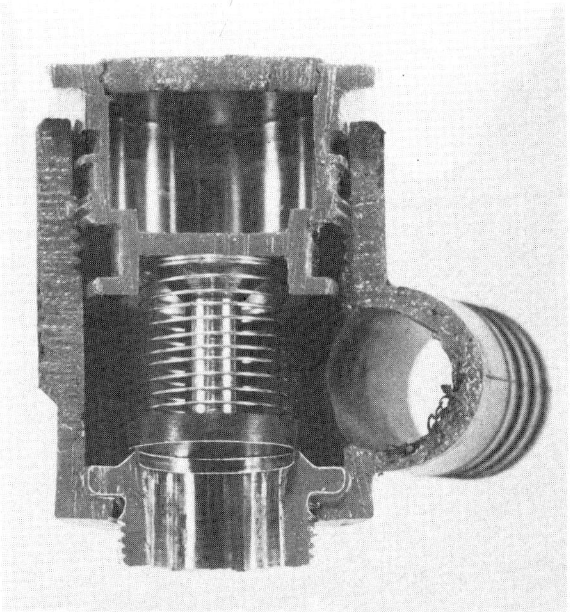

8/FIG. 5(*b*).—Shows a cross-section of the valve.

related to anesthetic vapour", since the rate of spontaneous abortion was lower among physician anaesthesiologists and nurse anaesthetists than among operating room nurses and technicians. Levels of anaesthetic exposure are agreed to be higher for physician anaesthesiologists and nurse anaesthetists than for operating room nurses and technicians.

It should also be remembered that, to such a restrospective study there are certain fundamental objections:

1. Only survivors, and less than 50 per cent of them, replied to the questionnaire.
2. It is difficult to avoid bias in the title. The questionnaire was headed "Effects of waste anesthetics on health".
3. Women are known to vary in what they consider to be abortions, between 8–25 per cent.

Later work, in Sweden,[37] claiming "unbiased data collection", showed that there were "no differences in the incidence of threatened abortions, in birth weight, in perinatal death rate, or in the incidence of congenital malformations", in a group of 494 women who worked throughout pregnancy in operating rooms. This study group was compared with a reference population composed of all women employed in medical work in Sweden who were delivered during the same period.

It would, of course, be prudent to minimise the amount of anaesthetic vapours inhaled by those who work in operating rooms, provided that this does not add a significant risk to the patient or staff. Two approaches to this problem are being used. One is to confine the anaesthetic gases to the patient's body and the anaesthetic apparatus, by the use of totally closed systems of anaesthesia. This has the logical advantage of vaporising a minimal amount of anaesthetic and is being studied by several authors.[38–41] It is also extremely economical in both capital and running costs, as well as conserving body fluid and heat. It is so economical in running costs that piped gas systems, with their own problems of mistaken identity and supply, would probably become unnecessary.

The other method involves "scavenging" waste gases, and this may be done by *passive* or *active* systems. *Passive* systems involve the use of pipes which allow the patient's expirations to pass by their own energy to a suitable discharge point, and various problems can arise. These include obstruction to outflow,[42] misconnection,[43] infection and final disposal. Unusual outside air pressures can cause back-flow, and as mentioned earlier there has already been one explosion, where a blowlamp ignited ether coming from a scavenging exhaust pipe. This was the first anaesthetic explosion in England and Wales reported since 1968.

*Active* systems involve power units to assist the passage of waste gases to their disposal point. This is usually achieved by connecting the circuit outlet valve (Fig. 5*a* and *b*) to some form of wall suction. Such systems require an air inlet to prevent subatmospheric pressure from being applied to the outlet valve. If the air inlet becomes occluded, subatmospheric pressure is applied to the outlet valve with consequent malfunction. Sharrock and Leith[44] have shown that this can result in dangerously high or low pressures in the anaesthetic circuit.

Furthermore, it is not recommended that flammable gases are vented to such systems, as their power supply may not be spark-proof.

It would appear unreasonable at present to insist on the use of scavenging apparatus with *known* potential risks, before a risk to staff has been shown to exist from breathing trace concentrations of anaesthetic gases. It would, however, appear to be very reasonable to employ closed circuit anaesthesia, or scavenging devices which are shown to be clearly "fail safe".

## REFERENCES


1. H.M.S.O. (1956). *Report of a Working Party on Anaesthetic Explosions, including safety code for equipment and installations*. London: H. M. Staty. Office.
2. Schön, G. and Steen, H. (1968). Explosion limits and ignition temperatures of some inhalation anaesthetics in mixtures with various oxygen carriers. *Anaesthesist*, **17**, 6.
3. Hazards Research Corporation (1974). Lower explosion limits of three anesthetics in mixtures of oxygen and nitrous oxide. *Hazards Research Corporation Report 3296* to Ohio Medical Products, Madison, Wisconsin.
4. Burns, T. H. S., Hall, J. M., Bracken, A. and Gouldstone, G. (1961). An investigation of new fluorine compounds in anaesthesia. (3) The anaesthetic properties of hexafluorobenzene. *Anaesthesia*, **16**, 333.
5. Garmer, N. L. and Leigh, J. M. (1967). Some effects of hexafluorobenzene in cats. *Brit. J. Pharmacol.*, **31**, 345.
6. Hall, L. W. and Jackson, S. R. K. (1973). Hexafluorobenzene. Further studies as an anaesthetic agent. *Anaesthesia*, **28**, 155.
7. Miller, G. L. and Dornette, W. A. L. (1961). Flammability studies of Fluoromar-Oxygen mixtures used in anesthesia. *Anesth. Analg. Curr. Res.*, **40**, 232.
8. Vickers, M. D. (1970). Explosion hazards in anaesthesia.*Anaesthesia*, **25**. 482.
9. Krantz, J. C., Jr., Carr, C. J. C., Lu, G. and Bell, F. K., (1953). Anesthesia XL. The anesthetic action of trifluoroethyl-vinyl ether. *J. Pharmacol. exp. Ther.*, **108**, 488.
10. Artusio, J. F., Jr. (1963). *Halogenated Anesthetics*. Philadelphia: F. A. Davis Co.
11. Leonard, P. F. (1975). The lower limits of flammability of halothane, enflurane and isoflurane. *Anesth. Analg. Curr. Res.*, **54**, 238.
12. Fabian, L. W., Dewitt, H. and Carnes, M. A. (1960). Laboratory and clinical investigation of some newly synthesized fluorocarbon anesthetics. *Anesth. Analg. Curr. Res.*, **39**, 456.
13. Bracken, A. and Wilton-Davies, C. C., (1963). Explosion risk in a "non-flammable" system. *Anaesthesia*, **18**, 439.
14. Vickers, M. D. (1965). The duration of the explosion hazard following induction with ether or cyclopropane. *Anaesthesia*, **20**, 315.
15. Nicholson, M. J. and Crehan, J. P. (1967). Fire and explosion hazards in the operating room. *Anesth. Analg. Curr. Res.*, **46**, 412.
16. Carroll, K. J. (1964). Unusual explosion during electrosurgery. *Brit. med. J.*, **2**, 1178.
17. Woodward, N. W. (1961). Prevention of explosion while fulgurating polyps of the colon. *Dis. Colon Rect.*, **4**, 32.
18. Cameron, B. G. D. and Ingram, G. S. (1971). Flammability of drape materials in nitrous oxide and oxygen. *Anaesthesia*. **26**, 281.
19. Lu, G., Ling, J. S. L. and Krantz, J. C., Jr. (1953). Anesthesia XLI. The anesthetic properties of certain fluorinated hydrocarbons and ethers. *Anesthesiology*, **14**, 466.
20. Burns, T. H. S., Hall, J. M., Bracken, A. and Gouldstone, G. (1982). An investigation of new fluorine compounds in anaesthesia. (9) Examination of six aliphatic compounds and four ethers. *Anaesthesia*, **37**, 278.
21. Raventós, J. (1956). The action of Fluothane—a new volatile anaesthetic. *Brit. J. Pharmacol.*, **11**, 394.
22. Artusio, J. F., Van Poznak, A., Weingram, J. and Sohn, Y. J. (1967). Teflurane. A nonexplosive gas for clinical anesthesia. *Anesth. Analg. Curr. Res.*, **46**, 657.
23. Pauca, A. L. and Dripps, R. D. (1973). Clinical experience with isoflurane (Forane). *Brit. J. Anaesth.*, **45**, 697.
24. Ubbelohde, A. R. (1935). Investigations on the combustion of hydrocarbons. I. The influence of molecular structure on hydrocarbon combustion. II. Absorption spectra and chemical properties of intermediates. *Proc. roy. Soc. A*, **152**, 354 and 378.
25. Hinshelwood, C. N. (1940). *The Kinetics of Chemical Change*. London: Oxford Univ. Press.
26. Jones, G. W. and Scott, G. S. (1942). U.S. Bureau of Mines, Report of Investigation 3666. Washington.
27. Coward, H. F. and Jones, G. W. (1952). Limits of flammability of gases and vapours. Washington: U.S. Bureau of Mines, Bulletin 503.
28. Coleman, E. H. (1952). Effect of fluorinated hydrocar-

bons on the inflammability limits of combustible vapours. *Fuel*, **31**, 445.
29. Quinton, A. (1953). Safety measures in operating theatres and the use of a radioactive thallium source to dissipate static electricity. *Brit. J. appl. Phys.*, Suppl. No. 2, S 92.
30. Wainwright, A. C., Moody, R. A. and Carruth, J. A. S. (1981). Anaesthetic safety with the carbon dioxide laser. *Anaesthesia*, **36**, 411.
31. Dobbie, A. K. (1975). Paper at Symposium on Environmental Hazards. Faculty of Anaesthetists, London.
32. Kerr, D. R. and Malhotra, I. V. (1981). Electrical design and safety in the operating room and intensive care unit. *Internat. Anesthesiol. Clin.* **19**, 27.
33. Hull, C. J. (1972). Symposium on Hazards in the operating theatre. Royal College of Surgeons at Newcastle upon Tyne.
34. Whitcher, C. D., Cohen, E. N. and Trudell, J. R. (1971). Chronic exposure to anesthetic gases in the operating room. *Anesthesiology*, **35**, 348.
35. American Society of Anesthesiologists (1974). Report of an Ad Hoc Committee on the effect of Trace Anaesthetics on the Health of Operating Room Personnel. *Anesthesiology*, **41**, 321.
36. Walts, L. F., Forsythe, A. B. and Moore, J. G. (1975). Occupational disease among operating room personnel. *Anesthesiology*, **42**. 608.
37. Ericson, A. and Kallen, B. (1979). Survey of infants born in 1973 or 1975 to Swedish women working in operating rooms during their pregnancies. *Anesth. Analg. Curr. Res.*, **58**, 302.
38. Aldrete, J. A., Lowe, H. J. and Virtue, R. W. (1979). *Low Flow and Closed System Anaesthesia*. New York: Grune & Stratton.
39. Burns, T. H. S. (1980). Closed circuit anaesthesia. *Anaesthesia*, **35**, 114.
40. Hughes, T. J. (1980). Closed system anaesthesia. *Anaesthesia*, **35**, 614.
41. Lin, C. Y., Mostert, J. W. and Benson, D. W. (1980). Closed circle systems. A new direction in the practice of anaesthesia. *Acta anaesth. Scand.*, **24**, 354.
42. Morgan, B. A. and Nott, M. R. (1980). Wear in plastic exhaust valves. *Anaesthesia*, **35**, 717
43. Tavakoli, M. and Habeeb, A. (1978). Two hazards of gas scavenging. *Anesth. Analg. Curr. Res.*, **57**, 286.
44. Sharrock, N. E. and Leith, D. E. (1977). Potential pulmonary barotrauma when venting anaesthetic gases to suction. *Anesthesiology*, **46**, 152.

## FURTHER READING

Dobbie, A. K. (1972). Electricity in Hospitals. *Bio-Medical Engineering*, **7**, 12.

CHAPTER 9

# Artificial Ventilation



## INTRODUCTION AND HISTORY

For centuries it has been realised that failure to breathe need not necessarily lead to death. In the Second Book of Kings there is a vivid description of successful mouth-to-mouth resuscitation which the Prophet Elisha performed on a child who appeared to be dead.

Towards the end of the eighteenth century there developed a great interest in resuscitating people rescued from drowning. The "Society for the Recovery of Drowned Persons" was formed in Amsterdam in 1767, and seven years later Dr. William Hawes, John Hunter and thirty enthusiasts with similar interests founded the Humane Society (later the Royal Humane Society). Medals and prizes were offered for new ideas and new apparatus for resuscitation. Many designs based on pumps, bellows and tubes were introduced, developing the suggestions that Vesalius and Paracelsus had put forward two hundred years previously.

Unfortunately, failure to appreciate the dangers of high airway pressure lead to deaths from tension pneumothorax. Leroy demonstrated that it was possible to rupture alveoli and reported his findings to the French Academy of Science in 1827. He believed that "many patients who would otherwise have recovered were speedily dispatched by over-enthusiastic use of the bellows equipment then issued by the Prefecture of Police".[1] Magendie's report of 1829 confirmed Leroy's findings and resuscitation using bellows fell into disrepute. After 1837, the Royal Humane Society recommended manual compression of the chest if artificial ventilation was necessary.

Resuscitation by bellows was to reappear sporadically during the next 100 years but only regained wide acceptance when Kreiselman introduced his apparatus during the Second World War. The Rubens' self-refilling bag was a later development based on the same principle.

Elisha's mouth-to-mouth resuscitation was rediscovered by Tossach in 1743 but the method was later condemned as unhygienic by the newly-founded Royal Humane Society. It was shown to be physiologically sound by Elam in 1954 and in 1958 Safar demonstrated that the ventilation provided was superior to that obtained by manual chest-pressure arm-lift manoeuvres. Expired air resuscitation is now regarded as the method of choice when equipment is not available.

In 1754, Benjamin Pugh described an air-pipe for the resuscitation of the newborn. One end of the pipe was placed next to the baby's larynx and the lungs could be inflated by mouth or bellows. During the nineteenth century, the obstetricians at the Maternité Hospital in Paris continued to use this method even though the positive pressure principle had been temporarily abandoned for ventilating adults.

During the period 1840–1940, most of the mechanical aids to artificial ventilation depended on applying a subatmospheric pressure to the outside of the thorax. Dr. Alfred F. Jones of Lexington, Kentucky, patented the first American tank ventilator in 1864. He claimed cures for "paralysis, neuralgia, rheumatism, seminal weakness, bronchitis, dyspepsia and many other diseases, including deafness".[2] The inventors of subsequent tank and cuirass ventilators only claimed successful treatment of respiratory diseases! Alexander Graham Bell invented a vacuum jacket for resuscitation of the newborn and in 1889, Dr. Egon Braun of Boston described a small tank ventilator for the same purpose.

In the 1920's, the gas and electricity supply industries, dissatisfied with the methods then available for treating victims of electric shock and gas poisoning, asked Philip Drinker of Harvard for advice on resuscitation. In 1929, Drinker and his colleagues introduced their tank ventilator for prolonged artificial respiration which subsequently became known as the "iron lung". Poliomyelitis was the main cause of respiratory failure in children and young adults during the first half of the present century, and the first patient to be treated in the "iron lung" was a victim of paralytic poliomyelitis. Modifications to the basic design were introduced over the next 25 years. Further developments of the cuirass ventilator proved useful during recovery from the acute phase of the disease.

In 1952, Denmark was struck by a particularly severe epidemic of paralytic poliomyelitis. At Blegdam Hospital in Copenhagen, the apparatus available consisted of one tank and six cuirass ventilators and these facilities were rapidly overwhelmed by the number of patients requiring respiratory assistance. By this time "controlled respiration" was well established in anaesthesia and almost as a last resort the technique was extended to patients needing long-term ventilation. At one time, 70 patients were receiving respiratory assistance from "ventilators" which consisted of medical students squeezing the bag of a to-and-fro system with carbon dioxide absorption. The medical students were paid for each eight-hour shift. Lassen and Ibsen established the basic principles of long-term ventilation: careful airway control and protection, humidification, avoidance of high inspired oxygen concentrations and meticulous physiotherapy. Once the acute phase of the disease was over, weaning was accomplished by a forerunner of intermittent mandatory ventilation (IMV). Adequacy of ventilation was assessed by oximetry and by end-tidal carbon dioxide concentration measurements.

A dramatic fall in mortality occurred after the new technique had been introduced, and this ensured that intermittent positive-pressure ventilation (IPPV) was to become the standard method of artificial ventilation. The superiority of IPPV was confirmed during the Stockholm epidemic in the following year and during the New England epidemic of 1955.

After the introduction of the Salk and Sabin vaccines the incidence of poliomyelitis fell sharply. However, the skills which had been developed were put to good use in the ventilatory management of polyneuritis, drug overdose and chest trauma. During the 1960's, the indications for IPPV were broadened further and the cardiovascular effects were investigated. Improvements in the immediate management of the injured showed that a group of patients who had been successfully resuscitated went on to develop a lung condition characterised by certain radiological changes and severe impairment of gas exchange. Shock lung and adult respiratory distress syndrome (ARDS) were two of the many names for this condition which proved to be particularly serious in septic patients.

The pathophysiology of ARDS was studied intensively during the 1970's. Positive end-expiratory pressure (PEEP) was added to IPPV to aid gas exchange in patients with ARDS but recognition of the adverse effects of PEEP on the circulation started the quest for an "ideal" PEEP level which would balance the respiratory advantages against the circulatory disadvantages. In spite of increased understanding of ARDS, the mortality rate of this condition remained (and remains) disappointingly high. For patients with overwhelming pulmonary failure, the 1970's saw the development of extracorporeal techniques which could ensure adequate gas exchange for several weeks. A few centres experimented with high-frequency ventilation (HFV), although the true role in long-term artificial ventilation of this interesting technique has yet to be established.

The benefits of long-term ventilation have not always been universally accepted. In the 1960's, the term "respirator lung" was introduced to describe radiological and pathological changes in the lungs of some patients who had received artificial ventilation. In restrospect, pulmonary oxygen toxicity was probably responsible for many cases of "respirator lung". The toxic effects on the lung of pure oxygen at standard atmospheric pressure had been recognised for over 50 years and an inspired oxygen concentration of 50 per cent or less was considered safe. After 1955, most ventilators in use in North America were powered by compressed oxygen and employed a venturi device to entrain air. It was erroneously assumed that these ventilators would deliver gas whose oxygen concentration was below 50 per cent. Several years later it was shown that the venturi device was not performing as expected: as a result, oxygen concentrations in the toxic range were being delivered to patients. Subsequent animal experiments using carefully controlled oxygen concentrations freed the respirator from blame. This evidence, together with the experience already gained with polio patients, established that IPPV with modest levels of oxygen in the inspired gas may be continued indefinitely without adverse effect on the lung.

Some still view long-term artificial ventilation with deep suspicion even though its value in intensive care is now beyond doubt. The prosecution's case is based on the following warped logic: "very sick patients often need a ventilator—very sick patients often die—this proves that ventilators eventually kill sick patients".[3] Other false arguments may be put forward in an attempt to limit use of the technique. There is still a widespread belief that satisfactory blood gas values, considered in isolation, indicate that artificial ventilation is unnecessary.

The first attempts to use artificial ventilation in anaesthesia were devoted to solving the "pneumothorax problem" in thoracic surgery. At the very end of the nineteenth century, the French surgeons Tuffier and Hallion, and the American surgeon Matas, performed thoracic operations while rhythmic ventilation of the lungs was carried out by bellows. The apparatus used by the French surgeons was strikingly advanced. The airway was maintained by a cuffed endotracheal tube and even PEEP could be applied by placing the end of the expiratory limb under water. Unfortunately these promising innovations were eclipsed by Sauerbruch's negative-pressure operating chamber which was introduced in 1904. One year later, Brauer introduced a helmet-like device which could apply positive pressure to the patient's head. Between 1909 and 1913, the American surgeons Green and Janeway devised a brilliant series of ventilators, but there was little interest in further development once the immediate surgical problem had been solved.

During the 1930's, the technique of "controlled respiration", was introduced. Artificial ventilation was carried out by rhythmically squeezing the reservoir bag of a circle and absorber system. The combination of hyperinflation and general anaesthesia suppressed the patient's spontaneous respiration. Guedel and Treweek used ether and called the technique "ether apnoea". A little later, Waters used cyclopropane and first suggested the term "controlled respiration". This method of artificial ventilation was used when curare was introduced into anaesthesia in the early 1940's.

When reviewing the history of artificial ventilation, it is salutary to remember that Vesalius solved the pneumothorax problem in 1555, that Brodie and Waterton employed the "curare plus bellows" principle in experimental animals in 1811, and that Brodie had also suggested "bellows breathing" could be used to treat opium poisoning.

After the Second World War, there were two stimuli to the development of mechanical ventilators for IPPV. The first was the introduction of curare into anaesthesia. The second was the fear of health authorities that if another poliomyelitis epidemic occurred, large numbers of patients might require artificial ventilation.

In 1940 the first commercial ventilator for anaesthesia, the Spiropulsator, was manufactured in Sweden by the AGA Company. The main features of this ventilator had been developed by the pioneers Giertz, Frenckner and Crafoord, but the commercial design involved the collaboration of Anderson, an engineer. The first British ventilator in commercial production was manufactured by Blease. This prototype was followed by the Blease "Pulmoflators" and these further developments were also the result of fruitful collaboration between doctors and a practical engineer.

The value of mechanical ventilators in anaesthesia was soon recognised in Sweden, Britain and some other European countries, but was disputed in the United States where reliance on manual assistance persisted. The more stringent ventilatory requirements of cardiac surgery were later to change this view.

Subsequent evolution of ventilators was to take two paths. One was to fulfil the need for cheap, simple and reliable models which could be used for anaesthesia and for the majority of patients needing long-term ventilation. The other was to provide increasingly sophisticated and versatile ventilators with the facilities necessary for treating patients with severe respiratory failure.

The development of high-frequency ventilation (HFV) has already been mentioned. This technique offers distinct advantages during anaesthesia for laryngeal and tracheal surgery but at present its use is still confined to relatively few centres.

More detailed accounts of the history of artificial ventilation are listed under "Further Reading—Historical" at the the end of this chapter.

## ARTIFICIAL VENTILATION DURING RESUSCITATION

Artificial ventilation is often necessary when equipment is not to hand. Many investigations have shown that the sooner resuscitation is started after ventilatory or circulatory arrest, the better the chance of survival. Immediate resuscitation will usually require action by the lay public, and it is essential to teach as many people as possible methods which will be effective without the use of equipment.

In 1968, the World Federation of Societies of Anaesthesiologists (WFSA) produced an excellent manual on cardiopulmonary resuscitation. The second edition has now been prepared by Dr. Peter Safar, a pioneer in resuscitation.[4] The original 48-page manual has expanded to 240 pages, and the new edition gives a comprehensive account of current practice in the management of respiratory and cardiac emergencies and the preservation of brain function. The concept of resuscitation has been extended from the site of the incident right through to the intensive care unit. The manual also discusses the educational, financial, ethical and legal implications of resuscitation; these will vary from country to country and Baskett has stressed the need in the United Kingdom for training programmes in resuscitation for paramedical staff and the general public.[5]

### Artificial Ventilation Requiring no Apparatus—Expired Air Resuscitation

Simple analysis shows that by doubling alveolar ventilation, a resuscitator can effectively "breathe for two". The presence of the resuscitator's dead space improves matters as the gas first delivered to the patient with each breath is room air. In 1954, Elam confirmed that during expired air resuscitation, arterial $Pco_2$ values were between 30–40 mm Hg (4 and 5·3 kPa) in the patient and between 20–30 mm Hg (2·7 and 4 kPa) in the resuscitator: arterial $Po_2$ values of over 75 mm Hg (10 kPa) were found in patients with normal lungs.

In 1958, Safar showed that other methods of resuscitation recommended at that time, such as the Holger-Nielsen and Silvester, failed to provide adequate ventilation for two reasons; first because they did not generate adequate inspiratory force, and second because they did not leave the resuscitator's hands free to control the airway. Since that time, expired air resuscitation has become the method of choice, *except for those who have inhaled toxic gases or who are the victims of cyanide poisoning.*

Teaching the method to the lay public has been shown to save lives.

Safar[4] has emphasised the following points of technique:

1. If possible, the patient is placed horizontal, supine and face-up, and the resuscitator approaches the patient's head from the side.
2. The airway must be cleared of foreign material and then maintained using any necessary components of the "triple manoeuvre" (head-tilt, mouth open, jaw thrust). Moderate backward head-tilt should be used when neck injury is suspected.
3. The resuscitator's mouth seals around the patient's mouth. Air leakage through the patient's nose can be prevented by pinching the nostrils with one hand or compressing the nose with the resuscitator's cheek. In children, the resuscitator's mouth can seal around both mouth and nose.
4. The resuscitator's expiration should be forceful into adults and gentle into children; puffs are used for infants. During inflation, the patient's chest is observed to see whether it rises; once chest movement is seen to occur, the resuscitator's head is turned to one side and passive expiration occurs.
5. Recommended inflation rates are about 12 per minute for adults and 20 per minute for children.
6. Mouth-to-nose is an alternative, and both techniques should be taught as there are occasions when one will be preferable. If trismus prevents opening of the mouth or if resuscitation is started during rescue from water, mouth-to-nose is the appropriate technique.
7. Expired air resuscitation may inflate the stomach. This may impede lung inflation and provoke regurgitation and aspiration. Decompression by gentle pressure on the epigastrium may be necessary, preferably with the patient in the "stable side position" to reduce risk of aspiration.

The technique may be made more aesthetically acceptable by placing a handkerchief over the patient's mouth and nose. However, experience has shown that in an emergency suitably trained bystanders rarely hesitate to use mouth-to-mouth or mouth-to-nose resuscitation.

### Artificial Ventilation Using Simple Apparatus

Simple apparatus may make resuscitation more acceptable and more effective. Nevertheless, artificial ventilation should never be delayed because apparatus is not immediately available.

**Mouth-to-mask.**—The Laerdal pocket mask makes expired air resuscitation more pleasant to perform. If oxygen is available, oxygen-enriched air can be used to ventilate the patient. The device looks like a transparent anaesthetic mask, but the angle-piece is replaced by a short, straight tube to which the resuscitator's lips can be applied. A nipple is placed on the body of the mask so that oxygen can be added to the inspired gas. The inspired oxygen concentration depends on the oxygen flow supplied.

The Laerdal pocket mask is no more effective than mouth-to-mouth resuscitation but it does make the procedure more hygienic and enables additional oxygen to be given. It has also proved useful when training the general public in the technique of expired air ventilation.

**Mouth-to-airway.**—These devices make expired air resuscitation more pleasant and the pharyngeal portion helps to maintain a patent airway. However gagging, vomiting and laryngospasm may be induced if the laryngeal and pharyngeal reflexes are still intact.

The *Safar S-tube* resembles a double Guedel airway; one of the airways is used as a pharyngeal airway for the patient, the other as a blow-tube by the resuscitator.

The *Brook Airway* (Fig. 1) is more sophisticated and has a non-return valve so that expired air from the patient does not pass out through the resuscitator's mouthpiece.

The *Oesophageal Obturator Airway*[6] has a mask and blow-tube to facilitate expired air resuscitation and a large, cuffed tube designed to obstruct the oesophagus and prevent reflux of gastric contents. Once inserted, the device must only be removed when the patient's airway is suitably protected from aspiration.

Although the oesophageal obturator airway is easier to insert than an endotracheal tube, its usefulness is not universally accepted.

The *Oesophageal (gastric tube) Airway*[120] is a development of the oesophageal obturator

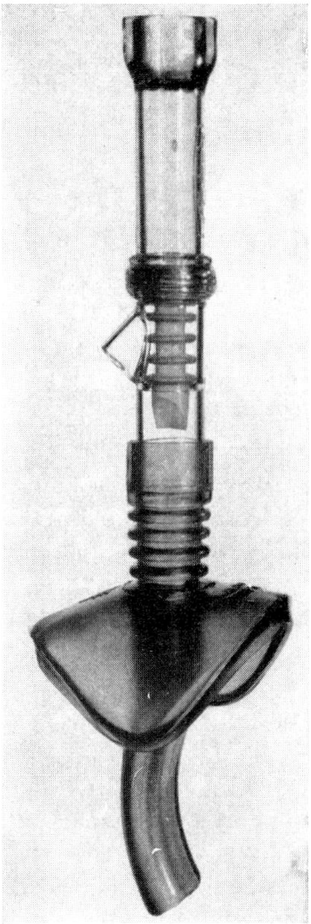


9/Fig. 1.—The Brook Airway. This mouth-to-airway device makes expired air resuscitation more pleasant. (Courtesy of Dr. M. H. Brook and the Editor of the *British Medical Journal*)

airway. It allows gastric suction to be carried out with the oesophageal airway in place. Its usefulness in resuscitation is being investigated at present.

**Bag-Valve-Mask.**—These devices have three components; a self-refilling bag, a non-rebreathing valve and an anaesthetic mask. Oxygen can be administered if available but a reservoir tube is necessary to deliver 100 per cent oxygen.

One hand compresses the bag during inspiration, leaving only the other hand available to maintain the patient's airway and a tight seal between mask and face. Leakage around the edges of the mask reduces the effective tidal volume.

Those without special training find it difficult to use these devices effectively; they are, however, particularly valuable for ventilating intubated patients. The Ambu resuscitator made to the Rubens' design is shown in Fig. 2.

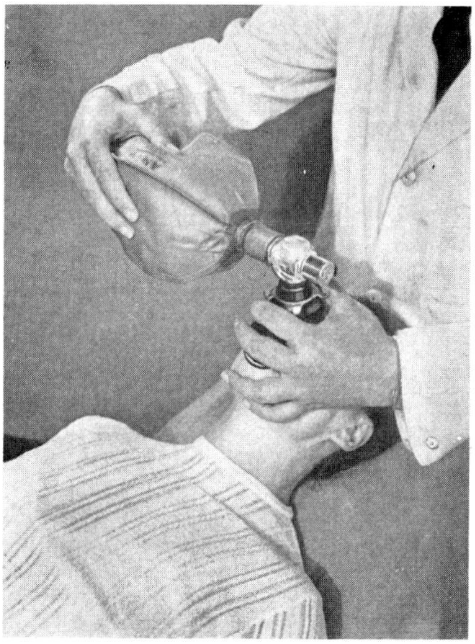

9/Fig. 2.—The Ambu Resuscitator based on the Rubens' design. (Courtesy of Medical and Industrial Equipment Ltd.)

## TANK AND CUIRASS VENTILATORS

These machines ventilate patients by applying a subatmospheric pressure to the outside of the thorax. This type of artificial ventilation is often called intermittent negative-pressure ventilation (INPV). The first tank ventilator was described in 1832 and the first cuirass in 1874. The development of apparatus for INPV has been reviewed by Woollam.[2]

### Tank Ventilators

The patient is placed on a mattress inside an air-tight cabinet from which only his or her head protrudes. A padded collar round the neck forms an effective seal. The pressure inside the cabinet is lowered rhythmically by a system of pumps or a set of bellows and is then allowed to return to atmospheric.

The first power-driven tank ventilator, the "iron lung", was introduced by Drinker, McKhann and Shaw in 1929. There were port-holes in the sides of the tank through which the patient could be observed and sealed ports to allow the use of manometers, blood pressure cuffs and stethoscopes. Many modifications of the original design were made over the next 25 years to make the patient more accessible and to add a "positive" phase to assist expiration. The Kelleher Rotating Tank Ventilator is shown in Figs. 3 and 4. The cabinet of this ventilator can rotate about its long axis so that the back of the patient's chest becomes accessible for auscultation and physiotherapy.

The two main disadvantages of tank ventilators are that access to the patient for nursing care and physiotherapy is restricted, and that the airway is not usually protected. Vomiting and regurgitation are particularly hazardous during INPV, even for patients who have normal laryngeal and pharyngeal reflexes. Should vomiting occur, a port should be opened immediately to equalise pressures inside and outside the tank and so reduce the risk of aspiration. Patients who have a tracheostomy can be ventilated in tank ventilators but the padded collar makes management difficult.

After 1952, IPPV became the standard method for long-term artificial ventilation. However, tank ventilators still have a role in treating patients who have normal laryngeal and pharyngeal reflexes and only minimal secretions. They are useful in the long-term management of those with chronic weakness of the respiratory muscles who need assistance during sleep or during an acute respiratory infection.

Nowadays, few anaesthetists have experience of either tank or cuirass ventilators. This is unfortunate as a small group of patients who might benefit from this alternative technique are being subjected to prolonged intubation or tracheostomy unnecessarily. Woollam and Houlton[7] describe the management of a case of respiratory failure in pregnancy using a tank ventilator. The patient had a severe kyphoscoliosis due to poliomyelitis; the pregnant uterus had splinted the diaphragm and caused further impairment of respiratory function.

### Cuirass Ventilators

Cuirass ventilators are named after a piece of 15th century body armour which consisted of a breastplate and backplate fastened together. A rigid shell fits over the thorax and upper abdomen and the padded rim makes contact with the skin to form an airtight seal. A bellows is connected by flexible tubing to the airspace between the skin and shell; expansion of the bellows creates a subatmospheric pressure in this airspace during inspiration.

Cuirass ventilators leave patients' arms and legs free and cause less circulatory embarrassment than tank ventilators. They are less efficient than tank ventilators and the tidal volume obtained by a given subatmospheric pressure will be smaller. The larger the cuirass shell, the more the performance approaches that of the tank ventilator.

Cuirass ventilators are used as assisters for patients who have chronic respiratory impairment or who are recovering from some episode of paralysis. Figure 5 shows a cuirass ventilator in use in a patient's home.

The Tunnicliffe Jacket, introduced in 1955, was a development of the standard cuirass. This device is discussed by Woollam,[2] who also describes belt ventilators such as the Bragg-Paul "Pulsator", and the cuirass-belt designed by Pinkerton.

## ARTIFICIAL VENTILATION BY IPPV

### INSTRUMENTATION

#### Ventilators

An automatic lung ventilator has to perform four functions:

1. To inflate the lungs during inspiration.
2. To change over from inspiration to expiration.

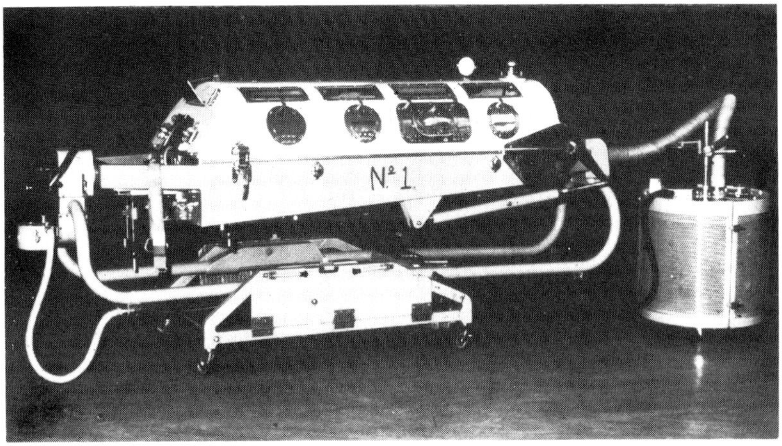


9/Fig. 3.—The Kelleher rotating tank ventilator. (Courtesy of Dr. W. H. Kelleher)

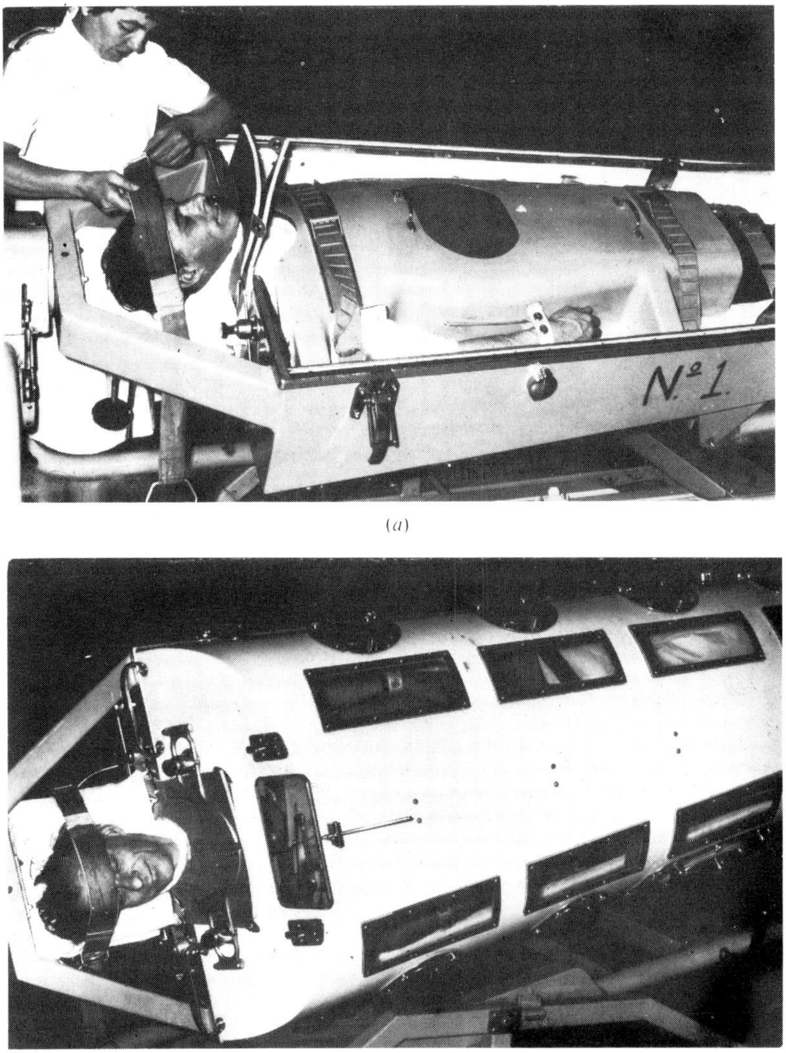


(*a*)

(*b*)

9/Fig. 4.—The Kelleher rotating tank ventilator in use.
(*a*) Before rotating the patient, a body-shaped shell is strapped into position inside the ventilator;
(*b*) the ventilator is rotated about its long axis whilst a forehead strap holds the patient's head. (Courtesy of Dr. W. H. Kelleher)

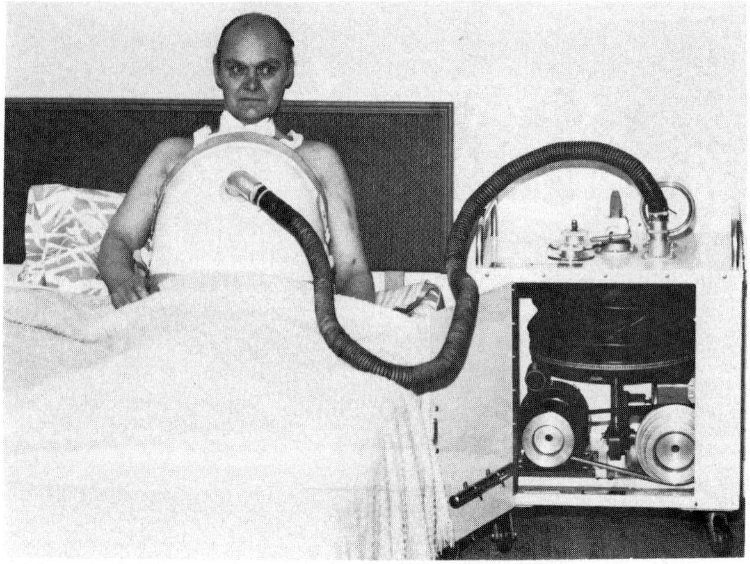

9/FIG. 5.—This patient with primary alveolar hypoventilation syndrome uses a cuirass ventilator for respiratory support at night. (Photograph by courtesy of Dr. B. D. W. Harrison and Dr. C. H. M. Woollam.)

3. To allow deflation of the lungs during expiration.
4. To change over from expiration to inspiration.

The changes from inspiration to expiration, and from expiration to inspiration, are referred to as "cycling".

**Inspiration**

During inspiration a ventilator may behave as a pressure generator or a flow generator.

A pressure generator applies a set pressure pattern to the upper airway during inspiration. As a result of the difference between upper airway pressure and alveolar pressure, gas flows into the lungs. The pattern of gas flow will depend on the pressure pattern produced by the ventilator, lung compliance, airway resistance and the time allowed for inspiration. Since the added tidal volume is given mathematically by the integral of the flow pattern with respect to time, the tidal volume will also depend on all the factors which affect flow. The maximum pressure generated by this type of ventilator is relatively low (25–30 cm $H_2O$).

A flow generator delivers a set flow pattern to the lungs during inspiration. The alveolar and upper airway pressures developed will depend on the flow pattern delivered by the ventilator, lung compliance, airway resistance and the time allowed for inspiration. However, since the tidal volume depends on the integral of the flow pattern, and the flow pattern is fixed, tidal volume is independent of lung compliance and airway resistance.

*Pressure generators* can be thought of as "weak" ventilators because the tidal volume delivered will change as the patient's lung characteristics change. In these ventilators airway pressure is the independent variable; flow and tidal volume are dependent variables and are affected by changes in lung compliance and airway resistance.

*Flow generators* can be thought of as "strong" ventilators because the tidal volume delivered will not change as the patient's lung characteristics change. In these ventilators flow and tidal volume are the independent variables; airway and alveolar pressure are the dependent variables and are affected by changes in lung compliance and airway resistance.

Pressure generators are adequate for artificial ventilation during anaesthesia or for long-term ventilation of patients with normal lungs. Flow generators are used on intensive care units for ventilating patients with low lung compliance and high airway resistance. Flow generators ensure that constant tidal volume is delivered in spite of changing lung characteristics.

In the past the distinction between pressure generators and flow generators was important. Cheap and simple ventilators used a weighted

9/Fig. 6.—Some waveforms which have been used when studying the effect of different inspiratory flow patterns on gas exchange and the circulation. (*a*) sine-wave; (*b*) ramp, or accelerating flow; (*c*) top-hat, or constant flow; (*d*) reverse ramp, or decelerating flow.

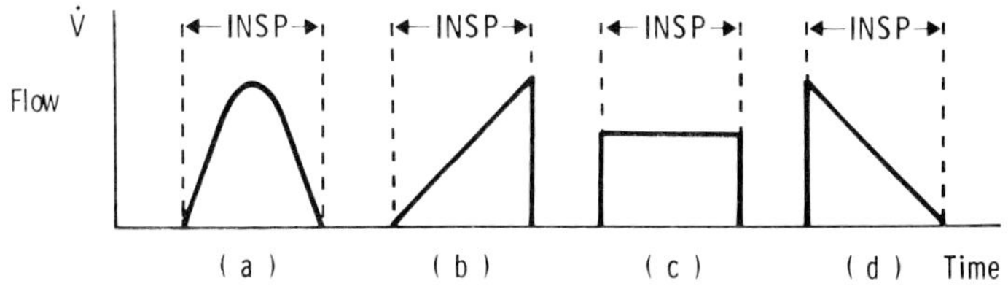


concertina bag to generate a constant pressure pattern during inspiration. Even today these ventilators remain adequate for the majority of patients who require artificial ventilation.

The more sophisticated modern ventilators are fitted with devices which measure the instantaneous flow of gas during inspiration. This information can be incorporated into a feedback loop to ensure delivery of some pre-determined flow pattern. As a result, there is now greater emphasis on the flow pattern produced by a ventilator during inspiration. In theory these ventilators could be designed to deliver any flow pattern, but when investigating the effects of various patterns on gas exchange, the four waveforms shown in Fig. 6 have attracted most interest.

No matter what flow pattern is chosen, the inspiratory flow can be modified further by adding an end-inspiratory pause (EIP). Towards the end of inspiration, the flow of gas ceases but the lungs are held inflated for a variable period called the "pause time". Figure 7 shows how flow and alveolar pressure vary with time when an end-inspiratory pause is added.

**Inspiratory-to-Expiratory Cycling (I→E)**

The changeover from inspiration to expiration may be:

1. Time-cycled, occurring after a pre-determined duration of inspiration.
2. Volume-cycled, occurring after a pre-determined volume has been delivered to the patient.

The use of any one mode of cycling implies that the changeover will occur no matter what the values of any other variables. For example, if a ventilator is time-cycled the change to expiration will occur no matter what airway pressure has been reached or tidal volume delivered.

*Time-cycling* is popular with ventilator designers. The timing mechanism may be electronic, mechanical or pneumatic.

*Volume-cycling*.—There is some confusion as to what volume-cycling really means. Ideally, a volume-cycled ventilator would change over to expiration when the desired tidal volume had been delivered to the patient's lungs. Unfortunately, lung expansion is not easy to measure and volume-cycled ventilators rely on measuring the volume of gas leaving the ventilator. If there are leaks in the apparatus, or if the connecting tubes are distensible, the volume leaving the ventilator may be very different from the volume which reaches the lungs.

It has been suggested that "true" volume-

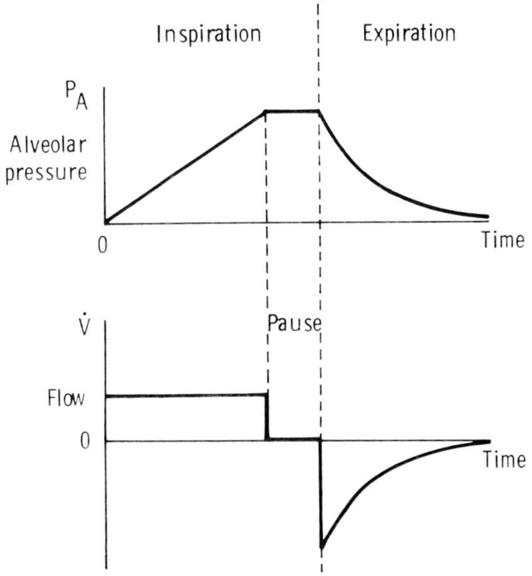


9/Fig. 7.—The variation of alveolar pressure and flow with time when an end-inspiratory pause is used. During the first part of inspiration this particular ventilator acts as a constant flow generator. The exponential flow pattern during expiration is characteristic of a constant pressure generator.

cycling should apply to those ventilators which measure the gas volume leaving the ventilator and compare it with the volume which the patient exhales. This would be better regarded as a form of monitoring during ventilation.

Further confusion arises because many ventilators have an adjustable tidal volume control which limits the excursion of the inflating bellows. Many such ventilators create the optical illusion of being volume-cycled, though in fact they are time-cycled: they can be classified as "volume pre-set". To ensure delivery of a pre-set volume, the ventilator must have sufficient power to overcome increases in airway resistance or decreases in lung compliance.

*Other forms of cycling*.—Both pressure-cycling and flow-cycling are possible, but neither is commonly used. If an adjustable pressure safety valve is set to a low value, the changeover from inspiration to expiration may become pressure-cycled in some ventilators that would otherwise be time-cycled or volume-cycled.

### Expiration

The majority of ventilators allow passive expiration to the atmosphere. The ventilator therefore behaves as a constant pressure generator during expiration, the generated pressure being atmospheric.

Simple passive expiration to atmosphere can be modified by applying:

1. Negative end-expiratory pressure, NEEP.
2. Expiratory retard, ER.
3. Positive end-expiratory pressure, PEEP.

**NEEP.**—During the early development of IPPV the use of a subatmospheric (negative) pressure phase during expiration was advocated to aid expiratory gas flow and reduce mean intrathoracic pressure. Many ventilators still provide this facility. The way in which the subatmospheric pressure is generated will determine the exact waveform of the applied pressure during expiration. Nevertheless, to maintain the analogy with PEEP, NEEP tends to be used as a blanket acronym whenever a subatmospheric pressure is applied during expiration.

**Expiratory retard.**—A variable resistance is placed in the expiratory limb of the ventilator. Expiratory flow rate is reduced and this may help to prevent peripheral airway collapse in chronic lung disease with air-flow obstruction; the effect is probably the same as that of "pursed-lip breathing" which some patients with chronic lung disease employ. The expiratory time may have to be prolonged to allow adequate lung deflation. The effect of ER on the fall of alveolar pressure during expiration is shown in Fig. 8(*a*).

**PEEP.**—Positive end-expiratory pressure increases alveolar pressure throughout the respiratory cycle. The ventilator still acts as a pressure generator during expiration but the generated pressure is some pre-set value (the PEEP level) above atmospheric pressure. PEEP is usually applied by plugging a spring-loaded valve into the expiratory port of the ventilator. The ideal PEEP valve should offer no resistance to flow until the pressure has fallen to the pre-set level.

The effect of PEEP on alveolar pressure during expiration is shown in Fig. 8(*b*).

### Expiratory-to-Inspiratory Cycling (E→ I)

The changeover from expiration to inspiration is nearly always time-cycled, though in theory other modes of cycling could be used.

It is important to know exactly which time interval is used to cycle the ventilator. Some ventilators cycle after a pre-set duration of expiration, others after a pre-set duration of the entire respiratory cycle. If the latter interval is used for cycling, any increase in the inspiratory time will lead to a corresponding decrease in the expiratory time. These changes may have a profound effect on inspiratory/expiratory time ratio.

### Inspiratory /Expiratory Time Ratio (I:E)

The I:E ratio can have an important effect on the changes in mean intrathoracic pressure

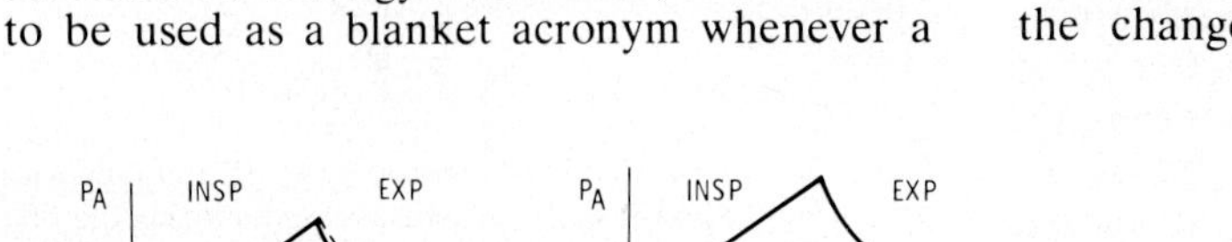

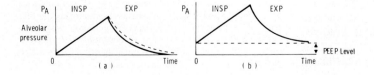


9/FIG. 8.—The variation of alveolar pressure with time: (*a*) with expiratory retard; (*b*) with PEEP. The fall in pressure during expiration with expiratory retard is shown by a dotted line.

which accompany IPPV. In some ventilators the I:E ratio is fixed at about 1:2. Where the ratio can be varied, expiration should normally occupy at least half the respiratory cycle.

**Minute Volume Divider**

Some ventilators are powered by pressure of the gas which will ultimately be delivered to the patient. The amount of gas which is delivered to the ventilator each minute therefore becomes the patient's minute volume. The minute volume is given by the product of the tidal volume and the frequency, so that only one of these variables can be chosen independently.

**Triggering**

Triggering allows control of the ventilator frequency by the patient's own respiratory rhythm. A triggering device detects the fall in pressure in the ventilator tubing as the patient starts to breathe and initiates an automatic inflation of the lungs. A safety mechanism ensures adequate minute volume should the patient become apnoeic.

**Intermittent Mandatory Ventilation (IMV)**

This technique combines spontaneous respiration and artificial ventilation. The intubated patient may breathe as he wishes but his own respiratory efforts are supplemented by "mandatory" inflations of constant volume from the ventilator. The ventilator frequency can be varied so that artificial ventilation forms a variable proportion of the total minute volume.

Two circuits are required for IMV, one for artificial ventilation and one for spontaneous respiration. Though they are both connected to the patient, they are separated functionally by two non-return valves. The design of these valves must ensure that little additional resistance is experienced by the patient when breathing spontaneously. The expiratory limb of the combined circuits can be modified to provide PEEP.

Whatever its advantages and virtues, IMV undoubtedly increases the complexity of the apparatus required for artificial ventilation.

**Mandatory Minute Volume (MMV)[8]**

This technique is a further development of IMV and ensures that the patient achieves a certain minimum minute volume. This minimum is delivered to the apparatus each minute and should the patient fail to achieve the required minute volume by spontaneous respiration, the deficit is delivered to the ventilator circuit to be supplied as mandatory ventilation. However, the patient is able to exceed the mandatory minute volume by spontaneous respiration.

**Dead Spaces**

Some conscious patients will not tolerate IPPV unless large tidal volumes are used. To avoid excessive reduction in arterial $P_{CO_2}$, artificial dead spaces consisting of tubes of different internal volumes (50–250 ml) can be inserted between the patient and the Y-piece of the ventilator tubing.

**Oxygen Enrichment**

Most patients receiving IPPV require some oxygen enrichment of the inspired gas to ensure adequate arterial $P_{O_2}$. Ventilators used for anaesthesia may draw their gas supply from an anaesthetic machine so that the inspired gas composition will be determined by the rotameter settings. If the ventilator applies a back pressure, the rotameters may not give a true indication of gas flows.

Other ventilators use gas mixing valves to provide air/oxygen or nitrous oxide/oxygen mixtures of known composition from sources of compressed gas. It is important that the oxygen concentration of the gas delivered by the ventilator remains constant throughout inspiration.

**Monitoring and Alarms**

Every ventilator must have facilities for measuring airway pressure, and expired tidal and minute volumes. It is important to measure the tidal volume *expired* by the patient: this may be less than the volume leaving the ventilator. A safety valve should be fitted to guard against excessive airway pressures; ideally this valve should be adjustable to take account of different clinical circumstances.

The following features will increase patient safety:

1. High and low value alarms for:
   - airway pressure
   - expired minute volume
   - oxygen concentration
2. Failure alarms for:
   - power source
   - oxygen supply

### Choice of Ventilator

This will be determined by clinical requirements and by cost. Whilst a simple ventilator may suffice for routine anaesthesia, a more sophisticated machine will be necessary for long-term ventilation of a patient with ARDS. Many modern ventilators offer a bewildering number of options for modifying the inspiratory and expiratory phases; unfortunately this gain in sophistication is often at the expense of reliability and simplicity.

The International Standards Organisation (ISO) and the American National Standards Institute have suggested tests which enable comparisons to be made between the performance of different ventilators. Loh and his colleagues[9] describe the four main tests which are carried out using a standard lung model whose resistance and compliance can be varied. These tests are:

1. Endurance test, to assess the ventilator's reliability over a period of 2000 hours.
2. Waveform test, to enable a functional analysis of the ventilator to be made, and to detect leakage through mechanical valves.
3. Volume performance, to show the maximum volumes of gas which can be delivered over a wide range of frequencies.
4. Internal compliance measurement, to measure the volume of gas compressed in the ventilator, humidifier and tubing.

Three ventilators with different specifications are shown in Figs. 9–11.

In the past, anaesthetists were expected to know how their ventilators worked. The technology of many modern ventilators is so complex that this requirement is no longer reasonable. Robinson[10] has suggested that the user should know *what the ventilator does*, not *how it does it*. Those who wish to know *how their ventilators do it* should consult the comprehensive account of the technical aspects of artificial ventilation given by Mushin and his colleagues;[11] they also give functional analyses of some 80 ventilators which are currently in use.

## Artificial Airway

To perform effective IPPV a cuffed tube must be placed in the trachea to ensure a gas-tight seal and to prevent aspiration of material into the lungs.

**Route.**—During the early development of IPPV, any patient who required ventilation for more than a few hours underwent tracheostomy. The red-rubber endotracheal tubes in use at that time were likely to cause laryngeal damage if left in place for too long and the length of an endotracheal tube made it difficult to aspirate secretions from the lungs.

Since the introduction of plastic tubes, the decision to perform tracheostomy can be delayed. Most centres are now prepared to consider 2 to 3 weeks of endotracheal intubation, but much longer periods have been used without subsequent evidence of permanent laryngeal damage.

The advantages and disadvantages of prolonged endotracheal intubation compared with tracheostomy are shown in Table 1. Some of the disadvantages of prolonged oral endotracheal intubation are overcome by nasal intubation. The advantages and disadvantages of the nasal route are shown in Table 2.

Though the trend is towards longer periods of endotracheal intubation,[121] there are undoubted practical advantages to early tracheostomy if IPPV is to be continued for several weeks or if the return to spontaneous respiration

9/Table 1

Prolonged Endotracheal Intubation Compared with Tracheostomy

| *Advantages:* | *Disadvantages:* |
|---|---|
| Intubation is an everyday procedure and may be repeated indefinitely on the same patient. | Heavy sedation may be required to tolerate an endotracheal tube. Tracheostomy tubes are more easily tolerated. |
| Operative complications of tracheostomy are avoided. | Laryngeal damage may occur. |
| Infection via stoma from adjacent wounds is avoided. | Fixation of the tube is more difficult and there is risk of endobronchial intubation. |
| No permanent scar is left. | The tube may become kinked in the pharynx. |
| | The long tube makes aspiration of secretions more difficult. |

(Courtesy of Seeley, H. F. (1981). Artificial Ventilation and Artificial Lungs. In *Thoracic Medicine*, Ed. Emerson, P. London: Butterworth.)

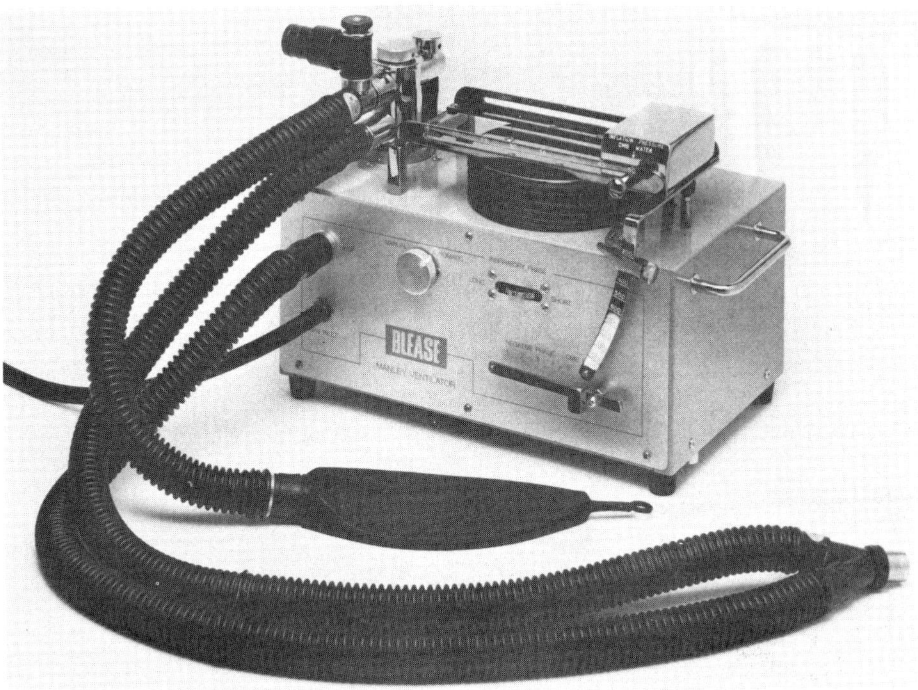


9/Fig. 9.—The Manley Anaesthetic Ventilator. This time-cycled pressure generator, a minute volume divider, is adequate for the majority of patients who require IPPV during anaesthesia. (Photograph courtesy of Blease Medical Equipment Ltd.)

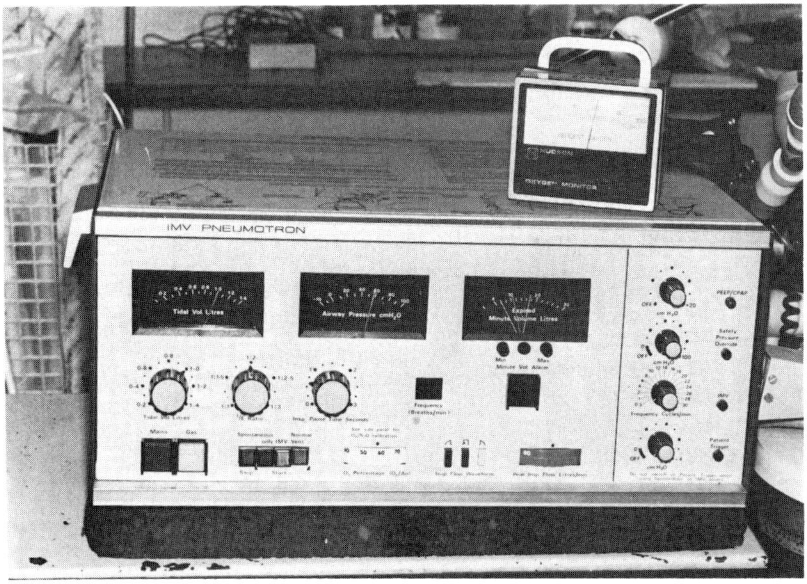


9/Fig. 10.—The IMV Pneumotron Ventilator (BOC Medishield) shown in use on the Intensive Care Unit at St. George's Hospital, London. This volume-cycled flow generator provides a wide range of facilities including IMV, end-inspiratory pause, PEEP/CPAP, and a choice of inspiratory flow waveform.

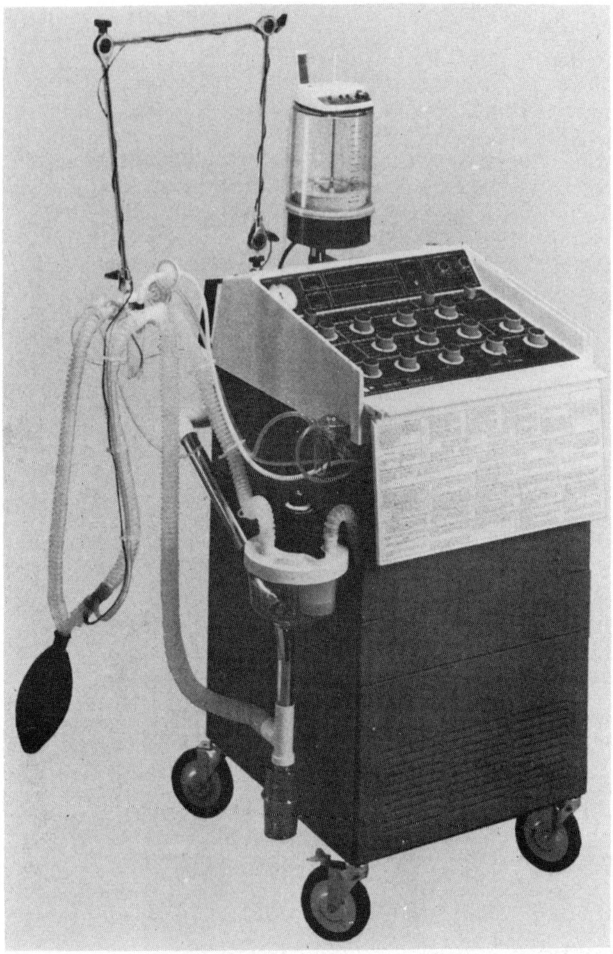

9/Fig. 11.—The Bennett MA-2 Ventilator. This volume-cycled constant flow generator provides facilities for IMV, end-inspiratory pause, PEEP/CPAP, artificial sigh and triggering. It is fitted with a comprehensive system of adjustable alarms. (Photograph courtesy of Simonsen and Weel Ltd. and Puritan-Bennett Corporation.)

9/Table 2
Nasotracheal Compared with Orotracheal Intubation

| *Advantages:* | *Disadvantages:* |
|---|---|
| Fixation of the tube is easier. | Damage to nose and nasopharynx can occur. |
| Less sedation required to tolerate tube. | Greater length of tube hinders aspiration of secretions. |
| Mouth care more easily performed. | |

(Courtesy of Seeley, H. F. (1981). Artificial Ventilation and Artificial Lungs. In: *Thoracic Medicine*, Ed. Emerson, P. London: Butterworth.)

is likely to be difficult or prolonged. Consideration of the merits of each route in an individual case is more valuable than relying on fixed time limits for one particular route.

There may, however, be surgical indications for performing a tracheostomy, such as neoplasia of the head and neck.

### Laryngeal and Tracheal Damage

The trachea and larynx are delicate structures and endotracheal and tracheostomy tubes are rigid foreign bodies. It is hardly surprising that damage can occur.

Laryngeal damage may follow oral or nasal intubation. Damage may be reduced by avoiding large diameter tubes, by preventing laryngeal movement, and by using tubes whose shape conforms to that of the upper airway. The shape of most endotracheal tubes available at present means that the posterior laryngeal structures are at greatest risk.[12] Close inspection of the larynx after extubation frequently reveals pathological changes. Hoarseness and some difficulty in swallowing are not uncommon but significant morbidity lasting more than a few days is rare.

Some degree of damage to the tracheal mucosa is inevitable and varies from microscopic hyperaemia to frank ulceration. If the underlying cartilage becomes eroded healing occurs by fibrosis, and subsequent contracture leads to tracheal stenosis. After tracheostomy stenosis may occur at three sites; at the stoma, at the site of the cuff, or at the position once occupied by the tip of the tube. The incidence of stenosis at the three sites differs in various surveys; this probably reflects the varying skill and experience of the surgeons performing the tracheostomy and the different standards of nursing care in the long-term management of the patients.

Radiographic evidence of tracheal stenosis after prolonged IPPV is common, but considerable reduction in the cross-sectional area of the trachea can occur without interference with respiratory function.[13] Patients who do develop symptoms complain initially of dyspnoea during moderate exercise, irritating cough, and an inability to clear the throat. In patients with chronic lung disease, these symptoms may be unjustly ascribed to the lung disease rather than to tracheal stenosis. Stridor is usually a late development and indicates a serious loss of tracheal area. In established stenosis, temporary relief may be afforded by tracheal dilatation, but tracheal resection or permanent tracheostomy offers the only hope of prolonged relief.

Corticosteroid therapy and the use of high inflation pressures during IPPV increase the risk of the opposite complication, tracheal dilatation.[14]

Considerable attention has been paid to cuff design, particularly for long-term intubation. Unfortunately, many studies have relied on measuring intra-cuff pressures which may not necessarily reflect tracheal wall pressures. It is now established that the use of large volume cuffs reduces the incidence of tracheal stenosis at the cuff site. When large volume cuffs are used, intra-cuff pressure gives a reasonable estimate of tracheal wall pressure and there are theoretical arguments for the greater preservation of mucosal blood flow when the cuff pressure is more evenly distributed. Unfortunately, the benefits of large volume cuffs are to some extent offset by the following disadvantages:

1. Difficulty of insertion and removal.
2. Increased incidence of laryngeal damage and sore throat.
3. Increased incidence of tracheal dilatation.
4. Increased incidence of aspiration along folds in the cuff.

The inflation of the cuff against the tracheal wall is tested at the peak airway pressure to which the patient will be subjected. The aim is to provide conditions of "minimal occlusion" or "minimal leak". The difference between occlusion and leak is one of intent rather than practice because the volume of gas in the cuff may change with temperature and with the diffusion of oxygen, carbon dioxide and nitrous oxide across the cuff membrane. The diameter of the trachea changes with the position of the head and in response to drugs. Thus management regimes based on attention to intracuff *pressure* are likely to be more successful than those which measure intracuff *volume*.

Large volume cuffs are sometimes called low pressure cuffs. This is misleading as overinflation can still lead to excessive pressure on the tracheal wall. As the intracuff pressure of large volume cuffs varies with airway pressure during IPPV, intracuff pressure measurements are quoted at some specific point in the respiratory cycle. An end-expiratory intracuff pressure of 25 cm $H_2O$ (2·5 kPa) has been proposed as a minimum to prevent aspiration of material which collects above the cuff.[15]

Various pressure-limiting devices have been proposed to guard against excessive cuff pressure but none has proved completely satisfactory in use. At present, constant surveillance to ensure correct cuff inflation is the best safeguard against tracheal damage.

In the past, cuff deflation was allowed at regular intervals in an attempt to rescue the ischaemic mucosa for short periods during each hour. This technique has now been shown to be either of no benefit or positively harmful and has been almost universally abandoned.[16,17]

Endotracheal tubes with small volume cuffs are still used widely in anaesthesia, where the long-term complication of tracheal stenosis is less likely and the problems of post-extubation stridor and sore throat are more troublesome. However, new developments in cuff design may make large volume cuffs more acceptable for short-term intubation. Recommendations for cuff design have been made recently by Mehta;[18,19] the problems of measuring cuff pressures have been reviewed by Black and Seegobin.[20] A selection of cuffed tubes and a gauge for measuring intracuff pressure are shown in Figs. 12 and 13.

## PHYSIOLOGY OF IPPV

### Gas Exchange

Gas exchange during IPPV is governed by two principles:

1. Minute volume is adjusted to give the required arterial $P_{CO_2}$.
2. Inspired $O_2$ concentration is adjusted to give the required arterial $P_{O_2}$.

The most efficient use of IPPV occurs when:

1. Ratio of physiological dead space/tidal volume ($V_D/V_T$) has a minimum value.
2. Alveolar/arterial (A-a) $P_{O_2}$ difference has a minimum value.

Since the introduction of IPPV, many studies have been carried out to try and identify the most efficient ventilatory pattern. These studies are technically difficult to perform and some of the results have been conflicting. The experimental subjects have usually been dogs or fit humans under anaesthesia and the extension of any findings to patients with severe respiratory disease should be made with caution. A summary of the major factors affecting the efficiency of gas exchange will now be given; more detailed accounts are those of Nunn,[21] Sykes,[22] and Baker and his colleagues.[23,24]

**Duration of Inspiration and Expiration**

An inspiratory time of 1·0–1·3 seconds is probably the minimum for efficient gas exchange but prolonging inspiration beyond this seems to offer no benefit. Expiratory time must allow full expiration and an inspiratory/expiratory ratio of about 1:2 is the most

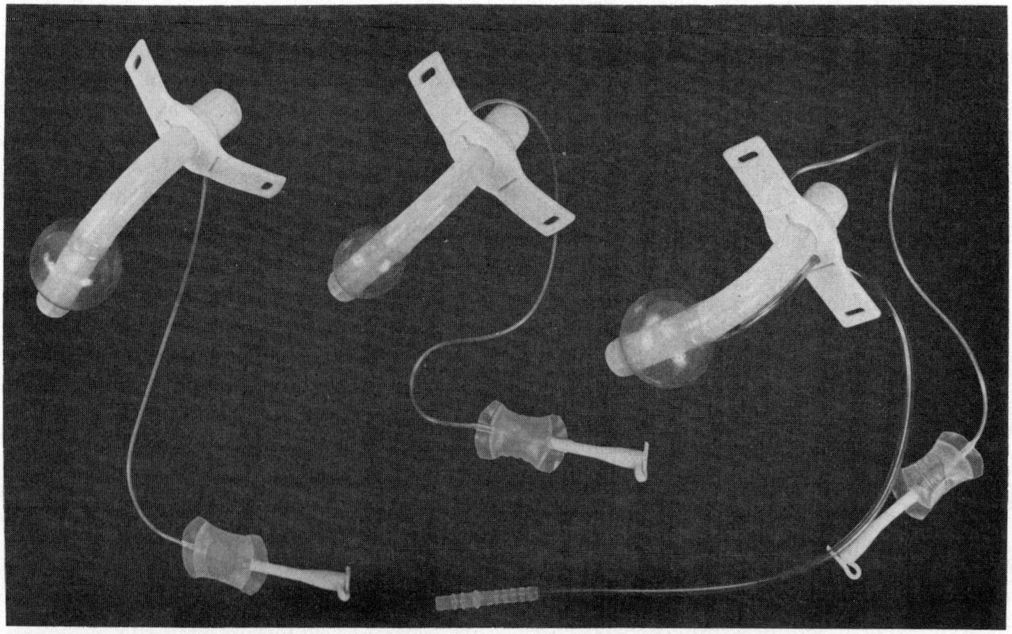

9/Fig. 12.—Disposable plastic tracheostomy tubes: (left) with large volume cuff; (centre) with small volume cuff; (right) with large volume cuff and an air/oxygen line which terminates just above the cuff—this line enables a flow of gas to be passed through the larynx so that the patient can speak. (Photograph courtesy of Portex Ltd.)

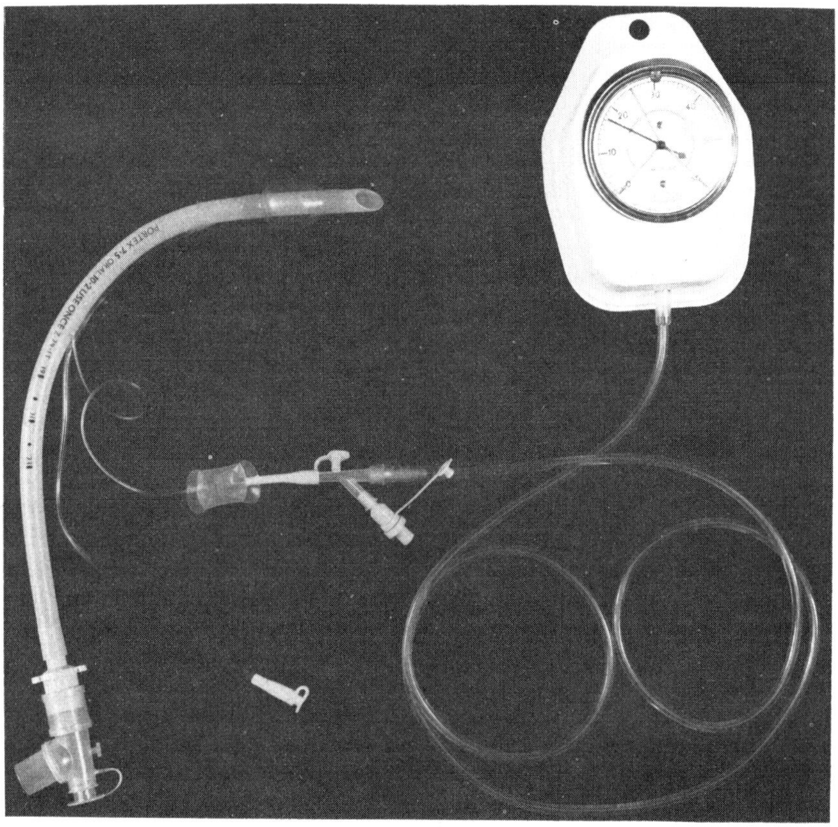

9/FIG. 13.—Disposable plastic endotracheal tube with large volume cuff. The tube is fitted with a $CO_2$ monitoring line to facilitate sampling of expired gas. A double swivel connector is in place: this connector can rotate through 360° in two planes so that drag from ventilator tubing is reduced, and a port allows suction without disconnection. Tubes are supplied uncut; before use they must be cut to suitable lengths depending on the size of the patient. A gauge for measuring intracuff pressure is also shown. (Photograph courtesy of Portex Ltd.)

common pattern. If expiration is made shorter than inspiration, the resulting increase in mean intrathoracic pressure may have adverse effects on the circulation.

### Flow Waveform

Recent studies suggest that the reversed ramp flow pattern is the most efficient for gas exchange[24] (see Fig. 6). The ramp waveform is the least efficient, and the top-hat and sine waveforms occupy an intermediate position. However, these differences are small and of little significance in patients with normal lungs. Some improvement in gas exchange is reported when an end-inspiratory pause is used.

### Tidal Volume

During the period 1959–1963, there were reports that IPPV with small tidal volumes led to a progressive fall in lung compliance and an increase in (A-a) $Po_2$ difference. These unwelcome changes could be prevented by administering deep breaths every 5–10 minutes. As a result, some ventilators incorporated a "sigh" mechanism to provide hyperinflation at regular intervals. Alternatively, the changes in the lungs could be prevented by using tidal volumes of at least 7 ml/kg body weight.

Subsequent work has cast doubt on the validity of the original reports and the value of sighing during IPPV is not universally accepted. Today, most anaesthetists use tidal volumes in excess of 7 ml/kg. Conscious patients rarely tolerate tidal volumes less than 10–15 ml/kg during artificial ventilation, in spite of satisfactory arterial blood gas values.

The value of maintaining "optimal mechanical lung function"[22] by removal of secretions, treatment of bronchospasm and re-expansion of areas of collapse is not disputed. Regular physiotherapy is essential during long-term ventilation but even during anaesthesia every opportunity should be taken to re-expand the lungs, especially after endotracheal suction.

Though ventilator function may affect $V_D/V_T$ and (A-a) $Po_2$, other factors are likely to be of greater practical importance during IPPV.

### Factors Affecting Ratio of Physiological Dead Space/Tidal Volume ($V_D/V_T$)

When comparing values of $V_D/V_T$ ratio, appropriate compensation must be made for changes in dead space introduced by apparatus. During IPPV values of $V_D/V_T$ ratio are increased by:

1. Increasing age of the patient.
2. Smoking and pulmonary disease.
3. Pulmonary hypoperfusion, whether intentional (deliberate hypotension) or unintentional (haemorrhage, myocardial infarction).
4. Anaesthesia.

The value of $V_D/V_T$ ratio is normally around 0·3. In 1967, Cooper showed that much higher values were present during anaesthesia with IPPV. An approximate formula relating the value of the ratio to age in patients with normal lungs is:

$$V_D/V_T \text{ (as percentage)} = 33 + (\text{Age}/3)$$

The reasons for the increase in $V_D/V_T$ ratio seen during anaesthesia with IPPV are discussed by Nunn[21] and Conway.[25]

Large increases in physiological dead space can usually be ascribed to increases in alveolar dead space. Any increase in alveolar dead space causes an increase in arterial/end-expiratory $Pco_2$ difference; this is of practical importance if end-tidal $CO_2$ measurements are used to estimate arterial $Pco_2$. In the presence of severe respiratory disease, the difference is large and unpredictable. Nunn[21] quotes the following findings during general anaesthesia in healthy patients:

1. The mean value of arterial/end-expiratory $Pco_2$ difference is 5 mm Hg (0·7 kPa) with a range of 0–10 mm Hg (0–1·3 kPa).
2. The value is uninfluenced by actual $Pco_2$ level, and is similar for both artificial ventilation and spontaneous respiration.

Higher values have been reported during thoracic surgery.

Continuous end-tidal $CO_2$ measurement can still be a valuable monitoring aid even when the arterial/end-tidal $Pco_2$ difference is unknown: the technique can provide useful qualitative information on respiratory and circulatory function.

End-tidal $Pco_2$ measurements have been used in automated systems for the control of artificial ventilation. A feedback loop permits the adjustment of minute volume to maintain the end-tidal $Pco_2$ within set limits.[26] Safeguards must be built into the system as there are many possible causes of a change in end-tidal $Pco_2$.

### Optimum Arterial $Pco_2$

Patients tolerate long-term artificial ventilation more satisfactorily when the arterial $Pco_2$ is maintained at 3·8–7·5 mm Hg (0·5–1·0 kPa) below its usual value. For those accustomed to an elevated $Paco_2$, this may result in a level which is still considerably above "normal".

The body stores of carbon dioxide are considerable so that changes in arterial $Pco_2$ due to alteration in alveolar ventilation are relatively slow. Measurement of $Paco_2$ at intervals of less than 30 minutes is rarely indicated. For a given change in ventilation, the fall in $Paco_2$ due to hyperventilation occurs much more rapidly than the equivalent rise in $Paco_2$ due to hypoventilation.

### Factors Affecting Alveolar/Arterial $Po_2$ Differences

These are:

1. Alveolar $Po_2$ (which in practice is determined mainly by the inspired $Po_2$).
2. Degree of right-to-left shunt, $\dot{Q}s/\dot{Q}_T$.
3. Increased ventilation/perfusion mismatch, $\dot{V}/\dot{Q}$ scatter.
4. Cardiac output, through its effect on (a) arterial/mixed venous oxygen content difference, and (b) distribution of pulmonary blood flow.

5. Oxygen consumption, through its effect on arterial/mixed venous oxygen content difference.
6. Shape of the haemoglobin dissociation curve ($P_{50}$ value).

It is possible to predict the effect of changes in any one of these factors provided the others remain constant. In practice, they are liable to interact in a non-linear mathematical relationship so that the final effect on alveolar/arterial $Po_2$ difference is unpredictable.

Fortunately the following generalisations can be made:

1. Intensive care:
   The majority of patients receiving artificial ventilation on intensive care units will have substantial increases in alveolar/arterial $Po_2$ difference. The highest values will be seen in patients with conditions such as adult respiratory distress syndrome (ARDS). Much smaller values are seen in those with normal lungs during prolonged IPPV. Many such patients can be ventilated satisfactorily with room air.
2. Anaesthesia:
   Alveolar/arterial $Po_2$ difference is nearly always increased during anaesthesia; this increase is least marked in children and young adults undergoing brief operations. Nunn[21] quotes pooled data from a number of studies which indicate close correlation between arterial $Po_2$ and inspired $Po_2$, the *mean* arterial $Po_2$ having a value of about half the inspired $Po_2$. However, the wide dispersion of arterial $Po_2$ values about each mean shows that some patients with apparently normal cardio-respiratory function have a surprisingly low $Pao_2$. To ensure adequate arterial $Po_2$ during anaesthesia using IPPV, inspired oxygen concentrations of 30–50 per cent are normally used. The unpredictability of the alveolar/arterial $Po_2$ difference during anaesthesia and intensive care means that no measurements made on inspired or expired gas can be used to infer the adequacy of arterial $Po_2$. Non-invasive means of assessing arterial oxygenation are discussed on page 286.

### Optimum Arterial $Po_2$

The inspired oxygen concentration should be set to the minimum value that gives adequate haemoglobin saturation. It is often forgotten that because of the shape of the haemoglobin-oxygen dissociation curve, the $Pao_2$ need not be maintained at the oft-quoted "normal" value of 100 mm Hg (13 kPa). When the $Pao_2$ is 60 mm Hg (8 kPa) haemoglobin is still about 90 per cent saturated with oxygen.

In contrast to carbon dioxide, the oxygen stores of the body are small. Very rapid changes in arterial $Po_2$ occur as a result of changes in alveolar $Po_2$; the timing of blood gas analysis should reflect this fact. The iso-shunt diagram[27] is useful for adjusting the inspired oxygen concentration to give a required level of arterial $Po_2$. Use of this diagram helps to reduce the number of blood gas analyses required for patient management.

During IPPV, increases in $V_D/V_T$ ratio can nearly always be compensated for by increasing alveolar ventilation. Unfortunately, compensation for an increased alveolar/arterial $Po_2$ difference cannot rely solely on raising alveolar $Po_2$. When selecting an inspired oxygen concentration, a course must be steered between arterial hypoxaemia on the one hand and pulmonary oxygen toxicity on the other.

The reasons for the increase in alveolar/arterial $Po_2$ difference seen during anaesthesia with IPPV are discussed by Nunn.[21]

## Circulatory Effects of IPPV

During quiet spontaneous respiration, mean intrathoracic pressure is about 5 cm $H_2O$ (0·5 kPa) below atmospheric pressure. The actual intrathoracic pressure swings about this mean value, decreasing some 3 cm $H_2O$ (0·3 kPa) below the mean during inspiration, and increasing by the same amount above the mean during expiration. A subatmospheric pressure within the thorax (often referred to as "negative pressure") aids venous return to the right side of the heart.

During IPPV, the cyclical pressure swings during inspiration and expiration are reversed and the application of positive pressure during inspiration causes a rise in mean intrathoracic pressure which impedes venous return. Any increase in airway resistance or fall in pulmonary compliance tends to exacerbate this increase in mean intrathoracic pressure.

The effects of different patterns of lung inflation on cardiac output were studied over thirty years ago by Cournand and his colleagues. Although Cournand's work was carried out on conscious volunteers ventilated by mask, his findings had a profound effect on the practice of artificial ventilation and on the design of ventilators. Negligible changes in cardiac output were reported when the inflation pattern was designed to reduce the inevitable rise in intrathoracic pressure to a minimum. This pattern consisted of a slow pressure rise during inspiration, a fast fall of pressure during expiration, and an expiratory time which exceeded the inspiratory time (Cournand Type III Curve). Not surprisingly, an adverse effect on cardiac output was seen when inspiration took longer than expiration, and a positive pressure was applied during expiration (Cournand Type II Curve).

Subsequent studies of the circulatory response to changing inspiratory waveform and inspiratory/expiratory time ratio have yielded conflicting results. These studies have simultaneously examined the effect of different ventilator settings on both gas exchange and the circulation. Recent work indicates that the reversed ramp waveform (Fig. 6) causes most interference with the circulation.[24] However, the differences are small and of doubtful practical importance in most cases. It is interesting that the pattern which promotes the best gas exchange has the worst effect on cardiac output, and vice versa.

The effects of raised airway pressure on the circulation have been studied for many years by performing the Valsalva manoeuvre. IPPV may be regarded as a train of Valsalva manoeuvres limited in the airway pressure achieved and the length of the inspiratory phase.

During the classical Valsalva manoeuvre, mean arterial pressure is well maintained in awake subjects with normal circulatory reflexes, whilst anaesthetised subjects usually show some decrease in arterial pressure. The changes in mean intrathoracic pressure which occur during "normal" IPPV are much less, so that mean arterial pressure is usually unaffected. Right atrial pressure is maintained by constriction of venous capacitance vessels. At high inflation pressures, the maintenance of arterial pressure also involves arteriolar constriction.

The ability of the circulation to withstand the adverse effects of IPPV depends on the integrity of various reflexes. Anything which interferes with transmission of impulses in the peripheral nervous system or which depresses the central nervous system, may result in the "blocked Valsalva" response: when positive airway pressure is applied, the arterial pressure falls; when the airway pressure is released, the recovery of arterial pressure is slow.

Factors likely to interfere with reflex compensation are:

1. Hypovolaemia.
2. Spinal cord transection, polyneuritis or peripheral neuropathy.
3. Ganglion blockade, $\alpha$-or $\beta$-adrenergic blockade.
4. Extensive intradural or extradural anaesthesia.
5. Moderate to deep general anaesthesia.
6. Head-up tilt.
7. Patient's general condition: old age, intrinsic myocardial disease, acute pancreatitis, septicaemia.

Some of these factors may be employed in techniques for producing deliberate hypotension. Many fit patients maintain their blood pressure in spite of a combination of these adverse factors: however, one additional physiological insult may then precipitate profound falls in cardiac output and arterial pressure.

Spontaneous respiration is accompanied by cyclical variations in right and left ventricular pressures. During inspiration, there is a rise in right ventricular output due to an increase in right ventricular diastolic filling and a decrease in right ventricular outflow impedance; there is a corresponding fall in left ventricular output as the increased capacitance of the pulmonary vascular bed during inspiration reduces the flow of blood to the left atrium.

This asynchrony of the cyclical changes of stroke volume with respiration is also seen during IPPV but the changes seen with inspiration and expiration during spontaneous respiration are reversed. During IPPV there is a transient rise in systemic arterial pressure during inspiration; this can often be detected by increased deflections of an oscillotonometer needle if the occluding cuff is inflated to just below systolic pressure. An identical transient increase in systemic arterial pressure is seen at the beginning of the Valsalva manoeuvre.

The circulatory effects of IPPV are normally ascribed to changes in mean intrathoracic pressure, but it would seem that cyclical variations in pulmonary vascular resistance and pulmonary blood volume also play a significant role. In clinical practice, effects of IPPV on the circulation are further complicated by changes in arterial $P_{CO_2}$ which occur. The actual value of $Pa_{CO_2}$ will have important effects on both pulmonary and systemic haemodynamics.

Detailed accounts of the effects of IPPV on the circulation are given by Conway[25] and Foëx.[28]

## PEEP AND NEEP

### Positive End-Expiratory Pressure (PEEP)

The application of PEEP can reduce alveolar/arterial $P_{O_2}$ difference for a given value of alveolar $P_{O_2}$. In practical terms, a higher arterial $P_{O_2}$ can be achieved at any given inspired oxygen concentration.

There are many experimental reports on the use of PEEP, but some of the results are conflicting. For detailed analysis and assessment the reader should consult the reviews by Stoddart,[29] Adams,[30] Pontoppidan and his colleagues,[31] and Fairley.[32]

The true importance of PEEP is difficult to assess. Some regard it as one of the greatest advances in respiratory therapy of the 1970s. Others point out that evidence for improved survival since the widespread introduction of PEEP is remarkably sparse.

PEEP probably produces its effects by three mechanisms:

1. An increase in functional residual capacity (FRC) and prevention of terminal airway closure.
2. A shift in interstitial pulmonary water.
3. Increased production and reduced inactivation of surfactant.

The first mechanism accounts for the increase in $Pa_{O_2}$ seen after a few breaths; the other mechanisms could account for the further increase which may be seen after 12–48 hours.

Mean intrathoracic pressure and pulmonary vascular resistance are increased during IPPV and further increases will occur when PEEP is used. Cardiac output tends to fall even though arterial pressure may remain unchanged. Additional factors which may contribute to this fall in cardiac output are:[33]

1. Reduced left ventricular stroke volume. Right ventricular loading modifies the configuration of the left ventricle as both structures are contained within the non-distensible pericardium.
2. Presence of a humoral factor with negative inotropic effects. A prostaglandin, whose metabolism is impaired when the lungs are stretched, is one suggestion.

Fortunately the adverse effects of PEEP on cardiac output are less marked in patients with ARDS, possibly because "stiff lungs" buffer the transmission of raised airway pressures to the great veins.

The falls in cardiac output which PEEP causes can usually be corrected by increases in blood volume. However, adverse effects of this relative circulatory overload may be seen if PEEP is subsequently removed.

PEEP reduces hepatic and renal blood flow, but the extent to which PEEP may contribute to a deterioration in hepatic and renal function in the critically ill is not known. PEEP may cause a rise in intracranial pressure and should be used with great caution in patients with head injuries or space-occupying lesions.

PEEP is used mainly in the treatment of ARDS and cardiac pulmonary oedema. It may be dangerous in asthma and offers no consistent benefit in the treatment of chronic obstructive airway disease, unless hypoxaemia is the result of large intrapulmonary shunt.[34]

Although a reduction in FRC occurs during general anaesthesia, PEEP has proved disappointing as a means of reducing the expected alveolar/arterial $P_{O_2}$ difference.[35] PEEP may have a place in thoracic anaesthesia; otherwise, in patients with normal lungs undergoing general anaesthesia, any benefits are outweighed by possible complications.

The following indications for PEEP have been suggested:

1. Inability to maintain an acceptable $Pa_{O_2}$ (60 mm Hg or 8 kPa) in spite of an inspired oxygen concentration of 50 per cent ($F_{IO_2}$ of 0·5).
2. Degree of pulmonary shunt ($\dot{Q}s/\dot{Q}_T$ ratio) greater than 10–15 per cent.
3. Conditions such as pulmonary aspiration where terminal airway closure would be expected.

Measurements of $Pa_{O_2}$ and $F_{IO_2}$ are easy to carry out and the first criterion is used more commonly. If the second indication is followed, then PEEP will be instituted more often.

It is customary to add PEEP in 3–5 cm $H_2O$ (0·3–0·5 kPa) increments and assess the effect of each addition after 20–30 minutes. The ultimate aim of artificial ventilation is to ensure adequate tissue oxygenation; since PEEP improves gas exchange whilst reducing cardiac output, a suitable compromise must be sought.

Suter and colleagues proposed that "best PEEP" is the PEEP level at which oxygen flux (cardiac output×arterial oxygen content) has a maximum value.[36] Experimentally they found that when the level was adjusted to "best PEEP", $V_D/V_T$ ratio had a minimum value. At "best PEEP" the highest value of total pulmonary compliance was observed.

Kirby and colleagues[37] believe that "optimal PEEP" coincides with the greatest reduction in $\dot{Q}s/\dot{Q}_T$ ratio in the absence of "detrimental effect" on cardiac output. They have used "high-level PEEP" (50–60 cm $H_2O$) in conjunction with IMV. Spontaneous breaths helped to limit the rise in intrathoracic pressure but the technique demands careful cardiovascular monitoring.

The following measurements have been suggested to assess the usefulness of PEEP:[38]

1. Inspired $O_2$ concentration.
2. Arterial $Po_2$.
3. Right atrial pressure.
4. Mixed venous $O_2$ content.
5. Pulmonary compliance.
6. Cardiac output.

Blood pressure, $Pao_2$ and $FIO_2$ are easily measured. Unfortunately, the information they provide is not sufficient to assess the therapeutic benefit of PEEP. Certainly PEEP demands close monitoring. Gas exchange may remain unchanged, and in some patients may actually deteriorate when PEEP is used. In any one patient, the need for PEEP and the appropriate PEEP level should be reassessed frequently. The problems of using PEEP in patients who are haemodynamically unstable have been reviewed by Hanson.[39]

Complications associated with the use of PEEP are:

1. Increases in ratio of volume of dead space/tidal volume ($V_D/V_T$) may occur.
2. Measurements of right and left atrial pressures and pulmonary capillary wedge pressure are more difficult to interpret.
3. Incidence of surgical emphysema and tension pneumothorax probably increases.
4. Complexity of the apparatus (and therefore the degree of hazard to the patient) is increased.

**Negative End-Expiratory Pressure (NEEP)**

During the early development of IPPV, negative end-expiratory pressure was advocated to increase the rate of expiratory gas flow and reduce the inevitable rise in intrathoracic pressure. It soon became apparent that any favourable effect on cardiac output was offset by decreases in both lung compliance and FRC. The decrease in FRC lead to air-trapping. However, adverse effects on arterial oxygenation are least when NEEP would be of greatest benefit, namely in hypovolaemia.[30]

Although NEEP has been abandoned, recent work shows that it improves renal function during artificial ventilation.[40] Whether preservation of function in other organs leads to a resurgence of interest in NEEP remains to be seen.

## SPECIFIC CLINICAL APPLICATIONS

### Indications for IPPV

IPPV may be indicated in the following circumstances:

1. During clinical anaesthesia, when drugs causing neuromuscular block or profound respiratory depression have been used deliberately as part of the anaesthetic technique.
2. When hypoxia and hypercapnia might be especially hazardous: after neurosurgery or cardiac surgery, or during the immediate treatment of head injuries.[41]
3. In primary ventilatory failure where there is interference with the nervous, muscular or skeletal mechanisms of normal breathing: poliomyelitis, myasthenia gravis, Guillain-Barré syndrome, and drug overdose. Initially, at least, lung function is normal in these patients.
4. In acute lung conditions which call for a great increase in respiratory work to maintain gas exchange: ARDS, cardiac pulmonary oedema, status asthmaticus, and

acute respiratory failure in chronic lung disease with air-flow obstruction.

These categories are not mutually exclusive. Patients with chest injuries may have bony cage fractures together with underlying lung contusion which causes gross ventilation/perfusion mismatch.

The value of "prophylactic" artificial ventilation has been recognised increasingly over the last 15–20 years. In many patients the risk of developing respiratory failure in the immediate postoperative period is so great that IPPV is continued for 24 to 48 hours after surgery. The technique may be regarded as an extension of anaesthetic management into the recovery period. It ensures adequate gas exchange, allows the liberal administration of narcotic analgesics and abolishes respiratory work.

Patients who should be considered for prophylactic ventilation include the obese, the cachectic, the septic, the hypothermic and those with previous history of cardiac or respiratory illness. The technique is of greatest value after thoracic, upper abdominal and major vascular operations.

Prophylactic ventilation can be useful in the management of certain patients; the extent to which it is truly "prophylactic" against pulmonary complications is debatable.

If full curarisation is used as part of an anaesthetic technique, the need for artificial ventilation is not in doubt. When patients have less extreme degrees of respiratory impairment the criteria for starting artificial ventilation are less clearly defined.

Three approaches have been used:

1. Tests of lung function together with blood gas analysis.
2. Careful clinical assessment of respiratory distress and use of an associated scoring system.
3. Experience and clinical judgment.

Using the first approach, the findings which suggest that IPPV is indicated are:[42]

| | |
|---|---|
| Respiratory rate | >35/min |
| Vital capacity | <15 ml/kg bodyweight |
| Maximum inspiratory force | <25 cm $H_2O$ |
| Forced expiratory volume in 1 second (FEV 1·0) | <10 ml/kg bodyweight |
| Arterial $Po_2$ | <70 mm Hg (9·5 kPa) breathing 35–40 per cent oxygen mixture |
| Alveolar/arterial $Po_2$ difference | >450 mm Hg (60 kPa) when breathing 100% oxygen |
| Arterial $Pco_2$ | >56 mm Hg (7·6 kPa) in absence of chronic hypercapnia |
| Ratio of physiological dead-space/tidal volume ($V_D/V_T$ ratio) | >0·6 |

No one test is conclusive; a whole spectrum should be considered before a final decision is taken. The trend of changing values is of greater significance than any absolute value at one particular time.

Gilston strongly advocates the second approach.[43,44] He has pointed out that the face is a rich source of information about the respiratory, cardiovascular and neurological state of the patient. The clinical signs of respiratory distress are closely related to respiratory work, whereas blood gas values and the indices quoted above are measures of respiratory function. Actual measurement of the work of breathing is not easy; in any case it is the individual patient's capacity for work which is important.

Figure 14 shows some clinical signs of respiratory distress. The nine signs underlined form the basis of a scoring system which can be used as a guide to starting artificial ventilation.[45] Though Gilston's work has been carried out in patients who have undergone cardiac surgery, the clinical signs are common to other conditions involving an increase in respiratory work.

Whatever criteria are used for starting IPPV, there is no doubt that excessive reliance is often placed on arterial blood gas analysis. Arterial $Pco_2$ may be below normal in severe ARDS and a slightly raised arterial $Pco_2$ in patients with status asthmaticus is often taken as a sign of impending exhaustion. Many factors affect alveolar/arterial $Po_2$ difference, and blood gas values give no indication of respiratory work. A certain number of patients with satisfactory blood gas values will need IPPV, whilst others with unsatisfactory values may not.

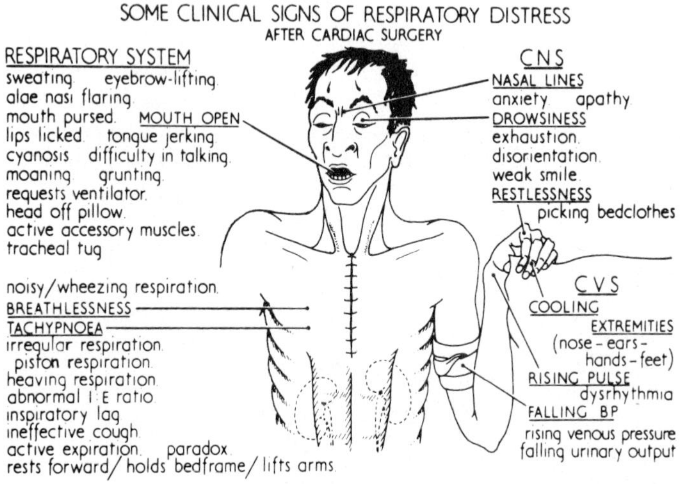


9/Fig. 14.—The clinical signs of respiratory distress after cardiac surgery can be classified under three systems: respiratory, cardiovascular and central nervous. (Courtesy of Dr. A. Gilston and Churchill-Livingstone, publishers.[44])

## Return to Spontaneous Respiration

### After Clinical Anaesthesia[21]

Adequate reversal of neuromuscular block is essential before any attempt to restore spontaneous respiration. During anaesthesia with IPPV, arterial $Pco_2$ often lies in the range 20–30 mm Hg (2·7–4·0 kPa). However, after light anaesthesia with rapid return of consciousness, spontaneous respiration will usually return even though arterial $Pco_2$ is below normal. If anaesthesia has been deeper, the administration of 5 per cent carbon dioxide during the last few minutes of IPPV will restore arterial $Pco_2$ to the range 40–50 mm Hg (5·3–6·7 kPa); spontaneous respiration usually returns even though the patient remains unconscious.

If spontaneous respiration is depressed by a slight overdose of narcotic analgesics, judicious use of a respiratory stimulant such as doxapram may stimulate breathing without reversing analgesia.

If adequate spontaneous respiration is not restored then IPPV must be continued. Difficulties and delays may be encountered in patients who are grossly obese, cachectic or critically ill. Such patients would be candidates for prophylactic ventilation.

### After Long-term Ventilation[46]

After prolonged ventilation the full return to spontaneous respiration may take some time. The gradual process of gaining independence from the ventilator is usually referred to as "weaning". Criteria for weaning are essentially the reverse of those for starting IPPV. The original condition for which the patient was ventilated should have shown significant improvement though complete resolution is not necessary. The patient should be able to withstand mild hypoxia and hypercapnia. The cardiovascular state should be stable and satisfactory. Renal failure and abdominal distension usually delay weaning. Patients in coma may be weaned successfully but an endotracheal or tracheostomy tube will be needed to ensure a patent airway and guard against aspiration.

Many objective criteria for starting to wean have been suggested and investigated. Hilberman and his colleagues[47] found that the most useful predictors were a vital capacity of at least 15 ml/kg body weight and a maximum inspiratory force of at least 28 cm $H_2O$. A ratio of physiological dead-space to tidal volume ($V_D/V_T$) greater than 0·6 usually precludes successful weaning.[48] Sahn and Lakshminarayan[49] reported that three further criteria were useful: adequate arterial oxygenation when breathing 40 per cent inspired oxygen concentration, resting minute ventilation less than 10 l/min, and the ability to double minute ventilation for a short period if requested.

The extent to which these criteria are the reverse of those for initiating IPPV is striking.

These objective criteria are based on pooled data from a number of patients. They do not assess factors such as endurance and motivation which may play an important role in an individual patient's attempt to sustain spontaneous respiration. There is no evidence that objective criteria are more valuable than experience and sound clinical judgment when deciding to start weaning.

The following methods are available for weaning:

1. *Changeover from total IPPV to total spontaneous respiration.* This method is routine after anaesthesia and is often used after several days ventilation in the young and previously fit. It is usually successful after 24–48 hours prophylactic ventilation.
2. *Alternating periods of IPPV and spontaneous respiration.* Starting with 5–10 minutes of spontaneous respiration each hour, these periods are gradually increased at a rate which depends on the patient's response. This classical method has been successful in the majority of patients, although it has been described as the "sink or swim" approach and compared to the medieval torture of "ducking".[56]
3. *Intermittent mandatory ventilation (IMV).* The frequency of mandatory ventilation is progressively reduced until respiration is entirely spontaneous. A trigger mechanism can be introduced to synchronise the mandatory ventilation with the patient's own inspiratory effort.[50] IMV has certain theoretical advantages during weaning. Less sedation is required and the abrupt effects on the circulation during the transition from IPPV to spontaneous respiration are buffered. The technique may permit earlier weaning and it has been claimed that weaning time is shortened. However, some reports on the use of IMV as an aid to weaning have not been entirely favourable.[51, 44]
4. *Mandatory minute volume.* There are few reports on the value of this technique but it has been used successfully in the management of a case of myasthenia gravis.[52]

Continuous positive airway pressure (CPAP) is exactly analagous to PEEP but is used during spontaneous respiration; an alternative name is $PEEP_{spont}$. CPAP may be beneficial during weaning for patients who have high closing capacities and for patients who are prone to develop alveolar collapse during weaning.[51] Such patients usually show a marked increase in alveolar/arterial $Po_2$ difference on switching to spontaneous respiration; this increase can be greatly reduced by the use of CPAP. Improvements in vital capacity and maximum inspiratory force have also been reported.

While the patient remains intubated, humidification must be provided even during spontaneous respiration.

No matter which method is used, all patients being weaned need reassurance and a full explanation of what is expected of them. A biofeedback technique whereby the patient can monitor his own performance may be useful. Close watch is kept for signs of hypoxia and carbon dioxide retention but too frequent pulse and blood pressure measurements may merely lead to anxiety. Clinical signs of respiratory distress are usually more valuable than blood gas analysis as a guide to progress.

Weaning should never be an endurance test and it is often helpful to ventilate or increase IMV rate overnight after the first full day off the ventilator. Some increase in alveolar/arterial $Po_2$ difference and arterial $Pco_2$ is usual after successful weaning, and oxygen enrichment of the inspired gas is often necessary.

Weaning is more difficult if an endotracheal tube is used as the artificial airway because:

1. *Intolerance of the tube* may be misinterpreted as adequate respiration.
2. *The heavy sedation* often necessary to tolerate an endotracheal tube causes respiratory depression.
3. *Laryngeal obstruction* may occur after extubation.

An endotracheal tube should not be removed unless facilities for immediate reintubation are available.

Cuffed tracheostomy tubes can be replaced by silver speaking tubes after 48 hours of spontaneous respiration. As can be seen in Fig. 15, the inner tube has a small hinged flap. The patient breathes in through the tracheostomy tube but during expiration the flap closes and directs the flow of air through the larynx. This half-way house allows aspiration of secretions and keeps the stoma open. If progress is satisfactory decannulation can follow after 48 hours or so. The stoma usually heals spontaneously. Until healing is complete, pressure

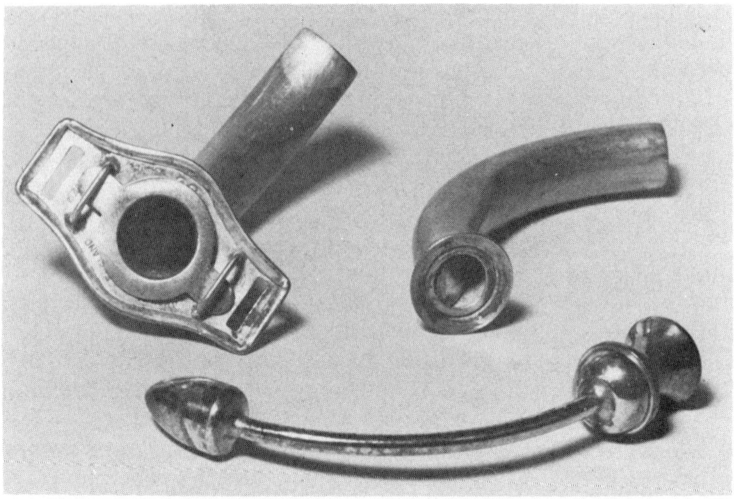

9/Fig. 15.—A silver tracheostomy speaking tube. The inner tube is fitted with a hinged flap which closes during expiration, thus diverting the expired gas through the larynx. The obturator is used during insertion.

should be applied to the stoma dressing when coughing to ensure an air-tight seal.

Satisfactory spontaneous respiration does not guarantee adequate laryngeal and swallowing reflexes. The latter may take days to return though sucking ice cubes often speeds the process. Until natural protection of the airway is adequate only small volumes of water should be given by mouth.

Though most patients can be weaned successfully, a small number remain obstinately dependent on the ventilator in spite of techniques such as IMV. Persistent failure to wean may be caused by the following problems:

1. Raised $V_D/V_T$ ratio.
2. Increased $CO_2$ production rate due to fever, shivering or feeding regimes which rely exclusively on glucose as an energy source.[53]
3. Reduced muscle strength due to low phosphate, high potassium or poor nutrition.
4. Dysco-ordinated breathing, a failure to synchronise the thoracic and diaphragmatic components of normal respiration.[42]
5. Increased work of breathing due to low compliance, high airway resistance or narrow endotracheal tube.

## Anaesthesia

Many ventilator settings have been recommended for anaesthesia. Typical values are:

1. Tidal volume: 10–15 ml/kg body weight
2. Frequency: 8–15 breaths/minute

If the ventilator used is a minute volume divider, then minute volumes of 6–11 l/min are typical. These settings usually result in hyperventilation and arterial $P_{CO_2}$ usually lies between 20–35 mm Hg (2·7–4·7 kPa) during anaesthesia with IPPV. Hypocarbia has long been held to enhance the effects of inhalational anaesthetic agents but more recent experimental work does not confirm this.

A more rigorous approach depends on selecting tidal volume and frequency with the aid of the nomogram which Radford introduced in 1954. This nomogram is based on certain assumptions and now that techniques for measuring $P_{CO_2}$ are widely available, blood gas analysis should be performed if the arterial $P_{CO_2}$ has to be controlled within defined limits.

Alveolar/arterial $P_{O_2}$ difference is increased during anaesthesia and an inspired oxygen concentration of 30–50 per cent is normal practice. Higher inspired oxygen concentrations can be used but the concentrations of nitrous oxide which can then be given as part of the anaesthetic technique will be limited.

## Long-term IPPV in Patients with Normal Lungs

A tidal volume of 10 ml/kg body weight and

a respiratory rate of 12 breaths/minute are suitable values to start IPPV; further changes can be made if arterial $Pco_2$ is unsatisfactory. An inspired oxygen concentration of 30–35 per cent should prove adequate. After prolonged IPPV, many of these patients can be ventilated satisfactorily with room air.

### Acute Respiratory Failure in Chronic Lung Disease with Air-flow Obstruction

IPPV in these patients usually follows one of two courses:

1. A short, sharp period of 24–48 hours ventilation using an endotracheal tube, allowing relief from exhaustion, effective physiotherapy and treatment with antibiotics and bronchodilators.
2. Several weeks ventilation via a tracheostomy, a prolonged and difficult weaning period and repeated acute chest infections due to increasingly bizarre organisms which are sensitive only to increasingly toxic antibiotics.

As a group, these patients are easy to ventilate and very difficult to wean, and this prolonged and often uncomfortable treatment may cause further deterioration in already damaged lungs. There is general agreement therefore that IPPV should only be used for patients who can be expected to return to a reasonable respiratory existence. Unfortunately they are often admitted to hospital *in extremis* and are put on to a ventilator before full clinical appraisal can be made.

These patients are ventilated using the following guide lines:

1. Adequate oxygenation can be achieved with moderate inspired oxygen concentrations (30–35 per cent).
2. These patients are at risk from drastic reduction in arterial $Pco_2$ when starting IPPV.
3. Once IPPV is established, modest tidal volumes and respiratory frequencies usually result in adequate $CO_2$ removal.
4. PEEP offers no benefit unless a large intrapulmonary shunt is present.
5. The risk of pneumothorax is greater in these patients.

There is a theoretical risk of inducing $CO_2$ coma during weaning if the patient is dependent on hypoxic drive. Serious problems are unlikely because observation is close and continuous. In any case, these patients may lose their dependence on hypoxic drive once the acute episode is over.[54] Blood gas analysis may be particularly unhelpful during weaning unless the patient's normal values are known.

Other aspects of the treatment of respiratory failure in chronic chest disease are discussed by McNicol.[55]

### Status Asthmaticus

These patients may be very difficult to ventilate. Large tidal volumes increase the tendency to dangerous hyperinflation and high flow rates dissipate energy in narrowed airways.

Therefore ventilator settings are based on:

1. Low tidal volume, 6–8 ml/kg body weight.
2. Low frequency, 8–12 breaths/minute.
3. Long inspiratory time which nevertheless allows adequate time for expiration.

A flow generator will be necessary.

These recommendations may need to be modified if further hyperinflation occurs. Using these settings, a rise in arterial $Pco_2$ is likely and heavy sedation and possibly neuromuscular block will be required.

High pressures will be generated in the large airways but fortunately these are not transmitted to the large veins. However, acute right heart failure may result from the increased vascular resistance of hyperinflated lungs.

PEEP is contra-indicated as it increases the tendency to hyperinflation. In theory, expiratory retard would be helpful but the correct adjustment is critical and a slightly excessive resistance will prevent full expiration and increase hyperinflation.

Asthmatics are difficult to wean because they are anxious and the endotracheal tube may precipitate bronchospasm if sedation is light.

Branthwaite[56] has written a very helpful guide to IPPV and weaning in the asthmatic patient. Further aspects of the treatment of status asthmaticus are discussed by Emerson[57] and McNicol.[55]

### Acute Alveolar Pathology

This term was introduced by Branthwaite[56] to describe a number of varied conditions which require the same ventilatory management. It includes pulmonary oedema of cardiac origin, thoracic injuries and the adult respiratory distress syndrome (ARDS). The term adult respiratory distress syndrome has been criticised because it lumps together many conditions of different aetiology; indeed there is no general agreement as to which conditions should be included in the syndrome. Table 3 gives a list of disorders which could reasonably be classified as ARDS.

Whatever the finer points of classification, all these patients have a large alveolar/arterial $Po_2$ difference and require:

1. Large tidal volumes.
2. Slow respiratory rate.
3. High inspired oxygen concentrations.
4. High airway pressures.
5. Heavy sedation and possibly neuromuscular block.

They *usually* benefit from PEEP, and *may* benefit from an end-inspiratory pause and suitable choice of inspiratory flow pattern.

A flow generator will be necessary.

A comprehensive account of all aspects of the management of patients with pulmonary failure following sepsis and trauma is given by Hanson.[58] She also describes the management of the pulmonary aspiration syndrome.[59] The treatment of chest injuries is discussed by Coppel[60] and by Dobb in Chapter 10. Recent reviews of the adult respiratory distress syndrome include those of Fein and colleagues,[114] Boggis and Greene,[115] and Wallace and Spence.[116]

9/Table 3
Adult Respiratory Distress Syndrome

Acute respiratory insufficiency associated with:

| | |
|---|---|
| Major surgery or trauma<br>Haemorrhage or shock<br>Cardiopulmonary bypass<br>Transplantation<br>Burns<br>Blast injury<br>Septic shock—Gram-negative<br>—Clostridial | Adult respiratory distress syndrome due to shock and trauma—*"Shock lung"* |

Acute pancreatitis
Fat embolism
Amniotic fluid embolism
Heroin-induced pulmonary oedema (also seen with other drugs)
High-altitude pulmonary oedema
Acute viral infections, whether confined to the lung or not
Pulmonary oxygen toxicity
Secondary drowning
Aspiration of gastric contents (Mendelson's syndrome)
Inhaled noxious gases
Oil contrast medium embolism

(Courtesy of Emerson, P. (1981). Acute respiratory failure in adults. In: *Thoracic Medicine*. London: Butterworth[57])

## PRACTICAL MANAGEMENT

### Respiratory Management

#### Pulmonary Oxygen Toxicity[61, 117]

High partial pressures of oxygen are toxic to the human lung. At one time manned American space craft provided an environment of pure oxygen at a pressure of one-third of an atmosphere. The absence of adverse effects on the lung after prolonged exposure confirmed that it is the partial pressure rather than the concentration which is toxic. However, breathing high concentrations of oxygen increases the tendency to alveolar collapse.

It is usual to quote inspired oxygen concentrations rather than inspired partial pressures. The distinction is important to those working at high altitude. At sea level the percentage concentration and the partial pressure expressed in kPa have almost the same numerical value. Thus 50 per cent inspired oxygen concentration corresponds to an inspired $Po_2$ of about 50 kPa (375 mm Hg).

The safe upper limit of inspired oxygen concentration is not known precisely; 60 per cent is a figure commonly quoted. When breathing pure oxygen the first signs of toxicity take 24 hours to develop. There is some evidence that a low arterial $Po_2$ offers protection to the lungs, but this is not universally accepted.[62] It would be fortunate if this were true for there are occasions when high inspired concentrations are necessary to achieve adequate haemoglobin saturation. However, these high concentrations may cause increased shunting in the lung and lead to a paradoxical fall in arterial $Po_2$.[63] It cannot be assumed, therefore, that increasing the inspired $Po_2$ will necessarily lead to a higher arterial $Po_2$.

Bleomycin, a drug used in cancer chemotherapy, appears to sensitise the lung to the toxic effects of oxygen. Lung damage may occur at oxygen concentrations that would normally be considered safe and this sensitisation may persist after bleomycin has been discontinued. The successful anaesthetic management of a patient who had received this drug is described by Allen and his colleagues.[64]

**Rate of Reduction of Arterial $Pco_2$**

It is easy to cause a profound fall in arterial $Pco_2$ when starting IPPV, particularly if the patient was previously *in extremis*. Hypotension may occur as sympathetic drive is withdrawn and any relative hypovolaemia exposed. Rapid changes in arterial pH can cause cardiac dysrhythmias as potassium shifts across cell membranes.

**Humidification[65, 66]**

Endotracheal and tracheostomy tubes bypass the structures which normally warm and humidify inspired gas. Lack of humidity causes ciliary paralysis in the tracheal mucosa and the normal upward flow of mucus ceases. Drying mucus is more viscous and the formation of tenacious secretions containing encrusted material may lead to blockage of small airways.

The need to humidify inspired gases during long-term ventilation is generally accepted. Although air normally reaches the carina fully saturated with water vapour, a relative humidity of 70 per cent at 37° C seems to be regarded as adequate during artificial ventilation. This level of humidity corresponds to the output of a number of heated water-bath humidifiers in current use.

Although adverse effects on mucus clearance have been demonstrated in patients breathing dry anaesthetic gases, deliberate humidification during routine anaesthesia is not common practice. Until the recent study of Chalon and colleagues,[67] there was little evidence that humidification during anaesthesia reduced the incidence of postoperative pulmonary complications. However, there is no doubt that humidification reduces the heat loss which is associated with prolonged operations and its use should be considered during vascular surgery where substantial falls in body temperature can occur. Other patients such as the elderly or the extensively burned may benefit from the heat conservation which humidification provides.

Methods of humidification include:

1. Heated water baths.
2. Heat and moisture exchangers (condenser humidifiers, artificial noses).
3. Nebulisers.

It has been argued that nebulisers should not be classed as humidifiers because they deliver some water in the form of fine droplets.

As long as the inspired gas already contains some moisture, disposable heat and moisture exchangers provide a convenient means of humidification during spontaneous respiration. They cannot provide adequate humidity when dry gases are used. However the addition of an hygroscopic element increases moisture retention and the combined device is capable of humidifying dry gases during anaesthesia and prolonged artificial ventilation.[68]

A disposable condenser humidifier is shown attached to a tracheostomy tube in Fig. 16; the hygroscopic version of this device, in use during anaesthesia with IPPV, is shown in Fig. 17.

**Intermittent Mandatory Ventilation (IMV)**

IMV was formally introduced as a technique for weaning patients from IPPV.[69] The concept has since been extended to long-term respiratory support and may be regarded as an alternative to conventional artificial ventilation.

IMV has certain theoretical advantages. The retention of spontaneous respiratory activity may:

1. Reduce mean intrathoracic pressure.
2. Provide more uniform pulmonary gas distribution.
3. Prevent dysco-ordination between chest wall and diaphragmatic function.[42]

The problem has been to demonstrate that these advantages are seen in clinical practice. However, IMV for long-term respiratory support has many enthusiastic advocates: the technique would seem to be more popular in North America than in Europe.

**Triggering**

Triggering has never been universally popular and its true value has been even harder to define since the introduction of IMV. A rapid respiratory rate may lead to a fight between man and machine with wild swings in alveolar ventilation. Triggered ventilators are used extensively by physiotherapists and respiratory therapists for "ventilatory assistance" rather than true artificial ventilation.

**Sedation for Patients on Long-term Ventilation**

Few conscious patients will tolerate artificial

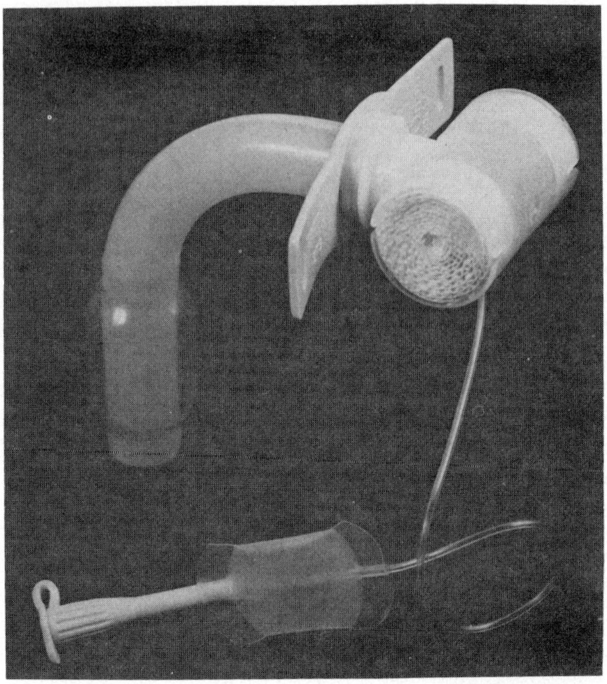

9/FIG. 16.—A tracheostomy tube with small volume cuff fitted with a condenser humidifier. (Photograph courtesy of Portex Ltd.)

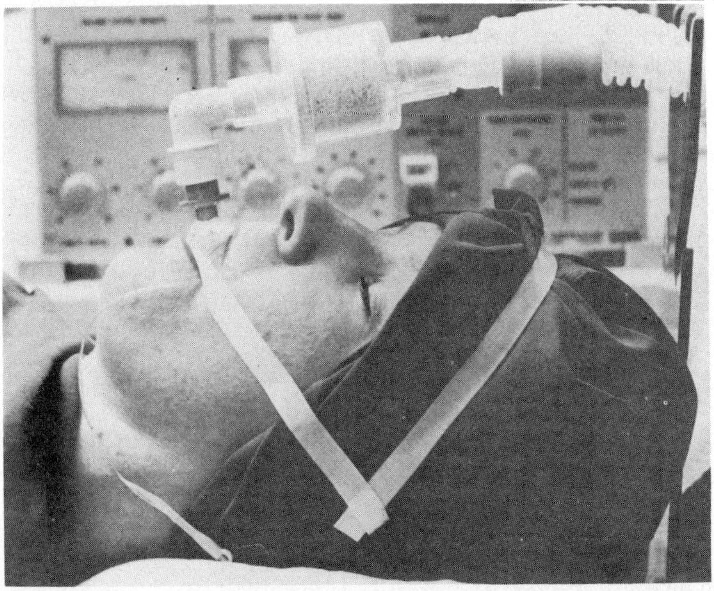

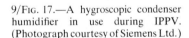

9/FIG. 17.—A hygroscopic condenser humidifier in use during IPPV. (Photograph courtesy of Siemens Ltd.)

ventilation without some help from drugs. This is especially true during the first few hours when the patient may need to be "settled" on the ventilator. Patients who retain their respiratory drive and resist artificial ventilation are said to be "fighting" the ventilator. Settling and sedation are euphemisms for the pharmacological suppression of natural reflexes. Before drugs are administered every effort must be made to ensure that blood gas values are satisfactory, that conditions such as a full bladder are not responsible for any restlessness, and that mechanical problems such as a pneumothorax or blocked tube have been excluded.

Four groups of drugs are commonly used:
1. Narcotic analgesics.
2. Drugs which relieve anxiety.
3. Neuromuscular blocking agents.
4. Intravenous anaesthetic agents.

Nitrous oxide-oxygen mixtures have the advantages of rapid onset and recovery, profound analgesia and minimal cardiovascular depression. However ventilation with nitrous oxide for 24 hours or longer is associated with megaloblastic changes in the bone marrow.[70] The safe use of nitrous oxide may therefore be limited to periods of only a few hours.

**Narcotic analgesics.**—Drugs such as morphine and phenoperidine provide analgesia and suppress respiratory drive and cough reflex. Their ability to relieve anxiety is insufficient for many patients. Hypotension can occur, often unpredictably. There is a risk of addiction, but this is rarely a practical problem as prolonged IPPV is usually followed by a period of weaning from both ventilator and drugs.[118]

**Drugs which relieve anxiety.**—Benzodiazepines are often prescribed: some members of this group (such as diazepam) are markedly cumulative. They have useful sedative and amnesic properties but provide neither analgesia nor useful respiratory depression.

**Neuromuscular blocking agents.**—These drugs create the semblance of calm by paralysing muscles. They may be useful during the first few hours or if cerebral depression must be avoided (for example to record an EEG or make a neurological assessment). Curarisation forms part of the treatment of severe tetanus.

Unless specifically contra-indicated, heavy sedation should be prescribed in addition, as patients report that paralysis when alert can be extremely unpleasant.

Neuromuscular blockade prevents the outward expression of pain and mental distress. It also suppresses the normal reflex motor responses to hypoxia, hypercapnia and airway obstruction. These responses still provide some measure of safety even in heavily sedated patients.

Neuromuscular blocking drugs have other disadvantages during long-term ventilation:
1. Coughing is totally suppressed.
2. Deep vein thrombosis may be more common.
3. Peripheral nerve injuries are more likely.

**Intravenous anaesthetic agents.**—Continuous infusion provides a light level of general anaesthesia. Only drugs which are rapidly metabolised and non-cumulative are satisfactory:
1. Alphaxalone-alphadolone (Althesin)[71]
2. Chlormethiazole (Heminevrin)[72]
3. Etomidate (Hypnomidate)[73]

This approach is useful for difficult patients but the long-term effects of these drugs after many days' infusion are unknown (see Footnote).

The final choice of drug will depend on the projected duration of IPPV, the type of patient, the nature of the underlying illness and whether IMV is used. No matter which drugs are chosen, control is usually smoother with continuous administration. The grossly obese and the aggressive are often difficult to sedate as are those accustomed to high alcohol consumption. Patients with head injuries and patients with stiff lungs may have an abnormally marked respiratory drive.

Although drugs for patients on ventilators are prescribed by doctors, the final choice of agent is often made by a nurse on an intensive care unit. A recent survey suggests that prescribers' intentions may be misinterpreted.[74] In particular, neuromuscular block is often confused with sedation. Pancuronium is popular with nurses, probably because it produces apparent calm with little risk of hypotension. It is essential to indicate clearly the drugs which should only be given when the patient is on the ventilator. Pancuronium, prescribed on an "as required" basis, has been administered to an extubated patient as night sedation with disastrous result.[75]

### Respiratory Monitoring[119]

Satisfactory arterial blood gas values provide the ultimate test of adequate artificial ventilation. Blood gas estimations are necessary during long-term ventilation and during anaesthesia for cardiac and neurosurgery; they are rarely performed during other operations unless an arterial cannula has been inserted for blood pressure monitoring.

The techniques for measuring arterial pH, $Po_2$ and $Pco_2$ are well established but depend on intermittent blood sampling. The intervals

Reports in *The Lancet* have drawn attention to the possible hazards of long-term infusions of etomidate[124] and Althesin.[125] Those who wish to use long-term infusions of intravenous anaesthetic agents are advised to check the current recommendations of the appropriate pharmaceutical company and the Committee on Safety of Medicine for the particular drug concerned.

between estimations may be unsatisfactory when conditions are changing rapidly and methods which allow continuous intravascular measurement have been developed. These advances have been particularly valuable in paediatrics but the same methods are useful in adults for observing changes in blood gas values during manoeuvres such as endotracheal suction. $Po_2$ may be measured by a miniature version of the Clark electrode; both $Po_2$ and $Pco_2$ may be measured by a technique based on mass spectrometry.[76]

The morbidity associated with arterial cannulation or repeated arterial puncture has prompted the development of non-invasive techniques which can give continuous indication of blood gas values. These include:

1. End-tidal $CO_2$ monitoring (see p. 272).
2. Ear oximetry, which measures the percentage saturation of haemoglobin with oxygen in arterial blood (Hewlett-Packard 47201A ear oximeter).
3. Transcutaneous $Po_2$ and $Pco_2$ ($P_{tc}o_2$ and $P_{tc}co_2$). This technique is well established for babies where the correlation between $Pao_2$ and $P_{tc}o_2$ is quite good. In anaesthetised adults transcutaneous $Po_2$ must be interpreted with caution:[77] anaesthetic gases may interfere with sensor performance.[78] As with many non-invasive techniques, observed changes may be more significant than absolute values.[79]
4. Mass spectrometry has been used in intensive care[80] and during anaesthesia.[81] This sophisticated technique permits measurement of the partial pressures of each and every inspired and expired gas. The addition of a microprocessor to the system enables calculations of metabolic gas exchange, lung volume, pulmonary blood flow and pulmonary tissue volume (lung water) to be performed.

The introduction of microprocessors has permitted rapid calculation of derived quantities such as $CO_2$ production rate, $V_D/V_T$, lung compliance and airway resistance from measurements of expired $CO_2$ concentration, tidal volume, airway pressure and arterial $Pco_2$. Monitoring units which will perform these calculations are available for use with sophisticated modern ventilators such as the Servo (Siemens-Elema Ltd.) and Engström series.

Inspired oxygen concentration should be measured whenever blood gas analysis is performed. The paramagnetic oxygen analyser is a somewhat delicate instrument and polarographic electrodes are available which are robust and simple to use. During anaesthesia inspired oxygen concentrations can be measured to check the accuracy of gas delivery systems. However the polarographic electrode may show an unpredictable sensitivity both to nitrous oxide[82, 83] and halothane.[84]

Expired tidal and minute volume, and peak airway pressure are observed continuously by the anaesthetist during anaesthesia. On intensive care units the following measurements are typical:

Every 15 minutes:
- Respiratory frequency.
- Exhaled tidal and minute volume.
- Peak airway pressure and PEEP levels.

Every 30 minutes:
- Humidifier water and inspired gas temperatures.

Every hour:
- Inspired oxygen concentration.

These measurements can be performed without disturbing the patient. Routine observations at regular intervals do not guard against hazards such as disconnection or mechanical obstruction: constant vigilance is essential.

### Care of the Lungs

Successful long-term ventilation depends on the skilled assistance of physiotherapists. Many patients receiving IPPV have excessive bronchial secretions and ineffective coughing. Loss of the natural "sigh" and interference with normal mucus transport predispose to sputum retention and infection.

Clearance of secretions by endotracheal suction is helped by postural drainage and the "artificial cough". The patient is usually treated lying on alternate sides. The lungs are hyperinflated with oxygen by slow compression of a reservoir bag ("bag squeezing"). After a brief end-inspiratory pause the raised airway pressure is suddenly released and the chest is shaken until expiration is complete. This manoeuvre mimics the natural cough and helps to move secretions from the periphery of the lung to the large airways. Thick secretions can be loosened by injecting 2–3 ml of normal saline down the endotracheal or tracheostomy tube before bag squeezing. Suction is carried out after about six hyperinflations and the whole process is repeated until the chest is clear to auscultation.

Modified chest physiotherapy must be performed cautiously (if at all) in the presence of air leaks or surgical emphysema, or in patients with low cardiac output. Bronchospasm may be precipitated in any patient and if already present may be made worse. Patients with recent chest wounds need effective analgesia before physiotherapy. The brief but intense analgesia given by 50 per cent oxygen/50 per cent nitrous oxide mixtures (Entonox) is very useful.

Physiotherapy for ventilated patients is reviewed by Johnston.[85]

Despite tracheal suction and vigorous physiotherapy, some patients retain secretions and suffer pulmonary collapse. Fibre-optic bronchoscopy is a valuable aid to the management of these patients.[86,87] The technique can also be used to examine the trachea and large airways, and to confirm the presence of a fistula between the oesophagus and upper respiratory tract.[88]

### Complications

**Pneumothorax.**—The positive pressures developed in the airways during IPPV increase the likelihood of gas escaping into the pleural cavity through any break in the visceral pleura. Whether PEEP increases this risk and whether IMV reduces it are subjects of debate. Chest drains must be readily available on any ward where IPPV is performed.

**Surgical emphysema.**—Gas under pressure may leak from the pleural cavity or from a misplaced tube into the subcutaneous tissues of the thorax and neck. This complication is usually less serious than its often hideous appearance might suggest. Once the source of the leak is treated, the gas is slowly absorbed. In extreme cases of surgical emphysema, the tracheostome cannot be found if accidental disconnection or extubation occurs; if mediastinal emphysema causes respiratory or circulatory embarrassment, surgical decompression may be necessary.

## NON-RESPIRATORY MANAGEMENT

### General Management

This will include treatment of the underlying condition. During the first few days of long-term ventilation the following daily investigations are suggested:

1. Chest X-ray.
2. Arterial blood gas analysis.
3. Hb estimation.
4. Urea and electrolyte estimations.

If the patient is unconscious, the usual nursing care of the eyes, mouth and skin will be required.

### Fluids and Feeding

Accurate fluid balance charts are essential. The nature, volume, and rate of administration of necessary fluids will depend on the underlying condition of the patient. An intravenous line is often useful for drug administration.

Feeding (whether by enteral or parenteral routes) is a neglected aspect of patient care. Malnutrition is frequently seen in patients receiving long-term artificial ventilation.[89]

Hypoalbuminaemia and heavy urinary losses of potassium and magnesium are common. A metabolic alkalosis may be a sign of potassium deficiency. Hyperkalaemia[90] and hypophosphataemia[91] may cause muscle weakness which could delay the return to spontaneous respiration.

Dehydration and hypoalbuminaemia should be corrected very carefully when treating ARDS. Leakage of protein-rich fluid from damaged capillaries into the alveoli may cause further deterioration in respiratory function.

### Anaemia

'Respirator anaemia' is often seen and may be due to:

1. Toxic bone marrow depression.
2. Unrecognised disseminated intravascular coagulation (DIC).
3. Unrecognised gastro-intestinal bleeding.
4. Folate deficiency, common in ITU patients.[92]
5. Frequent and numerous blood tests.

Transfusion is usually required.

### Gastro-intestinal Abnormalities

Ileus is common during long-term ventilation and a nasogastric tube is often needed, particularly during the first few days.

Gastro-intestinal bleeding is frequently seen and is usually put down to stress ulceration. Antacids and cimetidine are often given as prophylaxis.

### Infection[93]

Lower respiratory tract infection is a constant threat to the intubated patient. The ventilator and its associated equipment may act as reservoirs of bacteria and careless nursing technique may transfer organisms from one patient to another. Natural immunity is often compromised by severe illness, steroid therapy, malnutrition and prior treatment with broad-spectrum antibiotics.

The mouths of patients on intensive care units usually become colonised by Gram-negative bacteria and the artificial airway provides a route by which these organisms can reach the lungs. Anaerobes are important in aspiration pneumonia.

Tracheal aspirates and wound swabs from the tracheal stoma often grow pathogenic organisms and there may be a temptation to start antibiotic therapy. This should be resisted unless there is additional evidence of clinical infection such as fever, leucocytosis and purulent sputum.

The methods available for decontaminating ventilators and other anaesthetic equipment are discussed by Lumley.[94]

### Psychological Care

Many patients who have received long-term ventilation on an intensive care unit have written personal accounts of their experience.[95,96]

Conscious patients on ventilators need constant reassurance and even simple procedures such as taking blood pressure should be carefully explained beforehand. Bedside discussion of the patient's condition should be guarded and discreet; many patients who were apparently in coma or heavily sedated can subsequently recall in embarrassing detail conversations held by doctors or nurses in their presence.

Some patients can communicate successfully using their lips but for others a large pad of paper and a crayon, or a chart on which a few simple needs are illustrated, will be useful. Frequent visits from friends and relatives help to maintain contact with the outside world and windows, preferably looking out over trees and sky, help to establish normal diurnal rhythm.[97]

The patient should be kept informed of progress and told the likely programme for the next few days.

Depression and temper tantrums are not uncommon and represent a natural psychological reaction to serious illness and total dependence. Depressive illness may manifest itself more subtly as an acute confusional state which cannot be explained by metabolic disturbance or toxaemia.[98]

## HIGH FREQUENCY VENTILATION (HFV)[99, 122, 123]

There are at least three distinct types of high frequency ventilation:

1. High frequency positive-pressure ventilation (HFPPV), using frequencies of 60–100 breaths per minute.
2. High frequency jet ventilation (HFJV), using frequencies of 60–600 breaths per minute.
3. High frequency oscillations (HFO), using frequencies of 600–3000 breaths per minute.

### High Frequency Positive-Pressure Ventilation (HFPPV)[100]

During the late 1960s, a group of Swedish investigators was studying carotid sinus baroreceptor reflexes. The normal swings of blood pressure which accompany respiration were interfering with measurement and an alternative method of artificial ventilation had to be devised.

The first technique which was developed depended on high-flow endotracheal insufflation through a narrow-bore catheter. This catheter was mounted in the centre of an endotracheal tube and the gas flow down the catheter was pulsed by a solenoid valve at frequencies of 60–100 per minute. PEEP was applied by a variable resistance attached to the outlet of the endotracheal tube.[101]

This system of artificial ventilation was found to have interesting properties. As intended, systemic blood pressure did not vary with respiration, and heart rate and mean central venous pressure remained constant. Spontaneous respiration ceased within a few seconds of starting HFPPV yet returned within 10–15 seconds when it was stopped. At frequencies above 100 per minute, spontaneous respiration was less suppressed. This reflex suppression was not total as spontaneous respiration returned if the chemoreceptors were stimulated. An initial study performed on a small number of patients during routine surgery showed that adequate alveolar ventilation could be achieved with only minor variations in mean intrathoracic pressure.

The development of a pneumatic valve utilising the Coanda effect[11] has made the insufflation catheter unnecessary. Although the system is open, significant air entrainment need not occur and PEEP can still be applied. It is therefore possible to perform endotracheal suction while PEEP is maintained.

The chest movements of a patient receiving HFPPV have been compared to those of a panting dog.

The main features of HFPPV can be summarised as follows:

1. Positive airway pressures and negative intrathoracic pressures throughout the respiratory cycle.
2. Higher functional residual capacity (FRC) without the adverse circulatory effects of IPPV plus PEEP.
3. Reflex suppression of spontaneous respiratory activity, thus reducing the need for sedation or paralysis.
4. A more efficient gas distribution within the lung than is seen with IPPV, or IPPV plus PEEP.
5. Renal function may be better preserved.
6. Because of the constant efflux of gas, risk of aspiration is reduced without the need for an inflated cuff.

Many of these are also features of high frequency jet ventilation and high frequency oscillation.

HFPPV would seem to offer considerable advantages as an anaesthetic technique for bronchoscopy, laryngoscopy, microlaryngeal surgery and resection of tracheal stenosis. These operations have always presented major problems to the anaesthetist. A few trials and considerable anecdotal evidence suggest the technique may be useful in the treatment of infant and adult respiratory distress syndromes, severe asthma and pulmonary oedema; it has also been used to ventilate patients with bronchopleural fistulae and to assist weaning from long-term artificial ventilation.

### High Frequency Jet Ventilation (HFJV)

This technique was introduced by Klain and Smith in 1977.[102] The ventilating gas is delivered as small jets of high velocity through a narrow tube, usually a 14-gauge intravenous cannula. This cannula can be placed inside an endotracheal tube or inserted through the cricothyroid membrane; the latter route may permit emergency oxygenation in cases of acute upper airway obstruction.

HFJV has been used in anaesthesia for laryngoscopy,[103] in the management of a patient with a bronchopleural fistula,[104] and as an aid to weaning patients from artifical ventilation.[105]

### High Frequency Oscillation (HFO)

In 1972, Lunkenheimer described the technique of high frequency pressure oscillation (1,400–3,000 breaths per minute) to modify diffusion respiration.[106] More recently, successful HFO at lower frequencies (600–900 breaths per minute) has been described both in humans[107] and animals.[108]

Although IPPV is often regarded as "unphysiological", the tidal volumes and respiratory rates used are similar to those seen during spontaneous respiration. Movement of gas in the larger airways can be explained by convective bulk flow, and the tidal volume must exceed the volume of the anatomical dead-space.

During HFV the tidal volumes generated may be considerably less than the volume of the anatomical dead-space, and traditional concepts cannot account for the observed gas exchange. The phenomenon of facilitated or augmented diffusion has been invoked to explain gas exchange during HFV.[122,123]

A word of caution is therefore appropriate. With the exception of blood gas analysis, many of the standard measurements which aid management during IPPV will not have the same significance during HFV. At present HFV should be regarded as a separate and fundamentally different technique.

Until recently the use of high frequency ventilation has been confined to a few centres. Now that commercial ventilators suitable for HFV are available there is no doubt the technique will be more widely used. Once the means of delivering inspired gas to the upper airway are standardised further trials should soon establish the true place of this fascinating development in artificial ventilation. A commercial ventilator designed for high frequency jet ventilation is shown in Fig. 18.

## EXTRACORPOREAL GAS EXCHANGE

In spite of modern management the mortality

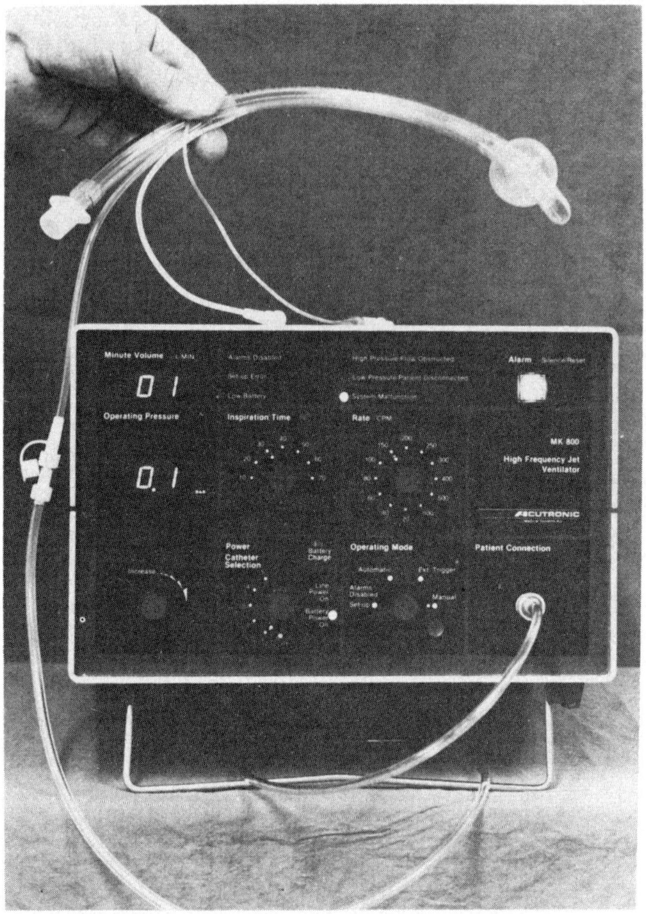


9/FIG. 18.—The Acutronic MK 800 Ventilator designed for high frequency jet ventilation (Acutronic Ltd.). The cuff on the specially designed endotracheal tube is shown inflated, but this is not always necessary during HFJV.

from respiratory failure due to acute alveolar pathology remains distressingly high.

After successful use of the extracorporeal circulation in cardiac surgery it was natural that the technique would be extended to patients whose primary problem was a severe impairment of pulmonary gas exchange. Many of the technical problems of long-term extracorporeal membrane oxygenation (ECMO) have now been solved; the complication rate is acceptably low, and patients can be supported successfully for as long as 2–3 weeks.

When introduced ECMO had two aims. The first was to maintain adequate oxygenation and carbon dioxide removal when diseased lungs were no longer able to maintain adequate gas exchange. The second was to place the lungs "at rest" and increase the chances of recovery by avoiding the high tidal volumes, high airway pressures and high oxygen concentrations which form part of conventional therapy. Early experience with ECMO suggested that patients whose failure was secondary to trauma or fat embolism responded better than those with severe bacterial or viral pneumonia.[109]

The therapeutic role of ECMO has been investigated during a multicentre trial sponsored by the National Heart, Lung and Blood Institute of the United States. The results of this trial, reported by Zapol and his colleagues in 1979,[110] confirm that ECMO works well as a support device but fails to influence the course of the lung disease in the majority of patients. It has been suggested, however, that the criteria for inclusion in the Trial may have been too rigid, thus excluding a group of patients with less severe lung disease whose chance of survival was greater.[31]

In future, ECMO may be used as a temporary measure until lung transplantation can be performed. Even then it is a technique which is likely to be confined to a few specialised centres. There are a number of detailed accounts of the technical aspects of ECMO.[51,111,112]

Extracorporeal carbon dioxide removal ($ECCO_2R$) is a modification of ECMO which has been introduced recently.[113] Carbon dioxide is removed from the blood through a membrane lung by low-flow veno-venous bypass. Oxygen is supplied by diffusion through the patient's lungs (apnoeic mass-movement oxygenation) which are either kept motionless or ventilated at a rate of 2–3 times per minute. Weaning criteria are based on increases in lung compliance rather than improvement in gas exchange.

First reports of the use of this technique in severe respiratory failure are very encouraging: the results of further experience are awaited with interest.

## REFERENCES


1. Rendell-Baker, L. (1963). History of thoracic anaesthesia. In: *Thoracic Anaesthesia*. Ed. by W. W. Mushin. Oxford: Blackwell Scientific Publications.
2. Woollam, C. H. M. (1976). The development of apparatus for intermittent negative pressure respiration. *Anaesthesia*, **31**, 537 and 666.
3. Gilston, A. (1980). Anaesthetists, mechanical ventilation and the training of surgeons. *Anaesthesia*, **35**, 919.
4. Safar, P. (1981). *Cardiopulmonary Cerebral Resuscitation*. Stavanger: Laerdal.
5. Baskett, P. J. F. (1982). The need to disseminate knowledge of resuscitation into the community. *Anaesthesia*, **37**, 74.
6. Don Michael, T. A. and Gordon, A. S. (1980). The oesophageal obturator airway: a new device in cardiopulmonary resuscitation. *Brit. med. J.*, **281**, 1531.
7. Woollam, C. H. M. and Houlton, M. C. C. (1976). Respiratory failure in pregnancy. *Anaesthesia*, **31**, 1217.
8. Hewlett, A. M., Platt, A. S. and Terry, V. G. (1977). Mandatory minute volume, a new concept in weaning from mechanical ventilation. *Anaesthesia*, **32**, 163.
9. Loh, L., Sykes, M. K. and Chakrabarti, M. K. (1978). The assessment of ventilator performance. *Brit. J. Anaesth.*, **50**, 63.
10. Robinson, J. S. (1978). Respiratory care. In: *Medical Management of the Critically Ill*. Ed. Hanson, G. C. and Wright, P. L. London: Academic Press.
11. Mushin, W. W., Rendell-Baker, L., Thompson, P. W. and Mapleson, W. W. (1980). *Automatic Ventilation of the Lungs*, 3rd edit. Oxford: Blackwell Scientific Publications.
12. Lindholm, C. E. and Grenvik, Å. (1977). Flexible fibreoptic bronchoscopy and intubation in intensive care. In: *Recent Advances in Intensive Therapy*., No. 1. Ed. Ledingham. Edinburgh: Churchill Livingstone.
13. Friman, L., Hedenstierna, G. and Schildt, B. (1976). Stenosis following tracheostomy. *Anaesthesia*, **31**, 479.
14. Fryer, M. E. and Marshall, R. D. (1976). Tracheal dilatation. *Anaesthesia*, **31**, 470.
15. Bernhard, W. N., Cottrell, J. E., Sivakumaran, C., Patel, K., Yost, L. and Turndorf, H. (1979). Adjustment of intracuff pressure to prevent aspiration. *Anesthesiology*, **50**, 363.
16. Jenicek, J. A., Danner, C. A. and Allen, C. R. (1973). Continuous cuff inflation during long-term intubation and ventilation: Evaluation of technic. *Anesth. Analg. Curr Res.*, **52**, 252.
17. Bryant, L. R., Trinkle, J. K. and Dubilier, L. (1971). Reappraisal of tracheal injury from cuffed tracheostomy tubes. Experiments in dogs. *J. Amer. med. Ass.*, **215**, 625.
18. Mehta, S. (1982). Performance of low pressure cuffs. An experimental evaluation. *Ann. roy. Coll. Surg. Engl.*, **64**, 54.
19. Mehta, S. (1982). Aspiration around high-volume, low pressure endotracheal cuff. *Brit. med. J.*, **284**, 115.
20. Black, A. M. S. and Seegobin, R. D. (1981). Pressures on endotracheal tube cuffs. *Anaesthesia*, **36**, 498.
21. Nunn, J. F. (1977). *Applied Respiratory Physiology*, 2nd edit. London: Butterworth.
22. Sykes, M. K. (1982). Respiratory mechanics. In: *Scientific Foundations of Anaesthesia*, 3rd edit. Ed. by Scurr, C. F. and Feldman, S. A. London: Wm. Heinemann Medical Books Ltd.
23. Baker, A. B., Babington, P. C. B., Colliss, J. E. and Cowie, R. W. (1977). Effects of varying inspiratory flow waveform and time in intermittent positive pressure ventilation. I. Introduction and methods. *Brit. J. Anaesth.*, **49**, 1207.
24. Baker, A. B., Colliss, J. E. and Cowie, R. W. (1977). Effects of varying inspiratory flow waveform and time in intermittent positive pressure ventilation. II. Various physiological variables. *Brit. J. Anaesth.*, **49**, 1221.
25. Conway, C. M. (1975). Haemodynamic effects of pulmonary ventilation. *Brit. J. Anaesth.*, **47**, 761.
26. Jonson, B. and Prakash, O. (1980). Feedback control of mechanical ventilation by end-tidal $P_{CO_2}$. Experience, problems and prospects from use in a thoracic surgical unit. In: *Artificial Ventilation. Technical, Biological and Clinical Aspects*. Ed. Payne, J. P. and Bushman, J. A. London: Academic Press.
27. Benatar, S. R., Hewlett, A. M. and Nunn, J. F. (1973). The use of iso-shunt lines for control of oxygen therapy. *Brit. J. Anaesth.*, **45**, 711.
28. Foëx, P. (1980). The mechanical effects of raised airway pressure. In: *The Circulation in Anaesthesia. Applied Physiology and Pharmacology*. Ed. Prys-Roberts, C. Oxford: Blackwell Scientific Publications.
29. Stoddart, J. C. (1979). Controlled ventilation. In: *Recent Advances in Anaesthesia and Analgesia, No. 13*. Ed. by Langton Hewer, C. and Atkinson, R. S. Edinburgh: Churchill Livingstone.
30. Adams, A. P. (1980). Physiological responses to pressure patterns during mechanical ventilation of the lungs. In *Artificial Ventilation. Technical, Biological and Clin-*

*ical Aspects*. Ed. Payne, J. P. and Bushman, J. A. London: Academic Press.
31. Pontoppidan, H., Wilson, R. S., Rie, M. A. and Schneider, R. C. (1977). Respiratory intensive care. *Anesthesiology*, **47**, 96.
32. Fairley, H. B. (1982). Physiology of mechanical ventilation. In *Scientific Foundations of Anaesthesia*, 3rd edit. Ed. Scurr, C. F. and Feldman, S. A. London: Heinemann Medical Books Ltd.
33. *British Medical Journal* (1981). Leading article: Artificial ventilation and the heart. **283**, 397.
34. Barat, G. and Asuero, M. S. (1975). Positive end-expiratory pressure. Effect on arterial oxygenation during respiratory failure in chronic obstructive airway disease. *Anaesthesia*, **30**, 183.
35. Whyche, M. Q., Teichner, R. L., Kallos, T., Marshall, B. E. and Smith, T. C. (1973). Effects of continuous positive-pressure breathing on functional residual capacity and arterial oxygenation during intra-abdominal operations. *Anesthesiology*, **38**, 68.
36. Suter, P. M., Fairley, H. B. and Isenberg, M. D. (1975). Optimum end-expiratory airway pressure in patients with acute pulmonary failure. *New Eng. J. Med.*, **292**, 284.
37. Kirby, R. R., Downs, J. B., Civetta, J. M., Modell, J. H., Dannemiller, F. J., Klein, E. F. and Hodges, M. (1975). High level positive end-expiratory pressure (PEEP) in acute respiratory insufficiency. *Chest*, **67**, 156.
38. Bennett, E. D. and Hanson, G. C. (1979). Monitoring in shock. In: *Medical Management of the Critically Ill*. Ed. Hanson, G. C. and Wright, P. L. London: Academic Press.
39. Hanson, G. C. (1980). Ventilating the haemodynamically unstable patient. In: *Artificial Ventilation. Technical, Biological and Clinical Aspects*. Ed. Payne, J. P. and Bushman, J. A. London: Academic Press.
40. Bevan, D. R. and Gammanpilot, S. (1977). Is NEEP dead? *Anaesthesia*, **32**, 405.
41. Horton, J. M. (1976). The anaesthetist's contribution to the care of head injuries. *Brit. J. Anaesth.*, **48**, 767.
42. Pontoppidan, H., Geffin, B. and Lowenstein, E. (1973). *Acute Respiratory Failure in the Adult*. Boston: Little, Brown & Co.
43. Gilston, A. (1976). Facial signs of respiratory distress after cardiac surgery. *Anaesthesia*, **31**, 385.
44. Gilston, A. (1979). Techniques and complications in cardiac surgery. In: *Recent Advances in Anaesthesia and Analgesia, No. 13*, Ed. Langton Hewer, C. and Atkinson, R. S. Edinburgh: Churchill Livingstone.
45. Gilston, A. (1976). A clinical scoring system for adult respiratory distress. Preliminary report of its use in heart disease. *Anaesthesia*, **31**, 448.
46. Barnett, M. B. (1980). Weaning patients from ventilators. *Brit. J. Clin. Equipment*. **5**, 151.
47. Hilberman, M., Kamm, B., Lamy, M., Dietrich, H. P., Martz, K. and Osborn, J. J., (1976). An analysis of potential physiological predictors of respiratory inadequacy following cardiac surgery. *J. Thorac. Cardiovasc. Surg.*, **71**, 711.
48. Teres, D., Roizen, M. F. and Bushnell, L. S. (1973). Successful weaning from controlled ventilation despite high deadspace-to-tidal volume ratio. *Anesthesiology*, **39**, 656.
49. Sahn, S. A. and Lakshminarayan, S. (1973). Bedside criteria for discontinuation of mechanical ventilation. *Chest*, **63**, 1002.
50. Harboe, S. (1977). Weaning from mechanical ventilation by means of intermittent assisted ventilation (IAV). *Acta anaesth. Scand.*, **21**, 252.
51. Hedley-Whyte, J., Burgess, III, G. E., Feeley, T. W. and Miller, M. G. (1976). *Applied Physiology of Respiratory Care*. Boston: Little, Brown and Co.
52. Higgs, B. D. and Bevan, J. C. (1979). Use of mandatory minute volume ventilation in the perioperative management of a patient with myasthenia. *Brit. J. Anaesth.*, **51**, 1181.
53. Askanazi, J., Nordenström, J., Rosenbaum, S. H., Elwyn, D. H., Hyman, A. I., Carpentier, Y. A. and Kinney, J. M. (1981). Nutrition for the patient with respiratory failure. *Anesthesiology*, **54**, 373.
54. Rudolf, M., Banks, R. A. and Semple, S. J. G. (1977). Hypercapnia during oxygen therapy in acute exacerbations of chronic respiratory failure. Hypothesis revisited. *Lancet*, **2**, 483.
55. McNicol, M. W. (1978). Respiratory failure in chronic and acute chest disease. In: *Medical Management of the Critically Ill*. Ed. Hanson, G. C. and Wright, P. L. London: Academic Press.
56. Branthwaite, M. A. (1978). *Artificial Ventilation for Pulmonary Disease*. Obtainable from Anaesthetic Department, Brompton Hospital, London, SW3.
57. Emerson, P. (1981). Acute respiratory failure in adults. In: *Thoracic Medicine*. Ed. Emerson, P. London: Butterworth.
58. Hanson, G. C. (1978). Pulmonary failure following sepsis and trauma. In: *Medical Management of the Critically Ill*: Ed. Hanson, G. C. and Wright, P. L. London: Academic Press.
59. Hanson, G. C. (1978). The pulmonary aspiration syndrome. In: *Medical Management of the Critically Ill*. Ed. Hanson, G. C. and Wright, P. L. London: Academic Press.
60. Coppel, D. L. (1978). The Management of Chest Injuries. In: *Medical Management of the Critically Ill*. Ed. Hanson, G. C. and Wright, P. L. London: Academic Press.
61. Winter, P. M. and Smith, G. (1972). The toxicity of oxygen. *Anesthesiology*. **37**, 210.
62. Smith, G. W. (1978). Oxygen toxicity. *Anaesthesia*, **33**, 274.
63. Kerr, J. H. (1975). Pulmonary oxygen transfer during IPPV in man. *Brit. J. Anaesth.*, **47**, 695.
64. Allen, S. C., Riddel, G. S. and Butchart, E. G. (1981). Bleomycin therapy and anaesthesia. *Anaesthesia*, **36**, 60.
65. Barnes, P. K. (1982). Principles of lung ventilators and humidification. In: *Scientific Foundations of Anaesthesia*. 3rd edit. Ed. Scurr, C. F. and Feldman, S. A. London: Heinemann Medical Books Ltd.
66. Hayes, B. (1980). Humidification during artificial ventilation. In: *Artificial Ventilation. Technical, Biological and Clinical Aspects*. Ed. Payne, J. P. and Bushman, J. A. London: Academic Press.
67. Chalon, J., Patel, C., Ali, M., Ramanathan, S., Capan, L., Tang, C-K and Turndorf, H. (1979). Humidity and the anesthetized patient. *Anesthesiology*, **50**, 195.
68. Gedeon, A. and Mebius, C. (1979). The hygroscopic condenser humidifier. *Anaesthesia*, **34**, 1043.
69. Downs, J. B., Klein, E. F., Desautels, D., Modell, J. H. and Kirby, R. R. (1973). Intermittent mandatory ventilation: A new approach to weaning patients from mechanical ventilators. *Chest*, **64**, 331.

70. Amess, J. A. L., Burman, J. F., Rees, G. M., Nance-kievell, D. G. and Mollin, D. L. (1978). Megaloblastic haemopoiesis in patients receiving nitrous oxide. *Lancet*, **2**, 339.
71. Ramsay, M. A. E., Savege, T. M., Simpson, B. R. J. and Goodwin, R. (1974). Controlled sedation with alphaxalone-alphadolone. *Brit. med. J.*, **2**, 656.
72. Scott, D. B., Beamish, D., Hudson, I. N. and Jostell, K-G. (1980). Prolonged infusion of chlormethiazole in intensive care. *Brit. J. Anaesth.*, **52**, 541.
73. Edbrooke, D. L., Newby, D. M., Hebron, B. S., Mather, S. J. and Dixon, A. M. (1981). Etomidate infusion: a method of sedation for the intensive care unit. *Anaesthesia*, **36**, 65.
74. Miller-Jones, C. M. H. and Williams, J. H. (1980). Sedation for ventilation. A retrospective study of fifty patients. *Anaesthesia*, **35**, 1104.
75. Medical Defence Union (1976). *Annual Report*. London: Medical Defence Union.
76. Foëx, P., Burt, G., Maynard, P., Ryder, W. A. and Hahn, C. E. W. (1979) Continuous measurement of blood-gases *in vivo* by mass spectrometry. *Brit. J. Anaesth.*, **51**, 999.
77. Whitesell, R. C., Dhamee, M. S. and Munshi, C. (1980). Transcutaneous $Po_2$ monitoring in adults. *Anesthesiology*, **53**, S372.
78. Forrester, P. C. (1981). Transcutaneous oxygen monitoring during anaesthesia. *Anaesthesia*, **36**, 66.
79. Tremper, K. K. (1982). Transcutaneous oxygen monitoring during anaesthesia. *Anaesthesia*, **37**, 222.
80. Gothard, J. W. W., Busst, C. M., Branthwaite, M. A., Davies, N. J. H. and Denison, D. M. (1980). Applications of respiratory mass spectrometry to intensive care. *Anaesthesia*, **35**, 890.
81. Gillbe, C. E., Heneghan, C. P. H. and Branthwaite, M. A. (1981). Respiratory mass spectrometry during general anaesthesia. *Brit. J. Anaesth.*, **53**, 103.
82. Orchard, C. H. and Sykes, M. K. (1980). Errors in oxygen concentration analysis: sensitivity of the IMI analyser to nitrous oxide. *Anaesthesia*, **35**, 1100.
83. Piernan, S., Roizen, M. F. and Severinghaus, J. W. (1979). Oxygen analyser dangerous-senses nitrous oxide as battery fails. *Anesthesiology*, **50**, 146.
84. Douglas, I. M. S., McKenzie, P. J., Ledingham, I. and Smith, G. (1978). Effect of halothane on $Po_2$ electrode. *Lancet*, **2**, 1370.
85. Johnston, V. (1977). Physiotherapy care of a ventilated patient. In: *Tracheostomy and Artificial Ventilation in the Treatment of Respiratory Failure*. Ed. Feldman, S. A. and Crawley, B. E. London: Edward Arnold.
86. Milledge, J. S. (1976). Therapeutic fibreoptic bronchoscopy in intensive care. *Brit. med. J.*, **2**, 142.
87. Barrett, C. R. jr. (1978). Flexible fibreoptic bronchoscopy in the critically ill patient; methodology and indications. *Chest*, **73**, 746.
88. Santiago, S. M. jr., Miranda, L. G., Feld, G. K. and Fisher, H. K. (1982). Fibreoptic bronchoscopy during mechanical ventilation. *Anaesthesia*, **37**, 219.
89. Driver, A. G. and LeBrun, M. (1980). Iatrogenic malnutrition in patients receiving ventilatory support. *J. Amer. med. Ass.*, **244**, 2195.
90. Barker, G. L. (1980). Hyperkalaemia presenting as ventilatory failure. *Anaesthesia*, **35**, 885.
91. Newman, J. H., Neff, T. A. and Ziporin, P. (1977). Acute respiratory failure associated with hypophosphataemia. *New Eng. J. Med.*, **296**, 1101.
92. Ibbotson, R. M., Colvin, B. T. and Colvin, M. P. (1975). Folic acid deficiency during intensive therapy. *Brit. med. J.*, **4**, 145.
93. Gaya, H. (1976). Infection control in intensive care. *Brit. J. Anaesth.*, **48**, 9.
94. Lumley, J. (1976). Decontamination of anaesthetic equipment and ventilators. *Brit. J. Anaesth.*, **48**, 3.
95. Henschel, E. O. (1977). The Guillain-Barré syndrome, a personal experience. *Anesthesiology*, **47**, 228.
96. Shovelton, D. S. (1979). Reflections on an intensive therapy unit. *Brit. med. J.*, **1**, 737.
97. Keep, P. J. (1977). Stimulus deprivation in windowless rooms. *Anaesthesia*, **32**, 598.
98. Brock-Utne, J. G., Cheetham, R. W. S. and Goodwin, N. M. (1976). Psychiatric problems in intensive care. *Anaesthesia*, **31**, 380.
99. Klain, M. (1981). High frequency ventilation. *Respiratory Care*, **26**, 427.
100. Sjöstrand, U. (1980). High frequency positive-pressure ventilation (HFPPV): a review. *Critical Care Medicine*, **8**, 345.
101. Jonzon, A., Őberg, P. Å., Sedin, G. and Sjöstrand, U. (1971). High-frequency positive-pressure ventilation by endotracheal insufflation. *Acta anesth. Scand.*, Supp. **43**, 1.
102. Klain, M. and Smith, R. B. (1977). High frequency percutaneous transtracheal jet ventilation. *Critical Care Medicine*, **5**, 280.
103. Babinski, M., Smith, R. B. and Klain, M. (1980). High frequency jet ventilation for laryngoscopy. *Anesthesiology*, **52**, 178.
104. Carlon, G. C., Ray, jr., C., Klain, M. and McCormack, P. M. (1980). High frequency positive-pressure ventilation in management of a patient with bronchopleural fistula. *Anesthesiology*, **52**, 160.
105. Kalla, R., Wald, M. and Klain, M. (1981). Weaning of ventilator-dependent patients by high frequency jet ventilation. *Critical Care Medicine*, **9**, 162.
106. Lunkenheimer, P. P., Rafflenbeul, W., Keller, H., Frank, I., Dickhut, H. H. and Furhmann, C. (1972). Application of transtracheal pressure oscillations as a modification of "diffusion respiration". *Brit. J. Anaesth.*, **44**, 627.
107. Butler, W. J., Bohn, D. J., Miyasaka, K., Bryan, A. C. and Froese, A. B. (1979). Ventilation of humans by high-frequency oscillation. *Anesthesiology*, **51**, S368.
108. Bohn, D. J., Miyasaka, K., Marchak, B. E., Thompson, W. K., Froese, A. B. and Bryan, A. C. (1980). Ventilation by high frequency oscillation. *J. Appl. Physiol*, **48**, 710.
109. British Medical Journal (1975). Extracorporeal oxygenation for acute respiratory failure. Leading Article. *Brit. med. J.*, **2**, 340.
110. Zapol, W. M., Snider, M. T., Hill, J. D., Fallat, R. J., Bartlett, R. H., Edmunds, L. H., Morris, A. H., Converse Peirce II, E., Thomas, A. N., Proctor, H. J., Drinker, P. A., Pratt, P. C., Bagniewski, A. and Miller, R. G. (1979). Extracorporeal membrane oxygenation in severe acute respiratory failure. *J. Amer. med. Ass.*, **242**, 2193.
111. Zapol, W. M., Snider, M. T. and Schneider, R. C. (1977). Extracorporeal membrane oxygenation for acute respiratory failure. *Anesthesiology*, **46**, 272.
112. Roberts, K. D. (1978). Mechanical support for the treatment of severe pulmonary failure, the membrane

oxygenator. In: *The Medical Management of the Critically Ill*. Ed. Hanson, G. C. and Wright, P. L. London: Academic Press.

113. Gattinoni, L., Pesenti, A., Rossi, G. P., Vesconi, S., Fox, U., Kolobow, T., Agostoni, A., Pelizzola, A., Langer, M., Uziel, L., Longon, F. and Damia, G. (1980). Treatment of acute respiratory failure with low frequency positive pressure ventilation and extracorporeal removal of $CO_2$. *Lancet*, **2**, 292.
114. Fein, A. M., Goldberg, S. K., Lippmann, M. L., Fischer, R. and Morgan, L. (1982). Adult respiratory distress syndrome. *Brit. J. Anaesth.*, **54**, 723.
115. Boggis, C. R. M. and Greene, R. (1983). Adult respiratory distress syndrome. *Brit. J. Hosp. Med.*, **29**, 167.
116. Wallace, P. G. M. and Spence, A. A. (1983). Adult respiratory distress syndrome. *Brit. Med. J.*, **286**, 1167.
117. Deneke, S. M. and Fanburg, B. L. (1982). Oxygen toxicity of the lung: an update. *Brit. J. Anaesth.*, **54**, 737.
118. Morgan, R. J. M. (1983). Rapid and safe withdrawal of intravenous papaveretum after prolonged continuous infusion. *Anaesthesia*, **38**, 492.
119. Mortimer, A. J. and Sykes, M. K. (1983). Monitoring of ventilation. In: *Recent Advances in Critical Care Medicine*, No. 2. Ed. Ledingham, I. McA. and Hanning, C. D. Edinburgh: Churchill Livingstone.
120. Merrifield, A. J. and King, S. J. (1981). The oesophageal obturator airway. *Anaesthesia*, **36**, 672.
121. Gilston, A. (1982). Prolonged nasotracheal intubation. *Anaesthesia*, **37**, 209.
122. Smith, R. B. (1982). Ventilation at high respiratory frequencies. High frequency positive-pressure ventilation, high frequency jet ventilation and high frequency oscillation. *Anaesthesia*, **37**, 1011.
123. Noel Gibney, R. T. and Wilson, R. S. (1983). High frequency ventilation. In: *Recent Advances in Critical Care Medicine*, No. 2. Ed. Ledingham, I. McA. and Hanning, C. D. Edinburgh: Churchill Livingstone.
124. Ledingham, I. McA. and Watt, I. (1983). Influence of sedation on mortality in critically ill multiple trauma patients. *Lancet*, **1**, 1270.
125. Lawler, P. G. P., McHutchon, A. and Bamber, P. A. (1983). Potential hazards of prolonged steroid anaesthesia. *Lancet*, **1**, 1270.

## FURTHER READING

Branthwaite, M. A. (1978). *Artificial Ventilation for Pulmonary Disease*. Obtainable from Anaesthetic Department, Brompton Hospital, London, SW3.

Hanson, G. C. and Wright, P. L. (1978). *Medical Management of the Critically Ill*. London: Academic Press.

Hedley-Whyte, J., Burgess, III, G. E., Feeley, T. W. and Miller, M. G. (1976). *Applied Physiology of Respiratory Care*. Boston: Little, Brown and Co.

Mushin, W. W., Rendell-Baker, L., Thompson, P. W. and Mapleson, W. W. (1980). *Automatic Ventilation of the Lungs*, 3rd edit. Oxford: Blackwell Scientific Publications.

Nunn, J. F. (1977). *Applied Respiratory Physiology*, 2nd edit. London: Butterworth.

Payne, J. P. and Bushman, J. A. (1980). *Artificial Ventilation. Technical, Biological and Clinical Aspects*. London: Academic Press.

Pontoppidan, H., Geffin, B. and Lowenstein, E. (1973). *Acute Respiratory Failure in the Adult*. Boston: Little, Brown and Co.

Pontoppidan, H., Wilson, R. S., Rie, M. A. and Schneider, R. C. (1977). Respiratory intensive care. *Anesthesiology*, **47**, 96.

Sykes, M. K., McNicol, M. W. and Campbell, E. J. M. (1976). *Respiratory Failure*, 2nd edit. Oxford: Blackwell Scientific Publications.

## FURTHER READING—HISTORICAL

Armstrong Davison, M. H. (1971). The History of Anaesthesia. In: *General Anaesthesia*, 3rd edit. Eds. Cecil Gray, T. and Nunn, J. F. London: Butterworth.

Lassen, H. C. A. (1953). A preliminary report on the 1952 epidemic of poliomyelitis in Copenhagen with special reference to the treatment of acute respiratory insufficiency. *Lancet*, **1**, 37.

Mushin, W. W., Rendell-Baker, L., Thompson, P. W. and Mapleson, W. W. (1980). *Automatic Ventilation of the Lungs*, 3rd edit. Oxford: Blackwell Scientific Publications.

Pontoppidan, H., Wilson, R. S., Rie, M. A. and Schneider, R. C. (1977). Respiratory intensive care. *Anesthesiology*, **47**, 96.

Rendell-Baker, L. (1963). History of thoracic anaesthesia. In: *Thoracic Anaesthesia*. Ed. W. W. Mushin. Oxford: Blackwell Scientific Publications.

Shackleton, R. P. W. (1962). In my end is my beginning. *Ann. Roy. Coll. Surg. Engl.* **30**, 229.

Woollam, C. H. M. (1976). The development of apparatus for intermittent negative pressure respiration. *Anaesthesia*, **31**, 537 and 666.

CHAPTER 10

# Intensive Therapy



## INTENSIVE THERAPY

The Intensive Care Unit (ICU) is designed for patients who need and can benefit from facilities and services which are not available in general hospital wards. Such patients usually have failure, or potential failure, of one or more major systems. They therefore need continuous support, monitoring, nursing care and availability of medical staff. In 1967[1] it was recognised that an ICU was an "economic arrangement for the treatment of grave illness" and "not only improves the chances of a patient with a desperate illness but was also likely to promote an improvement in the general level of medical and nursing care". Since then, intensive care or critical care medicine has developed enormously and it is uncommon in developed countries to find any but the smallest hospitals without their own ICU.

It has been said that the direct antecedent of the ICU was the postoperative recovery room[2] which dates back to the time of Florence Nightingale, but intensive care is not limited to postoperative patients and many would regard modern intensive care as dating from the poliomyelitis epidemic of the early 1950's. This provided the stimulus for provision of long-term artificial ventilation, with an immediate reduction in mortality,[3] and through this the development of mechanical ventilators. At first, most ventilated patients were nursed in general wards but the high complication rate, largely because of mechanical failure of airway equipment and ventilators, resulted in several centres establishing respiratory units in the late 1950's.[4] During the early 1960's Coronary Care Units (CCU's) were established for continuous electrocardiographic monitoring of patients with myocardial infarction[5,6] and to make the best use of the equipment which had become available for cardioversion,[7] and electrical pacing.[8] Continuous haemodynamic monitoring provided early warning of complications occurring in these patients and in patients who had undergone open heart surgery. Modern intensive care has developed from an amalgam of the lessons learnt from respiratory and coronary care with continued momentum provided by the clinical and technological developments in cardiopulmonary resuscitation, pharmacological and mechanical circulatory support, advances in the treatment of renal failure, respiratory failure, cerebral oedema, multiple organ failure and patient monitoring systems.

## DESIGN OF THE INTENSIVE THERAPY UNIT

### Organisation and Bed Numbers

In most hospitals the design of the ICU reflects its developmental history, pre-existing architecture, available space and the limitations imposed by financial restrictions. There is, however, no lack of helpful advice for those who are fortunate enough to be establishing a new ICU in a new building[9–11] or modernising an old one.[433]

Estimates of the proportion of intensive care beds required by a general hospital vary from 1 per cent[9] to 4 per cent[12] but in hospitals with a major cardiothoracic unit, trauma centre and neurosurgical unit the proportion of intensive care beds may be as high as 10 per cent.

Adult ICU's of up to 15 beds have been described,[13] but with increasing size the problems of day-to-day administration and logistical support become more complex. It also becomes difficult for any one person to keep up with the changes and progress of the patients in an active unit much above this in size. Perhaps even more important is the loss of identity and sense of personal contribution to each patient's progress that can occur in its staff if a unit is too large. Intensive Care Units of less than 6 beds make less efficient use of both staff and equipment. The optimum size for an ICU is therefore between 8 and 12 beds. This is large enough to justify its own medical, nursing and ancillary staff and make efficient use of expensive items of equipment.

Not all hospitals will be large enough to justify a major ICU. This has lead to the concept of regionalisation of ICU's. In both the USA[14] and Australia[15] four levels of provision of intensive care are recognised ranging from category 1 units in large comprehensive regional hospitals, which are fully equipped and staffed by full-time specialists, to category 4 units in small hospitals equipped for resuscitation and from which patients can be transferred to a larger centre. The organisation and work of a small ICU in a district general hospital[16] lies between categories 2 and 3 and provides both general and coronary care to a level required by the majority of patients, though occasionally patients may require transfer to a regional centre for facilities or investigations not available on site.

On the other hand, some large teaching hospitals with regional specialties and acting as secondary referral centres will need more intensive care beds than can be managed within a single unit. Unfortunately, the intensive care areas in these hospitals usually reflect the political muscle of individual departments and the fragmentation of intensive care areas into medical ICU, surgical ICU, cardiothoracic ICU, neurosurgical ICU, coronary care unit, respiratory care unit and so on shows a lack of understanding of problems in critical care medicine. Sometimes these units are just glorified nursing care areas which result in costly duplication of expensive equipment and inefficient use of resources. Concentrating critically ill but potentially salvagable patients in multidisciplinary ICU's or critical care centres (for example, combinations of adjacent medical, surgical and cardiac ICU's) has both patient care and economic advantages over purely department-specialty-organ orientated ICU's.[13,14] Published mortality figures support the creation of ICU's staffed by specially trained nurses and full-time ICU physicians. In one University hospital when specialty ICU's were replaced with a single multidisciplinary ICU (both staffed by physician specialists) mortality from respiratory insufficiency decreased from 30 per cent to 10 per cent and mortality from myocardial infarction decreased from 30 per cent to 15 per cent.[14] Division of a large critical care area into separate units can then be based on patient requirements rather than by specialty. For example, division into "clean" surgical, burns, coronary care and general units may be found suitable and reflects the different patient and nursing requirements for these groups.

Whether coronary care should be considered part of intensive care is open to dispute. While it is true that in the majority of hospitals the CCU is under the direction of a cardiologist there is much to be said for including it within the critical care area. Some of the patients with myocardial infarction, for example, those with severe pulmonary oedema and those who develop cardiogenic shock, can benefit from the facilities of an ICU and in some places intensive and coronary care have been very successfully carried out within the same unit.[17,18] Such an arrangement certainly offers considerable advantages in terms of the variety of experience it can offer medical and nursing staff in training and in the sharing of trained nursing, medical and ancillary staff and equipment.

The siting of the ICU within the hospital is important. It is one of the most active areas in the hospital and ideally it needs to be in close proximity to operating theatres, recovery room, casualty department and general wards for easy transfer of patients. It also needs to have ready access to the radiology department and laboratories to facilitate collection of samples and the conduct of investigations (Fig. 1). These considerations are not just academic. During a prospective clinical study into the effects of moving patients to and from an ICU, one patient a month suffered a major cardiorespiratory collapse or death as a direct result of movement.[19] The doors and corridors leading to and from the ICU must of course be big enough to allow easy access of beds and other bulky items such as portable image intensifiers.

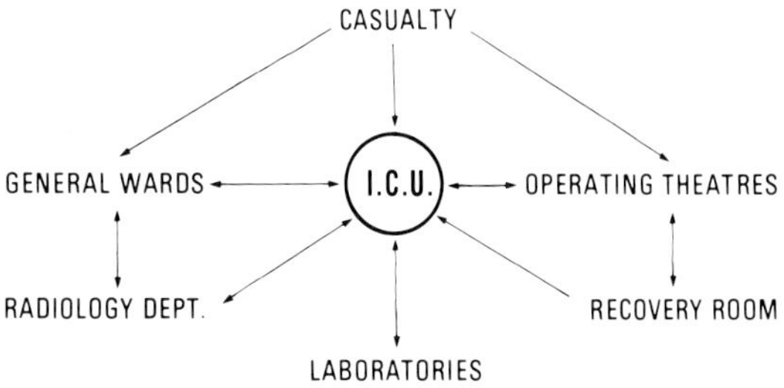


10/FIG. 1.—Relationship of the intensive care unit to other hospital departments.

The final constraint on the organisation and number of intensive care beds is that of availability and occupancy. Table 1 shows the effect of size of unit on the occupancy rates for two policies. One, that a bed will be unoccupied and available for admission of a patient 90 per cent of the time and the other that a bed will be available 99 per cent of the time.[20] This emphasises the relative cost efficiency of larger units and has suggested that by combining ICU's and CCU's under one management organisation the availability of beds can be enhanced without individual units becoming too large. In order to

10/TABLE 1
BED AVAILABILITY RELATED TO SIZE AND OCCUPANCY OF AN ICU

| *Average Census of Unit* | *90% Availability* | | *99% Availability* | |
|---|---|---|---|---|
| | *Beds Needed* | *% Av. Census* | *Beds Needed* | *% Av. Census* |
| 3 | 6 | 200 | 9 | 300 |
| 9 | 14 | 155 | 18 | 200 |
| 27 | 35 | 130 | 42 | 155 |

(Courtesy of Dr. M. H. Weil and Dr. H. Shubin and Harper Medical[20])

achieve a high bed availability in smaller units a low occupancy rate is necessary, but the occupancy rates proposed in most planning documents are in the range of 70 to 85 per cent with 75 per cent being the most quoted figure.[10]

### Space and Layout

Most ICU's have both multi-bed areas and single bed rooms in a ratio of between 1 and 2 to 1. While open-bed areas make observation of patients easier and allow for economies in nursing staff, single rooms are essential for segregation of infectious cases and those patients with an increased susceptibility to cross-infection. Single rooms are also useful for providing visual and auditory isolation for some patients and a degree of privacy for those patients who are conscious but require long-term ICU management, e.g. those with the Guillain-Barré syndrome (see below). Some of the advantages of single rooms can be gained by using mobile bed dividers while retaining the flexibility of an open plan area.

Planning documents vary widely in the minimum recommended floor space per bed, estimates ranging from 12 to 100 m$^2$. For single rooms 26 to 30 m$^2$ is satisfactory and in multi-bed areas 18·5 to 20 m$^2$ with at least 3·3 to 3·6 metres between bed centres. This allows enough room for doctors, nurses and equipment to get to the patient without overcrowding. The central nursing station should be located so that all patients in the unit can be seen from it. This is usually the most convenient site for a central patient monitor, storage of patient records and a medication cupboard.

The patient and central staff areas should have natural light and clear windows to provide a feeling of spaciousness, an awareness of the world outside the ICU and the passage of time. It has been convincingly demonstrated that lack of natural light increases the already high levels of stress experienced by staff in an ICU.[21] When the incidence of postoperative delirium was compared in two ICU's in the same town which were identical except for the absence of windows in one of them, it was found that more than twice as many episodes of delirium occurred in the windowless unit.[22]

In general, the area needed for supporting services and storage is at least as great as that allowed for the patient area and central nursing and monitoring station. The nature and purpose of the areas needed are well described in planning documents. A list of some of these areas is given in Table 2. A seminar room is useful in larger units because of the educational role they usually have. In many units the staff of an ICU change into lightweight uniforms and visitors must wear gowns and overshoes. If this practice is followed changing rooms will be needed for male and female staff, but there is no evidence that it gives any bacteriological protection whatsoever.

10/TABLE 2
ROOMS AND AREAS ASSOCIATED WITH AN ICU

| |
|---|
| Clean utility area |
| Dirty utility/sluice room |
| Charge sister's room |
| Doctor's room |
| "On call" room |
| Staff rest room/coffee room |
| Staff lavatories and cloakroom |
| Equipment storage areas |
| —electrical and monitoring |
| —respiratory |
| —disposable |
| Workshop for repair and maintenance |
| Laboratory |
| Linen store |
| Cleaners' room |
| Plant room |
| —emergency gas supplies |
| —air conditioning |
| Visitors' waiting room |
| Reception area |
| Distressed relatives' room |

Other requirements for the patient area include some provision for ensuring patient to patient visual and auditory privacy, adequate hand-washing facilities and storage space. The whole area should be air conditioned, well lit and decorated as harmoniously as possible. The materials used on walls and floors should be washable and help to reduce noise. Each bed space needs at least 8 power points, overhead lighting, a spot light, piped oxygen, compressed air and suction. In case of power or equipment failures the electrical circuits of an ICU should be connected to the hospital's emergency power supply and an emergency supply of oxygen and a portable suction apparatus should also be available. As far as possible equipment and apparatus should be kept off the floor to help

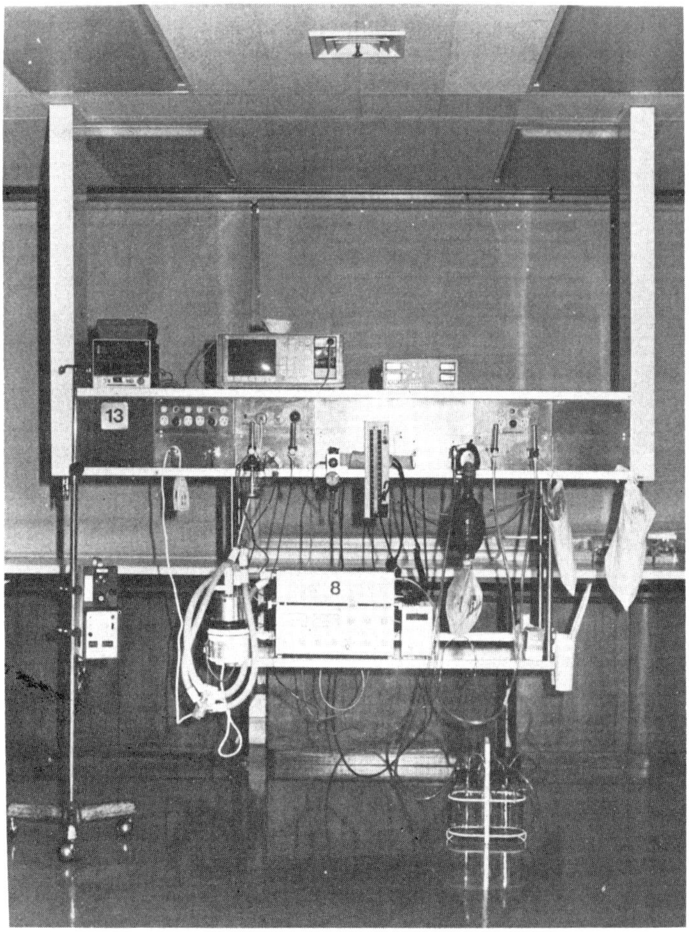


10/Fig. 2.—Attaching items of equipment to the wall helps to keep the floor clear for cleaning and improves access to the patient.

with cleaning and avoid unnecessary clutter. This is most easily done by attaching as many items as possible to the wall (Fig 2).

**Equipment**

The level and quantity of equipment in an ICU will vary considerably from hospital to hospital. What is appropriate for the ICU of a major teaching and referral centre will be inappropriate for a small district general hospital. The essential equipment for providing a minimal level of intensive care for trauma patients[23] is listed in Table 3. In larger units some or all of the equipment listed in Table 4 may be found. The patient's electrocardiogram as well as being displayed at the bedside, should also be seen on a central monitor with alarms and facilities for obtaining a permanent record of any dysrhythmias seen. Many other items can be monitored and recorded without recourse to electrical equipment. These include temperature, blood pressure, central venous pressure, and urine output, all of which should be regularly charted. In unstable patients with a variety of problems, electronic monitoring equipment will display and record all of these and so free nursing staff for other tasks. However, not all systems are so easily monitored and despite intracranial pressure monitoring and the cerebral function monitor, clinical assessment remains the best guide to a changing neurological disorder.

The different types of ventilator are discussed in Chapter 9. Factors such as reliability, ease of operation and the provision of alarms have a much greater effect on the choice of ventilator

10/Table 3
Equipment Required to Provide a Minimal Level of Intensive Care for Trauma Patients

| |
|---|
| Airway control and ventilation devices |
| Oxygen source with concentration controls |
| Cardiac emergency trolley |
| Temporary transvenous pacemaker |
| Electrocardiograph—oscilloscope—defibrillator |
| Mechanical ventilator |
| Patient weighing devices |
| Pulmonary function measuring devices |
| Pressure distribution beds |
| Drugs, intravenous fluids and supplies |

10/Table 4
Some Equipment that may be Found in a Large ICU Serving as a Regional or Subregional Centre.

| |
|---|
| Volume cycled ventilators |
| Provision of PEEP, IMV, etc. |
| Fibreoptic bronchoscope |
| Expired air $CO_2$ monitoring |
| Electronic pressure monitoring |
| —haemodynamic |
| —intracranial |
| Cardiac output computer |
| Intra-aortic balloon pump |
| Portable x-ray machine |
| Image intensifier |
| Infusion pumps |
| Equipment for dialysis |
| —peritoneal |
| —haemodialysis |
| Cerebral function monitor |

for use in an ICU than they would for a ventilator used solely in the operating theatre. Volume cycled ventilators are generally found easier to manage than the pressure cycled variety because changes in resistance and compliance of the patient's lungs with time or change of position have less effect on ventilation. Fibreoptic bronchoscopy is a useful adjunct to respiratory care, especially for patients with sputum retention and lobar collapse[24] and it has been suggested that this should be available as a routine service in ICU's. Certainly the risks of fibreoptic bronchoscopy seem small as long as some basic precautions are taken.[25]

While a unit may use more than one model of ventilator, pressure monitor, etc., some degree of standardisation is desirable so that nurses and other new staff coming to the unit can become familiar with their use as quickly as possible.

### Electrical Safety

In an area where so much electrical equipment is used electrical safety becomes particularly important, especially as patients with cardiac pacing electrodes, intracardiac ECG electrodes and fluid-filled catheters passing to or through the heart are commonly found in an ICU. These patients are at risk from microelectrocution (see Chapter 8). Standards for the electrical wiring and supply systems,[26] and the equipment used in an ICU[27,28] have been drawn up and all installations and equipment must meet these or similar standards.

### Computers

Increasing use is being made of computers in ICU's. Some, such as cardiac output computers and computer ECG analysis for monitoring of dysrhythmias, are based on single function systems. Micro-computers and programmable calculators[29] can be used for simple data collection and storage and for calculation of haemodynamic or respiratory profiles and parenteral nutrition requirements. More flexible systems based on mini-computers provide comprehensive patient data management including on-line analysis, charting and trend recording of arterial, central venous and pulmonary artery pressures, temperature and fluid balance and can store the patient's history, clinical examination and the pathology results.[30,31] The extent to which such systems become more widely used will depend on the results of evaluations of cost and benefit being made at present.

### Cross-Infection

Infection is a major hazard to patients in an ICU and, in the critically ill, may materially affect survival.[32] Unfortunately, these patients have a reduced ability to resist infection because of depression of a variety of both non-specific resistance mechanisms and specific immune responses.[33,34] However, many of the patients requiring intensive care do so because of some life-threatening infection. Avoidance of cross-infection therefore becomes a major concern especially when indiscriminate use of broad-spectrum antibiotics has led to selection of antibiotic-resistant bacteria.

Bacteria may be spread within an ICU by

airborne dissemination, direct personal contact or via fomites, such as food, drinks, instruments, equipment, catheters or contaminated cream lotions or solutions.[35,36] The presence of intravascular cannulae and catheters for infusion of fluids and monitoring adds to the risks and potential sources of infection.[37] Pressure transducers are also a potential source of infection, even when disposable domes are used.[38]

Airborne cross-infection can be largely eliminated by adequate room ventilation. Patients who are obviously infected or heavily colonised with a potentially epidemic organism can be nursed in exhaust-ventilated (negative-pressure) rooms while those who are immune suppressed or for other reasons may be particularly susceptible to infection are nursed under plenum ventilation (positive-pressure). An alternative approach is the provision of separate "clean" and "dirty" ICU's or separate areas within the one unit[18] but the effect that this will have on bed requirements must be remembered (see above). At least as important in the control of infection, are the policies for disinfection and sterilisation of equipment, the limitation of staff movements between patients and personal hygiene. Cross-infection is more likely when the ICU is busy and there are reservoirs of organisms such as *Pseudomonas aeruginosa*.[434] It must also be remembered that in the ICU patient with diminished resistance to infection his endogenous bacterial population is the most likely source of any infection. Several studies have shown that, in patients with severe acute illness, a failure of the delayed hypersensitivity skin test response—anergy—is associated with a significant mortality from septicaemia.[39] Reduced host resistance as reflected by anergy is almost certainly the reason these patients become infected rather than exposure to potential sources of infection *per se*.[40]

### Bed

A comfortable, functionally designed bed is an important but often forgotten item of ICU equipment. Ideally, the ICU bed should be mobile, easy to operate and allow all procedures to be performed with a minimum of disturbance to the patient and effort from the staff. Other important features are ease of cleaning, provision for patient's charts and a radiolucent base and mattress so that an image intensifier can be used for insertion of transvenous pacing catheters and so on without moving the patient. For selected patients it can be useful to have access to special beds such as the Egerton-Stoke Mandeville and fluidised bead beds.[41]

## STAFFING

### Medical

Who should be in charge of the ICU? Clearly the Director must have administrative abilities and the qualities of leadership to direct the large team of medical, nursing and ancillary staff an ICU requires and at the same time should be able to inspire confidence in the sick patients and anxious relatives he will be dealing with. In addition, he needs to have an expert knowledge of the problems encountered in ICU patients. In a large unit the director will need to be supported by other consultant staff with similar abilities to provide expert coverage twenty-four hours a day throughout the year while allowing for holidays, study leave, teaching and research commitments.[42] In many countries, including much of Europe, Latin America, Australia, Japan and South Africa these requirements have led to the development of critical care or intensive care medicine as a specialty or sub-specialty of anaesthesia or internal medicine.[43] In the past, doctors attracted to this field have had to seek knowledge about particular problems from various sources outside their basic specialty. Now advanced training schemes in intensive care for doctors with a background in anaesthesia, internal medicine or both[44] are available. An outline of such training within the structure of the NHS was proposed in 1976[45] but this has not been developed. A survey conducted by the Intensive Care Society in England and Wales[46] showed that only about half the ICU's are largely supervised by consultants with a heavy commitment to it and most did not believe intensive care work should be restricted to separate career specialist "intensivists". This contrasts with the situation in, for example, the USA and Australia where it is usual for the ICU director and, frequently, other senior staff to devote the whole of their time to intensive care. In the survey of practice in England and Wales there were only two completely full-time specialists in intensive care.

Most of the junior staff in British ICU's are anaesthetists[46] and intensive care and related topics form a large part of the questions in the final fellowship of the Faculty of Anaesthetists. However, junior medical cover can also be provided as part of medical or surgical rotations at SHO or registrar level with benefits to trainees that include gaining confidence in the management of seriously ill patients, resuscitation and appreciating the role of intensive care in patient management in terms of both the techniques available and its limitations.

### Nursing

The nature of intensive care implies constant nursing attention for each patient throughout each day, i.e. a nurse:patient ratio of 1:1, though in practice a single nurse may be able to observe a number of the less acutely ill patients if they are grouped together, or for example, in a specialised CCU. An establishment of 4·25 nurses per bed has been found adequate, allowing for holidays, sickness, etc.[47] At least 70 per cent of the nurses should be experienced so that the untrained nurse is given the opportunity to learn and accept responsibility at her own pace.[48] Many larger ICU's run courses for state registered or state enrolled nurses approved (in England) by the joint Board of Clinical Nursing Studies. Successful completion of such a course is recognised as demonstrating competence and familiarity with ICU nursing. An organised nurse orientation programme significantly improves the integration of new staff into the ICU.

The increased stress experienced by ICU nurses has been well documented.[49] This may be the result of internal unrelieved tension from constantly nursing critically ill patients, excessive emotional involvement with patients or the repetitive exposure to death. Other sources of stress experienced by ICU nurses include the problems in communicating with intubated patients, supporting distressed relatives, a sense of isolation from the rest of the hospital and a relationship with a nursing administration that may appear to understand little of the nursing problems peculiar to the ICU. Nowhere else in a hospital is a patient so totally dependent on the quality of the nursing care.

### Physiotherapists, Technical Staff and others

The smooth running of ICU depends on a large team of people. Some of these are listed in Table 5. In any but the smallest ICU a 24-hour physiotherapy and radiography service will be available. Servicing, sterilisation and repair of the respiratory and electrical equipment demands a high degree of skill and attention to detail. Technicians trained in these fields may be attached to the ICU or be a part of a department of medical physics, clinical measurement or anaesthetics with responsibilities extending to the ICU. This latter arrangement makes it easier to arrange cover for nights, weekends and holidays.

10/Table 5
Some of the Non-medical or Nursing Staff Required in an ICU

| | |
|---|---|
| Physiotherapists | Respiratory technicians |
| Radiographers | Electronics technicians |
| Dietitians | Cleaners |
| Pharmacists | Porters |
| Chaplains | |
| Social workers | |

## PATIENT SELECTION

Intensive care is expensive. In a district general hospital the cost of a bed in an ICU is about four times that of a bed in a general ward.[50] At present the indications for admission to an ICU are poorly defined. Selection of patients for admission may reflect the prejudices of the referring physician, the interests of the ICU and the level of the care available in the ward rather than defined medical criteria, but in most instances a number of factors are taken into consideration. Patients in the terminal phase of any chronic disease or with disseminated malignancy are usually excluded. Increasing age, while not the sole reason for determining admission, must be taken into account because of the decreased physiological reserves and a worse prognosis for most conditions that require intensive care.[51] Medical admissions may be an exception to this trend[435] because the prognosis for this group of diseases in an ICU does not appear to worsen with age. Attempts to predict the outcome of intensive care from the medical complications after 48 hours of ICU management have had some success[51] but such general considerations do not necessarily apply to an individual patient and do not take account of improvements in the delivery of intensive care, the understanding of disease processes and new treatments that become available over a period of time. More specific predictors of complications and mortality are needed[52] but in the meantime clinical judgment, including assessment of the patient's previous health, age-related mortality and the significance of particular complications, taken with the availability of ICU beds, are the basis for deciding whether or not a patient will be admitted.

Most reports have shown that between 16 and 24 per cent of patients admitted to an ICU die there, increasing to 30–33 per cent in those who require ventilation.[50] Some of the factors that affect the outcome and costs of intensive care have been reviewed by Cullen[53] and Detsky and colleagues.[54]

## PRINCIPLES OF INTENSIVE THERAPY

In many ways the approach to management of a patient in ICU has more in common with the management of a patient during anaesthesia, particularly anaesthesia for a major operation or as an emergency, than it does with conventional medical or surgical ward management, although this becomes less true as the patient's condition improves. The experience of anaesthetists in resuscitation, monitoring techniques and intensive management of one or just a limited number of patients at a time has undoubtedly made the transition from anaesthesia to intensive care or their joint practice easier for many. The components of ICU management are:

1. Resuscitation
2. Diagnosis
3. Monitoring
4. Specific therapy
5. Systems support

with a dynamic relationship existing between these components (Fig. 3). In addition, all patients will need the general care, including nursing, physiotherapy, sedation, analgesia, psychological and nutritional support and prophylaxis against complications that are fundamental to competent intensive care. The relative importance of these components of ICU management will vary between different patients

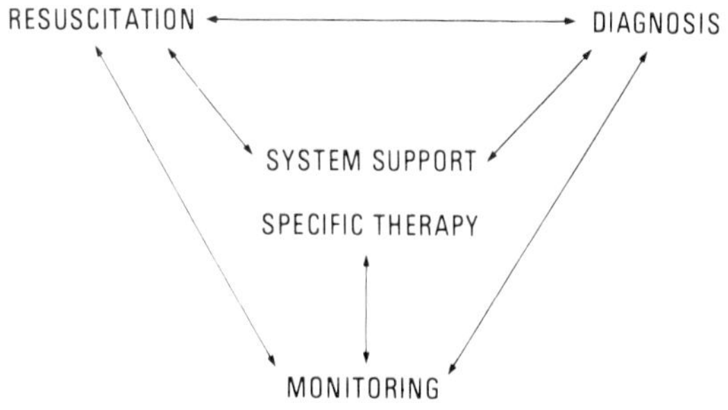


10/Fig. 3.—The components of patient management in the intensive care unit.

and for any one patient from time to time. Most patients will fall into one of two categories:

1. Those who are seriously ill on admission to hospital or whose condition deteriorates while in hospital and require resuscitation, specific diagnosis and specific treatment on admission to ICU. Continued monitoring and system support are needed while they recover from the underlying disease process.
2. Those admitted after major surgery or for coronary care. In these the major requirement is for monitoring so that resuscitation or specific therapy can be started at the earliest signs of any complication. Admission policies vary between hospitals but the surgical patients might include those who have had cardiac, major vascular or thoraco-abdominal surgery and those with serious medical problems such as recent myocardial infarction, cardiac dysrhythmias or respiratory failure.

The components of management should be carried out within the context of an overall plan that begins with the present situation and ends with discharge from ICU and eventually full rehabilitation. Clearly this plan needs to be flexible and, particularly in the early stages, it may need to be changed on an hour to hour basis as priorities change or new complications develop. In the seriously ill patient it is important to know exactly what effect an intervention is having and this is why careful haemodynamic, respiratory, biochemical and other monitoring is so important, succinctly expressed in the principle "measure, correct, remeasure". In this way it is possible to know not only that your patient is improving (or not) but, almost as important, why he is improving and what intervention is responsible. This counsel of perfection is rarely completely obtainable, but the aim should be to get as close to it as possible, to understand as fully as possible the nature of the patient's illness.

In nearly all ICU patients the different components of management will proceed simultaneously. In particular, steps should be taken to diagnose the underlying disease and start specific therapy while resuscitation and system support help to keep the patient alive.

**Resuscitation**

Cardiopulmonary resuscitation (Chapter 14) and blood transfusion (Chapter 17) are considered elsewhere while management of the "shocked" patient is considered below.

**Diagnosis**

Diagnosis in an ICU patient may be made in either physiological terms—decreased pulmonary compliance and increased intrapulmonary shunt, low cardiac output with elevated indirect left atrial pressure—or in specific pathological terms—pneumococcal lobar pneumonia, extensive anterior myocardial infarction. Correction of the abnormalities implied by the physiological diagnosis is the aim of resuscitation and systems support, while the specific pathological diagnosis is needed to direct treatment of the underlying disease.

The usual stages in making a diagnosis: taking a medical history, careful physical examination and investigation to confirm or make a differential diagnosis, applies as much to ICU patients as to those anywhere else in the hospital, but there may be unusual difficulties. A proportion of the patients admitted to ICU will be unconscious as a result of coma, injury or anaesthesia. These patients will be unable to give a history so it is important that as much information as possible is obtained from their family, friends, police, ambulance staff and previous medical attendants. Even if the patient is transferred from elsewhere in the hospital with a medical record, this should be carefully reviewed and confirmed as far as possible to reveal the events that led to them requiring admission to ICU.

Physical examination may be difficult to interpret because of the effects of drugs given before admission to ICU, the limitation of access due to skeletal traction, dressings, drains and so on, and the effects of artefacts introduced by intermittent positive-pressure ventilation or intra-aortic balloon pumping. It is nevertheless important that the results of the physical examination on admission are recorded. These difficulties in history taking and physical examination may make it appear that diagnosis of ICU patients depends more on the investigations and invasive monitoring methods than anything else; but it is even more true that in these patients attention to the history and examination may save unnecessary investigations and save time when the patient is already seriously ill.

Reaching the correct diagnosis is all important in starting specific therapy aimed at reversing the disease process. It is unusual for the ICU patient to have a single diagnosis or medical problem; combinations, such as recent duodenal perforation, sub-phrenic abscess, septicaemia, adult respiratory distress syndrome, acute renal failure with a past history of angina and hypertension, are common. In these patients the interaction between the different problems must be considered.

**Monitoring**

Clinical patient monitoring of such things as body temperature, respiratory rate, pulse, blood pressure, colour, skin temperature, urine output, level of consciousness, and muscle power can of course be performed on a general ward and with the greater nurse:patient ratio in ICU these can potentially be followed more closely. However, electrical monitoring equipment has a number of advantages in the seriously ill patient:

1. Continuous display so that changes can be detected immediately.
2. Greater accuracy, provided always that the apparatus is properly calibrated and that there are no artefacts.
3. Provision of measurements that cannot be made non-invasively, such as Pulmonary Artery Wedge Pressure (PAWP).
4. Release of nurses' time to other tasks.
5. Automatic alarms to attract the immediate attention of staff if a measurement exceeds preset limits.

The potential disadvantages include:

1. Sepsis associated with catheters and transducer systems.[55,56]

2. Inaccurate measurements caused by poor calibration, trapped air bubbles in catheter transducer systems or long connecting tubing.[57,58]
3. Local complications of the monitoring catheter or other items invading or in contact with the patient.
4. Electrical and other potential hazards to patient and staff from the equipment.

Undue reliance should never be placed on the monitoring equipment and if a measurement seems out of keeping with the patient's clinical condition the equipment should be checked and if possible the measurement repeated by a second method.

**Respiratory monitoring.**—Respiratory and ventilatory function of spontaneously breathing patients is adequately monitored in most cases by clinical observation[59] supplemented when necessary by intermittent spirometry, arterial blood gas analysis and chest x-rays. More sophisticated devices for measuring tidal and minute volume, respiratory rate and detection of apnoea are available[60,61] but have not been widely used.

In ventilated patients *tidal* and *minute volume* should be monitored continuously. Many ventilators have built-in mechanical respirometers or pneumotachographs to facilitate measurement and display of this data, and all should display *airway pressure*. A change in airway pressure can be the first indication of a number of potentially serious complications such as kinking or blocking of an endotracheal tube, the tube being pushed too far down so that it lies in the right main bronchus or development of a pneumothorax as well as demonstrating the changes in lung compliance with time and/or therapeutic interventions. *Arterial blood gas analysis* is a valuable guide to the adequacy of ventilation and oxygen therapy, though development of non-invasive methods of assessing these, such as transcutaneous measurement of oxygen tension,[62,63] end-tidal carbon dioxide levels and mass spectrometry,[64] may decrease the frequency with which blood gas analysis is required, while catheter tip oxygen electrodes allow continuous measurement of arterial or mixed venous oxygen tension[65] in unstable patients.

**Cardiovascular monitoring.**—It is usual for patients in ICU/CCU to have a continuous display of the *electrocardiogram* from chest leads on a bedside or central station oscilloscope. This can be combined with a display of the heart rate and facilities for "freezing" or recording any dysrhythmias that are seen on the screen. Computer analysis can detect and record the frequency of dysrhythmias in any individual patient. The methods and significance of haemodynamic monitoring in ICU have been extensively reviewed.[60,61,66–68] Automatic non-invasive methods of *blood pressure measurement* facilitate frequent measurements, but they tend to be affected by patient movement and are unreliable in hypotensive patients with a low cardiac output. In seriously ill patients undoubtedly the most accurate method is direct measurement from an intra-arterial catheter remembering the potential pitfalls with this method (see above).

In the "normal" patient the atrial pressures on the two sides of the heart are closely related and *central venous pressure* (CVP) may be used as a guide to the changes in effective blood volume. However, in the presence of lung disease or impaired myocardial function, which will be the case in many ICU patients, the CVP gives little guide to changes occurring in left atrial pressure (LAP). In ICU the LAP may be measured indirectly by using a flow-directed balloon-tipped catheter passed through the right side of the heart into the pulmonary artery so that with the balloon inflated it becomes wedged in a branch of the pulmonary artery (Fig. 4).[69] In general it has been found that there is a good agreement between the pressure obtained from such a catheter—the *pulmonary artery wedge pressure* (PAWP)—and LAP, although severe lung disease and high levels of PEEP may increase the differences. Measurement and monitoring of PAWP is particularly useful in patients with left ventricular dysfunction and low cardiac output in whom the PAWP can be increased to improve cardiac output but maintained below the level at which pulmonary oedema will occur. Further development of these catheters has permitted monitoring of CVP and measurement of *cardiac output* by thermodilution with a single catheter,[70] while the pulmonary artery pressure lumen may also be used for obtaining samples of mixed venous blood. A variety of complications, including dysrhythmias, infection, pulmonary artery perforation and pulmonary infarction have been

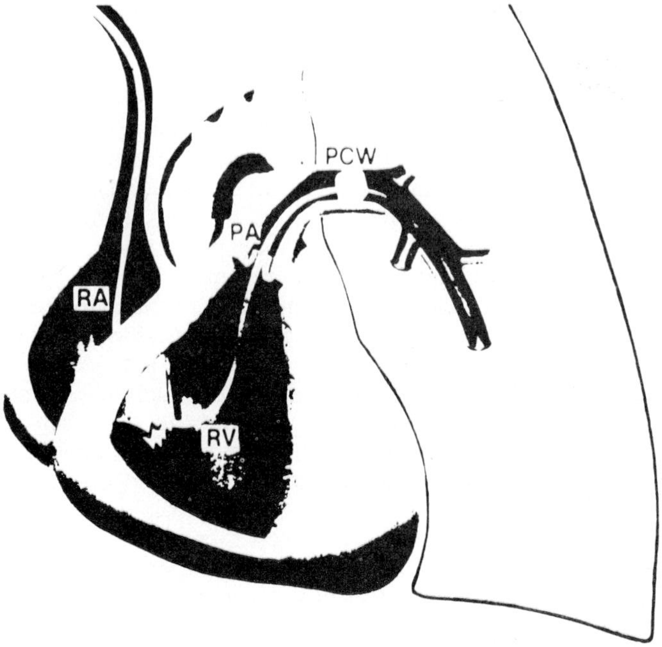


(*a*)

(*b*)

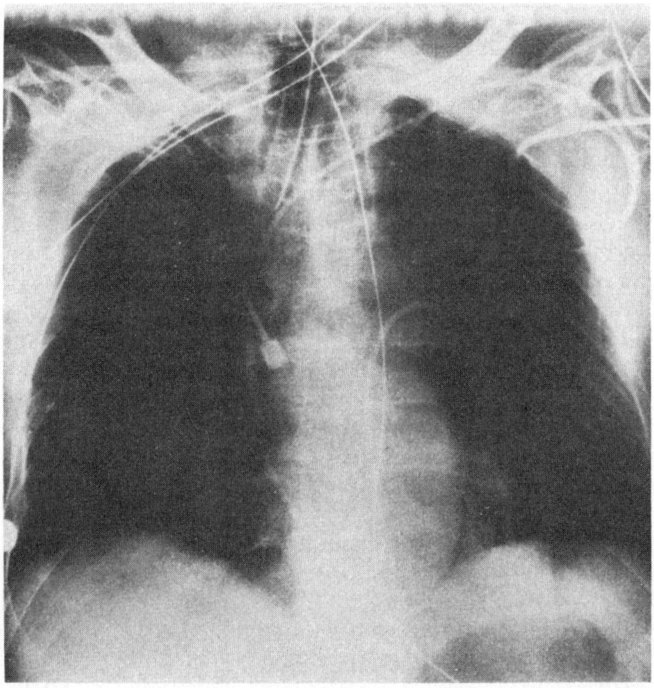

10/Fig. 4.—Left atrial pressure may be measured indirectly by inserting a pulmonary artery balloon flotation catheter.

reported from the use of pulmonary artery catheters, but the incidence of both these and the local complications such as pneumothorax, arterial puncture and haematoma formation is low.[71,72]

Thermodilution is the most commonly used method of *cardiac output* measurement in ICU. While there are a number of potential errors in its use[73] it has been found to be accurate enough to guide management in clinical practice and the ease with which repeated estimations may be made at the patient's bedside, particularly with the aid of small computers, have led to it being preferred to alternatives such as dye dilution or the Fick method. Non-invasive methods of cardiac output estimation have been developed and potentially offer a continuous measurement of cardiac output on a beat-to-beat basis. The transthoracic electrical impedance method, in which a high frequency current is passed between electrodes placed around the neck and chest and the changes in impedance with each systole are measured between two intervening electrodes (Fig. 5), has been reasonably accurate in normal volunteers and in patients during cardiac catheterisation[74,75] but disappointingly inaccurate in both ventilated and non-ventilated patients in ICU. Transcutaneous aortovelography, in which aortic blood flow velocities and acceleration are measured by an ultrasonic Doppler method, appeared promising in early investigations[76] and techniques such as pulse volume analysis and two dimensional echocardiography have also been described, but none of these non-invasive methods has as yet achieved wide application.

**Intracranial pressure monitoring.**—Intracranial pressure (ICP) can be measured through an intraventricular catheter or from devices inserted through a burr hole into the subdural or extradural spaces.[77,78] Pressure monitoring from an intraventricular catheter is the most accurate and because it allows CSF to be removed or fluid inserted, changes in brain compliance can also be followed. However, a ventricular catheter may be difficult to insert, especially if the ventricles are small or shifted, and there is a small risk of intracranial haemorrhage and infection. ICP monitoring can make a significant contribution to the management of patients with head injuries, after neurosurgical operations, in cases of Reye's syndrome or hypoxic brain damage.

**Fluid balance** charts on which are recorded all the fluids going into and coming out of the patient as measured by the nursing staff may give a guide to fluid balance but are notoriously inaccurate because of the problems in measuring all the volumes of fluid infused, drinks, drugs given, fluid content of food, etc., and in any case they do not take insensible losses into consideration. For these reasons daily weighing of the patient is a more accurate guide to changes in body water but, while daily weighing is a desirable ideal, it is not always a practicable proposition.

**Biochemical monitoring.**—Renal function, acid base status, liver function, glucose utilisation, and electrolyte balance all require biochemical monitoring. The frequency with which such tests are needed will depend on the nature and the severity of the patient's illness. In most hospitals work from the ICU accounts for a large proportion of the work performed outside normal office hours. Some ICU's have a small laboratory attached to them for performing arterial blood gas, blood glucose, sodium and potassium and other frequently needed estimations. The introduction of automated, self-calibrating equipment has made such a service easier in some cases but it is important to ensure that the same quality control standards are maintained as in the main laboratory. In the future intravascular monitoring, for example of

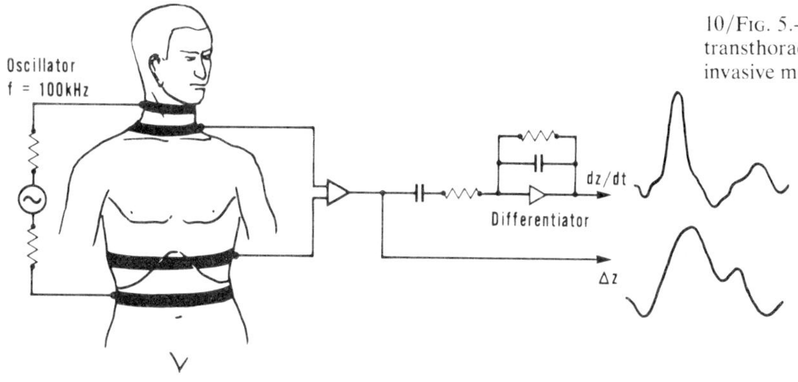


10/FIG. 5.—Measurement of changes in transthoracic electrical impedance is one non-invasive method of estimating cardiac output.

potassium, may be possible for patients with rapidly changing levels.[79]

Monitoring of the *plasma levels of drugs* is important in critically ill patients because subtherapeutic levels may perpetuate the condition it is wished to treat while at the same time the risks of accumulation or toxicity are increased because of impaired excretion or metabolism. Such monitoring may be the responsibility of either a biochemistry department or a department of clinical pharmacology.

**Bacteriological monitoring.** — Systematic bacteriological monitoring of ICU patients can identify developing colonisation or infection at an earlier stage than is normally achieved.[80] The frequency with which specimens need to be sent for culture to be of benefit is unclear, but most ICU's have a policy for regular collection of urine from catheterised patients, sputum from intubated patients and those with a productive cough, and peritoneal dialysis fluid. Blood cultures should be sent from any patient who develops a fever and pressure monitoring catheters should always be considered as the source of a "pyrexia of unknown origin" in the ICU patient.

The same considerations apply to antibiotics as discussed above for other drugs. Monitoring of plasma levels is particularly important for antibiotics with a low therapeutic ratio, such as the aminoglycosides.

**Haematological monitoring** (see also Chapter 17).—Severe acute illness is frequently associated with bone marrow depression and anaemia. This should not be accepted as the cause of a falling haemoglobin until other causes for this, such as occult bleeding, folate deficiency, drug-induced marrow depression, haemolysis or the anaemia associated with the use of "Intralipid",[81] have been excluded.

Changes in white cell count can provide a guide to the presence of sepsis but in the critically ill, bone marrow depression may prevent the normal response. The platelet count also reflects non-specific marrow depression but this may also be drug induced and sudden drops in platelet count can occur in disseminated intravascular coagulation (DIC). Measurement of prothrombin time, partial thromboplastin time, fibrinogen and fibrin degradation products aid the diagnosis of DIC and the monitoring of its severity. Clotting tests are also needed for the monitoring of anticoagulant therapy with heparin or warfarin and during infusion of streptokinase.

**Radiological monitoring.**—The most frequently requested x-ray in ICU is that of the chest. This is not only to monitor the progress of pulmonary pathology, pulmonary oedema and so on, but also to assess the positioning of endotracheal tubes, monitoring catheters, etc., and detect new complications such as pneumothorax, intrapleural fluid, atelectasis or pulmonary embolism that may otherwise progress insidiously. The ICU patient is not the ideal subject for high quality radiography, being often helpless, immobile or breathless and attached to apparatus that further restricts movements and may produce artefacts on the film. These difficulties are compounded by the technical problems of mobile x-ray machines, non-standard distance from machine to patient and the problems of interpretation of antero-posterior views especially if taken with the patient supine. The effects of all these problems can be minimised by sorting and numbering the films as they are taken, keeping a record of the exposure details for each patient and trying to keep them the same from time to time and, most importantly, reporting of the films in the ICU so that they remain with the patient. Problems of interpretation can then be discussed between the radiologist and the ICU staff.

Other radiological investigations are much less commonly needed, though in some patients serial CAT scans of the head may be needed to follow the progress of intracranial collections or cerebral oedema, or to detect new complications such as internal hydrocephalus.

Storage of all the information that is collected on ICU patients together with drug charts, fluid charts and nursing records becomes a major problem, both in terms of the mass of material to be kept and later in retrieval of information for reports, audit or research. "Problem orientated medical records" can create as many problems as they solve. Most ICU's use the ordinary hospital notes with perhaps a summary of the main events being made at the time of discharge of a patient from the ICU, recognising that this is less than ideal. In the future computer storage and retrieval may provide a better answer, if the problems of cost and confidentiality can be overcome.

### Specific Therapy

Specific therapy of underlying diseases or conditions should follow normal principles. It is, however, particularly important to recognise the need to avoid delay and take account of the way in which different diseases and their treatments may interact. The specific therapy of some of the conditions seen in the ICU is considered later in this chapter.

### System Support

The principles of support in cardiovascular, respiratory, renal and hepatic failure are considered in the appropriate chapters (Chapters 12, 9, 36, 35 respectively). In the ICU, failure of more than one major organ system is common. It is in balancing the requirements and priorities of different failing systems that the ICU doctor comes into his own. Treating a single system, rather than the whole patient, can only lead to disaster.

## GENERAL CARE

**Nursing.**—In the presence of high technology medicine it is all too easy to forget the importance of good basic nursing care. Lack of such care will rapidly cause new complications to appear. This can be seen most clearly in the unconscious, ventilated patient when such care is additional to maintaining the airway, ensuring adequate humidification of inspired gas, care of the endotracheal cuff, care of dressings, monitoring catheters and infusions, avoiding trauma to the patient and continuous monitoring of the patient's condition so that complications are detected quickly. The basic nursing care of unconscious ventilated patients includes care of the eyes, mouth, general hygiene, bowel treatment and positioning of the patient in the bed. Care of the pressure areas is vital if pressure sores are to be prevented especially in those patients who are unable to move by themselves because of sedation, paralysis or coma, or those with a reduced supply of oxygen to the skin, i.e. the hypoxaemic and hypotensive. It will be appreciated that many of the patients in an ICU are included in these groups. For patients who are less dependent, psychological aspects of nursing management become more important. Even if the patient appears to be unconscious all staff should talk to them and explain what is going on.

**Physiotherapy.**—A large part of an ICU physiotherapist's time is spent in preventing and treating chest complications. This is particularly important in patients who are intubated and therefore unable to clear secretions from their lungs by coughing. Postural drainage, vibration and percussion may all be helpful in clearing secretions from some patients, though there is remarkably little evidence on which to base treatment recommendations. There are a number of problems that may occur during chest physiotherapy in ventilated patients. These include transient hypoxaemia, though this is not invariable,[82,83] a decrease in cardiac output,[84] and the problems associated with endotracheal suction which include trauma of the tracheal mucosa and cardiac dysrhythmias. Careful design of the suction catheter can minimise damage to the tracheobronchial mucosa[85] but this does not entirely overcome the problem because angle tip catheters, more prone to causing mucosal damage, are needed to enter the left main bronchus. Bronchial anatomy favours entry to the right main bronchus if only straight catheters are used.[86]

The cardiac dysrhythmias seen during tracheal suction may be secondary to vagal stimulation or hypoxia. The danger of hypoxia can be reduced by careful attention to technique and in particular ensuring that the suction catheter is not more than half the diameter of the endotracheal tube and suction lasts for less than 15 seconds.[87] In some ICU's a simulated cough is used with chest physiotherapy and suction, the so-called "bag squeezing" technique.[88] (See also Chapter 9.)

Chest physiotherapy in non-ventilated patients can use standard techniques within the constraints of the patient's other problems. Some unintubated patients may also need help to clear secretions by tracheal suction through an oral or nasopharyngeal airway. Incentive spirometry can be used as an adjunct to physiotherapy[89] and may be particularly useful if there is a shortage of trained therapists.

It is usually the physiotherapists who ensure that the patients joints are put through a full range of either active or passive movements at least once a day. As much active movement as possible is desirable to prevent muscle wasting and active movements of the legs may reduce the risk of venous thrombosis. In unconscious patients passive movements will help to prevent contractures and stiffening of joints. Other tasks usually performed by the physiotherapist include monitoring of bedside respiratory function tests, neurological assessment with charting of muscle function, preparation of splints to reduce contractures or deformities and help in the management of concurrent problems in the ICU patient such as fractures, arthritis and so on.

**Sedation and analgesia.**—Some patients find intensive care a painful and unpleasant experience.[90] Apart from the pain from the injuries, surgical incisions or disease that might have precipitated admission to the ICU, many of the procedures that are carried out there, e.g. insertion of central venous catheters, urinary catheters, nasogastric tubes, etc, are uncomfortable and patients may find the regular turning and chest physiotherapy an agonising ordeal without adequate sedation and analgesia. With pain relief and sedation patients' recollection of their stay in ICU can be vastly improved, as many as 70 per cent even regarding their period in ICU as "pleasant".[91]

In conscious patients attention to their psychological needs (see below) and constant reassurance will help the patient to relax and reduce the amount of pain they feel. Simple measures, such as finding the most comfortable position and tending to urinary retention, flatulence and nausea will often make a great difference. Giving an effective dose of an analgesic *before* procedures that are expected to cause discomfort will do much to gain the patient's confidence and co-operation. Narcotics, oral analgesics, and regional anaesthetic techniques such as epidural or intercostal blocks can all be used. The effectiveness is more important than the technique. Nitrous oxide 50 per cent with oxygen 50 per cent is used in some ICU's to supplement analgesia. This may allow patients to breathe deeper and cough during physiotherapy without the respiratory depression and cough suppression seen with larger doses of narcotics.[92] Some patients prone to anxiety find a small dose of a minor tranquilliser such as diazepam, makes their stay in the ICU much more bearable while those who react to severe illness and intensive care by becoming depressed may benefit from an antidepressant.

Nitrous oxide has been used to provide sedation and analgesia for ventilated patients[92] but it cannot be used for more than 48 hours because marrow suppression occurs.[93] Potent analgesics, sedatives, anaesthetic agents, and neuromuscular blocking drugs have all been used in ventilated patients. Neuromuscular blocking agents should not be used alone to "settle" patients on ventilators, although there is evidence that this may be a common practice,[94] and should only be used when it is certain that the patient is asleep. Narcotic analgesics may be given as either intermittent bolus injections or by continuous infusion. Large doses are often needed to achieve satisfactory sedation, as opposed to analgesia, and other disadvantages include hypotension after bolus doses in acutely ill patients, inhibition of gastro-intestinal motility, the development of tolerance with long-term use and the risk of physical dependence if use is prolonged. Benzodiazepines, of which diazepam has been the most popular, tend to have a cumulative effect over repeated doses and in some patients recovery can be very prolonged, a disadvantage shared with the barbiturates. Althesin (alphaxalone/alphadolone) given by continuous infusion has been used successfully to provide sedation in ICU patients for up to 20 days.[95] Satisfactory sedation was achieved for 86 per cent of the time with minimal side-effects, lack of development of tolerance and a rapid recovery time. Its use in this way has, however, been found to cause a dyslipoproteinaemia,[96] and dose-dependent changes in arterial pressure and systemic vascular resistance.[97] Continuous infusion of etomidate shares many advantages with Althesin,[98] but involuntary movements and venous complications seem more frequent and there is evidence of increased mortality of patients sedated with etomidate (see also p. 635).

The sedation of patients requiring prolonged ventilation in the ICU is a difficult problem and no single agent has so far emerged as being entirely satisfactory.

**Psychological support.**—Intensive Care Units are often regarded as very frightening places by members of the medical and nursing profession as well as by the general public. It has been suggested that the atmosphere of a busy ICU is the opposite of the peace and quiet required for recovery from serious illness. For example, Redding and co-workers[99] studied the background noise levels in four ICU's and found them to be comparable to the hospital cafeteria at noon, and only slightly less noisy than the boiler room. This problem is not unique to the ICU[100] and may play a part in the sleep disturbance seen in hospitalised patients.[101] Indeed, lack of sleep is the commonest complaint, affecting about a quarter of the patients who have been in an ICU.[91,102]

Schroeder[49] considered the psychoreactive problems of the ICU under three headings:

1. *Anxiety, panic* and *apprehension* related to both the disease process and the new and strange environment. Explanations and frequent reassurance tend to allay these feelings and can help patients to accept the reality of the ICU environment quite calmly and so make sedative drugs unnecessary.
2. *Exhaustion, disorientation* and *confusion*: the problem of noise and sleep disturbance has been discussed. When prolonged over a period of days sleep deprivation can lead to disorientation, delirium and confusion. Active measures must be taken to ensure adequate sleep and maintain normal day/night orientation.
   Newspapers, radio, television and visitors can all help in achieving this and may reduce the incidence of delirium.
3. *Problems of communication*: patients with endotracheal tubes may feel insecure because they cannot speak and are unable to communicate their fears, anxieties or requests. Media such as a pencil and paper, "magic slates", alphabet boards and so on are useful, though many patients become irritated by the slowness of communicating by these means. Lip reading is a useful skill for ICU staff to acquire and can greatly alleviate this problem.

Some groups of patients seem particularly prone to delirium. After open heart surgery the reported incidence of delirium varies from 13 to 67 per cent. It has been suggested that this is related to biochemical changes that effect brain function[103] and certainly profound biochemical changes are seen in patients with severe shock, liver failure and renal failure, all of which may be associated with an altered mental state or delirium. Fortunately major and persisting psychological morbidity requiring psychiatric intervention is less common. In a surgical ICU, which included cardiac surgery, 7 per cent of patients required psychiatric consultation for depression, anxiety, psychosis or organic brain syndrome.[104] In a general ICU serious psychological breakdowns were much less common, affecting only 0·5 per cent of the patients. The most frequently seen disorder was a simple reactive depression occurring after five or six days in the ICU and disappearing spontaneously after a further week or ten days.[105]

Visitors can be a huge help in maintaining the morale of the patient in the ICU but their psychological needs must not be forgotten. Again, explanation of the patient's illness and the nature of the treatment they are receiving help to reduce anxiety, and involving the family in the patient's care by getting them to help with washing, feeding, turning and so on help them to feel a part of the intensive care the patient is receiving rather than a nuisance from being "in the way". Families confronted by the stress associated with severe illness in one of their number appear to go through phases of high anxiety, denial, anger, remorse, grief and reconciliation.[106] Social workers and other ICU staff can help the family to cope with this stress and help them to understand their reactions to it.[107] Inevitably some of the patients in the ICU will die. Encouragement of anticipatory grief within the family when it becomes clear that a fatal outcome is inevitable can help them come to terms with this. Once death has occurred the ICU staff can help to initiate the bereavement process in the family which will inevitably have to go through a period of readjustment.[108]

**Nutrition.**—Malnutrition is common in hospitalised patients[109] and is frequently seen in patients sick enough to be admitted to ICU, particularly those who are admitted after a period on a general ward where for some time it has been hoped they will be better and therefore able to eat "tomorrow". Patients should be tempted to eat by serving appetising food and having small snacks available between meals. For those patients too sick to eat normal food, systems for nutritional support using either enteral or parenteral routes have been developed that can meet the needs of nearly all patients.

Further details of these methods are given later in this chapter. It has long been known that if a patient loses more than 30 per cent of his initial body weight during an acute illness, his chance of survival is remote. Loss of the responses of delayed hypersensitivity skin test reactions to common antigens—anergy—has been found to correlate with weight loss, and it is known that such anergic patients have an increased mortality from sepsis.[39] Restoring the body weight to normal is usually followed by a return of skin reactivity.[110] Other problems associated with poor nutrition include specific deficiency syndromes, poor wound healing and a weakened, often apathetic patient.

**Prophylaxis.**—Prophylactic treatment may be given to patients in the ICU to reduce the incidence of known complications. These treatments include:

1. *Prophylactic antibiotics*: while there is no place for routine prophylactic antibiotics in patients admitted to ICU, in practice it is found that many patients are receiving antibiotics either prophylactically, e.g. after insertion of a prosthetic heart valve,[111] or as specific treatment, e.g. for pneumonia.

2. *Prophylactic anticoagulants*: low dosage heparin (5000 units) given subcutaneously two or three times a day is effective in reducing the incidence of deep venous thrombosis in surgical patients and probably after myocardial infarction.[112] It has also been shown to reduce the incidence of fatal pulmonary emboli in surgical patients.[112,113] Low dose heparin may therefore reduce the risk of deep venous thrombosis and pulmonary embolism in ICU patients, many of whom are particularly at risk because of prolonged immobility. The results of a retrospective study of patients admitted to a respiratory ICU support this conclusion.[436]

3. *Gastro-intestinal bleeding*.—In different series between 4 and 15 per cent of critically ill patients had gastro-intestinal bleeding severe enough to require transfusion of more than a litre of blood.[114] There is some evidence that either antacids given frequently enough to keep the gastric pH above 3·5[115] or cimetidine 300 mg 4-hourly[116] will reduce the risk of gastro-intestinal bleeding. Of the two methods, antacids appear to be more reliable[117] and in at least some comatose patients cimetidine is ineffective in raising the gastric pH.[118] These findings have lead to the recommendation that all acutely ill patients at risk from stress ulceration should be given antacids to keep the pH of their gastric aspirate above 3·5.[119]

## TOPICS IN INTENSIVE THERAPY

### SHOCK

The term "shock" is commonly used but poorly defined. It is applied to conditions which differ in aetiology, pathology and presentation, but common to all is a syndrome associated with inadequate oxygen transport to tissues and abnormal cellular metabolism. A number of classifications have been proposed but aetiological classification remains the most commonly used:

| | |
|---|---|
| Hypovolaemic | Septicaemic |
| Traumatic | Cardiogenic |

Such terms aid the description of the *early* cardiorespiratory changes and their management if a particular aetiology predominates but many shocked patients have more than one underlying factor, e.g. relative hypovolaemia and myocardial depression are common features of the septic shock syndrome. In addition, if the condition progresses or fails to respond to treatment the physiological alterations merge into a small group of common pathways.[120]

#### Pathophysiology

Common to all forms of shock is arterial hypotension. Arteriolar vasoconstriction tends to restore arterial pressure by increasing systemic vascular resistance but at the expense of reducing tissue perfusion. In part this is caused by the massive release of catecholamines that occurs in shock[121] and is accentuated by the effect of increased levels of angiotensin II, a very potent vasoconstrictor released in response to hypovolaemia.[122] Some vascular beds are affected more than others so that blood flow to the brain and coronary circulation tends to be preserved while flow to other organs is greatly reduced. Maldistribution of blood flow within individual organs and tissues also occurs because flow is directed through "preferred route" capillaries rather than nutrient vessels or even bypasses the capillary beds completely by shunting through arteriovenous anastomoses.[123]

The cells in areas of poor perfusion receive reduced amounts of both oxygen and substrate so energy production is severely impaired. Instead of 38 moles of ATP being formed as occurs during aerobic metabolism of a mole of glucose, only two moles of ATP are produced during anaerobic metabolism of a mole of glucose.

Lactic acid is produced during anaerobic metabolism. This is reflected by increased blood lactate concentrations and both local and systemic acidosis.

Without sufficient ATP to maintain normal activity in cell membrane ionic pumps, sodium and potassium ions move down concentration gradients. Water moves into cells, increasing the intracellular volume and ultimately causing swelling of mitochondria and other intracellular organelles including lysosomes. If this process continues cell membranes break down and enzymes are released, causing destruction of the cell and local tissue damage. Proteolytic enzymes released from damaged cells may then initiate or perpetuate formation of plasma kinins, activation of intravascular coagulation and the activation of complement (see below). Many of the changes occurring at the cellular level in shock have been brought together in the hypothesis proposed by Baue and others[124] as shown in Fig. 6.

**Role of Kinins, Prostaglandins, Complement and MDF** (Myocardial depressant factor)

Kinins are polypeptides which increase capillary permeability, dilate small blood vessels and depress myocardial function. They are formed from inactive precursors (kininogens) which form part of the alpha II globulin fraction of plasma protein.[125] Hageman factor (factor XII), initially thought to relate solely to the intrinsic coagulation system, has been shown to have a central role in the activation of kinins, initiation of coagulation and fibrinolytic systems and the activation of complement, particularly during septic shock (Fig. 7). In patients with sepsis the degree of complement depletion has been shown to equate with the clinical course, being greatest in those who become shocked[126] while the haemodynamic changes parallel changes in kinin levels.[127]

The predominantly vasodilator E-series prostaglandins (PGE) are also released during haemorrhage or endotoxaemia, contributing to the haemodynamic changes. Other important

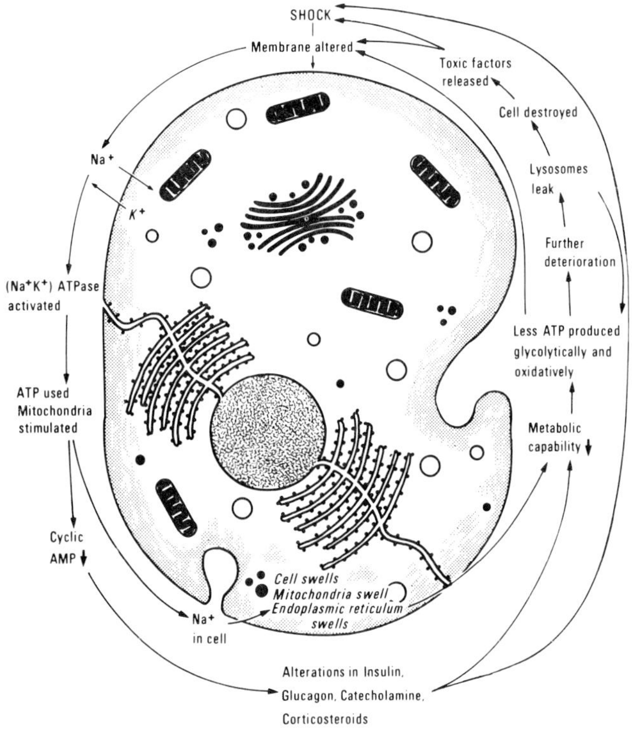


10/FIG. 6.—Diagram of a cell illustrating the hypothesis of changes in function at the cellular level occurring in shock. (Courtesy of Drs. A. E. Baue, I. H. Chaudry, M. A. Wurth and M. M. Sayeed and Williams and Wilkins Co.[124])

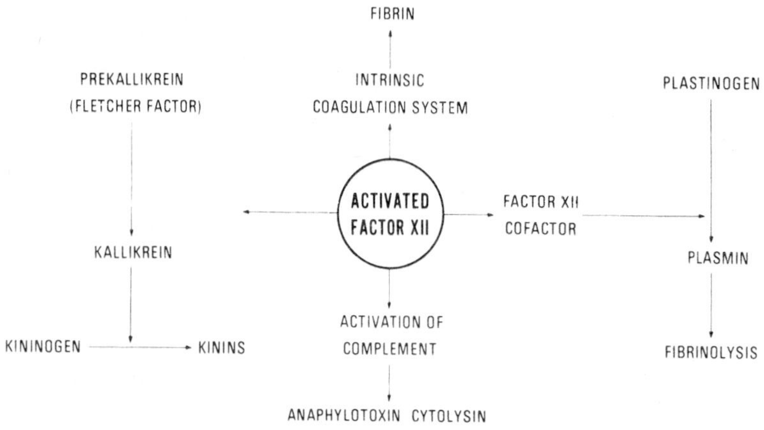


10/FIG. 7.—Interactions between activated factor XII and coagulation, fibrinolytic and inflammatory mechanisms. (Courtesy of Dr. F. E. Preston and Hospital Medicine Publications Ltd.[131])

effects of prostaglandins include platelet aggregation ($PGE_2$), increasing vascular permeability ($PGE_2$, $PGD_2$) and in some species $PGF_2$ alpha has been implicated in the pulmonary vasoconstriction, decrease in lung compliance and increase in airways resistance that occurs in shock. On the other hand, $PGE_1$ has a protective effect in experimental haemorrhagic shock[128] and inhibits platelet aggregation. At present the interaction between the different prostaglandins in shock is unclear and the therapeutic implications of either infusing them or inhibiting their production has still to be defined.

Myocardial depressant factor (MDF) was first described by Brand and Lefer.[129]. It is thought to be a peptide with a molecular weight of 800–1000 released from hypoxic pancreatic acinar cells.[130] As shock persists the plasma MDF level increases, increasing the degree of myocardial depression.

### Haematological Disturbances

The commonest haematological disturbance in shock results from activation of the coagulation system. This may cause *Disseminated Intravascular Coagulation* (DIC). For DIC to occur two separate factors are required:

1. Slow moving, acid capillary blood: factors such as high catecholamine levels, sympathetic stimulation, haemorrhage, etc. seen in shock produce this state.
2. The presence of a thrombogenic agent in the blood stream. Tissue thromboplastin, thought to be a large lipoprotein complex widely distributed in many body tissues, activates the coagulation cascade directly. Its release into the circulation activates factor VII so that it triggers the extrinsic coagulation system with consumption of factors V and X, generation of thrombin and the formation of fibrin. This process is accompanied by platelet consumption and enhanced fibrinolysis.[131] Coagulation may also be initiated indirectly by endotoxin and antigen-antibody complexes, both through activation of factor XII[132] and by causing endothelial cell damage.

Minor changes in coagulation tests are common in the conditions that cause shock. The most sensitive tests are those that involve fibrinogen. In particular the levels of Fibrin Degradation Products (FDP's) may be increased, reflecting secondary fibrinolysis and the thrombin clotting time may be prolonged because FDP's interfere with the action of thrombin on fibrinogen. In some cases a consumption coagulopathy occurs. This is more common when shock is associated with sepsis, extensive tissue injury, amniotic fluid embolism and other obstetric emergencies or incompatible blood transfusion. The result is a pronounced bleeding tendency with oozing from venepuncture sites and other wounds, purpura and bruising and occasionally severe haemorrhage. Laboratory tests will show reduced numbers of platelets and fibrinogen levels together with prolonged partial thromboplastin and prothrombin times while fibrinolysis is reflected by a short clot lysis time. Deposits of fibrin and intravascular clot formation increase the problem of tissue and cell hypoxia that occurs in shock and this may be responsible, at least in part, for the severe functional impairment of the lungs, kidneys, and other organs that occurs in established shock. The inter-relationships between the components of the coagulopathy that occurs in shock are summarised in Fig. 8.

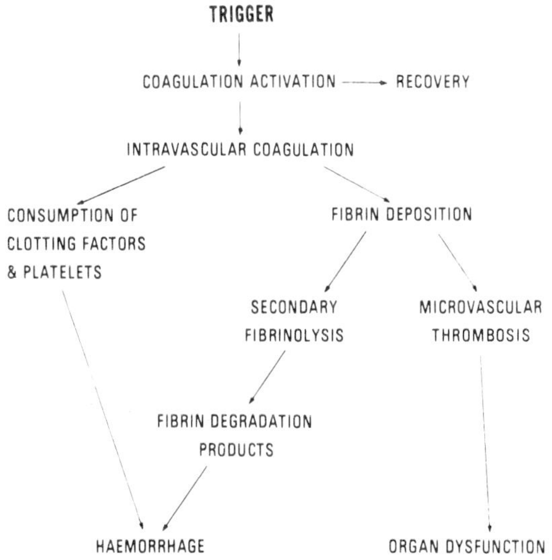


10/FIG. 8.—The interrelationships between the different components of the coagulation system. (Courtesy of Dr. F. E. Preston and Hospital Medicine Publications Ltd.[131])

## Effects on Pulmonary Function

Abnormalities of pulmonary function are common in shock from any cause. Unfortunately, a large number of names including "shock lung", "adult respiratory distress syndrome", "acute respiratory insufficiency", "post-traumatic pulmonary insufficiency" and others have been used to describe the same clinicopathological syndrome. Similar changes are also seen in patients with disseminated intravascular coagulation, following massive blood transfusion, fat embolism, aspiration of stomach contents, intracranial injury, oxygen toxicity or opiate overdose, so the response of the lung to shock is non-specific.

The Adult Respiratory Distress Syndrome (ARDS) has been divided into four phases.[133]

Phase 1: Hyperventilation and hypocapnia despite the lungs being clinically clear and a normal chest x-ray.

Phase 2: Persisting hyperventilation and hypocapnia but with increasing venous admixture (shunting) within the lungs causing progressive arterial hypoxaemia.

Phase 3: Increasing clinical signs of respiratory distress accompanied by an increasing alveolar-arterial oxygen gradient. The chest x-ray shows widespread areas of consolidation. Intensive respiratory care is required including intubation and intermittent positive-pressure ventilation or intermittent mandatory ventilation, perhaps with positive end-expiratory pressure.

Phase 4: Increasing hypoxaemia with rising lactate levels and a falling pH in arterial blood. Carbon dioxide retention may occur despite high tidal volumes, reflecting the increase in the dead space/tidal volume ratio. Death may follow from profound hypoxaemia and acidosis. In the past, 30–50 per cent of patients who died after trauma and shock had significant pulmonary involvement and in most of these this was the cause of death.[134]

Pulmonary hypertension and increased pulmonary vascular resistance are virtually universal features of ARDS.[135] These may be important additional factors limiting survival in severe ARDS.

The pathological changes in the lungs include:[136]

1. Interstitial and intra-alveolar oedema.
2. Interstitial and intra-alveolar haemorrhages.
3. Hyaline membrane formation.
4. Superimposed bronchopneumonia. This does not always occur, but is very common in those who die as a result of ARDS.[137]
5. Diffuse pulmonary fibrosis if the patient survives for a number of weeks.

The effect of these changes is to cause a reduction in lung compliance (they get "stiffer"), there is a reduction in functional residual capacity so that it falls within the closing volume and the work of breathing is increased (see Chapter 2). The evidence suggests that there are a number of factors (discussed below) that contribute to the development of ARDS.[138,139]

In general terms these factors act either to increase pulmonary capillary hydrostatic pressure or to increase capillary permeability (Fig. 9).

*Resuscitation*.—Inadvertent fluid overload during resuscitation has been considered an important factor in the aetiology of ARDS.[136] Fluid overload alone, particularly in the presence of a low colloid osmotic pressure,[140] may cause pulmonary oedema but the left atrial pressure has to be high (greater than 20 mm Hg) for this to be clinically significant. When this is the only cause for respiratory problems there is usually a rapid response to diuretics or vasodilators. Characteristically, ARDS occurs in the presence of relatively normal left atrial or pulmonary artery wedge pressure (PAWP) (less than 15 mm Hg) and reducing the left atrial pressure produces a much less dramatic response. High left atrial pressures, and other factors increasing capillary hydrostatic pressure (Fig. 9), will of course increase the rate of oedema formation, but there is no evidence that a low colloid osmotic pressure alone increases the pulmonary dysfunction.[141]

The role of fluid used in resuscitation, that is, whether crystalloid or colloid solutions should be used, has been the source of considerable controversy and has stimulated a lot of research. Despite this, the issue of which is more likely to increase the severity of ARDS, remains unresolved.[142] Pulmonary capillary injury, rather than the type of fluid given during resuscitation, is more likely to be the underlying problem and other factors, such as the rate of transfusion, may be as important as the nature of the fluid used.[143]

*Coagulopathy*.—Small vessel thromboemboli and intra-alveolar haemorrhage are among the histological features of ARDS. In animal models, fibrin-platelet aggregates have been demonstrated in the blood of those animals that went on to develop ARDS after shock. It has been shown that coagulation mechanisms are activated during shock (see above) and it seems likely that this is an important factor in initiating the pulmonary damage that leads to ARDS.[144] Some support for this comes from the finding that the use of filters during massive blood transfusion or cardiopulmonary bypass reduces the incidence of ARDS.

*Lung ischaemia*.—Decreased perfusion during shock has been proposed as a factor leading to lung damage. The type II alveolar cells, which produce surfactant, may be particularly sensitive to ischaemic damage. However, in animal experiments there are fewer changes in the lungs that have been excluded from the circulation during shock than those which have been perfused throughout[136] so that lung ischaemia alone is unlikely to be a major factor.

*Neurogenic factors*.—Pulmonary oedema and respiratory insufficiency after head injury are well documented. Moss and associates[145] have suggested that poor perfusion of the brain during shock is the cause of ARDS. Perfusing the brains of a variety of animals with anoxic blood caused pulmonary lesions that both anatomically and physiologically resembled ARDS. This response was thought to be mediated

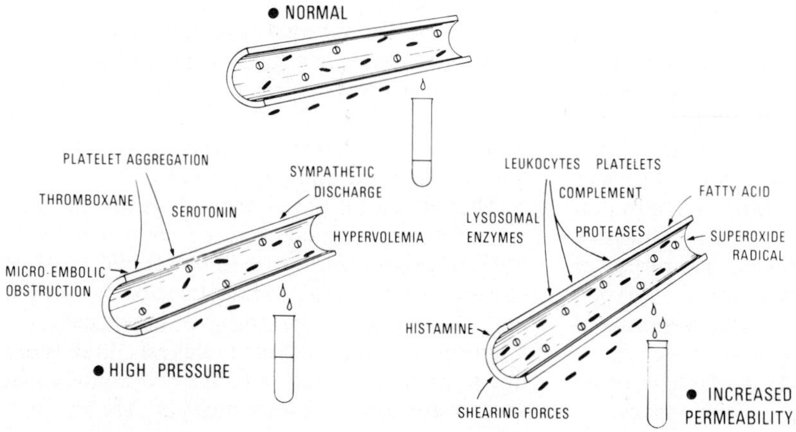


10/Fig. 9.—Factors that act to increase pulmonary capillary hydrostatic pressure or increase capillary permeability cause pulmonary oedema. Many ARDS states are a combination of these two forms of injury, but one form usually predominates. (Courtesy of Dr. R. H. Demling and W. B. Saunders Company.[139])

through the sympathetic nervous system but denervation experiments have not given uniform results.[144]

*Humoral factors.*—The role of complement, kinins, prostaglandins and other circulating substances in shock has been discussed. Complement activation has been shown to cause injury to the lungs[146] probably by promoting the clumping of granulocytes and through direct granulocyte mediated endothelial damage.[147] The other factors can also cause changes to the lung that correspond with the physiological and pathological findings in ARDS.

*Sepsis.*—ARDS is often seen in association with severe sepsis and animal studies have demonstrated that the lesion of ARDS can be precipitated by the injection of endotoxin or living bacteria. However, these injections do not produce ARDS in isolated, perfused lungs suggesting that some other mediator is required.

*Other factors.*—Aspiration, fat embolism and the effects of recent anaesthesia and surgery may contribute to the respiratory failure of shocked patients. It has been suggested that shock renders the lungs susceptible to injury and if there is a further insult such as sepsis or one of the above factors progressive pulmonary failure occurs.[138]

### Effects on Cardiac Function

Even if myocardial damage is not the primary cause for shock developing, cardiac function is found to be impaired. The possible role of myocardial depressant factor has been mentioned already. Other causes for reduced cardiac function include dysrhythmias, myocardial ischaemia (both as the result of alterations in blood flow and secondary to systemic hypotension) and focal myocardial lesions induced by high circulating levels of catecholamines and angiotensin.[148] Experimental work suggests that myocardial oedema also contributes to the decreased cardiac compliance and increased left ventricular end-diastolic pressures seen in shocked patients.[149]

### Effects on Renal Function

Renal function frequently becomes impaired during or soon after a period of shock. Sepsis, crush injury, shock related to obstetric catastrophes and pre-existing renal disease increase the incidence of acute renal failure for a given haemodynamic insult. Hypotension is associated with a reduction in renal blood flow and particularly the flow to the renal cortex. When the mean arterial pressure falls below about 50 mm Hg, urine production stops and certainly renal ischaemia is a major factor in the initiation of non-nephrotoxic forms of acute renal failure.[150] This observation has led to attempts to discover whether changes in the levels of endogenous vasodilator and vasoconstrictor substances play a role in the initiation or maintenance of acute renal failure. Much of the early work, reviewed by Brown and colleagues[151] suggested that the renin-angiotensin system might play a key part in precipitating renal failure. Plasma renin and angiotensin levels are increased in some patients with renal failure but more recent investigations suggest that they have at most a minor role. Other substances that have been investigated include the prostaglandins, antidiuretic hormone and the kallikreins but their contribution has not been defined.

Intratubular cast formation and necrosis of the wall of the tubule have been demonstrated by nephron dissection techniques in patients with acute renal failure[150] and these are probably significant in the persistence of acute renal failure after shock has been reversed.

The relationship between the different postulated mechanisms for causing acute renal failure in shock are summarised in Fig. 10.[152]

### Effects on Hepatic and Gastro-Intestinal Tract Function

Blood flow to the liver and gastro-intestinal tract is reduced in low cardiac output states. Liver dysfunction after shock is well recognised and persisting jaundice tends to be associated with a poor prognosis, perhaps reflecting the severity of end-organ damage caused by shock since the liver's ability to regenerate is greater than most other organs.

A paralytic ileus is common in shock and may persist for some time. Severe, prolonged hypotension, particularly in patients with atherosclerosis, may cause "water-shed" necrosis of the bowel in the area where the parts supplied by the inferior and superior mesenteric arteries meet. Patchy areas of bowel necrosis or necrosis of the bowel mucosa may also be seen after prolonged shock and carry an equally bad prognosis because of the almost invariable overwhelming sepsis that accompanies them.

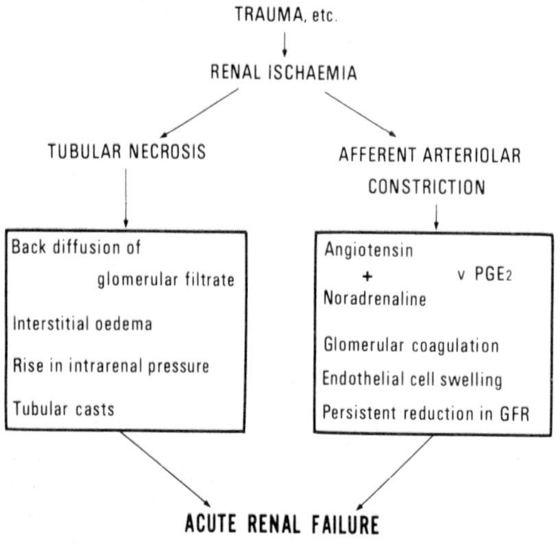


10/FIG. 10.—Mechanisms leading to the development of acute renal failure. (Courtesy of Professor J. S. Robson and Churchill Livingstone.[152])

## Classification

The shortcomings of classifying shock according to its aetiology have been discussed. The broad groupings of hypovolaemic, cardiogenic and septicaemic shock are, however, widely used. The term "traumatic shock" is also frequently used to include the components of hypovolaemia, direct tissue injury and central stress response that follow trauma. The clinical features of the three main types of shock are summarised in Table 6.

10/TABLE 6
CLINICAL FEATURES OF THE THREE MAIN TYPES OF SHOCK

| | *Hypovolaemic* | *Cardiogenic* | *Septic* |
|---|---|---|---|
| Arterial pressure | ↓ | ↓ | ↓ |
| Heart rate | ↑ | ↑↓ | ↑ |
| Central venous pressure | (N) ↓ | ↑ | N/↑/↓ |
| Pulmonary artery wedge pressure | ↓ | ↑ | N/↑/↓ |
| Cardiac output | ↓ | ↓ | N/↑/↓ |
| Core-periphery temperature gradient | ↑ | ↑ | N/↑ |

(Courtesy of Dr. I. McA. Ledingham and Dr. G. S. Routh and Hospital Medicine Publications Ltd.[125])

**Hypovolaemic shock.**—Hypovolaemia is still one of the commonest causes of circulatory inadequacy. Hypovolaemic shock occurs when the intravascular volume is decreased by 15–25 per cent. The fluid loss may be overt or concealed and consist of blood, plasma, or extracellular fluid. The clinical conditions associated with hypovolaemic shock include trauma, gastro-intestinal haemorrhage, burns, severe diarrhoea and the uncontrolled diuresis of diabetes insipidus. Relative hypovolaemia, in which marked vasodilatation is accompanied by low venous and arterial pressures, occurs when the normal blood volume is inadequate to fill the dilated vascular bed. This may occur with barbiturate overdosage, certain neurological injuries, acute adrenal steroid depletion and is a factor in some cases of septicaemia.

**Cardiogenic shock.**—Myocardial infarction is the commonest cause of cardiogenic shock. Shock occurs when at least 45 per cent of the ventricular myocardium has been damaged[153] and is frequently associated with an elevated PAWP. The onset of clinical hypoperfusion corresponds to a cardiac index of 1·8–2·2 l/min/m$^2$ and true cardiogenic shock is seen when the cardiac index is less than 1·8 l/min/m$^2$.[154] Shock secondary to failure of the heart to pump sufficient blood around the body, even though the venous pressures may be normal or high, also occurs with dysrhythmias or extremes of cardiac rate, valvular regurgitation caused by a ruptured cusp or papillary muscle dysfunction, acute septal perforation, cardiac tamponade, pulmonary embolism, atrial myxoma and following direct myocardial trauma.

**Septicaemic shock.**—Septic shock is associated with a high mortality. Ledingham and McArdle[155] found postoperative general surgical patients to be particularly vulnerable with most of the deaths from septic shock occurring in the first three postoperative days as a result of continuing hypotension and acute respiratory failure in the presence of uncontrolled sepsis. In their study of 113 patients admitted to an ICU with septic shock over a three-year period the mortality was reduced from 71 per cent to 47 per cent by initiating a program of aggressive antishock treatment.

The mechanisms of septicaemic shock have been reviewed[156] as have the effects on the cardiovascular system.[157] The clinical and haemodynamic findings are exceedingly variable. It used to be thought that there was a difference between the physiological responses to Gram-positive and Gram-negative septicaemia.[158] More recent investigations have shown that the usual response to septicaemia is a hyperdynamic state with a bounding pulse, wide pulse pressure and warm skin. Myocardial depression and a decrease in cardiac output may occur later as a result of the metabolic changes seen in prolonged severe sepsis or the effect of a specific myocardial depressant factor. In one study in which the clinical and physiological responses to septicaemia caused by Gram-positive or Gram-negative organisms, anaerobes or fungi were evaluated, the clinical and haemodynamic findings were similar no matter what the organism group or specific organism.[159]

Considerable attention has been directed to the role of endotoxin in Gram-negative septicaemia. The toxic part of the endotoxin complex is lipid-A, normally attached to the surface of the bacterium and hidden under a shield of hydrophilic polysaccharide. Endotoxaemia may occur after absorption of endotoxin from the bowel or from destruction of Gram-negative organisms in the blood. The small amounts of endotoxin that are normally absorbed from the bowel are inactivated by the Kupffer cells of the liver. This defence may be bypassed if there are portasystemic shunts or overwhelmed if there is a massive release of endotoxin as may occur in septicaemia. Lipid-A is the component detected by the Limulus test for endotoxin.[160] This test uses the ability of very small amounts of endotoxin to coagulate the protein of the white cells of the horseshoe crab, *Limulus polyphemus*, into a gel.

Some of the properties of endotoxin are listed in Table 7.[156]

### Treatment

The aims of treatment in shock are firstly to increase tissue blood flow and thereby increase the supply of oxygen and metabolites to the cells and secondly to maintain an adequate perfusing pressure within the limits of autoregulation of the brain and kidneys.

The methods of treatment available include:

1. Treatment of the underlying cause
   —haemorrhage
   —pump failure
   —sepsis
2. Correction of metabolic disturbances.
3. Optimising ventricular preload.
4. Improving myocardial contractility.
5. Reducing ventricular afterload.
6. Miscellaneous drugs.
7. Management of impaired end-organ function.

10/Table 7
Some Properties of Endotoxins

1. Pyrogens—direct and indirect via leucocyte endogenous mediators.
2. Cause a Schwartzman reaction with neurogenic vasoconstriction, catecholamine release and renin activation.
3. Activate coagulation and fibrinolysis.
4. Cause non-complement dependent necrosis of blood vessel endothelium.
5. Activate release of complement, kinins, prostaglandins and histamine.
6. Act as adjuvants, activators of macrophages and B-lymphocyte mitogens.
7. Stimulate production and release of prostaglandin by macrophages.
8. Antagonise glucosteroids.
9. Damage mitochondria.
10. Alter liver mitochondria, reduce liver glutathione levels and cause cholestasis.
11. Damage cell-surface phospholipids.

(Courtesy of Dr. N. Wardle and Hospital Medicine Publications Ltd.[156])

### Treatment of the Underlying Cause

*Haemorrhage.*—Most cases of haemorrhagic shock will require surgical intervention to identify and ligate the responsible vessel. Other methods that may be applicable to particular circumstances include balloon tamponade with a Sengstaken-Blakemore tube for bleeding from oesophageal varices,[161] therapeutic embolization,[162] or local infusion of vasoconstrictors.[163]

*Pump failure.*—Correction of dysrhythmias or mechanical lesions of the heart such as tamponade, acute valvular regurgitation or septal defect may have a dramatic effect on cardiac function. Cardiogenic shock associated with infarction is a more intractable problem, though therapeutic interventions designed to reduce infarct size offer some hope of reducing the incidence of this complication. Pump failure after heart surgery is seen less frequently since the advent of improved methods of myocardial preservation during cardiopulmonary bypass.[164]

*Sepsis* is sometimes associated with collections of pus such as subphrenic, diverticular or wound abscesses. These should be drained as soon as possible and the patient may not improve until this has been done. In other cases debridement or excision of an infected area may be required. Not all cases of septicaemia are amenable to surgery. This occurs when septicaemia is associated with pneumonia or a urinary tract infection and in those cases where the source of the septicaemia is unclear. The mainstay of treatment is then antibiotics.

If the organism and its sensitivities are known the choice of antibiotic is relatively straightforward. A bacteriocidal antibiotic should be given intravenously to ensure adequate absorption in doses sufficient to achieve therapeutic concentrations. Frequently however, antibiotics are started after appropriate cultures have been taken but before the results are available, because of the obvious life-threatening nature of the infection. The choice of antibiotic is made easier if the source of infection, the common organisms at this site and their local sensitivities, are known. Some guidelines for such an approach have been suggested by Geddes.[165] Additional help can be provided by a Gram stain of infected material when this is available.

On occasions broad-spectrum cover to include Gram-positive, Gram-negative and anaerobic organisms is required. A combination of gentamicin, ampicillin and lincomycin has been used[166] but there are problems in giving gentamicin safely to patients with renal failure because of its low therapeutic ratio and lincomycin may cause pseudomembranous colitis.[167] Ticarcillin with cefamandole, cefuroxime or cefoxitin is an alternative regimen while the role of the newer cephalosporins and cephamycins has still to be assessed. In the future, a better understanding of the way in which antibiotics interact with the host's immune defences may have an important effect on the choice of drug in sepsis.[168]

Current opinion favours using antibiotics promptly and in maximal doses. In theory, at least, this may cause a massive amount of endotoxin to be released from lysed organisms and trigger a haemodynamic crisis.[169] In the future, the administration of IgG antibody to lipid-A may limit the end organ damage associated with endotoxaemia.[437]

### Correction of Metabolic Disturbances

Hypoxaemia is common in the conditions associated with shock. Oxygen therapy using a face-mask or nasal cannulae may be sufficient to keep the arterial oxygen saturation above 90 per cent but, if not, intubation and continuous positive airway pressure (CPAP), intermittent mandatory ventilation (IMV), or intermittent positive-pressure ventilation (IPPV) using positive end-expiratory pressure (PEEP) if necessary, may be required to ensure an adequate arterial oxygen content.

Gross electrolyte abnormalities and acidosis should be corrected. A metabolic acidosis is common in shock and if severe it may further impair cardiac function. If the arterial pH is less than 7·2, 50 mmol aliquots of sodium bicarbonate should be given with measurement of pH between each aliquot, but the sodium load caused by this can be considerable.

### Optimising Ventricular Preload

Many shocked patients, from whatever cause, have a reduction in their effective circulating blood volume. Clinically this may be suspected from observation of the neck veins and confirmed by a low CVP. Rapid infusion of 200 ml of fluid should be followed by repeat measurement of heart rate, blood pressure and CVP.[170] If hypotension persists and the CVP remains low more fluid is given at a rate of 200 ml every 10 to 15 minutes until the systolic blood pressure is about 100 mm Hg or the CVP 10 mm Hg. If the patient remains hypotensive and the CVP is 10 mm Hg or more, a balloon flotation catheter may be inserted into the pulmonary artery so that the PAWP can be made optimal. A pulmonary artery catheter should be inserted earlier in patients with a history of left ventricular failure or acute myocardial infarction. Patients with haemorrhagic shock, particularly if the bleeding is uncontrolled must have fluids infused much more rapidly. Large bore intravenous cannulae are essential for this, but even maximum rates of fluid infusion may fail to increase the arterial pressure or CVP.

The MAST (Military Anti-Shock Trousers) suit can be life-saving under these circumstances. Inflating the MAST suit rapidly redistributes intravascular fluid so that between 600 and 2000 ml of blood are compressed from the veins of the legs and abdomen and made available to perfuse the heart, lungs and brain. The effect on arterial blood pressure can be dramatic and occurs almost immediately.[171]

An algorithmic approach to fluid administration in shock has been suggested by Shoemaker.[172] While providing guidelines this may not be appropriate for all cases. In particular, while a PAWP of 18 mm Hg may be optimal for patients with myocardial infarction[173] it may cause pulmonary oedema in a patient with increased capillary permeability or a low colloid oncotic pressure.[140] In patients with hypovolaemic and septic shock there is little to be gained by increasing the PAWP above 12 mm Hg.[438]

The fluid chosen for infusion depends on:

1. The patient's haemoglobin concentration: maximal oxygen transport occurs with a haematocrit of around 30 per cent,[174] unless cardiac output is severely depressed, in which case oxygen availability may be improved by higher haemoglobin concentration.
2. The need to correct coagulopathy, if present.
3. The need to maintain colloid osmotic pressure.
4. The need to maintain normal electrolyte concentrations and acid base balance.

If neither blood nor clotting factors are needed, plasma, salt-poor albumin, dextran or gelatin solutions have proved effective.[175]

If too much fluid is given or there is left ventricular failure the PAWP may be greater than optimum so predisposing to pulmonary oedema. In the absence of established renal failure the raised PAWP can be corrected by giving a potent diuretic such as frusemide or bumetanide. Venodilators such as nitroglycerine[176] or methods to reduce ventricular afterload can also be used to help reduce the PAWP.

### Improving Myocardial Contractility

If hypoperfusion and hypotension persist after the filling pressures are optimum the next step is to augment myocardial contractility. A positively inotropic drug will nearly always increase cardiac output, whether this is inadequate because of a primary disorder of the heart or because myocardial function has become impaired during severe or prolonged shock. Catecholamines are the most widely used inotropic drugs. Adrenaline, noradrenaline, isoprenaline, dopamine, dobutamine and salbutamol fall within this category. Some of their properties are summarised in Table 8. Much of the information about the pharmacological properties of these drugs is derived from work in healthy volunteers and many of the clinical investigations have used patients with chronic congestive heart failure. The response to drugs in shocked patients will not necessarily be similar.

*Dopamine* has been said to offer distinct advantages over other inotropic drugs in shock.[177] At low administration rates in the range 0·5 to 5 μg/kg/min its main effect is to stimulate dopaminergic receptors and cause vasodilatation of renal and mesenteric vascular beds. Infusion at 5 to 10 μg/kg/min results in inotropic and chronotropic effects by stimulation of beta-adrenergic receptors. At maximal effect dopamine may triple the work of the heart (and also the myocardial oxygen consumption). Infusion at rates greater than 10 μg/kg/min results in a progressive increase in alpha-adrenergic effects with vasoconstriction. Other aspects of the pharmacology of dopamine have been reviewed by Goldberg and co-workers.[178]

In patients with septic shock dopamine has

10/TABLE 8
PROPERTIES OF CATECHOLAMINES

| *Catecholamine* | *Effect on Receptors* | | | | *Effect on Blood Flow* | | | |
|---|---|---|---|---|---|---|---|---|
| | *Beta$_1$* | *Beta$_2$* | *Alpha* | *Dopaminergic* | *Coronary* | *Renal* | *Mesenteric* | *Skin/Muscle* |
| Adrenaline | ++ | ++ | +−++ | 0 | ↑ | ↓ | ↓ | ↓ |
| Noradrenaline | ++ | 0 | ++ | 0 | ↑ | ↓ | ↓ | ↓ |
| Isoprenaline | ++ | ++ | 0 | 0 | ↑ | → | ↑ | ↑ |
| Dopamine | ++ | 0 | +−++ | ++ | ↑ | ↑ | ↑ | ↓ |
| Dobutamine | ++ | + | + | 0 | ↑ | → | → | ↑ |
| Salbutamol | 0−+ | ++ | 0 | 0 | ↑ | ?→ | ?→ | ↑ |

been shown to increase cardiac output by a mean of 37 per cent and increase peripheral vascular resistance by 6 per cent.[179] Holzer and associates[180] have shown that dopamine is effective in treating patients with cardiogenic shock after myocardial infarction or cardiac surgery. It must be remembered that an inotropic effect is accompanied by increased myocardial oxygen requirements. If the myocardium is already ischaemic or in the presence of recent infarction, dopamine may worsen the myocardial oxygen supply:demand ratio and so increase the degree of ischaemia or increase infarct size. Comparisons of dopamine with other catecholamines in shock are few, reflecting the difficulties of such investigations. In a comparison with isoprenaline and noradrenaline, dopamine caused less tachycardia than isoprenaline and, at least in lower doses, the urine flow was greater during dopamine infusion than with the other two drugs.[177]

*Dobutamine*. The pharmacology of dobutamine has been reviewed by Sonnenblick and colleagues.[181] Its main effect is on $beta_1$ adrenergic receptors with only little effect on $beta_2$- or alpha- receptors. In moderate doses its main effect is on myocardial contractility, with little effect on peripheral vascular resistance (PVR) or heart rate. In higher doses the effects more closely resemble those of isoprenaline and a tachycardia and fall in PVR may occur. Dobutamine has been used by intravenous infusion at rates of 2–40 μg/kg/min in patients with septic shock,[182] after myocardial infarction[183,184] and following cardiac surgery.[185] It seems to be most useful when the atrial pressures are high. Prolonged infusion, i.e. 3-4 days, of dobutamine may result in tolerance developing.[186]

*Adrenaline* acts on both alpha- and beta-adrenergic receptors. It is useful during the resuscitation phase of shock when its potent vasoconstrictor and inotropic effect may produce an adequate cerebral perfusion pressure when all else has failed.

*Noradrenaline* is the most potent vasoconstrictor of the catecholamines.

*Isoprenaline* was more widely used in the management of shock before dopamine became available. It is a potent beta-adrenergic stimulant and may be infused at rates of 0·5 to 10 μg/min. Its use tends to be limited by tachycardia or dysrhythmias.

*Salbutamol* is predominantly a $beta_2$-stimulant so its major effect is to cause a reduction in PVR. Its role in shock is therefore similar to that of other drugs that reduce ventricular afterload. When compared with dopamine in the management of cardiogenic shock[187] salbutamol was preferred for improving cardiac output, but when correction of hypotension was of overriding importance dopamine was more useful.

The choice of catecholamine in a given clinical situation may be guided by the patient's haemodynamic profile but for most instances dopamine will be the drug of first choice. This is because it selectively maintains or increases renal blood flow, *an action which is not shared by any of the other catecholamines*. If the patient has high filling pressures dobutamine may be preferred. The factors affecting the choice of catecholamine have been considered in detail by Kuhn,[188,189] Scallan and associates,[190] Tinker[175] and Herbert & Tinker.[191]

Infusions of catecholamines should be given through a central venous catheter to ensure a constant infusion rate and avoid the local complications that may occur when catecholamine infusions are given through peripheral veins. On occasions two catecholamines may be infused simultaneously to achieve the desired mix of alpha and beta effects, or catecholamines may be given with a vasodilator or in conjunction with intra-aortic balloon pumping.[192] This should be done only when sophisticated haemodynamic monitoring is available.

*Digoxin* is still used widely, but it has a relatively slow onset of action and a long half-life. These, together with its low therapeutic ratio, make it less suitable as an inotropic drug in shock but it is still useful in the treatment of supraventricular dysrhythmias.

*Glucagon* has a positive inotropic effect and can be infused 4-12 mg/hr. It may cause hyperglycaemia, nausea and vomiting.

*Vasopressor amines* such as ephedrine, metaraminol and methoxamine produce their effects by acting on adrenergic receptors either directly, or indirectly by releasing noradrenaline from stores in adrenergic nerve terminals. *Except for resuscitation in profound hypotension they have little to offer in the management of shock.*

### Reducing Ventricular Afterload

Ventricular afterload reduction may be useful if the blood pressure is adequate but there is evidence of a low cardiac output and peripheral vasoconstriction. Afterload reduction therapy is of greatest use in cardiogenic shock whether from pump failure or associated with acute mitral incompetence or septal perforation. The vasodilator drugs used to reduce ventricular afterload include:

*Alpha-adrenergic blocking drugs*: phentolamine, chlorpromazine, prazosin.

*Ganglion blocking agents*: trimetaphan, hexamethonium.

*Direct vasodilators*: hydralazine—mainly on arterioles;

sodium nitroprusside—arterioles and venules;

glyceryl trinitrate and isosorbide dinitrate—mainly on venules.

*Beta$_2$-adrenergic agonists*: salbutamol—see above.

The use of a number of these drugs in chronic congestive heart failure has been well documented[193,194,195] but their role in shock has been less well defined. Potential benefits include:

1. Reduction of myocardial work and hence myocardial oxygen requirements.
2. Pooling of blood on the venous side of the circulation and therefore a decrease in atrial pressures.
3. Possible redistribution of blood flow within organs and tissues to improve the supply of oxygen and metabolites at cellular level.

The greatest danger with the use of vasodilators is a precipitous fall in the systemic blood pressure because of the fall in the PVR (peripheral vascular resistance) and reduction of preload. The blood pressure must therefore be closely monitored during vasodilator therapy. The vasodilators sodium nitroprusside and glyceryl trinitrate have recently been the subject of some interest as adjuncts to the management of circulatory failure. Their major advantage is their rapid onset of action and short half-lives so that the dose can be closely titrated against the response.

*Sodium nitroprusside* causes dilatation of both arterioles and venules by a direct action on vascular smooth muscle.[196] The effects are apparent within about 2 minutes of starting an infusion and wear off equally rapidly due to its rapid metabolism to cyanide and thiocyanate.[197] The thiocyanate is excreted almost exclusively by the kidneys with a half-life of 4 to 7 days when renal function is normal. If an infusion of sodium nitroprusside is continued for more than 48 hours the plasma thiocyanate level should be monitored at least every alternate day and more frequently if high infusion rates are used. Thiocyanate levels of 1·7 mmol/l (10 mg per cent) should not be exceeded.[198] Plasma cyanide is probably the major determinant of toxicity,[193] the cyanide causing inhibition of cytochrome oxidase and other enzymes with a shift to anaerobic metabolism and accumulation of lactate. Plasma cyanide levels should be kept to less than 3 μmol/l (8·1 μg per cent) and, other than during long-term infusions, are a more reliable guide to toxicity than the thiocyanate concentration.[199] It has been suggested that hydroxocobalamin be given during nitroprusside infusions to decrease the potential toxicity[200] but very large doses may be required to achieve a significant effect.[201]

Infusion rates of 20 to 500 μg/min have been used. Generally, it is best to start with the lower dose and gradually increase it until the desired effect is achieved. The higher infusion rates should be used for as short a time as possible and the patients closely monitored for signs of toxicity. Sodium nitroprusside is light sensitive. Solutions should be discarded if they darken and in any case after 8 hours. The infusion container should be protected from light by a paper bag or wrapping in aluminium foil.

After myocardial infarction, sodium nitroprusside infusion consistently increased cardiac output in patients with signs of left ventricular failure or shock, but had little effect on those without these signs.[202] In one investigation the mortality from cardiogenic shock was reduced from 85 to 40 per cent[203] by the use of nitroprusside, but this degree of improvement has not been experienced by others.

*Glyceryl trinitrate* is predominantly a venodilator, particularly when given by intravenous infusion. Its effects are seen within seconds of intravenous administration and it has a plasma half-life of around 4 minutes.[176] It can be given intravenously by infusion at 10–400 μg/min or by intermittent bolus injection. Infusion should be started at the lowest rate and increased until the desired effect is achieved. Nitroglycerine may be useful in the management of left ventricular failure after myocardial infarction but its precise role has still to be defined.

Ventricular afterload reduction is one of the major effects of intra-aortic balloon pumping (see Chapter 12).

### Miscellaneous Drugs

*Steroids.*—Large doses of steroids, for example, methylprednisolone 30 mg/kg body weight, are widely used in the management of shock but their precise rôle, mode of action and effect on morbidity and mortality remain controversial. The beneficial effects that have been claimed include positive inotropic action, peripheral and pulmonary vasodilatation, stabilisation of cell and lysosomal membranes and specific anti-endotoxin properties.

Not all investigators have been able to demonstrate any beneficial haemodynamic effect. For example, Piepenbrock and colleagues[204] found that methylprednisolone 30 mg/kg had no effect on left ventricular dp/dt max (the maximum rate of increase in pressure in the left ventricle during contraction), systemic blood pressure, cardiac index or peripheral vascular resistance. On the other hand, Dietzman and Lillehei[205] found that methylprednisolone 30 mg/kg, dexamethasone 6 mg/kg or hydrocortisone 150 mg/kg decreased the peripheral vascular resistance and increased cardiac output in patients with cardiogenic shock. In an experimental model, pre-treatment with methylprednisolone helped to preserve myocardial contractility in dogs subjected to haemorrhagic shock.[206] At present, the most convincing evidence for a useful effect of high doses of steroids is in septic shock[207] and the prevention of the adult respiratory distress syndrome seen after shock or trauma.[208,209]

*Naloxone* has been found to increase blood pressure in some patients with septic shock.[210] The effect was most marked in patients who had not received exogenous steroids.

### Management of Impaired End-Organ Function

The mechanisms of organ damage in shock have been considered. The optimum method for reducing such damage is to reverse the shock state as rapidly as possible. If this cannot be done, multiple organ failure may occur. The principles of management of organ failure are considered in the appropriate chapters.

### Conclusion

Shock may be produced by a variety of aetiologies but the ultimate effects on the body and on tissue perfusion are similar. Non-controversial methods of management are to remove the cause and optimise ventricular preload. Most of the other aspects of management are based on investigations performed in animal models, chronic rather than acute circulatory failure or short-term haemodynamic studies. There is at present a great need for controlled studies to evaluate the effects of different treatment methods on patient survival.

An approach to management of the shocked patient is summarised in Table 9.

10/Table 9
Management of Shock

1. Establish aetiology and institute appropriate therapy
2. Correct abnormalities of oxygenation, haematocrit, electrolytes or acid-base balance.
3. Measure CVP (PAWP).
4. Infuse fluid if necessary to optimise CVP (PAWP).

| *Improve cardiac performance* | *Consider* | *Support other systems especially:* |
|---|---|---|
| (a) Specific measures | (a) Steroids | (a) Kidneys |
| (b) Non-specific measures | (b) Vasodilators | (b) Lungs |

## IMMEDIATE MANAGEMENT OF TRAUMA

In a recent survey on mortality and morbidity following major trauma from road accidents, at least a third of deaths in hospital occurred within six hours, and more than half within 24 hours after admission.[211] How many of these may have been preventable is unknown, but clearly intensive early management may reduce mortality and minimise morbidity. The commonest causes of death soon after injury are severe brain damage, hypoxia and exsanguination. As soon as a severely injured patient arrives in an emergency department the main lines of management outlined below should be instituted and may in many cases proceed simultaneously. The highest levels of efficiency are achieved when all the equipment likely to be needed is readily available, there is sufficient space for several procedures to be carried out simultaneously and preliminary investigations such as x-rays can be performed without moving the patient.

**Initial Assessment**

This must be rapid but accurate because delay in commencing resuscitation may be crucial. The level of consciousness should be determined, and the patency of the *airway*, adequacy of *breathing*, and the state of the *circulation* assessed.

**Resuscitation**

**Airway.**—Following major injury, the two principles of management are firstly to ensure that the airway is clear at all times and secondly, to protect the lungs from contamination by stomach contents. If either of these objectives is in danger of being compromised, then intubation should be performed with a cuffed endotracheal tube. In this context, it should be remembered that head injuries are often associated with neck injuries and the heads of unconscious patients should not be rotated or flexed until fracture of the cervical spine has been excluded. In general the most stable position for most neck fractures is slight extension, but forced or hyperextension must be avoided. During intubation the head should be held absolutely still by an assistant. Acute gastric dilatation is extremely common in patients with severe trauma. The stomach should be decompressed through a naso- or oro-gastric tube. If urgent intubation is necessary, the technique should follow that used for "crash induction" including the use of cricoid pressure to reduce the risk of regurgitation of stomach contents.

If the injuries have caused obstruction of the upper respiratory tract so that translaryngeal intubation is impossible, cricothyroidotomy offers the quickest and easiest way of providing an airway[439] (Fig. 11).

**Breathing.**—As soon as a patent airway has been established inspection and auscultation will reveal the ability of the patient to breathe satisfactorily and ventilate both lungs. The decision whether to assist ventilation is a matter of judgment based on the nature of the injuries and clinical signs of respiratory difficulty supported by arterial blood gas analysis at the earliest possible time. In head injuries, failure to prevent hypercapnia and hypoxaemia will exacerbate the primary injury and will have a significant effect on prognosis and the long-term results in those who recover. Added oxygen should be given to all patients, particularly those with cyanosis or hypotension. Intermittent positive-pressure ventilation in patients with chest injuries may result in the development of a tension pneumothorax, and the *possibility of this complication must be constantly borne in mind.* Treatment consists of insertion of a chest drain following confirmation of the diagnosis with a chest x-ray, but if the patient's condition is critical, *immediate decompression should be performed.*

**Circulation.**—Access to the circulation should preferably be established by at least two large-bore cannulae inserted percutaneously or by cut-down. There is thus a spare line which can be used for infusion of drugs, and also for volume replacement should the other line become blocked. The rate and volume of initial fluid replacement will depend on the amount of blood lost and the response to replacement. A guide to the amount of blood loss which may be associated with particular fractures is shown below:

| | | |
|---|---|---|
| Pelvis: | bilateral | 2000 ml |
| | unilateral | 1000–1500 ml |
| Femur | | 1000 ml |
| Tibia | | 500 ml |
| Humerus | | 350 ml |
| Ribs | | 125 ml/rib |

Virtually all severely injured patients will have lost more than 20 per cent of their blood volume and will present the clinical features of shock with tachycardia and hypotension. Treatment of such cases should follow the principles outlined previously in the section on "Shock".

Careful and frequent monitoring during infusion of large volumes of fluid is essential, and a central venous pressure line should be inserted. Where appropriate, measurement of PAWP with a pulmonary artery balloon flotation catheter will allow more precise haemodynamic assessment. Persistent hypotension with a high CVP (and PAWP) may be due to tension pneumothorax or cardiac tamponade. Acute haemorrhage of as little as 150 ml into the pericardium can seriously impair cardiac function and should be treated by pericardial aspi-

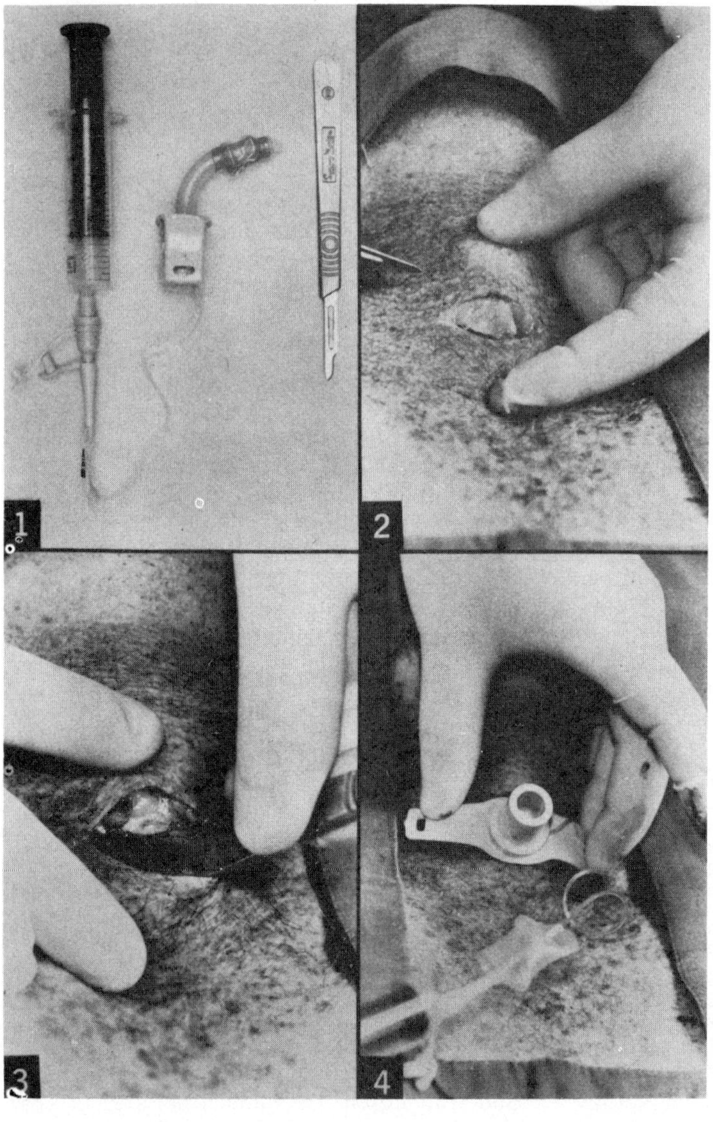

10/Fig. 11.—Cricothyroidotomy. (1) The equipment needed is a scalpel blade and handle, a 24 F.G. (8 mm OD) tracheostomy tube and a 10 ml syringe to inflate the cuff. (2) Run the index finger down the thyroid cartilage until the cricothyroid membrane is palpated, then make a transverse skin incision to reveal the membrane. (3) Incise the lower border of the membrane, insert the butt end of the scalpel handle and turn it through 90° to open the wound. (4) The tracheostomy tube is then inserted and the cuff inflated.

ration. Re-accumulation of blood in the pericardial space is an indication for urgent thoracotomy, drainage and exploration to control the source of the haemorrhage. The adequacy of renal perfusion can be assessed by measurements of hourly urine flow and an indwelling urinary catheter should be inserted.

### Detailed Assessment

**History.**—If the patient is conscious it may be possible to obtain a lot of information directly, but often the severely injured patient is unable to give a clear and coherent account of his medical history and the events leading to the incident. In the case of the latter, useful information may be obtained from available relations, eye-witnesses and ambulance attendants.

**Examination.**—The patient must be completely undressed, cutting clothes off when necessary. Until the examination is complete, movement should be kept to an absolute minimum. When it is necessary to turn the patient for examination or treatment this should be achieved with the spine kept as straight as possible. After evaluating the major and obvious injuries, a thorough and methodical examination will avoid missing any less obvious injuries. This examination must include the following areas, even in the absence of related symptoms: head and neck, as complete a neurological assessment as is possible, chest, abdomen, pelvis, genitalia, rectum and extremities. If it is forgotten that every patient has a back as well as a front, important injuries will be missed.

**Investigation.**—The initial investigations required in a case of severe trauma include a full blood picture, urea and electrolytes, blood grouping and cross-matching, arterial blood gases, ECG, and x-rays of the chest and other parts of the body as indicated. In addition, more specialised techniques such as CAT scanning, arteriograms, excretion urography and ultrasound examination may be required.

### Diagnosis and Treatment

Assessment and investigation will result in diagnosis of the nature and extent of the patient's injuries. As diagnoses are reached, specific treatments can be started, although management of the different problems may change as the investigation proceeds. For example, after signs of increasing intracranial pressure develop, it will be necessary to control ventilation and hyperventilate the patient to buy a short amount of time until pressure can be relieved surgically. The diagnosis of continued profuse intra-abdominal haemorrhage will be an indication for immediate surgery, perhaps delaying full assessment and investigation.

**Chest injuries.**—Trauma to the chest may produce instability of the thoracic cage and contusion of the lungs. This may be associated with a haemo- and/or pneumothorax, and there may be concomitant injuries to other organs such as the heart and great vessels, oesophagus and diaphragm. Emergency treatment should be directed towards maintenance of a clear airway and adequate ventilation, circulatory support, drainage of the pleural cavity with appropriately sited chest drains, and relief of pain. Subsequent treatment will depend on the nature and extent of the injuries. Patients with extensive lung or chest wall damage, pre-existing lung disease and associated head or abdominal injuries will usually need IPPV. The great enthusiasm for IPPV splintage of flail chests has more recently been tempered by results suggesting that over-enthusiastic ventilator therapy, with a high incidence of tracheostomy, may actually increase morbidity and mortality. It has been suggested that patients with less severe injuries may benefit from a conservative regime based on adequate analgesia, humidified oxygen, fluid control and careful tracheobronchial toilet.[212,213] Avoiding fluid overload is particularly important in patients with pulmonary contusion.[214]

**Head injuries.**—The three major factors causing death after severe head injury are intracranial haematoma, cerebral hypoxia, and increase in brain bulk.[215] The aims of treatment are (1) early diagnosis and treatment of intracranial haematoma; (2) prevention of hypoxia and hypercapnia; and (3) maintenance of adequate cerebral perfusion by limiting cerebral oedema and maintaining the blood pressure. All patients must be carefully and continually assessed, paying particular attention to the level of consciousness and focal neurological signs. Assessment of the former may be facilitated by the use of scoring systems such as the Glasgow coma scale.[216] Where available, the direct measurement of intracranial pressure[217] will indicate the need for, and effectiveness of, decompressive measures. If there are signs suggestive of an intracranial haematoma, it must be sought either by CAT scanning or angiography (depending on the facilities available) and relieved surgically. In urgent cases it may be necessary to perform emergency burr holes without prior investigations. Hypertonic agents may be used to help reduce brain oedema, and more recently, it has been suggested that high-dose barbiturates may protect the brain from hypoxia.[218] The practical value of the latter has yet to be fully established.

**Abdominal injuries.**—Abdominal injuries may occur as the result of either penetrating or non-penetrating injuries. Diagnosis, particularly in the latter, may be difficult and demands the highest skill from the surgeon. Investigations which may help include abdominal x-rays (looking in particular for gas under the diaphragm suggesting a ruptured hollow viscus; fractured ribs which may be associated with a lacerated spleen or kidney, and obliteration of the psoas shadow suggesting a retro-peritoneal collection of fluid), barium studies, angiography, intravenous pyelogram, and in some cases, diagnostic peritoneal lavage. Most would agree that early exploration should be undertaken where there are reasonable suspicions of intra-abdominal damage. Where possible, adequate resuscitation should be carried out before a general anaesthetic is administered for laparotomy, but where this is impossible because of continued bleeding, adequate access to the circulation must be secured before induction. The absolute indications for immediate exploration have been summarised by Petty[219] as follows:

(1) shock occurring immediately after successful resuscitation or later in a patient with suspicion of an abdominal injury;
(2) the presence of free gas in the abdomen on x-ray;
(3) the splenic rupture syndrome—persistent tenderness under the left costal margin, left shoulder pain, fracture of the lower left ribs;
(4) increasing abdominal distension;
(5) gradually increasing abdominal pain, tenderness or rigidity.

## ANAPHYLAXIS

The term "anaphylaxis" was introduced by Poitier and Richet in 1902 to describe the profound shock and subsequent death that occurred in some dogs on re-injection of the poison of the sea anemone.[220] Anaphylaxis was later used to describe an acute clinical syndrome that followed repeated antigenic challenge[221] but it is now known that similar clinical syndromes can be produced by direct histamine release, complement-mediated reactions and IgG antibodies without previous sensitisation. It has been suggested, that on the basis of clinical observation alone, hypersensitivity reactions are better described as "anaphylactoid" and the term "anaphylaxis" reserved for those reactions that can be shown to be antibody-mediated.[222]

### Clinical Features

The clinical course of anaphylaxis is extremely variable in severity, the time from exposure to the antigen to symptoms developing and the duration of the reaction.[223] After parenteral injection most reactions will occur within 30 minutes and nearly all within 3 minutes if the intravenous route is used. After oral ingestion of antigen, symptoms may take hours to appear but in other cases the symptoms appear within minutes.

The symptoms of anaphylaxis are summarised in Table 10. Severe bronchospasm is associated with an increased risk of death[224] and is usually the most difficult feature to treat.[225] Bronchospasm occurs more frequently in patients with a history of asthma or hay fever. In the series of 116 cases of anaphylaxis reported by Fisher & More[225] the first clinical feature noted was as shown in Table 11.

A wide variety of different antigens may cause anaphylaxis including drugs, heterologous sera such as equine tetanus antitoxin, pollen extracts, venoms and stings, and foods. Anaphylaxis may occur with a frequency as high as 1 in 5000 general anaesthetics and in New Zealand intravenous drugs used in anaesthesia were the fourth most common cause of reported anaphylaxis[226]. Almost all of the agents that may be given intravenously during anaesthesia have been implicated. Atopic patients, that is, those with a history of asthma, hay fever or eczema[220] and patients with a history of previous drug reactions[225] are more prone to anaphylactic reactions. In different series the mortality from anaphylaxis during anaesthesia has been 4 per cent[227] and 3·4 per cent.[225]

### Mechanisms in Anaphylaxis

The type I immune response or immediate hypersensitivity reaction most closely resembles that seen in anaphylaxis. This response is classically linked with the production of an IgE immunoglobulin or reagenic antibody in response to a previous antigenic challenge. Once produced, the reagenic antibodies adhere to mast cells and basophils. Subsequent exposure to the antigen causes the release of histamine and other mediators of anaphylaxis from these cells. IgG reagenic antibodies are also known, but unlike the IgE they require the interaction of complement for the mediators to be released.[222] A number of other stimuli can trigger release of the mediators of anaphylaxis from mast cells and basophils. These include the complement-derived products C3a and C5a, certain kinins, a histamine releasing lymphokine and lysosomal basic proteins derived from neutrophils.[228]

At one time histamine was the only known mediator of anaphylaxis but now about 20

10/TABLE 10
SYMPTOMS IN ANAPHYLAXIS

| *System* | *Reaction* | *Symptoms* | *Signs* |
|---|---|---|---|
| Respiratory tract | Rhinitis | Nasal congestion and itching | Mucosal oedema |
| | Laryngeal oedema | Dyspnoea | Laryngeal stridor<br>Oedema of cords |
| | Bronchospasm | Cough<br>Wheezing<br>Sensation of retrosternal oppression | Cough<br>Wheezing<br>Râles<br>Respiratory distress<br>Tachypnoea |
| Cardiovascular system | Hypotension | Syncope<br>Feeling of faintness | Hypotension<br>Tachycardia |
| | Dysrhythmia | | Electrocardiographic changes:<br>Non-specific ST segment and T-wave change<br>Nodal rhythm<br>Atrial fibrillation |
| | Cardiac arrest | | Absent pulse<br>Electrocardiographic change:<br>Asystole<br>Ventricular fibrillation |
| Skin | Urticaria | Pruritus<br>Hives | Typical urticarial lesion |
| | Angioedema | Nonpruritic swelling of an extremity, perioral or periorbital region | Oedema frequently asymmetrical |
| Gastro-intestinal system | | Nausea<br>Vomiting<br>Abdominal pain<br>Diarrhoea | |
| Eye | Conjunctivitis | Ocular itching<br>Lacrimation | Conjunctival inflammation |

(Courtesy of Dr. J. F. Kelly and Dr. R. Patterson and the American Medical Association[223])

different mediators are known.[228] Histamine has been shown to dilate terminal arterioles and increase the permeability of venules, causing a contraction of endothelial cells so that gaps appear through which plasma extravasates. Histamine also causes an increase in airway resistance which is reduced by atropine and is thought to be mediated through a vagal reflex initiated by bronchial irritant receptors rather than a direct effect on the smooth muscle. In the skin, histamine produces vasodilatation (flushing), pruritus and urticaria. The actions of some other mediators include:

**Eosinophil Chemotactic Factor of Anaphylaxis** (ECF-A) selectively attracts eosinophils. Eosinophils contain a number of enzymes capable of degrading the mediators of anaphylaxis and may therefore control and limit the response.

**Slow Reacting Substance of Anaphylaxis (SRS-A) and Leukotrienes.** SRS-A is now known to form part of the group of leukotrienes. These are substances produced by leucocytes from arachidonic acid (prostaglandins are also formed from arachidonic acid). SRS-A causes sustained contraction of pul-

10/TABLE 11
FIRST FEATURE OF ANAPHYLACTOID REACTION NOTED

| *Feature* | % |
|---|---|
| Flush | 38 |
| Bronchospasm | 14 |
| Impalpable pulses | 13 |
| Transient difficulty in inflation | 8 |
| Coughing | 6 |
| Urticarial rash | 5 |
| Others | 16 |

(Courtesy of Dr. M. McD. Fisher and Dr. D. G. More and the Australian Society of Anaesthetists[225])

monary smooth muscle, particularly in peripheral airways, hypotension and increased vascular permeability.

**Platelet Activating Factor (PAF)** is released from basophils and mast cells. It causes platelet aggregation and release of vaso-active amines from platelets.

**Prostaglandins.** $PGD_2$ and $PGF_2$ cause bronchoconstriction.

### Treatment

The treatment of cardiovascular collapse caused by anaphylaxis includes:

**Adrenaline**—0·3 to 1 ml of 1 in 1000 solution—300 to 500 $\mu$g—should be given intramuscularly or intravenously. Its alpha adrenergic vasoconstriction opposes the vasodilatation seen in anaphylaxis and the beta$_2$-adrenergic activity promotes bronchodilatation. Adrenaline impairs further release of the mediators of anaphylaxis.[229] Further adrenaline should be given at intervals until clinical improvement occurs.

**Cardiopulmonary resuscitation,** if this is indicated, with external cardiac compression and intermittent positive-pressure ventilation.

**Intubation** will be required if laryngeal oedema causes respiratory obstruction. If it is impossible to insert an oral endotracheal tube the patient needs a cricothyroidotomy (p. 326).

**Infusion of colloid.**—Fisher[230] has shown that large volumes of fluid are needed to restore the circulating blood volume. Colloid solutions (plasma, Haemaccel, dextran) were the most effective in achieving this, at least in the early stages. Central venous pressure measurement facilitates volume replacement.

**Oxygen** should be given to relieve hypoxia.

**Antihistamines,** for example chlorpheniramine 10–20 mg by slow intravenous injection, will alleviate the histamine-$H_1$-receptor mediated effects such as angio-oedema, pruritus and urticaria. Antihistamines have not been shown to be of benefit in established anaphylaxis.

**Steroids** have little place in the immediate treatment of anaphylaxis because their effects are delayed for some hours. In more severe cases hydrocortisone 200 mg intravenously should be given.

The majority of patients with anaphylaxis or an "anaphylactoid" reaction will respond to a combination of adrenaline, antihistamine and a colloid infusion tritrated against the patient's arterial pressure.

### Prevention

An accurate history of previous drug reactions and allergy, a knowledge of cross-reactions between different agents and intradermal skin testing should reduce the chance of exposing patients to drugs to which they are sensitive.[231] If such exposure is unavoidable, pretreatment with steroids and antihistamines, with subcutaneous adrenaline in high-risk cases, gives the best protection.

## TOXIC-SHOCK SYNDROME

The toxic-shock syndrome (TSS) was described by Todd and colleagues[232] in a group of seven children aged 8 to 17 years. The clinical features included fever, generalised erythroderma, conjunctival hyperaemia, subcutaneous oedema, hypotension, renal dysfunction and liver injury. The occurrence of hypotension was often sudden and relatively refractory to treatment. Headache, sore throat and diarrhoea are clinical features that have subsequently been described. About 95 per cent of cases have been in menstruating women in whom TSS has been associated with tampon usage, though the role of tampons in the pathogenesis of the syndrome is unclear. Such cases have been reported from England,[233] the U.S.A.[234,235] and Australia.[236] More recently, an increasing proportion of reported cases have not been associated with menstruation and it appears that staphylococcal infections of virtually any type can cause TSS.[237] A toxin produced by phage group I

*Staphylococcus aureus* appears to cause the syndrome, but the nature of the toxin is, as yet, unknown.

*Staph. aureus* can be isolated from vaginal cultures in the majority of cases but not from blood cultures.[238] The risk of recurrence can be considerably reduced by treatment with beta-lactamase-resistant antibiotics such as cloxacillin. It is also recommended that women who have had an episode of TSS should not use tampons for several menstrual cycles or until *Staph. aureus* has been eradicated from the vagina.

The management of toxic-shock syndrome includes antibiotics and the measures outlined for the management of shock. Most of the strains of *Staph. aureus* isolated from patients with this syndrome have been resistant to penicillin so it is important that the chosen antibiotic is resistant to beta-lactamases. Large volumes of fluid may be needed to return the CVP to normal because vasodilatation is a prominent feature of TSS. In the more severe cases, catecholamines may be needed to support the systemic blood pressure. The reported mortality has been 10–15 per cent.[238]

## CORONARY CARE

There has been some dispute over the advantages of hospital as against home care for patients with suspected myocardial infarction,[239–241] but the majority of such patients and those with life-threatening dysrhythmias are admitted to hospital.[240] In one epidemiological survey the incidence of myocardial infarction was 4·9 per thousand population with a 28-day fatality rate of 50·5 per cent. Seventy per cent of deaths occurred within 3 hours of the onset of symptoms. The frequency of early deaths lead to the recommendation that coronary care ambulances be established to give patients the benefit of advanced life support systems from the earliest possible time.[242] These ambulances have proved successful in a number of cities both in the United Kingdom and overseas.[243] They also provide a service for patients with "sudden coronary death" (SCD) in the community. Resuscitation from SCD is associated with a relatively favourable long-term prognosis[244] and in the majority of cases is not associated with myocardial infarction.[245]

In the majority of hospitals, patients with suspected recent infarction are admitted to a coronary care or intensive care unit. Most units have no definite age limit for admission but patients aged over 70 years are often managed elsewhere when intensive measures seem inappropriate or if the unit's capacity to accept young patients would be jeopardised. While many are convinced that the mortality from myocardial infarction can be reduced with the facilities available in a specialised unit,[246] by no means all studies have succeeded in demonstrating such a benefit.[247,248]

### Mechanisms of Acute Infarction

Myocardial infarction usually occurs in the presence of significant atherosclerotic coronary artery disease. Epidemiological studies have shown that cigarette smoking, hyperlipidaemia, hypertension,[249] use of oral contraceptives by women[250] and psychological factors[251,252] are important risk factors in the development of atherosclerosis and myocardial infarction. Opinions are divided on the effects of physical activity on coronary heart disease. Rather than this being a direct effect of exercise the reported reduction in coronary disease may just reflect a lower incidence of the other known risk factors[253] though other studies suggest that vigorous exercise has a distinct protective effect on its own.[254]

Myocardial infarction occurs when there is a sustained decrease in the supply of blood to an area of heart muscle. Important causes of this are:[255]

1. Coronary artery thrombosis: several post-mortem studies have shown a strong correlation between occlusive thrombus in a coronary vessel and an infarcted area.
2. Haemorrhage into an atherosclerotic plaque or plaque rupture predisposing to thrombus formation.
3. Coronary artery spasm may be superimposed on an already stenotic vessel or occur in apparently normal vessels. It has been suggested that this is the likely immediate cause of acute infarction,[256] but this is probably a minority view.[257] Spasm may be the major factor when infarction occurs in the absence of significant coronary atherosclerosis.

Prolonged systemic arterial hypotension can cause infarction because coronary perfusion is dependent on mean and diastolic blood pressure. This may be a factor in peri-operative infarction of patients at risk.

### Presentation and Diagnosis

Chest or epigastric pain is by far the commonest presenting symptom in myocardial infarction, being present in over 80 per cent of cases[258] and usually lasting for more than 30 minutes. Classically it is severe and crushing in character and may radiate to the jaw, neck or arms. Autonomic reactions such as profuse sweating, pallor and nausea or vomiting are common. Additional symptoms may be caused by complications such as dysrhythmias or ventricular failure. Occasionally infarction occurs without chest pain, the so-called "silent infarct" and in these cases symptoms may be non-specific or related solely to any complications.

The clinical diagnosis is supported by changes in the electrocardiogram and serum enzymes. In only half of the patients who have had an infarct can the diagnosis be made from the first electrocardiogram but this rises to 83 per cent with serial traces.[259] Enzymes are released from necrotic myocardium. Those most commonly measured in the diagnosis of myocardial infarction are creatinine kinase (CK), aspartate transaminase (formerly glutamic oxaloacetic transaminase) and lactic dehydrogenase. A raised CK is suspicious of myocardial infarction until proved otherwise. Plasma CK activity rises rapidly after acute infarction and reaches a maximum after 16 to 24 hours. Recent vigorous exercise or intramuscular injections may cause a rise in total CK activity.[260] Cases of doubt can be resolved by measurement of CK isoenzyme activity. Skeletal muscle contains CK-MM. The myocardium contains 10–20 per cent CK-MB, the remainder being CK-MM. The third isoenzyme, CK-BB, occurs mainly in brain tissue. The finding of significant CK-MB activity therefore confirms myocardial infarction.

There are occasions on which the ECG is uninterpretable because of previous myocardial infarction or disorders of electrical activation. Enzyme measurements can give borderline, or later in the evolution of infarction, normal results. Radioisotope imaging with $^{99m}$technetium-labelled imidodiphosphonate which is selectively concentrated in necrotic areas of myocardium[261] may be useful in these cases.

### Management

A large proportion of the patients admitted to a CCU or ICU with definite or suspected infarction follow an uncomplicated course and require only general care and observation. Complications are more commonly seen in the elderly.[262]

### General Care

*Analgesia.*—Patients frequently describe the pain of myocardial infarction as the worst they have known. Their first need is for effective analgesia. Diamorphine (heroin) is most effective but is unavailable in many countries. Morphine is widely used but occasionally causes bradycardia and hypotension and the side-effects of nausea and vomiting may be troublesome. Pethidine is much less effective in relieving the severe pain of myocardial infarction.

*Bed rest.*—Periods of bed rest as long as six weeks used to be advised for patients who had had a myocardial infarct. During the 1970's a number of studies of early mobilisation after myocardial infarction were published[263,264] and since then the period of complete bed rest has been limited to 24–48 hours in the absence of complications. Some patients develop late complications and require readmission to coronary care after initial discharge. It is difficult to identify which patients these will be although recurrence of ischaemic pain for the first time 24 hours or more after admission is one risk factor.[265] The policy of shorter periods of bed rest has been accompanied by a policy of shorter hospital stay during which the patient is progressively mobilised. A hospital stay as short as eight days appears to be acceptable in the absence of complications, pre-existing disease of social constraints.[266]

*Oxygen* is given routinely to patients in many units but there is no evidence that patients with uncomplicated infarction derive any benefit from this practice.[267] On the other hand, supplemental oxygen should be given to patients with left ventricular failure or shock to correct hypoxaemia.

*Monitoring and observation* is the major purpose of modern coronary care. In addition to the detection of life-threatening dysrhythmias serious complications may be prevented by early therapy for minor dysrhythmias and haemodynamic abnormalities.

*Psychological.*—Myocardial infarction can have a profound psychological effect on the patient and their spouse.[268] Sedatives may be useful for reducing anxiety in the initial phase. Often, however, a careful explanation of the situation to the patient and his family is all that is needed. It should be emphasised that the first hours are the period of greatest risk and that after an infarct most patients are able to return to work and all their former activities. This is also a good opportunity to discuss some aspects of secondary prevention.

*Anticoagulants.* — Subcutaneous heparin, 5000 units tds, may be given to reduce the incidence of deep venous thrombosis.[269] Prophylactic anticoagulation may also reduce the risk of stroke, particularly for those who have had a large infarct.[270] Whether there are any additional benefits from using anticoagulants in acute myocardial infarction is controversial.[271]

*Previous drug therapy* can generally be continued, though particular care may be needed with antihypertensive drugs, beta-adrenergic blocking agents and calcium antagonists. Patients receiving these should be observed closely for bradycardia, heart block, hypotension or signs of ventricular failure. Myocardial infarction causes a transient impairment of glucose tolerance. Diabetics may need increased doses of insulin and those who have been satisfactorily controlled by diet or oral hypoglycaemics frequently require insulin to prevent hyperglycaemia.

### Limitation of Infarct Size

In experimental animals it has been shown that myocardial infarction progresses over several hours in a wave-front fashion with cell death beginning in the core of the ischaemic area and spreading with time. A number of different methods have been proposed to limit infarct size.[272] These include glucose-insulin-potassium infusions, hyaluronidase, steroids, cobra venom factor, aprotinin, propranolol, sodium nitroprusside and nitroglycerine. More recently, both experimental and clinical investigations have been reported into the effects of intra-aortic balloon pumping alone[273] or in combination with various pharmacological agents,[274] prostacyclin,[275] coronary artery reperfusion[276,277] and lysis of intracoronary thrombus by intracoronary infusion of streptokinase,[278,279] on indices of infarct size or local myocardial blood flow. Many of these proposed treatments require invasive haemodynamic monitoring or facilities unlikely to be available outside a large regional or teaching hospital. The widespread use of any of these treatments should therefore depend on the results of trials designed to determine their effect on the morbidity and mortality of infarction. Such trials are being carried out for some of these treatments but the results are, as yet, unavailable.

## COMPLICATIONS

### Persisting or Recurrent Ischaemic Pain

Persisting or recurrent ischaemic pain must be differentiated from other causes of chest pain after myocardial infarction. These include pericardial pain, pulmonary emboli and musculoskeletal pains. Ischaemic pain may be caused by extension of the area of infarction or the onset of unstable angina. In some patients the pain subsides with analgesia or with moderate doses of nitrates but in others the pain is more difficult to control. In these patients more aggressive measures may be indicated as for other patients with unstable angina (see below), recognising that coronary artery surgery carries a higher risk within the first month after infarction.[255]

### Dysrhythmias and Heart Block

*Sinus bradycardia* occurs in 10–20 per cent of patients with myocardial infarction. It is most common in the early stages and tends to be associated with inferior infarction. Treatment is unnecessary unless it is accompanied by hypotension or ventricular ectopic beats (VEB's) when atropine should be given in 0·3 mg aliquots to return the heart rate to normal.

*Sinus tachycardia* in the period immediately after infarction is associated with sympathetic overactivity. The tachycardia can be controlled by giving a beta-adrenergic blocker such as practolol in 5–10 mg aliquots.[280] Persisting sinus tachycardia is associated with left ventricular failure or a large area of infarcted myocardium.

*Atrial fibrillation or flutter* occurs in about 20 per cent of patients, but is usually transient. A rapid ventricular response may be associated with recurrence of ischaemic pain, hypotension or cardiac failure. Digoxin is useful for controlling the ventricular response but acts too slowly to have an immediate effect. In the period before digoxin becomes effective practolol or verapamil may be given cautiously to control the rate, remembering that both of these drugs have a negative inotropic effect. Electrical cardioversion should be used if there is marked haemodynamic deterioration. This can be done using either a synchronised direct current shock from a defibrillator or, in the case of type 1 atrial flutter, by rapid atrial pacing through a transvenous pacing catheter.[281]

*Ventricular dysrhythmias.* — Ventricular ectopic beats (VEBs) occur in over 90 per cent of patients during the first 24 hours after a myocardial infarct and in most cases are benign. Ventricular fibrillation (VF) occurs in about 8 per cent of patients admitted directly to a CCU, about two-thirds of these being associated with cardiac failure or shock.[282] The incidence decreases with time from infarction. Of the patients who have ventricular fibrillation in the absence of cardiac failure or shock ("primary VF"), 16 per cent have recurrent VF.[283]

It was thought that frequent, multifocal or R-on-T VEBs—the so-called "warning" dysrhythmias—were predictors of VF and that pharmacological suppression of these would reduce the incidence of VF. More recent work has shown that warning dysrhythmias are not reliable predictors of VF, that they occur frequently in patients who do not develop VF and that they do not occur frequently enough or long enough before to be useful in all patients who do develop VF during the first 48 hours after infarction.[284] This has lead to the suggestion that patients with definite or suspected infarction should be given prophylactic antidysrhythmic drugs during the period of greatest risk for VF, i.e. the first 24–48 hours. Lignocaine has been the most commonly used antidysrhythmic, but attention must be paid to the method of administration. Aps and associates[285] found that a lignocaine bolus of 1–2 mg/kg followed by an infusion at 4 mg/min for 30 minutes, 2 mg/min for 2 hours and 1 mg/min thereafter would usually maintain levels within the therapeutic range in patients with uncomplicated infarcts. A review of 13 trials of lignocaine prophylaxis for primary VF found only one that was free from major defects in trial design.[286] In this double blind randomised study[287] lignocaine was highly effective in preventing primary VF but careful observation of patients and infusion rates were required to prevent side-effects.

The management of VF, if it occurs, is that of cardiac arrest (see Chapter 14). Direct current cardioversion should be used to treat the dysrhythmia.

Ventricular tachycardia (VT) is defined as three or more consecutive ventricular ectopic beats occurring at a rate greater than 100/min. Short runs of VT or more prolonged runs with a rate of less than 130–140/min are unlikely to cause significant haemodynamic disturbance. More prolonged or rapid runs of VT may cause hypotension, cardiac failure or loss of consciousness and may degenerate into VF. Drugs may be used to treat and suppress VT. Lignocaine, given according to the regimen outlined above, is the drug of choice. If lignocaine is ineffective, alternatives include procainamide, disopyramide, mexilitine, bretylium, phenytoin, amiodarone and others. The pharmacology and application of these drugs has been reviewed by Harrison and co-workers[288] and Singh and associates.[289] An alternative method for reverting VT is by using a temporary ventricular pacing catheter to insert single or paired paced beats, overdrive the ventricle (i.e. briefly pace at a rate faster than the VT), or pace the ventricle asynchronously. Sometimes pacing the ventricle at a rate faster than the patient's spontaneous rate will prevent VT recurring.[281] Unless it responds very quickly to either drugs or pacing, VT associated with hypotension or loss of consciousness should be treated by direct current cardioversion.

*Heart block.*—Various kinds of atrioventricular or intraventricular block may occur after myocardial infarction. First degree heart block is usually associated with inferior infarction and, by itself, requires no treatment. Second degree Mobitz I or Wenckebach block is also most commonly associated with inferior infarction and even if it progresses to complete heart block this is usually only a temporary problem. It is unusual for profound bradycardia to occur when complete heart block is associated with inferior infarction. Ventricular pacing is considered for treatment of hypotension, cardiac failure or recurrent ischaemic pain. Atropine or an isoprenaline infusion may be given as an interim measure to increase the ventricular rate.

Mobitz II second degree heart block, on the other hand, is often associated with anterior infarcts, the site of block being below the atrioventricular node. Complete heart block may occur suddenly with profound bradycardia or ventricular asystole. A pacing catheter should therefore be inserted into all patients with Mobitz II second degree heart block and those that progress to complete heart block. The management of atrioventricular block complicating myocardial infarction is considered in greater detail by Gazes and Gaddy.[290]

New bundle-branch blocks are usually associated with large anterior infarcts and for this reason tend to be associated with a greater than average mortality. There is also, depending on the nature of the bundle-branch block (BBB), a variable risk of progression to a high degree atrioventricular block[291] as shown as Table 12. Practices vary, but many would insert a temporary pacing catheter prophylactically in all those with a high risk of progression to high degree block.[292]

10/TABLE 12
MORTALITY AND RISK OF PROGRESSION TO HIGH DEGREE ATRIOVENTRICULAR BLOCK IN PATIENTS WHO DEVELOP BUNDLE-BRANCH BLOCK AFTER MYOCARDIAL INFARCTION (EXCLUDES PATIENTS WITH CARDIAC FAILURE IN SHOCK).

| *Type of Block** | *Hospital Mortality* | *Progression to High Degree Block* |
|---|---|---|
| LBBB | 24% | 13% |
| RBBB | 22% | 14% |
| RBBB+LAHB | 29% | 27% |
| RBBB+LPHB | 38% | 29% |
| Alternating BBB | 44% | 44% |

* LBBB—Left bundle-branch block
RBBB—Right bundle-branch block
LAHB—Left anterior hemiblock
LPHB—Left posterior hemiblock

*Hypertension.*—Patients without pre-existing hypertension may have raised arterial blood pressures in the period following myocardial infarction, perhaps as a result of sympathetic overactivity. This is associated with a worse prognosis.[293] If the hypertension does not respond to analgesics or nitroglycerine, sodium nitroprusside can be used to return the blood pressure to normal levels.

*Left ventricular failure.*—Left ventricular failure (LVF) in acute myocardial infarction is usually associated with an increased left atrial pressure. The symptoms include dyspnoea, tachypnoea and orthopnoea and the signs include tachycardia, a gallop rhythm and basal crepitations on auscultation of the lung fields. The chest x-ray confirming the diagnosis will show upper lobe diversion of blood flow and evidence of interstitial or alveolar oedema. Occasionally these features are found in the absence of an elevated left atrial pressure.[294] This may reflect delayed resolution after the left atrial pressure has returned to normal.

Severe pulmonary oedema can cause life-threatening hypoxaemia. Supplemental oxygen should be given by face mask or, if this is insufficient, intubation and ventilation with PEEP may be indicated. The treatment of LVF consists of:

1. Diuretics
2. Venodilators, e.g. nitroglycerine
3. Ventricular afterload reduction.

Patients with moderate or severe LVF and those that are hypotensive should have this therapy monitored, using a pulmonary artery flotation catheter to measure indirectly left atrial pressure and estimate cardiac output because the clinical findings often lag behind the haemodynamic changes. Sodium nitroprusside is both a venodilator and reduces ventricular afterload. Patients given sodium nitroprusside achieve an optimum left atrial pressure more rapidly than those given diuretics,[295] but this seems to have little effect on overall morbidity or mortality.

The prognosis for patients who develop LVF after myocardial infarction depends on their cardiac output, as shown in Table 13.[154]

10/TABLE 13
MORTALITY RATES FOR HAEMODYNAMIC SUBSETS AFTER MYOCARDIAL INFARCTION.

| *Subset* | *Pulmonary Artery Wedge Pressure > 18 mm Hg* | *Cardiac Index < 2·2 l/min/m²* | *Mortality* |
|---|---|---|---|
| I | – | – | 3% |
| II | + | – | 9% |
| III | – | + | 23% |
| IV | + | + | 51% |

(Courtesy of Drs. J. S. Forrester, W. Ganz, G. Diamond, T. HcHugh, D. W. Chonette and H. J. C. Swan and the Massachusettes Medical Society[70]).

*Cardiogenic shock.*—Aspects of the pathogenesis and management of cardiogenic shock are considered in the section on "Shock" and have been reviewed by Kuhn[188,189] and Gunnar and associates.[272]

*Papillary muscle dysfunction and septal perforation.*—Both of these conditions present with haemodynamic deterioration and a new systolic murmur. Complete rupture of a papillary muscle causes massive mitral regurgitation and severe LVF which can be fatal within minutes or hours. Less complete involvement of the supporting structure of the mitral valve can be tolerated for longer, so giving time for diagnosis, medical treatment and, when indicated, surgical correction.

A clinical diagnosis of either papillary muscle dysfunction or ventricular septal perforation can be confirmed by inserting a pulmonary artery flotation catheter. In patients with mitral regurgitation a large V-wave is seen on the wedged pressure tracing. Blood samples for measurement of oxygen saturation should be taken from each heart chamber as the catheter is advanced. If septal perforation has occurred there is an increase in oxygen saturation at the level of the ventricle. The extent of the left to right shunt can also be calculated.

Treatment is similar for both conditions. The first aim is to improve the cardiac output through the systemic circulation. This is achieved by reducing ventricular afterload with sodium nitroprusside and/or intra-aortic balloon pumping. The definitive management of these lesions is by surgical repair after defining the lesion and coronary anatomy by angiography. Surgery used to be delayed as long as possible in the hope that the infarct would "mature" and that this would reduce the operative mortality. A high incidence of sudden deterioration or death while waiting for surgery has lead to early operation, in some centres as soon as the diagnosis has been established.[272] The mortality from these conditions, however, remains high.

*Pericarditis.*—Pericarditis with an audible friction rub occurs in about 7 per cent of patients after myocardial infarction[296] and a larger number have typical pericardial pain without a rub being heard. The occurrence of pericarditis does not affect the prognosis. Simple analgesics such as aspirin or paracetamol are often effective in reducing the pain.

*Myocardial rupture.*—Rupture of the heart causes between 2 and 15 per cent of deaths from myocardial infarction. Usually there is sudden collapse and loss of palpable pulses while the electrocardiogram may continue to show normal sinus rhythm. Occasionally the leak is slow and it presents as a rapidly increasing pericardial infusion or tamponade. The only available treatment is surgical repair.

### After Care

After they have been discharged from the intensive care or coronary care unit patients who have had a myocardial infarct are gradually mobilised before being sent home from hospital. At this stage consideration may be given to therapeutic modes of secondary prevention, such as beta blockers, sulfinpyrazone, aspirin and so on and whether referral for exercise testing or angiography is appropriate. Other aspects of the after care have been reviewed by Pentecost.[297]

## Patients Without Proven Infarcts

Patients are admitted for coronary care because of definite or suspected infarction. A proportion of these, in some series 50 per cent or more, will prove not to have had an infarct. These patients fall into one of three groups:

1. Patients with unstable angina.
2. Patients with an alternative cause for their symptoms which is positively identified.
3. Patients with chest pain of unknown aetiology.

### Patients with Unstable Angina

Unstable angina, also referred to as coronary insufficiency, crescendo angina, accelerating angina and intermediate coronary syndrome, includes several clinical patterns:

(i) New onset angina associated with minimal stress.
(ii) An increase in the frequency, severity or duration of previously stable angina.
(iii) Prolonged ischaemic pain indistinguishable clinically from myocardial infarction but without ECG or enzyme changes.

There has been considerable controversy concerning the optimum management of these patients and in particular the merits of medical treatment as opposed to urgent angiography and coronary artery bypass grafting. It now appears that there is a relatively low incidence of early infarction and death in patients with unstable angina and that this incidence is unaffected by urgent surgery.[298]

The main elements of medical treatment are bed rest, nitrates and either beta-adrenergic blockers or calcium antagonists. Nitrates can be given sublingually, orally or topically in the form of nitroglycerine ointment. In the more refractory cases intravenous nitroglycerine can be used.[176]

Beta-adrenergic blocking drugs such as propranolol are used to decrease cardiac work, reduce ischaemia and so relieve the symptoms of unstable angina. Doses of at least 80 mg and occasionally more than 640 mg of propranolol per day are used. The dose is adjusted according to the relief of symptoms and appearance of side-effects, bradycardia being the dose-limiting factor. More recently there has been considerable interest in the use of calcium antagonists such as verapamil and nifedipine in unstable angina. They are highly effective in angina associated with coronary artery spasm and have been shown to be effective in the management of chronic stable angina. When coronary artery spasm is an important contributory factor in unstable angina, calcium antagonists would appear to be the logical adjunct to nitrate therapy, but whether they offer any advantage over beta blockers in the management of unstable angina in general is, at present, uncertain.

With medical therapy pain will be controlled in over half the patients within 24 hours.[299] If pain persists despite optimum medical therapy and correction of dysrhythmias, anaemia or hypertension, consideration should be given to transferring the patient to a regional cardiothoracic centre where further investigation and treatment can be performed.

It seems that urgent angiography can be performed safely in patients with unstable angina[299] but many centres prefer to use the intra-aortic balloon pump (IABP) to control the pain first and then proceed with investigation and surgery on a semi-elective basis. The IABP increases coronary perfusion pressure and, by reducing ventricular afterload, reduces myocardial oxygen demand. On occasion it is dramatically effective in controlling unstable angina[298] and its use may reduce the risks of angiography and surgery. Coronary angiography should be followed by coronary artery grafting unless there is inoperable coronary disease. Surgery usually results in the patient becoming symptom free.[299]

The patients with unstable angina whose pain is controlled by nitrates and beta blockers or calcium antagonists may be discharged from the coronary or intensive care unit to be mobilised and further investigated by exercise testing and angiography on an elective basis.

#### Alternative Causes

Pulmonary embolism, aortic dissection, pericarditis, cholelithiasis and other conditions can cause pain similar to that of myocardial infarction.

#### Chest Pain of Unknown Aetiology

Some of the patients admitted with suspected infarction will have this excluded and have no other cause found for their pain. Further investigations such as exercise testing or angiography may demonstrate ischaemic heart disease but there remains a proportion for whom no satisfactory explanation can be found. The prognosis for patients without infarcts that have been admitted to a CCU is similar to those with a proven infarct,[300] for both death and subsequent infarction. This suggests that a significant proportion of these patients in fact have myocardial ischaemia even though their coronary arteries may be normal. Suggested aetiologies for the chest pain include coronary artery spasm, coronary embolism with subsequent lysis of the clot, abnormal haemoglobin-oxygen dissociation, disease in vessels too small to display on angiography or a cardiomyopathy, but none has been proven.[301]

The chest pain may be recurrent and can be very difficult to treat. In different series 23 per cent had their symptoms reduced by propranolol and 50 per cent by perhexiline. Nitrates are usually ineffective. Until the cause or causes of this syndrome are known the treatment is likely to remain unsatisfactory.

### TETANUS

Tetanus is most frequently seen in underdeveloped countries where it is a significant public health problem estimated to cause many thousands of mostly neonatal deaths each year. In countries with a high active immunisation rate against tetanus it has become an uncommon disease. During 1977 only 70 cases were reported from the whole of the USA[302] and 16 cases from England and Wales.[303] In Australia, during the decade ending 1975, 207 cases of tetanus were notified.[304]

Tetanus is caused by *Clostridium tetani*, an anaerobic Gram-positive spore-forming rod. The spores only germinate under conditions of relative anoxia, that is, where there is extensive tissue damage, necrosis, infection or in the vicinity of foreign bodies. In approximately 50 per cent of tetanus cases the wounds were considered too trivial to require medical treatment.[304] The organism produces two toxins:

1. Tetanolysin produces haemolysis *in vitro*. This plays no significant part in the development of clinical tetanus.
2. Tetanospasmin is a potent double-stranded protein neurotoxin that produces the clinical syndrome of tetanus.

Tetanospasmin is distributed throughout the body in the blood stream and then travels mainly via peripheral motor neurones, to reach the central nervous system where it binds to gangliosides. The symptoms of tetanus develop after the toxin has crossed the synaptic cleft to thc pre-synaptic terminals of spinal interneurons.[302] Its main effect is to interfere with the inhibition of spinal reflexes. Both alpha and gamma motor neurons are affected causing an increase in muscle tone with paroxysmal exacerbations causing the spasms that occur spontaneously or when provoked by external stimuli. The autonomic nervous system may also be affected.[305,306]

The usual incubation period is from 3 days to 3 weeks, though it may range from one day to several months.[307] In 90 per cent of cases it is less than 15 days.

### Prevention

Tetanus is a preventable disease. The methods available for its prevention include:

1. Active immunisation.
2. Management of wounds in patients.
3. Passive immunisation.

**Active immunisation.**—This is achieved by giving a course of injections of tetanus vaccine which is tetanus toxin made non-toxic by the action of formalin. The course consists of 3 doses of 0·5 ml given at an optimal interval of 6–12 weeks between the first and second doses and 6–12 months between second and third doses,[304] though intervals as short as 4 weeks may be sufficient to provide immunity.[307] The patient responds by making antibodies to tetanus toxin, the immunity taking several weeks to develop. A booster injection at 10-year intervals will maintain immunity.

**Management of wounds in patients.**—Wounds should be thoroughly cleaned, any necrotic material excised and foreign bodies removed. Patients with tetanus-prone wounds should be given adequate antibiotic treatment with penicillin, or erythromycin for those with a history of penicillin sensitivity, though some feel this is unnecessary if tetanus immunoglobulin is given. If the last dose of tetanus toxoid was given more than 5 years before, a booster dose of toxoid should be given.[308]

**Passive immunisation.**—Passive immunisation with human tetanus immunoglobulin should be given to those with tetanus-prone wounds who have either never received a course of tetanus toxoid or whose last injection was more than 10 years ago.[308] The recommended prophylactic dose is 250 units by intramuscular injection or 500 units if the wound is grossly contaminated or more than 24 hours have passed since the injury.[304] Adsorbed tetanus toxoid may be given at the same time to start a course of active immunisation, as long as it is given in the opposite limb with a separate syringe and not more than 250 units of tetanus immunoglobulin have been given.

### Diagnosis

The diagnosis of tetanus is essentially clinical. Patients with tetanus commonly present with trismus, difficulty in swallowing or back pain. Examination will confirm jaw stiffness and show increased tone in the trunk muscles and anterior abdominal wall. Reflex spasms, which may be provoked by external stimuli, occur in 70 per cent of patients and are accompanied by trismus, spinal extension perhaps progressing to opisthotonos and sometimes respiratory difficulty.[309] Local tetanus, in which there is rigidity of the muscle groups near the site of infection, is rare but may be seen in partially immunised patients.

Laboratory investigations are of little help in

reaching a diagnosis. Wound cultures are positive in less than 50 per cent of patients.[307] It has been suggested that serum cholinesterase levels are reduced in tetanus[310] but this has not been confirmed as being of diagnostic value.[311] The levels of tetanus antibody do not increase during an attack of tetanus so this cannot be used as a diagnostic test for the disease.[311]

Localised conditions causing trismus, dyskinetic symptoms caused by drugs such as phenothiazines or metoclopramide, tetany caused by hysterical hyperventilation or hypocalcaemia and strychnine poisoning can mimic the symptoms of tetanus.[312] Differentiation may be difficult, particularly since very few clinicians in developed countries see more than an occasional case.

### Management

Tetanus can progress very rapidly and sudden severe spasms needing immediate paralysis and intubation are well recognised. For this reason, patients with tetanus should be managed in an ICU. Cases of tetanus have been graded as:

*Mild (grade 1)* with no dysphagia or respiratory difficulty.

*Moderate (grade 2)* with more pronounced spasticity and some interference with swallowing or respiration.

*Severe (grade 3a)* with gross spasticity and major spasms requiring paralysis and artificial ventilation.

*Very severe (grade 3b)* with evidence of autonomic dysfunction as well.

**Neutralisation of toxin.**—Human tetanus immunoglobulin (HTIG) is given to neutralise toxin that is outside the nervous system. HTIG 500–1000 units is given intramuscularly or by slow intravenous injection. The usual doses of HTIG have no effect on the toxin that is causing clinical effects or has already penetrated the central nervous system. Therefore, it acts only on toxin present or subsequently formed in the wound or that which has yet to be taken up by the central nervous system.[313] Some studies have suggested that some of the unbound toxin within the central nervous system may be neutralised by large doses (10,000 units) given intravenously or by smaller doses given intrathecally.[304] Gupta and others[314] found that 250 units of HTIG given intrathecally reduced the incidence of progression of the disease and also the number of deaths when given to patients with symptoms of early tetanus but it appears to have little effect when given later.

**Wound treatment.**—The wound is debrided to remove toxin-producing organisms and the anaerobic environment in which they can survive and multiply. HTIG must be given before débridement because toxin will be released into the blood stream during surgical manipulation. The material excised is sent for bacteriological culture.

Antibiotics are given to destroy any remaining organisms. Benzyl-penicillin 10 megaunits per day for at least 4 days is the drug of choice. Erythromycin, tetracycline and chloramphenicol are also effective.[307]

**Control of rigidity and spasms.**—Spasms may be provoked by noise, movement or injections and all of these should be kept to a minimum. Traditionally, patients with tetanus are nursed in a quiet, semi-darkened room with the minimum of interference.

Diazepam has been considered by many to be the drug of choice for the muscular rigidity seen in tetanus. The dose is titrated against its effect, the range being 2–20 mg every 1 to 8 hours.[307] In mild cases, sedation with diazepam may be all that is required. The long-acting barbiturates have also been used to provide sedation and chlorpromazine may be used with either barbiturates or diazepam. Sedation will not prevent reflex spasms and treating more severe cases with sedatives alone results in an oversedated patient unable to protect his airway.

Paralysis and ventilation is indicated when rigidity and spasms are not controlled by sedation. A tracheostomy is required for long-term ventilation and may be performed early if dysphagia is a prominent problem. A tracheostomy also protects against the effects of laryngeal spasm.

Paralysis is maintained by regular doses of tubocurarine. Alcuronium and pancuronium have also been used and may be preferred in patients with a tendency to hypotension. Pancuronium, however, may provoke tachycardia and hypertension.[315] Adequate sedation during the period of paralysis and ventilation is essential both for humanitarian reasons and to reduce the incidence of autonomic disturbance.

**Autonomic disturbance.**—A variety of autonomic disturbances have been described in patients with severe tetanus. These include tachy- and bradycardia, labile hypertension, peripheral vasoconstriction, cardiac dysrhythmias, profuse sweating and hyperpyrexia. Other causes for these symptoms and signs, such as pulmonary embolism, sepsis, pneumothorax, haemorrhage or an acute abdomen from perforation of a viscus, must first be excluded. The manifestations of sympathetic overactivity can be treated by alpha- and beta-adrenergic blocking drugs, the dosage being titrated against the cardiovascular effects. Propranolol has been widely used to control tachycardia, but has been associated with a number of fatal or near fatal episodes of excessive bradycardia.[302] Phentolamine or phenoxybenzamine can be used in the control of hypertensive episodes.

Labetolol, a drug with both alpha- and beta-adrenergic blocking activity, may be particularly suited for controlling the effects of sympathetic overactivity in tetanus and has been shown to be effective.[316]

An alternative approach, also used with success, has been to use morphine in either high[317] or low[315] doses as an adjunct to sedation. The reason for its success is not entirely clear but it is probable that it acts centrally to reduce sympathetic tone.

Hypotension and bradycardia are also well-recognised complications of tetanus.[318] Hypotension will usually respond to simple measures such as stimulating the patient, tilting the patient head-down or increasing the arterial carbon dioxide tension by a reduction in alveolar ventilation. Episodes of bradycardia usually respond to atropine, but if recurrent and profound, temporary demand pacing is safer.[306]

**Nutrition and fluid balance.**—Oxygen consumption rises significantly in tetanus, reflecting an increase in metabolic rate.[319] At the same time there is often an ileus or failure of gastric emptying caused by drugs or perhaps secondary to disturbances of autonomic function. Parenteral nutrition has been used to overcome this problem and prevent malnutrition[320] but in practice it is nearly always possible to provide adequate nutrition by the enteral route.

Problems with fluid balance may occur due to the unmeasured losses of profuse sweating, or sodium and water retention may cause severe peripheral oedema.[303]

**Physiotherapy and general care.**—Patients with tetanus may require prolonged periods of sedation and ventilation. Respiratory complications are particularly common, in one series accounting for three-quarters of the deaths.[303] Chest physiotherapy is essential to keep the chest clear of secretions and prevent atelectasis.

Patients with tetanus require the full range of general care available in an intensive care unit (see above).

### Prognosis

With the full facilities of a modern intensive care unit the prognosis for even severe tetanus is relatively good. Results from England have shown a 10 per cent mortality related to the episode of tetanus from one centre[303] and two deaths in 34 cases from another.[302] Higher mortality rates are associated with the extremes of age, a short incubation and the occurrence of autonomic dysfunction.[307] From other countries, higher mortality rates in the range 40–60 per cent have been reported[307] but most of these date from the 1960s and early 1970s. In a more recent series of 233 cases from Venezuela the mortality was only 11 per cent.[321]

Patients who have had tetanus do not develop immunity and a full course of active immunisation must be given to prevent recurrence.

## GUILLAIN-BARRÉ SYNDROME

The Guillain-Barré syndrome—a number of synonyms are used including Landry Guillain-Barré-Strohl syndrome, acute post-infective polyneuritis or post-infective polyradiculopathy—is an acute diffuse disorder of the nervous system involving the spinal roots, peripheral nerves and sometimes the cranial nerves. Some of the more controversial aspects and recent developments were discussed at a conference devoted to the syndrome in 1980.[322]

The history of the syndrome was reviewed by Ravn.[323] Ten cases of a syndrome were described by Landry in 1859 with clinical features similar to those described by Guillain, Barré and Strohl in 1916, who were the first to demonstrate the characteristic elevation of cerebrospinal fluid protein levels in the absence of increased cellularity. Guillain-Barré syndrome (GBS) is thought to be a lymphocyte-mediated hypersensitivity reaction to peripheral nervous system antigens.[324] The trigger for the hypersensitivity reaction is unclear but it may be viral. After the 1976 influenza vaccination programme in the USA which employed A-

New Jersey (swine) vaccine there was an excess of cases of the Guillain-Barré syndrome with an onset 2 to 3 weeks after vaccination. This has not been seen after subsequent influenza vaccination programs.[325]

Guillain, and subsequently others[326] have suggested that the syndrome should be restricted to those who satisfy the following clinical criteria:

1. The syndrome often, but not invariably, begins 1 to 3 weeks after an infective episode.
2. Dysaesthesias of the feet, hands, or both precede the onset of paralysis.
3. Rapid onset of symmetrical loss of power, sometimes involving cranial nerves, with loss of or diminished tendon reflexes.
4. Minimal objective sensory loss, usually of "glove and stocking" distribution.
5. Sparing of direct involvement of the bladder.

It was also suggested that recovery should begin within 3 weeks and continue without relapse to be complete by 6 months, but clinically identical cases with similar laboratory findings are seen in which recovery is more prolonged and less complete than is strictly compatible with the criteria.

### Diagnosis

The clinical diagnosis is supported by a cerebrospinal fluid protein content greater than 0·4 g/l with a cell count less than $10\times10^3$/l. Electromyography shows a reduced interference pattern in affected muscles with fibrillation potentials developing after 3 to 4 weeks. Nerve conduction studies showed marked slowing where the segment of nerve investigated was affected by the disease.[327] Pathologically, the syndrome is characterised by segmental demyelination of peripheral nerves.

### Management

The natural history of the disease is to run a self-limiting course followed by improvement and the value of any specific treatment is at present unproven. Management therefore consists largely of supportive and symptomatic measures. It might be expected that the mortality from such a self-limiting condition would approach zero but this has not been the case. Review of 10 reported series, totalling 425 patients, showed a mortality as high as 22 per cent,[323] but more recently this has been considerably reduced, mainly because of improved management of those requiring artificial ventilation. The majority of patients with GBS have a relatively mild form and can be managed perfectly adequately in a general ward. In one series this comprised 57 per cent of the total.[328] Intercostal, phrenic or cranial nerve involvement causing difficulty in breathing or swallowing due to centripetal spread of paralysis is an indication for admission to an ICU.

The ICU management of these more severely affected patients consists of:

1. **Monitoring of respiratory function.**—Clinical assessment and repeated measurement of vital capacity will show when ventilatory failure is becoming imminent. If the vital capacity falls below 1·5 ml/kg body weight patients experience difficulty in producing an effective cough. This predisposes to the retention of secretions and lobar collapse or infection. Frequently it is apparent to both patient and doctor that ventilation is becoming progressively less adequate and that intubation and ventilation are indicated. The chest x-ray and arterial blood gas analysis provide further information about respiratory problems.
2. **Monitoring of bulbar function.**—Bulbar weakness causes difficulty with swallowing and laryngeal function. These patients are at risk of aspirating food, drink or other material from the pharynx into the lungs. They may also be unable to cough effectively because the vocal cords do not fully adduct, this being necessary to achieve the ejection velocity of a proper cough.
3. **Monitoring of skeletal muscle function.**—This is most easily done by muscle charting, and performed at intervals provides a guide to the patient's progress.
4. **Intubation and ventilation when necessary.**—The indications being respiratory failure or airway protection. The form of assisted ventilation, that is, IMV or IPPV and whether PEEP is required, will depend on the nature and extent of the patient's respiratory problems. Although these patients can be managed with an endotracheal tube they are generally considered for early tracheostomy because this is more comfortable for the patient, reduces the need for sedation, is easier to aspirate and facilitates weaning from ventilation.
5. **General care, monitoring and prophylactic**

**measures:** as outlined in the relevant sections. Skin care and physiotherapy for both chest and skeletal muscles and joints is particularly important. Psychological problems are common. Patients with GBS require a lot of reassurance and must get adequate rest and sleep. The frustration of being unable to communicate easily can be imagined, as the fully conscious patient may require intubation for a period of weeks while their limbs are too weak for writing messages or using indicator boards. Where possible, the patient should be involved in decision making and occupational therapy, television, music, radio programmes and visitors are all of tremendous importance.

6. **Steroids** have been used but most reports show that they do not significantly alter the course of the disease,[328] although they may be useful in the small group of patients who develop a relapsing polyneuropathy.[329]
7. **Plasmapheresis** has been used with encouraging results in some cases. The theoretical reason for using plasma exchange is the demonstration of antibody and complement activity against peripheral nerves in the patients with GBS. Controlled, multicentre trials are currently being performed to assess this method of treatment.

### Complications

Major complications are most common in those who develop respiratory failure[328] Those related to respiratory failure include *pneumonia*, *atelectasis*, *pulmonary barotrauma* and the *complications of intubation and tracheostomy*. Prolonged immobilisation predisposes to *thromboembolism* so that heparin prophylaxis is particularly important.

The other reported complications associated with GBS have been reviewed by King & Jacobs.[330] These include:

*Poor nutrition* because of general malaise and difficulty in swallowing. A fine-bore feeding tube should be passed if it is clear that the amount of food and drink that can be managed is inadequate.

*Autonomic dysfunction* with an abnormally labile blood pressure[331] or hypertension and tachydysrhythmias.[328] Autonomic dysfunction may be a cause for sudden death in patients with GBS.[332]

*Diabetes insipidus*.[333]

*Inappropriate ADH secretion*.[328, 334]

*Acute glomerulonephritis*.[335]

*Painful paraesthesiae* are not uncommon, particularly during the recovery period, and may be difficult to treat. Mild analgesics, anti-inflammatory agents, opiate analgesics, benzodiazepines and transcutaneous nerve stimulation can be tried but on occasions the pain fails to respond to any of these. Carbamazepine is sometimes effective in more resistant cases.

### Prognosis

As originally defined, persistent neurological deficit would exclude a diagnosis of GBS, but in most series of patients with a clinically indistinguishable syndrome some patients have been left with residual neurological deficit. If very minor abnormalities are included this proportion may be as high as 57 per cent,[336] but only about 5 per cent have significant neurological damage.

Occasional cases of a similar polyneuropathy follow a relapsing course.[329]

## POISONING AND OVERDOSE

Poisoning and drug overdose are among the most common causes for hospital admission. In depressed urban areas intentional drug overdose may be the single most common cause for admission to an ICU. In the majority of cases the effects of the drug wear off as it is eliminated from the body. In these patients a conservative approach with careful monitoring and management of circulatory or respiratory failure is all that is required.[337] Other drugs and poisons, such as cyanide, paracetamol and paraquat, have a toxic effect on one or more body tissues. A more aggressive approach to treatment, including measures to increase the rate of elimination or giving a specific antidote, must be considered when these have been taken.

Many countries now have a poisons information service based on major regional centres. The telephone number of the nearest office of this service should be available in every accident and emergency department and every ICU. Often the poisons information service is able to supply information about the contents of commercial products and the management of the less common causes of poisoning, such as plants and fungi.

**Principles of Management**

The principles of management of poisoning and drug overdose have been considered by Wright,[337] Vale[338] and Locket.[339]

**Diagnosis.**—Poisoning or drug overdose should be suspected in any unconscious patient. Other causes for coma must be excluded, but often the circumstances under which the patient is found will suggest that poisoning or drug overdose are likely. While empty bottles can be helpful they may also be misleading as when planted deliberately by a patient making a serious suicide attempt.

Samples of blood, urine and gastric contents should be taken for toxicological analysis and may help to identify the drug or poison involved. This analysis rarely needs to be done as an emergency but paracetamol and salicylate overdose are two examples where such analysis and estimation of plasma levels will affect management. The toxic concentrations of some of the drugs most commonly taken in overdose are shown in Table 14. Frequently, more than one drug has been taken, often in combination with alcohol.

10/TABLE 14
TOXIC PLASMA LEVELS OF SOME OF THE DRUGS MORE COMMONLY TAKEN IN OVERDOSE.

| *Drug* | *Toxic plasma concentration (mg/l)* |
|---|---|
| Amitriptylline | > 1 |
| Short-acting barbiturates | >10 |
| Medium-acting barbiturates | >30 |
| Long-acting barbiturates | >70 |
| Diazepam | > 5 |
| Paracetamol | Time dependent—see text |
| Salicylates | >400 |

**Initial management.**—The first steps are to ensure that the patient has a clear airway, is breathing adequately and has an adequate blood pressure. If the patient is unable to protect his airway or is breathing inadequately he should be intubated with a cuffed endotracheal tube and ventilated. All but the least affected patients should have an intravenous cannula inserted so that drugs can be given quickly if their condition deteriorates.

More detailed clinical examination must include:

- measurement of body temperature: hypothermia is common in prolonged unconsciousness caused by sedatives;
- a search for venepuncture marks;
- a search for pressure lesions or blisters;
- examination of the lips and mouth for signs of burns caused by corrosives;
- smelling for the characteristic odour of alcohol, organophosphates or petroleum products.

**Measures to Decrease Absorption**

*Induced emesis* should only be used in a fully conscious patient and is contra-indicated if corrosives or petroleum products have been swallowed. Ipecacuanha syrup is the most commonly used emetic in a dose ranging from 15 ml at 1 year to 50 ml in adults. The dose can be repeated after 30 minutes if the patient fails to vomit.

*Gastric lavage* should not be performed if corrosives have been swallowed because of the risk of perforation. Petroleum products may cause a severe pneumonitis if aspirated into the lungs. If there is any impairment of consciousness whatsoever an endotracheal tube is inserted to protect the airway before a lubricated wide-bore tube is passed into the stomach. About 250 to 300 ml of tap water is run into the stomach and then allowed to drain out. This is repeated until the drain fluid is clear. Gastric lavage is usually unnecessary if the poison or overdose has been taken more than 4 hours before the patient is seen. Exceptions are salicylates and amitriptyline overdose because of delayed gastric emptying, and paracetamol and paraquat because of the importance of reducing the total amount absorbed.

*Adsorption*: 50 grams of powdered activated charcoal mixed with water and washed in through the gastric lavage tube will bind to any residual drug. An extensive list of drugs adsorbed by activated charcoal has been compiled by Greensher and colleagues.[340]

*Faecuresis* can be used to clear the small bowel before absorption is complete. Mannitol 20 per cent solution may be used with 500 ml being given through a nasogastric tube over 5–10 minutes followed by a further 500 ml over the next hour. If this method is used the patient must be observed closely for fluid and electrolyte imbalance.

*Chelating agents*, such as desferrioxamine 5

grams in 50 ml of water for iron poisoning or dimercaprol for heavy-metal poisoning, chelate the toxic substance in the bowel so making it unavailable for absorption.

*Topical methods*: contaminated clothing is removed and the skin thoroughly washed if the toxic substance can be absorbed by this route. Examples of such substances are the organophosphate compounds and chlorinated insecticides.

**Measures to Increase Elimination**

*Forced diuresis* is rarely necessary and for most cases the hazards of this method of treatment outweigh the benefits. It may, however, have a place in the management of severe long-acting barbiturate overdose and a moderate induced diuresis should be used for cases of salicylate poisoning. Excretion of barbiturates and salicylates can be increased by alkalinising the urine to a pH of 7·5–8·5 by giving bicarbonate. Acidification of urine to a pH of 5·5–6·5 by intravenous arginine hydrochloride or ammonium chloride has a limited application in severe amphetamine poisoning.

*Dialysis* is rarely indicated but can be useful in patients with renal failure and to increase the elimination rate of lithium and other dialysable poisons particularly if there is evidence of clinical deterioration despite adequate treatment.[341]

*Haemoperfusion* may be used in cases of a very severe poisoning but *should be reserved for those that fail to improve despite maximal supportive measures* and those that develop serious complications.[342] Early attempts at haemoperfusion through activated charcoal columns caused complications such as embolism, coagulopathy, leukopaenia and fever. These are largely overcome by coating the charcoal with an acrylic hydrogel, similar to that from which soft contact lenses are made. Haemoperfusion appears to be the best method available for increasing the elimination of barbiturates, glutethamide, methaqualone, paraquat and salicylates.

*Oxygen* should be given in the highest possible concentration to patients with carbon monoxide poisoning. In severe cases hyperbaric oxygen therapy may be useful.[343]

**Antidotes and Agents to Decrease Toxicity**

Specific antidotes or agents that decrease toxicity are available for some poisons or drug overdoses. When these are available they should be used. Some examples are shown below and are considered more fully in the section on specific drugs and poisons.

Paracetamol—N-acetylcysteine or methionine
Narcotic analgesics—naloxone
Organophosphates—atropine and pralidoxime
Methyl alcohol—ethyl alcohol
Heavy metals—chelating agents

**Supportive Measures and Management of Complications**

*Endotracheal intubation* should be performed if an adequate airway cannot be maintained, ventilation is inadequate or if the patient is drowsy and is to have a gastric lavage. If the patient does not require intubation but is drowsy or unconscious they should be nursed in the "coma" or "recovery" position.

*Ventilation*.—The most common indications for artificial ventilation are respiratory failure or severe pulmonary aspiration. Occasionally patients who have taken a drug overdose develop pulmonary oedema. This has been reported in association with aspirin and narcotic overdose and must be differentiated from pulmonary oedema caused by fluid overload during forced diuresis, myocardial depression and pulmonary aspiration. Ventilation of patients who have taken a drug overdose should follow normal principles.

*Correction of hypotension*.—Mild hypotension is common after a variety of drug overdoses. If the patient is warm, well perfused and passing adequate amounts of urine no specific treatment is needed. Moderate or severe hypotension should be treated on the same principles as "shock" from any other cause (p. 319). Usually the hypotension responds to intravenous infusion of fluids. This should be monitored in the more severe cases by CVP measurements. Pulmonary wedge pressure measurements are more reliable than the CVP if there is clinical or radiological evidence of pulmonary oedema.

*Dysrhythmias*.—The ECG should be monitored if a dysrhythmogenic drug or poison has been taken. This includes tricyclic antidepressants, chloral hydrate, digoxin and cholinesterase inhibitors. If dysrhythmias occur they are treated in the usual way.

*Renal dysfunction* is usually secondary to hypotension but can also be caused by nephrotoxic drugs and poisons.

*Hepatic dysfunction* may be caused by prolonged hypotension, hypoxaemia or by direct toxic effects such as those produced by paracetamol metabolites.

*Convulsions*. — Tricyclic antidepressants, methaqualone with diphenhydramine—"Mandrax", phenothiazines and antihistamines when taken in overdose can cause convulsions. Convulsions can usually be controlled with diazepam or clonazepam. In the more resistant cases phenytoin or barbiturates may be used.

Physostigmine 1–2 mg intravenously can stop convulsions associated with an overdose of tricyclic antidepressants.

The oculogyric crises and bizarre extrapyramidal side-effects of phenothiazine overdose may resemble convulsions. These can be controlled with benztropine.

*Hypothermia*: coma, vasodilatation, lowered metabolic rate and exposure can all contribute to this problem. Passive rewarming with a "space blanket", warmed infusion fluids and warmed humidified gases are usually sufficient.

*Hyperthermia* may occur when an overdose of tricyclic antidepressants, salicylates or atropine has been taken. The patient should be actively cooled.

*General care*.—Patients who have taken a drug overdose need the full care afforded to any other comatose patient. This includes skin, eyes, mouth and bladder care and regular physiotherapy.

### Poisoning and Overdose in Children

Most cases of poisoning and drug overdose in children occur in the under 4 age group. Plants and berries are responsible for some of the cases of poisoning but given the natural curiosity of children this can be difficult to prevent. Poisoning with household products or drugs on the other hand should be preventable by storing these out of the reach of children, in child proof cabinets and having "child proof" seals on the containers.

Poisoning or drug overdose in older children is more likely to be a manifestation of serious psychopathology.[344]

### Psychiatric Aspects

Psychiatric aspects of drug overdose in adults have been reviewed by Burrows and Harari.[345] A majority of cases are associated with personality disorders or are a reaction to an acute personal crisis. Affective and psychotic disorders are found in less than half of the patients referred because of self poisoning.

In many cases the objective of self poisoning was not suicide but a reaction to a situation seen as being intolerable. The term "parasuicide" has been used to describe these cases.

In Britain the Department of Health has recommended that all cases of deliberate self poisoning should be referred to a psychiatrist for assessment. In practice there appears to be no particular advantage in doing this[346] but obviously patients should be referred to a psychiatrist for further treatment if they have a mental disorder.

Patients admitted to an intensive care unit because of self poisoning may evoke feelings of hostility from the medical and nursing staff particularly since they may be noisy, aggressive and unco-operative and are rarely appreciative of the efforts being made on their behalf. While these feelings of hostility can be difficult to overcome it is important that the patients are not denied normal standards of care. Drug overdose is now such a common cause for admission to an ICU that all those working there should understand something of the psychopathology of self poisoning and try to develop a sympathetic attitude to these patients, difficult as it may be.

## Prognosis

The prognosis for patients admitted to hospital after a drug overdose is excellent unless hypoxic brain damage has occurred before admission or there is serious intercurrent disease. In one series of 1,166 admissions the mortality was 0·4 per cent.[337] The more severe cases requiring admission to an ICU have a higher mortality, but the prognosis is still good unless the patient has hypoxic brain damage.[347]

The psychiatric prognosis is that of the underlying condition. About 30 per cent of patients make further attempts at suicide or "parasuicide" within a year.[346]

Some poisons are associated with a poor

prognosis if tissue damage occurs. Paracetamol and paraquat are examples of this.

### Specific Treatment

Information concerning the specific treatment of drugs taken in overdose and ingested poisons can often be found in the manufacturer's product literature. Further information is available from Poisons Information Centres and is reviewed for some of the more common drugs and poisons by Krapez and Cole.[348]

**Barbiturates**

Hypotension, hypothermia and blistering of the skin are common complications. The hypotension is usually caused by peripheral vasodilatation and responds to infusion of colloid. Coma and respiratory depression are treated with full supportive measures until the drug is excreted. Forced alkaline diuresis is rarely needed (see p. 344).

**Benzodiazepines**

The benzodiazepines are among the more common causes of self poisoning. They have a high therapeutic ratio and no specific measures other than general supportive treatment are needed.

**Chloral Hydrate**

Chloral compounds are being used more commonly as hypnotics because of the reduction in prescribing barbiturates. Respiratory and central nervous system depression are seen, but the more serious complications of chloral overdose are hypotension and cardiac dysrhythmias. Hypotension may be severe and is associated with marked depression of myocardial function. Pulmonary oedema can occur if too much fluid is infused so that the CVP or PAWP should be carefully monitored. If the patient is hypotensive with a high CVP/PAWP a dopamine infusion should be started to maintain cardiac output and urine output.

Ventricular dysrhythmias are managed in a conventional manner. Lignocaine will usually suppress them.

**Corrosives**

Ingestion of strong acids and alkalies causes burns of the lips, mouth, tongue, pharynx, oesophagus and upper gastro-intestinal tract. These can be very mutilating and painful. Early complications include upper airway obstruction, and gastric necrosis, perforation and generalised chemical peritonitis. The patient may become shocked because of the extensive tissue damage.

Gastric lavage and emesis are contra-indicated. The corrosive should be diluted by drinking water or milk as soon as possible but intractable vomiting can make it hard to keep it down. Milk of magnesia can be given to neutralise acid and 1 per cent acetic acid or vinegar for alkalies but most authorities do not advocate the use of neutralising agents because of the danger of further damage from the heat of reaction.[349] Steroids—prednisolone 2 mg/kg body weight per day—have been recommended to reduce late stricture formation. Early fibreoptic oesophago-gastroscopy can be useful in assessing the extent of the injury.[350,351] Even if the whole stomach has become necrotic early aggressive surgical treatment can result in survival.[352]

Late complications include oesophageal stricture and pyloric stenosis.

Complications seen with some corrosives include:

- Oxalic acid—found in bleaches and metal cleaners may cause hypocalcaemia.
- Ammonia—pulmonary oedema is common because of its high volatility.
- Phenol
  - salicylate-like effects;
  - methaemoglobinaemia;
  - renal and hepatic dysfunction.

**Cyanide**

Potassium and sodium cyanides are corrosive. The onset of cyanide poisoning is very rapid and it is likely that a patient will be drowsy or unconscious on admission to hospital if a significant amount has been swallowed. The odour of "bitter almonds" is characteristic. Other diagnostic clues are a high oxygen saturation in venous blood and lactic acidosis. General management includes maintaining the airway, adequate oxygenation and correction of hypotension. Specific treatment includes:

*Amyl nitrite inhalation*: ampoules are crushed into gauze and one ampoule given over 15 sec. every 2 to 3 minutes, while a sodium nitrite infusion is prepared.

*Sodium nitrite*: 300 mg intravenously over 3 minutes for adults followed by:

*Sodium thiosulphate*: 12·5 g infused over 10 minutes in adults. About 250 mg/kg is used in children.

*Dicobalt tetracemate* ("Kelocyanor"): 300 mg is given intravenously in cases of definite cyanide poisoning and repeated after 2 minutes if there are no adverse effects. It may cause respiratory and cardiovascular depression.

Blood must be taken for methaemoglobin estimation as soon as these drugs have been given. A methaemoglobin level of 26 per cent is optimum. If the level is greater than 40 per cent, 1 mg/kg body weight of methylene blue is given over 5 to 10 minutes and the methaemoglobin level remeasured. The blood pressure must be measured frequently during treatment, particularly while the nitrites are being given. Nitrite treatment should be stopped if the systolic blood pressure falls below 80 mm Hg.

Cyanide poisoning can cause a profound lactic acidosis. This should be corrected by sodium bicarbonate and monitored by arterial blood gas measurements. As much as 500 ml or more of 8·4 per cent sodium bicarbonate may be needed.

The management of cyanide poisoning is considered in more detail by Naughton.[353]

**Monoamine Oxidase Inhibitors**

The clinical presentation of monoamine oxidase inhibitor (MAOI) overdose is very variable. While tachycardia, sweating, hyperpyrexia, and signs of CNS stimulation usually predominate, CNS depression and coma can occur. Similarly, while hypertension is more common, patients may become hypotensive.

Hypertension can be produced by deliberate eating of a tyramine-containing food that patients taking MAOI's are instructed to avoid. Diazoxide 150–300 mg intravenously or sodium nitroprusside infusion can be used to return the blood pressure to normal levels.

Gastric lavage and activated charcoal are useful in reducing absorption of MAOI's. Management is otherwise limited to general supportive measures and the treatment of complications as they arise. Problems can occur because of interactions between MAOI's and other drugs. All CNS depressants, including barbiturates, narcotics and phenothiazines are potentiated by MAOI's. If a patient becomes hypotensive and a catecholamine infusion is needed, the response must be very closely monitored. Indirect pressor amines should be avoided.

**Organophosphates**

Organophosphates are widely available as insecticides. Poisoning may occur chronically or acutely. Chronic poisoning usually occurs through inhalation of insecticide spray by agricultural workers. The symptoms and signs of poisoning are those of cholinergic stimulation: intense salivation, lachrymation, abdominal cramps, diarrhoea and pin-point pupils. There may be progression to respiratory failure, flaccid paralysis, severe bradydysrythmias, coma, convulsions and death. The plasma and red cell cholinesterase are very low or undetectable.

The management of organophosphate poisoning has been reviewed by Ganendran.[354] Contaminated clothing must be removed and the skin washed to prevent further absorption. Atropine is given in increments of 0·6 mg intravenously until signs of atropine toxicity appear. Surprisingly high doses can be needed to achieve this. Protopam chloride (Pralidoxime; PAM) 1 gm is given intravenously over 10 minutes, and repeated after 30 minutes if there is no improvement in symptoms. Further doses are then given 6-hourly.

Asystole and life-threatening bradycardia can occur without warning, even if the patient has a tachycardia for most of the time. It is therefore important to ensure that adequate amounts of atropine are given. Recurrent bradydysrhythmias may be managed more easily by inserting a transvenous pacing electrode.

**Narcotic Analgesics**

Naloxone is an example of a true pharmacological antagonist. Given intravenously in a dose of 0·2–1·2 mg it reverses the effects of narcotic analgesics including pentazocine, codeine and dextropropoxyphene. Naloxone has a short half-life so patients must be closely observed and further doses given as required.

If naloxone is given to narcotic addicts it can precipitate an acute withdrawal reaction.

**Paracetamol**

Paracetamol is a widely available analgesic. There are many proprietary preparations that contain paracetamol and it forms part of the compound analgesic tablets with codeine and dextropropoxyphene that are so frequently prescribed. The most serious and potentially fatal complication of paracetamol overdose is acute centrilobular hepatic necrosis. Hepatic damage may follow absorption of 10 grams or more in adults.

Paracetamol is metabolised by the liver, only 4 per cent being excreted unchanged in the urine. During metabolism a highly reactive intermediate metabolite is formed. Normally this is only present in small amounts and is rapidly conjugated with glutathione. When an overdose of paracetamol has been taken the hepatocyte is unable to synthesise glutathione quickly enough and the toxic metabolite binds irreversibly to cell components causing necrosis.[355]

During the first hours after an overdose of paracetamol the only symptoms are anorexia, nausea and vomiting, but early assessment of the severity of poisoning is vital because treatment becomes less effective with time. The risk of liver damage can be assessed from the plasma paracetamol level as shown in Fig. 12.

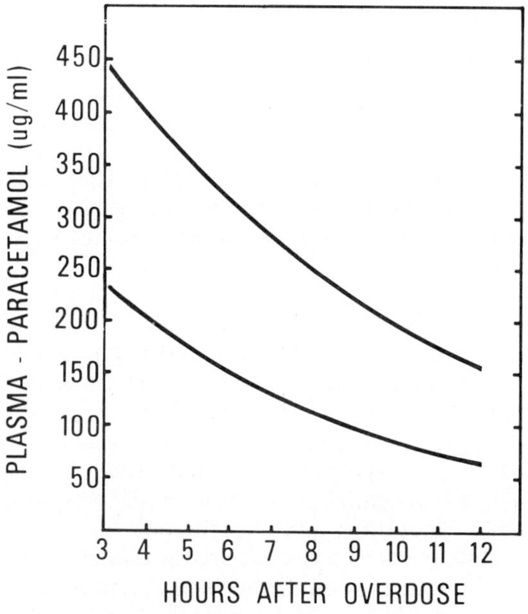


10/Fig. 12.—The risk of liver damage to plasma paracetamol levels and the time from ingestion. (Courtesy of Drs. L. F. Prescott, J. Park, G. R. Sutherland, I. J. Smith and A. T. Proudfoot, 1976, and the Editors of the *Lancet*.[432])

Paracetamol is rapidly absorbed from the stomach and upper gastro-intestinal tract but all those who are seen within a few hours of taking an overdose and those in coma should have gastric lavage. Currently, the treatment of choice is intravenous N-acetylcysteine.[356] This acts as a sulphydryl donor to conjugate the toxic metabolite. The initial dose is 150 mg/kg body weight diluted in 200 ml of 5 per cent dextrose and infused over 15 minutes followed by 50 mg/kg in 500 ml of 5 per cent dextrose over 4 hours and 100 mg/kg in 1000 ml of 5 per cent dextrose over the next 16 hours, this amounting to 300 mg/kg body weight over 20 hours. N-acetylcysteine is most effective when given less than 8 hours after the paracetamol has been taken, but still offers some protection up to 15 hours. If there is any doubt about the timing of the overdose, N-acetylcysteine should be given because it has few side-effects but is potentially of great benefit.

Other compounds that have been used in paracetamol overdose include cysteine, cysteamine, methionine, penicillamine and dimercaprol. These have been less effective or had more side-effects than N-acetylcysteine. Early intervention with specific therapy has meant that severe liver damage should be confined to those who present late.[357] If hepatic failure occurs it is treated in the conventional way.

**Paraquat**

Paraquat is a herbicide. When sprayed on green foliage it acts only in the presence of sun light to kill the plant. It has no residual action and is deactivated on contact with soil. Two formulations are available: a solution containing 20 per cent paraquat ("Gramoxone") and granules containing 2·5 per cent paraquat in a base consisting mainly of magnesium sulphate. Paraquat can be absorbed through the skin or bronchial mucosa but serious poisoning is only seen when it has been swallowed. The 20 per cent solution is corrosive and causes burns to the lips, mouth, pharynx and oesophagus when taken by mouth.

The clinical course depends on the amount taken. If a large volume of the concentrate is swallowed shock, convulsions, metabolic acidosis, pulmonary oedema and cardiac failure cause death within 6 to 24 hours. When smaller amounts of concentrate are swallowed vomiting, abdominal discomfort, dysphagia and diarrhoea usually follow. Occasionally there are few early symptoms even though a lethal dose has been swallowed.[358] The early symptoms settle within 24 hours or so and are followed by desquamation of the mouth and pharynx, deteriorating renal and hepatic function and increasing breathlessness. Renal function can be affected within 12 hours of paraquat ingestion. Excretion of paraquat is dependent on renal tubular function, so renal tubular damage effectively limits or prevents elimination of the poison. Liver function is affected by hepatocellular damage but is not a major problem. The most serious complication of paraquat poisoning is its effect on the lungs. Within two to three days a chemical alveolitis develops with alveolar oedema and haemorrhage. This is followed within 5 to 40 days by proliferation of fibroblasts within the alveoli and progressive lung fibrosis.[355] Increasing respiratory failure usually ends in death from hypoxaemia. Such severe symptoms are unusual if the granular form of paraquat has been taken though there may be transient mild renal failure. Lung fibrosis and death have occurred up to six weeks after ingestion of only 60 grams of granules, equivalent to 1·5 grams of paraquat.

All cases of paraquat poisoning must be regarded seriously and treated vigorously no matter how small the quantity thought to have been swallowed. A simple urine test will confirm that poisoning has occurred.[359] Gastric aspiration and lavage is followed by purging of the gastro-intestinal tract. It is important that this is done as soon as possible and preferably within four hours of ingestion. Adults are given 200 ml of 20 per cent mannitol followed by 1 litre of a 15–30 per cent suspension of Fuller's earth in water (or 70 grams of bentonite in 100 ml of glycerol made up to 1000 ml with water, if Fuller's earth is unavailable). These solutions must be made up freshly. Additional 100 ml doses of Fuller's earth are given hourly with 15 grams of magnesium sulphate until the stools are seen to contain Fuller's earth. Considerable amounts of fluid and electrolytes can be lost with this treatment. These losses should be replaced by intravenous infusion. Other treatments that have been used in paraquat poisoning include:

- forced diuresis.[359] This is often ineffective and more than usually hazardous because of the high incidence of renal failure;
- dialysis,
- haemoperfusion through activated charcoal or a cation exchange resin.[360]

Haemoperfusion seems the most promising of these methods and should be used within 48 hours if significant amounts of paraquat have been absorbed. Plasma paraquat concentrations provide a guide to the outcome[361] but with haemoperfusion, survival has been reported despite considerably higher plasma levels.[362] Overall mortality rates after ingestion have been 70 per cent for concentrate and 10 per cent for granules.

Renal failure can be managed by peritoneal dialysis or haemodialysis. Respiratory failure is a more difficult management problem because oxygen appears to enhance the pulmonary toxicity of paraquat. Some authors have recommended the use of hypoxic gas mixtures but this can be hazardous and it is preferable to delay the use of oxygen as long as possible and use the lowest possible concentrations.

**Salicylates**

As little as 10 grams of aspirin can be fatal but survival has been reported after 150 grams have been taken. Symptoms of poisoning such as tinnitus, deafness, sweating, hyperventilation and vasodilatation and pyrexia become increasingly common with plasma salicylate concentrations above 350 mg/litre. Salicylates rarely cause loss of consciousness so if the patient is comatose it is likely that more than one drug has been taken.

The acid-base disturbances caused by salicylate are complex. In children there is usually a metabolic acidosis. In adults a mixed metabolic acidosis and respiratory alkalosis is the usual finding with the latter predominating.[355]

Salicylates also have a complex effect on blood sugar concentrations. Both hyper- and hypoglycaemia have been reported. Hypoglycaemia, which may be profound, is especially common in children. Treatment is guided by blood sugar measurements but children who loose consciousness or become drowsy after aspirin poisoning should be given dextrose immediately.

Most patients who have taken salicylates alone are fully conscious. Absorption can be decreased by inducing the patient to vomit or by gastric aspiration and lavage.

If the patient is hyperventilating or the plasma

salicylate level is greater than 500 mg/litre forced alkaline diuresis should be considered as a means of increasing the rate of excretion. This is contra-indicated if there is renal failure or pulmonary oedema but can generally be used safely in otherwise healthy patients. A regimen that has been used successfully is:

- 4 per cent dextrose with 0·18 per cent saline 1·5 litres/hour
- 8·4 per cent sodium bicarbonate 150 ml/hour
- added potassium to maintain a normal plasma concentration.

The aim is to achieve a urine pH greater than 7 but the blood pH should not exceed 7·6. The CVP should be kept to less than 12 cm of water. Elderly patients and those with a history of heart disease must be observed carefully for signs of left heart failure. The forced diuresis is stopped when the patient clinically improves or the plasma salicylate level falls below 450 mg/litre.

### Tricyclic Antidepressants

There is a wide range of susceptibility to tricyclic antidepressants but as little as 500 mg has caused death in an adult.[363] Tricyclics are rapidly converted to active metabolites which are not measurable. Blood and urine levels therefore do not reflect the severity of the overdose but may be useful in confirming the diagnosis. Potentially serious complications include cardiac dysrhythmias, hypotension, convulsions, coma, respiratory depression and hyperpyrexia.

After gastric aspiration and lavage activated charcoal can be given to absorb any drug remaining in the gastro-intestinal tract. Sinus tachycardia with T-P conjunction is common in tricyclic overdose and needs no specific treatment. Other ECG abnormalities that are seen include widening of the QRS complex and ST and T wave changes. Both tachy- and brady-dysrhythmias can occur with both being seen within a few minutes of one another in some patients. Hypoxia, acidosis and hypokalaemia predispose to dysrhythmias. A mild alkalosis, induced by giving 50 to 100 ml of 8·4 per cent sodium bicarbonate, and giving potassium to keep the level within the normal range, reduces the incidence of dysrhythmias. If dysrhythmias still occur they are treated in the usual way. When particularly troublesome a temporary pacing electrode can be inserted to prevent bradycardia and help to control tachydysrhythmias. Patients who have taken significant quantities of tricyclics should have their ECG monitored for at least 24–48 hours. Occasionally dysrhythmias are seen even later.

The central anticholinergic effects of tricyclic antidepressants can be reversed by physostigmine.[364] The side-effects of physostigmine include convulsions, bradycardia, excessive salivation and bronchorrhoea so it should not be used routinely. In practice, most patients with tricyclic antidepressant overdosage make a full recovery with conservative supportive management so a case can be made for limiting the use of physostigmine to the management of convulsions.

## NUTRITION

Starvation is a common and serious complication of acute illness. The body's reserves of different nutrients are shown in Table 15. For amino acids and carbohydrates the immediate reserves are limited to a few hours. Lawson[365] found that loss of 30 per cent of initial body weight after major surgery or trauma was invariably fatal. Poor nutrition causes poor wound healing, coagulation disorders, altered drug metabolism, reduced enzyme synthesis, decreased tolerance to radiotherapy and chemotherapy[366] and an increased susceptibility to infection.[367]

10/Table 15
Body Reserves of Different Nutrients

| | |
|---|---|
| Amino acids | a few hours |
| Carbohydrate (mainly liver glycogen) | about 12 hours |
| Fat | 27–90 days |
| Thiamine | 30–60 days |
| Ascorbic acid | 60–120 days |
| Niacin | 60–180 days |
| Vitamin A | 90–365 days |
| Iron | 750 days (less if depleted) |
| Iodine | 1000 days |
| Vitamin $B_{12}$ | about 3 years |

The ICU patient almost always has anorexia, gastro-intestinal dysfunction or other problems that make it difficult to maintain a normal food intake. In addition, many will have increased metabolic demands because of the illness or injury that precipitated their admission to the ICU. Surgery, trauma or serious illness are accompanied by endocrine and metabolic changes which, in general, reflect the severity of the illness.[368,369,370] This is reflected by an increase in energy consumption, impaired glucose tolerance and abnormal responses to starvation as compared to healthy or mildly stressed patients.[371] These changes are seen at their most extreme in patients with septicaemia or severe burns.[372,373] The metabolic responses to surgery can be modified by beta-adrenergic blockade[374] and naftidrofuryl.[375] Whether the effect of either of these agents is clinically significant has still to be determined.

Whenever possible adequate nutrition should be encouraged by presenting wholesome appetising meals in a form that can be managed by the patient. However, it may be obvious that eating is impossible or nutritional assessment may show that food intake has been inadequate. Inadequate nutrition for a short period may be preferable to complicated attempts to feed the patient, but the short period must be emphasised. Three or four days should be regarded as a maximum. After this time patients should receive nutritional support.

Three groups of patients may be distinguished:

1. *Malnourished patients with normal or only mildly altered metabolic pathways*.—This group will include:
   - patients with pre-existing disease, for example malabsorption or anorexia nervosa;
   - patients with social or ethnic malnourishment caused, for example, by poverty or religious belief;
   - patients with neurological disorders causing dysphagia;
   - patients with obstruction of the upper gastro-intestinal tract caused by carcinoma of the oesophagus or pylorus;
   - patients with prolonged coma.

   The carbon dioxide production in these patients (a measure of their metabolic rate) is less than 4 ml/kg body weight/minute and urine nitrogen excretion about 10 g/day. Adequate enteral or parenteral feeding can result in a positive nitrogen balance and weight gain.
2. *Moderately stressed patients*.—This group includes many of the patients who will be admitted to an ICU, including those with serious illness, recent trauma or major surgery. Their carbon dioxide production is in the range 4–6 ml/kg/min and urinary nitrogen excretion 10–20 g/day. Without nutritional support these patients will have a period of marked negative nitrogen balance. With optimal nutritional support this can be minimised, but in practice it is found impossible to maintain nitrogen balance until they enter the recovery phase of their illness.
3. *Highly stressed patients* including those with continuing sepsis or major burns. Carbon dioxide production is in excess of 6 ml/kg/min and urinary nitrogen excretion more than 24 g/day. These patients have marked glucose and fat intolerance and appear unable to utilise these fully as energy substrates.[373] If they are given glucose in excess of their ability to metabolise, then in addition to the problem of hyperosmolality caused by the hyperglycaemia, they develop hepatomegaly because of fatty infiltration and produce increased amounts of carbon dioxide.[372] As increased amounts of glucose are infused the respiratory quotient (RQ) rises and beyond an RQ of 1 a relatively small increase in intravenous glucose delivery rate causes a marked increase in RQ and a marked increase in carbon dioxide production in relation to oxygen consumption. To avoid a respiratory acidosis the patient's alveolar ventilation must be increased either spontaneously or by increasing mechanical ventilation with all the consequent effects on other systems. It is impossible to avoid a negative nitrogen balance in these patients and because of the potential dangers of excessive exogenous energy substrates, great care must be taken not to exceed the tolerated quantities.

**Nutritional Assessment**

Up to 50 per cent of patients on surgical wards have been found to be moderately or severely malnourished.[109] Goode[366] has reviewed the available methods of nutritional assessment. In practice, a recent loss of more than 10 per cent of body weight, a serum albumin less than 32 g/l and loss of delayed hypersensitivity reactions to common antigens have identified those with an increased morbidity and mortality after surgery. Serum transferrin levels may also provide a useful guide[376] if direct estimations rather than those derived from measurement of total iron-binding capacity are used.[377] In most cases, however, such measurements are unnecessary, a nutritional history and clinical examination being all that are needed.[378]

Approximate daily requirements for protein, nitrogen, energy and electrolytes are shown in Table 16, but clearly the actual intake may need to be modified to suit the patient, particularly in renal and hepatic failure. A means for estimating the daily nitrogen losses is shown in Table 17.

10/TABLE 16
DAILY REQUIREMENTS FOR PROTEIN NITROGEN, ENERGY AND ELECTROLYTES FOR AN AVERAGE ADULT

| | |
|---|---|
| Nitrogen 8–20 g | |
| Energy 1500–4000 kcal (6·3–16·8 MJ) | |
| Electrolytes and trace elements | |
| Sodium | 70–220 mmol |
| Potassium | 60–120 mmol |
| Chloride | 70–220 mmol |
| Calcium | 5–10 mmol |
| Magnesium | 5–20 mmol |
| Phosphate | 20–40 mmol |
| Zinc | 2–7 mg |
| Copper | 1–6 mg |
| Selenium | 120 μg |
| Iodine | 120 μg |
| Chromium | 5–10 μg |

(Courtesy of J. Powell-Tuck and A. W. Goode and MacMillan Journals Ltd[416])

10/TABLE 17
CALCULATION OF DAILY PROTEIN NITROGEN LOSSES
(* Extrarenal losses include gastric aspirate or intestinal fistulae and protein loss into peritoneal dialysis).

| | | |
|---|---|---|
| Protein catabolism | = urine urea (g)×0·56<br>= urea (mmol)×0·0336 | = A |
| Blood urea correction | rise in urea (g/l)×body weight×0·28<br>rise in urea (mmol/l)×body weight×0·0168 | = B |
| Urinary protein loss | = g×0·16 | = C |
| Daily nitrogen loss | = A+B+C (g)+any extrarenal losses* | |

## ENTERAL FEEDING

Some form of enteral nutrition should be considered for all patients who are unable to eat but have a functioning or potentially functioning gastro-intestinal tract. The advantages of using the enteral route rather than parenteral nutrition are:

1. It does not require a central venous catheter so the problems of sepsis and other complications of these catheters are avoided.
2. It does not require the same degree of nursing supervision as parenteral nutrition.
3. Intestinal structure and enzyme activity is maintained whereas prolonged parenteral nutrition is associated with loss of intestinal mucosa and reduced disaccharidase activity.[379]
4. There is a greater insulin response to enteral than to parenteral glucose.[379]
5. There is less tendency to retain salt and water.[380]
6. Experimental evidence of greater resistance to infection.[381]
7. Cost: enteral feeding is between 1/8th and 1/25th as expensive as parenteral nutrition for the same protein and calorie intake, the exact ratio depending on the formulations chosen.

Enteral feeding should not be regarded as an easy option however. It is just as important to pay attention to fluid balance, providing balanced amounts of protein, carbohydrate and fat, trace elements and vitamins by careful clinical and biochemical monitoring as it is during parenteral feeding.

### Methods

Enteral feeding has a long history. In 1598 Capivacceus fed a patient through a tube attached to an animal bladder and in the 1770's and 80's John Hunter used tube feeds in patients recovering from near drowning and in a patient with paralytic dysphagia.

*Naso-enteric tubes.*—Large-bore rubber tubes are now obsolete. They tended to cause oesophageal inflammation or ulceration with oesophageal stricture being a serious late complication. Modern plastic nasogastric tubes are much less irritating but oesophageal and gastric erosions can still be a problem and, particularly with larger-bore tubes, rhinitis, pharyngitis and otitis media may be troublesome. A tube passing through the pharynx stimulates the swallowing reflex. Normally the amount of air swallowed equals the volume of food and drink but the presence of a tube may double the amount of air swallowed with subsequent gaseous distension and abdominal discomfort.[382]

Fine-bore enteral feeding tubes such as the "Dobbhof" (Biosearch Medical Products), "Clinifeed" (Roussel) and "Keofeed" (Health Development Inc.) or locally fabricated fine-bore polyethylene catheters are tolerated better than normal nasogastric tubes for long-term feeding. Fine-bore tubes are, however, more difficult to insert. Some brands are supplied with a flexible wire guide but this increases the theoretical risks of perforation and certainly increases the ease with which they can be passed into the trachea, even if a cuffed endotracheal tube is in place. Endoscopy facilitates insertion of a fine-bore tube in cases of difficulty and can be particularly useful for getting the distal end of nasoduodenal or naso-intestinal tubes through the gastric pylorus.[383] The position of the feeding tube should always be checked before feeding starts. The most reliable way of doing this is with an x-ray to demonstrate its course and position of the distal end.

*Tube enterostomy.*—Torosian and Rombeau[384] have reviewed the methods of tube enterostomy that are available. Pharyngostomy, oesophagostomy, gastrostomy, duodenostomy and jejunostomy have been described but the stomach and jejunum are the most usual sites. Some have advocated inserting a needle catheter jejunostomy at the time of surgery in all patients having extensive emergency or elective procedures on the upper gastro-intestinal or pancreatico-biliary tracts.[385] This is because small bowel motility and absorption are only briefly affected by surgery whereas gastric emptying takes much longer to recover. These patients can therefore be fed enterally some time before it would be possible by conventional means. On the other hand, Yeung and colleagues[386] found that needle jejunostomy feeding was not of any significant benefit and was associated with a number of complications. They therefore suggest it should be reserved for selected cases rather than being used routinely.

*Administration.*—Gastro-intestinal motility and absorptive capacity can be assessed by starting with 30 ml of water each hour. Feeds are started at 30–50 ml/hour at half strength. The volume and finally the strength of the feed are then increased in steps over a couple of days until the fully daily requirement is being given. If a conventional nasogastric tube is being used, the stomach can be aspirated before each feed to ensure that they are being absorbed. This should only be necessary during the early stages and once it is clear that the feeds are being tolerated it can be changed for a fine-bore tube through which the feeds are delivered by continuous gravity infusion. The features of some of the available tubes and delivery systems were considered by Brown.[387] When problems are encountered with bolus feeds or gravity infusion an infusion pump may help to overcome them.[388] This ensures a steadier delivery of feeds, and can overcome some of the gastro-intestinal complications, such as diarrhoea, as well as saving nursing time, ensuring that the tube remains patent and facilitating control in diabetic patients.

**Feeds**

*Liquidised food* can be strained and syringed down a feeding tube. In theory this should be nutritionally adequate and well tolerated. In practice such feeds tend to be deficient in water-soluble vitamins and meat fibres are retained by the strainer, so reducing the protein content. If the feeds are not strained, the feeding tube is likely to become blocked.

*Commercially available feeds* in both powder and liquid form have been devised to supply the protein, energy, electrolyte, vitamin and trace element needs of the "average" patient. At full strength they contain about 1 cal/ml (4·2 kJ/ml). The composition of some of these feeds is shown in Table 18. All provide an appropriate calorie:nitrogen ratio. Ideally, such a feed should be close to iso-osmolar with plasma, lactose-free because of problems with lactose intolerance, of low viscosity and as cheap as possible. Whole protein, fat and glucose polymer containing feeds such as "Isocal" (Mead Johnson) and "Ensure" (Abbott) are suitable for most patients. They are also cheaper and more physiological than elemental diets.

*Elemental diets.*—Such as "Flexical" (Mead Johnson) and "Vivonex" (Norwich Eaton) contain oligosaccharides, oligopeptides and amino acids and a variable amount of fat as medium chain triglycerides. An elemental diet has been advocated for patients with the short-bowel syndrome, bowel fistulae, inflammatory bowel disease and pancreatic insufficiency.[389] It has also been used for early postoperative feeding after abdominal surgery.[390] There are, however,

10/TABLE 18
MAJOR CONSTITUENTS OF SOME ENTERAL FEEDS. (* LOW LACTULOSE; † CONTAINS MCT; ‡ SHOULD BE ADDED TO MILK).

| *Supplier* | *Name* | *Quantity* | *Energy (keal)* | *Protein (g)* | *Fat (g)* | *Na (mmol)* | *K (mmol)* | *Ca (mmol)* | *Mg (mmol)* | *P (mmol)* |
|---|---|---|---|---|---|---|---|---|---|---|
| | Cow's milk | 1000 ml | 650 | 33 | 38 | 22 | 38 | 30 | 5 | 31 |
| Carnation Ltd | ‡ Build up | 1 pkt | 132 | 25·6 | 0·2 | 5·4 | 9·8 | 8·3 | 0·9 | 7·9 |
| Glaxo Ltd | Complan | 100 g | 444 | 20 | 16 | 15·2 | 21·8 | 18·3 | 2·9 | 18·7 |
| Scientific Hospital Supplies Ltd | Albumaid* | 100 g | 305 | 76 | — | 54 | 3·8 | 7·5 | 8·5 | 10·7 |
| | Maxipro* | 100 g | 352 | 88 | — | 10 | 11·5 | 7·5 | | 12·5 |
| | Metabolic Mineral mix* | 100 g | — | — | — | 172 | 212 | 205 | 40 | 192 |
| BDH Pharmaceutical Ltd | Triosorbon*† | 85 g (1 pkt) | 400 | 16·2 | 16·2 | 17 | 17 | 5·1 | 3 | 7·7 |
| Roussel Laboratories Ltd | Clinifeed 400 Vanilla | 375 ml (1 tin) | 400 | 15 | 13·4 | 10·5 | 12·4 | 5 | 2 | 7·4 |
| | Clinifeed 400 Chocolate | 375 ml (1 tin) | 400 | 15 | 13·4 | 10·5 | 21 | 5 | 5·7 | 9·4 |
| | Clinifeed 500 Vanilla | 375 ml (1 tin) | 500 | 30 | 11·0 | 12·8 | 21·6 | 3·3 | 1·9 | 9·0 |
| | Clinifeed LLS* | 375 ml (1 tin) | 500 | 22·5 | 15·0 | 7·0 | 12·9 | 3·4 | 0·9 | 6·5 |
| Abbot Laboratories Ltd | Ensure* | 235 ml (1 tin) | 241 | 8·7 | 8·7 | 7·6 | 7·7 | 3·1 | 2·0 | 1·6 |
| Mead Johnson Laboratories | Portagen*† | 100 g | 464 | 16·5 | 22·5 | 9·6 | 15 | 11 | 3·9 | 10·7 |
| | Isocal*† | 355 ml (1 tin) | 375 | 12·1 | 15·7 | 8·1 | 12 | 5·6 | 3·1 | 6·1 |
| | Flexical*† | 100 g | 441 | 9·9 | 15 | 6·7 | 14·1 | 6·6 | 3·7 | 7·1 |
| Eaton Laboratories Ltd | Vivonex Standard* | 80 g (1 pkt) | 300 | 6·3 | 4 | 11·2 | 9 | 3·3 | 2·4 | 1·4 |
| | Vivonex HN* | 80 g (1 pkt) | 300 | 12·5 | 0·3 | 10·1 | 5·4 | 2·0 | 1·4 | 0·8 |

(Courtesy of J. Powell-Tuck and A. W. Goode and MacMillan Journals Ltd.[416])

no controlled studies to demonstrate any advantage from giving an elemental diet rather than using one of the cheaper preparations.

*Special requirements.*—The commercially available products may need to be modified or a feed made up specifically for patients with abnormal plasma electrolytes, renal or hepatic failure and those with high energy requirements. Usually a dietitian is responsible for meeting these special requirements. "Calo-nutrin" (Geistlich Ltd) or "Calorine" (Scientific Hospital Supplies Ltd) both of which are glucose polymers, can be used as the carbohydrate source; "Aminutrin" (Geistlich Ltd), "Forceval" (Unigregg Ltd) or "Casilan" (Glaxofarley Health Products) to supply protein and amino acids; and medium chain triglycerides to supply additional calories in the form of fat.

**Complications**

The complications of enteral feeding and their management are summarised in Table 19 and have been reviewed by Heymsfield and co-workers.[379] Of these, diarrhoea is the most common and can be a difficult problem to solve. The factors that contribute to diarrhoea include:

*Over-rapid introduction of feeds* by increasing either volume or concentration too quickly. The volume and/or concentration of feeds should be reduced and then slowly increased again.

*Hyperosmolarity*, particularly with elemental diets. Continuous infusion may help patients to tolerate hyperosmolar feeds.

*Bacterial contamination* should be avoided by care during preparation, sterilisation of con-

10/TABLE 19
COMPLICATIONS OF ENTERAL HYPERALIMENTATION AND THEIR MANAGEMENT

| Complication | Frequency % | Management |
|---|---|---|
| *Mechanical* | | |
| Tube blocked | Infrequent (< 10) | Flush with water<br>Replace if necessary |
| Pulmonary aspiration | Rare (< 1) | Head of bed should be elevated<br>Discontinue if regurgitated or vomited. |
| Oesophageal erosion | Rare (< 1) | Change to soft fine bore tube if possible<br>Remove if not |
| Local rhinitis, otitis media | Rare | Change nostril or remove |
| Leak from 'ostomy | Variable, about 3 | Cease feeds, consider surgical repair |
| Inadvertent intravenous administration | V. rare | Avoid compatible connections |
| *Gastro-intestinal symptoms* | | |
| Halitosis | Common especially with elemental | Change feed |
| Bloating & vomiting | 10–15 | Reduce flow rate |
| Diarrhoea | 10–20 | See text |
| *Metabolic or electrolyte* | | |
| Hyperglycaemia | 10–15 | Reduce flow rate and/or give insulin |
| Hypernatraemia, kalaemia, calcaemia | < 5 | Adjust electrolyte content |
| Essential fatty acid deficiency | Feeds may need to be supplemented with linoleic acid or intravenous "Intralipid" given if linoleic acid is lacking in the formula. | |
| Vitamin K deficiency | Unusual | Check prothrombin ratio; give Vit. K. |

(Courtesy of Drs. S. B. Heymsfield, R. A. Bethel, J. D. Ansley, D. W. Nixon and D. Rudman and the American College of Physicians[379])

tainers or by using a pre-packaged sterile liquid diet such as "Isocal" (Mead Johnson).

*Lactose intolerance* can be overcome by changing to a lactose-free preparation (see Table 18).

*Factors unrelated to the feeds* including antibiotic-associated diarrhoea, aperients given to relieve constipation because of the low residue of enteral feeding or magnesium trisilicate mixture given to reduce the risk of stress ulceration.

## PARENTERAL NUTRITION

Parenteral nutrition is used to supplement or replace enteral feeding when this is either inadequate or impossible. Successful parenteral nutrition has become widely practised since the development of suitable nutrient solutions and central venous catheters. The foundations were laid in the 1930's and 1940's with clarification of the metabolic responses to starvation, and in particular the responses to trauma and surgery. Elman and Weiner[391] described the intravenous use of protein hydrolysates in 1939, but the first successful report of parenteral nutrition was by Helfrik and Abelson in 1944.[392] During the next seventeen or so years, most attempts to repeat this success failed because of difficulties in maintaining venous access, but in 1961 Schuberth and Wretlind[393] reported the use of a stable fat emulsion which could be given through peripheral veins without difficulty. With this as a calorie source, and amino acid and low osmolarity sugar solution to provide protein and cardohydrate, the basic nutritional needs could be met but thrombophlebitis tended to limit the use of any single infusion site to 24–48 hours. These early methods were reviewed by Peaston.[394]

Modern parenteral nutrition may be said to date from 1968 when Dudrick and his associates[395] described the administration of a hypertonic glucose and protein hydrolysate mixture into a central vein for long periods of time in children with continued growth, development and positive nitrogen balance.

### Indications

Most patients will tolerate a short period, perhaps three or four days, of inadequate nutrition, but feeding should be started earlier in those of poor nutritional status. Parenteral nutrition should only be considered when enteral nutrition is either impossible using any of the methods discussed or proves to be inadequate. Other indications are:

- preparation of cachectic patients for major surgery, for example, before oesophageal resection;
- management of patients with enterocutaneous fistulae;
- possibly in the management of inflammatory bowel disease, although a controlled trial has failed to show any benefit from parenteral nutrition in acute colitis.[396]

### Administration

**Vascular access.**—Peripheral veins can and have been used but this effectively restricts the choice of solutions to fat emulsions and low concentration glucose and amino-acid solutions. Hypertonic solutions rapidly cause phlebitis and thrombosis of peripheral veins. Arteriovenous shunts or fistulae have been used for long-term parenteral nutrition but are also prone to thrombosis. A central venous catheter therefore represents the best route for parenteral nutrition. Any method of insertion can be used, but the infraclavicular subclavian approach is generally chosen because it is easy to secure the catheter in this position and it is well tolerated by the patient. Powell-Tuck,[397] has described a method for inserting a soft silicone rubber catheter infraclavicularly with a 5–10 cm skin tunnel before its exit point on the anterior chest wall. With this technique a caval catheter can be maintained for long periods. Alternatively, the internal jugular vein can be used and the end of the catheter tunnelled subcutaneously to emerge below the clavicle. The caval catheter used for parenteral nutrition should not be used for blood sampling or injection of intravenous medications.

**Infusion sets.**—The most simple arrangement possible should be used with the minimum connections. Luer-lock connectors reduce the risk of inadvertent disconnection. The infusion set should be changed every 48 hours.[398] The rate of infusion is most conveniently controlled by an infusion pump which may require a specially designed infusion set.

*Preparation.*—Whenever possible each patient's daily requirements of carbohydrates, protein, electrolytes and trace elements should be prepared by the hospital pharmacy in a sterile area with full aseptic precautions and placed into sterile plastic bags ready for infusion. Unused solution should be discarded after 24 hours. In addition to the reduced risk of bacterial contamination, this system provides an opportunity for cross-checking on the compatibility of additives and simplifies the ward management of parenteral nutrition.[399,400] Fat emulsions are usually infused separately because of the danger of "cracking" the emulsion, though this risk may have been overemphasised.

### Components

The components of some of the solutions available for parenteral nutrition are shown in Table 20.

*Carbohydrates.*—Dextrose is the best carbohydrate source for parenteral nutrition. A gram of dextrose provides 3·76 cal (0·016 MJ) so that hypertonic dextrose solutions with 250 g per litre or more are necessary to keep the total volume within reasonable limits. Fructose, sorbitol and alcohol are no longer recommended because they have a higher incidence of side-effects. The most common complication when using dextrose as an energy source is hyperglycaemia. Urine testing for glycosuria at regular intervals allows early detection of this complication. Glucose intolerance can be reduced by slowly increasing the rate of an infusion during the early stages. If the dextrose infusion is suddenly stopped for any reason the patient is likely to become hypoglycaemic because of the high rate of endogenous insulin production. This problem is avoided by slowly reducing the rate of dextrose infusion when parenteral nutrition is no longer needed.

*Protein.*—Casein hydrolysates such as "Aminosol" were widely used but have been criticised because of their high sodium content and the high proportion of the total protein that is in the form of oligopeptides, these being less well utilised than free amino acids. Laevo-form amino-acid solutions are the most efficient means of providing for protein synthesis. A large number of l-amino-acid solutions are now

10/TABLE 20
COMPONENTS OF SOME SOLUTIONS AVAILABLE IN THE U.K. FOR PARENTERAL NUTRITION

| | *Constituents of 1 litre* | *Energy (kcal)* | *N (g)* | *mmol of* | | | | | |
|---|---|---|---|---|---|---|---|---|---|
| | | | | *Na* | *K* | *Mg* | *Ca* | *$PO_4$* | *HCO* |
| Aminoplex 5 | L Amino Acids (LAA) Sorbitol 1·00% Ethanol 5% | 1000 | 5 | 35 | 15 | — | — | — | — |
| Aminoplex 14 | LAA | 340 | 13·4 | 35 | 30 | — | — | — | — |
| Vamin glucose | LAA 10% glucose | 650 | 9·4 | 50 | 20 | 1·5 | 2·5 | — | — |
| Vamin N | LAA | 250 | 9·4 | 50 | 20 | 1·5 | 2·5 | — | — |
| Aminosol 10% | Casein hydrol. | 310 | 12–15 | 135 | 1·4 | — | — | 5 | — |
| Travasol Synthamin 7S | LAA Sorbitol 15% | 760 | 6·6 | 38 | 30 | 2·5 | — | 15 | — |
| Synthamin 9 | LAA | 250 | 9·3 | 73 | 60 | 5 | — | 30 | — |
| 14 | LAA | 375 | 14·3 | 73 | 60 | 5 | — | 30 | — |
| 17 | LAA | 450 | 16·9 | 73 | 60 | 5 | — | 30 | — |
| Aminofusin L600 | LAA Sorbitol 10% | 600 | 8·8 | 40 | 30 | 5 | — | — | — |
| Electrolyte in dextrose A | 20% Glucose | 800 | — | — | — | 28 | 26 | — | — |
| B | 20% Glucose | 800 | — | — | 60 | — | — | 60 | — |
| Glucoplex 1000 | 24% Glucose | 1000 | — | 50 | 30 | 2·5 | — | 18 | — |
| 1600 | 40% Glucose | 1600 | — | 50 | 30 | 2·5 | — | 18 | — |
| Glucose 20% | | 800 | — | — | — | — | — | — | — |
| Intralipid 10% | Soya bean oil 10% Glycerol | 1000 | — | — | — | — | — | 15 | — |
| Intralipid 20% | Soya bean oil 20% Glycerol | 2000 | — | — | — | — | — | 15 | — |

(Courtesy of J. Powell-Tuck and A. W. Goode and MacMillan Journals Ltd.[416])

available with some marked differences in the proportions of different amino acids that they contain.

Conventionally, eight amino acids are regarded as "essential". These are isoleucine, leucine, lysine, methionine, phenylalanine, threonine, tryptophan and valine. Of the other amino acids:

- Histidine is essential in infants and uraemic patients
- Tyrosine and cystine are essential in premature babies.
- Arginine occupies a central role in the urea cycle and should be present to protect against hyperammonaemia.
- Alanine, proline and glutamic acid should be given because their synthesis from other amino acids is comparatively slow.
- Too high a proportion of glycine may cause hyperammonaemia.
- The essential amino acids should comprise 40–50 per cent of the total quantity.
- Isoleucine, leucine and valine, that is the branched chain amino acids, should be present in amounts relatively greater than the other amino acids.
- Excessive amounts of cationic amino acids should be avoided to reduce the risk of metabolic acidosis.[401]

There have been two major approaches to the balance of different amino acids provided in a solution. One has been to provide a mixture similar to egg protein and the other has had as its major objective maintenance of the normal plasma amino-acid profile. Which of these is better, or whether it makes any difference in the majority of cases, is unknown but in infants[402] and patients with hepatic failure or severe sepsis[403] the amino-acid composition is more critical. For the l-amino-acid preparations listed in Table 20 the differences in composition are summarised in Table 21.

*Fat* provides 9 cal (0·038 MJ) per gram. "Intralipid", the most widely available intravenous fat preparation, consists of a 10 per cent or 20 per cent emulsion of soya bean oil, 2·5 per

10/TABLE 21
Comparison of Amino-acid Solutions (EAA's: Essential Amino Acids; BCAA's: Branched Chain Amino Acids)

| *Solution* | *Contains No* | *High in (%)* | *EAA's %* | *BCAA's %* |
|---|---|---|---|---|
| Aminoplex | Cystine<br>Glutamate<br>Serine<br>Tyrosine | Alanine } 33%<br>Glycine } | 45% | 15·7% |
| Vamin | | | 41% | 19% |
| Synthamin (Travasol) | Aspartate<br>Cystine<br>Glutamate<br>Serine | Alanine } 42%<br>Glycine } | 39% | 16% |
| Aminofusion | Aspartate<br>Cystine<br>Serine<br>Tyrosine | Alanine } 32%<br>Glycine }<br>Glutamate 18% | 27% | 11% |

cent glycerol and 1·2 per cent egg-lecithin phosphatides and is approximately isosmolar with plasma. The diameter of the fat droplets is similar to that of chylomicrons. "Intralipid" may be used on a daily basis to supply a significant proportion of the energy requirement or used only intermittently to prevent essential fatty acid deficiency, with the energy requirement being met by dextrose. It provides a very concentrated energy source, 500 ml of 20 per cent "Intralipid" supplying 1000 cal (4·2 MJ), with only 375 ml of water, but it is recommended that a maximum of 50 per cent of the total non-protein energy come from this source. On the first day of infusion the total should not exceed 1 g per kilogram body weight, this being increased to no more than 3 g per kilogram body weight subsequently if more energy is needed. When used regularly, plasma samples must be checked before the next bottle is to be infused to ensure that the fat is being cleared. If the plasma is still strongly opalescent or milky, further infusions should be postponed. Fat tolerance is reduced in patients with sepsis or shock, so greater care is needed.

Carnitine facilitates the transport of fatty acids into mitochondria and the development of a relative deficiency of this metabolite may be partly responsible for the development of intolerance.[404] Heparin infused concurrently increases the rate at which fat is cleared from the plasma. Mild anaemia, with morphological changes in red cells, granulocytes and platelets and changes in plasma lipids, occur when "Intralipid" is used regularly.[81] Excessive amounts of "Intralipid" cause gastro-intestinal disturbances, hepatosplenomegaly, impaired liver function, thrombocytopenia and a coagulopathy.[405]

The role of essential fatty acids in nutrition is incompletely understood,[406] but signs of deficiency with skin changes can develop within a week in infants and after several weeks in adults if no fat is given. A litre of 10 per cent "Intralipid" or its equivalent each week is enough to prevent essential fatty acid deficiency developing.[407]

*Water and electrolytes.*—Daily fluid requirements vary considerably from patient to patient. Fluid balance charts are notoriously inaccurate but daily weighing, clinical observation and measurement of venous pressures can provide a guide to over- or under-hydration. The volume infused may have to be restricted but most patients are given 2–3 litres a day of parenteral nutrition solution.

Sodium, 1–2 mmol/kg/day and potassium about 1 mmol/kg/day, are given to replace losses and maintain plasma levels. The actual amounts given may need to be adjusted on a daily basis as a result of biochemical monitoring. Calcium, magnesium and phosphate levels must also be monitored and supplied in the parenteral nutrition solution in amounts sufficient to maintain plasma levels within normal limits. On average, 5–10 mmol of calcium, 5–10 mmol of magnesium and 20–30 mmol of phosphate per day are given. When these are added to the parenteral nutrition solution, care must be taken to avoid exceeding the solubility limits for calcium phosphate. This problem has been reviewed by Nedich.[408]

*Vitamins.*—Bradley and associates[409] have shown that an ampoule of water-soluble vitamins daily, supplemented by weekly intramuscular injections of folic acid 15 mg, vitamin $B_{12}$ 1 mg and vitamin K 10 mg, was adequate to maintain tissue levels of the water-soluble vitamins and folate. Available vitamin preparations include:

"Parenterovite" (Beecham) contains vitamins of the B group and vitamin C in a pair of ampoules. There are different formulations for intravenous and intramuscular use.

"Multibionta" (Merck) contains vitamin A, B group vitamins and vitamins C and E.

"Dayamin" (Abbot) contains vitamins A, B group, C, D and E in a form suitable for intramuscular injection.

"MVI" (USV) contains vitamins A, B group, C, D and E in a form suitable for intravenous infusion.

None of the formulations contains folate or vitamin K. Only "Dayamin" contains vitamin $B_{12}$, 20 μg per ampoule. These vitamins have to be given separately. For most patients a weekly dose is sufficient, but patients with renal failure who are being dialysed need extra folate—5 to 10 mg/day—because of increased losses into the dialysate. The water-soluble vitamins are infused over at least 30 minutes to prevent excessive urinary losses, but if they are added to the parenteral nutrition infusion the container must be protected from light to prevent significant losses of potency. Fat-soluble vitamin deficiencies are unlikely before two or three weeks of total parenteral nutrition so that for the first two weeks one of the cheaper preparations containing the water-soluble vitamins alone is sufficient.

*Trace elements.*—At least 14 trace elements are necessary for normal growth and development of one or more animal species but only seven—cobalt, copper, fluoride, iodine, iron, manganese and zinc—have been regarded as important in human nutrition.[410] More recent evidence suggests that selenium is also essential.[411] Iron deficiency is treated with one of the parenteral iron preparations ("Imferon", Fisons; "Jectofer", Astra). Deficiency of the other trace elements is unlikely during short-term parenteral nutrition but may appear during long-term therapy and in patients with enterocutaneous fistulae or prolonged diarrhoea. Plasma zinc and copper levels can be measured fairly easily and provide evidence of the need for trace element supplements. Small amounts of trace elements are found in parenteral nutrition solutions.[412,413] During prolonged parenteral nutrition the trace element intake can be supplemented using one of the preparations available from either Travenol or Vitrium A. B.

## Insulin in Parenteral Nutrition

Glucose intolerance is common in patients requiring parenteral nutrition, particularly those in an ICU. Exogenous insulin may be given to prevent hyperglycaemia. If insulin is added to the nutrition infusion a variable amount is adsorbed to the plastic or glass container and the giving set so that precise requirements are unknown. Another disadvantage is that the container may need to be discarded if there are marked changes in glucose tolerance during the time between it being made up and completely infused. An alternative is to give insulin separately either by infusion or subcutaneously. When given by infusion the insulin can be diluted in a colloid solution such as "Haemaccel", plasma protein solution or albumin to prevent adsorption to glass or plastic.

In catabolic patients with a urea production greater than 15 g/day, glucose given with insulin had a greater protein sparing effect than glucose alone[414] but this effect of insulin was not seen in non-catabolic patients. The mechanism for this is uncertain but it may be a direct effect of insulin on muscle protein breakdown. More severely catabolic patients, particularly those with sepsis, may have marked glucose intolerance. Using large doses of insulin to correct the hyperglycaemia does not increase the rate of glucose oxidation.[372] The excess glucose is converted to fat. Over a period of time this causes marked fatty infiltration of the liver. Instead of increasing the dose of insulin the amount of dextrose infused should be reduced.

**Parenteral Nutrition Regimens**

Numerous parenteral nutrition regimens can be devised making use of the range of products now available. This allows the regimen to be designed around the individual patient's needs. The questions to be answered in designing a regimen are:

1. What are the constraints imposed by cardiac, renal or hepatic failure?
2. How much protein is needed? Generally this is 1–2 g/kg body weight/day.
3. What product is to be used as the protein/amino acid source
4. How much energy must be supplied? About 200 calories (0·84 MJ) for each gram of protein nitrogen is usually recommended, but under some circumstances as much as 450 calories (1·89 MJ) may be needed to make the most efficient use of the protein supplied.[415]
5. Is fat to be used as a significant energy source and if so what proportion of the energy requirement will it supply? Fat emulsions are considerably more expensive than dextrose, but a controlled trial has shown that protein repletion occurred in patients who received both fat and dextrose but not in those who received dextrose alone as the non-protein energy source.[396] It is usually recommended that no more than 50 per cent of the energy requirement is supplied by fat but proportions as high as 80 per cent have been used without any obvious harmful effects. It is probably wise to provide a minimum of 500 calories (2 MJ) a day as carbohydrate to cover cerebral requirements even though the brain is capable of adapting to ketone metabolism.[416] The energy requirements not met by fat are supplied as dextrose.
6. What electrolyte additives are needed? The electrolyte content of the protein and energy source must be taken into account together with the electrolytes contained in drugs such as antibiotics.
7. Which vitamins and trace elements are needed? Are these to be added to the infusion or given separately?

Parenteral nutrition infusions should be spread evenly over each 24-hour period and the protein and energy sources given simultaneously. Examples of two regimens suitable for short-term parenteral nutrition in a patient without major complications are shown in Table 22. Alternative regimens are described in manufacturer's product literature and by Ellis and his co-workers.[417]

**Special Situations**

*Renal failure.*—A combination of essential amino acids and glucose was shown to reduce the mortality of acute renal failure when compared to hypertonic glucose alone.[418] Generally a high calorie, low protein mixture is used for patients in renal failure but the total volume infused may be limited by oliguria. To some

10/TABLE 22

ALTERNATIVE PARENTERAL NUTRITION REGIMENS SUITABLE FOR SHORT-TERM USE IN A PATIENT ESTABLISHED ON PARENTERAL NUTRITION. (See section on monitoring.)

| | |
|---|---|
| 1. Synthamin 10% 1000 ml<br>Dextrose 50% 1500 ml<br>+ Sodium 100 mmol<br>Potassium 70 mmol<br>Calcium 5–10 mmol<br>Magnesium 5–10 mmol<br>Phosphate 20–30 mmol | = 100 G protein or 16 G nitrogen<br>= 3000 nonprotein kcal (12·6MJ)<br>i.e. 188 kcal (0·8MJ)/G $N_2$<br>Water soluble vitamins supplied as "Parenterovite" 2 amps infused over 30 minutes.<br>Folate 10 mg, Vit K 10 mg weekly |
| 2. Synthamin 10% 1000 ml<br>Dextrose 50% 1000 ml<br>+ Sodium 100 mmol<br>Potassium 70 mmol<br>Calcium 5–10 mmol<br>Magnesium 5–10 mmol<br>Phosphate 20 mmol<br>Intralipid 20% 500 mmol | = 100 G protein or 16 G nitrogen<br>Dextrose supplies 2000 kcal (8·4MJ)<br>Intralipid supplies 1000 kcal (4·2MJ)<br>Vitamins as for 1.<br>Also gives 188 kcal (0·8MJ)/G $N_2$<br>(+Phosphate 7·5 mmol in "Intralipid") |

extent this problem can be overcome by dialysis, and frequent dialysis also allows increased amounts of protein to be given.

*Hepatic failure.*—Intravenous fat emulsions should not be given to patients with hepatic failure. When the standard amino-acid solutions are given to patients with hepatic failure they develop abnormalities of the plasma amino-acid profile.[419] A special mixture has been developed which is high in branched chain amino acids. When used in hepatic failure the plasma amino-acid profile remained normal and there was an improvement in encephalopathy.[420]

*Infants and children.*—The problems of parenteral nutrition in infants and children have been reviewed by Harries[421] and in an Editorial.[422] While the principles of parenteral nutrition are similar to those followed in adults even greater care is needed in designing the regimen. The fluid and electrolyte requirements must be calculated with care and monitored closely (see also Chapter 42).

*Malignant disease.*[423]—Anorexia is a common problem in malignant disease, both from the effects of the disease itself and also because of the effect of radiotherapy and chemotherapy. Parenteral nutrition is used to reduce the amount of weight loss during treatment and improve the patient's sense of well being.

10/Table 23
Routine Investigations for Patients on Parenteral Nutrition.

| |
|---|
| *Daily* |
| Urea and electrolytes |
| Blood sugar (more often if glycosuria > 2%) |
| Urine urea and electrolytes for balance studies |
| Visual inspection of plasma (if "Intralipid" used). |
| *Twice Weekly* |
| Calcium, phosphate |
| Liver function tests |
| Haemoglobin, full blood count |
| Prothrombin time |
| *Weekly* |
| Zinc |
| Magnesium |
| *As indicated* |
| Blood cultures |
| Arterial blood acid-base analysis |
| Iron and iron binding capacity |
| Folate |
| Vitamin $B_{12}$ |

*Long-term parenteral nutrition* has been described from a number of centres. Most of the patients requiring this have had extensive bowel resection. Ladefoged and Jarnum[424] described their experience with 19 patients who received parenteral nutrition for 6 to 63 months. For most of this time the patients were at home. Most complications were related to the central venous catheter rather than nutritional deficiencies.

## Peripheral Amino-Acid Infusion

The work of Blackburn and his colleagues[425]

10/Table 24
Some Complications of Parenteral Nutrition.

| | |
|---|---|
| *Catheter related* | |
| Complications of insertion: pneumothorax, haematoma, etc. | |
| Sepsis | |
| Air embolism | |
| Venous thrombosis | |
| *Pharmaceutical* | |
| Contamination of infusion fluid | |
| Incompatability of additives | |
| Precipitation of calcium salts | |
| *Metabolic* | |
| From glucose | —hyperglycaemia<br>—hypoglycaemia |
| From fat | —hyperlipidaemia<br>—pyrogenic and "allergic" reactions<br>—anaemia, thrombocytopenia |
| From protein | —acidosis<br>—prerenal azotaemia<br>—amino acid imbalance<br>—hyperammonaemia |
| Electrolyte disturbances | —sodium, potassium, calcium, magnesium, phosphate |
| Vitamins | —hypervitaminosis, especially of fat-soluble vitamins |
| Other | —cholestasis and jaundice<br>—hyperosmolality<br>—fluid overload |
| *Deficiencies* | |
| Inadequate protein and/or energy | |
| Essential fatty-acid deficiency | |
| Vitamin deficiencies | |
| Trace element deficiency<br>—zinc the most common | |

suggested that infusing an isotonic amino-acid solution into peripheral veins minimised the negative nitrogen balance of postoperative patients unable to eat. Others have confirmed the response to this "protein-sparing therapy";[426–428] but have not supported its routine use for postoperative patients who make an uneventful recovery. In patients with a greater degree of metabolic stress, peripheral amino-acid infusion alone had no effect on nitrogen balance.[429] An energy source must also be provided in these patients and it must be noted that while "protein-sparing therapy" may reduce the negative nitrogen balance of some patients it does not prevent it or reverse it. Full parenteral nutrition can do this and should not be withheld when needed.

## Monitoring

Many of the potential complications of parenteral nutrition can be avoided by regular biochemical monitoring. This is particularly important during the early stages in patients with sepsis, and renal, hepatic or cardiac failure. A protocol for routine investigations is shown in Table 23.

## Complications

Although there are numerous potential complications from parenteral nutrition, most are avoidable with careful attention to detail and regular monitoring. Ausman and Hardy,[430] Sheldon and Baker[431] and Michel and associates[378] have reviewed aspects of this topic in depth and provide guidelines for the management of complications if they occur. Table 24 shows some of the complications that have occurred during parenteral nutrition. There is evidence that the incidence of complications can be reduced by a "parenteral nutrition team" consisting of a clinician, pharmacist, and nurse supplemented by a dietitian and microbiologist.[399, 400]

## REFERENCES


1. BMA Planning Unit Report (1967). *Intensive Care*. London: British Medical Association.
2. Hilberman, M. (1975). The evolution of intensive care units. *Crit. Care Med.*, **3**, 159.
3. Lassen, M. C. A. (1953). A preliminary report on the 1952 epidemic of poliomyelitis in Copenhagen with special reference to the treatment of acute respiratory insufficiency. *Lancet*, **1**, 37.
4. Pontoppidan, H., Wilson, R. S., Rie, M. A. and Schneider, R. C. (1977). Respiratory intensive care. *Anesthesiology*, **47**, 96.
5. Brown, K. W. G., MacMillan, R. L., Forbath, N., Mel'Grano, F. and Scott, J. W. (1963). Coronary unit, an intensive care centre for acute myocardial infarction. *Lancet*, **2**, 349.
6. Shillingford, J. P. and Thomas, M. (1964). Organisation of unit for intensive care and investigation of patients with acute myocardial infarction. *Lancet*, **2**, 1113.
7. Lown, B., Amarasingham, R. and Neuman, J. (1962). New method for terminating cardiac arrhythmias—use of synchronised capacitor discharge. *JAMA*, **182**, 548.
8. Portal, R. W., Davies, J. G., Leatham, A. and Siddons, A. H. M. (1962). Artificial pacing for heart block. *Lancet*, **2**, 1369.
9. Great Britain Department of Health and Social Security (1974). Hospital building note: 27 *Intensive Therapy Unit*. London: H.M. Stationery Office.
10. U.S. Department of Health, Education and Welfare (1979). *Planning for general medical and surgical intensive care units: a technical assistance document for planning agencies*. (Health Planning Methods and Technology Series, No. 11.) Springfield, Virginia: National Technical Information Service.
11. Health Services and Promotion Branch, Department of National Health and Welfare (1979). *Evaluation and space programming, methodology series* No. 15: special care units. Department of Health and Welfare, Canada.
12. Campbell, D., Reid, J. M., Telfer, A. B. M. and Fitch, W. (1967). Four years of respiratory intensive care. *Brit. Med. J.*, **2**, 255.
13. Gilbert, A. E. and Hoffman, T. C. (1980). Unified CCU benefits patients and staff. *Hospitals* (Feb. 16th), **54**, 137.
14. Safar, P. and Grenvik, A. (1977). Organization and physician education in critical care medicine. *Anesthesiology*, **47**, 82.
15. Committee on Applications and Costs of Modern Technology in Medical Practice (1978). *Report*, p. 139. Canberra: Australian Government Publishing Service.
16. Tanser, A. R. and Wetten, B. G. (1973). Multi-purpose Intensive Care Unit in a District General Hospital. *Brit. Med. J.*, **2**, 227.
17. Robinson, J. S., Hopkins, B. E. and Clarke, G. M. (1970). Combined respiratory and coronary care. *Med. J. Aust.*, **2**, 124.
18, Bell, J. A., Bradley, R. D. Jenkins, B. S. and Spencer, G. T. (1974). Six years of multi-disciplinary intensive care. *Brit. Med. J.*, **2**, 483.
19. Waddell, G. (1975). Movement of critically ill patients within hospital. *Brit. Med. J.*, **1**, 417.
20. Weil, M. H., Shubin, H. and Carlson, R. W. (1976). The new practice of critical care medicine. In: *Critical Care Medicine, Current Principles and Practices*, p. 1. Ed. Weil, M. H. and Shubin, H. Hagerstown, Maryland: Harper and Row.
21. Keep, P. J. (1977). Stimulus deprivation in windowless rooms. *Anaesthesia*, **32**, 598.

22. Wilson, L. M. (1972). Intensive care delirium. *Arch. Int. Med.*, **130**, 225.
23. Committee on Trauma of the American College of Surgeons (1976). Optimal hospital resources for care of the seriously injured. *Bull. Amer. Coll. Surgs.* (Sept. 1976).
24. Milledge, J. S. (1976). Therapeutic fibreoptic bronchoscopy in intensive care. *Brit. Med. J.*, **2**, 1427.
25. Editorial (1979). Hazards of fibreoptic bronchoscopy. *Brit. Med. J.*, **1**, 212.
26. Standards Association of Australia (1976). Australian standard 3003. *SAA code for electrical installations in electromedical treatment areas.* S.A.A., Sydney, N.S.W.
27. Standards Association of Australia (1978). Australian standard 3200. *Approval and test specification for electromedical equipment: general requirements.* S.A.A., Sydney, N.S.W.
28. British Standards Institution (1979) B.S. 5724. *Specification for safety of medical electrical equipment.* Part 1: General requirements. London: British Standards Institution.
29. Kenny, G. N. C. (1979). Programmable calculator: a program for use in the intensive care unit. *Brit. J. Anaesth.*, **51**, 793.
30. Manzano, J. L., Villalobos, J., Church, A. and Manzano, J. J. (1980). Computerised information system for ICU patient management. *Crit. Care Med.*, **8**, 745.
31. Norlander, O. (1979). Computer systems to facilitate the management of the critically ill. In: *Handbook of Critical Care Medicine*, p. 35. Eds. Weil, M. H. and Henning, R. J. Chicago: Year Book Medical Publishers.
32. Meakins, J. L., Wicklund, B., Forse, R. A. and McLean, A. P. H. (1981). The surgical intensive care unit: current concepts in infection. *Surg. Clin. N. Am.*, **60**, 117.
33. Walton, B. (1979). Effects of anaesthesia and surgery on immune status. *Brit. J. Anaesth.*, **51**, 37.
34. Parkes, R. P. F. (1982). Immunology. In: *Intensive Care*. Ed. Sherwood-Jones E. Lancaster: M.T.P. Press.
35. LaForce, F. M. and Eickhoff, T. C. (1977). The role of infection in critical care. *Anesthesiology*, **47**, 195.
36. Gaya, H. (1976). Infection control in intensive care. *Brit. J. Anaesth.*, **48**, 9.
37. Maki, D. G., Goldmann, D. A. and Rhame, F. S. (1973). Infection control in intravenous therapy. *Ann. Intern. Med.*, **79**, 867.
38. Buxton, A. E., Anderson, R. L. Klimek, J. and Quintiliani, R. (1978). Failure of disposable domes to prevent septicemia acquired from contaminated pressure transducers. *Chest*, **74**, 508.
39. Clumeck, N. and George, C. (1981). Immunological aspects of severe bacterial sepsis. *Intens. Care Med.*, **7**, 109.
40. Bradley, J. A., Ledingham, I. McA. and Hamilton, D. N. H. (1981). Assessment of host resistance in critically ill surgical patients by the response to recall skin antigens. *Intens. Care Med.*, 7, 105.
41. Thomson, C. W., Ryan, D. W., Dunkin, L. J., Smith, M. and Marshall, M. (1980). Fluidised bead bed in the intensive therapy unit. *Lancet*, **1**, 568.
42. Smallwood, R. W., Sands, M. J. W. and Holland, R. B. (1981). Medical staff needed in a hospital to service anaesthesia and intensive care. *Anaesth. Intens. Care*, **9**, 3.
43. Grenvik, A., Leonard, J. J., Arens, J. F., Carey, L. C. and Disney, F. A. (1981). Critical care medicine: certification as a multidisciplinary subspeciality. *Crit. Care Med.*, **9**, 117.
44. Worthley, L. I. G. (1981). Training in intensive care: an Australian view. *Crit. Care Med.*, **9**, 69.
45. Chew, H. E. R. and Hanson, G. C. (1976). A case for the medical administrator of an intensive therapy unit to be trained in intensive therapy. *Europ. J. Intens. Care Med.*, **2**, 107.
46. Gilston, A. (1981). Intensive care in England and Wales: A survey of current practice, training and attitudes. *Anaesthesia*, **36**, 188.
47. Tinker, J. (1976). The staffing and management of intensive therapy units. *Brit. J. Hosp. Med.*, **16**, 399.
48. Porter, S. W. (1977). Intensive therapy nursing. *Intens. Care Med.*, **3**, 99.
49. Schroeder, H. G. (1971). Psycho-reactive problems of intensive therapy. *Anaesthesia*, **26**, 28.
50. Nunn, J. F., Milledge, J. S. and Singaraya, J. (1979). Survival of patients ventilated in an intensive therapy unit. *Brit. Med. J.*, **1**, 1525.
51. Civetta, J. M. (1977). Selection of patients for intensive care. In: *Recent Advances in Intensive Therapy*, No. 1, p.9. Ed. Ledingham, I. McA. Edinburgh: Churchill Livingstone.
52. Thibault, G. E., Mulley, A. G., Barnett, G. O., Goldstein, R. L., Reder, V. A., Sherman, E. L. and Skinner, E. R. (1980). Medical intensive care: indications, interventions and outcomes. *New Engl. J. Med.*, **302**, 938.
53. Cullen, D. J. (1977). Results and costs of intensive care. *Anesthesiology*, **47**, 203.
54. Detsky, A. S., Stricker, S. C., Mulley, A. G. and Thibault, G. E. (1981). Prognosis, survival and the expenditure of hospital resources for patients in an intensive care unit. *New Engl. J. Med.*, 305, 667.
55. Editorial (1979). Monitoring devices and septicaemia. *Brit. Med. J.*, **1**, 1747.
56. Maki, D. G. and Hassemer, C. A. (1981). Endemic rate of fluid contamination and related septicemia in arterial pressure monitoring. *Am. J. Med.*, **70**, 733.
57. Shinozaki, T., Deane, R. S. and Mazuzan, J. E. (1980). The dynamic responses of liquid-filled catheter systems for direct measurement of blood pressure. *Anesthesiology*, **53**, 498.
58. Rothe, C. F. and Kim, K. C. (1980). Measuring systolic arterial blood pressure; possible errors from extension tubes or disposable transducer domes. *Crit. Care Med.*, **8**, 683.
59. Gilston, A. (1976). A clinical scoring system for adult respiratory distress. Preliminary report on its use in heart disease. *Anaesthesia*, **31**, 448.
60. Hill, D. W. and Dolan, A. M. (1976). *Intensive Care Instrumentation*. London: Academic Press.
61. Hill, D. W. and Dolan, A. M. (1976). Respiratory Measurements. In: *Intensive Care Instrumentation*, Chap. 4, p. 76. London: Academic Press.
62. Rooth, G., Hedstrand, U., Tyden, H. (1976). The validity of the transcutaneous oxygen tension method in adults. *Crit. Care Med.*, **4**, 162.
63. Rithalia, S. V. S., Rozkovec, A. and Tinker, J. (1979). Characteristics of transcutaneous oxygen tension monitors in normal adults and critically ill patients. *Intens. Care Med.*, **5**, 147.
64. Gothard, J. W. W., Busst, C. M., Branthwaite, M. A., Davies, N. J. H. and Denison, D. M. (1980). Applications

of respiratory mass spectrometry to intensive care. *Anaesthesia*, **35**, 890.
65. Armstrong, R. F., Southorn, P. A., Secker-Walker, J., Lincoln, J. C. R. and Soutter, L. (1976). Continuous monitoring of mixed venous oxygen tension. *Brit. Med. J.*, **2**, 282.
66. Buchbinder, N. and Ganz, W. (1976). Hemodynamic monitoring: invasive techniques. *Anesthesiology*, **45**, 146.
67. Poole-Wilson, P. A. (1978). Interpretation of haemodynamic measurements. *Brit. J. Hosp. Med.*, **20**, 371.
68. Editorial (1980). Haemodynamic monitoring in the intensive care unit. *Brit. Med. J.*, **1**, 1035.
69. Swan, H. J. C., Ganz, W., Forrester, J. S., Marcus, H., Diamond, G. and Chonette, D. (1970). Catheterization of the heart in man with use of flow-directed balloon tipped catheter. *N. Engl. J. Med.*, **283**, 447.
70. Forrester, J. S., Ganz, W., Diamond, G., McHugh, T., Chonette, D. W. and Swan, H. J. C. (1972). Thermodilution cardiac output determination with a single flow-directed catheter. *Am. Heart J.*, **83**, 306.
71. Elliott, C. G., Zimmerman, G. A. and Clemmer, T. P. (1979). Complications of pulmonary artery catheterization in the care of critically ill patients. *Chest*, **76**, 647.
72. Dobb, G. J. (1980). The Swan-Ganz catheter: a prospective study of use and complications in a general intensive care unit. *Anaesth. Intens. Care*, **8**, 97.
73. Levitt, J. M. and Replogle, R. L. (1979). Thermodilution cardiac output: a critical analysis and review of the literature. *J. Surg. Res.*, **27**, 392.
74. Naggar, C. Z., Dobnik, D. B., Flessas, P., Kripke, B. J. and Ryan, T. J. (1975). Accuracy of the stroke index as determined by the transthoracic electrical impedance method. *Anesthesiology*, **42**, 201.
75. Denniston, J. C., Maher, J. T., Reeves, J. T., Cruz, J. C., Cymerman, A. and Grover, R. F. (1976). Measurement of cardiac output by electrical impedance at rest and during exercise. *J. Appl. Physiol.*, **40**, 91.
76. Hanson, G. C. and Bilton, A. H. (1978). Clinical experience with transcutaneous aortovelography: preliminary communication. *J. Roy. Soc. Med.*, **71**, 501.
77. Miller, J. D. (1978). Intracranial pressure monitoring. *Brit. J. Hosp. Med.*, **19**, 497.
78. Moss, E. and McDowall, D. G. (1979). Monitoring of Intracranial Pressure. In: *Management of Acute Intracranial Disasters*. Ed. Trubuhovich, R. V. *Internat. Anesth. Clin.*, **17**, Nos. 2 & 3, p. 375.
79. Treasure, T. (1978). The application of potassium selective electrodes in the intensive care unit. *Intens. Care Med.*, **4**, 83.
80. Shield, M. J., Hammill, H. J., Neale, D. A. (1979). Systematic bacteriological monitoring of intensive care unit patients. The results of a 12-month study. *Intens. Care Med.*, **5**, 171.
81. Gibson, J. C., Simms, L. A., Raik, E. and Barton, L. (1978). Haematological and biochemical abnormalities associated with intralipid hyperalimentation. *Anaesth. Intens. Care*, **6**, 350.
82. Gormezano, J. and Branthwaite, M. A. (1972). Effects of physiotherapy during intermittent positive pressure ventilation. *Anaesthesia*, **27**, 258.
83. Mackenzie, C. F., Shin, B. and McAslan, T. C. (1978). Chest physiotherapy: the effect on arterial oxygenation. *Anesth. Analg.*, **57**, 28.
84. Barrell, S. E. and Abbas, H. M. (1978). Monitoring during physiotherapy after open heart surgery. *Physiotherapy*,**64**, 272.
85. Sackner, M. A., Landa, J. F., Greeneltch, N. and Robinson, M. J. (1973). Pathogenesis and prevention of tracheobronchial damage with suction procedures. *Chest*, **64**, 284.
86. Kubota, Y., Magaribachi, T., Ohara, M., Fujita, M., Toyoda, Y., Asada, A., Harioka, T. (1980). Evaluation of selective bronchial suctioning in the adult. *Crit. Care Med.*, **8**, 748.
87. Rosen, M. and Hillard, E. K. (1960). The use of suction in clinical medicine. *Brit. J. Anaesth.*, **32**, 486.
88. Clement, A. J. and Hübsch, S. K. (1968). Chest physiotherapy by the "bag squeezing" method: a guide to technique. *Physiotherapy*, **54**, 355.
89. Belman, M. and Mittman, C. (1981). Incentive spirometry: the answer is blowing in the wind. *Chest*, **79**, 254.
90. Shovelton, D. S. (1979). Reflections on an intensive therapy unit. *Brit. Med. J.*, **1**, 737.
91. Bradburn, B. G. and Hewitt, P. B. (1980). The effect of intensive therapy ward environment on patients' subjective impressions: a follow-up study. *Intens. Care Med.*, **7**, 15.
92. Parbrook, G. D. (1972). Entonox for postoperative analgesia. *Proc. Roy. Soc. Med.*, **65**, 8.
93. Editorial (1978). Nitrous oxide and the bone marrow. *Lancet*, **2**, 613.
94. Miller-Jones, C. M. H. and Williams, J. H. (1980). Sedation for ventilation: a retrospective study of fifty patients. *Anaesthesia*, **35**, 1104.
95. Ramsay, M. A. E., Savege, T. M., Simpson, B. R. J. and Goodwin, R. (1974). Controlled sedation with alphaxalone-alphadolone. *Brit. Med. J.*, **2**, 656.
96. Stewart, G. O., Dobb, G. J. and Craib, I. A. (1983). Clinical trial of continuous infusion of alphaxalone/alphadolone in intensive care patients. *Anaesth. Intens. Care*, 11, 107.
97. Sear, J. W. and Prys-Roberts, C. (1979). Dose-related haemodynamic effects of continuous infusions of althesin in man. *Brit. J. Anaesth.*, **51**, 867.
98. Edbrooke, D. L., Newby, D. M., Mather, S. J., Dixon, A. M. and Hebron, B. S. (1982). Safer sedation for ventilated patients. A new application for etomidate. *Anaesthesia*, **37**, 765.
99. Redding, J. S., Hargest, T. S. and Minsky, S. H. (1977). How noisy is intensive care? *Crit. Care Med.*, **5**, 275.
100. Bentley, S., Murphy, F. and Dudley, H. (1977). Perceived noise in surgical wards and an intensive care area: an objective analysis. *Brit. Med. J.*, **2**, 1503.
101. Murphy, F., Bentley, S., Ellis, B. W. and Dudley, H. (1977). Sleep deprivation in patients undergoing operation: a factor in the stress of surgery. *Brit. Med. J.*, **2**, 1521.
102. Jones, J., Hoggart, B., Withey, J., Donaghue, K. and Ellis, B. W. (1979). What the patients say: a study of reactions to an intensive care unit. *Intens. Care Med.*, **5**, 89.
103. Dubin, W. R., Field, H. L. and Gastfriend, D. R. (1979). Postcardiotomy delirium: a critical review. *J. Thorac. Cardiovasc. Surg.*, **77**, 586.
104. Hale, M., Koss, N., Kerstein, M., Camp, K. and Barash, P. (1977). Psychiatric complications in a surgical ICU. *Crit. Care Med.*, **5**, 199.
105. Tomlin, P. J. (1977). Psychological problems in intensive care. *Brit. Med. J.*, **2**, 441.

106. Epperson, M. M. (1977). Families in sudden crisis: process and intervention in a critical care centre. *Social Work in Health Care*, **2**, 265.
107. Williams, C. C. and Rice, D. G. (1977). The intensive care unit: social work intervention with the families of critically ill patients. *Social Work in Health Care*, **2**, 391.
108. Pattison, E. M. (1977). The family matrix of dying and death. In: *The Experience of Dying*, p. 28. Englewood Cliffs, N.J.: Prentice-Hall.
109. Hill, G. L., Blackett, R. L., Pickford, I., Burkinshaw, L., Young, G. A., Warren, J. V., Schorah, C. J. and Morgan, D. B. (1977). Malnutrition in surgical patients. *Lancet*, **1**, 689.
110. Sheukin, A. (1979). Monitoring the nutritional status of critically ill patients. *Intens. Care Med.*, **5**, 165.
111. Keighley, M. R. B. (1980). Prophylactic antibiotics in surgery. *Brit. J. Hosp. Med.*, **23**, 465.
112. Editorial (1975). Low-dose heparin and the prevention of venous thromboembolic disease. *Brit. Med. J.*, **3**, 447.
113. Sagar, S., Massey, J. and Sanderson, J. M. (1975). Low-dose heparin prophylaxis against fatal pulmonary embolism. *Brit. Med. J.*, **4**, 257.
114. Croker, J. R. (1979). Acute gastrointestinal bleeding in the critically ill patient. *Intens. Care Med.*, **5**, 1.
115. Hastings, P. R., Skillman, J. J., Bushnell, L. S. and Silen, W. (1978). Antacid titration in the prevention of acute gastrointestinal bleeding. *New Engl. J. Med.*, **298**, 1041.
116. Halloran, L. G., Zfass, A. M., Gayle, W. E., Wheeler, C. B. and Miller, J. D. (1980). Prevention of gastrointestinal complications after severe head injury: a controlled trial of cimetidine prophylaxis. *Am. J. Surg.*, **139**, 44.
117. Priebe, H. J., Skillman, J. J., Bushnell, L. S., Long, P. C. and Silen, W. (1980). Antacid versus cimetidine in preventing acute gastrointestinal bleeding. *New Engl. J. Med.*, **302**, 426.
118. Martin, L. F., Staloch, D. K., Simonwitz, D. A., Dellinger, E. P. and Max, M. H. (1979). Failure of cimetidine prophylaxis in the critically ill. *Arch. Surg.*, **114**, 492.
119. Menguy, R. (1980). The prophylaxis of stress ulceration. *New Engl. J. Med.*, **302**, 461.
120. Shoemaker, W. C. (1978). Treatment of shock and trauma states: use of cardiorespiratory patterns to define therapeutic goals, predict survival and tritrate therapy. In: *Critical Care Medicine Manual* Ed. Weil, M. H. and DaLuz, P. L. New York: Springer Verlag.
121. Benedict, C. R. and Graham-Smith, D. G. (1978). Plasma noradrenaline and adrenaline concentrations and dopamine-B-hydroxylase activity in patients with shock due to septicaemia, trauma and haemorrhage. *Quart. J. Med.*, **47**, 1.
122. Morton, J. J., Semple, P. F., Ledingham, I. McA., Stuart, B., Tehrani, M. A., Garcia, A. R. and McGarrity, G. (1977). Effect of angiotensin-converting enzyme inhibitor (SQ 20881) on the plasma concentration of angiotensin I, angiotensin II and arginine vasopressin in the dog during hemorrhagic shock. *Circulation Res.*, **41**, 301.
123. Silver, I. A. (1977). Local factors in tissue oxygenation. *J. Clin. Path.*, Suppl. 11, p. 7.
124. Baue, A. E., Chaudry, I. H., Wurth, M. A. and Sayeed, M. M. (1974). Cellular alterations with shock and ischaemia. *Angiology*, **25**, 31.
125. Ledingham, I. McA. and Routh, G. S. (1979). The pathophysiology of shock. *Brit. J. Hosp. Med.*, **22**, 472.
126. Whaley, K., Yee Khong, T., McCartney, A. C. and Ledingham, I. McA. (1979). Complement activation and its control in gram negative endotoxic shock. *Clin. Lab. Immunology*, **2**, 117.
127. O'Donnell, T. F., Clowes, G., Talamo, R. C. and Colman, R. W. (1976). Kinin activation in the blood of patients with sepsis. *Surg. Gynec. Obstet.*, **143**, 539.
128. Machiedo, G. W., Brown, C. S., Lavigne, J. E. and Rush, B. F., Jnr. (1973). Prostaglandin $E_1$ as a therapeutic agent in hemorrhagic shock. *Surg. Forum*, **24**, 12.
129. Brand, E. C. and Lefer, A. M. (1966). Myocardial depressant factor in plasma from cats in irreversible post-oligemic shock. *Proc. Soc. Exp. Biol. (N.Y.)*, **122**, 200.
130. Lefer, A. M. (1978). Properties of cardio-inhibitory factors produced in shock. *Fed. Proc.*, **37**, 2734.
131. Preston, F. E. (1979). Haematological problems associated with shock. *Brit. J. Hosp. Med.*, **21**, 232.
132. Morrison, D. C. and Cochrane, C. G. (1974). Direct evidence for Hageman factor (factor XII) activation by bacterial lipopolysaccharides (endotoxins). *J. Exp. Med.*, **140**, 797.
133. Barkett, V. M., Coalson, J. J. and Greenfield, L. J. (1968). Protective effects of pulmonary denervation in haemorrhagic shock. *Surg. Forum*, **19**, 38.
134. Dowd, J. and Jenkins, L. C. (1972). The lung in shock: a review. *Canad. Anaesth. Soc. J.*, **19**, 309.
135. Zapol, W. M. and Snider, M. T. (1977). Pulmonary hypertension in acute respiratory failure. *New Engl. J. Med.*, **296**, 476.
136. Blaisdell, F. W. and Schlobohm, R. M. (1973). The respiratory distress syndrome: a review. *Surgery*, **74**, 251.
137. Fulton, R. L., Rayner, A. V. S., Jones, C. and Gray, L. A. (1978). Analysis of factors leading to post-traumatic pulmonary insufficiency. *Ann. Thorac. Surg.*, **25**, 500.
138. Beyer, A. (1979). Shock lung. *Brit. J. Hosp. Med.*, **21**, 248.
139. Demling, R. H. (1980). The pathogenesis of respiratory failure after trauma and sepsis. In: *Respiratory Care in Surgery*. Ed. Bartlett, R. H. *Surg. Clin. N. Amer.*, **60**, 1373.
140. Weil, M. H., Henning, R. J. and Puri, V. K. (1979). Colloid osmotic pressure: clinical significance. *Crit. Care Med.*, **7**, 113.
141. Kohler, J. P., Rice, C. L., Zarins, C. K., Cammack, B. F. and Moss, G. S. (1981). Does reduced colloid oncotic pressure increase pulmonary dysfunction in sepsis? *Crit. Care Med.*, **9**, 90.
142. Shoemaker, W. C. and Hauser, C. J. (1979). Critique of crystalloid versus colloid therapy in shock and shock lung. *Crit. Care Med.*, **7**, 117.
143. Jelenko, C., Williams, J. B., Wheeler, M. L., Callaway, B. D., Fackler, V. K., Albers, C. A. and Barger, A. A. (1979). Studies in shock and resuscitation, I: Use of a hypertonic, albumin-containing, fluid demand regimen (HALFD) in resuscitation. *Crit. Care Med.*, **7**, 157.
144. Blaisdell, F. W. and Lewis, F. R. (1977). Respiratory distress syndrome of shock and trauma. In: *Major Problems in Clinical Surgery*, **21**, Philadelphia: Saunders.
145. Moss, G. Staunton, C. and Stine, A. A. (1972). Cerebral etiology of the shock lung syndrome. *J. Trauma*, **12**, 885.
146. Hammerschmidt, D. E., Weaver, L. J., Hudson, L. D., Craddock, P. R. and Jacob, H. S. (1980). Association of

complement activation and elevated plasma-C5a with adult respiratory distress syndrome. *Lancet*, **1**, 947.
147. Jacob, H. S., Craddock, P. R., Hammerschmidt, D. E. and Moldow, C. F. (1980). Complement-induced granulocyte aggregation. *New Engl. J. Med.*, **302**, 789.
148. Gavras, H., Kremer, D., Brown, J. J., Gray, B., Lever, A. F., MacAdam, D., Medina, A., Morton, J. J. and Robertson, J. I. S. (1975). Angiotensin and norepinephrine-induced myocardial lesions: experimental and clinical studies in rabbits and man. *Am. Heart J.*, **89**, 321.
149. Peyton, M. D., Hinshaw, L. B., Greenfield, A. J. and Elkins, R. C. (1976). The effects of coronary vasodilatation on cardiac performance during endotoxin shock. *Surg. Gynec. Obstet.*, **143**, 533.
150. Smolens, P. and Stein, J. H. (1981). Pathophysiology of acute renal failure. *Am. J. Med.*, **70**, 479.
151. Brown, J. J., Gleadle, R. I., Lawson, D. H., Lever, A. F., Linton, A. L., MacAdam, R. F., Prentice, E., Robertson, J. I. S. and Tree, M. (1970). Renin and acute renal failure: studies in man. *Brit. Med. J.*, **1**, 253.
152. Robson, J. S. (1977). Pathogenesis of acute renal failure. In: *Recent Advances in Intensive Therapy*, p. 203. Ed. Ledingham, I. McA. Edinburgh: Churchill Livingstone.
153. Caulfield, J. B., Dunkman, W. B. and Leinbach, R. C. (1972). Cardiogenic shock. *Arch. Pathol.*, **93**, 532.
154. Forrester, J. S., Diamond, G., Chatterjee, K. and Swan, H. J. C. (1976). Medical therapy of acute myocardial infarction by application of hemodynamic subsets. *New Engl. J. Med.*, **295**, 1356 & 1404.
155. Ledingham, I. McA. and McArdle, C. S. (1978). Prospective study of the treatment of septic shock. *Lancet*, **1**, 1194.
156. Wardle, N. (1979). Bacteraemic and endotoxic shock. *Brit. J. Hosp. Med.*, **21**, 223.
157. Hess, M. L., Hastillo, A. and Greenfield, L. J. (1981). Spectrum of cardiovascular function during gram-negative sepsis. *Prog. Cardiovasc. Dis.*, **23**, 279.
158. Blain, C. M., Anderson, T. O., Pietras, R. J. and Gunnar, R. M. (1970). Immediate hemodynamic effects of gram-negative *vs* gram-positive bacteremia in man. *Arch. Intern. Med.*, **126**, 260.
159. Wiles, J. B., Cerra, F. B., Siegel, J. H. and Border, J. R. (1980). The systemic septic response: does the organism matter? *Crit. Care Med.*, **8**, 55.
160. Levin, J., Poore, T. E., Young, N. S., Margolis, S., Zauber, N. P., Townes, A. S. and Bell, W. R. (1972). Gram-negative sepsis: detection of endotoxaemia with the Limulus test. *Ann. Int. Med.*, **76**, 1.
161. Pitcher, J. L. (1971). Safety and effectiveness of the modified Sengstaken-Blakemore tube: a prospective study. *Gastroenterology*, **61**, 291.
162. White, R. I., Barth, K. H., Kaufman, S. L., DeCaprio, V. and Strandberg, J. D. (1980). Therapeutic embolization with detachable balloons. *Cardiovasc. Intervent. Radiol.*, **3**, 229.
163. Thomson, K. R. and Goldin, A. R. (1979). Angiographic techniques in interventional radiology. *Radiol. Clin. N. Am.*, **17**, 375.
164. Editorial (1981). Cardioplegia. *Lancet*, **1**, 24.
165. Geddes, A. M. (1978). Use of antibiotics: septicaemia. *Brit. Med. J.*, **2**, 181.
166. Goodwin, C. S. (1980). Antibiotics: their administration, choice and prophylactic use. *Anaesth. Intens. Care*, **8**, 34.
167. Editorial (1979). Antibiotic-associated colitis—a bacterial disease. *Brit. Med. J.*, **2**, 349.
168. Miller, T. E. and North, D. K. (1981). Clinical infections, antibiotics and immunosuppression: a puzzling relationship. *Am. J. Med.*, **71**, 334.
169. Buxton Hopkin, D. A. (1978). Frapper fort ou frapper doucement: a gram-negative dilemma. *Lancet*, **2**, 1193.
170. Weil, M. H. and Henning, R. J. (1979). New concepts in the diagnosis and fluid treatment of circulatory shock. *Anesth. Analg.*, **58**, 124.
171. Shine, K. I., Kuhn, M., Young, L. S. and Tillisch, J. H. (1980). Aspects of the management of shock. *Ann. Int. Med.*, **93**, 723.
172. Shoemaker, W. C. (1975). Algorithm for resuscitation: a systematic plan for immediate care of the injured or postoperative patient. *Crit. Care Med.*, **3**, 127.
173. Crexells, C., Chatterjee, K., Forrester, J. S., Dikshit, K. and Swan, H. J. C. (1973). Optimal level of filling pressure in the left side of the heart in acute myocardial infarction. *New Engl. J. Med.*, **289**, 1263.
174. Messmer, K. (1975). Hemodilution. *Surg. Clin. N. Am.*, **55**, 659.
175. Tinker, J. (1979). A pharmacological approach to the treatment of shock. *Brit. J. Hosp. Med.*, **21**, 261.
176. Hill, N. S., Antman, E. M., Green, L. H. and Alpert, J. S. (1981). Intravenous nitroglycerin: a review of pharmacology, indications, therapeutic effects and complications. *Chest*, **79**, 69.
177. Thompson, W. L. (1977). Dopamine in the management of shock. *Proc. Roy. Soc. Med.*, **70** (Suppl. 2), 25.
178. Goldberg, L. I., Hsich, Y-Y. and Resnekov, L. (1977). Newer catecholamines for treatment of heart failure and shock: an update on dopamine and a first look at dobutamine. *Prog. Cardiovasc. Dis.*, **19**, 327.
179. Loeb, H. S., Winslow, E. B. J., Rakimtoola, S. H., Rosen, K. M. and Gunnar, R. M. (1971). Acute hemodynamic effects of dopamine in patients in shock. *Circulation*, **44**, 163.
180. Holzer, J., Karliner, J. S., O'Rourke, R. A., Pitt, W. and Ross, J. (1973). Effectiveness of dopamine in patients with cardiogenic shock. *Am. J. Cardiol.*, **32**, 79.
181. Sonnenblick, E. H., Frishman, W. H. and LeJemtel, T. H. (1979). Dobutamine: a new synthetic cardioactive sympathetic amine. *New Engl. J. Med.*, **300**, 17.
182. Jardin, F., Sportiche, M., Bazin, M., Bourokba, A. and Margairaz, A. (1981). Dobutamine: a haemodynamic evaluation in human septic shock. *Crit. Care Med.*, **9**, 329.
183. Gillespie, T. A., Ambos, H. D., Sobel, B. E. and Roberts, R. (1977). Effects of dobutamine in patients with acute myocardial infarction. *Am. J. Cardiol.*, **39**, 588.
184. Keung, E. C. H., Siskind, S. J., Sonnenblick, E. H., Ribner, H. S., Schwartz, W. J. and LeJemtel, T. H. (1981). Dobutamine therapy in acute myocardial infarction. *JAMA*, **245**, 144.
185. Sakamoto, T. and Yamada, T. (1977). Hemodynamic effects of dobutamine in patients following open heart surgery. *Circulation*, **55**, 525.
186. Unverferth, D. V., Blanford, M., Kates, R. E. and Leier, C. V. (1980). Tolerance to dobutamine after a 72 hour continuous infusion. *Am. J. Med.*, **69**, 262.
187. Timmis, A. D., Fowler, M. B. and Chamberlain, D. A. (1981). Comparison of haemodynamic responses to dopamine and salbutamol in severe cardiogenic shock

complicating acute myocardial infarction. *Brit. Med. J.*, **282**, 7.
188. Kuhn, L. A. (1978). Management of shock following acute myocardial infarction. Part I. Drug Therapy. *Am. Heart J.*, **95**, 529.
189. Kuhn, L. A. (1978). Management of shock following acute myocardial infarction. Part II. Mechanical circulatory assistance. *Am. Heart J.*, **95**, 789.
190. Scallan, M. J. H., Gothard, J. W. W. and Branthwaite, M. A. (1979). Inotropic agents. *Br. J. Anaesth.*, **51**, 649.
191. Herbert, P. and Tinker, J. (1980). Inotropic drugs in acute circulatory failure. *Intens. Care Med.*, **6**, 101.
192. Sturm, J. T., Fuhrman, T. M., Sterling, R., Turner, S. A., Igo, S. R. and Norman, J. C. (1981). Combined use of dopamine and nitroprusside therapy in conjunction with intra-aortic balloon pumping for the treatment of postcardiotomy low-output syndrome. *J. Thorac. Cardiovasc. Surg.*, **82**, 13.
193. Editorial (1978). Controlled intravascular sodium nitroprusside treatment. *Brit. Med. J.*, **2**, 784.
194. Editorial (1978). Imbalanced ventricles and cardiac failure. *Brit. Med. J.*, **1**, 324.
195. Editorial (1981). Long term vasodilator therapy for heart failure. *Lancet*, **1**, 1350.
196. Palmer, R. F. and Lasseter, K. C. (1975). Sodium nitroprusside. *New Engl. J. Med.*, **292**, 294.
197. Tinker, J. H. and Michenfelder, J. D. (1976). Sodium nitroprusside: pharmacology, toxicology and therapeutics. *Anesthesiology*, **45**, 340.
198. Cole, P. (1978). The safe use of sodium nitroprusside. *Anaesthesia*, **33**, 473.
199. Vesey, C. J., Cole, P. V. and Simpson, P. J. (1976). Cyanide and thiocyanate concentrations following sodium nitroprusside infusion in man. *Br. J. Anaesth.*, **48**, 651.
200. Fahmy, N. R. (1981). Consumption of vitamin $B_{12}$ during sodium nitroprusside administration in humans. *Anesthesiology*, **54**, 305.
201. Cottrell, J. E., Casthely, P., Brodie, J. D., Patel, K., Klein, A. and Turndorf, H. (1978). Prevention of nitroprusside-induced cyanide toxicity with hydroxocobalamin. *New Engl. J. Med.*, **298**, 809.
202. Franciosa, J. A., Guiha, N. H., Limas, C. J., Rodriguera, E. and Cohn, J. N. (1972). Improved left ventricular function during nitroprusside infusion in acute myocardial infarction. *Lancet*, **1**, 650.
203. Chatterjee, K., Parmley, W. W., Ganz, W., Forrester, J., Walinsky, P., Crexells, C. and Swan, H. J. C. (1973). Hemodynamic and metabolic responses to vasodilator therapy in acute myocardial infarction. *Circulation*, **48**, 1183.
204. Piepenbrock, S., Hempelmann, G. and Westermann, C. (1977). Massive doses of methylprednisolone (30 mg/kg) in man: immediate haemodynamic effects in "low output state". *Intens. Care Med.*, **3**, 69.
205. Dietzman, R. H. and Lillehei, R. C. (1968). The treatment of cardiogenic shock. V. The use of corticosteroids in the treatment of cardiogenic shock. *Am. Heart J.*, **75**, 274.
206. Merin, G., Eimerl, D., Raz, S., Tzironi, D. and Gotsman, M. S. (1978). Preservation of myocardial contractility in hemorrhagic shock with methylprednisolone. *Ann. Thorac. Surg.*, **25**, 536.
207. Schumer, W. (1976). Steroids in the treatment of clinical septic shock. *Ann. Surg.*, **184**, 333.
208. Sladen, A. (1976). Methylprednisolone. pharmacologic doses in shock lung syndrome. *J. Thorac. Cardiovasc. Surg.*, **71**, 800.
209. Cheney, F. W., Huang, T. H. and Gronka, R. (1979). Effects of methylprednisolone on experimental pulmonary injury. *Ann. Surg.*, **190**, 236.
210. Peters, W. P., Johnson, M. W., Friedman, P. A. and Mitch, W. E. (1981). Pressor effects of naloxone in septic shock. *Lancet*, **1**, 529.
211. Hoffman, E. (1976). Mortality and morbidity following road accidents. *Ann. Roy. Coll. Surg. Engl.*, **58**, 233.
212. Trinkle, J. K., Richardson, J. D., Franz, J. L., Grover, F. L., Arom, K. V. and Holmstrom, F. M. G. (1975). Management of flail chest without mechanical ventilation. *Ann. Thorac. Surg.*, **19**, 355.
213. Shackford, S. R., Smith, D. E., Zarins, C. K., Rice, C. K. and Virgilo, R. W. (1976). The management of flail chest: a comparison of ventilatory and non-ventilatory treatment. *Amer. J. Surg.*, **132**, 759.
214. Richardson, J. D., Adams, L. and Flint, L. M. (1982). Selective management of flail chest and pulmonary contusion. *Ann. Surg.* **196**, 481.
215. Lewin, W. (1976). Changing attitudes to the management of severe head injuries. *Brit. med. J.*, **2**, 1234.
216. Teasdale, G. and Jennett, B. (1974). Assessment of coma and impaired consciousness. *Lancet*, **2**, 81.
217. McDowall, D. G. (1976). Monitoring the brain. *Anesthesiology*, **45**, 117.
218. Steen, P. A. and Michenfelder, J. D. (1980). Mechanisms of barbiturate protection. *Anesthesiology*, **53**, 183.
219. Petty, A. H. (1973). Abdominal injuries. *Ann. Roy. Coll. Surg. Engl.*, **53**, 167.
220. Austen, K. F. (1974). Systemic anaphylaxis in the human being. *New Engl. J. Med.*, **291**, 661.
221. Lichtenstein, L. M. and Norman, P. S. (1969). Human allergic reactions. *Am. J. Med.*, **46**, 163.
222. Watkins, J. (1979). Anaphylactoid reactions to I.V. substances. *Br. J. Anaesth.*, **51**, 51.
223. Kelly, J. F. and Patterson, R. (1974). Anaphylaxis: course, mechanisms and treatment. *JAMA*, **227**, 1431.
224. Fisher, M. McD. (1977). The management of anaphylaxis. *Med. J. Aust.*, **1**, 793.
225. Fisher, M. McD. and More, D. G. (1981). The epidemiology and clinical features of anaphylactic reactions in anaesthesia. *Anaesth. Intens. Care*, **9**, 226.
226. Fisher, M. McD. (1975). Severe histamine mediated reactions to intravenous drugs and in anaesthesia. *Anaesth. Intens. Care*, **3**, 180.
227. Clarke, R. S. J., Dundee, J. W., Garrett, R. T., McArdle, G. K. and Sutton, J. A. (1975). Adverse reactions to intravenous anaesthetics. *Br. J. Anaesth.*, **47**, 575.
228. Altman, L. C. (1981). Basic immune mechanisms in immediate hypersensitivity. *Med. Clin. N. Am.*, **65**, 941.
229. Editorial (1981). Treatment of anaphylactic shock. *Brit. Med. J.*, **282**, 1011.
230. Fisher, M. (1977). Blood volume replacement in acute anaphylactic cardiovascular collapse related to anaesthesia. *Br. J. Anaesth.*, **49**, 1023.
231. Fisher, M. McD. (1981). The prevention of second anaphylactoid reactions to anaesthetic drugs. *Anaesth. Intens. Care*, **9**, 242.
232. Todd, J., Fishaut, M., Kapral, F. and Welch, T. (1978).

Toxic shock syndrome associated with phage-group I staphylococci. *Lancet*, **2**, 1116.

233. Holt, P. (1980). Tampon-associated toxic shock syndrome. *Brit. Med. J.*, **281**, 1321.
234. Davis, J. P., Chesney, J., Wand, P. J. and LaVenture, M. (1980). Toxic-shock syndrome: epidemiologic features, recurrence, risk factors and prevention. *New Engl. J. Med.*, **303**, 1429.
235. Shands, K. N., Schmid, G. P., Dan, B. B., Blum, D., Guidotti, R. J., Hargrett, N. T., Anderson, R. L., Hill, D. L., Broome, C. V., Band, J. D. and Fraser, D. W. (1980). Toxic-shock syndrome in menstruating women: association with tampon use and *Staphylococcus aureus* and clinical features in 52 cases. *New Engl. J. Med.*, **303**, 1436.
236. Hosking, N., Bolitho, L. E., Bhardwaj, N., Sloman, R., Ryan, A. and Newman, W. (1981). Toxic shock associated with tampon usage. *Med. J. Aust.*, **1**, 638.
237. Reingold, A. L., Dan, B. B., Shands, K. N. and Broome, C. V. (1982). Toxic shock syndrome not associated with menstruation. *Lancet*, **1**, 1.
238. Glasgow, L. A. (1980). Staphyloccocal infection in the toxic-shock syndrome. *New Engl. J. Med.*, **303**, 1473.
239. Mather, H. G., Morgan, D. C., Pearson, N. G., Read, K. L. Q., Shaw, D. B., Steed, G. R., Thorne, M. G., Lawrence, C. J. and Riley, I. S. (1976). Myocardial infarction: a comparison between home and hospital care for patients. *Brit. Med. J.*, **1**, 925.
240. Colling, A. (1974). Home or hospital care after myocardial infarction: is this the right question? *Brit. Med. J.*, **1**, 559.
241. Hill, J. D., Hampton, J. R. and Mitchell, J. R. A. (1978). A randomised trial of home-versus-hospital management for patients with suspected myocardial infarction. *Lancet*, **1**, 837.
242. Working Party of the Royal College of Physicians of London and the British Cardiac Society (1975). The care of the patient with coronary heart disease. *J. Roy. Coll. Phys. Lond.*, **10**, 5.
243. Briggs, R. S., Brown, P. M., Crabb, M. E., Cox, T. J., Ead, H. W., Hawkes, R. A., Jequier, P. W., Southall, D. P., Grainger, R., Williams, J. H. and Chamberlain, D. A. (1976). The Brighton resuscitation ambulances: a continuing experiment in prehospital care by ambulance staff. *Brit. Med. J.*, **2**, 1161.
244. Mackintosh, A. F., Crabb, M. E., Grainger, R., Williams, J. H. and Chamberlain, D. A. (1978). The Brighton resuscitation ambulances: review of 40 consecutive survivors of out-of-hospital cardiac arrest. *Brit. Med. J.*, **1**, 1115.
245. Tresch, D. D., Grove, J. R., Keelan, M. H., Siegel, R., Bonchek, L. I., Olinger, G. H. and Brooks, H. L. (1981). Long term follow up of survivors of pre-hospital sudden coronary death. *Circulation*, **64** (Suppl. II), 1.
246. O'Rourke, M. F., Walsh, B., Fletcher, M. and Crowley, A. (1976). Impact of the new generation coronary care unit. *Brit. Med. J.*, **2**, 837.
247. Astvad, K., Fabricius-Bjerre, N., Kjaerulff, J. and Lindholm, J. (1974). Mortality from acute myocardial infarction before and after establishment of a coronary care unit. *Brit. Med. J.*, **1**, 567.
248. Hill, J. D., Holdstock, G. and Hampton, J. R. (1977). Comparison of mortality of patients with heart attacks admitted to a coronary care unit and an ordinary medical ward. *Brit. Med. J.*, **2**, 81.
249. Khosla, T., Newcombe, R. G. and Campbell, H. (1977). Who is at risk of a coronary? *Brit. Med. J.*, **1**, 341.
250. Mann, J. I., Inman, W. H. W. and Thorogood, M. (1976). Oral contraceptive use in older women and fatal myocardial infarction. *Brit. Med. J.*, **2**, 445.
251. Jenkins, C. D. (1976). Recent evidence supporting psychologic and social risk factors for coronary disease. *New Engl. J. Med.*, **294**, 987 and 1033.
252. Heller, R. F. (1979). Type A behaviour and coronary heart disease. *Brit. Med. J.*, **2**, 368.
253. Hickey, N., Mulcahy, R., Brurke, G. J., Graham, I. and Wilson-Davis, K. (1975). Study of coronary risk factors related to physical activity in 15 171 men. *Brit. Med. J.*, **3**, 507.
254. Morris, J. N., Everitt, M. G., Pollard, R., Chave, S. P. W. and Semmence, A. M. (1980). Vigorous exercise in leisure-time: protection against coronary heart disease. *Lancet*, **2**, 1207.
255. Willerson, J. T. and Buja, L. M. (1980). Cause and course of acute myocardial infarction. *Am. J. Med.*, **69**, 903.
256. Hellstrom, M. R. (1979). Coronary artery vasospasm: the likely immediate cause of acute myocardial infarction. *Br. Heart J.*, **41**, 426.
257. Ganz, W. (1981). Coronary spasm in myocardial infarction: fact or fiction? *Circulation*, **63**, 487.
258. Kinlen, L. J. (1973). Incidence and presentation of myocardial infarction in an English community. *Br. Heart J.*, **35**, 616.
259. McGuiness, J. B., Begg, T. B. and Semple, T. (1976). First electrocardiogram in recent myocardial infarction. *Brit. Med. J.*, **2**, 449.
260. Scott, B. B., Simmons, A. V., Newton, K. E. and Payne, R. B. (1974). Interpretation of serum creatinine kinase in suspected myocardial infarction. *Brit. Med. J.*, **4**, 691.
261. Joseph, S. P., Pereira-Prestes, A. V., Ell, P. J., Donaldson, R., Somerville, W. and Emanuel, R. W. (1979). Value of positive myocardial infarction imaging in coronary care units. *Brit. Med. J.*, **1**, 372.
262. Williams, B. O., Begg, T. B., Semple, T. and McGuiness, J. B. (1976). The elderly in a coronary care unit. *Brit. Med. J.*, **2**, 451.
263. Tucker, H. H., Carson, P. H. M., Bass, N. M., Sharatt, G. P. and Stock, J. P. P. (1973). Results of early mobilization and discharge after myocardial infarction. *Brit. Med. J.*, **1**, 10.
264. Hayes, M. J., Morris, G. K. and Hampton, J. R. (1974). Comparison of mobilisation after two and nine days in uncomplicated myocardial infarction. *Brit. Med. J.*, **3**, 10.
265. Singer, D. E., Mulley, A. G., Thibault, G. E. and Barnett, G. O. (1981). Unexpected readmissions to the coronary care unit during recovery from acute myocardial infarction. *New Engl. J. Med.*, **304**, 625.
266. Gelson, A. D. N., Carson, P. H. M., Tucker, H. H., Phillips, R., Clarke, M. and Oakley, G. D. G. (1976). Course of patients discharged early after myocardial infarction. *Brit. Med. J.*, **1**, 1555.
267. Rawles, J. M. and Kenmure, A. C. F. (1976). Controlled trial of oxygen in uncomplicated myocardial infarction. *Brit. Med. J.*, **1**, 1121.
268. Skelton, M. and Dominian, J. (1973). Psychological stress in wives of patients with myocardial infarction. *Brit. Med. J.*, **2**, 101.

269. Emerson, P. A. and Marks, P. (1977). Preventing thromboembolism after myocardial infarction: effect of low-dose heparin or smoking. *Brit. Med J.*, **1**, 18.
270. Thompson, P. L. and Robinson, J. S. (1978). Stroke after acute myocardial infarction: relation to infarct size. *Brit. Med. J.*, **2**, 457.
271. Goldman, L. and Feinstein, A. R. (1979). Anticoagulants and myocardial infarction. *Ann. Int. Med.*, **90**, 92.
272. Gunnar, R. M., Loeb, H. S., Scanlon, P. J., Moran, J. F., Johnson, S. A. and Pifarre, R. (1979). Management of acute myocardial infarction and accelerating angina. *Prog. Cardiovasc. Dis.*, **22**, 1.
273. O'Rourke, M. F., Norris, R. M., Campbell, T. J., Chang, V. P. and Sammel, N. L. (1981). Randomised controlled trial of intra-aortic balloon counter-pulsation in early myocardial infarction with acute heart failure. *Am. J. Cardiol.*, **47**, 815.
274. Jett, G. K., Dengle, S. K., Barnett, P. A., Platt, M. R., Willerson, J. T., Watson, J. T. and Eberhart, R. C. (1981). Intra-aortic balloon counter-pulsation: its influence alone and combined with various pharmacological agents on regional myocardial blood flow during experimental acute coronary occlusion. *Ann. Thorac. Surg.*, **31**, 144.
275. Ribeiro, L. G. T., Brandon, T. A., Hopkins, D. G., Reduto, L. A., Taylor, A. A. and Miller, R. R. (1981). Prostacyclin in experimental myocardial ischemia: effects on hemodynamics, regional myocardial blood flow, infarct size and mortality. *Am. J. Cardiol.*, **47**, 835.
276. Baughman, K. L., Maroko, P. R. and Vatner, S. F. (1981). Effects of coronary artery reperfusion on myocardial infarct size and survival in conscious dogs. *Circulation*, **63**, 317.
277. Campbell, C. D., Takanashi, Y., Laas, J., Meus, P., Pick, R. and Replogle, R. L. (1981). Effect of coronary artery reperfusion on infarct size in swine. *J. Thorac. Cardiovasc. Surg.*, **81**, 288.
278. Mathey, D. G., Kuck, K-H., Tilsner, V., Krebber, H-J. and Bleifeld, W. (1981). Non-surgical coronary artery recanalisation in acute transmural myocardial infarction. *Circulation*, **63**, 489.
279. Rentrop, P., Blanke, H., Karsch, K. R., Kaisor, H., Köstering, H. and Leitz, K. (1981). Selective intracoronary thrombolysis in acute myocardial infarction and unstable angina pectoris. *Circulation*, **63**, 307.
280. Pantridge, J. F. and Geddes, J. S. (1976). Diseases of the cardiovascular system. Management of acute myocardial infarction. *Brit. Med. J.*, **2**, 168.
281. Waldo, A. L., Wells, J. L., Cooper, T. B. and MacLean, W. A. H. (1981). Temporary cardiac pacing: applications and techniques in the treatment of cardiac arrhythmias. *Prog. Cardiovasc. Dis.*, **23**, 451.
282. Lawrie, D. M., Higgins, M. R., Godman, M. J., Oliver, M. F., Julian, D. G. and Donald, K. W. (1968). Ventricular fibrillation complicating acute myocardial infarction. *Lancet*, **2**, 523.
283. Logan, K. R., McIlwaine, W. J., Adgey, A. A. J. and Pantridge, J. F. (1981). Ventricular fibrillation and its recurrence in early acute myocardial infarction. *Lancet*, **1**, 242.
284. Editorial (1979). Anti-dysrhythmic treatment in acute myocardial infarction. *Lancet*, **1**, 193.
285. Aps, C. A., Bell, J. A. Jenkins, B. S., Poole-Wilson, P. A. and Reynolds, F. (1976). Logical approach to lignocaine therapy. *Brit. Med. J.*, **1**, 13.
286. Noneman, J. W. and Rogers, J. F. (1978). Lignocaine prophylaxis in acute myocardial infarction. *Medicine (Baltimore)*, **57**, 501.
287. Lie, K. I., Wellens, H. J., Van Capelle, F. J. and Durrer, D. (1974). Lidocaine in the prevention of primary ventricular fibrillation. *New Engl. J. Med.*, **291**, 1324.
288. Harrison, D. C., Meffin, P. J. and Winkle, R. A. (1977). Clinical pharmokinetics of antiarrhythmic drugs. *Prog. Cardiovasc. Dis.*, **20**, 217.
289. Singh, B. N., Collett, J. T. and Chew, C. Y. C. (1980). New perspectives in the pharmacologic therapy of cardiac arrhythmias. *Prog. Cardiovasc. Dis.*, **22**, 243.
290. Gazes, P. C. and Gaddy, J. E. (1979). Bedside management of acute myocardial infarction. *Am. Heart J.*, **97**, 782.
291. Hindman, M. C., Wagner, G. S., Jaro, M., Atkins, J. M., Scheinman, M. M., DeSanctis, R. W., Hutter, A. H., Yeatman, L., Rubenfire, M., Pujura, C., Rubin, M. and Morris, J. J. (1978). The clinical significance of bundle branch block complicating acute myocardial infarction. 1. Clinical characteristics, hospital mortality and one-year follow-up. *Circulation*, **58**, 679.
292. Hindman, M. C., Wagner, G. S., Jaro, M., Atkins, J. M., Scheinman, M. M., DeSanctis, R. W., Hutter, A. H., Yeatman, L., Rubenfire, M., Pujura, C., Rubin, M. and Morris, J. J. (1978). The clinical significance of bundle branch block complicating acute myocardial infarction. 2. Indications for temporary and permanent pacemaker insertion. *Circulation*, **58**, 689.
293. Fox, K. M., Tomlinson, I. W., Portat, R. W. and Aber, C. P. (1975). Prognostic significance of acute systolic hypertension after myocardial infarction. *Brit. Med. J.*, **3**, 128
294. Timmis, A. D., Fowler, M. B., Burwood, R. J., Gishen, P., Vincent, R. and Chamberlain, D. A. (1981). Pulmonary oedema without critical increase in left atrial pressure in acute myocardial infarction. *Brit. Med. J.*, **283**, 636.
295. Hockings, B. E. F., Cope, G. D., Clarke, G. M. and Taylor, R. R. (1981). Randomized controlled trial of vasodilator therapy after myocardial infarction. *Am. J. Cardiol.*, **48**, 345.
296. Thadani, U., Chopra, M. P., Aber, C. P. and Portal, R. W. (1971). Pericarditis after acute myocardial infarction. *Brit. Med. J.*, **2**, 135.
297. Pentecost, B. L. (1978). Aftercare of acute myocardial infarction. *Brit. J. Hosp. Med.*, **20**, 252.
298. Amsterdam, E. A., Lee, G. and Mason, D. T. (1981). Management of unstable angina: current status and new perspectives. *Am. Heart J.*, **102**, 144.
299. Brooks, N., Warnes, C., Cattell, M., Balcon, R., Honey, M., Layton, C., Sturridge M. and Wright, J. (1981). Cardiac pain at rest: management and follow-up of 100 consecutive cases. *Br. Heart J.*, **45**, 35.
300. Schroeder, J. S., Lamb, I. H. and HU, M. (1980). Do patients in whom myocardial infarction has been ruled out have a better prognosis after hospitalization than those surviving infarction? *New Engl. J. Med.*, **303**, 1.
301. Editorial (1980). Chest pain with normal coronary arteries. *Lancet*, **1**, 130.
302. Kerr, J. (1979). Current topics in tetanus. *Intens. Care Med.*, **5**, 105.
303. Edmonson, R. S. and Flowers, M. W. (1979). Intensive care in tetanus: management, complications and mortality in 100 cases. *Brit. Med. J.*, **1**, 1401.
304. Trinca, J. C. Ed. (1979). *CSL Medical Handbook*,

p. 36. Commonwealth Serum Laboratories, Parkville, Vic.
305. Kerr, J. H., Travis, K. W., O'Rourke, R. A., Sims, J. K. and Uhl, R. R. (1974). Autonomic complications in a case of severe tetanus. *Am. J. Med.*, **57**, 303.
306. Hollow, V. M. and Clarke, G. M. (1975). Autonomic manifestations of tetanus. *Anaes. Intens. Care*, **3**, 142.
307. Alfrey, D. D. and Rauscher, L. A. (1979). Tetanus: a review. *Crit. Care Med.*, **7**, 176.
308. Smith, J. W. G., Laurence, D. R. and Evans, D. G. (1975). Prevention of tetanus in the wounded. *Brit. Med. J.*, **3**, 453.
309. Editorial (1980). The diagnosis of tetanus. *Lancet*, **1**, 1066.
310. Porath, A., Acker, M. and Perel, A. (1977). Serum cholinesterase in tetanus. *Anaesthesia*, **32**, 1009.
311. Stoddart, J. C. (1979). The immunology of tetanus. *Anaesthesia*, **34**, 863.
312. Stoddart, J. C. (1979). Pseudotetanus. *Anaesthesia*, **34**, 877.
313. Editorial (1976). Antitoxin in treatment of tetanus. *Lancet*, **1**, 944.
314. Gupta, P. S., Kapoor, R., Goyal, S., Batra, V. K. and Jain, B. K. (1980). Intrathecal human tetanus immunoglubulin in early tetanus. *Lancet*, **2**, 439.
315. Buchanan, N., Cane, R. D., Wolfson, G. and DeAndrade, M. (1979). Autonomic dysfunction in tetanus: the effects of a variety of therapeutic agents, with special reference to morphine. *Intens. Care Med.*, **5**, 65.
316. Dundee, J. W. and Morrow, W. F. K. (1979). Labetolol in severe tetanus. *Brit. Med. J.*, **1**, 1121.
317. Rie, M. A. and Wilson, R. S. (1978). Morphine therapy controls autonomic hyperactivity in tetanus. *Ann. Int. Med.*, **88**, 653.
318. Corbett, J. L., Spalding, J. M. K. and Harris, P. J. (1973). Hypotension in tetanus. *Brit. Med. J.*, **3**, 423.
319. Femi-Pearse, D., Afonja, A. O., Elegbeleye, O. O. and Odusote, K. A. (1976). Value of determination of oxygen consumption in tetanus. *Brit. Med. J.*, **1**, 74.
320. Heurich, A. E., Brust, J. C. M. and Richter, R. W. (1973). Management of urban tetanus. *Med. Clin. N. Am.*, **57**, 1373.
321. Trujillo, M. J., Castillo, A., Espana, J. V., Guevara, P. and Eganez, H. (1980). Tetanus in the adult: intensive care and management experience with 233 cases. *Crit. Care Med.*, **8**, 419.
322. Conference (1981). Guillain-Barré syndrome. *Ann. Neurol.* **9** (Suppl.).
323. Ravn, H. (1969). The Landry-Gullain-Barré syndrome: a survey and clinical report of 127 cases. *Acta Neurol. Scand.*, **43** (Suppl. 30), 9.
324. Sheremata, W., Colby, S., Lusky, G. and Cosgrove, J. B. R. (1975). Cellular hypersensitization to peripheral nervous antigens in the Guillain-Barré syndrome. *Neurology*, **25**, 833.
325. Hurwitz, E. S., Schonberger, L. B., Nelson, D. B. and Holman, R. C. (1981). Guillain-Barré syndrome and the 1978–1979 influenza vaccine. *New Engl. J. Med.*, **304**, 1557.
326. Osler, L. D. and Sidell, A. D. (1960). The Guillain-Barré syndrome: the need for exact diagnostic criteria. *New Engl. J. Med.*, **262**, 964.
327. Editorial (1975). Guillain-Barré syndrome. *Brit. Med. J.*, **3**, 190.
328. Moore, P. and James, O. (1981). Guillain-Barré syndrome: incidence, management and outcome of major complications. *Crit. Care Med.*, **9**, 549.
329. Editorial (1971). Relapsing polyneuropathy and corticosteroids. *Brit. Med. J.*, **1**, 62.
330. King, E. G. and Jacobs, H. (1971). "Complications" of the Landry-Guillain-Barré-Strohl syndrome. *Canad. Med. Assoc. J.*, **104**, 393.
331. Davis, A. G. and Dingle, H. R. (1972). Observations on cardiovascular and neuroendocrine disturbance in the Guillain-Barré syndrome. *J. Neurol. Neurosurg. Psychiat.*, **35**, 176.
332. Lichtenfeld, P. (1971). Autonomic dysfunction in the Guillain-Barré syndrome. *Am. J. Med.*, **50**, 772.
333. Pessin, M. S. (1972). Transient diabetes insipidus in the Landry-Guillain-Barré syndrome. *Arch. Neurol.*, **27**, 85.
334. Posner, J. B., Entel, N. H. and Kossmann, R. G. (1967). Hyponatraemia in acute polyneuropathy. Four cases with the syndrome of inappropraite secretion of antidiuretic hormone. *Arch. Neurol.*, **17**, 530.
335. Rodriguez-Iturbe, B., Garcia, R., Rubio, L., Zabala, J., Moros, G. and Torres, R. (1973). Acute glomerulonephritis in the Guillain-Barré-Strohl syndrome. *Ann. Int. Med.*, **78**, 391.
336. Löffel, N. B., Rossi, L. N., Mumenthaler, M., Lütschg, J. and Ludin, H-P. (1977). The Landry-Guillain-Barré syndrome. Complications, prognosis and natural history in 123 cases. *J. Neurol. Sci.*, **33**, 71.
337. Wright, R. C. (1974). A simple plan for the management of drug overdosage. *Anaesth. Intens. Care*, **2**, 228.
338. Vale, J. A. (1977). The immediate care of cases of poisoning. *Anaesthesia*, **32**, 483.
339. Locket, S. (1978). Overdose. *Brit. J. Hosp. Med.*, **19**, 200.
340. Greensher, J., Mofenson, H. C., Picchioni, A. L. and Fallon, P. (1979). Activated charcoal updated. *JACEP*, **8**, 261.
341. Graham, J. D. P. and Webb, D. B. (1979). The place of dialysis in the treatment of poisoning. In: *Advanced Medicine 15*, p. 323. Ed. Harper, P. S. and Muir, J. R. Tunbridge Wells: Pitman Medical.
342. Vale, J. A., Rees, A. J., Widdop, B. and Goulding, R. (1975). Use of charcoal haemoperfusion in the management of severely poisoned patients. *Brit. Med. J.*, **1**, 5.
343. Myers, R. A. M., Linberg, S. E. and Cowley, R. A. (1979). Carbon monoxide poisoning: the injury and its treatment. *JACEP*, **8**, 479.
344. Brown, T. C. K., Bishop, F. I. and Mullins, G. C. (1974). Drug overdosage in children. *Anaesth. Intens. Care*, **2**, 303.
345. Burrows, G. D. and Harari, E. (1974). Psychiatric aspects of drug overdose in adults. *Anaesth. Intens. Care*, **2**, 310.
346. Gardner, R., Hanka, R., O'Brien, V. C., Page, A. J. F. and Rees, R. (1977). Psychological and social evaluation in cases of deliberate self-poisoning admitted to a general hospital. *Brit. Med. J.*, **2**, 1567.
347. Morgan, E. B. (1975). Severe drug overdose: results of treatment. *Anaesth. Intens. Care*, **3**, 131.
348. Krapez, J. R. and Cole, P. (1977). The management of acute poisoning. *Anaesthesia*, **32**, 494.
349. Knopp, R. (1979). Caustic ingestions. *JACEP*, **8**, 329.
350. Chung, R. S. K. and DenBesten, L. (1975). Fibreoptic endoscopy in treatment of corrosive injury of the stomach. *Arch. Surg.*, **110**, 725.

351. Campbell, G. S., Burnett, H. F., Ransom, J. M. and Williams, D. (1977). Treatment of corrosive burns of the esophagus. *Arch. Surg.*, **112**, 495.
352. Berry, W. B., Hall, R. A. and Jordan, G. L. (1965). Necrosis of the entire stomach secondary to ingestion of a corrosive acid. Report of a patient successfully treated by total gastrectomy. *Am. J. Surg.*, **109**, 652.
353. Naughton, M. (1974). Acute cyanide poisoning. *Anaesth. Intens. Care*, **2**, 351.
354. Ganendran, A. (1974). Organophosphate insecticide poisoning and its management. *Anaesth. Intens. Care*, **2**, 361.
355. Proudfoot, A. T. and Prescott, L. F. (1977). Poisoning with paraquat, salicylate and paracetamol. In: *Recent Advances in Intensive Therapy*, **1**, p. 217. Ed. Ledingham, I. McA. Edinburgh: Churchill Livingstone.
356. Prescott, L. F., Illingworth, R. H., Critchley, J. A. J. H., Stewart, M. J., Adam, R. D. and Proudfoot, A. T. (1979). Intravenous N-acetylcysteine: the treatment of choice for paracetamol poisoning. *Brit. Med. J.*, **2**, 1097.
357. Breen, K. J., Burg, R. W., Desmond, P. V., Forge, B. H. R., Mashford, M. L. and Whelan, G. (1982). Paracetamol self poisoning. *Med. J. Aust.*, **1**, 77.
358. ICI Australia (1980). *The Treatment of Paraquat Poisoning: a Guide for Doctors.*
359. Kerr, F., Patel, A. R., Scott, P. D. R. and Tompsett, S. L. (1968). Paraquat poisoning treated by forced diuresis. *Brit. J. Med.*, **3**, 290.
360. Maini, R. and Winchester, J. F. (1975). Removal of paraquat from blood by haemoperfusion over sorbent materials. *Brit. Med. J.*, **3**, 281.
361. Proudfoot, A. T., Stewart, M. S., Levitt, T. and Widdop, B. (1979). Paraquat poisoning: significance of plasma-paraquat concentrations. *Lancet*, **2**, 330.
362. Okonek, S., Baldamus, C. A. and Hofmann, A. (1980). Survival despite potentially fatal plasma paraquat concentrations. *Lancet*, **2**, 589.
363. Callaham, M. (1979). Tricyclic antidepressant overdose. *JACEP*, **8**, 413.
364. Newton, R. W. (1975). Physiostigmine salicylate in the treatment of antidepressant overdose. *JAMA*, **231**, 941.
365. Lawson, L. J. (1965). Parenteral nutrition in surgery. *Brit. J. Surg.*, **52**, 795.
366. Goode, A. W. (1981). The scientific basis of nutritional assessment. *Br. J. Anaesth.*, **53**, 161.
367. Rhoads, J. E. (1980). The impact of nutrition on infection. *Surg. Clin. N. Amer.*, **60**, 41.
368. Egdahl, R. H., Meguid, M. M. and Aun, F. (1977). The importance of endocrine and metabolic responses to shock and trauma. *Crit. Care Med.* **5**, 257.
369. Dahn, M., Kirkpatrick, J. R. and Bouwman, D. (1980). Sepsis, glucose intolerance and protein malnutrition. A metabolic paradox. *Arch. Surg.*, **115**, 1415.
370. Traynor, C. and Hall, G. M. (1981). Endocrine and metabolic changes during surgery: anaesthetic implications. *Br. J. Anaesth.*, **53**, 153.
371. Birkhahn, R. H., Long, C. L., Fitkin, D. L., Busnardo, A. C., Geiger, J. W. and Blakemore, W. S. (1981). A comparison of the effects of skeletal trauma and surgery on the ketosis of starvation in man. *J. Trauma*, **21**, 513.
372. Burke, J. F., Wolfe, R. R., Mullany, C. J., Mathews, D. E. and Bier, D. M. (1979). Glucose requirements following burn injury. *Ann. Surg.*, **190**, 274.
373. Cerra, F. B., Seigel, J. H., Coleman, B., Border, J. R. and McMenamy, R. R. (1980). Septic autocanabalism. A failure of exogenous nutritional support. *Ann. Surg.*, **192**, 570.
374. Tsuji, H., Asoh, T., Shirasaka, C. and Takeuchi, Y. (1980). Inhibition of metabolic responses to surgery with $\beta$-adrenergic blockade. *Br. J. Surg.*, **67**, 503.
375. Burns, H. J. G., Galloway, D. J. and Ledingham, I. McA. (1981). Effect of naftidrofuryl on the metabolic response to surgery. *Brit. Med. J.*, **283**, 7.
376. Eriksson, B. and Douglass, H. O. (1980). Intravenous hyperalimentation. An adjunct to treatment of malignant disease of upper gastrointestinal tract. *JAMA*, **243**, 2049.
377. Miller, S. F., Morath, M. A. and Finley, R. K. (1981). Comparison of derived and actual transferrin: a potential source of error in clinical nutritional assessment. *J. Trauma*, **21**, 548.
378. Michel, L., Serrano, A. and Malt, R. A. (1981). Nutritional support of hospitalised patients. *New Engl. J. Med.*, **304**, 1147.
379. Heymsfield, S. B., Bethel, R. A., Ansley, J. D., Nixon, D. W. and Rudman, D. (1979). Enteral hyperalimentation: an alternative to central venous hyperalimentation. *Ann. Int. Med.*, **90**, 63.
380. Yeung, C. K., Smith, R. C. and Hill, G. L. (1979). Effect of an elemental diet on body composition. A comparison with intravenous nutrition. *Gastroenterology*, **77**, 652.
381. Peterson, S. R., Kudsk, K. A., Carpenter, G. and Sheldon, G. (1981). Malnutrition and immunocompetence: increased mortality following an infectious challenge during hyperalimentation. *J. Trauma*, **21**, 528.
382. Bateman, E. C. (1977). Tube feeding. *J. Human Nutr.*, **31**, 85.
383. Atkinson, M., Walford, S. and Allison, S. P. (1979). Endoscopic insertion of fine-bore feeding tubes. *Lancet*, **2**, 829.
384. Torosian, M. H. and Rombeau, J. L. (1980). Feeding by tube enterostomy. *Surg. Gynec. Obstet.*, **150**, 918.
385. Page, C. P., Carlton, P. K., Andrassy, R. J., Feldtman, R. W. and Shield, C. F. (1979). Safe, cost-effective postoperative nutrition. Defined formula diet via needle-catheter jejunostomy. *Am. J. Surg.*, **138**, 939.
386. Yeung, C. K., Young, G. A., Hackett, A. F. and Hill, G. L. (1979). Fine needle catheter jejunostomy—an assessment of a new method of nutritional support after major gastrointestinal surgery. *Br. J. Surg.*, **66**, 727.
387. Brown, J. (1981). Enteral feeds and delivery systems. *Brit. J. Hosp. Med.*, **26**, 168.
388. Jones, B. J. M., Payne, S. and Silk, D. B. A. (1980). Indications for pump-assisted enteral feeding. *Lancet*, **1**, 1057.
389. Koretz, R. L. and Meyer, J. H. (1980). Elemental diets—facts and fantasies. *Gastroenterology*, **78**, 393.
390. Sagar, S., Harland, P. and Shields, R. (1979). Early postoperative feeding with elemental diet. *Brit. Med. J.*, **1**, 293.
391. Elman, R. and Weiner, D. O. (1939). Intravenous alimentation with special reference to protein (amino acids) metabolism. *JAMA*, **112**, 796.
392. Helfrick, F. W. and Abelson, N. M. (1944). Intravenous feeding of a complete diet in a child. *J. Pediatrics*, **25**, 400.
393. Schuberth, O. and Wretlind, A. (1961). Intravenous infusion of fat emulsions, phosphatides and emulsifying

agents. Clinical and experimental studies. *Acta Chir. Scand.*, **278** (Suppl. 278).

394. Peaston, M. J. T. (1968). Parenteral nutrition in serious illness. *Hosp. Med.*, **2**, 708.
395. Dudrick, S. J., Wilmore, D. W., Vars, H. M. and Rhoads, J. E. (1968). Long term total parenteral nutrition with growth, development and positive nitrogen balance. *Surgery*, **64**, 234.
396. Hill, G. L. (1981). Controlled clinical trials of parenteral nutrition. Presented at the 8th Annual Scientific Meeting of the Australian Society of Parenteral and Enteral Nutrition.
397. Powell-Tuck, J. (1978). Skin tunnel for central venous catheter: non-operative technique. *Brit. Med. J.*, **1**, 625.
398. Band, J. D. and Maki, D. G. (1979). Safety of changing intravenous delivery systems at longer than 24-hour intervals. *Ann. Int. Med.*, **91**, 173.
399. Powell-Tuck, J., Nielsen, T., Farwell, J. A. and Lennard-Jones, J. E. (1978). Team approach to long-term intravenous feeding in patients with gastrointestinal disorders. *Lancet*, **2**, 825.
400. Nehme, A. E. (1980). Nutritional support of the hospitalised patient. The team concept. *JAMA*, **243**, 1906.
401. Heird, W. C., Dell, R. B., Driscoll, J. M., Grebin, B. and Winters, R. W. (1972). Metabolic acidosis resulting from intravenous alimentation mixtures containing synthetic amino acids. *New Engl. J. Med.*, **287**, 943.
402. Ste.-Marie, M. T. (1978). Use of Travasol in paediatric patients. In: *Advances in Parenteral Nutrition*, p. 293. Ed. Johnston, I.D.A. Lancaster: M.T.P. Press Ltd.
403. Freund, H. R., Ryan, J. A. and Fischer, J. E. (1978). Amino acid derangements in patients with sepsis: treatment with branched chain amino acid rich infusions. *Ann. Surg.*, **188**, 423.
404. Editorial (1980). Carnitine metabolism in man. *Nutr. Rev.*, **38**, 338.
405. Belin, R. P., Bivens, B. A., Jona, J. Z. and Young, V. L. (1976). Fat overload with a 10 per cent soybean oil emulsion. *Arch. Surg.*, **111**, 1391.
406. Rivers, J. P. W. and Frankel, T. L. (1981). Essential fatty acid deficiency. *Br. Med. Bull.*, **37**, 59.
407. Barr, L. H., Dunn, G. D. and Brennan, M. F. (1981). Essential fatty acid deficiency during total parenteral nutrition. *Ann. Surg.*, **193**, 304.
408. Nedich, R. L. (1978). The compatibility of extemporaneously added drug additives with Travasol (amino acid) injection. In: *Advances in Parenteral Nutrition*, p. 415. Ed. Johnston, I. D. A. Lancaster: M.T.P. Press Ltd.
409. Bradley, J. A., King, F. R. J. G., Schorah, C. J. and Hill, G. L. (1978). Vitamins in intravenous feeding: a study of water-soluble vitamins and folate in critically ill patients receiving intravenous nutrition. *Br. J. Surg.*, **65**, 492.
410. Fell, G. S. and Burns, R. R. (1978). Zinc and other trace elements. In: *Advances in Parenteral Nutrition*, p. 241. Ed. Johnston, I.D.A. Lancaster: M.T.P. Press Ltd.
411. Young, V. R. (1981). Selenium: a case for its essentiality in man. *New Engl. J. Med.*, **304**, 1228.
412. Kartinos, N. J. (1978). Trace element formulations in intravenous feeding. In: *Advances in Parenteral Nutrition*, p. 233. Ed. Johnston, I. D. A. Lancaster: M.T.P. Press Ltd.
413. Van Caillie, M., Degenhart, H., Luijendijk, I. and Fernandes, J. (1978). Zinc content of intravenous solutions. *Lancet*, **2**, 200.
414. Woolfson, A. M. J., Heatley, R. V. and Allison, S. P. (1979). Insulin to inhibit protein catabolism after injury. *New Engl. J. Med.*, **300**, 14.
415. Chen, W-J., Ohashi, E. and Kasai, M. (1974). Amino acid metabolism in parenteral nutrition: with special reference to the calorie:nitrogen ratio and blood urea nitrogen level. *Metabolism*, **23**, 1117.
416. Powell-Tuck, J. and Goode, A. W. (1981). Principles of enteral and parenteral nutrition. *Br. J. Anaesth.*, **53**, 169.
417. Ellis, B. W., Stanbridge, R. de L., Fielding, L. P. and Dudley, H. A. F. (1976). A rational approach to parenteral nutrition. *Brit. Med. J.*, **1**, 1388.
418. Abel, R. M., Beck, C. H., Abbott, W. M., Ryan, J. A., Barnett, O. and Fischer, J. E. (1973). Improved survival from acute renal failure after treatment with intravenous essential l-amino acids and glucose. *New Engl. J. Med.*, **288**, 695.
419. Fischer, J. E., Yoshimura, N., Aguirre, A., James, J. H., Cummings, M. G., Abel, R. M. and Deindoerfer, F. (1974). Plasma amino acids in patients with hepatic encephalopathy. Effects of amino acid infusions. *Am. J. Surg.*, **127**, 40.
420. Fischer, J. E., Rosen, H. M., Ebeid, A. M., James, J. H., Keane, J. M. and Soeters, P. B. (1976). The effect of normalization of plasma amino acids on hepatic encephalopathy in man. *Surgery*, **80**, 77.
421. Harries, J. T. (1978). Aspects of intravenous feeding in childhood. In: *Advances in Parenteral Nutrition*, p. 267. Ed. Johnston, I. D. A. Lancaster: M.T.P. Press Ltd.
422. Editorial (1977). Intravenous feeding in infancy. *Brit. Med. J.*, **1**, 1490.
423. Brennan, M. F. (1981). Total parenteral nutrition in the cancer patient. *New Engl. J. Med.*, **305**, 375.
424. Ladefoged, K. and Jarnum, S. (1978). Long term parenteral nutrition. *Brit. Med. J.*, **2**, 262.
425. Blackburn, G. L., Flatt, J. P., Clowes, G. H. A., O'Donnell, T. E. and Hensle, T. B. (1973). Protein sparing therapy during periods of starvation with sepsis or trauma. *Ann. Surg.*, **177**, 588.
426. Craig, R. P., Davidson, H. A., Tweedle, D. and Johnston, I. D. A. (1977). Intravenous glucose, amino acids and fat in the post-operative period. A controlled evaluation of each substrate. *Lancet*, **2**, 8.
427. Collins, J. P., Oxby, C. B. and Hill, G. L. (1978). Intravenous amino acids and intravenous hyperalimentation as protein-sparing therapy after major surgery. A controlled clinical trial. *Lancet*, **1**, 788.
428. Rowlands, B. J. and Clark, R. G. (1978). Post-operative aminoacid infusions: an appraisal. *Br. J. Surg.*, **65**, 384.
429. Ching, H., Mills, C. J., Crossi, C., Angers, J. W., Jham, G., Zurawinsky, H. and Nealon, T. F. (1979). The absence of protein-sparing effects utilizing crystalline amino acids in stressed patients. *Ann. Surg.*, **190**, 565.
430. Ausman, R. K. and Hardy, G. (1978). Metabolic complications of parenteral nutrition. In: *Advances in parenteral nutrition*, p. 403. Ed. Johnston, I.D.A., Lancaster: M.T.P. Press Ltd.
431. Sheldon, G. F. and Baker, C. (1980). Complications of nutritional support. *Crit. Care Med.*, **8**, 35.
432. Prescott, L. F., Park, J., Sutherland, G. R., Smith, I. J. and Proudfoot, A. T. (1976). Cysteamine, methionine

and penicillamine in the treatment of paracetamol poisoning. *Lancet*, **2**, 110.
433. Ryan, D. W., Copeland, P. F., Miller, J. and Freeman, R. (1982). Replanning of the intensive unit. *Brit. Med. J.*, **285**, 1634.
434. Noone, M. R., Pitt, T. L., Bedder, M. and Hewlett, A. M. (1983). *Pseudomonas aeruginosa* colonisation in an intensive therapy unit: role of cross infection and host factors. *Brit. Med. J.*, **286**, 341.
435. Fedullo, A-J. and Swinburne, A. J. (1983). Relationship of patient age to cost and survival in a medical ICU. *Crit. Care Med.*, **11**, 155.
436. Pingleton, S. K., Bone, R. C., Pingleton, W. W. and Ruth, W. E. (1981). Prevention of pulmonary emboli in a respiratory intensive care unit. *Chest*, **79**, 647.
437. Wardle, E. N. (1982). The importance of anti-lipid A (anti-endotoxin): prevention of "shock lung" and acute renal failure. *World J. Surg.*, **6**, 616.
438. Packman, M. I. and Rackow, E. C. (1983). Optimum left heart filling pressure during fluid resuscitation of patients with hypovolaemic and septic shock. *Crit. Care Med.*, **11**, 165.
439. Walton, R. L., Hagan, K. F., Parry, S. H. and Deluchi, S. F. (1982). Maxillofacial trauma. *Surg. Clin. N. Amen.*, **62** (1), 73.

## FURTHER READING

Berk, J. L., Sampliner, J. E., Artz, J. S. and Vinocur, B. (1976). *Handbook of Critical Care*. Boston: Little, Brown and Co.

Hanson, G. C. and Wright, P. L. (Eds) (1978). *The Medical Management of the Critically Ill*. London: Academic Press.

Ledingham, I. McA. (Ed) (1977). *Recent Advances in Intensive Therapy*, No. 1. Edinburgh: Churchill Livingstone.

Oh, T. E. (Ed) (1981). *Intensive Care Manual*. London: Butterworths.

Phillips, G. D. and Odgers, C. L. (1981). *Parenteral and Enteral Nutrition. A Practical Guide*. University Relations Unit, Flinders University, South Australia.

Rinaldo, J. E. and Rogers, R. M. (1982). Adult respiratory distress syndrome. Changing concepts of lung injury and repair. *New Engl. J. Med.*, **306**, 900.

Society of Critical Care Medicine. *Critical Care: State of the Art*. Annual volumes from 1981, SCCM, 223E. Imperial Highway, Suite 110, Fullerton, CA92635, USA.

Trunkey, D. D. (Ed.) (1982). Symposium on trauma. *Surg. Clin. N. Amer.*, **62** (1).

CHAPTER 11

# Thoracic Anaesthesia

## Including Postoperative Pulmonary Complications



## THORACIC ANAESTHESIA

### Introduction

In developed areas of the world thoracic, non-cardiac surgery, is mainly carried out for the treatment and diagnosis of malignant disease, although benign lung disease and oesophageal conditions may also require thoracotomy.

During the period 1935–45 pulmonary tuberculosis and bronchiectasis were the major lung diseases treated surgically. Florid, "wet", cases of pulmonary tuberculosis and bronchiectasis are now rarely seen in developed countries because of an improvement in socio-economic conditions and the introduction of effective chemotherapy. However, several anaesthetic techniques, which were developed to deal with these diseases at operation and therefore allowed thoracic surgery to progress, are still in use today. These techniques, many of which have been improved over the years, are discussed in the appropriate sections of this chapter. The development of thoracic anaesthesia has recently been reviewed by Rendell-Baker.[1]

## Anaesthesia for Diagnostic Procedures

The diagnosis of pulmonary and intrathoracic disease may require invasive investigation such as rigid bronchoscopy, mediastinoscopy and oesophagoscopy carried out under general anaesthesia. Information can also be obtained from fibreoptic bronchoscopy and bronchography carried out under local anaesthesia, although in some circumstances it may be necessary to employ general anaesthesia for these procedures. Anaesthesia for bronchography and bronchoscopy is discussed below.

### Bronchography

Bronchography, a method of delineating the bronchial tree with radio-opaque contrast medium, is used mainly for the diagnosis and evaluation of bronchiectasis and is now a relatively uncommon investigation in developed countries. It is safer to undertake bronchography using local anaesthesia in the majority of patients, but children or unusually nervous adults may require a general anaesthetic for the procedure.

General anaesthesia for bronchography presents three problems; firstly the patient's respiratory function is unlikely to be optimal in the presence of increased sputum and is further impaired with the introduction of contrast medium into the tracheobronchial tree; secondly, anaesthetic requirements during and after the procedure are in conflict with a need for abolition of the cough reflex *during* the procedure but an equally important need for a rapid return of reflexes *afterwards*. Finally, there are the hazards associated with anaesthesia in a poorly illuminated x-ray room.

The iodine-containing radio-opaque substance Dionosil (Propyl iodine B.P.) is used in its oil-based form for bronchography. Dionosil oil is a relatively inert compound although sensitivity reactions, usually manifest as an acute asthmatic response, can occur. A powder of tantalum pentoxide is ideal for coating bronchi and gives excellent proximal bronchograms if inhaled through the upper airways. However, it has to be introduced selectively into each lobe to demonstrate peripheral airways and therefore tantalum bronchography is time-consuming and only applicable to research at present.

Hypoxia and some degree of obstruction to the airway are inevitable during bronchography with conventional media. This is much more of a hazard in children under one year and so bronchography should be avoided in this age group if at all possible or, if regarded as essential, confined to one lung only and the dose of contrast medium kept to a minimum.

Anaesthesia for bronchography in small children has been fully discussed by Ryan[2] and is also outlined below.

**General anaesthesia for bronchography in children.**—Pre-operative preparation of the child with bronchiectasis is aimed at assessing the extent of any respiratory disability and clearing infected sputum from the respiratory tract by physiotherapy and postural drainage. Light premedication with a sedative and atropine can be given in the majority of cases but the sedative should be omitted in children under the age of one year or those with bronchospasm.

Anaesthesia can be induced intravenously but an inhalational induction may be preferred. Following induction, endotracheal intubation is carried out after the administration of intravenous suxamethonium. Anaesthesia is then maintained with halothane added to an oxygen and nitrous oxide mixture. This carries the theoretical risk of contributing to segmental or even lobar collapse if the bronchi are totally blocked by contrast, because nitrogen will have been replaced by a much more soluble gas. Most anaesthetists prefer to employ gentle manual intermittent positive-pressure ventilation at this point, maintaining muscle relaxation with a non-depolarising drug or intermittent suxamethonium. Some radiologists prefer maintenance of spontaneous respiration, however, because in this way the contrast medium is inhaled smoothly into the respiratory tract.

Once anaesthesia has been established, contrast medium is introduced through a catheter placed down the endotracheal tube via a suitable inlet in the endotracheal tube connector. The right side is studied first when both lungs are to be examined during one procedure, because a lateral view is needed to demonstrate the bronchial anatomy on this side and this will be confused if there is residual contrast material on the left side. The patient is placed in the right lateral position initially to favour filling of the right upper lobe and then the catheter is advanced until its tip is opposite the opening of the right middle lobe. A slight head-up tilt at this stage aids filling of both the middle and lower lobes but it may be necessary to turn the patient semi-prone to achieve satisfactory films of the right middle lobe. As much contrast as possible is cleared from the right lung by suction and then the patient is turned into the left lateral position so that the second side can be studied. A single oblique view is sufficient to demonstrate the entire bronchial tree on the left.

At the end of the procedure the anaesthetic is terminated and non-depolarising muscle relaxants reversed if necessary. Suction and physiotherapy are used to remove contrast material from the respiratory tract but often very little is obtained. The endotracheal tube should remain in place until there is an active cough reflex and the patient should be nursed flat or head down with the healthier lung uppermost. Humidified oxygen should be given in the recovery period as laryngospasm is an occasional complication of this procedure.

### Bronchoscopy

Bronchoscopy is a common investigation required for the diagnosis of chest disease and can be carried out under local or general anaesthesia. Rigid bronchoscopy is favoured for the immediate pre-operative location of tumours and surgical assessment and is the method of choice for extraction of foreign bodies. Most endoscopists and virtually all patients prefer general anaesthesia for this procedure (different types of adult rigid bronchoscopes are shown in Fig. 1).

The smaller flexible fibreoptic bronchoscope can penetrate to the sub-segmental bronchi and is now used routinely to bronchoscope patients under local anaesthetic for general diagnostic purposes.

**Local anaesthesia for bronchoscopy.**—The nerve supply to the larynx is principally derived from the ninth (glossopharyngeal) cranial nerve through its pharyngeal, tonsillar and lingual branches and from the tenth (vagus) nerve via the superior laryngeal and recurrent laryngeal nerves.

In a suitably pre-medicated patient the back of the throat is first sprayed with 2 ml of 4 per cent lignocaine. Alternatively, an amethocaine lozenge can be given to the patient to suck prior to the administration of any vagolytic drug. It is then necessary to pass a small swab soaked in lignocaine into each pyriform fossa using suitably curved forceps (Krause). The trachea can then be anaesthetised by injecting lignocaine over the back of the tongue, because, although injection of lignocaine by cricothyroid punc-

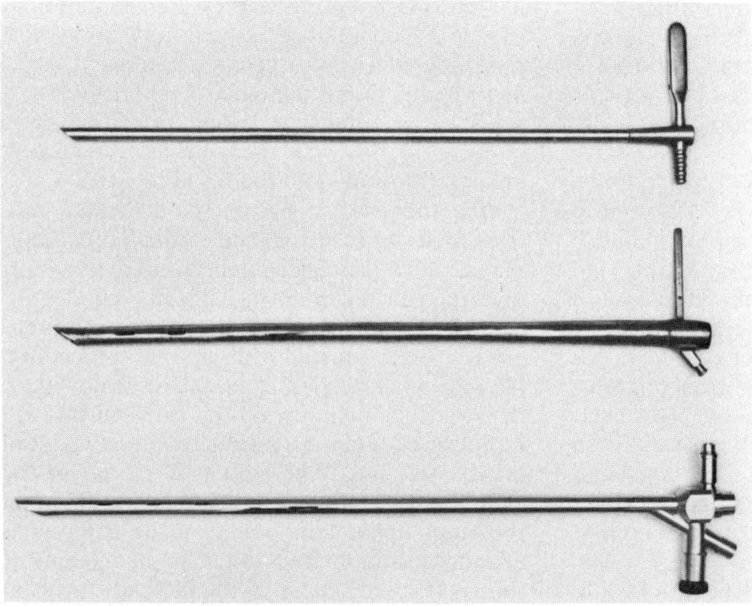

11/Fig. 1.—Three types of adult bronchoscope. From top to bottom: (i) an intubating bronchoscope; (ii) Negus bronchoscope; (iii) adult Storz bronchoscope.

ture was popular at one time, it can cause surgical emphysema or infection along the needle track. After a few minutes the local anaesthetic effect should be at its maximum and bronchoscopy can proceed. It must be noted, however, that the maximum safe dose of lignocaine (3 mg/kg) should not be exceeded during this procedure.

The fibreoptic instrument has simplified the whole procedure of local anaesthesia for bronchoscopy because after introduction through an anaesthetised nose, lignocaine can be sprayed directly on the larynx and bronchi as the instrument is advanced.

**General anaesthesia for rigid bronchoscopy.**—The specific problems of rigid bronchoscopy under general anaesthesia can be summarised thus:

1. There is competition between the bronchoscopist and anaesthetist for control of the airway;
2. Instrumentation of the respiratory tract is a potent cause of bronchospasm, laryngospasm and cardiac dysrhythmias;
3. The procedure is sometimes indicated as an emergency on an unprepared patient who has impaired cardiovascular or respiratory function;
4. Ventilation can be further impaired during or after the procedure if a lobar bronchus is obstructed by the bronchoscope or haemorrhage is caused by a biopsy.

Despite these problems there are few unequivocal contra-indications to rigid bronchoscopy although it should be avoided, if possible, in the presence of severe acute hypoxia, respiratory obstruction, massive bronchopleural fistula and marked superior vena caval obstruction.

General anaesthesia for bronchoscopy must provide unconsciousness, sufficient relaxation to allow easy passage of the instrument, abolition of reflexes from the respiratory tract, maintenance of adequate gas exchange and, if possible, a rapid recovery at the end of the procedure.

Bronchoscopy can be carried out under deep inhalational anaesthesia but this is only indicated if there is a specific reason for preserving spontaneous respiration, for example, respiratory obstruction in a child. The most widely used technique is light anaesthesia with an intravenous anaesthetic agent and muscle relaxant. Some anaesthetists also spray the vocal cords with lignocaine to minimise postoperative laryngospasm. Patient awareness is a great problem using this type of technique but in a recent report[3] recall was eliminated when methohexitone was given in a standard manner with an initial dose of 1·5 mg/kg followed by 25 per cent of this dose every two minutes.

The incidence of dysrhythmias is low (4 per cent) if adequate gas exchange is maintained during bronchoscopy (see below) and specific drug therapy is rarely required. Atropine should be to hand, however, in case a bradycardia results from the use of intermittent suxamethonium.

Ventilation during bronchoscopy in the paralysed patient can be carried out by means of apnoeic oxygenation, high frequency positive-pressure ventilation (HFPPV), a ventilating bronchoscope or a venturi injector device.[4] These methods are considered in more detail below.

*Apnoeic oxygenation.*—A fine catheter is passed into the trachea and oxygen insufflated at six litres per minute throughout bronchoscopy. Satisfactory arterial oxygenation is maintained because oxygen is taken up from the alveoli where the concentration remains high because of mass movement of oxygen from the insufflating catheter. However, there is a progressive rise in arterial carbon dioxide tension (mean rise 3 mm Hg per minute—0·4 kPa) and therefore this method is unsuitable for prolonged bronchoscopy.

*High frequency positive-pressure ventilation (HFPPV)* rates between 60 and 100 per minute have been found to provide adequate alveolar ventilation at a low airway pressure. The principle has evolved from systems designed for use during endoscopy[5] and a particular benefit during bronchoscopy is that there is no entrainment of air and so anaesthetic gases can be delivered at known concentrations.

*Ventilating bronchoscope.* — Anaesthetic gases are administered through a side-arm and the proximal lumen is occluded by a glass window. The window is usually discarded in practice to permit the passage of telescopes and biopsy forceps and even when in place satisfactory ventilation is rarely possible because the bronchoscope is a poor fit within the trachea.

*Venturi injector device.*—Its use during bronchoscopy was first described by Sanders in

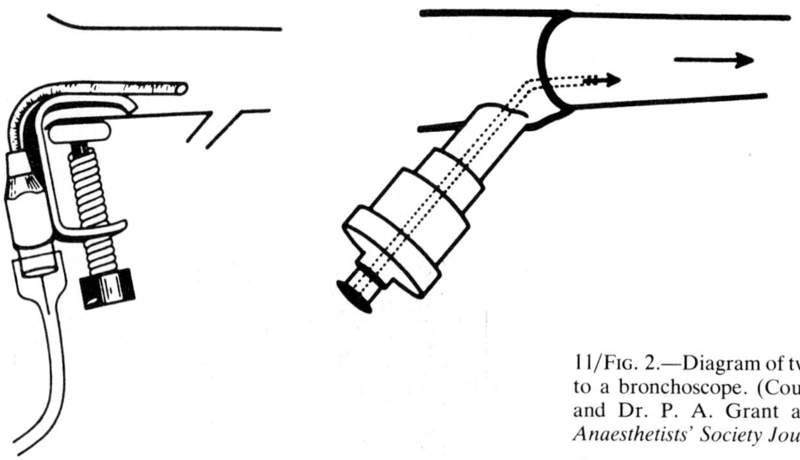

11/Fig. 2.—Diagram of two types of injector for attachment to a bronchoscope. (Courtesy of Professor W. E. Spoerel and Dr. P. A. Grant and the Editor of the *Canadian Anaesthetists' Society Journal*[7])

1967.[4] Oxygen from a high pressure source is injected intermittently through a narrow needle (Fig. 2) placed at the proximal end of the bronchoscope. The venturi effect which this creates entrains atmospheric air so that the lungs can be inflated with oxygen-enriched air as long as the distal end of the bronchoscope is beyond the larynx.

The system consists of a high pressure source of oxygen (usually pipeline pressure at 410 kPa; approximately 60 psi), an on-off tap, high pressure tubing and a needle of suitable size. It is essential that the size of the needle should match that of the bronchoscope so that good air entrainment is achieved without creating excessive airway pressure.[6] A 16 SWG needle coupled to a driving gas pressure of 410 kPa (approximately 60 psi) is usually used with an adult Negus bronchoscope (Fig. 1) and gives a maximum inflation pressure of 25–30 cm water (2·5–3·0 kPa). Typical maximum pressures achieved with various sizes of needle and bronchoscope are summarised in Table 1.

Using this system it is possible not only to maintain arterial oxygenation but also keep arterial carbon dioxide values within normal limits in a normal subject. However, excessive pressure can be created if the proximal end of the bronchoscope is obstructed and the distal end is a tight fit at the larynx or elsewhere in the tracheobronchial tree. Complications can also occur if the driving gas pressure and venturi needle size are not matched appropriately.

11/Table 1
Maximum Inflation Pressure Achieved With Various Venturi Bronchoscope Injector Systems
(Driving Pressure 410 kPa or 60 psi)

| *Negus Bronchoscope* | *Injector Needle Size* | | *Typical Max. Pressure* |
|---|---|---|---|
| | *SWG* | *Internal Diameter (mm)* | *cm $H_2O$* |
| Adult | 14 | 1·2 | 50 |
| Adult | 16 | 1·2 | 25–30 |
| Adult | 17 | 1·10 | 23–25 |
| Child | 19 | 0·69 | 14–18 |
| Suckling | 19 | 0·69 | 15 |

**General anaesthesia for fibreoptic bronchoscopy.**—In an adult it is a simple matter to pass a fibreoptic bronchoscope through an 8·0 or 9·0 mm endotracheal tube. Ventilation and anaesthesia can then be continued without difficulty provided the bronchoscope is inserted through a diaphragm which seals the endotracheal tube connector.[8] In children the fibreoptic bronchoscope will be too large to pass down an endotracheal tube. In these circumstances ventilation can be continued using the apnoeic oxygenation technique or a modified injector method with a catheter through the vocal cords. This latter method is usually used but, if the catheter impacts in a bronchus or against the side wall of the trachea or there is obstruction to passive expiration, then pneumothorax and fatal air embolism can occur,[9] when gas is delivered at high pressure. It is, therefore, recommended that the oxygen driving pressure is lowered in this type of system or that some form of blow-off valve is incorporated.[10]

## General Principles of Anaesthesia for Thoracotomy

### Pre-Operative Assessment and Preparation

Pre-operative assessment is carried out on the general lines appropriate for any operation. Particular note should be taken of symptoms and signs relevant to anaesthetic management during thoracotomy and to any pathology which can be treated prior to surgery. Stridor, a history of haemoptysis and signs of superior vena caval (SVC) obstruction should alert the anaesthetist to possible problems during induction of anaesthesia and endobronchial intubation. Airways obstruction may be reversible and drugs which achieve this include oral or, preferably, inhaled $\beta$-sympathomimetics, oral theophylline derivatives, ipratropium bromide (Atrovent) and inhaled corticosteroids. Sputum retention can be treated by physiotherapy, postural drainage and the administration of appropriate antibiotics.

Pre-operative investigations of particular relevance to the anaesthetist are the chest x-ray and lung function tests. Inspection of a postero-anterior and lateral chest x-ray may demonstrate the lesion for which thoracotomy is indicated and any distortion of the trachea and main bronchi should be noted in case endobronchial intubation proves difficult. The presence or absence of a pneumothorax should also be ascertained, especially if chest drains have recently been removed or a needle biopsy has been carried out.

Complex lung function tests (see page 60), including arterial blood gas analysis, are unnecessary in the majority of fit patients without symptoms or signs of respiratory disability. However, specific enquiry should be made regarding dyspnoea and exercise tolerance and a test of climbing two or three flights of stairs is informative. Bedside measurements of vital capacity (VC), forced expired volume in one second ($FEV_1$), and peak expiratory flow rate (PEFR) are so easy to record that they could be carried out as a routine in all patients. In those patients with significant clinical impairment of respiratory function or where lung resection may cause further deterioration, more complex lung function testing is required so that the risks of operation can be weighed against possible benefits. However, although it is possible to identify high risk groups of patients, who may have inadequate reserves of pulmonary function following lung resection none of these functional studies provides a reliable prognosis in individual patients (see Table 2). The final factor affecting outcome is often one that cannot be foreseen, namely the occurrence of operative and postoperative complications.

11/Table 2
Criteria Considered to Indicate a Greater Than Normal Risk of Morbidity or Mortality After Lung Resection

| |
|---|
| Forced Vital Capacity (FVC) less than 50 per cent of predicted value |
| Forced Expiratory Volume in one second ($FEV_1$) less than 50 per cent of FVC |
| Maximum Breathing Capacity (MBC) less than 50 per cent of predicted value |
| $Paco_2$ more than 45 mm Hg (6·0 kPa) |
| Gas transfer (TLCO-Transfer factor for the lung for carbon monoxide) less than 50 per cent of predicted value |
| Pulmonary artery pressure (mean), during unilateral occlusion of left or right main pulmonary artery, greater than 30 mm Hg (4·0 kPa) |

Adapted from Tisi, 1979[11] and Olsen *et al.*, 1975.[12]

### Control of Secretions. Use of Posture

During surgery infected secretions can spread within a lung or from one lung to the other despite pre-operative physiotherapy. Early attempts at controlling secretions by posture utilised both secretion-*draining* and secretion-*retaining* positions. Beecher (1940)[13] used a steep head-down tilt to drain secretions from the upper lung of patients in the lateral position into the trachea and Overholt and associates (1946)[14] described a prone position with the diseased lung dependent, to retain secretions. Posture is now rarely used to control excessive sputum intra-operatively although some centres in the United Kingdom still use the prone, secretion-draining position described by Parry Brown (1948).[15] In this posture (see Fig. 3) padded rests support the pelvis and shoulders to allow free diaphragmatic movement. The arm on the operated side hangs freely over the edge of the operating table so that the scapula

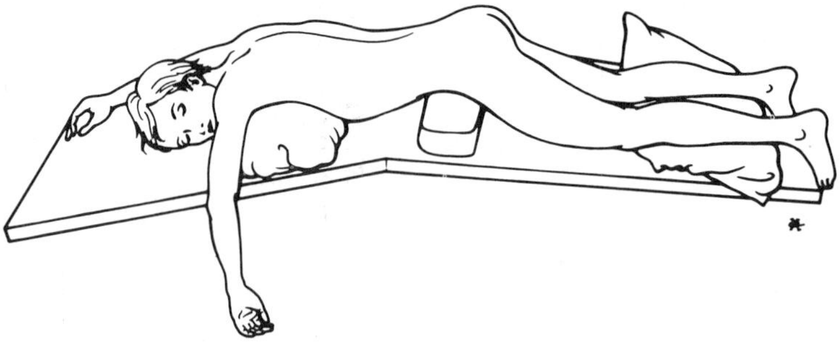

11/FIG. 3.—The prone Parry-Brown thoracotomy position.

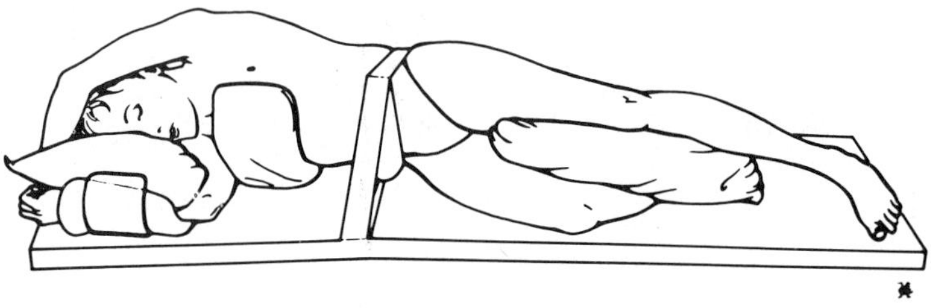

11/FIG. 4.—Lateral thoracotomy position.

is drawn away from the site of surgery, and the head is supported in a flexed position with the face turned towards the diseased side. The trachea and main bronchus on the non-operated side are then as nearly in as straight a line as possible and the trachea is inclined at an angle of 45° from carina to larynx so that secretions drain freely and are easily accessible to suction. This provides drainage without the use of endobronchial apparatus and with little risk of aspiration into the opposite lung.

The upright sitting position is used to prevent spillover from a pneumonectomy space in patients with a bronchopleural fistula. The use of this posture is discussed in the relevant section below.

The most commonly used posture for thoracotomy is the *lateral* position shown in Fig. 4. For this posture the patient lies with the operative side uppermost and the lower shoulder is pulled through anteriorly so allowing the flexed arm to be tucked under the pillow supporting the head. The upper arm is extended, and placed over and in front of the head to pull the scapula away from the site of operation without stretching the brachial plexus. Stability of the pelvis can be achieved by flexing the lower leg at the hip and knee while the upper leg is kept straight. In addition, it is preferable to support the patient with padded rests in front of the sternum and pelvis. A wide strap provides additional support if placed around the pelvis, pelvic support and table, and pressure from one leg on the other is avoided by placing a pillow between the knees.

In the lateral position infected secretions can spread from the diseased upper lung to the dependent lung. Control of secretions, therefore, is mainly achieved by isolating one lung from the other with specialised endobronchial apparatus as described below.

## ENDOBRONCHIAL APPARATUS

Methods for selectively intubating or blocking main or lobar bronchi have been practised for at least 50 years and many early items of equipment are no longer available. Some have been superseded because of improvements in design and production and others are required so infrequently now that their manufacture is uneconomic. Endobronchial apparatus largely of historical interest is listed in Table 3, which also includes the date of the original description. Accounts of the development of endobronchial apparatus are provided by White,[16] and Pappin.[17]

Figures 5 and 6 show two types of bronchial blocker. These blockers are now rarely used even in specialised centres. They are placed

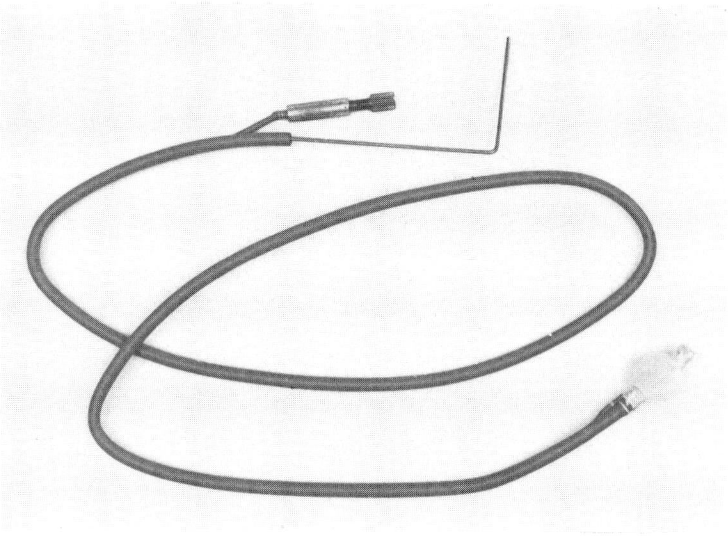

11/FIG. 5.—Vernon Thompson bronchial blocker. (Courtesy of Dr. J. W. W. Gothard and M. A. Branthwaite and the publishers of *Anaesthesia for Thoracic Surgery*, 1982, Blackwell Scientific Publications.)

under direct vision via a rigid bronchoscope and used in combination with an endotracheal tube intra-operatively (Fig. 7).

Table 4 lists endobronchial apparatus in current use and a more detailed description of these items follows.

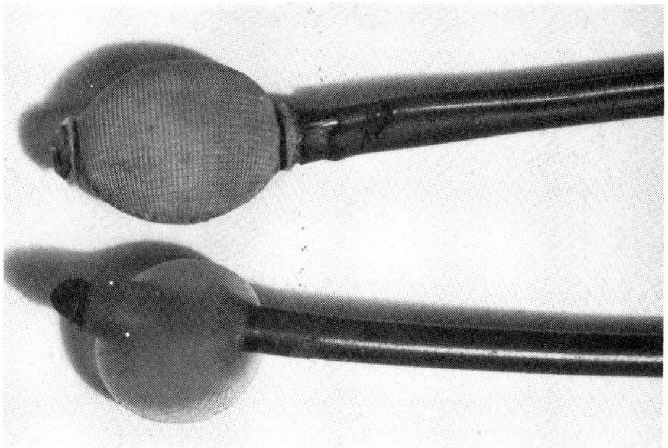

11/FIG. 6.—Comparison of inflated cuffs on the Thompson (above) and Magill blockers.

11/TABLE 3
ENDOBRONCHIAL APPARATUS MAINLY OF HISTORICAL INTEREST

| | | |
|---|---|---|
| *Bronchus Blockers* | | |
| Magill | 1934 | Latex/rubber bronchial cuff |
| Crafoord | 1938 | Bronchial tamponage |
| Vernon Thompson | 1943 | Gauze covered bronchial cuff |
| *Single Lumen Endobronchial Tubes* | | |
| Gale and Waters | 1932 | Single lumen tube with detachable carinal cuff |
| Magill | 1936 | Single lumen tube. Later development included wire spiral extension of right-sided tube |
| Machray | 1958 | Short, single bronchial cuff |
| *Combinations* | | |
| Sturtzbecher | 1953 | Endotracheal tube combined with bronchus blocker |
| Vellacot | 1954 | Single lumen tube designed to control right upper lobe bronchopleural fistula |
| Green | 1958 | Similar function to Vellacot tube |

See references White,[16] Pappin.[17]

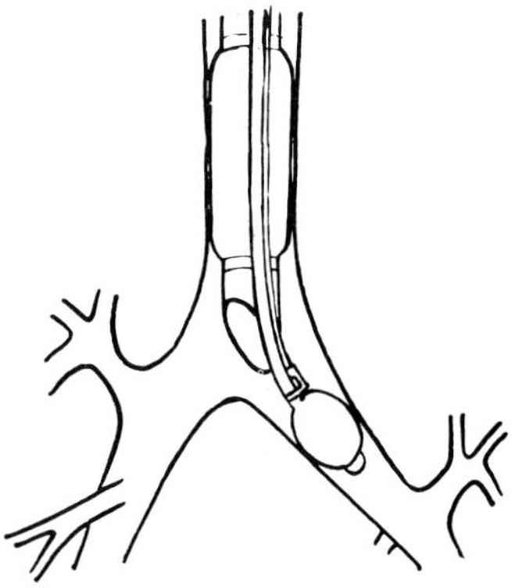

11/FIG. 7.—Diagram to show relationship of blocker to endotracheal tube.

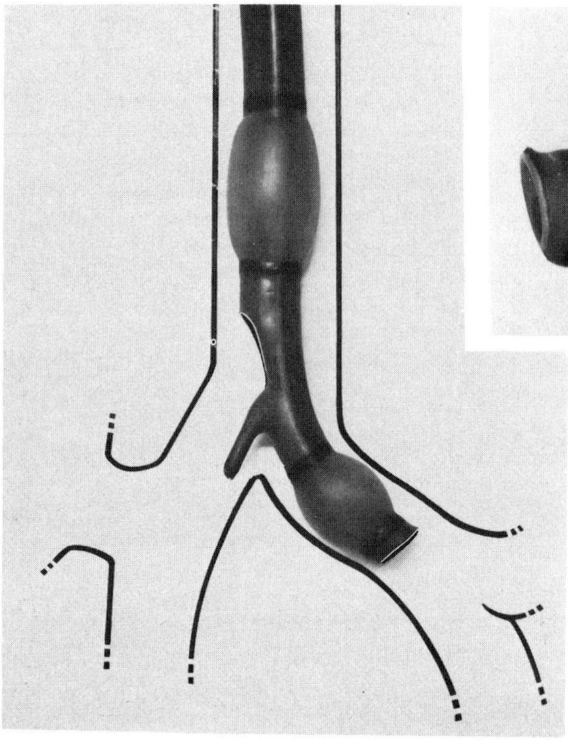

11/FIG. 8(*a*).—Carlens double lumen endobronchial tube.

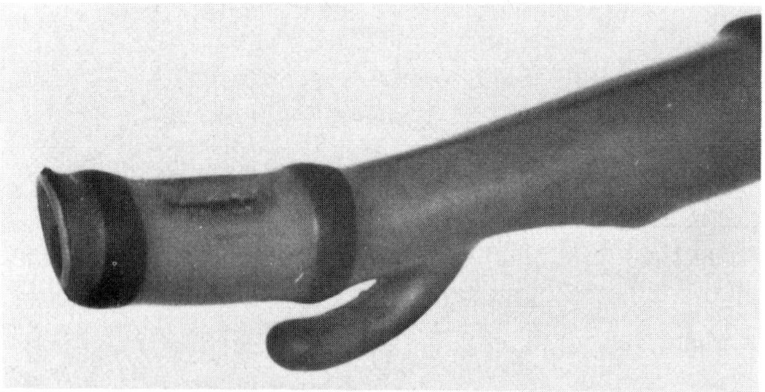

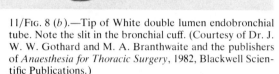

11/FIG. 8 (*b*).—Tip of White double lumen endobronchial tube. Note the slit in the bronchial cuff. (Courtesy of Dr. J. W. W. Gothard and M. A. Branthwaite and the publishers of *Anaesthesia for Thoracic Surgery*, 1982, Blackwell Scientific Publications.)

11/TABLE 4
ENDOBRONCHIAL APPARATUS IN CURRENT USE

| | |
|---|---|
| *Single Lumen Endobronchial Tubes* | |
| Gordon and Green | 1955 |
| Macintosh and Leatherdale | 1955 |
| Brompton-Pallister | 1959 |
| *Double Lumen Endobronchial Tubes* | |
| Carlens | 1950 |
| Bryce-Smith | 1959 |
| Bryce-Smith and Salt | 1960 |
| White | 1960 |
| Robertshaw | 1962 |
| Bronchocath* | 1978 |
| Portex | 1981 |
| *Combination of Endotracheal Tube and Bronchus Blocker* | |
| Macintosh and Leatherdale | 1955 |

* National Catheter Co. (USA)

## Double Lumen Endobronchial Tubes

Double lumen tubes are designed to provide independent channels for suction or ventilation to both lungs and the lumen on one side is extended at an angle which favours its entry into one of the main bronchi. The other lumen terminates in the trachea distal to a tracheal cuff so that the non-intubated lung can also be ventilated. These tubes also have a secondary curve which fits the oropharynx.

*Carlens tube* (Fig. 8*a*).—This tube, available in four sizes, was designed originally for differential bronchospirometry and has both oropharyngeal and bronchial curves with the endobronchial extension entering the left lung. The thick wall and D-shaped lumen interfere with the passage of suction catheters and provide a noticeable resistance to gas flow. A carinal hook is intended to ensure correct placement but it makes the tube difficult to pass through the larynx. A double lumen tube of similar pattern but with the endobronchial extension angled to the right and a slit in the bronchial cuff to allow inflation of the right upper lobe is available as the *White* double lumen tube (Fig. 8*b*). This modification to the bronchial cuff is necessary because the right upper lobe bronchus arises much nearer the carina than that on the left (Fig. 9) and therefore a conventional cuff placed in the right main bronchus would block off the upper lobe.

*Bryce-Smith double lumen tube* (Fig. 10*a*).—The largest size of this tube has a 7 cm endobronchial limb which curves posteriorly and to the left to enter the left main bronchus. The other lumen ends just above the carina at a fenestrated aperture on the anterior aspect of the tube, just below the tracheal cuff. There is an oropharyngeal curve as well as an endobron-

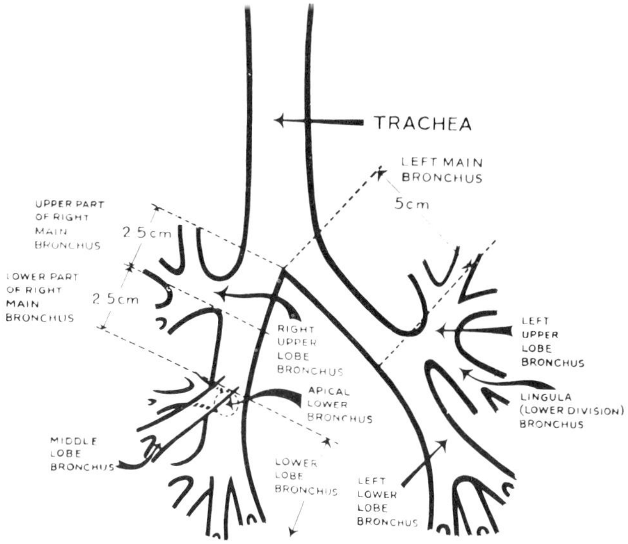


11/Fig. 9.—The anatomy of the tracheobronchial tree. (Courtesy of Drs. R. E. Mansfield and R. Jenkins and the publishers, Baillière, Tindall and Cassell.[18])

chial curve but no carinal hook. The double lumen portion of the tube is oval in cross-section and, when in place, the tracheal lumen lies anterior to the endobronchial lumen so that the long axis of the oval lies in the long axis of the larynx. These tubes are manufactured in four sizes ranging from 5 to 7 mm, designated by the diameter of each limb, and are considered to be less traumatic to the larynx than either a Carlens or Robertshaw tube.

*Bryce-Smith and Salt double lumen tube* (Fig. 10*b*).—This is a right-sided version of the Bryce-Smith tube with an endobronchial portion directed to the right at an angle of 17° and a slit in the bronchial cuff to allow ventilation of the right upper lobe.

*Robertshaw double lumen tubes* (Fig. 11).—Right and left patterns of this tube are produced and their general design is similar to other double lumen tubes with twin limbs, tracheal and bronchial cuffs, and oropharyngeal and endobronchial curves. They are designed and manufactured to achieve the maximum possible internal diameter in each lumen and, in the double lumen portion, each lumen is D-shaped in cross section. The two channels are arranged side by side so that the double lumen portion of the tube is oval in cross section with a long axis which lies at right angles to the long axis of the larynx. The angle between the endobronchial and tracheal sections is 45° and 20° respectively on the left and right, there is no carinal hook, and the bronchial cuff on a right sided tube has a slit to allow ventilation to the right upper lobe. These tubes are manufactured in large, medium and small sizes which correspond to the old Magill sizes 12, 10 and 8. Disposable, plastic left-sided double lumen tubes are now available; the Bronchocath, as illustrated in Fig. 12, which is of a similar design to the Robertshaw tube and also a Portex endobronchial tube.

**Insertion of double lumen tubes.**—Laryngoscopy is carried out as usual. With the larynx in view the tube is turned through 90° so that the concavity of the endobronchial extension faces upwards and then it is inserted between the cords. Once within the trachea the tube is turned back through 90° so that the endobronchial extension will enter the appropriate bronchus as it is advanced towards the carina. Both tracheal and bronchial cuffs are inflated once the tube is in place and ventilation can be commenced via a double catheter mount attached to separate connectors previously placed in each limb of the tube. It is important not to over-distend the bronchial cuff and therefore it is inflated just far enough to achieve an airtight seal when ventilation is confined to that side. Correct placement of the tube is confirmed by both inspection and auscultation particularly over the upper lobes, while ventilation is restricted to first one side and then the

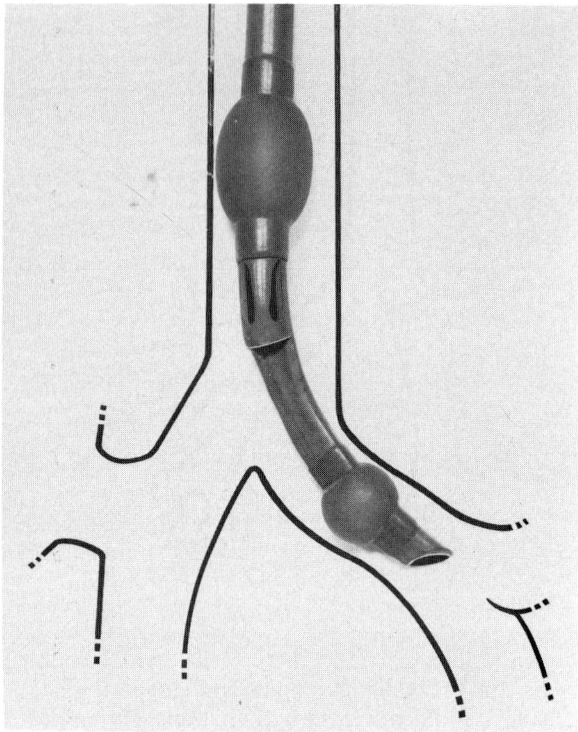

11/FIG. 10(*a*)

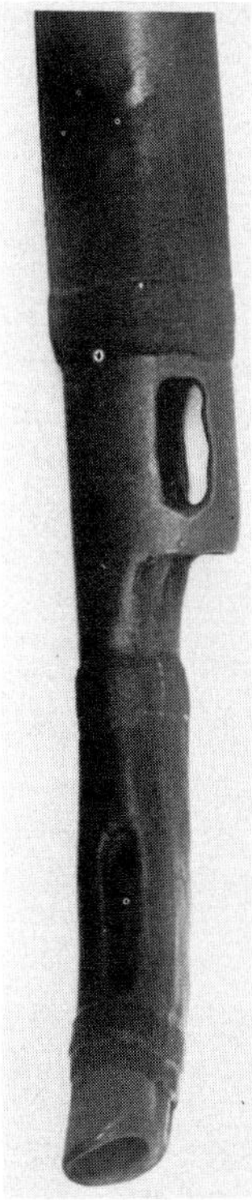

11/FIG. 10(*b*)

11/FIG. 10(*a*).—A Bryce-Smith double lumen LEFT endobronchial tube.

11/FIG. 10(*b*).—The tip of a Bryce-Smith and Salt RIGHT double lumen endobronchial tube. (Courtesy of Dr. J. W. W. Gothard and M. A. Branthwaite and the publishers of *Anaesthesia for Thoracic Surgery*, 1982, Blackwell Scientific Publications.)

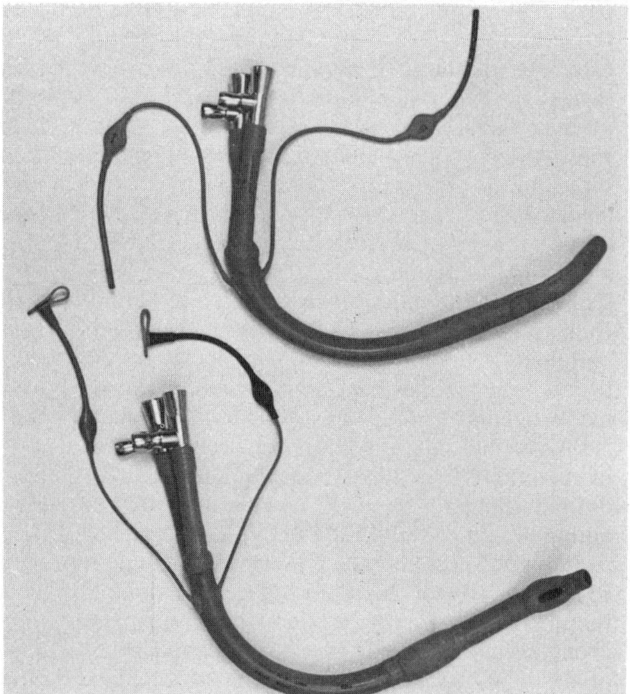

11/FIG. 11.—Left (upper) and right Robertshaw double lumen endobronchial tubes. (Courtesy of Dr. J. W. W. Gothard and M. A. Branthwaite and the publishers of *Anaesthesia for Thoracic Surgery*, 1982, Blackwell Scientific Publications.)

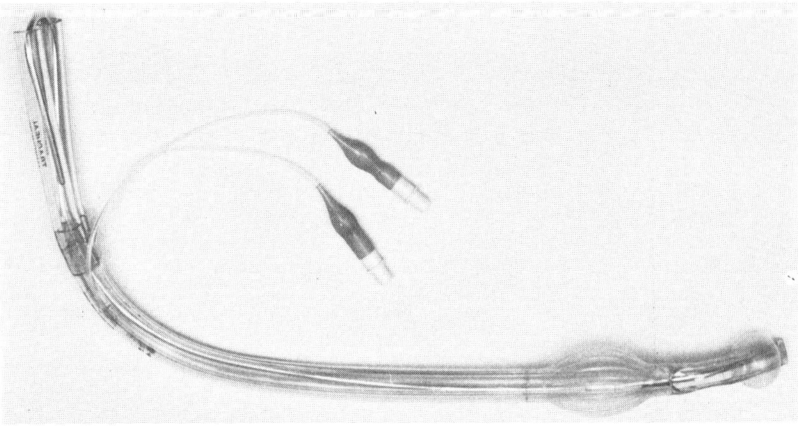

11/Fig. 12.—A Bronchocath (National Catheter Co.) double lumen left endobronchial tube (note stylette in position). (Courtesy of Dr. J. W. W. Gothard and M. A. Branthwaite and the publishers of *Anaesthesia for Thoracic Surgery*, 1982, Blackwell Scientific Publications.)

other side. Both cuffs can remain inflated during surgery and one-lung anaesthesia is achieved by clamping one limb of the catheter mount and opening the suction cap on the tube connector on that side to atmosphere to allow the lung to deflate. This limb should be suctioned after surgery before ventilation is re-established.

### Single Lumen Endobronchial Tubes

The configuration of some single lumen endobronchial tubes is such that they can be passed blindly into the trachea and will enter the correct bronchus because of their shape. Others are designed with only a slight curve similar to that of an endotracheal tube and are intended to be mounted on the outside of an intubating bronchoscope and placed under direct vision. The distal cuff on all endobronchial tubes is short by comparison with the cuff on an endotracheal tube, and current patterns also have a longer cuff on the shaft to make a seal in the trachea. The two cuffs are supplied by separate channels, each with its own pilot balloon which is either labelled or colour coded to identify which cuff it supplies. The tubes are made of red rubber with a wall thickness which is slightly less than that of an endotracheal tube of comparable diameter, and the bevel is designed to face the side which the tube will enter.

*Gordon-Green or Green-Gordon tube* (Fig. 13).—The 4 cm endobronchial section of this tube is designed to enter the right main bronchus and is set at an angle of 15° to the rest of the tube. The bronchial cuff inflates asymmetrically around a 2 cm slit in the side wall which should be opposite the right upper lobe orifice when the tube is correctly positioned. A rubber hook at the junction between the endobronchial and tracheal sections of the tube is intended to engage on the carina when the tube is passed blindly and so ensure its correct placement. The tube is manufactured in four sizes and the design of the cuff on modern tubes has been streamlined so that the larger two sizes can be mounted on the outside of an intubating bronchoscope. This means that the tube can be introduced under direct vision and in this instance it is preferable to cut off the carinal hook.

*Pallister (Brompton) triple-cuffed left endobronchial tube* (Fig. 14).—This tube was designed for use during sleeve resection of the right upper lobe when surgery very close to the carina threatens the integrity of a balloon in the left main bronchus. There are, therefore, two bronchial cuffs as well as one tracheal cuff. Each of the three cuffs is supplied by a separate inflating channel with a pilot balloon on those supplying the tracheal and outer bronchial cuffs. The tube is unremarkable in shape, with a single gentle curve in the long axis; it is usually introduced under direct vision mounted on an intubating bronchoscope but it can be positioned with the aid of a fibreoptic bronchoscope.[19] The tube is available in 8·0 and 9·0 mm sizes only.

*Macintosh-Leatherdale left endobronchial tube* (Fig. 15).—The proximal and distal ends of this tube are angled to fit the oropharynx and left main bronchus respectively and it is intended to be passed blindly into the left side,

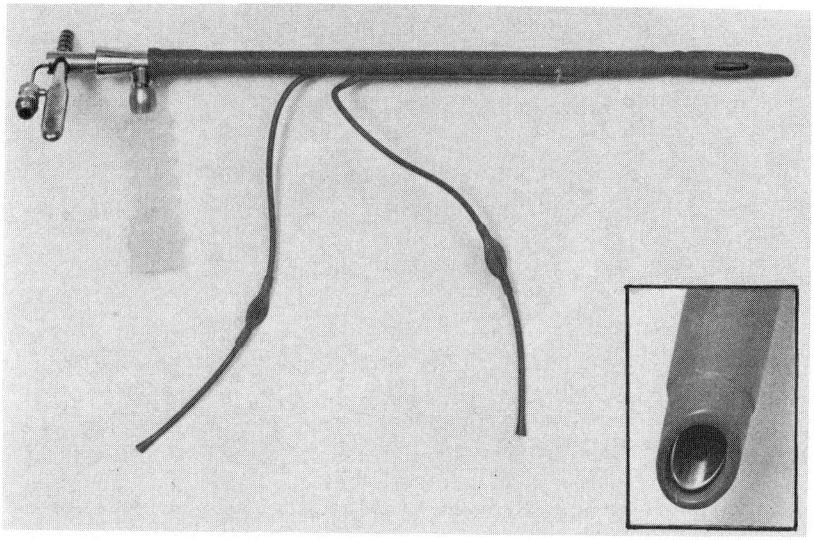

11/Fig. 13.—A Gordon and Green right-sided single lumen endobronchial tube mounted on an intubating bronchoscope. Note that the carinal hook has been cut off. Inset shows alignment of the bevels of the tube and bronchoscope. (Courtesy of Dr. J. W. W. Gothard and M. A. Branthwaite and the publishers of *Anaesthesia for Thoracic Surgery*, 1982, Blackwell Scientific Publications.)

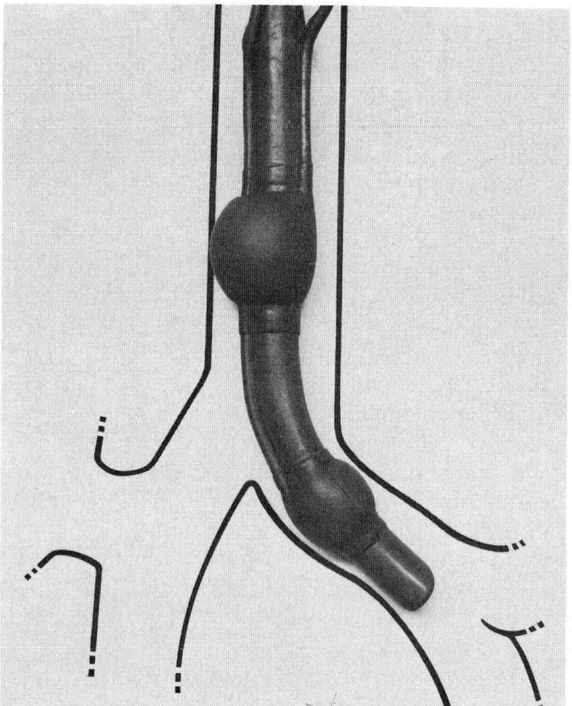

11/Fig. 14.—A Brompton-Pallister single lumen, left, endobronchial tube.

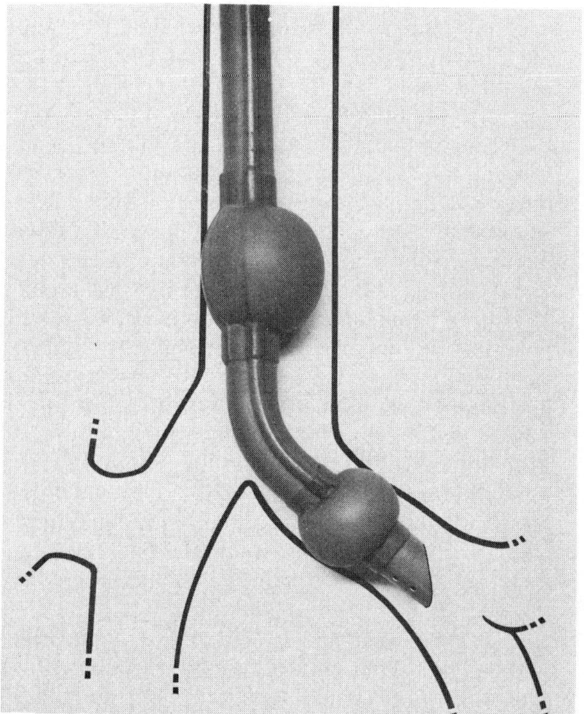

11/Fig. 15.—A Macintosh-Leatherdale left endobronchial tube (note perforations at the tip).

stiffened with a firm rubber introducer if necessary. There are a number of perforations in the wall of the endobronchial section beyond the endobronchial cuff which permit free ventilation of the left lung, even if the bevel of the tube is partly obstructed because it lies against the wall of the bronchus. As well as channels for inflating the tracheal and bronchial cuffs, there is a separate suction catheter fused to the posterior aspect of the outer wall of the tube, with its distal aperture located just above the junction between the bronchial and tracheal sections of the tube. This provides a means of suction to the right lung during left lung anaesthesia, or can be used to insufflate oxygen to the right side. This tube is available in four sizes from 7 to 10 mm.

*Macintosh-Leatherdale combined endobronchial blocker and endotracheal tube* (Fig. 16).—A thick-walled, semi-rigid suction catheter is fused to the wall of an endotracheal tube at an angle which allows it to enter the left main bronchus when the tube is passed blindly into

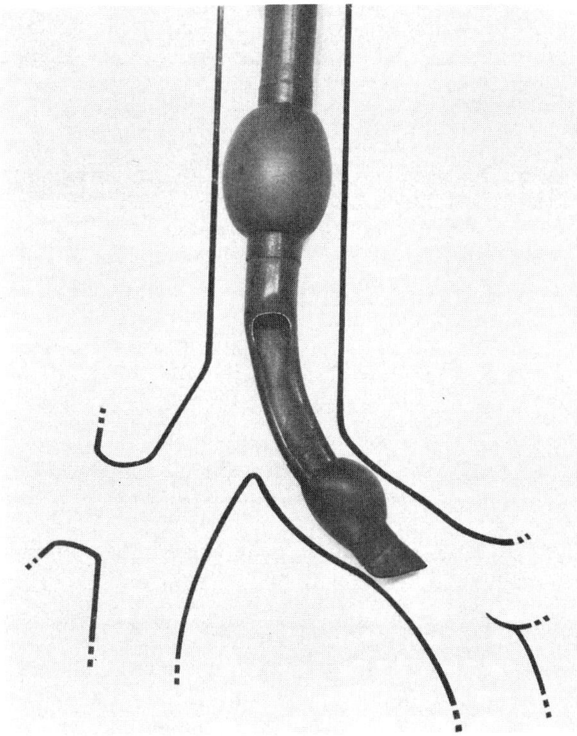

11/Fig. 16.—A Macintosh-Leatherdale combined endotracheal tube and bronchus blocker.

the trachea. It is difficult to dislodge, unlike isolated endobronchial blockers, and its correct placement is helped by a curve at the proximal end which fits the oropharynx. It is available in four sizes from 7 to 10 mm and is inserted blindly through the trachea.

*Insertion of single lumen tubes under direct vision.*—The endobronchial tube is placed on an intubating bronchoscope previously lubricated with a sterile water-soluble agent. The tube is aligned on the bronchoscope so that their bevels coincide. There is no advantage in cutting the tube to the exact distance between the major bronchi and the front teeth and it is better to have the tube a little too long than too short. Bronchoscopy is then performed and the bronchoscope placed within the trachea. With the head of the operating table lowered the bronchoscope is advanced until the carina is seen, the proximal end is then angled laterally and the patient's head rotated away from the side to be entered so that the tip of the bronchoscope is directed towards the appropriate bronchus. The tube and bronchoscope are then advanced a further one or two cm and positioned so that on the left the tip lies above the left upper lobe orifice and on the right the tip is beyond the upper orifice. Final positioning, especially relative to the right upper lobe orifice, should be checked by auscultation.

During one-lung anaesthesia the bronchial cuff is inflated only, but prior to this it may be possible to ventilate both lungs with only the tracheal cuff inflated (see below). At the end of surgery it is usually necessary to withdraw the tube into the trachea and inflate the tracheal cuff only so that the bronchial stump on the operated side can be tested or remaining lobes inflated. Once the tube has been withdrawn in this manner it is almost impossible to re-position.

### Choice of Endobronchial Apparatus

Bronchial blockers can be used to isolate a lobe or lung and permit suction to it during resection. In general, they have been superseded by double lumen tubes which are less likely to be displaced or damaged during operation and which allow the operated lung to be ventilated if required, as well as isolated and drained. The great majority of anaesthetists in the United Kingdom use Robertshaw double lumen tubes when selective ventilation or isolation of a lung is indicated.[17] Occasionally, it may still be desirable on theoretical grounds to choose a bronchial blocker to isolate a single lobe but, because few anaesthetists today have sufficient experience to use them reliably, attempts to do so may cause more problems than accepting isolation of the whole lung with a single or double lumen endobronchial tube.

Single lumen endobronchial tubes have the advantage that they can be introduced over a bronchoscope in adults and so placed under direct vision. This is particularly helpful if the bronchial anatomy is distorted, especially if it is essential that the endobronchial apparatus be placed correctly at the first attempt as in the management of a bronchopleural fistula. Ventilation to both lungs may be possible with a single lumen tube if the tracheal cuff is inflated and the bronchial cuff is deflated, provided the tube is not a tight fit in the bronchus. However, this cannot be guaranteed. In addition, it is not possible to use suction to the operated side so in general single lumen endobronchial tubes do not provide such flexible control over ventilation and suction as double lumen tubes.

## Ventilation during Thoracotomy and the Physiology of One-Lung Anaesthesia

The consequences of an open thorax namely pulmonary collapse, paradoxical respiration, pendulum air (Pendelluft), mediastinal displacement and reflex disturbances are largely avoided if intermittent positive-pressure ventilation (IPPV) is employed. If controlled ventilation is used in the lateral position the high dependent diaphragm does not have the mechanical advantage it has during spontaneous respiration. The upper lung is ventilated preferentially because the compliance of the lung and chest wall on this side is greater than on the dependent side, because of compression by the weight of the mediastinum. This inequality of compliance and hence tidal ventilation becomes even more marked as soon as the chest is opened. In addition, the poorly ventilated dependent lung will be receiving a greater proportion of pulmonary blood flow than the upper lung because of the effect of gravity on the low pressure pulmonary circulation. As a result of this mismatch of blood flow and ventilation, gas exchange is inefficient.

**One-lung anaesthesia.**—If only the dependent lung is ventilated intra-operatively the preferential distribution of gas to the upper lung is eliminated, improving access for the surgeon and ensuring the well-perfused dependent lung is well ventilated. However, the upper lung is still perfused and this blood flow through an unventilated lung is an important source of venous admixture which is a temporary increase in "true" shunt ($V/Q = O$). The dependent lung in this situation will be receiving the effective minute volume and a high proportion of the cardiac output. In some areas of this lung there will be areas with excess of perfusion relative to ventilation (alveoli with *low* V/Q ratios) and this will also contribute to venous admixture. Reported figures for total venous admixture during one-lung anaesthesia range from 30–40 per cent[20] but individual values greater than this are seen from time to time.

Arterial hypoxaemia is the most important consequence of venous admixture, carbon dioxide elimination rarely being a problem. The extent of hypoxia during one lung anaesthesia has been documented in many studies.[21–26] Mean values for arterial oxygen varying from 60 to 120 mm Hg (8–16·3 kPa) have been reported during one-lung anaesthesia with inspired oxygen concentrations between 40–50 per cent and figures of 115 to 213 mm Hg (15·3–24·8 kPa) with 100 per cent oxygen. However, individual values far lower than this have been reported. Severe hypoxaemia is particularly likely in several circumstances:

1. Where thoracotomy is carried out for disease other than in the lung (e.g. oesophageal surgery where the upper non-ventilated lung is often normal).
2. The cardiac output, and hence mixed venous oxygen content, is low.
3. There is disease in the dependent lung.
4. Ventilation to the dependent lung is inadequate because of misplaced endobronchial apparatus (e.g. an upper lobe is not ventilated).
5. The function of the dependent lung has deteriorated because of prolonged surgery and anaesthesia.

The lower level of arterial oxygenation acceptable during one-lung anaesthesia is debatable and depends on many factors such as pre-operative arterial blood gas values, the age of the patient, the cardiac output and so on. A practical solution is to ventilate with 40–50 per cent oxygen during one-lung anaesthesia and then measure arterial blood gas values. If the arterial oxygen concentration is below say 70 mm Hg (9·3 kPa) the inspired oxygen concentration can be increased once all other measures have been taken to ensure adequate ventilation of the dependent lung. In these circumstances increasing the inspired oxygen concentration will improve arterial oxygenation largely by its effect on the alveoli with low V/Q ratios in the dependent lung. This manoeuvre cannot obviously affect the "true" shunt through the upper, non-ventilated lung. Other measures which can be taken to minimise hypoxia during one-lung anaesthesia include the use of an optimal ventilatory pattern, early clamping of pulmonary vessels, insufflation of oxygen to the upper lung and cessation of two-lung ventilation as late as possible.

*Optimal ventilatory pattern*.—Carbon dioxide elimination is not a problem if the same minute volume is continued during one-lung anaesthesia as was employed to achieve normocapnia during two-lung ventilation. This minute volume should be delivered to the dependent lung in such a way that there is not an excessive rise in intra-alveolar pressure, as this will only divert blood flow away to the upper non-ventilated lung. Khanam and Branthwaite[21,22] recommended a small tidal volume (7 ml/kg body weight) delivered at an increased respiratory rate (20 breaths per minute). They also used a fairly short inspiratory time, with an inspiratory to expiratory ratio of 1:2, to avoid increases in mean intra-alveolar pressure created by long inspiratory times. Positive end-expiratory pressure may prevent atelectasis in the dependent lung but this is achieved at the expense of diverting blood flow away from that lung and also reducing cardiac output. Most studies have failed to demonstrate any benefit when positive end-expiratory pressure is used during one-lung anaesthesia.

*Early clamping of pulmonary vessels* will eliminate most of the venous admixture during one-lung anaesthesia but this is not always technically possible.

*Insufflation of oxygen to the upper lung* will improve oxygenation if carried out at a positive pressure of 10 cm $H_2O$.[26] This method is particularly applicable to oesophageal surgery where hypoxia is more likely and where insufflation is less likely to hinder surgery.

*Cessation of ventilation to the upper lung*. Ventilation should be continued to both lungs for as long as possible. Hypoxic pulmonary vasoconstriction does not play a significant part in minimising the shunt through the non-ventilated lung during an average length thoracotomy and it has been shown that many anaesthetic agents inhibit this process.[27,28] There is no benefit, therefore, from collapsing the upper lung early during thoracotomy and if it is ventilated up to the last possible minute oxygen is taken up from this lung for approximately 10 minutes after ventilation has ceased, thus decreasing the period and extent of possible hypoxia.

## Anaesthetic Technique and Intra-operative Management

### Maintenance of Anaesthesia

Light general anaesthesia with muscular relaxation and controlled ventilation is an ideal combination for the majority of thoracotomies. If 60 per cent nitrous oxide is used throughout a thoracotomy, intravenous supplements of natural or synthetic opiates can be given to provide analgesia both during and after the procedure. The addition of a low concentration of an inhalational agent such as halothane, enflurane or methoxyflurane, may be needed to control excessive rises in blood pressure and ensure a satisfactory depth of anaesthesia. If the inspired oxygen concentration is increased during thoracotomy steps must be taken to eliminate the possibility of patient awareness. This can usually be achieved with adequate concentrations of an inhalational agent, but an infusion of a suitable intravenous anaesthetic agent such as Althesin or etomidate can be used.

### Monitoring

For the majority of thoracic operations it is mandatory to measure blood pressure non-invasively and display the ECG. Arterial cannulation permits continuous display of the blood pressure and also provides a source of samples for blood gas analysis. Cannulation of the radial artery, following all the usual precautions, is justified in those patients considered particularly prone to hypoxaemia or vulnerable to its consequences, or if considerable haemorrhage or extensive dissection and retraction of the mediastinum are anticipated.

The measurement of central venous pressure is unnecessary during the majority of thoracotomies but cannulation of a central vein allows rapid transfusion of blood and plasma substitutes and can therefore be very helpful during extensive procedures. The internal jugular vein is a popular site for central venous cannulation[29] but it is wise to cannulate the vein on the side of the thoracotomy because pneumothorax is a known complication of this technique.

### Heat Loss

Heat loss can be substantial during thoracotomy. This can be minimised if the inspired gas is warmed and humidified and large transfusions of cold fluids are avoided. Temperature monitoring and the use of a warming blanket are sensible precautions in infants and children.

### Chest Closure and Drainage

The aim at the end of any operation in the thoracic cavity is to achieve full expansion of all remaining lung tissue with the mediastinum approximately central. For this reason it is usually necessary to drain the pleural cavity so that air or fluid cannot accumulate, although the situation is somewhat different after pneumonectomy (see below).

A drain must allow the escape of air or blood and wide-bore tubing is chosen to prevent obstruction by clot. Two tubes are usually used to drain both air and fluid from the anterior and posterior aspects of a thoracotomy space after lobectomy, one at the apex favouring the escape of air and the other at the base draining accumulating fluid. These drains are usually inserted through separate incisions just before the chest is closed. The lung is then re-expanded by manual ventilation once the drains are *in situ* and before the chest is closed. Gentle re-expansion can also be repeated just prior to extubation of the patient when the chest is closed and the drains are connected to an underwater seal drain.

An *underwater seal* drain is merely a simple and reliable one-way valve which allows air to be expelled from the pleural space but not to enter during the next inspiration. The volume of blood or fluid draining from the chest can also be measured accurately if a graduated bottle is used.

The space above the water in an underwater seal is usually vented to atmosphere through a short tube. Suction can be applied here to assist the escape of air or fluid from the pleural space and hence promote expansion of the lung. Opinions differ on the role of suction in the management of chest drains but many surgeons apply a low suction pressure of 20 cm of water to all chest drains (except after pneumonectomy—see below) and increase this to 50 cm of water if the lung does not expand fully. It could be argued that high pressures would potentiate a leak from a raw lung surface; alternatively it is hoped that the leak will seal if the lung is fully expanded and held against the chest wall.

Following lung resection chest drains are removed when there is no appreciable air leak and blood loss has ceased. Patients require additional analgesia for this procedure.

## The Immediate Post-operative Period

At the end of surgery, anaesthesia is terminated and muscle relaxation reversed in the usual way. The lungs are then suctioned and any remaining lung tissue on the side of operation re-inflated with the chest drains open before the endobronchial tube is removed once a satisfactory pattern of respiration has been established. In general, mechanical ventilation is contra-indicated after pulmonary surgery because of the added risks of infection, problems with continuing air leaks from lung surfaces, and because bronchial suture lines are vulnerable to the effects of both positive pressure and the trauma which follows repeated endotracheal suction. However, a patient's ability to breathe adequately must be judged on conventional grounds and mechanical ventilation may be necessary in a small number of patients in the immediate post-operative period. If controlled ventilation is necessary inflation pressures should be kept as low as possible.

Following extubation humidified oxygen is delivered by face-mask and patients should be sat up as soon as possible so that abdominal contents do not interfere with diaphragmatic movement.

### Post-operative Pain Relief

Pain is a prominent feature after thoracic surgery and analgesia needs to be effective as it may improve respiratory function and will certainly aid a patient's ability to cough and clear secretions.

Parenteral narcotics, administered as required, still form the basis of pain relief after thoracotomy, but newer techniques with intravenous infusions and patient-controlled therapy can be applied. Inhalational agents such as 50 per cent nitrous oxide in oxygen (Entonox) can be used to provide additional analgesia for painful procedures such as chest drain removal or physiotherapy and, in addition, the very nature of the thoracic cage lends itself to a number of local anaesthetic techniques which can be used to complement or supplant drug therapy.

The majority of patients will benefit from intra-operative local anaesthetic intercostal blocks[30,31] although these may have to be repeated in the post-operative period. Freezing of the intercostal nerves with a cryoprobe utilising the Joule Thompson principle affects long-lasting analgesia for a period of two or three weeks and has been shown to alleviate post-thoracotomy pain substantially.[32,33] The more difficult local anaesthetic techniques of paravertebral block and thoracic epidural block can be considered in those patients at risk of post-operative sputum retention or after particularly painful operations such as pleurodesis. However, thoracic epidural block in particular has a high complication rate.[34]

Epidural and spinal opiates may also be used to provide analgesia after thoracotomy but the possibility of producing respiratory depression must be considered.[35]

## Anaesthetic Implications of Specific Surgical Procedures

### Lobectomy

It is desirable to isolate the operated lung for lobectomy in the lateral position so that exposure is as good as possible and secretions can be controlled if necessary. A double lumen tube with the endobronchial extension in the dependent lung is preferable unless distortion of the bronchial tree makes its introduction difficult. An unacceptable degree of arterial hypoxaemia occurs occasionally during one-lung anaesthesia in those with generalised pulmonary disease who are, nevertheless, judged capable of withstanding lobectomy. Both lungs can be ventilated throughout in these circumstances, but a double lumen tube is still useful because it isolates both lungs.

It is usual to test the integrity of bronchial suture lines prior to closing the chest by pouring saline into the pleural cavity to cover the stump while a positive pressure of 30–40 cm of water is held within the tracheobronchial tree by manual compression of the rebreathing bag. General intra-operative management of the lobectomy patient and the principles of chest drainage are as described above.

### Pneumonectomy

Pneumonectomy is a high-risk procedure for which there is a significant morbidity and mortality because of the inevitable reduction in pulmonary function post-operatively. Criteria considered to indicate patients having greater than normal risk of morbidity or mortality after lung resection have already been summarised in Table 2.

Good pre-operative preparation is essential and it is important to familiarise the patient with manoeuvres which will be required during post-operative physiotherapy. Prophylactic antibiotics and subcutaneous heparin are frequently used and many surgeons digitalise the patient pre-operatively. The incidence of dysrhythmias, usually atrial in origin, is high following pneumonectomy. Pre-operative digitalisation has been shown to decrease the incidence of these dysrhythmias and in any case controls the ventricular rate in fast atrial rhythm disturbances, thus preventing a catastrophic drop in cardiac output.

It is quite feasible to carry out pneumonectomy using endotracheal anaesthesia but it is preferable to use a double or single lumen endobronchial tube placed in the dependent lung to aid surgical access and, more importantly, to isolate both lungs and prevent the spread of infected secretions. Blood loss can be considerable and a minimum of four units of blood should be available for transfusion. Intra-operative dysrhythmias are more common than during lobectomy.

Post-operatively a pneumonectomy space gradually fills with a sero-sanguinous fluid over a period of days and over a longer period of time becomes obliterated and eventually fibrosed. Some surgeons close the chest with a basal drain *in situ* in order to manipulate the position of the mediastinum and drain excessive bleeding. Others do not drain the space but manipulate the position of the mediastinum so that it is approximately central or slightly towards the operated side by injecting air into, or aspirating air from, the pleural space on the operated side. This is preferably carried out via a system including a manometer or pressure gauge.

If the chest is drained after pneumonectomy the drainage tube is joined to an underwater seal bottle and clamped once the patient is breathing spontaneously in a supine position and it has been ascertained that the mediastinum is central. Thereafter it is unclamped for one to two minutes in every hour for the first twelve to twenty-four hours so that the nature and volume of the drainage can be noted and any build-up of pressure in the space avoided. It is usually possible to remove the drain on the first post-operative day when the risk of serious bleeding has passed.

### Bronchopleural Fistula

A bronchopleural fistula is a communication between the tracheobronchial tree and pleural cavity which can result from trauma, a neoplasm in the bronchial tree or rupture of an inflammatory lesion. It is most commonly seen, however, when a bronchial stump leaks after pneumonectomy, although its overall incidence is very low.

A fistula usually presents within two weeks of a pneumonectomy but can occur at any time. If the fistula is small, symptoms are unobtrusive with a low-grade fever, tachycardia and a persistent cough with expectoration of small amounts of blood-stained sputum. A large bronchopleural fistula usually presents dramatically, although it is often preceded by the symptoms described above. There is an abrupt onset of dyspnoea after a bout of coughing which may have been precipitated by a change of posture which allows the operated side to be uppermost. Thin brown fluid characteristic of the space contents is inhaled into the remaining lung causing broncho-constriction, respiratory distress and hypoxaemia. Signs of circulatory failure rapidly ensue. If confirmation of the diagnosis is required a chest x-ray will show a considerable fall in the space fluid-level and possibly consolidation and collapse in the remaining lung.

General resuscitative measures should be instituted and the patient sat up and supported so that the pneumonectomy side is dependent. A basal chest drain is then inserted to drain fluid from the space and thus prevent further spillover. Urgent surgery is required to repair a large bronchopleural fistula.

**Anaesthetic management.**—The anaesthetic requirements for repair of a bronchopleural fistula are that further hypoxaemia must be avoided, that entry of more space fluid into the remaining lung must be prevented and that positive-pressure ventilation should be withheld until the fistula has been isolated. Positive-pressure ventilation is likely to be ineffective with a large fistula and will aid the spillover of fluid. Endobronchial intubation is therefore mandatory to isolate the fistula. Double lumen endobronchial tubes are satisfactory for this purpose but an experienced operator placing a single lumen endobronchial tube under direct vision is probably more likely to site the tube correctly at the first attempt.

Endobronchial intubation under local anaesthesia is theoretically attractive because spontaneous ventilation and the ability to cough are retained until positive-pressure ventilation can be instituted safely. Similar advantages can be claimed for an inhalational general anaesthetic which is deepened to the point where intubation can be achieved without muscle relaxants.

In practice these methods are difficult to use. Local anaesthetics penetrate the mucosa poorly if viscid and purulent secretions are present and if absorption is rapid, toxic reactions are more likely in the sick hypoxic patient. Deep inhalational anaesthesia is also unsatisfactory as hypotension is likely in the upright position and spontaneous ventilation may fail before a sufficient depth of anaesthesia is reached to prevent coughing during intubation. The majority of experienced anaesthetists, therefore, choose to use general anaesthesia in patients with a bronchopleural fistula.

With the chest drain open and the patient in a sitting position pre-oxygenation is carried out. Anaesthesia is then induced intravenously with the minimum dose of a suitable agent, followed by complete muscular relaxation achieved with suxamethonium. This provides perfect conditions for atraumatic endobronchial intubation, with no risk of coughing or straining, but is only safe if the tube is sited correctly. Following endobronchial intubation the patient can be safely placed in position for thoracotomy.

In the future high frequency positive-pressure ventilation may have a role to play in the ventilatory management of bronchopleural fistula both during surgery and in the post-operative period.[36,37]

### Drainage of Empyema

An empyema or purulent effusion within the pleural space occurs as a complications of an inflammatory process in the underlying lung or following pneumonectomy. Adequate drainage is essential and in the acute stage can be carried out by inserting an intercostal drain under local anaesthesia. After this has been done, then rib resection may be necessary at a later date to ensure adequate drainage.

It is unreasonable to carry this out under local anaesthetic as extensive infiltration is neither particularly safe nor reliable in the presence of infection.

An empyema is often associated with a bronchopleural fistula particularly after pneumonectomy. Although the fistula may be small it is safer to manage general anaesthesia for drainage of empyema on the lines discussed above.

### Lung Cysts

In adults surgery to plicate and obliterate air-filled lung cysts is usually only advised when they are large enough to interfere with pulmonary function. Anaesthetic management of these patients may prove hazardous for several reasons,[38] especially if positive-pressure ventilation is used via an endotracheal tube. Four complications may arise:

1. The cyst may be preferentially ventilated.
2. A valvular communication with the airway may allow the cyst to enlarge and increase the tension.
3. The cyst may rupture causing a tension pneumothorax.
4. Nitrous oxide may be taken up by the cyst causing it to enlarge considerably.

In adults, it is reasonable to intubate the lung contralateral to the cyst endobronchially following pre-oxygenation of the patient and an intravenous induction. Positive-pressure ventilation can then be applied to the healthy lung with 100 per cent oxygen[39] thereby avoiding the use of nitrous oxide and positive pressure to the cyst. Theoretically, spontaneous respiration could be maintained until the chest is opened, but spontaneous ventilation is likely to be inefficient in the presence of a large lung cyst especially in those who have widespread emphysema.

Occasionally a tumour within the bronchial tree can cause a one-way ball-valve effect (see Figs. 17*a*, *b*) either for a lobe or the whole lung. In this instance it is safer to isolate that lobe or lung as described above until such time as the chest is open, when the lung can be controlled surgically.

If asymptomatic lung cysts are seen on the chest x-ray of a patient presenting for general surgery, conventional anaesthetic techniques for the procedure in question can usually be used without disastrous consequences. Local anaesthesia is obviously useful and spontaneous respiration can be employed if it is appropriate to the procedure. Few anaesthetists would choose to avoid nitrous oxide if general anaesthesia is essential (although this is easy to do) but if positive-pressure ventilation is used the pattern should be adjusted to minimise inflation pressures. The anaesthetist should remain alert to possible complications relating to the cyst during and after the procedure and facilities for prompt drainage of the pleural space should be available.

## POST-OPERATIVE PULMONARY COMPLICATIONS

### Introduction

Disordered respiratory function, resulting in hypoxaemia, is a universal finding following major surgery and anaesthesia. Post-operative pulmonary complications are also common and may be evident on chest x-ray as atelectasis, pneumonia and lobar collapse, or clinically as fever with or without production of purulent sputum. Overt pulmonary complications do not necessarily accompany disorders of respiratory function but the two are interrelated. Pulmonary complications will exacerbate changes in respiratory function and are probably an extension of the factors which contribute to these changes, namely micro-atelectasis and airway closure. Post-operative pulmonary function has been the subject of several reviews[40–42] and

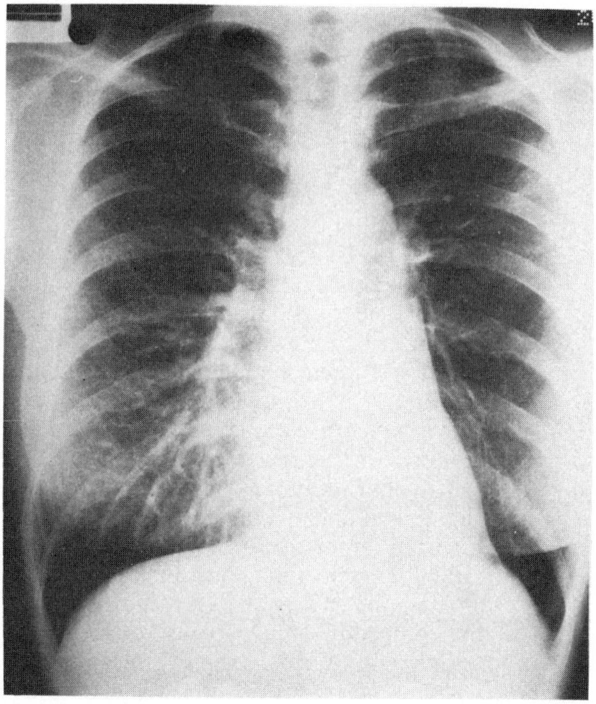

(*a*)

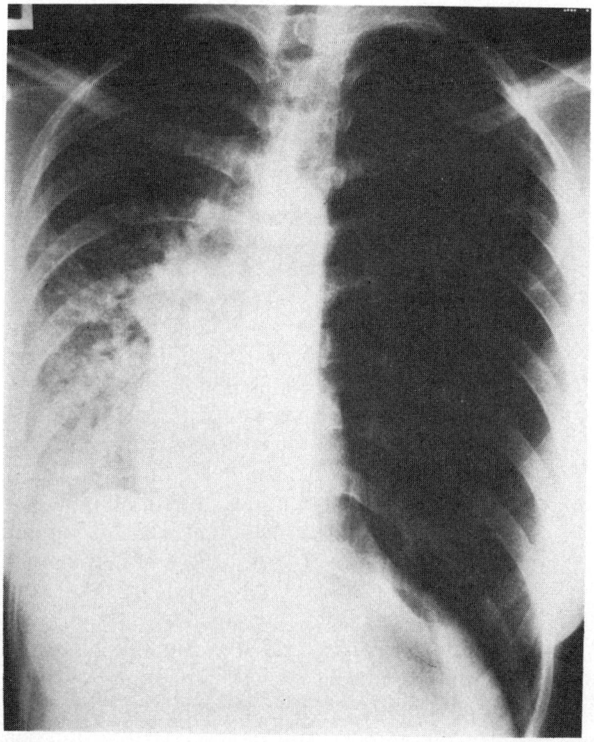

(*b*)

11/Fig. 17.—Chest x-rays (*a*) in inspiration, (*b*) in expiration, of a female patient with a ball-valve adenoma in the left main bronchus. Note the hyper-expanded lung and deviated trachea on the expiratory film.

factors affecting lung function during anaesthesia are considered in Chapter 3, p. 100.

In order to understand the mechanisms which may lead to pulmonary complications it is helpful to outline current knowledge of respiratory function following anaesthesia and surgery. This is followed by a more detailed discussion of post-operative pulmonary complications. Pulmonary embolus and aspiration pneumonitis are considered in Chapters 14 and 40 respectively.

### Respiratory Function Following Anaesthesia and Surgery

Immediately following surgery hypoxaemia occurs for a variety of reasons including inadequate reversal of muscle relaxants, respiratory depression, increased oxygen consumption associated with shivering, a low cardiac output and the diffusion of highly soluble nitrous oxide into the alveoli (Fink effect). Other mechanisms have to be invoked to explain the hypoxia which may last several hours following even a minor anaesthetic and the hypoxaemia lasting several days following upper abdominal and thoracic surgery.

The main pulmonary changes during general anaesthesia, irrespective of the technique used, are an increase in the alveolar component of the respiratory dead space; an increase in the alveolar-arterial (A-a) oxygen tension difference, quantified as increased pulmonary venous admixture; and a decrease in functional residual capacity.[43] Following major surgery these changes persist and functional residual capacity (FRC) may remain depressed for several days, gradually returning to normal between 9 to 14 days. In addition vital capacity (VC) may initially be reduced to 40 per cent of preoperative values with a concomitant decrease in maximum inspiratory and expiratory flow rates.

### Lung Volumes

A reduction in FRC following laparotomy was first documented by Beecher as early as 1933;[44] subsequently it has been demonstrated that changes in FRC occur during anaesthesia whether spontaneous or mechanical ventilation is employed.[45,46] A change in FRC relative to closing capacity (CC) is probably the most important factor contributing to post-operative hypoxaemia. Closing capacity is the lung volume at which small airway closure begins to occur in normal subjects. In conscious normals FRC is greater than CC and airway closure does not occur during normal tidal breathing. Recent evidence suggests that CC may decrease during anaesthesia,[47] but this change is probably relatively smaller than the decrease in FRC. However, in the post-operative period hypoxaemia occurs as FRC decreases below CC so that airway closure occurs during tidal breathing. Alexander and his co-workers[48] found a significant correlation between changes (decrease) in FRC and an increase in A-a gradient after abdominal surgery and also a significant correlation between changes in FRC minus CC and A-a gradient. Changes in FRC relative to CC can also explain the decrease of $Pa_{O_2}$ with increasing age and the correlation between increasing age and degree of post-operative hypoxaemia.

The primary reason for changes in FRC during anaesthesia and the post-operative period remains obscure. Post-operatively abdominal distension, pneumoperitoneum, spasm of abdominal muscle as a result of wound pain and the collapse of lung tissue have all been suggested as causes of hypoxaemia. Adequate pain relief might be expected to mitigate changes in FRC and hence the extent and duration of hypoxaemia following abdominal surgery; to some extent the study of Spence and Smith,[49] which compared intramuscular morphine and extradural block for analgesia following abdominal surgery, confirmed this. In this study, the extradural group were better off in terms of their clinical state and arterial oxygenation than the morphine group, but there was no significant difference in the degree of vital capacity impairment. Subsequent studies, however, have shown that larger doses of narcotics, compared with the doses used by Spence and Smith, provide better analgesia and that extradural block is not necessarily more effective in reducing post-operative hypoxaemia.[48,50,51] There is little evidence, therefore, that FRC is restored towards normal if extradural analgesia is used following upper abdominal surgery and it may be significant that forced expiratory volume ($FEV_1$), forced vital capacity (FVC) and peak expiratory flow rate (PEFR) are all reduced following thoracic extradural blockade ($T_2$–$T_{12}$) in patients awaiting surgery, possibly because of thoracic and abdominal muscle weakness.[52] A recent study[53] has also demonstrated a significant fall in FRC during thoracic extradural analgesia.

### Pulmonary Blood Flow

A reduction in pulmonary blood flow may, in certain circumstances, be more important than a reduction in ventilation as a contributing factor to post-operative hypoxaemia. The pulmonary circulation is a low pressure system and therefore blood flow and distribution is greatly affected by gravity. As a result a decrease in cardiac output can lead to a large increase in the amount of unperfused and over-ventilated alveoli (increased physiological dead space). An increase in physiological dead space also occurs if micro-aggregates of white cells, platelets and fibrin accumulate in the pulmonary vascular bed as a result of large transfusions of unfiltered, stored blood. Amniotic and fat embolism have a similar effect..

### Post-operative Pulmonary Complications

Despite improvements in anaesthetic techniques the majority of studies show that there has been little decrease in the incidence of post-operative pulmonary complications in recent years. Most series show an overall incidence of 5 per cent for all types of surgery and Garibaldi and his colleagues[54] reported an incidence of 17·5 per cent in high-risk patients, particularly in those undergoing elective thoracic (40 per cent) and abdominal surgery. A pulmonary complication rate of this magnitude is similar to figures obtained by investigators thirty years ago using comparable criteria and an equally high-risk group of patients. The reason why this complication rate remains high, despite a greater understanding of pulmonary pathology and improved methods of prophylaxis and management, is unclear. It is likely that patients are now operated upon who would formerly be rejected on grounds of age, poor respiratory function or other debilitating disease.

Post-operatively pulmonary complications may easily be recognised as an overwhelming pneumonic process leading to respiratory failure or as distinct lobar collapse (Fig. 18). Ninety per cent of complications reported, however, fall in the atelectasis/bronchopneumonia category and criteria used for their diagnosis in most studies include pyrexia, increased sputum production with or without microbiological confirmation of infection, an abnormal clinical examination of the chest, and x-ray evidence of atelectasis. Tisi[11] defines atelectasis as closure of lung units. This covers a spectrum from being diffuse at sublobular levels, and therefore not visible radiographically (micro-atelectasis), to localised collapse of a segment, lobe or lung that is apparent on chest x-ray.

### Risk Factors

**Pulmonary defence mechanisms.**—Normally secretions are removed from the lower to the upper bronchial tree by ciliary activity, while at a higher level an active cough reflex leads to effective expulsive efforts. These defence mechanisms also protect the lung against inhaled particles and bacteria. Disease, smoking, surgery, anaesthesia and many other factors can alter these mechanisms thus leading to inadequate clearance of mucus and particulate matter.

General anaesthesia may impair these processes in several ways. Mechanical stimuli such as an airway or endotracheal tube can provoke an increase in salivary and bronchial secretions, as does neostigmine. Agents such as atropine and hyoscine may cause sputum to become viscid and tenacious and mucus transport is impaired if dry gases are inhaled.[55] There is also evidence that some anaesthetic agents depress ciliary activity.[56] All these factors predispose to atelectasis.

**The patient.**—Males are more prone to pulmonary complications than females[57] and post-operative pneumonias occur more frequently in the elderly and obese.

The preponderance of complications in males is related to the greater incidence of smoking in this group. Smoking increases the risk of pulmonary complications proportionately with the number of cigarettes consumed.[58] This is not surprising when one considers its deleterious effect on cilial activity and normal mucus production.

Pre-existing lung disease greatly increases the risk of pulmonary problems and in Wightman's study[57] complications were found in approximately 26 per cent of patients with respiratory disease and in only 8 per cent of patients with normal lungs. A recent upper respiratory tract infection may also increase the incidence of pulmonary problems. The increased incidence of pre-existing respiratory problems in the elderly and obese may, to some extent, explain the

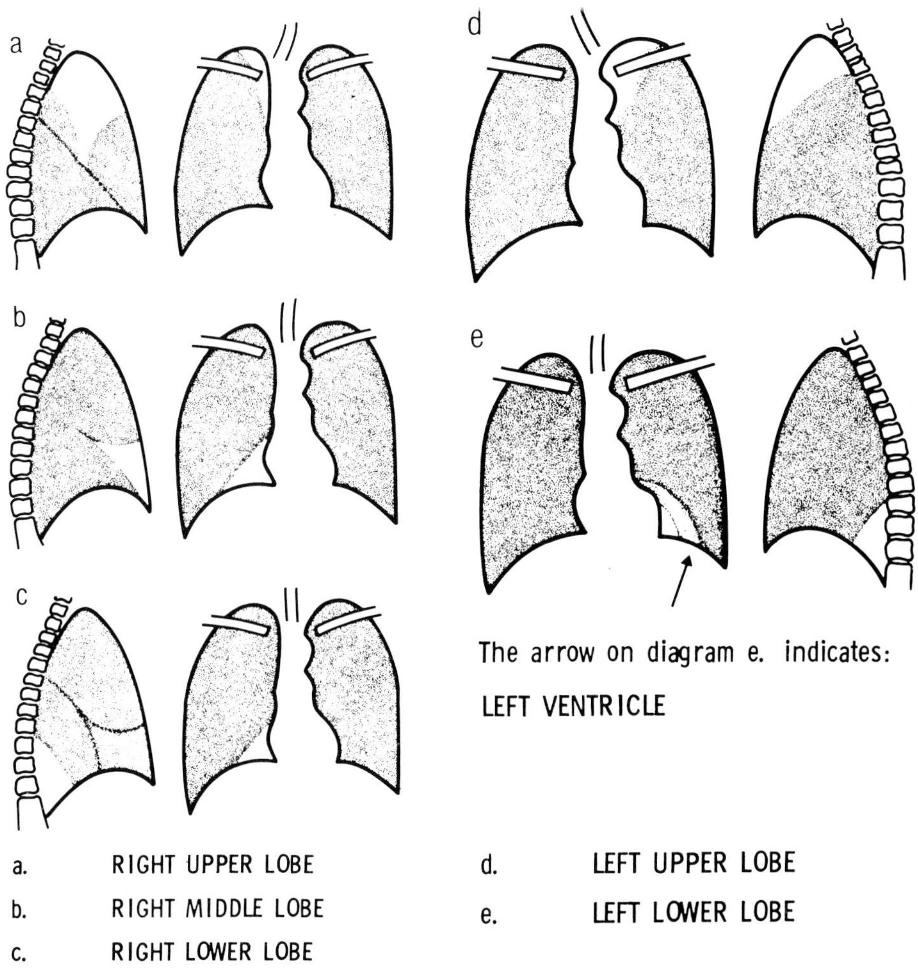


11/FIG. 18.—Diagrams of the radiographic changes produced by lobar collapse.

increased occurrence of pulmonary complications post-operatively in these patients. However, both these groups are relatively hypoxic as normal conscious subjects and there are physiological reasons, again partly because of changes in FRC relative to CC, which account for this. This may also explain the patient's propensity to post-operative chest infections.

Lung disease may in some cases be iatrogenic and more patients are now being referred for surgery following irradiation or cytotoxic drug therapy. These forms of treatment can cause pulmonary fibrosis and a restrictive lung defect. The effects of bleomycin on the lung[59] and the possible "sensitising" action of high inspired oxygen concentrations are now well known but other cytotoxic drugs can also cause lung damage.[60]

Finally, one must consider the patient as a whole. A patient starved because of oesophageal obstruction or immunosuppressed as a consequence of drug therapy is obviously at risk from developing a post-operative chest infection. In more general terms it is interesting to note that Garibaldi and colleagues[54] found that patients with a high American Society of Anesthesiologists (ASA) pre-anaesthesia physical status classification and those with low serum albumin concentrations were at increased risk of developing post-operative pneumonia.

**The operation.**—As previously stated the site of operation is the most important factor affecting the incidence of pulmonary complications and patients are particularly at risk following upper abdominal and thoracic surgery where post-operative pain is marked and pulmonary mechanics most deranged. Prolonged surgery and the effects of posture, particularly the steep head-down Trendelenburg and lithotomy positions, which limit total lung capacity because of pulmonary venous congestion and displacement of abdominal contents, are also potentiating factors.[61]

### Prevention and Treatment

**Pre-operative assessment and preparation.**—This should include a full history and a detailed clinical examination. An estimate of risk can then be made with reference to the points discussed above and it is sometimes possible to eliminate some risk factors. For example, it is always worthwhile stimulating a patient to lose weight or stop smoking, although the latter must cease several weeks before surgery to have a beneficial effect on lung function.[62]

Patients over the age of 50,[63] those undergoing major abdominal or thoracic surgery and those at risk of developing complications should have a pre-operative chest x-ray. Lung function tests are a useful baseline in those with significant respiratory disease and also allow the hazards of surgery and anaesthesia to be more clearly defined in individual cases.[11,64]

Subjects with established lung disease will benefit from pre-operative physiotherapy, particularly those with excessive quantities of sputum.[65] Postural drainage may be useful if sputum is excessive, particularly in diseases such as bronchiectasis and cystic fibrosis. In addition, most patients will benefit from preoperative instructions regarding breathing exercises.

A pre-operative chest infection, proven on culture, should be vigorously treated with an appropriate antibiotic and surgery postponed, if possible, until the sputum is clear. The place of prophylactic antibiotics commenced just prior to surgery remains controversial. On general principles, it would seem sensible not to prescribe prophylactic antibiotics for a previously fit patient solely to cover or prevent a post-operative chest infection, but rather to treat a proven infection with an appropriate antibiotic as the occasion arises. In the case of bronchitic subjects Lazlo and his colleagues[66] found there was no benefit to be gained from giving this group antibiotic cover prior to minor surgery but that a broad spectrum antibiotic did appear to reduce the incidence and morbidity of post-operative pulmonary infections in patients undergoing upper abdominal surgery.

Bronchodilator drugs may be prescribed preoperatively in patients with reversible airways obstruction and drug therapy, including corticosteroids, where previously prescribed, should be continued in asthmatic subjects.

Finally, a sympathetic pre-operative visit is a proven method of reassuring the anxious patient and is a factor in decreasing the severity of post-operative pain.

### Anaesthetic Technique

**Premedication.**—Many anaesthetists now omit atropine from premedication regimes because of the unpleasant and unnecessary dry mouth that it creates. Atropine also causes sputum to become more viscid and has been established as a contributory factor to post-operative hypoxaemia. If secretions are copious in the first place, however, and endotracheal or endobronchial instrumentation is planned it is logical to include atropine or a similar drug in the premedication. In addition Jones and Drummond[67] failed to show that atropine, as a premedicant has any influence on the frequency of pulmonary complications.

**General anaesthesia or local anaesthesia.**—It has not been clearly demonstrated that any particular anaesthetic technique, either general or local, influences the incidence of pulmonary complications. This only applies if anaesthesia is conducted in an optimal fashion and pre- and post-operative care is meticulous. Evidence for this is to be found in the classic study of Dripps and Deming (1946).[68] Local anaesthetic techniques can, however, sensibly be used for peripheral and superficial surgery particularly in patients with significant respiratory disease.

Local anaesthetic techniques, applied safely and without compromising patient comfort, can be beneficial if used intra-operatively in other situations. McLaren and his co-workers[69] compared the use of spinal anaesthesia and general anaesthesia in elderly patients undergoing surgery for fractured neck of femur and, although there was no significant difference in post-operative morbidity of the two groups, long-term survival was significantly higher in the spinal group. McKenzie and others[70] in a similar study, could not confirm this effect of spinal anaesthesia on survival after major orthopaedic surgery but did find that their spinal group had a significantly higher $Pao_2$ than the general anaesthetic group in the post-operative period. Fox and his colleagues[71] have also found extradural analgesia combined with light general anaesthesia to be a useful technique in the morbidly obese.

*General anaesthesia.*—During general anaesthesia inspired gases should be humidified in order to prevent drying of secretions and the mucosa of the tracheobronchial tree. Inspired oxygen concentrations should be kept below 100 per cent, if possible, as this favours the production of absorption collapse and if mechanical ventilation is used ventilation should be adjusted to prevent pulmonary collapse. In practice, a ventilatory pattern with an increased inspiratory time and an inspiratory pause may be appropriate, but there is no sound evidence that any particular mode of ventilation, including the use of positive end-expiratory pressure (PEEP), influences the incidence of pulmonary complications.

### The Post-Operative Period

In the immediate post-operative period it should be ascertained that any muscle relaxant drugs are adequately reversed and that some form of analgesia is continued so that a patient can breathe in an effective pain-free manner. Controlled oxygen therapy is continued and the patient sat up as soon as possible to aid diaphragmatic movement. If adequate muscle tone cannot be re-established, either because of an overdose of muscle relaxant or biochemical imbalance, then it is preferable to continue mechanical ventilation until respiratory effort is satisfactory. A short period of mechanical ventilation in the post-operative period can also be beneficial for patients with very poor lung function.

**Pain relief.**—Adequate analgesia is an essential part of post-operative care. Studies by Simpson and others[72] and Bromage[73] suggested that epidural analgesia was more effective than conventional analgesic regimes in preventing the occurrence of pulmonary complications. This was not confirmed, however, by Pflug and his colleagues.[51] Simpson and his associates[72] also emphasised the importance of vigorous physiotherapy in the post-operative period because they were only able to demonstrate an increase in lung compliance in extradural patients after effective coughing manoeuvres had been carried out. Several authors have pointed out that any analgesic regime must, to be successful, allow a "stir-up" programme including change in position, deep breathing and coughing to be instituted without causing respiratory depression or disability.

**Physiotherapy.**—Chest physiotherapy plays an essential part in the prevention and treatment of pulmonary complications, particularly in patients with respiratory disease. Physiotherapy may include breathing exercises, percussion and shaking the chest to loosen secretions and aid expectoration and, in certain circumstances, postural drainage. Intermittent positive-pressure breathing (IPPB) instituted via a "Bird" ventilator may be useful particularly in those with bronchospasm, to whom bronchodilator drugs can be administered via the nebuliser of the system. Incentive spirometers have also been designed to encourage patients to inspire a predetermined volume and thus improve the effectiveness of voluntary deep breathing. Forced expiratory manoeuvres contribute to lung collapse and should be avoided.

**Drug therapy.**—Ideally antibiotics should be administered with regard to sputum culture results. Bronchodilator therapy is indicated in patients with bronchospasm. The therapeutic value of respiratory stimulants in the post-operative period is less certain. Gawley and his colleagues[74] found that the use of doxapram hydrochloride reduced the incidence of pulmonary complications in previously fit patients undergoing abdominal surgery. In contrast, Sebel and his co-workers,[75] concluded that doxapram had no effect on post-operative pulmonary complications in patients with lung disease undergoing thoracic surgery.

## REFERENCES


1. Rendell-Baker, L. (1981). History of anesthesia for thoracic surgery: a chronology. *Anesthesiol. Rev.*, **7**, 8.
2. Ryan, D. W. (1980). Anaesthesia for bronchography in small children. *Ann. Roy. Coll. Surg. Engl.*, **62**, 223.
3. Newell, J. P. and Collis, J. M. (1980). Anaesthesia for bronchoscopy: examination of a standard technique. *Proc. roy. Soc. Med.*, **73**, 241.
4. Sanders, R. D. (1967). Two ventilating attachments for bronchoscopes. *Delaware med. J.*, **39**, 170.
5. Borg, U., Eriksson, I., Lyttkans, L., Lars-Goran, N. and Sjostrand, U. (1977). High frequency positive pressure ventilation applied in bronchoscopy under general anaesthesia. *Acta Anaesth. Scand. (Suppl.)*, **64**, 69.
6. Bethune, D. W. and Collis, J. M. (1979). Anaesthesia for bronchoscopy. *Anaesthesia*, **34**, 210.
7. Spoerel, W. E., and Grant, P. A. (1971). Ventilation during bronchoscopy. *Canad. Anaesth. Soc. J.*, **18**, 178.
8. Lett, Z. and Ong, G. B. (1974). Anaesthesia for fibreoptic bronchoscopy. *Brit. J. Anaesth.*, **47**, 1219.
9. Vivori, E. (1980). Anaesthesia for laryngoscopy. *Brit. J. Anaesth.*, **52**, 638.
10. Mette, P. J. (1980). Avoiding complications during jet ventilation. *Anesthesiology*, **52**, 451.
11. Tisi, G. M. (1979). Pre-operative evaluation of pulmonary function. *Amer. Rev. Resp. Dis.*, **119**, 293.
12. Olsen, G. N., Block, A. J., Swenson, E. W., Castle, J. R. and Wynne, J. W. (1975). Pulmonary function evalution of the lung resection candidate: a prospective study. *Amer. Rev. Resp. Dis.*, **111**, 379.
13. Beecher, H. K. (1940). Some controversial matters of anesthesia for thoracic surgery. *J. Thorac. Surg.*, **9**, 202.
14. Overholt, R. H., Langer, L., Szypulski, J. T. and Wilson, N. T. (1946). Pulmonary resection in the treatment of tuberculosis. *J. Thorac. Surg.*, **15**, 384.
15. Parry Brown, A. I. (1948). Posture in thoracic surgery *Thorax*, **3**, 161.
16. White, G. M. J. (1960). A new double-lumen tube. *Brit. J. Anaesth.*, **32**, 232.
17. Pappin, J. C. (1979). The current practice of endobronchial intubation. *Anaesthesia*, **34**, 57.
18. Mansfield, R. E. and Jenkins, R. (1967). *Practical Anaesthesia for Lung Surgery*. London: Baillière Tindall and Cassell.
19. Aps, C. and Towey, R. M. (1981). Experiences with fibre-optic bronchoscopic positioning of single-lumen endobronchial tubes. *Anaesthesia*, **36**, 415.
20. Torda, T. A., McCulloch, C. H., O'Brien, H. D., Wright, J. S. and Horton, D. A. (1974). Pulmonary venous admixture during one-lung anaesthesia. *Anaesthesia*, **29**, 272.
21. Khanam, T. and Branthwaite, M. A. (1973). Arterial oxygenation during one-lung anaesthesia (1). *Anaesthesia*, **28**, 132.
22. Khanam, T. and Branthwaite, M. A. (1973). Arterial oxygenation during one-lung anaesthesia (2). *Anaesthesia*, **28**, 280.
23. Kerr, J. H., Crampton Smith, A., Prys-Roberts, C. and Meloche, R. (1973). Observations during endobronchial anaesthesia I: Ventilation and carbon dioxide clearance. *Brit. J. Anaesth.*, **45**, 159.
24. Kerr, J. H., Crampton Smith, A., Prys-Roberts, C. and Meloche, R. (1974). Observations during endobronchial anaesthesia II: Oxygenation. *Brit. J. Anaesth.*, **46**, 84.
25. Katz, J. A., Laverne, R. G., Fairley, H. B. and Thomas, A. N. (1980). Pulmonary oxygen exchange during endobronchial anaesthesia. *Anesthesiology*, Suppl., **53**, 411.
26. Capan, L. M., Turndoff, H., Patel, C., Ramanathan, S., Acinapura, A. and Chalan, J. (1980). Optimization of arterial oxygenation during one-lung anaesthesia. *Anesth. Analg. Curr. Res.*, **59**, 847.
27. Benumof, J. L. and Wahrenbrock, E. A. (1975). Local effects of anesthetics on regional hypoxic pulmonary vasoconstriction. *Anesthesiology*, **43**, 525.
28. Sykes, M. K., Hurtig, J. G., Tait, A. R. and Chakrabarti, M. K. (1977). Reduction of hypoxic pulmonary vasoconstriction during diethyl ether anaesthesia in the dog. *Brit. J. Anaesth.*, **49**, 293.
29. English, I. C. W., Frew, R. M., Piggott, J. F. and Zaki, M. (1969). Percutaneous catheterisation of the internal jugular vein. *Anaesthesia*, **24**, 521.
30. Kaplan, J. A., Miller, E. D. and Gallagher, E. G. (1975). Post-operative analgesia for thoracotomy patients. *Anesth. Analg. Curr. Res.*, **54**, 773.
31. Moore, D. C. (1975). Intercostal nerve block for postoperative somatic pain following surgery of thorax and upper abdomen. *Brit. J. Anaesth.*, **47**, 284.
32. Katz, J. and Nelson, W. (1980). Cryoanalgesia for postthoracotomy pain. *Lancet*, **1**, 512.
33. Maiwand, O., and Makey, A. R. (1981). Cryoanalgesia for relief of pain after thoracotomy. *Brit. med. J.*, **282**, 1749.
34. Griffiths, D. P. G., Diamond, A. W. and Cameron, J. D. (1975). Post-operative extradural analgesia following thoracic surgery: a feasibility study. *Brit. J. Anaesth.*, **47**, 48.
35. Bromage, P. R. (1981). The price of intraspinal narcotic analgesia: basic constraints. *Anesth. Analg. Curr. Res.*, **60**, 461.
36. Carlon, G. C., Ray, C., Klain, M., McCormack, P. M. (1980). High frequency positive pressure ventilation in management of a patient with broncho-pleural fistula. *Anesthesiology*, **52**, 160.
37. Malina, J. R., Nordström, S. G., Sjöstrand, U. H. and Wattwil, L. M. (1981). Clinical evaluation of high frequency positive pressure ventilation (HFPPV) in patients scheduled for open-chest surgery. *Anesth. Analg. Curr. Res.*, **60**, 234.
38. Cullum, A. R., English, I. C. W. and Branthwaite, M. A. (1973). Endobronchial intubation in infancy. *Anaesthesia*, **28**, 66.
39. Caseby, N. G. (1981). Anaesthesia for the patient with coincidental giant lung bulla. *Canad. Anaesth. Soc. J.*, **28**, 272.
40. Hewlett, M. and Branthwaite, M. A. (1975). Postoperative pulmonary function. *Brit. J. Anaesth* , **47**, 102.
41. Stoddart, J. C. (1978). Post-operative respiratory failure: an anaesthetic hazard? *Brit. J. Anaesth.*, **50**, 695.
42. Craig, D. B. (1981). Post-operative recovery of pulmonary function. Review article. *Anesth. Analg. Curr. Res.*, **60**, 46.
43. Nunn, J. F. (1981). Anesthesia and the lung. *Anesthesiology*, **52**, 107.
44. Beecher, H. K. (1933). Effect of laparotomy on lung volume. Demonstration of a new type of pulmonary collapse. *J. Clin. Invest.*, **12**, 651.
45. Hewlett, A. M., Hulands, G. H., Nunn, J. F. and Heath, J. R. (1974*a*). Functional residual capacity during anaes-

thesia II: Spontaneous respiration. *Brit. J. Anaesth.*, **46**, 486.
46. Hewlett, A. M., Hulands, G. H., Nunn, J. F. and Milledge, J. S. (1974*b*). Functional residual capacity during anaesthesia III: Artificial ventilation. *Brit. J. Anaesth.*, **46**, 495.
47. Juno, P., Marsh, H. M., Knopp, T. J. and Rehder, K. (1978). Closing capacity in awake and anesthetized-paralysed man. *J. Appl. Physiol.*, **44**, 238.
48. Alexander, J. I., Spence, A. A., Parikh, R. K. and Stuart, B (1973). The role of airway closure in post-operative hypoxaemia. *Brit. J. Anaesth.*, **45**, 34.
49. Spence, A. A. and Smith, G. (1971). Post-operative analgesia and lung function: a comparison of morphine with extradural block. *Brit. J. Anaesth.* **43**, 144.
50. Spence, A. A. and Logan, D. A. (1975). Respiratory effects of extradural nerve block in the post-operative period. *Brit. J. Anaesth.*, **47**, 281.
51. Pflug, A. E., Murphy, T. M. Butler, S. H. and Tucker, G. T. (1974). The effects of post-operative peridural analgesia on pulmonary therapy and complications. *Anesthesiology*, **41**, 8.
52. Sjögren, S. and Wright, B. (1972). Respiratory changes during continuous epidural blockade. *Acta Anaesth. Scand.*, **46**, 27.
53. Takasaki, M. and Takahashi, T. (1980). Respiratory function during cervical and thoracic extradural and analgesia in patients with normal lungs. *Brit. J. Anaesth.*, **52**, 1271.
54. Garibaldi, R. A., Britt, M. R., Coleman, M. L., Reading, J. C. and Pace, N. L. (1981). Risk factors for post-operative pneumonia. *Amer. J. Med.*, **70**, 677.
55. Forbes, A. R. (1974). Temperature, humidity and mucus flow in the intubated trachea. *Brit. J. Anaesth.*, **46**, 29.
56. Nunn, J. F., Sturrock, J. E. and Willis, E. J. (1974). The effect of inhalational anaesthetics on the swimming velocity of *Tetrahymena pyriformis*. *J. Cell Sci.*, **15**, 537.
57. Wightman, J. A. K. (1968). A prospective study of post-operative pulmonary complications. *Brit. J. Surg.*, **55**, 85.
58. Chalon, J., Tayyab, M. A. and Ramanthan, S. (1975). Cytology of respiratory epithelium as a predictor of respiratory complications after operation. *Chest*, **67**, 32.
59. Goldiner, P. L., Carlon, G. C., Cvitkovic, E., Schweizer, O. and Howland, W. S. (1978). Factors influencing post-operative morbidity in patients treated with bleomycin. *Brit. med. J.*, **1**, 1664.
60. Selvin, B. L. (1981). Cancer chemotherapy. Implications for the anesthesiologist. *Anesth. Analg. Curr. Res.*, **60**, 425.
61. Schiller, W. R. (1978). The Trendelenburg position. In: *Positioning in Anesthesia and Surgery*, Ed. J. T. Martin. Philadelphia: W. B. Saunders Co.
62. Otto, C. W. (1980). Respiratory morbidity and mortality. An "Anesthetic Side Effects and Complications". Ed. W. D. Owens. *Internat. Anesthesiology Clinics*. Vol. 18, No. 3, Little, Brown and Company, Boston.
63. Kerr, I. H. (1974). The pre-operative chest x-ray. *Brit. J. Anaesth.*, **46**, 558.
64. Rigg, J. R. A. and Jones, N. L. (1978). Clinical assessment of respiratory function. *Brit. J. Anaesth.*, **50**, 4.
65 Gracey, D. R., Divertie, M. B. and Didier, E. P. (1979). Pre-operative pulmonary preparation of patients with chronic obstructive pulmonary disease. *Chest*, **76**, 123.
66. Lazlo, G., Archer, G. G., Darrell, J. H., Dawson, J. M. and Fletcher, C. M. (1973). The diagnosis and prophylaxis of pulmonary complications of surgical operation. *Brit. J. Surg.*, **60**, 129.
67. Jones, G. C. and Drummond, G. B. (1981). Effect of atropine premedication on respiratory complications. *Brit. J. Anaesth.*, **53**, 441.
68. Dripps, R. D. and Deming, M. V. (1946). Post-operative atelectasis and pneumonia. *Ann. Surg.*, **124**, 94.
69. McLaren, A. D., Stockwell, M. C. and Reid, V. T. (1978). Anaesthetic techniques for surgical correction of fractured neck of femur. A comparative study of spinal and general anaesthesia in the elderly. *Anaesthesia*, **33**, 10.
70. McKenzie, P. J., Wishart, H. W., Dewar, K. M. S., Gray, I. and Smith, G. (1980). Comparison of the effects of spinal anaesthesia and general anaesthesia on post-operative oxygenation and perioperative mortality. *Brit. J. Anaesth.*, **52**, 49.
71. Fox, G. S., Whalley, D. G. and Bevan, D. R. (1981). Anaesthesia for the morbidly obese. *Brit. J. Anaesth.*, **53**, 811.
72. Simpson, B. R., Parkhouse, J., Marshall, R. and Lambrechts, W. (1961). Extradural analgesia and the prevention of post-operative respiratory complications. *Brit. J. Anaesth.*, **33**, 628.
73. Bromage, P. R. (1967). Extradural analgesia for pain relief. *Brit. J. Anaesth.*, **39**, 721.
74. Gawley, T. H., Dundee, J. W. and Jones, C. J. (1975). The role of doxapram in the reduction of pulmonary complications following surgery. *Brit. J. Anaesth.*, **47**, 906.
75. Sebel, P. S., Kershaw, E. J. and Rao, W. S. (1980). Effects of doxapram on post-operative pulmonary complications following thoracotomy. *Brit. J. Anaesth.*, **52**, 81.

## FURTHER READING

Gaskell, D. V. and Webber, B. A. (1980). *The Brompton Hospital Guide to Chest Physiotherapy*, 4th edit. Oxford: Blackwell Scientific Publications.

Gothard, J. W. W. and Branthwaite, M. A. (1982). *Anaesthesia for Thoracic Surgery*. Oxford: Blackwell Scientific Publications.

Nunn, J. F. (1977). *Applied Respiratory Physiology*, 2nd edit. London: Butterworth.

Sykes, M. K., McNicol, M. W. and Campbell, E. J. M. (1976). *Respiratory Failure*, 2nd edit. Oxford: Blackwell Scientific Publications.

*Section Two*

# THE CARDIOVASCULAR SYSTEM

CHAPTER 12

# The Cardiovascular System



## Circulatory Innervation and Anatomy

The function of the heart and the tone of the blood vessels are controlled by a variety of neuronal and chemical mechanisms. Generally autonomic nervous system activity predominates, but there are circumstances in which chemical mechanisms take over—for example, in the physiological autoregulating response improving muscle and myocardial blood flow during exercise or in pathological states such as phaeochromocytoma.

### Innervation of the Heart

The parasympathetic outflow via the vagi is the dominant influence in the normal rate control of the heart, which is achieved by a reduction in the rate of discharge from the sino-atrial (SA) node. Atrioventricular (AV) conduction is impaired with increased vagal tone, but there is no direct vagal effect upon ventricular contractility. Vagal tone is responsible for the normal resting heart rate which can, of course, be abolished by atropine. Sympathetic innervation via the cardio-accelerator fibres from five thoracic segments, increases the rhythmicity of the SA node (positive chronotropic action) and enhances the force and rate of ventricular contraction. This sympathetic supply plays little part in the control of the heart rate at rest.

### Innervation of the Blood Vessels

This is mainly via the sympathetic vasoconstrictor fibres from the thoracolumbar outflow and controls vascular tone in most vessels, excluding the coronary and cerebral circulations (see Fig. 1). Innervation to the arterioles, the capillary sphincters and post-capillary venules provides adjustment of resistance vessel calibre, whilst efferents to larger veins increase capacitance tone Table 1).

Vasodilatation occurs either from a reduction in sympathetic tone, for example with carotid sinus compression, or from the activation of vasodilator receptors, such as the beta adrenergic and cholinergic receptors in skeletal muscle.

Autoregulating processes independent of neuronal influences play a more important part in the control of certain vascular beds, for example, the coronary and cerebral vasculature. These are discussed elsewhere.

The autonomic nerves are the final pathway for a number of reflexes that control arterial pressure. The medullary centres, from which they arise, are subject to influences from:

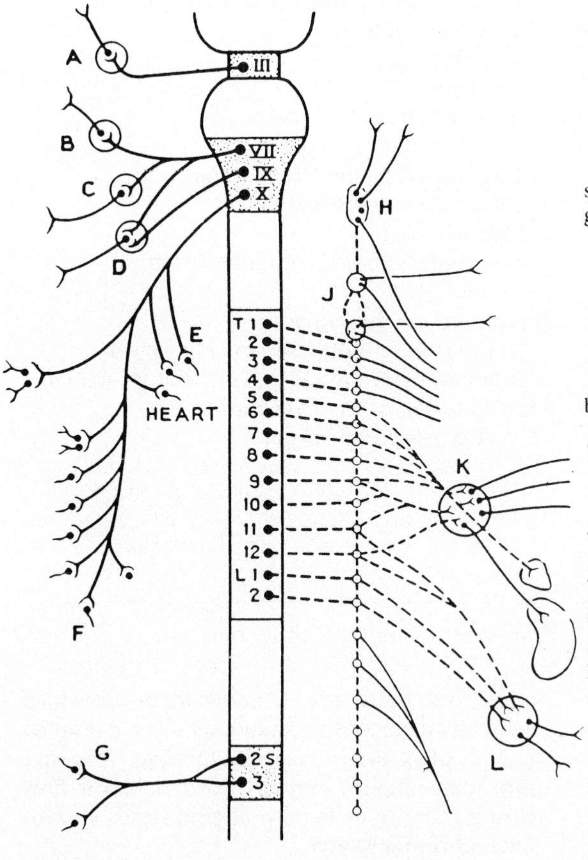


12/Fig. 1.—The Autonomic Nervous System

*On left*: Cranial and sacral autonomic (parasympathetic) system. Thick lines from III, VII, IX, X, and S2, 3 are preganglionic (connector fibres).

A—ciliary ganglion.
B—sphenopalatine ganglion.
C—submaxillary and sublingual ganglia.
D—otic ganglion.
E—vagus excitor cells in nodes of heart.
F—vagus excitor cells in wall of bowel.
G—sacral autonomic ganglion cells in pelvis. Thin lines beyond—post-ganglionic (excitor) fibres to organs.

*On right*: Sympathetic nervous system. Dotted lines from T 1–12, L 1, 2 are preganglionic fibres.

H—superior cervical ganglion.
J—inferior cervical and 1st thoracic ganglia (stellate ganglion).
k—coeliac and other abdominal ganglia (note preganglionic fibres directly supplying the adrenal medulla).
L—lower abdominal and pelvic sympathetic ganglia. Continuous lines beyond—post-ganglionic fibres.

(Courtesy of Samson Wright from *Applied Physiology*, published by Oxford Medical Publications.)

12/Table 1
Cardiovascular Responses to Autonomic Stimuli

| *Organ* | *Adrenergic Response* | *Cholinergic Response* |
|---|---|---|
| **Heart** | | |
| SA node | $\beta_1$ adrenergic increases rate | rate decrease or sinus arrest (vagus) |
| Atria | $\beta_1$ adrenergic increases contractility and conduction velocity | decrease in contractility (vagus) |
| A-V node | $\beta_1$ adrenergic increases automaticity and conduction velocity | AV block (vagus) |
| His Purkinje | $\beta_1$ adrenergic increases automaticity and conduction velocity | — |
| Ventricles | $\beta_1$ adrenergic: increases contractility, increases conduction velocity, increases automaticity, increases idioventricular pacemaker discharge. | — |
| **Blood Vessels** | | |
| Coronary | $\alpha$ adrenergic constricts<br>$\beta_2$ adrenergic dilates<br>(autoregulation predominates) | — |
| Skin | $\alpha$ adrenergic constricts | — |
| Skeletal muscle | $\alpha$ adrenergic constricts<br>$\beta_2$ adrenergic dilates | sympathetic cholinergic fibres dilate |
| Cerebral | $\alpha$ adrenergic may constrict<br>dopaminergic dilates<br>(autoregulation predominates) | — |
| Pulmonary | $\alpha$ adrenergic constricts<br>(autoregulation predominates) | —<br>infused acetylcholine dilates |
| Splanchnic and renal | $\alpha$ adrenergic constricts<br>dopaminergic dilates<br>$\beta_2$ adrenergic dilates | — |
| Systemic veins | $\alpha$ adrenergic constricts<br>$\beta_2$ adrenergic dilates | — |

(After Goodman and Gilman, 1980[1])

(*a*) *Higher centres.*

(*b*) *Vascular stretch receptors.*—Baroreceptors in the carotid sinus and aortic arch send afferents to the medulla and control vasomotor discharge in a negative feedback response to a raised arterial pressure. Other stretch receptors exist in the vena caval/right-atrium junction, and in the pulmonary artery trunk.

(*c*) *Chemoreflexes.* — Vasoconstriction is induced following carotid and aortic body stimulation caused by hypoxaemia or hypercarbia.

(*d*) *Skeletal muscle.*—Contraction of even small muscle groups produces an almost instantaneous rise in cardiac output and blood pressure.

These reflexes are often obtunded during anaesthesia and limit the capability of the circulation to adapt in response to hypovolaemia, posture or intermittent positive-pressure ventilation.

### The Anatomy of the Coronary Vasculature

The heart is supplied with blood by two coronary arteries which arise from the root of the aorta immediately above the aortic valve (Fig. 2). Their detailed anatomy is variable, but the left coronary artery always gives rise to the left anterior descending branch which supplies the anterior wall of the left ventricle and a major portion of the interventricular septum. The continuation of the left coronary, now called the circumflex, is more variable but usually supplies the lateral part of the left ventricle. In ten per cent of the population the left coronary is dominant and the circumflex supplies the inferior and posterior parts of the left ventricle, but in 90 per cent of the population this territory, including the atrioventricular

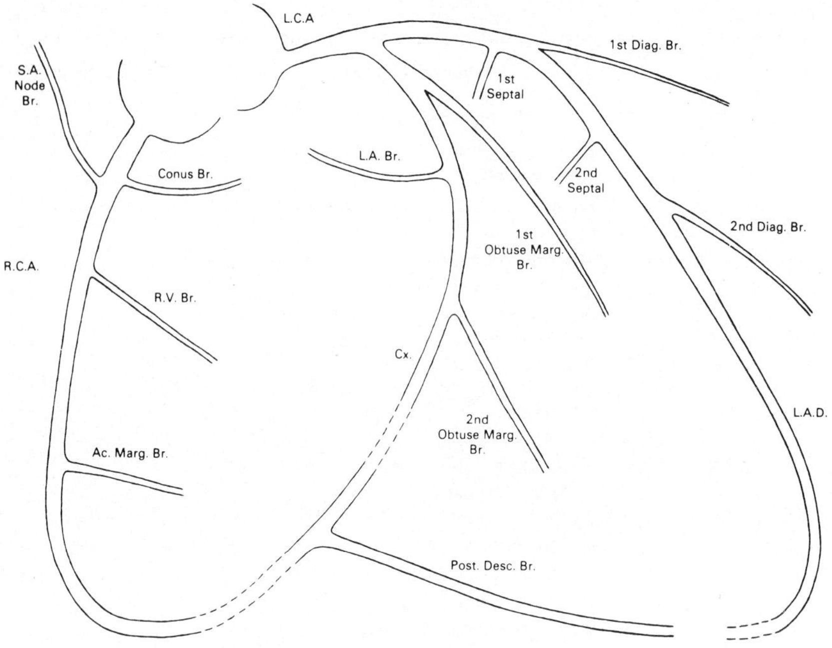


12/FIG. 2.—THE CORONARY ARTERIES.
This is a diagram used in reporting the results of coronary angiography.
*RCA*—The right coronary artery continues as the posterior descending artery anastomosing in a variable fashion with vessels from the left. *LCA*—The left coronary artery divides into two major vessels, the circumflex (Cx) and left anterior descending (LAD) artery. *S.A. Node Br.*—Sino-atrial node branch. *Diag. Br.*—Diagonal branch. *L.A. Br.*—Left atrial branch. *Obtuse Marg. Br.*—Obtuse marginal branch. *R.V. Br.*—Right ventricular branch. *Ac. Marg. Br.*—Acute marginal branch. *Post. Desc. Br.*—Posterior descending branch.

node, is supplied by the right coronary, another smaller branch of the right supplying the right ventricle.

The main venous return from the heart muscle is via the coronary sinus which drains to the right atrium. Some myocardial drainage does occur directly into the ventricles and that direct to the left ventricle accounts for part of the right-to-left shunt which exists normally.

### The Conducting System of the Heart

The specialised conducting tissues of the heart are of importance to the anaesthetist in relation to dysrhythmias and disorders of conduction which may be apparent in patients prior to anaesthesia, or which may arise during anaesthesia (Fig. 3). The particular tissues are the sino-atrial node – the atrial pacemaker, specialised conducting pathways in the atrium, the atrioventricular node, bundle of His—which divides into right and left bundles, and the anterior and posterior subdivisions of the left bundle. The ultimate ramification of this specialised conducting tissue are the fibres of Purkinje. The time taken for an impulse to traverse this pathway is seen on the ECG as the P-R interval which, in adults, varies between 0·12 to 0·20 seconds. (Electrocardiography is discussed later in this chapter.)

## CARDIAC OUTPUT

### THE MEASUREMENT OF CARDIAC OUTPUT

In the experimental animal and during human cardiac surgery it is possible to measure cardiac output by electromagnetic flow probes placed around the aorta. Under most other circumstances cardiac output is determined either by the direct Fick method or by indicator dilution. Non-invasive methods have become less inaccurate and therefore more popular.

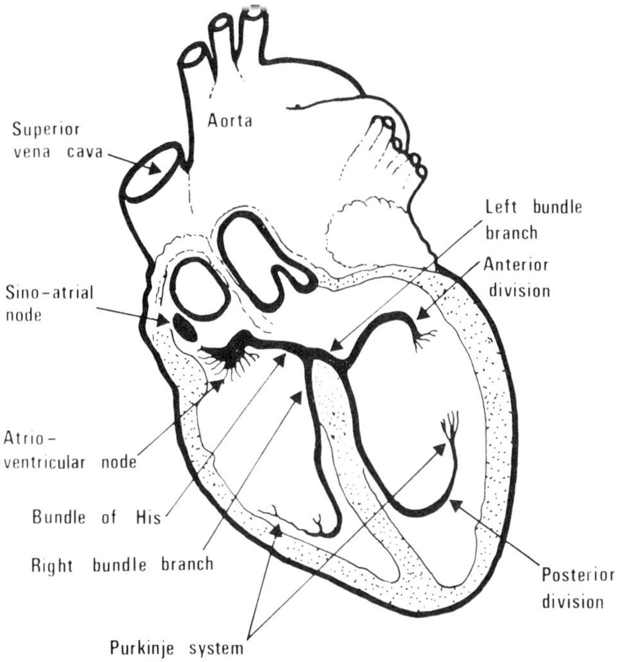


12/FIG. 3.—The conducting system of the heart. (Adapted from *Principles of Clinical Electrocardiography* by Mervyn J. Goldman, published by Lange Medical Publications.)

(a) **The direct Fick method** is the most accurate method and remains the standard by which other methods are judged. The information required is the oxygen uptake from the lungs in unit time and the oxygen content of arterial and mixed venous blood. The technique implies right heart catheterisation to obtain mixed venous blood from the pulmonary artery and requires considerable skill with the van Slyke apparatus for the measurement of oxygen content in blood. The relationship of flow to oxygen consumption is then given by the equation:

$$Q = \frac{O_2 \text{ consumption}}{(A\text{-}V)O_2 \text{ content difference}}$$

The technical difficulties of the Fick method have resulted in a general acceptance of less accurate but easier methods of which the commonest are the indicator dye and thermal dilution methods. Both involve a bolus injection of indicator proximal to the heart and the measurement of a concentration-time curve distal to the heart which is assumed to be a uniform mixing chamber.

(b) **Indocyanine green** has superseded other dyes. It has the advantage that the concentration is measured by spectrophotometry in the infrared region at 805 Å (80·5 nm) at which wave length both oxygenated and reduced haemoglobin have identical optical densities. The value is therefore unaffected by changes in the haemoglobin saturation. Originally, the concentration of dye in arterial blood was measured by the withdrawal of arterial blood through a cuvette densitometer (Fig. 4). More recently, an end-catheter densitometer has been evolved which enables the concentration curve to be determined at different sites within the vascular system. If a non-invasive technique is required, an earlobe densitometer is available which is sufficiently accurate for comparative determinations in the same patient.

(c) **The thermodilution** technique uses cold saline or dextrose and its negative heat (relative to body temperature) as the indicator. The advantages of thermodilution as a method are that the problems of recirculation on the concentration-line curve are insignificant and that the harmless indicator is speedily excreted making frequent estimations possible. The accuracy of the method is greatest when the injection is made just proximal to the right atrium and the change of temperature monitored by a thermistor in the pulmonary artery. The transit time is thus kept to a minimum and extravascular heat loss diminished.

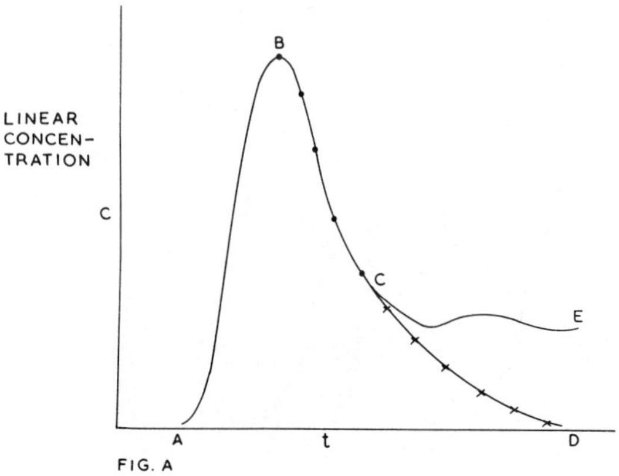


12/FIG. 4(*a*).—Curve A B C E is that produced by the output of a cuvette densitometer.

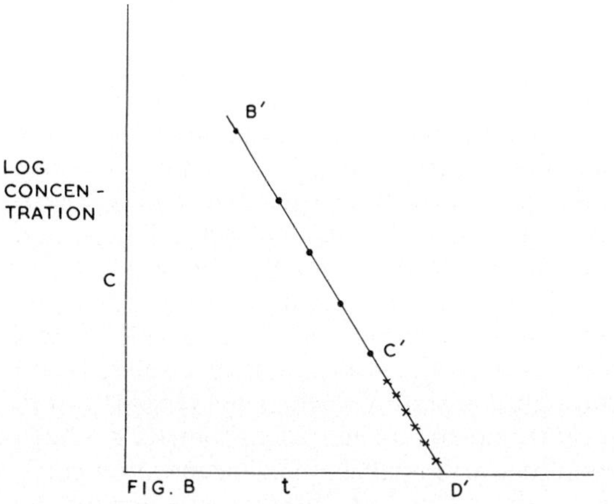


12/FIG. 4(*b*).—This is the downslope portion of the curve in Fig. 4(*a*) redrawn on semi-logarithmic paper.

The concentration of dye (C) in Fig. 4(*a*) does not fall to zero after one passage through the body due to the effect of recirculation of the dye. The effect of recirculation is ignored by re-plotting the downslope portion of the curve (BC) on a semi-logarithmic scale (B′C′). Since the downslope is an exponential decay, B′C′ will be linear and may be extrapolated to D′. Points along the line CD on the original curve may thus be obtained by reference to the semi-logarithmic plot. Thus the area beneath the curve A B C D may be obtained, free of the effects of recirculated dye. In practice, this calculation is normally integrated electronically, producing an instantaneous readout, although the actual curve is always inspected for artefact or other variation which the computer would be unable to recognise as making the curve unsuitable for cardiac output calculation.

The thermistor is commonly combined in a catheter which can be flow-directed into the pulmonary artery and which can be used to measure pulmonary artery or wedge pulmonary-capillary pressures at the same time as the cardiac output is determined.

### THE DETERMINANTS OF CARDIAC OUTPUT

The cardiac output is a function of heart rate and stroke volume (the output per beat). The stroke volume is itself influenced by three variables, the preload, the myocardial contractility and the afterload.

#### (*a*) **Heart Rate and Rhythm**

When in sinus rhythm the cardiac rate is determined by the rhythmicity of the sino-atrial node. Other sites in the heart also exhibit this rhythmicity but under normal circumstances the sino-atrial node has the fastest rate and the quickest transmission route enabling it to override the other slower sites. In the sinus node there is a steady continuous decay of resting-membrane potential resulting from an increase of cell membrane conductivity for potassium and an influx of sodium. This phase IV depolarisation (Fig. 5) continues until the potential has declined from −80 mV to a threshold at around −40 mV, when a rapid spontaneous depolarisation spike occurs. This intrinsic rhythmicity is enhanced by factors such as

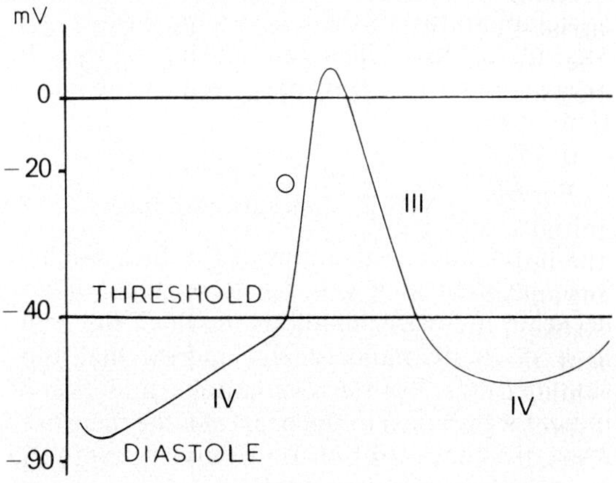


12/FIG. 5.—The action current of a pacemaker fibre recorded by an intracellular electrode. (Adapted from figure in *British Journal of Hospital Medicine* by Dr. Peter Stock.)

increased stretch, pyrexia and hyperthyroidism but is depressed by cold, hypothyroidism and by ischaemia. The sinus node is strongly influenced by nervous impulses. The rate of the denervated sinus is about 120/min and most variation in pulse rate below this level, that is most normal rate control, is the result of variations in the dominant parasympathetic influence. In heart failure, the adrenergic control is more important, and during exercise, the increased sympathetic activity is responsible both for an increase in cardiac rate and in myocardial contractility.

Despite the fact that the cardiac output is the resultant of cardiac rate and stroke volume, these latter two variables do not necessarily vary inversely to maintain a given cardiac output constant. While many physiological and drug effects are able to produce increases in both factors, the normal heart itself has a mechanism to maintain stroke volume in the face of moderate increases in rate. At the same time, the importance of cardiac rate is seen in the decline of cardiac output at very slow heart rates and in the inability of patients with complete heart block with a fixed heart to increase their cardiac output appropriately on demand.

Although cardiac rhythm is commonly considered with rate since abnormal rhythms frequently result in abnormal rates, it is equally important in the consideration of ventricular preload. Firstly, because of the contribution which atrial contraction makes to ventricular filling (atrial transport mechanism) and secondly, because in abnormal rhythms the atrial pressure may no longer accurately reflect the ventricular end-diastolic pressure (see below).

(*b*) **Preload**

Force of contraction is proportional to the initial (end-diastolic) fibre length—the greater the initial fibre length, the greater the shortening and therefore the output. In clinical practice, stroke-work or stroke-output is a more convenient measurement than force of contraction, while initial fibre length is more simply expressed as proportional to diastolic volume. This, in turn, is more conveniently expressed as a function of end-diastolic pressure. The relationship between end-diastolic volume and end-diastolic pressure is an expression of ventricular compliance. When making assumptions about stroke output or stroke work in relation to end-diastolic pressure, the ventricular compliance has to be taken into account for three main reasons. Firstly, the relationship between ventricular volume and ventricular diastolic pressure is very alinear. Secondly, chronic change in compliance occurs in ventricular hypertrophy, in aortic stenosis or hypertension and, finally, acute change in compliance occurs in myocardial infarction and after extracorporeal circulation. Thus, in some circumstances, a falling end-diastolic ventricular pressure may represent an altering compliance rather than an increasing myocardial contractility. However, under most circumstances end-diastolic pressure changes accurately reflect changes in initial fibre length. Provided the atrioventricular valve is open and unobstructed, the diastolic pressures in the atrium and ventricle are the same and in most clinical situations the mean atrial pressure is a sufficiently accurate reflection of ventricular preload. This relationship is true for both sides of the heart and the cardiac output can normally be increased by raising the preload usually by transfusion. The limits to which preload can be increased, are determined on the right side of the heart, by dilatation of the right ventricle with development of tricuspid incompetence and, on the left side of the heart, by increases in pulmonary blood volume leading to a progressive decrease in lung compliance and the eventual development of pulmonary oedema. Furthermore, over-distension of either ventricle compromises contractility and myocardial oxygenation so that ventricular function may actually worsen.

**The determinants of ventricular preload.**—If it is accepted that mean atrial pressure is a good reflection of ventricular preload, the factors which determine its value are:

1. Blood volume
2. Venous tone
3. Ventricular compliance
4. Myocardial contractility
5. Ventricular afterload.

If the other factors are kept constant the atrial pressure will reflect the ability of the ventricle to contract, thus when the heart develops left ventricular failure, the left atrial pressure rises and when the right ventricle fails the right atrial pressure rises. Interpretation of a venous pressure value must, therefore, include some consideration of the state of the myocardium.

The preload is also affected by acute changes in afterload. The right atrial pressure is commonly raised in pulmonary embolism and the left atrial pressure raised in the hypertension caused by the administration of a pure vasoconstrictor such as phenylephrine, both examples representing increased afterload on the respective ventricle. When the acute load is relieved, the atrial pressure necessary for the ventricle to produce a normal cardiac output falls.

During anaesthesia and surgery the venous pressure may vary following changes in ventricular compliance or myocardial contractility according to the action of anaesthetic agents, vasoactive drugs and alterations in physiological variables (see below). The effect of endogenous catecholamine secretion is complex as not only may it raise the afterload but it will also affect cardiac rate, myocardial contractility and venous tone.

However, the commonest causes of variation in ventricular preload during anaesthesia and surgery are alterations either in blood volume or venous tone which may be accentuated by alterations in posture.

Blood volume may be depleted either by haemorrhage or by fluid loss due to fluid restriction, diuresis, sweating, gastro-intestinal losses or losses from raw surfaces. The commonest cause of increased blood volume is undoubtedly over-enthusiastic fluid replacement particularly when not accurately monitored and when given to a vasodilated patient. When the anaesthetic-induced vasodilatation wears off, or if it is replaced by postoperative vasoconstriction induced by pain, acidosis or hypothermia, then the relative blood volume may be much too great and the atrial pressure rise excessively.

### The Venous System

The large capacity venous reservoir contains approximately 70 per cent of the total blood volume and the greater proportion of this is accommodated in the splanchnic bed. The compliance of this system is determined by venomotor tone which, like arterial tone, is controlled by autonomic impulses from the vasomotor centre in the floor of the fourth ventricle. The effect of sympathetic stimulation is to increase the venous tone which increases atrial pressures and consequently ventricular preload. Under normal circumstances, variations in venous tone will cope with the effect of altered posture and increases in venous tone will maintain ventricular filling pressure when blood volume falls due to haemorrhage. This compensatory ability may be affected by disease or by drugs. In certain conditions which affect the nervous system (diabetes, peripheral neuritis) the vasomotor outflow is inactive and the patient suffers from postural hypotension due to venous pooling in the unconstricted veins in the upright condition. Autonomic neuropathy often results in a failure to increase the venous tone during positive-pressure ventilation so that both effective filling pressure and thus the cardiac output falls. A similar effect can occur during anaesthesia, following barbiturate overdose, after ganglionic blockade and with the administration of opiates, sodium nitroprusside and glyceryl trinitrate, all of which produce impaired vasomotor activity, either by interrupting the nervous pathway or by direct action on the the vessels themselves and which, therefore, impair the ability of the patient to compensate either for alterations in posture or reversal of intrathoracic pressures. The integrity of the circulatory reflex may be tested by the Valsalva manoeuvre (see Figs. 6–7). In patients with blocked cardiovascular reflexes the Valsalva produces a progressive fall in blood pressure with a slow recovery and no overshoot when the expiratory pressure is withdrawn. In low cardiac output states, the sympathetic activity is increased and the venous tone high, hence paralysis of the vasomotor response by anaesthesia in such patients produces dramatic falls in blood pressure and cardiac output.

The ability of changes in venous tone to compensate for changes in blood volume, and body posture, may be inadequate if the alterations are excessive. The effective ventricular preload will also be affected by factors affecting venous flow, such as venous compression by skeletal muscle, intrapleural and intrapericardial pressure and the atrial contribution to ventricular filling.

### The Relationship Between Left- and Right-Sided Filling Pressures

The filling pressure of each ventricle depends on the venous pressure (blood volume/venous

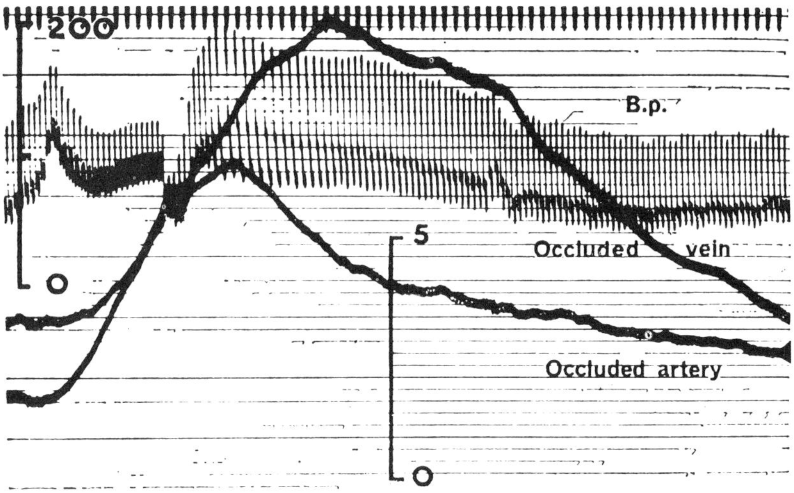


12/Fig. 6.—Effect of Valsalva Manoeuvre on Arterial and Venous Pressure.

Upper margin: time-scale (sec).

Upper record (Bp) is that of the arterial pressure in the left brachial artery and shows the usual changes with the Valsalva manoeuvre in a subject with a normal circulation.

The two curves are the right brachial artery pressure (occluded artery) and the right antecubital venous pressure (occluded vein). The limb has been cut off from the rest of the circulation by a high-pressure cuff on the upper arm, so that only nervous impulses can influence the vessels. The blood is stationary in the limb. After seven seconds of the Valsalva manoeuvre, reflex arterial and venous constriction is shown by the rise of pressure in both sets of vessels. Reflex dilatation occurs after the overshoot.

Calibrations in mm Hg. (Courtesy of the Editor of the *British Medical Bulletin*)

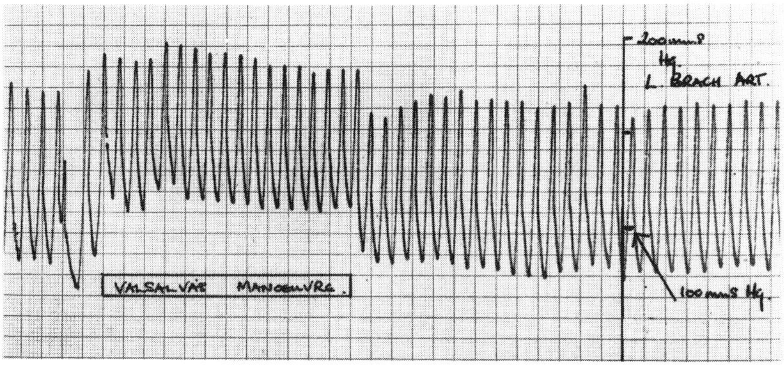


12/Fig. 7(*a*).—Square wave response to the Valsalva manoeuvre in a patient with left ventricular failure.

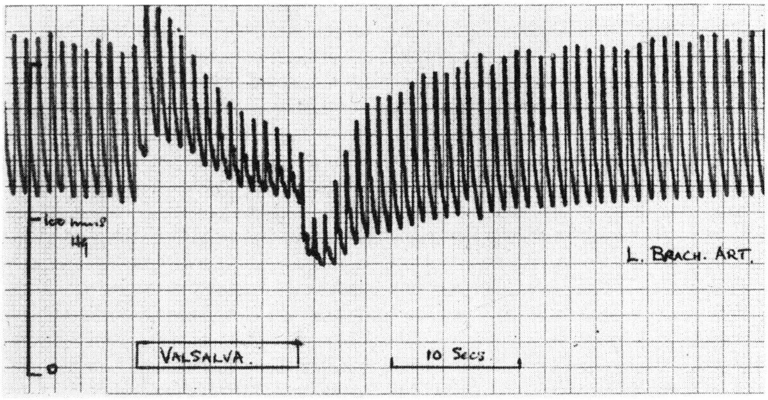


12/Fig. 7(*b*).—Effect of Valsalva manoeuvre in a patient with blocked circulatory reflexes.

tone), the ventricular compliance, the myocardial contractility and the afterload. The left ventricle is less compliant with a greater afterload than the right ventricle and the left-sided filling pressure is normally higher than the right. If the right-sided filling pressure is raised by transfusion the increase in pressure is greater on the left than on the right. Under all normal circumstances the right side of the heart and the lungs are merely passive conduits for the blood and it is possible to discern a relationship between right-sided filling pressure (central venous pressure) and left-sided cardiac output. This is the common clinical situation in which the circulation is manipulated by transfusion according to measurements of central venous pressure and if the left atrial pressure is measured it would alter passively, reflecting left ventricular compliance, contractility and afterload.

In Fig. 8 at a right-sided filling pressure of 0 mm Hg the right ventricle has a stroke output of 70 ml/beat while the left ventricle has the same stroke output from an initial filling pressure of 7 mm Hg (0·9 kPa). If the patient is transfused to raise the right ventricular filling pressure to 4 mm Hg (0·5 kPa) the stroke output rises to 90 ml/beat. There is a transient disequilibrium with the right ventricular output higher than the left, resulting in an increase in central blood volume. The left ventricular output rises until a new equilibrium is reached with left and right ventricular outputs the same, but now the left ventricular end-diastolic pressure is 16 mm Hg (2·1 kPa) and the pulmonary blood volume is higher than it was. As the left atrial pressure rises there is a progressive increase in lung stiffness, a progressive diminution in arterial oxygen tensions due to the development of interstitial oedema and ultimately pulmonary oedema. The disadvantage of manipulating the circulation according to measurements of the central venous pressure is that it pre-supposes knowledge of the relationship between left and right ventricular compliance, contractility and afterload. In health it may be possible to make reasonable assumptions about these relationships and it is probably true that any patient whose central venous pressure is less than 5 cm $H_2O$ (0·5 kPa) relative to the sternal angle is not overfilled. However, in disease, no such assumptions can be made and under the conditions of anaesthesia and surgery, when the circulatory function may be modified by anaesthetic and other drugs and by the effects of blood/gas, electrolyte and auto-

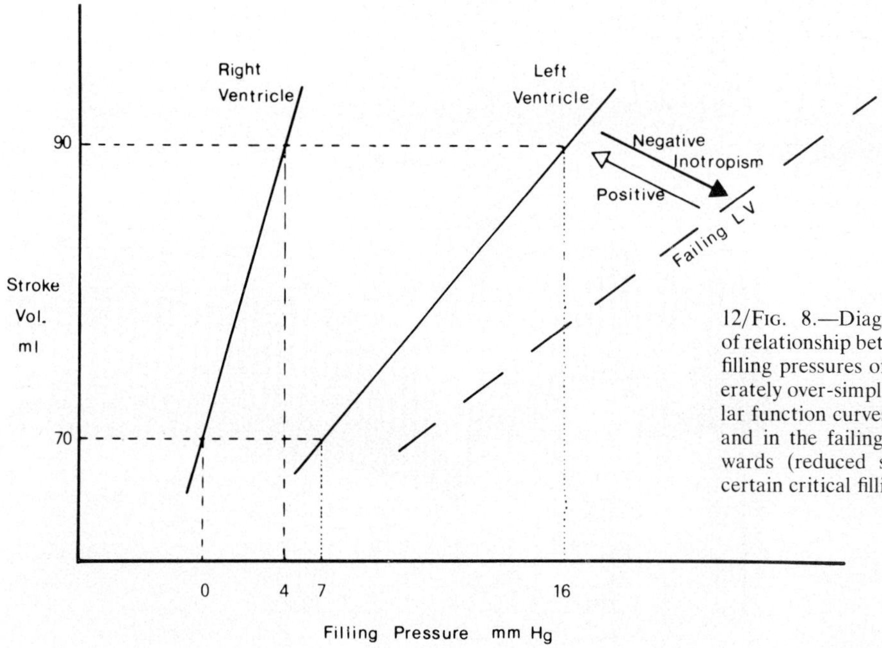


12/Fig. 8.—Diagrammatic representation of relationship between left- and right-sided filling pressures of the heart. This is deliberately over-simplified for clarity. Ventricular function curves in reality are not linear, and in the failing heart may curve downwards (reduced stroke volume) above a certain critical filling pressure.

nomic nervous system disturbances, conclusions about the left heart based on measurements of the central venous pressure may well be invalid. In this case it is much safer to manipulate the circulation according to the filling pressure of the left side of the heart. This may be estimated using the pulmonary capillary wedge pressure, measured with a flow-directed pulmonary artery catheter, although a directly measured LA pressure may be available following cardiac surgery.

### (*c*) Myocardial Contractility

Contractility refers to the intrinsic muscle fibre shortening property of the myocardium. The simplest approach is to consider that an increase in cardiac output with an unchanged filling pressure represents increased contractility, but this takes no account of the effect of afterload which must also remain constant. Because afterload is itself related to ventricular function (see below) this is a difficult concept to apply in practice and among the many efforts made to quantitate contractility an important approach is to consider the ventricle only during its isovolaemic phase before the aortic valve opens and the fibres start to shorten. The experimental approach to problems of myocardial contractility, as far as possible, is to reduce each experiment to only two variables by maintaining a constant cardiac rate by electrical pacing and constant pre- and after-load by reservoir adjustment. Even then, correlation between the various indices of contractility is poor. In the non-experimental situation of clinical anaesthesia the simpler concept of the slope of the curve defining the relationship between stroke work and ventricular filling pressure usually suffices as an index of cardiac performance, as it represents the integrated response of the heart in its role of the central component of the intact circulation. A steep slope (i.e. moved up and to the left) implies good myocardial performance, a flatter curve (i.e. moved downwards and to the right) a worse ventricle, but there is no doubt that this seriously understates the complexity of the relationship between contractility and cardiac output.

### (*d*) Afterload

After the isovolaemic phase is over and the aortic valve opens, the left ventricle is interacting with the peripheral circulation which now becomes an important determinant of the rate of rise of aortic pressure, the size, duration and velocity of ejection and the shape and volume of the ventricles during systole. Thus, afterload is a function both of the impedance to blood flow, that is the compliance of the aorta and the arteriolar run off, and the ventricular wall tension. Tension is dependent not only on the intracavity pressure but on mean ventricular radius (see Myocardial oxygen consumption, p. 417). This of course means that afterload changes as the heart contracts and the ventricle changes size. In heart failure, when the heart is dilated, ventricular wall tensions (and afterload and oxygen consumption) increase above normal. Hypertrophy of the ventricle, however, reduces the stress on each unit of the myocardium and tends to maintain the afterload of each myocardial cell close to normal.

After the administration of a vasodilator, and provided that the ventricular filling pressures are maintained, the cardiac output often rises as the afterload decreases. This ability to increase cardiac output secondary to a reduction in afterload does not depend on a normal heart but can also be observed in patients with aortic or mitral incompetence and in the failing heart when this effect forms the rationale for vasodilator therapy.

Afterload, by being both a determinant and a consequence of stroke volume, plays an important role in circulatory equilibrium. The normal heart continually adjusts its contractile state to compensate for changes in afterload (Anrep effect).

### (*e*) The Arterial System and Blood Pressure

The arterial system, which contains 15 per cent of the blood volume, is the distributive and resistive element of the circulation. The interaction between this resistive element and the cardiac output results in the development of the blood pressure whose function is to ensure a forward flow of blood to all parts of the body and to provide a general pressure background against which local alterations in resistance can affect the distribution of flow.

During exercise, blood pressure may change very little although cardiac output increases enormously implying a large drop in systemic vascular resistance and hence in afterload. Most of this occurs in the vessels supplying the exercising muscle and if the rise in cardiac output is inadequate to supply the demand for flow in the muscle then resistance rises in those areas, such as the mesenteric bed, which are uninvolved in the exercise.

### Control Mechanism of the Arterial Bed

The control of individual arteriolar resistance is both by intrinsic and extrinsic mechanisms. The intrinsic mechanism is the inherent myotonic activity of the smooth muscle in the precapillary resistance vessels which accounts for most of the basal vascular tone. This activity is modified by the dilator influences of hypoxia and metabolites and by the constrictor effect of the distending blood pressure within the lumen. If extrinsic factors are abolished the intrinsic factors tend to maintain appropriate tissue flow despite wide perfusion pressure changes. The extrinsic factors are neural and humoral, of which the latter is less important. The innervation is predominantly sympathetic but, depending on the the tissue, may be vasoconstrictor or vasodilator. The contribution which the constrictor fibres make to basal vascular tone is minimal provided the heart is normal. The main function of the neural extrinsic mechanism is to provide speedy or even anticipatory response to an instantaneous demand for increased blood flow as part of the general neural control of the circulation.

### Determinants of Blood Pressure

When blood is ejected into the aorta the systolic pressure depends partly on the stroke volume and partly on the impedance. Impedance is defined as the ratio of the instantaneous rate of change of aortic pressure to the instantaneous aortic flow. It depends on the compliance of the aorta and large arteries and the rate of run off from the arterial bed during systole. This explains the systolic hypertension of slow heart rates (large ejection volume), of senile atherosclerosis (decreased aortic and large vessel compliance), and of essential hypertension (decreased run off). While resistance is mainly a function of arteriolar radius which may be altered structurally or by variations in vascular tone, it is also influenced by blood viscosity which may alter during anaesthesia and surgery. The same factors affect diastolic pressure but not to an identical degree so that the two pressures normally vary independently of each other with diastolic pressure being mainly influenced by the rate of peripheral arteriolar runoff.

## The Coronary Blood Flow and Myocardial Oxygen Consumption

Under most circumstances, coronary autoregulation adjusts the coronary blood flow according to myocardial oxygen demand. Autoregulation, however, only occurs at arterial pressures between 70 and 160 mm Hg (9·3–21·3 kPa) and at pressures less than this the flow may be inadequate, while at higher pressures, the oxygen consumption rises disproportionately. The flow may be locally or generally insufficient, even within the normal pressure range in the presence of coronary artery disease or if the ventricular wall tension is high.

Both $\alpha$ and $\beta$-receptor sites exist in the coronary arterial tree. However, the systemic administration of vasoactive drugs affects coronary blood flow mainly by their indirect effects on myocardial oxygen consumption, subsequent to changes in arterial pressure and ventricular work. The coronary arteries are sensitive to changes in carbon dioxide tension, and hypocapnia may reduce coronary blood flow below a critical level especially in ischaemic heart disease.

### The Measurement of Coronary Blood Flow

Accurate measurement of the CBF is difficult and requires coronary sinus cannulation. The classic method is that of Katz using nitrous oxide uptake but more recently thermodilution has been used. These methods give a coronary blood flow of approximately 250 ml/minute and an oxygen consumption of 25 ml oxygen/minute. Thus the myocardial blood flow is approximately 5 per cent of the cardiac output whereas the myocardial oxygen consumption is about 10 per cent of the minute oxygen uptake. This implies a high oxygen extraction by the heart and coronary sinus blood is more desaturated than other venous blood.

### The Determinants of Myocardial Oxygen Supply and Consumption

(*a*) **Supply.**—Coronary blood flow occurs mainly during diastole when the ventricular muscle tone is low. The driving force, the coronary artery perfusion pressure, is the diastolic blood pressure minus the left ventricular end-diastolic pressure. In the subendocardial layer, the transmitted cavity pressure may directly compress the subendocardial capillaries. Thus a generalised reduction of diastolic pressure, occurring at the same time as a raised end-diastolic pressure in the ventricle, may result in myocardial ischaemia.

The duration of diastole is also a significant factor. While in healthy hearts, tachycardia is usually achieved predominantly by a shortening of systole with a smaller reduction in the duration of diastole, in a diseased heart with a reduced capacity for increase in contractility, tachycardia produces significant reduction in the duration of diastole and, hence, in the time available for myocardial blood flow. The integrated product of coronary perfusion pressure and time, known as the diastolic pressure-time index (DPTI), is a useful concept in considering myocardial oxygen supply. The other two factors of practical importance to the anaesthetist are the haemoglobin concentration and the carbon dioxide tension. The latter because of the vasoconstrictive response of the coronary arteries to hypocapnia and the former because of the high extraction rate of oxygen from the blood during its passage through the myocardium, bearing in mind that polycythaemia will reduce flow due to an increase in viscosity.

(*b*) **Consumption.**—There are three main factors which affect myocardial oxygen consumption:

1. *Left ventricular wall tension.*—Oxygen consumption is related to the wall tension; under Laplace's law the wall tension (T) is a function of the ventricular pressure (P) and the size of the chamber (radius = r) such that $T = \frac{Pr}{2}$.

The important implications of this are that tension and therefore oxygen consumption increase (i) as ventricular pressure increases, (ii) as the ventricle dilates (bigger radius), even if the pressure stays constant as in the failing heart.

The oxygen consumption will be related to the time during which the tension is excited, and the integrated product of wall tension and its duration (the tension-time index, TTI) is a close correlate of myocardial oxygen consumption. This is more commonly measured as the product of ventricular pressure and time, when it is more correctly referred to as the systolic pressure-time index (SPTI).

2. *Myocardial contractility.*—The disadvantage of the tension-time and systolic pressure time indices is that they fail to pick up major increases in myocardial oxygen consumption associated with increases in myocardial contractility. Increase in the rate of rise of ventricular pressure and hence in the acceleration of blood flow may have little effect on the size of the cardiac output but produce striking increase in myocardial oxygen consumption. $\beta$-adrenergic blocking drugs reduce myocardial contractility and, without necessarily affecting the cardiac output, decrease myocardial oxygen consumption except in the presence of cardiac failure with left ventricular dilatation.

3. *Heart rate.*—Increases in heart rate have a trebly deleterious effect on myocardial oxygen supply and demand. As increases in heart rate are accompanied by shortening of the diastolic period, particularly in the diseased heart, the proportion of time that the wall tension is high is increased, while, due to the diminution in time available for coronary perfusion, the diastolic pressure time index falls and there is thus a worsening of the relationship between SPTI and DPTI (the demand-supply ratio). In most instances, tachycardia is also associated with an increase in myocardial contractility, itself producing a rise in oxygen consumption.

In the production of blood flow to the tissues, cardiac work (and hence oxygen consumption) is much greater when a moderate cardiac output is produced at a high blood pressure than when a greater cardiac output is produced at a low pressure. A clinically useful, but very rough approximation, as an index of myocardial oxygen consumption is the product of systolic arterial pressure and cardiac rate (the rate pressure product) which, in a very simple index, combines the most significant factors both in myocardial oxygen supply and demand.

## ELECTROPHYSIOLOGY

### The Electrocardiogram

The electrocardiogram (ECG) is a graphic display of the electrical activity of the heart, in which the major deflections represent the depolarisation and repolarisation of atrial and ventricular muscle. The activity of the specialised conducting tissue is deduced from the timing and spatial orientation of the electrical activity

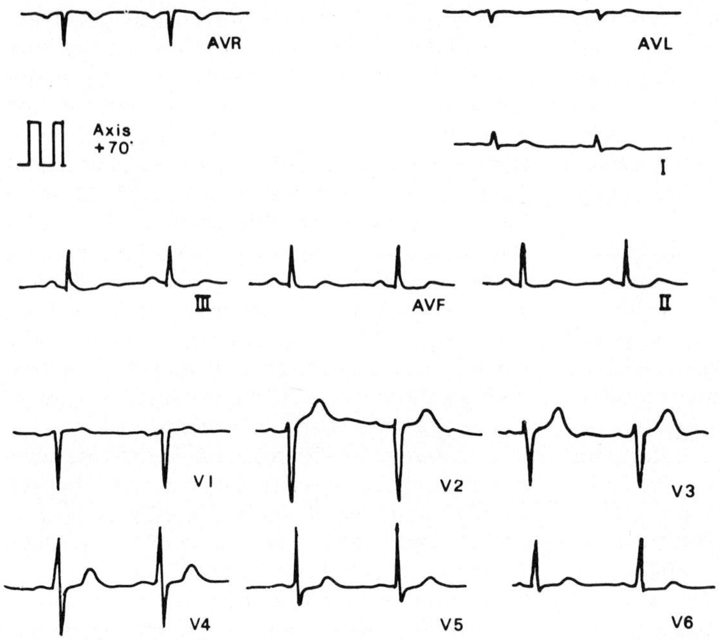


12/Fig. 9.—Normal standard 12-lead ECG.

but no such similar deduction can be made from the ECG about the ability of the heart to contract and to generate pressure.

The standard 12-lead ECG (Fig. 9) consists of three bipolar limb leads, three unipolar limb leads and six chest leads, positioned as in Fig. 10.

Standard limb lead II is normally chosen for continuous monitoring during anaesthesia when disorders of rhythm are thought the most likely complication. With the electrical axis parallel to the electrical axis of the heart, the P wave is clearly shown and the differentiation of ventricular and supraventricular dysrhythmias is facilitated.

Evidence of anterior or lateral wall ischaemia, however, is more apparent in those leads which lie in the horizontal plane. Chest lead $V_5$ is the better lead in the continuous monitoring of those patients thought to be at risk of cardiac ischaemia when ST segment changes will appear but, at the same time, will enable good representation of atrial activity.

In systems with only three electrodes, the $V_5$ electrode can be obtained by placing the left arm electrode on the $V_5$ position and selecting lead AVL.[2] With simpler three-lead cables and no switching selector, a similar result can be obtained if the three leads are arranged around the heart in the coronal plane.

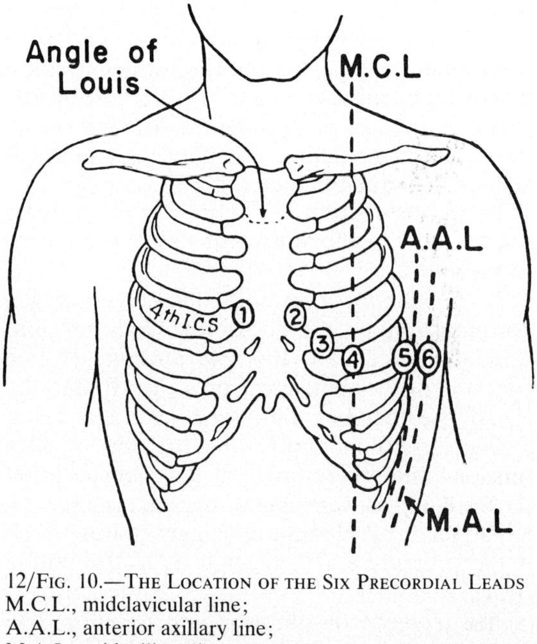


12/Fig. 10.—The Location of the Six Precordial Leads
M.C.L., midclavicular line;
A.A.L., anterior axillary line;
M.A.L., midaxillary line.
(Courtesy of E. Goldberger and the publishers Lea and Febiger and reproduced from *Unipolar Lead Electrocardiography and Vectorcardiography*.)

The normal electrocardiograph is recorded at a paper speed of 2·5 cm/sec and a sensitivity of 10 mm deflection = 1 mV. If the ECG is displayed on an oscilloscope the sweep speed and sensitivity should be adjusted to these values.

**The normal electrocardiogram.** — The impulse that initiates a normal heart beat arises from specialised tissue—the sino-atrial node—situated at the junction of the superior vena cava and right atrium (Fig. 3).

The time taken for this impulse to reach the ventricles is seen as the PR interval which, in adults, varies between 0·12 to 0·20 seconds (Fig. 11), but in children the time is shorter (0·10–0·18 seconds). To a small extent the value varies inversely with the heart rate.

The P wave is the resultant of the electrical current produced by atrial muscle depolarisation. Atrial hypertrophy increases the size of this wave and delays in its passage across the atrium will prolong it.

Sinus rhythm may be inferred from the finding of normal P waves (indicating the expected pattern of atrial muscle depolarisation) and their constant relationship with the QRS complexes. During sinus rhythm the cardiac rate will show minor variations in response to a variety of normal physiological stimuli and in particular may show a periodic variation with respiration. This sinus dysrhythmia results from the increase in vagal tone which accompanies inspiration producing cardiac slowing, the heart speeding up again during expiration.

The QRS complex represents the depolarisation of the ventricular muscle. In a normal heart the mean frontal QRS vector lies between −30° and +100° (Fig. 12) and the width of the complex is narrow (less than 0·09 second). Widening of the QRS occurs if the conduction velocity through the specialised pathways is slower than normal or if the pathway is abnor-

12/TABLE 2

SHOWING POSITION OF BIPOLAR AND UNIPOLAR LIMB LEADS

| | | | | |
|---|---|---|---|---|
| Lead | I | Right arm—left arm | aVR . | Right arm lead |
| | II | Right arm—left leg | aVL . | Left arm lead |
| | III | Left arm — left leg | aVF . | Left leg lead |
| | | Right leg lead—earth lead | | |

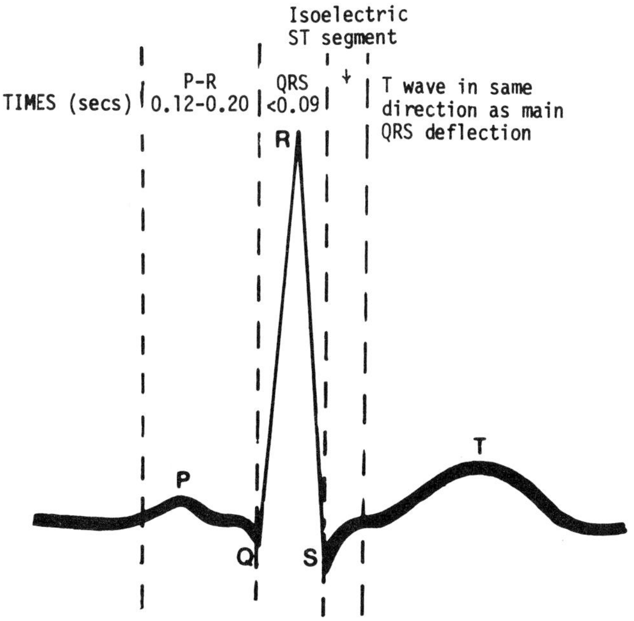


12/FIG. 11.—Normal lead II.

The normal ECG is defined by:

(1) P waves of normal size, direction and shape at an appropriate rate and each followed by a QRS complex.

(2) The PR interval less than 0·20 seconds (0·18 seconds in children).

(3) A QRS of less than 0·09 seconds and with a frontal axis between −30° and +100°.

(4) An isoelectric S-T segment.

(5) The T waves in the limb leads in the same direction as the corresponding QRS complex.

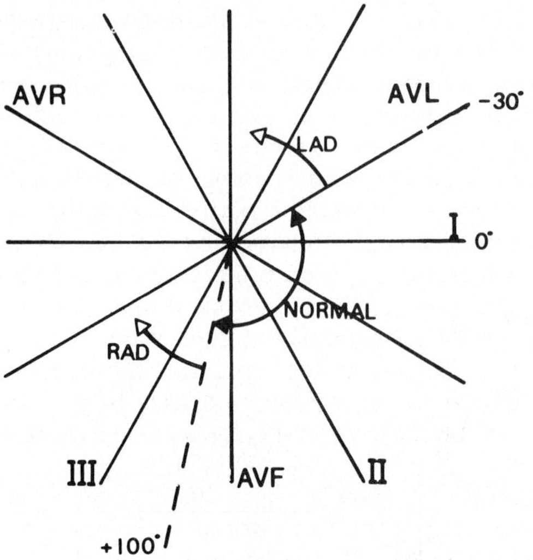


12/Fig. 12.—Frontal QRS vector diagram.

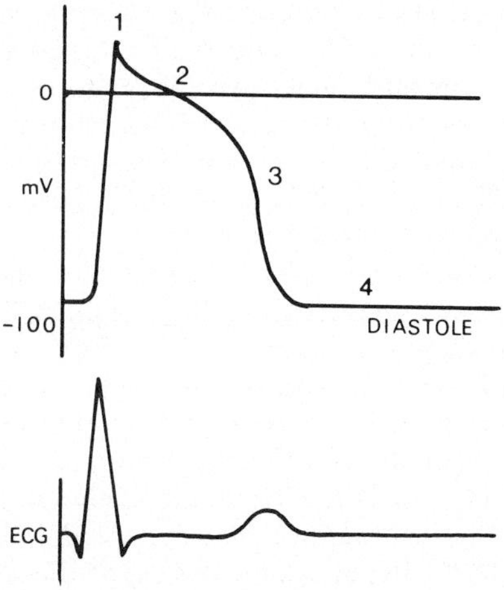


12/Fig. 13.—The action current of a ventricular muscle fibre recorded by an intracellular electrode and simultaneous external ECG.

mally long. The height of the QRS complex represents the net resultant of the electrical forces generated by the muscle in a number of different directions. When in a normal heart the muscle depolarises simultaneously in all areas, a considerable cancellation of electrical forces occurs and the QRS is relatively small. An increase in the size of the QRS occurs not only in the presence of ventricular hypertrophy but also when conduction is altered. Thus in right or left bundle-branch block, or in a ventricular ectopic beat, not only is the QRS prolonged but it is larger than usual.

The ST segment of the ECG is usually iso-electric. It corresponds to the plateau phase of the intracardiac action potential (Fig. 13). A shift in the ST segment reveals the presence of an abnormal current in the heart.

The T wave portrays the repolarisation (phase 3) of the ventricular muscle and is normally orientated in the same direction in the frontal plane as the preceding QRS complex. Abnormalities of repolarisation either flatten or invert this T wave.

The duration of depolarisation and repolarisation (Q-T interval) is directly related to cardiac rate—becoming shorter at faster rates provided the heart is normal.

(For discussion of the abnormal ECG see Chapter 13, p. 463 *et seq.*)

**Effect of Drugs upon the Electrocardiogram**

*Digitalis* principally produces alterations in the S-T segment and the T wave. With early digitalisation there is a depression of the S-T segment in all leads in the opposite direction to the main deflection of the QRS complex. As digtalis therapy proceeds, first the T wave becomes reduced in amplitude and then the S-T segment moves above or below the base line in the opposite direction to the QRS complex. The result is an ECG with a typical "sagging" effect (Fig. 14).

These changes can be observed within a few minutes of an intravenous dose of digoxin during anaesthesia. Over-digitalisation affects not only the rate and the rhythm of the heart by means of vagal stimulation and a direct depressant action on the conductive system, but it is capable of reproducing every known type of dysrhythmia and heart block. The effects of digitalis therapy may be observed in some cases 2–3 weeks after cessation of therapy and they are exaggerated in the presence of a low serum potassium (see Digoxin, p. 466).

*Quinidine* tends to depress the electrical activity of the heart. The P wave and the QRS are increased in duration. The S wave widens and the T wave is lowered and widened. In excessive dosage all types of cardiac irregularities may be observed.

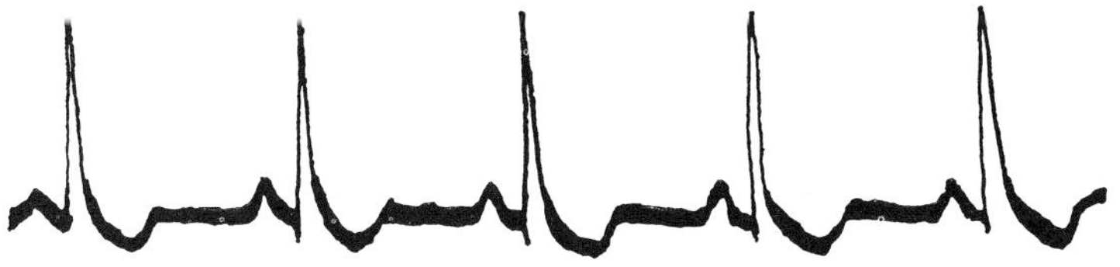

12/Fig. 14.—Effect of digitalis. Note that S-T segment is depressed and "sagging" is present. There is a low-voltage T wave. (Courtesy of M. Bernrieter and the publishers of *Electrocardiography*, J. B. Lippincott Co.)

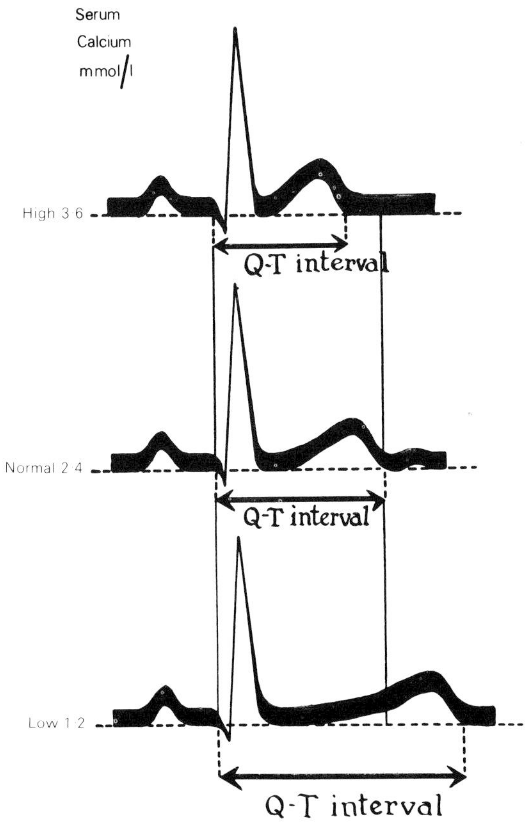


12/Fig. 15.—Effect of alteration in serum calcium level on ECG. (Adapted from *A Primer of Electrocardiography* by G. E. Burch and T. Winsor, published by Lea and Febiger.)

*Adrenergic drugs*, adrenaline, ephedrine, etc. lower the amplitude of T waves and may reverse their direction. Cholinergic drugs may have the same effect.

### The Effect of Electrolytes on the Electrocardiogram and Cardiovascular System

(*a*) **Calcium.**—The calcium ion influences the phase 2 component of the cardiac action potential, the effective refractory period, conduction velocity and excitability of ventricular muscle.[3] The normal total plasma calcium concentrations lie within the range 2·25–2·55 mmol/l, although total plasma concentration does not give a true indication of the ionised fraction. It is, of course, the ionised calcium that is responsible for its electrocardiographic and haemodynamic effects. Scheidegger and Drop[4] confirmed that the inverse relationship between serum calcium and the Q-T interval (hypercalcaemia shortened the QT interval) was due to the *ionised* moiety (Fig. 15). These workers also demonstrated that the haemodynamic effects of calcium were related to the pre-existing ionic concentration, so that an infusion of calcium during hypocalcaemia increased blood pressure, primarily due to an improvement in ventricular function, whilst increasing plasma calcium from normal, raised blood pressure by an effect on systemic vascular resistance. Low plasma calcium concentrations occur in hypoparathyroidism after prolonged vomiting and during cardiopulmonary bypass if calcium is not added to the priming fluid. Hypercalcaemia is seen in hyperparathyroidism but a more common cause is the administration of calcium salts during cardiopulmonary resuscitation.

Untoward effects of intravenous calcium administration include superficial vein thrombosis, ventricular dysrhythmias, especially in the presence of hypokalaemia, and an increase in fibrinolytic activity.[5]

Despite the theoretical differences in calcium ionisation of the various salts available for intravenous administration (chloride, gluconate or gluceptate), the increases in plasma ionised calcium concentration produced appear, for all practical purposes, to be similar if equimolar dosages of the different preparations are employed.[3,6]

(*b*) **Magnesium.**—Magnesium is of vital importance for the maintenance of myocardial structure and function, but its importance tends to have been overshadowed in the literature by the effects of other ions, such as calcium and potassium. In the myocardial cell, magnesium is essential for the activation of ATPase and subsequent oxidative phosphorylation. Deficiency leads to an inhibition of this process, a reversal of the cellular ionic pump causing mitochondrial swelling, which may then lead ultimately to myocardial fibre necrosis. High magnesium concentrations, that may occur with over-enthusiastic magnesium therapy for example, also inhibits myocardial metabolism and may have a negative inotropic effect (see Cardioplegia, p. 562).

*The effects on the electrocardiogram* of a low magnesium are a progressive widening of the QRS with ST depression and peaking of the T waves. Other ionic deficiences may also be present and can modify these ECG signs. Of more significance to the anaesthetist is the lengthening of the QTc interval (measured from the beginning of the Q to the end of the T wave and corrected for rate) which represents the whole of ventricular systole. An increase in the QTc interval (normal 0·42 seconds), implies delay in repolarisation, a situation which makes these patients particularly susceptible to dysrhythmias. Sudden death in magnesium deficiency can be precipitated by just those factors that are associated with surgery, such as hypoxia, hyperventilation, acid-base changes, anaesthetic (depressant) drugs, haemodilution, as well as the pre-operative state of the patient. Krasner and his associates[7] demonstrated in patients undergoing mitral valve replacement an increase in QTc intervals that were associated with dysrhythmias following surgery. Another group of patients who were pretreated with oral magnesium, however, had significantly less prolongation of the QTc interval and developed no serious dysrhythmias. No correlation was made in this study between the ECG changes and the serum magnesium, because blood concentrations do not necessarily equate with myocardial magnesium, especially in cardiac disease. The increase in QTc interval was probably enhanced, on top of a diuretic-induced magnesium deficiency, by the dilutional effect of cardiopulmonary bypass[8] combined with the other conditions related to surgical procedures.

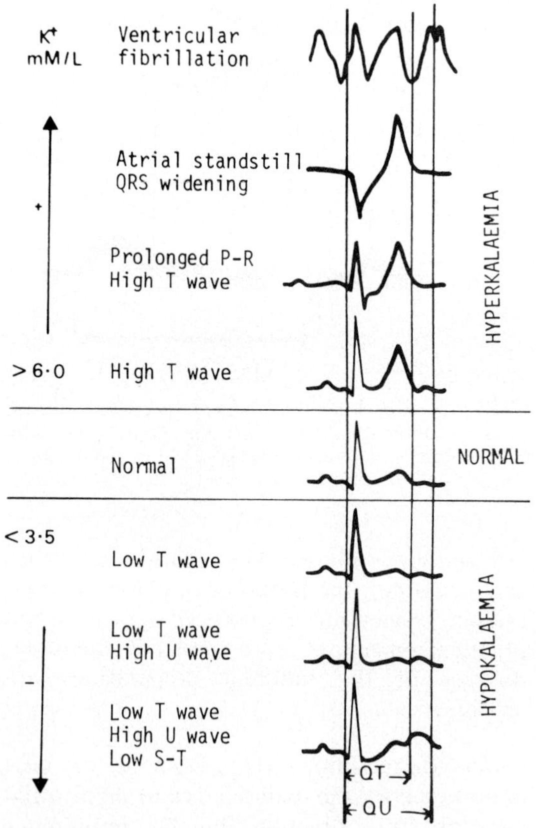

12/Fig. 16.—Effect of serum potassium levels on ECG.

*Causes of Magnesium Deficiency*[9]

1. Gastro-intestinal problems:
   malabsorption states
   diarrhoea
   nasogastric suction
2. Endocrine disorders:
   parathyroid disease
   hyperaldosteronism
   diabetic coma
3. Renal disease
4. Diuretic therapy
5. Alcoholism and alcoholic cirrhosis
6. Extracorporeal circulation (may be modified by magnesium-containing cardioplegic solutions)
7. Porphyria with inappropriate ADH secretion

(*c*) **Potassium.**—Serum potassium concentrations influence the whole of the action potential and also the character of the ST segment. Under normal conditions, the plasma potassium concentration lies between 3·5 to 5 mmol/l, but this does not necessarily equate with total body or intracellular potassium concentrations. When the level drops to around 3·5 mmol/l or lower, the T wave becomes broader and flatter, and a U wave may be seen to fuse with the T wave (Fig. 16). Dysrhythmia potential is enhanced in *hypokalaemia*, especially in patients with pre-existing cardiac disease, and this may lead to ventricular fibrillation. Hypokalaemia is provoked by enhanced potassium loss during diuretic therapy, intestinal obstruction, or nasogastric suction, and may also be induced by respiratory alkalosis during hyperventilation.[10,11] Intravenous potassium replacement in severe hypokalaemia should be performed cautiously under ECG monitoring, and should rarely exceed a rate of 40 mmol per hour. Too rapid a rate may enhance, rather than reverse, cardiac irritability, particularly in chronic hypokalaemia, and produce ventricular fibrillation.[12] Classically, however, *hyperkalaemia* depresses myocardial electrophysiology and if severe may lead to asystole.

With an increasing serum potassium from about 6 mmol/l, peaked T waves and a prolonged P-R interval are followed by complete heart block, atrial asystole, widened or bizarre QRS complexes and, ultimately, asystole or ventricular fibrillation. It is probably the rate of change of extracellular potassium concentration that causes profound cardiac effects rather than merely the serum potassium concentration itself. Hyperkalaemia may be seen in acidosis, tissue trauma, renal failure or following suxamethonium administration in susceptible patients.

*Acute treatment of hyperkalaemia* is directed towards maintaining the circulation while lowering the serum potassium. If the cardiac output is satisfactory, intravenous calcium chloride and sodium bicarbonate will both combat the physiological effects of hyperkalaemia and lower serum potassium. Elimination of potassium may be further enhanced by active diuresis or the administration of calcium resonium enema. Dialysis may be required in renal failure. Insulin lowers serum potassium by promoting its entry to the intracellular compartment and should be administered with glucose in order to prevent hypoglycaemia. If the circulation is compromised by severe bradydysrhythmias, it may be necessary artificially to pace the heart[13] whilst serious tachydysrhythmias will need specific treatment until the serum potassium is corrected.

## THE CARDIOVASCULAR EFFECTS OF ANAESTHETIC DRUGS

### General Considerations

The cardiovascular effects of agents used in anaesthesia are described in the sections dealing with individual agents in this book. These haemodynamic actions are normally described in relation to healthy patients, and the response of the patient to the variations imposed by the administration of anaesthetic agents may be quite different in the presence of cardiovascular disease. Commonly, a choice of anaesthetic agent or technique can be made which will maintain or improve the pre-anaesthetic state of the circulation and those agents or techniques which are deleterious can be avoided. To do so requires a knowledge of the effects of anaesthetic agents in the abnormal (as well as the normal) circulation, and an understanding of the haemodynamic abnormality in specific cardiovascular disease. As an example, cyclopropane, by reducing right ventricular infundibular tone, may reduce right-to-left shunting and improve pulmonary perfusion and arterial oxygenation in Fallot's tetralogy, but may increase pulmonary vascular resistance and dramatically reduce cardiac output in acute pulmonary embolism.

Some drugs commonly used in anaesthetic practice are briefly discussed below with particular reference to their effects in patients with cardiovascular disease.

### Intravenous Agents

The **barbiturates** cause hypotension as a result of three effects. A capacitance venodilatation, producing a fall in ventricular preload, a reduction in systemic vascular resistance and a reduction in myocardial contractility. Both methohexitone and thiopentone have similar actions. Their careful use is not necessarily contra-indicated in cardiac disease.

The **benzodiazepines**, diazepam and the newer midazolam, may be preferable for the induction of anaesthesia in sick patients. Neither drug produces much change in cardiac index or systemic vascular resistance, although midazolam may cause tachycardia[14] and perhaps more hypotension[15] than diazepam. Pain on injection and thrombophlebitis is less common with the water soluble midazolam, which has a shorter half-life than diazepam. A new preparation of diazepam as an emulsion (Diazemuls) has a lower incidence of local vascular complications.

In normal patients, **etomidate** produces quantitatively similar effects on the cardiovascular system to other intravenous induction agents.[16] In patients with a decreased cardiac reserve, the effects are less than in similar patients receiving thiopentone. Hypotension, when it occurs, is due mainly to a reduction in systemic vascular resistance associated with a reduction in left ventricular work.[17] Myocardial contractility is also reduced.[16]

**Althesin** has a very short duration of action, but a reputed incidence of anaphylactoid response following intravenous administration.[18] The cardiac output is usually maintained, despite a reduction in ventricular function and stroke index, by a compensatory tachycardia. There is a variable effect on the systemic vascular resistance and hence the blood pressure.[19]

**Ketamine**, by producing an increase in cardiac rate, myocardial contractility and afterload, causes a large increase in myocardial oxygen consumption and is unsuitable for patients with coronary insufficiency. In other situations, as for instance following trauma with blood loss, when other intravenous induction agents might provoke decompensatory collapse, it may be particularly indicated. In patients with acquired valve disease, Spotoft and his colleagues[20] found ketamine to produce deleterious increases in pulmonary and systemic arterial pressures associated with increases in atrial filling pressures, systemic and pulmonary vascular resistances and ventricular work.

The hypertension, though not the tachycardia, can be prevented by the calcium antagonist, verapamil, and Johnstone[21] suggests that ketamine has a direct myocardial stimulating action through an effect on the transmembrane calcium flux.

**Opiates** and other narcotic drugs are used both for induction and maintenance of anaesthesia for cardiac cases. Morphine, which may be used in varying dose ranges, is associated in most patients with cardiovascular stability, although the reduction in vasomotor tone, affecting mainly the capacitance vessels, may produce hypotension unless the filling pressure is maintained by volume expansion. A reduction in systemic vascular resistance also occurs, and in patients with a fixed cardiac output (constrictive pericarditis, aortic stenosis) the blood pressure may fall dangerously. It is probable that morphine induced hypotension is mediated by endogenous histamine release and that cardiovascular changes following morphine can be attenuated by the administration of $H_1$ with $H_2$ histamine receptor antagonists.[22]

**Pethidine** (meperidine) largely superseded by phenoperidine or fentanyl, has a mild anticholinergic action which may increase heart rate, a negative inotropic effect, and produces a dose-dependent reduction of systemic vascular resistance.[23]

**Fentanyl** may produce hypotension with a reduction in cardiac index and left ventricular work.[24,25] However, fentanyl is also associated with a reduction in heart rate and has been shown in dogs with experimentally induced coronary artery stenosis to produce negative inotropism.[26] Provided the coronary perfusion pressure is maintained, the reduction in myocardial oxygen demand under fentanyl anaesthesia makes it an advantageous agent in coronary insufficiency and Stanley and colleagues[27] have recommended high-dose fentanyl for anaesthesia in patients undergoing coronary revascularisation. This drug may produce myoclonic movements and chest wall rigidity, which can embarrass those with poor cardiorespiratory reserve.[28] Alfentanil and Sufentanil have similar properties.

**Phenoperidine** has a longer duration of action than fentanyl, with an elimination half-life of 1–2 hours. It is partially metabolised to pethidine (meperidine) and nor-pethidine.[29] Its cardiovascular effects have been less extensively studied than those of fentanyl, but its effects are similar, with a fall in systemic arterial pressure due to a reduction in systemic vascular resistance and a rate-dependent decrease in cardiac output.[30] While severe cardiovascular collapse following phenoperidine administration in the seriously ill has been reported—with reversal by naloxone[31]—minor falls in blood pressure may be restored by volume expansion.

**Droperidol** in combination with an opiate—usually fentanyl—is reputed to provide cardiovascular stability in patients with compromised cardiac reserve, although the alpha adrenoreceptor blocking action of droperidol will add to the vasodilator action of the opiate with which it is being used. During high dose fentanyl-droperidol anaesthesia for coronary artery surgery, Quintin and colleagues[32] observed a fall in systemic vascular resistance and a rise in cardiac index, but no increase in ventricular work or rate-pressure product. Volume expansion, however, was necessary to compensate for the venodilatation in order to maintain ventricular filling pressure. Droperidol attenuates the cardiovascular response to intubation[33] and has useful antidysrhythmic properties.

**Suxamethonium** produces alterations in cardiac rate and rhythm by two mechanisms. Its acetylcholine-like molecule is vagomimetic and it also has significant effects on potassium flux, especially in the presence of a low cardiac output and acidosis. Both these effects are potentially dysrhythmic.

**Pancuronium** possesses sympathomimetic and vagolytic activity increasing arterial pressure, ventricular rate and cardiac output[34–36] with a venoconstrictor effect on capacitance vessels.[37] These apparent disadvantages, which can lead to an increase in myocardial oxygen consumption, are attenuated by depressant or vasodilating anaesthetic agents or by beta-blockade.

**Tubocurarine** has a minimal effect on cardiac rate[38] but may produce arterial hypotension, an effect which is principally due to histamine release[39] rather than to other mechanisms such as ganglionic blockade.

**Metocurine** reduces systemic vascular resistance and venocapacitance tone but produces hypotension less often than tubocurarine. The incidence of hypotension is, however, greater than with pancuronium[40] and its potentially beneficial effect on rate-pressure products suggests that it might be a better agent during coronary artery surgery.

In clinical practice, the choice of neuromuscular blocker in respect of haemodynamic stability depends on the combined effects of all drugs in any one technique rather than of the individual effects on the circulation of a given relaxant[41] (see also Chapter 23).

### Inhalational Agents and Vapours

**Nitrous oxide** has always been considered a benign drug in relation to the circulation. It is possible to demonstrate that it produces an increase in both systemic and pulmonary vascular resistance, a reduction in pulmonary hypoxic vasoconstrictor response and a direct negative inotropic effect. The significance of these effects is negligible although under certain circumstances, such as in myocardial ischaemia, nitrous oxide may prove deleterious.

**Halothane** and **enflurane** may be conveniently discussed together as their effects on the cardiovascular system are similar, any differences being of degree only. Both depress myocardial contractility and reduce cardiac output, especially in those with poor ventricular function,[42,43] in which case ventricular filling pressures may rise. Both have a negative chronotropic effect on the SA node. Halothane has only a small effect on systemic vascular resistance, despite cutaneous vasodilatation, while enflurane has a much greater effect.[44] The cardiac output and arterial pressure may be further reduced by peripheral venous pooling secondary to venodilatation. Atrioventricular conduction is depressed, especially in the presence of pre-existing conduction defects, but enflurane is less likely to provoke catecholamine-induced dysrhythmias than halothane.

Both halothane and enflurane have a potential for improving the myocardial oxygen supply-demand ratio. Provided the ventricular size does not increase, and that any reduction in coronary perfusion pressure is not disproportionate, the decrease in myocardial oxygen consumption, secondary to the reduction in contractility, may exceed the reduction in oxygen supply. Smith and his colleagues[45] have demonstrated in dogs an increase in regional myocardial oxygen availability/consumption in experimentally induced areas of ischaemia in the presence of halothane. This myocardial sparing action of halothane in the presence of ischaemia is probably the result of a general reduction in myocardial contractility, combined with effects on the peripheral circulation.[46] (See also Chapter 6.)

**Isoflurane** which provides more cardiovascular stability, is fully discussed on page 212.

### Antisialagogues

**Atropine** has pronounced vagolytic activity and promotes a dose-related tachycardia. An initial bradycardia, which is rarely seen after intravenous injection, has been attributed to a central action, or to a peripheral or bimodel action on the SA node. The central action appears unlikely since atropine methylbromide, which does not cross the blood-brain barrier, shows the same biphasic action.[47] Bradycardia, impaired conduction and reduced cardiac output, due to the cardiac effects of acetylcholine, are reversed by atropine, but dysrhythmias may be provoked, especially in the presence of inhalation anaesthetics. At the same time, atropine may be useful as a therapy for some dysrhythmias associated with depressed A-V conduction and may convert nodal to sinus rhythm, or abolish ventricular ectopic beats complicating ventricular bradycardia.

**Hyoscine** produces much less effect on the heart rate. An initial accelerator phase is followed by bradycardia with concomitant changes in cardiac output, systemic vascular resistance and central venous pressure.

**Glycopyrrolate** (glycopyrronium), a quaternary ammonium anticholinergic agent has minimal effects on the cardiovascular system. At normal heart rate a bradycardia follows small intravenous (0·1 mg) doses and no change in rate occurs after 0·2 mg.[48] Dysrhythmias are uncommon but junctional (nodal) rhythm with associated wandering pacemaker or atrial extrasystoles, may follow its administration. Glycopyrrolate appears to be quite useful in the treatment of sinus bradycardia during anaesthesia. (See also Chapter 44.)

## CARDIOVASCULAR RESPONSES TO ANAESTHETIC MANOEUVRES AND TO SURGERY

The cardiovascular responses observed during anaesthesia and surgery, as well as being a consequence of the administration of anaesthetic and other drugs, may be modified by other aspects of anaesthetic and surgical technique. These changes are grouped briefly here, although some are described elsewhere in greater detail.

### 1. Pre-anaesthetic Techniques and Monitoring

Apart from the changes produced in the patient's circulation by pre-operative apprehension, the initial observation in the anaesthetic room will reflect the patient's response to the type and strength of the premedication given. It may be considered normal practice to measure the pulse rate and blood pressure and perhaps attach an ECG prior to induction. Significant changes in circulatory state may arise when infusion or monitoring cannulae are introduced under local anaesthesia prior to induction and Lunn and colleagues[49] showed marked heart rate and arterial pressure rises during cannulation which were not observed if the patient was anaesthetised first. Waller and associates[50] stressed that significant cardiovascular responses can be avoided by the presence of $\beta$-adrenergic blockade, particularly in combination with adequate premedicant sedation and the liberal use of local anaesthetic. Intravenous diazepam, given prior to cannulation under local anaesthesia, provides good conditions with little effect on blood pressure or rate. Dysrhythmias may be provoked during central venous cannulation if the catheter enters the right ventricle, or indeed by a flow-directed catheter during its passage to the pulmonary artery (see p. 480).

### 2. Laryngoscopy and Intubation

Tachycardia, hypertension and dysrhythmias all occur during laryngoscopy and intubation, and the consequent rise in rate/pressure product may result in a myocardial oxygen demand which exceeds the oxygen supply and, under these circumstances, may induce myocardial ischaemia. This response is sympathomimetically mediated and can be attenuated by $\beta$-adrenergic blockade.[51,52] Alternative or additional techniques to avoid this response, which may be dangerous, not only to the heart, but also in raising intracranial pressure, are the provision of an adequate depth of anaesthesia before attempted intubation, the addition of a potent analgesic, such as fentanyl[53] and the prior administration of lignocaine topically or intravenously.[54,55] Other drugs, such as phentolamine, sodium nitroprusside, labetalol and $\beta$-blockers have also been recommended.

### 3. Alterations in Ventilatory Function

Alterations in ventilatory function during anaesthesia may provoke changes consequent on variations in blood oxygen and carbon dioxide tensions, either of which may be independently raised or lowered while other changes may follow the introduction of intermittent positive-pressure ventilation with or without the addition of positive end-expiratory pressure.

Hypoxia initially produces sympathetic stimulation, but continuous hypoxia with metabolic acidosis results in myocardial depression, falling blood pressure and cardiac output, and the development of dysrhythmias or extreme bradycardia. In the anaesthetised patient, the signs of initial sympathetic stimulation may be absent and bradycardia and hypotension appear as the first signs. Although a linear, but rather flat relationship exists between carbon dioxide tension and cardiac output, signs of sympathetic stimulation as a response to hypercarbia during anaesthesia are frequently absent. However, with certain volatile anaesthetics, a higher incidence of dysrhythmias occurs when carbon dioxide tension is raised.

An excessively high arterial oxygen tension is associated with a rise in systemic vascular resistance and a diminution in cardiac output. A reduction in cardiac output and a diminution in tissue blood flow, which may lead to the development of a metabolic acidosis, also follows maintained hypocapnia, and in low cardiac output states, an attempt should be made to keep $Paco_2$ near normal.

The introduction of positive-pressure ventilation with its effect of raising mean intrathoracic pressure and diminishing venous return, normally results in a diminution of cardiac output to a degree which depends on the mechanical characteristics of the ventilation, the state of the autonomic nervous system and the innervated vessels and the blood volume. Appreciation of the greater complexity of this relationship has followed researches into the effects of positive end-expiratory pressure on the circulation and which have emphasised the part played by the pericardium in determining the relationship between right and left heart filling, the effect on right ventricular afterload, and in the appearance in the plasma of substances, perhaps prostaglandins, which exert a negative inotropic effect, and which may arise in stretched lung.[56]

4. **Posture**

With anaesthetically induced impairment of the autonomic control of the cardiovascular system, substantial alterations may occur when the patient's position is altered from the horizontal. In particular, with steep head-up or sitting position, venous pooling in the dependent parts will cause a decrease in cardiac output. Conversely, the head-down position, particularly if associated with elevation of the legs in the lithotomy position, will maintain and may mask the effects of hypovolaemia until the patient is returned to the horizontal at the end of the operation. The face down position, apart from the effects which it produces on ventilation, may augment or diminish venous pooling in the splanchnic bed, depending on the degree of abdominal compression.

5. **Surgical Haemorrhage**

The circulatory responses to blood loss—increase of venous tone, tachycardia, reduction of pulse pressure—will be superimposed on, and modified by, the circulatory changes produced by anaesthesia. In many instances, the compensatory mechanism to haemorrhage may be impaired. Quite small changes in blood volume, in the presence of reduced compensatory mechanisms in the venous system, may produce large changes in ventricular filling pressure and thus in cardiac output and blood pressure.

6. **Surgical Stimulation**

Sympathetic response to surgical stimulation during anaesthesia can be frequently observed due principally to variations in the intensity of stimulation at different stages in the operation and can usually be obtunded by deepening the level of anaesthesia. Roizen and colleagues[57] were able to reverse the increases in systolic blood pressure, pulmonary capillary wedge pressure, systemic vascular resistance and plasma nor-adrenaline that followed surgical manipulation by simply increasing the inspired concentrations of enflurane or halothane. Although high dose fentanyl is recommended for its cardiovascular stability and amelioration of the metabolic stress response in surgery, Edde[58] demonstrated that even 50 $\mu$g/kg failed to prevent the increase in systemic vascular resistance and arterial pressure provoked by sternotomy prior to cardiac surgery, and that only direct vasodilator therapy could prevent it completely. Surgical stimulation may also manifest itself via the vagus, usually the consequence of pulling on the mesentery, particularly in relation to the gall bladder, or gastro-oesophageal junction or from the oculo-cardiac reflex, when bradycardia and hypotension occur despite the absence of hypovolaemia. A third form of surgical stimulation occurs from the handling of actively secreting glands—e.g. phaeochromocytoma—when sudden rises in the blood level of their active ingredient may produce large variations in cardiovascular function.

### 7. Mechanical Interference with the Circulation

Direct mechanical interference with the heart itself, impairing its ability to fill during diastole, is a situation usually confined to cardiac surgery. Substantial alterations in arterial afterload are more common, principally during vascular surgery when arterial impedance may be altered by aortic cross-clamping. In the extreme case of high aortic clamping in coarctation surgery, myocardial depressant drugs and vasodilator therapy may be necessary to prevent excessive hypertension in the proximal segments at the time of cross-clamping. Following the release of arterial obstruction and the removal of arterial cross-clamps, the sudden decrease in arterial impedance may be aggravated by excessive flows through the dilated hypoxic channels which have been re-established and severe falls in blood pressure may occur. This can be further aggravated if the patient is hypovolaemic at the time.

Interference with venous return to the heart is, however, the commonest of the mechanical interferences with the circulation, and may be seen even in the absence of anaesthesia and surgery in the compression of the inferior vena cava by the gravid uterus. It may occur as a deliberate surgical technique—ligation of the inferior vena cava to prevent pulmonary embolism—as a consequence of position, the lateral nephrectomy position with pronounced "break", or as a consequence of excessive abdominal packing or injudicious placing of deep retractors. In thoracic surgery, and particularly in tension pneumothorax, extreme displacement of the mediastinum may obstruct the vena cavae.

### 8. Dysrhythmias

Dysrhythmias are considered in detail elsewhere, but although they are common during anaesthesia, they are usually haemodynamically unimportant. However, an acute change in a circulatory variable, usually pulse rate but often blood pressure, is frequently a sign of a change in cardiac rhythm.

### 9. Blood Viscosity

An infrequently considered component of systemic vascular resistance is the part played by the blood viscosity, of which the main determining factor is the packed cell volume. Quite large alterations in blood viscosity may occur during surgery, particularly if substantial quantities of crystalloid infusion or hyperosmolar solutions are made at a time of blood loss. The decreased viscosity may actually enhance tissue perfusion[59] and be associated with a rise in cardiac output, although arterial pressure may fall.

## DRUGS AND THE CARDIOVASCULAR SYSTEM

This section deals with agents specifically employed for circulatory control and includes the vasodilators, vasoconstrictors, inotropes, beta-blockers and antidysrhythmic agents. Certain other drugs which are used in cardiac disease, for example digoxin, are discussed elsewhere.

### Vasoconstrictors

Clearer understanding of the principles of circulatory management has, in general, resulted in the treatment of hypotension proceeding along physiological lines, with the aetiology of the hypotension being identified before appropriate corrective therapy. So far have concepts changed that, in some instances, a vasodilator may be more appropriate therapy for hypotension than a vasoconstrictor. While the maintenance of cardiac output is commonly considered more important than the blood pressure, there remains a number of situations, usually related to arteriolar dilatation in the presence of a fixed cardiac output (mitral stenosis, aortic stenosis) or severe coronary artery disease, in which elevation of the systemic vascular resistance may be indicated. The choice of vasoconstrictors may well then depend on its additional actions upon the cardiovascular system.

**Methoxamine** has actions which are almost exclusively due to direct $\alpha$-receptor agonism and which produce a rise in systemic vascular resistance. Provided cardiac output is maintained—and it is usually little affected—blood pressure rises while pulse rate slows, partly due to a reflex mechanism and partly from direct $\alpha$ effect on the SA node. Coronary blood flow varies according to myocardial work load but cerebral splanchnic and renal perfusion are directly reduced. Methoxamine can be used to reverse paroxysmal atrial tachycardia. It may be given intravenously in 0·5–1·0 mg increments.

**Phenylephrine**, while structurally similar to adrenaline, has almost entirely direct $\alpha$-agonist activity. There is very little $\beta$ or indirect sympathomimetic action. The arteriolar constriction is similar to that caused by methoxamine but, in contrast, there is less venoconstriction. Pulmonary artery pressure rises secondary to pulmonary vasoconstriction and this may be disadvantageous in pulmonary hypertensive states. The intravenous dose is similar to methoxamine.

**Ephedrine** has both direct $\alpha$- and $\beta$-receptor agonist activity as well as indirect actions due to the release of noradrenaline peripherally. The pressor response is mainly attributable to an increase in myocardial contractility together with arterial vasoconstriction. The consequent maintenance of cardiac output makes the drug attractive in the management of hypotension complicating obstetric epidural analgesia. The intravenous dose is 1–5 mg.

**Metaraminol** also has direct $\alpha$ and $\beta$ and indirect sympathomimetic actions. The increase in blood pressure is mainly due to arteriolar vasoconstriction as reflex bradycardia tends to limit any increase in cardiac output. In common with most vasoconstrictors, metaraminol may significantly reduce renal blood flow. The intravenous dose is 0·5–1·0 mg.

## Vasodilators

### (a) Smooth Muscle Dilators

**Sodium nitroprusside**, presumably due to its nitroso-moiety, is a potent smooth muscle vasodilator. Its major effect is on the arterioles, thus reducing systemic vascular resistance, but it also reduces venocapacitance tone and ventricular filling pressure. The consequent fall in blood pressure is dose dependent.

The physiological effects of sodium nitroprusside have been extensively studied. Not all the data obtained is readily translatable to the clinical situation, partly because the experimental evidence is often obtained in animals and partly because variation in response to the nitroprusside infusion in respect of smooth-muscle dilatation is complicated by variation in degree of the reflex response evoked in the whole organism.

The commonest observation is the development of a tachycardia which occurs subsequent to increased plasma catecholamine concentration, presumably produced by increased carotid sinus baroreceptor activity.[60] In the presence of the reduced afterload, the effect of this tachycardia is to maintain, or even increase, the cardiac output, unless the venous return is markedly reduced. Cardiac output may also be raised as a result of increased myocardial contractility,[61] although Vance and colleagues[62] showed a dose-dependent reduction in left ventricular dp/dt max (the maximum rate of increase in pressure in the left ventricle during contraction). The effect of this maintenance of cardiac output may be to prevent a reduction in blood pressure, unless the tachycardia is reduced by administration of a $\beta$-adrenergic blocker. A further mechanism acting on the blood pressure during sodium nitroprusside infusion may well be enhanced renin angiotensin activity,[63] as the rebound hypertension which follows discontinuation of sodium nitroprusside in rats can be prevented by saralasin, a competitive inhibitor of angiotensin I.

Blood flow to organs is well maintained with a normal body and myocardial oxygen consumption.[62] Behnia and associates[64] demonstrated unimpaired renal medullary oxygenation in neurosurgical patients whose mean arterial pressure was reduced by half although the endogenous creatinine clearance fell. In a group of dogs which were resistant to the effects of nitroprusside and which required large doses to produce a reduction in blood pressure, a redistribution of blood was seen towards the brain and myocardium at the expense of liver, kidney and spleen blood flows.[61]

Under normal circumstances, sodium nitroprusside has little effect on pulmonary vascular resistance; however, in those circumstances when the pulmonary vascular resistance is reversibly increased, usually in response to hypoxia or acidosis, the administration of nitroprusside will reduce pulmonary hypertension by inhibition of the pulmonary hypoxic vasoconstriction.[65,66]

Sodium nitroprusside is converted to cyanmethaemoglobin and free cyanide in the red cell, the cyanide is then metabolised to thiocyanide in the liver and subsequently eliminated via the kidney. Nitroprusside overdose causes an increased plasma cyanide and consequent histotoxic hypoxia. It is recommended that the total dose of sodium nitroprusside should be less than 1·5 mg/kg[67] and that plasma cyanide should not exceed 300 $\mu$mol per cent. Nitroprusside should be avoided in those patients in whom cyanide metabolism is compromised, e.g. Leber's optic atrophy, tobacco amblyopia and vitamin $B_{12}$ deficiency.[68] In practice the desired haemodynamic effect can be obtained quite easily within the dose range if tachycardia is controlled by the administration of a $\beta$-adrenergic blocker. If continued control of blood pressure is required which might lead to a large dose being used, a change can be made to a longer-acting drug such as hydralazine.

Sodium nitroprusside is normally given intravenously from a microdrip buretrol or constant infusion pump via a venous cannula, reserved solely for the administration of that drug. During anaesthesia, accurate monitoring of the arterial blood pressure is mandatory if appreciable hypotension is to be induced.

**Glyceryl trinitrate** was originally employed as an oral, or rather sublingual, anti-anginal agent when its mode of action was attributed to coronary and systemic vasodilator effects, with reduction in coronary vasospasm and improvement in myocardial collateral blood flow. With the introduction of a stable intravenous preparation, its action to reduce venocapacitance tone, with a lesser though important reduction in arteriolar resistance[69,70] has become valuable in peri-operative treatment of heart failure and ischaemia. The venodilatation reduces ventricular filling pressures and volume and thus ventricular wall tension. Effective emptying of the heart is enhanced by the reduction in systemic vascular resistance, but because the principal action to improve cardiac performance is by reduction in preload, there is less reflex tachycardia than occurs with agents acting mainly on systemic arteriolar resistance. Optimum improvement in myocardial function can be obtained with glyceryl trinitrate only if the vascular volume is carefully adjusted with monitoring of the ventricular filling pressure at the same time as the drug is given.

Glyceryl trinitrate reduces pulmonary vascular resistance, but also causes a fall in arterial oxygen tension due to alterations in ventilation/perfusion relationships and abolition of the hypoxic vasoconstrictor effect.

In the management of hypertension following myocardial revascularisation, Tobias[71] compared glyceryl trinitrate and sodium nitroprusside and found both to have similar effects on systemic vascular resistance, cardiac output and heart rate. Trinitrate administration was easier to control with less overshoot hypotension and more effect on the pulmonary vascular resistance. On pharmacological principles, it would seem logical to employ glyceryl trinitrate in vasodilator therapy when an action is required principally on cardiac preload, and sodium nitroprusside when the main benefit is to be derived from arteriolar dilatation and reduction in afterload.

**Hydralazine**, a phthalazine derivative, is a useful anti-hypertensive agent which acts directly on vascular smooth muscle. Systemic vascular resistance is reduced, but there is less reduction in veno-capacitance tone and the incidence of significant postural hypotension during long-term therapy is low. There is a variable effect on cardiac output and heart rate which tend to increase in response to the vasodilatation. An increase in myocardial oxygen consumption may provoke angina in some patients with ischaemic heart disease. Oral hydralazine has proved useful in the treatment of primary pulmonary hypertension, presumably by reducing pulmonary vascular resistance.[72] The systemic hypotensive action appears 20–30 minutes after intravenous injection, the dose being 5–30 mg. The plasma half-life is about 2–6 hours and varies between individuals.

### (b) The $\alpha$-Adrenergic Antagonists

The main clinical applications for $\alpha$-adrenergic antagonists in relation to anaesthesia are the intra-operative control of blood pressure, reduction in pulmonary vascular resistance and the attenuation of the effects of high catecholamine levels as in phaeochromocytoma.

**Tolazoline** and **phentolamine** are imidazoline related drugs which have similar actions on the cardiovascular system producing arteriolar and veno-dilatation, a reduction in pulmonary vascular resistance and a reflex tachycardia. As well as blocking the $\alpha$-receptors, there is a direct action on vascular smooth muscle, similar to that produced by histamine. Endogenous noradrenaline release causes more increase in cardiac output than might be expected from reflex activity alone and in the case of tolazoline, the blood pressure may rise. The overall response in the patient will depend both on the pre-existing level of sympathetic activity and the amount of volume replacement made to compensate for the venodilatation.

Phentolamine is given intravenously in incremental doses of 1 mg. An infusion may be employed but tachyphylaxis occurs.

**Phenoxybenzamine** is a longer-acting drug used in the pre-operative preparation of patients with phaeochromocytoma and in the treatment of Raynaud's disease although during anaesthesia the duration of action may be disadvantageous. Generalised arteriolar and venodilatation, a reflex tachycardia and a variable effect on cardiac output and blood pressure can be seen.

### The Inotropes

#### (a) $\beta$-receptor agonists

The main indication for the use of beta-receptor agonists is to produce a positive inotropic effect. All of them will also have other effects on the cardiovascular system which will influence the choice of agent to suit a particular clinical situation. Pure pharmacological effects are often modified by the circulatory state of the patient so that an increase in cardiac output and improvement in peripheral flow may, for example, attenuate direct drug-induced vasoconstriction (Table 3).

**Isoprenaline** stimulates both $\beta_1$ and $\beta_2$ receptors producing positive inotropic and chronotropic effects, an improvement in atrio-ventricular conduction, an increase in myocardial irritability and a reduction in systemic vascular resistance. It is useful in situations associated with bradydysrhythmias, in left ventricular failure, in the presence of $\beta$-blockade and when reduction in systemic vascular resistance would be advantageous. In fixed cardiac output states, isoprenaline may produce hypotension. Isoprenaline is relatively contra-indicated in the presence of tachydysrhythmias. It is best administered as a constant infusion in the dose range 0·01–0·1 mg/kg/min.

**Adrenaline** has a similar powerful action on $\beta_1$ and $\beta_2$ receptors, producing inotropic and chronotropic effects with an increase in myocardial irritability, and an additional effect on $\alpha$-receptors. Although this effect on skin and skeletal muscle vessels may, in the normal circulation, slightly reduce total systemic vascular resistance, in therapeutic doses in the abnormal circulation arteriolar resistance frequently rises. Usually, the blood pressure rises secondary to the increase in cardiac output, but inadequate improvement of cardiac output may be associated with a decrease in peripheral blood flow and a reduction in renal and splanchnic perfusion. Although improvement in myocardial contractility might be expected to result in a fall of ventricular filling pressure, in practice the intense constriction of capacitance vessels results in large increases in atrial pressure and concomitant vasodilator therapy may be necessary both to reduce the venous pressure and by reducing systemic vascular resistance, limit the rise in myocardial oxygen consumption.

Adrenaline, unlike isoprenaline, produces coronary vasoconstriction, but this effect is normally overridden by the local vasodilator response, secondary to the rise in myocardial oxygen demand. Continuous infusion of adrenaline is made in the dose range 0·05–0·5 $\mu$g/kg/min.

**Noradrenaline** has potent $\alpha$-agonist, but only moderate $\beta$-agonist, activity, which causes systemic vascular resistance and blood pressure to rise with a reflex reduction in heart rate. Direct coronary vasoconstriction is overwhelmed by coronary vasodilatation occurring secondary to the increase in ventricular work while skin, muscle, splanchnic and renal flows decrease. Noradrenaline is twenty times weaker as an inotrope than isoprenaline, but may be useful in the presence of tachydysrhythmias, particularly if the vasoconstrictor effects are modified by the simultaneous infusion of sodium nitroprusside or glyceryl trinitrate. Noradrenaline infusion is given at 0·05–0·5 $\mu$g/kg/min.

**Dopamine** is a catecholamine-like agent with moderate inotropic properties. Its effects on the cardiovascular system are *variable and dose-*

*related*, partly due to its flexible molecular configuration which allows it to act on a number of receptor sites and partly due to its role as a noradrenaline precursor at adrenergic nerve endings. It is possible to demonstrate a mixed effect on $\alpha$- and $\beta$-receptors, a specific agonist action on dopaminergic receptors and a noradrenaline effect.

At low infusion rates—1–5 μg/kg/min—the drug produces a moderate inotropic effect with vasodilator activity. At high infusion rates—10–20 μg/kg/min the more powerful inotropic action is accompanied by vasoconstriction and, at these doses, is similar to adrenaline so that additional vasodilator therapy may become necessary. The improvement in myocardial function is associated with less tachycardia and dysrhythmogenic effects than with isoprenaline but a poorer response on A-V conduction and ventricular rate in the presence of conduction defects. Increase in venocapacitance tone may result in rises of left ventricular filling pressure despite improvement in contractility in left ventricular failure. Coronary, renal, mesenteric and cerebral blood flow all increase at low infusion doses, but this may be replaced by vasoconstriction when the dose is increased.

Although dopamine produces direct renal vasodilatation, the increase in cardiac output further improves renal blood flow and glomerular filtration with a resultant diuresis. A diuresis and natriuresis which occurs independently of the renovascular effects[73] is possibly mediated via stimulation of tubular adenylcyclase with subsequent effects on sodium readsorption.[74]

**Dobutamine** is a $\beta$-agonist structurally similar to dopamine, but lacking dopaminergic properties, as it has no specific reno-vasodilating effect. It exerts its main action via the $\beta_1$ receptors with little $\beta_2$ or $\alpha$ effect. Thus it is a potent inotrope with little chronotropic and vasodilator properties except at higher doses.

Reports on its haemodynamic effects vary according to the clinical situation in which it is employed. Generally cardiac output improves with no change or a fall in left ventricular filling pressure and only moderate changes in heart rate and peripheral resistance. In patients with high ventricular filling pressures, dobutamine may be preferable to dopamine.

Dobutamine tends to increase ventricular rate in complete heart block and may improve conduction in supra-His bundle block by increasing SA node automaticity, and reducing conduction time and refractory period in the atrioventricular node. At the same time, dysrhythmogenicity is less than with isoprenaline. It is given intravenously in the dose range 1–10 μg/kg/min.

**Prenalterol** is a new high selective $B_1$ agonist with marked inotropic, but minimal chronotropic and dysrhythmogenic, properties. The increase in cardiac output is produced by an increase in contractility and stroke volume. The effect on systemic vascular resistance is attributed to a reflex response to an improvement in cardiac index[121] although, in contrast to low dose dopamine following cardiac surgery, prenalterol has been shown significantly to lower both the systemic and pulmonary vascular resistances.[122]

(b) **Other Inotropes**

**Aminophylline**, while used most commonly for its smooth muscle relaxing effect in the treatment of bronchospasm, also has significant effects on the cardiovascular system which may be particularly useful in the presence of $\beta$-adrenergic blockade. Myocardial contractility and cardiac rate increase with a rise in stroke volume and cardiac output and a fall in ventricular filling pressures, and a reduction in pulmonary and systemic vascular resistances. Ventricular dysrhythmias may occur, particularly in the presence of halothane. Although coronary vascular resistance is reduced, myocardial oxygen demand increases and the net effect is unpredictable. In low cardiac output states, its action on the cerebral vessels may reduce cerebral blood flow.

The mode of action of aminophylline is largely by the inhibition of cyclic nucleotide phosphodiesterase, the enzyme responsible for the intracellular breakdown of cyclic 5-AMP. Thus synergism occurs with catecholamines and glucagon, which promote the formation of cyclic AMP.[75] Because aminophylline is very largely metabolised by hepatic biotransformation and is about 50 per cent bound to plasma proteins (mechanisms which are disturbed in liver disease), it should be used with caution in hepatic disorders.

**Glucagon**, a single chain polypeptide secreted by the pancreas, raises blood sugar by increasing hepatic glycogenolysis and gluconeogenesis during the stress response. The cardiovascular actions are due to its stimulation of adenyl

12/TABLE 3
QUALITATIVE CARDIOVASCULAR EFFECTS OF CATECHOLAMINES

| | *Adrenaline* | *Noradrenaline* | *Isoprenaline* | *Dobutamine* | *Dopamine* Lower Dose 2·5–7·5 mcg/kg/min | *Dopamine* High Dose 10–25 mcg/kg/min | *Salbutamol* |
|---|---|---|---|---|---|---|---|
| Receptor Activity | $\alpha\ \beta_1\ \beta_2$ | $\alpha\ (\beta_1)$ | $\beta_1+\beta_2$ | $\beta_1\ (\beta_2)\ (\alpha)$ | Dopaminergic $\beta_1\ (\alpha+\beta_2)$ | Dopaminergic $\alpha\ \beta_1\ (\beta_2)$ | $\beta_2\ (\beta_1)$ |
| Inotropic Effect | strong | slight to moderate | strong | strong | moderate | moderate to strong | slight |
| Chronotropic Effect | strong | slight or negative | strong | moderate | slight | moderate | moderate to strong |
| Enhancement of AV Conduction | strong | may be vagally depressed | strong | moderate | slight | moderate | slight |
| Dysrhythmic Potential | strong | moderate | strong | moderate | slight | strong | slight |
| Total Systemic Vascular Resistance | may be increased | increased | reduced | little change | reduced | increased | reduced |
| Pulmonary Vascular Resistance | increased | increased | reduced | little change | little change | increased | reduced |
| Direct Effect on Renal Arterioles | constriction | constriction | no effect | no effect | dilatation | constriction | no effect |
| Direct Effect on Veno-Capacitance Tone | constriction | constriction | no effect | little effect | may constrict | constricts | no effect |
| Dilution for Infusion | 0·5–2 mg in 500 ml | 4–8 mg in 500 ml | 1–4 mg in 500 ml | 250–500 mg in 500 ml | 200–400 mg in 500 ml | | 5–20 mg in 500 ml |
| Normal Dose Range (Adult) | 1–15 mcg/min | 1–15 mcg/min | 0·5–5 mcg/min | 100–500 mcg/min | 175–515 mcg/min | 700–1750 mcg/min | 5–20 mcg/min (bronchodilating & vasodilating dose) |

(Compiled by A. Wielogorski, 1982) mcg = μg

It should be noted that the actual effects are modified by the clinical state of the patient. The use of catecholamines, in the clinical context, usually precludes a normal circulation and the responses to these drugs may differ from those predicted on pure pharmacological grounds. This table makes an attempt to indicate the circulatory changes likely to be induced under those circumstances in which these agents are often employed.

cyclase to increase myocardial cyclic AMP with a positive inotropic and chronotropic result. As this mechanism bypasses the $\beta_1$-receptor effects on adenyl cyclase, glucagon has proved useful in improving cardiac function in the presence of $\beta$-adrenergic blockade.[76] Conduction defects, following myocardial revascularisation surgery in patients who are on $\beta$-blockers, have been successfully treated with glucagon—an effect that is enhanced by aminophylline. Glucagon may be given in the dose range of 1–10 mg i.v., but the effect is of relative short duration and an infusion may be required.

**Amrinone** is a synthetic inotropic agent that

may be given orally or parenterally. It appears to have a unique mode of action quite dissimilar to other inotropes. Although not fully elucidated, it is possible that an effect on calcium activity within the myocardial sarcoplasm may explain its potent effect on contractility.[123] It also possesses marked vasodilator activity which, in heart pump failure, augments the improvement in cardiac function.

**Calcium** is discussed on page 421.

### Beta-adrenergic Blockers

The beta-adrenergic antagonists are drugs which specifically and competitively block the action of isoprenaline on the $\beta$-receptors in a dose dependent agonist-antagonist relationship.[77] Certain drugs, for example *metoprolol*, *acebutolol* and *atenolol*, are termed cardioselective as their action is principally on the $\beta_1$ receptors and are particularly useful when $\beta_2$ antagonism is contra-indicated, as in reversible airway obstruction. Others, such as *oxprenolol* and *practolol* have intrinsic sympathomimetic activity (ISA), in which partial $\beta$-agonist activity can be demonstrated, although the drugs are employed clinically for their $\beta$-blocking action. *Propranolol* is not cardioselective and also does not possess ISA, but is in widespread use both as an anti-angina agent and to assist in the control of the circulation during anaesthesia (Table 4).

The pharmacological effects of $\beta$-receptor blockers depend both on the degree of block produced and the type of receptor blocked. They produce a reduction in cardiac contractility and heart rate (and thus cardiac output) a central reduction in vasomotor activity and an action on the renin-angiotensin system. The increase in plasma renin activity which follows hypotension caused by sodium nitroprusside, can be reduced by propranolol.[66] Atrioventricular conduction defects may be worsened but ventricular dysrhythmias are suppressed, although in the case of propranolol this latter action is partly due to a local anaesthetic membrane stabilising effect.

The clinical effects observed in patients depend on the level of sympathetic activity prior to the administration of $\beta$-receptor blockers. For patients in whom sympathetic overactivity predominates, as in thyrotoxicosis, anxiety states or phaeochromocytoma, the circulation can be markedly improved by $\beta$-receptor blockade, which may also be useful in the control of both acute and chronic hypertensive states. $\beta$-receptor blockade may, however, produce a deterioration in the circulation when sympathetic activity is necessary for the maintenance of effective function, as in cardiac failure.

Initial fears that $\beta$-adrenergic blockade would inhibit an intact sympathetic nervous system which would be essential during anaesthesia in the event of uncontrollable myocardial depression or cardiac arrest, have been superseded by an appreciation of the beneficial effects of $\beta$-blockade in certain diseases, the deleterious effects of the sudden withdrawal of therapy, and a better understanding of the pharmacology and interaction of the $\beta$-blockers.[77,78] Furthermore, the '$\beta$-blocked' patient is still capable of cardiovascular stimulation, either by the administration of larger than usual doses of sympathomimetic drugs, on the grounds that clinical $\beta$-blockade is seldom complete, or with drugs that use some alternative pathway. Atropine, by its vagolytic action, is often effective in increasing heart rate, calcium chloride will improve cardiac contractility, as will glucagon, which stimulates intramyocardial adenyl cyclase independent of $\beta_1$ activity, and aminophylline which inhibits the phosphodiesterase breakdown of cyclic AMP (see p. 432). Despite this facility to overcome the action of $\beta$-blockers, caution must be exercised during the administration of any anaesthetic agent whose actions are likely to be potentiated by $\beta$-blockade. Obvious examples are those agents which rely on sympathetic stimulation—cyclopropane, isoflurane and ether—for the maintenance of a stable cardiovascular state. Moreover the myocardial depressant actions of halothane and enflurane, the bradycardia following succinylcholine or neostigmine, the vasodilatation following tubocurarine, may all exaggerate hypotension in the presence of $\beta$-blockade and the dose and rate of administration of the drug should be adjusted accordingly.

This greater understanding of the advantages and limitations of concurrent $\beta$-receptor blockade and anaesthesia stem from experience in patients with ischaemic heart disease. In these patients, abrupt withdrawal can cause serious rebound hypertension and may provoke angina or myocardial infarction. By optimising myocardial oxygen supply/demand ratios and

12/Table 4

| *Drug* | *Intrinsic sympathomimetic activity* | *Cardio-selective (mainly $\beta_1$)* | *Elimination plasma half-life (h)* | *Typical dose for angina therapy (oral)* | *Typical dose for treatment of tachydysrhythmias (slow i.v.)* |
|---|---|---|---|---|---|
| Propranolol | No | No | 1–6 | 20–80 mg qds | 1–5 mg |
| Oxprenolol | Yes | No | 2 | 20–80 mg qds | 1–2 mg |
| Metoprolol | No | Yes | 3 | 50 mg tds | – |
| Acebutolol | Yes | Yes | 3 | 200 mg tds | 10 mg |
| Practolol | Yes | Yes | 13 | Oral therapy absolutely contra-indicated because of eye damage and retroperitoneal fibrosis. | 1–10 mg |

(after Roberts, 1980,[77] Opie, 1980[79]).

by obtunding the sometimes significant increase in rate/pressure product associated with anxiety, laryngoscopy and intubation and other stresses of the pre, intra and postoperative areas, continuation of $\beta$-blockade reduces the likelihood of acute myocardial ischaemia.[124]

The elimination half-lives of $\beta$-adrenergic blockers are relatively short. Discontinuation of a morning dose on the day of operation may, in some patients, result in previously adequate control being replaced by an uncontrolled hypertensive or ischaemic state (see Table 4).

*Labetalol* hydrochloride is an amide possessing both $\alpha$- and $\beta$-receptor blocking activity and which is used clinically in the control of hypertensive states. Following intravenous administration, its $\beta$-antagonistic effect is about seven times more powerful than its $\alpha$-blocking effect.[79] Following oral administration, first-pass clearance from the liver is high and the oral dose (100–300 mg) is much higher than the intravenous (5–35 mg). Plasma half-life is 3–4 hours.

12/Table 5
Comparative Doses Giving Similar Degrees of Antagonism

| | | |
|---|---|---|
| $\beta_1$ antagonism | 3 mg propranolol | 15 mg labetalol |
| $\beta_2$ antagonism | 1 mg propranolol | 15 mg labetalol |
| $\alpha$ antagonism | 2 mg phentolamine | 15 mg labetalol |

(after Cope and Crawford, 1979[80])

The main interest in labetalol has been in the control of blood pressure and haemorrhage during surgery.[80] Increments of 5–10 mg intravenously, will rapidly lower the blood pressure by a reduction in cardiac output, systemic vascular resistance and heart rate. The latter is probably the main determinant in the reduction of output, as arterial pressure can be improved with atropine. Labetalol, as with other beta blockers, is synergistic with halothane in its myocardial depressant activity, and profound hypotension may be provoked,[81,82] although induced hypotension is readily controlled by adjusting the halothane concentration.

### Antidysrhythmic Agents

**Lignocaine** (Lidocaine USP) is used primarily in the treatment of ventricular dysrhythmia. Unlike quinidine and procainamide, it produces lengthening of the active potential duration[83] and no widening of the QRS complex, there being no change in heart rate or conduction velocity. In *normal therapeutic doses* there is no change in myocardial pump action.

Intravenously administered lignocaine has also been used to obtund the tachycardia and hypertension caused by intubation.[55] While Donnegan and Beford[84] failed to observe this action in barbiturate-treated patients with closed head injuries, they did demonstrate a fall in intracranial pressure which they attributed to a reduction in cerebral oxygen demand, blood flow and cerebral volume.

Due to its high lipid solubility and rapid rate of absorption, therapeutic plasma levels of lignocaine may occur after topical laryngeal spray,[85] after peritoneal dialysis, after topical application to the epicardium during open heart surgery, and following subcutaneous infiltration during neurosurgery.[86]

Lignocaine exerts a local (but not a systemic) effect on vascular smooth muscle and, in common with other local anaesthetics,[87,88] lignocaine causes localised vasodilatation after intradermal injection in direct proportion to the concentration of drug used. Aberg[89] has suggested that local anaesthetics in high concentrations relax smooth muscle by membrane stabilisation which inhibits calcium release.

Systemic toxicity from local anaesthetic agents causes, with increasing plasma concentrations, sedation, disorientation, inebriation, anxiety, restlessness, tremors, paraesthesiae and ultimately convulsions. The severe hypoxia and acidosis which can occur compound the drug-induced medullary depression and aggravate depressed myocardial function so that profound cardiovascular collapse ensues.

For therapeutic effectiveness, plasma lignocaine concentrations need to be instantly raised, and then maintained at 2–4 $\mu$g/ml. Such an effect can be produced by an intravenous bolus of 75–100 mg, followed by an infusion at the rate of 4 mg/min for 30 minutes, 2 mg/min for the next two hours and, thereafter, at 1 mg/min. The more common regime of a bolus followed by a 1 mg/min infusion will not produce therapeutic levels in under 4 hours.[90] With prolonged infusion, it is possible to reach toxic blood levels, particularly if the hepatic clearance is reduced due to a decrease in cardiac output.

**Mexiletine** is a local anaesthetic similar in structure and electrophysical properties to lignocaine. Its main use is in controlling ventricular dysrhythmias, secondary to acute or chronic myocardial ischaemia. Like lignocaine, it is highly lipid soluble and widely distributed to the tissues and, thus, for intravenous administration, a bolus followed by a high and then declining rate of infusion, is suitable.[91] The therapeutic ratio is lower, the plasma therapeutic concentration lying between 0·75–2·0 $\mu$g/ml, and the elimination half-life is longer than lignocaine, so that side-effects are not uncommon. These affect the central nervous system (drowsiness, confusion, tremor, nystagmus) and the cardiovascular system (hypotension, sinus bradycardia, conduction defects and widening of the QRS complexes). There appears to be a higher incidence of side-effects[83] in patients following myocardial infarction who have obtunded cardiac function and who may have already received other myocardial depressant therapy. The haemodynamic effects appear to depend on the pre-existing cardiovascular status of the patient and may be minimal or produce hypotension by a reduction in myocardial contractility or systemic vascular resistance. The main contra-indication to its use is in the presence of severe left heart pump failure with cardiogenic shock or bradydysrhythmias.

The advantage of mexiletine over lignocaine is that it can be administered orally as its first-pass hepatic clearance is low. Absorption can be delayed by slow gastric emptying, but normally peak plasma concentrations occur after about three hours.

**Quinidine**, an optical isomer of quinine, is a myocardial depressant with anticholinergic properties. Thus it prolongs the effective refractory period, increases the threshold potential for excitability, and reduces the conduction velocity throughout the cardiac muscle. In atrial flutter or fibrillation, the atrial rate is slowed, but its vagolytic effect on the AV node may produce a "paradoxical" increase in ventricular rate in the undigitalised patient. However, its main antidysrhythmic uses are for those atrial dysrhythmias which may be converted to sinus rhythm. Ventricular ectopics may be controlled and it is occasionally of benefit in suppressing intractable ventricular fibrillation in the ischaemic heart during open-heart surgery. The ECG signs of overdosage are an increasing PR interval and widening of the QRS and T wave, with T wave inversion. Idiosyncratic and hypersensitivity reactions infrequently occur and may include cardiorespiratory collapse, central nervous system changes and immunologically-induced coagulation defects.

**Procainamide** differs from procaine in the replacement of the vulnerable ester leakage with an amide. Essentially similar in cardiac action to quinidine, it depresses cardiac output, conduction and atrial and ventricular excitability. There is less anticholinergic activity, although the heart rate may be increased. The effect on myocardial contractility is less than that of quinidine. Widening of the PR interval and QRS complexes on the ECG may be followed by complete AV block and breakthrough idioventricular beats or ectopics, leading to ventricular fibrillation. There is occasionally a fall in systemic vascular resistance, which may be additive to a reduction in cardiac output in susceptible patients. It may be given orally in doses of 500 mg to 1 g, although absorption varies enormously between individuals and renal excretion is high. Intravenously the dose is approximately 500 mg given slowly, and should be administered with full ECG and systemic arterial pressure monitoring.

**Disopyramide** is a recently introduced Class I antidysrhythmic agent that also possesses anticholinergic (atropinic) activity.[92] Many of the physiological effects on cardiac muscle are similar to those produced by procainamide and quinidine. The anticholinergic actions may cause dryness of the mouth and urinary retention and may also increase the heart rate. However, its inherent ability to depress sinus or nodal automaticity competes with the vagolytic effects and may account for the inconsistencies in some of its reported actions.[83] In the normal heart, disopyramide tends to provoke a tachycardia whilst having no effect on AV conduction. In cardiac disease, conduction defects are often further impaired by disopyramide. A negative inotropic effect can be demonstrated particularly in the abnormal myocardium. This may be associated with an increase in systemic and coronary vascular resistance that is attributed to a direct drug effect. The main indications for its use are in the treatment and prophylaxis of ventricular dysrhythmias, especially those provoked by myocardial ischaemia, or those resistant to other antidysrhythmic therapy. Supraventricular dysrhythmias are less effectively and less predictably suppressed with disopyramide. The oral dose is 100 mg, 6-hourly, and intravenous dosage 50 mg given slowly, or by infusion 10 mg/hour. The elimination half-life after intravenous administration is between 4 and 8 hours.

**Bretylium tosylate.**—Bretylium was introduced as an antihypertensive agent in 1959 and was subsequently shown to have potent antidysrhythmic properties, especially in the management of ventricular dysrhythmias following acute myocardial ischaemia and infarction. Its mechanisms of action seem to vary with the dose and duration of exposure to the drug. In lower concentrations there is an increase in rate and conduction velocity and a reduction in the effective refractory period. At higher concentrations, its antidysrhythmic properties are due to an inhibition of adrenergic neurotransmitter release and a direct effect on the electrophysiology of heart muscle which prolongs the duration of the action potential and increases the effective refractory period.[83] It appears that bretylium is effective in the infarcted heart by reducing the disparity in action potential duration between the infarcted and normal myocardium, thus reducing the propensity to ventricular tachydysrhythmia. Its antihypertensive effect is similar to that of guanethidine in preventing adrenergic noradrenaline release and will obtund effects due to indirectly acting sympathomimetics such as amphetamine. Hypotension, which may also be postural, may be controlled by noradrenaline or volume infusion.

### Calcium Antagonists

**Verapamil**, a class IV antidysrhythmic agent, is a synthetic derivative of papaverine, and hence has vasodilator properties on both the peripheral and coronary vasculature. Clinically its major use lies in the treatment of supraventricular dysrhythmias, an effect due to its actions on transmembrane calcium flux. The action on the phase IV depolarisation in the SA node, together with a depressant effect on AV nodal function reduces atrioventricular conduction, and slows the ventricular rate in atrial fibrillation and flutter and in nodal re-entry supraventricular tachycardia.[83] Myocardial function is depressed by the impairment of calcium ionic flux but this can be reversed with calcium or glucagon. The total haemodynamic change will also be influenced by changes in systemic arteriolar tone and reflex alteration in heart rate and cardiac output.

**Nifedipine**, like verapamil, is a calcium antagonist that has smooth muscle vasodilator properties. It is a potent coronary artery dilator and is useful in angina associated with coronary artery spasm. It has much less effect than verapamil on the A-V node and is of no use in the treatment of supraventricular dysrhythmias, although dysrhythmias may diminish subsequent to an improvement of myocardial oxygen supply/demand ratio in the ischaemic heart. Its main action to reduce systemic arteriolar resistance has led to its use in hypertension, angina and pulmonary oedema.[93] The absence of much effect on the atrioventricular conduction may make it a suitable alternative to the use of $\beta$-adrenergic blockade when this is contra-indicated.

Nifedipine is administered orally, but not intravenously, due to light sensitivity, in the dose 5–20 mg tds. It is well absorbed from the gastro-intestinal tract and the duration of action is 8–12 hours.

## MANIPULATION OF THE CIRCULATION

The alteration in cardiovascular variables previously described, which occur during anaesthesia and surgery, are seldom of great clinical significance in healthy patients. In patients with cardiovascular disease (discussed in the next chapter) the responses may have a much greater importance. It is also possible to produce deliberate alteration in cardiovascular variables.

The manipulation of the circulation refers either to the deliberate production of an abnormal circulatory state, as in the technique of induced hypotension for the reduction of surgical bleeding, or to a therapeutic intervention in order to improve or optimise a compromised cardiovascular system.

Correct circulatory manipulation must be preceded by an accurate assessment of the patient's circulatory state.

### Circulatory Assessment

Circulatory assessment occurs at three levels. The simplest is clinical observation when deductions about tissue and organ perfusion can be made from the appearance of the skin, its dryness, colour, peripheral temperature and the speed of capillary flow. An idea of kidney function may be taken from the urine output and of brain function from the level of consciousness. Limited information about the circulatory and respiratory system may be inferred from the cardiac rate and rhythm and the pattern of breathing. These findings may be supplemented by measurement of the blood pressure. The shape of a trace derived from intra-arterial monitoring may add to information about the cardiac output, measurement of the right atrial pressure and observation of the ECG. Although these variables, particularly of the blood pressure, pulse and central venous pressure, may enable the observer to make some estimate of circulatory change within a patient, a more complete knowledge of the circulation requires cardiac output measurement as well as pulmonary artery and left heart filling pressures. Then it is possible to calculate systemic and pulmonary arteriolar resistance and to make some estimate of the function of the two ventricles.

### Hypotension

#### Pre-operative Hypotension

The absolute value of a patient's immediate pre-operative blood pressure must be considered against the patient's general condition and knowledge, if any, of his previous blood pressure. Thus a "normal" blood pressure may represent hypotension, as may occur following a myocardial infarct in a hypertensive patient, or alternatively, a "normal" blood pressure may be being sustained only by extreme vasoconstriction when the abolition of this compensatory mechanism by anaesthesia will result in a profound fall in pressure.

The induction of anaesthesia in a patient with a naturally low systemic pressure presents no special problems beyond the normal precaution against the indiscriminate use of drugs which are likely to lower it still more. However, where for example the hypotension is the result of a fixed low-output cardiac disease, which is usually associated with vasoconstriction in the peripheral vessels, the induction of anaesthesia and the consequent peripheral vasodilatation may be fatal.

#### Hypotension during Anaesthesia and Operation

During normal sleep, blood pressure falls. In a small series of patients who had normal blood pressure when awake[94] it was demonstrated that systolic pressures of 90 or 80 mm Hg (12·0 or 10·7 kPa) were normal while asleep. Littler and his colleagues[95] investigated 18 subjects and found an almost equal fall of about 20 per cent in both systolic and diastolic pressure in normotensive, hypertensive and treated hypertensive groups although they did not elucidate the mechanism of this fall. A blood pressure lower than the pre-operative value might perhaps be considered physiological during anaesthesia. A satisfactory blood pressure is not the cardinal sign of circulatory well-being and it needs to be correlated with other physical signs in an attempt to judge the state of the circulation. The systolic blood pressure is, however, one index upon which the anaesthetist can calibrate his impression of circulatory change.[96]

Superimposed upon this physiological tendency towards hypotension during anaesthesia are other, more potent, causes of circulatory derangement which include:

(i) effects of anaesthetic agents (see p. 423)
(ii) effects of IPPV
(iii) surgical compression of vessels
(iv) posture
(v) haemorrhage
(vi) dysrhythmias.

It is essential to decide whether the final degree of hypotension is significant as, in some cases, hypotension associated with vasodilatation may actually enhance tissue perfusion provided that the cardiac output is maintained. Vasodilatation can, by a number of mechanisms, improve output (see p. 415) and, thus, moderate hypotension *per se* is not necessarily a disadvantage.

### Postoperative Hypotension

One of the most illogical situations, that to a certain extent still exists in present day anaesthesia, is the immense amount of expert skill and care that is lavished upon the patient in the operating theatre, often only to be abruptly abandoned the moment the anaesthetic is stopped. During a period when a rapid physiological transition is taking place, the patient may be submitted to major alteration in posture and environment and transported to some far corner of the hospital where, although observed for the gross complication, may not be tested for the earliest premonitory signs of them.

Hypotension (or indeed hypertension) in the postoperative period is common. Its occurrence should lead to a careful appraisal of the patient's circulation and the appropriate therapy instituted.

Probably the two commonest causes of hypotension are hypovolaemia and the residual action of anaesthetic agents—the two frequently combining. A further contributory factor may be the variations in cardiac rate and rhythm, with bradycardia being a not infrequent cause of hypotension. The amount of blood lost is frequently underestimated and in the event of postoperative hypotension the blood loss and replacement figures should be re-examined, consideration also being given to concealed losses, and the central venous pressure measured. Most patients respond to correct replacement therapy although the residual action of drugs such as halothane or morphine may result in a low pressure despite a normal blood volume. In this case, when oligaemia has been treated or excluded, moderate hypotension can be safely treated expectantly by keeping the patient flat or by raising the foot of the bed. Hypotension may be precipitated if the patient is rolled over onto his side or sat up prematurely before the return of his vascular control.

Myocardial insufficiency due to cardiac disease will produce hypotension secondary to a low cardiac output, while quite severe hypotension may follow an operation and anaesthetic if a patient fails to compensate by the normal output of adrenocortical hormones which may occur following adrenalectomy in patients on long-term steroid therapy or in prolonged or severe disease.

Unrelieved pain may cause hypotension, but before administering potentially hypotensive—narcotic—drugs other causes of hypotension should be eliminated. The essentials of postoperative care therefore are the proper relief of pain, the correct replacement of fluid and the ensuring that respiration, both oxygenation and $CO_2$ elimination, is adequate.

## Manipulation of the Compromised Circulation

Hypotension may be produced by either a reduction in cardiac output or by a reduction in systemic vascular resistance, or both. Despite the advantages of vasodilatation in the face of a normal cardiac output, arterial pressure may fall below critical perfusion levels and certain organs, such as the heart, kidney, brain and liver may be jeopardised. Logical treatment under these circumstances would be to restore or increase arteriolar resistance with a vasoconstrictor. In patients with relatively healthy cardiovascular systems, in whom the fall in arteriolar resistance is thought to be self-limiting, it may be permissible to produce an abnormal rise in cardiac output by relative overtransfusion with a crystalloid solution. The danger in this technique lies in the inappropriate rise in left atrial pressure, coinciding with a fall in plasma oncotic pressure secondary to the haemodilution. This is particularly so if reliance is being placed only on right atrial pressure monitoring, when such a situation leads to the unexpected development of pulmonary oedema.

Usually, under anaesthesia, there is also an element of myocardial depression and, if it becomes necessary to use a vasoconstrictor, it is a good general principle to use one that also has beta-agonist properties, in order to avoid the potential further impairment of contractility in the face of increased afterload.

The more common and worrying problem is when the cardiac output is reduced; this may or may not be associated with hypotension.

*The methods for increasing cardiac output are:*

1. removal of iatrogenic causative factors (e.g. enflurane-negative inotropism, surgical impairment of the circulation or inappropriately high intrathoracic pressures)
2. control of rate and rhythm
3. adjustment of ventricular preload
4. improvement of myocardial performance.

Consideration of all four possibilities proceeds simultaneously. Reduced cardiac output is particularly amenable to diagnosis and treatment during cardiac surgery when there is adequate monitoring and good access to the circulation.

**Rate and rhythm.**—Rate is one determinant of cardiac output and optimal rate in any one patient will vary. In most patients, reversal of a bradycardia with atropine, or sometimes isoprenaline, will improve cardiac output and blood pressure. In certain circumstances, too fast a rate will reduce output, for example in mitral stenosis or hypertrophic obstructive cardiomyopathy. The atrial transport mechanism plays an important part in ventricular filling. Dysrhythmias, such as nodal rhythm or atrial fibrillation, impair diastolic filling and may produce catastrophic falls in output and blood pressure in cardiac disease. The treatment of dysrhythmias is discussed on page 492.

**Alterations in ventricular preload.**—Ventricular filling pressures may be too low or too high, and are influenced by blood volume, venocapacitance tone, intrathoracic pressure, posture and myocardial function. Interpretation of central venous (right atrial) pressure in the absence of left-sided information can be difficult in left ventricular dysfunction, as a quite modest raise in right atrial pressure may result in a large increase in left atrial pressure leading to pulmonary oedema. Low-filling pressures are best managed with suitable infusions, bearing in mind that there may be an abnormal venocapacitance tone (high or low) and, therefore, the change in venous pressure in response to infusions will need to be carefully monitored. Venodilating drugs, such as nitroprusside, glyceryl trinitrate and morphine, will also influence ventricular preload. In other situations, venoconstriction with an alpha-adrenergic agonist may be required, although volume loading is the more practical approach to this problem. Venomotor tone is increased by pain, the stress response, acidosis, hypoxia and reduced cardiac output. Management of preload under these circumstances should also include treatment of the cause of the venoconstriction.

**Myocardial performance** may be impaired by a number of treatable factors which include:

1. hypoxia
2. acidosis
3. electrolyte imbalance
4. metabolic defects, e.g. diabetic acidosis
5. drugs, e.g. halothane
6. acute myocardial ischaemia
7. hypothermia.

Improvement in myocardial performance in cardiac disease is further discussed on page 483.

Direct therapeutic intervention by *inotropic therapy* is indicated when these, and all other determinants of cardiac output, are optimised. Inotropic agents are described on page 431, and the choice between them made with regard to the clinical state of the patient. Bradydysrhythmias and depressed myocardial function, for example, may be best managed with an isoprenaline infusion (1–4 $\mu$g/min) which will improve both contractility and heart rate and reduce ventricular afterload. If a tachycardia is to be avoided, or ventricular dysrhythmias are a problem, then dopamine or dobutamine may be preferable, whilst in the heavily beta-blocked and depressed myocardium, glucagon, aminophylline and calcium could prove more successful.

## HAEMORRHAGE DURING SURGERY

One of the functions of anaesthesia and the anaesthetist is to provide optimum operating conditions for the surgeon. Blood loss, by obscuring the surgical field, or even by the sheer magnitude of the loss, may make surgery difficult or even impossible and it is a part of good anaesthesia to provide as bloodless a field as possible. In the past this has too often been considered under the heading of "induced hypotension". The term "deliberate hypotension" is both misleading and poorly descriptive, because in the production of a bloodless field a specific degree of hypotension is not required. It also obscures the concept that much blood loss is venous in origin and therefore Eckenhoff[97] suggested the use of the term "circulatory control" to cover all those points of technique which are used to ensure a good operating field.

The factors which give rise to increased wound bleeding usually result from either venous engorgement, an increased cardiac output or sudden raised blood pressure.

(a) **Hypercapnia.**—In this instance, the raised carbon dioxide tension increases both the blood pressure and cardiac output by stimulation of the sympathetic nervous system whilst the capillary flow is increased by a local effect of the carbon dioxide on the vessel wall itself.

(b) **Hypoxia.**—A low arterial oxygen tension produces vasodilatation and chemoreceptor stimulation increases the cardiac output.

Anaesthesia tends to produce deleterious alterations in the lung ventilation-perfusion ratios, changes which are accentuated by reduction in blood pressure or cardiac output. The anaesthetist must compensate for these alterations, which usually implies controlled ventilation with, sometimes, an increased $F_{IO_2}$.

(c) **Respiratory obstruction.**—Besides the effect on blood oxygen and carbon dioxide levels the alterations in intrathoracic pressure can result in a raised central venous pressure. With spontaneous respiration any resistance to expiration can increase venous pressure and the amount of bleeding.

(d) **Improper posture** is the most important factor in promoting venous bleeding (see below).

(e) **Inadequate analgesia and anaesthesia** results in a raised cardiac output as a consequence of peripheral somatic stimulation causing an increase in catecholamines.

(f) **Ether and cyclopropane** both cause secretion of catecholamines and a raised cardiac output.

(g) **Very deep anaesthesia**, now seldom used, to the point of myocardial depression produces hypoxia and venous engorgement.

(h) **Certain drugs** employed in anaesthesia may produce tachycardia (gallamine, atropine) or cause hypertension (pancuronium, ketamine) both of which may increase surgical haemorrhage.

### Reduction in Blood Loss during Surgery

In seeking to reduce the amount of bleeding during surgery the first principle is to avoid those factors, discussed above, which give rise to an increase in bleeding.

The good anaesthetist thus provides unobstructed ventilatory exchange, adequate anaesthesia with full analgesia, and avoids those agents which provoke catecholamine secretion in a properly postured patient. Larson[98] in an excellent review, comments that induced hypotension must never be considered a panacea for indifferent anaesthesia but rather that anaesthesia must first be perfect in all respects and hypotension induced as a complementary measure only. This view holds true today.

Further reduction of blood supply to the operative field can then be produced in a number of different ways.

(a) *Tourniquet.*—Obviously restricted in its application but producing complete ischaemia for a limited period.

(b) *Use of local vasoconstrictor solutions.*—Used mainly for skin infiltration before operation (thyroidectomy) or topically, during eye or ear, nose and throat operations. Systemic effects produced by intravascular absorption of injected adrenaline, noradrenaline or phenylephrine, can occasionally cause hypertension or tachycardia which may offset the initial attempt to reduce bleeding.

(c) *The use of induced hypotension.*

## Induced Hypotension and Circulatory Control

The reduction of blood pressure and cardiac output must be considered together because of their interdependence. The blood pressure can be reduced by lowering the systemic vascular resistance but if the patient remains flat the cardiac output is usually unchanged or may even rise due to the reduction in afterload. Of itself, this hypotension will not necessarily produce a good operating field, but if the operative site is elevated, blood flow and loss is reduced.

Thirty years ago Enderby[99] stressed the importance of taking into account the effect on the brain of any tilt away from the horizontal. For example, the blood pressure is usually measured in the arm, with the limb on a level with the heart; if the patient is tilted into the head-up position the pressure in the arm may remain the same, but the effect of the weight of the column of blood must be taken into account on both the head and the feet. Thus, in this position, the pressure in the feet may be 180 mm Hg (24·0 kPa) or more, yet in the head it may be only 80 mm Hg (10·7 kPa).

As a general rule the difference in pressure in a particular area may be calculated on the basis of allowing + or − 2 mm Hg (0·25 kPa) for every one inch (2·5 cm) vertically below or above the level of the heart. This is one reason why posture has come to play such an important part in reducing bleeding during surgery. If the operation site is raised above the level of the heart the effect of gravity not only reduces the pressure in the arterial system but also encourages local venous emptying.

Often improved operating conditions are only produced if the hypotension is also accompanied by a reduction in cardiac output.

A reduction in cardiac output is achieved by:

(1) decreasing cardiac preload by a combination of reduction in venous tone and posture;
(2) decreasing cardiac contractility;
(3) blocking sympathetic stimulation;
(4) utilising mechanical and chemical changes of controlled ventilation.

### Reduction in Vascular Tone

As has been discussed above, a reduction in arteriolar resistance will lower blood pressure and reduce, to a certain degree, operative bleeding. The main mechanism in the control of surgical haemorrhage lies in the reduction of venous tone which, combined with suitable posture, reduces ventricular filling and cardiac output. Reduction in venous tone is achieved by ganglionic blockade, spinal or epidural analgesia, specific venodilating drugs, such as sodium nitroprusside or glyceryl trinitrate, and by the effect of some anaesthetic agents. To a varying extent, a drop in arteriolar resistance will also occur, but the means by which the circulation is largely controlled depends upon the effects on ventricular preload.

The basic mechanism of this technique results in a vascular tree which is unresponsive to the effects of low cardiac output or haemorrhage. With dilated inelastic capacitance vessels quite small blood losses can produce large alterations in the filling pressure of the heart, and thus the cardiac output. More prompt action is required than in the normal patient to raise the filling pressure by alteration in posture or by blood transfusion in the event of haemorrhage.

1. **Subarachnoid and epidural block.**—The circulatory effects of these are entirely due to their actions on the sympathetic nervous system, either by direct preganglionic sympathetic blockade, an interruption of the adrenal sympathetic nerve supply, or by sensory blockade to the operative site which obtunds the haemodynamic sympathetic response to pain. The exact mechanisms whereby surgical haemorrhage is reduced vary with the degree of block and the type of procedure, but generally rely upon hypotension produced by a reduction in systemic vascular resistance and by an impaired cardiac output following a reduction in venous capacitance tone. High thoracic block can also reduce cardiac performance which can be modified with inotropic therapy.[100] Compensatory vasoconstriction in non-blocked areas tends to modify the overall haemodynamic effects, but does not necessarily offset the regional reduction in bleeding. Indeed, other factors play an important part in controlling the surgical haemorrhage under epidural or spinal block, not the least of which is suitable posture. Marked head-down tilt during prostatectomy, for example,

encourages prostatic venous emptying with a concomitant fall in blood loss, aided by arterial hypotension. However, this position also encourages venous return and ventricular filling, attentuating the expected fall in cardiac output due to venodilatation. The value of regional block and the analgesia thus produced is extended into the postoperative period where rebound hypertension due to pain on awakening is avoided.

2. **Ganglion blockade.**—Opinions differ about the technique for induced hypotension by ganglion blockade. There are those who recommend posturing the patient for the surgical operation—even though this necessitates the use of the head-up position—before giving any hypotensive drug, and there are others who induce vasodilatation in the horizontal position and only make use of posture should it be needed to reduce the cardiac output. The latter technique is safer and to be preferred, and should normally be combined with an initial small dose of the hypotensive drug to assess the reaction of the patient.

Young, normotensive people are more resistant to induced hypotension than the aged or those with hypertension. An initial fall in blood pressure may be quickly followed by a rise to the normal level in the former; further doses of ganglion-blocking agent may then have little effect even with the aid of posture. For such people halothane or controlled respiration can assist in controlling the level of blood pressure. It is essential to have some reliable method of measuring the blood pressure and most anaesthetists, in the absence of direct intra-arterial manometry, prefer the use of the oscillotonometer. A reliable intravenous infusion is also essential.

**Hexamethonium** is usually given initially in a small intravenous test dose (10 mg) in the horizontal position before proceeding with the main injection, as occasionally a patient will be found to be hypersensitive, in which case the hypotension will be profound. Provided this is not so an intravenous dose of 25–50 mg should be given. Thereafter these doses can be repeated after five minutes if the extent of the fall in systolic pressure is not sufficient. In fit, young, healthy adults, it may be difficult to induce or maintain hypotension with hexamethonium on account of a tachycardia which often follows the use of this drug.

**Pentolinium**, or pentamethylene-1:5 bis-(1-methylpyrrolidinium hydrogen tartrate), has about five times the activity of hexamethonium bromide and a longer duration of action. The initial intravenous dose varies from 3 to 20 mg depending upon the age and physical state of the patient. Enderby[101] notes that pentolinium causes a slow fall in blood pressure, that the hypotension it produces is more easily potentiated by posture and controlled respiration than that of hexamethonium, and that a single dose is effective for up to 45 minutes and rarely leads to tachycardia. But in fact the blood pressure may take several hours to return to normal.

**Trimetaphan**, one of the short-acting thiophanium group of drugs, has a marked ganglion-blocking effect but it also has a direct vasodilator action in dogs, while its intravenous injection leads to the release of histamine. The latter could account for some of the hypotension that trimetaphan produces. The extremely short length of action of this drug is believed to be partly due to its destruction by the enzyme cholinesterase. It can be given either as a continuous steady infusion (0·5–1 mg/ml) or by the intermittent injection of 2·5 to 5 mg. Continuous infusions should be monitored carefully since it is possible to reach steady state conditions in which the blood pressure falls no further, so that an inappropriately high total dose may be given which will greatly delay recovery. Rarely it may appear from the rate of administration that the total dose of trimetaphan is likely to exceed 1 g due to the patient's resistance. Prolonged neuromuscular blockade has been described as following this dose of trimetaphan and if it appears that the patient is probably resistant (usually due to tachycardia) a $\beta$-blocker should be added or a change made to another drug.

3. **Direct vascular smooth muscle dilators.**—*Sodium nitroprusside, glyceryl trinitrate and hydralazine* are discussed on page 429.

Profound arterial hypotension is employed by some anaesthetists, but in general, good surgical conditions can be just as readily and more safely achieved by a modest reduction in blood pressure, in conjunction with good posture and correct anaesthetic technique. Vasodilators are usefully employed in order to prevent hypertension which itself can increase bleeding. Sodium nitroprusside infusion

(10–50 μg/min), by its major action on arteriolar resistance, rapidly controls blood pressure and has a short duration of action. Beta-blockade is often necessary to obtund the reflex tachycardia, but only relatively small doses need be given, for example propranolol 0·5 mg or practolol 2 mg intravenously.

Some patients, especially the young fit adult, require doses of nitroprusside that are either in excess of the recommended dose or have an insignificant effect on blood pressure. MacRae and his associates,[102] described a technique for inducing hypotension with a mixture of trimetaphan 125 mg with sodium nitroprusside 12·5 mg in 500 ml dextrose solution which was administered by intravenous infusion. True synergism between these two agents contributed to the success of this method and the extremely low total doses required.

**Glyceryl trinitrate** would be expected to be less effective as an arteriolar vasodilator, but combined with posture would be the logical agent to use for the production of venous pooling and reduced cardiac output. This approach deserves more study.

**Hydralazine** is less attractive for rapid control of the circulation because of its delay in onset and long duration of action. It may be used in doses of 5–20 mg intravenously in order to obtund hypertensive episodes as part of a total anaesthetic technique.

4. **Inhalational anaesthetics.**—Both halothane and enflurane are used as adjuvants in various hypotensive techniques. They may be used to potentiate the effects of other agents, and small alterations in their inspired concentrations can achieve fine control in blood pressure. Myocardial depression predominates with a subsequent reduction in cardiac output. Peripheral vascular effects vary and both preload and afterload may be altered depending on the individual circumstances. Distribution of flow is altered so that with halothane, for example, cutaneous vasodilatation may even increase surgical bleeding in superficial procedures. The hypotensive action of these agents are enhanced by posture, intermittent positive-pressure ventilation and beta blockade. Very occasionally, hypotension resistant to preload, afterload and rate adjustment, may only be reversed with an inotropic agent such as calcium chloride.

### Sympathetic Stimulation and Tachycardia

*Tachycardia* can be a troublesome complication of drug-induced hypotension particularly in younger fit patients in whom the tachycardia may be sufficient to prevent much fall in the blood pressure. The exact mechanism of this response is not clear. It may represent an attenuation of vagal control by the ganglion blocker or more probably be the result of carotid and aortic baroreceptor stimulation. Other causative factors are atropine premedication, gallamine used as a muscle relaxant, surgical stimulus under too light anaesthesia, and carbon dioxide retention or hypoxia. In a healthy patient the tachycardia may be troublesome only in that it prevents much fall in the blood pressure as the cardiac output tends to be maintained. In the presence of coronary artery disease or certain cardiac diseases—when induced hypotension is probably contra-indicated anyway—tachycardia in the face of a lowered blood pressure may be dangerous and must be promptly controlled.

Halothane may control tachycardia and facilitate the reduction of the blood pressure in the middle-aged and elderly but in the young and particularly in children the cardiac rate can often only be controlled by the use of β-blockade.

### β-Adrenergic Blockade During Hypotensive Anaesthesia

Propranolol[103,104] was the first drug used in this way but practolol which has a longer duration of action and is more cardioselective is often preferred. In old patients (55 years or more) these drugs are seldom necessary and when used the dose should be small (propranolol 0·25–0·50 mg; practolol 0·5–1·0 mg). There is an increasing requirement for these drugs in younger patients and the dose is increased to 1·0–2·5 mg, repeated as necessary. In children and young adults below the age of 25, Enderby[105] has recommended the slow intravenous use of both drugs (propranolol 0·035 mg/kg and practolol 0·14 mg/kg) before the production of ganglionic blockade. Oxprenolol 0·5–2 mg which, like practolol, has intrinsic sympathomimetic properties, may control rate with less effect on myocardial contractility, especially in the presence of halothane. Labetalol, which possesses both alpha- and beta-adrenergic blocking properties, reduces afterload and pulse rate. It has a short duration of action and the hypotensive effects can largely be reverted with atropine. Beta-blockers are discussed on page 434.

### Controlled Ventilation and Hypotensive Anaesthesia

Spontaneous ventilation under anaesthesia tends to be inefficient. Changes in functional residual capacity, closing volume and physiological dead space superimposed upon drug-induced respiratory depression may lead to hypoxaemia and hypercarbia. Hypotension, a reduced cardiac output and posture exacerbate the deleterious effects upon arterial oxygenation by a further increase in dead space[106] and in venous admixture.

For those reasons, most authorities consider that induced hypotension, to a significantly low level, is an indication for controlled ventilation. This has the added advantage that cardiac output can be controlled by alterations in intrathoracic pressure and that arterial gases, particularly $Paco_2$ can be optimised.

### Dangers of Induced Hypotension

The most serious complications are those involving the brain, heart and kidneys. While the circulation to these organs is usually capable of adaptation to alterations in blood pressure and cardiac output, these compensatory mechanisms may fall down in the face of abnormally low perfusion pressures. Atherosclerotic disease compromises distal flow still further in the presence of low perfusion pressures. Autoregulation of the cerebral blood vessels becomes inadequate when the mean arterial pressure falls below 60–70 mm Hg (8·0–9·3 kPa) and cerebral blood flow declines rapidly below these levels.[107] The level at which cerebral ischaemia becomes manifest depends on the patient's previous blood pressure. In conscious man, signs of ischaemia (confusion, etc.) appeared at mean arterial pressure of 29 mm Hg (3·9 kPa) in normotensive subjects, but at mean arterial pressure of 90 mm Hg (12·0 kPa) in patients with severe hypertension. Cerebral thrombosis is sometimes encountered, and this may either prolong unconsciousness, appear as a hemiplegia, or even develop after consciousness has been regained. Thrombosis of the central artery of the retina, leading to unilateral blindness, may also occur. These cerebrovascular complications are almost all confined to patients with signs of arteriosclerosis, and the few in normal patients only occur when excessive degrees of hypotension (i.e. 60 mm Hg (8·0 kPa) and below) have been produced. If the patient has been observed to have an excessive drop in blood pressure during hypotensive anaesthesia and then shows signs of a delayed return to consciousness it is advisable to assume that he is suffering from cerebral oedema and institute appropriate treatment.

Bedford[108] drew attention to the possible psychological changes that may occur in the elderly after the use of this technique. Unfortunately, such changes are known to occur even in the absence of hypotension, when old people undergo major surgical operations, and therefore it is difficult to assess the precise part played by the low blood pressure.

Other factors, such as hyperventilation and hypocarbia exacerbate cerebral hypoxia in the presence of hypotension, which may put certain groups of patients especially at risk. The effects of posture on regional arterial pressure have already been discussed.

Acute myocardial ischaemia may be provoked during hypotension, but the fact that the generalised vasodilatation reduces the work of the heart will in some measure compensate for any reduction in blood flow. This may however be offset by the development of a tachycardia. If there is any doubt about the state of the myocardium, the ECG should be monitored continuously and particular attention should be paid to those factors influencing myocardial oxygen supply and demand (see p. 416).

Oliguria suggests a renal lesion, but one of the fundamental points that must be borne in mind when assessing the complications of hypotension is that these lesions may arise from other causes such as the surgical trauma, haemorrhage, or the anaesthetic itself. The complete absence of figures on a well-controlled series of cases with and without induced hypotension makes it difficult to arrive at any definite conclusions.

Reactionary haemorrhage may arise if particular care is not taken to ligate any vessel seen to be bleeding; the use of induced hypotension does not excuse the surgeon the task of tying all bleeding-points, but by removing the persistent ooze it makes this work much easier.

McLaughlin[109] using meticulous haemostasis at the time of operation, reports an incidence of only one reactionary haemorrhage in 1,000 cases of controlled hypotensive anaesthesia.

Much depends on the rate of rise of the blood pressure in the postoperative period. In some cases only a transient fall in systemic pressure is required at particular stages of an operation as during resection of coarctation of the aorta or ligation of a big patent ductus arteriosus. Much more commonly, the beneficial effects are required for some time afterwards and a sustained fall in blood pressure with a gentle protracted return to normal values reduces the incidence of reactionary haemorrhage and haematoma formation. Postoperative rebound hypertension can be prevented by the judicious use of pentolinium, hydralazine or, sometimes, beta-blockers. However, the adequate management of pain, temperature and acidosis must also be considered.

### Indications for Induced Hypotension

In one sentence the indication for induced hypotension has been described as where the advantages are of certain benefit and likely to outweigh the accepted risks.[110] That is to say that there are no absolute indications. McLaughlin[111] has emphasised that the technique needs to be considered in relation to each patient and that both surgeon and anaesthetist must understand the implications of the technique and that if either feels incapable of mastering these, hypotension should not be induced.

The claimed benefits in induced hypotension are a reduced blood loss, thus avoiding the dangers of massive blood transfusion, a more accurate surgical technique, and in cases where large raw areas are produced, as in reconstructive surgery, better wound healing. Cancer surgery is an indication as any improvement in operating conditions may directly benefit the patient. At one time or another every operation has been advocated as suitable for induced hypotension but the decision must be made consciously each time.

### Contra-indications to Induced Hypotension

Most contra-indications are not particularly well substantiated and depend on logical thought rather than positive evidence.

Any patient with a history of myocardial ischaemia, hypertension or cerebrovascular disease is unsuitable for this technique. Sudden or profound changes in blood pressure are unwise in patients with obvious disease of any vital organ; in hepatic and renal disease, hypotension may reduce parenchymal perfusion to critically low levels and precipitate acute organ failure. Diabetes, asthma and pre-existing neurological disease have been cited as contra-indications.

Conditions which interfere with the transport of oxygen, such as anaemia, respiratory insufficiency, hypovolaemia and cardiac failure, are all contra-indications. Obstructive airway disease is probably also a contra-indication as the high inflation pressures required may severely reduce the cardiac output. Due to the need for special postoperative care (see below) absence of good immediate postoperative supervision may well be a contra-indication.

### Postoperative Care after Induced Hypotension

To avoid the danger of reactionary haemorrhage, blood pressure is usually allowed to rise gently, although the return to consciousness normally causes some elevation. If the cardiac output and blood pressure are low, pain and restlessness may increase the body oxygen demand above the level of supply, a situation which is aggravated by respiratory obstruction or lung dysfunction in a patient breathing air.

With a vascular system still unresponsive to haemorrhage quite small blood losses will result in acute drops in blood pressure. Blood loss and replacement need to be as carefully monitored and controlled, using central venous pressure measurement if necessary, as they were during the operation.

Combining the results of 16 papers representing 13,264 cases of induced hypotension, 110 deaths (97·3 per cent of the total deaths) were reported to have occurred in the post-operative period.[98]

### Discussion

The arguments for and against induced hypotension,[112,113] have continued unabated since its introduction. Many feel that this technique only adds an unjustifiable risk to the patient's life and intellectual capacity. Others argue that in skilled hands it carries no great risk. Wyman[114] reported on its use in 1,000 patients with 5 deaths. Two were believed to be due to the patient's disease and three to faulty technique. If the technique is understood he claims it should not offer any additional risks at an operation. Larson[98] in a comprehensive review of controlled hypotension points out that though the complication risk is higher than normal, in skilled hands a very high degree of proficiency with a low morbidity can be obtained. Among the factors which he lists as militating against success are inexperience with the technique and lack of teamwork between surgeon and anaesthetist. The best results are obtained by careful selection of patients, control of ventilation, sustained gentle changes in blood pressure, the careful maintenance of blood volume and adequate postoperative care.

One of the great difficulties in assessing results is that like is not always compared with like. Ideally, we should consider operations with and without hypotension performed by the same surgeon and anaesthetist, using the same technique for blood loss measurement and replacement, but, as was discussed at the start of this chapter, the aim of the technique is to produce good operating conditions by reducing haemorrhage and with so many other factors influencing wound bleeding there is no constant relationship between blood pressure and the amount of haemorrhage. As Eckenhoff[97] has pointed out, there is very little data on the surgical benefits of hypotension so it is hard to know how much one can offset an increased morbidity.

Figures for mortality and morbidity need to be accepted with caution. If some of the early large series are examined in the light of current thought about technique, about monitoring of blood loss and blood replacement, about the relationship of flow and pressure, about proper selection of cases and postoperative care, then one may arrive at quite different conclusions from the original authors.

Eckenhoff and his colleagues[115] have compared 18 patients undergoing hypotension with 18 patients operated on at normal pressures and have been unable to show any change in brain function as demonstrated by psychometric testing. This study was on young patients but Rollason and colleagues[116] reached a similar conclusion in a group of elderly men undergoing prostatectomy. In another comparison involving 301 patients Eckenhoff and Rich[117] demonstrated an appreciable saving in blood loss with no death directly attributable to deliberate hypotension.

Later, Rollason and associates[118] compared mental function assessed by psychometric tests in elderly patients who were given spinal anaesthesia with or without a vasopressor to prevent hypotension and could find no difference.

Lindop[119] using pooled data found an incidence of non-fatal complications of 1 in 39, and of fatal complications of 1 in 167 cases, although he added a rider that no conclusion could be drawn as to whether these complications were directly caused by the hypotensive technique. However, unreported personal series by anaesthetists with much experience of the technique suggest a low complication rate is attainable.

The final assessment and decision on the use of induced hypotension must rest with a balance of the relative risks and merits to a particular patient. The size of that risk depends on the state of that patient's vascular tree, the degree of hypotension attained, and the skill of the administrator. It would be unwise however, to dismiss completely a most useful adjunct to the anaesthetist's armamentarium, but it is imperative to proceed with circumspection.

Finally, we must consider whether induced hypotension to pressures that leave little margin for safety is really essential in order to provide good surgical conditions. There are a few, usually highly specialised, circumstances (e.g. intracranial aneurysmectomy) where severe hypotension is necessary. A safer and more physiological approach to the control of the circulation is appropriate for the majority of surgical procedures that require attenuation of blood loss. Moderate reduction in pressure, cardiac output and heart rate, combined with adequate ventilation and a sensible anaesthetic technique, provide the required conditions in most cases.

## MANIPULATION OF THE CIRCULATION FOR MICROVASCULAR SURGERY

Microvascular surgery (excluding neurosurgical procedures) is a relatively new technique which involves the transplanting of a free graft of skin or bone, together with its blood vessels, to a new site and the anastomosing of its vessels to the local blood supply. It has also been employed in the repair of amputated limbs or other extremities and involves the anastomosis of very small vessels under an operating microscope. Conventional anaesthetic management includes the use of epidural, and hence sympathetic, blockade in order to promote peripheral vasodilatation. However, small vessel spasm is still easily induced by surgical manipulation, acidosis and hypothermia which combine to make anastomoses technically difficult. The procedures frequently take many hours to perform and may be associated with appreciable fluid and blood loss.

These problems have led to a reappraisal of the anaesthetic management[120] which involves the manipulation of the circulation aimed at enhancing peripheral flow and avoiding microvascular spasm by the use of smooth muscle vasodilators.

Peripheral vasoconstriction is minimised by the control of temperature and arterial blood gases during a balanced neurolept-anaesthetic technique. Core temperature is maintained at 37° C using an efficient humidifier and warming mattress. The $Paco_2$ is kept near normal by adjusting ventilation and monitoring end-tidal $Paco_2$; metabolic acidosis, if it occurs, is treated with sodium bicarbonate. Regional blockade with local anaesthesia is not employed, but intrathecal morphine is administered for the prevention of postoperative vasoconstriction due to pain. During the micro-anastomoses, sodium nitroprusside is infused via a central line with a view to promoting arteriolar vasodilatation, and the arterial pressure is monitored from a radial artery cannula. Under those circumstances cardiac output, and hence tissue perfusion, is enhanced, provided that the ventricular filling pressures are maintained. Only a moderate fall in systemic pressure is allowed, as is a relative tachycardia, which helps the increase in cardiac output. Unlike vasodilatation induced in other surgical manoeuvres, here it is provided to *increase* operative blood flow. Blood loss is initially replaced with colloid (plasma) as the fall in PCV and viscosity will enhance graft blood flow, but too much crystalloid may encourage graft oedema. For this reason, dexamethasone and mannitol may also be given. The sodium nitroprusside infusion is continued until the operation is completed. During the immediate post-operative phase, significant vasoconstriction seems not to occur as the properly managed patient is optimally warm, pain free, well perfused and awake.

Using this aggressive technique, many of the undesirable side-effects of prolonged surgery are avoided, small vessel spasm eliminated and free graft survival appears to be enhanced.

## REFERENCES


1. Mayer, S. E. (1980). Chapter in *The Pharmacological Basis of Therapeutics*, 6th edit. ed by Goodman, A., Goodman, L. S. and Gilman, A. New York: Macmillan Publishing Co.
2. Kaplan, J. A., and King, S. B. (1976). The precordial electrocardiographic lead ($V_5$) in patients who have coronary-artery disease. *Anesthesiology*, **45**, 570.
3. Drop, L. J. and Cullen, D. J. (1980). Comparative effects of calcium chloride and calcium gluceptate. *Brit. J. Anaesth.*, **52**, 501.
4. Scheidegger, M. D. and Drop, L. J. (1979). The relationship between duration of Q-T interval and plasma ionised concentration. *Anesthesiology*, **51**, 143.
5. Fahmy, N. R. and Lappas, D. G. (1979). Intravenous calcium chloride and the coagulation—fibrinolytic system. *Anesthesiology*, **51**, S117.
6. Bull, J. and Band, D. M. (1980). Calcium and cardiac arrest. *Anaesthesia*, **35**, 1066.
7. Krasner, B. S., Girdwood, R. and Smith, H. (1981). The effect of slow releasing magnesium chloride on the $QT_c$ interval of the electrocardiogram during open heart surgery. *Canad. Anaesth. Soc. J.*, **28**, 329.
8. Westhorpe, R. N., Varghese, Z., Petrie, A., Willis, M. R. and Lumley, J. (1978). Changes in ionised calcium and other plasma constituents associated with cardiopulmonary bypass. *Brit. J. Anaesth.*, **50**, 951.
9. Krasner, B. S. (1979). Cardiac effects of magnesium with special reference to anaesthesia: a review. *Canad. Anaesth. Soc. J.*, **26**, 181.
10. Sanchez, M. G. and Finlayson, D. C. (1978). Dynamics of serum potassium change during acute respiratory alkalosis. *Canad. Anaesth. Soc. J.*, **25**, 495.
11. Hassan, H. (1979). Hypercapnia and hyperkalaemia. *Anaesthesia*, **34**, 897.
12. Wong, K. C., Kawamura, R., Hodges, M. R. and Sullivan, S. P. (1977). Acute intravenous administration of potassium chloride to furosemide pre-treated dogs. *Canad. Anaesth. Soc. J.*, **24**, 203.
13. Browning, J. J. and Channer, K. S. (1981). Hyperkalaemic cardiac arrhythmia caused by potassium citrate mixture. *Brit. med. J.*, **283**, 1366.
14. Reves, J. G., Samuelson, P. N. and Lewis, S. (1979). Medazolam maleate induction in patients with ischaemic heart disease—haemodynamic observations. *Canad. Anaesth. Soc. J.*, **26**, 402.
15. Samuelson, P. N., Reves, M. D., Kouchoukos, N. T.,

Smith, L. R. and Dole, K. (1980). Midazolam versus diazepam: haemodynamic comparison. *Anesthesiology*, **53**, S9.
16. Criado, A., Maseda, J., Navarro, E., Escarpa, A. and Avello, F. (1980). Induction of anaesthesia with etomidate: haemodynamic study of 36 patients. *Brit. J. Anaesth.*, **52**, 803.
17. Colvin, M. P., Savege, T. M., Newland, P. E., Weaver, E. J. M., Waters, A. F., Brookes, J. M. and Inniss, R. (1979). Cardiorespiratory changes following induction of anaesthesia with etomidate in patients with cardiac disease. *Brit. J. Anaesth.*, **51**, 551.
18. Watkins, J. (1979). Anaphylactoid reactions to intravenous substances. *Brit. J. Anaesth.*, **51**, 51.
19. Spotoft, H., Korshin, J. D., Sorenson, M. B., Skovsted, P. (1979). Cardiovascular haemodynamics after induction of anaesthesia with althesin in patients with valvular heart disease. *Canad. Anaesth. Soc. J.*, **26**, 468.
20. Spotoft, H., Korshin, J. D., Sorenson, M. B., Skovsted (1979). The cardiovascular effects of ketamine used for induction of anaesthesia in patients with valvular heart disease. *Canad. Anaesth. Soc. J.*, **26**, 463.
21. Johnstone, M. (1976). The cardiovascular effects of ketamine in man. *Anaesthesia*, **31**, 893.
22. Philbin, D. M., Moss, J., Akins, C. W., Rosow, C. E., Kono, K., Schneider, R. C., Verlee, T. R. and Savarese, J. J. (1981). Use of $H_1$ and $H_2$ histamine antagonists with morphine anaesthesia: a double-blind study. *Anesthesiology*, **55**, 292.
23. Priano, L. L. and Vatner, S. F. (1981). Generalised cardiovascular and regional effects of meperidine in conscious dogs. *Anesth. Analg. Curr. Res.*, **60**, 649.
24. Hicks, H. C., Mowbray, A. G., Yhap, E. O. (1981). Cardiovascular effects of and catecholamine responses to high dose fentanyl—$O_2$ for induction of anaesthesia in patients with ischaemic coronary artery disease. *Anesth. Analg. Curr. Res.*, **60**, 563.
25. Prakash, O., Verdouw, J. D., de Jong, J. W., Meij, S. H., Van Der Borden, S. G., Dhasmana, K. H. and Saxena, P. R. (1980). Haemodynamic and biochemical variables after induction of anaesthesia with fentanyl and nitrous oxide in patients undergoing coronary artery surgery. *Canad. Anaesth. Soc. J.*, **27**, 223.
26. Van der Vusse, G. J., Van Belle, H., Van Gerven, W., Kruger, R. and Reneman, R. S. (1979). Acute effect of fentanyl on haemodynamics and myocardial carbohydrate utilisation and phosphate release during ischaemia. *Brit. J. Anaesth.* **51**, 927.
27. Stanley, T. H., Philbin, D. M. and Coggins, C. H. (1979). Fentanyl-oxygen anaesthesia for coronary artery surgery: cardiovascular and antidiuretic hormone responses. *Canad. Anaesth. Soc. J.*, **26**, 168.
28. Comstock, M. K., Carter, J. G., Moyers, J. R. and Stevens, W. C. (1981). Rigidity and hypercarbia associated with high dose fentanyl induction of anaesthesia. *Anaesth. Analg. Curr. Res.*, **60**, 362.
29. Milne, L., Williams, N. E., Calven, T. N., Murray, G. R. and Chan, K. (1980). Plasma concentrations and metabolism of phenoperidene in man. *Brit. J. Anaesth.*, **52**, 537.
30. Prys-Roberts, C. and Kelman, G. R. (1967). The influence of drugs used in neuroleptanalgesia on cardiovascular and ventilatory function. *Brit. J. Anaesth.* **39**, 134.
31. Green, D. W. (1981). Severe cardiovascular collapse following phenoperidene. *Anaesthesia*, **36**, 617.
32. Quintin, L., Whalley, D. G., Wynands, J. E. Morin, J. E. and Mayer, R. (1981). Oxygen–high dose fentanyl—droperidol anesthesia for aortocoronary bypass surgery. *Anesth. Analg. Curr. Res.*, **60**, 412.
33. Curran, J., Crowley, M. and O'Sullivan, G. (1980). Droperidol and endotracheal intubation. *Anaesthesia*, **35**, 290.
34. Domenach, J. S., Garcia, R. C., Sasiain, J. M. R., Loyola, A. Q. and Oroz, J. S. (1976). Pancuronium bromide: an indirect sympathomimetic agent. *Brit. J. Anaesth.*, **48**, 1143.
35. Kumar, S. M., Kothary, S. P. and Zsigmond, E. K. (1978). Effect of pancuronium on plasma-free norepinephrine and epinephrine in adult cardiac surgical patients. *Acta Anaesth. Scand.*, **22**, 423.
36. Kreul, J. F. and Atlee, J. L. (1979). Pancuronium enhances A-V conduction in anaesthetised dogs. *Anesthesiology*, **51**, S.86.
37. Lee, C., Yang, E. and Lippmann, M. (1980). Constrictive effect of pancuronium on capacitance vessels. *Brit. J. Anaesth.*, **52**, 261.
38. Stoelting, R. K. (1972). The haemodynamic effects of pancuronium and *d*-tubocurarine in anesthetized patients. *Anesthesiology*, **36**, 612.
39. Moss, J., Rosow, C. E. Savarese, J. J., Philbin, D. M. and Kniffen, K. J. (1981). Role of histamine in the hypotensive action of *d*-tubocurarine in humans. *Anesthesiology*, **55**, 19.
40. Heinonen, J. and Yrjölä, H. (1980). Comparison of haemodynamic effects of metocurine and pancuronium in patients with coronary artery disease. *Brit. J. Anaesth.*, **52**, 931.
41. Pauca, A. L. and Skovsted, P. (1981). Cardiovascular effects of pancuronium in patients anaesthetised with enflurane and halothane. *Canad. Anaesth. Soc. J.*, 28, 39.
42. Wilkinson, P. L., Hamilton, W. K., Moyers, J. R. Graham, B. G., Ports, T. A., Ullyot, D. J. and Chaterjee, K. (1981). Halothane and morphine—nitrous oxide anesthesia in patients undergoing coronary artery bypass operation. *J. Thorac. cardiovasc. surg.*, **82**, 372.
43. Cockings, E., Prasad, K., Bharadivaj, B. and O'Neil, C. L. (1980). Effects of enflurane on cardiovascular function in dogs with induced chronic mitral valve disease. *Brit. J. Anaesth.*, **52**, 1087.
44. Shimosato, S., Iwatsuki, N. and Carter, J. G. (1979). Cardio-circulatory effects of enflurane anaesthesia in health and disease. *Acta anaesth. Scand.* Suppl. **71**, 69.
45. Smith, G., Rogers, K. and Thorburn, J. (1980). Halothane improves the balance of oxygen supply to demand in acute experimental myocardial ischaemia. *Brit. J. Anaesth.*, **52**, 577.
46. Behrenbeck, T., Nugent, M., Quash, A., Koffman, E., Ritman, E. and Tinker, J. (1980). Halothane and ischaemic regional myocardial wall dynamics. *Anesthesiology*. **53**, S, 140.
47. Shutt, L. E. and Bowes, J. B. (1979). Atropine and hyoscine. *Anaesthesia*, **34**, 476.
48. Mirakhur, R. K. (1979). Intravenous administration of glycopyrronium. Effects on cardiac rate and rhythm. *Anaesthesia*, **34**, 458.
49. Lunn, J. K., Stanley, T. H., Webster, L. R. and Bidwai, A. V. (1979). Arterial blood-pressure and pulse rate

responses to pulmonary and radial artery catheterisation prior to cardiac and major vascular operations. *Anesthesiology*, **51**, 265.

50. Waller, J. L., Zaiden, J. R., Kaplan, J. A. and Bozeman, R. (1980). Hemodynamic responses to vascular cannulation before coronary bypass surgery. *Anesth. Analg. Curr. Res.* **59**, 563.
51. Manners, J. M. and Walters, F. J. M. (1979). Beta-adrenoreceptor blockade and anaesthesia *Anaesthesia*, **34**, 3.
52. Coleman, A. J. and Jordan, C. (1980). Cardiovascular responses to anaesthesia. *Anaesthesia*, **35**, 972.
53. Dahlgreen, N. and Messeter, K. (1981). Treatment of stress response to laryngoscopy and intubation with fentanyl. *Anaesthesia*, **36**, 1022.
54. Abou-Madi, M., Keszler, H. and Yacoub, O. (1975). A method for prevention of cardiovascular reactions to laryngoscopy and intubation. *Canad. Anaesth. Soc. J.*, **22**, 316.
55. Abou-Madi, M., Keszler, H. and Yacoub, J. M. (1977). Cardiovascular reactions to laryngoscopy and tracheal intubation following small and large intravenous doses of lidocaine. *Canad. Anaesth. Soc. J.*, **24**, 12.
56. Editorial (1981). Artificial ventilation and the heart. *Brit. med. J.*, **283**, 397.
57. Roizen, M. F., Hamilton, W. K. and Sohn, Y. J. (1981). Treatment of stress-induced increases in pulmonary capillary wedge pressure using volatile anaesthetics. *Anesthesiology*, **55**, 446.
58. Edde, R. R. (1981). Hemodynamic changes prior to and after sternotomy in patients anesthetised with high-dose fentanyl. *Anesthesiology*, **55**, 444.
59. Cundy, J. (1980). The perioperative management of patients with polycythaemia. *Ann. Roy. Coll. Surgs.(Engl.)*, **62**, 470.
60. Rawlinson, W. A. L., Loach, A. B. and Benedict, C. R. (1978). Changes in plasma concentrations of adrenaline and noradrenaline in anaesthetised patients during sodium nitroprusside-induced hypotension. *Brit. J. Anaesth.*, **50**, 937.
61. Fan, F. C., Kim, S., Simchon, S., Chen, R. Y. Z., Schuessler, G. B. and Chien, S. (1980). Effects of sodium nitroprusside on systemic and regional hemodynamics and oxygen utilization in the dog. *Anesthesiology*, **53**, 113.
62. Vance, J. P., Brown, D. M., Smith, G. and Thorburn, J. (1979). Effect of hypotension induced with sodium nitroprusside on canine coronary arterial flow. *Brit. J. Anaesth.* **51**, 297.
63. Delaney, T. J. and Miller, E. D. (1980). Rebound hypertension after sodium nitroprusside prevented by saralasin in rats. *Anesthesiology*, **52**, 154.
64. Behnia, R., Siqueira, E. B. and Brunner, E. A. (1978). Sodium nitroprusside-induced hypotension—effect on renal function. *Anesth. Analg. Curr. Res.*, **57**, 52.
65. Pace, J. B. (1978). Pulmonary vascular response to sodium nitroprusside in anesthetized dogs. *Anesth. Analg. Curr. Res.*, **57**, 551.
66. Marshall, W. K., Bedford, R. F., Arnold, W. P., Miller, E. D., Longnecker, D. E., Sussman, M. D. and Hakala, M. W. (1981). Effects of propranolol on the cardiovascular and renin-angiotensin systems during hypotension produced by sodium nitroprusside in humans. *Anesthesiology*, **55**, 277.
67. Vesey, C. J., Cole, P. V. and Simpson, P. J. (1976). Cyanide and thiocyanate concentrations following sodium nitroprusside infusion in man. *Brit. J. Anaesth.*, **48**, 651.
68. Cole, P. (1978). The safe use of sodium nitroprusside. *Anaesthesia*, **33**, 473.
69. Opie, L. H. (1980). Drugs and the heart: II. Nitrates. *Lancet*, **1**, 750.
70. Brown, M. J. (1980). Vasodilator drugs: systemic and regional considerations. *Anaesth. Intens. Care.*, **8**, 310.
71. Tobias, M. A. (1981). Comparison of nitroprusside and nitroglycerine for controlling hypertension during coronary artery surgery. *Brit. J. Anaesth.*, **53**, 891.
72. Rubin, L. J. and Peter, R. H. (1980). Oral hydralazine therapy for primary pulmonary hypertension. *New Eng. J. Med.*, **302**, 69.
73. Hilberman, M., Maseda, J., Spencer, R. J., Derby, G. C., Jyers, B. D. and Stinson, E. B. (1980). The renal effects of dopamine and dobutamine. *Anesthesiology*, **53**, S 119.
74. Schoeppe, W. (1977). Effects of dopamine on kidney function. *Proc. roy. Soc. Med.*, **70**, Suppl. **2**, 36.
75. Scallan, M. J. K., Gothard, J. W. W. and Branthwaite, M. A. (1979). Inotropic agents. *Brit. J. Anaesth.*, **51**, 649.
76. Opie, L. H. (1980). Drugs and the heart: V. Digitalis and sympathomimetic stimulants. *Lancet*, **1**, 912.
77. Roberts, J. G. (1980). Beta-adrenergic blockade and anaesthesia with reference to interactions with anaesthetic drugs and technique. *Anaesth. Intens. Care*, **8**, 318.
78. Chung, D. C. (1981). Anaesthetic problems associated with the treatment of cardiovascular disease: II. beta-adrenergic antagonists. *Canad. Anaesth. Soc. J.*, **28**, 105.
79. Opie, L. H. (1980). Drugs and the heart. *Lancet*, **1**, 693.
80. Cope, D. H. P. and Crawford, M. C. (1979). Labetolol in controlled hypertension. *Brit. J. Anaesth.*, **51**, 359.
81. Hunter, J. M. (1979). Synergism between halothane and labetolol. *Anaesthesia*, **34**, 257.
82. Scott, D. B., Buckley, F. P., Littlewood, D. G., Macrae, W. R., Arthur, G. R. and Drummond, G. B. (1978). Circulatory effects of labetolol during halothane anaesthesia. *Anaesthesia*, **33**, 145.
83. Singh, B. N., Collett, J. T. and Chew, C. Y. C. (1980). New perspectives in the pharmacologic therapy of cardiac arrhythmias. *Progr. Cardiovasc. Dis.*, **XXII**, 243.
84. Donegan, M. F. and Bedford, R. F. (1980). Intravenously administered lidocaine prevents intracranial hypertension during endotracheal suctioning. *Anesthesiology*, **52**, 516.
85. Rosenberg, P. H., Heinonen, J. and Takasaki, M. (1980). Lidocaine concentration in blood after topical anaesthesia of the upper respiratory tract. *Acta anaesth. Scand.*, **24**, 125.
86. Kanto, J., Jalonen, J., Laurikainen, E., Nieminen, V. and Salo, M. (1980). Plasma concentrations of lidocaine (lignocaine) after cranial subcutaneous injection during neurosurgical operations. *Acta anaesth. Scand.*, **24**, 178.
87. Aps, C. and Reynolds, F. (1978). An intradermal study of the local anaesthetic and vascular effects of the isomers of bupivacaine. *Brit. J. Clin. Pharmacol.*, **6**, 63.
88. Aps, C. and Reynolds, F. (1976). The effect of concentration on vasoactivity of bupivacaine and lignocaine. *Brit. J. Anaesth.*, **48**, 1171.
89. Aberg, G. (1972). Myogenic action of local anaesthetics on smooth muscle; role of $Ca^{++}$ and cyclic AMP. *Acta Pharmac. Tox.*, **31**, Suppl. 1. 46.

90. Aps, C., Bell, J. A., Jenkins, B. S., Poole-Wilson, P. A. and Reynolds, F. (1976). Logical approach to lignocaine therapy. *Brit. Med. J.*, **1**, 13.
91. Prescott, L. F., Pottage, A. and Clements, J. A. (1977). Absorption, distribution and elimination of mexiletine. *Postgrad. Med. J.*, **53**, Suppl., 1, 50.
92. Carson, I. W., Lyons, S. M. and Shanks, R. G. (1979). Anti-arrhythmic drugs. *Brit. J. Anaesth.*, **51**, 659.
93. Opie, L. H. (1980). Drugs and the heart: III. Calcium antagonists. *Lancet*, **1**, 806.
94. Richardson, D. W., Honour, H. J., Fenton, G. W., Stott, F. N. and Pickering, G. W. (1964). Variation in arterial pressure throughout day and night. *Clin. Sci.*, **26**, 445.
95. Littler, W. A., Honour, A. J., Carter, R. D. and Sleight, P. (1975). Sleep and blood pressure. *Brit. med. J.*, **3**, 346.
96. Prys-Roberts, C. (1974). Editorial. *Anesthesiology*, **40**, 1.
97. Eckenhoff, J. E. (1966). Circulatory control in the surgical patient. *Ann. roy. Coll. Surg.*, **39**, 67.
98. Larson, A. G. (1964). Deliberate hypotension. *Anesthesiology*, **25**, 682.
99. Enderby, G. E. H. (1954). Postural ischaemia and blood pressure. *Lancet*, **1**, 185.
100. Reiz, S., Nath, S. and Rais, O. (1980). Effects of thoracic epidural block and prenalterol on coronary vascular resistance and myocardial metabolism in patients with coronary artery disease. *Acta anaesth. Scand.*, **24**, 11.
101. Enderby, G. E. H. (1954). Pentolinium tartrate in controlled hypotension. *Lancet*, **2**, 1097.
102. Macrae, W. R., Wildsmith, J. A. W. and Dale, B. A. B. (1981). Induced hypotension with a mixture of sodium nitroprusside and trimetaphan camsylate. *Anaesthesia*, **36**, 312.
103. Hellewell, J. and Potts, M. W. (1966). Propranolol during controlled hypotension. *Brit. J. Anaesth.*, **38**, 794.
104. Hewitt, P. B., Lord, P. W. and Thornton, H. L. (1967). Propranolol in hypotensive anaesthesia. *Anaesthesia*, **22**, 82.
105. Enderby, G. E. H. (1974). Pharmacological blockade. *Postgrad. med. J.*, **50**, 572.
106. Eckenhoff, J. E., Enderby, G. E. H., Larson, A., Edridge, A. and Judevine, D. E. (1963). Pulmonary gas exchange during deliberate hypotension. *Brit. J. Anaesth.*, **35**, 750.
107. Locke, G. E., Yashon, D. and Hunt, W. E. (1971). Cerebral tissue lactate in trimetaphan induced hypotension. *Amer. J. Surg.*, **122**, 818.
108. Bedford, P. D. (1955). Adverse cerebral effects of anaesthesia on old people. *Lancet*, **2**, 259.
109. McLaughlin, C. R. (1961). Hypotensive anaesthesia in plastic surgery: a surgeon's view. *Brit. J. plast. Surg.*, **14**, 39.
110. Gillies, J. (1959). In: *General Anaesthesia*, p. 55. Ed. by Evans, F. T. and Gray, T. C. London: Butterworth.
111. McLaughlin, C. R. (1966). Hypotensive anesthesia. A surgeon's view. *Anesthesiology*, **27**, 239.
112. Enderby, G. E. H. (1958). The advantages of controlled hypotension in surgery. *Brit. med. Bull.*, **14**. 49.
113. Davison, M. H. A. (1958). The disadvantages of controlled hypotension in surgery. *Brit. med. Bull.*, **11**, 52.
114. Wyman, J. B. (1953). Discussion on hypotension during anaesthesia. *Proc. roy. Soc. Med.*, **46**, 605.
115. Eckenhoff, J. E., Crompton, J. R., Larson, A. and Davies, R. M. (1969). Assessment of the cerebral effects of deliberate hypotension by psychological measurements. *Lancet*, **2**, 711.
116. Rollason, W. N., Robertson, G. S. and Cordiner, C. M. (1968). Effect of hypotensive anaesthesia on mental function in the elderly. *Brit. J. Anaesth.*, **40**, 477.
117. Eckenhoff, J. E. and Rich, J. C. (1966). Clinical experiences with deliberate hypotension. *Anesth. Analg. Curr. Res.*, **45**, 21.
118. Rollason, W. N., Robertson, G. S., Cordiner, C. M. and Hall, D. J. (1971). A comparison of mental function in relation to hypotensive and normotensive anaesthesia in the elderly. *Brit. J. Anaesth.*, **43**, 561.
119. Lindop, M. J. (1975). Complications and morbidity of controlled hypotension. *Brit. J. Anaesth.*, **47**, 799.
120. Aps, C., Plantevin, O. M., Barrett, R. F. and Walton, D. P. (1983). A logical anaesthetic approach to anaesthesia for microvascular surgery. (In preparation.)
121. Scott, D. M. T., Arthur, G. R., Boyes, R. N. and Scott, D. B. (1979). Cardiovascular effects on prenalterol H133/22 in normal man. *Brit. J. Clin. Pharmacol*, **7**, 365.
122. Tyden, H., Johansson, L. and Nystrom, S. O. (1982). The haemodynamic effects of dopamine and prenalterol in patients after cardiac valve surgery. *Acta anaesth. Scand.*, **26**, 468.
123. Hayward, R. (1983). Amrinone-promising innovation for treatment of the failing heart. *Intens. Care Med.*, **9**, 1.
124. Pontén, J., Haggendal, J., Milocco, I. and Waldenstrom, A. (1983). Long-term metoprolol therapy and neurolept-anaesthesia in coronary artery surgery: withdrawal versus maintenance of $B_1$-adrenoreceptor blockade. *Anesth. Analg.*, **62**, 380.

CHAPTER 13

# Anaesthesia and Cardiac Disease



CARDIAC disease covers a wide spectrum of both anatomical and physiological disturbance. How cardiac disease affects and is affected by anaesthesia and surgery is discussed in the following pages. However, the basic principles for successful management of cardiac patients derive, in the first place, from a proper understanding of the haemodynamic effects and complications of the patient's lesion. The anaesthetist needs, therefore, to be able to diagnose the lesion and to assess correctly the effects that it has on the patient's haemodynamic state.

## THE ASSESSMENT OF THE PATIENT WITH CARDIAC DISEASE

**Objects.**—The main objects in the assessment of patients with cardiac disease are:

(a) to determine the capability of the heart and circulation to withstand the stresses which accompany anaesthesia and surgery, not only during the operative period but equally in the post-operative period;

(b) to make a logical choice of anaesthetic techniques and supportive therapy, based on an understanding of the patient's haemodynamic state.

**Diagnosis.**—Assessment involves firstly the diagnosis of the nature and severity of the specific lesion present. From this the haemodynamic consequences and likely complications can be predicted and therefore sought. The complications of a lesion are often more important than the actual disease itself.

An assessment, therefore, includes consideration of:

(a) the state of the myocardium—which may be shown by low cardiac output, congestive cardiac failure, or by the occurrence of dysrhythmias;

(b) the state of the vessels—particularly in respect of the cerebral, renal and peripheral vessels, coronary arteries or the presence of systemic hypertension;

(c) the condition of the lungs—both the ventilatory function which may be impaired by pulmonary oedema, chronic bronchitis and emphysema, and the pulmonary vascular tree in which pulmonary arterial obstructive disease can occur;

(d) the function of other organs—particularly of the liver and kidneys—which may be affected by tricuspid valve disease, venous engorgement or a low cardiac output.

(e) neurological function which may be obtunded by atherosclerotic disease, emboli, or chronic low cardiac output.

**Clinical assessment.**—A thorough history and clinical examination of the patient will provide most of the information needed in the assessment of the fitness of patients to withstand the operation and post-operative period.

### Observation of the Patient

The important part of assessment is in the evaluation of the functional status of the circulation, rather than in establishing the fine points of cardiological diagnosis. A simple estimation of what the patient can do is valuable. The ability to carry out housework normally in the case of a woman, to climb a flight of stairs without stopping, to walk up a hill or even to dress, in some measure gives an indication of whether or not the heart can increase its output in response to demand.

### Symptoms

The symptoms of cardiac disease result from physiological disturbances. The likely symptoms can be predicted if the diagnosis is known and the patient specifically questioned for them. The haemodynamic alterations, their causative factors and the resulting symptoms are:

**Angina.**—Angina is due to an imbalance between myocardial oxygen supply and demand and is the pain produced by myocardial ischaemia. This may follow narrowing of the coronary arteries, severe anaemia, thyrotoxicosis, or increased myocardial demands for oxygen which exceed the supply, as may occur in the hypertrophic ventricle of aortic stenosis or in the rapid heart rates of paroxysmal tachycardia. There are four major features of anginal pain:

i. it is situated maximally behind the sternum or across the front of the chest:
ii. the pain is described as "crushing" or as a "tight constricting sensation";
iii. it radiates characteristically to the angle of the jaw and down the inside of the left arm, but may also spread into the shoulders and neck and down the other arm to the hand;
iv. the pain comes on during exertion, anger or excitement, and is exacerbated by cold weather. When the stimulus is discontinued the pain wears off in two to three minutes or is relieved by glyceryl trinitrate.

**Dyspnoea.**—Dyspnoea is a common symptom of cardiac disease and is usually the result of a raised pulmonary venous pressure. Rises of pressure in the left atrium and pulmonary veins are transmitted back to the pulmonary capillaries increasing the transudation of fluid from the capillaries into the interstitial tissues of the lungs. These spaces drain via the lymphatics which can be seen to be engorged both at operation and in the chest x-ray (Kerley's lines). The excess fluid reduces compliance, increases

13/Table 1
Symptoms in Cardiovascular Disease

| *Abnormality* | *Causes* | *Symptoms* |
|---|---|---|
| 1. Raised left atrial pressure | left ventricular failure<br>mitral valve disease<br>aortic valve disease | dyspnoea<br>cough<br>recurrent bronchitis<br>haemoptysis<br>palpitations |
| 2. Raised systemic venous pressure | tricuspid valve disease<br>constrictive pericarditis<br>right heart failure<br>secondary to:<br>lung disease<br>pulmonary hypertension<br>pulmonary stenosis<br>left heart failure | hepatic pain:<br>symptoms related to<br>peripheral oedema<br>ascites |
| 3. Low cardiac output | ventricular failure<br>mitral stenosis<br>aortic stenosis<br>obstructive cardiomyopathy<br>pulmonary hypertension<br>constrictive pericarditis<br>pulmonary stenosis<br>heart block | fatigue<br>syncope<br>palpitations<br>dyspnoea<br>weight loss |
| 4. Dysrhythmias | myocardial ischaemia<br>ventricular failure<br>atrial distension<br>electrolyte disturbances<br>digoxin<br>ventricular hypertrophy<br>mitral valve disease<br>congenital | palpitations<br>syncope |
| 5. Myocardial ischaemia | coronary artery disease<br>coronary spasm<br>aortic regurgitation<br>aortic stenosis<br>tachydysrhythmias<br>ventricular hypertrophy | angina<br>palpitations<br>syncope<br>dyspnoea |

respiratory work and may reduce arterial oxygenation.

Orthopnoea and paroxysmal nocturnal dyspnoea are specific types of dyspnoea. Orthopnoea is dyspnoea which occurs when lying flat and which is relieved by sitting up. Paroxysmal nocturnal dyspnoea is orthopnoea which wakens the patient from sleep forcing him to sit upright or stand out of bed for relief. In either case the effect is due to the increased output from the right heart secondary to the increased right atrial pressure in the horizontal position. The left ventricle is unable to cope with the increased supply of blood, so the left ventricular end-diastolic, left atrial and pulmonary capillary pressures rise.

Should the pressure in the pulmonary veins rise above the plasma oncotic pressure pulmonary oedema will occur; dyspnoea is then acute and is accompanied by a cough and copious pink or white frothy sputum. The adoption of the upright position lowers the right atrial pressure which in turn diminishes the right ventricular output and leads to a decrease in pulmonary congestion and consequently ventilation becomes easier with less dyspnoea. Chronic congestion leads to fibrosis in the interstitial tissue of the lung between the alveoli and the capillaries, and tends to prevent transudation into the alveoli so that frank pulmonary oedema is less evident at this stage. Pulmonary oedema is therefore more readily provoked early in the progress of cardiac disease and can be precipitated by the stress of effort or emotion or by the onset of uncontrolled atrial fibrillation or tachycardia.

Useful information about the severity of heart disease is obtained by grading the severity of the dyspnoea:

Grade 1. Dyspnoea while undertaking unusual exertion (running, walking up hill, scrubbing).
Grade 2. Dyspnoea on normal exertion: moderate walking on the level causing breathlessness.
Grade 3. Dyspnoea on minimal exertion: unable to continue walking, even slowly, on the level. All but the lightest housework has to be given up.
Grade 4. Dyspnoea at rest: the patient is practically confined to bed by dyspnoea.

A history of nocturnal dyspnoea or acute pulmonary oedema places the patient in grade 4 irrespective of effort tolerance. Dyspnoea may also occur in conditions which give rise to a low cardiac output when tissue anoxia may be responsible for mild dyspnoea. Breathlessness on exertion is present in all right-to-left intracardiac shunts as the reduced oxygen content of the arterial blood stimulates the chemoreceptors at the carotid body. Dyspnoea occurring in patients with cardiac disease may also be due to some incidental lung disease.

**Cough** may be precipitated by a rise in pulmonary venous pressure during exertion, causing engorgement of the bronchial mucosa. This gives rise to a troublesome dry cough. Recurrent bronchitis is a common symptom of raised left atrial pressure or increased pulmonary blood flow.

**Haemoptysis.**—Haemoptysis is an important symptom in cardiac disease. It commonly occurs from the rupture of a small engorged vein in conditions which give rise to a raised left atrial pressure. The source of bleeding may be a pulmonary infarct and haemoptysis is common in chronic bronchitis. The patient may also describe "coughing up blood" when suffering from acute pulmonary oedema.

**Palpitations.**—This is a commonly used term for any awareness of an irregular heart beat, for example ventricular ectopic beats. Sudden fast palpitations may represent the onset of an attack of paroxysmal tachycardia or of atrial fibrillation.

**Syncope.**—Fainting occurs when cerebral perfusion is inadequate. This symptom arises from more than one mechanism. Syncope on effort occurs as a symptom of a low fixed cardiac output due to severe aortic or pulmonary stenosis or to mitral stenosis with severe pulmonary hypertension.

Syncope also occurs as Stokes-Adams attacks during rhythm changes, particularly at the onset of complete heart block. Sudden loss of consciousness is not uncommon in children with Fallot's tetralogy. These attacks are often precipitated by emotional stress when they are thought to be due to spasm of the infundibulum of the right ventricle. If the attack is prolonged, death may occur. Transient attacks of cerebral ischaemia may also be due to cerebrovascular disease or to emboli.

**Peripheral oedema.**—Congestive cardiac failure is one of the causes of peripheral oedema and is due to an abnormal retention of salt and water. The fluid tends to settle under the influence of gravity into the most dependent parts of the body and the patient usually complains of swollen ankles.

**Hepatic pain** follows the enlargement and distension of the hepatic capsule which is secondary to a high systemic venous pressure in right heart failure. It causes a dull ache in the epigastrium and right hypochondrium and is often aggravated by exertion which further increases the systemic venous pressure. Sustained liver engorgement and reduced cardiac output lead to hepatic dysfunction, which may lead to jaundice or coagulopathies.

**Medication history.**—It is not unusual for patients with circulatory disease to be receiving some form of medication which may influence anaesthetic and peri-operative management. A specific enquiry concerning therapy should be made with particular reference to:

(a) *Digoxin* (see p. 466). The therapeutic range is narrow and toxicity may lead to serious dysrhythmias during surgery. Hypokalaemia and hyperventilation, acidosis, hypoxia and sympathetic overactivity exacerbate digitalis-induced dysrhythmias.

(*b*) *Diuretics* (see p. 468). Chronic diuretic therapy may lead to electrolyte deficiencies and, in extreme cases, may critically reduce blood volume and ventricular filling pressures.

(*c*) *Beta blockers* (see p. 434). Withdrawal of therapy leads to more problems than the maintenance of treatment, and may occur if specific orders to administer the drug are not given, especially if it is an oral drug and the patient is fasting before anaesthesia.

(*d*) *Calcium antagonists* (see p. 437). Significant myocardial depression may occur when halogenated anaesthetics are used.

(*e*) *Anti-hypertensive drugs* (see p. 470). As with beta blockers, therapy is normally continued.

(*f*) *Warfarin*. It may be unwise to discontinue anticoagulation completely over the operative period, for example in patients with mechanical heart valve prosthesis. The prothrombin time ratio should be measured and if necessary heparin is substituted for warfarin. Fresh frozen plasma or vitamin K is occasionally required to correct coagulation deficiencies during surgery.

(*g*) *Other drugs*. Tricyclic antidepressants may predispose towards dysrhythmias and changes in arterial pressure in association with anaesthesia. Bronchodilator therapy may have to be continued intra-operatively. Diabetes is not uncommon in the elderly or in patients with ischaemic heart disease, and the appropriate peri-operative management will need to be considered (see p. 995).

(*h*) *Drug allergies*. A history of allergy or atopy must be checked. This is especially important in patients with cardiac disease who might be expected to receive a variety of drugs, including antibiotics, and who are particularly at risk should a serious drug reaction occur.

### Examination of the Patient

Examination of the cardiovascular system is carried out in a standard order so that no detail is missed. The patient is placed reclining against the pillows of the bed so that the thorax is at an angle of 45° to the horizontal and the head is supported so that the sternomastoid muscles are relaxed.

**General appearance.**—The general appearance of the patient is noted, especially emaciation which might accompany chronic heart failure, stunted growth which may be the result of congenital cyanotic heart disease, or obesity which may aggravate cardiac disease. Patients with a chronically low cardiac output have a dusty mauve flush with telangiectases on their cheeks known as a malar flush, most commonly seen in mitral valve disease complicated by pulmonary hypertension. A cool periphery with poor capillary filling may also be due to a low cardiac output.

Cyanosis indicates an excess of reduced haemoglobin in the blood and the critical distinction must be made between peripheral and central cyanosis. Peripheral cyanosis due to increased oxygen extraction by the tissues as a compensation for low cardiac output is best seen in the lobes of the ear, the nose, and in the fingers. Central cyanosis, which is caused by reduction in oxygen content of the systemic arterial blood due to intracardiac or pulmonary right-to-left shunts, is characteristically seen in warm mucous membrane, such as the tongue, lips and conjunctivae. Although clubbing of the fingers occurs with a variety of diseases, it may be seen in cyanotic heart disease, bacterial endocarditis or left atrial myxoma. Polycythaemic states may exaggerate the cyanosis.

The signs of anaemia and thyrotoxicosis are sought for as these two conditions both aggravate cardiac disease or may even precipitate cardiac failure.

**Arterial pulse.**—The arterial pulse is analysed for the four characteristics of rate, rhythm, amplitude and wave form. The brachial is a larger and more convenient artery for study than the radial, but wave form is best appreciated in the carotid. At the same time the quality of the vessel wall is noted for evidence of thickening. The main peripheral pulses are palpated to confirm their presence and to exclude the diagnosis of a coarctation of aorta. A very rapid rate is likely to lead to cardiac failure, whereas a slow rate of 60 per minute or less in the absence of heart block is the most frequent precursor of ventricular extrasystoles, and this may slow even further after anaesthetic premedication. A sinus bradycardia is common in patients who are taking beta blocking drugs. If a dysrhythmia is present it will require ECG confirmation of its type.

*Pulsus alternans* should be sought as this is good evidence of left ventricular failure. *Pulsus paradoxus* is an accentuation of the normal reduction in systemic arterial blood pressure during inspiration. This occurs either with huge swings in intrathoracic pressure (e.g. asthma or stridor) or when there is mechanical impairment of ventricular filling (e.g. tamponade and constrictive pericarditis). Two mechanisms combine to reduce left ventricular filling and output during inspiration. Firstly, right ventricular filling is enhanced with the fall in intrathoracic pressure which distorts the intraventricular septum and impairs the filling on the left side. Secondly, pulmonary venous pressure falls, effectively reducing left atrial pressure. These changes are modified or reversed during IPPV.

**Blood pressure.**—The blood pressure, systolic and diastolic, is measured with particular attention being paid to the width of the sphygmomanometer cuff which has to be appropriate to the circumference of the arm. Hypertension, and especially hypotension, are significant in cardiac disease, although the presence of normotension does not necessarily imply that the cardiac output is normal.

**Jugular venous pressure.**—The jugular venous pressure is assessed with the patient lying at 45° to the horizontal and the pulsations in the internal jugular vein are sought. The venous pulse is analysed for its height above the sternal angle and for its wave form (Fig. 1). The normal mean pressure is −5 to +3 cm of water above the sternal angle and the wave form reveals both "a" and "v" waves of approximately equal heights. A raised JVP will be apparent in right ventricular failure. The "a" and "v" waves may be replaced by fast flutter waves in atrial flutter. Large "v" waves will occur if there is tricuspid incompetence and these may be confused with "cannon waves" which will be regular if due to nodal rhythm or irregular if due to atrioventricular dissociation. A high venous pressure occurs with cardiac tamponade (note the systolic descent) and constrictive pericarditis (note the post-systolic descent). Non-pulsatile veins may simulate a raised central venous pressure

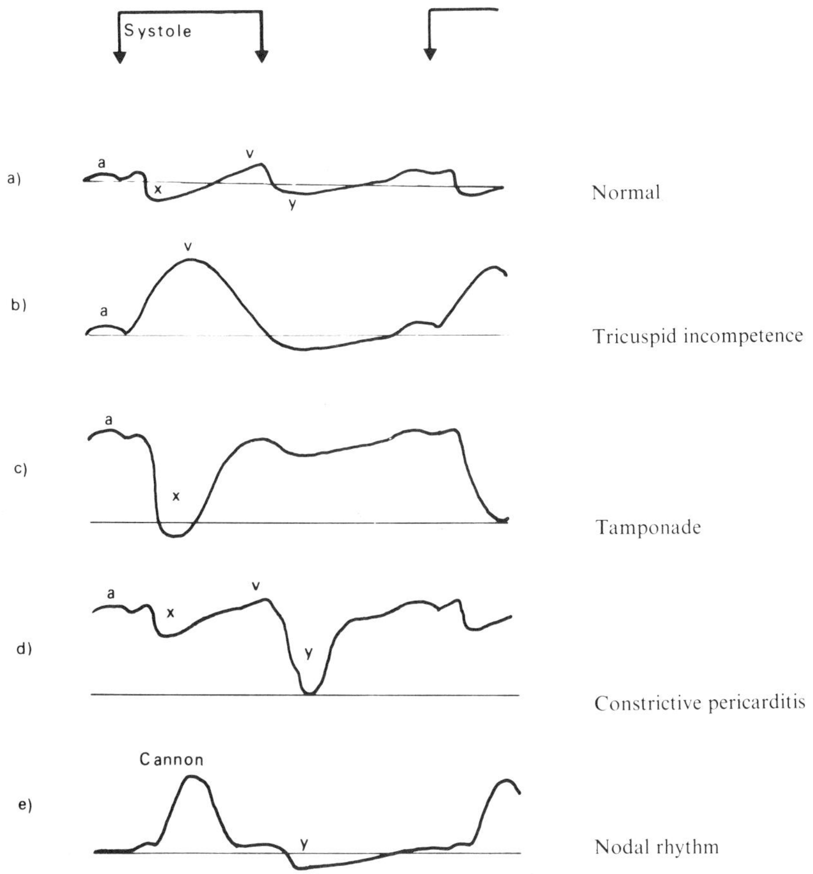


13/Fig. 1.—Characteristic jugular venous wave forms.

and result from superior vena caval obstruction, perhaps due to bronchial or thyroid carcinomas.

**Cardiac palpation.**—The most reliable evidence of cardiac enlargement comes from the chest radiograph, but a good estimate of the heart size can be made by palpating the apex beat which should lie in the fifth intercostal space within the mid-clavicular line. Apex beats outside these boundaries indicate cardiac enlargement provided the heart is not displaced by pulmonary disease or thoracic deformity. The characteristic of the apical impulse is assessed to estimate left ventricular hypertrophy while the left sternal edge is palpated with the flat of the hand to assess right ventricular hypertrophy. Loud murmurs may be felt as palpable vibrations (thrills) which are maximal where the murmur is loudest. Loud heart sounds can also be felt—in mitral stenosis the loud first sound (the tapping impulse) and the second sound in the pulmonary area if the pulmonary arterial pressure is raised.

**Cardiac auscultation.**—In each area the appropriate heart sound is listened to individually and separately and additional heart sounds—ejection click, opening snap, third and fourth heart sounds—are sought. When the timing and characteristics of the heart sounds have been clearly established, murmurs are sought. A full description of any murmur includes its timing—systolic or diastolic (Fig. 2), the site of its maximal intensity and conduction, its loudness and quality, and the influence on it of respiration. Mitral murmurs are heard loudest in the region of the apex beat with the patient turned on the left side with the breath held in expiration. Tricuspid murmurs are localised to the fourth left interspace at the sternal edge and are accentuated by inspiration which increases flow across the valve. Aortic murmurs are heard loudest in the aortic area, at the apex and over the carotid arteries in the neck. The diastolic murmur of aortic regurgitation is heard at the left sternal edge during full expiration with the patient leaning forward. Sounds from the pulmonary valve are usually localised and

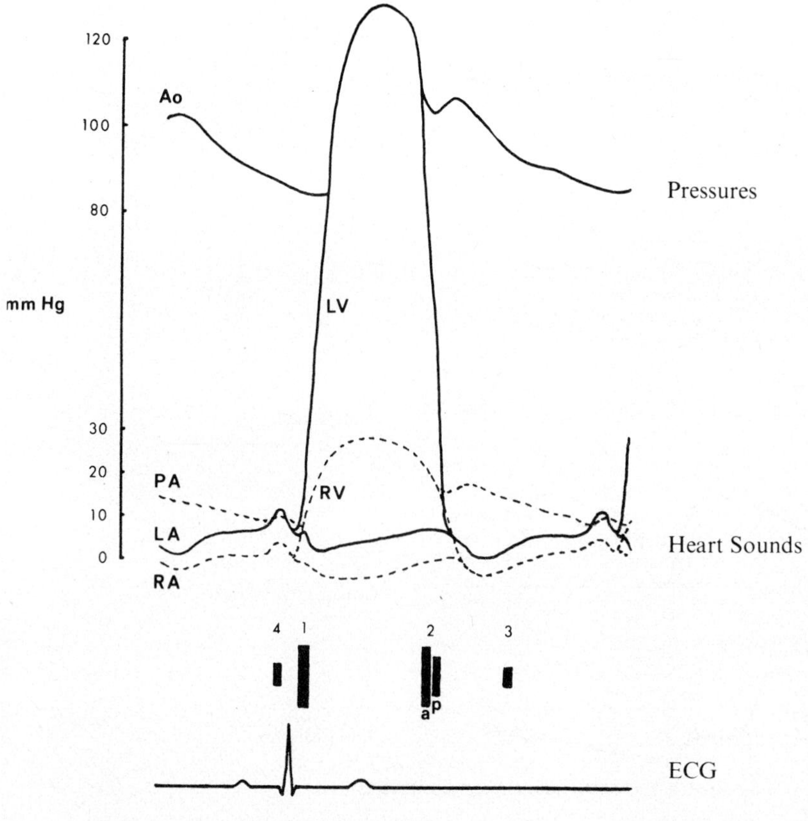


13/Fig. 2.—Typical normal pressure tracings for the various chambers of the heart superimposed on a common scale. From the relative pressures, the time of aortic and pulmonary valve movement and the opening and closing of the atrioventricular valves can be predicted. The diagram also enables the timing of murmurs in the heart to be understood.

heard best over the pulmonary area and are accentuated during inspiration with the increased blood flow into the lungs.

**Lungs.**—The lungs are examined for the presence of a pleural effusion, which is not uncommon in heart failure, and for the presence of crepitations or râles at the lung bases. Left ventricular failure does not always give rise to crepitations and the absence of these sounds does not exclude the diagnosis. Sounds will also frequently be suppressed by positive-pressure respiration. Increased bronchial secretions caused by a high left atrial pressure may cause widespread rhonchi. Widespread crepitations caused by fluid in the bronchi and alveoli are heard in pulmonary oedema.

**Liver.**—The liver is examined to determine whether it is palpable below the costal margin and whether it is tender as well as enlarged. Frank jaundice may be apparent, and is of serious prognostic significance.

The *oedema* fluid of cardiac failure is most commonly found as pitting oedema of the ankles and feet in ambulant patients, or as a pad of oedema overlying the sacrum in patients who have been confined to bed. Ascites and pleural effusions are also a reflection of salt and water retention that occurs in severe congestive cardiac failure, although ascites may sometimes be produced primarily by hepatic failure.

### Signs of Cardiac Failure

(*a*) *Left ventricular failure.*—The physical signs of early left ventricular failure are sinus tachycardia, a jugular venous pressure which is usually normal or only slightly raised and a third heart sound heard at the apex. The congestion of the pulmonary capillaries leads to dyspnoea and orthopnoea and, on auscultation, moist sounds can be heard at the bases of the lungs. More severe left ventricular failure may be associated with pulsus alternans, Cheyne-Stokes respiration and poor peripheral tissue perfusion.

(*b*) *Right ventricular failure.*—The signs of right ventricular failure may exist by themselves or be superimposed on those of left ventricular failure. The main sign of right-sided failure is a raised jugular venous pressure with a large "v" wave. A right ventricular third sound may be audible. The enlarged and sometimes tender liver may be associated with abnormal hepatic function. Oedema collects at the ankles and sacrum, and pleural effusions and ascites may be present.

## Special Tests

### Chest Radiography

Clinical examination of the patient continues with an interpretation of the straight x-ray of the heart in the standard posterior-anterior view. Penetrated posterior-anterior and penetrated left lateral chest x-rays may also be valuable for the detection of valvular or pericardial calcification, or left atrial enlargement (Fig. 3).

Having checked that the patient is not rotated and that the film is straight, the heart is scrutinised in an orderly fashion. First, the right border working from above downwards. The superior vena cava is seen as a vertical line at the upper border of the heart medial to the sterno-clavicular angle. Below this lies the ascending aorta which if dilated bulges to the right and distorts the normal smooth line of the SVC. This suggests post-stenotic dilatation, due to aortic valve disease, or an aneurysm of the ascending aorta. Below the ascending aorta the right atrium forms the right border of the heart, terminating at the diaphragm. A prominent or bulging right wall of the heart may be due to right atrial enlargement, to enlargement of the left atrium which lies behind the right atrium, or to a pericardial effusion.

Second, the left border of the heart. At the top, this is composed of the arch of the aorta, seen as a rounded knuckle at the upper left margin of the cardiac silhouette. This may be prominent in aortic incompetence or lesions causing dilatation of the aorta (e.g. aortic aneurysm, post-stenotic dilatation in aortic stenosis), or it may be inconspicuous in low cardiac output states such as severe mitral stenosis (Fig. 4). The pulmonary trunk lies immediately below the aortic knuckle and is dilated in pulmonary valve stenosis or in conditions leading to an increased flow or pressure in the pulmonary artery. Below the pulmonary artery is the left atrial appendage and this is not normally visible on chest radiography unless enlarged. Enlargement of the left atrium usually accompanies enlargement of the appendage and this chamber can usually be seen as a circular shadow lying centrally behind the heart or to the right of the

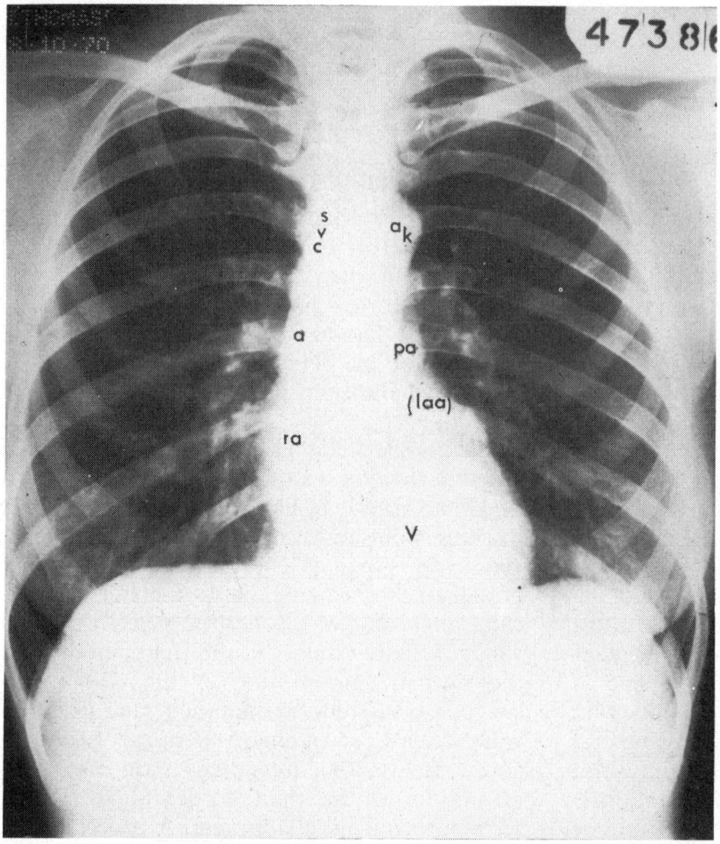


13/FIG. 3.—NORMAL CHEST X-RAY
V—Ventricular mass
r.a.—Right atrium
a—Ascending aorta
S.V.C.—Superior vena cava
a.k.—Aortic knuckle
p.a.—Pulmonary artery
(laa)—Position of left atrial appendage

right atrium and of a slightly higher density. This is seen on a penetrated posterior-anterior picture, or more clearly in a lateral film. A large left atrium may compress the left lower lobe bronchus leading to distal collapse.

Differentiation between left and right ventricular hypertrophy is impossible on a chest x-ray, being better appreciated by palpation of the precordium and by characteristic ECG changes.

Examination of the chest radiograph is completed by consideration of the lung fields and bony structures. The larger branches of the pulmonary arteries and main pulmonary veins, responsible for the normal lung markings, dilate and the smaller vessels become visible when the blood flow through the lungs is increased. This is a characteristic of a left-to-right cardiac shunt.

If the pulmonary vascular resistance is raised (pulmonary hypertension) the proximal pulmonary arteries are large but the peripheral vessels become almost invisible leaving the lung fields abnormally clear and translucent. With decreased pulmonary blood flow (pulmonary atresia, pulmonary stenosis, Fallot's tetralogy) the vascular markings are small and sparse and the lung fields abnormally clear. In pulmonary venous congestion, secondary to a raised left atrial pressure, the veins are dilated and the upper lobe pulmonary veins more easily seen (upper-lobe diversion). The increased interstitial fluid and engorgement of the lymphatics produces an overall ground-glass appearance, a peri-hilar flare and fine horizontal lines in the costophrenic angle (Kerley B lines). Chronic congestive heart failure may cause pleural effusions while pulmonary oedema represents extreme pulmonary venous congestion and patchy shadowing is seen around the hilum extending out into the surrounding lung. Rib notching may be seen in coarctation of the aorta

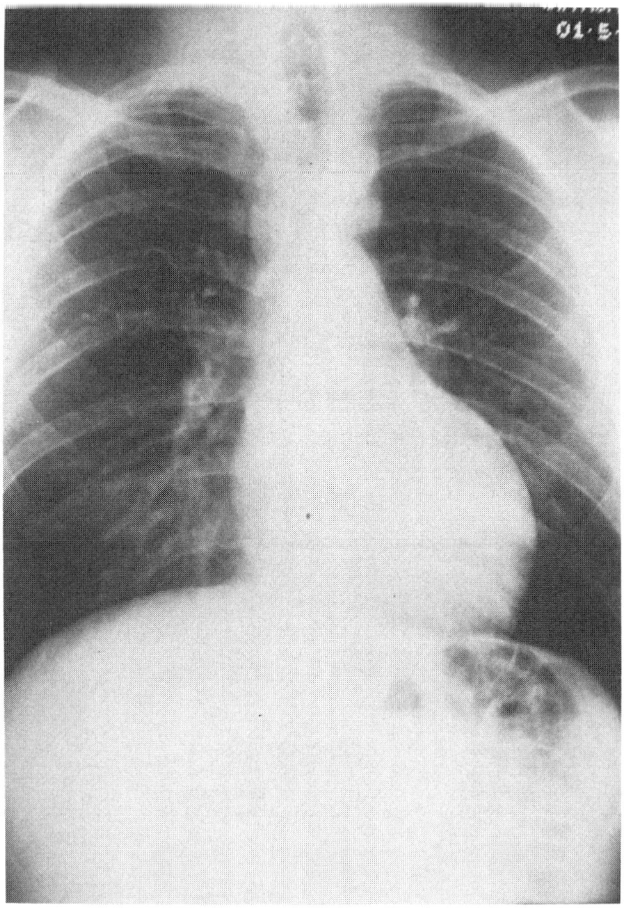

13/FIG. 4.—MITRAL STENOSIS. Note the pulmonary venous engorgement and the enlarged pulmonary artery shadow. The left atrium is enlarged and can be seen bulging to right behind the right atrium. (Courtesy of Dr. M. M. Webb-Peploe, St. Thomas' Hospital.)

and alteration in skeletal anatomy may suggest previous surgery. Artefacts may be evident such as sternal wires, pacemaker apparatus or prosthetic cardiac materials.

### Blood Tests

Abnormal blood tests which may be a direct result of the cardiac disease process or its therapy are often of anaesthetic significance.

(*a*) *Haemoglobin.*—By reducing oxygen carrying capacity, anaemia requires a higher than normal cardiac output to maintain oxygen supply, resulting in an increase in myocardial work and hence oxygen consumption. If the cardiac output is not capable of adequate increase, oxygen supply is reduced to levels which may produce tissue hypoxia. Polycythaemia raises the viscosity of blood, increasing afterload and myocardial work and reducing tissue blood flow.

(*b*) *Potassium* (see p. 422).—Hypokalaemia, often the consequence of diuretic therapy, enhances the potential for the production of dysrhythmias. Hyperkalaemia is less common and may be an indication of renal failure or metabolic acidosis secondary to a low cardiac output.

(*c*) *Liver function tests* may be abnormal in congestive or right heart failure. Hypoalbuminaemia encourages extravascular fluid shifts and may allow pulmonary oedema to develop at only moderately raised left atrial pressures. It will also influence drug binding to plasma proteins. Decreased liver function may indicate a relative inability to metabolise certain anaesthetic agents or to manufacture clotting factors.

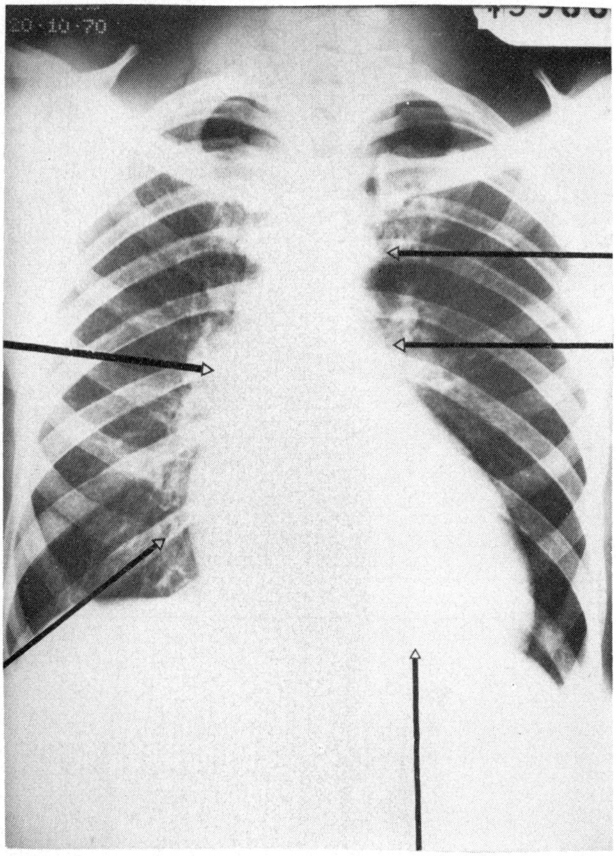


13/Fig. 5.—Predominant Aortic Stenosis with regurgitation
The ventricular mass is enlarged due to left ventricular hypertrophy and an increase in end-diastolic volume in the presence of aortic regurgitation. Left heart failure eventually occurs as a late manifestation of aortic stenosis.

(*d*) *Coagulation studies* and *platelet count*.—Difficulties with clotting are often encountered following open heart surgery with extracorporeal circulation; whatever the operation, pre-existing coagulation defects should be corrected where possible, or replacement therapy (fresh donor blood, fresh frozen plasma, platelet concentrates) made available intra-operatively.

(*e*) *Creatinine and urea*.—An assessment of renal function is valuable as the combination of kidney disease and poor renal perfusion (which may occur intra- or post-operatively) may lead to acute renal failure.

(*f*) *Thyroid function* (see p. 992).—Hypo- or hyperthyroidism may mimic or accentuate some forms of cardiac disease, and may lead to cardiovascular difficulties under anaesthesia.

(*g*) *Arterial blood gases*.—These should be performed if hypoxia, hypercarbia or acidosis is suggested by clinical examination: pre-operative values may assist in postoperative assessment and management. Pathological results are normally encountered only in severe cardio-respiratory disease.

(*h*) *Australia antigen* (Hepatitis B antigen—HBAg).—This should be a standard test for every patient at risk and is especially important before cardiac surgery where there is increased

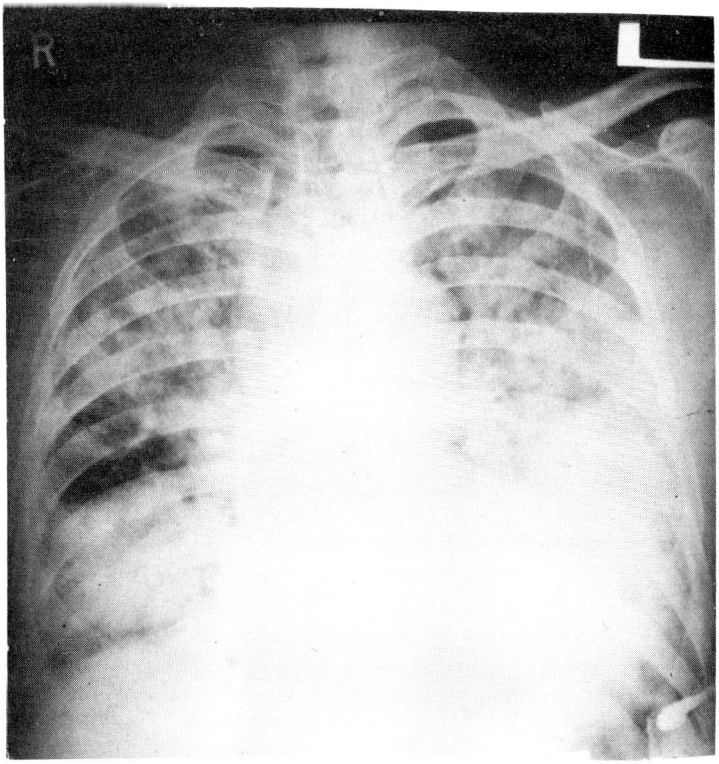

13/Fig. 6.—Severe bilateral pulmonary oedema, particularly marked in the lower lobes, following a myocardial infarction. Note that the heart is quite small. Physical signs at this time:
Patient dyspnoeic, sweating, confused, cyanosed, hypotensive.
Moist sounds all over chest.
Copious pink frothy sputum.
pH 7·31, $Pa_{CO_2}$ 30 mm Hg (4·0 kPa), $Pa_{O_2}$ 46 mm Hg (6·1 kPa)

likelihood of staff contact with the patient's blood.

(*i*) *Sickle haemoglobin* (see p. 603).—Extracorporeal circulation is particularly hazardous in patients with sickle-cell disease, and may even produce sickling in patients who only exhibit the trait.

### Electrocardiography

The ECG is examined for information on cardiac rate and rhythm, electrical axis, hypertrophy, strain or ischaemia, atrioventricular conduction and drug and electrolyte effects, remembering that a normal ECG does not exclude cardiovascular disease. Frequent atrial or ventricular ectopic beats of a rhythm other than sinus are associated with an increased cardiac risk during and after surgery.[1] (The normal ECG is described on page 417 *et seq*., the diagnosis and treatment of dysrhythmias on page 487 *et seq*., the ECG appearances of acute myocardial infarction on page 473.)

*Right ventricular hypertrophy:* during early childhood the right is the dominant ventricle. However, after this period, the following are the signs of pathological right ventricular hypertrophy (Fig.7*a*):

Tall peaked P waves in lead II (right atrial hypertrophy).

Right axis deviation—that is, a mean frontal QRS greater than 100°.

Dominant R waves in leads $V_{1-3}$.

*Left ventricular hypertrophy:* this cannot be dianosed on the ECG in the presence of left bundle-branch block. The signs suggestive of left ventricular hypertrophy are (Fig. 7*b*):

Bifid P waves in lead II (left atrial hypertrophy).

Large voltage R waves in leads I, aVL, $V_{2-7}$.

More severe disease results in the appearance of abnormal repolarisation and the development of a strain pattern evidenced by depression of the ST segments and T wave inversion (Fig. 7*c*). Ischaemia is suggested by flat ST depression greater than 1 mm in any lead, while an old infarct may be recognisable by Q waves greater than 0·3 mm.

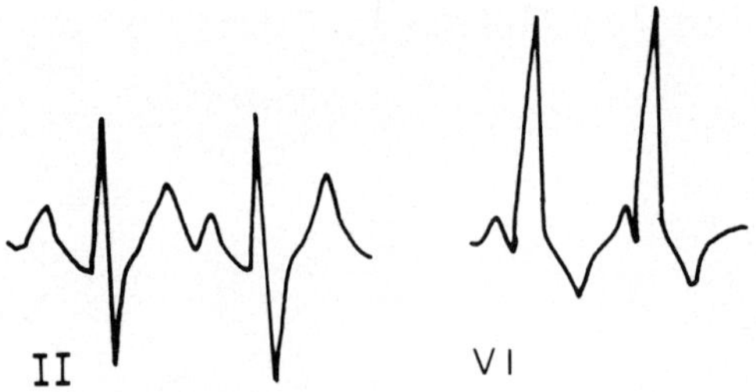


(a) Right ventricular hypertrophy

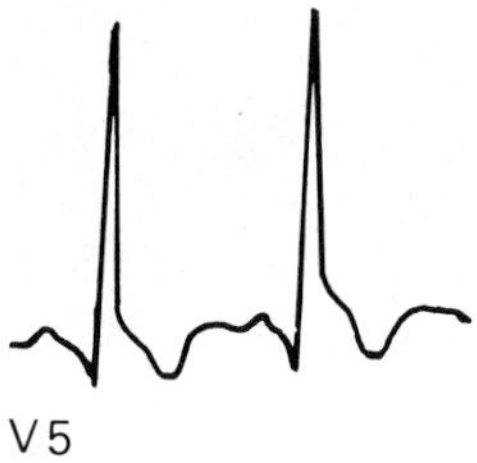


(b) Left ventricular hypertrophy

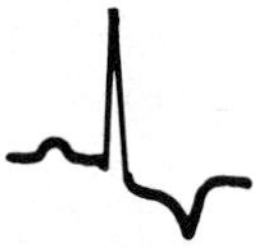

(c) Strain

13/Fig. 7

### Specific Diagnostic Tests

In certain circumstances the clinical work-up must be supplemented by specialised investigations such as echocardiography or cardiac catheterisation.

#### Cardiac Catheterisation and Angiocardiography

A thorough history and clinical examination supplemented by examination of the ECG and chest radiograph will enable the diagnosis to be made in most cases of cardiovascular disease. In many instances, however, the diagnosis may remain in doubt and in other cases the diagnosis may be known but its quantitative effects not be clearly apparent. Cardiac catheterisation and angiocardiography are undertaken to confirm the diagnosis accurately and to provide the information on which future treatment, particularly surgical, can be based. Complications include cardiac tamponade, ventricular fibrillation, peripheral artery thrombosis and systemic embolisation.

In right heart catheterisation a catheter is passed through a vein, usually in the groin or elbow via the vena cava to the right atrium. It can then be passed through the tricuspid valve to the right ventricle and out through the pulmonary valve into the pulmonary arteries. An indirect measurement of left atrial pressure can be taken from the pulmonary artery occlusion pressure. The coronary sinus can also be entered from the right atrium.

Left heart catheterisation can be performed in three ways. The left heart may be entered in the presence of a septal defect or patent foramen ovale during right-sided cardiac catheterisation. If there is no communication it is possible to perforate the inter-atrial septum with a special needle during right-sided catheterisation and a catheter can then be threaded over the needle into the left atrium and thence to the left ventricle (trans-septal approach). Alternatively, aortic catheterisation can be performed by the retrograde passage of a catheter up the aorta from a peripheral artery and thence across the aortic valve and into the left ventricle.

The coronary arteries are entered from the aorta. During cardiac catheterisation and angiocardiography the information derived is either anatomical or physiological. Anatomical information includes the normality of the superior vena caval drainage, intracardiac communications, the size and movement of the ventricles and heart valves, the anatomy and patency of the coronary arteries and the anatomy of the great vessels. Angiography also yields physiological data in that assessment of ventricular volume can be made in systole and in diastole and an estimation of ventricular performance may be derived from the ejection fraction.

Physiological information (see Table 2) can support the anatomical evidence in intracardiac shunts: serial oxygen saturations taken at separate points along the SVC-right atrial-IVC axis may demonstrate a "step-up" in saturation at, say, the mid-right atrium, which would suggest a left-to-right shunt of oxygenated blood through an atrial septal defect.

Pressure measurements are made in all chambers and the great vessels. Ventricular end-

13/TABLE 2
NORMAL VALUES OBTAINED AT CARDIAC CATHETERISATION

**PRESSURE IN mm. OF MERCURY**

| Site | Phasic | Mean | Remarks |
|---|---|---|---|
| RA | a 1 v 2 | 1 | reference point |
| RV | 15/1 | | at sternal angle, |
| PA | 15/5 | 11 | supine, spont. resp. |
| PCWP | | 5 | |
| LA | | 5 | |
| LV | 120/5 | | LVEDP 5 |
| AO | 120/30 | 93 | |

**BLOOD SAMPLES**

| Site | % Sat. | Remarks |
|---|---|---|
| SVC | 76 | no shunt at atrial |
| RA | 75 | level |
| IVC | 75 | |
| PA | 75 | |
| AO | 97 | |

**ANGIOGRAPHIC DATA**

| | | | | | | |
|---|---|---|---|---|---|---|
| End-diastolic Volume | 110 | ml ( 61 ml/M² ) | Ejection Fraction | 0.66 | |
| End-systolic Volume | 37 | ml ( 21 ml/M² ) | Ejection Rate | | ml/sec |
| Stroke Volume | 73 | ml ( 40 ml/M² ) | Normalised Ej. Rate | | EDV/sec |

**CORONARY SINUS FLOW DATA**

| Heart Rate bt/min | C.S. Flow ml/min | C.S. Flow /100 g | L.V. $O_2$ content ml/100ml | C.S. $O_2$ content ml/100ml | A–V Difference ml/100ml | Myoc $O_2$ uptake ml/min |
|---|---|---|---|---|---|---|
| 71 | 120 | 109 | 18,3 | 8.1 | 10.2 | 12.2 |

**DYE CURVES**

| Injec. Site | Sample Site | App. Time | Flow L/min | Remarks |
|---|---|---|---|---|
| | THERMODILUTION | | | |
| PA | dist PA | | 5.2 | |
| | INDOCYANINE GREEN DYE | | | |
| PA | AO | | 5.4 | |

40 year old male 70kg. surface area 1.8 m²

**BLOOD GAS TENSIONS**

| Time | Site | $pO_2$ | $pCO_2$ | pH |
|---|---|---|---|---|
| | AO | 93 | 36 | 7.41 |
| | breathing room air | | | |

**FICK CALCULATIONS**

| | | |
|---|---|---|
| Oxygen Consumption | 220 | cc/min |
| Oxygen Capacity | 18.6 | vols % |
| Systemic Art. Content | 18.3 | vols % |
| Systemic Ven. Content | 14.1 | vols % |
| Systemic A-V Difference | 4.2 | vols % |
| SYSTEMIC FLOW | 5.2 | L/min |
| | 2.9 | L/min/M² |
| Pulmonary Ven. Content | | vols % |
| Pulmonary Art. Content | | vols % |
| Pulmonary A-V Difference | | vols % |
| PULMONARY FLOW | | L/min. |
| | | L/min./M² |
| Pulm./Syst. Flow Ratio | | |

| | | |
|---|---|---|
| Pulmonary Arteriolar Resistance | 6/5.2 = 1.15 | units |
| Systemic Arteriolar Resistance | 92/5.2 = 17.6 | units |
| Pulm./Syst. Resistance Ratio | | |

diastolic (or atrial) pressures may help in the assessment of ventricular performance while pressure gradients across valves assist in the estimation of valve orifice size. Cardiac output may be measured in a variety of ways (see p. 408) and, with the appropriate pressure measurements, calculations of systemic and pulmonary vascular resistances are made. Sometimes cardiac catheterisation is performed as an emergency in life-threatening situations, such as pulmonary embolism and aortic dissection. Here, only the minimum of investigation necessary to define the lesion is performed as the effects of the contrast medium (vasodilatation and hypotension) may decompensate an already compromised circulation.

Finally, muscle biopsy of the ventricular wall may be indicated in cardiomyopathic disease and is performed using a special catheter.

Anaesthesia for cardiac catheterisation and angiocardiography is considered on page 510.

**Comment**

The difficulty in pre-operative assessment lies not in diagnosing the specific lesion or complication, nor perhaps in estimating its anatomic severity. The problems lie in deciding how far the disease has encroached on the patient's cardiovascular reserves and how much the patient's disease increases his risk during anaesthesia and surgery. The presence or absence of heart failure, pulmonary hypertension or coronary artery disease and the patient's response to exercise may help resolve the first problem and enable some comparison to be made with the stresses of anaesthesia, surgery and the post-operative period.

At the extremes of cardiac disability, severe heart failure, fixed low cardiac output, or recent myocardial infarction, the risks are obvious, but there is evidence that any form of cardiovascular disease, even asymptomatic changes in the ECG, increase the risk over the normal population. Goldman and his colleagues[1] identified nine significant correlates of life-threatening or fatal circulatory complications in 1001 patients undergoing non-cardiac surgical procedures. These included the presence of a third heart sound and raised jugular venous pressure, myocardial infarction within the previous six months and frequent ectopic beats or a rhythm other than sinus. Complications occurred more commonly in patients who were over the age of 70 or who were in poor general condition. Morbidity was higher in major intrathoracic, intraperitoneal and great vessel surgery. While careful intra-operative anaesthetic management may temporarily improve the circulatory state, such intensive care may not be available in the subsequent postoperative period when the demands made on the patient's heart and circulation may be much greater than those occurring during an appropriately administered anaesthetic.

The other benefit in careful pre-operative assessment is in ensuring that the patient presents for surgery in his optimum condition having received the correct therapy for his disease, suitably modified for surgery.

## PRE-OPERATIVE TREATMENT

Pre-operative treatment depends both on the nature of the cardiac disease and the nature of the operation to be performed. Treatment prior to cardiac or major vascular surgery is different in emphasis from that prior to some incidental operation. All treatment should be considered under two headings: first, the treatment which is necessary to gain control of the patient and to render him in the best possible condition for surgery, and second, how this treatment should be modified in the immediate peri-operative period.

In general, such treatment is directed to the correction of cardiac failure, the prevention or treatment of dysrhythmias, the symptomatic management of coronary artery disease, and the treatment of hypertension. Abnormal haemoglobin, prothrombin time, serum potassium, together with co-existing pulmonary disease, may also need appropriate therapy.

### Chronic Cardiac Failure

Uncontrolled cardiac failure should normally be considered a contra-indication to anaesthesia and the operation postponed to allow ample time for the medical treatment of the patient. Sometimes the operation is urgent and postponement is not possible but even then much can be done to improve the condition of the patient in the short interval available.

(*a*) **Bed rest** is the mainstay of treatment. As long as failure continues there should be strict bed rest and the patient only allowed up very cautiously once control has been gained.

(*b*) **Reduced salt diet.**—A normal diet contains 50 to 60 mmol of salt per day. Patients being treated for cardiac failure are advised not to add salt to their food and to avoid salty dishes. This reduces the intake to around 40 mmol per day.

(*c*) **Digoxin.**—Digoxin, a cardiac glycoside, is used mainly to control supraventricular dysrhythmias and also to improve myocardial function in chronic heart failure.

*Action and uses.*—Improvement in myocardial contractility probably depends upon the ability of digoxin to inhibit the membrane-bound Adenosine Triphosphate-ase (ATPase) which is responsible for intracellular sodium and potassium transport. Inhibition of this enzyme depletes intramyocardial potassium and increases the intracellular sodium. The latter becomes available for exchange with extracellular calcium so that sarcoplasmic calcium concentration is increased and contractility improved.[2]

Clinically, the more important effects of digoxin are on the SA node, the atrial fibres and the AV node. A direct effect decreases conduction velocity and prolongs the effective refractory period of the AV node (which may lead to AV block) to decrease the ventricular rate in atrial flutter or fibrillation. Indirect effects via the autonomic nervous system include enhanced vagal activity which slows the sino-atrial rate. This vagomimetic action may also be the mechanism whereby digoxin converts atrial flutter to fibrillation and terminates paroxysmal supraventricular tachycardia. The improvement in cardiac output that occurs following the control of ventricular rate in cardiac failure leads also to a reduction in sympathetic tone and systemic vascular resistance. This effect may be offset by a direct peripheral vasoconstrictor effect of digoxin which may account for the increase in arterial pressure observed after intravenous administration and which may sometimes be deleterious to cardiac function.

In the acute situation the value of digoxin as an inotropic agent remains controversial[3] and intravenously administered digoxin compares poorly with the use of catecholamines in the management of acute low cardiac output states. Goldstein and his co-workers[4] studied the haemodynamic effects of dobutamine (8·5 μg/kg/min) and digoxin (12·5 μg/kg) in patients with cardiac failure following acute myocardial infarction. Only dobutamine reduced pulmonary capillary wedge pressures and systemic vascular resistance and, although digoxin increased cardiac index by 9 per cent, dobutamine improved this by 33 per cent. Moreover, patients with myocardial ischaemia appear to be unduly sensitive to the toxic effects of digitalis,[5] which may be a reflection of the increased susceptibility to dysrhythmia formation in coronary artery disease, or to a direct coronary vasoconstrictor effect of the cardiac glycosides themselves.

*Administration and toxicity.*—Digoxin may be administered orally or intravenously, the intramuscular route being too unpredictable. In acute cases, intravenous digoxin 0·065 mg is given every 20–30 minutes until the desired effect is achieved or to a maximum dose of between 0·25–0·75 mg, depending on the size, age and general condition of the patient. Caution should be observed as there is a delay before full clinical improvement is seen. The main disadvantage of digoxin lies in the narrow margin between therapeutic and toxic concentrations. The therapeutic range is 1·3–2·6 nmol/litre (1–2 ng/ml) and while toxic symptoms are common at levels over 4 ng/ml, they may occur at lower concentrations in the presence of hypokalaemia. Toxicity is also enhanced by hyperkalaemia, alkalosis, hypoxaemia, hypercalcaemia and hypomagnesaemia. Despite the ease of measurement of blood levels, toxicity is not uncommon and is associated with a high mortality.

Symptoms of toxicity include nausea, vomiting, diarrhoea, giddiness, sweating, visual defects and syncope. The signs of digoxin toxicity are typically related to rhythm disturbances and may present as a sinus bradycardia, SA block, A-V block, atrial dysrhythmia (including atrial tachycardias), junctional rhythms, ventricular ectopics, tachycardia or fibrillation. The changes induced in the electrocardiogram are discussed on page 420.

Patients for major cardiac surgery who present already digitalised will usually have their digoxin stopped two days pre-operatively, their cardiac failure being controlled by bed rest. The half-life of digoxin averages 30–40 hours (which is dependent upon renal function) so that problems in controlling ventricular rate in atrial fibrillation during this pre-operative period rarely occur. Patients having minor or incidental surgery will often omit their dose only on the morning of operation, but note should be taken of the dose the patient has been receiving previously, the resting cardiac rate and any symptoms which might suggest digoxin toxicity so that the treatment may be amended. An unexplained pre-operative bradycardia in a patient on digoxin is suspicious of toxicity until proved otherwise. If it is not discovered until the patient is in the anaesthetic room, a small dose of atropine may be useful to determine whether the pulse rate is capable of increase.

As a general rule, if there is any doubt about the advisability of continuing or administering digoxin, the best course is to withhold it.

(*d*) **Diuretics.**—The other mainstay in the treatment of chronic cardiac failure is the use of diuretics. The best index of fluid retention is a change in the weight of the patient, and daily weighing is the most accurate chart of progress in the treatment of cardiac failure. The jugular venous pressure and ankle or sacral oedema are less reliable because pure left ventricular failure can exist in the presence of an almost normal right atrial pressure, although sinus tachycardia and apical gallop (3rd sound) may point to the diagnosis. Diuretics are prescribed initially to reduce the weight and thereafter to maintain it constant, while keeping the haematocrit, serum sodium, potassium and blood urea at normal levels.

*Thiazides*.—These are potent non-mercurial diuretics which are well tolerated and which can be given by mouth. Their mode of action is to inhibit proximal tubular reabsorption of sodium and chloride, in contrast to mercurials which act primarily by inhibiting chloride reabsorption. There are now a number of these drugs whose effectiveness is comparable and which differ only in dose and price. *Bendrofluazide* is cheap and effective. The dose is initially 5–10 mg with a maintenance of 2·5–5·0 mg daily. Diuresis starts two hours after ingestion and lasts for twelve hours.

*Frusemide* is a monosulphanyl diuretic which acts in a similar fashion to the thiazides but is much more potent. It is both quicker-acting and of shorter duration and possesses the advantage that it can be given intravenously. The initial oral dose is 40 mg but up to 160 mg can be given daily. The intravenous dose is 20 mg but much larger doses may sometimes be required.

*Bumetanide* is an alternative diuretic for patients who are unresponsive to frusemide. Given orally the dose is up to 10 mg daily.

*Ethacrynic acid* is a desulphanyl compound which is even more potent and can be given intravenously in a dose of 50 mg.

Both frusemide and ethacrynic acid have been advocated for use in the treatment of acute pulmonary oedema. Given intravenously, both produce a response within 10 minutes which may be very effective. Their potency gives rise to two dangers—the diuresis is accompanied by potassium loss and the very size of the diuresis after intravenous ethacrynic acid may produce hypovolaemic hypotension. Hypovolaemia is a danger with all diuretic therapy and care must be taken that, in encouraging the excretion of excess fluid, the filling pressure of the heart is not reduced below that level necessary to produce an adequate cardiac output.

(*e*) **Potassium and diuretics.**—All the above diuretics, besides causing inhibition of salt and water retention, lead to excessive loss of body potassium and magnesium. This may be a chronic state following long-continued diuretic therapy, an acute response to a sudden diuresis, or, most dangerously, an acute loss superimposed on a chronic deficiency. Many patients who have been on continued diuretic therapy will have a total body potassium content which may be reduced, although this probably relates more to the reduction in total muscle mass superimposed upon a decreased ability of the cells to retain potassium which accompanies chronic cardiac failure. A low serum potassium or an otherwise unexplained metabolic alkalosis suggests a very severe deficiency. Both potassium and magnesium depletion potentiate dysrhythmia formation, particularly those due to digoxin, and may lead to ventricular tachycardia or fibrillation.

Patients who are receiving diuretic therapy should receive potassium supplements in some form which contains chloride, such as "Slow K" (8 mmol/tablet). The dose depends slightly on diet, but because not all is absorbed and the minimum loss in urine is about 30 mmol/day, patients may require 50–100 mmol daily. If the potassium level falls below 3·5 mmol/l as a result of an acute diuresis and the patient develops ventricular dysrhythmias, intravenous potassium is given in 5 mmol increments until the dysrhythmia disappears, when a slow infusion of potassium 50–100 mmol/day can be used to restore the potassium balance (see p. 423). Because of the loss of potassium which accompanies the use of the diuretics already described, three other diuretics—spironolactone, triamterene and amiloride—which promote potassium reabsorption are sometimes prescribed in conjunction with the thiazides.

*Spironolactone* is an aldosterone antagonist. Aldosterone, secreted by the adrenal cortex, promotes the retention of sodium and excretion of potassium. Spironolactone reverses this effect and when used in conjunction with the thiazides, frusemide or ethacrynic acid, increases the diuresis as well as reducing the potassium loss. The minimum effective dose is 100–150 mg daily, but due to its blocking action further increments do not enhance its effect.

*Triamterene* which is an aminopteridine, increases excretion of sodium and chloride but it also acts on the distal tubule to decrease potassium loss, but not by antagonism of alder-sterone (dose 50 mg b.d.).

*Amiloride* acts on the distal tubule producing potassium retention in a similar manner to triamterene. A more powerful diuretic than spironolactone it is sometimes given in combination with frusemide, dose 5–10 mg daily.

**Effusions.**—In the medical treatment of cardiac failure, pleural effusions or ascites are rarely tapped. However, large pleural effusions may embarrass cardiac and pulmonary function, particularly if the patient is to be placed in the lateral position on the operating table. These are best removed the day before operation so that the patient has 24 hours to readjust, as on rare occasions acute pulmonary oedema may develop when the fluid is removed too quickly. There is also the possibility of causing a pneumothorax during the aspiration, and a chest x-ray should be performed following pleurocentesis.

## Hypertension

The hypertensive patient represents an increased risk for anaesthesia and surgery. This is the result of two factors, the much greater lability of the blood pressure, which is due to the systemic vascular resistance changing markedly for small alterations in vessel tone and the fact that patients with hypertension show earlier and more widespread arteriosclerosis than do comparable normotensive patients. It is possible that left ventricular cavity size may be abnormally small in the presence of ventricular hypertrophy: this would tend to limit stroke volume and may contribute to the instability of arterial pressure under anaesthesia. The two particular dangers to which the hypertensive subject is liable under anaesthesia are hypotension and an exacerbation of hypertension. Hypotension produces serious reduction in flow in the arteriosclerotic renal, cerebral and myocardial vessels with the danger of renal failure, cerebral ischaemia and myocardial infarction. Conversely, hypertension may also cause myocardial ischaemia leading to cardiac failure, or produce intracranial haemorrhage.

### Assessment and Treatment

Patients with hypertension need careful assessment before anaesthesia and surgery. This should include a full medical history and examination together with chest x-ray and an ECG. An attempt must also be made to assess the extent of arteriosclerosis in the important vessels; myocardial ischaemia may be apparent from the history or the ECG; laboratory tests may demonstrate renal impairment; the fundal vessels should be inspected by ophthalmoscopy for direct evidence of arteriosclerosis. Any cardiac failure should be treated prior to surgery.

Prys-Roberts and his colleagues[6] in their study showed a high incidence of myocardial ischaemia in patients with high initial arterial pressure exposed to anaesthesia, and suggested that even symptom-free hypertensive patients should receive therapy to lower their pressure before anaesthesia and surgery. Mauney and his colleagues[7] and Breslin and Swinton[8] also concluded that pre-operative stabilisation of high arterial pressures should be achieved before elective surgery.

The usual aim of medical treatment is to produce a diastolic pressure of 100 mm Hg (13·3 kPa) or lower although this aim is not always possible.

According to the severity of the hypertension, different drug combinations are employed.

**Diuretics.**—The thiazide diuretics promote salt and water excretion and, by reducing plasma volume, may be sufficient therapy for some mild hypertensives. They also have some direct vasodilator action because the blood pressure remains low when the plasma volume returns to normal. In mild hypertension, diuretics alone may be used but in more severe cases they may also be employed to potentiate the anti-adrenergic drugs.

**Beta-adrenergic blockade.**—Various $\beta$-

blockers are widely used in the treatment of hypertension, frequently in combination with a diuretic. Beta-adrenergic blockade sometimes reveals a high degree of spontaneous $\alpha$-adrenergic vasoconstrictor activity which may be treated with a vasodilator such as hydralazine. By their negative chronotropic and inotropic effects, by the lowering of plasma renin activity and by central effects, the $\beta$-blockers lower blood pressure both in the standing and lying positions. Sudden withdrawal may lead to a rebound hypertensive state.

**Methyldopa.**—More severe hypertension is treated with methyldopa which inhibits vasoconstrictor impulses mainly by a central action and also possibly by the interruption of the normal synthesis of noradrenaline. After oral administration an effect is achieved in three to five hours and lasts up to twenty-four hours. Renal blood flow and glomerular filtration are well maintained but fluid retention, tiredness and depression are complications and drug tolerance often develops. A diuretic is usually added to combat fluid retention.

**Anti-adrenergic drugs.**—*Bethanidine, guanethidine* and *debrisoquine* are used infrequently. All act on post-ganglionic adrenergic neurones and deplete catecholamine stores. They have different rates of onset and duration of action but all produce a postural hypotension which may be troublesome in the morning and on exercise. Hot weather and factors which deplete blood volume will potentiate their effects. Side-effects are bradycardia, dry mouth, impotence, diarrhoea and fluid retention.

**Other drugs.**—*Clonidine* is a centrally-acting hypotensive drug which may have two disadvantages. Firstly, sudden withdrawal of clonidine may lead to an exacerbation of the hypertension. Secondly, when given with digitalis it provokes digitalis toxicity.

*Diazoxide* is a thiazide derivative which causes hypotension and hyperglycaemia. It is only used intravenously in the acute treatment of uncontrolled hypertension where it has tended to replace pentolinium and trimetaphan. Intra-venous anti-adrenergic drugs should not be used for this purpose as they produce an initial transitory rise in blood pressure.

**Antihypertensive drugs and anaesthesia.**—Once antihypertensive drugs have been started, even temporary discontinuation may be dangerous. Discontinuation may precipitate renal failure, myocardial failure or a cerebrovascular accident and the patient with a high blood pressure is much more liable to large alterations in blood pressure with the particular danger of producing myocardial ischaemia or infarction. Ominsky and Wollman[9] considered that most intra-operative hypotension is related to the patient's disease or the anaesthetic and not to the antihypertensive therapy which should be continued throughout the peri-operative period.

Fortunately, with the wide variety of anaesthetic techniques available, continued therapy is quite compatible with anaesthesia. At the same time, care must be taken to avoid those drugs which will potentiate the hypotensive action, particularly by direct depression of the myocardium, and the circulation must be properly monitored and supported. An ECG is an obvious requirement. Blood loss is measured and replaced to maintain adequate ventricular filling pressures.

Should a vasoconstrictor be required, it must be one which is effective in the face of the antihypertensive therapy, and the dose must be restricted to that necessary to restore the blood pressure to its previous level since, in excess, it may impose an overwhelming afterload on a potentially depressed myocardium particularly if the anaesthetic includes such direct myocardial depressants as halothane or enflurane.

Extreme variations in pressure are a particular hazard to the arteriosclerotic hypertensive due to the dangers of ischaemia or thrombosis, and Prys-Roberts and his colleagues[10] have shown that whereas the well-controlled hypertensive patient tends to behave like his normotensive counterpart, the untreated or badly treated hypertensive patient is at considerable risk during anaesthesia. This risk occurs not only during steady state anaesthesia but is accentuated during induction, when severe hypotension may be precipitated by intravenous agents including tubocurarine, and during laryngoscopy and intubation which usually cause hypertension. A hypertensive episode may also follow the use of pancuronium which must be used with caution in these patients, although the use of tubocurarine may produce a disastrous fall in blood pressure: metocurine may be a safer alternative. The immediate awakening period may also provoke a hypertensive reaction. Although an increase in blood pressure might be expected to improve coronary flow, the resulting increase in ventricular wall tension raises myocardial oxygen consumption and diminishes circulation in the subendocardial collaterals which may cause subendocardial ischaemia or necrosis. S-T segment deviation may often be seen on the ECG under these circumstances.

## Coronary Artery Disease

The incidence of coronary artery disease (CAD) has been estimated at 20 per cent in the male population under the age of 60[11] and is a potent cause of morbidity and sudden death. Many causative factors have been examined including diet, stress, lack of physical exercise and ethnic origin. Probably the most relevant factors that appear to predispose towards CAD are tobacco smoking, a family history of myocardial ischaemia, obesity, diabetes and abnormal serum lipids.

*Symptoms of CAD*

(1) There may be none. Indeed, the presenting sign of critical coronary artery stenosis (see Fig. 8) may be sudden death, often following a period of increased physical effort.
(2) Angina pectoris (see p. 453). Atypical pains may or may not be ischaemic in origin and could be confused with referred vertebral pain, peptic ulceration, hiatus hernia, pulmonary disease or mitral valve leaflet prolapse.
(3) Palpitations or syncope. Supraventricular, or more particularly, ventricular dysrhythmias, are common in ischaemic heart disease and may be associated with mitral valve dysfunction and atrioventricular conduction defects.
(4) Symptoms may result from ventricular failure secondary to myocardial ischaemia.
(5) Symptoms can be caused by other diseases which are related to ischaemic heart disease; for example, those due to bronchitis and emphysema (cigarette smoking), generalised arterial disease (transient ischaemic attacks, limb pain), diabetes and perhaps peptic ulceration.

*Signs of CAD*

There may be none. Cardiovascular examination may however reveal hypertension, dysrhythmias, ventricular hypertrophy or

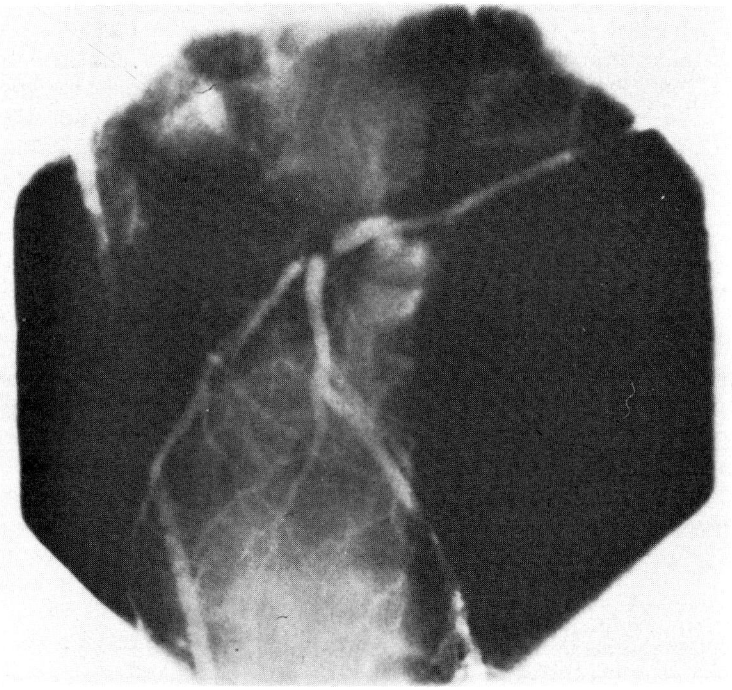

13/Fig. 8.—Critical Left Main-stem Coronary Artery Stenosis. Left coronary angiogram demonstrating a filling defect in the main-stem at the junction between the left anterior descending and circumflex vessels. (Courtesy of Dr. B. S. Jenkins, St. Thomas' Hospital.)

enlargement, signs of pump failure, peripheral vascular disease (including carotid bruits), valve dysfunction and retinal changes. The physical examination should also include a thorough assessment of the respiratory and neurological systems.

*Special Investigations*

(*a*) The chest x-ray may demonstrate an enlarged heart with pulmonary venous congestion, or a dilated left atrium secondary to left ventricular failure. The lung fields may show evidence of coincidental bronchitis and emphysema; sometimes bullae are present. Calcification of the aorta will give a clue as to the state of the arterial system in general. More often, the chest x-ray is normal.

(*b*) The electrocardiogram taken at rest can also be normal despite the presence of significant coronary artery disease, although ischaemic changes are usually provoked during exercise which provides the rationale for the exercise ECG (see Fig. 9). There may be signs of left ventricular hypertrophy or strain, pathological Q waves, prolonged P-R interval (>0·20 sec), bundle-branch block and ST changes. Ventricular ectopics are often present, but rhythms other than sinus (for example, atrial fibrillation) carry a more serious prognostic significance.

(*c*) Blood tests of particular relevance to the anaesthetist are the haemoglobin, which may indicate polycythaemia (increased viscosity)

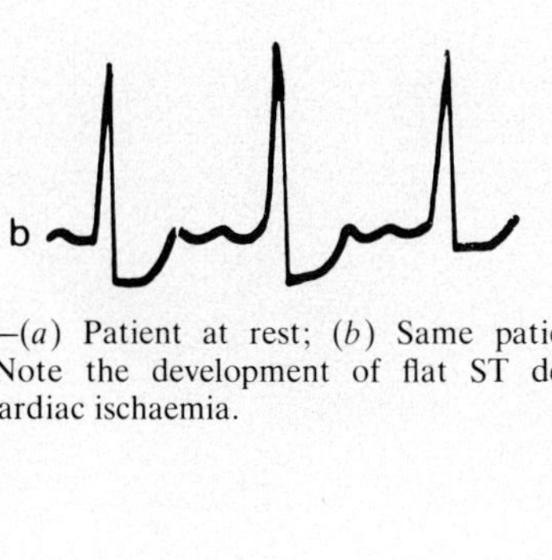

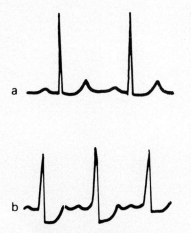


13/Fig. 9.—(*a*) Patient at rest; (*b*) Same patient after exercise. Note the development of flat ST depression denoting cardiac ischaemia.

or anaemia (exacerbation of angina), blood glucose and glucose tolerance test, cardiac enzymes (recent infarction), creatinine and liver function tests. Recently, abnormalities in blood lipids have been clarified, and a correlation with coronary artery disease has been demonstrated, with raised plasma concentrations of low-density lipoprotein cholesterol and with lowered high-density lipoprotein concentrations.[12]

(*d*) Cardiac catheterisation and coronary angiocardiography. This special investigation is mandatory before cardiac surgery for coronary revascularisation, its prime value being to delineate by angiography the anatomy and disease of the coronary arteries. An assessment of ventricular function will be assisted by cine-angiography (ventricular wall motion, ejection fraction), by pressure measurements (left atrial, ventricular end-diastolic, or pulmonary capillary wedge pressure) and by cardiac output estimations. Mitral valve dysfunction, due to papillary muscle ischaemia or rupture may also be demonstrated.

**The Treatment of Coronary Artery Disease**

**Medical.**—The aim of treatment is to reduce angina and hopefully to prevent myocardial infarction with drugs which either act upon the heart in order to improve the relationship between myocardial oxygen supply and demand, or which act upon the systemic vasculature in order to reduce ventricular afterload and improve cardiac efficiency.

The *nitrates*, either short-acting sublingual or longer-acting oral preparations, exert their effects primarily on peripheral vessels. The effects on venomotor tone and on arteriolar resistance reduce ventricular volume, pressure and afterload, and thus improve the balance between myocardial oxygen availability and consumption. When coronary spasm exists, the nitrates relieve angina by direct coronary vasodilator activity.

*Nitroglycerine* as the sole treatment for angina has been largely replaced by beta-adrenergic blocker therapy.[13] This group of drugs is discussed on page 430. *Beta blockade* diminishes myocardial oxygen demands by reducing heart rate and contractility and also lowers the blood pressure in hypertension. It prevents the rise in myocardial work during emotion and stress, as well as limiting the haemodynamic responses to anaesthesia and surgery.

*Calcium antagonists* (see p. 437) are increasingly used in angina as an alternative to beta blockade. Nifedipine or verapamil are the two drugs most commonly used and have varying degrees of vasodilator, myocardial depressant and antidysrhythmic activity.

Other drugs employed in patients with coronary artery disease are aimed at the management of related symptoms and pathology and include antidysrhythmics—such as disopyramide or mexiletine; antihypertensives, in addition to the beta blockers; hypoglycaemics; antiplatelet and antilipid drugs. In heart failure, digoxin and diuretics replace drugs with negative inotropic activity and improve angina by reducing ventricular size and wall tension.

**Surgical.**—A number of surgical procedures may be indicated for cardiac problems secondary to ischaemic heart disease.

(i) Coronary revascularisation. Reversed saphenous vein aorto-coronary bypass grafts, and more rarely, internal mammary—coronary artery grafting.
(ii) Excision of ventricular aneurysm.
(iii) Mitral valve replacement. Mitral regurgitation due to ischaemic papillary muscle dysfunction or rupture carries a high operative mortality if associated with poor left ventricular function. Rendering the mitral valve competent increases the forward-flow work of the ventricle and sometimes precipitates irreversible pump failure.
(iv) Repair of ventricular septal defect. This is an emergency procedure to correct a VSD produced by anteroseptal infarction.
(v) Heart transplantation may eventually be required for intractable ventricular failure from gross myocardial infarction.

### Myocardial Infarction

Those patients who do not die immediately from an infarct present with either severe chest pain, which lasts more than half-an-hour in the absence of exertion or emotion, or as sudden left ventricular failure, which may develop into cardiogenic shock and which is associated with severe dysrhythmias. The diagnosis of myocardial infarction is made primarily on the history, supported by serial electrocardiograms and enzyme studies, although the changes in these tests may take some time to develop. In contrast, an infarct occurring in the postoperative period is frequently "silent", the patient experiencing no pain and the diagnosis is only confirmed by the serial ECGs which are usually recorded in an attempt to elucidate the cause of postoperative hypotension or cardiac failure.

The earliest change in the ECG is elevation of the T wave over the site of the infarct. This is followed by ST segment elevation, T wave inversion and, if the infarct is transmural, the development of a Q wave. If the infarct is not full thickness, the Q wave does not appear but the amplitude of the R wave is diminished.

The site of the infarct is revealed by the leads in which the changes are best developed:

Left Coronary Artery Occlusion:
  Anteroseptal $V_{1-3}$  Anterior $V_{1-5}$
  Anterolateral $V_{5-7}$  High lateral I, aVL
Right Coronary Artery Occlusion:
  Inferior  II III aVF
  Posterior  $V_{1-2}$ (tall R waves).

### Fixed Low Cardiac Output

In fixed cardiac output states there is a limited, or even absent, ability to increase the cardiac output in response to vasodilatation, exercise or stress. Under these circumstances, cerebral perfusion may suffer and syncope result. During anaesthesia (*vide infra*) such patients are particularly liable to develop severe hypotension. In some valvular lesions, such as aortic or mitral stenosis (see p.503), a fixed cardiac output initially results from mechanical limitations imposed by the orifice size rather than from ventricular pump failure, which may ultimately occur in these and other lesions. Thus a fixed low cardiac output may be the common end-point from a number of circulatory disease states, which include:

Pulmonary hypertension
Aortic stenosis
Mitral stenosis
Pulmonary stenosis
Constrictive pericarditis
Complete heart block
Severe ventricular (pump) failure from any cause

Acute conditions – cardiac tamponade
– pulmonary embolus
– massive haemorrhage.

In this state, the patient is particularly vulnerable to certain events occurring during anaesthesia. These are:

1. *Bradycardia or dysrhythmias*—the stroke output is small and a faster cardiac rate must be maintained. Loss of atrial transport in rhythms other than sinus (see pp. 411 and 487) may aggravate the reduction in cardiac output which occurs at slow heart rates.
2. *Vasodilatation*—ventricular filling pressures may fall below the critical levels required to maintain an adequate cardiac output in response to venodilatation or to reduction in sympathetic tone. At the same time, any reduction in systemic arteriolar resistance enhances the fall in arterial pressure in the face of a fixed cardiac output.
3. *Myocardial depression*.—These patients are particularly susceptible to drugs that further impair myocardial performance.
4. *Myocardial ischaemia*.—Falls in arterial pressure or cardiac output in the presence of an increased ventricular wall tension may result in myocardial ischaemia, itself a myocardial depressant, and are extremely hazardous.

At the same time, skilful anaesthesia which avoids these hazards may improve the patient by controlling ventricular afterload and preload, and by abolishing the work of breathing with intermittent positive-pressure ventilation, reduce the total body oxygen consumption.

### Changes in Ventilatory Function Associated with Heart Disease

Patients with cardiac disease frequently suffer from associated respiratory problems. The cardiac disease itself may be secondary to chronic lung disease (cor pulmonale). The lungs may have interstitial oedema from an acute rise in left atrial pressure or long-standing congestion may have led to thickening and fibrosis in the lung. Thus the pulmonary vasculature may be abnormal both in the quality of the vessels and in the distribution of blood flow. These effects lead to a reduced lung compliance and therefore an increase in the work of breathing and hence in oxygen demand and cardiac output. At the same time the efficiency of gaseous exchange is reduced by an increased $V_D/V_T$ ratio and increased ventilation-perfusion mismatch, so that arterial oxygenation may be incomplete. This arterial hypoxaemia will be aggravated if the cardiac output is reduced.

Pleural effusions in congestive cardiac failure further compromise respiratory reserve and it may be necessary to aspirate them before anaesthesia.

If there is confusion as to whether the patient's dyspnoea is of pulmonary or cardiac origin it may be necessary to perform preoperative lung function tests both to define the respiratory limitation and to show to what extent it can be reversed by bronchodilator drugs or alterations in inspired oxygen tension. Ventilation during anaesthesia is discussed on page 482 and postoperative ventilation in cardiac patients on page 496.

## ANAESTHESIA FOR PATIENTS WITH CARDIAC DISEASE

To a certain extent the management of patients with cardiac disease undergoing anaesthesia and surgery depends on the particular operation being performed. The most fundamental distinction lies between cardiac and non-cardiac surgery. In the latter the stresses of surgery and, more especially, of the postoperative period will be placed on an abnormal circulation which will almost certainly be further compromised by the alterations produced by anaesthesia, pain or pyrexia and blood volume changes. In contrast, one may reasonably expect that cardiac surgery, as a procedure designed to improve cardiac status, should have a beneficial effect on the patient's heart. In practice, intensive care is necessary following heart surgery in order to monitor and correct a variety of complications, and also to prevent the deleterious circulatory changes that usually follow surgery of any type. Thus, in some respects, patients with cardiac disease who undergo incidental surgery are put at a disadvantage when compared with others who have corrective heart operations.

Irrespective of the particular disease, a given operation may dictate specific anaesthetic techniques which are beneficial to circulatory states and which provide good operating conditions. Open cardiac surgery with extracorporeal circulation is the extreme example and is discussed in a later chapter.

To a considerable degree the choice of anaesthesia, of monitoring, of circulatory management depends on the cardiac state of the patient. The pre-operative assessment defines the nature and severity of the haemodynamic alteration in the patient's cardiovascular system. The consequences of anaesthesia and surgery on the normal circulation are known. The difficulty lies in predicting how the intact but abnormal circulation, which is limited in its physiological reserves, will respond to the stresses imposed upon it.

There is now considerable information on the effects of anaesthetic agents on the abnormal heart. Whereas halothane produces moderate depression of the normal myocardium, in ventricular failure the additive effect of the anaesthetic combined with the cardiac pathology produces severe depression of myocardial contractility, and similar effects may be seen with other agents. This true functional state of the depressed myocardium produced by a conjunction of myocardial pathology and anaesthetic agent may only be revealed when the heart is challenged by an increase in preload and afterload or by a demand for an increased cardiac output, when it may be unable to respond appropriately.

Some conclusions can be drawn from knowledge of the patient's lesion. Specific lesions are considered in detail later but a few examples may be cited in brief here. In mitral stenosis a long diastolic period is needed for adequate ventricular filling and anaesthetic-induced tachycardia will depress cardiac output, while at the same time, due to the relatively small left ventricle in mitral stenosis, severe bradycardia will also reduce cardiac output.

In aortic stenosis the thick-walled left ventricular cavity needs the extra distension of atrial contraction to produce a good cardiac output and the small intracavity volume limits stroke output. Rhythm disturbances and slow rates will severely depress the cardiac output which will be enhanced by increased filling pressure, tachycardia and by inotropic stimulation. In the apparently similar subaortic stenosis of hypertrophic obstructive cardiomyopathy, inotropic stimulation will aggravate the obstruction and in this condition which is commonly treated with $\beta$-adrenergic blockade, a reasonable case can be made for the use of a myocardial depressant anaesthetic as well as preventing the exacerbation of the ventricular obstruction by endogenous catecholamine secretion. In subaortic stenosis a well-maintained filling pressure is important to reduce the obstruction and the effect of a maintained blood pressure and afterload is to prevent the ventricle contracting down at the end of systole and aggravating the obstruction. A similar effect may be seen in severe right ventricular infundibular stenosis. When this is associated with a ventricular septal defect in Fallot's tetralogy, the magnitude of the right-to-left shunt will depend on the relative resistances to the outflow down the pulmonary artery and aorta. The right-to-left shunt will be aggravated either by systemic arteriolar dilatation or by an increase in right ventricular infundibular tone, which may follow increased contractility induced by fear, stress or ketamine anaesthesia.

Thus the haemodynamic effects of the patient's lesion may suggest that some particular state, perhaps tachycardia or low filling pressure or catecholamine secretion, is undesirable and the anaesthetic technique chosen to avoid this factor, whether it be produced by the anaesthetic agent itself, by ventilatory or reflex effects or by any other way. And similarly the correct supportive measures, the ideal cardiac rate, the state of the preload and afterload are defined by an understanding of the patient's cardiovascular state.

The other factor of importance in dealing with the abnormal circulation and particularly with the failing heart, is the extent to which the maintenance of such a circulation depends on elevated sympathetic drive. Any interference by anaesthesia with this increased activity, either by depressing it or by depressing the ability of the end-organ to react to it, will have more profound effects than in the normal circulation.

This small amount of information when set against the infinite variety of patient response dictates the four principles of successful anaesthesia in cardiac disease.

(a) Meticulous continuous accurate monitoring of the patient's circulation.
(b) A choice of anaesthetic agents and techniques which produces the least alteration in cardiovascular performance.

(c) Manipulation of the patient's circulation to produce the most efficient situation in respect of satisfying tissue metabolic demands at minimum cardiac cost.

(d) Continuation of these principles into the postoperative phase when cardiorespiratory assessment and manipulation has a tendency to be relatively neglected.

## MONITORING DURING ANAESTHESIA FOR CARDIAC PATIENTS

The minimum acceptable monitoring for any patient with cardiac disease is frequent recording of the pulse and blood pressure and a continuous electrocardiographic display. Perhaps, considering the ease with which it can be measured, the central venous pressure could be added to this list.

For cardiac surgery or major general surgery in cardiac patients, full monitoring could include:

ECG: pulse rate: arterial blood pressure: central venous pressure: pulmonary capillary wedge pressure: arterial oxygen and carbon dioxide tensions: acid-base state: urine output: thermo-dilution cardiac output measurement: core and peripheral temperature: serum potassium: blood balance.

In monitoring one only measures "what one measures" (Kirklin). This truism implies that even with accurate measuring apparatus the greatest care must be taken in the interpretation of values obtained. For example, the numerical value of the central venous pressure is just that: of itself, it conveys no information whatsoever about the left atrial pressure, the function of the left ventricle, the need for blood replacement or the size of the circulating volume. Some of this information may be deduced by comparison with earlier values for CVP and considered in relation to the other information about the patient, but of itself, a numerical value is only evidence about that value. Further when taken by itself with no other knowledge of the patient's condition, the value may suggest therapy which is wrong or even dangerous.

The second point of importance about monitoring is that the evidence must fit together logically and no piece of information must be discarded on the grounds that it must be wrong unless the most careful scrutiny shows this to be so. Otherwise the first sign of some disorder will frequently be overlooked.

Most measurements have to be interpreted both against the patient's general condition and all the factors known to affect that measurement. Thus the arterial oxygen and carbon dioxide tensions are relevant only when considered against the cardiac output, the patient's metabolic state, the composition of the inspired gas, the mechanical factors of ventilation (tidal volume, airway pressure, expiratory pressure, ventilatory pattern) and the state of the patient's heart and lungs.

The difficulty in monitoring and assessing the cardiovascular system is that there is no one measurement of cardiovascular well-being. Because of the ease with which it is measured, the blood pressure has always been accorded a degree of importance. Certainly, extremes of blood pressure are potentially lethal in hypertension, coronary artery and other vascular or valve disease but, equally, the blood pressure can be substantially normal a few seconds before terminal cardiovascular collapse. It is often assumed that the cardiac output is a more important value and inferences are made about the output from the appearance of the patient's skin and temperature, the urine output, the arterial pressure and the blood gas values. Again, the cardiac output can be normal at a time when the blood pressure or the ECG suggest a far from normal state. Only very limited inferences can be made about ventricular function from the blood pressure. In the presence of valvular disease particularly, the added knowledge of left atrial pressure only marginally assists in the assessment of left ventricular function, which certainly cannot be estimated from arterial and central venous pressures alone. Absolute circulatory assessment is therefore difficult but the more frequently a clinician calibrates his impressions and observations against the results of extreme monitoring, the more able he will become to make statistically probable interpretations on limited or inadequate data. It is, however, fairly easy to monitor change and frequently this is more important than defining an absolute state, most circulatory support during anaesthesia and surgery being aimed at maintaining a given state constant.

**Technical Considerations**

All monitoring techniques must be carefully examined to ensure that they do not add to the risks to the patient, particularly in relation to electrical hazards and to sepsis. Because much monitoring relies on electricity (ECG, EEG, pressure monitoring, temperature) it brings the dangers of electric shock producing ventricular fibrillation and a potential for burns, particularly in conjunction with faulty diathermy apparatus. With the increasing tendency to leave monitoring catheters in for several days, sterility at the time of insertion and whenever fluids are added, particularly through 3-way taps, must be maintained. A potential hazard exists if foreign material, air, sterilising fluids or caustic substances (KCl, $CaCl_2$, antibiotics) are injected, particularly with arterial cannulae.

**ECG.**—Ideally the ECG amplifier should have an electrically isolated power supply. Although this will render unnecessary subsequent precautions it is good practice to use them due to the frequency of mixed electrical apparatus in use. The precautions include ECG plates rather than needle electrodes, a common earth (right leg lead) attached to the diathermy plate, and the use of high-resistance leads.

Lead II is the most useful for long-term observation of cardiac rhythm and $V_5$ for the detection of cardiac ischaemia (see p. 418).

**Central venous pressure.**—Accurate values for central venous (right heart filling) pressure can be obtained only if the tip of the catheter lies within the thorax, preferably in the right atrium or intrathoracic portion of either vena cava. The innominate vein is less satisfactory, particularly if the chest is open, when compression may produce inaccurate readings. Confirmatory signs that the catheter tip is in the correct place are that it is possible to aspirate blood easily, that the blood level falls freely and, having settled, fluctuates with respiration. Visual display of the venous waveform should depict a dynamic rather than a mean trace. The central venous pressure is measured against a stated reference point, which is usually either the sternal angle or mid-axillary line. The position of the patient is important, as is the type of ventilation (spontaneous or positive pressure). The normal CVP in the supine, spontaneously breathing patient, referred to the sternal angle, lies between −4 and +2 cm $H_2O$.

Access to an intrathoracic site may be via an antecubital, jugular, subclavian or femoral vein. Using the antecubital approach, only about 70 per cent of catheters can be expected to reach a suitable intrathoracic position, although an improved technique described by Bridges and his colleagues[14] has reported a 98 per cent success rate.

The femoral vein, entered below the inguinal ligament medial to the femoral artery is less satisfactory for long-term monitoring due to difficulty in avoiding bacterial contamination. The right side is preferred as the catheter runs up more easily than on the left. If the catheter catches on the bifurcation or a renal vein, it may kink and advance with a loop. This can be detected by difficulty in aspirating blood and partial withdrawal of the catheter usually straightens the loop, so that the catheter can be readvanced. At certain stages of cardiopulmonary bypass, when the venous drainage of the upper and lower halves of the body are separated, it may be necessary to monitor pressure in the inferior vena cava using the femoral vein approach.

Subclavian venous cannulation by the infraclavicular approach provides catheter stability with good long-term patient acceptance. In inexperienced hands, it has the highest incidence of serious complications, principally haemorrhage and pneumothorax. In cardiothoracic surgery, it is less suitable as the catheter may intrude on the operative field.

External jugular cannulation is safe and easy but it is often difficult or impossible to thread the catheter to an intrathoracic position. If the catheter tip remains within the external jugular, it will only give an approximate central venous pressure if the head is positioned so that the neck vein is in unobstructed communication with the intrathoracic veins.

The most satisfactory vessel to use is the right internal jugular vein. Although there are complications with its use, these are minimised by meticulous attention to technique and, especially, with experience. Either the cannula-over-needle method or the Seldinger technique is suitable.

1. The use of the right internal jugular vein is preferable to the left as there is a more direct communication with the superior vena cava.
2. The patient lies supine, and if possible in a Trendelenburg tilt, with the head turned fully

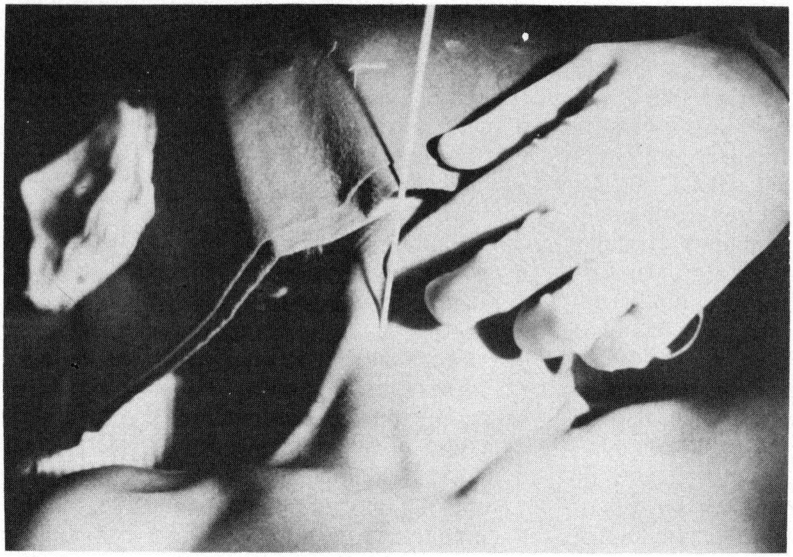

13/Fig. 10.—Right internal jugular venous cannulation. Note: the aseptic precautions and the direction of the cannula. This female patient was in congestive cardiac failure secondary to mitral valve disease. The external jugular vein is readily visible lateral to the bulge made by the internal jugular vein. The anaesthetist's left index finger is applying slight skin traction and is not palpating the carotid artery.

to the left and unsupported by pillows (see Fig. 10).

3. The anaesthetist stands at the head of the table and the patient's skin is prepared with iodine. The hair should be covered with a sterile towel.
4. An imaginary line is drawn from the sternal head of the sternomastoid muscle to the mastoid process, and a skin puncture is made halfway along this line. This is usually just above or below the point at which the external jugular vein crosses the sternomastoid and palpation briefly confirms that the common carotid artery lies medial to this point. There is no need to attempt to retract the artery, as retraction tends to distort the internal jugular vein.
5. Observation and palpation usually reveal the position and course of the internal jugular vein which, at the level of the skin puncture, tends to lie just posterior or slightly lateral to the sternomastoid muscle.
6. A 5½ in teflon 16 G cannula with its indwelling needle is attached to a syringe. The cannula is inserted through the skin puncture and directed caudally towards the internal jugular vein; usually this direction is slightly lateral, and backwards at an angle of about 25° (see Fig. 11).
7. The cannula is advanced slowly whilst aspirating with the syringe. When the needle enters the vein, blood should freely fill the syringe. Without altering the position of the needle, the cannula is slid off the needle into the vein. There should be no resistance, but sometimes rotating the cannula as it is advanced prevents it becoming kinked.
8. The cannula is tested for free aspiration of blood and then firmly secured, taking appropriate precautions against contamination.
9. More than one cannula can be inserted into the same jugular vein.

**Complications of central venous cannulation.**—The complications of central venous cannulation fall into two groups: those which arise from the act of cannulation and those secondary to the continued presence of the indwelling cannula.[15] The first group includes complications that are usually the result of trauma to nearby structures, such as the carotid artery, pleura and brachial plexus (Fig. 11). These may arise from initial misplacement of the cannula, or from correct placement followed by perforation. The immediate consequences are haemorrhage with haematoma formation (which in extreme circumstances may cause hypovolaemia), haemothorax, local compression or cardiac tamponade, the development of pneumothorax or surgical emphysema and the production of intimal damage with subsequent

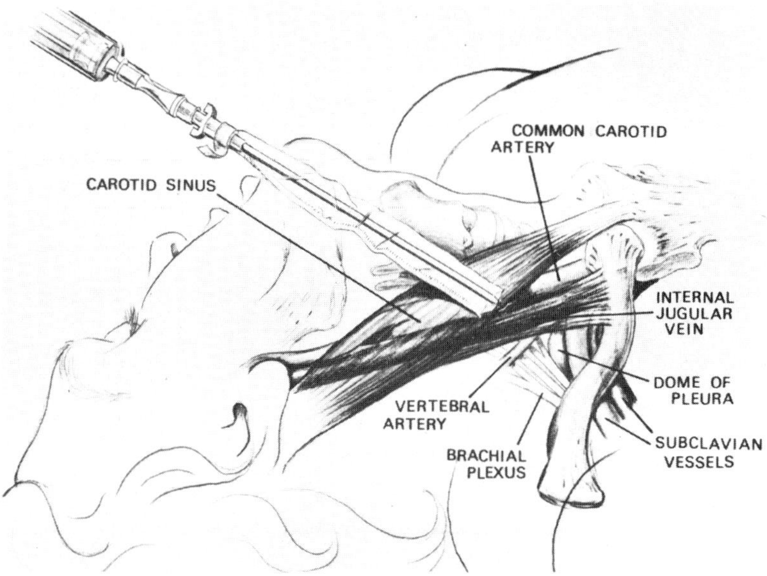


13/FIG. 11.—Right internal jugular venous cannulation. The 16G, 12-cm teflon cannula illustrated is protected from bacteriological contamination by a plastic sheath that is removed after cannulation. (Courtesy of H. G. Wallace Ltd., Colchester, England and Dr. Alan Gilston, National Heart Hospital.)

thrombosis. Cannulae lying within the atria or, more particularly, the right ventricle, may cause dysrhythmias.

The second group of complications are due to:

(i) Misconnections, leading to haemorrhage, air embolism, or failure of supportive intravenous therapy.

(ii) Infusion of fluids or drugs through a malpositioned catheter causing skin necrosis, hydrothorax, hydromediastinum or inadvertent intra-arterial injections.

(iii) Infection. The incidence of central venous cannula contamination is potentially high; Opie[16] reported a 65 per cent incidence of bacterial contamination of internal jugular catheters used in cardiac surgery. Usually bacterial infection is caused by the patient's own skin or nasal flora, but only occasionally does this become pathogenic. If it is evident, however, extremely virulent organisms, resistant to many antibiotics, may produce serious infection, particularly in the already sick patient. Cannula contamination can be minimised by meticulous aseptic technique, with careful skin preparation at the time of cannulation, the prophylactic use of nasal antiseptic ointments and subsequent care when handling stop-cocks and manometer lines.

### Arterial Pressure

If the arterial pressure is measured with a cuff, either manually or by an automated process, the size of cuff must be appropriate for the arm; the thicker the arm, the wider the cuff, or spurious readings will be obtained. The oscillotonometer, although very accurate in conditions associated with peripheral vasodilatation (induced hypotension) is more difficult to read if the circulation is inadequate. For sick patients undergoing major or cardiac surgery, or during profound hypotensive anaesthesia, direct arterial pressure monitoring with continuous display is preferable.

The left radial is the most commonly chosen for cannulation, after adequate collateral flow via the ulnar artery has been demonstrated by Allen's test or one of its modifications. The frequency of subsequent radial artery occlusion is between 30 per cent[17] and 40 per cent[18] with a higher incidence in women. Complications can be reduced by the use of smaller bore (20 G) non-tapered, teflon cannulae.

Other arteries, such as the brachial, femoral or dorsalis pedis may also be used. The femoral artery should probably be cannulated only when other sites are unavailable or when the cardiac output is so low as to make more peripheral measurements inaccurate. The dorsalis pedis artery is convenient for direct arterial pressure monitoring when access to the arm is difficult, as in neurosurgery. However, its routine use is not recommended by Husum, Palm and Eriksen[19] because of the inadequacy of collateral circulation to the foot and the frequency of arterial thromboses.

With practice, arterial cannulation is no more difficult than venepuncture, and there is no need to puncture the back wall of the artery as this will result in further intimal damage and unnecessary haematoma. Meticulous technique will minimise complications, but the advantages of direct arterial pressure monitoring and availability of arterial blood samples must always be weighed against the potential disadvantages.

**Pulmonary Artery Catheterisation**

The Swan Ganz multi-lumen catheter incorporates a balloon at its distal end. This has two functions: when inflated with air it encourages the passage of the catheter through the right ventricle into the pulmonary artery; subsequently, once the catheter tip has entered a distal pulmonary artery, inflation of the balloon occludes this vessel so that the pressure recorded by the catheter changes from a pulmonary arterial trace to that of the pulmonary capillary. This "wedge" pulmonary artery trace can, in most circumstances, be regarded as representing the left atrial pressure.

The catheter is first inserted via a jugular or antecubital vein to the right atrium and, after the balloon has been inflated with 0·5–1·0 ml air, advanced while the ECG and cannula tip pressure are monitored. If available, radiographic control may facilitate placement. Ventricular extrasystoles, which are common during the passage of the cannula through the right ventricle, may be effectively suppressed by intravenous lignocaine (1 mg/kg).[20] The final position of the catheter is inferred by the change in character of the pressure trace when the balloon is inflated. This should only be maintained for short periods to obviate the risk of pulmonary infarction.[21]

The extra lumena of the catheter can be used for the simultaneous measurement of right atrial pressure or, depending on the type of catheter, for the measurement of cardiac output, electrocardiography or cardiac pacing.

The complications of flow-directed pulmonary artery catheterisation are:

(1) *At insertion*—trauma to SVC, right atrium, right ventricle and pulmonary artery, production of dysrhythmias, ventricular fibrillation, heart block, accidental knotting of the catheter.
(2) *During use*—failure to wedge, thrombus function, pulmonary infarction, balloon rupture with air embolus, infection.

**Drips and Drug Administration**

The maintenance of adequate ventricular filling pressures is important in most cardiac disease states. Haemorrhage, fluid loss or venodilatation may necessitate rapid infusion in order to restore cardiac output, and for this reason an absolute requirement is a large intravenous cannula, preferably connected to blood warming apparatus. Blood loss during cardiac surgery is often less than in many other forms of major surgery; however, when it occurs, it can be quick and massive and facilities for rapid transfusion (e.g. pressure infusion bags) are essential.

At critical moments during surgery, it may be necessary to transfuse quickly, measure the central venous pressure and administer drugs simultaneously. There are disadvantages to injecting irritant drugs (KCl, $CaCl_2$) into peripheral veins and to injecting potent drugs into lines whose rate of flow is dependent on some other factor. For these reasons, one or two extra venous lines reserved for the administration of drugs are often useful.

## CHOICE OF ANAESTHETIC AGENTS AND TECHNIQUES IN CARDIAC DISEASE

(a) **Anaesthetic Agents**

Anaesthetic agents may possess one or more actions which are undesirable of which the most important are depression of myocardial contractility and reduction in peripheral venous tone. When these two are combined together in a drug such as thiopentone, its quick administration can be lethal to severely incapacitated patients. Reduction in venous tone is perhaps less dangerous than myocardial depression as it can be compensated for by fluid infusion, provided the venous pressure is monitored. However, sudden venodilatation can lead to a dangerous reduction in cardiac output before adequate replacement can be achieved. Myocardial depression caused by anaesthetic agents could be treated with inotropic drugs but this would postulate an unnecessarily complicated anaesthetic technique, very dependent on accurate monitoring and prompt correction of anaesthetic side-effects with other potent drugs. The better rule in the choice of drugs for cardiac patients is to select those agents which produce minimal myocardial depression and which do not significantly alter peripheral venous tone. Within these restrictions the actual choice of drugs probably does not matter and it is the skill of the administrator in the careful maintenance of the circulation which is important. The many papers which attest to the value of one technique over another and the difficulty in substantiating the claims, confirm this view. The most popular techniques are variations of balanced anaesthesia with paralysis, IPPV, nitrous oxide and oxygen supplemented by opiates, or minimal concentrations of volatile anaesthetic agents. For the spontaneously ventilating patient, neuroleptanaesthesia may provide more stable cardiovascular conditions than the more traditional halothane or enflurane anaesthesia. The requirements for and limitations of, the latter two agents can be reduced by the addition of regional or systemic analgesia.

### (b) Premedication

Adequate sedation is necessary for patients with cardiac disease and although careful preoperative psychological support and explanation should always be given, this does not obviate the need for premedicant drugs. A generous premedication reduces the dose of induction agent and diminishes the likelihood of violent alterations, in either direction, of the blood pressure. An increase in sympathetic tone due to fear and apprehension may provoke untoward haemodynamic changes leading to angina, dysrhythmias or pulmonary oedema. In certain patients, such as those with critical coronary artery stenoses, mild sedation in the form of lorazepam or diazepam may be administered for several days prior to operation. $\beta$-adrenergic blocking drugs, if indicated, will normally be continued or administered with the premedication and while antibiotics are often given at the same time, their intramuscular injection is painful and they are equally effective given intravenously, following induction.

Morphine is particularly suitable and the dose given can be generous as large doses can usually be used safely in patients with minimal cardiac reserves. In low cardiac output states which are sensitive to alteration in ventricular filling pressure, the reduction in venocapacitance tone in previously vasoconstricted patients may lead to hypotension. Morphine or papaveretum is mostly given in combination with hyoscine, which has the advantage of having an antisialogogue effect with amnesic, anti-emetic and sedative properties.

Atropine has the disadvantage of producing no sedative action and may cause a tachycardia. The latter is undesirable in mitral stenosis and in coronary artery disease, particularly if the blood pressure is also raised. The use of atropine as a sole premedicant in cardiac patients may be positively harmful. Glycopyrrolate would appear to offer little advantage over atropine as it has no sedative or anti-emetic actions, although it would be less likely to produce a tachycardia. Both valium and morphine-scopolamine premedication may be associated with significant arterial hypoxaemia[22,23] and some authorities recommend the administration of oxygen following pre-operative sedation.

### (c) Induction

Except in the most ill patients, induction is usually performed in the anaesthetic room; it is usually easier to bring the operating table into the anaesthetic room and place the patient on it before induction. Some patients, particularly children, may need to be induced sitting up. Such patients should be moved from their ward in a sitting up position and not forced to lie down on a trolley.

The ECG should be attached before induction. Most patients will be presented in their optimum condition, not in cardiac failure and then, provided manual measurement of pulse and blood pressure is normal, induction may proceed, to be followed by arterial, venous and central venous cannulation. In other patients, more extensive invasive monitoring may need to be established before induction, either because the patient's pre-induction state is unsatisfactory, or because of the possibility of rapid deterioration during, or immediately after, induction. In these cases, intravenous diazepam or midazolam accompanied by oxygen administration reduces untoward cardiovascular responses induced by fear and anxiety while arterial, central venous and/or pulmonary catheters, and infusion cannulae are inserted under local anaesthesia. Increasing familiarity with this technique and hence high success rate with cannulation, encourages many anaesthetists to adopt it in all cardiac cases, both high and low risk.

Certain cardiovascular changes are to be expected at induction. Usually a reduction in blood pressure and cardiac output secondary to a reduction in arteriolar and venous tone and a depression of myocardial contractility depending on the agents employed, followed by a rise in blood pressure and heart rate during intubation. Moderate variations may be acceptable in most patients, but in others they may be dangerous and while the choice of technique should be aimed at preventing these changes, it is prudent to have available drugs such as metaraminol, calcium, lignocaine and phentolamine to reverse them if they become excessive.

In the extremes of a low fixed cardiac output, the use of intravenous barbiturates is potentially lethal and induction is better performed with diazepam and small doses of a suitable opiate. Gaseous induction is no longer popular, although cyclopropane has enjoyed popularity in the past on the grounds that it ensures a quick induction in a high oxygen atmosphere and in patients in gross cardiac failure, produces significantly less cardiac depression than the fluorinated hydrocarbons.

In the majority of cardiac patients, however, a *small* sleep dose of thiopentone, given slowly to allow for increased circulation time, is remarkably well tolerated and any hypotension can usually be treated with volume replacement or, more rarely, a mixed $\alpha$ and $\beta$ agonist (metaraminol). As most cardiac patients will be ventilated during anaesthesia and hence require a long-acting muscle relaxant, intubation will usually be performed under this rather than after suxamethonium. While in certain cases tubocurarine may be indicated, the more common choice is pancuronium and the effect of this drug and the vasopressor effect of intubation tends to offset the hypotensive effect of thiopentone. Metocurine is advocated as an alternative to pancuronium and although it is less likely to provoke an increase in rate or pressure, it may very occasionally be associated with hypotension. Intubation must be delayed until the patient is fully relaxed, being preceded by first, assisted, and then controlled, ventilation with nitrous oxide in oxygen. In patients with coronary artery disease in whom hypertension and tachycardia may be more dangerous than hypotension, the use of $\beta$-blockers and vasodilators may be necessary at induction, although the addition of halothane may prove equally effective.

### (d) **Ventilation during Anaesthesia**

Respiratory dysfunction is commonly found in association with cardiac disease, particularly those which cause high left atrial pressure or increased pulmonary blood flow. These patients may exhibit mechanical difficulties with respiration due to decreased compliance or obstructive airway disease and have an increase in the mechanical work of breathing. They may also have clinical or subclinical hypoxia when breathing air due to an increase in ventilation-perfusion mismatch which is aggravated by any reduction in cardiac output. The carbon dioxide tension may be altered in either direction but is commonly low in cardiac dyspnoea. For these reasons, IPPV during anaesthesia is particularly advisable and allows greater control of arterial blood gas tensions, while eliminating the respiratory and cardiac work of breathing.

In the normal patient, the introduction of IPPV will have little effect on the cardiovascular system provided that the inspiratory-expiratory time ratio is short, the airway pressure low and severe hypocapnia is avoided. In cardiac disease, haemodynamic changes due to IPPV may become significant. The rise in mean intrathoracic pressure has two main effects which lead to a reduction in stroke volume and cardiac output. Firstly, the venous return is impaired which lowers right ventricular output, secondly the pulmonary vascular impedance increases. This imparts an increased afterload on the right ventricle which may increase the dimensions of the right ventricle, distorting the intraventricular septum to impair left ventricular diastolic filling. The impairment of venous return may not always be disadvantageous and may prevent a patient with high venous pressure developing pulmonary oedema when laid flat on the operating table. Oxygenation may also improve in conditions with high pulmonary capillary pressures after the introduction of

IPPV, particularly when combined with a positive end-expiratory pressure.

Apart from the mechanical effect of ventilation on the cardiac output, a separate chemical mechanism has been postulated[24] which may partially explain the inappropriately large reductions in ventricular performance observed in some patients undergoing IPPV with the chest opened. These mechanisms include a modification of pulmonary prostaglandins produced by the stretch response which may exhibit a negative inotropic effect. The mechanical effects, however, are usually of more clinical significance.

In conditions of reduced pulmonary blood flow, pulmonary embolism, severe pulmonary stenosis or pulmonary hypertension, IPPV may lead to catastrophic falls in pulmonary blood flow and cardiac output. More commonly, attempts to avoid IPPV have even greater disadvantages. In Fallot's tetralogy, the reduction in pulmonary blood flow, secondary to appropriately applied IPPV, is much less than that caused by the rise in pulmonary vascular resistance, secondary to hypercapnia, in the spontaneously breathing anaesthetised patient.

## CIRCULATORY COMPLICATIONS DURING ANAESTHESIA

### Low Cardiac Output and Hypotension

Hypotension during surgery has been discussed in the context of circulatory manipulation and induced hypotension in the previous chapter. In patients with cardiac disease, the stability of the circulation is often precarious and while circulatory deterioration should be avoided during anaesthesia, in many patients, by careful assessment and therapy it may be possible actually to improve or optimise the circulation.

Mild hypotension by itself, if the cardiac output is maintained, may not be serious. In cardiac failure, arteriolar dilatation tends to improve cardiac output and reduce myocardial oxygen consumption. In general terms, however, a significant lowering of blood pressure in cardiac patients usually implies a worsening of, rather than an improvement in, circulatory status. Rapid assessment is then required to elucidate the cause or causes of the circulatory deterioration so that subsequent management is possible on a sound logical base, which will take into account the haemodynamic problems of the particular cardiac disease from which the patient is suffering.

The causes of intra-operative hypotension and reduced cardiac output are conveniently considered according to the determinants of cardiac output and blood pressure, namely ventricular filling pressure, cardiac rate and rhythm, myocardial contractility and arteriolar resistance, together with the additional possibility of an iatrogenic cause.

(a) **Iatrogenic causes.**—During cardiac surgery, the cardiac output may be affected by surgical manipulation of the heart and great vessels. This can compromise ventricular filling, induce dysrhythmias or reduce contractility. Cardiac output may also be reduced secondary to changes produced by the introduction of positive-pressure ventilation or by the inappropriate use of drugs, including anaesthetic agents which have a circulatory effect.

(b) **Ventricular filling pressure** may be reduced by drug-induced reductions in venomotor tone (common at the time of induction) or by true hypovolaemia. Frequently these two conditions may co-exist when otherwise mild changes may summate to produce a serious effect. Effective ventricular filling pressure may also be reduced by mechanical distortion of the heart and great vessels, changes in cardiac rhythm or elevation of the mean intrathoracic pressure. Maintenance of the optimal filling pressure is more important in cardiac disease than in the normal patient and monitoring of the central venous or pulmonary capillary wedge pressure may be essential.

Equally circulatory deterioration may be associated with a high venous pressure in pump failure, valve disease, dysrhythmias or increased venocapacitance tone and will be aggravated by overtransfusion and inadequate depth of anaesthesia. Inappropriately high ventricular end-diastolic pressure may provoke pulmonary oedema and by overdistending the ventricle, reduce ventricular function and coronary perfusion, leading to further deterioration. While therapy is normally directed to the initial cause, it may be necessary to reduce the effective filling pressure either by drug-induced venodilatation in conjunction with posture, or by venesection.

(c) **Arteriolar resistance.**—In those patients

with a relatively fixed cardiac output (stenotic valve lesions, pulmonary hypertension, complete heart block), arteriolar dilatations may exceed the compensatory ability of the heart and the blood pressure will fall. Many anaesthetic agents produce arteriolar dilatation either by direct action or by a centrally mediated reduction in sympathetic tone, as may some drugs used in cardiac disease (isoprenaline, salbutamol). Provided the other determinants of cardiac output are maintained and the cardiac output itself has not been further reduced, management of this form of hypotension is achieved by restoring systemic vascular resistance.

(d) **Cardiac rate and rhythm.** — The extremes of cardiac rate, both bradycardia and tachycardia, may result in hypotension, particularly in the presence of a cardiac lesion whose effect is very dependent on cardiac rate. Thus, in mitral stenosis, tachycardia is associated with a reduction in cardiac output due to impaired ventricular filling. Dysrhythmias may have a two-fold effect on cardiac output, one due to the variation in cardiac rate and a second, often more serious, due to the loss of the atrial transport mechanism. Treatment is directed at restoring the cardiac rate to normal with the elimination of the precipitating causes of the dysrhythmia (cardiac manipulation, acidosis, hypokalaemia, ischaemia) before specific anti-dysrhythmic agents are employed.

(e) **Myocardial contractility.**—Poor ventricular function is often a feature of cardiac disease and inotropic support may be required in order to maintain the cardiac output. However, positive inotropic therapy is no substitute for avoiding these factors associated with anaesthesia which lead to a reduction in myocardial contractility, nor as compensation for neglect of the other factors discussed above.

### Inotropic Agents

If elimination of the precipitating causes and correction of hypoxia and acidosis does not restore the circulation, then an inotropic agent may be required. *Isoprenaline*, infused at a rate of 0·5–5 μg/min, has strong $\beta$-stimulating actions on the heart; it increases the cardiac rate and produces peripheral vasodilatation, reducing the afterload on the left ventricle. It will frequently convert nodal rhythm back into sinus control, and may be useful in heart-block as it increases the ventricular rate. However, in fixed cardiac output states (mitral or aortic stenosis, pulmonary hypertension or cardiac tamponade) isoprenaline may merely reduce the systemic vascular resistance and aggravate hypotension. Isoprenaline may also be inappropriate in the presence of ventricular tachydysrhythmias. *Dopamine* has less of an effect on arteriolar resistance than isoprenaline, and is more suitable in situations which require only minimal effects in vasomotor tone. In high doses the systemic vascular resistance may actually be increased. Dopamine, like noradrenaline and adrenaline, can increase veno-capacitance tone, and raise ventricular diastolic pressure despite an improvement in contractility. This action may prove disadvantageous in myocardial ischaemia, when it can upset the delicate myocardial oxygen supply/demand balance. Dopamine, in low doses, enhances renal blood flow and is unlikely to cause the renal ischaemia that can occur with adrenaline.

Cardiogenic shock is usually accompanied by intense vasoconstriction which only relaxes following an improvement in cardiac output; under these circumstances even inotropic drugs with a vasoconstrictive action tend to enhance renal blood flow, subsequent to an improvement in cardiac performance. *Dobutamine* is a powerful inotrope which produces less tachycardia and vasodilatation than isoprenaline and is a useful alternative where less of an effect on heart rate and systemic vascular resistance is required, as in mitral stenosis. *Prenalterol*, a pure $\beta_1$-agonist, has less of an effect on peripheral resistance and minimal chronotropic properties. *Noradrenaline* actually possesses moderate inotropic activity and, combined with a vasodilator (see below) so as to avoid intense veno- and arteriolar constriction, is sometimes effective in severe myocardial dysfunction following cardiopulmonary bypass.

Under certain circumstances, relative contra-indications to the use of an inotropic drug may exist:

(i) in myocardial ischaemia when an increase in rate and contractility may be detrimental and an improvement in cardiac output and blood pressure should be achieved by other means;

(ii) in hypertrophic obstructive cardiomyopathy when an inotropic drug can increase outflow tract obstruction or provoke serious dysrhythmias;

(iii) in situations where there is inadequate patient monitoring;

(iv) when the reduced cardiac output is not due to poor myocardial contractility.

### Vasodilator Therapy

Vasodilator therapy is occasionally necessary in severe ventricular dysfunction, when the improvement in ventricular function occurs secondary to changes in preload and afterload. *Glyceryl trinitrate* has a predominant action upon preload and is discussed on page 430.

Vasodilator therapy with *sodium nitroprusside* has proved valuable in improving left ventricular performance in the presence of left ventricular failure, in valvular regurgitation and in selective cases following myocardial infarction.[25] The circulation is affected by actions mainly on the arteriolar resistance but also on the venous capacitance (Table 3).

(i) *Afterload reduction*: Ventricular wall tension during systole is reduced by the effect on arterial tone. Sodium nitroprusside increases the compliance of the great vessels and the peripheral arterioles so that the aortic input impedence (the rate of change of aortic pressure/instantaneous aortic flow) is reduced and ventricular wall tension (afterload) falls. The increase in forward flow (that is cardiac output) encourages the left ventricle to empty more effectively so that ventricular end-systolic volume falls, leading to a reduction in ventricular size and a further reduction in wall tension.

(ii) *Preload reduction*: Lowering of venocapacitance tone, reduces atrial pressure, effective ventricular filling pressure and chamber size. This also reduces wall tension, so that an effect on preload becomes interrelated with an effect on afterload. For example in patients with severe left ventricular failure, secondary to cardiomyopathy or ischaemic heart disease, Thompson and his colleagues[26] showed that sodium nitroprusside caused a reduction in left ventricular end-systolic and end-diastolic pressures and in systemic vascular resistance. These effects produced an increased cardiac output and, despite the increase in ventricular minute work, the myocardial oxygen consumption fell due to improved myocardial efficiency. In some cases the improvement in cardiac output following the administration of sodium nitroprusside may be limited by the fall in effective filling pressure to a lower than optimal level. Stone and his colleagues[27] used crystalloid infusions to maintain ventricular filling pressure during sodium nitroprusside administration and found greater increases in cardiac output than when the filling pressures were allowed to fall. A further problem arises in the use of sodium nitroprusside in ventricular failure secondary to ischaemic heart disease, due to the effect on coronary artery perfusion pressure. While a reduction in myocardial oxygen consumption will follow the decrease in wall tension, secondary to the reduction in afterload, if systemic hypotension produces a critical reduction in coronary perfusion pressure, reduction in oxygen supply may exceed reduction in oxygen demand and subendocardial ischaemia may result.[28]

## Pulmonary Oedema

Pulmonary oedema results from an exaggeration of the normal physiological process that continually produces and removes extravascular pulmonary fluid.[29] An increased pulmonary capillary pressure tends to drive water into the interstitial tissues of the lung, an effect which is largely opposed by the plasma colloid osmotic pressure. Normally lymphatic drainage removes excess lung water, but this mechanism is limited and can be overwhelmed. Damage to pulmonary capillaries can increase permeability and leakage, when the increase in extravascular colloid further upsets the osmotic transcapillary gradients and accentuates the fluid loss.

In cardiac disease, pulmonary oedema is principally due to an increase in pulmonary capillary pressure, secondary to an abnormally high left atrial pressure. Haemodilution will lower plasma oncotic pressure and increase the susceptibility to oedema formation, whilst pulmonary capillary endothelial damage due to sepsis, inhalational damage, drugs or anaphy-

13/TABLE 3
THE USES OF SODIUM NITROPRUSSIDE IN CARDIAC DISEASE

| *Condition* | *Mechanism of Effect* |
|---|---|
| (1) Ventricular failure | Reduces afterload and increases cardiac output. Reduces ventricular filling pressures. |
| (2) Aortic regurgitation | Encourages forward aortic flow reducing regurgitant diastolic fraction and lowering left ventricular end-diastolic volume. Enhanced by an increase in rate. |
| (3) Mitral regurgitation | Encourages forward aortic flow in systole. |
| (4) Ischaemic heart disease | Reduces myocardial oxygen demand by lowering wall tension due to a fall in systemic vascular resistance and a drop in left ventricular end-diastolic pressure. Also controls hypertension. |
| (5) Coarctation, dissection or transection of aorta | Controls aortic blood pressure, preventing further damage or allowing surgical control of haemorrhage. |
| (6) Following cardiopulmonary bypass | Vasodilatation improves rewarming, ventricular function and efficiency, and controls hypertension. |

laxis, may provoke non-cardiogenic pulmonary oedema (see p. 566).

**The treatment of acute cardiogenic pulmonary oedema during anaesthesia.**—The aim is to reduce the pulmonary capillary pressures by:

(a) *Reduction in right ventricular output and pulmonary blood volume*
- anti-Trendelenburg position to encourage venous pooling;
- veno-capacitance dilatation with morphine or glyceryl trinitrate;
- intermittent positive-pressure ventilation and PEEP to reduce right ventricular filling and increase right ventricular afterload, as a result of the increase in intrathoracic pressure. Reduction in cardiac output may occur but can be largely offset by the beneficial effects on oxygenation, and the elimination of the increased work of breathing;
- diuresis—frusemide is usually the appropriate choice, whereas osmotic diuretics (such as mannitol) are contra-indicated;
- venesection—the above measures usually suffice but rapid control of blood volume can be achieved by removal of blood into a blood-donor bag which can be used subsequently for re-transfusion.

(b) *Reduction in left atrial pressure*

The reduction in right ventricular output will tend to reduce left atrial pressure and this effect will be enhanced if left ventricular function is improved. This is achieved by the appropriate measures which include:
- treatment of acidosis and hypoxia;
- control of heart rate and rhythm;
- inotropic and/or vasodilator therapy;
- removal of negative inotropic drugs (e.g. halothane, enflurane);
- treatment of acute myocardial ischaemia.

Removal of the oedema fluid by suction is quite useless. Fluid merely accumulates as fast as it is removed and the action of sucking impairs ventilation. Continuous positive-pressure ventilation must not be discontinued until the measures to lower left atrial pressure have had time to work.

In general, good anaesthesia decreases the risk of acute pulmonary oedema, but in those patients whose circulatory equilibrium is finely balanced, even a change of posture—from the upright to the horizontal—may induce failure. Patients who are on the borderline of pulmonary oedema may need to be induced in the upright position. Pregnant women with cardiac disease are especially liable to this complication after delivery of the placenta at the moment when the contracting uterus displaces a large volume of blood into the general circulation. The intravenous use of ergometrine enhances the risk.

Occasionally acute pulmonary oedema occurs in association with radiological procedures, such as trans-lumbar aortography for the investigation of arterial disease. Here, left ventricular function may be compromised by coronary artery disease and the patient unable to tolerate the hypervolaemic response to the injection of contrast medium.

**Cardiac arrest.**—This is discussed in Chapter 14

### The Diagnosis and Treatment of Cardiac Dysrhythmias Occurring During Anaesthesia

In normal patients, cardiac dysrhythmia is not uncommon during anaesthesia and surgery. They occur most frequently during induction and intubation, and less frequently during stable anaesthesia. Somewhat surprisingly they are common during regional anaesthesia but the overall incidence of dysrhythmia which is either haemodynamically significant or precursors of dangerous dysrhythmia, is very low.

In cardiac disease, dysrhythmias are both more frequent and more important. Their significance is two-fold:

Firstly, the presence of dysrhythmias may be the only indication of underlying cardiovascular disease, particularly premature ventricular contractions which, when frequent, may indicate myocardial ischaemia. Premature atrial contractions or atrial dysrhythmias may indicate a marginal cardiac reserve. The onset of dysrhythmias may represent either the cause or the effect of progressive deterioration in myocardial performance.

Secondly, whereas the normal myocardium will tolerate dysrhythmias well and maintain a reasonable output in the face of a continued abnormal rate, even minor dysrhythmias may be haemodynamically significant in the presence of myocardial or valvular disease.

#### Haemodynamic Implications

Dysrhythmias produce alterations in the haemodynamic state, the importance of which varies with the underlying disease.

1. *Lack of atrial transport mechanism.* Atrial contraction is particularly important for adequate ventricular filling under three circumstances:

(*a*) Where obstruction exists between atrium and ventricle. Commonly in mitral stenosis, rarely in tricuspid stenosis.

(*b*) Where the ventricle is hypertrophied or non-compliant and requires a higher than normal filling pressure to fill it adequately, e.g. aortic or pulmonary stenosis, systemic or pulmonary hypertension, hypertrophic cardiomyopathy.

(*c*) Where the unhypertrophied ventricle is suddenly stressed, e.g. pulmonary embolism.

2. *Effects of bradycardia.* Patients with low fixed stroke volumes depend on an adequate rate for their cardiac output. Bradycardia causes a serious drop in cardiac output in constrictive pericarditis, cardiac tamponade, pulmonary hypertension and cardiac failure. It is also deleterious in both aortic incompetence and stenosis.

3. *Effects of tachycardia.* There are two main effects of tachycardia:

(*a*) Lack of time for diastolic filling of ventricle. This is most obvious in patients with mitral stenosis but even normal hearts are embarrassed if the rate is fast enough.

(*b*) An increase in the tension-time index demonstrating an increase in myocardial oxygen consumption, usually unaccompanied by any increase in coronary blood flow. Tachycardia is thus bad both in coronary artery disease and in ventricular hypertrophy.

4. *Effects of abnormal pattern of ventricular contraction.* The abnormally propagated excitatory impulse in ventricular dysrhythmias produces a less efficient contraction. This is particularly disadvantageous in aortic and pulmonary stenosis, systemic and pulmonary hypertension.

#### Predisposing Factors

Dysrhythmias may result from direct stimulation of the heart at surgery or by intravascular catheters but more commonly, rhythm disturbances are produced by the summation of a number of factors which, taken singly, would not necessarily cause the same effect. During anaesthesia dysrhythmias are common in patients with heart disease and in patients with pre-existing dysrhythmias. Predisposing factors include:

*Increased catecholamine levels* which may be due to exogenous catecholamines from local infiltration or intravenous inotropic agents, or to excessive endogenous catecholamine liberated in response to painful stimuli under too light anaesthesia, ether or cyclopropane anaesthesia, hypercarbia or hypoxia.

*Hypoxia*, besides stimulating catecholamine secretion, has a direct action on the heart muscle cells. While general hypoxia may result from ventilatory or circulatory defects, local areas of hypoxia in the heart arise from discrepancies between oxygen delivery and oxygen consumption.

*Reflex stimulation* can arise from pharynx, larynx, abdominal and thoracic organs and the eye muscles. It may both provoke catecholamine release and stimulate the vagus so that the development of escape beats is more likely. At the same time, excessive parasympathetic blockade with atropine leaves the way for unopposed sympathetic action and a higher incidence of dysrhythmias. Dysrhythmias are frequently provoked by laryngoscopy and endotracheal intubation.

*Electrolyte changes*, particularly of extracellular potassium and magnesium, predispose to the development of dysrhythmias. Alterations in potassium may follow direct administration or result from alterations in pH, usually the consequence of change in ventilation or metabolic state, or occur following the administration of intravenous succinylcholine.

*Drugs*—certain anaesthetic agents are associated with the development of dysrhythmias, particularly cyclopropane, halothane, atropine and suxamethonium. Other drugs include digoxin and the tricyclic antidepressants. Hypercarbia potentiates drug-induced dysrhythmias.

*Physical factors* such as ventricular dysrhythmias are more common if the arterial pressure rises while atrial tachycardias are more common when the atrial pressures are high.

*Specific cardiac diseases* are frequently associated with dysrhythmic formation, i.e. cardiomyopathy, myocarditis, ventricular hypertrophy, coronary artery disease and low cardiac output states.

*Endocrine disorders* can now show an increased liability to dysrhythmias as seen in phaeochromocytoma and thyrotoxicosis.

**Mechanism of Dysrhythmias**

There are three mechanisms of dysrhythmia production:

(*a*) *Enhancement of phase 4 depolarisation* (see 12/Fig. 5, p. 410) may occur in any part of the heart which has rhythmic activity. It is characteristic of the rhythm disturbances caused by hypoxia or overdistension such as atrial fibrillation.

(*b*) *Electrical re-entry* in tissues where there are disparities in refractory period. This occurs in cardiac disease, digoxin toxicity and at slow heart rates. Typical dysrhythmias are supraventricular tachycardia, atrial flutter, ventricular tachycardia and certain ventricular ectopic beats.

(*c*) *Atrioventricular dissociation*, when the atria and ventricles contact independently of each other.

**Classification and Diagnosis of Dysrhythmias**

Dysrhythmias are most conveniently considered according to their site of origin, namely those which arise above the atrioventricular node, at the node itself, and below the node. The particular diagnosis is made on the ECG appearance although this will not identify the cause. Diagnosis may be assisted by a knowledge of the pulse rate and its rhythm and by the appearance or disappearance of normal or abnormal wave forms in the venous pulse. If the heart is exposed during cardiac surgery, direct observation may help elucidate the time relationship between atrial and ventricular contraction.

SUPRAVENTRICULAR DYSRHYTHMIAS

1. **Atrial Ectopic Beats**

These are due to premature atrial depolarisation in some site other than the sinus node. Isolated atrial ectopics are not particularly common but multiple ectopics may herald the onset of atrial fibrillation. The P wave configuration is abnormal and different to the existing P wave shape. It is followed by a normal QRS complex (Fig. 12*a*).

2. **Atrial Tachycardias**

(*a*) *Atrial fibrillation* is due to totally disorganised atrial depolarisation which results in the atrioventricular node being bombarded with impulses which are irregular both in time and strength. The ventricular response is, therefore, irregular and ECG diagnosis depends on irregular QRS complexes and the absence of P waves. The recognition of atrial electrical activity is not necessary for diagnosis (Fig. 12*e*).

(*b*) *Atrial flutter* is due to regular atrial depolarisation at some site other than the sinus node. The atrial rate is usually near 300/min and is commonly associated with 2:1 block giving a ventricular rate of 150, although other fixed block may occur and variable block is common in the presence of digoxin. The diagnosis may be difficult but is suggested by the absence of P waves, a regular fixed ventricular rate of approximately 150/min having normal QRS complexes. Flutter waves, so-called saw tooth appearance, may or may not be obvious (Fig. 12*b* and *c*).

(*c*) *Paroxysmal atrial tachycardia* is due to fast depolarisation at a site other than the sinus node which has a rate between 140–200/min (faster in children) and which is not accompanied by block so that the ventricles have the same rate. ECG shows normal QRS at approximately 140–200 beats/min preceded by an abnormal P wave.

A varying degree of block with paroxysmal atrial tachycardia is suggestive of digoxin toxicity (Fig. 12*d*).

3. **Atrial Bradycardias**

(*a*) *Sinus bradycardia* may result from vagal stimulation. The extreme example is sinus arrest with no electrical activity until it is terminated by a junctional or lower escape beat. It may also occur in pathological states such as the "sick sinus syndrome" in coronary artery disease.

(*b*) *Sino-atrial block*: the activity of the SA node is not transmitted to the atrium and no P wave occurs. Some lower rhythm establishes itself.

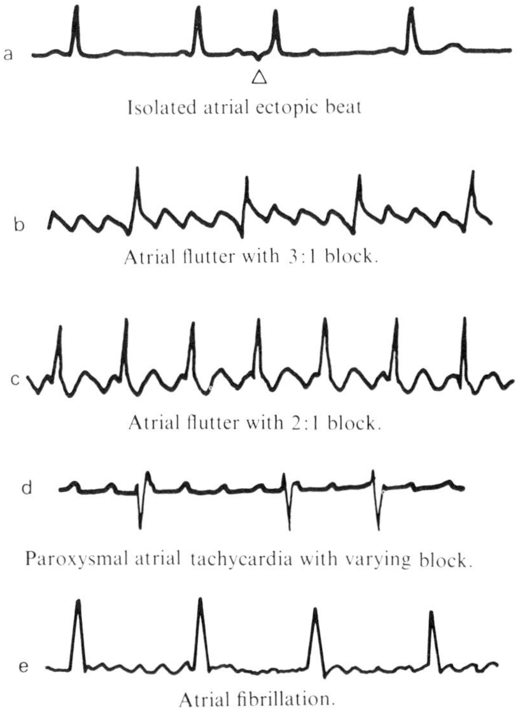


13/FIG. 12.—Supraventricular dysrhythmias.

### JUNCTIONAL DYSRHYTHMIAS

1. **Nodal ectopics** are isolated beats arising in the atrioventricular node and which are premature, in contrast to escape beats which occur after a long pause. The P waves may not be recognisable, being buried in the QRS complex which is normal.

Inverted P waves due to retrograde atrial activation may be seen immediately before or after the ventricular complex (see Fig. 13).

2. **Tachycardia.**—*Nodal tachycardia* is characterized by regular depolarisation at approximately 120–150/min arising in the AV node; this is faster than the natural sinus rate. The retrogradely activated P waves are either buried in the normal QRS or appear inverted before or after the ventricular complex. It is a common rhythm after cardiac surgery and in digoxin intoxication. The diagnosis may be assisted by the observation of regular cannon waves in the venous pulse.

*Atrioventricular dissociation* may exist between the atria under the control of the sinus node and the ventricles responding to a slightly faster rate arising in the atrioventricular node. The ECG diagnosis depends on recognising the regular but differing atrial and ventricular rates. (Normal P waves "walking through" normal QRS complexes). An occasional sinus beat may capture the atrioventricular node and thus the ventricles causing an occasional irregularity in

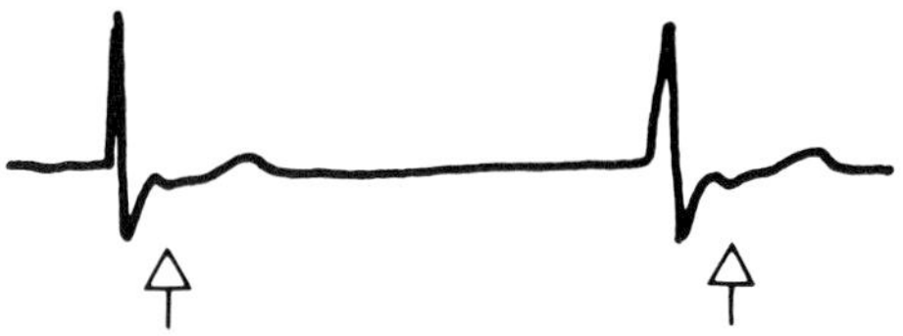

13/FIG. 13.—Nodal rhythm; note inverted P waves following the ventricular complex side.

the ventricular rate. The venous pulse will show irregular cannon waves.

3. **Nodal bradycardia** has the ECG characteristics of a nodal rhythm but occurs at between 40–60/min. Spontaneous sinus node activity must be absent or slower than the nodal rate. Cannon waves are apparent in the venous trace.

### Ventricular Dysrhythmias

1. **Ventricular ectopics** are premature beats arising somewhere within the ventricle. The ECG is characterised by a wide QRS complex whose voltage is usually greater than the normal complexes and which is not preceded by an associated P wave. The ectopic may or may not be followed by a compensatory pause. The shape of the QRS complex may suggest the site of origin (left bundle-branch block configuration suggests origin in right ventricle) and different shaped complexes suggest more than one site of origin (Fig. 14*a*).

Ventricular ectopic beats are very common and often benign. Those arising in the left ventricle may, perhaps, be more serious than those from the right ventricle.

Features of ventricular ectopic beats which give rise to concern are:

i. Multifocal origin as shown by varying QRS shapes which suggest more widespread disease.

ii. Runs of two or more which may herald ventricular tachycardia or ventricular fibrillation.

iii. Ectopics which are close to the preceding beat. Should the ectopic fall on the peak of the preceding T wave (R on T phenomenon), ventricular fibrillation may occur.

iv. Frequency is less significant than the first three factors, but ventricular ectopics predispose to further dysrhythmias, therefore the more frequent the ectopics the greater the possibility of some other rhythm disturbance. This is the particular significance of bigeminy in digitalis therapy.

2. **Ventricular tachycardia.**—This is always a dangerous rhythm. It usually drops the cardiac output and frequently precedes ventricular fibrillation. The ECG diagnosis is given by wide bizarre complexes occurring at 150–200/min, which may be slightly irregular. The P waves are usually not seen being buried in the ventricular complex from which they are dissociated, although regular retrograde activation of the atria may occur (Fig. 14*b*).

Confusion may exist between ventricular tachycardia and supraventricular or nodal tachycardia may be associated with wide QRS complexes. The widening of the QRS complex may result from right or left bundle-branch block or to aberrant conduction secondary to drugs or hyperkalaemia, or to the fast rate itself which overloads the normal conduction system causing it to be refractory to the next impulse. This difficult differential diagnosis may only be resolved after intracardiac electrocardiography, but it is important as the treatment for the two conditions is different.

3. **Ventricular fibrillation** is due to multiple areas of re-entry in the ventricular muscle. Diagnosed on the ECG by the totally random appearance (Fig. 14*c*). The bigger the amplitude of the complexes the better the prognosis for restarting the heart.

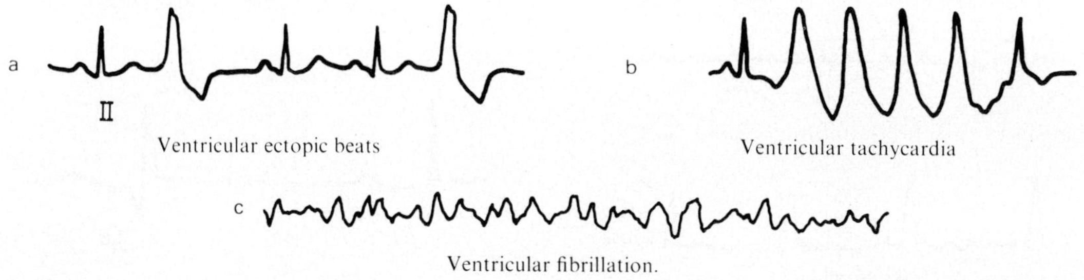


Ventricular ectopic beats

Ventricular tachycardia

Ventricular fibrillation.

13/Fig. 14.—Ventricular dysrhythmias.

### Wolff-Parkinson-White Syndrome

An ECG pattern characteristic of the Wolff-Parkinson-White syndrome is found in approximately 0·1 per cent of the population. Patients with this syndrome have a propensity to develop supraventricular tachycardia, ventricular tachycardia or ventricular fibrillation and these dysrhythmias may be induced during anaesthesia and surgery.[30] The underlying defect is an alternative atrioventricular pathway so that ventricular events occur earlier than would be expected if atrioventricular conduction were normal, hence the ECG shows a short PR interval and a broadened QRS complex with an initial slur (the delta wave). Less commonly, the ECG may appear normal except when conduction is down the aberrant fasciculus.

Prophylactic therapy is directed to preventing tachydysrhythmias either by depressing A-V nodal conduction (verapamil or $\beta$-blockers) or by slowing conduction in the alternative pathway (quinidine, disopyramide or procainamide). In patients with a known history of dysrhythmias, these agents should be continued over the operative period and anaesthetic agents which produce tachycardia or have vagolytic actions should be avoided. The ECG should be monitored and verapamil, disopyramide or practolol may be needed to treat intra-operative tachydysrhythmias. Rarely is DC cardioversion necessary.

### Romans Ward Syndrome
### (Congenital prolongation of the QT interval)

Prolongation of the QT interval increases the likelihood of ventricular dysrhythmias or even ventricular fibrillation. QT prolongation may occur secondary to electrolyte imbalance or secondary to a congenital imbalance of the cardiac sympathetic tone, which leads to a delay in ventricular repolarisation. Ventricular dysrhythmias may then be precipitated by exertion, stress, surgery or anaesthesia (atropine and pancuronium should be avoided). Treatment includes the use of $\beta$-blockers or an interruption of sympathetic nervous supply to the heart by surgical sympathectomy or stellate ganglion blockade.

### Heart Block

1. **First degree.**—The bundle continues to conduct all impulses but at a slower rate than normal. It may be a sign of digoxin toxicity or of the presence of atrioventricular node disease. On the ECG the PR interval is greater than 0·22 seconds in adults, only changing slightly with alterations in cardiac rate. In children there is more variability with rate and the upper limit is shorter (see Fig. 15*b*).

2. **Second degree.**—(*a*) *Wenckebach phenomenon.* There is a progressive increase in the PR interval until an impulse is not transmitted. This pause allows the AV node time to recover and the cycle is repeated starting with the shortest PR interval. It may occur in digoxin therapy or as a result of atrioventricular node ischaemia.

(*b*) *Regular 2 to 1 or 3 to 1 heart block.* ECG shows normal P waves and QRS complexes but only alternate (or third etc.) P waves are followed by the ventricular complex.

3. **Complete heart block.**—The electrocardiographic appearance is one of complete dissociation of atrial and ventricular complexes, with the ventricular rate slower than the atrial rate. If the block is high the QRS complex will appear normal and confusion may exist with 2:1 heart block as the sinus rate is often 80/min

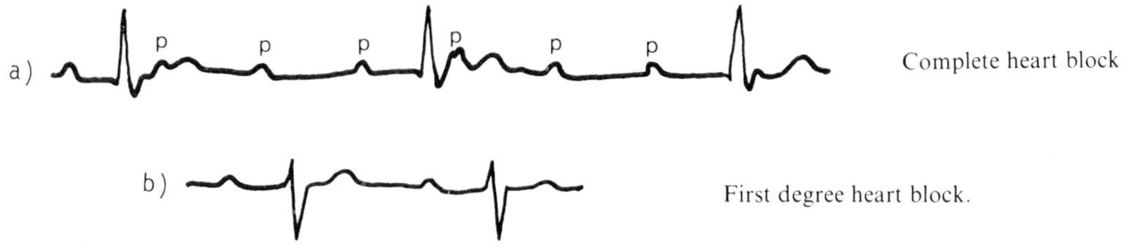


13/Fig. 15.—Conduction defect.

and the idioventricular rate 40. If the block is lower, the QRS complex will appear widened (see Fig. 15*a*).

**Bundle-Branch Block**

If one or two of the three main fasciculi (see 12/Fig. 3, p. 409) are interrupted, although the electrical impulse down the unaffected bundles will activate its related area of ventricle normally, the part of the ventricle no longer supplied by its bundle will be activated by some other slower route. The QRS will therefore be widened and the bundle that is interrupted can be recognised by the complex shape in different leads (see Fig. 16).

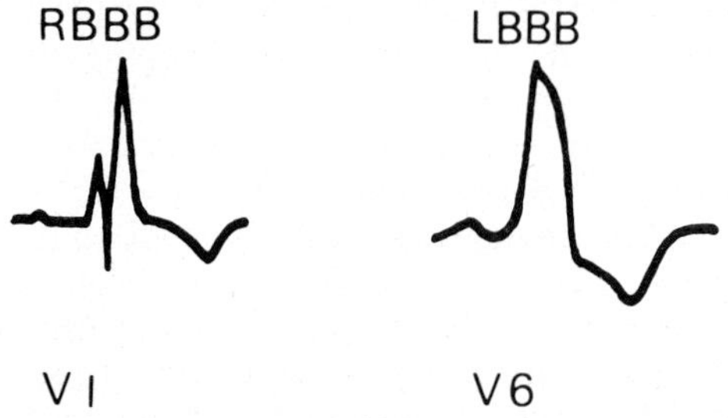


13/Fig. 16.—Right and left bundle-branch block.

**Right bundle-branch block.**—QRS greater than 0·12 seconds. Delay in right ventricular activation produces a late R wave in leads $V_{1-2}$.

**Left bundle-branch block.**—QRS greater than 0·12 seconds. Delay in left ventricular activation produces late R wave in leads I, AVL, $V_{5-7}$.

**Left anterior hemiblock.**—QRS up to 0·10 seconds with the appearance of left axis deviation.

**Left posterior hemiblock.**—QRS up to 0·10 seconds with appearance of right axis deviation.

Hence the association of either left or right axis deviation with right bundle-branch block suggests that two of the three fasciculi are interrupted ("bi-fascicular block") and that there is a danger of complete heart block developing. This may be an indication for elective transcutaneous electrode placement prior to surgery.

**Prevention and Treatment**

The prevention of dysrhythmias lies in the avoidance of those factors known to predispose towards their production and the first stage in the treatment of any dysrhythmia is the elimination of predisposing factors before proceeding to further therapy.

Any rhythm disturbance, including the commonest sinus tachycardia, may be a sign that there is some defect in anaesthetic or circulatory management.

If a dysrhythmia occurs during anaesthesia it must be decided if the disturbance is immediately life-threatening because of inadequate cardiac output either because the heart is arrested (asystole, ventricular fibrillation) or because the cardiac output has been severely lowered by one or more of the haemodynamic consequences of the dysrhythmias listed above. The second possibility is either that the dysrhythmia is the precursor of a rhythm which is life-threatening or that it may indicate acute myocardial ischaemia. Tachydysrhythmias are particularly dangerous in the presence of coronary artery disease. In either case, immediate treatment is needed to restore the rhythm to normal and, if necessary to support the circulation until that happens.

The great majority of dysrhythmias will not fall into these categories,[31] in which case specific treatment may not be needed and care must be taken that therapy does not introduce a greater hazard.

Once the predisposing factors have been eliminated, the number of serious dysrhythmias remaining is small and in the short term, as during anaesthesia, the selection of drugs for their treatment is relatively limited.

Ventricular fibrillation and ventricular tachycardia associated with an inadequate cardiac output are both emergency situations requiring immediate DC cardioversion. Ventricular ectopics are treated in two ways. In patients already on digoxin, a high proportion are due to hypokalaemia and will disappear if a small amount (up to 5 mmol) KCl is given intravenously over one minute. This may need to be repeated. If, however, the patient is not hypokalaemic, then the treatment is to suppress ventricular excitability. The drug of first choice is lignocaine (1 mg/kg intravenously) which can, if necessary, be followed by a sequential intravenous infusion.[32] Other antidysrhythmic drugs may be required if ventricular irritability is not suppressed by lignocaine. Beta-blockers, such as propranolol 0·5–2 mg or practolol 1–5 mg are particularly effective for the treatment of tachydysrhythmias associated with sympathetic overactivity but may, in combination with halothane or enflurane, produce an unacceptable degree of myocardial depression. Disopyramide or quinidine may occasionally be required, but caution must be observed as inappropriate doses may slow A-V conduction or reduce ventricular contractility. While it is doubtful that droperidol can be used as an antidysrhythmic drug, it does offer some protection against intra-operative dysrhythmias, and its use tends to reduce the anaesthetic requirements for dysrhythmogenic agents such as halothane. In the treatment of ventricular ectopic beats, one must be certain that the ectopics are not, in fact, ventricular escape beats secondary to supraventricular bradycardia for which the treatment is with isoprenaline or atropine. Classically the sudden onset of any supraventricular tachycardia may be treated either by DC cardioversion or with digoxin. If the rate has a very deleterious effect on the cardiac output and if the factors provoking it are temporary, then cardioversion is the treatment of choice. This may be accompanied by digitalisation to control the rate of ventricular response should the dysrhythmia recur. If, however, the cardiac output is adequate and it is thought that cardioversion is unlikely to be successful, then digitalisation alone is indicated. However, during surgery, DC cardioversion may be impractical and digitalisation during anaesthesia may be ineffective or dangerous. Thus the acute control of ventricular rate may have to be achieved by the cautious use of $\beta$-blockers.

Sinus arrest, sinus or nodal bradycardia, will usually revert to sinus rhythm after intravenous atropine or an infusion of isoprenaline. Isoprenaline may be useful in nodal tachycardia, the rate seldom increases, but P waves appear, capture the node, and when the infusion is slowed, the patient continues in sinus rhythm. Rarely, cardioversion of nodal tachycardia may be necessary. Paroxysmal atrial tachycardia may respond to a vagal-stimulating action.

### The Treatment of Heart Block

Isoprenaline, dobutamine or atropine can improve conduction in A-V dissociation and may prevent the conversion of less significant degrees of A-V conduction defects to complete heart block. Sudden deterioration in A-V conduction may occur during surgery following cardiopulmonary bypass. In the presence of an adequate ventricular rate, attention should be drawn towards those factors that enhance heart block, for example, myocardial ischaemia, electrolyte imbalance, acidosis or drug effects. An infusion of isoprenaline may be required in order to improve the ventricular rate, but may induce hypotension in refractory block due to vasodilatation. When the cardiac output is compromised because the ventricular rate is too slow, despite drug therapy, then electrical pacing is indicated.

Ventricular pacing, rather than atrial, is the obvious approach in heart block and can be performed in four ways:

(*a*) *Direct epicardial pacing*. This can be easily performed by the surgeon when the chest is open. One temporary pacing wire is lightly sutured to the right ventricle (active) and another to the surrounding tissues (indifferent).

(*b*) *Transvenous endocardial pacing*. A sterile pacing wire is threaded from the subclavian or internal jugular vein to rest against the endocardial surface of the right ventricle. This wire is bipolar and requires no separate "indifferent" lead. Ideally this is performed under x-ray image intensifier control, although in an emergency it can be introduced in a blind fashion until the required pacing effect is achieved. Severe ventricular tachydysrhythmias may occur during insertion of the wire, and full resuscitation facilities must be available.

(*c*) *Transoesophageal cardiac pacing*. Recently, this approach has been re-examined[33] and would appear particularly suitable in acute situations such as sudden complete heart block occurring following cardiac arrest or during anaesthesia. A transoesophageal pacing catheter ("Oesocath", Vygon, UK Ltd.) is passed via the nasopharynx into the oesophagus, and connected via an amplifier to a pacemaker box. The amplifier is required to increase the voltage to around 30 v dc, which is necessary under these circumstances.

(*d*) *Permanent epicardial or endocardial pac-*

*ing* requires the insertion of a pacing box into the rectus sheath and is connected to the heart by a suitable wire. (Heart block and anaesthesia are discussed on page 512).

**Cardioversion.**—Cardioversion is used to terminate both supraventricular and ventricular tachycardias. Conversion of ventricular tachycardia and ventricular fibrillation are considered elsewhere, only supraventricular dysrhythmias being considered here.

Cardioversion may be performed as an emergency procedure when some rhythm is life-threatening and other treatment will take too long to be effective. Thus the sudden onset of fast atrial fibrillation in a patient with heart disease may reduce cardiac output severely and cardioversion is performed while drug therapy takes effect.

More commonly, cardioversion is performed where a dysrhythmia has persisted after the precipitating cause has been removed and it is thought likely that sinus rhythm, if restored, will be stable. Thus it is sometimes performed post-operatively after cardiac surgery, or after pneumonia or thyrotoxicosis which have been treated. Quinidine is no longer used to attempt conversion of atrial fibrillation to sinus rhythm. Digoxin is normally stopped 24 to 48 hours prior to cardioversion.

The contra-indications to attempted cardioversion are when the tachycardia is sinus in origin or when the patient is suffering from digoxin toxicity. Fast atrial fibrillation itself, paroxysmal atrial tachycardia with block, and nodal tachycardia may all be manifestations of digoxin toxicity and further administration of digoxin or cardioversion may be dangerous as they may precipitate ventricular fibrillation which on further attempted cardioversion changes to a refractory asystole. If a shock is deemed life-saving it is preceded by intravenous lignocaine (1 mg/kg) and is of smaller amplitude than usual. Sometimes reversion to sinus rhythm may bring out latent digoxin toxicity and rapid administration of intravenous potassium and lignocaine is then necessary. $\beta$-adrenergic blockade is normally considered a contra-indication to attempted cardioversion as a refractory asystole may follow the shock.

Cardioversion is not usually performed if the patient has had a recent history of systemic embolism unless he has been anticoagulated for a month. A large heart, long-standing fibrillation and ischaemic heart disease are relative contra-indications and decrease the chance of successful reversion.

A DC shock of 75–300 joules is administered with two electrodes so positioned that the shock passes through the atria. The principal danger is the production of ventricular fibrillation should the shock fall on the T-wave upstroke although this should be avoided by proper synchronisation with the R wave. Other complications are the appearance of digoxin toxicity, sudden development of cardiac failure with acute pulmonary oedema and electrical failures which can lead to the patient's attendants being shocked should they be touching him.

(Anaesthesia for cardioversion is considered on p. 510).

## THE POSTOPERATIVE CARE OF CARDIAC PATIENTS

The immediate postoperative period is perhaps the commonest time for patients to suffer serious complications. These can only be anticipated and prevented if the standard of care postoperatively is as high as during the operation. After major surgery, and particularly after cardiac surgery, the journey between theatre and the intensive care or recovery area is frequently hazardous—monitoring is discontinued temporarily, the supervision of blood balance and the control of potent inotropic drugs may be less than adequate, and alteration in the position of the patient may encourage venous pooling. For these reasons the journey should be speedy and carried out according to a routine. Where possible, some degree of cardiovascular monitoring should be continued; the ECG can be displayed on a battery powered instrument and the blood pressure measured on a portable oscilloscope or aneroid gauge, or assessed by movement of an air bubble in the arterial line. A battery powered defibrillator should be readily available and may form part of the portable ECG apparatus.

There is a good case for not extubating the patient until after he has been allowed time to restabilise in the intensive care or recovery unit. During the transfer, ventilation is continued using Entonox (50% $N_2O$/50% $O_2$ in a single cylinder), but to ensure proper sedation with protection against a sympathetic response occurring at this time, an adequate supplement of intravenous sedation or analgesic may be given a short while before the end of the operation.

*Circulatory Support*: Once the patient has an adequate and stable cardiovascular system, as seen by a good cardiac output achieved at low ventricular filling pressures, an absence of dysrhythmias and normal tissue perfusion with a good urinary output, an absence of metabolic acidosis and warm well-perfused extremities with a minimal temperature gradient between the periphery and the centre, it may be possible to withdraw circulatory support. This should be performed slowly by a process of incremental reduction allowing adequate time between each reduction for reassessment and taking care not to change more than one factor at a time. Only after the circulation has demonstrated its capacity for adequate function over a period without circulatory support should the frequency and extent of monitoring be reduced towards a simpler routine. Those patients who do not intra-operatively require circulatory support (and in non-cardiac procedures this will be in the majority of patients) may, however, deteriorate after the operation when increased demands are made on the heart by the circulatory responses to pain, cold and reversal of anaesthetic agents. This potential state of affairs requires close monitoring of cardiorespiratory status in the immediate recovery period.

### Postoperative Respiratory Care

(*a*) *Prophylactic.*—Post-operative ventilatory problems are reduced if the patient presents in his optimum respiratory and cardiovascular state. Smoking should be stopped and adequate time allowed for pre-operative physiotherapy to clear the lungs of excess secretions. Cardiac failure, particularly left ventricular failure, must be correctly treated.

(*b*) *Pulmonary venous engorgement.*—Lung compliance and oxygen transfer is facilitated if pulmonary venous congestion is minimised by keeping the left atrial pressure as low as is compatible with an adequate cardiac output. Low cardiac output is better managed with inotropic or vasodilator therapy rather than by overtransfusion resulting in high left-sided filling pressures which may not only fail to improve output, but may even produce cardiovascular deterioration.

(*c*) *Pain relief.*—Inadequate pain relief fails to prevent a rise in oxygen consumption and cardiac output, while at the same time inhibiting respiration and discouraging deep breathing so that retained secretions and lung collapse become more likely. The catecholamine secretion which accompanies pain raises venous tone and, transferring blood from the systemic to the pulmonary vascular tree, tends to raise the left atrial pressure.

Pain relief tends to be inadequate for a number of reasons:

(i) the "time rule"—analgesia is better given in frequent small doses rather than by adhering to a 3- or 4-hour rule;

(ii) carbon dioxide tension—an undue obsession with maintaining a normal arterial carbon dioxide tension may cause analgesia to be withheld. Provided the patient is not hypoxic and has a good cardiovascular function, free from dysrhythmias, then it is probably unimportant if the $Pco_2$ rises to 50 or even 55 mmHg (6·7–7·3 kPa). Sometimes the administration of morphine may result in a reduction in $CO_2$ tension following the relaxation of the inhibition of breathing caused by pain.

(iii) hypotension—a fall in blood pressure may follow the administration of morphine and is usually due to a relaxation of tone in the venous capacitance vessels resulting in a fall in cardiac filling pressure. It responds to transfusion. There are two implications of this effect: (a) the capacitance vessels must have been constricted previously, perhaps due to lack of analgesia or to hypovolaemia, (b) if the analgesia is allowed to wear off and pain recurs the vessels will again constrict and the left atrial pressure rise, perhaps this time even higher due to the infused fluid. This "yo-yo" effect of analgesia on the cardiovascular system dictates that stability is best achieved by frequent small or continuous doses of analgesia with careful maintenance of the blood volume.

Epidural or intrathecal opiate administration may provide good pain relief, particularly after cardiac surgery when there is commonly an initial period of artificial ventilation. Under these conditions, the analgesia (but not the sedation) persists after extubation and enhances the ability of the patient to breathe deeply and obtain maximum benefit from physiotherapy. Mathews and Abrams[34] using intrathecal morphine, reported a good effect in patients who were extubated immediately following cardiac surgery. Against the cardiorespiratory advantages of this method must be considered the risks of delayed respiratory depression, although under the intensive monitoring of post-cardiac surgical patients, this should be an avoidable hazard.

Although less suitable for patients with a median sternotomy, continuous thoracic epidural or paravertebral block are useful alternative forms of pain control in patients who have a lateral thoracotomy. Caution should be exercised with the thoracic sympathetic blockade that occurs after epidural block in some cardiac patients. The provision of adequate analgesia without central respiratory depression does not necessarily imply the absence of a need for positive-pressure ventilation and, indeed, patients receiving such ventilation will equally still require proper sedation.

(*d*) *Temperature control*.—Excessive respiratory (and cardiac) work may develop secondary to a metabolic demand as a patient attempts to restore his temperature to normal if he has been allowed to waken while hypothermic. Careful intra-operative temperature control should ideally ensure that the patient is completely rewarmed both centrally and peripherally by the end of the operation. This will also avoid the circulatory complications which arise as hypothermic vasoconstriction gives way to normothermic vasodilatation.

**Postoperative Artificial Ventilation**

After surgery, there is an increase in metabolism which dictates both a rise in cardiac output and an increase in respiratory work in order to supply tissue oxygen demands. The increase in metabolism may be aggravated by catecholamine release secondary to hypoxia, hypercapnia, pain or fear.

At the same time, the efficiency of ventilation and gas exchange may be impaired. Lung compliance is decreased by high left atrial pressures which cause pulmonary engorgement, by retention of secretions causing bronchial obstruction with segmental lung collapse and by the mechanical effects of surgery on the thoracic cage.[35]

Oxygen uptake is reduced by the development of areas of arteriovenous shunt within the lungs which, in severe cases, may account for up to 30 per cent of the cardiac output. However, the cardiac performance and output is often impaired and any reduction in cardiac output will exaggerate the fall in arterial oxygen tension caused by the lung shunt. This hypoxaemia will have a more pronounced effect on the already compromised myocardium leading to a further deterioration in its performance. Paradoxically, venous admixture may be worsened by those drugs which may be used to improve the circulation[36] such as glyceryl trinitrate, dopamine and isoprenaline.[37]

In patients with *severe* cardiac disease, the rise in oxygen consumption which occurs when spontaneous ventilation is restored, is not the normal 3·5 per cent, but can be as high as 30 per cent. Even if gas transfer is adequate, the compromised circulation may be unable to raise the cardiac output proportionately to satisfy this demand and the patient will become hypoxic, developing signs of cardiovascular instability, particularly dysrhythmias and acute ventricular failure.

While it is possible to improve the cardiac output with inotropic or vasodilator therapy, to reduce pulmonary engorgement and to treat lung collapse, the immediate improvement of the hypoxic low cardiac output patient is best achieved by removing the excessive but unproductive work of breathing and employing positive-pressure ventilation until the cardiovascular status has been improved. Therefore, the two principal indications for ventilation in the postoperative period are the relief of cardiorespiratory work in low cardiac output states, and the optimisation of gas exchange in patients with pulmonary disease. Continued ventilation has the added advantages of allowing generous administration of analgesics without concern over respiratory depression, of allowing time for the complete excretion of anaesthetic agents and complete return to normothermia and allowing the best conditions for the prompt institution of cardiopulmonary resuscitation or the treatment of pulmonary complications. In practice, the great majority of patients will only be ventilated for the first few hours of the postoperative period while the circulation is stabilised.

**Management**

Most patients will be ventilated via the plastic oro-tracheal tube inserted at the time of operation. Even for long-term ventilation, tracheostomy tends to be avoided as long as possible because of the particular danger of infection in a tracheostomy wound, so adjacent to a median sternotomy and the tissue spaces of the mediastinum. An alternative for longer-term continued ventilation, which is both more comfortable and more stable, is nasotracheal intubation, although the long-term effects of this technique as compared with tracheostomy have yet to be fully elucidated.[38]

Minute volume is normally adjusted to produce a just sufficient reduction in arterial carbon dioxide tension that respiratory drive is eliminated, but not so low that cardiac output and tissue perfusion is reduced secondary to hypocapnia. A further argument against over-ventilation is the mechanical effects of altered intrathoracic pressure on the circulation when raised mean intrathoracic pressure may severely reduce cardiac output. A similar reduction in cardiac output may follow the use of positive end-expiratory pressure and the use of this technique in cardiac patients should be with caution.[36] The advantage of improved arterial oxygenation subsequent to the re-expansion of atelectatic areas of lung is often offset by the reduction in cardiac output. Certain patients, especially those with pulmonary hypertension, tolerate this procedure very badly.

The $Pa_{O_2}$ can usually be maintained at a satisfactory level by manipulation of the inspired oxygen content. The $F_{IO_2}$ should, if possible, not exceed 0·6 in order to avoid the potential problems of oxygen toxicity. Rarely, higher inspired oxygen concentrations may be needed although other manoeuvres—improvement in cardiac output, re-expansion of collapsed area of lung, cautious imposition of PEEP—are often more successful.

**Sedation**

Sedation and analgesia are almost always necessary. *Nitrous oxide* has the advantage of instant control, but has the disadvantage associated with air-cavity distension, marrow depression and is not without effect on the cardiovascular system (see p. 425); its use also increases the chance of ventilator accidents. The *opiates* provide both analgesia and sedation, and reduce respiratory drive—venocapacitance tone may be lowered, but this should be considered a beneficial effect as it reverses abnormal venoconstriction. *Diazepam* leads to a satisfactory objective and subjective state of sedation and amnesia,[39] although its accumulation and long elimination time may lead to an unacceptable degree of central depression by the time extubation is considered. Shorter-acting benzodiazepines such as midazolam may be more suitable. Infusions of rapidly eliminated anaesthetic agents, such as Althesin or etomidate, are very satisfactory in some situations and allow a rapid return to consciousness after they are discontinued.

The only indications for the use of muscle relaxants during postoperative ventilation are:

(*a*) If the patient is severely hypoxic and his respiratory drive comes not from his $CO_2$ tension but from his hypoxia, when control may be very difficult to achieve without paralysis. This hypoxia may be the result of a ventilatory derangement or the consequence of a severely reduced cardiac output.

(*b*) If due to neurological damage the patient has either excessive CNS drive to respiration or uncontrollable fits which make mechanical ventilation impossible.

Postoperative confusion, whether pharmacological or organic, may also contribute to difficulties with IPPV. This may be compounded by excessive sedation and often a compromise therapy with short-acting sedatives and muscle relaxants will have to be used.

*Chest physiotherapy* during postoperative ventilator support should be administered appropriately rather than routinely. Indiscriminate "bag-squeezing" may merely cause cardiovascular upset—either a reduction in cardiac output or, conversely, severe hypertension and tachycardia. Bag-squeezing should be reserved

(*a*) for the re-expansion of collapsed areas of lung;

(*b*) as an "artificial cough" in order to shift excessive secretions which cannot be removed by endotracheal suction alone.

### Discontinuation of Artificial Ventilation and Extubation

The duration of artificial ventilation in the postoperative period depends on a number of factors. Firstly, there are certain criteria to be reached before extubation can be considered and these are discussed below. How quickly these conditions obtain depends on the operation performed, the previous haemodynamic state of the patient, the type and conduct of anaesthesia and the circulatory management during the operation. It also depends to a large extent on the philosophy adopted by the particular anaesthetist and surgical team. At one extreme, there may be a policy of immediate extubation at the end of the operation, at the other extreme, a policy may exist to ventilate all cardiac surgery patients for a minimum of 24 hours. A sensible progressive policy would be to ventilate all patients in the first few hours of the postoperative period while circulatory stability is achieved, haemostasis assured, level of support assessed and complete normothermia achieved. Extubation is performed at the *earliest point that these criteria for extubation are satisfied.* Although the advantages of postoperative mechanical ventilation have been described, the long-term continuation of such therapy must be associated with a progressive increase in its complications; in particular to mechanical problems associated with the use of a ventilator and endotracheal tube, to the likelihood of pulmonary infection and to problems relating to the excretion of sedative or narcotic drugs when it is ultimately decided to restore spontaneous ventilation.

Although each case needs to be considered individually, or for some reason may be considered to differ from the usual (e.g., pulmonary hypertension), the normal criteria for discontinuing ventilatory support are:

1. *An intact neurological system.* If it is thought that the patient has suffered neurological damage at the time of operation, ventilatory support tends to be continued because of the risk to recovery of the neurological system by any degree of hypoxia or hypercarbia. Assessment of neurological status can be delayed until cardiovascular stability is reached, and the decision is then made whether to extubate or not. Confusion leads to an impaired ability to cough or co-operate with the physiotherapist and increases the chances of alveolar collapse following extubation. Such obtunded neurology may be an indication for a further period of ventilation.

2. *A stable cardiovascular system.* This implies a reasonable cardiac output achieved at low ventricular filling pressures with adequate tissue perfusion and absence of significant dysrhythmias. If the periphery is warm, the CVP normal or low, the arterial pressure satisfactory, urine output good and the patient not acidotic, then circulatory status can be presumed satisfactory. Sometimes this state can only be achieved with pharmacological or mechanical support. A moderate degree of inotropic or vasodilator therapy is not necessarily a contra-indication to extubation, although such therapy should be maintained during the transition from IPPV to spontaneous ventilation. Intra-aortic balloon counter pulsation itself is not a contra-indication to extubation provided the cardiac output is adequate. Massive or increasing circulatory support implies poor ventricular performance that would benefit from continued artificial ventilation.

3. *Haemostasis.* Cardiovascular stability is at risk if there is excessive postoperative haemorrhage. Re-operation may be necessary to stop the bleeding; after cardiac surgery, tamponade is always a possibility and may be apparent at an early or late stage postoperatively. Extubation is normally delayed until it is obvious that the patient is not suffering from continuing blood loss.

4. *Adequate mechanical and gas exchange function in the lung.*

(*a*) The alveolar-arterial oxygen tension gradient should be small. The patient ought to be capable of an arterial oxygen tension greater than 100 mm Hg (13·3 kPa) when receiving 40 per cent oxygen in the inspired air—this being the concentration available from a facemask after extubation.

(*b*) The minute volume of ventilation to produce a normal carbon dioxide tension should be approximately that expected for the size of the patient.

(*c*) The tidal volume should be achieved at a low inflation pressure implying a compliant chest so that the work of breathing will be small.

5. *The chest X-ray should be clear and the patient pain free.*

Because a patient is on a ventilator there may be a tendency to reduce the analgesic dose and once he is extubated the pain of breathing with a chest wound, particularly a lateral thoracotomy, will be such that considerable amounts of narcotics, regional blockade or spinal opiate administration may be needed. The gas tensions should be carefully monitored in the post-extubation period and deterioration in their values or in the cardiovascular state (as evidenced by dysrhythmias, tachycardia, rising venous pressure, falling blood pressure and diminution in urine output) or the appearance of respiratory distress (tiredness, the use of the accessory muscles of respiration) are indications to reintubate the patient (*vide infra*).

### Weaning

Weaning from the ventilator is seldom required in most cardiac patients. However, in a small proportion, some form of weaning may be necessary; this can be achieved by a variety of techniques such as intermittent mandatory ventilation (IMV), mandatory minute volume (MMV), high frequency jet pressure ventilation (HFJPV) or continuous positive airway pressure (CPAP). The latter is particularly appropriate in small children and can also be used to prevent atelectasis in the intubated, spontaneously breathing adult.

In general, a weaning process should be considered:

(*a*) in patients with neurological problems and impaired ability to cough.
(*b*) in patients with co-existing pulmonary disease.
(*c*) in patients with multi-system pathology and cachexia.
(*d*) in patients with a permanently poor ventricular performance.

Gradually increasing periods of spontaneous breathing, alternating with IPPV is a simple and satisfactory alternative to the more sophisticated methods available for weaning, provided that progressive alveolar collapse is prevented and treated.

### Reintubation and Reinstitution of Ventilation

After resumption of spontaneous respiration it may become obvious that further artificial ventilation is required when, provided the patient has not yet been extubated, he can easily be reconnected to the ventilator. Essentially the conditions for the reintroduction of controlled ventilation are that the criteria for extubation listed above are no longer satisfied. There is usually a greater reluctance to recommence artificial ventilation once the patient has been extubated but, in general, once reintubation is considered, it is usually overdue. Gilston[40] has described the facial signs of respiratory distress following extubation after cardiac surgery which provide a rich source of information regarding the inter-relationships between increased respiratory work and the cardiovascular and central nervous systems. He states "it is usually possible to make a firm decision about mechanical ventilation simply by watching the patient from the end of the bed and feeling his feet". Reintubation at this time may well be hazardous, particularly if there is circulatory deterioration, and needs to be speedy and atraumatic. The patient is pre-oxygenated with 100 per cent oxygen through a good fitting mask, unconsciousness obtained by the administration of a small dose of diazepam and relaxation produced with pancuronium. Suxamethonium is best avoided as in the potential presence of hypoxia, acidosis or abnormal serum potassium, there is a real danger of this drug provoking dangerous dysrhythmias.

## SOME ASPECTS OF DIFFERENT CARDIAC DISEASES IN RELATION TO ANAESTHESIA AND OPERATION

It is not possible in a general anaesthetic textbook to describe in detail a large number of individual cardiac lesions and, omitting many rarer congenital lesions for which a specialised textbook should be consulted, discussion is limited to certain commonly encountered lesions and their special aspects, which are of particular concern to the anaesthetist. The principles of anaesthesia previously described apply irrespective of the particular disease in the heart, but certain lesions may suggest a variation of technique or the use of an ancillary such as induced hypotension, hypothermia, or the extracorporeal circulation. Moreover, increasing experience of the behaviour of patients with certain lesions during anaesthesia and operation gives a clue to expected morbidity and mortality. Such facts as these and brief descriptions of those rarer diseases and operations, which are only likely to be seen in specialised clinics, are included to give the anaesthetist a broad background to the subject.

The particular problems of infants and children are not discussed here and the reader is referred to the paediatric section of this book (Chapter 42).

### Coarctation of the Aorta

Coarctation is a common form of congenital heart disease occurring once in every 1500 births. When it occurs proximal to the ductus arteriosus (preductal) it is almost always associated with an open duct and the lower limbs are perfused with desaturated blood from the pulmonary artery. The children usually have other congenital cardiac abnormalities and often present in cardiac failure.

The more common adult (post-ductal) coarctation has a very varied anatomy and 25 per cent of all cases have associated lesions. Most patients are asymptomatic and the diagnosis may well be made at a routine clinical examination when radial to femoral artery delay is noticed or because rib-notching has been observed on the chest x-ray. The patients have a labile hypertension above the constriction with a lower pressure below. The left ventricle is hypertrophied and the dilated aorta above the coarctation is thick-walled (Fig. 17).

The lower part of the body is supplied by a collateral circulation, principally via the internal mammary, subscapular and intercostal arteries. These anastomotic vessels are thin-walled, tortuous and easily damaged at operation, particularly the intercostals which are often aneurysmal at their origins from the aorta.

If the disease is untreated, premature death occurs due to heart failure, aortic rupture, intracranial haemorrhage from the commonly associated berry aneurysm, or bacterial infection. Most patients fall in the age group 10–30 years, but prophylactic resection is now advocated at any age over 5 years unless uncontrollable cardiac failure makes earlier operation necessary.

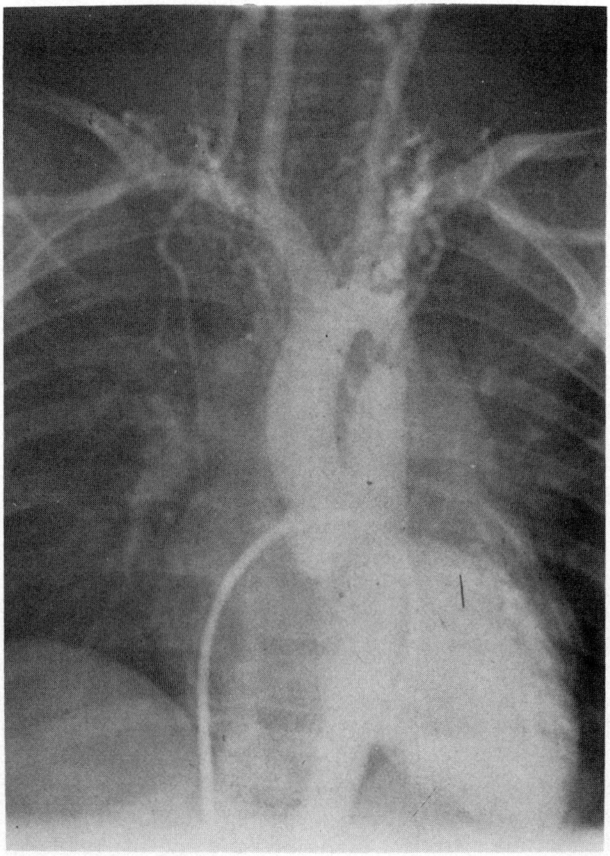

13/Fig. 17.—Aortogram demonstrating adult (post-ductal) coarctation of the aorta. The radio-opaque cannula has been inserted from the right heart into the left ventricle by a trans-atrioseptal approach. Note the collateral vessels and rib notching which is best seen in the lower right quadrant. (Courtesy of Dr. M. M. Webb-Peploe, St. Thomas' Hospital.)

The choice of operation lies between resection of the stricture with end-to-end anastomosis, insertion of a dacron gusset or tube grafting if the gap between the ends, after resection, is too great. Unless heart failure has already ensued, the patient will be physically fit and the mortality rate low.

The special factors to be noted are:

1. Excessive bleeding may be encountered from the dilated arteries in the chest wall during the thoracotomy.
2. The intercostal arteries are easily torn during the mobilisation of the aorta.
3. The left subclavian may be anatomically abnormal or may be clamped during the operation and cannot be used for blood pressure measurements. On rare occasions, the right subclavian may arise from the aorta below the coarctation.
4. During the period of resection and anastomosis the aorta is clamped above and below the coarctation. The proximal blood pressure may rise depending on the degree of the collateral circulation. If the subclavian, which through its branches normally carries a large proportion of the anastomotic flow, is also clamped, the proximal hypertension is aggravated.
5. When the clamps are removed the sudden decrease in resistance causes a considerable drop in blood pressure.
6. Haemorrhage is likely to occur to some degree from the anastomosis in the period immediately after the clamps are removed.

Control of blood pressure is usually achieved using sodium nitroprusside or trimetaphan, short-acting agents that allow a rapid return of perfusion pressure should it be required. While the aorta is cross-clamped, reduction of proximal hypertension may be difficult with vasodilators alone, and myocardial depressants (halothane, enflurane, beta-blockers) may be required in addition.

If the coarctation is mild and hypertension only develops on exercise, or if the patient is being re-operated upon for restenosis or inadequate primary resection, the anastomatic vessels may be inadequate and clamping of the aorta, besides producing dangerous hypertension in the upper part of the body, will endanger the spinal cord and kidneys. In these patients, left atrio-femoral bypass or a temporary jump graft will be needed to protect the spinal cord.

Postoperatively the patients often develop a rebound hypertension which may place the aortic anastomoses in jeopardy. This effect is probably reflexly mediated and is associated with high endogenous catecholamine levels. Normothermia and adequate analgesia will help minimise this response but vasodilators in association with a head-up posture may be required. Hydralazine is a useful agent. Abdominal colic is occasionally observed and has been attributed to mesenteric vasospasm.

### Left-to-Right Shunt

The three common congenital conditions which lead to an increased flow through the lungs are patent ductus arteriosus, atrial septal defect and ventricular septal defect. The enhanced pulmonary blood flow, which may be twice or three times the systemic flow, results in rapid uptake of oxygen and inhalational anaesthetic agents. As any left-to-right shunt may have a small right-to-left component at certain moments in the cardiac cycle, intravenous injections must be scrupulously sterile and free from air bubbles. Patent ductus leads to an overload of the left ventricle, atrial septal defect to an overload of the right ventricle, while a ventricular septal defect loads both ventricles. Anaesthesia for all three types of case presents no problem unless the patient is suffering from a complication and they can be treated as relatively healthy patients with good cardiorespiratory reserve.

The complications which may occur are:

(i) *Cardiac failure*. This may often be precipitated by the patient changing from sinus rhythm to atrial fibrillation or flutter. Failure must be treated with the appropriate measures before surgery. Sometimes in neonates the size of shunt is so large that only repair of the defect will enable the failure to be controlled. Frequently severe cardiac failure in neonates with left-to-right shunts is complicated by the presence of multiple circulatory abnormalities.

(ii) *The development of pulmonary hypertension*. When the pulmonary vascular resistance exceeds that of the systemic circuit the shunt will be reversed (Eisenmenger syndrome) and corrective surgery is no longer possible. With lesser degrees of pulmonary hypertension anaesthesia must be conducted with care (see above).

(iii) *Chest infections*. The vascularity of the pulmonary circulation leaves these patients very prone to recurrent chest infections and bronchitis.

Although most left-to-right shunts are congenital in origin, there are acquired lesions. A ventricular septal defect may appear after myocardial infarction involving the septum. Aorto-atrial shunts may follow rupture of an aneurysm of sinus of Valsalva.

Atrial and ventricular septal defects accompanied by a significant left-to-right shunt are repaired during extracorporeal circulation at an early age to prevent the development of complications.

**Patent ductus arteriosus.**—A narrow or long ductus is easily ligated but a broad short one requires careful dissection to avoid a tear, and its tense pulsations can be reduced at the time of ligation with a short-acting hypotensive agent such as sodium nitroprusside. After ligation the patient develops a rise in diastolic pressure and a bradycardia (Bramham phenomenon). Surgical difficulties may be associated with massive haemorrhage from the aorta or pulmonary artery and, therefore, adequate access to the circulation should always be available for infusion and monitoring. The left recurrent laryngeal nerve may be damaged at the time of operation and give rise to postoperative respiratory problems.

## Right-to-Left Shunts

This group includes Fallot's tetralogy, pulmonary stenosis with atrial septal defect and transposition of the great vessels. The common features are central cyanosis, which is unrelieved by increasing the inspired oxygen concentration, and an increased haemoglobin concentration. They frequently have a metabolic acidosis, abnormal cerebral vessels and coagulation defects.

Due to their reduced lung blood flow, the rate of rise of the arterial concentration of poorly soluble anaesthetics is much reduced, although the more soluble agents are less affected. The speed of induction will, of course, still depend to a large extent on the potency of the inhalational agent used and, despite its poor solubility, cyclopropane will produce a speedy induction. High concentrations of inhalational induction agents are well tolerated because of the slow rise of blood level. Arm-brain circulation time is very short and intravenous agents act quickly. Meticulous care is required both in sterile technique and in preventing air from being accidentally injected.

**Fallot's tetralogy.**—In this combination of pulmonary stenosis, patent ventricular septal defect, overriding aorta and hypertrophied right ventricle, the defect between the ventricles is usually large and the pressures in the right and left ventricles are identical. The degree of shunt, which is normally right to left, depends on the balance between the resistance due to the obstruction in the pulmonary outflow and the systemic vascular resistance. The pulmonary obstruction will be fixed if due to valve stenosis but pulmonary infundibular stenosis may be aggravated by hypoxia or catecholamines. The dangers of infundibular shutdown are lessened by the use of generous opiate premedication or by the prophylactic administration of $\beta$-blockers. Cyclopropane has been recommended as an induction agent, but ketamine is totally contraindicated. The shunt will be increased if the systemic vascular resistance drops on induction of anaesthesia and the resulting hypoxia will further reduce pulmonary flow by increasing pulmonary vascular resistance. Therefore hypotension must be promptly treated with a peripheral vasoconstrictor such as methoxamine. Positive-pressure ventilation may further reduce pulmonary blood flow and aggravate the shunt although reduction in the carbon dioxide tension, if this was previously raised, may relax infundibular spasm and prevent the adverse effects of hypoventilation on pulmonary arteriolar tone. The functional effects of infundibular shutdown are aggravated if ventricular volume is reduced by hypovolaemia, and right-sided filling pressures should be well maintained.

Normally the packed cell volume (haematocrit) is high, leading to a marked rise in viscosity of the blood. There is a danger of spontaneous thrombosis occurring if the patient becomes dehydrated. As a consequence of the small plasma volume there is a low renal plasma flow and renal problems occur. To compensate for the danger of spontaneous thrombus formation these patients develop a very active fibrinolytic mechanism and blood loss is higher and coagulation difficulties more common at surgery.

In the management of cyanotic patients with a high haematocrit, fluid balance must be well maintained to avoid dehydration. Initially, lost blood can be replaced with plasma or plasma-substitute with frequent checks made of the packed cell volume, although the oxygen carrying capacity of the blood must not be seriously reduced until the haemodynamic defect is corrected. Coagulation difficulties are best dealt with by meticulous surgical haemostasis, as use of antifibrinolytic drugs may be accompanied by serious thrombus formation in the vascular tree.

Correction of Fallot's tetralogy is achieved by closure of the ventricular septal defect and relief of the right ventricular outflow tract obstruction. In very severe tetralogy, with gross cyanosis and small pulmonary arteries, a first stage operation—either pulmonary valvotomy without closure of the VSD or the formation of a palliative shunt between a systemic artery and the pulmonary artery—may be necessary to allow development of the child until the definitive correction is considered feasible. The particular postoperative problems following the corrective operation are haemorrhage, heart block, and pulmonary valve incompetence.

## Valve Disease

Alterations of valve function may occur as a result of rheumatic fever, as a consequence of congenital abnormality or following functional dilatation of the valve ring, as occurs in the tricuspid incompetence that follows right ventricular failure. In the United Kingdom, rheumatic fever was formerly the principal cause of heart disease, although its position has now been superseded by coronary artery disease; in many other parts of the world, however, rheumatic fever still remains the most prevalent form of heart disease and is seen in a particularly florid form in younger people. It is important to remember that rheumatic fever is a disease, not only of the valves, but also of the heart muscle, and that although alterations in ventricular function will follow any long-standing valve disease, the effects may be seen earlier in rheumatic heart disease.

While valve disease is discussed under individual valves and stenosis and regurgitation are considered separately, the symptoms and signs are frequently confused as both stenosis and incompetence can occur at the same time in a given valve, although one of the lesions will usually be the more haemodynamically dominant. Equally, the haemodynamic effects may be altered or masked by disease occurring in two or more valves simultaneously.

### Pulmonary Stenosis

*Pulmonary stenosis* produces little effect until it becomes severe, the cardiac output being maintained by a higher than normal right ventricular pressure. Once right ventricular failure occurs or the rhythm changes from sinus to nodal or atrial fibrillation then the cardiac output falls. Normally the non-compliant hypertrophied right ventricle requires a high filling pressure and the additional filling of atrial contraction to distend it adequately in diastole. The right ventricular output can be increased with inotropic drugs if the stenosis is valvular but these drugs must be avoided if the obstruction is infundibular, as the increase in right ventricular tone aggravates the obstruction. Under this circumstance, $\beta$-blockade is the preferred treatment. The output is better sustained at faster heart rates and the filling pressure should be well maintained.

Once the stenosis is severe or cardiac failure occurs, anaesthetic management falls under the heading of fixed low output (*q.v.*) and operative intervention at this stage is associated with a high mortality. Patients with severe pulmonary stenosis are very vulnerable to right ventricular depression secondary to anaesthetic or drug action and to the mechanical effects of positive-pressure respiration.

### Mitral Valve Disease

*Mitral stenosis* is undoubtedly a more difficult problem for the anaesthetist to cope with than mitral regurgitation. Dyspnoea is the main symptom and is caused by pulmonary venous engorgement secondary to elevation of the left atrial pressure. Cardiac output is limited by the impaired left ventricular filling across the stenosed valve, and is very dependent on the heart rate. Fast rates reduce the time available for diastolic filling, while a change in rhythm to atrial fibrillation impairs atrial transport and further reduces stroke volume. This disease is often associated with a small-cavity left ventricle so that too slow a rate also produces a low output. With time, the pulmonary artery and right ventricular pressures rise, ultimately the right ventricle fails and the patient develops a fixed low cardiac output state.

In severe mitral stenosis the patient may have all the signs of a low output state—cachexia, malar flush, feeble pulses with peripheral vasoconstriction—and of congestive cardiac failure with peripheral oedema, ascites and hepatic dysfunction. In the early states of haemodynamically significant mitral stenosis, the problem is to maintain the cardiac output without provoking pulmonary oedema either by overtransfusion or by increasing the right ventricular output. During anaesthesia, hypotension is frequently provoked by a fall in systemic vascular resistance, in veno-capacitance tone or a change in heart rate. Improving arteriolar tone with a vasoconstrictor, such as metaraminol, usually restores arterial pressure. Knowledge of the left atrial or wedge pulmonary artery pressure is valuable, but is not always safe or practical; right-sided venous pressure monitoring may be useful in order to avoid gross swings in ventricular filling pressure. Inotropic therapy should be reserved for ventricular pump failure, in the absence of which isoprenaline may produce hypotension by an increase in heart rate and a fall in systemic vascular resistance. Severe hypotension, induced by tachydysrhythmias should be treated by measures aimed at reducing cardiac rate—digoxin is not perhaps the most satisfactory agent for intra-operative use, and small doses of beta-blockers may be a cautious alternative.

The induction of anaesthesia may be complicated by the slow circulation time, so that a considerable interval may elapse between the administration of intravenous drugs and their action. Hepatic venous congestion may impair the liver's ability to eliminate certain drugs. Once severe right ventricular failure has developed, particularly if associated with pulmonary vascular disease, hypotension is in part due to reduced myocardial performance. At this stage, inotropic therapy may improve right ventricular function and output, although care must be taken at the same time to maintain or improve right-sided filling pressures. Thiopentone, as an induction agent, is particularly dangerous in this late stage of the disease.

*Closed mitral valvotomy* via a left thoracotomy is performed to open the commissures of non-calcified valves with pure stenosis, once it has become haemodynamically significant as shown by a raised left atrial pressure. The stenosed valve is split with a dilator passed through the apex of the left ventricle. At the time of cardiac manipulation, clot may be thrown off and the anaesthetist is called on to compress the carotid arteries temporarily. Cardiac manipulation produces acute falls in blood pressure, particularly when the surgeon's fingers or the dilator are blocking the stenosed orifice, so that continuous ECG and arterial pressure monitoring is essential. Immediately the valvotomy has been performed, the circulation usually improves but, if not, the surgeon is requested not to manipulate the heart further until the cardiac output, which is now more responsive to inotropic drugs, has improved. Before awakening the patient, the peripheral pulses should be palpated to exclude embolism at the time of surgery.

A complication of this operation is the production of acute mitral regurgitation; alternatively, re-stenosis may occur after some years. Open mitral valvotomy or mitral valve replacement performed on cardiopulmonary bypass is now the more common specific surgical treatment for severe mitral stenosis. Here the morbidity of open heart surgery is combined with the problems of myocardial dysfunction, cachexia and pulmonary hypertension that are seen in gross long-standing mitral stenosis, and the operation has a significant mortality.

*Mitral regurgitation* is a disease of the left ventricle and although the patients develop cardiac failure they seldom present for surgery in the low output state seen with the stenotic valve. The mean left atrial pressure is lower in mitral incompetence than in a comparable degree of mitral stenosis and the heart is less embarrassed by increases in right ventricular output or by tachycardia. Mitral incompetence will, however, produce severe pulmonary congestion when it is of sudden onset, as following ruptured chordae tendinae or acute papillary muscle dysfunction secondary to myocardial infarction. Under these conditions, left atrial pressure is high and pulmonary oedema common. Myocardial depressant anaesthetic agents will depress cardiac output but vasodilatation is less hazardous than increases in systemic vascular resistance, which aggravates the mitral regurgitation. Stone and his colleagues[27] have demonstrated an improvement in left ventricular dynamics and forward flow, when patients with mitral incompetence have their afterload reduced with sodium nitroprusside. The cardiac output is better maintained at faster heart rates and bradycardia should be avoided.

Again, the development of pulmonary hypertension or the presence of other lesions, particularly aortic valve disease, increase the operative risks.

### Aortic Valve Disease

*Aortic stenosis.*—Valvular aortic stenosis occurs as a congenital abnormality, as the result of rheumatic fever, or as the result of calcification in a congenital bicuspid valve. Outflow obstruction to the left ventricle also occurs in hypertrophic obstructive cardiomyopathy.

Patients develop a thickened hypertrophied ventricle which is called on to perform more work. Despite this, cardiac output and myocardial oxygenation are depressed resulting in angina, syncopal attacks and left ventricular failure leading to pulmonary oedema.

The small cavity of the thickened, poorly compliant, ventricle is only filled with difficulty to produce an adequate cardiac output and it is essential to maintain a good filling pressure and sinus rhythm. Atrial fibrillation is uncommon in early aortic stenosis but the development of dysrhythmias, particularly nodal rhythm, may result in an acute drop in cardiac output and is a common cause of sudden death in these patients. If cardiac arrest occurs, resuscitation is difficult due to the ineffectiveness of external cardiac compression in producing an adequate coronary perfusion.

During anaesthesia, the particular concern is to maintain the balance between myocardial oxygen demand and supply in the presence of a hypertrophied ventricle and a reduced coronary flow.

Hypertension secondary to inadequate anaesthesia, hypoxia, catecholamine secretion or injudicious administration of vasopressor agents during anaesthesia is dangerous and by increasing the work load of the heart can precipitate acute myocardial ischaemia. At the same time, hypotension may seriously reduce coronary blood flow. Under anaesthesia, provided the cardiac rate and rhythm is well maintained, the patient not hypovolaemic, and the ventricular muscle not depressed, the most likely cause of hypotension is drug-induced vasodilatation, in which case the judicious use of a vasoconstrictor to restore vascular tone to normal levels is the most appropriate therapy.

*Hypertrophic obstructive cardiomyopathy* produces a subvalvar stenosis so that hypovolaemia, $\beta$-adrenergic stimulation or reduction in systemic vascular resistance will aggravate its effects. Hence filling pressure and systemic vascular resistance must be well maintained and inotropic drugs are contra-indicated. Patients are commonly treated with propranolol which should be continued during anaesthesia and surgery.

*Aortic regurgitation.*—Aortic regurgitation normally leads to a dilated left ventricle with a rise in left ventricular end-diastolic pressure which causes breathlessness. The decreased cardiac output and arterial diastolic blood pressure may result in a diminished coronary artery perfusion pressure but as the ventricle is only slightly hypertrophied and the afterload is not increased, angina only occurs in 5 per cent of cases of pure aortic incompetence and then only when the leak is severe. These patients are vulnerable to changes in rate and rhythm and to the effects of myocardial depressants. In contrast to aortic stenosis, a reduction in systemic vascular resistance (e.g. nitroprusside) promotes forward flow and reduces ventricular size. A relative tachycardia also reduces the regurgitant fraction and helps minimise the fall in diastolic pressure which, in some cases, may jeopardise coronary filling.

### Cardiac Valve Prosthesis and Re-operation

Many patients with cardiac valve disease will present subsequently for surgery after the insertion of a valve prosthesis. Maillé and colleagues[41] review their anaesthetic problems and comment that they will still have many of the problems associated with their original disease. Further, they will have acquired new restrictions and problems (e.g. anticoagulation) and will still require careful management. Before surgery, prophylactic antibiotics should be started at the time of the premedication. These patients may also present with failure of their prosthetic valve with a view to its replacement. In addition to the hazards already discussed, there is a great danger of structural damage to the heart in the initial dissection and of haemorrhage from adhesions within the pericardium.

## Coronary Artery Disease

Patients with coronary artery disease may present either for incidental surgery or for an operation, most commonly saphenous vein aortocoronary bypass grafting, designed to improve myocardial blood supply. The mortality of this operation in low-risk cases is now around 1 per cent and is thus no greater than the incidence of cardiac death in patients over 40 years old following non-cardiac surgery.[1]

In the pre-operative evaluation of the patient with coronary artery disease, it is necessary to consider, not only the extent of the vessel disease, but also the degree of left ventricular dysfunction.[42] However, even those patients without symptoms or signs of ischaemic heart disease or ventricular dysfunction at rest may develop them during the haemodynamic stimulation which can occur during anaesthesia and surgery. Equally, they may be seen in the postoperative period when shivering, pain or vasoconstriction place an unacceptable demand on myocardial oxygenation.[43] Later, myocardial oxygenation may be threatened by dehydration, hypercoagulability, increased metabolic rate, hypoxaemia and the effects of starvation.

Recent myocardial infarction complicates surgery, mainly because of the risk of reinfarction at the time of operation—a risk which is associated with pre-operative hypertension, intra-operative hypotension and non-cardiac thoracic or abdominal operations of more than three hours duration.[44] Reinfarction may be hard to diagnose as intra-operative infarcts are frequently silent and present only as sudden hypotension or heart failure, but a study by Steen and his colleagues confirms earlier observations that reinfarction is both frequent and associated with a high mortality. Of his 587 patients with a previous infarct, 36 reinfarcted and of those 25 (nearly 70 per cent) died. The incidence of repeat infarction diminishes as the time interval between the original infarct and surgery increases (Table 4) and as a general principle, elective operations that can be delayed should not be performed within six months of myocardial infarction. Although the time interval is the most obvious factor, the

13/Table 4
Relationship of Reinfarction Rate to Infarct/Surgery Interval

| *Time from previous MI* | *Reinfarction rate* |
|---|---|
| within 3 months | 27% |
| 3–6 months | 11% |
| over 6 months | 4–5% |

(Steen *et al.*, 1978[44])

type and extent of the infarction and, more particularly, the condition of the patient since then are also important. Left ventricular failure, angina and an unstable ECG increase the risk of anaesthesia and surgery.

The management of patients with coronary artery disease is directed towards the improvement of myocardial oxygen supply relative to the demand not only during anaesthesia, but also in the pre- and postoperative periods. The choice of therapy must depend on the aetiology of the myocardial ischaemia which will vary from patient to patient. The impossibility of a universally applicable therapeutic manoeuvre is demonstrated by the incompatibility inherent in the two old adages "maintain a good head of pressure" and "give the heart a rest". Whereas ischaemia, secondary to tachycardia and hypertension, may respond to vasodilatation and beta-blockade, it will be aggravated by the combination of vasodilatation with inotropic therapy. This would be more appropriate for ischaemia secondary to left ventricular failure with raised left ventricular end-diastolic pressure and volume.

**Anaesthesia.**—Following pre-operative assessment (see p. 471), a generous premedication should be prescribed in order to obtund the haemodynamic responses to anxiety, although the significant hypoxaemia which may occur after premedication[22,23] may require oxygen administration. Beta-blockade should be continued and, if some time has elapsed since the last maintenance dose, it is advisable to add a small *oral* supplement such as 20 mg propranolol, one hour before the intramuscular premedication. Beta-blockade has revolutionised the management of severe ischaemic heart disease and reduces swings in myocardial oxygen demand, provoked by anaesthesia and surgery. Papaveretum, or morphine, with hyoscine proves generally satisfactory for sedation and may be combined with a prior dose of a benzodiazepine orally.

The subsequent choice of anaesthetic agents and techniques is perhaps less important than the ability to control the cardiovascular responses to anaesthesia and surgery which may provoke ischaemia. Edde[45] demonstrated that even during high dose fentanyl anaesthesia, increased myocardial oxygen demand occurred following median sternotomy, which could not be prevented by deeper anaesthesia and which could only be reversed by vasodilator therapy. At the same time, the actual choice has some relevance in that, by their actions on heart rate, contractility and blood pressure, most agents used in anaesthesia have some effect on myocardial oxygen balance.

**Monitoring** in ischaemic heart disease should provide, where possible, information on the determinants of myocardial oxygen balance. In cardiac surgery, pulmonary artery occlusion pressure, cardiac output, right atrial and direct arterial pressure measurements are routinely employed. For non-cardiac operations, the sickness of the patient and the extent of the operative technique will tend to dictate the degree of invasive monitoring employed. However, indirect blood pressure measurements and ECG alone may be insufficient in some cases. Lead $V_5$ (precordial) ECG monitoring (see p. 477) is preferred over limb lead II for the detection of ST changes from ischaemia. The development of ST changes characteristic of ischaemia during surgery could be considered an indication of failure of management of the circulation, which should have been prevented.[43] In severe coronary artery disease, an attempt should be made to monitor the circulation before induction of anaesthesia so that untoward haemodynamic effects can be controlled rapidly. Estimates of rate pressure product (systolic pressure × rate) and triple index (systolic pressure × rate × pulmonary capillary wedge pressure) give a useful indication of myocardial oxygen demand, whilst diastolic pressure-time index (if available) correlates with myocardial oxygen supply. Temperature monitoring aids control of core and peripheral temperatures with a view to producing a normothermic recovery period.

The manoeuvres which influence variables affecting myocardial oxygenation can be considered under the heading of each determinant:

**Prevention of reduction in myocardial oxygen supply** (see Table 5)

1. *Arterial oxygen tension*: The arterial oxygenation may be impaired by lung disease, by pulmonary engorgement secondary to a raised left atrial pressure, by a reduction in cardiac output, or by a reduction in ventilation due to respiratory depressant drugs. Lung disease should be treated, cardiac failure corrected and oxygen may need to be given following premedication and in the postoperative period.

2. *Haemoglobin:* The haemoglobin should be maintained at normal levels to maintain oxygen transport but polycythaemic states may need correction because of the concomitant increase in blood viscosity.

13/TABLE 5
FACTORS INFLUENCING MYOCARDIAL OXYGENATION

| | | | | | |
|---|---|---|---|---|---|
| MYOCARDIAL OXYGEN SUPPLY (AVAILABILITY) | $PaO_2$ | Hb | CORONARY VESSEL CALIBRE | CORONARY ARTERY PERFUSION PRESSURE (Diastolic aortic BP minus left ventricular diastolic pressure) | DIASTOLIC CORONARY PERFUSION TIME |
| ↑ VERSUS ↓ | | | | | |
| MYOCARDIAL OXYGEN DEMAND (CONSUMPTION) | VENTRICULAR RATE | | CONTRACTILITY (and Hypertension) | | VENTRICULAR WALL TENSION<br>1. Aortic input impedence<br>2. Arteriolar run off<br>3. Ventricular cavity radius |

3. *Coronary vessels:* Coronary artery spasm can be relieved by intravenous, sublingual or paste glyceryl trinitrate, which may be taken sublingually by the patient himself up to the moment of induction. During intermittent positive-pressure ventilation, the carbon dioxide tension should be only slightly reduced to avoid the coronary vasoconstriction which hypocarbia provokes.

4. *Coronary perfusion pressure:* The coronary perfusion pressure depends both on the maintenance of the arterial diastolic pressure at reasonable levels and on a low ventricular end-diastolic pressure. In the presence of an adequate cardiac output the former will depend on the degree of arteriolar tone, and vasoconstrictive drugs such as methoxamine or metaraminol may be required. A high ventricular end-diastolic pressure is a result of venoconstriction or ventricular failure and requires treatment with glyceryl trinitrate, sodium nitroprusside or, somewhat cautiously, with inotropes.[46]

5. *Diastolic coronary perfusion time:* The time available for coronary perfusion is reduced during tachycardia, particularly in diseased hearts in which tachycardia is achieved mainly by shortening of diastole. The rate should be optimised to allow adequate coronary perfusion time (while preventing a low cardiac output secondary to bradycardia) by the use of intravenous increments of beta-blockers such as oxprenolol 0·5 mg, propranolol 0·25 mg or practolol 1 mg.

**Prevention of an increase in myocardial oxygen demand** (see Table 5)

1. *Heart rate:* Tachycardia is associated with an increased oxygen demand. Apart from the avoidance of drugs which produce this (atropine, gallamine, isoprenaline) and the elimination of other causes, such as pain, by an adequate depth of anaesthesia, particularly with an anaesthetic agent that tends to control rate such as fentanyl or halothane, persistent tachycardia can be controlled by the use of $\beta$-blockers.
2. *Contractility:* Increases in cardiac contractility and cardiac output occur secondary to stress responses during anaesthesia, at times such as laryngoscopy and intubation or in the postoperative period, secondary to shivering or uncontrolled pain. These rises can be prevented by beta-blockade or by the use of adequate quantities of halothane or enflurane. Acute rises in blood pressure can also be treated with droperidol, phentolamine or continuous infusions of sodium nitroprusside, or glyceryl trinitrate as enhanced contractility in the face of hypertension is particularly significant in terms of myocardial oxygen consumption.
3. *Ventricular wall tension:* Where cardiac failure is an aetiological factor in myocardial ischaemia, a further depression of ventricular function by drugs, such as halothane, enflurane, verapamil or as a result of acidosis, may cause an increase in ventricular size so that wall tension rises and ischaemia is aggravated. More commonly, the wall tension in ischaemic heart disease is high because of decreased arteriolar runoff, together with a reduced ejection fraction and a raised end-diastolic pressure. Sodium nitroprusside or similar vasodilators will improve arteriolar runoff, encourage left ventricular emptying and reduce ventricular end-diastolic pressure. The maintenance of normocarbia will avoid the venoconstriction associated with hypocapnia. Volume overloading leading to a rise in left ventricular end-diastolic pressure and wall tension as a consequence of venoconstriction may be treated with alpha-blockers, morphine or glyceryl trinitrate, although too slow a heart rate may itself increase ventricular volumes from exaggerated ventricular filling.

**Post-operative care** for patients with coronary artery disease should be taken as seriously as the intra-operative management, and maintenance beta-blockers or other therapy continued or reinstated as soon as possible. Prevention of heat loss (shivering) and removal of pain are important factors to take into consideration.[43] Parenteral opiates may be substituted by intrathecal or extradural opiates in selected, well-monitored patients, provided respiratory depression is avoided. Postoperative hypo- or hypertension should be managed promptly, because myocardial infarction is likely to occur at this stage of the peri-operative period. Ganglion blockers or hydralazine may be easier to administer than infusions of potent vasodilators such as SNP in some recovery areas. Finally, prevention of hypoxia is important, especially during this period of increased myocardial oxygen demands.

### Dysrhythmias in Coronary Artery Disease

Ventricular and supraventricular dysrhythmias are common in coronary artery disease, and are often associated with atrioventricular conduction defects, particularly after open-heart surgery. Ventricular dysrhythmias occur more frequently during periods of myocardial ischaemia and may indicate actual infarction. The primary approach in treatment is the correction of myocardial oxygen supply/demand imbalance. Severe bradycardia, which occurs during acute cardiac ischaemia often precedes ventricular extrasystoles and fibrillation and should be managed with atropine or electrical pacing, while manoeuvres to improve myocardial oxygenation are instituted. Dysrhythmic potential may be accentuated by low serum potassium or magnesium (which are commonly seen following cardiopulmonary bypass or during diuretic therapy), acid-base changes, hypothermia and exogenous or endogenous catecholamines. Lignocaine intravenously as a bolus (1 mg/kg) followed by a sequential infusion regime[32] proves useful, but refractory dysrhythmias may require treatment with disopyramide, bretylium, quinidine or beta-blockers (see p. 435). The presence of halothane is associated with a higher incidence of dysrhythmias than are seen with enflurane, while droperidol-fentanyl is said to offer some protective effect. Conduction defects are sometimes improved by atropine, isoprenaline or dobutamine, but in the presence of beta-blockade, glucagon with aminophylline is more successful; ventricular pacing may be necessary.

## Chronic Constrictive Pericarditis

The essential effect of this disease is a limitation of the diastolic expansion of all chambers of the heart leading to a reduction in stroke output and pulsus paradoxus (see p. 456). Eventually the pressure rises in the right atrium and systemic venous congestion occurs. Pulmonary congestion is, however, rare. Because of the limitation on stroke volume, the cardiac output is very dependent on cardiac rate and the maintenance of ventricular filling pressure, while with a relatively fixed cardiac output, the blood pressure is markedly altered by variations in arteriolar tone.

The risk during anaesthesia is essentially similar to that of other diseases in which the cardiac output is reduced to a stage at which compensation for sudden falls in peripheral resistance cannot take place. These patients must be treated in a manner similar to those with mitral stenosis and great caution exercised in the use of thiopentone.

Central venous pressure monitoring is essential during pericardectomy, both for the maintenance of right ventricular filling pressure and also to observe the fall in central venous pressure that follows the adequate surgical relief of the constriction. Haemorrhage during the operation may be considerable. The rotation of the heart necessary during the approach to the pericardium around the base of the heart and right atrium results in frequent dysrhythmias and hypotension. Besides an ECG, a continuous display of arterial pressure is mandatory. The left ventricle is normally decompressed before the right, otherwise there is a danger of pulmonary oedema. Two other complications are the development of cardiac failure, as a result of myocardial involvement in the disease, and the possibility of damage to the coronary arteries during the operation.

In the pre-operative preparation, despite their high venous pressure and frequent oedema, patients with constrictive pericarditis must not be given an excessive diuresis as they are very dependent on an adequate right-sided filling pressure to maintain the cardiac output.

## Tamponade

Cardiac tamponade is often an acute life-threatening event in which a severely limited cardiac output is only maintained by a tachycardia and a high right ventricular filling pressure. When tamponade immediately follows the causative event, the diagnosis is usually obvious, but if the onset is delayed, the diagnosis may be more difficult and is frequently confused with congestive cardiac failure. Tamponade should always be considered when circulatory deterioration follows chest trauma or surgery, cardiac catheterisation or the passage of any catheter or cannula near the heart.

The diagnosis is made on the discovery of a low cardiac output (oliguria, metabolic acidosis, cold poorly perfused peripheries) with pulsus paradoxus in association with a high right atrial pressure showing a marked systolic descent. The combination of tachycardia, a small stroke volume and severe peripheral vasoconstriction may result in an impalpable peripheral pulse.

The immediate treatment of tamponade is the percutaneous aspiration of the accumulation in the pericardial sac. Then anaesthesia and surgery can be more safely performed. If, however, anaesthesia is required before pericardial decompression as for instance in stab wounds of the heart, the cardiac rate and sinus rhythm must be maintained and vasodilatation actively prevented if necessary with a vasoconstrictor. Induction with diazepam and maintenance with nitrous oxide and oxygen following paralysis with pancuronium produces less circulatory depression than more traditional techniques. The effect of the introduction of positive-pressure ventilation is variable depending on the extent of the impairment of right ventricular filling. Anaesthesia for patients with cardiac tamponade ranks with severe pulmonary hypertension and pulmonary embolism as a dangerous procedure.

**Raised pulmonary vascular resistance** (Pulmonary hypertension).—The pulmonary artery pressure may be raised, with no change in the pulmonary vessels, as a result of a raised left atrial pressure. A raised pulmonary vascular resistance is due to medial hypertrophy and intimal thickening in the walls of the pulmonary arterioles. This change, which may be irreversible, occurs in 30 per cent of those conditions which are characterised by a chronically raised left atrial pressure or a large left-to-right shunt. A similar effect may be produced by recurrent pulmonary emboli. Pulmonary hypertension is aggravated by anoxia or respiratory acidosis. These patients are existing at the limits of their right ventricular function and need a high right ventricular end-diastolic pressure to maintain their output. They are, therefore, if anything, even more sensitive to vasodilatation than patients whose fixed cardiac output is due to left ventricular limitation.

### Extracorporeal Circulation

The general principles for anaesthesia and management of patients with cardiac disease, paying particular attention to the problems of specific lesions, apply to operations performed with the aid of extracorporeal circulation. One of the many peculiar problems posed is that of keeping the patient unconscious during the period of bypass and this is discussed in greater detail in Chapter 15.

## CARDIOVERSION

Electrical countershock for the conversion of tachydysrhythmias may be performed as an elective procedure or as an emergency if the cardiac output is severely depressed. Unless the patient is already unconscious, it is too painful to be performed without anaesthesia. The cardioversion of chronic atrial fibrillation to sinus rhythm is a relatively safe procedure provided there is no danger of digoxin toxicity and the serum potassium is normal.

Although inhalational anaesthesia or amnesia/analgesia have been described, intravenous anaesthesia is the usual method. It is, however, worth continuing with nitrous oxide:oxygen, perhaps with a low dose of inhalational agent, so as to restrict the dose of intravenous agent should more than one shock be required. Neither premedication nor succinylcholine are necessary. Diazepam has been frequently advocated due to its benign effect on the circulation. It should not be administered in the absence of facilities for artificial ventilation and because of its variable effect and dosage, occasional patients may remain somnolent for some hours. The more predictable effects of thiopentone or methohexitone are to be preferred.

An open vein is mandatory because of the risk of ventricular fibrillation and of post-conversion dysrhythmias. The standard resuscitative and antidysrhythmic drugs, particularly atropine, potassium chloride, lignocaine and $\beta$-blockers should be to hand. Acute pulmonary oedema and peripheral circulatory embolism are two uncommon post-conversion complications.

## CARDIAC CATHETERISATION AND ANGIOCARDIOGRAPHY

Cardiac catheterisation is not a painful procedure except for the introduction of the catheter through the skin and this can be adequately covered by local anaesthesia. The passage of the catheter through the vessels should provide no sensation, but the mental strain and the discomfort of lying continuously in the dark X-ray room on a hard table for any length of time may make it unacceptable to the patient. Angiocardiography may be less pleasant, the injection of the contrast medium is followed by a hot sensation spreading over the body and a bursting sensation in the head.

The choice for cardiac catheterisation is either local analgesic, local analgesic combined with sedation, or general anaesthesia. The argument in favour of avoidance of general anaesthesia is mainly on the grounds that changes in cardiorespiratory function during anaesthesia are unpredictable and that unpremedicated, unanaesthetised patients breathing air are likely to be in a more physiological condition. The technique of cardiac catheterisation without sedation produces satisfactory results in most adults, if the staff work hard at reassuring the patient beforehand and avoid upsetting him during the procedure.

Sedation or anaesthesia tends to be indicated for the following groups of patients:

1. Those patients in whom catheterisation without sedation is impossible due to the presence of a language barrier or the patient having such a low mentality that one is unable to communicate with him properly.

2. If the patient has had a previous catheterisation of which he has unpleasant memories, he may express unwillingness to have a second performance without the benefits of general anaesthesia.

3. Children.

Moffit and colleagues[47] reviewing eleven years' experience of anaesthesia in children, found it satisfactory both for child and physician. The exposure to the process of diagnosis made the anaesthetist better able to manage the same child at the subsequent operation.

### Special Considerations

(*a*) A steady state is required because the various measurements at different sites are often made consecutively, not simultaneously.

(*b*) The cardiovascular state (pulse, resistance, cardiac output, etc.) should be altered as little as possible. Although cardiac output is normally measured at some time during the catheterisation, this is not always so. Deductions can only be made from the measurements on the assumption that the cardiovascular state is substantially unchanged by the anaesthetic technique.

(*c*) Ventilation. Alterations in oxygen or carbon dioxide tension have circulatory effects as do the mechanical factors of positive-pressure respiration. Again, the requirement is to maintain the patient as near normal as possible. In small children it is particularly easy to overventilate, producing substantial reductions in carbon dioxide tension, although this is preferable to hypercarbia with its effects on pulmonary vascular resistance and intracardiac shunting.

(*d*) In small children, hypothermia and hypoglycaemia must be avoided.

(*e*) Fluid balance. Blood samples and unnoticed haemorrhage may add up to large fluid deficits while enthusiastic flushing of catheters can result in considerable fluid administration.

(*f*) Contrast medium. The dye used for angiography has a transient depressive action on the heart and is also a powerful vasodilator. Although the volume is usually strictly limited, the fluid is hypertonic and leads to an expansion in the circulatory blood volume which may overload the heart.

(*g*) Acidosis. A metabolic acidosis may develop if the cardiac output is low, particularly if the reduction is aggravated by dysrhythmias provoked during the catheterisation. The acidosis will itself impair cardiac contractility.

(*h*) The pre-investigation clinical diagnosis may turn out to be entirely incorrect and the patient suffering from some quite different haemodynamic process. Any method of sedation or anaesthesia needs to be as universally applicable as possible to allow for this contingency.

### Techniques

*Sedation*.—The principal advantage of sedation is that patients breathe air spontaneously. The obvious danger is respiratory depression to the point of hypoxia with changes in the circulation secondary to hypoxia and hypercapnia.

Between the ages of six months and 12 years, good results with heavy sedation can be obtained for catheterisation and angiocardiography using the schedule recommended by Nicholson and Graham.[48] Sodium phenobarbitone 2 mg/kg is given the previous evening and again three hours before the procedure or alternatively trimeprazine tartrate 3–4 mg/kg given four hours before. Half an hour before the procedure an intramuscular injection of 1 ml/10 kg body weight of a compound injection of pethidine, of which 1 ml contains chlorpromazine 6·25 mg, promethazine 6·25 mg and pethidine 25 mg.

The dose is halved in children below the age of six months or those who are ill. If the child becomes restless towards the end of a long procedure the sedation is supplemented with small doses of intravenous diazepam.

*Neuroleptanalgesia.*—Innovar (droperidol 2·4 mg with fentanyl 0·05 mg in 1 ml) has been shown to have minimal effects on the cardiac output and work, although the blood pressure and vascular resistance declined. However, in a study by Tarhan and his colleagues[49] all patients had decreases in arterial oxygen tension, sometimes to hypoxic levels and the effects of hypercapnia and hypoxia may have masked cardiovascular depression. Graham and colleagues[50] recommend Innovar 0·025 ml/kg body weight to a maximum of 1 ml. This gave good results but the dose must not be exceeded.

*Ketamine.*—Bovill and colleagues[51] regarded cardiac catheterisation as being a specific indication for the use of ketamine, although Tweed and associates[52] described it as unsuitable in the presence of coronary artery disease, severe myocardial disease or aortic stenosis. There is respiratory depression and rise in blood pressure which usually returns to normal after 15 minutes. It does not appear to affect the pulmonary vascular resistance.[53] Atropine premedication is necessary and Brandus and colleagues[54] recommend ketamine intramuscularly 5 mg/kg in children, 3–4 mg/kg in infants, 1–2 mg/kg in neonates and thereafter adjusting the dose of small intravenous increments to the response of the patient. The principal danger in the use of ketamine lies in its inotropic effect which may lead to exacerbation of infundibular stenosis resulting in a drastic fall in cardiac output or oxygenation. The use of ketamine does not dispense with the need to have an anaesthetist present.

*General anaesthesia.*—A suitable technique in children is premedication with trimeprazine 3 mg/kg given 2 hours before the procedure followed by a generous dose of papaveretum: hyoscine to be given an hour later. Vagolytic agents should always be administered in order to prevent excessive secretions and to avoid bradycardias caused by succinylcholine or halothane. Atropine is satisfactory for babies and should preferably be given intramuscularly, but hyoscine is the drug of choice in larger children as it provides more sedation and amnesia without a tendancy towards a tachycardia. Induction, which may be gaseous or intravenous, is followed by succinylcholine, which may be safely used to facilitate intubation. Ventilation may then be continued with nitrous oxide, oxygen and a minimal concentration (0·3 per cent) halothane, with just enough hyperventilation to eliminate respiratory drive. Alternatively, intubation can be performed after pancuronium when no volatile agent will be required. The pain of cannulation is usually covered by local infiltration so that nitrous oxide in the presence of a heavy premedication is sufficient to maintain unconsciousness. The minor deviations of cardiorespiratory performance induced by positive-pressure ventilation are more than offset by the avoidance of other agents which affect myocardial contractility, peripheral resistance and the likelihood of dysrhythmias.

## HEART BLOCK AND ANAESTHESIA

Complete heart block is defined as a condition in which there is atrioventricular dissociation and the ventricular rate is slower than the atrial rate.

Complete atrioventricular block most commonly results from degeneration of the conducting tissue of the heart. It may also be the result of surgery or drug therapy, occur as a congenital abnormality, or be due to ischaemic disease. Block may be complete or affect only one or two of the three main fasciculi. Complete block occurring high in the bundle produces a fairly fast ventricular rate and Stokes-Adams attacks are unusual. Low block is associated with slow and unreliable spontaneous ventricular activity.

Stokes-Adams attacks occur:

(*a*) When partial block becomes complete.

(*b*) During established block with unreliable ventricular activity (low block).

(*c*) As attacks of ventricular tachycardia or fibrillation.

Partial or unstable block is a more dangerous condition than stable complete block and a history of Stokes-Adams attacks, giddiness, collapse or fainting suggests an unstable block.

Patients present for anaesthesia in two states:

1. They may present in partial or complete block for pacemaker insertion or for incidental surgery.
2. Patients may appear for anaesthesia and surgery with an indwelling pacemaker already in use.

Patients with stable complete block have a very fixed cardiac output which can only be altered marginally by increases in stroke volume. They are, therefore, very vulnerable both to myocardial depressant drugs and to vasodilatation, although it may be possible to increase their rate with atropine or isoprenaline (the treatment of heart block is discussed further on page 493). If isoprenaline does not speed up the heart the blood pressure is liable to fall due to its vasodilator action. Provided the patient's cardiac output is sufficient to sustain him normally, he can probably be safely anaesthetised using techniques which avoid myocardial depression or peripheral dilatation.

Patients with block of recent onset or with unstable block and a history of Stokes-Adams attacks need a temporary transvenous pacemaker inserted prior to anaesthesia and surgery. This will probably apply to patients presenting for their first permanent pacemaker insertion.

When any patient with a conduction defect is being anaesthetised, a continuous ECG display is mandatory. A pacing box and sterile transvenous leads must also be available in the theatre. If a transvenous pacemaker is in use any sudden or violent movement may dislodge the pacing contact. Failure to pace may also arise from increases in pacemaker threshold due to alterations in serum electrolytes or myocardial depression due to anaesthetic agents such as halothane. The efficacy of pacing must be judged not by the ECG but by an adequate peripheral pulse so that in some patients, radial artery cannulation with continuing blood pressure monitoring is valuable. Sudden cessation of pacing is an emergency and if the spontaneous cardiac output is inadequate and shows no response to isoprenaline, external cardiac compression may be necessary until an adequate ventricular rate is achieved.

## DIATHERMY AND THE PACEMAKER

The dangers of diathermy used on a patient with a pacemaker are twofold. The diathermy may affect the rate of pacemaker discharge—most commonly this is apparent as total inhibition of demand pacing but it may also result in high discharge rate (200–600 impulses/min) which may provoke ventricular tachycardia or fibrillation.[55] Alternatively diathermy may induce currents in the circuit at an inappropriate moment and provoke ventricular fibrillation. The safest course if a patient has an indwelling pacemaker, is to forbid the use of the diathermy. If the patient is being paced with an external box, the pacer can be disconnected briefly each time the diathermy is used—it may not be sufficient merely to turn it off. As the ECG will also be inhibited by the diathermy at this moment, the pulse must be monitored continuously while the diathermy is used.

## REFERENCES


1. Goldman, L., Caldera, D. L., Nussbaum, S. R., Southwick, F. S., Krogstad, D., Murray, B., Burke, D. S., O'Malley, T. A., Goroll, A. M., Caplan, C. M., Nolan, J., Carabello, B., Slater, E. C. (1977). Multifactorial index of cardiac risk in non cardiac surgical procedures. *New Eng. J. Med.*, **297**, 845.
2. Hoffman, B. F. and Bigger, J. T. (1980). In: *The Pharmacological Basis of Therapeutics*, 6th edit., p. 732, edited by Gilman, A. G., Goodman, L. S., Gilman, A. New York: Macmillan Publishing Co.
3. Scallon, N. J. H., Bothard, J. W. W. and Branthwaite, M. A. (1979). Inotropic agents. *Brit. J. Anaesth.*, **51**, 649.
4. Goldstein, R. A., Passaman, E. R., Roberts, R. (1980). A comparison of digoxin and dobutamine in patients with acute infarction and cardiac failure. *New Eng. J. Med.*, **303**, 846.
5. Hebert, P. and Tinker, J. (1980). Inotropic drugs in acute circulatory failure. *Intens. Care Medicine*, **6**, 101.
6. Prys-Roberts, C., Meloche, R. and Foëx, P. (1971). Studies of anaesthesia in relation to hypertension: I.

Cardiovascular responses of treated and untreated patients. *Brit. J. Anaesth.*, **43**, 122.
7. Mauney, F. M., Ebert, P. A. and Sabiston, D. C. (1970). Postoperative myocardial infarction: a study of predisposing factors, diagnosis and mortality in high risk group of surgical patients. *Ann. Surg.*, **172**, 497.
8. Breslin, D. J. and Swinton, N. W. (1970). Elective surgery in hypertensive patients—pre-operative considerations. *Surg. Clin. N. Amer.*, **50**, 585.
9. Ominsky, A. J. and Wollman, H. (1969). Hazards of general anaesthesia in the reserpinised patient. *Anesthesiology*, **30**, 443.
10. Prys-Roberts, C., Foëx, P., Greene, L. T. and Waterhouse, T. D. (1972). Studies of anaesthesia in relation to hypertension: IV. The effect of artificial ventilation on the circulation and pulmonary gas exchanges. *Brit. J. Anaesth.*, **44**, 335.
11. Foex, P. (1978). Pre-operative assessment of patients with cardiac disease. *Brit. J. Anaesth.*, **50**, 15.
12. Miller, N. E., Hammett, F., Saltisi, S., Rao, S., Van Leller, H., Coltart, J., Lewis, B. (1981). Relation of angiographically defined coronary artery diseases to plasma lipoprotein subfractions and apolipoproteins. *Brit. med. J.*, **282**, 1741.
13. Opie, L. H. (1980). Drugs and the heart. *Lancet*, **1**, 693.
14. Bridges, B. B., Carden, E., Takas, F. A. (1979). Introduction of central venous pressure catheters through arm veins with a high success rate. *Canad. Anaesth. Soc. J.*, **26**, 128.
15. Csànky-Treels, J. (1978). Hazards of central venous pressure monitoring *Anaesthesia*, **33**, 172.
16. Opie, J. C. (1980). Contamination of internal jugular lines. *Anaesthesia*, **35**, 1060.
17. Davis, F. M. and Stewart, J. M. (1980). Radial artery cannulation. *Brit. J. Anaesth.*, **52**, 41.
18. Palm, T. (1977). Evaluation of peripheral arterial pressure on the thumb following radial artery cannulation. *Brit. J. Anaesth.*, **49**, 819.
19. Husum, B., Palm, T. and Erikson, J. (1979). Percutaneous cannulation of the dorsalis pedis artery. *Brit. J. Anaesth.*, **51**, 1055.
20. Shaw, T. J. I. (1979). The Swan-Ganz pulmonary artery catheter. *Anaesthesia*, **34**, 651.
21. Prys-Roberts, C. (1980). *The Circulation in Anaesthesia* p. 129. Oxford: Blackwell Scientific Publications.
22. El-Mikatti, N. (1981). The effects of oral diazepam premedication in blood gases. *Ann. roy. Coll. Surg. Engl.*, **63**, 429.
23. Kopman, E. A. and Ramirez-Inawat, R. C. (1980). Arterial hypoxaemia following premedication in patients with coronary artery disease. *Canad. Anaesth. Soc. J.*, **27**, 132.
24. Editorial (1981). Artificial ventilation and the heart. *Brit. med. J.*, **283**, 397.
25. Opie, L. H. (1980). Drugs and the heart. VI. Vasodilating drugs. *Lancet*, **1**, 966.
26. Thompson, D. S., Juul, S. M., Wilmshurst, P., Naqvi, N., Coltart, D. J., Jenkins, B. S., Webb-Peploe, M. M. (1981). Effects of sodium nitroprusside upon cardiac work, efficiency and substrate extraction in severe left ventricular failure. *Brit. Heart J.*, **46**, 394.
27. Stone, G. J., Hoar, P. F., Calabro, J. R., Depetrillo, M. A., Bendixen, H. K. (1980). Afterload reduction and preload augmentation improve the anesthetic management of patients with cardiac failure and valvular regurgitation. *Anesth. Analg.*, **59**, 737.
28. Meretoja, D. A. and Laaksonen, V. O. (1978). Haemodynamic effects of preload and sodium nitroprusside in patients subjected to coronary artery surgery. *Circulation*, **58**, 815.
29. Noble, W. M. (1980). Pulmonary oedema: a review, *Canad. Anaesth. Soc. J.*, **27**, 286.
30. Klepper, I. (1981). Cardioversion in late pregnancy: the anaesthetic management of a case of Wolff-Parkinson-White syndrome. *Anaesthesia*, **36**, 611.
31. Katz, R. L. and Bigger, J. T. (1970). Cardiac arrhythmias during anesthesia and operation. *Anesthesiology*, **33**, 193.
32. Aps, C., Bell, J. A., Jenkins, B. S., Poole-Wilson, P. A. and Reynolds, F. (1976). Logical approach to lignocaine therapy. *Brit. med. J.*, **1**, 13.
33. Hartley, J. M. F. (1982). Transoesophageal cardiac pacing. *Anaesthesia*, **37**, 192.
34. Mathews, E. and Abrams, L. D. (1980). Intrathecal morphine in open heart surgery. *Lancet*, **2**, 543.
35. Gale, G. D., Teasdale, S. J., Sanders, D. E., Bradwell, P. J., Russell, A., Solaric, B., York, J. E. (1979). Pulmonary atelectasis and other respiratory complications after cardiopulmonary bypass and investigation of aetiological factors. *Canad. Anaesth. Soc. J.*, **26**, 15.
36. Hinds, C. J. (1982). Current management of patients after cardiopulmonary bypass. *Anaesthesia*, **37**, 170.
37. Marin, J. L. B., Orchard, C., Chakrabati, M. K., Sykes, M. K. (1979). Depression of hypoxic pulmonary vasoconstriction in the dog by dopamine and isoprenaline. *Brit. J. Anaesth.*, **51**, 303.
38. Gilston, A. (1982). Prolonged nasotracheal intubation. *Anaesthesia*, **37**, 209.
39. Paiemont, B., Boulanger, M. Jones, C. W. and Roy, M. (1979). Intubation and other experiences in cardiac surgery: the consumer's views. *Canad. Anaesth. Soc. J.*, **26**, 173.
40. Gilston, A. (1976). Facial signs of respiratory distress after cardiac surgery. *Anaesthesia*, **31**, 385.
41. Maillé, J., Dryda, I., Paiement, B. and Boulanger, M. (1973). Patients with cardiac valve prosthesis: subsequent anaesthetic management for non-cardiac surgical procedures. *Canad. Anaesth. Soc. J.*, **20**, 207.
42. Waller, J. L. and Kaplan, J. A. (1981). Anaesthesia for patients with coronary artery disease. *Brit. J. Anaesth.*, **53**, 759.
43. Tinker, J. H. (1981). Myocardial oxygenation during anaesthesia. *Curr. Rev. in Clin. Anaesth.*, Lesson 26, Vol **1**, p. 210.
44. Steen, P. A., Tinker, J. H. and Tarhan, S. (1978). Myocardial reinfarction after anaesthesia and surgery. *J. Amer. med. Ass.*, **239**, 2566.
45. Edde, R. R. (1981). Hemodynamic changes prior to and after sternotomy in patients anesthetised with high-dose fentanyl. *Anesthesiology*, **55**, 444.
46. Fletcher, R. (1980). Coronary disease and anaesthesia. *Anaesthesia*, **35**, 27.
47. Moffit, E. A., McGoon, D. C. and Ritter, D. G. (1970). The diagnosis and correction of congenital cardiac defects. *Anesthesiology*, **33**, 144.
48. Nicholson, J. R. and Graham, G. R. (1969). Management of infants under six months of age undergoing cardiac investigation. *Brit. J. Anaesth.*, **41**, 417.
49. Tarhan, S., Moffitt, E. A., Lundborg, R. O. and Frye,

R. L. (1971). Hemodynamic and blood-gas effects of "Innovar" in patients with acquired heart disease. *Anesthesiology*, **34**, 250.
50. Graham, T. P., Atwood, G. F. and Werner, B. (1974). Use of droperidol-fentanyl sedation for cardiac catheterisation in children. *Amer. Heart. J.*, **87**, 287.
51. Bovill, J. G., Coppell, D. L., Dundee, J. W. and Moore, J. (1971). Current status of ketamine anaesthesia. *Lancet*, **2**, 1285.
52. Tweed, W. A., Minuck, M. and Mymin, D. (1972). Circulatory responses to ketamine anaesthesia. *Anesthesiology*, **37**, 613.
53. Gassner, S., Cohen, M. Aygen, M., Levy, E., Ventura, E. and Shashdi, J. (1974). The effect of ketamine on pulmonary artery pressure. *Anaesthetic*, **29**, 141.
54. Brandus, V., Benoit, C. and Koch, L. (1971). Ketamine anaesthesia. *Lancet*, **2**, 543.
55. Orland, H. J. and Jones, D. (1975). Cardiac pacemaker induced ventricular fibrillation during surgical diathermy. *Anaesth. Intens. Care*, **3**, 321.

CHAPTER 14

# Circulatory Arrest, Pulmonary and Systemic Embolism



## CIRCULATORY ARREST

Hypoxia and hypovolaemia are the most common causes of cardiac arrest during surgery. Occasionally cardiac disease or interference with the heart or great vessels may be responsible. In a small proportion of patients, circulatory arrest occurs when death is expected in the immediate future from some terminal illness. Then, even though temporary resuscitation may be possible, it is neither reasonable nor desirable.

Most cases of circulatory arrest can be successfully treated provided action is efficient and prompt. In general, cardiac arrest falls into two categories. It may be the end result of a progressive derangement of physiology which has gone unnoticed or unheeded for some time and which usually includes respiratory or metabolic acidosis and electrolyte disturbances. Alternatively, it may result from some sudden catastrophic event superimposed on an otherwise normal background. Camarata and colleagues[1] confirmed the impression of intensive care physicians that in the latter group one may expect initial and long-term success but that in the former group success will be rare and that cardiac arrest is better prevented than treated.

### Diagnosis

The most important point in the diagnosis is that no pulse can be felt in a large artery (femoral or carotid). In a surgical case this disappearance of an effective circulation may be noted by the sudden cessation of bleeding. An absent pulse indicates that the circulation is inadequate and that immediate treatment is needed.

Unconsciousness and cessation of respiration occur and, usually within one minute, the pupils dilate. The absence of heart sounds is an unreliable sign and unless an ECG is already connected no time should be wasted in so doing before starting treatment.

The usually accepted time interval between circulatory arrest and the death of tissue in the *normal, previously well-oxygenated* central nervous system is approximately three-and-a-half minutes. Because of the rapidity with which this time can pass in an emergency, the prime factor influencing the outcome of circulatory arrest is the speed at which effective resuscitation is instituted.

The implication of this is that cardiopulmonary resuscitation should be as simple as possible, easily taught to the layman and applicable almost anywhere without complex equipment. The outcome may also be affected not merely by the speed and efficiency of the initial resuscitation, but by the quality of circulatory and neurological care in the post-arrest period. Some cases have been reported of recovery from protracted cerebral ischaemia, but these are usually associated with hypothermia produced during drowning, commonly in children, but sometimes in adults who have cooled quickly due to high blood alcohol levels.

## CARDIOPULMONARY RESUSCITATION

Once circulatory arrest has been diagnosed and whatever the initial cause, the immediate treatment must be aimed at providing an artificial circulation of oxygenated blood to the brain and myocardium, followed by a rapid return to an adequate circulatory state. Treatment falls under three headings which must be performed logically and promptly.

**Phase 1:** *First Aid* (the artificial circulation of oxygenated blood). Artificial ventilation together with external cardiac massage (ECM). This is continued *with as little interruption as possible* at least until Phase 2 is completed.

**Phase 2:** *Restoration of cardiac function and adequate cardiac output.* (i) Diagnosis—underlying causes, ECG; (ii) Drug therapy and defibrillation.

**Phase 3:** *After-treatment.* Subsequent management(i) maintenance of the circulation and adequate gas exchange; (ii) treatment of the underlying cause; (iii) treatment of complications.

### PHASE 1: FIRST AID

**Artificial ventilation.**—Of the many methods of artificial ventilation advocated over the years, only those involving intermittent positive-pressure ventilation produce sufficient volume exchange. In the hospital environment there will usually be to hand either a face mask or an endotracheal tube with oxygen supply, or an Ambu bag or Brook airway. Every anaesthetist should, however, be familiar with the technique of mouth-to-mouth or mouth-to-nose ventilation. The use of the oesophageal obturator, however, is probably best reserved for paramedical personnel who are not experienced in endotracheal intubation.

In all cases, the first step is to clear the airway, and then maintain its clarity while ventilation is carried out. Endotracheal intubation is the eventual aim so that the lungs can be easily inflated with less likelihood of gastric distension, regurgitation of gastric contents and potential lung soiling and obstruction from inhalation. Intubation must, however, be speedy, so as not to interrupt ventilation or external cardiac compression. Under these conditions, which may well be difficult, the inexperienced will do better to ventilate with a face mask until skilled assistance is to hand.

Due to the low cardiac output produced by external cardiac compression and the deterioration which occurs in ventilation-perfusion relationships in the lung, ventilation with 100 per cent oxygen should be substituted as soon as possible and even this may not produce fully saturated blood. Expired air (mouth-to-mouth) ventilation, with an $F_{IO_2}$ of around 0·16, is obviously even less satisfactory. Respiratory acidosis is not uncommon, despite apparent hyperventilation, because of the abnormal distribution of the reduced blood flow through the lungs. Where possible, however, a normal $Pa_{CO_2}$ should be aimed for, remembering also that extreme hypocarbia may further compromise cerebral blood flow in the face of a low perfusion pressure.

Classically, ventilation alternates with cardiac compression in the ratio of 1:5.

**External (closed-chest) cardiac compression.**—Compression is applied through the heel of one hand which is placed over the lower half of the sternum while the operator's other hand rests on the top of the hand directly on the chest. No force is transmitted through the fingers so that compression of the lateral part of the thorax, which produces rib fractures, is avoided. In an adult the sternum is depressed for 4–6 cm towards the spine—this requires a force of 50–70 lb (23–32 kg) and it is necessary for the operator to be well above the patient, kneeling on the bed if necessary, so as to use his body weight rather than the arm muscles alone, which is both fatiguing and ineffective. The cardiac output produced is less than normal. Cardiac compression should be applied at a rate of around 60 per minute, allowing for ventilatory pauses. The *quality* of sternal compression is important, and an equal time should be allowed for compression and relaxation in order to produce optimal flows.

Taylor and his colleagues[2] made detailed studies on eight patients during cardiopulmonary resuscitation in which they were able to alter independently, the compression rate and compression duration (expressed as a percentage of the cycle time), while measuring relative changes in forward flow. At a constant compression duration, alterations in compression rate between 40 and 80 beats per minute caused no variation in forward flow. This was in marked contrast to the effect observed when compression duration was increased whilst maintaining compression rate constant. Here, each increase in compression duration resulted in an increase in forward flow and a smaller parallel increase in mean arterial pressure. It would appear that whereas in the normally beating heart peak forward flow occurs early in systole and then falls off rapidly, during a prolonged cardiac compression, flow continues perhaps due to delayed opening of poorly perfused capillary vascular beds (in patients who have already received large doses of vasoconstrictor), or to alterations in venous pressure during the compression cycle. The implication is straightforward, chest compression should be delivered at 60/min with at least half of each cycle spent in systole. In order to perform massage correctly, a pause should be made at maximal compression and quick punching compressions should be avoided.

In children compression is with one hand only, producing proportionately less sternal displacement, and is at a faster rate. In babies the whole chest may be grasped with one hand and the sternum displaced with the thumb while the fingers support the spine.

To be effective, external cardiac compression must produce a palpable pulse in the carotid or femoral artery. In cases where a direct arterial pressure recording is possible systolic pressures of 100 mm Hg (13·3 kPa) are commonly seen during massage, although of course this near normal pressure does not signify a near normal cardiac output. Mean arterial pressure is a better indication of flow than systolic pressure.

External cardiac massage is briefly interrupted after every fifth compression to allow ventilation to be performed. When working single-handed, a ratio of two inflations to fifteen compressions is easier.

The exact technique of cardiac compression which produces the optimum output is unfortunately only learnt with experience. Too quick a compression while producing a good systolic pressure results in little forward flow, too slow a compression results in a low systolic pressure and too slow a rate, thus producing a low output. Practice on a "Ressussi-anne" or similar manikin with an experienced teacher is invaluable.

### "New" Cardiopulmonary Resuscitation

Recent studies have shown that the raised intrathoracic pressure produced by sternal compression can, itself, enhance forward blood flow, and that this mechanism may hold equal importance to the compression of the heart against the spine.[3] The increase in intrathoracic pressure is transmitted to all the vascular structures within the thorax, and this is transmitted in turn to the extrathoracic arteries. However, the rise in extrathoracic *venous* pressure is limited by valves and the collapse of the veins at the thoracic inlets, so that a pressure gradient is set up between the extrathoracic arteries and veins, encouraging anterograde flow. Relaxation of compression lowers intrathoracic venous pressure and venous return. This mechanism has led to a new approach in cardiopulmonary resuscitation, namely the simultaneous application of positive-pressure ventilation with sternal compression, to raise the intrathoracic pressure even more. "New CPR" has been demonstrated to provide significant increases in mean systolic artery pressure and carotid flow.[4] This apparent improvement in technique may not, however, reflect an improvement in cerebral perfusion, as carotid blood flow does not necessarily equate with cerebral blood flow. Furthermore, a raised intrathoracic pressure may also increase intracranial pressure thus minimising any improvement in cerebral perfusion caused by an increase in carotid flow.[5]

Until investigations have yielded the true value in terms of patient survival and neurological recovery using "new CPR", it is probably wiser to adopt the standard technique of alternating IPPV with properly administered compression. It would also appear possible that simultaneous compression-ventilation under less than ideal conditions in relatively inexperienced hands could lead to complications associated with inappropriate gas-exchange, pulmonary baro-trauma and actual impairment of cerebral perfusion.

### Internal Cardiac Massage

External cardiac compression has replaced internal cardiac massage in the majority of cases of cardiopulmonary arrest. There are, however, certain indications for the internal, rather than external, technique:

(*a*) if the chest is already opened during surgery;
(*b*) following cardiac surgery, when the presence of intrathoracic pathology must be excluded (e.g. cardiac tamponade, compression of aortocoronary grafts);
(*c*) abnormalities of the chest wall which prevent effective external compression;
(*d*) associated problems that themselves require thoracotomy, e.g. trauma, tension pneumothorax, haemorrhage.

Unless there is a surgical wound that can be re-opened, an incision is made in the fourth left interspace lateral to the internal mammary artery and the space pulled open with the hands. In the absence of a rib spreader an anaesthetic mouth gag can be used. After the pericardium has been incised, the heart is compressed between two hands or, failing this, with the flat of one hand behind the heart and the thumb and thenar eminence in front, taking care not to perforate the chambers with the fingers.

The comparative efficiencies of internal versus external cardiac massage can only be considered in the light of the presenting clinical situation. In general an adequate circulation can usually be achieved using external massage without the disadvantages associated with a thoracotomy performed under difficult circumstances.

### Sedation

Adequate initial resuscitation should, by definition, restore cerebral oxygenation and a return to consciousness. Sedation must be administered at this stage in order to obtund patient awareness during a frightening and unpleasant procedure. Intravenous diazepam is satisfactory and, in sensible doses (10–30 mg), is unlikely to have adverse cardiovascular effects.

## PHASE 2: RESTORATION OF CARDIAC FUNCTION

In cases of transient circulatory arrest such as Stokes-Adams attacks, or dysrhythmias associated with myocardial infarction, the prompt institution of external cardiac compression and artificial ventilation may result in the return of an effective spontaneous heart beat. In a coronary care unit with the patient already connected to an ECG, it may be possible to have one attempt at defibrillation as a first manoeuvre if this is within seconds of the arrest.

If the circulation is not restored immediately, definitive therapy is required as an emergency because the chances of success diminish as time passes.

*Cardiac massage and IPPV are continued whilst:*

1. Access to the circulation via a suitable vein is secured. This is essential for the administration of therapeutic agents and is best performed by internal or external jugular venous cannulation (see p. 477), which is usually easy in the presence of venous distension. Cannulation of a peripheral vein is less satisfactory as there is a delay in onset of action following drug administration.
2. An ECG is applied for the diagnosis of cardiac rhythm.
3. Other equipment (defibrillator, drug trolley and suction apparatus) is prepared by separate personnel.
4. Arterial blood is withdrawn for estimation of acid-base status and for serum electrolytes, especially potassium. Femoral artery cannulation can be performed for pressure monitoring and further sampling.

At this diagnostic stage of cardiopulmonary resuscitation the following questions should be considered:

—is the patient severely hypothermic?
—is there concealed haemorrhage?
—is there a tension pneumothorax?
—is the patient a diabetic?
—is there evidence for a cerebrovascular accident?
—was the arrest drug-induced?
—is the resuscitation justified?

The continuation of cardiac massage and IPPV are mandatory if there is no palpable carotid or general pulsation, regardless of the ECG appearance. Interruption of resuscitation for diagnostic purposes is inevitable, but these periods should be kept as short as possible and for no longer than a few seconds.

### Drug Therapy

1. **Correction of metabolic acidosis.**—The circulatory stagnation of cardiac arrest always leads to metabolic acidosis and this may be so severe that it not only depresses myocardial contractility, but also reduces the action of catecholamines, lowers the ventricular fibrillation threshold and impairs the restoration of a normal beat. In an intensive or coronary care unit where cardiac arrest may be treated within thirty seconds and a normal circulation is quickly restored no alkalinising agent may be required, but generally an initial dose of 1–2 mmol/kg body weight of sodium bicarbonate is necessary. Thereafter the correction of metabolic acidosis is best controlled by serial estimations of the acid-base state of the arterial blood bearing in mind that the fluid compartment accessible for correction under the conditions of cardiac massage may be quite small. Excessive administration of sodium bicarbonate besides leading to an alkalosis which may itself depress the heart, leads to large shifts in potassium so that the patient may become severely hypokalaemic. The fluid and sodium load may also contribute to the development of pulmonary oedema and may accentuate the development of a hyperosmolar state if 8·4 per cent bicarbonate is used. Further bicarbonate generates carbon dioxide in the body and the pH is only corrected once this is eliminated, hence good ventilation is as important as bicarbonate in the correction of metabolic acidosis. Once a normal beat is restored and the tissues become re-perfused, a much larger acidosis is revealed which may often require further correction.

2. **Inotropic drugs.**—Inotropic drugs may be required:

(*a*) in asystole in order to provoke ventricular contraction;
(*b*) to improve myocardial contractility;
(*c*) for their chronotropic action in bradycardia or heart-block;
(*d*) to improve myocardial tone before defibrillation in feeble ventricular fibrillation.

The two inotropes most frequently employed in cardiopulmonary resuscitation are calcium and adrenaline. The latter is given via a central vein in a dose of 1 mg (10 ml of 1:10,000 solution). Repeated injections may be necessary before the required effect is produced. Occasionally, after the cardiac output is restored, hypertension and tachydysrhythmias persist as a result of over-enthusiastic adrenaline therapy. These usually subside fairly quickly, but sometimes vasodilators and antidysrhythmic agents are needed (Fig. 1).

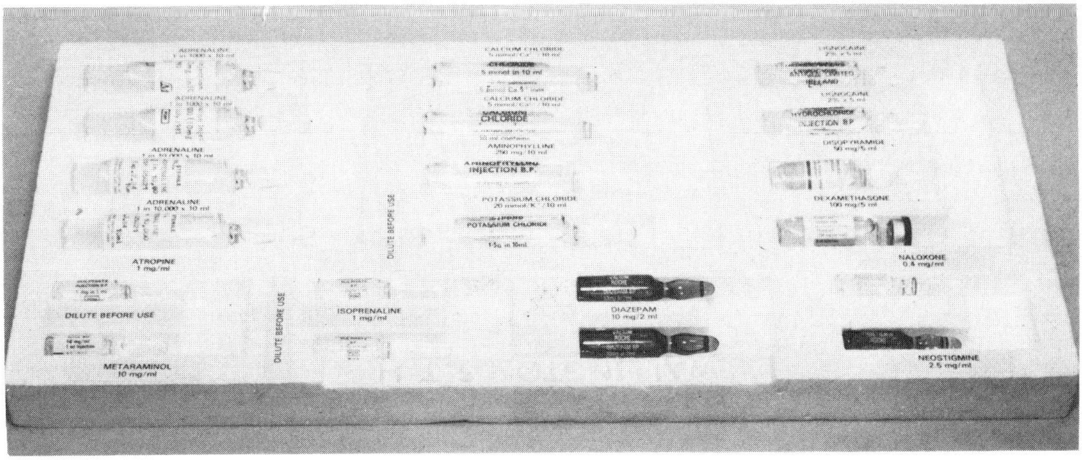


14/Fig. 1.—Polystyrene tray containing drugs, in a readily accessible fashion, which are likely to be needed during cardiopulmonary resuscitation. The used tray is replaced immediately after use, and there is an alternative drug-tray for paediatric use. (Tray designed by P. Wallington, Cardiac Arrest Technician, St. Thomas' Hospital.)

Calcium is given as an intravenous injection in doses of up to 1 g (9 mmol), but with caution if the arrest is thought to be hypokalaemic in origin. Adrenaline will produce intense veno- and arteriolar constriction and, although this tends to distribute blood flow to the cerebral and coronary arteries, ventricular filling pressures may become too high. However, until a spontaneous rhythm and cardiac output is produced, vasodilators are not indicated. In this context, isoprenaline may be positively harmful. Vasoconstrictors *per se* (methoxamine, metaraminol), should not be used unless the arrest was due to hypotension, secondary to massive arteriolar dilatation. The catecholamines may have little effect in the beta-blocked, arrested patient; glucagon (1–10 mg) improves myocardial performance under these circumstances, the effect of which is enhanced by aminophylline (see p. 432).

3. **Treatment of asystole.**—Asystole will usually respond to effective cardiac massage and ventilation together with correction of the acidosis and the administration of inotropic drugs. In cases of complete heart block or refractory bradycardia which do not respond to chronotropes, it may be necessary to resort to electrical pacing. Emergency ventricular pacing can be performed using a transvenous pacing catheter inserted via a subclavian or jugular vein into the right ventricle. Recently, transoesophageal pacing has been re-appraised (see p. 493).

4. **Treatment of ventricular dysrhythmias.**—Ventricular fibrillation may be present as the initial form of circulatory arrest or it may arise during the emergency treatment. Spontaneous defibrillation with the development of a normal beat may follow the initial external cardiac compression but more commonly defibrillation is required with a direct current machine once the myocardial tone has been improved with adequate oxygenation by good massage, drug therapy and the correction of acid-base and electrolyte abnormalities. The two electrode paddles are positioned so that the heart lies between them. One is placed over the apex, and it is convenient if the other can be placed under the right scapula as it can be left there during cardiac compression.

Direct current defibrillation through the closed chest requires an energy release of between 200–400 joules (50–200 joules in children). For direct defibrillation of the exposed heart 20–50 joules may be required according to the size of the heart.

Antidysrhythmic drugs are usually needed. Lignocaine (1 mg/kg) should be administered intravenously before defibrillation and further doses may be needed if this manoeuvre fails. Recurrent dysrhythmias are frequently a problem, and an infusion of lignocaine 1 mg/min is a sensible precaution. In intractable ventricular fibrillation or tachycardia, alternative drugs should be considered (see p. 435 *et seq.*). Quinidine or procainamide are rarely used and can be associated with myocardial depression. Beta-blockers in moderate doses can also depress myocardial contractility but are sometimes necessary when other antidysrhythmic drugs fail, and practolol (1–2 mg increments) is preferable to propranolol as it exhibits less negative inotropism. Disopyramide (25–100 mg) is a useful alternative to beta-blockers but, unlike lignocaine, may cause a reduction in conduction or contractility.

Two other factors must be taken into account. Firstly, in cardiac patients or patients with *electrolyte imbalance*, disturbances of serum potassium may cause cardiac arrest, and defibrillation may not be possible until this has returned to normal. Hypokalaemia is easily treated with intravenous potassium. The effects of hyperkalaemia can be partially antagonised by administration of $CaCl_2$, or the level of serum potassium may be reduced by increasing the cellular uptake of $K+$ either by giving glucose and insulin intravenously (100 ml 50 per cent dextrose with 12·5 units soluble insulin) or by bicarbonate administration and hyperventilation, while cardiac massage is continued. Even in the absence of electrolyte imbalance, calcium is frequently used to increase the tone of the myocardium prior to defibrillation and acid base derangement will itself enhance the dysrhythmia potential independent of its effects on potassium flux.

Secondly, *severe hypothermia* will prevent a return to normal rhythm. This problem may be encountered in cases of drowning, exposure or in the elderly, and resuscitation cannot be deemed to have failed until the core temperature is restored by active rewarming.

5. **"Cerebral prophylaxis."**—Dexamethasone (0·5–1 mg/kg) offers some protection against the effects of cerebral hypoxia, and should probably be administered to all cases early in the resuscitation procedure.

## PHASE 3: AFTER TREATMENT

Initial resuscitation can be considered successful if the patient is able to maintain a viable cardiac output, albeit with inotropic support and controlled ventilation. Further management depends on the consideration of the following:

1. **Inotropic support.**—Catecholamine administration via a central vein may need to be continued. Those with vasodilator properties (isoprenaline, low-dose dopamine) are, in principle, more suitable as they tend to encourage forward flow and tissue perfusion. Not infrequently cardiac output is dependent upon more powerful inotropes, such as adrenaline, and these may cause the intense vasoconstriction to persist.

2. **Intermittent positive-pressure ventilation.**—Ventilation is often inadequate following cardiopulmonary resuscitation due to ventilation perfusion abnormalities (made worse by a low output), pulmonary oedema, trauma and cerebral depression. IPPV would be expected to reduce cardiac output, but this is more than offset by the improvement in arterial oxygenation, control of the $Pa{CO_2}$ and the elimination of the work of breathing.

3. **Antidysrhythmic therapy.**—If the arrest was associated with gross ventricular dysrhythmias, an infusion of lignocaine should be continued for some hours.[3] An infusion rate of 1 mg/min may be insufficient to maintain therapeutic plasma concentrations in those patients with a good cardiac output (see p. 436) and a sequential regime should be adopted.

4. **Sedation.**—This is essential for the conscious patient who requires IPPV; fear, pain, stress and difficulty with ventilator synchronisation will tend to predispose towards catecholamine-induced tachydysrhythmias and vasoconstriction. Diazepam is satisfactory and may need to be combined with an opiate such as morphine.

5. **Renal function.**—Prolonged low cardiac output, hypotension, vasoconstriction and acidosis predispose towards acute renal damage. These factors should be eliminated during the period following the arrest and renal function should return. A continued low urinary output is an indication for urgent treatment and strenuous efforts made to improve renal blood flow and to encourage a diuresis with frusemide. Dopamine, in low to moderate doses, enhances cardiac output and has specific renal vasodilating and natriuretic effects. Osmotic diuretics, such as mannitol, should be used with caution if the ventricular filling pressure is high.

6. **Cerebral salvage.**—Hypoxic cerebral damage may follow a cardiac arrest despite an apparently successful resuscitation. It is vital in these cases to minimise the oedematous response to the ischaemic insult in order to

avoid a further rise in intracranial pressure and reduction in cerebral perfusion.

### Management of Cerebral Ischaemic Damage

(*a*) *Arterial pressure.*—This should be maintained where possible at near normal levels. Hypotension lowers cerebral perfusion pressure and hypertension may increase intracranial pressure.

(*b*) *Posture.*—A slight head-up tilt lowers cerebral venous pressure and reduces intracranial pressure.

(*c*) $Paco_2$.—Mild hypocarbia (around 30 mm Hg) reduces intracranial pressure by a vasoconstrictor effect on cerebral vessels. However, in the presence of hypotension, hypocarbia can cause inadequate cerebral perfusion.[6]

(*d*) *Diuretics.*—Overhydration aggravates cerebral oedema and a moderate diuresis is desirable. Following a cardiac arrest, maintenance of optimal filling pressures may be difficult if either a massive diuresis is induced, or a hyperosmotic circulatory load is imposed with agents such as mannitol. The latter may reduce cerebral oedema partly by its osmotic effect on the brain and is suitable for use in the presence of an adequate cardiac output.

(*e*) *"Specific" drugs.*—

(i) *Steroids* have been shown to modify cerebral oedema following an ischaemic insult.[7] Classically, dexamethasone (0·5–1 mg/kg) is given initially, followed by 4–8 mg 6-hourly, but methylprednisolone may prove to be as effective.

(ii) *Barbiturate therapy.*—The efficacy of barbiturates in enhancing neurological recovery after cerebral hypoxia is controversial. There is some evidence that barbiturates, if given early and in suitable dosage may, in combination with the other measures discussed, offer cerebral protection against the secondary events that follow an anoxic episode.[8] The postulated mechanism of action of the barbiturates are

- anaesthesia, preventing intracranial pressure rises associated with endotracheal suction and other manoeuvres;
- reduction in cerebral metabolism and brain oxygen requirements;
- free-radical scavenging preventing lipid peroxidation;
- anticonvulsant activity;
- direct reduction in intracranial pressure.

Thiopentone is a convenient drug to use. Following cardiac arrest, therapeutic blood levels may lead to inappropriate cardiovascular depression, so barbiturate therapy, in this context, may be limited. Ideally, dosage should be adjusted to give an isoelectric EEG, but this is not always feasible. Approximate thiopentone dosages are, a loading dose of 25–50 mg/kg followed by an infusion of 2–10 mg/kg/hour, to give plasma concentrations of 10–50 mg/l. Accumulation occurs and recovery may be prolonged over a period of days before neurological assessment can be made.

### Comment

All too often, cardiac arrest is the end-result of a derangement of physiology which has been either unnoticed or untreated for some time. It is much better to prevent a cardiac arrest than to treat it, however effectively.

Also, the treatment defined above covers only the essential practical details of resuscitation. Resuscitation will often be ineffective if the precipitating cause is not recognised and treated. It requires a calm logical mind with a good understanding of medicine to sort out and treat the underlying condition while at the same time performing emergency resuscitation.

However, accepting that cardiac emergencies may arise suddenly, the successful treatment must depend to some extent on the provision of proper facilities and the adequate training of personnel.

Basic resuscitation kits should be kept available in all wards and departments of the hospital. There should be a well-rehearsed plan of action so that no time is wasted on inessential manoeuvres. The ultimate result for a patient will depend on the brevity of the interval between cardiac arrest and the restoration of an effective circulation, and every anaesthetist should know what can and what should be done in that period.

## POST-OPERATIVE VENOUS THROMBOSIS AND PULMONARY EMBOLISM

There has been a continuous absolute increase in deaths from pulmonary embolus since 1943 and, for example, in 1975 an estimated 21,000 patients died annually in the United Kingdom from this cause.[9] Of those patients 60 per cent might have been expected to return to normal life had it not been for their embolus.[10]

## Deep Vein Thrombosis

**Aetiology.**—The actual "trigger" mechanism of deep vein thrombosis is unknown. The thrombosis starts as a small area of platelet deposition within a valve cusp and then propagates. Although the calf is the commonest site of thrombosis, it can begin in any part of the peripheral venous system and may develop in more than one site simultaneously.[11]

Deep vein thrombosis is associated with bedrest, major surgical procedures, cerebrovascular accidents and malignancy. The middle-aged and elderly are more at risk than the young, although the use of the contraceptive pill is tending to change this distribution. Chest, abdomen and hip operations have a greater incidence than head, neck and breast surgery.

Anaesthesia and operation are conducive to venous stasis. Certain positions on the operating table and some anaesthetic techniques favour venous pooling. The removal of all skeletal muscle tone and the direct effects of surgical trauma—as in pelvic operations—are normal accompaniments of many operations. These may be accentuated by oligaemia and by changes in coagulability which occur in the postoperative period.

Deep venous thrombosis may start at the time of operation or in the first 24–48 hours after surgery but if the predisposing factors existed pre-operatively, the thrombotic process may already have been established by the time the patient comes to surgery. Pulmonary embolism may then be precipitated when the femur is manipulated or an Esmarch tourniquet applied.

**Diagnosis.**—The diagnosis is often not obvious, an estimated 70 per cent of deep vein thromboses having neither signs or symptoms. The most reliable sign when it occurs is ankle oedema; less reliable but much commoner are tenderness of the calf accompanied perhaps by an increase in calf diameter or a slight rise in temperature. Early diagnosis depends on a suspicious mind in the doctor.

The Doppler ultrasound technique, which has the merits of simplicity and cheapness, is accurate in diagnosing occlusive thrombosis above the knee. It cannot detect thrombosis in the calf veins which may be diagnosed using $^{125}I$-labelled fibrinogen uptake. More recently labelled platelet-scanning has been introduced to detect small thrombi after they have developed. Fortunately, calf vein thrombosis, although commonest, seldom gives rise to pulmonary embolism. Ultimate definition of the thrombus is obtained by phlebography which in the long run gives the most reliable and diagnostic information about deep vein thrombosis.

**Prophylaxis.**—The best treatment for deep vein thrombosis is obviously prophylactic, and there are two main approaches—prevention of stasis and alteration of blood coagulability.

*Prevention of stasis.*—This can be passive—elastic stockings and elevation of the leg—or active. The evidence that passive measures are effective is only marginal. The active measures include regular electrical stimulation of the calf muscle, mechanical movement of the feet and intermittent pneumatic compression of the calf muscles. These measures produce benefit except in high-risk patients and there are logistic difficulties about applying them in the postoperative period.

*Alteration in blood coagulability.*—The most popular and effective methods are small-dose heparin and intravenous dextran-70. Infusion of dextran-70 reduces the incidence of deep venous thrombosis compared with control patients undergoing general surgery but not to the same extent as heparin.[12] Normally, 500 ml dextran-70 is given at the time of operation followed by 500 ml in the next 24 hours. This dose should not give rise to circulatory overload unless administered too quickly in a susceptible patient. The other important complication of dextran is the development of a dextran-induced anaphylactoid reaction. The incidence of this complication, which can occur in anaesthetised or unanaesthetised patients is put at 0·07 per cent, based on the number of units infused.[13] The reaction may range in severity from mild skin manifestations, through mild to moderate hypotension, gastro-intestinal disturbance and respiratory distress to the severest form of bronchospasm, respiratory arrest, severe hypotension and even cardiac arrest. The earlier the reactions occur in the administration, the more severe they are likely to be.[14]

Low-dose subcutaneous heparin is undoubtedly effective in reducing the incidence of calf vein thrombosis detectable by $^{125}$I-labelled fibrinogen uptake. Several dose schedules are recommended, the commonest being 5,000 units twice daily for one week, starting two hours before operation. This 12-hourly regimen will have a lower incidence of bleeding complications, but a higher failure rate than heparin given 8-hourly.[15] Because of the variability of effect of heparin in individual patients this schedule may be ineffective in some patients, particularly those undergoing hip operations, but may give rise to bleeding problems in others. Up to 1974, subcutaneous heparin had been shown to reduce the frequency of calf vein thrombosis, but no study had shown that it also reduced the incidence of pulmonary embolism. The results of the International Multicentre Trial[16] showed low-dose heparin to be effective in preventing fatal postoperative pulmonary embolism, and subsequent re-analysis of the data, in the light of certain criticisms, supported this conclusion.[17] In a further multicentre trial, Gruber and his colleagues[18] compared the incidence of fatal postoperative pulmonary embolism after prophylaxis with dextran-70 and low-dose heparin and showed no statistically significant difference between the two treatment groups after a full course of prophylaxis. Doubts about the true value of low-dose heparin continue to be expressed, however, and in their preliminary results, Immelman and colleagues[19] could not substantiate the value of heparin and thought its routine use in patients aged over 40 not necessarily advisable.

### Treatment of Simple Deep Vein Thrombosis

Once diagnosed, the treatment is with anticoagulants. Intravenous heparin is given either as 6,000 units 4-hourly or as a continuous infusion giving 40,000 units over 24 hours. At the same time oral warfarin or phenindione is started. The heparin is usually discontinued after 2–3 days but continued for 5–6 days if there is a pulmonary embolus. Oral anticoagulants are continued for at least 3 months with the blood prothrombin time increased two or threefold.

Surgical removal of vein clot in the upper femoral or iliac vein is only successful if there is recent non-adherent clot. Thrombus may be prevented from embolising to the lungs by plication of the inferior vena cava or iliac vein, or ligation of the femoral vein below the profunda, which may be indicated if anticoagulation fails to prevent recurrent pulmonary embolism and if phlebography reveals a large, loose, life-threatening thrombus.

### Pulmonary Embolism

The common sites of origin for a pulmonary embolism are the veins of the pelvis and lower extremities—small emboli arising from the calves while large emboli come from the ilio-femoral venous segment. In cardiac disease thrombi may originate on the right side of the heart. The total incidence of pulmonary embolism is very high—in unselected post-mortem examinations as many as 70 per cent of cases can be shown to have some degree of pulmonary emboli—but the incidence of clinically detectable pulmonary embolism in post-operative patients is probably less than 1 per cent. This incidence is of course much higher in groups of patients particularly at risk, notably those with a previous history of thrombo-embolism and those undergoing orthopaedic operations or splenectomy.

The common time of occurrence is some days—3 to 21—after an operation, but this depends on the patient being fit and well previously. If the predisposing factors have existed for some time pre-operatively the time scale is shifted—the embolism may even occur at the time of operation. Fractured neck of femur followed by late reduction in an elderly patient—a situation full of predisposing factors—may well result in a pulmonary embolus at the time of reduction.

**Diagnosis.**—sudden pleuritic pain in the chest and dyspnoea are the classical symptoms, and if the blood clot is large enough to obstruct the pulmonary arterial circulation materially, death may rapidly follow from acute cor pulmonale. Smaller degrees of obstruction produce a less catastrophic picture but evidence of right ventricular failure—dyspnoea, tachycardia, venous engorgement, hypotension—may be present to some degree. The ECG may show right ventricular strain and the chest x-ray may show "pruning" of the affected pulmonary vessels, consolidation, elevation of the diaphragm or pleural effusion. Chest x-ray is rarely diagnostic and a lung scan may be more helpful. Pulmonary angiography is the definitive diagnostic test, but is not without its own inherent dangers (*vide infra*).

Small emboli usually cause little more than pain and dyspnoea in the first place, but these symptoms may be followed after twenty-four hours by haemoptysis, fever, and signs of pulmonary infarction. The ultimate circulatory result of a simple pulmonary embolus in a given patient is influenced partly by the size of the embolus and partly by the preceding state of the patient's heart and pulmonary vasculature—thus some patients may survive a single large pulmonary embolism, while others die from the effects of repeated small ones.

### Treatment of Deep Vein Thrombosis with Pulmonary Embolism

As with simple deep vein thrombosis the initial treatment is with heparin. A phlebogram is performed to define the thrombi. If the thrombus appears old and well fixed, long-term anticoagulation is the only treatment necessary; if however the clot appears fresh and loose and is thought likely to cause further emboli then more radical treatment is required. Thrombectomy is possible for thrombi lying in the major vessels, but where the smaller vessels, such as the calf veins, are affected, then either peripheral vein ligation or streptokinase therapy are indicated, although recent surgery may prohibit the latter. Thrombectomy or peripheral vein ligation may be performed under general anaesthesia when the anaesthetist may be called upon to perform a Valsalva manoeuvre to reverse the flow in the inferior vena cava at the moment the vein is opened. The anaesthetist should also remember that positioning on the table, perhaps even the muscle fasciculations of succinylcholine, may precipitate a further larger pulmonary embolus during anaesthesia and careful monitoring of the patient is necessary despite the apparent simplicity of the surgical procedure.

### Treatment of Pulmonary Embolism

Patients with small pulmonary emboli are treated with anticoagulants and the deep vein thrombosis considered separately for special treatment as defined above. The difficulty in choice of treatment lies in those patients who have had major pulmonary emboli but who are not so ill as to require immediate pulmonary embolectomy. These are probably best investigated with a pulmonary angiogram and then treated with streptokinase. An improvement in haemodynamic status may not be seen for many hours, so that streptokinase therapy is inappropriate in patients whose circulation is severely compromised by pulmonary embolism.[20] Streptokinase may also produce haemorrhage, especially in the immediate post-operative period. Routine phlebography should always follow a pulmonary embolism to identify, and treat, the patient who remains at risk of a further, possibly fatal, embolism.

## MAJOR PULMONARY EMBOLISM

In major pulmonary embolism, a single large embolus may obstruct the main pulmonary artery, or several slightly smaller emboli may obstruct all but one of the major arterial subdivisions, leading to an acute restriction in right ventricular output and a resultant left ventricular hypovolaemia. Thus major pulmonary embolism results in acute circulatory failure (hypotension, tachycardia, acidosis and oliguria) associated with hypoxia. Initially, left ventricular contractility is maintained, the cardiac output being determined by left ventricular filling pressure, but eventually left ventricular failure ensues in the face of persistent hypotension and hypoxia. The right ventricle fails as its afterload is increased, and its function is very dependent upon an adequate right ventricular filling pressure, so that venodilatation must be avoided. Sometimes an infusion of plasma may enhance right ventricular performance, but if the right ventricle has become over-distended a volume load will not improve output and is likely to further compromise its function.

The acute circulatory management in major pulmonary embolism is therefore:

1. Administration of oxygen in an attempt to minimise hypoxia.
2. Maintenance of an adequate right ventricular filling pressure and the avoidance of venodilating drugs.
3. Improvement in right ventricular contractility with inotropes. Adrenaline is useful as it tends to maintain systemic vascular resistance in the presence of a low cardiac output, unlike isoprenaline which may, due to vasodilatation, cause hypotension. Dopamine and calcium are useful alter-

natives, but digoxin in the acute situation is of little use and may provoke dangerous dysrhythmias.

4. Correction of acidosis and measures to preserve renal and cerebral integrity.

Urgent pulmonary angiography is usually indicated (Fig. 2), but is often performed on a desperately ill patient in difficult circumstances. It causes a further deterioration in the haemodynamics due to the adverse vasodilating effects of the contrast media, so there is a good case for performing this in, or near, the prepared operating room. Cardiac arrest should be managed by closed cardiac massage and IPPV and urgent pulmonary embolectomy performed.

### Pulmonary Embolectomy

The type of operation is dictated by the urgency of the situation and the facilities available. There are two main approaches:

(i) *In-flow occlusion arrest*.—The chest is opened, and the vena cavae clamped. The pulmonary artery is rapidly opened under relatively avascular conditions and the thrombus removed. This requires a high degree of surgical competence as the time taken to perform the embolectomy and to secure the pulmonary arteriotomy, determines the duration of cerebral ischaemia in an already hypoxic patient. The anaesthetist is asked to time the periods of circulatory arrest, and heavy demands are made upon him to correct the circulatory chaos and to minimise the cerebral damage.

(ii) *Pulmonary embolectomy using extracorporeal circulation*.—Cerebral perfusion and adequate oxygenation can be maintained on cardiopulmonary bypass, which can be established either by a formal median sternotomy with aortic and right atrial cannulation, or by femoro-femoral bypass. The femoral vessels can be cannulated if necessary under local anaesthesia before thoracotomy, or during cardiopulmonary resuscitation. Pulmonary embolectomy is performed through the pulmonary arteriotomy using forceps or a sucker, and quite considerable amounts of thrombus are often removed. A timely inflation of the lungs will often dislodge peripheral clots into more proximal vessels.

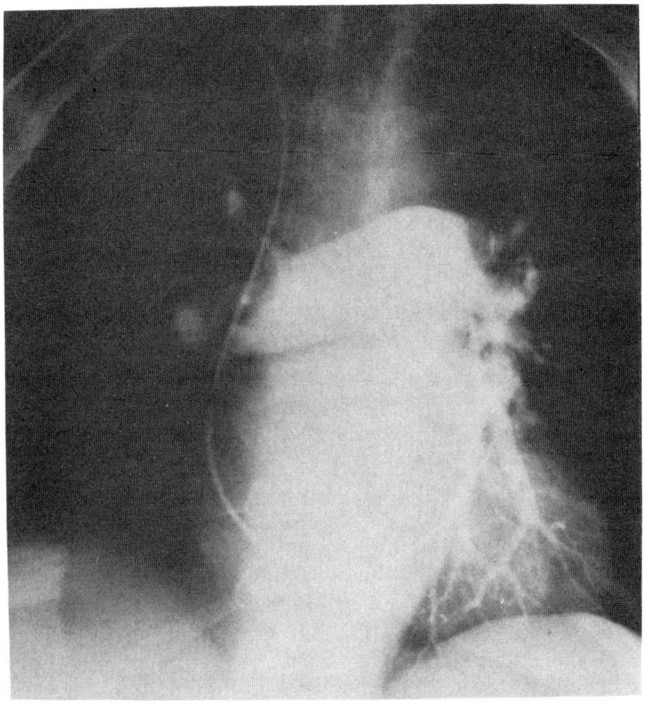

14/Fig. 2.—Pulmonary angiogram in major pulmonary embolism. The radio-opaque cannula has been inserted from an arm vein into the main pulmonary artery. The injected contrast fails to fill all but the left lower lobe vessels. (Photograph supplied by Dr. M. Webb-Peploe, St. Thomas' Hospital.)

### Anaesthetic Management for Pulmonary Embolectomy

A thorough understanding of the haemodynamic implications of pulmonary embolus will dictate the anaesthetic management, so that inotropic and vasoconstrictor drugs must be available, together with heparin and full resuscitation equipment. Access to the circulation for monitoring and intravenous therapy should be rapidly established under local anaesthesia before induction, and an ECG applied. Induction agents should not include cyclopropane (which dramatically increases pulmonary vascular resistance), the opiates, droperidol or thiopentone (which have variable vasodilating effects) or myocardial depressants such as halothane or enflurane. Pre-oxygenation followed by intravenous diazepam (10–30 mg) and pancuronium (8–12 mg) produce satisfactory and relatively stable conditions for asleep intubation. The institution of IPPV (with 100 per cent oxygen) unfortunately increases right ventricular afterload even more, so that a profound fall in arterial pressure may ensue. Vasoconstriction and inotropic therapy may temporarily improve the situation, but cardiac arrest may precede the institution of cardiopulmonary bypass. There is therefore a good case, in severe circulatory collapse, for establishing femoral cannulae under local anaesthesia and for "painting up" and towelling the patient before intubation is performed.

Following the embolectomy, right ventricular function may be inadequate either because overdistension has damaged the ventricle or because the pulmonary vascular resistance remains high. The latter seems to be a chemical response to the original insult and may, in part, be reduced by pulmonary vasodilators. Inotropic therapy may therefore be required, and efforts should also be made to restore cerebral and renal function and to correct an acidosis. Some centres routinely give large doses of dexamethasone for cerebral protection before severe hypotension occurs, and occasionally other forms of cerebral salvage may be necessary. For these and other reasons a prolonged period of support may be required postoperatively.

When cardiac output is satisfactory an effort must be made to deepen anaesthesia and nitrous oxide with suitable adjuvants may be administered.

## OTHER EMBOLIC PHENOMENA

Embolus translated literally means a plug. Various substances other than thrombus may be carried along in the blood stream until they ultimately obstruct one or more blood vessels but those of particular interest are fat, air, tumour, and amniotic fluid.

### Fat Embolism

This usually follows fracture of a bone—typically a long bone or rib—or rupture of the liver or kidney. It may result from an operative procedure on a bone and rarely may follow sudden decompression in a deep-sea diver or high-altitude flier. The origin of the fat is generally considered to be the fat at the site of trauma. Hallgren and his colleagues[21] showed that emboli recovered from the lungs of dogs with fractured legs have a similar triglyceride composition to bone marrow and depot fat but dissimilar to the normal chylomicron fat found in suspension in the blood.

Pulmonary fat embolism is very common after injury and is believed to be almost universal after fracture of a marrow bone. Fat emboli may be released during surgical procedures involving bone, and has been observed in non-orthopaedic operations such as median sternotomy in open-heart surgery. Clinically fat embolism can be divided into three groups; first the fulminating case, secondly the classical syndrome with cerebral, neurological and respiratory symptoms, and thirdly the incomplete or partial case. *A fulminating embolus* may occur within a few hours or days of a severe traumatic injury and is generally only diagnosed when the brain is sectioned after a post-mortem. Fat embolism may be suspected when the patient fails to respond to adequate resuscitation therapy, and when a period of normal consciousness subsequent to the injury is followed by coma. *The classical syndrome* can be expected to occur suddenly some twenty-four hours after an injury, and is typified by a mixture of mental confusion, often with localising neurological symptoms and signs, respiratory distress with pyrexia, and a petechial rash mainly over the upper chest, shoulders and lower neck. *An incomplete or partial case* is mild in course showing only some of the symptoms of the classical case.

In fracture patients with signs of fat embolism, hypoxaemia is often clinically important. Gurd and Wilson[22] found the arterial oxygen tension below 50 mm Hg (6·7 kPa) in 24 of 50 cases and between 51 and 80 mm Hg (6·8 and 10·7 kPa) in another 17. Studies of other fracture patients with no other evidence of fat embolism frequently reveal subclinical hypoxaemia ($Pa_{O_2}$ circa 70 mm Hg–9·3 kPa), and although other causes such as post-traumatic pulmonary microthrombo-emboli may be responsible, fat embolism as the cause would accord with the high rate of histologically proven lung embolism after fractures.

The diagnosis is usually made on clinical grounds[23] but fat globules may be seen in the retinal vessels or in the urine or sputum. Histological examination of petechiae may demonstrate fat. The discovery of fat globules larger than 10 $\mu$m in diameter in the serum is said to be pathognomonic of fat embolism.

The hypoxaemia following pulmonary fat embolism is due partly to an increase in alveolar dead space and to an increase in pulmonary veno-arterial admixture of between 20 and 50 per cent of the cardiac output.[24] Sevitt[25] has postulated two routes for the fat emboli to gain access to the systemic circulation and thus the brain. Minor systemic embolism may occur by small fat globules passing through the pulmonary capillaries but when there is serious blockage of the pulmonary vascular bed, blood might be diverted via pulmonary-bronchial anastomoses to the left side of the heart without passing through a fine capillary bed.

**Treatment.**—The efficacy of many of the advocated treatments is not proven. The respiratory system should be treated symptomatically which will usually mean a raised inspired oxygen concentration or positive-pressure ventilation. Circulatory support is not often needed provided the hypoxia is eliminated but dysfunction in other organ systems may require the appropriate treatment.

## Air Embolism

The first recorded case of air embolism in the medical literature is that occurring in a French locksmith in 1818.[26] Sporadic reports followed this and Hunter[27] remarked that air embolism as a complication during anaesthesia was not common until the advent of controlled respiration (for neurosurgery in the sitting position). Others[28] have felt that this increase was secondary to the introduction of muscle relaxants and the low venous pressure which followed their use in the upright patient. More recently the true and much larger incidence of air embolism has been revealed in prospective studies[29] and by the use of the Doppler ultrasound device.[30]

Although air embolism has been most commonly described in relation to posterior fossa neurosurgery performed in the sitting position[31] there are a large number of other situations in which it can occur (Table 1). Indeed when one

14/Table 1
The Principal Sources of Air Embolus

| | |
|---|---|
| 1. Surgical —danger increased by low central venous pressure. | Operations involving veins of head, neck, thorax, abdomen, pelvis<br>Heart—particularly open heart operations. |
| 2. Obstetric and Gynaecological | Delivery in presence of placenta praevia<br>Insufflation of fallopian tubes.<br>Criminal abortion.<br>Laparoscopy. |
| 3. Diagnostic | Air encephalogram.<br>Angiocardiography.<br>Air myelography.<br>Venturi ventilation during bronchoscopy. |
| 4. Therapeutic | I.V. therapy.<br>Antral washouts.<br>Pneumothorax.<br>Pneumoperitoneum.<br>IPPV.<br>Transfusion.<br>Monitoring apparatus.<br>Haemodialysis.<br>Extracorporeal circulation. |
| 5. Accidental | Rapid decompression. |

considers how often a low central venous pressure and an open vein must exist, e.g. cervical laminectomy, the surprise is how seldom it actually gives rise to trouble and that there must be other aetiological factors. There is a suggestion that children may be more at risk than adults in some circumstances. Gardner[32] reports 13 cases of gas embolism during diagnostic radiology of which nine occurred in children. Perhaps this is due to the large volume of air used relative to the child's size. Intraperitoneal insufflation with a gas during laparoscopic procedures is now commonly undertaken, and the effects of inadvertent systemic gas embolism is minimised by using carbon dioxide.

**Effects of Air Embolism**

In some cases air enters the arterial system directly—usually during open heart surgery or extracorporeal circulation—and passes to the periphery causing effects according to the vessel entered and the position of the patient at the time. The air causes obstruction to flow in the arterioles and also acts as an endothelial irritant producing segmental arteriolar spasm. In the cerebral vessels air can be found 48 hours after experimental air embolism.

More commonly air enters the venous system. The effect depends partly on the total volume and perhaps more importantly on the rate of entry, although precise quantitation of these factors is lacking. The air bubbles may collect in the right atrium, from where they can often be aspirated, but, depending on the right atrial pressure, the flow rate of blood through it and the position of the patient, may be passed into the right ventricle and be churned up into froth before being ejected into the pulmonary artery. Pulmonary hypertension (with right ventricular strain) develops partly due to mechanical blockage of the pulmonary vessels and partly through a neurogenic effect. The churning action of the foam may lead to fibrin deposits in the pulmonary artery and damage may occur to blood elements at the blood gas interface. The cardiac output and blood pressure fall and dysrhythmias, including ventricular fibrillation, may be precipitated. Respiration is stimulated (becoming laboured) and respiratory efforts may break through controlled ventilation. The large inspiratory pressure swings thus generated may enhance the entrainment of air.

Air will pass from the right side of the heart to the systemic circulation either through the pulmonary vascular bed or across intracardiac defects. Knowledge of an intracardiac defect in a patient demands even more scrupulous care about intravenous therapy than normal. The particular dangers of systemic air are that very small quantities of air entering the coronary arteries can provoke ventricular fibrillation and that air entering the cerebral vessels can produce permanent neurological damage.

The effect of air embolism is aggravated if the patient is receiving nitrous oxide at the time. Nunn[33] was the first to suggest than $N_2O$ which is thirty times more soluble than $N_2$, would diffuse quickly into the bubbles and appreciably increase their size, a complication which may be particularly important when air has reached the systemic circulation. Munson and Merrick[34] have shown experimentally that venous air embolism is more likely to be fatal if nitrous oxide is being administered at the time, and Munson[35] has shown that as the bubbles pass through the pulmonary capillaries very rapid direct gas exchange occurs between the alveolus and the bubble which emphasises the need to *discontinue* the $N_2O$ if air embolism is suspected.

**Monitoring Techniques**

In an anaesthetic situation in which air embolism is an expected complication—such as posterior fossa neurosurgery, careful prospective monitoring using the techniques described below must be undertaken. In less likely situations if a patient suddenly develops hypotension, dysrhythmias, and irregular respirations, the possibility of air embolism should be considered and auscultation of the heart will confirm the diagnosis. Sometimes, of course, the noise of air entering the vein may have been heard.

1. ***Doppler ultrasound technique***

Doppler cardiac auscultation[30] is the most sensitive qualitative method for detecting intravascular air embolism. The receiver is placed over the tricuspid valve and its function confirmed with a small injection of $CO_2$ or the forceful injection of a small quantity of saline. "It is the only diagnostic technique which is not dependent on a pathophysiological alteration in vital functions and thus allows preventative and therapeutic measures to be instituted before cardiorespiratory collapse develops."[36]

The Doppler is not a quantitative instrument, it being impossible to determine the volume of air from the character and loudness of the air artefact, but it will detect very small amounts of air. Thus vanguard bubbles which may herald a larger air embolism may be detected. Electrical interference occurs between the diathermy and the ultrasound device, which is worse with spark gap (rather than valve operated) diathermy, but this is a transient effect and could, if necessary, be excluded.

2. ***Auscultation***

The first effect of air entering the heart is to produce faintly audible transitory high-pitched tinkling sounds; as the volume of air increases the heart sounds become resonant and drum-like. 30 ml of air produces the characteristic harsh mill-wheel murmur which denotes a worse prognosis. These changes are better and earlier appreciated through an oesophageal stethoscope than via a precordial instrument. Michenfelder and associates,[28] writing in 1969 before the use of the Doppler, reported that in 90 per cent of cases the first observed sign was a cardiac murmur.

The oesophageal stethoscope being simple and inexpensive, should be standard practice where air embolism is possible.

3. ***Electrocardiogram***

The ECG changes which follow air embolism are best seen in lead $V_1$ and comprise signs of right heart strain (right bundle-branch block, inverted T waves and tall peaked P waves in the right chest leads) and the development of ventricular dysrhythmias which may lead to ventricular fibrillation. Small amounts of air may, on occasion, produce ECG abnormalities before alterations in heart sounds are noted.

4. ***Cardiovascular monitoring***

(*a*) *Arterial pressure.* A fall in arterial pressure, secondary to a low cardiac output usually accompanied by tachycardia, and best seen on a continuous display of directly measured pressure, is not necessarily the first sign of significant air embolism.

(*b*) *Right atrial line.* A catheter whose tip is in the right atrium[28]—confirmed by radiography or by intracardiac electrocardiography—can be used for therapy (see below) and diagnosis. The two diagnostic signs are that the central venous pressure rises when the right ventricle comes under strain, and it may be possible to aspirate air from the right atrium. The catheter needs to be long enough that it can be advanced into the right ventricle if necessary.

(*c*) *Pulmonary artery pressure.* Marshall and colleagues[37] described the advantages of pulmonary artery cannulation in neurosurgical procedures. An increase in pulmonary artery pressure occurred during significant air embolism often before systemic circulatory changes were observed. Air can also be removed from the right atrium and pulmonary artery through triple-lumen flow-directed catheters.

5. ***End-tidal carbon dioxide***

Pulmonary air embolism results in a sudden fall in alveolar carbon dioxide content due to an increase in alveolar dead space secondary to the development of veno-arterial shunts in the lung and this can be picked up as a sudden diminution in the end-expiratory $CO_2$ content measured with an infra-red rapid $CO_2$ analyser.[38]

Edmonds-Seal and Maroon[39] compared different methods of detecting air embolism and found the ultrasonic method to be the most sensitive, followed by the measurement of end-tidal $CO_2$. Changes in BP, ECG, CVP, and respiratory pattern occurred only after quite large emboli, and the changes in these variables due to small amounts of air may be indistinguishable from those due to alterations in surgical stimulation or level of anaesthesia.

**Prevention.**—There are a number of factors which either encourage or worsen air embolism. Obviously the first is a portal of entry for the air, and in those operations where air embolism is a known hazard, special care must be taken by the surgeon and adequate monitoring with facilities for specific therapy should be available to the anaesthetist.

The next most important factor is a low central venous pressure, and while this applies particularly in respect of head and neck veins while in the upright posture it also applies during such conditions as lacerated liver. The low venous pressure may be caused by posture, haemorrhage, the effect of vasodilator drugs, and perhaps the effects of muscle relaxants. It will be aggravated by violent or obstructed respiratory movements. It has been suggested that the CVP should be maintained at a level which is just less than that which causes troublesome oozing. This may be achieved by infusion of plasma expanders, by the use of an antigravity suit, by the adjustment of the intrathoracic pressure with IPPV, PEEP or CPAP, and local venous congestion can be caused by intermittent compression with an inflatable collar or an intravenous balloon catheter.

The use of air as a contrast medium in radiology should be replaced by a more soluble gas such as carbon dioxide, or perhaps nitrous oxide.

In view of the diffusion of $N_2O$ into air bubbles, with consequent increase in size, this gas should be avoided as part of the anaesthetic technique when the complication is considered likely. At the same time it has to be remembered that the mortality of air embolism is low and that the methods used for its detection and prevention must not introduce a greater hazard of their own.

**Treatment.**—The most important factor in treatment is speedy recognition of the complication. Treatment can be considered under three headings—prevention of entry of more air, removal of the embolised air, and support of the circulation.

(*a*) *Prevention of further entry of air*

The first act is to compress or ligate the open vessel: if it cannot be identified then flooding the wound with saline or packing it with saline-soaked swabs may suffice. Identification of the vessel may be helped, and further air entry prevented, if the central venous or local venous pressure can be raised by altering the posture of the patient, by inflation of a balloon catheter or antigravity suit, by local venous compression, or by raising the intrathoracic pressure using positive pressure applied to the airway.

(*b*) *Support of the circulation*

If the circulation is obviously inadequate, the patient is placed supine and external cardiac massage and IPPV with 100 per cent oxygen are started. Not infrequently these two measures are sufficient to restore a circulation. If not, massage must be continued, vasopressors administered, and acid/base imbalance corrected. Ventricular fibrillation will require electrical defibrillation.

(*c*) *Removal of air*

The classical description is that turning the patient on the left side head down places the right atrium and tricuspid valve above the right ventricle and tends to delay the passage of air into the pulmonary artery. The foam stays uppermost with liquid blood flowing underneath it and the air can be aspirated through the right atrial monitoring catheter which can be advanced into the right ventricle if required. However, the posture of the patient is often dictated by the clinical circumstances, so that if external cardiac massage is required, the supine position is mandatory. With facilities for central venous cannulation, aspiration of air is relatively simple (if incomplete) and in Michenfelder's large series successful aspiration was actually performed with the patient still in the upright position and the table was lowered in only 13 per cent of cases. It is rare for direct aspiration of the heart to be necessary.

The natural absorption of the air is hastened by ventilation of the patient with pure oxygen which reduces the amount of nitrous oxide (and nitrogen) in the blood.

Whole body compression at greater than atmospheric pressures may be valuable to force the gas into solution, particularly in cases of systemic air embolism involving the brain, or when gas bubbles form in the blood following rapid decompression. Calverley and his colleagues[40] discuss this in some detail and describe a technique which employs rapid compression to six ATA. If the patient responds favourably after 10–20 minutes the pressure is reduced to three ATA. At this level 100 per cent oxygen can then be used for progressive decompression over the next few hours.

## Tumour Embolism

Tumour embolism may occur spontaneously or at operation, and, should the pieces of growth be big enough, can obstruct the pulmonary (arterial) or the systemic circulation, depending upon the site of the growth. Sudden death may occur from pulmonary obstruction or obstruction of the outflow tract of the left heart. Probert[41] described a patient who died suddenly during exploration of a carcinoma of the bronchus due to tumour embolism in the pulmonary veins, but a more common cause is that of a hypernephroma invading the inferior vena cava that can embolise during nephrectomy.

## Amniotic Fluid Embolism[42]

This is considered in Chapter 38.

## REFERENCES


1. Camarata, S. J., Weil, M. H., Hanashiro, P. K. and Shubim, H. (1971). Cardiac arrest in the critically ill. A study of predisposing causes in 132 patients. *Circulation*, **44**, 688.
2. Taylor, G. J., Tucker, W. M., Greene, H. L., Rudikoff, M. T. and Weisfeldt, M. L. (1977). Importance of prolonged compression during cardiopulmonary resuscitation in man. *New Eng. J. Med.*, **296**, 1515.
3. Donegan, J. H. (1981). New concepts in cardiopulmonary resuscitation. *Anesth. Analg.*, **60**, 101.
4. Chandra, N., Rudikoff, M. and Weisfeldt, M. L. (1980). Simultaneous chest compression and ventilation at high airway pressure during cardiopulmonary resuscitation. *Lancet*, **1**, 175.
5. Editorial (1981). Cerebral blood flow during cardiopulmonary resuscitation. *Anesth. Analg.*, **60**, 73.
6. Leven, R. M. Zadigian, M. E. and Hall, S. C. (1980). The combined effect of hyperventilation and hypotension on cerebral oxygenation in anaesthetised dogs. *Canad. Anaesth. Soc. J.*, **27**, 264.
7. Bremer, A. M., Yamada, K. and West, C. R. (1980). Ischaemic cerebral edema in primates: effects of acetazolamide, phenytoin, surbitol, dexamethasone and methylprednisolone on "brain" water and electrolytes. *Neurosurgery*, **6**, 149.
8. Belopavlovic, M. and Buchthal, A. (1980). Barbiturate therapy in cerebral ischaemia. *Anaesthesia*, **35**, 235.
9. Kakkar, V. V. (1975). Deep vein thrombosis. Detection and prevention. *Circulation*, **51**, 8.
10. Evans, D. S. (1971). The early diagnosis of thromboembolism by ultrasound. *Ann. roy. Coll. Surg. Engl.*, **49**, 225.
11. Browse, N. L. and Thomas, M. L. (1974). Source of non-lethal pulmonary emboli. *Lancet*, **1**, 258.
12. Vasilescu, C. and Ruckley, C. N. (1974). A multi-unit trial of dextran and heparin in prophylaxis of deep vein thrombosis. *Brit. J. Surg.*, **61**, 320.
13. Ring, J. and Messmer, K. (1977). Incidence and severity of anaphylactoid reactions to colloid volume substitutes. *Lancet*, **1**, 466.
14. Hedin, H., Richter, W. and Ring, J. (1976). Dextran induced anaphylactoid reactions in man: role of dextran reactive antibodies. *Int. Arch. Allergy Appl. Immunol.*, **52**, 145.
15. Browse, N. L. (1977). Personal views on published facts. What should I do about deep vein thrombosis and pulmonary embolism? *Ann. roy Coll. Surg. Engl.*, **59**, 136.
16. Kakkar, V. V., Corrigan, T. P., Sutherland, I., Shelton, M. and Thirlwall, J. (1975). Prevention of fatal postoperative pulmonary embolism by low doses of heparin. International Multicentre Trial. *Lancet*, **2**, 45.
17. Kakkar, V. V., Corrigan, T. P., Fossard, D. P. Sutherland, I. and Thirwell, J. (1977). Prevention of fatal postoperative pulmonary embolism by low doses of heparin. Reappraisal of results of International Multicentre Trial. *Lancet*, **1**, 567.
18. Gruber, U. F., Saldeln, T., Brokop, T., Eklöf, B., Eriksson, I., Goldie, I., Gran, L., Hohl, M., Jonsson, T., Kristersson, S., Ljungstrom, K. G., Lund, T., Maartman Moe, H., Svensjö, E., Thomson, D., Torhorst, J., Trippestad, A. and Ulstein, M. (1980). Incidences of fatal postoperative pulmonary embolism after prophylaxis with dextran-70 and low-dose heparin: an international multicentre study. *Brit. med. J.*, **1**, 69.
19. Immelman, E. J., Jeffery, P., Benatar, S. R., Elliot, M. S., Smith, J. A., Funston, M. R. Shepstone, B. J., Ferguson, A. D., Jacobs, P., Pretorius, J. P. and Louw, J. H. (1979). Failure of low dose heparin to prevent significant thromboembolic complications in high risk surgical patients: interim report of prospective trial. *Brit. med. J.*, **1**, 1447.
20. Branthwaite, M. A. (1980). In: *Anaesthesia for Cardiac Surgery*, 2nd edit. Oxford: Blackwell Scientific Publications.
21. Hallgren, B., Kerstell, J., Rudenstan, C. M. and Svanbong, A. (1966). Chemical analysis of fat emboli in experimental bone fractures. *Acta chir. scand.*, **132**, 613.
22. Gurd, A. R. and Wilson, R. I. (1974). The fat embolism syndrome. *J. Bone Jt. Surg.*, **56B**, 408.
23. Wright, B. D. (1971). Diagnostic features of fat embolism—results in six cases. *Anesthesiology*, **34**, 290.
24. Prys-Roberts, C., Greenbaum, R., Nunn, J. F. and Kelman, G. R. (1970). Disturbances of pulmonary function in patients with fat embolism. *J. clin. Path.*, 23, Suppl., **4**, 143.
25. Sevitt, S. (1973). The significance of fat embolism. *Brit. J. hosp. Med.*, **9**, 784.
26. Magendie, F. (1821). Sur l'entree accidentelle de l'air dans les veins. *J. de Physiologie Experimentale (Paris)*, **1**, 190.
27. Hunter, A. R. (1962). Air embolism in the sitting position. *Anaesthesia*, **17**, 467.
28. Michenfelder, J. D., Martin, J. T., Altenburg, B. M. and Rehoer, K. (1969). An evaluation of right atrial catheter for diagnosis and treatment of air embolism during neurosurgery. *J. Amer. med. Ass.*, **208**, 1353.
29. Tateishi, H. (1972). Prospective study of air embolism. *Brit. J. Anaesth.*, **44**, 1306.
30. Michenfelder, J. D., Miller, R. H. and Gronert, G. A. (1972). Evaluation of an ultrasonic device (Doppler) for the diagnosis of venous air embolism. *Anesthesiology*, **36**, 164.
31. O'Higgins, J. W. (1970). Air embolism during neurosurgery. *Brit. J. Anaesth.*, **42**, 459.
32. Gardner, L. G. (1971). Air embolism during arterial air myelography. *Brit. J. Anaesth.*, **43**, 807.
33. Nunn, J. F. (1959). Controlled respiration in neurosurgical anaesthesia. *Anaesthesia*, **14**, 413.
34. Munson, E. S. and Merrick, H. C. (1966). Effect of $N_2O$ on venous air embolism. *Anesthesiology*, **27**, 783.
35. Munson, E. S. (1971). Effect of nitrous oxide on the pulmonary circulation during venous air embolism. *Anesth. Analg. Curr. Res.*, **50**, 785.
36. Maroon, J. C. (1973). Venous air embolism. *Lancet*, **1**, 605.
37. Marshall, W. K. and Bedford, R. F. (1980). Use of a pulmonary-artery catheter for detection and treatment of venous air embolism. *Anesthesiology*, **52**, 131.
38. Brechner, V. L. and Bethune, R. W. M. (1971). Recent advances in monitoring pulmonary air embolism. *Anesth. Analg. Curr. Res.*, **50**, 255.
39. Edmonds-Seal, J. and Maroon, J. C. (1971). Air embol-

ism. A comparison of various methods of detection. *Anaesthesia*, **26**, 202.

40. Calverley, R. K., Dodds, W. A., Trapp, W. G. and Jenkins, L. C. (1971). Hyperbaric treatment of cerebral air embolism. *Canad. Anaesth. Soc. J.*, **18**, 665.

41. Probert, W. R. (1956). Sudden operative death due to massive tumour embolism. *Brit. med. J.*, **1**, 435.

42. Editorial (1979). Amniotic fluid embolism. *Lancet*, **2**, 398.

CHAPTER 15

# Extracorporeal Circulation and Hypothermia

### The Place of Hypothermia and Extracorporeal Circulation in Cardiac and Vascular Surgery

Some operations can be performed on the heart or arterial system without the need for any special ancillary technique. Ligation of patent ductus arteriosus or coarctation of the aorta is carried out under normal anaesthesia, while closed mitral valvotomy is performed on the beating heart which continues to supply the circulation throughout the operation.

Other operations may interrupt the circulation either in its entirety as in a heart operation, or locally, as in thoracic aneurysm, for periods which, in the absence of some support technique, would lead to the death of an organ or of the whole patient. The techniques used are:

1. **Simple hypothermia.** Body temperature is reduced to approximately 30° C resulting in a 25 per cent decrease in metabolic rate which enables whole body or organ circulatory interruption to be prolonged proportionately.
2. **Deep or profound hypothermia.** Body temperature is reduced to approximately 15–20° C in a technique which usually necessitates some form of extracorporeal circulation and which allows much longer circulatory arrest.
3. **Bypass techniques.**
   (*a*) Simple bypass—the temporary insertion of a conduit, e.g. into the carotid artery, while a segment of artery supplying a vital organ is disobliterated.
   (*b*) Extracorporeal circulation—
      i. without a gas-exchange apparatus (e.g. left atriofemoral bypass in surgery of the descending thoracic aorta).
      ii. with a pump oxygenator with or without some degree of hypothermia (e.g. most open heart surgery).

## HYPOTHERMIA

### Introduction and Historical Note

During hypothermia the body temperature is reduced below its normal value so that therapeutic use can be made of the concomitant reduction in metabolic rate. Hypothermia is described as mild (35–28° C), moderate (27–21° C) and deep or profound (below 20° C) and can be achieved either by surface cooling or by core cooling—the latter implying the use of some extra-corporeal circuit.

Cold therapy for a variety of conditions attracted the intermittent attention of physicians from the 15th century onwards until in 1940 Smith and Fay[1] reported on the use of general hypothermia in the treatment of malignant disease. This followed their histological findings that cold led to a regression and degeneration of neoplastic tissue. The importance of this contribution did not lie in its effectiveness as a cancer cure but rather it revealed the essential secret of achieving hypothermia, namely that sedation or anaesthesia (including muscle relaxants) must be used to control shivering.

In 1950, Bigelow[2] and his colleagues demonstrated survival in experimental dogs after 15 minutes circulatory arrest at 20–25° C and this observation was applied clinically by Lewis and Tauffic[3] during the correction of an atrial septal defect. Surface hypothermia became widely applied in cardiac surgery but its usefulness was limited by the incidence of ventricular fibrillation at temperatures below 28° C. The safe temperature limit of 30° C allows only ten minutes of circulatory interruption which restricts the surgery to easily repaired defects. Despite experiments with various drugs to depress myocardial irritability, no reliable method of surface cooling to deeper levels was found and the impetus to further research was diminished by the successful development of the pump-oxygenator for extracorporeal circulation. Later, mild and moderate hypothermia were introduced into bypass practice but dissatisfaction with the pump oxygenator system and its results led Drew and colleagues[4] to develop the technique of profound hypothermia to 13–15° C. The unsuccessful results of conventional bypass in neonates caused a group of Japanese surgeons[5] to re-examine the possibilities of surface-induced deep hypothermia and a technique developed which enabled 50–60 minutes circulatory interruption.[6] This technique has been recently reviewed by Niyazaki and his colleagues[7] from Kyoto University, who reported on the anaesthetic management during profound hypothermia induced by surface cooling for cardiac surgery in babies and small children. Core temperatures of approximately 20° C allowed circulatory arrest for over an hour. Interestingly, ventricular fibrillation at such low temperatures was not observed, this being attributed to the circulatory stability obtained with deep ether anaesthesia. The overall mortality was less than 8 per cent and the incidence of neurological complication less than 6 per cent. In many hands this has now been modified to include some degree of extracorporeal circulation particularly in the rewarming phase.

The late 1950s were probably the heyday of surface-induced hypothermia when it was widely applied in cardiac and great vessel surgery, in neurosurgery, as an ancillary technique to induced hypotension, and as a treatment for anoxic cerebral damage. In the latter condition, mild hypothermia is employed as an adjuvant to other forms of cerebral salvage and seldom as a sole technique. Hypothermia during neurosurgery is now rarely used, but profound hypothermia with circulatory arrest using a cardiopulmonary bypass technique is occasionally needed for operations on the great vessels involving the blood supply to the brain.

## PHYSIOLOGY OF HYPOTHERMIA

### Temperature Regulation and Shivering

Heat production in the body comes from two main sources; the metabolism in ordinary cells, particularly the very active ones (e.g. liver) and from the effect of muscle contraction, most of which is voluntary, but some of which (e.g. heart) is continuous and involuntary. This heat is dissipated through the skin and exhaled air and there is a temperature gradient between the body core and the surface. The amount of heat dissipation through the skin is controlled by variations in skin blood flow and this is normally sufficient to maintain the body temperature within its physiological range. Major decreases in environmental temperature may be too great for the adaptive power of the skin and blood temperature falls. When the temperature of the blood reaching the brain is reduced by about 0·5° C the thermal nucleus in the hypothalamus is stimulated. This nucleus is concerned with co-ordinating the peripheral response to changes in skin and blood temperature. The effect of this stimulation is to provoke the shivering reflex producing a massive increase in metabolism and cardiac output.

It is not possible to induce hypothermia in man unless the shivering reflex is obtunded either by central depression of the thermal nucleus or by preventing the muscle activity by the use of muscle relaxants.

### Metabolic Rate: Oxygen Consumption and Utilisation

Experimental work on metabolic rate during hypothermia has been confused by:

1. Difficulties in temperature measurement—the site at which the temperature is measured (e.g. oesophageal) may not accurately reflect the temperature of the whole body.
2. Temperature gradients within the body—calculations have been based on the assumption that the body has been uniformly cooled whereas a steady state has not been achieved and some highly metabolic organs are still not hypothermic.
3. Drug and metabolic effects: early work was often made with the patient breathing spontaneously. The effects of hypercarbia and of anaesthetic agents in stimulating the autonomic nervous system were not eliminated. When these defects are corrected it appears that the oxygen consumption and metabolic rate are depressed to 75 per cent of basal at 30° C to 45 per cent at 25° C and to 17 per cent at 20° C.

The possibility exists that this reduction in oxygen consumption represents a failure in supply and utilisation rather than a true depression of metabolism. This could result from inhibition of enzymatic processes by hypothermia, changes in the oxygen dissociation curve or alterations in the circulation. The latter two effects may be offset by increased dissolved oxygen in plasma at low temperatures, which may not, however, be enough to supply the metabolic needs of the cells. The effect of hypothermia is to displace the oxygen dissociation curve to the left (Chapter 3) producing a reduction in oxygen release by haemoglobin in the tissues. This effect can be compensated by the creation of a respiratory acidosis, which has the added advantage of preventing cerebral vasoconstriction. Poor tissue perfusion consequent on hypothermia may depress oxygen availability to the cells. However, if the circulation is interrupted at a low temperature so that an oxygen debt occurs, when the circulation is restored there is a rise in oxygen consumption until the oxygen debt is paid off. This effect occurs even if the patient is maintained hypothermic suggesting that the capacity for utilisation of oxygen at these temperatures is not the limiting factor.

### Acid-base Balance

Interpretation of acid-base balance during hypothermia is complicated by the problem of measurement. Most measuring electrodes are maintained at 37° C and when blood, removed anaerobically from a hypothermic patient, is put into the electrode, the change in carbon dioxide solubility produced by the alteration in temperature affects the observed $Paco_2$ and pH. Thus the $Paco_2$ will be higher and the pH will be lower at 37° C than the values would be if the measurement was made at the temperature of the patient. There are three schools of thought on how to act upon blood gas measurements during hypothermia.[8]

1. Using "uncorrected" values, that is basing further management upon acid-base values measured at 37° C, irrespective of the patient's temperature.
2. Correcting the observed values to a computed estimate of the values expected at the patient's temperature—this being easier than altering the temperature of the electrode system.
3. Refusing to act upon such result until the patient is normothermic.

If the first option is taken, then correction of the apparent respiratory acidosis will tend to produce a condition which by interpretation according to the second option would represent an alkalotic state with hypocarbia in the hypothermic patient, a situation which appears to optimise enzyme function.[9] However, this might be expected to compromise cerebral perfusion and further shift the oxygen dissociation curve to the left. In practice, these effects are largely offset by the reduction in tissue metabolic requirements during hypothermia. The correct physiological approach to this conundrum has yet to be fully elucidated. The third option is impractical when faced with the necessity to make a decision on the minute ventilation to be delivered to the patient. Fortunately, the quantitation of fixed acids is only slightly affected by this problem of temperature difference.

**Respiratory effects.**—During spontaneous respiration the minute volume progressively decreases and ventilation will cease at about 23° C. Gas transfer is not impaired but an increase in anatomical and physiological dead space occurs due to cold-induced bronchial dilatation. The overall effect is the development of a respiratory acidosis. Respiration is normally controlled during hypothermia and with the decreased carbon dioxide production and increased carbon dioxide solubility, a respiratory alkalosis is easily produced. The minute volume of artificial ventilation during hypothermia must therefore be reduced according to the blood gas tension values.

**Metabolic effects.**—The development of a metabolic acidosis is common, although less so during surface hypothermia than during core cooling. It results from a decrease in the availability of oxygen due to a reduction in tissue perfusion, associated with a breakdown of autoregulatory systems and an increase in blood viscosity with intracapillary sludging so that the reduction in blood flow is greater than the reduction in cellular metabolism. Lactic acidosis is inevitable during periods of circulatory occlusion, but may not become apparent until rewarming when tissue blood flow is re-established. If the circulation is intact and liver function returns to normal, this acidosis is often self-correcting and the administration of sodium bicarbonate may lead subsequently to a metabolic alkalosis.

### Carbohydrate Metabolism

Hypothermia causes an increase in plasma glucose. This is thought to be due to reduced insulin activity, depressed liver function and inhibition of enzymes concerned with glucose metabolism. If glucose is given intravenously the blood sugar rises steeply and exerts an osmotic effect on the cells, increasing blood volume and lowering serum electrolyte levels. Small infants undergoing surface hypothermia who receive no intravenous glucose during the procedure show satisfactory and stable blood glucose levels throughout,[10] although this does not obviate the necessity for monitoring blood sugar.

### Fluid Balance and Electrolytes

Studies of water balance and electrolyte levels during hypothermia often show completely divergent findings due either to methodological differences or to alterations in respiratory or circulatory function predominating over the minor changes consequent on the effects of hypothermia itself. Serum sodium and potassium and packed cell volume estimations are, however, valuable to assist intra-operative management.

### Circulatory System

Heart.—Myocardial oxygen uptake is reduced as temperature falls and this facilitates longer periods of interruption to the coronary circulation with better preservation of myocardial function. During surface cooling there is a small fall in blood pressure and a more marked slowing of the pulse until about 25–26° C. Below 26° C the blood pressure falls more quickly as the cardiac output declines and then at 20° C, as the peripheral vascular resistance, which has initially increased, gives way to vasodilatation with venous pooling the blood pressure drops more quickly.

Once the temperature falls below 32°–30° C dysrhythmias are common. The most frequent are ventricular extrasystoles and there is a progressive increase in the development of atrioventricular dissociation. In the ECG, prolongation of P–R, QRS and QT intervals are seen and below 25° C ST segment and T wave changes occur. It is common for patients to develop ventricular fibrillation below 28° C. The cause of this increased myocardial irritability is unknown. It occurs later in children who can often be cooled below 25° C particularly if the serum potassium level is carefully controlled.[11] Possible factors are temperature or pH gradients in the myocardium and disproportion in alteration of conduction velocities. A large number of apparently contradictory methods have been advocated for its prevention, but severe dysrhythmias should always be anticipated in the hypothermic patient.

### Blood Elements and the Microcirculation

Blood viscosity increases and platelets and white cells diminish during hypothermia but these changes are small above 28° C. However, at temperatures below this the alteration in the blood and in haemodynamics result in poor tissue perfusion. These effects can be reversed by mechanical augmentation of the circulation, by the use of vasodilator drugs, and most importantly by the reduction in blood viscosity in the haemodilution technique which significantly increases tissue blood flow and oxygen availability.

### Liver

Hypothermia reduces splanchnic blood flow and liver metabolism in direct proportion to the fall in body temperature. The detoxication of drugs such as barbiturates, morphine and adrenaline is reduced and the coagulation time of the blood is prolonged. However, the liver will then tolerate increased periods of circulatory occlusion provided these are not accompanied by a high venous pressure with consequent engorgement of the liver parenchyma.

### Kidneys

Blood flow, oxygen consumption and glomerular filtration decrease during hypothermia and urine production usually ceases around 20° C. Hypothermia appears to protect the kidneys well against circulatory interruption both in the intact patient during cardiac and great vessel surgery where post-operative renal failure is uncommon, and in the isolated kidney where hypothermia is used to protect the organ during the interval between removal from a donor and implantation in a recipient.

### The Central Nervous System and Tolerance to Cold and Circulatory Interruption

It was suggested initially that cold itself might induce damage in brain and nerve. In many of the early experiments it is possible to incriminate either low-flow perfusion or the existence within the brain of temperature gradients usually the result of too rapid cooling. The large body of recent clinical evidence suggests that reducing brain temperature to 10° C *per se* is not a cause of brain injury. Nervous tissue metabolism appears to fall with temperature in the normal way and, despite the absence of any stored metabolic substrate, the brain appears to be able to tolerate circulatory arrest for periods which are proportionate to the reduction in temperature. The practitioners of deep hypothermia, by paying meticulous attention to cerebral blood flow and to slow cooling with an absence of temperature gradients, allow 60 minutes total arrest at 15° C with apparent complete recovery. Fisk and his colleagues[12] when examining the brains of piglets which had clinically shown no lesions after experimental deep hypothermia with circulatory arrest, found histological evidence to suggest that damage had occurred and, with other authors, have cautioned that circulatory interruption times during hypothermia should be the minimum possible, not the longest practicable.

## CLINICAL TECHNIQUE OF MILD SURFACE HYPOTHERMIA

(i) **Anaesthesia.**—The anaesthetic requirement is that the shivering reflex is prevented so that the patient allows his temperature to fall. Due to the inadequacy of spontaneous ventilation during hypothermia, patients will normally be intubated and ventilated, thus muscle relaxants will assist in the prevention of shivering. The volume of ventilation is adjusted to maintain the carbon dioxide tension approximately at normal values after the appropriate temperature correction has been made. The natural response to a cold environment is vasoconstriction and the drop of body temperature is facilitated by the production of vasodilatation.

Ether was originally a popular drug, both for its vasodilatory action and for its benign effect on the circulation, but is contra-indicated with the widespread use of the diathermy, and vasodilatation is usually achieved with drugs such as chlorpromazine, which can be given intravenously at the time or may be included in the premedication. The latter should also include a vagal blocking drug to modify cold-induced bradycardia.

(ii) **Monitoring.**—Temperature is best monitored by thermistors which can display mid-oesophageal temperature as representative of heart temperature and nasopharyngeal or tympanic membrane temperature as representative of brain temperature. The heart temperature is obviously important in respect of the development of dysrhythmias while the brain temperature dictates the safe duration of circulatory arrest. Rectal temperature is useful as an index of temperature gradient within the body as it tends to lag behind core temperature measured elsewhere and, particularly during rewarming, to indicate when this can be safely discontinued without danger of recooling. An electrocardiogram is mandatory and most anaesthetists would insist upon direct arterial and venous pressure monitoring in addition to a reliable infusion site. Arterial cannulation also provides easy access for samples for blood gas and electrolyte estimation.

(iii) **Cooling Techniques.**

(*a*) *Immersion.*—Once anaesthetised, the patient is lowered on a canvas stretcher into a bath of water at 4° C. The toes and fingers are normally held out of the bath to guard against frostbite. Sudden movement, particularly elevation of a cold limb, may lead to the arrival of a quantity of supercooled blood at the heart causing ventricular fibrillation. The limbs must either be left stationary or massaged continuously. This will speed the cooling process and reduce the amount of "after-drop" and the average adult will cool from 37° C to 30° C in an hour.

(*b*) *Evaporation.*—Although less efficient than immersion, it is easier to perform. The patient is positioned on the operating table. Ice bags are placed over the groin, neck and axilla, but not over the precordium. The skin is thoroughly wetted and heat loss by evaporation is encouraged by creating a wind tunnel with fans around the patient. Although the rate of cooling is slightly slower, this method has the advantage that the patient is positioned for surgery before cooling commences and unlike the immersion method, there is not the danger of having to move the patient once the temperature is low.

(*c*) *Cooling blanket.*—This is the least satisfactory. The area of contact between patient and blanket is often small but the solution in the pipes must not be below 0° C for danger of localised ice-burns. Cooling is therefore slow.

### Level of Hypothermia and Rate of Cooling

In simple hypothermia, cooling is usually to a temperature of not less than 30° C which will protect the brain from up to ten minutes circulatory interruption. The rate of cooling is such that the temperature usually falls to this level in about an hour. Active cooling stops some way above 30° C because the peripheral tissues are cooled below this level and their continued perfusion causes the central temperature to continue to drop. This "afterdrop" or "overshoot" depends partly on the speed of cooling, being greater when the temperature has dropped rapidly, and partly on the size and shape of the patient. It is unwise to allow the surgeon to start operating until one is quite certain that the temperature drop has plateaued. In the cool environment of the theatre, the patient will usually stay cold unless active rewarming is undertaken. The most satisfactory solution is to have a water mattress under the patient and this can be circulated to provide fine control of the temperature, to check the afterdrop or to prevent rewarming. However, it is important to be thinking and planning well ahead as the application of warmth under such conditions is rarely followed by a rise in body temperature for at least half-an-hour. At the same time, the warm water must not exceed the skin temperature by too much because of the danger of skin burns. An efficient humidifier in the ventilator circuit has the advantage of providing active rewarming from the core.

Safety in a hypothermia technique depends on continued careful monitoring. If the electrocardiogram shows signs of dysrhythmias which are not due to hypoxia, acid-base or electrolyte disturbance, then the technique must be stopped at a temperature short of that which gives rise to the disturbance.

*Infusion.*—Care is needed both in the type of solution and its temperature. During hypothermia glucose metabolism is inhibited and glucose administration leads to high blood sugar levels. Quite satisfactory levels are maintained if Ringer lactate is used and its temperature should be adjusted to that of the patient. In particular, very cold blood should not be given quickly to already hypothermic patients. Metabolic destruction of citrate is retarded and ACD blood must be carefully covered with the correct quantities of calcium salts.

**Rewarming.**—There is usually no hurry about rewarming which can be allowed to occur slowly with a hot water blanket over the top of several normal blankets. This will prevent localised areas of heating which might lead to burns. If speedy rewarming is very necessary reimmersion in a warm bath is quickest. The anaesthesia must not be discontinued until the temperature has returned to normal otherwise shivering will occur placing a tremendous load on the still hypothermic cardiovascular system.

### Indications

Simple surface hypothermia was at one time widely practised, but today the commonest indication is probably during the correction of congenital cardiac abnormalities in small children, but even here extracorporeal circulation is often required for active rewarming. Hypothermia is rarely used during coarctation of the aorta or aneurysm surgery to protect the kidneys or spinal cord, or during carotid disobliteration to protect the brain. More commonly, some form of bypass technique (local shunt or extracorporeal circulation) is employed in order to preserve distal-organ integrity.

When used in cardiac surgery the technique was to expose the heart after cooling to 30° C then to clamp off both vena cava and aorta thus isolating the heart from the rest of the circulation. Within an eight-minute period, the heart was opened, the defect repaired, the heart closed and all air evacuated from it. Few intracardiac lesions can be repaired in this time and the better operating conditions provided by extracorporeal circulation, together with the comparable operative risk has resulted in inflow occlusion with mild hypothermia being generally abandoned in favour of extracorporeal circulation.

## THE EXTRACORPOREAL CIRCULATION

**Definition.**—Extracorporeal circulation, or cardiopulmonary bypass, refers to a technique whereby blood is totally or partially diverted from the heart into a machine with gas exchange capability and subsequently returned to the arterial circulation at appropriate pressures and flow rates. In total bypass techniques the patient's heart and lungs are largely excluded from the circulation, and tissue perfusion and oxygenation is maintained artificially.

### Introduction

The widespread use of extracorporeal circulation, usually for cardiac surgical procedures, has led to a remarkably low mortality as a result of the technique itself. Barring accidents, mortality is usually attributable to the pre-existing cardiac disease state superimposed upon the operative risks associated with major cardiac surgery. Morbidity, however, remains appreciable.

Although physiological derangement during extracorporeal circulation is both better understood and corrected, coagulation difficulties need further elucidation with a fresh rather than an empirical approach. Neurological impairment, however mild, is common following extracorporeal circulation,[13] and may not merely be a reflection of micro-emboli. Finally, morbidity associated with the degree of invasive monitoring must be considered, together with iatrogenic manoeuvres that may in some cases threaten, instead of improve, patient welfare.

## Historical Note

In 1812 Legallois[14] wrote "If one could substitute for the heart a kind of injection of artificial blood, either naturally or artificially made, one would succeed in maintaining alive indefinitely any part of the body whatsoever." This armchair experimentation became a near-reality nearly fifty years later, when the physiologist Brown-Séquard (1858)[15] attempted, with moderate success, to perfuse the decapitated head of a dog. He was one of the first workers to emphasise the importance of cerebral blood flow and, in fact, showed that a period of five minutes' ischaemia of the brain was sufficient to cause death in dogs.

The development of the various methods of oxygenating blood has been a slow process and those in use today are similar to many that were tried over ninety years ago. The difference between the present-day success and the failures of yesterday seems to lie in the realisation of the enormous surface of blood that must be exposed if adequate oxygenation is to occur. Amongst the first reports of a mechanical oxygenator is that of Ludwig (1865),[16] who tried shaking blood in a balloon filled with air. Later, other workers tried bubbling air through blood but although they achieved adequate oxygenation they were hampered by foaming.[17–19]

Frey and Gruber (1885)[20] were amongst the first to exploit the idea of a thin film of blood exposed to oxygen. Their apparatus consisted of a cylinder and the blood was allowed to flow along the inner walls and thus take up oxygen on its way. This principle of a thin film of blood was brilliantly adapted by Gibbon[21] and became the basis of one of the most successful early heart-lung machines.

## Discovery of Heparin and Protamine

An inability to prevent clotting of the blood was one of the principal causes of failure in the early experiments on the extracorporeal circulation. The discovery of *heparin* represents one of the rare "accidental finds" in modern medicine. Before 1916 there was no known substance which could prevent coagulation of the blood. Howell, who is well-known for his contribution to the theories on the clotting mechanism, assigned the task of purifying certain phosphatides to a second-year medical student—one Jay McLean—at Johns Hopkins University, Baltimore. At that time, Howell was looking for a substance that would speed up rather than slow down the clotting process. McLean found that one phosphatide (cuorin) extracted from the heart muscle of dogs actually prevented coagulation. Howell recognised immediately the importance of this substance and in the following year, at a Harveian Oration in London, he described this substance as an anti-prothrombin. Later, it was found that this substance could be extracted in abundance from dog's liver, and thus it came to be called *heparin*.

More recent work has shown that heparin originates in the granules of mast cells of both animals and man; these cells are found not only in the liver and lungs, but also in the connective tissue surrounding capillaries and in the walls of blood vessels throughout the body.

The role of protamine in restoring the coagulating mechanism after the use of heparin was soon identified. As long ago as 1880 Schmidt-Mulheim[22] described the effect of "peptone shock" in dogs; this condition is characterised by circulatory collapse followed by a temporary loss of clotting power in the blood. This later effect was believed to be due to the release of heparin from the mast cells. Waters and his colleagues[23] conclusively demonstrated the value of protamine when they showed that it prevented the failure of clotting which is the characteristic of this condition.

## BYPASS PUMPING CIRCUITS AND CANNULATIONS

The pumping circuits to be considered are:

(i) Normal extracorporeal circulation with a pump oxygenator.
(ii) Supportive bypass.
(iii) Left atriofemoral bypass.
(iv) Profound hypothermia techniques
—with normal extracorporeal circulation
—with homologous lung gas exchange.

### Normal Extracorporeal Circulation with a Pump Oxygenator

This is currently the commonest method of choice for supporting the circulation during the performance of open intracardiac and great vessel surgery (Fig. 1).

The heart is most commonly approached through a midline sternal split (median-sternotomy) incision although rarely a left or right thoracotomy may be specially indicated.

*Venous cannulation*.—The superior vena cava and inferior vena cava are normally cannulated with catheters inserted through the right atrium although when operating on the left heart a single tube in the right atrium is sometimes used.

The size of the venous catheters is chosen by prior calibration to be adequate for the drainage of blood through them during bypass but, at the same time, to be not so large as to obstruct the venous return before the onset of perfusion (Fig. 2). Once bypass has commenced, venous drainage is achieved with a gravity siphon, which can be impeded by an adjustable clamp on the main venous line. If the venae cavae of the patient are 20–30 cm higher than the oxygenator or venous reservoir, siphonage produced by this difference in height is sufficient to maintain a good flow. In some cases, the siphonage may become excessive when it only defeats its own end by collapsing the vessel walls against the orifice of the tubes. If the right side of the heart, or the left side in the presence of a septal communication, is opened air will enter the tubes and stop the siphon flow. This is prevented by tightening snares around the two cavae once bypass is established (Fig. 3), a condition traditionally termed "total" bypass. In this state venous blood is prevented from flooding around the vena caval cannula to enter the heart, where it may cause ventricular distension with subsequent myocardial damage.

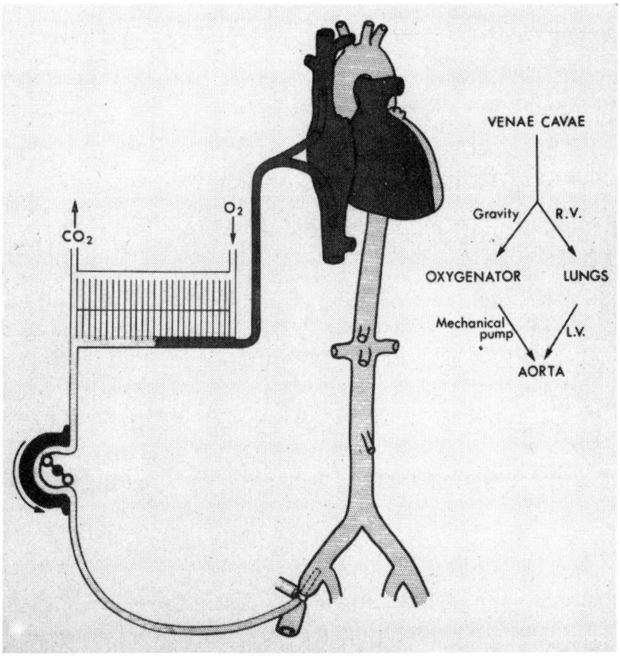


15/Fig. 1. "*Partial*" *bypass*. It is still possible for blood to enter the right heart and lungs if the free venous return to the oxygenator is at all impeded. If no blood enters the heart, the circulation is totally maintained by the extracorporeal apparatus.

For simplicity, this and subsequent figures do not illustrate the usual site for arterial cannulation in the ascending aorta. (Courtesy of Dr. J. S. Fleming, Mr. M. V. Braimbridge and Blackwell Scientific Publications)

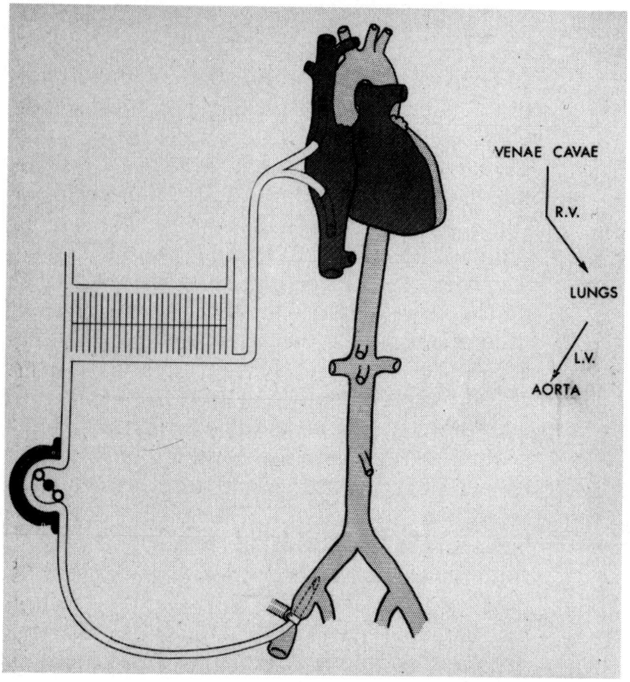


15/FIG. 2.—Before the establishment of extracorporeal circulation.

The heart and lungs are functioning in the normal way, despite aortic and venous cannulation. Mechanically induced impairment of venous return by the vena caval cannulae and induced dysrhythmias may compromise cardiac output at this stage. (Courtesy of Dr. J. S. Fleming, Mr. M. V. Braimbridge and Blackwell Scientific Publications)

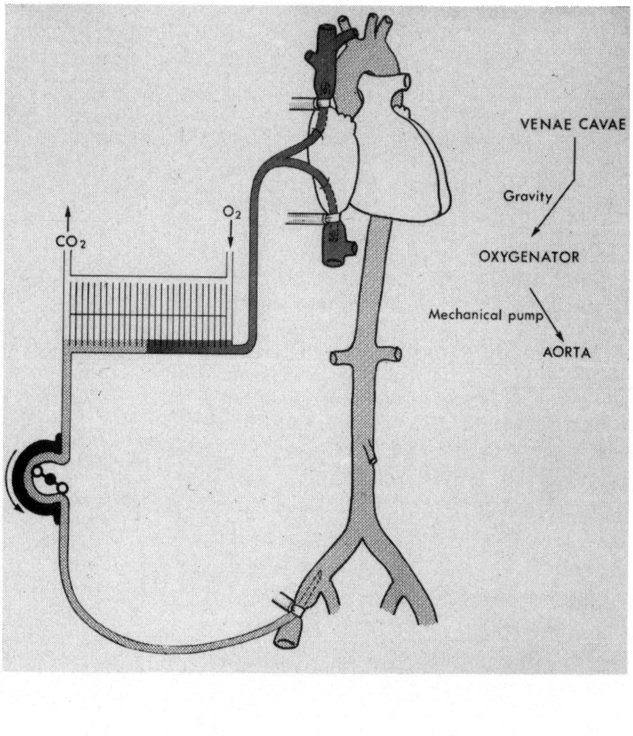


15/FIG. 3.—"Total" bypass. Left ventricular venting has yet to be performed. (Courtesy of Dr. J. S. Fleming, Mr. M. V. Braimbridge and Blackwell Scientific Publications)

Blood may also enter the heart from three other sources (Fig. 4).

1. Coronary venous return mostly re-enters the heart through the coronary sinus which drains into the right atrium. If the venous pressure is low, this blood then flows backwards into the venae cavae and down the main tubes. Alternatively, if the venous pressure is high or the venae cavae are snared, this blood may be aspirated with coronary suckers, usually from the right atrium. During aortic cross-clamping (see p. 560), there is virtually no return through the coronary sinus.
2. The bronchial arteries (which in Fallot's tetralogy can take up to 20 per cent of cardiac output) anastomose with the pulmonary circulation and drain via the pulmonary veins into the left atrium where the blood is aspirated with suckers or with the left ventricular vent (see below). During cardioplegic arrest, when the myocardium is ischaemic and protected by local hypothermia, excessive bronchial venous return can provoke dangerous local rewarming. This "vent-return" can be diminished by reducing pump flow and systemic arterial perfusion pressure while the patient is maintained at low, whole body, temperatures.
3. In the presence of aortic incompetence, blood can also pass retrogradely across the aortic valve and will have to be aspirated from the left ventricle by the vent.

During the period that the patient is heparinised the blood aspirated by the suckers is passed with the venous return to the oxygenator, and returned to the circulation. Prolonged suction in this fashion promotes haemolysis and excessive levels of plasma free haemoglobin can cause renal damage.

*Arterial cannulation.*—Direct return of blood to the aorta is standard except where special consideration indicates use of the femoral or iliac vessels. Size is less critical than for the venous cannula because the arterial cannula is unlikely to obstruct the aorta. It must, however, be large enough that the pressure drop across it at the expected flow is small. Thus damage to the red cells caused by high velocity flow is decreased and the possibility of cavitation with bubble formation in the blood flow after entry to the aorta is avoided.

**Left heart venting.**—The left heart vent has a number of functions:

1. As a simple sucker to keep the operative field clear of blood.
2. To maintain low left atrial and pulmonary venous pressures in order to avoid pul-

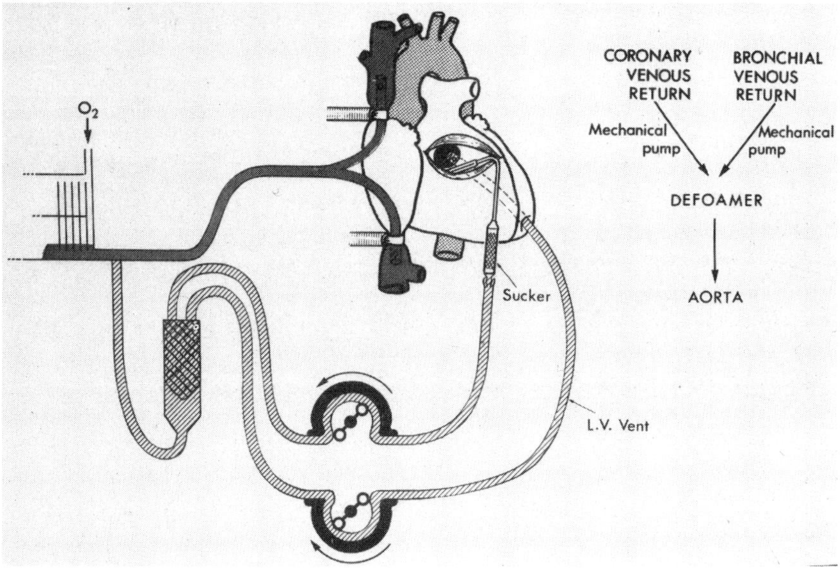


15/Fig. 4.—Return of blood from bypassed heart. (Courtesy of Dr. J. S. Fleming, Mr. M. V. Braimbridge and Blackwell Scientific Publications)

monary capillary engorgement and pulmonary oedema.

3. To reduce ventricular distension when the heart cannot eject, as in ventricular fibrillation. Establishing cardiopulmonary bypass in aortic incompetence relies upon ventricular contraction to eject the regurgitant fraction, and ventricular fibrillation or failure at this stage can rapidly result in overdistension and damage the heart.
4. When the aorta is cross-clamped during cold-ischaemic arrest, adequate left heart venting is essential to prevent myocardial rewarming.
5. The vent also provides a route through which air may be removed from the cardiac chambers prior to allowing the heart to eject.

Left heart venting is most commonly achieved by the insertion of the vent sucker directly into the left ventricle through a stab wound at the apex. Occasionally the left atrium, the aorta or the pulmonary outflow tract may be used instead. The blood is returned to the pump oxygenator. The vent must be clamped or removed before attempting to discontinue bypass.

**Supportive Bypass**

This refers to an extracorporeal circulation which provides a proportion of the required blood flow supplementing the patient's own cardiac output, and is employed in clinical situations in which the patient's circulation is severely compromised (Fig. 5). Supportive bypass can be converted to complete extracorporeal circulation if the patient's own circulation declines further.

Other situations in which this technique may be useful are:

(i) in difficult re-operations when there is a danger of damaging the heart or vessels while opening the chest; the femoral vein and artery are cannulated before starting the main incision and bypass instituted if the circulation is jeopardised by manipulation or haemorrhage;

(ii) in life-threatening pulmonary embolism, supportive bypass can be established after cannulation of the femoral vessels under local anaesthesia. If necessary this can be performed before pulmonary angiography, as the latter frequently

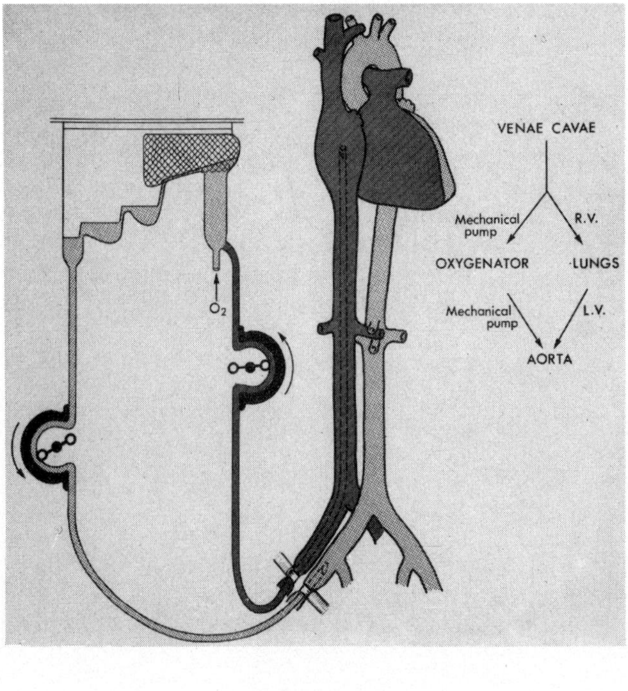


15/Fig. 5.—Supportive bypass. Thoracotomy is not necessarily performed. (Courtesy of Dr. J. S. Fleming, Mr. M. V. Braimbridge and Blackwell Scientific Publications)

causes a severe deterioration of the circulation to the point of cardiac arrest.

### Left Atriofemoral Bypass

During operations for aneurysms of the descending thoracic aorta (or coarctation of the aorta) the arterial supply to the kidneys and spinal cord may be temporarily interrupted, leading to renal failure or paraplegia. These organs can be supported by taking oxygenated blood from the left atrium and returning it, at arterial pressure levels, to the aorta below the clamp. The blood pressure is measured continuously in the major vessels of the upper part of the body which are supplied normally by the beating heart (Fig. 6).

The pump is run at such a speed that the arterial pressure remains constant. If there is proximal hypertension the pump is speeded up to lower left atrial pressure and thus reduce the output of the left ventricle to the upper part of the body and vice versa. With adequate flow, the pressure in the lower half of the body seems unimportant. Gas exchange occurs normally in the patient's lungs, but an oxygenator can be incorporated in the extracorporeal circuit if patient oxygenation becomes compromised.

An alternative means whereby distal perfusion can be maintained, involves the use of a bypass shunt inserted above and below the aortic cross-clamps.

### Profound Hypothermia Techniques

In 1963, Horiuchi and his colleagues[5] described a technique for inducing profound hypothermia in neonates by surface cooling. However, profound hypothermia, in which the aim is to reduce the body temperature to 10–15° C permitting circulatory arrest for up to an hour, is more commonly achieved with extracorporeal circulation. This can be performed in one of two ways.

(*a*) In a normal extracorporeal circuit removing blood from the right side of the heart, passing it through an oxygenator and a heat exchanger, and returning it to a systemic artery.

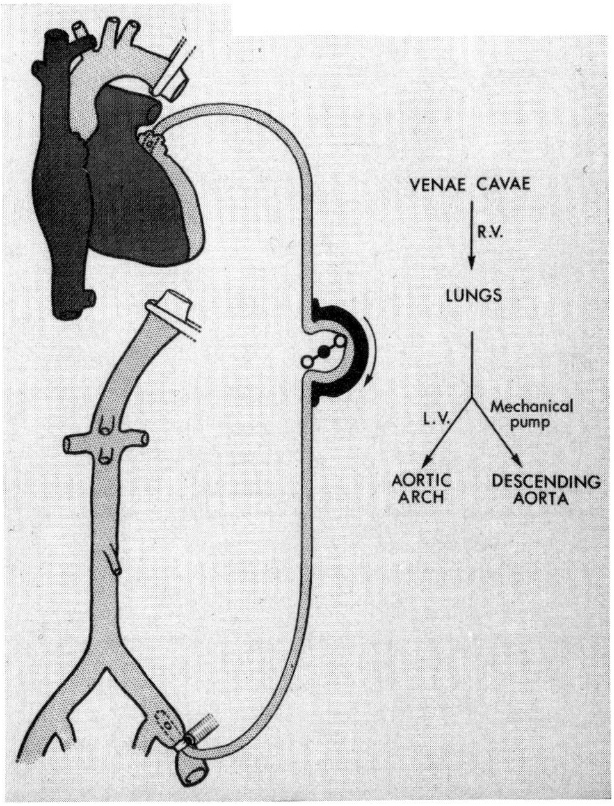

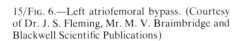

15/Fig. 6.—Left atriofemoral bypass. (Courtesy of Dr. J. S. Fleming, Mr. M. V. Braimbridge and Blackwell Scientific Publications)

This method has the advantage of considerable flexibility. It is sometimes indicated for operations on the great vessels where continuous perfusion would involve multiple cannulations of the aorta, carotid and subclavian arteries, and it is particularly suitable for complex congenital heart surgery.

(*b*) The Drew technique[4, 24] (Fig. 7) involved cannulation of the right atrium and pulmonary artery to bypass the right ventricle and of the left atrium and a systemic artery to bypass the left ventricle. The patient's own lungs were used for oxygenation and carbon dioxide elimination. This method achieved considerable success, particularly in the treatment of congenital heart disease, but has been superseded either by standard extracorporeal hypothermic techniques or by profound surface hypothermia particularly in neonates. It had the disadvantages of requiring multiple vessel cannulations, of being time-consuming, as both cooling and rewarming were slow to avoid the development of temperature gradients within the body and yet, at the same time, placing a restriction on intracardiac operating time. It was also technically difficult in the presence of severe aortic incompetence. The merit of this method lay in the very good oxygenation of the patient's blood when compared with the performance of early oxygenators but with the development of machines capable of fully oxygenating high flows of blood the need for this type of profound hypothermia has disappeared.

## APPARATUS

Anaesthetised adult patients consume approximately 110–130 ml $O_2$ per square metre of body surface area per minute, with a higher rate in infancy. To provide a full flow of completely oxygenated blood, an oxygenator needs to be capable of adding this quantity of oxygen to the venous blood for an indefinite period. Sufficient reserve capacity is also needed to cope with the patients who initially are

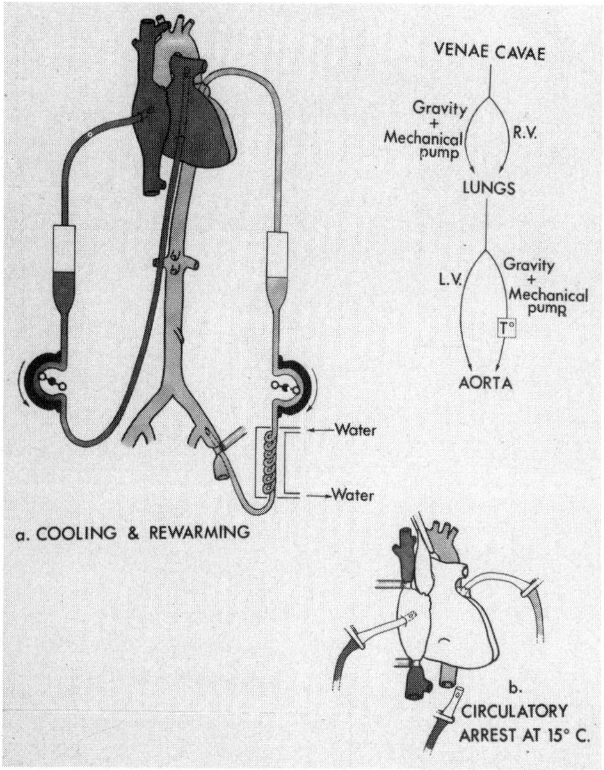


15/Fig. 7.—Profound hypothermia (Drew technique). (Courtesy of Dr. J. S. Fleming, Mr. M. V. Braimbridge and Blackwell Scientific Publications)

hypoxic or who develop an oxygen debt before bypass or during rewarming.

In the human lung, blood is efficiently oxygenated because of the huge surface area and the very intimate contact between the red cells and the alveolus. Thus oxygenation is achieved despite a low oxygen tension difference between alveolus and capillary (100−40 = 60 mm Hg or 13·3−5·3 = 8·0 kPa), a short exposure time (0·1 sec to 0·3 sec) and a low lung blood volume. The principal problem in the design of oxygenators has been the production of a sufficiently thin film of blood with an adequate surface area. In bubble oxygenators, adequate oxygenation is achieved by creating a large surface area from the many bubbles and then exposing this to an oxygen tension, which increases the normal gradient tenfold, for several seconds. The problem of the distance which oxygen has to diffuse through plasma to reach the red cells is diminished by the turbulence in the oxygenating column, which throws the red cells up to the surface of the bubbles.

## Oxygenators

Despite the large number of types of oxygenators which have been described and used at different times, today there are only two basic types in common use: those in which oxygen is dispersed in blood and those which seek to re-create normal lung relationships.

(*a*) **Dispersal of Oxygen in Blood** (Bubble oxygenators)

Blood and gas flow together at the bottom of a column which is thus filled with ascending froth and which has a very large area of blood gas interface. The size of the bubble is important. Small bubbles produce a large surface area and thus good oxygenation, but are difficult to eliminate before the blood is returned to the patient. A proportion of larger bubbles is necessary for the adequate elimination of carbon dioxide. At the top of the column the froth comes into contact with a large surface area coated with silicone-type anti-foam, which alters the surface tension of the bubbles causing them to burst. Any residual bubbles are trapped at the surface of settling reservoirs or helices before the blood is returned to the patient. Modern bubble oxygenators which are highly efficient and can cope with large flows of blood are generally made of plastic, and are supplied pre-sterilised and designed to be used only once. Because of their small priming volume, the use of blood is often unnecessary. This oxygenator was originally described by De Wall and colleagues[25] and is widely available in a variety of slightly different forms.

(*b*) **The Recreation of Normal Lung Relationships** (The membrane oxygenator)

Bubble oxygenators depend for their efficiency on the existence of a large blood-gas interface to which the blood is repeatedly exposed, which is in direct contrast to the normal lung where blood and air are separated by pulmonary endothelium. The physical forces at the interface cause denaturation of the plasma proteins with an alteration in their physicochemical properties which ultimately limits the safe duration of extracorporeal circulation. This, and the other haematological problems associated with bypass (haemolysis, platelet aggregation) prompted the development of an oxygenator that mimics normal blood-alveolar relationships by the diffusion of gases across a semipermeable membrane.

Initial attempts to design a successful membrane oxygenator were hampered in two ways.

(i) *Membrane availability*.—Early membranes were either too fragile and ruptured easily or were robust but had poor gas transfer characteristics. The current silicone elastomer membrane is thin but robust, can be unsupported over suitable surface areas and has good oxygen transfer properties.

(ii) *Haemodynamic design*.—As with film oxygenators the initial problem was that of obtaining a thin film, but later it became apparent that the limiting factor to diffusion is the existence of a stable boundary layer of plasma through which oxygen passes slowly.

The semipermeable membrane is folded into layers in such a way that the blood and gas phases remain separated. Gas exchange has become very efficient and oxygen transfer is of the order of 150 ml $O_2$ $min^{-1}$ $m^{-2}$ membrane area at clinically acceptable flow rates.

The advantages of membrane over bubble oxygenators lie principally in their more benign effect upon blood constituents. As these effects become more pronounced with the duration of bypass, membrane oxygenation has been employed with variable success for the non-surgical management of acute respiratory failure, in which arterial oxygenation is achieved by long-term (days) extracorporeal circulation while the original pulmonary pathology is corrected. In open-heart surgery with limited bypass duration, there is some evidence that haemolysis is less, platelet preservation better and peri-operative blood loss smaller with membrane, rather than bubble, oxygenators.[26] However, the extent of damage to blood does not entirely depend on the type of oxygenator used, and as mortality is more importantly related to factors other than the choice of oxygenator, the greater cost of the disposable membrane oxygenator has deterred many centres from adopting it for routine cardiac surgery.

The third type of oxygenator, now of historical interest only, relies upon the dispersal of blood in oxygen.

(*c*) **Dispersal of Blood in Oxygen** (Screen and disc oxygenators)

This principle is exemplified by the first generation stationary screen and rotating disc oxygenators. Their popularity has declined due to their high initial cost, the difficulty in re-sterilisation and their high priming volume and thus they have been widely abandoned in favour of the disposable bubble oxygenators.

## Pumps

Pumps are used in the extracorporeal circuit to return the oxygenated blood to the systemic arterial tree at high pressure levels and to provide suction to remove blood from the operative field. Pumps need to be simple, robust, easily calibrated and adjusted, and atraumatic to blood. Those parts actually in contact with the blood are usually disposable.

Of the many types of pump described, only the roller pump has survived for widespread use. These may have single, double (Fig. 8) or triple arms. Correctly adjusted for minimal occlusion with good quality tubing, they are relatively atraumatic to blood. The rate of haemolysis is directly related to the number of passages the roller makes over the tube and large-bore tubing in a slow running pump is to be preferred.

**Blood flow, pulsatile or continuous.**—Most pumps in use today, which are robust and simple, produce a predominantly continuous flow, which is physiologically inefficient in terms of tissue perfusion compared with normal pulsatile flow.

An approximation to pulsatile perfusion can be produced by devices superimposed on the action of the continuous flow roller pump. The latter can be electronically triggered to rotate in a jerky fashion so that rapid alternating acceleration and deceleration of flow are achieved. A similar device to an aortic counter-pulsation balloon pump can be placed between the roller and the patient and triggered by a suitable signal to produce intermittent-pressure swings proximal to the aortic cannula. Pressure gradients across the arterial cannula must not be excessive as high velocity jets may cause cavitation with bubble formation and damage to blood constituents, and one of the disadvantages of attempting to achieve pulsatile flow lies in the high proximal pressure swings required. For short-term clinical perfusions, the attendant problems still outweigh the benefits. The advantages, however, of pulsatile over continuous flow techniques are attractive, and are due to the improved tissue perfusion achieved with pulsatile flow which results in a higher whole body oxygen consumption, a lower systemic vascular resistance and better preservation of organ function (notably the brain and kidneys).

### Filters

A filter, often combining the function of a bubble trap, is usually incorporated into the circuit. A pore size of 40 $\mu$m is necessary to catch the microaggregates of leucocytes and platelets which pass freely through the standard 200 $\mu$m filters and which can cause embolic neurological dysfunction. As these emboli arise mainly in the oxygenator the filter needs to lie between the oxygenator and the patient.

**Disposable apparatus.**—In the past, great difficulty has been encountered in cleaning extracorporeal apparatus that has been in contact with blood. Every surface becomes filmed with protein and minute scratches encourage the deposition of fibrin and platelets. This problem has been eliminated by the use of extracorporeal circuits and oxygenators that are disposable.

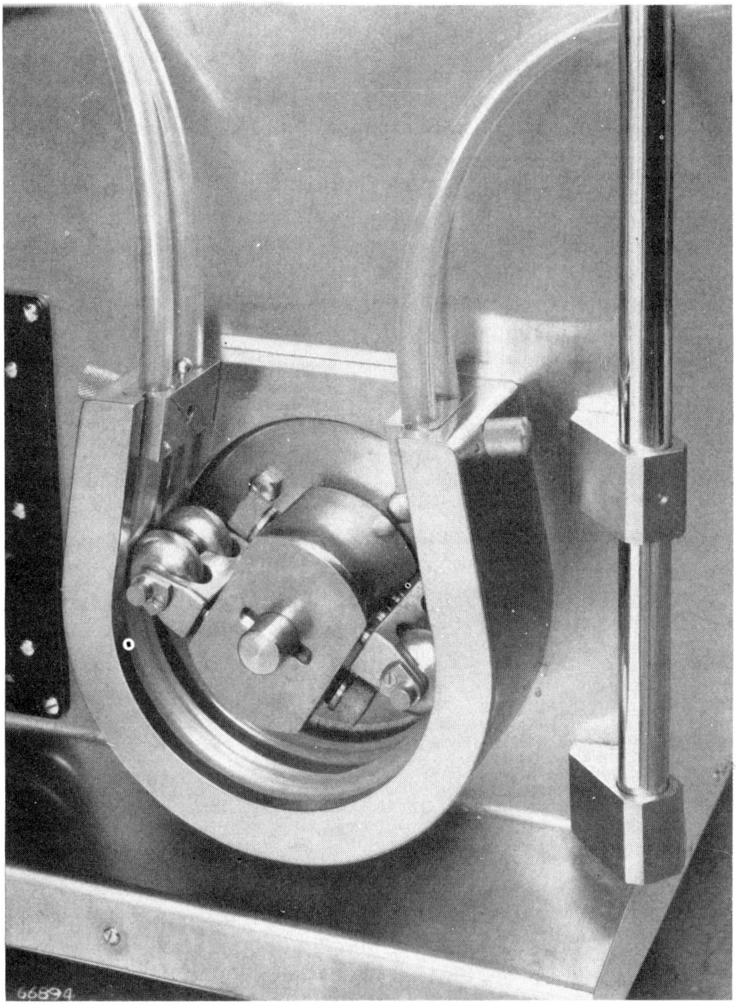

15/Fig. 8.—Roller pump. (Courtesy of Dr. G. Melrose and Honeywell Controls Ltd.)

## ANAESTHESIA AND MONITORING FOR OPERATIONS PERFORMED DURING EXTRACORPOREAL CIRCULATION

### Anaesthesia

Virtually all operative procedures performed using extracorporeal circulation involve surgery on the heart and great vessels. The underlying pathological and clinical state of the patient largely determines the type of anaesthetic technique that will be adopted, and the choice of anaesthetic drugs will be made in the light of their particular effects on the circulation. Thus induction and maintenance of anaesthesia can be achieved using a variety of drugs, intravenous or inhalational, the actual choice being made of the technique either least likely to further compromise, or perhaps even to improve, the patient's cardiovascular system and the dosages adjusted in the normal fashion according to the response of the patient. A consideration, peculiar to operations performed with extracorporeal circulation bypass, arises due to the exclusion of the patient's lungs from the extracorporeal circuit once bypass is established. The use of inhalational agents to maintain unconsciousness during bypass is difficult and while it is possible to vaporise certain agents such as halothane or trichloroethylene in the gas supply to the oxygenator, the use of intravenous anaesthetic techniques which are based upon high-dose opiates are more common. The degree of hypothermia which is a common feature of bypass, reduces cerebral metabolism and, presumably, central anaesthetic requirements. This, however, does not itself guarantee sleep, especially prior to cooling and during the rewarming period, and thus particular care must be taken in administering adequate amounts of anaesthetic. Before bypass, extra doses of opiates and neuromuscular blockers are added to the primary solution of the oxygenator—for example, 0·05 mg/kg pancuronium with 0·05 mg/kg phenoperidine, or 5–10 μg/kg fentanyl.

The benzodiazepines are useful adjuncts, potentiating the effect of the opiates and providing a degree of anterograde amnesia. Thiopentone 250–500 mg can safely be given at the start of bypass when plasma concentrations of other anaesthetic agents may be low. Examples of anaesthetic techniques that appear to fulfil these two major considerations in open-heart surgery are:

1. Adequate premedication (see p. 481) with pre-oxygenation.
2. Induction: intravenous diazepam 0·1–0·4 mg/kg; midazolam 0·05 mg/kg fentanyl 5–20 μg/kg or phenoperidine 0·1 mg/kg pancuronium 0·15 mg/kg

   *alternatively*:

   a small dose of thiopentone or etomidate may be administered following the diazepam and before a smaller dose of opiates.
3. Maintenance: Nitrous oxide (50–66 per cent) in oxygen before and after bypass, with supplemental doses of opiates. Before bypass it is sometimes appropriate to add halothane, for example in the hypertensive patient with ischaemic heart disease.
4. During extracorporeal circulation: Further doses of opiates and pancuronium and, occasionally, diazepam or thiopentone.

**Patient Monitoring and Access to the Circulation**

The extent is dictated by the severity of the disease and the type of operation and should be sufficient to cover anticipated or potential problems.

(*a*) Access to the circulation is required for fluid, blood and drug administration, and for the withdrawal of blood samples. It is fulfilled by central venous and arterial cannulation together with a peripheral venous cannula of adequate size to allow rapid infusion when required.

(*b*) Monitoring:

(i) *Central venous* ("right atrial") *pressure monitoring*.—At least two cannulae should be inserted, preferably via the right internal jugular vein, thus allowing pressure monitoring to continue uninterrupted by the need to administer potent drugs via a central line.

(ii) *Radial or brachial arterial cannulation*.—Traditionally this is performed in the left arm, as inadvertent misplacement of the aortic cannula may be suspected by abnormal arterial pressure swings during bypass. For operations on the aorta, right arm arterial pressure monitoring is necessary to avoid problems which occur should the left subclavian artery be clamped.

(iii) *Electrocardiogram*.—This is mandatory and should be connected to the defibrillator so that a synchronised DC shock is obtainable if required. Lead II or $V_5$ is normally used in continuous monitoring.

(iv) *Temperature*.—Core temperature must be continuously displayed. A number of sites are available, the most logical being nasopharyngeal or tympanic membrane. Oesophageal temperatures may not record true core temperature if pericardial cooling techniques are employed and rectal temperature changes lag behind nasopharyngeal temperatures. Peripheral (toe) temperatures are sometimes monitored (see p. 562).

(v) *Urinary catheter*.—Urine output, in the face of a crystalloid load, is a useful index of renal perfusion and hence cardiac output.

(vi) *Peripheral perfusion monitor*.—As an adjunct to peripheral temperature monitoring, a photo-electric pulse monitor can be applied to a finger. This, when connected to an oscilloscope, gives a waveform, the amplitude of which varies with cardiac output and arteriolar resistance: contraction of this waveform is noticed with vasoconstriction, a low cardiac output and extreme hypotension.

(vii) *Pulmonary artery, pulmonary capillary wedge (occlusion) pressure and cardiac output* estimations are routinely performed in many units for major and cardiac surgery, and give valuable information on left heart performance and systemic and pulmonary vascular resistances.

(viii) *Cerebral function monitor* (see below).

(ix) *End-tidal carbon dioxide tension*. This is valuable before and after bypass to optimise ventilatory control, with particular reference to the effects of $Paco_2$ on the peripheral, coronary and cerebral circulations.

### Investigations During Bypass

Repeated estimations of packed cell volume, arterial (and sometimes mixed venous) blood gas tensions and pH, serum sodium and potassium are essential during extracorporeal circulation.

Occasionally blood glucose measurements and comprehensive coagulation studies are required at some stage during open-heart surgery, while urinalysis for potassium may help predict total potassium loss via that route. Free plasma haemoglobin estimations were, in the past, considered necessary, but in the properly managed, short bypass with minimal surgical suction, haemolysis is now much less of a problem. Anticoagulation monitoring is discussed below.

### Cerebral Function Monitor

Patients undergoing open-heart surgery on cardiopulmonary bypass are particularly susceptible to cerebral damage, either because of periods of haemodynamic upset and inadequate perfusion, or from emboli. Postoperative neurological problems are compounded by low plasma oncotic pressures, raised cerebral venous pressure, periods of hypotension, intracranial pressure swings secondary to IPPV and coughing, drugs and changes in $Paco_2$.

The cerebral function monitor enables serious change in the cerebral state to be detected and treated more promptly.

The cerebral function monitor[27] is a heavily filtered 2-channel EEG that records cortical activity as a slow moving graph. Either a change in mean level of activity or alterations in amplitude denote disturbance in cortical function. Abnormal recordings may indicate impaired activity secondary to cerebral hypoperfusion, and are observed during periods of cardiac arrest, hypotension and at the onset of cardiopulmonary bypass. Schwartz and associates[28] were able to predict with approximately an 80 per cent accuracy neurological outcome following significant cerebral function monitor abnormalities observed during surgery. Other factors that appear to influence CFM changes are certain anaesthetics (notably thiopentone and nitrous oxide), $Paco_2$, temperature and haematocrit. Although it has been suggested that the cerebral function monitor merely reflects the changes in cerebral function which might be expected following observed events, experience with this device reveals that cerebral activity varies between individuals. Patients with chronic, severe heart disease, for example, appear to have lower levels of cortical function that may be particularly vulnerable to intraoperative upsets.

## PHYSIOLOGY OF THE EXTRACORPOREAL CIRCULATION

At first sight, the withdrawal of blood from a patient with subsequent oxygenation and then retransfusion would appear to be a simple matter, but in practice it is fraught with difficulties. The most important single factor for success is the organisation of the team, which should be fully conversant with all the aspects of extracorporeal circulation. Some of these problems are considered individually below.

### Anticoagulation

The passage of blood through the heart lung machine and its tubing could lead either to sudden massive coagulation with frank clots developing in the tubing or, more commonly, to an insidious microscopic process leading to complete depletion of coagulation factors and subsequent intractable haemorrhage. To prevent this, complete reversible inhibition of the clotting process must be achieved before extracorporeal circulation is instituted. Despite the limitations of the method, which are discussed below, heparin remains the current anticoagulant of choice and is normally administered prior to aortic and vena caval cannulation. At the end of bypass, following removal of the vena caval line, the action of heparin is reversed by the administration of protamine.

**Heparin**

(1) *Mechanism of action*.—Heparin exerts its anticoagulant effect by a number of mechanisms which depend principally upon ionic protein binding. A major mechanism of action appears to be binding to and activation of circulating antithrombin (AT3 or heparin co-factor) which then inhibits thrombin activity.[29] Deficiencies in existing antithrombin levels which reduce the anticoagulant action of heparin can occur with haemodilution, sepsis and intravascular coagulation. Under these circumstances, greater than normal doses of heparin may be required in an attempt to produce adequate anticoagulation.[30] Alternatively, substrate (antithrombin) concentrations can be restored with whole blood, fresh frozen plasma or antithrombin concentrates. Heparin has other actions, including an enhanced deactivation of certain clotting factors, which contribute to its effect. The complex interactions between heparin and the coagulation proteins has yet to be fully elucidated and, in certain pathological states, its anticoagulant activity may be unpredictable and can, under rare circumstances, actually enhance thrombogenic potential.[29] Furthermore, heparin has a variable effect upon platelets, either upon their half-lives, aggregation or total numbers. In situations where platelet aggregation is stimulated (e.g. cardiopulmonary bypass) platelet factors are released which directly interfere with heparin activity.

(2) *Elimination*.—The plasma half-life of heparin is approximately 1·5 hours, but varies considerably between individuals. The elimination of heparin from the plasma does not appear to occur by renal excretion, hepatic biotransformation or plasma enzymatic processes. The most likely explanation is that it is removed from the vascular compartment by the reticulo-endothelial system. Due to its binding affinity, non-specific sequestration may possibly occur, leading to a subsequent heparin "rebound" effect, although this phenomenon may eventually prove to be influenced by alternative mechanisms such as changing antithrombin concentrations.

(3) *Cardiovascular effects*.—The cardiovascular effects of heparin are minimal particularly with modern purified preparations with which hypersensitivity and anaphylactoid reactions are rare. Heparin has been reported to have a mild vasodilatory action and could be a cause of pre-bypass hypotension,[31] although there are other more significant reasons for haemodynamic changes at this moment. In experimental use in animals at very high concentrations, heparin may cause myocardial depression.

Heparin also affects the free, unbound plasma concentrations of haemodynamically active drugs. By activation of liproprotein lipase in the capillary endothelium, heparin raises circulating free fatty acids which then bind to albumin, displacing highly-bound drugs such as quinidine, phenytoin, diazepam,[32] or propanolol.[33]

**Anticoagulation During Bypass**

The certain production of adequate anticoagulation during cardiopulmonary bypass is difficult. A number of interrelated but unpredictable factors, including patient variability, alter the effect of heparin which means that heparin dosage calculated against patient weight or surface area may result in inadequate control. It is therefore necessary to adopt some form of intra-operative anticoagulation monitoring, not least because anticoagulation is affected as much by deficiencies in target enzymes as by inadequacies of heparin level. Some of these problems are illustrated in Fig. 9. Platelet aggregation which occurs during cardiopulmonary bypass, particularly in relation to blood filters, causes the release of platelet factor 4, which has anti-heparin activity. Other platelet factors are released that tend to stimulate the clotting system which, in the presence of incomplete anticoagulation, can lead to a subclinical intravascular coagulation; this in turn may produce microvascular occlusion and a depletion of clotting factors. *Prostacyclins* are potent inhibitors of platelet aggregation and have been shown to improve platelet preservation and reduce heparin requirements during cardiopulmonary bypass;[34] fibrinogen concentrations are also better maintained with prostacyclins and heparin than with heparin alone. Because of its ultra-short plasma half-life, prostacyclin is administered as a continuous infusion in the dose range

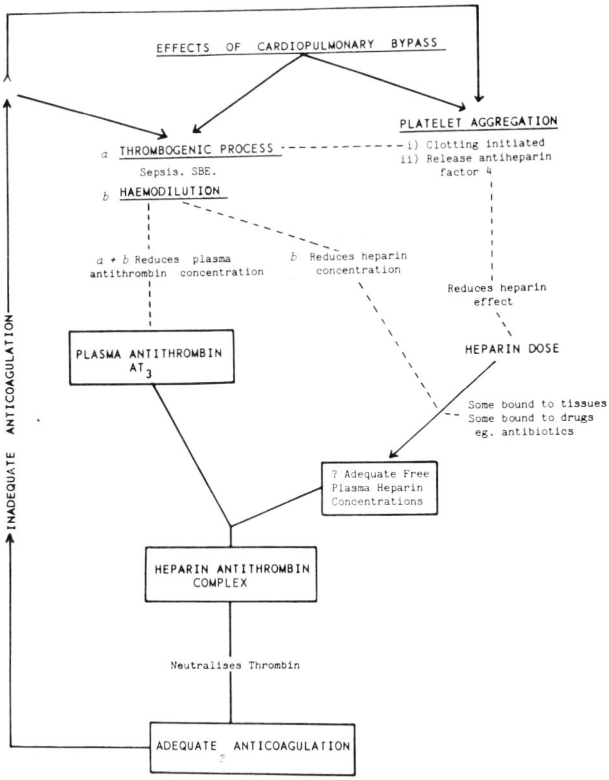


15/FIG. 9.—Relationship between heparin and antithrombin during CPBP.

10–50 ng/kg/min. It is a potent vasodilator and hypotension may have to be attenuated by $\alpha$-agonists. Prostacyclins may, in the future, provide some of the answers to a number of coagulation problems during extracorporeal circulation. In the meantime, the drawbacks associated with heparin anticoagulation can be minimised by a better understanding of its actions and by an attempt to monitor the adequacy of anticoagulation intra-operatively.

*Monitoring of anticoagulation* during cardiac surgery can be performed using one of the various methods to determine activated-clotting time. Whole blood activated clotting time (WBACT; Haemochron) or blood activated recalcification times (BART) are convenient methods and give a reasonable estimation of the clotting ability (or lack of it) of the blood. Comparative studies using the WBACT and direct fluorometric techniques show a poor correlation between prolongation of clotting time and true plasma heparin concentrations. Moreover, activated clotting times are subjected to inaccuracies caused by sample temperatures as well as the method of sampling so that absolute values do not necessarily equate with the degree of "heparinisation". Studies are in progress which it is hoped will clarify the discrepancies between WBACT, heparin and antithrombin concentrations, in an attempt to improve anticoagulant monitoring in bypass.

Meanwhile, activated clotting time measurements are both convenient and rapid and in the clinical context provide at least a guide for the control of anticoagulation.

An initial sample is taken prior to heparinisation which is then usually performed on an empirical basis giving a dose of 2–3 mg/kg body weight or 6000–9000 units/m² body surface area. This dose should raise the clotting time which should then be maintained at a value in excess of three times the control level. A degree of overheparinisation is less dangerous than underheparinisation. Monitoring of clotting time is particularly necessary when bypass is prolonged, necessitating repeated administration of heparin or during hypothermia when the elimination of heparin is altered.

### Heparin Reversal after Cardiopulmonary Bypass

The coagulability of the blood is normally restored following the completion of the operation once it has been established that the circulatory state is stable and satisfactory and that there is no continuing surgical haemorrhage. The vena caval cannulae are removed and protamine is administered. The dose of protamine may be based either on the patient's surface area or body weight (e.g. 3–6 mg/kg) or as a multiple of the initial dose of heparin. In either case, the activated clotting time is subsequently determined to establish its return to control values. Further doses of protamine may be required in order to maintain adequate clotting. This heparin "rebound" effect has been attributed to tissue sequestration, enzymatic breakdown of the heparin-protamine complex or an increase in antithrombin levels caused by blood transfusion. Postoperatively, the reappearance of free heparin should always be proved before more protamine is given as a similar effect clinically is produced by the breakdown of fibrinogen. The continued exact correction of the coagulation mechanism is required for minimal blood loss.

Major coagulation deficiencies following extracorporeal circulation are rarely due to inadequate reversal of heparin activity, and are frequently encountered following long bypass procedures associated with surgical haemorrhage and overuse of suction. Haemodilution with platelet and clotting factor reduction are primarily responsible and may be superimposed upon a subclinical intravascular coagulopathy. Here the management lies best in replacing the missing factors with fresh donor whole blood, fresh frozen plasma and platelet concentrates. Poor clot stability may be due to enhanced fibrinolytic activity. If fibrinolysis is suspected and, more particularly if it can be demonstrated by coagulation tests, antifibrinolytic agents such as tranexamic acid (Cyklokapron) 0·5–1·0 g may be given. Vitamin K seems of little use in the immediate therapy of coagulation deficiencies when replacement therapy with fresh frozen plasma is so effective.

### Autotransfusion in Cardiac Surgery

One or two units of the patient's own blood (9–18 per cent blood volume) may be withdrawn into donor bags before cardiopulmonary bypass is instituted. These will contain a sensible number of platelets (if kept at room temperature) and a useful quantity of clotting factors for replacement therapy after the finish of cardiopulmonary bypass when the coagulation is being returned to normal. A compensatory transfusion of stored blood, plasma or crystalloid is necessary in order to maintain ventricular filling pressures, PCV, plasma oncotic pressure and antithrombin concentrations.

### The Cardiovascular Effects of Protamine

A variety of haemodynamic effects have been attributed to protamine[35, 36] varying from vasodilatation and myocardial depression to actual improvement in cardiac function and output. However, clinically the most commonly observed effect is hypotension which is usually attributed to vasodilatation. The degree of hypotension can be minimised by administering the protamine slowly over a period of several minutes and by coupling this with volume expansion. The observed hypotension is less in patients who are vasodilated and adequately filled prior to protamine administration as compared with patients who have a reduced vascular volume with vasoconstriction.

In the dog, protamine produces a significant fall in ionised calcium concentration,[37] which precedes the maximum observed fall in cardiac output and blood pressure. While Conahan[35] has suggested that dogs may be more susceptible to the effects of protamine than man, a clinical observation is that calcium can sometimes reverse the hypotension which follows protamine administration in man.

Protamine may also cause a delayed increase in pulmonary vascular resistance. This action, which can be largely reversed by pulmonary vasodilators such as aminophylline, salbutamol, sodium nitroprusside or tolazoline, appears to be caused by the heparin-protamine complex. It is a particularly hazardous effect in patients with pre-existing high pulmonary vascular resistance in whom the increase can be prevented with a low dose (1 mg/min) aminophylline infusion.

Despite the fact that protamine is derived from a fish protein, allergic phenomena are very rare. Immunologically mediated reactions have, however, been occasionally reported, for example, in a patient allergic to fish[38] and in a diabetic receiving protamine zinc insulin.[39]

**Priming Solutions**

(*a*) **Volume.**—It is possible to construct an oxygenator system with a minimal priming blood volume. In such a system, however, any interference with the venous return results either in the reduction of flow or in the almost instantaneous emptying of the oxygenator into the patient with consequent risk of air embolism. For safety, therefore, most open systems have a reserve volume of about 25 per cent of the minute volume flow over and above the volume in the connecting tubes, and thus priming volumes of around two litres for adults are usual.

(*b*) **Composition.**—The factors which have to be taken into consideration include oxygen carrying capacity, viscosity, tonicity, electrolyte balance and clotting ability.

*Oxygen carrying capacity.*—Provided the flow rate is adequate, it is quite possible to maintain a near-normal mixed venous oxygen tension in the face of a reduced oxygen carrying capacity. The lower limit for packed cell volume once mixing between patient and prime has occurred, is usually put at about 25 per cent, although lower levels are tolerated in those units which feel strongly about the need to avoid the use of stored blood. In an adult patient with, say, a blood volume of 4600 ml and 2000 ml r.b.c. it is usual to prime a machine with 2000 ml of clear fluid which will reduce the haematocrit to around 25 per cent. The reduction in viscosity (see below) compensates for the reduction in haematocrit so that the relative oxygen transport capacity is maximised at a haematocrit of around 25–29 per cent.

*Blood.*—Whereas blood was originally thought to be the most physiological fluid to prime a heart lung machine, today the opposite view is more common. Blood is only used to raise the oxygen carrying capacity of the priming solution to an acceptable minimum. It has fallen out of favour, partly because of the immense difficulties of finding the quantities of blood required each day for the many operations performed. The homologous blood syndrome, although seen only in dogs in its most florid form, also occurs to some extent in humans. Post-operatively there is a much greater incidence of poor lung function after a blood prime than if the prime is with nonsanguinous fluid. Coagulation difficulties are also provoked by the use of large quantities of blood. These dangers are added to all the normal problems (incompatibility, serum hepatitis, etc.) of blood transfusion in general.

When blood is required, and this occurs most commonly in infants in whom the ratio of priming volume to patient's blood volume is large, this is provided as normal ACD or preferably CPD blood that is less than 7 days old and which is heparinised before use.

**Haemodilution technique.**—The reduction in viscosity achieved by using isotonic solutions leads, under the artificial conditions of extracorporeal circulation, to a better tissue perfusion: there is also very little difficulty in obtaining the venous return sufficient to attain the ideal flow rate. Where hypothermia is used, this decrease in viscosity also offsets the rise in viscosity which normally occurs when the temperature drops.

The very multiplicity of fluids advocated and actually used indicates that no one priming solution is ideal. The large molecular dextrans are not used because of the interference with the clotting mechanisms and this is true also of low molecular dextrans in amounts in excess of 20 ml/kg body weight. A lactated Ringer's solution or 5 per cent dextrose plus certain electrolytes (usually calcium and potassium) are the most common. If the solution is to be fully re-infused, the water load is usually restricted to 30–40 ml/kg body weight; this fluid is usually rapidly excreted and the haematocrit returns to normal in the early postoperative phase. Some cardiac centres use gelatin colloid solutions (Haemaccel) or add albumin or plasma substitutes to maintain plasma oncotic pressure.

**Changes in Plasma Constituents**

Both the volume and nature of the priming fluid will influence electrolyte and protein concentrations. Westhorpe *et al.*[40] demonstrated the following changes during and after extracorporeal circulation using an initial 2-litre

15/TABLE 1.—CHANGES IN ELECTROLYTE AND PROTEIN CONCENTRATIONS WITH CARDIOPULMONARY BYPASS
(after Westhorpe *et al.*[40])

| *Change From Control* | *During Bypass* | *30 minutes after Bypass* | *20 hrs after Bypass* |
|---|---|---|---|
| Total calcium | lower | no change | no change |
| Ionised calcium | higher | higher | higher |
| Complexed calcium | higher | higher | no change |
| Magnesium | lower | lower | lower |
| Inorganic phosphate | no change | no change | no change |
| Total proteins | lower | lower | lower |

prime of lactated Ringer's solution with added calcium (Table 1).

The dilutional effect of a crystalloid prime was responsible for a fall in magnesium and plasma proteins, whilst the calcium concentrations were altered by haemo-(plasma) dilution and by the addition of calcium chloride both to the prime and following bypass to the patient. In situations in which calcium is not added to the priming fluid, deficiencies in that ion will need to be corrected in order to maintain myocardial contractility after CPBP. Furthermore, considerable chelation of calcium by citrated blood transfusions may temporarily reduce available calcium ions until hepatic function is restored and adequate citrate metabolism takes place. The reduction in magnesium may be especially significant in chronic heart failure and prolonged diuretic therapy (see p. 421), although the use of magnesium-containing cardioplegic solutions reverses the tendency towards magnesium deficiency.[41] Hypoalbuminaemia produced by haemodilution has a profound effect on colloid oncotic pressure, which may be reduced to 40 per cent of normal.[42] This in turn increases the susceptibility towards extravascular fluid shifts and organ oedema. This increased vulnerability to oedema is particularly relevant to the brain, heart and lungs.

Other protein fractions include the clotting factors which are also influenced by haemodilution; both quantitative and qualitative decreases occur. Replacement therapy with fresh frozen plasma following bypass is designed to replace clotting factor deficiencies, and this will be enhanced by haemo-concentration secondary to a diuresis.

Sodium and potassium are predictably influenced by the effects of extracorporeal circulation. The former is maintained with sodium-containing priming fluids, and tends to be increased with bicarbonate therapy or renal dysfunction. A natriuresis induced by diuretics or dopamine may occasionally lower plasma sodium. Potassium replacement is often necessary for the following reasons:

1. pre-existing potassium depletion
2. bicarbonate therapy
3. renal excretion
4. fluid and electrolyte shifts
5. changes in cell function
6. following insulin administration.

Catecholamine release may also be associated with changes in serum potassium, initially a rise due to alpha-adrenergic release from the liver followed by a $\beta_2$-adrenergic stimulation of muscle-cell uptake. Beta blockade may alter such changes which are often induced during cardiopulmonary bypass. Propranolol, unlike more cardioselective beta-adrenergic antagonists, tends to maintain serum potassium concentrations by blocking muscle uptake.[43]

The effect of cardiopulmonary bypass on blood glucose is variable, although hyperglycaemia predominates. Raised blood glucose often reflects the stress response to surgery, the effect of hypothermia as well as the intravenous administration of glucose-containing fluids. Latent diabetes is often unmasked during cardiac surgery so that even diet-controlled diabetes may require insulin peri-operatively. Hypoglycaemia, however, is occasionally seen; this may be due to a combination of prolonged starvation, beta blockade and a depression of the normal hyperglycaemic response to surgery by modern anaesthetic techniques.

The normal stress response to surgical stimulus appears to be accentuated by extracorporeal circulation. This is generally reflected by a rise in plasma catecholamines, cortisol, vasopressin and growth hormone concentrations observed during open-heart surgery.[44] The degree of the stress hormonal response is influenced by a number of factors which include hypotension, haemodilution, depth of anaesthesia, hypothermia, changes in carbohydrate metabolism and the type of extracorporeal pump flow. These changes continue into the postoperative period so that blood sugar, vascular resistances and susceptibility to dysrhythmias may be increased as a result of the pathophysiological responses to cardiopulmonary bypass.

### Control of Perfusion and Flow Rates

In the early days of heart surgery, due to the inadequacy of oxygenators, only a low flow of blood was used. With the advent of oxygenators capable of adding 250 to 300 ml of oxygen per minute to the blood flow, low flow has become unacceptable. As flow rate is increased the oxygen consumption rises until it reaches a near plateau at approximately 2·4 l $min^{-1}m^{-2}$ body surface area. Further increase in flow rate does not increase oxygen consumption but causes more blood destruction in the oxygenator.

This rate of oxygen consumption is maintained or enhanced by haemodilution and may be increased by pulsatile flow. Perfusion at this rate should not result in an oxygen debt or the development of a metabolic acidosis but does depend on normal distribution of flow through the body. This tends to fail during hypothermia when a metabolic acidosis develops despite a high flow. It is not uncommon for the flow rate to be reduced once the patient is hypothermic, thus reducing flow via bronchial and coronary collaterals which otherwise tends to obscure the surgical field. Tissue perfusion is impaired by excessive reduction in carbon dioxide tension and systemic vascular resistance rises with duration of bypass and with high oxygen tensions. Unfortunately, venous oxygen tension is not a good index of the quality of tissue oxygenation as a high venous oxygen tension may be associated with arteriovenous shunts and a low oxygen consumption.

### Gas Flow

The gas flow through the oxygenator is only roughly predictable. In theory a relatively low oxygen flow should be adequate to oxygenate the blood and by careful monitoring to remove the carbon dioxide. In practice, the control of carbon dioxide tension is much easier if the oxygenator is flushed out with a flow of gas two to three times that of the flow of blood, and which contains approximately 2½ to 3 per cent carbon dioxide. Fine adjustment of carbon dioxide tension to physiological values is made after blood gas measurements once bypass has achieved a steady state. The disadvantages of a low carbon dioxide tension in shifting the oxygen dissociation curve and in reducing tissue and cerebral blood flow are so great that a slightly raised carbon dioxide level is to be preferred during bypass.

Now that oxygenators are capable of producing oxygen tensions of the order of 300 mm Hg (40 kPa) the effect of high oxygen tension in raising peripheral vascular resistance and impairing tissue perfusion becomes relevant, and the oxygen tension should perhaps be limited to that which produces full oxygen saturation of the blood.

### Arterial Pressure

During cardiopulmonary bypass, the arterial pressure is generally considered to be less important than the flow rate. Low perfusion pressures, either accidental or deliberate, are not uncommon, the result partly of anaesthetic drugs and partly from the low viscosity of the blood in the haemodilution technique. It is desirable to maintain the mean arterial pressure between 50 and 100 mm Hg (6·7–13·3 kPa) depending slightly on the patient's previous blood pressure and tending towards the upper figure when the ischaemic myocardium is being reperfused. At fixed flow rates, control of arterial pressure can only be achieved by agents that alter systemic vascular resistance. Methoxamine, metaraminol or noradrenaline, increase perfusion pressure, whilst phentolamine or sodium nitroprusside are sometimes required to lower it. A combination of a low flow rate and vasoconstriction may be more hazardous to organ perfusion than accepting a mild degree of hypotension. Hypotension is, of course, better tolerated at low core temperatures.

### Blood Volume

The volume in the oxygenator reservoir is dependent on the patient's blood volume and venocapacitance tone. It is also altered by the venous return to the oxygenator and the efferent flow back into the aorta. Further additions of fluid to the pump are often required, the choice of which (e.g. lactated Ringers, blood or plasma) will be determined by the particular circumstances in that operation. Excess volume is usually seen in crystalloid overload and heart failure, and is best managed by promoting a diuresis.

## THE STATE OF THE HEART DURING EXTRACORPOREAL CIRCULATION

At certain periods of extracorporeal circulation while surgery is being performed within the heart or on the coronary vessels, myocardial perfusion may be compromised by two interrelated factors:

1. The co-ordinated cardiac contraction may be changed to either asystole or ventricular fibrillation to improve operating conditions and thus to facilitate the surgery.

2. Coronary blood flow may be interrupted especially during aortic valve or coronary artery surgery.

### Methods of Induced Cardiac Arrest

Cardiac arrest may be induced electrically, by drug therapy or occur as a result of the development of myocardial ischaemia secondary to aortic cross-clamping.

**Drug induced arrest.**—In the earliest days of cardiac surgery, *potassium arrest* was used to stop the heart. A potassium-rich solution was injected into the root of the aorta following aortic cross-clamping. Although relieved of the work of contraction, the oxygen consumption of the normothermic heart remained high, so that the myocardium soon suffered anoxic damage leading to poor recovery and the technique fell into disrepute. A developed concept of drug induced arrest, termed *cardioplegia*, is now extensively used and combines the reduction in oxygen consumption secondary to the cessation of contraction, with a further reduction of the oxygen consumption of the resting heart to normal levels by the inclusion of localised myocardial hypothermia. This technique provides excellent operating conditions and is described in detail below.

**Electrically induced ventricular fibrillation.**—Ventricular fibrillation may be induced electrically in the presence or absence of aortic cross-clamping. In the absence of aortic cross-clamping, even though the aortic valve is competent and the perfusion pressure satisfactory, myocardial oxygenation is commonly inadequate. The fibrillating heart has an increased oxygen consumption and high muscle tone so that the distribution of the coronary blood flow is altered with the development of ischaemia, with the threat of infarction, in the subendocardial region. The fibrillating heart also loses potassium from its cells and develops interstitial oedema which is accentuated by the low colloid plasma oncotic pressure associated with cardiopulmonary bypass.[40]

**Aortic cross-clamping.**—Ischaemic cardiac arrest will occur following aortic cross-clamping with interruption of the coronary flow. It may be combined with electrical fibrillation or with mild whole body hypothermia (25–30° C). While remaining an anoxic technique, it appears to produce relatively little long-term damage to the myocardium provided the periods of clamping are short compared with the periods of perfusion.

The effects of aortic cross-clamping are:

(i) the myocardium is no longer perfused
(ii) the cessation of coronary arterial perfusion stops blood pouring out of the coronary sinus to flood the operative field
(iii) if there is aortic regurgitation, it prevents blood tipping through the aortic valve
(iv) if there is any danger from air embolism from a beating heart, cerebral air complications can be prevented by the application of an aortic clamp.

### Myocardial Protection During Open-Heart Surgery

Myocardial ischaemia leads to structural and functional changes that may be reversible or fatal. A number of methods have been employed in order to reduce the degree of muscle damage, and these can be divided into two groups.

1. *Intermittent periods of myocardial perfusion*
   (i) intermittent aortic cross-clamping
   (ii) intermittent coronary perfusion with arterialised blood from the heart lung machine via two small cannulae inserted into the coronary ostia (e.g. aortic valve surgery—see Fig. 10).
   (iii) alternating ventricular fibrillation with defibrillation to allow the heart to beat intermittently.

These methods are designed to limit, rather than prevent myocardial damage. Success depends upon adequate periods of coronary

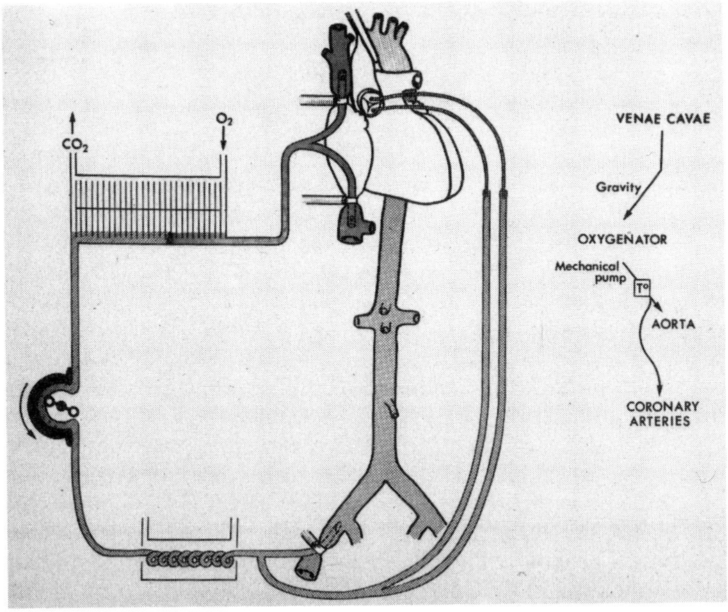


15/Fig. 10.—Circuit for aortic valve surgery, with direct coronary perfusion cannulae. (Courtesy of Dr. J. S. Fleming, Mr. M. V. Braimbridge and Blackwell Scientific Publications.)

perfusion with a beating heart, low circulating blood temperature to reduce myocardial metabolic demands, and adequate time on supportive bypass to allow the heart to recover. During coronary artery grafting, the recovery time of the post-ischaemic myocardium tends to become shorter as subsequent areas are surgically revascularised, despite an increasing accumulative cross-clamp time.

2. *Cardioplegic arrest*

This is a common method for the majority of cardiac operations as both the operating conditions and degree of myocardial protection are good.

**Method.**—After the establishment of extracorporeal circulation and temperature reduction to a core temperature of 25–32° C, the left heart is vented and the aorta is cross-clamped proximal to the aortic cannula. The myocardium is now ischaemic.

*First phase* (induction of cardiac arrest and hypothermia). Asystolic arrest is induced by the rapid infusion under pressure of one litre of cold (0–4° C) cardioplegic solution through a 14 g needle inserted into the aortic root below the cross-clamp. In the presence of aortic incompetence, the infusion is directly through cannulae inserted into each coronary ostium—each of which receives 500 ml of solution.

Points to remember are:

1. Both the low temperature and the high potassium content of the solution rapidly arrest the heart, reducing metabolic demand while the full thickness of the myocardium is cooled.
2. Adequate cardioplegic infusion pressure must be maintained in order to ensure rapid distribution throughout the myocardium. An aortic root or coronary artery infusion pressure of approximately 100 mm Hg is recommended.
3. The final temperature of myocardium and septum determines the success of the myocardial protection. A septal temperature of 6–15° C should be achieved.
4. Arrest must be total. Any electrical activity while the aorta is clamped implies that oxygen-demanding metabolism is present and that ischaemic muscle damage may follow.
5. This cardioplegic infusate will reappear through the coronary sinus and will enter the circulating blood volume where it will represent a further crystalloid and electrolyte load, unless it is separately aspirated and discarded. If the vena cavae are snared, the solution will be prevented from draining out of the right atrium and could cause right ventricular distension and pulmonary damage unless the atrium is decompressed.

## Cardioplegic Solution

A number of different cardioplegic solutions have been described. The St. Thomas' Hospital solution is supplied in 20 ml ampoules containing:

| | |
|---|---|
| $MgCl_2 . 6H_2O$ | 16 mmol |
| KCl | 16 mmol |
| Procaine | 272·8 mg |
| Water | to 20 ml |

This ampoule is added to one litre of a solution such as the non-lactated Ringer's (which has a more physiological pH than Hartmann's solution) which has been previously stored at 4° C in a blood bank refrigerator. The diluted cardioplegic solution is then stored in ice water ready for use.

*Second phase* (the maintenance of a low myocardial temperature by topical cooling).

Maintenance of myocardial hypothermia while the aorta is cross-clamped is of vital importance, and follows the cardioplegic arrest.

The simplest technique involves flooding the pericardial cavity with ice-cold Hartmann's solution so that the ischaemic heart lies in a pool of isotonic cold solution. The postero-inferior aspect of the heart is separated from warmer structures, such as the descending aorta and the diaphragm overlying the liver, by swabs or corrugated rubber. As the cold Hartmann's is run into the pericardial cavity (about 6 l/hour) a sucker removes and discards the surplus volume which is not allowed to enter the circulation.

Points to remember are:

1. Monitor the ECG. Returning electrical activity implies inadequate protection and the heart should be recooled by a repeat of phase I using a smaller volume.

2. Blood can still enter the heart even on full bypass with the aorta cross-clamped. Firstly, if the venae cavae are not snared around the venous cannulae, blood may enter the right heart and passively reappear in the left ventricle. This is prevented by taking care that the venous return to the pump is perfect, in order to keep the right atrium empty or by snaring the venae cavae (so-called "total" bypass). Secondly, the systemic bronchial arteries drain most of their venous blood into the pulmonary veins and, hence, to the left heart. Thirdly, pericardial vessels may sometimes feed the coronaries which may bleed during coronary revascularisation. Both of these effects may be reduced by lowering the pump flow rate and arterial perfusion pressure. During ischaemic cardioplegic arrest it is therefore important to lower the circulating blood temperature to avoid rewarming the myocardium and to remove this unwanted blood (which may also distend and damage the ventricles) with a suitable vent. This is classically inserted into the left ventricular apex, or sometimes in the left atrium or pulmonary artery.

### The Myocardial Effects of Cardioplegic Techniques

The effects of cardioplegia have been widely assessed by the study of biochemical, structural and functional changes. The common aim is to *limit* myocardial energy requirements and *reduce* intracellular derangement produced by ischaemia.

The variety of cardioplegic solutions reflect the potential advantages of the particular chemical ingredients they contain. Potassium paralyses the cellular membrane transport system, preserving energy reserves for the maintenance of cell membranes. Magnesium inhibits intracellular metabolism and procaine has membrane stabilising properties and both have an effect on membranes to block depolarisation.[45] Other additives that are used include hyperosmotic solutions, such as mannitol, which may limit oedema, or plasma proteins that may be added in order to maintain oncotic pressure. Buffering agents (bicarbonate, THAM, phosphates) may reduce the extent of ischaemic injury as cellular metabolic processes are pH dependant. Substrate addition (glucose, insulin) is employed in some centres.

Any period of ischaemic arrest will produce some change in myocardial integrity, and cardioplegic arrest is no exception. Such changes are claimed to be less with a properly conducted cardioplegic technique than with other ischaemic methods. Intracellular ATP stores are better maintained, intracellular damage and myocardial oedema is less and myocardial function better preserved. An ischaemic time during cardioplegia should be less than 90 minutes, however, if myocardial damage is to be minimised. Some authorities maintain that it is difficult to ensure global cardioplegic cooling in severe coronary artery disease, and are reappraising this form of myocardial protection compared with other techniques (e.g. intermittent aortic cross-clamping) for coronary artery revascularisation.

## Hypothermia During Extracorporeal Circulation

The aims of selective hypothermia of the heart and of mild whole body hypothermia, that is down to between 25° C and 30° C as a part of an extracorporeal technique, are the same, namely to reduce metabolic demands so that inadequate or interrupted perfusion can be better tolerated.

Although in theory greater reductions of temperature might be desirable as providing better protection, hypothermia itself produces complications. Vascular spasm occurs and leads to underperfusion of tissue, viscosity of the blood increases, and below 30° C there is a marked increase in the incidence of bleeding in the post-operative period.

Temperature control during extracorporeal circulation is normally effected by the passage of blood through heat exchangers, which are large surface areas of a high conductivity material over which the blood is filmed. The temperature in the water jacket can then be altered to affect the temperature of the blood. Commonly the heat exchanger is incorporated into some other piece of apparatus usually the oxygenator. Cooling can usually be effected more rapidly than rewarming because of the larger temperature gradient possible between blood (37° C) and the circulating fluid (0° C), whereas during rewarming the highest possible water temperature is approximately 40° C.

### Rewarming Before the Discontinuation of Bypass

Slow rewarming is desirable to avoid islets of cold tissue remaining in the body which cause the patient to cool again, perhaps dangerously, after bypass has been discontinued. The maintenance of normothermia following extracorporeal circulation can be influenced in two ways. Firstly rewarming is more efficient in the presence of vasodilators and high pump flows. Noback and Tinker[46] used sodium nitroprusside and achieved a smaller afterfall in nasopharyngeal temperatures, presumably because a more homogeneous body rewarming had taken place. Secondly, the loss of body heat subsequent to extracorporeal circulation can be minimised by the active addition of core heat using a Bennett-Cascade humidifier, which supplies a measured inspired gas temperature in excess of 40°C[47], by the use of a heated water mattress beneath the patient, and by careful temperature control of infused fluids. Cool extremities in the postoperative patient are therefore not only a sign of low cardiac output, but may also reflect a normal physiological response to heat loss. Moreover, a cold, constricted periphery imposes an increased afterload on a recovering myocardium.

### Renal Preservation

Although disturbances of renal function during and after extracorporeal circulation are now uncommon they may still occur in patients with pre-existing renal disease, low cardiac output states and in association with massive haemolysis. Under conditions of high flow, particularly when associated with haemodilution, urine output is normally sustained at a high level during cardiac surgery. This is particularly so if dextrose is used in the priming solution due to its osmotic effect. If the urine output falls below 30 ml of urine per hour, mannitol (25 g) is commonly added to the perfusate. A high urine output also helps to excrete the products of haemolysis. The urine production commonly ceases if the patient becomes acidotic and then returns to normal on correction of the metabolic acidosis. Post-operative renal problems appear to stem not so much from the bypass procedure but from a low cardiac output produced by the patient after surgery which is aggravated by vasoconstriction and acidosis. A low-dose dopamine infusion encourages renal blood flow, even in the face of low cardiac output and may thus offer some protection against acute tubular damage.

## THE DISCONTINUATION OF BYPASS

Once the cardiac repair has been completed, maintenance of the circulation is transferred from the heart lung machine to the patient's own heart—a process termed "coming off bypass". Before the heart is allowed to assume this load, the patient must be normothermic, free of acid-base or electrolyte disturbance and the heart must be beating at an adequate rate, preferably in sinus rhythm but at least free from frequent or serious dysrhythmias. Lung ventilation is resumed and the venous return to the oxygenator is impeded so that the heart fills with blood. The distension of the heart with blood is monitored, both by direct observation and by measurement of the right and left sided filling pressures, and should lead to the appearance of an arterial pulse and an adequate arterial pressure. It is then possible to decrease and ultimately stop the arterial pump, at the same time completely discontinuing the venous flow so that the filling pressures remain constant. While it is possible to measure the cardiac output either by thermodilution or using an aortic electromagnetic flow pulse, it is more common to infer an adequate cardiac output from the appearance of the arterial pressure trace, the urine output and evidence of tissue perfusion.

An inadequate cardiac output, in the absence of mechanical problems, may be improved either by raising the filling pressure or by increasing the cardiac rate. If, however, the output remains inadequate despite reasonable filling pressures and cardiac rhythm and rate, the inference remains that ventricular pump action is unsatisfactory. It may then be necessary to improve the cardiac action by inotropic or vasodilator therapy (see p. 484). Coming off bypass may, in some patients, be extremely difficult and may require massive pharmacological intervention and mechanical support to achieve the transition from the extracorporeal to the physiological circulation. Very occasionally, for a variety of reasons, ventricular performance is so poor that despite maximum support, a viable cardiac output is never achieved.

After cardiopulmonary bypass has been discontinued, the venous cannulae are removed, and further additions to intravascular volume can be made through the aortic cannula. The latter is removed when ventricular filling pressures are adequate or the oxygenator reservoir is empty, and when the reversal of heparin by protamine has been started.

### Mechanial Support "The Balloon-pump"

Of the various forms of mechanically assisted devices that have been investigated, the aortic counter-pulsation balloon-pump remains the most applicable to the management of heart (pump) failure following extracorporeal circulation. A balloon, which is available in various sizes (average adult capacity 35 ml) is inserted usually via a femoral artery into the upper thoracic aorta. This is connected to a machine which, triggered by a signal from the ECG, alternately inflates and deflates the balloon. Inflation occurs during diastole after closure of the aortic valve and deflation occurs early in ventricular systole. The diastolic inflation augments coronary artery filling whilst the deflation reduces left ventricular afterload, so that balloon pumping improves ventricular performance in two ways: biventricular myocardial oxygenation is improved and left ventricular work is reduced so that forward flow increases. Aortic counter pulsation reduces ventricular tension and size and thus oxygen demand, while at the same time improving myocardial oxygen supply. This has led to its use in other contexts, namely the treatment of cardiogenic shock secondary to myocardial infarction. Indeed, the success of this technique will be enhanced in those patients in whom failure to discontinue extracorporeal circulation is primarily due to ventricular failure secondary to myocardial ischaemia.

## COMPLICATIONS

### Haemolysis

Trauma to the formed elements of the blood can be a major complication of extracorporeal circulation. The most easily measurable result is the appearance of free plasma haemoglobin, but other deleterious effects occur at the same time, particularly the denaturation of the plasma proteins which results from the presence of blood-gas interface in the oxygenator. Haemolysis can be reduced to a minimum by the use of high-quality tubing, by the siliconing of parts which come into contact with the blood, by the use of roller pumps which are carefully adjusted and which have large-bore tubing over which the roller only passes very slowly. Haemolysis is commoner in bubble oxygenators than in membrane oxygenators, but the principal source of haemolysis in fact lies in the suckers which are used to aspirate spilt blood from the heart. These should be of a wide bell-mouthed type and the surgical assistant should, wherever possible, suck pools of liquid blood, rather than a mixture of blood and air. Haemolysis normally increases almost linearly with the passage of time. With cardioplegic techniques, surgical suction tends to be minimised, and haemolysis is uncommon. However, with current-day well-maintained apparatus, it is rare for plasma haemoglobins to exceed approximately 100 mg per 100 ml blood even at the end of long perfusions. This is a level which is not normally associated with renal damage.

### Air Embolism

Air embolism is one of the major hazards of open heart surgery. The air normally gains access to the heart during an intracardiac manoeuvre and is then ejected out into the systemic circulation when the heart is reconnected to the general circulation. Every effort, therefore, is made to ensure that the heart is free of air before the heart is allowed to eject into the systemic circulation.

The following manoeuvres are employed:

1. Removal of air from the chambers of the heart is achieved while still on bypass. The apex of the heart is elevated so that the left ventricular vent site is uppermost and the venous return to the oxygenator is impeded. Blood enters the heart displacing the air which is released through the left ventricular apex. Timely inflation of the lungs empties blood (and air) from the pulmonary veins into the left side of the heart. Alternatively, aspirating needles are inserted into the chambers of the heart in order to remove sequestered air. Under no circumstances is ejection allowed to occur before the air has been adequately eliminated, and sometimes an electrical fibrillator is used to prevent premature contraction.
2. An aspirating needle is placed in the highest point of the aorta before the clamp is removed. This eliminates air already in the aorta and also tends to remove bubbles that may be ejected subsequently.

However meticulous the attempt at air removal, there is likely to be some degree of systemic (and cerebral) air embolism. The effects of this could be minimised by the use of pure oxygen for ventilation during the first 15 minutes after the heart begins to eject, and perhaps by offering cerebral (steroid) prophylaxis with an avoidance of raised intracranial pressure in all patients subjected to extracorporeal circulation.

Accidental air embolism during extracorporeal circulation can occur if there is inadequate attention to the blood level in the reservoir, accidental detachment of the oxygenator or if there is defective equipment. Mills and Ochsner[48] advocate for massive air embolism during bypass, a deep Trendelenburg position, a stab-wound in the aorta for retrograde drainage from the cerebrovascular bed and temporary retrograde cerebral perfusion through the superior vena cava. Subsequent management should include resumption of extracorporeal circulation with an elevated perfusion pressure, steroids and deep barbiturate anaesthesia. In the thirteen cases managed in this way who suffered massive extracorporeal air embolism, four died instantly, two had transient cerebral injury but the remainder had no neurological sequelae.

Micro-emboli of platelet and white cell aggregates can also cause neurological sequelse, the incidence of which can be reduced by adequate filtration in the efferent arterial line from the pump.

### Lung Dysfunction Following Extracorporeal Circulation

Post-perfusion lung is the name given to a collection of syndromes which result from different causes. The common feature is that lung function is disturbed and there is a large alveolar-arterial difference in oxygen tension. Whereas in normal lungs the venous admixture effect in the lung is approximately 3 per cent of the cardiac output, after extracorporeal circulation this figure may rise as high as 30 per cent.[49] In the face of a low cardiac output the alveolar-arterial (A–a) $O_2$ tension difference may be large enough to make the patient hypoxic despite ventilation with pure oxygen.

The causes of lung disburbance are:

i. *Simple lung collapse*, usually of the left or right lower lobe and much commoner than usually thought. This will always respond to physiotherapy but is better prevented than treated.

ii. *Overdistension of pulmonary capillaries* at operation. Before the routine use of a left heart vent to decompress the left heart at operation, damage used to occur to the lung capillaries and at post-mortem the lungs appeared liver-like with the alveoli filled with haemorrhagic exudate. Intra-operative manoeuvres can, however, distort the pulmonary veins and lead to huge, albeit temporary, increases in pulmonary capillary pressure.

iii. *High left atrial pressure*. Gross damage to the pulmonary capillaries is now rare but pulmonary engorgement due to an excessively high left atrial pressure is not uncommon. This results from inappropriate efforts to increase the cardiac output by raising the filling pressure of the ventricles while measuring only the right atrial pressure. Quite huge and unpredictable differences can exist between the functions of the two ventricles and quite small increases in right atrial pressure can produce increases in the left sided pressure which will result in pulmonary oedema.[50]

iv. *Low colloid plasma oncotic pressure.* This can be reduced to 40 per cent of normal during extracorporeal circulation, principally by the effects of haemodilution, but sometimes by the accidental aspiration of cardioplegic or cooling solutions. The tendency towards pulmonary oedema in the face of only moderately raised pulmonary venous pressures is increased, and certainly is the cause of the increase in lung water which follows bypass.

v. *Surgical trauma.* Pneumothorax with subsequent atelectasis is not infrequent, and may require specific treatment afterwards. Very occasionally, pulmonary lymphatic or venous drainage is inadvertently compromised by surgical interference, and this may lead to pulmonary oedema in a classical anatomical distribution.

vi. *Chemical effects of extracorporeal circulation.* A number of responses to extracorporeal circulation may lead to pulmonary dysfunction. Complement activation seems to be among these and is frequently observed.[51,52] It is thought to contribute to the development of so-called post-pump syndromes. Complement activation stimulates polymorphonuclear granulocyte aggregation, encouraging pulmonary leuco-emboli,[53] and increases pulmonary capillary permeability, leading to interstitial oedema. These effects become more significant during long bypass procedures, and are particularly significant in patients with high left atrial pressures. High dose corticosteroids are advocated in order to modify complement activation, and should be considered for prophylactic therapy in high-risk cases. Other chemical responses include reduction in lung-surfactant, lysosomal enzyme release and the effects of endogenous histamine release, which can be drug induced, all of which may contribute to unexplained pulmonary pathology following extracorporeal circulation. So-called noncardiogenic pulmonary oedema is not infrequently observed in patients with normal left heart function following open-heart surgery; this probably represents an individual manifestation of a multi-factorial picture of increased lung sensitivity to acute damage caused by the total effects of cardio-pulmonary bypass.

## REFERENCES


1. Smith, L. W. and Fay, T. (1940). Observations on human beings with cancer maintained at reduced temperatures of 75–90° Fahrenheit. *Amer. J. clin. Path.*, **10**, 1.
2. Bigelow, W. G., Callaghan, J. C. and Tupps, J. A. (1950). General hypothermia for experimental intracardiac surgery. *Ann. Surg.*, **132**, 531.
3. Lewis, F. J. and Tauffic, M. (1953). Closure of atrial septal defects with the aid of hypothermia. *Surgery*, **33**, 52.
4. Drew, C. E., Keen, G. and Benazon, D. B. (1959). Profound hypothermia. *Lancet*, **1**, 745.
5. Horiuchi, T., Koyamada, K. and Matamo, I. (1963). Radical operation for ventricular septal defect in infancy. *J. thorac. cardiovasc. Surg.*, **46**, 180.
6. Mohri, H., Nessel, E. A., Nelson, R. J., Matano, I., Anderson, N. H., Dillard, D. H. and Merendino, K. A. (1966). Use of rheomacrodex and hyperventilation in prolonged circulatory arrest under deep hypothermia induced by surface cooling. *Amer. J. Surg.*, **112**, 241.
7. Niyazaki, M., Yoda, K., Tanaka, Y., Tsukawaki, Y., Ogli, K. (1980). A study of profound hypothermia by surface cooling. *Canad. Anaesth. Soc. J.* **27**, 370.
8. Williams, J. J. and Marshall, B. E. (1982). A fresh look at an old question. *Anesthesiology*, **56**, 1.
9. Rahn, H., Reeves, R. B. and Howell, B. J. (1975). Hydrogen ion regulation, temperature and evolution. *Amer. Rev. Respir. Dis.*, **112**, 165.
10. Mohri, H. and Merendino, K. A. (1969). In: *Hypothermia With or Without a Pump Oxygenator in Surgery of the Chest.* Ed. by Gibbon, Sabiston and Spencer. Philadelphia: W. B. Saunders.
11. Brown, T. C. K., Dunlop, M. E., Stevens, B. J., Clarke,

C. P. and Shanahan, E. A. (1973). Biochemical changes during surface cooling for deep hypothermia in open heart surgery. *J. thorac. cardiovasc. Surg.*, **65**, 402.
12. Fisk, G. C., Wright, J. S., Turner, B. B., Baker, W. de C. and Hicks, R. G. (1974) Cerebral effects of circulatory arrest at 20° C in the infant pig. *Anaesth. Intens. Care*, **2**, 33.
13. Editorial (1982). Brain damage after open heart surgery. *Lancet*, **1**, 1161.
14. Legallois, J. J. C. (1812). *Expériences sur le principe de la vie, notamment sur celui des mouvements du coeur, et sur le siège de ce principe*. Paris.
15. Brown-Séquard, E. (1858). Du sang rouge et du sang noir, et de leurs principaux éléments gazeuses, l'oxygène et l'acide carbonique. *J. Anat. (Paris)*, **1**, 95.
16. Ludwig, C. F. W. (1865). *Die physiologischen Leistungen des Blutdrucks*. Leipzig: S. Hirzel.
17. Schroder, W. (1882). Über die Bildungstatte des Harnstoffs. *Naunyn-Schmiedeberg's Arch. exp. Path. Pharmak.*, **15**, 364.
18. Jacoby, C. (1890). Apparat zur Durchblutung isolirter überlebender Organe. *Naunyn-Schmiedeberg's Arch. exp. Path. Pharmak.*, **26**, 388.
19. Brodie, T. G. (1903). The perfusion of surviving organs. *J. Physiol. (Lond.)*, **29**, 266.
20. Frey, M. and Gruber, M. (1885). Ein Respirationsapparatus für isolirte Organe. *Arch. Anat. Physiol.*, **9**, 519.
21. Gibbon, J. H. (1937). Artificial maintenance of circulation during experimental occlusion of the pulmonary artery. *Arch. Surg.*, **34**, 1105.
22. Schmidt-Mulheim, A. (1880). Beitrage zur Kenntniss des Peptons und seiner physiologischen Bedeutung. *Arch. Anat. Physiol., Lpz.* (Physiol. Abt.). p. 33.
23. Waters, E. T., Markowitz, J. and Jaques, L. B. (1938). Anaphylaxis in the liverless dog, and observations on anticoagulant effect of anaphylactic shock. *Science*, **87**, 582.
24. Feldman, S. A. (1971). Profound hypothermia. *Brit. J. Anaesth.*, **43**, 244.
25. De Wall, R. A., Warden, H. E., Varco, R. L. and Lillehei, C. W. (1957). Helix reservoir pump oxygenator. *Surg. Gynec Obstet.*, **104**, 699.
26. Wright,.J. S., Torda, T. A. and Hicks, R. G. (1975). Some advantages of the membrane oxygenator for open-heart surgery. *J. Thorac. Cardiovasc. Surg.*, **69**, 884.
27. Branthwaite, M. A. (1973). Factors affecting cerebral activity during open-heart surgery. *Anaesthesia*, **28**, 619.
28. Schwartz, M. S., Colvin, M. P., Prior, P. F., Strunin, L., Simpson, B.R., Weaver, E. J. M. and Scott, D. F. (1973). The cerebral function monitor. *Anaesthesia*, **28**, 611.
29. Estes, J. W. (1980). Clinical pharmacokinetics of heparin. *Clin. Pharmacokinetics*, **5**, 204.
30. Chung, F., David, T. E. and Watt, J. (1981). Excessive requirement for heparin during cardiac surgery. *Canad. Anaesth. Soc. J.*, **28**, 280.
31. Seltzer, J. L. and Gerson, J. I. (1979). Decrease in arterial pressure following heparin injection prior to cardiopulmonary bypass. *Acta Anaesth. Scand.* **23**, 575.
32. Desmond, P. V., Roberts, R. K., Wood, A. J. J., Dunn, G. D., Wilkinson, G. R. Schenker, S. (1980). Effect of heparin administration on plasma binding of benzodiazepines. *Brit. J. Clin. Pharmacol.*, **9**, 171.
33. Wood, M., Shand, D. G., Wood, A. J. J. (1979). Propranolol binding in plasma during cardiopulmonary bypass. *Anesthesiology*, **51**, 512.
34. Longmore, D. B., Bennett, G., Gueirrara, D., Smith, M., Bunting, S., Moncada, S., Reed, P., Read, N. G. and Vane, J. R. (1979). Prostacyclin: a solution to some problems of extracorporeal circulation. *Lancet*, **1**, 1002.
35. Conahan, T. J., Andrews, R. W. and Macvaugh, H. (1981). Cardiovascular effects of protamine sulfate in man. *Anesth. Analg.*, **60**, 33.
36. Iwatsuki, N., Matsukawa, S. and Iwatsuki, K. (1980). A weak negative inotropic effect of protamine sulfate upon isolated canine heart muscle. *Anesth. Analg.*, **59**, 100.
37. Jones, R. M., Hill, A. B., Nahrwold, M. L. and Tait, A. R. (1981). Effect of protamine on plasma ionised calcium in the dog. *Canad. Anaesth. Soc. J.*, **29**, 65.
38. Knape, J. T. A., Schuller, J. L., deHaan, P., De Jong, A. P. and Bovill, A. P. (1981). An anaphylactic reaction to protamine in a patient allergic to fish. *Anesthesiology*, **55**, 324.
39. Moorthy, S. S., Pond, W. P. and Rowland, R. G. (1980). Severe circulatory shock following protamine. (An anaphylactic reaction.) *Anesth. Analg.*, **59**, 77.
40. Westhorpe, R. N., Varghese, Z., Petrie, A., Wills, M. R. and Lumley, J. (1978). Changes in ionised calcium and other plasma constituents associated with cardiopulmonary bypass. *Brit. J. Anaesth.*, **50**, 951.
41. Manners, J. M. and Nielsen, M. S. (1981). Magnesium flux during open heart surgery: the effect of St. Thomas' Hospital cardioplegia solution. *Anaesthesia*, **36**, 157.
42. deLeon, R. S., Paterson, J. L. and Sykes, M. K. (1980). Changes in colloid osmotic pressure and plasma albumin associated with extracorporeal circulation. *Brit. J. Anaesth.*, **52**, 630P.
43. Petch, M. C., McKay, R. and Bethune, D. W. (1981). The effect of beta$_2$ adrenergic blockade on serum potassium and glucose levels during open heart surgery. *European Heart J.*, **2**, 123.
44. Yamashita, M., Wakayama, S., Matsuki, A., Kudo, M. and Oyama, T. (1982). Plasma catecholamine levels during extracorporeal circulation in children. *Canad. Anaesth. Soc. J.*, **29**, 126.
45. Chatrath, R. R., Kaul, T. K. and Walker, D. R. (1980). Myocardial protection during cardioplegia in open-heart surgery: a review. *Canad. Anaesth. Soc. J.*, **4**, 381.
46. Noback, C. and Tinker, J. (1980). Hypothermia after cardiopulmonary bypass in man. *Anesthesiology*, **53**, 277.
47. Crawford, R. D. (1982). Hypothermia after cardiopulmonary bypass in man. *Anesthesiology*, **56**, 1234.
48. Mills, N. L. and Ochsner, J. L. (1980). Massive air embolism during cardiopulmonary bypass. *J. Thorac. Cardiovasc. Surg*, **80**, 708.
49. Fordham, R. (1965). Hypoxaemia after aortic valve surgery under cardiopulmonary bypass. *Thorax*, **20**, 505.
50. Sarin, C. L., Yalav, E., Clement, A. J. and Braimbridge, M. V. (1970). The necessity for measurement of left atrial pressure after cardiac valve surgery. *Thorax*, **25**, 185.
51. Chenoweth, D. E., Cooper, S. W., Hugli, T. E., Stewart, R. W., Blackstone, E. H. and Kicklin, J. W. (1981). Complement activation during cardiopulmonary bypass. *New Eng. J. Med.*, **304**, 497.
52. Haslam, P. L., Townsend, P. J. and Branthwaite, M. A. (1980). Complement activation during cardiopulmonary bypass. *Anaesthesia*, **35**, 22.
53. Hammerschmidt, D. E., Weaver, L. J., Hudson, L. D., Craddock, P. R. and Jacob, H. S. (1980). Association of complement activation and elevated plasma–C5a with adult respiratory distress syndrome. *Lancet*, **1**, 947.

CHAPTER 16

# Body Water, Electrolytes and Parenteral Fluid Therapy



FLUIDS given parenterally include water and electrolytes, blood and blood substitutes, and solutions used in parenteral nutrition. In this chapter only water and electrolytes are considered. The therapeutic use of blood and blood substitutes is discussed in Chapter 17, parenteral nutrition in Chapter 10 and fluid therapy in infants and children in Chapter 41.

## BODY FLUIDS

*Total body water* can be measured by dilutional techniques using deuterium oxide, tritiated water or urea.[1] The proportion of body weight as water is greatest at birth and decreases with age (Table 1). There is a lot of variation between individuals, but mean values are greater in men than women. This is probably related to differences in the proportion of adipose tissue which has a water content of only 25–30 per cent.[2] Body water is divided between the intracellular and extracellular fluid.

*Extracellular fluid* (ECF) volume is difficult to measure. Dilutional techniques, using either crystalloids such as mannitol, inulin or sucrose, or isotopic markers such as $^{82}Br$, $^{36}Cl$ or $^{35}S$ labelled thiosulphate and sulphate, have given widely varying results. The crystalloid methods underestimate the ECF because of slow equilibration within connective tissue, cartilage and bone, and are made more complex because allowance must be made for losses into the urine. Monovalent radioisotopes overestimate the ECF because some of the isotope also enters cells. Radioisotope labelled divalent or polyvalent ions probably offer the most accurate marker for dilutional methods of estimating the volume of the ECF, being widely distributed but remaining almost completely in the extracellular compartment.

Edelman and Liebman[3] in their classic review of the anatomy of body fluids called that part of the extravascular ECF that rapidly reached equilibrium with crystalloid markers the "interstitial lymph". This forms about 20 per cent of total body water and is that part of the ECF which is in dynamic equilibrium with plasma.

The transcapillary movement of water is governed by the balance of hydrostatic and osmotic forces. These were defined by Starling in 1896[4] and subsequently expressed in the form shown in Fig. 1. The four pressures in the

16/Table 1.
Variation of Total Body Water (Expressed as a Percentage of Body Weight) in Normal Man with Age and Sex.

| *Age* | *Males* | *Females* |
|---|---|---|
| 10–16 years | 58·9 | 57·3 |
| 17–39 years | 60·6 | 50·2 |
| 40–59 years | 54·7 | 46·7 |
| 60+ | 51·5 | 45·5 |

(Courtesy of Dr. M. W. B. Bradbury, and MacMillan Journals Ltd.[2])

equation—$P_c$, $P_{IF}$, $\pi_p$ and $\pi_{IF}$—are often called the "Starling forces". The balance of Starling forces usually leads to filtration of fluid from the capillaries to the interstitium. Fluid is returned to the vascular compartment through the lymphatics. The way in which alteration of the Starling forces affects fluid filtration has been considered in detail by Civetta.[5] Ions and small molecules can move rapidly between the interstitial fluid and plasma so changes in the composition of plasma, for example, are rapidly equilibrated throughout the ECF.

*Intracellular fluid volume* is estimated from the difference between total body water and the extracellular volume. Because of the difficulties in measuring ECF volume estimates of the ratio of intracellular to extracellular fluid vary from 3:1 to almost 1:1 with a ratio of 55:45 being widely quoted.[3] There are considerable differences in the composition of extracellular and intracellular fluid (ICF) as shown in Table 2. For the intracellular volume to remain constant ECF and ICF must be isotonic. In addition, both ECF and ICF must have the cationic and anionic charges in balance, but in ICF many of the anions are in the form of large molecules to

$$V = K_f S \left[ (P_c - P_{IF}) - \sigma(\pi_p - \pi_{IF}) \right]$$

| | | |
|---|---|---|
| $V$ | : | rate of movement of water |
| $K_f$ | : | capillary filtration coefficient |
| $S$ | : | area of the capillary bed |
| $P_c$ and $P_{IF}$ | : | capillary and interstitial fluid hydrostatic pressures |
| $\sigma$ | : | reflection coefficient for protein molecules |
| $\pi_p$ and $\pi_{IF}$ | : | the plasma and interstitial fluid oncotic pressure |

16/Fig. 1.—A mathematical expression of Starling's hypothesis.

16/Table 2
Comparison of the Composition of Extracellular and Intracellular Fluid.

| | *Extracellular fluid* | *Intracellular fluid* |
|---|---|---|
| Sodium | 140 mmol/l | 12 mmol/l |
| Potassium | 4 mmol/l | 155 mmol/l |
| Magnesium | 1 mmol/l | 28 mmol/l |
| Chloride | 100 mmol/l | 10 mmol/l |
| Bicarbonate | 28 mmol/l | 10 mmol/l |
| Phosphate | 1 mmol/l | 105 mmol/l |
| pH | 7·4 | 7·0 |

which the cell membrane is impermeable. The most abundant cations in the body are sodium and potassium. Cell membranes are relatively impermeable to sodium which is actively removed from cells by the sodium pump so that sodium is largely restricted to the ECF. On the other hand, cell membranes are freely permeable to potassium and also to chloride. Osmotic and electrical equality are achieved by having a relatively high intracellular concentration of potassium and a low concentration of chloride.

### Osmolality, Tonicity and Colloid Osmotic Pressure

Osmolality is a measure of the particle concentration in solution and strictly speaking should be expressed in terms of osmoles per kilogram of solvent. In clinical practice there is little difference between osmolality and osmolarity which refers to concentration per litre of solution. This is because of the small temperature range and low solute concentrations of body fluids. Adding the molar concentrations of the ions in plasma gives a calculated osmolality of 310 mOsm/kg. When measured directly the normal plasma osmolality is 285±5 mOsm/kg. The difference is a result of the number of "free" particles being less than the theoretical value because of interionic and other effects in the complex solution of plasma.[6]

A solution is isotonic if cells that are suspended in it do not change their volume. Isotonic fluids have similar particle concentrations but do not necessarily have the same chemical composition. Solutions that are isotonic with plasma include 0·9 per cent sodium chloride, 5 per cent dextrose and Hartmann's solution.

Normal plasma with a total protein concentration of approximately 70 g/l has a colloid osmotic or oncotic pressure (COP) of about 25 mm Hg.[7]

Albumin accounts for 67–75 per cent of COP with most of the remainder being due to globulin and fibrinogen.

### Maintenance of Extracellular Volume and Composition

The volume of ECF is kept remarkably constant despite large variations in salt and water intake. Homeostasis is achieved through mechanisms that act to maintain the osmolality of ECF. The reason for such vigorous defence of osmolality is not immediately clear, but may be related to the optimum performance of intracellular reactions involving protein and electron transfer.[8] The physiological mechanisms that control the osmolality of extracellular fluid also affect intracellular volume. That is, as long as the cellular content of osmotically active solutes remains constant, keeping the ECF osmolality constant stabilises cell volume. A number of physicochemical and biological mechanisms act to maintain the cellular content of osmotically active solutes[9] so if ECF osmolality decreases water must enter the cells. Conversely, if ECF osmolality increases due to an increase in solutes that penetrate cell membranes poorly, cellular volume will decrease.

The major determinant of ECF osmolality is sodium, so it is the quantity of sodium in the ECF that determines the volume of this compartment.[10] Control of ECF osmolality is integrated within the hypothalamus. The mechanisms through which this control is achieved include the following.

**Thirst.**—Social and personal habits rather than thirst usually determine the timing and quantity of fluid intake. This is normally greater than the minimum required, but an intake insufficient to replace losses or an increase in the solute load causes the sensation of thirst.[11,12]

**Antidiuretic hormone** is a nine amino-acid peptide with a molecular weight of 1,084 Daltons. It is formed in the cells of the supra-optic and paraventricular nuclei and subsequently passes down into the posterior pituitary.[13] Antidiuretic hormone (ADH) controls water excretion by regulating the water permeability of the renal tubular cells lining the collecting ducts. This allows urine to be produced with a wide range of osmolalities: 50 or 100—1000 or 1200 mOsm/kg. ADH release is modulated by changes in both the volume and osmolality of ECF.

Changes in ECF volume are sensed by a number of receptors.[10] Receptors sensitive to variations in either mechanical stretch or transmural pressure have been described in the atria, ventricles and great vessels. Stimuli from these receptors travel via cranial nerves IX and X to the hypothalamic and medullary centres that initiate the physiological responses of altered ADH release, altered renal sympathetic tone and changes in the tone of pre- and post-capillary resistance vessels. Other volume receptors have been described in the arteries, kidneys and central nervous system. The carotid sinus is sensitive to changes in arterial pressure. A decrease in arterial pressure causes an increase in sympathetic tone and activates the renin-angiotensin system.[14]

There are no volume receptors in the interstitium but under most circumstances the volume of interstitial fluid remains fairly constant. The volume of interstitial fluid is to a large extent self adjusting as a result of structural resistance to volume changes, self adjustment of the Starling forces and automatic adjustment of lymph according to local demands.[15] If, as a result of increased hydrostatic pressure or decreased plasma oncotic pressure, more fluid passes from capillaries to the interstitium, lymphatic flow is increased to remove the extra fluid. Oedema occurs when the lymphatics can no longer keep pace with the rate of fluid loss from the capillaries.

A series of experiments by Verney[16] and his associates led to the conclusion that osmoreceptors in the anterior hypothalamus or pre-optic area of the brain controlled the release of antidiuretic hormone. More recent review of this work has revealed some inconsistencies and while there is some additional evidence to support the existence of both cerebral and peripheral osmoreceptors their precise role and influence on ADH release remain uncertain.[17] Most authors, however, still believe that regulation of ADH is primarily by osmotic stimuli with non-osmotic factors affecting the threshold and sensitivity.

Other factors may stimulate ADH release and so interfere with the control of water excretion. These include pain, emotional stress, hyperthermia and drugs such as opiates, barbiturates and sulphonylureas.

**Renal sodium excretion.**—While thirst and antidiuretic hormone control the intake and excretion of water respectively the content of urine is largly determined by mechanisms acting within the kidney. These have been reviewed by Skorecki and Brenner.[10] Urinary sodium excretion is affected by both changes in glomerular filtration rate (GFR) and tubular reabsorption of sodium. Expansion of ECF volume causes an increase in GFR, probably by resetting the normal feed-back control of GFR,[18] so increasing the distal delivery of salt and water. However, ECF volume expansion causes large increases in sodium excretion even in the face of a reduced GFR, demonstrating the overriding effect of those factors that affect tubular reabsorption of sodium. These include:

*Renal sympathetic tone.*—Increased sympathetic tone results in diminished sodium excretion.

*Renin - angiotensin - aldosterone system.*—Angiotensin II may increase sodium reabsorption either directly or by effects on renovascular tone that change the Starling forces in peritubular capillaries. These forces, to a large extent, determine the amount of fluid reabsorbed from the proximal tubule. Angiotensin II also causes the release of aldosterone from the adrenal cortex. Aldosterone then acts on the collecting ducts to increase net sodium reabsorption.

**Prostaglandins** appear to have an important role in the control of renal blood flow and may also have an effect on sodium excretion as a result of changes in peritubular Starling forces.

**Kallikrein-kinin system.**—This also affects renovascular responses but its role in sodium excretion is unclear.

**Natriuretic hormone** has yet to be identified but is postulated to reduce tubular reabsorption of sodium and enhance its excretion.

To summarise, the GFR, sympathetic tone, and, through their effect on peritubular Starling forces, angiotensin II and perhaps prostaglandins, determine the volume and constitution of filtrate reaching the collecting ducts. Here the volume and composition are adjusted by the effects of ADH and aldosterone (Fig. 2). These mechanisms can vary urinary sodium excretion from 1 or 2 mmol/l if the body is depleted of sodium to 200 mmol/l after a sodium load.[19]

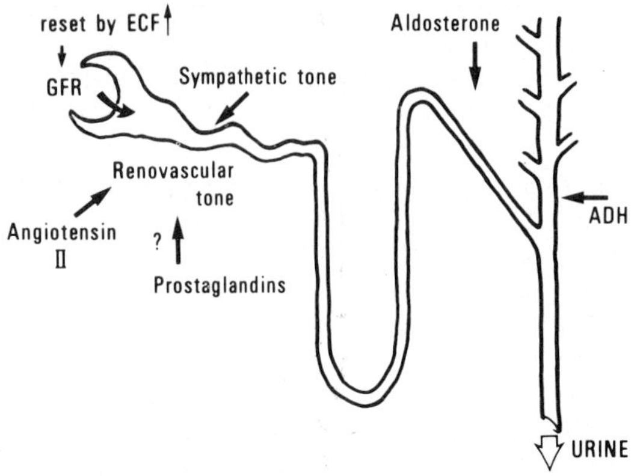


16/FIG. 2.—Factors determining salt and water excretion.

## WATER BALANCE

Water is gained from fluids, food and as an end product of metabolism. The water of metabolism is normally about 500 ml/day. Water intake is balanced by losses through the skin, lungs, faeces and urine. Losses from the skin are about 500 ml in a cool environment but increase considerably during sweating. Evaporative water loss from the respiratory tract accounts for about 700 ml and faeces for a further 50 ml/day. Healthy kidneys can increase the osmolality of urine to over 1000 mOsm/kg. Even during fasting the solute load to be excreted by the kidneys is of the order of 400 mOsm/day, demanding a urine volume of at least 400 ml. Therefore, to maintain water balance a minimum of about 1200 ml/day is required.

It follows that conventional "fluid balance" charts are a relatively poor guide to the true state of water balance. Changes in body weight and clinical assessment are often more useful.

### Water Overload

It is difficult to drink at a rate faster than water can be excreted by normal kidneys. Occasionally this happens in mental disorders associated with compulsive water or beer drinking, but the most common causes of "water intoxication" are inappropriate secretion of antidiuretic hormone, renal disease, glucocorticoid deficiency (Addison's disease) or anterior pituitary failure (see also p. 994). Inappropriate secretion of ADH may be associated with recent surgery, head injuries, malignant tumours, lung disease,[20] and positive-pressure ventilation.

Water overload reduces the osmolality of intracellular and extracellular fluids equally. The increase in cell volume has its greatest effect on the brain. The most prominent symptoms include nausea, vomiting, headache, drowsiness, and eventually coma, convulsions and death if treatment is not given. The serum sodium is generally less than 120 mmol/l by the time symptoms occur. Apart from correcting the underlying cause, when possible, the mainstay of treatment is water restriction. Obligatory water losses then ensure the osmolality of body fluids returns towards normal. Patients with prolonged inappropriate ADH secretion who will not restrict their fluid intake have been treated with lithium,[21] demeclocycline,[22] urea[23] and frusemide.[24]

### Water Depletion

Predominant water depletion is uncommon but may be seen:

- in those isolated in a waterless environment or when a patient is unable to respond to thirst because of impaired consciousness, sedation, severe illness or dysphagia;
- in those unable to compensate for the urinary water losses due to diabetes insipidus or an osmotic diuresis induced by hyperglycaemia, particularly in the absence of ketosis.

More commonly water and sodium depletion occur together (see below).

The major symptom of water depletion in a conscious person is thirst. Other clinical features occur only when dehydration is advanced. They include oliguria and a falling blood pressure because of reduced extracellular fluid volume, and cerebral disturbances including drowsiness, confusion and coma related to loss of intracellular water. Treatment is by oral fluids or 5 per cent dextrose infusion in those unable to drink. If the patient has been severely dehydrated with a plasma sodium 160–180 mmol/l, rehydration should be extended over 24 to 48 hours to avoid rapid changes in cerebral hydration which may lead to intracranial haemorrhages.

## SODIUM BALANCE

The sodium content of a man weighing 70 kg is about 4000 mmol. To maintain sodium balance an amount of sodium almost equal to that ingested is excreted in the urine. The mechanism by which this is achieved has been discussed above. The dietary intake in Australia is approximately 150 mmol/day[14] but there is a large variation between individuals and in different parts of the world.

The normal plasma concentration of sodium is 134–143 mmol/l.

### Sodium Excess

Sodium excess is usually associated with retention of an equivalent amount of water and chloride. The most common clinical feature is oedema reflecting the increased volume of ECF. Sodium excess occurs:

*in congestive cardiac failure*, a reduced cardiac output producing the same physiological responses as hypovolaemia, that is, salt and water retention.[25]

*in association with hypoalbuminaemia.* When plasma oncotic pressure falls the net Starling forces increase the loss of fluid from the capillaries to the interstitial space and therefore a fall in blood volume. The body responds by retaining salt and water. In many of the diseases in which hypoalbuminaemia and oedema coexist, such as the nephrotic syndrome, it is likely that increased capillary permeability contributes to the oedema.

*in renal failure* when sodium intake exceeds excretion.

*in primary hyperaldosteronism.*

*after infusion of excessive amounts of saline* or other salt solutions or when these have been used for resuscitation of hypovolaemic patients.

The plasma sodium may be normal, increased or decreased depending on the amount of water retained.

Treatment consists of correction of the underlying cause where possible, restriction of sodium intake and diuretics. When sodium excess is associated with hypoalbuminaemia diuretics must be used very carefully because the blood volume tends to be low and further loss of blood volume may reduce cardiac output causing hypotension and oliguric renal failure.

### Sodium Depletion

Sodium depletion is usually associated with loss of water and chloride so that ECF volume is reduced. The clinical features include loss of skin turgor, collapsed peripheral veins and postural hypotension. Hypovolaemic shock ultimately leads to death. Sodium depletion occurs:

*from excessive sweating* before acclimatisation

*from gastro-intestinal losses* during prolonged vomiting, diarrhoea or from small-bowel fistulae

*from excessive renal losses* in, for example, Addison's disease, after relief of urinary obstruction, diabetes mellitus or excessive use of diuretics.

The plasma sodium may be normal, or low if salt and water losses caused by excessive sweating or gastro-intestinal loss have been replaced by water alone. Plasma, urea and creatinine are increased, both as a result of haemoconcentration and reduced renal blood flow. The physiological responses include oliguria and sodium conservation. The low urinary sodium concentration helps to distinguish this from the oliguria of intrinsic renal failure.

Treatment is by saline infusion to correct the salt and water deficit. Patients with Addison's disease need steroid replacement therapy.

### Hyponatraemia

Kennedy and co-workers[26] found that hyponatraemia with a plasma sodium concentration of less than 125 mmol/l occurred in 0·9 per cent of medical admissions and 0·4 per cent of surgical admissions to a general hospital. The pathophysiology of hyponatraemia has been reviewed by Thompson.[19] It may be caused by sodium depletion, water retention or a combination of these (see above). In the study by Kennedy and associates[26] in hospital in-patients 41 per cent of cases of hyponatraemia were iatrogenic and caused by diuretics, postoperative infusion of 5 per cent dextrose (see below) or both. Of the others, 25 per cent were associated with chest disease and 23 per cent with gastro-intestinal or renal salt and water loss.

Severe acute hyponatraemia is associated with a mortality of up to 50 per cent. Rapid correction of the sodium concentration by giving both frusemide and hypertonic saline appears to reduce both mortality and persisting neurological damage from severe hyponatraemia.[27]

*"Sick cell syndrome."*—Hyponatraemia is very common in seriously ill patients. Flear and Singh[28] reviewed the evidence suggesting that "sick cells" caused this because of their increased membrane permeability to sodium and decreased active removal of sodium from the cells by the energy-dependent cation exchange pump. They suggest a number of clinical and biochemical features that enable the syndrome to be distinguished from inappropriate ADH secretion but note that plasma ADH levels may also be raised in patients with the "sick cell" syndrome. Certainly raised plasma ADH levels are common in hyponatraemic patients, whatever the underlying cause.[29]

## POTASSIUM BALANCE

Potassium is the major intracellular cation. Alterations in intracellular or extracellular potassium concentration affect nerve, muscle and other excitable tissues because the membrane potential varies directly with the intracellular : extracellular potassium ratio. An average daily diet contains 60–100 mmol of potassium and to maintain a balance a similar amount is excreted, mostly in the urine. Less than 2 per cent of the body's potassium content is in the ECF. Intracellular potassium may be considerably depleted in the presence of a normal or even a high plasma concentration. The normal plasma concentration of potassium is 3·5–5 mmol/l.

Absorption of potassium from the bowel into the ECF is passive. The total amount of potassium in the ECF is less than the average daily intake, so a potassium load must be cleared rapidly from this compartment. The physiological mechanisms that contribute to this are summarised in Fig. 3.

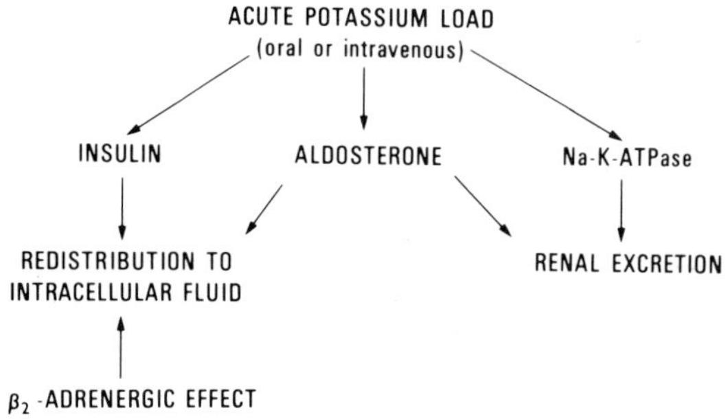


16/Fig. 3.—Summary of the factors which tend to prevent hyperkalaemia after an acute potassium load. (Courtesy of Dr. J. R. Stockigt and the Australian Society of Anaesthetists[38])

**Insulin.**—Potassium stimulates the release of both insulin and glucagon so that potassium is removed from the extracellular fluid without any marked change in blood sugar.[30] It is generally thought that the fall in potassium concentration is a result of glucose entry into cells, but there is some evidence that potassium influx or reduced efflux of potassium from cells is a direct effect of insulin.[31]

**$B_2$-adrenergic effects.**—Both adrenaline[32] and isoprenaline[33] have been shown to lower plasma potassium. This effect appears to be mediated through $B_2$-adrenergic receptors and has been used therapeutically in hyperkalaemic periodic paralysis managed by inhalation of salbutamol.[34]

**Aldosterone** is principally involved in sodium conservation, but an increase in plasma potassium concentration is also a potent stimulus to its release by an action independent of the renin-angiotensin system. Aldosterone increases potassium excretion mainly by stimulating the active transport of potassium from peritubular fluid into the cells of the distal convoluted tuble and enhancing the luminal permeability to potassium.[30]

**Sodium-Potassium-ATPase** in the collecting ducts is directly induced by potassium.

In contrast to the body's ability to clear potassium its ability to conserve potassium is very limited but if potassium intake is restricted the urinary potassium loss slowly reduces to 20–30 mmol/day.

### Effect of Acid-base Balance

It is well recognised that acidosis causes an increase in plasma potassium concentration and that in alkalosis potassium moves into the cells so the plasma concentration falls. A 0·6 mmol/l change in plasma potassium for each 0·1 unit change in pH is widely quoted.[35] More recent evidence suggests that a large number of factors other than just the change in hydrogen ion concentration affect the distribution of potassium between extracellular and intracellular fluid during acid-base disorders.[36]

During metabolic acidosis renal hydrogen ion excretion is usually increased and the excretion of potassium diminished. Conversely, metabolic alkalosis is associated with an increased loss of potassium into the urine until the body is potassium depleted and the plasma concentration falls. Potassium ions are then conserved and hydrogen ion excretion rises. This causes the paradoxical aciduria seen in severe hypokalaemic metabolic alkalosis.

### Hyperkalaemia

Hyperkalaemia is a potentially life-threatening clinical problem. It may occur:

- in acute or chronic renal failure
- in respiratory or metabolic acidosis
- in Addison's disease, usually only a small rise in potassium concentration
- iatrogenically because of an excessive rate of infusion of potassium salts, excessive oral or intravenous supplements, or from potasssium-sparing diuretics such as spironolactone, amiloride and triamterene
- as one of the manifestations of the "crush syndrome"
- during massive haemolysis caused, for example, by mismatched blood transfusion or during massive transfusion of old, stored blood
- during anaesthesia if suxamethonium is given to patients with burns, muscle trauma or spinal-cord lesions,[37] or if the patient develops malignant hyperpyrexia
- in the rare condition of hyperkalaemic periodic paralysis.

The effects of hyperkalaemia are on the neuromuscular system and the heart but patients can be completely asymptomatic with a plasma potassium concentration sufficient to cause cardiac arrest. It is unusual for neuromuscular effects to occur until the concentration is greater than 8mmol/l. The effects include paraesthesiae, decreased or absent tendon reflexes and muscular weakness which may be mild or severe enough to cause a flaccid quadriplegia.

The earliest change in the electrocardiogram resulting from hyperkalaemia is peaking of the T waves. This can occur with a concentration of 5·5 mmol/l but is not an invariable feature. As the potassium concentration rises the QRS complex widens and the P waves become lower and wider with a prolonged PR interval, ultimately becoming unidentifiable (Fig. 4). Hyperkalaemia may be complicated by ventricular fibrillation and cardiac arrest.

*Treatment* should be instituted immediately if the plasma potassium concentration is greater than 6–6·5 mmol/l. The plasma urea, electrolytes, blood sugar and acid-base balance should also be checked and it is important to exclude spurious hyperkalaemia caused by haemolysis, thrombocytosis, massive leukocytosis and forearm exercise during venous occlusion.[38] Apart from correcting the underlying cause when this is possible the specific treatment includes:

- *calcium*, as 10 ml of 10 per cent calcium gluconate given over 2–3 minutes, opposes the membrane depolarizing effects of hyperkalaemia and therefore reduces the risk of life-threatening dysrhythmias. Its effect is almost immediate but it does not alter the potassium concentration.
- *correction of systemic acidosis* with intravenous bicarbonate has been described as, "The fastest, safest and most reliable way of correcting hyperkalaemia".[38] The sodium load may, however, be a problem if the patient is already salt and water overloaded as commonly occurs in renal failure.
- *glucose loading*. 50 ml of 50 per cent dextrose with 5 units of soluble insulin injected over 10 minutes has proved effective but some would suggest that the insulin is unnecessary unless the patient is diabetic.
- *methods to increase potassium excretion*. These include:
  1. ion exchange resins in the sodium or calcium phase that may be given orally or in the form of enemas.
  2. an induced diuresis if fluid balance permits.
  3. peritoneal or haemodialysis.

### Hypokalaemia

Hypokalaemia is usually caused by increased losses of potassium from either the gastro-intestinal tract or in the urine. Gastro-intestinal potassium loss may come from prolonged vom-

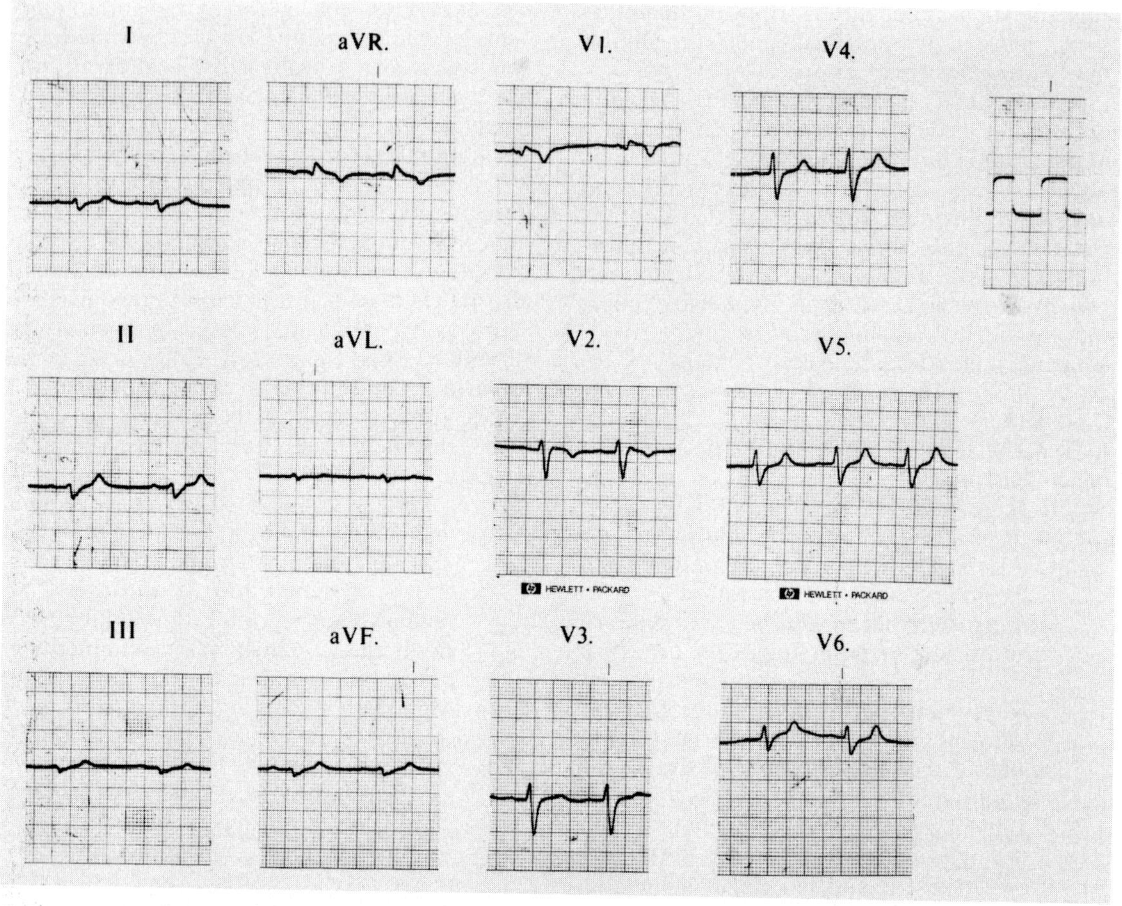


16/Fig. 4.—The electrocardiogram from a patient with a plasma potassium concentration of 7·3 mmol/l. The P waves are flattened, there is a prolonged PR interval and widening of the QRS complex. Peaking of the T waves is not an invariable feature of hyperkalaemia.

iting, diarrhoea, laxative abuse, uretero-sigmoidostomy and in rare cases from mucus-secreting neoplasms. The commonest cause of increased urinary loss is diuretic therapy with either thiazides or the potent loop diuretics such as frusemide. Excessive urinary loss also occurs in metabolic and respiratory alkalosis, uncontrolled diabetes mellitus, renal tubular acidosis, hyperaldosteronism and during treatment with high dose steroids or carbenoxolone. In severe cases the body potassium deficiency can amount to 1000 mmol.

Moderate hypokalaemia is often symptomless. When severe, and especially when the potassium concentration is less than 2·5 mmol/l, muscle weakness, abdominal distension with an ileus or pseudo-obstruction, impaired renal function with polyuria because of reduced concentrating ability and cardiac dysrhythmias become progressively more likely. The cardiac dysrhythmias, which may be the cause of sudden death in hypokalaemic patients, are potentiated by concurrent treatment with digoxin. Another important drug interaction is with non-depolarizing neuromuscular blocking drugs to which hypokalaemic patients are abnormally sensitive.

The plasma potassium concentration is, of course, reduced in hypokalaemia, but the plasma concentration may remain normal despite considerable depletion of the body potassium content. The other important biochemical finding is a raised plasma bicarbonate reflecting the extracellular alkalosis of potassium depletion.

The electrocardiogram is altered by hypokalaemia. The T waves become broader and flatter and the U waves more prominent. In severe hypokalaemia ST depression can be seen (see also Chapter 12, p. 422).

*Treatment.*—Hypokalaemia associated with diuretics can be prevented by giving oral potassium supplements or using a potassium-sparing diuretic such as amiloride, triamterene or spironolactone concurrently. These same oral potassium supplements can be used to treat mild or moderate hypokalaemia. A number of different preparations are available commercially in the form of elixirs and slow-release or effervescent tablets. Very severe cases require intravenous replacement of potassium both for rapidity of effect and because of the almost invariable altered bowel function. It must be remembered, however, that the extracellular potassium pool is very small and easily overloaded. For this reason it is desirable to monitor the electrocardiogram if potassium is to be infused at rates greater than 10 mmol/hour. An additional problem is the intense pain which may be caused when potassium salts are infused through a peripheral vein.

## CALCIUM BALANCE

Most of the calcium in the body, an average of about 25,000 mmol, is contained in bone. Calcium also has important roles in neuromuscular activity, coagulation and in the activation of a number of enzyme systems. Only about 35 mmol is in the extracellular fluid. The concentration of calcium in extracellular fluid is maintained by number of homeostatic mechanisms involving parathyroid hormone, 1,25-dihydroxycholecalciferol and calcitonin.[39] These act to control the rate of calcium absorption or deposition in bone, the absorption of calcium from the bowel and its excretion through the kidney. A normal daily diet contains about 25 mmol of calcium. The average losses amount to about 19 mmol in the faeces and 6 mmol in the urine.

A normal plasma calcium concentration is 2·25 to 2·65 mmol/l. This is present in more than one physical form. The metabolically active ionized fraction accounts for about 50 per cent and the remainder consists of protein bound (40 per cent) and complexed forms (10 per cent). Protein bound calcium can readily be dissociated by, for example, an increase in hydrogen ion concentration. Alkalosis on the other hand, causes a shift of calcium from the ionized to the protein-bound fraction. The total plasma calcium is affected by the plasma protein concentration, and particularly that of albumin. Formulae to allow the correction of plasma calcium for albumin concentration have been published with correction factors varying from 0·018 mmol calcium/g albumin to 0·025 mmol/g. Much of the controversy concerning calcium correction factors is probably accounted for by variation between individuals.[40]

### Hypercalcaemia

The symptoms of hypercalcaemia are non-specific and do not usually appear until the calcium concentration is greater than 3·5 mmol/l. They include general malaise, nausea, vomiting, constipation, polyuria and mental disturbances. The most common causes are bone metastases and hyperparathyroidism. Vitamin D intoxication, thyrotoxicosis and sarcoidosis account for most of the other cases.

Hypercalcaemia causes shortening of the Q–T interval on the electrocardiogram.

The treatment of hypercalcaemia was reviewed by Wills[41] and in an Editorial.[42] Calcium excretion can be increased by inducing a diuresis with frusemide and replacing the sodium, potassium and water losses. Corticosteroids reduce plasma calcium levels except in hyperparathyroidism. Grossly elevated plasma calcium levels may cause coma and cardiac dysrhythmias. The emergency treatment may include intravenous infusion of phosphate, EDTA,* mithramycin (an anti-tumour agent) or calcitonin.

### Hypocalcaemia

The classical symptom of a reduction in plasma ionized calcium concentration is tetany associated with positive Chvostek's and Trousseau's signs. Laryngeal stridor, mental changes and convulsions can occur in more severe cases. Hypocalcaemia causes a prolongation of the Q–T interval on the electrocardiogram and may cause hazardous ventricular dysrhythmias.

* EDTA—Ethylenediamine tetra-acetic acid.

True hypocalcaemia must be distinguished from that caused by a low plasma albumin concentration (see above). True hypocalcaemia may be caused by a lack of vitamin D, malabsorption syndromes, hypoparathyroidism, uraemia (associated with a high phosphate) or excision of the parathyroids during thyroid or parathyroid surgery. Transient hypocalcaemia may occur during very rapid blood transfusion. A decrease in ionized calcium while the total remains constant is caused by the alkalosis of hyperventilation. Partial rebreathing rapidly returns the plasma pH to normal.

Symptomatic hypocalcaemia may be treated by slow injection of 10–20 ml of 10 per cent calcium gluconate. It is important to avoid extravasation during injection because calcium salts are extremely irritant and can cause local tissue necrosis. Repeated injections can be given as often as necessary until long-term treatment takes effect. The longer-term treatment includes oral calcium supplements and vitamin D.

## MAGNESIUM BALANCE

Magnesium is the fourth most plentiful cation in the body. Like potassium, most of it is intracellular. It is important for a number of enzyme systems and neuromuscular function. There is some evidence that magnesium protects the heart against myocardial necrosis and dysrhythmias,[43] providing a theoretical basis for its inclusion in the cold cardioplegia solution used during cardiac surgery.

An average daily diet contains 10–20 mmol of magnesium. The normal plasma concentration is 0·7–1·1 mmol/l. The factors regulating magnesium balance have been reviewed.[44] They include alterations in both absorption from the gastro-intestinal tract and renal excretion but the precise control of plasma concentration is poorly understood.

### Hypermagnesaemia

Renal failure is the commonest cause of hypermagnesaemia which may be exacerbated by magnesium containing antacids. The clinical features include central nervous system depression progressing to coma, hypotension and abnormal cardiac conduction causing electrocardiogram changes similar to hyperkalaemia. Life-threatening complications can be treated by opposing the effects of magnesium with calcium given intravenously.

### Hypomagnesaemia

Hypomagnesaemia has been described in a large number of conditions.[44] Of particular importance to the anaesthetist are its association with long term diuretic therapy[45] and open heart surgery, though the incidence is lower if magnesium-containing cardioplegia solution is used.

The clinical features include nausea, vomiting, diarrhoea, weakness, tetany, mental confusion, convulsions and cardiac dysrhythmias. The electrocardiogram changes include shortening of the PR interval, ST depression, prolongation of the Q-T interval and abnormalities of repolarization.

Treatment with magnesium supplements can be given orally or intravenously depending on the urgency of the situation. Magnesium chloride can be infused intravenously at a rate not exceeding 0·5 mmol/minute but may cause pain when given through peripheral veins.

## ANAESTHESIA, SURGERY AND FLUID BALANCE

The characteristic response to anaesthesia and surgery is sodium and water retention. In general, the tendency to retain water is related to the severity of surgery, becoming greater with more extensive operations. A number of factors may contribute to this:

1. Effects of anaesthetic agents on renal blood flow and glomerular filtration rate[46] (Chapter 36)
2. Effects of intra-operative hypotension or hypovolaemia on renal function
3. Increased sympathetic tone and circulating adrenaline levels causing renal vasoconstriction
4. The salt- and water-retaining effects of increased plasma cortisol and aldosterone levels in response to the "stress" of surgery
5. Increased antidiuretic hormone (ADH) activity.

One of the most important of these is the increase in ADH activity. This is almost invariable and during surgery the ADH concentration may be 50–100 times greater than pre-operatively.[17] The concentrations fall at the end of surgery but do not return to normal for 3–5 days. This is similar to the period of postoperative oliguria. There is some controversy over the primary reason for this. Some, of whom Jenkins and his associates[48] provide an example, have maintained that ADH secretion is a physiological response to the loss of functional extracellular fluid into cells or by its sequestration and immobilization in damaged tissues—the so-called "third space". Others believe that the ADH response is multifactorial and caused by the drugs, pain and other factors related to the "stress" of surgery. The difference is important because on it depends the choice between fluid loading and fluid restriction as the most physiological approach to fluid therapy in the peri-operative period.

*The "third space" theory* arose from the work of Shires and co-workers[49] who, by using radioactive isotope dilution techniques, found that there was an apparent decrease in the functional ECF volume during surgery. This led to a reversal of peri-operative salt and water restriction and a vast increase in the quantity of salt-containing fluids, particularly Ringer lactate, infused during surgery[50] and the sporadic occurrence of pulmonary oedema. While it is true that urine output can be increased by fluid loading,[51] this is not an invariable finding.[52] Only about half of the extra fluid is excreted in the peri-operative period.[53] The greater urine output may be a result of the greater central venous pressure seen in fluid loaded patients when compared with fluid-restricted patients. Colloid infusion is arguably a more rational therapy[54] if the aim is simply to maintain a predetermined central venous pressure. There appears to be no difference in ADH levels between fluid-loaded and fluid-restricted patients undergoing surgery.[55]

The "third space" theory received a further setback from the investigations of Roth and his colleagues[56] which failed to confirm the original work of Shires and lead to the conclusion that, "Functional reduction of extracellular space is a myth and therapeutic regimens based upon it are accordingly irrational."[50]

## Peri-Operative Fluid Therapy

The frequency with which intravenous infusions are given during anaesthesia varies considerably between different countries and between individual anaesthetists. While some would hardly contemplate giving even the most simple anaesthetic without an intravenous infusion running, others would reserve this for more prolonged procedures and those in which blood loss may occur and use an indwelling needle or cannula to establish an "open vein" for repeated doses of intravenous drugs. There are, however, undoubted risks from infection, phlebitis and local complications related to infusion of fluids.[57] The risk of peri-operative deep venous thrombosis may also be increased.[58] The risks and benefits of intravenous infusion must therefore be weighed up in each individual case.

Evaporative water loss from the skin is unchanged during anaesthesia and surgery, but losses from the respiratory tract are increased, probably because of the additional water required to humidify dry inspired gases.[59] Additional water is lost by evaporation from the wound.

Patients having major surgery need intravenous fluids in the peri-operative period. During surgery it is customary to give 5–10 ml/kg/hour of a balanced salt solution to replace evaporative water losses and loss of fluid in the oedema of damaged tissues. There is some evidence that this may reduce the risk of intra-operative hypovolaemia and subsequent impairment of renal function. In patients having major vascular surgery such fluid therapy, monitored by pulmonary-artery wedge pressure meaurements to prevent fluid overload and pulmonary oedema, significantly improved postoperative renal function.[60] During the period after surgery the patient's water requirements can be met by giving about 30 ml/kg/body weight/day of 5 per cent dextrose. This will need to be increased by about 250 ml/day for each 1° C increase of body temperature in the pyrexial patient. Sodium excretion in the urine is reduced in the peri-operative period but it is usual to supply some sodium to compensate for the loss of extracellular fluid into the oedema of traumatized tissues in the operative field and the wound. Suitable fluid regimens for the early postoperative period in a patient without complications who is unable to eat or drink are shown in Table 3. Patients with additional fluid losses into the bowel because of ileus or from vomiting, diarrhoea, fistulae or nasogastric suction will need

16/TABLE 3
DAILY FLUID AND ELECTROLYTE REGIMENS FOR THE EARLY POSTOPERATIVE PERIOD.

| *Fluid* | *Volume (ml)* | *Sodium (mmol)* |
|---|---|---|
| 5% Dextrose | 2000 | – |
| Hartmann's Solution* | 500 | 65 |
| 5% Dextrose | 2000 | – |
| 0·9% Sodium Chloride* | 500 | 75 |
| 4·3% Dextrose with 0·18% Sodium Chloride | 2500 | 75 |

*Optional on the first day.

these replacing with an equal volume of 0·9 per cent sodium chloride or Hartmann's solution. If such losses are prolonged it is preferable to measure the electrolyte content of the fluid to enable more precise replacement of the ions lost.

It is usually unnecessary to add potassium to the intravenous fluids for the first 24–48 hours after surgery. After this time 1 mmol/kg body weight/day can be given with the amount being adjusted according to plasma levels.

In practice, it is found that previously healthy patients with an uncomplicated peri-operative course tolerate even the most bizarre fluid regimens. Fluid and electrolyte problems are much more common in those with pre-existing renal or cardiopulmonary disease and those who develop postoperative complications.

## SPECIAL SITUATIONS

### Blood Loss

The use of blood and blood substitutes is considered in Chapter 17. Patients with a normal pre-operative haemoglobin concentration and normal cardiopulmonary function can lose 10 per cent of their total blood volume before transfusion of blood needs to be considered. The fluid lost can be replaced with either crystalloids, such as normal saline or Hartmann's solution, or a colloid solution such as Haemaccel.

### Burns

Patients with severe burns may require general anaesthesia early in their course for associated injuries or incision of circumferential burns. Most Burns Units have adopted a formula as a guide to fluid resuscitation during the early period after a burn. A large number of different formulae have been proposed, using different amounts of crystalloid and colloid solutions.[61–63]

A comparative review of the different fluid regimens in use[64,65] showed that they resulted in similar amounts of sodium/kg body weight/% burns being given. A more recent formula using mainly plasma is derived from work in the Burns Unit of Mount Vernon Hospital.[66] This provides for infusion of a volume of plasma equal to:

$$\frac{\%\text{ area of burn} \times \text{body weight in kg}}{2}\ \text{ml}$$

during successive periods of 4, 4, 4, 6, 6 and 12 hours after the burn. Blood is used to replace some of the plasma in an amount equal to 1 per cent of the calculated blood volume for each 1 per cent deep burn. The "Mount Vernon" formula is based on infusion of plasma. Others have suggested that only crystalloids should be used during the first 24 hours because of the increased loss of protein into interstitial fluid during this period after a burn injury.[67] When more than 30 per cent of the body surface area is burned this increased vascular permeability occurs throughout the body, though most pronounced in the area of the burn. After the first 24 hours it was suggested that colloid be used to maintain the circulating volume as capillary integrity apparently returns to normal.

This debate on whether crystalloid or colloid infusion is better for resuscitation of burned patients is likely to continue, but a recent reviewer concluded that the composition of the fluid infused in the first 24 hours post burn probably makes very little difference and there is no evidence of any particularly beneficial effect of colloid-containing fluid as compared to colloid-free electrolyte solution.[68]

It must be emphasised that whichever formula is used it should serve only as a guide to the likely fluid requirements. The amount infused may need to be modified in response to the findings on repeated clinical assessment or measurement of serial haematocrits and urine output. The formulae only provide for the fluid losses caused by the burn.

If a recently burnt patient requires general anaesthesia fluid should continue to be given according to the locally used formula. Extra fluid and blood will need to be given to meet normal water and electrolyte requirements and replace any blood lost.

**Obstructive Jaundice**

Obstructive jaundice predisposes to post-operative renal failure. The reduction in post-operative creatinine clearance has been shown to correlate well with pre-operative bilirubin concentration. In the same study it was found that renal impairment can be prevented by maintaining a diuresis with mannitol from the time of premedication until 2 or 3 days after the operation.[69] After premedication 500 ml of 10 per cent mannitol can be infused and thereafter 5 per cent mannitol may be given to maintain the urine output at more than 1 ml/minute.

Frusemide has been advocated as an alternative means of maintaining urine output.[47] Whichever diuretic is used it is important to replace sufficient fluid to prevent hypovolaemia.

**Spinal and Extradural Analgesia**

Sympathetic blockade associated with spinal or extradural analgesia causes vasodilatation and a reduction in blood pressure. Fluid loading with up to a litre of Hartmann's solution is frequently used to maintain venous pressure and so prevent the fall in blood pressure. The same effect can be achieved with a smaller volume of a colloid solution such as Haemaccel.

**Water Intoxication during Transurethral Prostatectomy**

Water intoxication may occur during transurethral resection of the prostate as the result of absorption of large amounts of irrigating fluid through the opened prostatic venous sinuses.[70, 71, 72] The use of near iso-osmolar irrigating solutions containing glycine or mannitol has overcome the problems of haemolysis (which would otherwise occur if water is used), but the problem of excessive fluid absorption remains. The amount absorbed will depend on the hydrostatic pressure of the irrigating solution, the number and size of the venous sinuses opened, and the duration of resection. Excessive amounts absorbed into the circulation will lead to a fall in the plasma sodium concentration and may result in the development of acute heart failure, pulmonary oedema and cerebral oedema. The clinical syndrome seen differs with the type of anaesthetic employed; under regional anaesthesia, the main signs will consist of

1. mental confusion with nausea, retching and headache
2. a rise in systolic and diastolic pressures accompanied by an increase in pulse pressure
3. bradycardia
4. dyspnoea with or without cyanosis.

During general anaesthesia the subjective signs will obviously not be evident and the only signs may be those involving the cardiovascular or respiratory systems. Following these initial manifestations, the patient may become severely hypotensive and comatose, with the development of tetanus-like twitchings. Minor degress of absorption will be corrected by spontaneous diuresis, but more severe cases with cerebral or cardiovascular problems will need treatment with hypertonic saline solution.

**Oliguric or Anuric Patients**

Patients in established renal failure are particularly susceptible to fluid overload. Perioperative fluids should replace insensible losses and the measured blood and fluid loss. Extra fluid can be given if there are signs of hypovolaemia such as tachycardia, low venous pressure or a reduction in blood pressure.

## Administration of Intravenous Fluids

Intravenous therapy has a long history. In 1657 Sir Christopher Wren and Robert Boyle injected tincture of opium into a dog using a sharpened quill attached to a bladder. Metal needles, rubber tubing and glass syringes and needles were developed during the 19th and early 20th centuries, but it is only during the second half of this century with the development of plastics and later the revolution in plastic disposable equipment that intravenous fluid administration has become simple and routine. Today, modern intravenous cannulae coupled with a little manual dexterity permit ready access to the venous system for administration of drugs and fluids. However, volume overload, local damage to veins with resulting thrombosis, sepsis and air embolism remain well-recognised complications. Careful monitoring of fluid balance, venous pressure, aseptic technique during insertion of the cannulae and scrupulous nursing care help to reduce the incidence of these complications.

### Venous Cannulation Techniques

The techniques of peripheral and central venous cannulation have been described by Smith[73] but are best learnt by demonstration and supervised practice. Other descriptions of the techniques for venous cannulation at various sites include peripheral,[74] infraclavicular subclavian,[75] internal jugular,[76] basilic, external jugular, internal jugular, subclavian and femoral vein approaches.[77]

### Control of Infusion Rate

Most intravenous infusions are given through a standard gravity-fed administration set with the flow rate controlled by a simple plastic regulating clamp. The behaviour and problems of this system were investigated by Flack and Whyte[78] who showed that the major factor affecting flow rate is the variation in the patient's venous pressure. In practice, less than half the infusions given through this system are given over the correct period[79] but in most cases this has no clinical significance. There are some infusions, however, in which an accurate flow rate is more important. This applies particularly to infusions of intravenous drugs, concentrated electrolyte solutions and parenteral nutrition.

Paediatric infusion sets have a smaller drop size which is less subject to variation, usually have a screw-clamp to control the infusion rate and have a calibrated burette so it is easier to check the infusion rate. With these, more accurate control of the infusion rate can be achieved but it is still subject to changes in the patient's venous pressure and may need frequent adjustment.

A number of more sophisticated devices are now available to control intravenous infusion rates. These were reviewed by Rithalia and Tinker.[80] The simplest are manually controlled in line flow regulators such as the "Dial-A-Flow" (Simonson and Weel Ltd) or "Helix" (Van Leer Ltd.), but these tend to be inaccurate at low flow rates and flow varies with changes in infusion pressure or venous pressure. Drip rate controllers such as the Ivac 230 (Ivac UK Ltd.) can be used on standard administration sets and overcome the variation in flow rate with changes in venous pressure. Occlusion by the servo-driven clamp is varied according to the signals from a photoelectric drop detector and compared with the pre-set drip rate. These devices are very prone to malfunction alarms caused by movement of the drip chamber or sub optimal positioning of the detector on the drip chamber. The accuracy of these devices is limited by variation in drop size.

Volumetric pumps such as the Ivac 630, Imed (Imed Ltd.) and Valleylab 5000 (Valleylab UK Ltd.) are inherently more accurate and equipped with alarms to indicate if the infusion line has become blocked or air has entered the system. They are also considerably more expensive.

Syringe pumps[106] are best suited to accurate infusion of small volumes of fluid, for example, concentrated solutions of inotropic drugs, sodium nitroprusside or nitroglycerine. The infusion rate is not affected by venous pressure, cannula size or fluid viscosity. Some newer pumps incorporate an over-pressure alarm to warn if the infusion becomes blocked or occluded.

**Rapid Infusion.**—When very high flow rates are needed the most rapid infusion rates are achieved by placing a pressure infusion cuff around a collapsible plastic container of the fluid to be infused.[81]

### Phlebitis

Phlebitis is a common complication of peripheral infusions. The factors that have been implicated in its aetiology include:

1. *The duration* of cannula placement: the incidence of infusion phlebitis increases with time.[82, 83]
2. *The material* of which the cannula is made; fluoroethylenepropylene (FEP) cannulae are associated with a delay in the appearance of phlebitis as compared to polypropylene or Teflon.[83, 84]
3. *The pH* of the fluid infused, phlebitis being less with fluids of neutral pH[85]
4. *The infusion rate*, phlebitis being less with rapid intermittent infusions than slow infusions.[86]
5. *Particulate matter* in the infusion fluid or injections made into it; high numbers of particles are carried into the circulation by intravenous infusions. Studies have shown that an end-line filter with a 0·45 μm pore size reduces the incidence of infusion phlebitis.[87] Such a filter, the Pall "Ultipor", is

available commercially and because of its construction also markedly reduces the risk of air embolism. It appears, however, to be unsuitable for adult patients in the peri-operative period because of the limitation it imposes on maximal flow rates but it may have a place in long-term infusions and in those patients at risk from even a small air embolus.[88]

6. *Irritant drugs:* many intravenous drugs predispose to phlebitis; they include diazepam and many intravenous antibiotics.

The addition of heparin 1 unit/ml to the infusion fluid has been shown to produce a significant decrease in the incidence of phlebitis, perhaps by inhibiting fibrin clot formation around the tip of the cannula.[89]

### Complications of Central Venous Catheterisation

Many complications of central venous catheterisation have been reported, but most are rare. They include:

- arterial puncture
- haematoma formation
- pneumothorax
- infection
- venous thrombosis
- aberrant placement within the venous system[90]
- thoracic duct cannulation[91]
- hydrothorax[92, 93]
- cardiac tamponade[94, 95]
- neurological damage[96]
- phrenic nerve damage[97]
- catheter knotting[98]
- catheter embolisation: this was an ever present risk with "catheter-through-needle" designs of central venous catheter and has lead to these no longer being favoured. Embolised catheter fragments can be removed using a percutaneous transvenous technique with a catheter and snare.[99]

The incidence of the more common complications varies between different series and the route chosen for central venous cannulation.[77, 100–102] A total overall complication rate of 5–10 per cent is commonly experienced, with pneumothorax occurring in around 1 per cent of subclavian vein punctures. The incidence of complications may be reduced by proper tuition and should be less when catheters are inserted by experienced operators,[103] while newer materials and heparin bonding may reduce the incidence of catheter-related thrombosis.

### Intravenous Fluids

Intravenous fluids must be clear. If there is any haziness or particulate matter present the bottle should be kept for inspection and the hospital pharmacy contacted so that the rest of the batch can be checked.

When drugs are added to bags or bottles of intravenous fluid they must be thoroughly mixed. The amount of shaking required is much greater than might be expected: two or three turns is insufficient and it is more difficult to mix solutions in plastic than glass containers. Rarely should more than one drug be added to the same infusion. If it is unavoidable, confirmation of compatibility must be obtained. Many of the formulations of drugs for intravenous injection or infusion contain stabilisers, preservatives, solubilisers or unusual solvents and these materials are often the cause of unexpected incompatibility. Incompatibility can occur without a precipitate forming.

The position of the intravenous cannula should be checked before an infusion is started, especially if drugs have been added to the infusion or injections are to be made into the infusion tubing. Extravasation of intravenous fluids will at best result in local swelling and pain, but may result in severe local tissue damage that may even require skin grafting at a later stage. This is particularly likely to happen after extravasation of calcium salts, hypertonic glucose,[104] sodium bicarbonate, thiopentone, pressor amines or cytotoxic drugs.[105]

**5 per cent dextrose** contains 5 g of dextrose in each 100 ml of water. It is isotonic with plasma and has a pH of 4·55 (an acid load of 0·28 mmol/l). It is suitable for diluting drugs to be given by intravenous infusion except those that are acid labile such as the penicillins and amphotericin B. The dextrose is metabolised, leaving the free water.

Five per cent dextrose is the fluid of choice for patients who are likely to be retaining sodium or who are at risk of heart failure. During the first 24 hours after surgery, sodium retention is common and 5 per cent dextrose should account for most of the intravenous fluids.

**0·9 per cent or "normal" saline** contains 0·9 g of sodium chloride in each 100 ml of water or 150 mmol/l of sodium and chloride. It has a pH of 4·0 (an acid load of 0·8 mmol/l). It is "normal" in the physiological sense of being isotonic with extracellular fluid, not in the chemical sense of 1 mole/l.

An average patient requires 70–100 mmol of sodium each day or approximately 500 ml of 0·9 per cent saline. In addition any gastro-intestinal losses such as nasogastric aspirate should be replaced by saline.

**Hartmann's solution (Ringer lactate)** was designed to replace extracellular fluid losses and has a similar electrolyte content—sodium 131 mmol/l, potassium 5 mmol/l, calcium 2 mmol/l, chloride 112 mmol/l and lactate 28 mmol/l—but does not have the colloid osmotic effects to replace plasma. The lactate is included as a bicarbonate source but its metabolism may be delayed by hypovolaemia and other shock states, hypoxia or severe liver disease.

The high electrolyte content makes it unsuitable for routine use as the sole intravenous fluid in the postoperative patient.

**Dextrose/saline.**—Some anaesthetists favour the use of a compromise solution of 0·18 per cent sodium chloride in 4 per cent dextrose for infusion in the postoperative period. This combination is isotonic and gives 30 mmol/l of sodium, 30 mmol/l chloride and 40·0 g of anhydrous dextrose leading to approximately 150 cal/l.

**8·4 per cent sodium bicarbonate** contains 8·4 g of sodium bicarbonate/100 ml or 1 mmol/ml of both sodium and bicarbonate. It is used for the correction of acute metabolic acidosis but must be used with care because:

1. It can cause fluid to shift from the intracellular to the extracellular compartment and may precipitate pulmonary oedema.
2. It can cause a hyperosmolar state.
3. It can precipitate a cardiac arrest by unmasking hypokalaemia in the potassium-deficient patient.
4. A profound metabolic alkalosis may occur after organic acids have metabolised.

For these reasons it is best to give it in 50 ml aliquots with estimation of the patient's acid-base status by arterial blood sampling before and after each aliquot. It is not necessary to completely correct acidosis. Correction to a pH greater than 7·2 is all that is usually required.

## REFERENCES


1. Schloerb, P. R., Palaskas, C. L. and Mintun, M. A. (1981). Rapid computer prediction of total body water in fluid overload. *J. Trauma*, **21**, 757.
2. Bradbury, M. W. B. (1973). Physiology of body fluids and electrolytes. *Br. J. Anaesth.*, **45**, 937.
3. Edelman, I. S. and Leibman, J. (1959). Anatomy of body water and electrolytes. *Am. J. Med.*, **27**, 256.
4. Starling, E. H. (1896). On the absorption of fluids from the connective tissue spaces. *J. Physiol.* **19**, 312.
5. Civetta, J. M. (1979). A new look at the Starling equation. *Crit. Care Med.*, **7**, 84.
6. Bevan, D. R. (1978). Osmometry 1. Terminology and principles of measurement. *Anaesthesia*, **33**, 794.
7. Weil, M. H., Henning, R. J. and Puri, V. K. (1979). Colloid oncotic pressure: clinical significance. *Crit. Care Med.*, **7**, 113.
8. Bevan, D. R. (1978). Osmometry 2. Osmoregulation. *Anaesthesia*, **33**, 801.
9. MacKnight, A. D. C. and Leaf, A. (1977). Regulation of cellular volume. *Physiol. Rev.*, **57**, 510.
10. Skorecki, K. L. and Brenner, B. M. (1981). Body fluid homeostasis in man. A contemporary overview. *Am. J. Med.*, **70**, 77.
11. Phillips, P. J. (1977). Water metabolism: *Anaesth. Intens. Care*, **5**, 295.
12. Andersen, B. (1978). Regulation of water intake. *Physiol. Rev.*, **58**, 582.
13. Hays, R. M. (1976). Antidiuretic hormone. *New Engl. J. Med.*, **295**, 659.
14. Barratt, L. J. (1977). Sodium metabolism. *Anaesth. Intens. Care*, **5**, 305.
15. Aukland, K. and Nicholaysen, G. (1981). Interstitial fluid volume: local regulatory mechanisms. *Physiol. Rev.*, **61**, 556.
16. Verney, E. B. (1957). Renal excretion of water and salt. *Lancet*, **2**, 1237 and 1295.
17. Bie, P. (1980). Osmoreception, vasopressin and control of renal water excretion. *Physiol. Rev.*, **60**, 961
18. Wright, F. S. and Briggs, J. P. (1979). Feedback control of glomerular blood flow, pressure and filtration rate. *Physiol. Rev.*, **59**, 958.
19. Thompson, F. D. (1979). Hyponatraemia. *Br. J. Hosp. Med.*, **21**, 46.
20. Bartter, F. C. and Schwartz, W. B. (1967). The syndrome of inappropriate secretion of antidiuretic hormone. *Am. J. Med.*, **42**, 790.
21. White, M. G. and Fetner, C. D. (1975). Treatment of the syndrome of inappropriate antidiuretic hormone secretion. *New Engl. J. Med.*, **292**, 390.
22. Forrest, J. N., Cox, M., Hong, C., Morrison, G., Bia, M. and Singer, I. (1978). Superiority of demeclocycline over lithium in the treatment of chronic syndrome of inappropriate secretion of antidiuretic hormone. *New Engl. J. Med.*, **298**, 173.

23. Decaux, G., Brimioulle, S., Genette, F. and Mockel, J. (1980). Treatment of the syndrome of inappropriate secretion of antidiuretic hormone by urea. *Am. J. Med.*, **69**, 99.
24. Decaux, G., Waterlot, Y., Genette, F. and Mockel, J. (1981). Treatment of the syndrome of inappropriate secretion of antidiuretic hormone with furosemide. *New Engl. J. Med.*, **304**, 329.
25. Cannon, P. J. (1977). The kidney in heart failure. *New Engl. J. Med.*, **296**, 26.
26. Kennedy, P. G. E., Mitchell, D. M. and Hoffbrand, B. I. (1978). Severe hyponatraemia in hospital inpatients. *Brit. Med. J.*, **2**, 1251.
27. Ayus, J. C., Olivero, J. J. and Frommer, J. P. (1982). Rapid correction of severe hyponatraemia with intravenous hypertonic saline solution. *Am. J. Med.*, **72**, 43.
28. Flear, C. T. G. and Singh, C. M. (1973). Hyponatraemia and sick cells. *Br. J. Anaesth.* **45**, 976.
29. Thomas, T. H., Morgan, D. B., Swaminathan, R., Ball, S. G. and Lee, M. R. (1978). Severe hyponatraemia. *Lancet*, **1**, 621.
30. Stockigt, J. R. (1977). Potassium homeostasis. *Aust. N.Z. J. Med.*, **7**, 66.
31. Goldfarb, S., Cox, M., Singer, L. and Goldberg, M. (1976). Acute hyperkalaemia induced by hyperglycaemia: hormonal mechanisms. *Ann. Int. Med.*, **84**, 426.
32. Lockwood, R. H. and Lum, B. K. B. (1974). Effects of adrenergic agents and antagonists on potassium metabolism. *J. Pharmacol. Exp. Ther.*, **189**, 119.
33. Pettit, G. W. and Vick, R. L. (1974). An analysis of the contribution of the endocrine pancreas to the kalemotropic actions of catecholamines. *J. Pharmacol. Exp. Ther.*, **190**, 234.
34. Wang, P. and Clausen, T. (1976). Treatment of attacks in hyperkalaemic familial periodic paralysis by inhalation of salbutamol. *Lancet*, **1**, 221.
35. Burnell, J. M., Villamil, M. F., Uyeno, B. T. and Scribner, B. H. (1956). The effect in humans of extracellular pH changes on the relationship between serum potassium concentration and intracellular potassium. *J. Clin. Invest.*, **35**, 935.
36. Adrogué, H. J. and Madias, N. E. (1981). Changes in plasma potassium concentration during acute acid-base disturbances. *Am. J. Med.*, **71**, 456.
37. Gronert, G. A. and Theye, R. A. (1975). Pathophysiology of hyperkalemia induced by succinylcholine. *Anesthesiology*, **43**, 89.
38. Stockigt, J. R. (1977). Potassium metabolism. *Anaesth. Intens. Care*, **5**, 317.
39. Reeve, J. (1977). Disorders of plasma calcium. *Hosp. Update*, **3**, 19.
40. Ryan, G. D. and Masarei, J. R. L. (1979). Validity of "corrected" calcium values. *Clin. Chim. Acta*, **91**, 329.
41. Wills, M. R. (1973). Calcium homeostasis in health and disease. In: *Recent Advances in Medicine*, 16th edit., p. 57. Eds. Baron, D. N., Compston, N. and Dawson, A. M. London: Churchill-Livingstone.
42. Editorial (1978). Management of hypercalcaemic crisis. *Lancet*, **2**, 617.
43. Krasner, B. S. (1979). Cardiac effects of magnesium with special reference to anaesthesia: a review. *Canad. Anaesth. Soc. J.*, **26**, 181.
44. Graber, T. W., Yee, A. S. and Baker, F. J. (1981). Magnesium: physiology, clinical disorders and therapy. *Ann. Emerg. Med.*, **10**, 49.
45. Lim, P. and Jacob, E. (1972). Magnesium deficiency in patients on long-term diuretic therapy for heart failure. *Brit. Med. J.*, **3**, 620.
46. Cousins, M. J. and Mazze, R. I. (1973). Anaesthesia, surgery and renal function. *Anaesth. Intens. Care.*, **1**, 355.
47. Bevan, D. R. (1978). Intraoperative fluid balance. *Brit. J. Hosp. Med.*, **19**, 445.
48. Jenkins, M. T., Giesecke, A. H. and Johnson, E. R. (1975). The postoperative patient and his fluid and electrolyte requirements. *Brit. J. Anaesth.*, **47**, 143.
49. Shires, T., Williams, J. and Brown, F. (1961). Acute change in extracellular fluids associated with major surgical procedures. *Ann. Surg.*, **154**, 803.
50. Editorial (1969). Administration of crystalloids in shock and surgical trauma. *Lancet*, **1**, 1298.
51. Barry, K. G., Mazze, R. I. and Schwartz, F. D. (1964). Prevention of surgical oliguria and renal-hemodynamic suppression by sustained hydration. *New Engl. J. Med.*, **270**, 1371.
52. MacKenzie, A. L. and Donald, J. R. (1969). Urine output and fluid therapy during anaesthesia and surgery. *Brit. Med. J.*, **3**, 619.
53. Fieber, W. W. and Jones, J. R. (1966). Intraoperative fluid therapy with 5 per cent dextrose in lactated Ringer's solution. *Anesth. Analg.*, **45**, 366.
54. Irvin, T. T., Modgill, V. K., Hayter, C. J., McDowall, D. G. and Golligher, J. C. (1972). Plasma volume deficits and salt and water excretion after surgery. *Lancet*, **2**, 1159.
55. Sinnatamby, C., Edwards, C. R. W., Kitau, M. and Irving, M. H. (1974). Antidiuretic hormone response to high and conservative fluid regimes in patients undergoing operation. *Surg. Gynec. Obstet.*, **139**, 715.
56. Roth, E., Lan, L. C. and Maloney, J. V. (1969). Ringer's lactate solution and extracellular fluid volume in the surgical patients: a critical analysis. *Ann. Surg.*, **169**, 149.
57. Editorial (1975). A further hazard of intravenous therapy. *Brit. Med. J.*, **2**, 262.
58. Janvrin, S. B., Davies, G. and Greenhalgh, R. M. (1980). Postoperative deep venous thrombosis caused by intravenous fluids during surgery. *Brit. J. Surg.*, **67**, 690.
59. Reithner, L., Johansson, H. and Strouth, L. (1980). Insensible perspiration during anaesthesia and surgery. *Acta Anaesth. Scand.*, **24**, 362.
60. Bush, H. L., Huse, J. B., Johnson, W. C., O'Hara, E. T. and Nabseth, D. C. (1981). Prevention of renal insufficiency after abdominal aortic aneurysm resection by optimal volume loading. *Arch. Surg.*, **116**, 1517.
61. Cope, O. and Moore, F. D. (1947). The redistribution of body water and fluid therapy of the burned patients. *Ann. Surg.*, **126**, 1010.
62. Kyle, M. J. and Wallace, A. B. (1951). Fluid replacement in burnt children. *Brit. J. Plast. Surg.*, **3**, 194.
63. Evans, E. I., Purnell, O. J., Bobinett, P. W., Batchelor, A. D. R. and Martin, M. (1952). Fluid and electrolyte requirements in severe burns. *Ann. Surg.*, **135**, 804.
64. Davies, J. W. L. (1975). The fluid therapy given to 1027 patients during the first 48 hours after burning. I. Total fluid and colloid output. *Burns*, **1**, 319.
65. Davies, J. W. L. (1975). The fluid therapy given to 1027 patients during the first 48 hours after burning.

II. The inputs of sodium and water and the tonicity of therapy. *Burns*, **1**, 331.
66. Muir, I. (1981). The use of the Mount Vernon formula in the treatment of burn shock. *Intens. Care Med.*, **7**, 49.
67. Moncrief, J. A. (1973). Burns. *New Engl. J. Med.*, **288**, 444.
68. Pruitt, B. A., (1981). Fluid resuscitation for extensively burned patients. *J. Trauma*, **21**, (Suppl), 690.
69. Dawson, J. L. (1965). Post-operative renal function in obstructive jaundice: effect of a mannitol diuresis. *Brit. Med. J.*, **1**, 82.
70. Charlton, A. J. (1980). Cardiac arrest during transurethral prostatectomy after absorption of 1·5 per cent glycerine. *Anaesthesia*, **35**, 804.
71. Desmond, J. (1970). Complications of transurethral prostatic surgery. *Canad. Anaesth. Soc. J.*, **17**, 25.
72. Marx, G. F. and Orkin, L. R. (1962). Complications associated with transurethral surgery. *Anesthesiology*, **23**, 802.
73. Smith, B. L. (1978). Intravenous techniques. *Brit. J. Hosp. Med.*, **19**, 454.
74. Anderton, J. M. (1980). How to set up a peripheral drip. *Brit. J. Hosp. Med.*, **23**, 424.
75. Simon, R. R. (1978). A new technique for subclavian puncture. *JACEP*, **7**, 409.
76. Defalque, R. J. (1973). Percutaneous catheterization of the internal jugular vein. *Anesth. Analg.*, **53**, 116.
77. Burri, C. and Ahnefeld, F. W. (1978). *The Caval Catheter*. Berlin: Springer-Verlag.
78. Flack, F. C. and Whyte, T. D. (1974). Behaviour of standard gravity-fed administration sets used for intravenous infusion. *Brit. Med. J.*, **3**, 439.
79. Chaput de Saintonge, D. M., Dixon, J. and Newman, M. S. (1974). Variation in intravenous infusion rates. *Brit. Med. J.*, **4**, 531.
80. Rithalia, S. V. S. and Tinker, J. (1981). Recent developments in infusion devices. *Brit. J. Hosp. Med.*, **25**, 69.
81. Dula, D. J., Muller, A. and Donovan, J. W. (1981). Flow rate variance of commonly used IV infusion techniques. *J. Trauma*, **21**, 480.
82. Collin, J., Collin, C., Constable, F. L. and Johnston, I. D. A. (1975). Infusion thrombophlebitis and infection with various cannulas. *Lancet*, **2**, 150.
83. Frazer, I. H., Eke, N. and Laing, M. S. (1978). Is infusion phlebitis preventable. *Brit. Med. J.*, **2**, 232.
84. Thomas, E. T., Evers, W. and Racz, G. B. (1970). Post infusion phlebitis. *Anesth. Analg.*, **49**, 150.
85. Hessor, I. and Bojsen-Møller, M. (1976). Experimental infusion thrombophlebitis. Importance of the pH of glucose solutions. *Intens. Care Med.*, **2**, 97.
86. Hessor, I. and Bojsen-Møller, M. (1975). Experimental infusion thrombophlebitis. Importance of the infusion rate. *Intens. Care Med.*, **2**, 103.
87. Lowe, G. D. (1981). Filtration in IV therapy. Part I: clinical aspects of IV fluid filtration. *Brit. J. Intravenous Ther.*, **2** (3), 42.
88. Wood, G. J. and Ward, M. E. (1981). The Pall Ultipor IV filter and air eliminator. *Brit. J. Intravenous Ther.*, **2** (3), 15.
89. Tanner, W. A., Delaney, P. V. and Hennessy, T. P. (1980). The influence of heparin on intravenous infusions: a prospective study. *Brit. J. Surg.*, **67**, 311.
90. Dunbar, R. D., Mitchell, R. and Lavine, M. (1981). Aberrant locations of central venous catheters. *Lancet*, **1**, 711.
91. Majek, M., Malatinsky, J. and Kadlic, T. (1977). Inadvertent thoracic duct catheterization during transjugular central venous cannulation. A case report. *Acta Anaesth. Scand.*, **21**, 320.
92. Allsop, J. R. and Askew, A. R. (1975). Subclavian vein cannulation: a new complication. *Brit. Med. J.*, **4**, 262.
93. Rudge, C. J., Bewick, M. and McColl, I. (1973). Hydrothorax after central venous catheterization. *Brit. Med. J.*, **3**, 23.
94. Greenall, M. J., Blewitt, R. W. and McMahon, M. J. (1975). Cardiac tamponade and central venous catheters. *Brit. Med. J.*, **2**, 595.
95. James, O. F. and Tredrea, C. R. (1979). Cardiac tamponade caused by caval catheter—a radiological demonstration of an unusual complication. *Anaesth. Intens. Care*, **7**, 174.
96. Briscoe, C. E., Bushman, J. A. and McDonald, W. I. (1974). Extensive neurological damage after cannulation of internal jugular vein. *Brit. Med. J.*, **1**, 314.
97. Epstein, E. J., Quereshi, M. S. A. and Wright, J. S. (1976). Diaphragmatic paralysis after supra-clavicular puncture of subclavian vein. *Brit. Med. J.*, **1**, 693.
98. Nicolas, F., Fenig, J. and Richter, R. M. (1970). Knotting of subclavian central venous catheter. *JAMA*, **214**, 373.
99. Edwards, A. C. and Sowton, E. (1978). Management of embolised central venous catheters. *Brit. Med. J.*, **2**, 669.
100. Blackett, R. L., Bakran, A., Bradley, J. A., Halsall, A., Hill, G. L. and McMahon, M. J. (1978). A prospective study of subclavian vein catheters used exclusively for the purpose of intravenous feeding. *Brit. J. Surg.*, **65**, 393.
101. Ross, A. H. McL., Anderson, J. R. and Walls, A. D. F. (1980). Central venous catheterisation. *Ann. Roy. Coll. Surg. Eng.*, **62**, 454.
102. Padberg, F. T., Ruggiero, J., Blackburn, G. L. and Bistrain, B. R. (1981). Central venous catheterization for parenteral nutrition. *Ann. Surg.*, **193**, 264.
103. Woolfson, A. M. J. (1981). Central venous access. Proper tuition reduces complications. *Brit. J. Intravenous Ther.*, **2** (3), 5.
104. Editorial (1976). Dangerous drips. *Lancet*, **1**, 291.
105. Gaze, N. R. (1978). Tissue necrosis caused by commonly used intravenous infusions. *Lancet*, **2**, 417.
106. Dickenson, J. E. (1983). Syringe pumps. *Brit. J. Hosp. Med.*, **29**, 187.

## FURTHER READING

Pestana, C. (1980). *Fluids and Electrolytes in the Surgical Patient*, 2nd edit. Baltimore, Maryland: Williams & Wilkins Co.
Symposium on disorders of extracellular volume and composition (1982). Part 1. *Am. J. Med.*, **72**, 272; Part 2. *Am. J. Med.*, **72**, 473.

CHAPTER 17

# Blood Transfusion



## Introduction

The anaesthetist has frequently to use blood or blood products in treating the shocked or bleeding patient. It is important to choose the therapy rationally with reference to a minimum number of rapid laboratory tests. Whole stored or fresh blood and fractions or concentrates of either humoral or cellular elements, all have their optimal use. Component therapy also enables the transfusion services to make economical use of that valuable resource, human donor blood.

One of the most important principles in blood transfusion is to avoid stimulating the production of antibodies by the recipient. This is difficult with white cell, platelet and plasma protein antigens. Antibodies produced to these are frequently responsible for reactions, particularly in patients who have had multiple transfusions. Antibodies to red-cell antigens are potentially much more dangerous as they may cause fatal intravascular haemolysis (most commonly ABO incompatibility) or the rapid destruction of transfused red cells with concomitant jaundice and anaemia.

## BLOOD GROUPING

Donor and patients are routinely grouped as to their ABO and Rhesus (C,E,D,E, e) groups. Only if incompatibility appears on cross-matching or antenatal screening, or if it is thought vital to use accurately genotyped blood are the red cells typed as to the other blood group systems, e.g. Lewis, Kell, MNS, Duffy, Kidd, etc.

In *ABO grouping*, both red cells and serum are tested as the serum contains isohaemagglutinins to those group-specific substances which are not present on the red cells. The *in vitro* reactions produced are summarised in Table 1. The ABO groups are determined by the terminal sugars of large glycoprotein molecules which protrude from the red-cell membrane. The isohaemagglutinins are probably produced after exposure to gut flora (particularly *E. coli*) which have similar sugars in their membranes. Neonates and individuals raised in a germ-free environment have very low levels of these agglutinins.

17/Table 1
Reactions in ABO Groups

| *Blood Group* | *Red Cells React with* anti A | anti $A_1$ | anti B | *Serum reacts with* $A_1$ cells | B cells | O cells |
|---|---|---|---|---|---|---|
| O | − | − | − | ++ | ++ | − |
| $A_1$ | ++ | ++ | − | − | ++ | − |
| $A_2$ | + | − | − | −/+ (anti $A_1$) | ++ | − |
| B | − | − | ++ | ++ | − | − |
| $A_1B$ | ++ | ++ | ++ | − | − | − |

*Rhesus grouping* is usually done to determine the presence or absence of the D antigen. In Britain, 85 per cent of the population are rhesus (D) positive and 15 per cent negative. Many transfusion services also determine the presence of the other rhesus antigens C, c, E, e as these are commonly involved in transfusion incompatibilities. The other antigens associated with the rhesus system of which there are more than 38 described, are of limited clinical application. If there is any doubt about the rhesus (D) group, it is preferable to give D-negative blood, particularly to women of childbearing age. If D-positive blood or contaminated fractions (e.g. platelet concentrates) are given to a D-negative recipient, a suitable dose of intramuscular anti-D (calculated on the number of red cells given) should be administered as soon as possible, certainly within 72 hours, to try to prevent rhesus immunisation.

### Cross-matching

Cross-matching of patients serum against donor red cells is usually done by a variety of techniques designed to show up a range of different antibodies. Cells and serum are incubated in saline at room temperatures and 37° C for 2 hours with the addition of albumin. Incompatibility is indicated by lysis or agglutination of the red cells. Cells are also washed and treated with anti-human globulin antisera to show up the presence of antibody or complement components bound to their surface. A rapid cross-match in which incubation times are shortened may not reveal slow-reacting but still potentially haemolytic antibodies in the recipient's serum, although it should exclude major ABO incompatibility. The more widespread use of techniques employing low ionic strength saline (LIS) which facilitates antibody and complement fixation, gives improved reliability in cross-match after short incubation (20 minutes). All blood products contaminated with red cells should be cross-matched, e.g. buffy coats (this is the slightly opaque, narrow layer that lies above the red-cell mass after centrifugation of whole blood; it consists largely of white cells and platelets suspended in plasma).

### The Use of O (D) Negative Blood

The practice of giving un-crossmatched group O rhesus (D) negative blood to recipients of unknown blood group is not without risk. Group O individuals (25–50 per cent in different series) not uncommonly have a high titre of lytic anti-A or anti-B in their sera. This may cause rapid haemolysis in a group A, B or AB recipient. The recipient may also have been sensitised by previous transfusion or pregnancy and have an antibody to one of the other blood group antigens which may cause lysis of the transfused cells.

## BLOOD VOLUME

The total blood volume can be measured as the sum of the red-cell volume and plasma volume, or derived from one of the several nomograms available which depend on the individual's height and weight[1]. A simple ml/kg estimation of the red-cell volume (males up to 36 ml/kg and females up to 32 ml/kg) may be adequate for the majority of situations, but falls short when the individual is markedly over- or under-weight.

### Estimation of Red-Cell Volume (RCV)

This is commonly performed by an isotope dilution method employing $^{51}Cr$ (other isotopes such as $^{99m}$ Tc sodium pertechnate or sodium phosphate $^{32}P$ have also been used). A known volume of washed and labelled red cells are re-injected into the individual and samples taken after complete mixing. The red-cell volume can be calculated from the degree of dilution of the isotope.

### Estimation of Plasma Volume (PV)

This is usually also measured by an isotope dilution technique but its accuracy is adversely affected by diffusion of the radioactive label into the extravascular space. $^{125}I$ labelled albumin is commonly used but other substances have been used in the past (e.g. urea, $^{131}I$ and transferrin).

### Calculation of Blood Volume (BV)

Total blood volume is given by the equation:

$$BV = RCV + PV$$

The total body haematocrit (TBH) is given by:

$$TBH = \frac{RCV}{BV}$$

It is normally found to be less than the haematocrit of a venous blood sample (venous haematocrit—VH)

$$\frac{TBH}{VH} = 0{\cdot}91$$

Using this correction, it is possible to estimate the blood volume from the RCV or the PV and the venous haematocrit although, in practice, it is simpler to measure both simultaneously using two labels, $^{51}$ C and $^{125}I$.

$$BV = RCV \times \frac{100}{0{\cdot}91 \times VH}$$

also

$$BV = PV \times \frac{100}{100 - 0{\cdot}91\ VH}$$

Accurate estimation of red-cell and plasma volumes is probably only indicated for diagnostic purposes, primarily for the confirmation of polycythaemia and in practice it is adequate to use the nomogram mentioned above. Mollison[2] even goes so far as to suggest that five litres is a good enough estimate of blood volume for practical purposes!

Variations in blood volume can occur both physiologically and pathologically, and may be due to alterations in plasma volume, red-cell volume or both. The commonest example of a physiological increase in blood volume is *pregnancy*, where the plasma volume increases to a maximum at 32 weeks gestation, subsequently falling to its non-pregnant level two days post-partum. The red-cell volume also increases slowly throughout pregnancy, but to a lesser extent, thus producing an apparent anaemia with a fall in packed-cell volume (PCV) to 36 per cent.

### The Regulation of Blood Volume and Response to Haemorrhage

The response of the body to haemorrhage depends on both the volume and rate of blood loss, and the time over which it occurs. The condition of the patient before the bleeding begins, and whether he is anaesthetised, may well modify his response. When a healthy adult loses some 10 per cent of his blood volume (500 ml) over a few minutes, there will be no detectable alteration in his physical signs. Pulse rate, blood pressure, peripheral circulation and central venous pressure will all remain unchanged. Volume receptors in the right atrium will detect the reduction in circulating volume and cause the vasomotor centre to stimulate the sympathetic autonomic nervous system, resulting in widespread vasoconstriction. The reduced pressure at the arterial end of the capillary will allow less fluid to be lost to the interstitial space and the reduced renal perfusion will cause sodium and water retention so that within 12 hours the blood volume is restored, albeit somewhat diluted. The plasma protein concentration rapidly returns to normal, and over the next two weeks there will be extra haemopoiesis to make up for the lost red cells.

This compensatory process is an extremely effective one for increasing blood losses until some 30 per cent of the blood volume is lost, i.e. 1500 ml. At this point, the patient develops haemorrhagic or hypovolaemic "shock" (shock being defined as an inability to provide adequate perfusion to the tissues for their metabolic needs). If blood-volume replacement is not instituted immediately, irreversible shock will undoubtedly follow. Stimulation of the sympathetic nervous system, which for small volumes of blood loss is so effective, becomes progressively less appropriate as hypovolaemia proceeds. This is because, in the attempt to preserve blood flow to the brain and heart, profound vasoconstriction of the kidney, splanchnic circulation, lungs, skin and muscles occurs, which further compound the damage. Hence, the characteristic picture of hypotension, tachycardia, poor peripheral circulation, oliguria or anuria, hypoxia and acidosis. The state of irreversible shock occurs when tissue hypoxia can no longer be reversed by restoring the circulatory blood volume. One of the processes that is thought to occur in this state, is that the local build up of tissue metabolites causes the relaxation of the precapillary sphincter, but not the postcapillary sphincter and, consequently, large volumes of plasma leak into the tissues, which further exacerbate the hypovolaemia.

## PLASMA-VOLUME EXPANDERS

These are solutions with the same osmolarity as plasma which may be given instead of plasma or blood, in order to restore the circulating blood volume. The ideal plasma-volume expander should possess the following properties:

(i) be isosmotic with plasma
(ii) remain in the vascular compartment for some time
(iii) be easily eliminated by the body
(iv) not cause hypersensitivity reactions
(v) not interfere with blood group serology
(vi) remain liquid over a wide temperature range.

The more commonly used plasma-volume expanders are:

**Haemaccel.**—This is a 3·5 per cent solution of degraded gelatin with an average molecular weight of 35,000 and pH of 7·25. It has an intravascular half-life of about 4 hours and 85 per cent is excreted by the kidneys. Storage life at room temperature is indefinite. It does not interfere with cross-matching, but can occasionally cause an acute hypersensitivity reaction.

**Gelofusine.**—This is a newer preparation. It consists of modified, partially hydrolysed gelatin (with an average molecular weight of 30,000) in normal saline and, therefore, is isotonic and isosmotic. It has a longer half-life than Haemaccel and is hydrolysed by proteolysis before being excreted. It does not interfere with cross-matching and does not cause bleeding. Thus far no hypersensitivity reactions have been reported following its use.

**Dextran** consists of long chains of glucose units with a variable degree of branching. By hydrolysis and subsequent fractionation, preparations can be produced with the desired range of molecular weights. The available preparations are these:

*Dextran-40.* This has a molecular weight average of 40,000. It is supplied as a 10 per cent solution in either 5 per cent dextrose or normal saline, and has a rather short plasma half-life. Between 40–70 per cent is excreted by the kidneys within 24 hours and most of the remainder is metabolised. There is some evidence that dextran-40 has anti-sludging properties and can promote blood flow in small vessels. It has a much higher oncotic pressure than plasma and so causes an increase in plasma volume which may, in part, explain this effect. However, it has been shown that it can reverse erythrocyte aggregation *in vitro*[3]. Dextran-40 is contra-indicated in the treatment of "shock", and where there is known to be renal impairment as it may cause renal tubular obstruction.

*Dextran-70* has a molecular weight average of 70,000 and a rather longer half-life than dextran-40. It comes as a 6 per cent solution in either 5 per cent dextrose or normal saline.

A trial of dextran-70 for the prevention of deep-vein thrombosis and pulmonary embolism showed that it does reduce the risk, but not as effectively as low-dose heparin.[4–7]

*Dextran-110.* This has a molecular weight average of 110,000. It has a longer half-life than 40 or 70 but may produce rouleaux formation. All the dextran preparations may interfere with the red-cell surface, thus making cross-matching difficult.

## BLOOD COMPONENTS AVAILABLE FOR THERAPY AND INDICATIONS FOR THEIR USE

### Whole Blood

#### Selection of Donors

In the United Kingdom, all blood is collected from voluntary donors. They are excluded if they are found to be anaemic (Hb< 13·5 g/dl in males: 12·5 g/dl in females) or to have hepatitis B associated antigen ($Hb_sAG$), positive syphilis serology or a history of significant exposure to malaria or Chagas' disease because of the risk of transmitting infection to the recipient. In addition, potential donors with the following medical conditions are excluded: T.B., epilepsy, hypertension, renal disease, severe atopy, malignant disease or jaundice.

#### Collection and Preservation

Blood is collected into plastic bags containing preservative and stored at 4° C. Blood should never be frozen as this causes haemolysis which can result in severe transfusion reactions.

The preservative solutions in common use are acid citrate dextrose (ACD) and citrate phosphate dextrose (CPD). The composition of the two solutions is:

| | | |
|---|---|---|
| *ACD:* | Trisodium citrate | 2·2 g |
| | Citric acid | 0·8 g |
| | Dextrose | 2·5 g |
| | Water to | 100 ml |
| | pH | 5·0 to 5·1 |

67·5 ml ACD are mixed with 420–450 ml blood.

| | | |
|---|---|---|
| *CPD:* | Trisodium citrate | 26·3 g |
| | Citric acid | 3·27 g |
| | Sodium dihydrogen phosphate | 2·22 g |
| | Dextrose | 25·5 g |
| | Water to | 1 litre |

63 ml CPD are mixed with 450 ml whole blood.

Heparin is occasionally used as an anticoagulant, but because of its short half-life (4 hours), the blood must be transfused within 12 hours of its being taken. Its value is principally in neonatal transfusion and infant open heart surgery.

#### The Effects of Storage

The rate of glycolysis of the red cells is lowered both by the low temperature of storage and also by the lowered pH. The enzyme hexokinase is particularly sensitive to acid conditions, and the failure of glycolysis causes the loss of nucleotides and phosphate esters (of which 2–3 diphosphoglycerate (2–3 DPG) is the most important). CPD solution is preferable to ACD in that the final pH of the mixture is higher and thus glycolysis continues longer and, also, the presence of the phosphate ion in CPD encourages the preservation of phosphate esters. The number of viable red cells falls progressively on storage. After 14 days storage in ACD, viability within the first 24 hours of transfusion is 90 per cent and this falls to 70 per cent at 21 days, which is the limit for storage. However, post-transfusion survival of red cells stored in CPD is better maintained and the limit of storage is usually 32 days when 80 per cent viability is achieved.

*2–3 Diphosphoglycerate (2–3 DPG)* is derived from 3-phosphoglyceraldehyde which is an intermediate product of the Embden Meyerhof pathway. It facilitates the transition of oxyhaemoglobin to deoxyhaemoglobin. Therefore, the more 2–3 DPG present, the less the affinity of the red blood cell for oxygen and the more oxygen available to the tissues. The level of 2–3 DPG falls progressively during storage, resulting in a shift to the left of the oxygen dissociation curve. This is a reversible defect, but levels of 2–3 DPG are not restored to normal until 24 hours after transfusion. It might be expected that the low levels of 2–3 DPG in stored blood would cause problems of tissue hypoxia. However, in clinical practice, the restoration of the circulating blood volume is astonishingly effective, albeit with red cells reluctant to release their oxygen to the tissues.

As glycolysis ceases, *adenosine triphosphate (ATP)* levels fall and the red-cell membrane enzymes are no longer able to maintain the active transport of sodium and potassium. As a result, potassium leaks out of the cells causing high levels of plasma potassium (up to 25 mmol/l), and sodium and water pass into the cells causing swelling and even lysis. Membrane constituents, such as lipids, are also lost. The addition of many "conditioning" agents such as adenine, adenosine, inosine, guanosine and xanthosine have been recommended to improve maintenance of red-cell nucleotides and to "rejuvenate" stored blood. They are becoming more widely used, as the viability of red cells in CPD adenine is 75–80 per cent after 5 weeks storage.

### Indications for the Use of Whole Blood

Some would say that there is no longer any indication for the transfusion of stored whole blood, in that the plasma of stored blood is a poor source of clotting factors and its albumin rapidly disappears after transfusion. It could be said that the simultaneous transfusion of plasma-reduced red cells with normal saline or Hartmann's solution is just as effective clinically as the transfusion of stored whole blood and, furthermore, allows the plasma to be used for other purposes (this argument does not apply if fresh whole blood is to be used). However, old habits die hard and when faced with haemorrhage, most anaesthetists are still happiest when transfusing whole blood. The indications, therefore, for the transfusion of whole blood (or plasma-reduced blood plus normal saline) are:

*Trauma.*—Assessment of the volume of blood lost is always difficult in these cases. The restoration of blood volume is greatly aided by continuous measurement of the central venous pressure.

*Surgery.*—The decision as to when, whether, and how much to transfuse during surgical operations is often a difficult one. The measurement of blood loss at operation is fraught with inaccuracy. Swab weighing is certainly better than nothing, but usually underestimates by 25 per cent[8]. As well as the operative blood loss, the predicted postoperative loss from oozing, the pre-operative haemoglobin concentration and the cardiovascular status of the patient must all be taken into consideration. The benefit of replacing all blood lost in the perioperative period is debatable. The postoperative patient certainly looks better and there is some evidence that wound healing is faster if the haemoglobin concentration is restored to its pre-operative value. However, there are risks associated with any transfusion and particularly that of overtransfusion, if the loss has been estimated wrongly.

*Massive burns.*—The grossly burnt patient loses red cells as well as plasma, due to haemolysis of the cells on heating to temperatures above 50° C[9] at the time of the burn. During the subsequent 48 hours more red cells are lost if there is more than 20 per cent full thickness skin loss.

*Gastro-intestinal haemorrhage.* — Here again central venous pressure monitoring is an extremely valuable aid to assessing loss and monitoring replacement.

*Obstetrics.*—Antepartum and postpartum haemorrhage can be sudden, and large in volume, as can be the haemorrhage associated with threatened, incomplete or complete abortion. The massive bleeding of a ruptured ectopic pregnancy may be contained by a rigid abdomen, and become much worse as general anaesthesia is induced and abdominal relaxation occurs. This phenomenon is also seen with ruptured aortic aneurysms.

## Red-Cell Concentrates

There are several varieties of red-cell concentrates provided by different transfusion centres from which plasma and/or white cells and platelets have been removed.

*Concentrated red cells.*—These contain 70–90 per cent red cells, and have a high viscosity and consequently are slow to transfuse.

*Plasma-reduced red cells.*—These are produced by centrifugation and removal of the plasma and the buffy coat into an attached transfer pack. The resulting preparation contains between 60–80 per cent red cells but cannot be considered free of all white cells, plasma or platelets.

*Washed red cells.*—These are red-cell concentrates which are washed several times with sterile saline. This renders them almost free of contaminating white cells and the resulting preparation, when resuspended in a small volume of saline, has a lower viscosity than other red-cell concentrates.

*Frozen red cells*.—Various preservatives have been used to enable red cells to be frozen and stored at −20° C to −50° C, e.g. glycerol and hydroxy ethyl starch. After thawing, all the preservative must be completely removed by repeated washing.

### Indications for Use

*Concentrated red cells and plasma-reduced red cells*: As stated above, these can be used together with normal saline or balanced salt solution in the place of whole blood, for the treatment of haemorrhage.

Either of these is the product of choice for the treatment of chronic anaemia where transfusion is indicated.

*Washed red cells* are valuable for the patient who has had multiple transfusions who commonly has febrile or other allergic manifestations after transfusion with whole blood, due to antibodies to white cells, platelets or plasma proteins.

*Frozen red cells* are of great value for patients who have rare blood group antigens or antibodies to very common blood groups. Compatible blood, or the patient's blood, can be stored in preparation for surgery or delivery.

Their use in patients awaiting organ transplants (kidney, marrow, liver and heart) is not yet clear, although by using HLA (human leucocyte antigen) matched blood, the chances of raising anti-HLA antibodies are reduced.

All red-cell products which have been washed or manipulated are potentially infected and usually have a limit of 12 to 24 hours stipulated for their use.

### The Problem of Pre-operative Anaemia and Whether to Transfuse

Most anaesthetists are unwilling to administer a general anaesthetic for elective surgery to a patient with a haemoglobin concentration of less than 10 g/dl (the exception is a patient with chronic renal failure who is usually well adapted to his severe anaemia). If anaemia is discovered some weeks before operation, there is ample time to diagnose the cause and institute logical treatment. If, however, the operation cannot be postponed and pre-operative transfusion is deemed necessary, it should be given at least 48 hours prior to operation so that 2–3 DPG levels are restored to normal by the time of the anaesthetic. An ultrafilter should be used in order that the pulmonary capillaries may be kept free of microaggregates and pulmonary function compromised as little as possible.

## White Cells

Donor white cells may be obtained in a number of ways from normal donors or from patients with chronic granulocytic leukaemia.

### Indications for Use

The most important indication for their use is in the severely neutropenic patients with infection, particularly septicaemia, and in conjunction with antibiotics. White-cell concentrates should be given as soon as possible after collection and certainly within 24 hours.

## Platelets

### Collection and Storage

Platelets are usually collected as concentrates from donor bags of whole blood by centrifugation. Platelet concentrates usually contain white cells and red cells and, for this reason, platelets of the correct blood group should be given. Rhesus-negative subjects should be given anti-D specific immunoglobulin if it is necessary for them to receive rhesus-positive platelets in order to prevent sensitisation, especially if they are women of child-bearing age.

Platelets should be used within 12 hours of collection and, preferably, stored at 22° C with gentle agitation.

### Indications for Use

Thrombocytopenia with bleeding is an absolute indication for platelet transfusion. Severely thrombocytopenic patients ($<20\times10^9$/l platelet count) probably warrant platelet transfusion, especially in the presence of infection, even if there is no bleeding or purpura. Platelet cover is also necessary for surgery on thrombocytopenic patients or in patients with defective platelet function. Defective platelet function is most commonly an acquired lesion (myelo-proliferative disorders, cardiopulmonary bypass) but there are a few extremely rare congenital conditions in which it occurs. If splenectomy is being carried out as treatment for thrombocytopenia, it is advisable to withhold platelet transfusion until the splenic artery is clamped, provided haemostasis can be achieved; this prevents the transfused platelets being lost to the spleen. A dose of platelets—$2\times10^{11}$—will raise the platelet count by an anticipated $18\times10^{9}$/l in the recipient. In the presence of platelet antibodies, either in immune thrombocytopenia, or following multiple platelet transfusions, little or no rise in the count may be seen, although some clinical improvement in haemostasis may be achieved.

## Plasma

### Fresh Frozen Plasma (FFP)

This is obtained from the centrifugation of donor units followed by rapid freezing to −20° C. Clotting factors are well preserved, but are relatively too dilute for FFP to be very useful in the management of severe deficiencies. However, it may be used as a source of albumin. It cannot be regarded as entirely free of the risk of transmitting hepatitis.

*Indications for use.*—FFP is principally used in the treatment of multiple coagulation deficiencies, e.g. liver disease, reversal of warfarin and disseminated intravascular coagulation. Transfusion of stored blood in large volume usually results in coagulation deficiencies, even if not apparent clinically; therefore, *one unit of FFP should be given for every 4–6 units of stored blood*. FFP may also be used as a replacement fluid for plasmapheresis, usually in combination with plasma protein fraction (PPF), albumin, saline or synthetic plasma expanders.

### Dried Plasma

This is rarely produced in the United Kingdom nowadays as plasma is normally fractionated into more specific concentrates. There is a high risk of hepatitis transmission in its use.

*Indications for use.*—The only indication for its use is as a plasma expander when no safer preparation is available.

### Plasma Protein Fraction (PPF)

This fraction contains 95 per cent albumin and, because it is pasteurised (60° C for 10 hours) there is no risk of hepatitis transmission. The protein concentration is 46 g/l, sodium concentration 130–160 mmol/l and potassium and calcium, less than 2 mmol/l. It has a five-year shelf-life at room temperature.

*Indications for use.*—It may be used as a plasma expander and as a source of albumin.

### Albumin

This is concentrated from plasma and is available in liquid or freeze-dried form. Salt-poor albumin is also available and all are relatively expensive products.

*Indications for use.*—In hypo-albuminaemic states and as a plasma expander.

### Cryoprecipitate

Plasma which has been frozen rapidly to −40° C and then thawed, contains a precipitate rich in factor VIII (approximately 50 per cent of the original plasma concentration) and fibrinogen. It is stored at −20° C after removal of the supernatant plasma. It also contains anti-A and anti-B in concentrations similar to those in the donor unit and therefore only ABO-compatible cryoprecipitate should be used. Due to the lability of factor VIII, it is thawed at 37° C immediately prior to transfusion.

*Indications for use.*—The primary use of cryoprecipitate is in the treatment of haemophilia (although freeze-dried concentrates are preferred—see below) and in Von Willebrand's disease. It is occasionally used as part of the replacement therapy in disseminated intravascular coagulation (DIC) because of its high concentration of factor VIII and fibrinogen. ABO-compatible cryoprecipitate should always be used, as with large doses there is a risk of haemolysis.

### Factor VIII Concentrate

This freeze-dried material has a high concentration of factor VIII (20 units/ml). There is a risk of hepatitis transmission in its use.

*Indications for use.*—It is used for the treatment of bleeding episodes, and to cover surgery in haemophiliacs.

### Factor II, IX, X Concentrate

This is a freeze-dried material. There is evidence of clotting factor activation in some preparations and therefore it should not be used in disseminated intravascular coagulation (DIC). Large doses used therapeutically should probably be covered by the administration of heparin (10 units of heparin per 100 units of Factor IX) to prevent thrombosis.

*Indications for use.*—It can be used for the reversal of warfarin when a rapid restoration of normal coagulation is required, especially where there has been overdosage. It is also used for the treatment of Christmas disease.

### Fibrinogen Concentrates

These are available in freeze-dried form.

*Indications for use.*—Hypofibrinogenaemia in liver disease or DIC.

### Anti-thrombin III Concentrate

This can be isolated from plasma and is currently being evaluated in clinical trials. Anti-thrombin III is necessary for heparin action and low levels are commonly associated with thrombosis and DIC.

*Indications for use.*—It is used for the treatment of anti-thrombin III deficiency. This condition may occur during surgery or prolonged heparin treatment or be associated with liver disease. In rare instances, anti-thrombin III deficiency may be congenital.

## THE MONITORING OF THE TRANSFUSED PATIENT

### Massive Transfusion given in the Operating Theatre

Pulse, blood pressure, central venous pressure, central temperature and hourly urine output should all be monitored in the transfused patient. A continuous ECG monitor is also useful. If possible, the transfused patient should be kept on a warming blanket.

### Small-volume Transfusions Given in the Ward

These are the transfusions least monitored and most likely to cause problems, particularly if the patient is on the verge of left ventricular failure. The nursing staff should measure pulse, blood pressure and temperature as often as is practicable and central venous pressure as well, if possible. A careful fluid balance chart should be kept, although a urinary catheter is not normally indicated in these patients.

## THE HAZARDS OF BLOOD TRANSFUSION

### Haemolytic Transfusion Reactions

Fortunately, very few ABO-incompatible transfusions occur; when they do, mortality may be as high as 10 per cent. The commonest cause of an incompatible transfusion is a clerical error, i.e. the mixing up of names and labels on blood samples for cross-matching or on units of donor blood. Each patient should have a label with his name and hospital number attached to his wrist and the blood, which has been cross-matched for him, should also be labelled with his name, number and group. The greatest care should be afforded to checking the unit and its label against the patient before starting the transfusion.

Reactions to the transfusion of incompatible blood depend on the type of antibody which is involved. Immediate major reactions are the result of intravascular haemolysis. Delayed reactions occur over a longer period following transfusion, although there may be a febrile reaction while the incompatible blood is being transfused.

**Intravascular haemolysis** is usually associated with an IgM antibody which fixes complement and the majority are due to ABO incompatibility. The haemolysis causes a rise in plasma haemoglobin and methaemoglobin, and the liberation of intracellular contents may trigger off disseminated intravascular coagulation which is responsible for much of the morbidity and mortality. The clinical picture may include fever, rigors, chest pain, dyspnoea, loin pain, hypotension, oliguria and anuria. This can occur after as little as 100 ml blood.

*Management* the first priority is to stop the transfusion and resuscitate the patient. The circulating volume must be restored and maintained with plasma, a synthetic plasma expander or normal saline and, if hypotension and a poor peripheral circulation persist despite this, an inotrope such as dopamine may be necessary. The urinary output should be monitored and if oliguria or anuria continue in the presence of an adequate cardiac output, mannitol 25 g and frusemide in generous dosage should be given in order to provoke a diuresis. If there is no response to this, then it must be assumed that acute tubular necrosis has occurred and the patient managed accordingly.

The unused blood and giving set should be returned to the laboratory together with a sample of the patient's blood and urine (if available). The following investigations should be performed.

Full blood and platelet count
DIC screen (*vide infra*)
Regrouping and re-crossmatching of all blood transfused
Direct antiglobulin test (Coombs test)
Blood culture
Free plasma haemoglobin (degree of haemolysis)
Free haemoglobin in urine.

**Extravascular haemolysis** is the result of incomplete IgG antibodies which attach to the red cell without fixing complement and cause it to be destroyed by the reticulo-endothelial system over the next few hours or days (up to 7 days post-transfusion). This causes hyperbilirubinaemia, anaemia with a positive direct antiglobulin test, and an increased urinary urobilinogen. Renal failure is rare. Blood should be sent to the laboratory with, if possible, the empty transfusion bags.

Post-transfusion jaundice may also result from non-viable red cells, although this should not normally happen if blood has been preserved and stored correctly. Laboratory findings will confirm a haemolytic process and no evidence of hepatitis.

### Infection

**Transfusion of bacterially infected blood.**—This is the other major, though rare, cause of mortality following transfusion. Contamination may occur at the time of collection. In this case haemolysis usually results and the blood appears abnormal but occasionally this may not be obvious and, within minutes of the transfusion starting, the patient may develop pyrexia, dyspnoea, chest pain or hypotension. If contamination occurs at the time of administration, the signs of septicaemia may be delayed.

**Post-transfusion hepatitis.**—Rigorous testing of donated blood for $HB_s$ AG has not led to the eradication of post-transfusion hepatitis. Many cases are now due to non-A, non-B hepatitis which has an incubation period of about 30 days. This is particularly common following the use of plasma fractions which have been obtained from large pools of plasma.

**Infections transmitted in donor blood.**—Syphilis is excluded by screening of the donor and in addition, the spirochete rarely survives storage at 4° C for longer than 24 hours. Malaria may be transmitted for many years after clinical illness, depending on which organism is involved. Trypanosoma cruzi is also readily transmitted but this can be prevented by the addition of crystal violet to the blood.

Viruses, such as cytomegalovirus and the herpes viruses, survive storage and may be responsible for some cases of "post-cardiotomy syndromes".

The aetiology of the recently recognised acquired immune deficiency syndrome (AIDS) is as yet unproven, but may be viral. Haemophiliacs comprise one of the high risk groups who develop this immunological deficiency state with associated opportunistic infections or Kaposi's sarcoma, indicating that the causal agent may be transmitted by transfusion of blood products.

### Fever

This is the commonest complication of blood transfusion. It may be due to sensitivity to leucocytes, platelets, plasma proteins or, more rarely, caused by pyrogens. If there are no major signs of incompatibility or infection, transfusion may be continued with careful observation.

### Air Embolus

This complication has, fortunately, become extremely rare with the advent of plastic blood bags. Classically it used to be caused by pumping air into glass blood bottles.

### Haemolysed Blood

If blood has been inadvertently frozen or overheated, haemolysis may occur. Transfusion of this can cause signs and symptoms as severe as those of major incompatibility.

### Allergic or Anaphylactic Reactions

Urticarial reactions are not uncommon and normally respond to antihistamine therapy. Anaphylactic reactions are rare but are sometimes seen in congenitally IgA-deficient recipients or in those with sensitivity to plasma protein antigens.

## PARTICULAR PROBLEMS ASSOCIATED WITH MASSIVE TRANSFUSION

### Temperature

Large volumes of very cold stored blood will rapidly drop the recipient's temperature to as low as 27·5 °C[10,11] at which level fatal dysrhythmias may occur. Therefore, any patient who is to receive more than 2 or 3 units of blood over a short period of time, should have the blood warmed to body temperature prior to delivery. Blood may be warmed either by running it through a long coil immersed in a water bath at 37°—39° C or by the use of one of the newer electrically heated warmers. *At no time must the blood be exposed to temperatures above 40° C.*

### Biochemical Changes

*Citrate.*—The plasma concentration of citrate in stored whole blood (ACD or CPD) is 15 mEq/l at 10 days and 30 mEq/l at 28 days and consequently massive transfusions are associated with a high plasma level which has its deleterious effect by causing a lowering of the ionised calcium. This may result in cardiac arrest and will certainly impair clotting mechanisms. The maximum rate of citrate administration is 0·04 mmol/kg/min[12] which is equivalent to blood at a rate of 1 litre in 10 minutes to an adult. The administration of calcium reverses the adverse effects of citrate and doses of 10 ml of 10 per cent calcium gluconate for every litre of citrated blood are recommended.[2] Care should be exercised in the administration of intravenous calcium as a large bolus may induce dysrhythmia and even cardiac arrest (see also Calcium, below). Citrate toxicity is rare if there is normal tissue metabolism because citrate is rapidly broken down, but may occur in the presence of impaired liver function, hypotension or hypothermia. In this context the neonate is particularly susceptible and care should be exercised.

*Acid-base disturbance.*—The pH of fresh stored blood in CPD can be as low as 6·0 but, surprisingly, massive transfusions do not cause the expected acidosis provided the circulating blood volume is rapidly restored and maintained. The citrate is metabolised to bicarbonate producing a metabolic alkalosis within 24 hours.

*Calcium.*—As stated above, if supplements are not given, the ionised calcium tends to fall during massive transfusion, but some authorities believe that calcium supplements are not necessary.[13] There is an immediate rise in parathormone levels following transfusion, which mobilises ionised calcium from the bone.

### Microaggregates

During storage, aggregates of leucocytes and platelets with diameters up to 200 μm are formed. Standard giving sets have filters with a pore size of 170 μm and so permit the passage of quite sizeable microaggregates. With each unit of one-week-old ACD whole blood, 15 million 20–40 μm diameter microaggregates and 20 million with diameters over 40 μm can wash into the capillary bed.[14] If more than 20 per cent of the blood volume is transfused without ultrafiltration, significant increases occur in arteriovenous shunting and alveolar arterial oxygen differences,[15] and protection has been shown by the use of microfiltration.[16,17] On the other hand, there are instances of massive unfiltered transfusions causing no respiratory problems.[18]

Microfilters or ultrafilters are filters which do not allow the passage of aggregates larger than 20–40 μm (depending on the filter). The only disadvantage of the routine use of an ultrafilter is expense, and the possibility of red-cell trauma if undue pressure has to be exerted on the blood in order to force it through. Loong[19] recommends microfiltration of all blood more than four days old with a Pall 40 μm pore size screen filter. This will take 8–10 units of blood.

## HAEMOSTATIC MECHANISMS

The body is protected from excessive bleeding in response to injury and from spontaneous bleeding by the haemostatic mechanism. This will be discussed in terms of (a) mechanisms which promote haemostasis—*primary haemostasis, intrinsic coagulation mechanism, extrinsic coagulation mechanism*; (b) *naturally occurring inhibitors of haemostasis*; and (c) the mechanism which causes breakdown of formed clot—*fibrinolysis*.

*Primary haemostasis* (see Table 2).—This is the formation of a platelet plug at the site of vascular injury. Endothelial damage causes exposure of subendothelial collagen which

17/TABLE 2
DETAILS OF CLOTTING FACTORS

| *Number* | *Name* | *Half-life* in vivo | *Site of Production* | |
|---|---|---|---|---|
| I | Fibrinogen | 4–6 days | Liver | |
| II | Prothrombin | 3–4 days | Liver | (Vitamin K Dependent) |
| III | Tissue Thromboplastin | | Tissues | |
| IV | Calcium | | | |
| V | Proaccelerin | 24 hours | Liver | |
| VII | Proconvertin | 4–6 hours | Liver | (Vitamin K Dependent) |
| VIII | Antihaemophilic Factor/Globulin | 12 hours | Endothelial Cells | |
| IX | Christmas Factor | 18–24 hours | Liver | (Vitamin K Dependent) |
| X | Stuart Prower Factor | 60–70 hours | Liver | (Vitamin K Dependent) |
| XI | Plasma Thromboplastin Antecedent | 60–70 hours | Liver | |
| XII | Hageman Factor | | | |
| XIII | Fibrin Stabilising Factor | 6 days | | |

17/TABLE 3

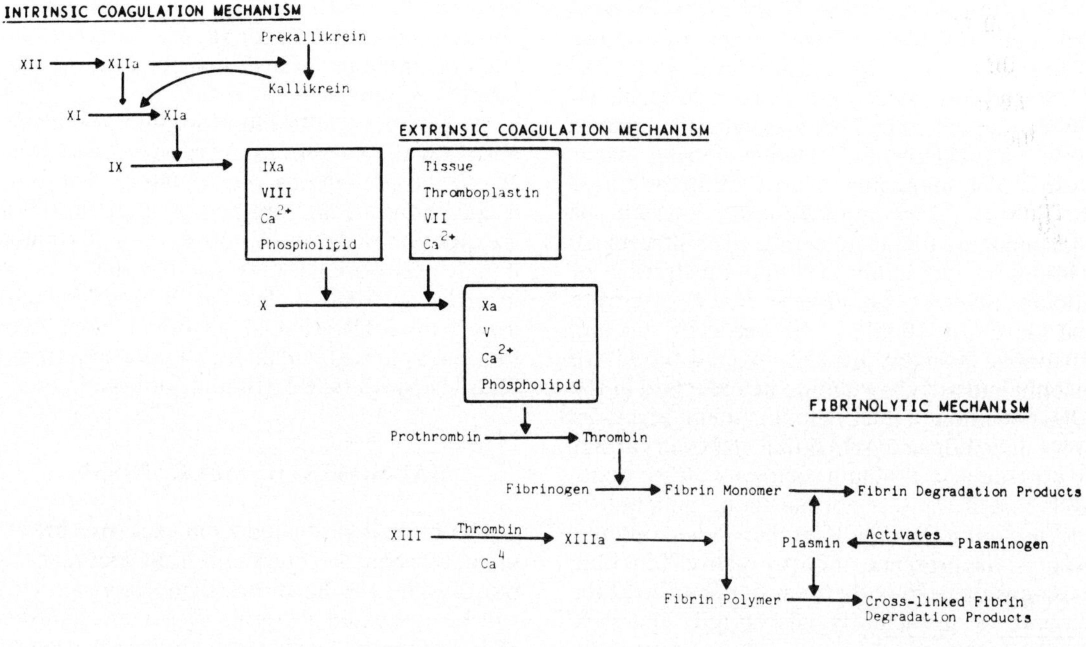


results in primary aggregation of platelets. ADP is released from platelet granules and causes secondary platelet aggregation and the formation of a firm haemostatic plug. Serotonin and thromboxane $A_2$ (a prostaglandin metabolite) are also released and cause local vasoconstriction.

*Intrinsic coagulation mechanism* (see Table 3).—This is a cascade mechanism whereby inactive coagulation factors are activated enzymically in succession in the presence of calcium ions and phospholipids. The initiation of this process is the activation of factor XII and factor XI by contact with collagen. The reactions then proceed as shown in Table 3 resulting in the formation of a cross-linked fibrin clot.

*Extrinsic coagulation mechanism* (see Table 3).—This is a much more rapid pathway whereby tissue thromboplastin, derived from injured cells, forms a complex with factor VII in the presence of calcium ions and activates factor X directly and hence the final common pathway.

*Naturally occurring inhibitors of haemostasis.*—The most powerful anti-platelet aggregatory agent known is prostacyclin ($PGI_2$). This is made in endothelial and smooth muscle cells and also causes powerful vasodilatation.

The coagulation cascade is controlled and modified by a number of plasmatic inhibitors and by removal of complexed activated clotting factors by the reticuloendothelial system. Antithrombin III inactivates thrombin and is a necessary cofactor for heparin activity. $\alpha_2$ antiplasmin, $\alpha_2$ macroglobulin and $\alpha_1$ antitrypsin are other inhibitors of coagulation factors and plasmin.

*Fibrinolysis.*—Plasminogen exists in the blood and all other body fluids. It is activated to the proteolytic enzyme plasmin by a variety of activators. Intrinsic activators include factor XII and prekallikrein. Extrinsic activators are produced by many different tissues including vascular endothelium, uterus, urinary tract (producing urokinase), gastric tissue and a variety of malignant tumours. Streptokinase is an extrinsic activator produced by $\beta$-haemolytic streptococci. A number of inhibitors to the system have been described. Plasmin proteolyses fibrin to give rise to a series of fibrin degradation products (FDP) and lysis of the clot.

### SCREENING TESTS FOR HAEMOSTATIC DEFECTS

*Bleeding time.*—This is a test of primary haemostasis and is dependent on normal numbers of normally functioning platelets and a normal vasoconstriction response.

*Prothrombin time ratio* (PTR).—The time taken for a fibrin clot to form in the presence of tissue thromboplastin and calcium is expressed as a ratio with the time taken for normal plasma. A ratio greater than one is caused by any defect in the extrinsic or final common coagulation pathways (i.e. factors VII, X, V, II, I).

*Partial thromboplastin time* (PTT).—This is an *in vitro* test of the intrinsic coagulation pathway, and is thus dependent on the presence of all coagulation factors except factor VII.

*Thrombin time* (TT).—The addition of thrombin to plasma in the presence of calcium, tests the rate of formation of fibrin from fibrinogen. It is prolonged by heparin, fibrin degradation products, dysfibrinogenaemia (congenital or acquired) and low fibrinogen concentrations.

*Arvin time* (AT).—The Malayan pit-viper's venom acts directly on fibrinogen to form fibrin. It is not affected by the presence of heparin but is prolonged in the presence of fibrin degradation products (FDP), enabling interpretation of a prolonged thrombin time.

*Fibrin degradation products* (FDP).—Increased levels are found in disseminated intravascular coagulation and in conditions of increased fibrinolysis.

*Fibrinogen concentration.*—This is dependent on the rate of production and rate of consumption of fibrinogen. In hepatocellular failure and in disseminated intravascular coagulation, it is reduced. Raised levels are found in most acutely or chronically ill patients and in pregnancy. Low to normal concentrations of fibrinogen in these individuals may suggest DIC.

*Platelet count.*—Reduced platelet counts may be due to a variety of bone-marrow disorders. A falling platelet count, however, in a patient developing a haemorrhagic diathesis is suggestive of DIC. The presence of normal numbers of platelets does not exclude a functional disorder. The bleeding time is a most useful screen in these circumstances.

*Antithrombin III.*—Low levels indicate patients at risk from thrombosis, and cause resistance to heparin anticoagulation.

## DISORDERS OF THE HAEMOSTATIC MECHANISM

### Platelet Abnormalities

**Thrombocytopenia.**—This may be caused by bone-marrow infiltration (e.g. leukaemia or other malignancy) or bone-marrow suppression (idiopathic or due to drugs, chemicals or irradiation). Increased platelet destruction giving rise to thrombocytopenia may also occur as a result of immune (anti-platelet antibodies, immune complex disease) or non-immune mechanisms (e.g. hypersplenism).

**Platelet function defects.**—Acquired defects of platelet aggregation are seen following administration of a number of drugs, for example, aspirin. Partial activation of platelets in cardiopulmonary bypass may lead to platelets circulating in a degranulated and unresponsive state. Abnormal platelets are sometimes produced in marrow disorders, especially the myeloproliferative syndromes and myelofibrosis. In uraemia, there is a circulating prostacyclin-like substance which prevents platelet aggregation. There are also a few very rare congenital defects of platelet function.

## Disorders of Clotting Factors

### Inherited Abnormalities

**Haemophilia** is a sex-linked recessive disorder characterised by reduced or absent levels of the coagulant activity of factor VIII (FVIIIC). There are normal levels of factor VIII related antigen (FVIIIR:AG). The severity of the disorder depends on the concentration of factor VIIIC. Patients with less than one International unit per 100 ml (1 iu/100 ml) are severely affected and suffer spontaneous haemorrhages into joints, muscles and other tissues. Patients with levels of 1–5 iu/100 ml are moderately affected, and those with greater than 5 iu/100 ml rarely have spontaneous bleeding.

Treatment of spontaneous haemorrhages is by intravenous factor VIII concentrates, usually freeze-dried material, but cryoprecipitate may also be used to raise factor VIII levels to 20–40 iu/100 ml. Prior to surgery, concentrates should be given to raise the factor VIII level to 100 iu/100 ml, and the level should be maintained between 50–100 iu/100 ml for a week to ten days postoperatively by twice-daily administrations of concentrate. This is necessary because of the short half-life of factor VIII. Because of their multiple exposure to plasma concentrates, haemophiliacs commonly have antibody to $HB_sAg$, while a few are chronic carriers of $HB_sAg$ and non-A and non-B hepatitis.

The development of anti-factor VIII antibodies in 5–10 per cent of haemophiliacs makes them resistant to normal doses of factor VIII concentrates. In these cases, either very high doses of factor VIII or a variety of activated prothrombin complexes may be used.

Occasionally, haemophilia carriers may have FVIIIC levels low enough to require concentrates prior to surgery.

**Von Willebrand's disease.**—This is an autosomal dominant defect of the production of factor VIII related antigen (FVIIIR:AG) which is characterised by low levels of both circulating FVIIIR:AG and the coagulant active factor VIII (FVIIIC). Added to this, there is a platelet aggregation abnormality which can be demonstrated *in vitro* by a failure to aggregate with ristocetin. Because of this latter defect, patients with Von Willebrand's disease—unlike haemophiliacs—have a prolonged skin bleeding time. Replacement therapy for surgery or spontaneous bleeding is with cryoprecipitate, which is richer in the Von Willebrand's factor than factor VIII complexes. Anti-fibrinolytic drugs are valuable, particularly for mucous-membrane bleeding (*vide infra*).

**Christmas disease** (Haemophilia B).—This is a sex-linked recessive defect of factor IX production. The incidence is 10 per cent that of haemophilia. Clinically, both present a similar picture. Treatment of spontaneous or traumatic bleeding is with factor IX (FIX) concentrates. It has been found that these are thrombogenic and, if given in large doses to cover surgery, should be accompanied by low doses of heparin (100 units heparin per 1,000 units factor IX) to prevent thromboembolic complications.

**Rare deficiencies** of factors V and VIII, fibrinogen, X, XI, XII. These do not usually give rise to serious problems, except during surgery or trauma, when replacement therapy should be given to keep the concentration of the relevant factor within the normal range.

### Acquired Abnormalities

**Hepatocellular disease.**—Acute hepatocellular failure due to hepatitis or drug overdose (e.g. paracetamol), or chronic liver damage from whatever cause, gives rise to coagulation factor deficiencies. The vitamin K dependent factors II, VII, IX and X may be partially or completely synthesised after therapeutic vitamin K, but low levels of factors XI and V and fibrinogen will not respond. Treatment of haemorrhagic symptoms is usually with fresh frozen plasma.

**Vitamin K deficiency.**—This occurs in neonates, or may be seen in starvation or malabsorption. Administration of parenteral vitamin K corrects the defect rapidly and is given routinely to many neonates (see Chapter 42).

**Massive transfusion** of stored blood is associated with coagulation defects because of the loss of clotting factors and platelets on storage. This is corrected with fresh plasma (see above).

### Excess Inhibitors of Coagulation

These disorders are rare and usually acquired.

*Anti-factor VIII* antibodies may be produced spontaneously, more often in the elderly and may also occur in association with autoimmune disorders such as systemic lupus erythematosus and rheumatoid arthritis, pregnancy and penicillin treatment. The antibodies are usually present in low titre, but may give rise to severe haemorrhagic symptoms. Treatment is usually by a combination of plasmapheresis and cytotoxic drugs, such as cyclophosphamide, to reduce the production of the antibody. For acute bleeding symptoms, high doses of factor VIII concentrate or activated complexes may be used as for haemophiliacs with acquired inhibitors. Patients with myeloma and macroglobulinaemia may have acquired coagulation defects because of the paraprotein: removal of this by plasmapheresis and chemotherapy is the most effective way to restore haemostasis.

### Disseminated Intravascular Coagulation (DIC)

(Defibrination Syndrome, Consumption Coagulopathy or Microangiopathic Haemolytic Anaemia)

This is a haemorrhagic disorder in which clotting factors and platelets are used up in a process of diffuse intravascular clotting. It is usually an acute condition caused by entry into the blood stream of factors which trigger the clotting mechanism and may occur as a complication of the conditions listed in Table 4.

The clinical features of defibrination are bleeding, which may be generalised or localised, and the effects of organ damage due to ischaemia caused by intravascular thrombosis. After laboratory confirmation of the diagnosis, treatment should be aimed at:

1. *Elimination of the precipitating cause.* This is often not possible, but, for example, septicaemia should be treated with the appropriate antibiotics.
2. *Replacement of coagulation factors and platelets.* Fresh blood (less than 12 hours old) or fresh frozen plasma should be given. In addition, in cases with severe bleeding, fibrinogen 5–10 g in 500 ml should be infused over 2–3 hours.
3. *Inhibition of the clotting process with heparin.* Heparin may be given after clotting factor replacement if the defibrination process is continuing or if intravascular thrombosis is causing organ damage. Careful laboratory monitoring is essential.

17/Table 4
Causes of DIC

| |
|---|
| Septicaemia. |
| Surgery, especially of heart and lungs. |
| Obstetric accidents: |
| (*a*) Abruptio placentae (premature placental separation). |
| (*b*) Amniotic fluid embolism. |
| (*c*) Abortion. |
| (*d*) Intra-uterine death. |
| Haemolytic transfusion reaction. |
| Pulmonary embolism. |
| Malignant disease. |
| Snake bite. |
| Hypersensitivity reactions. |
| Heat stroke. |
| Burns. |

#### Mechanism

Widespread intravascular activation of the clotting system gives rise to a haemorrhagic syndrome characterised by depletion of fibrinogen, other clotting factors and platelets. The meshwork of fibrin laid down in the microvasculature can lead to considerable tissue damage (the kidneys are particularly vulnerable) and to rapid intravascular haemolysis of red cells which are destroyed as they are forced over the fibrin strands. If the haemolytic process is the predominant feature, the term "microangiopathic haemolytic anaemia" is sometimes used. The plasmin system is activated to break down the fibrin, and fibrin degradation products circulate in high concentrations, interfering with further fibrin formation and increasing the risk of haemorrhage. The severity of the syndrome varies enormously. In some patients there may be uncontrolled haemorrhage, severe purpura and signs of renal failure—whereas in others there may only be laboratory evidence of the process. In some degree, compensated DIC is seen in many pathological states and it is by no means always necessary to treat it.

### Laboratory Findings

Classically these are:

(*a*) prolongation of prothrombin time ratio
(*b*) prolongation of partial thromboplastin test
(*c*) prolongation of the thrombin test
(*d*) prolongation of the arvin time
(*e*) low plasma fibrinogen
(*f*) low platelet count
(*g*) high level fibrin degradation products in plasma and urine

but it is unlikely that all of these defects will be demonstrated, particularly in the early stages of the disease.

In a rapidly changing situation, it is necessary to repeat screening tests every few hours and for this reason, the *platelet* count and the *thrombin* time are probably the most useful indicators of the progression of the disorder and the success of management.

Treatment is primarily directed at the underlying condition wherever possible, with intensive supportive measures such as the restoration of circulating volume and reversal of hypotension, hypoxia and acidosis. Replacement of clotting factors with fresh plasma will often lead to an improvement in the clinical condition and laboratory tests. Platelet transfusion is usually contra-indicated as this may tend to activate the process. Fresh blood transfusion may be life-saving especially in obstetric DIC. Intermediate-dose heparin therapy (approximately 500 u/kg body weight) is used in severe haemorrhagic DIC with skin gangrene and organ damage (sometimes referred to as purpura fulminans).

## Drugs Affecting the Haemostatic Mechanism

(*a*) **Coumarins.**—This group of drugs, which includes warfarin, phenindione, biscoumacetate, compete with vitamin K as a co-factor in the production of factors II, VII, IX and X in hepatic cells. They give rise to the presence of functionally inactive, but otherwise identical, molecules known as PIVKA (proteins induced by vitamin K absence or antagonists). Therapeutic anticoagulation is usually monitored by the prothrombin time ratio which is kept between 2·0 and 3·5. Alternatively, Thrombotest, a test also dependent on factor IX, is used (therapeutic range 5–15 per cent). The effect of coumarins on clotting should be checked regularly, particularly in the presence of cardiac or renal failure which prolong its action, or if other medication is changed. Other drugs interfere with the anticoagulant effect of warfarin in a variety of ways (see Table 5).

17/Table 5
Some of the Commoner Drug Interactions with Warfarin

| *Drug* | *Mechanism of action* | *Effect on warfarin* |
|---|---|---|
| Protein bound drugs: phenylbutazone aspirin sulphonamides | Displacement of warfarin from protein | Potentiation |
| Phenylbutazone | Inhibition of hydroxylation of warfarin | Potentiation |
| Barbiturates and hypnotics | Induction of warfarin hydroxylases | Reduction |
| Antibiotics<br>Paraffin<br>MAOI | Reduction of vitamin K absorption | Potentiation |
| Alcohol | Hepatotoxicity<br>Reduction of vitamin K absorption | Potentiation |

### Management of Surgery for Patients on Warfarin

*Dental extraction* or limited operative procedures. Because of its delayed action, warfarin should be stopped 48 hours pre-operatively. This usually gives a prothrombin time ratio less than 2·0, which is safe for limited surgery. Warfarin can be restarted on the evening of the operative day. Bleeding from dental extractions is reduced if a week's course of antifibrinolytic drugs is given, starting immediately pre-operatively.

*Major elective surgery.*—Warfarin should be stopped 48 hours pre-operatively. If the patient has a prosthetic heart valve, a continuous intravenous heparin infusion should be instituted (see below). Other patients may be given prophylactic low-dose subcutaneous heparin until warfarin can be restarted.

*Reversal of warfarin for emergency surgery or overdose.*—Vitamin K rapidly reverses the warfarin effect, especially if given intravenously. It will make the individual resistant to warfarin for some days and is, therefore, not the method of choice if anticoagulation is to be rapidly restarted. In these situations, fresh frozen plasma or factor II-IX-X concentrate should be given. Note that the concentrate is deficient in factor VII and the prothrombin time ratio will reflect this.

(*b*) **Heparin.**—Heparin is widely distributed in all animal tissues. The therapeutic preparations vary in their effects depending on the molecular size of the heparin involved. Smaller heparin molecules have a marked anticoagulant effect which is mediated by combining with antithrombin III to inhibit thrombin virtually instantaneously: other clotting factors are also inhibited. Larger molecular forms may have little antithrombin activity, but probably have a considerable antithrombotic effect by altering the surface charge of vascular endothelium. In the absence of antithrombin III heparin has no anticoagulant effect. The half-life of infused heparin is short—approximately 90 minutes in normal individuals—but the range is large and affected by the patient's clinical condition.

*Administration of heparin.*—Three different modes of heparin therapy are currently in use:

*Low-dose heparin.*—Prophylaxis for the prevention of thrombo-embolic disease is a regime of 5,000 units given subcutaneously twice or three times daily. The risk of bleeding is slight, especially if only 10,000 units per 24 hours are given, and there is no need for laboratory monitoring of the anticoagulant effect.

*Intermediate-dose heparin.*—This is principally used to prevent progression of thrombosis, or in DIC. The dose is usually 30,000–40,000 units per day given, if possible, by continuous intravenous infusion. Bolus therapy is difficult to control as immediately after injection the heparin levels are very high and the risk of bleeding is considerable, whereas just before the next dose is due (if doses are given 6-hourly) there may be very little measurable anticoagulation. Control of dosage for patients on continuous therapy is by the partial thromboplastin time. Blood should be tested as soon as possible after venepuncture, because of the short half-life of heparin. A value of the clotting time for the PTT of twice to three times the clotting time of normal plasma is recommended.

*High-dose heparin.*—Doses of 60,000 to 120,000 units per 24 hours have been used in the first day of treatment of massive pulmonary embolism with shock, reducing thereafter to the intermediate dose regime.

**Reversal of heparin.**—This is achieved with protamine sulphate on a weight for weight basis, i.e. 1 mg protamine neutralises 1 mg (100 usp units) heparin. If a continuous infusion of heparin is used, a dose of protamine should be given to neutralise the heparin given in the last hour and the thrombin time should be checked. Overdose of protamine is dangerous as it can give rise to an anticoagulant effect. New methods of direct heparin assay will give a more rapid and accurate estimate of the dose of protamine necessary for reversal.

**Complications.**—Apart from the major risk of haemorrhage, there are a few comparatively rare risks of prolonged heparin administration. These include reduction of antithrombin III levels leading to heparin resistance and hypercoagulability, especially after the heparin is stopped. Thrombocytopenia due to heparin-dependent anti-platelet antibodies is also seen, developing after 10 days administration of the drug.

(*c*) **Streptokinase** is a plasminogen activator and is used to lyse extensive clots. It is most effective if given within 24 hours of the formation of the clot.

## Sickle-cell Haemoglobin and Anaemia

Normal adult haemoglobin (Hb.A) contains two $\alpha$-polypeptide chains and two $\beta$-polypeptide chains. If the polypeptide chains are abnormal so is the haemoglobin, most haemo-

17/Table 6
Sickle-cell Syndromes

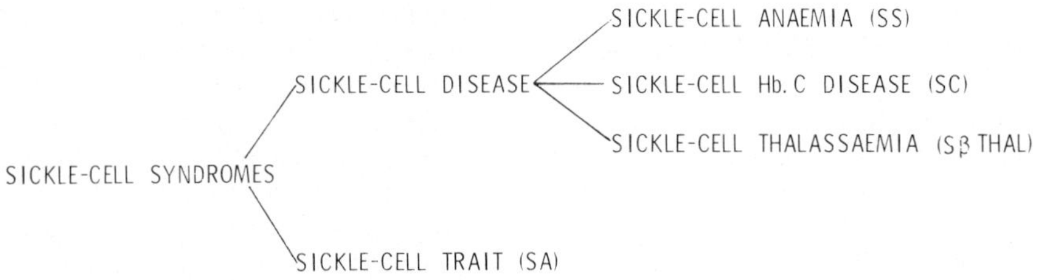


globinopathies resulting from substitution of one amino acid at a single position in either the α or β chain. In sickle-cell haemoglobin (Hb.S) glutamic acid in the 6th position of the normal β chain is replaced by valine, whereas in Hb.C it is replaced by lysine.

Alternatively, there may be defective production of qualitatively normal chains, resulting in α thalassamia (α-chain deficiency) or β thalassamia (β-chain deficiency).

For a subject to have sickle-cell anaemia (SS) a sickle-cell β-polypeptide chain gene must have been inherited from each parent. If such a gene has only been inherited from one parent, the subject being heterozygous for Hb.S, then the other gene is usually normal. This condition is called "sickle-cell trait" (SA). Rarely the other gene is abnormal, for example Hb.C or Hb β thalassaemia, giving rise to sickle-cell haemoglobin C disease or sickle-cell thalassaemia respectively.

In equatorial Africa the incidence of sickle-cell trait (SA) is 20–30 per cent, but the overall Negro Hb.S carrier rate is probably about 10 per cent. The condition is not confined to coloured races and occurs in parts of the Mediterranean littoral and the Middle East.

## Sickling

When Hb.S is deoxygenated it becomes much less soluble and forms long crystals or tactoids which distort the erythrocyte, producing the sickle shape (Fig. 1). These sickle cells tend to aggregate in the capillaries and venules obstructing the flow of blood and so causing zones of infarction. Reoxygenation of the Hb.S causes the red cells to revert to their normal form, although eventually sickling of any particular red cell may become irreversible due to damage to its membrane. The sickling phenomenon is dependent on:

1. Percentage of Hb.S in the red cell.
2. Oxygen tension.
3. pH.
4. Nature of the other haemoglobins present.

*Percentage of Hb.S in the red cell.*—The higher the proportion of Hb.S the more likely is the cell to sickle. A simplified table of the percentages of the haemoglobins present in the various sickle-cell syndromes is given in Table 7.

*Oxygen tension.*—A red cell will sickle at a particular level of deoxygenation, the $Po_2$ at which this occurs depending on the position of the haemoglobin-oxygen dissociation curve.

17/Table 7
Haemoglobins in various Sickle-Cell Syndromes

| *Genotype* | *per cent Hb.S* | *per cent Hb.C* | *per cent Hb.F (fetal)* | *per cent Hb.A (Normal adult)* | *Total Hb g/dl* |
|---|---|---|---|---|---|
| SS | 90–95 | — | 5–10 | — | 5–10 |
| SA | 25–45 | — | <3 | 55–75 | normal |
| SC | 50 | 50 | <3 | — | 10–14 |
| S β THAL | 70–100 | — | 5–10 | 0–30 | 8–14 |

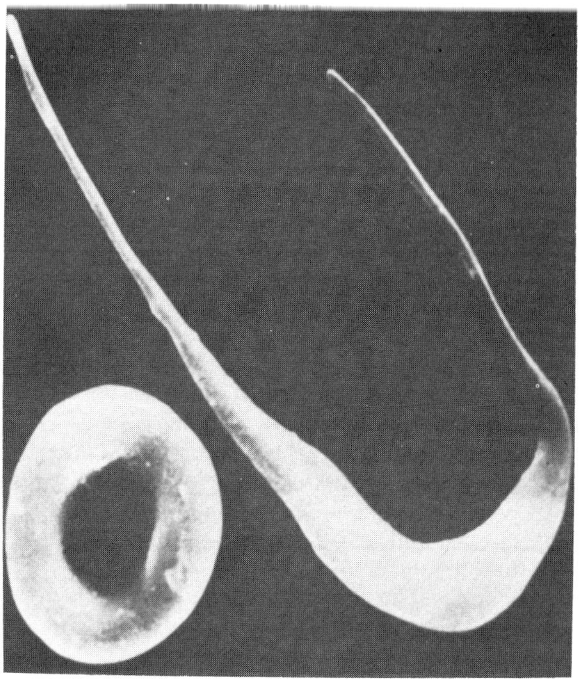

17/Fig. 1.—Electromyograph of a sickle cell and a normal erythrocyte. (Courtesy of Dr. B. F. Cameron and Dr. R. Zucker and *Current Reviews for Nurse Anaesthetists*.)

Approximate values of $Po_2$ at which sickling occurs are as follows:

| | |
|---|---|
| sickle-cell anaemia (SS) | 40 mm Hg (5·3 kPa) |
| sickle-cell Hb.C disease (SC) | 30 mm Hg (4·0 kPa) |
| sickle-cell trait (SA) | 20 mm Hg (2·7 kPa). |

The oxygen tension in some vascular beds may be considerably lower than the mixed venous $Po_2$.

*pH*.—A reduction in pH causes the haemoglobin-oxygen dissociation curve to shift to the right (Bohr effect) so that for a given $Po_2$ the haemoglobin is more deoxygenated.

*Nature of the other haemoglobins present*.—Sickling is more likely to occur in the presence of Hb.C than in the presence of Hb.A or Hb.F.

### Diagnosis of Sickle-Cell Syndromes

1. Anaemia with the presence of sickle cells or target cells in the blood film is suggestive of sickle-cell disease (SS, SC or S $\beta$ THAL).
2. *Sickledex* (Ortho Diagnostics). This is a commerically available test which detects Hb.S by a precipitation reaction.
3. Sodium metabisulphite. If erythrocytes which contain Hb.S are made grossly hypoxic by suspending them in a solution of the reducing agent sodium metabisulphite they will sickle.
4. Haemoglobin electrophoresis. This is the definitive test for the presence and concentrations of different haemoglobins.

### Clinical Features

Sickle-cell trait is usually asymptomatic though sickling can occur under hypoxic conditions, e.g. flying in unpressurised aircraft, and there is an increased incidence of pyelonephritis, haematuria and renal papillary necrosis.[20]

In the three forms of sickle-cell disease crises may be precipitated and take several forms.

*Haemolytic crisis*.—This is due to a sudden further reduction in the red cell lifespan, possibly precipitated by infection. In patients with sickle-cell anaemia (SS) the red cell lifespan may be as little as 7 days in the absence of a haemolytic crisis.

*Infarctive crisis*.—Sickling causes sludging of red cells within small vessels and leads to infarction especially of lungs, spleen and bones though any organ (including the brain) may be affected. Because of the circulatory stasis produced, increasing local hypoxia and acidosis predispose to further sickling.

The treatment and prevention of infarctive crisis is controversial. Oral bicarbonate (up to 20 g/day) is strongly recommended by Huntsman and Lehmann.[21] Intravenous magnesium sulphate, which is a vasodilator and mild anticoagulant, appears to be of benefit especially in the treatment of priapism.[22] Cyanate[23] and urea[24] are toxic and not very effective.

*Aplastic crisis.*—Marrow depression often associated with viral infection or folate deficiency causes an acute aplastic anaemia. This complication is relatively uncommon.

*Sequestration crisis.*—There is enlargement of the liver and spleen with pooling of red cells. This type of crisis mainly affects young children and infants and may necessitate immediate transfusion.

Features of sickle-cell anaemia (SS) which may be present include:

history of bone and joint pain, osteomyelitis
bossing of skull with overgrowth of maxilla
leg ulcers
enlarged liver (spleen usually not enlarged because of repeated infarction)
jaundice due to haemolysis, gallstones
haematuria
priapism.

**Anaesthesia and Sickle-cell Syndromes**

This subject is well reviewed by Howells,[25] Searle,[26] Bennett and Dalal.[27] The blood of all patients of African extraction and originating from countries bordering on the Mediterranean should be screened for Hb.S prior to anaesthesia. This is not necessary for neonates who still have a high concentration of fetal haemoglobin (Hb.F). If Hb.S is detected, electrophoresis must be carried out so that the potentially dangerous sickle-cell diseases, Hb.SS, Hb.SC and sickle-cell thalassaemia can be differentiated from sickle-cell trait (SA). If operative treatment is urgent there may not be time for conventional electrophoresis, although very rapid electrophoresis techniques are now available; as mentioned above, anaemia and the presence of target cells are indicative of one of the sickle-cell diseases rather than the trait. Abdominal pain may be caused by sickling.

1. *Sickle-cell trait.* No special precautions are needed, although gross hypoxia may cause sickling.[25]

2. *Sickle-cell disease.* Certain precautions should be taken in order to reduce the risk of anaesthesia to a minimum. Except for a life-saving operation, no patient should be anaesthetised during a crisis. Any infection should be treated and folate deficiency corrected if time permits.

Pre-operative transfusion is not indicated unless the haemoglobin level is less than 5–6 g/dl;[28,21] the dangers of an increased blood viscosity outweigh the advantages of increased oxygen capacity. If blood replacement is likely to be necessary during the operation fresh blood should be cross-matched. Old blood has a reduced 2:3 DPG content with a resulting shift to the left of the haemoglobin-oxygen dissociation curve; if this blood is transfused, then for a given oxygen delivery to the tissues the patient's Hb.S will be more desaturated.

The patient should be starved pre-operatively in the usual way but it is important to avoid dehydration because of the increased blood viscosity. The use of alkalis has been recommended.[21,29] It is difficult to achieve a significant alkalosis with oral sodium bicarbonate and its effect of shifting the haemoglobin-oxygen dissociation curve to the left is offset by a reduced production of 2:3 DPG, but it nevertheless increases the alkali reserve and so helps to prevent acidosis. The alternative is to give sodium bicarbonate intravenously at the start of anaesthesia and if at any stage a metabolic acidosis develops, this should be corrected.

For elective surgery, total red cell exchange is recommended, if possible by use of a cell-separator. The concentration of sickle haemoglobin should be less than 10 per cent and the haemoglobin concentration is raised to normal values. Exchange transfusion in the third trimester of pregnancy is also valuable. This can be simply achieved by 2 pint mini-exchanges at fortnightly intervals starting at 26–28 weeks gestation.

During anaesthesia it is important to avoid hypoxia, hypercapnia, vasoconstriction, reduction in cardiac output and cooling.[29] Moderate hyperventilation should be used to induce a respiratory alkalosis.

Post-operatively the patient should receive a raised inspired oxygen concentration by mask for at least 24 hours, and analgesic drugs must be used cautiously so as to avoid hypercapnia due to respiratory depression. Adequate hydration has been mentioned. Chest physiotherapy is important as post-operative chest infection is a special risk in these patients. Tourniquets should be avoided whenever possible.

## REFERENCES


1. Nadler, S. B., Hidalgo, J. V. and Bloch, T. (1972). Premotion of blood volume in normal human adults. *Surgery*, **51**, 224.
2. Mollison, P. L. (1979). Blood transfusion in clinical medicine, 6th edit. Oxford: Blackwell Scientific Publications.
3. Engest, J., Stalker, A. L. and Matheson, N. A. (1966). Effects of Dextran 40 on erythrocyte aggregation. *Lancet*, **1**, 1124.
4. Lambie, J. M., Barber, D. C., Chall, D. P. and Matheson, N. A. (1970). Dextran 70 in prophylaxis of postoperative venous thrombosis. A controlled trial. *Brit. Med. J.*, **2**, 144.
5. Bonnar, J. and Walsh, J. (1972). Prevention of thrombosis after pelvic surgery by British Dextran 70. *Lancet*, **1**, 614.
6. Kline, A., Hughes, L. E., Campbell, H., Williams, A., Zlosnick, J. and Leach, K. G. (1975). Dextran 70 in prophylaxis of thromboembolic disease after surgery: a clinically orientated randomized double blind trial. *Brit. med. J.*, **2**, 109.
7. Multi-Unit Controlled Trial (1974). Heparin versus Dextran in the prevention of deep vein thrombosis. *Lancet*, **2**, 118.
8. Caceres, E. and Whittembury, G. (1959). Evaluation of blood losses during surgical operations. Comparison of the gravimetric method with the blood volume determination. *Surgery*, **45**, 681.
9. Shen, S. C., Ham, T. H. and Fleming, E. M. (1943). Studies in the destruction of red blood cells III. Mechanism and complications of haemoglobinuria in patients with thermal burns. Spherocytosis and increased osmotic fragility of red blood cells. *New Eng. J. med.*, **229**, 701.
10. Maclean, L. D. and Van Tyn, R. A. (1961). Ventricular defibrillation. *J. Amer. med. Ass.*, **175**, 471.
11. Boyan, C. P. and Howland, W. S. (1963). Cardiac arrest and temperature of bank blood. *J. Amer. med. Ass.*, **183**, 58.
12. Howland, W. S., Bellville, J. W., Zucker, M. B., Boyan, P. and Clifton, E. E. (1957). Massive blood replacement. V: Failure to observe citrate intoxication. *Surg. Gynaec. Obstet.*, **105**, 529.
13. Cade, D. C., Donavan, J. E. O., Panelli, D. and Galbally, B. P. (1980). Volume replacement in shock. *Medicine*, **28**, 1463.
14. Solis, R. T. and Gibbs, M. B. (1972). Filtration of the microaggregates in stored blood. *Transfusion*, **12**, 245.
15. Barrett, J., Tahir, A. H., Litwin, M. S. (1978). Increased pulmomary arteriovenous shunting in humans following blood transfusion. *Arch. Surg.*, **113**, 947.
16. Goldiner, P. L., Howland, W. S. and Ray, C. (1972). Filter for prevention of microembolism during massive transfusions. *Anesth. Analg. Curr. Res.*, **51**, 717.
17. Reul, G. J., Beall, A. C. and Greenberg, S. D. (1974). Protection of the pulmonary micro-vasculature by fine screen blood filtration. *Chest*, **66**, 4.
18. Virgilio, R. W., Smith, D. E., Rice, C. L., Hobelman, C. F. and Peters, R. M. (1977). To filter or not to filter? *Europ. J. Int. Care Med.*, **3**, 144.
19. Loong, E. D. (1980). Microfiltration of stored blood. *Anaesth. and Intens. Care*, **VIII**, no. 2.
20. *British Medical Journal* (1976). Leading Article—Sickle cell trait. **1**, 1359.
21. Huntsman, R. G. and Lehmann, H. (1974). Treatment of sickle-cell disease. *Brit. J. Haemat.*, **28**, 437.
22. Hugh-Jones, K., Lehman, H. and McAlister, J. M. (1964). Some experiences in managing sickle-cell anaemia in children and young adults, using alkalis and magnesium. *Brit. med. J.*, **2**, 226.
23. Ranney, H. M. (1972). The clinical use of cyanate in sickling. *New Engl. J. Med.*, **287**, 98.
24. McCurdy, P. R. and Mahmood, L. (1971). Intravenous urea treatment of the painful crisis of sickle-cell disease. *New Engl. J. Med.*, **285**, 992.
25. Howells, T. H., Huntsman, R. G., Boys, J. E. and Mahmood (1972). Anaesthesia and sickle-cell haemoglobin. *Brit. J. Anaesth.*, **44**, 975.
26. Searle, J. F. (1973). Anaesthesia in sickle cell states. *Anaesthesia*, **28**, 48.
27. Bennett, E. J. and Dalal, F. Y. (1975). Haemoglobin S and its clinical application. In: *Oxygen Measurements in Biology and Medicine*. Ed. by J. P. Payne and D. W. Hill, London: Butterworth & Co.
28. Oduro, K. A. and Searle, J. F. (1972). Anaesthesia in sickle-cell states—a plea for simplicity. *Brit. med. J.*, **4**, 596.
29. Gilbertson, A. A. (1967). The management of anaesthesia in sickle cell states. *Proc. roy. Soc. Med.*, **60**, 631.

*Section Three*

# THE NERVOUS SYSTEM

CHAPTER 18

# General Pharmacological Principles



PRECISION in the use of drugs depends on knowledge not only of the effects they exert on tissues but also of how these effects are produced and influenced by the disposal of the drugs concerned. In this chapter the general principles of drug action and disposal are discussed with special, though not exclusive, reference to drugs used in anaesthesia. No mention is made of inhalational anaesthetics in the disposal of which some special factors are involved; these are considered in Chapter 6. Stress is placed on the simple physical laws which determine the ways in which drugs reach their target cells, exert their effects, interact with substances of physiological importance or with other drugs and are then removed from their site of action and from the body. The actions of individual agents are discussed only in relation to the general principles concerned. For details of such actions the reader is referred to the special chapters dealing with particular groups of drugs.

In what follows general pharmacological principles are discussed under separate headings:

- Drug action on receptors
- Drug concentrations in plasma, pharmacokinetics
- Passage of drugs across membranes
- Drug administration
- Drug distribution
- Drug metabolism
- Drug excretion
- Variation in drug response
- Adverse drug reactions

There is, however, much overlap in the principles involved and such a division is used only for convenience. Drug interactions, for example, may occur clinically in a number of ways; these are considered in the appropriate sections.

## DRUG ACTION ON RECEPTORS

Drugs exert many different effects on different tissues. These effects are, however, specific to a greater or lesser extent in that different drugs produce different effects. Living cells must therefore possess special sites of drug action, the properties of which are to react with drugs of a specific nature and to initiate a chain of events leading to the pharmacological effect. Such sites of action are receptors. For many years no more than a useful concept for explaining in qualitative and quantitative terms how drugs act, receptors are now known to exist in fact. In recent years, some receptor types have been purified and isolated by chomatographic techniques and subsequently analysed and counted. For detailed study, the reader is referred to a recent review volume.[1]

**Drug-receptor interactions.**—The attachment of drug to receptor has been the focus of much attention. Studies of the relative effects exerted by closely related drugs have shown that it involves physical bonding by a number of forces, ionic, van der Waal, hydrogen bonding and others. The extent to which each of these contributes to the drug-receptor attraction varies from one drug to another and from one receptor to another. The number of bonds involved is usually multiple and their steric arrangement critical. Thus it is usual to find among drugs which exist as two or more stereoisomers that one of these is much more potent than the other. It is well known, for example, that L-noradrenaline exerts many times the pressor effect of D-noradrenaline, presumably because the three-point attachment of the former is more favourable than that of the latter. Similarly, D-amphetamine is more powerful a stimulant than L-amphetamine and D-propoxyphene a more potent analgesic than L-propoxyphene. Stereoisomers may differ even qualitatively in their action, as found for example in the drug pairs, levorphanol: dextromethorphan and quinine: quinidine. Bonding arrangements have been most deeply studied for cholinergic[2] and adrenergic[3] receptors, for which optimal drug dimensions have been calculated. The relationship between receptor structure and bonding is the subject of a review.[4]

Drugs which stimulate receptors and induce a pharmacological effect are *agonists*; those which block them are *antagonists*. Drugs such as nicotine and nalorphine which have both actions are referred to as partial agonists.

Quantitative aspects of drug-receptor interaction were first studied by Clark,[5] who proposed that stimulant drugs occupied receptors and that the tissue response was proportional to the number occupied. He showed that the shape of the dose-response curve could be predicted from the law of mass action in a manner similar to that proposed by Michaelis and Menten[6] for the behaviour of enzymes. The effect of an antagonist could be shown theoretically and in practice to modify the action of the agonist in a way which shifted the log dose-response curve to the right without altering its shape or the size of the maximum response attainable (Fig. 1). This is competitive antagonism, seen clinically in a number of situations: atropine or tubocurarine acting against acetylcholine, cimetidine against histamine, phentolamine against noradrenaline, propranolol against adrenaline, and naloxone against morphine or pethidine. It is so-called because agonist and antagonist compete for the same receptor in a way which conforms with the law of mass action.

Clark's occupation theory as originally proposed is not entirely satisfactory for several reasons. First, one must assume that two types of receptor occupation are possible: one for agonists which exerts an effect, another for antagonists which does not do so. Secondly, how is it possible to achieve maximal agonist responses when many receptors are occupied by antagonist molecules? In Fig. 1 the curves reach the same height even though there is antagonist present. One must assume either that the agonist displaces the antagonist from the receptor or alternatively that there is a plentiful supply of extra receptors ("spare" receptors as proposed by Stephenson[7]) which are not needed for a maximum response. The former explanation is untrue; agonist does not displace antagonist. In anaesthetic practice, partial curarisation can be overcome by administering edrophonium, but when the edrophonium effect wears off one is left with just as much curarisation as if the edrophonium had never been given. Thirdly, how can one account for the action of partial agonists like nicotine and nalorphine which both stimulate and block receptors?

An alternative "rate" theory proposed by Paton,[8,9] went some way towards overcoming these and other objections. The assumption here was that receptors are stimulated not by occupancy but momentarily by the act of combination with the drug, the rate of impact being

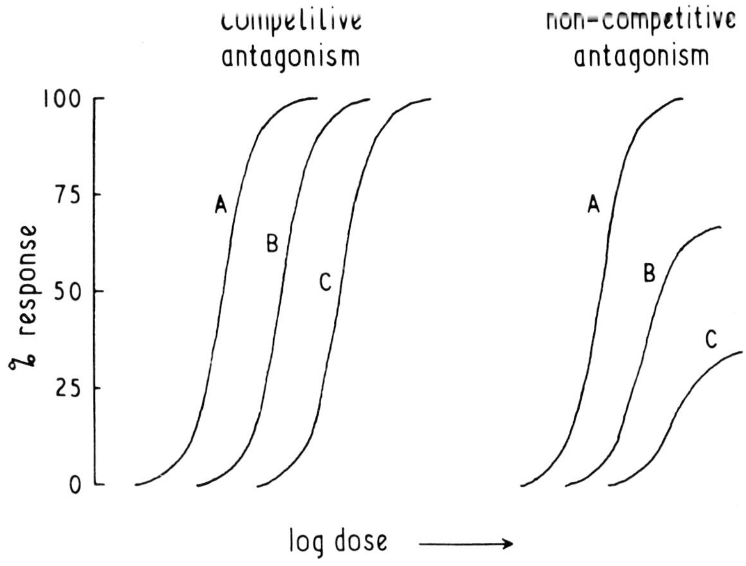


18/FIG. 1.—Theoretical log dose-response curves for drug action. Competitive antagonists shift the curve to the right. Non-competitive antagonists alter the slope and maximal response. A = response without antagonist, B and C with increasing doses of antagonist.

governed by the law of mass action. Once occupied, the receptor is unavailable for further stimulation. On this theory the critical difference between agonists and antagonists lies in the rates of dissociation of the drug-receptor complexes. An agonist should dissociate rapidly, thus freeing the receptor for a fresh act of combination. An antagonist, on the other hand, should dissociate slowly, thus reducing the availability of receptors to agonist impacts. A partial agonist should lie between these extremes. Rate theory does not explain why some agonists are more effective than others, why different ones produce maximal effects of different sizes or why log dose-response curves for the same receptor are not parallel for all agonists. Evidently agonists have other intrinsic properties which influence the effects they induce on the receptor containing tissue.

It is now generally accepted that Clark's original occupation theory is correct but that drugs exert their effects on receptors according to their efficacy. Agonists are assumed to have variable degrees of efficacy and to induce changes in their receptors which, in turn, initiate pharmacological responses. By contrast, antagonists have zero efficacy and induce no changes in their receptors, but they prevent access of agonists and therefore inhibit the pharmacological responses. In either case, however, the response is modified by a large population of spare receptors which permit maximal agonist responses even when most receptors are blocked. Thus, at the neuromuscular junction, for example, tubocurarine and pancuronium produce no discernible blockade until more than 90 per cent of the receptors are inactivated.

The action of competitive antagonists serves to verify predictions implied in drug receptor interaction theory. Other types of antagonism are also demonstrable at the tissue site. Non-competitive antagonism is shown under some conditions by phenoxybenzamine. It decreases the maximal effect of alpha adrenoceptor stimulants and flattens the log dose-response curve (Fig. 1). Physiological antagonism is that which occurs when two drugs have opposite actions without real interference.

For a number of reasons it is useful to have measures of potency and specificity of drug antagonists acting on particular receptors. This is achieved by the measurement of their affinity for the receptors concerned. This function is a constant and it is usually expressed in logarithmic form (i.e. log K). In practical terms log K is the negative decimal logarithm of the molar concentration of antagonist required to reduce the potency of an appropriate agonist two-fold. Drugs with powerful antagonist potency therefore have high values, those with weak potency low ones. For example, against histamine's action on guinea-pig ileum mepyramine has a log K value of 9·4, i.e. $10^{-9.4}$ mol/l reduces the potency of histamine two-fold. This and other values are given in Table 1.

18/TABLE 1
LOG AFFINITY CONSTANTS OF DRUG ANTAGONISTS ON GUINEA-PIG ILEUM (from Schild[10])

| *Antagonist* | *Against histamine* | *Against acetylcholine* |
|---|---|---|
| mepyramine | 9·4 | 4·8 |
| atropine | 5·7 | 8·6 |
| pethidine | 6·2 | 5·8 |

Such measurements indicate the considerable specificities of mepyramine (40,000 times greater against histamine than against acetylcholine) and atropine (1,000 times vice versa) and the negligible specificity of pethidine as antagonists. One can deduce from these results the obvious clinical implications that mepyramine is a useful antihistamine but a useless anticholinergic, that atropine has the opposite properties and that pethidine is both antihistaminic and anticholinergic. For more detailed study of drug receptors, the reader is referred to a review by Rang.[11]

When two drugs of similar action (either agonistic or antagonistic) act together, synergistically, the resultant effect is the sum of the individual components. If the log dose-response curves are steep this summation can result in a surprisingly large effect which is often though erroneously referred to as potentiation. It is well known, for example, that combinations of barbiturates with alcohol can produce dangerous cerebral depression, as can combinations of most central depressant drugs. The effects are the result of summation and not potentiation, the latter of which implies that the total is more than the sum of its components. Potentiation occurs almost exclusively when one drug alters the metabolism or the excretion of the other; this topic is discussed later.

## DRUG CONCENTRATIONS IN PLASMA PHARMACOKINETICS

The action of any drug at its receptor site is determined by its concentration in the biophase, that is the fluid bathing the receptor. Unfortunately this critical concentration can never be measured directly, though deductions about its time profile can be made from the time-course of its pharmacological action.[12] Over a longer period, equilibration of drug between plasma and biophase occurs, and the plasma concentration is then a direct determinant of the intensity of the pharmacological response. In turn the plasma concentration is influenced by the rates of drug absorption, distribution to various tissues, metabolism and excretion, and the extent to which the drug is bound to plasma protein (see below). The dynamic equilibrium established is influenced also by the extent to which the drug is ionised in each body fluid. A scheme of distribution is illustrated in Fig. 2. From measurements of drug and metabolite concentrations in plasma and urine, time courses of distribution have been simulated with the help of computers.[13] Such simulations can help to predict durations of drug action under certain circumstances (e.g. for tubocurarine[14]). In many clinical instances, however, particularly in anaesthetic practice, the intravenous route of drug administration results in concentrations which change too rapidly for equilibration to occur and, furthermore, the kinetics of drug disposition are complicated by binding to plasma protein and sequestration in tissue depots. Under such circumstances, plasma concentrations do not necessarily give direct indications of the pharmacologically active concentrations at the site of drug action and attempted correlations between plasma concentration and drug action become too complex to evaluate. Additionally, many drugs have active metabolites whose contribution to the overall action makes such correlation invalid.

Concentrations in plasma of drugs which are not significantly bound to plasma protein or sequestered in tissues decline by a simple exponential (first order elimination) whereby the concentration C at time t can be represented by the equation:

$$C = A.e^{-\beta t}$$

where A and $\beta$ are constants. This provides a straight line on a log concentration/time graph and gives a measure of the half-life of the drug in the plasma. For drugs administered intravenously, the decline is usually bi-exponential because disappearance from the plasma is a

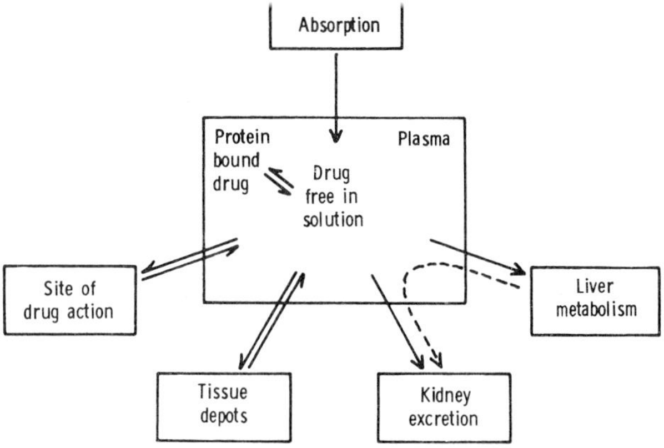


18/Fig. 2.—Distribution of drugs in the body.

function of distribution to body tissues as well as elimination by metabolism or excretion. In such instances, a curve such as that for buthalitone shown in Fig. 3 results. For kinetic analysis of such data, the simplified assumption can be made that the drug is distributed to two homogeneous compartments in the body—a central compartment to which the drug is administered and from which it is removed by metabolism and/or excretion, and a peripheral compartment into and out of which the drug moves from the central one (Fig. 4). Such a model can provide a precise fit to experimental data points of the type shown in Fig. 3, though in many situations more complex modelling is required. For further study, the reader is referred to the book by Gibaldi and Perrier.[15]

**Protein Binding**

In the circulation many drugs are bound to plasma proteins. Acidic drugs tend to be bound to albumin and basic drugs to $\alpha$-acid glycoprotein, but there is much overlap. The extent of binding varies from one drug to another and it

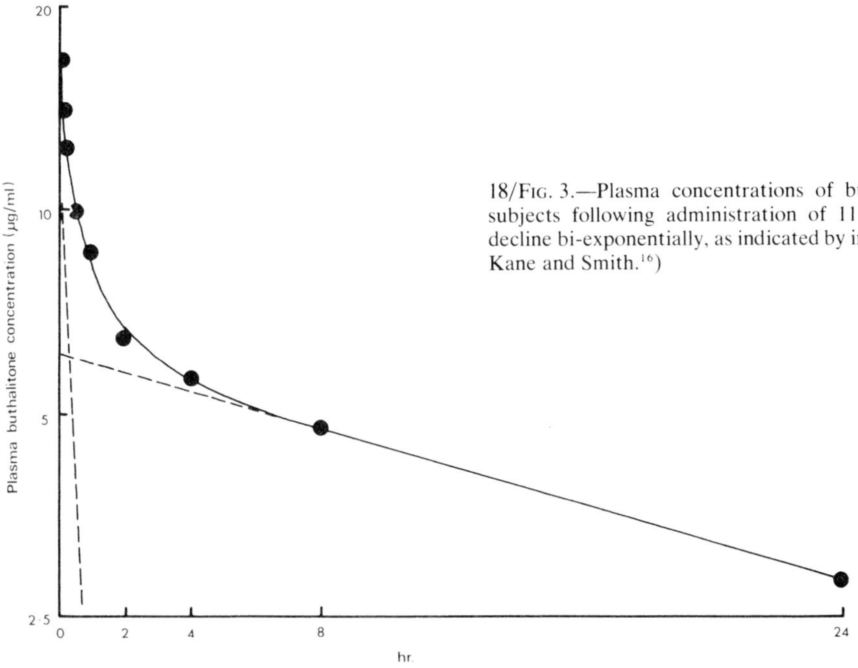


18/Fig. 3.—Plasma concentrations of buthalitone in healthy male subjects following administration of 11 mg/kg i.v. Concentrations decline bi-exponentially, as indicated by interrupted lines. (Data from Kane and Smith.[16])

is dependent on the drug concentration. The nature of the binding process is complex and probably involves a number of binding sites of variable specificity. Some of these involve van der Waal bonding, some ionic attractions and others lipophilic affinities. The latter probably account for the binding of barbiturate molecules and explain the fact that it is the ultra-short-acting drugs in the group (the most lipid-soluble) which are most highly bound. Other sites are specific for acidic drugs such as sulphonamides and coumarin anticoagulants.

The extent to which any drug is bound is influenced by its concentration, very high concentrations tending to swamp the binding sites and lower the proportion of bound drug. A rapid increase in effect and toxicity would be expected above this level. It is difficult, however, to predict the exact behaviour because at high concentrations subsidiary binding mechanisms may come into play. For example, thiopentone may then be bound in both its ionised and non-ionised forms. At low concentrations very high proportions of circulating drugs may be bound: thiopentone about 85–90 per cent, digitoxin 95 per cent and warfarin 98 per cent. Among such drugs only a small proportion remains available for diffusion to the tissues, where the drugs exert their pharmacological actions, and some of this is metabolically degraded or filtered by the kidneys. Extensive binding therefore has the effects of limiting potency and prolonging duration of action. Bound drug is thought to be pharmacologically inactive, though the bound fraction is in a state of dynamic equilibrium with that free in solution and can therefore exert effects once it is released.

Protein binding may vary in different individuals. It is diminished by low circulating albumin levels such as occur in liver disease and malnutrition. Patients with severe liver disease are therefore intolerant of drugs which are usually highly bound because much larger proportions of the drugs circulate free in solution in plasma and are avaiable for diffusion into the tissues. Binding of particular drugs may also be reduced by the presence of other drugs which compete for the same binding sites; this induces true potentiation. Clinically such interactions occur most obviously with acidic drugs such as sulphonamides, penicillins, salicylates, coumarin anticoagulants, sulphonylureas, phenylbutazone and methotrexate. In some instances interactions produced by concurrent administration of two or more of these drugs may be of minor importance. If they include sulphonylureas such as tolbutamide or anticoagulants such as warfarin, however, unexpected and often dangerous potentiation may occur. For further discussion of this subject the reader is referred to a survey by Prescott.[17]

Tissue proteins may also bind drugs. Barbiturates in particular are bound to homogenates of most tissues including brain,[18] the extent corresponding roughly with the distribution of these drugs *in vivo*. It is not, however, clear how this influences the effects of such drugs at their sites of action, because of the possibilities that drugs may be either drawn away from, or held in the vicinity of, the appropriate biophase. Tricyclic antidepressant drugs are exceptional in being bound very highly to tissues. The effect of this on their apparent volumes of distribution is considered below.

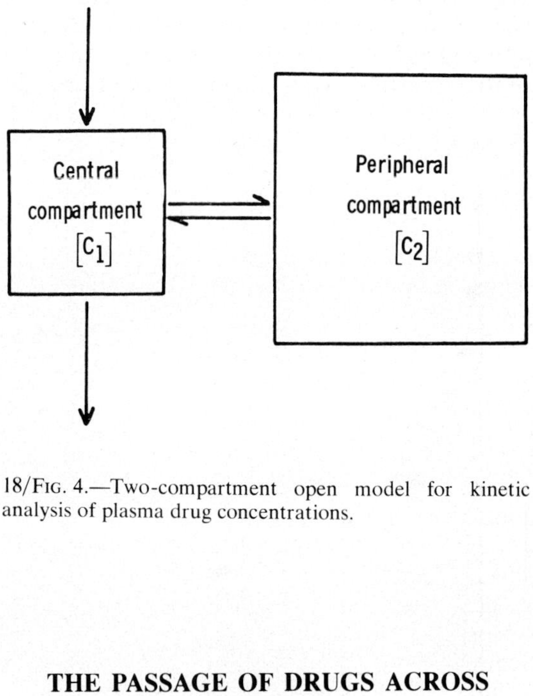


18/FIG. 4.—Two-compartment open model for kinetic analysis of plasma drug concentrations.

## THE PASSAGE OF DRUGS ACROSS MEMBRANES

The effect of a drug at its site of action in body tissues is dependent on its presence at critical concentration at that site. To achieve this, the drug must be absorbed from its site of administration and be distributed in the body in a suitable manner, such absorption and distribution being dependent on the ability of the drug to cross cellular membrane barriers. Because the physical properties of cell membranes are similar in different parts of the body, the factors involved in absorption and distribution into different tissues are also similar.

Drugs can cross cell membranes in three ways: by diffusion, by penetration through membrane pores and by means of active transport.[19]

### Diffusion

Most drugs used in medical practice and in anaesthesia are weak acids or bases. Acidic drugs such as barbiturates, salicylates, penicillins and sulphonamides in aqueous solution form salts with metal cations (e.g. $Na^+$ or $K^+$); such solutions are therefore alkaline. Basic drugs such as local anaesthetics, phenothiazines, opiate analgesics and adrenaline in aqueous solution form salts with inorganic acids (e.g. HCl); such solutions are therefore acidic. In body fluids, as indeed in any aqueous solution, such drugs exist in two forms in equilibrium, viz. non-ionised (undissociated) and ionised (dissociated). The extent to which a drug is ionised is dependent on the pH of the solution and on its dissociation constant, conventionally expressed as the pKa or negative logarithm of the acid dissociation constant. Thus:

$$\text{for acids: } pK_a - pH = \log \frac{C_n}{C_i}$$

$$\text{for bases: } pK_a - pH = \log \frac{C_i}{C_n}$$

where $C_i$ and $C_n$ are the concentrations of the ionised and non-ionised forms respectively. The $pK_a$ values of some important compounds are illustrated in Fig. 5.

The importance of these factors to drug absorption and distribution is that in the non-ionised (undissociated) state drugs have lipid solubility and are therefore able to diffuse across cell membranes, whereas in the ionised (dissociated) form they have no lipid solubility and therefore cannot diffuse across. Drugs such as barbiturates, which have $pK_a$ values close to

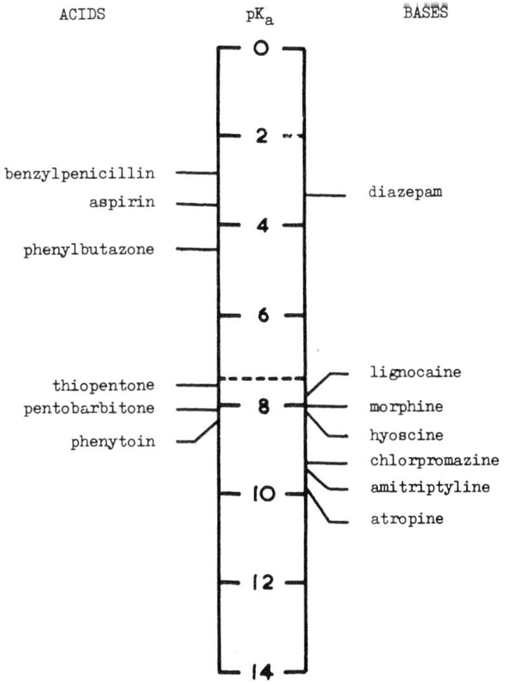


18/FIG. 5—$pK_a$ values of acids and bases (data from Smith and Rawlins[20]).

physiological pH are about 50 per cent ionised in the body and, having reasonable lipid solubility, are therefore well-absorbed from the gastro-intestinal tract, cross the blood-brain and placental barriers and are reabsorbed in the renal tubule. By contrast, quaternary ammonium compounds like tubocurarine and suxamethonium which are fully ionised at physiological pH have no lipid solubility and are therefore not absorbed from the gastro-intestinal tract, do not cross the blood-brain or placental barriers and are not reabsorbed in the renal tubule. They can, however, cross capillary walls and do therefore penetrate the extracellular spaces where they act. Drug transfer across the placenta is discussed further in Chapter 41.

Transfer of a drug by diffusion across a cell membrane proceeds at a rate which is proportional to its concentration. In theory this rate is unlimited and it requires no metabolic energy. The amount of drug absorbed from the gastro-intestinal tract is therefore a direct function of the dose administered; the amount that pene-

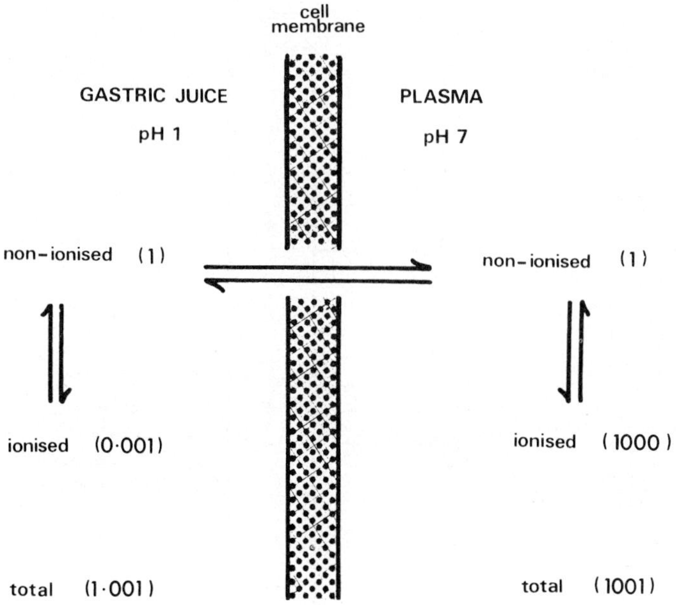


18/Fig. 6.—Theoretical distribution of a weak acid of $pK_a$ 4·5 (e.g. phenylbutazone) between gastric juice and plasma. Differences in ionisation produce a large concentration gradient. Theoretical relative concentrations are shown in parentheses.

trates into the brain, the fetus or any other organ is a direct function of the concentration of the drug free in solution in the plasma.

Surprisingly diffusion can set up concentration gradients such that one tissue may contain much more drug than another. If there is a marked pH difference across the membrane such as exists across the gastric mucosa, total drug concentrations differ considerably because the concentrations of non-ionised drug must be the same on the two sides. The equilibrium established is illustrated in Fig. 6, which shows that a weak acid like phenylbutazone is unevenly distributed in a way which leads to its absorption from the stomach into the gastric cells. By contrast, weak bases show the opposite distribution and are therefore excreted into the stomach. For the same reason, weak bases equilibrate to higher concentrations in intracellular water than in extracellular water; weak acids *vice versa*.

The same factors influence the reabsorption of weak acids and bases from the renal tubule (see below).

### Penetration Through Pores

Many substances which are lipid-insoluble can enter cells and penetrate membrane barriers. Such substances as water and urea do so by filtration through pores in the cell membrane. Their movement occurs by diffusion; the rate is usually slow because the pores occupy only a minute fraction of the cell surface (perhaps 0·2 per cent). Inorganic ions penetrate in the same way, though the rate of their movement is limited further by the polarisation of the membrane surface. Lipid-soluble substances may be absorbed from the gastro-intestinal tract in this manner by solution in chylomicrons.

### Active Transport

Many physiological substances and a few drugs are transferred across cell membranes by specialised transport systems. Such systems are thought to involve the use of carriers whose function is to combine reversibly with the substance at one surface of the membrane, transfer it to the opposite surface and release it there. Considerable concentration gradients may be set up and the process is energy-dependent, rate limited and susceptible to blockade by metabolic inhibitors. Special transport systems exist for sugars, amino acids, inorganic ions and neurohumoral transmitters such as noradrenaline, 5-hydroxytryptamine and gamma-aminobutyric acid. Some synthetic sympathomimetic amines are carried into nerve-endings in the same manner by use of the noradrenaline carrier.

Many drugs in common use are powerful inhibitors of these transport systems and their pharmacological actions are dependent on this property. Cocaine, for example, owes its sympathomimetic action to its ability to inhibit reuptake of noradrenaline back into nerve-endings.[21] Amitriptyline and other tricyclic antidepressants are powerful inhibitors of 5-hydroxytryptamine uptake by platelets; their antidepressant effect may result from the same action in the brain. The antithyroid action of potassium perchlorate depends on its ability to antagonise thyroid iodide transport.

## DRUG ADMINISTRATION

### Intravenous

In anaesthetic practice many drugs are administered intravenously. Concentrations of these drugs in the plasma and indirectly in the tissues rise almost instantaneously to a maximum and the time to onset of drug effect is reduced to a minimum. Mixing of the drug solution with the whole circulating plasma volume is relatively slow, however, and is not achieved for several circulation times. Until mixing has occurred, therefore, some blood contains much more drug than the remainder, this effect being most marked immediately following the drug's administration. The difference is exaggerated further if the injection is given quickly and reduced if it is given slowly. After rapid injection, a bolus of drug solution of high concentration may travel in the circulation almost unmixed for long enough to exert a powerful drug action; if the total amount of drug administered is mixed completely by slow injection no effect may result. This "bolus effect" was described by Paton[8] and is illustrated in Fig. 7.

In clinical practice such bolus effects have a profound influence on drug action. They explain, for instance, why a rapid injection of a small dose of an intravenous anaesthetic exerts a brief but powerful effect, whereas a slowly injected much larger dose has no effect at all. In patients with heart failure, of course, the time to onset of drug effect is greatly increased because of the slow circulation.

Measurements of plasma concentrations of intravenously administered drugs within 5 minutes or so of administration are therefore of doubtful value. They may produce higher or lower levels depending on the phase of mixing.

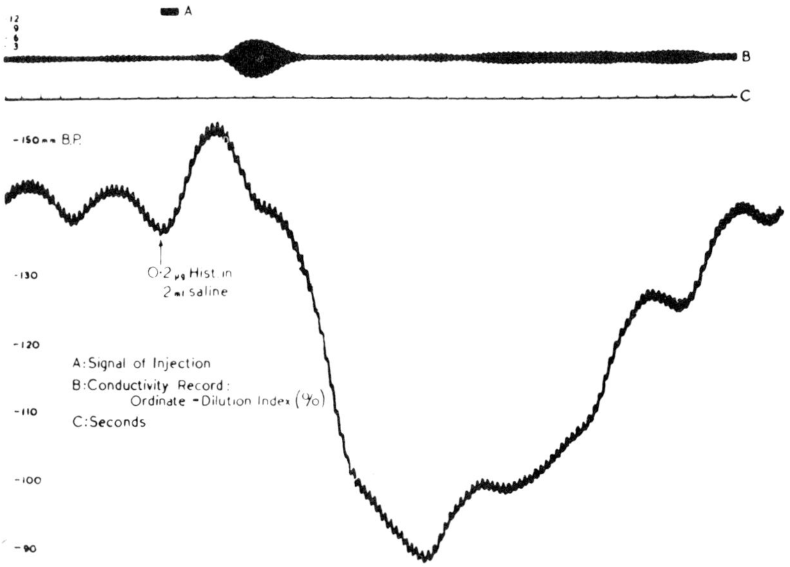


18/Fig. 7.—Bolus effect of rapid i.v. administration of histamine 0·2μg in 2 ml saline in an anaesthetised cat. Upper tracing: conductivity of carotid arterial blood gives a measure of drug concentration. Lower tracing: arterial blood pressure. The drug effect follows the bolus but wanes in spite of a rising drug concentration with recirculation. (Courtesy of Professor W. D. M. Paton and the Honorary Editors of the *Proceedings of the Royal Society of Medicine*[8].)

### Intramuscular, Subcutaneous and Intraperitoneal

Following drug administration by these routes, absorption into the circulation occurs at a rate which depends on the physico-chemical properties of the drug, the extent to which the drug solution spreads in the tissue and the state of the local circulation. Insoluble forms of drugs such as procaine, penicillin and depot preparations of insulin are only slowly absorbed because dissolution must first occur. Given intraperitoneally, drugs are very rapidly absorbed because of rapid spread of solution over the absorptive surface and the highly vascular nature of that surface. Intramuscular and subcutaneous routes allow slower absorption because of reduced spread and blood supplies in these regions. The rates are therefore further slowed if the regional blood supply is reduced as in states of shock or by the addition of vasoconstrictors to the drug solutions. The times to peak plasma concentrations, and indirectly to drug effects elsewhere, are therefore progressively prolonged.

### Oral

Absorption of drugs from the gastro-intestinal tract is influenced by the factors mentioned above and also by some special factors. Most rapid and effective absorption occurs at either end, from the oral and the rectal mucosae following local administration. Such mucosae are highly vascular and, provided the drug is lipid soluble, allow rapid transfer of the drug into the circulation. More importantly, such routes allow drug passage directly to the systemic circulation and not into the portal circulation, thus avoiding the immediate effect of the liver which in many cases inactivates drugs by metabolism. This is the so-called "first-pass" effect. Such drugs as glyceryl trinitrate or isoprenaline, given sublingually, exert systemic actions within 2 minutes. When swallowed, these drugs have no effect at all.

When swallowed, some drugs, mostly weak acids, can be absorbed from the stomach if they are largely in the non-ionised state at the pH of the stomach contents (see above). The most important consequence of this is that high drug concentrations are built up in the gastric mucosal cells, which may explain the erosions and haemorrhage associated with the use of aspirin and phenylbutazone. Such absorption is diminished if the subject has consumed antacids in quantity sufficient to raise the intragastric pH significantly.

Although the pH conditions are not always ideal, most drug absorption occurs from the small intestine because of the enormous available absorptive surface area. Absorption is limited by the presence of food in the lumen such that some drugs taken after, rather than before, meals may hardly be absorbed at all. Meals also impede absorption by delaying gastric emptying. Malabsorption states may of course hinder absorption of drugs as they do of foodstuffs.

Drugs which interfere with intestinal function can inhibit drug absorption. Thus atropine-like drugs and drugs such as phenothiazines and antidepressants which produce atropine-like effects delay gastric emptying and thus prevent intestinal absorption of other drugs. Similar effects may be produced by shock states when gastric motility is inhibited reflexly. Contrariwise, metoclopramide which accelerates gastric emptying into the duodenum accelerates intestinal absorption of other drugs given at the same time.

Many drugs are ineffective when administered by mouth because they are inactivated in the gastro-intestinal tract. Some penicillins are acid-labile and therefore degraded by gastric juice; polypeptides are hydrolysed by gastric and intestinal enzymes; many amines such as catecholamines, histamine and tyramine (e.g. cheese) are oxidised by amine oxidases in the gut wall. Drug interaction can occur within the lumen, limiting or preventing absorption. Thus, magnesium- and aluminium-containing antacids form complexes with tetracyclines and the resin cholestyramine with acidic drugs like warfarin and phenylbutazone. In each case absorption is prevented. Antibiotics may indirectly exert effects by inducing changes in bacterial flora, producing intestinal hurry and thus malabsorption. In addition, such changes can increase the effects of coumarin anticoagulants if absorption of vitamin K (with which the anticoagulants compete) is reduced.

## DRUG DISTRIBUTION

Once a drug enters the circulation it is distributed to a variety of compartments within the body, mostly by diffusion down concentration gradients. The rate and extent of such distribution depends on several factors: the physico-chemical properties of the drug (principally its lipid solubility), the binding of the drug to plasma and/or tissue protein, the regional distribution of blood flow, and in a few instances the presence of active transport mechanisms. The total amount of drug in the body (X) and its concentration in the plasma (C) are related as follows:

$$X = C.\,V_D$$

where $V_D$ is the volume of distribution. In a few instances drugs are distributed into strict anatomical spaces, e.g. heparin into plasma water (0·05 l/kg), alcohol into total body water (0·60 l/kg); the distribution volume is then a real volume which is readily envisaged. Drugs which are highly lipid-soluble or extensively bound to proteins are distributed quite differently; the distribution volume is then an apparent volume which does not conform to an anatomical space. It is merely that volume in which the drug would be dissolved were it all at the same concentration as in the plasma. It is largely independent of dosage and it is characteristic of the drug concerned. Some values of drugs which cover a wide range of distribution volume are indicated in Table 2. To the extent that drug effects must be related to drug concentrations at tissue sites and therefore indirectly to plasma concentrations, volumes of distribution are important determinants of drug action.

18/TABLE 2
DISTRIBUTION VOLUMES ($V_D$) AND PLASMA ELIMINATION HALF-LIVES ($T_{\frac{1}{2}}$) OF SELECTED DRUGS IN MAN.

| *Drug* | $V_D$ (l/kg) | $T_{\frac{1}{2}}$ (hr) |
|---|---|---|
| nortriptyline | 21·1 | 34·2 |
| pentobarbitone | 2·0* | 42·0 |
| buthalitone | 1·8 | 21·7 |
| thiopentone | 1·2* | 4·0 |
| tubocurarine | 0·14 | 0·8 |

(* approximate values)

## DRUG METABOLISM

The lipid solubility of many of the drugs in common use renders them incapable of excretion by the kidney because of back-diffusion in the tubules. Elimination of such drugs therefore requires hepatic biotransformation to render them more polar, less lipid-soluble and therefore more readily excretable. The metabolic processes involved are conveniently divisible into two categories: Phase I (oxidation, reduction, hydrolysis) and Phase II (conjugation). Some of the more important processes involved are summarised as follows.

### Oxidation

Oxidising or hydroxylating enzymes are responsible for the degradation and inactivation of many drugs. The processes, which require triphosphopyridine nucleotide and oxygen, may involve oxidation, dealkylation, deamination, ring or side-chain hydroxylation and sulphoxide formation. Drugs which are affected by oxidative reactions include barbiturates and thiobarbiturates, ethanol, phenothiazines, sympathomimetic and other amines, analgesics and antidepressants.

### Reduction

Reduction is important for only a small number of drugs and the alcoholic products which result are usually further oxidised, often quite rapidly. Adrenaline and noradrenaline are partly excreted as reduced products (phenylglycols) and chloral derivatives are reduced to yield the active metabolite trichloroethanol.

### Hydrolysis

Hydrolytic splitting is responsible for the destruction of a number of compounds such as cardiac glycosides, anthracene purgatives, procaine and choline esters. Drugs such as propanidid and suxamethonium are hydrolysed by cholinesterase in the plasma as well as in the liver.

### Conjugation

Synthetic processes in the liver are responsible for the formation of conjugates, particularly glucuronides and sulphates. Catecholamines, phenols, steroids, chloral derivatives and tribromethanol are all partly excreted in this form. Aromatic acids may be conjugated with glycine and some amines such as sulphonamides and histamine by acetylation.

Because of their reduced lipid solubility, most

drug metabolites are not only more readily eliminated but also less potent than their parent compounds. Potency may, however, be only partly lost in any one metabolic stage and total inactivation thus often depends on more than one stage. For example, diamorphine is degraded partly to morphine which has approximately half the potency. Thiobarbiturates are converted in part to their equivalent oxybarbiturates with similar result. In some cases metabolism activates the drug with the opposite effect that the metabolite is more potent than its precursor. Thus diazepam is converted into at least three active metabolites, one of which (N-desmethyldiazepam) is so slowly eliminated that it exerts much more effect than diazepam itself.

The metabolism of drugs in the liver occurs largely by microsomal enzymes which are located in the smooth-surfaced endoplasmic reticulum. Liver damage induced by acute or chronic disease suppresses the activity of these enzymes and induces intolerance to drugs which are normally inactivated by them. Thus patients with cirrhosis or some impairment of liver function may show exaggerated and prolonged effects to compounds like ethanol, benzodiazepines and opiates. There is a tendency for the rate of drug metabolism to decline also with age, though its importance is unclear at present. It is admittedly well known that many drugs such as nitrazepam, produce prolonged effects in the elderly, but these may be the result of increased dynamic sensitivity[22] or change in distribution volume[23] rather than failure of metabolism.

Microsomal enzymes can also be affected by drugs. Administration of cimetidine or of monoamine oxidase inhibitors inhibits the enzymes so that drug metabolism is slowed. Thus monoamine oxidase inhibitors render the patient intolerant not only of sympathomimetic amines which are metabolised by monoamine oxidase but also of drugs which are degraded in microsomes, amphetamine, pethidine, ethanol, phenothiazines and most hypnotics. MAO inhibitors are further considered in Chapter 21.

Drugs can also have the opposite effect. Administration of barbiturates, phenytoin, glutethimide, dichloralphenazone and some other compounds cause enzyme induction; there is proliferation of the hepatocellular endoplasmic reticulum, increased enzyme formation and resultant accelerated drug metabolism. Patients under this influence become tolerant of drugs which are metabolised by these enzymes. Pharmacological aspects have been reviewed by Conney[24] and clinical aspects by Burns and Conney[25] and Prescott.[17]

The clinical implications of enzyme induction are still under investigation. In many instances a two- or three-fold increase in drug metabolism is probably of little consequence. In two fields, however, important interactions can result with unfortunate effects if the patient stops taking the inducing drug (e.g. a barbiturate). The two fields concern the use of coumarin anticoagulants and oral hypoglycaemic agents, most of which are inactivated by microsomal enzymes. The danger is likely to arise in patients who are stabilised on these drugs while taking enzyme-inducing agents and who stop taking the inducer at a later date while continuing on the same daily dosage of the anticoagulant or hypoglycaemic. The induction wears off in about 2–3 weeks and the original dosage of anticoagulant or hypoglycaemic agent becomes too great. Enzyme induction by phenobarbitone is used to lower serum bilirubin concentrations in the newborn.

## EXCRETION

Drugs and their metabolites are excreted from the body largely by the kidney. Some compounds, however, appear in the faeces, either because they are incompletely absorbed after oral administration or because they are excreted into the intestine via the bile, sometimes as metabolites. Oral contraceptives and many antibiotics are re-cycled in this way with resultant prolongation of their actions. Some ions such as bromides, iodides and lithium are also secreted by mucous membranes and by sweat glands.

Disposal by the kidney depends on a balance of three processes:

### Glomerular Filtration

A drug free in solution in plasma enters the renal tubular lumen by filtration, whilst a protein-bound drug is retained unless albuminuria is present. The glomerular filtrate therefore contains drug or metabolite at the same concentration as is present free in the plasma.

### Tubular Reabsorption

During its passage down the tubule, the filtrate is reduced in volume by the removal of sodium, chloride and water, so that drug or metabolite concentration increases progressively to a very high level. Under the concentration gradient thus established between tubular fluid and blood stream the drug may then diffuse passively back into the circulation, limiting its excretion. Only non-ionised drug can cross the tubular cell membrane, however, with the result that the reabsorption of weak acids and bases is strongly pH dependent. This provides the basis for alteration of the urinary pH in cases of drug poisoning. In poisoning by weak acids like phenobarbitone and salicylates, alkalinisation of the urine with bicarbonate increases ionisation, limits reabsorption and therefore increases their excretion in the urine; the same effect is produced in poisoning by weak bases such as amphetamines and phenothiazines by acidification of the urine with ammonium chloride. The effectiveness of such manoeuvres is dependent on effective increases in the ionised fraction of the drugs in the urine. Drugs which are totally ionised, even at the extremes of urinary pH, are not reabsorbed at all. Thus drugs such as decamethonium and neostigmine, which are quaternary ammonium compounds and fully ionised, are relatively rapidly eliminated by the kidney.

Tubular reabsorption is diminished if the flow of urine is increased because tubular fluid becomes concentrated to a lesser degree and the drug gradient across the tubular cell membrane is reduced. Thus forced diuresis increases the elimination of many drugs in proportion to the urine flow. Forced diuresis is therefore potentially useful in the management of drug poisoning, though in practice not much benefit accrues often because the drugs taken have large distribution volumes leaving little at all for handling by the kidney. In practice, forced diuresis is helpful only in phenobarbitone and salicylate overdosage.

### Tubular Secretion

A number of compounds, mostly organic acids, are actively secreted by the tubular cells into the urine. The elimination of such compounds as penicillins and sulphonamides is thereby accelerated. A few weak bases are also secreted actively but it is doubtful whether the process is important quantitatively.

Tubular secretion is susceptible to inhibition by drugs. Thus probenecid which antagonises the secretion of organic acids has been used to delay the elimination of penicillins. Probenecid, salicylates and phenylbutazone also antagonise active tubular reabsorption of urates; hence their use in the treatment of gout.

The elimination of drugs by the kidney is retarded in renal insufficiency, largely because of the reduced glomerular filtration rate. Though this is not usually of clinical significance, with a few drugs it is important if they are liable to produce toxic effects at only moderately increased blood concentrations. Such drugs as gentamicin and kanamycin may accumulate in these circumstances to produce labyrinthine and auditory damage. Monitoring blood concentrations provides the only safeguard. Renal function declines also with age, to the extent that the 75-year-old patient usually has a glomerular filtration rate of no more than 60 ml/minute. Appropriate dose adjustments for potentially harmful drugs like digoxin or aminoglycoside antibiotics are necessary.

## VARIATIONS IN RESPONSE

Healthy normal individuals vary in their response to drugs. This variation is quantitative and sometimes qualitative. It can occur because of pharmacokinetic variation, i.e. from individual differences in drug disposition and disposal, or because of pharmacodynamic variation, i.e. from differences in the way the drug affects the tissue or its receptors. Part at least of this variability is inherent and is under genetic control. Pharmacogenetics is the subject of a monograph by Kalow,[26] and variability in drug response of a review.[20]

Much interest has centred on genetically-determined individual variations in drug metabolism. For the anaesthetist the most important of these are the variations in suxamethonium metabolism caused by atypical varieties of plasma cholinesterase (see Chapter 23). These varieties are determined by the presence or absence of particular genes of large effect. Similar factors affect the metabolism of isoniazid and sulphadimidine by acetylation in the liver. The rate of drug metabolism is also affected by multiple genes which influence the quantity of enzyme present. Information derived from twin studies suggests that inheritance greatly influences the half-lives of dicoumarol, antipyrine and phenylbutazone[27] and steady-state blood concentrations of nortriptyline.[28] More recent evidence,[29] however, casts some doubt on these findings. The exact extent to which inheritance determines the rates at which individuals metabolise drugs in the liver is therefore uncertain.

Pharmacodynamic variation may also be of genetic origin. The reader is referred to other chapters in this volume for explanations of the porphyrias and malignant hyperpyrexia (Chapter 26), both of which exert profound influences on the reaction to drugs used in anaesthesia.

## ADVERSE DRUG REACTIONS

It is beyond the scope of this chapter to discuss unwanted effects of drug therapy in detail. The reader is referred to the comprehensive textbook on the subject.[30]

In general terms, adverse effects occur as a consequence of particular properties of the drug, of the characteristics of the patient or of an interaction of the two. Many so-called side-effects arise as a logical consequence of the primary drug action, in which case they should be termed "secondary effects". Thus antihypertensive drug therapy tends to exaggerate the hypotensive effect of intermittent positive-pressure ventilation by impairment of the reflexes which usually compensate for the decline in venous return to the heart. Similarly, antibiotic therapy tends to result in the emergence of resistant bacterial species because of natural selection and other consequences of the drug's action. True side-effects may be linked to the primary drug action in being elicited by actions on the same receptor type or they may be independent of it. The former is exemplified by the respiratory depression which accompanies the action of most opiate analgesics; it is believed that the respiratory action involves opiate receptors of the same or closely similar type. The latter is exemplified by the sedation which occurs with many $H_1$-antihistamines such as promethazine. In this case, the side-effect is probably not mediated through $H_1$-histamine receptors and is therefore a manifestation of the multi-receptor activity of the drug. Many drugs have actions on more than one receptor type, with the result that side-effects are often multiple as well as unrelated to the primary drug action.

Many adverse effects occur because of particular characteristics of the patient's genetic make-up (*v.s.*), his or her sex and age, the disease present and past experience of the same or other drug therapy. Idiosyncratic reactions usually involve inherited factors, some of which are discussed above and elsewhere in this volume. Hypersensitivity reactions, such as anaphylaxis, skin rashes and bone marrow suppression, occur most readily in atopic individuals and are always linked to prior exposure to the same or closely related drugs. For consideration of the mechanisms involved, the reader is referred to the textbook of clinical pharmacology by Rogers, Spector and Trounce.[31]

The general level of drug response in any individual is determined by the size of the dose administered and by the degree of tolerance or intolerance set by the factors considered elsewhere in this chapter. In ideal circumstances, drug dosage should always be matched to the individual's requirements and careful monitoring used to ensure that dosage and action are appropriate to the clinical circumstances.

## REFERENCES

1. Lamble, J. W. Ed. (1981). *Towards Understanding Receptors. Current Reviews in Biomedicine I.* Amsterdam: Elsevier/North-Holland.
2. Waser, P. (1961). Chemistry and pharmacology of muscarine, muscarone and some related compounds. *Pharmacol. Rev.*, **13**, 465.
3. Belleau, B. (1963). An analysis of drug receptor interactions. *Proc. First International Pharmacological Meeting*, **7**, 75.
4. Ehrenpreis, S., Fleisch, J. H. and Mittag, T. W. (1969). Approaches to the molecular nature of pharmacological receptors. *Pharmacol. Rev.*, **21**, 131.

5. Clark, A. J. (1937). General pharmacology. In: *Heffter's Handbuch der experimentellen Pharmakologie*, Erg. Vol. 4. Ed. by Heubner, W. and Schüller, T. Berlin: Springer.
6. Michaelis, L. and Menten, M. L. (1913). Die Kinetik des Invertinwirkung. *Biochem. Z.*, **49**, 333.
7. Stephenson, R. P. (1956). A modification of receptor theory. *Brit. J. Pharmacol.*, **11**, 379.
8. Paton, W. D. M. (1960). The principles of drug action. *Proc. roy. Soc. Med.*, **53**, 815.
9. Paton, W. D. M. (1961). A theory of drug action based on the rate of drug-receptor combination. *Proc. roy. Soc., B*, **154**, 21.
10. Schild, H. O. (1947). pA, a new scale for the measurement of drug antagonism. *Brit. J. Pharmacol.*, **2**, 189.
11. Rang, H. P., Ed. (1973). *Drug Receptors* (Biological Council Symposium). London: Macmillan.
12. Hull, C. J., English, M. J. M. and Sibbald, A. (1980). Fazadinium and pancuronium: a pharmacodynamic study. *Brit. J. Anaesth.*, **52**, 1209.
13. Wiegand, R. G. and Sanders, P. G. (1964). Calculation of kinetic constants from blood levels of drugs. *J. Pharmacol. exp. Ther.*, **146**, 271.
14. Gibaldi, M., Levy, G. and Hayton, W. (1972). Kinetics of the elimination and neuro-muscular blocking effect of *d*-tubocurarine in man. *Anesthesiology*, **36**, 213.
15. Gibaldi, M. and Perrier, D. (1982). *Pharmacokinetics*., 2nd edit. New York: Marcel Dekker.
16. Kane, P. O. and Smith, S. E. (1959). Thiopentone and buthalitone: the relationship between depth of anaesthesia, plasma concentration and plasma protein binding. *Brit. J. Pharmacol.*, **14**, 261.
17. Prescott, L. F. (1969). Pharmacokinetic drug interactions. *Lancet*, **2**, 1239.
18. Goldbaum, L. R. and Smith, P. K, (1954). The interaction of barbiturates with serum albumin and its possible relation to their disposition and pharmacological actions. *J. Pharmacol. exp. Ther.*, **111**, 197.
19. Christensen, H. N. (1962). *Biological Transport*. New York: W. A. Benjamin.
20. Smith, S. E. and Rawlins, M. D. (1973). *Variability in Human Drug Response*. London: Butterworth & Co.
21. Iversen, L. L. (1967). *The Uptake and Storage of Noradrenaline in Sympathetic Nerves*. London: Cambridge Univ. Press.
22. Castleden, C. M., George, C. F., Marcer, D. and Hallett, C. (1977). Increased sensitivity to nitrazepam in old age. *Brit. med. J.*, **1**, 10.
23. Kangas, L., Iisalo, E., Kanto, J., Lehtinen, V., Pynnönen, S., Ruikka, I., Salminen, J., Sillanpää, M. and Sivälahti, E. (1979). Human pharmacokinetics of nitrazepam: effect of age and diseases. *Eur. J. clin. Pharmacol.*, **15**, 163.
24. Conney, A. H. (1967). Pharmacological implications of microsomal enzyme induction. *Pharmacol. Rev.*, **19**, 317.
25. Burns, J. J. and Conney, A. H. (1965). Enzyme stimulation and inhibition in the metabolism of drugs. *Proc. roy. Soc. Med.*, **58**, 955.
26. Kalow, W. (1962). *Pharmacogenetics: Heredity and the Response to Drugs*. Philadelphia: W. B. Saunders.
27. Vesell, E. S. and Page, J. G. (1968). Genetic control of dicoumarol levels in man. *J. clin. Invest.*, **47**, 2657.
28. Alexanderson, B., Evans, D. A. P. and Sjöqvist, F. (1969). Steady-state plasma levels of nortriptyline in twins: influence of genetic factors and drug therapy. *Brit. med. J.*, **4**, 764.
29. Blain, P. G., Mucklow, J. C., Wood, P., Roberts, D. F. and Rawlins, M. D. (1982). Family study of antipyrine clearance. *Brit. med. J.*, **284**, 150.
30. Davies, D. M. Ed. (1981). *Text Book of Adverse Drug Reactions*, 2nd edition Oxford: Oxford University Press.
31. Rogers, H. J., Spector, R. G. and Trounce, J. R. (1981). Allergy and immunosuppression, p. 758. In: *A Textbook of Clinical Pharmacology*, London: Hodder and Stoughton.

CHAPTER 19

# Intravenous Anaesthesia



ACCORDING to Price,[1] the first genuine attempt at intravenous anaesthesia was made in 1665, when Elsholtz injected an opiate to produce insensibility. Despite some transient acclamation for the use of chloral hydrate by Ore in the 1870s, however, intravenous anaesthesia did not enter routine anaesthetic practice until the introduction of thiopentone by Lundy in 1935.[2] Thereafter, its property of producing peaceful sleep easily led to its rapid acceptance and it remains to this day the commonest used induction agent. Within the last 25 years a number of alternative drugs have been introduced though not all have gained acceptance, because they showed few, if any, clear advantages over the parent drug either in ease of induction or in safety.

Intravenous agents differ from inhalational anaesthetics in that, once injected, there is nothing that can be done to facilitate the removal of the drug. Given the obvious dangers of respiratory and cardiovascular depression, there is still justification for the oft repeated adage "thiopentone is fatally easy to give". To a great extent, the properties of existing agents are similar. Their most important ones rest on their ability to penetrate the tissues of the body, particularly the central nervous system, without delay. Their rapid course of action is explained by their high lipid solubility coupled with a rich cerebral blood flow which ensures rapid penetration into the brain. This being so, the intensity and duration of this action is critically influenced, not only by the dose, but also by the speed at which that dose is injected. This is the bolus effect, for further discussion of which the reader is referred to Chapter 18. Once admixture with the circulating blood volume has occurred, the drug effect declines predominantly in most instances with redistribution of the drug into less richly perfused areas of the body, muscle, skin and finally fat depots. This decline reflects a rapid fall in plasma drug concentration defined pharmacokinetically as the $\alpha$-distributional phase, which is contrasted with the slower $\beta$-elimination phase. With most induction agents, distribution is so wide that elimination time plays little or no part in determining how quickly the anaesthetic effect wears off. Only after exceptionally large or repeated doses can elimination, mainly by metabolic degradation in the liver, exert a critical influence. The pharmacokinetics of intravenous anaesthetics are discussed in a paper by Ghonesin and Korttila.[3]

In this chapter, greatest space is given to thiopentone both because it is still the most widely used drug and also because it is the one whose pharmacokinetics and dynamics have been most intensely studied over the years. The principles involved are, however, applicable to all the agents used. Only the details differ. Brief mention is made of one or two agents which, introduced recently, are still subject to exploratory investigation. For a review of the whole topic the reader should consult the book by Dundee and Wyant.[4]

Intravenous anaesthetics can, of course, like all drugs, induce adverse reactions. At a time when many new induction agents are being introduced as potential replacements for the established ones like thiopentone and methohexitone, it is particularly important to appreciate the nature, frequency and severity of unwanted drug effects. The subject has been extensively reviewed by Whitwam.[5] Adverse reactions can usefully be described under four headings, namely:

1. *Reactions associated with induction.*—Muscle movements, cough, hiccup, respiratory and cardiovascular depression.
2. *Tissue complications.*—Local tissue damage, thrombophlebitis at the site of injection.
3. *Reactions associated with recovery.*—Psychic problems, motor disturbances, pain, nausea, prolonged somnolence.
4. *Hypersensitivity.*—Anaphylaxis, anaphylactoid reactions, skin rashes, bronchospasm.

It is beyond the scope of this text to review in detail all the spectra of reported reactions for each drug. The frequencies of reports of induction problems with propanidid, anaphylactoid reactions with Althesin, local pain with etomidate, thrombophlebitis with diazepam and psychic emergence problems with ketamine are, however, such that many anaesthetists continue to use thiopentone and methohexitone unless these are specifically contra-indicated. The adverse reactions to these barbiturates are for the most part dose-related and they can therefore be avoided by care in the anaesthetic technique. There is always merit in the use of those drugs which have been most used and which are best understood, and this branch of medicine provides no exception.

Anaphylactoid reactions to anaesthetic drugs are the subject of a recent review.[6]

**Thiopentone (Intraval, Pentothal)**

Thiopentone is a thiobarbiturate derivative, 5-ethyl, 5-(1-methylbutyl), 2-thiobarbiturate, the structural formula of which is:

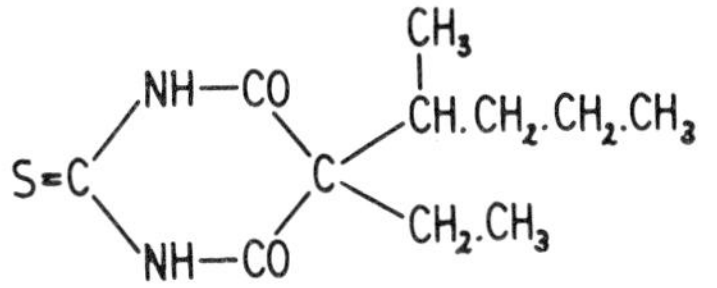


**Physical properties.**—Thiopentone is a weak acid of pKa 7·60 and therefore has optimal aqueous solubility at high pH values. At physiological pH where the drug is slightly more than half in the non-ionised state, it can precipitate from the solution. For this reason, in order to ensure total solution even in the presence of atmospheric carbon dioxide, it is presented commercially as sodium thiopentone containing 6 per cent sodium carbonate. Sodium thiopentone is a pale yellow powder with a bitter taste and a slightly sulphurous smell. The freshly made solution has a pH of 10·6.

**Pharmacological actions.**—Thiopentone rapidly crosses the blood-brain barrier and the concentration in the cerebrospinal fluid reaches a level almost as high as that of the unbound drug in the plasma. The depth of anaesthesia produced by the intravenous injection of thiopentone depends on its concentration in the blood, but the relationship is not a simple one, for the larger the initial dose the higher the brain concentration or plasma level at which the patient will awake.[7] This has been called acute tolerance, though the fact that a patient will wake sooner from a rapid injection than from a slow one is probably accountable on the basis of the bolus effect (see Chapter 18).

Thiopentone produces a progressive depression of the central nervous system. In clinical practice this is produced so rapidly that the classical signs of anaesthesia are of no value. Respiratory depression is marked, and a patient with apnoea may yet react to a surgical stimulus. The response to a surgical stimulus determines to a greater extent than with other agents the clinical signs of anaesthesia. The surgical stimulus may provide the "drive" to respiration and this may lead to fatal respiratory depression when the stimulus is removed.

Thiopentone has no analgesic properties—indeed hypersensitivity to pain and touch may be manifest.

The effect of thiopentone depends greatly on the premedication with analgesic drugs or the supplementation of thiopentone narcosis with analgesia—opiate or nitrous oxide with oxygen. These allow surgical intervention with no response at lower plasma levels of thiopentone and with less respiratory depression.

*Cerebral metabolism and blood flow.*—Cerebral oxygen consumption is reduced despite normal or even increased blood flow.[8] The latter is, however, probably more a consequence of increased arterial $Pco_2$ than of thiopentone itself.

*Respiratory system.*—The usual sequence of events when a dose of thiopentone is given slowly is for a few deeper breaths to be taken just prior to the loss of consciousness. There may then be a brief period of apnoea due to the direct effect of the thiopentone on the respiratory centre coinciding with a low carbon dioxide tension from the preceding deep breaths. Respiration returns gradually and then further fades away as more thiopentone is given.

The laryngeal reflexes are not depressed until the deep levels of thiopentone narcosis are reached, and stimulation, local or remote, may provoke laryngeal spasm at light levels of narcosis. If there is a predisposing cause present—such as a sensitive bronchial tree or stimulation of the larynx by mucus—the patient may develop bronchospasm or laryngospasm, but thiopentone does not of itself cause these conditions.

*Cardiovascular system.*—Under light anaesthesia there is widespread dilatation of the muscle and skin vessels but no obvious alteration in the total peripheral resistance.[9] The increase in peripheral flow is compensated for by constriction of the splanchnic and renal blood vessels so that the blood pressure and cardiac output remain relatively unchanged. In contrast, the rapid induction of deep anaesthesia leads to a fall in cardiac output due at least in part to peripheral vasodilatation causing pooling of the blood in the extremities and a reduction of the venous return to the heart. Thiopentone may also have a direct depressant action on the myocardium but probably only at very high drug concentrations.

Dysrhythmias occur in a proportion of cases, and are usually ventricular extrasystoles.

*Alimentary tract.*—In animals thiopentone produces some depression of intestinal motility, but this soon recovers and has returned to normal when the animal is awake.

*Liver and kidneys.*—There is no evidence that thiopentone adversely affects liver function unless hypoxia is present. Blood glucose concentrations are unaltered.

The effects of thiopentone on the kidneys are secondary to its actions on the circulation, and to the liberation of antidiuretic hormone that it causes. The urine output during thiopentone anaesthesia is decreased.

*Effect on muscles and myoneural junction.*—Thiopentone, in large doses in animals, prolongs the contraction of muscle, whether stimulated directly or indirectly, increasing the latency but decreasing the voltage of the action potential. This is consistent with a decreased rate of propagation of the potential on the surface of the muscle. In man there is no evidence that thiopentone in doses up to 1·5 g affects neuromuscular transmission.

*Reproductive system.*—In therapeutic doses, thiopentone does not alter the tone of the gravid uterus or the motility of the Fallopian tubes. Thiopentone, rapidly crosses the placental barrier, as do all lipid-soluble compounds, entering the fetal circulation in potentially active amounts. Neonatal respiration can be depressed by thiopentone, but the degree of depression depends upon the dose of the drug given to the mother and the duration of time that elapses between induction of anaesthesia and delivery of the baby, besides its maturity. The available evidence suggests that in operative obstetric practice, the intravenous injection of a small sleep dose of thiopentone to the mother is unlikely to impair respiration of the newborn baby to a significant extent. Thiopentone is therefore widely used in this context. For fuller discussion the reader should consult Chapter 41.

### Distribution, Metabolism and Excretion

Our understanding of what happens to a dose of thiopentone following its intravenous administration to man rests on the pioneer research of Brodie and his colleagues in the 1950s[10, 11] and of Price.[12] Though many of the observations were made in dogs, rather than man, the principles involved are universal in their application and are relevant, not only to thiopentone, but also to other intravenous anaesthetics in man. On first circulation, much of the drug is taken up from the injected bolus by tissues of high blood flow, particularly the central nervous system. The rate of drug transfer is known to be very fast, presumably because of the drug's lipophilic property, and this correlates with its rapid onset of anaesthetic action. Subsequent somewhat slower transfer of the drug from the plasma occurs to other tissues which are less well perfused, at first to muscle and later to fat depots, such that plasma drug concentrations fall markedly and quickly. As a result, the drug leaves the central nervous system for the periphery and recovery of consciousness ensues. At this time, most of the injected dose is still present in the body; it is merely redistributed to the tissues. Eventually, sequestration occurs to fat depots where the drug remains for many days in equilibrium with the relatively minute quantity in the plasma.

In the plasma, thiopentone is bound to protein, predominantly albumin, to a normal extent of 70–80 per cent. At high concentrations the proportion bound is markedly reduced,[13] indicating that the binding sites can become saturated.

This binding limits the concentration in free solution readily available for transfer to the brain. In old age and in severe liver disease or malnutrition, where protein binding is impaired, more drug is available for transfer and an exaggerated anaesthetic response may result. In such circumstances, thiopentone should be given in appropriately smaller doses. Similar potentiation has been reported with drug treatments which compete for mutual binding sites. Thus, sulphafurazole[14] and probenecid,[15] have both been shown to exaggerate the responses to standard doses of thiopentone, though they may not necessarily achieve this exclusively in the way that is described.

Thiopentone is ultimately eliminated almost entirely after metabolic degradation in the liver, less than 0·5 per cent being excreted unchanged in the urine. Metabolism renders the molecule less lipid and more water-soluble, thus depriving it of biological activity and rendering it less readily reabsorbed in the renal tubules. The pathways involved in the liver are threefold, namely:

(*a*) side-chain oxidation at $C_5$
(*b*) oxidative replacement of sulphur at $C_2$ to form a small quantity of the drug's oxy-equivalent, pentobarbitone, and
(*c*) ring cleavage to form urea and a three-carbon fragment.

Hepatic dysfunction slows elimination and can prolong recovery, though only after large doses.

The rates at which distribution and elimination occur have been the subject of several recent pharmacokinetic studies. The time course of the disappearance of thiopentone from the plasma (Fig. 1) shows obvious distribution and elimination phases, but mathematically it is best resolved into three exponentials

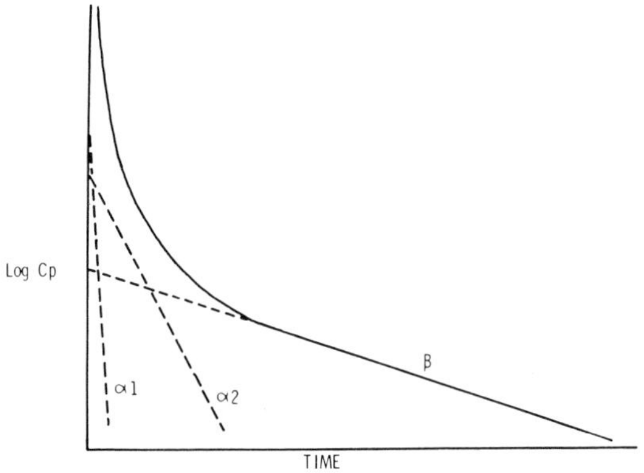


19/Fig. 1.—Time course of plasma thiopentone concentration resolved into three exponentials.

which possibly represent distribution to high blood-flow areas ($\alpha_1$), distribution to low blood-flow areas such as fat ($\alpha_2$) and elimination ($\beta$). Christensen and colleagues[16] have shown that a tri-exponential equation can be calculated which yields half-lives in young healthy patients within the ranges:

| | | | | |
|---|---|---|---|---|
| $\alpha_1$ | 1·7 | to | 6·5 | min |
| $\alpha_2$ | 23 | to | 71 | min |
| $\beta$ | 206 | to | 1321 | min |

True drug elimination is therefore very slow and this is confirmed by Morgan and associates.[13] However, total body clearance is high (82 to 288 ml/min) indicating that the reason underlying slow elimination is the large distribution volume which makes most of the drug inaccessible to the liver for its breakdown.

In the elderly, the concentration of drug present at sleep onset is lower than in the young, indicating increased sensitivity of the brain to the drug, and elimination is slower reflecting changes in volumes of distribution and possibly transfer constants.[17]

**Clinical use.**—Thiopentone can be used for several purposes—to induce anaesthesia, as a sole anaesthetic, as the principal anaesthetic but supplemented by other drugs, in conjunction with regional analgesia, to relieve acute convulsive states of differing aetiology, and to produce simple sedation.

Thiopentone leads to a rapid and pleasant loss of consciousness that can be produced with the minimum of apparatus. Herein lie its greatest advantages and its dangers—a fatal overdose is very easily administered. The safety of thiopentone—and indeed of all intravenous anaesthetics—is largely dependent upon the skill of the administrator in assessing, both before and during anaesthesia, the requirements of the patient, because when sensitivity to thiopentone is increased, both toxic and effective doses fall concomitantly. There are occasions therefore when it is necessary to use it with particular care and occasionally to avoid it altogether. These are:

1. *General.*—Out-patients who are unaccompanied are unsuitable for thiopentone because there is frequently a stage of euphoria for some time following the return of consciousness. In this stage, the patient is in no fit state to look after himself or to take responsible action. In no circumstances should he drive a car within 24 hours of the anaesthetic.

   Children are unsuitable for the administration of thiopentone as the sole or principal anaesthetic agent, since they need relatively large doses to produce a satisfactory depression of reflex activity. Provided venepuncture can be accomplished easily and painlessly, thiopentone is, however, an excellent induction agent for children.
2. *Respiratory disease.*—When the adequacy of the airway is in doubt, thiopentone must be used, if at all, with extreme caution. Factors which may affect the airway during induction, such as vomiting or bleeding, suggest either a special technique for the use of thiopentone or its avoidance. Thiopentone may be contra-indicated for an asthmatic patient, as it can lead to an aggravation of the condition.
3. *Cardiac and circulatory disease.*—The benefits of a smooth and pleasant induction with thiopentone must be balanced against the deleterious effects of vasomotor and respiratory depression. In fixed output cardiac diseases, such as mitral stenosis and constrictive pericarditis, vasodilatation and consequent hypotension—particularly if acute—may lead to cardiac arrest. Similarly in "shock" states, in which the blood pressure is maintained by peripheral vasoconstriction, the vasodilatation produced by even a small dose of thiopentone can prove fatal. Such conditions do not necessarily contra-indicate the use of thiopentone, unless the administrator is inexperienced and unable to assess the severity of the disease. With careful administration, the drug is safe to give even to patients whose cardiac performance is compromised by ischaemia.[18]
4. *Other diseases.*—For patients in whom coma is imminent due to diseases such as severe hepatic dysfunction, uraemia or uncontrolled diabetes, or due to over-sedation with drugs, thiopentone is either best avoided or used in minimal dosage so that recovery from its effect is rapid. Thiopentone is contra-indicated in the presence of any of the porphyrias because acute attacks may be precipitated and fatal respiratory paralysis can occur. It should be used with caution for patients with adrenocortical failure, in whom its action may be unduly prolonged. Abnormal respiratory depression may follow the use of thiopentone in dystrophia myotonica. Untreated myxoedematous patients are sensitive to most anaesthetics, thiopentone amongst them.

**Administration.**—Thiopentone should not be used as a stronger solution than 2·5 per cent—i.e. 0·5 g in 20 ml. Solutions should be freshly made, although they keep for a week in a refrigerator. Bottles of solution should be shaken before use to ensure adequate mixing.

The advantage of this concentration is that it is unlikely to cause serious harm if placed extravenously or intra-arterially.

*Intravenous.*—A vein should be chosen and palpated before the application of the tourniquet, which should be applied no more tightly than is necessary for occlusion of the venous system alone. When choosing a vessel for injection, so far as possible the medial aspect of the antecubital fossa should be avoided because of the occasional finding of an aberrant ulnar artery running superficial to the bicipital aponeurosis. Such a vessel may be found in up to 10 per cent of cases.

When the needle is firmly in the vein and the tourniquet released, 2 ml of thiopentone is injected with a pause after this so that an inadvertent intra-arterial injection may become manifest. Should this have occurred, the patient will complain of a severe burning sensation in the hand (see below). The estimated dose is given at a rate and in an amount that must depend upon the state of the patient and the purpose for which the thiopentone is being given. It may range from as little as 0·05 g for the induction of anaesthesia in a severely ill patient to 1·0 g as the sole anaesthetic for a fit adult. It is best to use the smallest effective dose, and to supplement this with more flexible and potent anaesthetic agents rather than to administer large doses of thiopentone.

*Rectal.*—The rectal administration of thiopentone is useful in children to produce basal narcosis, particularly for minor operations. It is unsuitable when a rapid return of reflexes is required immediately after the operation. If the expected stimulation is great then supplementation should be started before the operation to prevent such reactions as laryngeal spasm.

Atropine, or other suitable anti-sialogogues, should be given 1 hour before the thiopentone and the patient should have had nothing by mouth for at least five hours. Sleep comes on within 5 to 15 minutes and the maximum effect lasts for another 20 to 30 minutes, consciousness usually beginning to return one hour after the dose has been given.

The rectal injection of thiopentone by the anaesthetist provides a valuable, though somewhat slow, method for inducing sleep. No sterile precautions are necessary and the powder can be made up in a 5 per cent solution, the dose being assessed on the basis of 45 mg/kg body weight. When thiopentone is used some method for inflating the child's lungs with oxygen must be to hand, as central depression of the medulla may occur, particularly if the injection is made too quickly. The solution should be given over 10–20 minutes and only until the child is sleeping soundly.

**Local complications of thiopentone injections.**—Any intravenous injection carries a slight risk of causing a haematoma or losing the broken part of a needle. The incidence of haematomata can be lessened by early release of the tourniquet and the application of pressure to the site of venepuncture while the needle is being removed and for an adequate period of time afterwards. In thin patients, particularly the elderly, pressure should be maintained for three minutes, and elevation of the arm above the level of the heart is a valuable manoeuvre.

Needles break rarely but most commonly at the junction of the shaft with the hub and they should never be inserted as far as this so that, should one unfortunately break, the shaft can be grasped and removed. To avoid trouble, the arm should be gently but firmly held so that at the slightest movement the grip can be tightened. Movement is more likely to occur in the young and in unpremedicated patients. If a needle breaks, the arm must be held still and if the shaft cannot be grasped and removed, surgical removal with X-ray localisation of the needle must be undertaken. Even with immediate fixation of the arm it is surprising how far the needle may have travelled.

Solutions of thiopentone are alkaline and therefore irritant to the tissues. If enough of the solution is placed extravenously it may cause necrosis of the subcutaneous tissue with an ulcer. If the injection is attempted on the medial side of the antecubital fossa—a site that is not recommended—damage to the median nerve may occur: this is suggested by a shooting pain down the arm and movement of the hand or wrist.

*Intra-arterial injection.*—The incidence of this complication, which may have extremely severe sequelae for the patient, is unknown, though it has been variously estimated as 1:55,000 to 1:3,500. The number of permanent sequelae that follow intra-arterial injection is also unknown. Most of the reports of permanent damage refer to those that follow the use of stronger solutions than that now employed. No permanent sequelae have been reported following the use of a 2·5 per cent solution of thiopentone, and this concentration, therefore, has become the standard for clinical practice.

Intra-arterial injection occurs when insufficient attention is paid to the vessel chosen for puncture and to the initial response to a very small quantity of thiopentone. Absence of arterial pulsation may make difficult the normal differentiation between artery and vein, and this may be caused by excessive tourniquet pressure and even by bracing back the shoulders or rotating the neck in some patients.

Puncture of an arterial wall is usually painless, but the injection of 2 ml of solution into the vessel nearly always causes pain of a burning character which is radiated to the hand. Following the injection, spasm of the artery occurs and the pulse at the wrist may disappear. The immediate effect is probably due to the local release of noradrenaline in or near the vessel wall. Waters[19] has shown that arterial obstruction can be caused by crystallisation of the drug at the normal pH of plasma, due to the limited solubility of the non-ionised form of thiopentone. In a proportion of patients thrombosis takes place in the artery or its distal terminations. Blanching, and perhaps, cyanosis and gangrene of the distal part of the limb can therefore result, though this will depend to some extent on the state of the artery and circulation at the time.

When the accident occurs treatment must be aimed at diluting the thiopentone, overcoming the initial arterial spasm, and preventing thrombosis or extension of the clot. Operative removal of a thrombus may be necessary.

The needle must be kept in the artery—this may be difficult due to the intense pain that the patient feels—and 10 to 20 ml of 0·5 per cent procaine solution injected to dilute the thiopentone and encourage vasodilatation. When available 40–80 mg of papaverine in 10–20 ml of physiological saline is preferable. Alternatively, a potent vasodilator such as sodium nitroprusside may be used. It is also advisable to inject procaine or papaverine around the artery at the site of injection, and to remove other vasoconstrictor influences by performing a brachial plexus block and putting the patient on an alpha sympathetic blocking agent and considering anticoagulant therapy. When the damage is thought to have progressed to thrombus formation, then operative removal of the clot should be undertaken within six hours of the original injection, as it is doubtful whether muscle can survive more than this period of circulatory arrest.

*Venous thrombosis.*—The incidence of venous thrombosis has rarely been reported. The belief is that it is much more common after the use of 5 per cent thiopentone than after the use of 2·5 per cent solution. Usually the thrombosis is simple, but occasionally a chemical thrombophlebitis may occur with oedema and tenderness in the neighbourhood of the injected vein and its tributaries. Rest for the affected arm is the best treatment, as the condition settles in about seven to ten days: there is no specific therapy.

**General complications of thiopentone administration.**—These are usually due to an overdose of thiopentone having been given. This is often not a "large" dose but one too large for the patient due to an inaccurate assessment of his requirements, or attempting too much with thiopentone as the sole anaesthetic. The complications are mainly due to depression of respiration and the circulation, and have been described under the pharmacological actions of the drug.

### Methohexitone (Brietal, Brevital: Methohexital)

Methohexitone is an oxybarbiturate, $\alpha$-dl-1-methyl-5-allyl 5′-(1-methyl-2-pentynyl) barbiturate, the structural formula of which is:

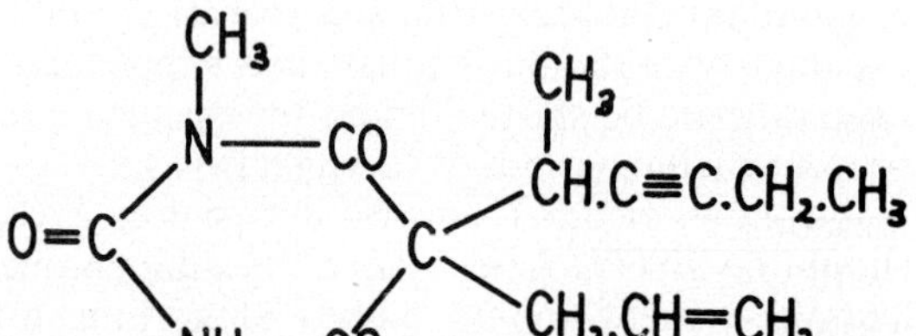


Because it has two asymmetrical carbon atoms, there are four possible isomers of this substance, which can be separated into two pairs: $\alpha$-dl (high melting point) and $\beta$-dl (low melting point). The $\alpha$-dl pair, which is methohexitone, produce hypnosis without stimulation of skeletal muscle. The mixture of all four isomers has been found to produce excessive skeletal muscle activity and even convulsions.[20]

**Physical properties.**—Methohexitone is a white powder. It is a weak acid of pKa values 7·9 and 8·3 and it therefore has optimal aqueous solubility at high pH values. As with thiopentone, the commercial solution incorporates sodium carbonate (6 per cent by weight of the powder) to ensure stabilisation even in the presence of atmospheric carbon dioxide. Such a solution is stable at room temperature for up to 6 weeks and is of pH 10–11.

**Pharmacology.**—Methohexitone is about twice as potent a cerebral depressant as thiopentone judging by the relative plasma concentrations of the two drugs required for equivalent electro-encephalographic responses. Estimates of relative potency based on clinical observation, however, have yielded slightly higher values though these depend very much on the conditions under which the drugs are used. Thus because the duration of action of methohexitone is shorter than that of thiopentone, it is less cumulative and larger total doses are required to maintain anaesthesia for a long time.

Most of the pharmacological actions of methohexitone are comparable to those of thiopentone though they are shorter lasting. Methohexitone produces dose-dependent cerebral depression. Following its intravenous administration, consciousness is lost somewhat more slowly than with thiopentone and the induction is frequently accompanied by transient twitching of skeletal musculature, hiccup and laryngospasm. Though the incidence of such complications is uncertain, they have been reported in up to 45 per cent of cases.[21] Premedication with cerebral depressants such as opiates or benzodiazepines reduces their incidence but, of course, prolongs the anaesthetic response to this otherwise short-acting drug. As with thiopentone, respiratory depression can occur though apnoea is usually only transient. Nevertheless, methohexitone reduces respiratory drive by up to 50 per cent for a few minutes after administration,[22] so it should not be used in patients with seriously compromised respiratory function.

Methohexitone should never be given to patients with a history of epilepsy, for convulsions, or even status epilepticus can be precipitated.[23] A recent electroencephalographic study[24] revealed serious disturbances in 5 out of 48 epileptics investigated. This potentially stimulant property of the drug is thought to involve the ring N-methyl group in its structure, a group which is absent from most other barbiturates which, therefore, are not contra-indicated.

Like thiopentone, methohexitone causes transient vasomotor depression with peripheral vasodilatation, but with a sleep dose given to a healthy patient, the blood pressure is unlikely to fall. At high concentration, methohexitone depresses myocardial contractility.[25]

Methohexitone does not cause bronchospasm, even in asthmatic subjects, and the total incidence of hypersensitivity reactions, as with all barbiturates, is very low, only 10 cases having been reported in over 20 years since the drug was introduced.

**Distribution, Metabolism and Excretion**

Like thiopentone, methohexitone is a lipid soluble drug which is 70 to 80 per cent bound to plasma protein and which shows qualitatively a similar pattern of distribution and elimination. It is, however, much less lipid soluble than thiopentone, consequently it has a smaller volume of distribution, is less sequestered in fat depots and is much more rapidly metabolised in the liver. The onset of anaesthesia is therefore less influenced by the bolus effect and the offset is determined more by the rate of drug metabolism than by distributional factors. Methohexitone is ultimately eliminated only after metabolic degradation in the liver, the pathways involving side-chain oxidation, N-demethylation and ring splitting.

A pharmacokinetic study[26] performed on a small number of healthy volunteers confirmed the relatively small distributional volume and the fast elimination of half-life 1–2 hours (*cf.* thiopentone 3·5–21 hours).

**Administration.**—Methohexitone is supplied as a powder in bottles containing 500 mg of methohexitone and 30 mg of anhydrous sodium carbonate, which should be made up as a 1 per cent solution. Solutions of methohexitone should not be mixed with acid solutions or precipitation of the sparingly soluble free acid will occur.

Methohexitone is administered intravenously. Sensations may occur at the site of injection or along the vein but they are usually mild and thrombophlebitis does not occur. The induction dose is approximately 1 mg/kg body weight, producing sleep lasting two or three minutes from which the patient makes a rapid recovery.

For out-patients requiring dental extractions, Coleman and Green,[27] using approximately 0·8 mg/kg of methohexitone, found that 90 per cent of patients were able to leave the dental chair within 6 minutes and 96 per cent were deemed to be safe to go home within half an hour. Recovery is of course dose-related and may be substantially slower after larger or repeated doses or in patients who are physically unfit. Even in healthy young subjects, driving skill is impaired for up to 8 hours after a dose of 2 mg/kg.[28] Patients should therefore not be allowed to drive on the same day.

**Indications.**—Methohexitone is recommended for any brief anaesthetic where rapid, complete recovery is required. It is especially useful for out-patients needing electro-convulsive therapy or dental extraction. It has a place in obstetrics, particularly for Caesarean section for which an induction dose of 1 mg/kg is appropriate. Such a dose does not affect neonatal blood gases, nor reduce the Apgar score.[29] As an induction agent in paediatric anaesthesia, an appropriate dose is 0·5 mg/kg.

### Other Ultra-short-acting Barbiturates

Other barbiturates such as buthalitone and hexobarbitone have been used in the past as intravenous induction agents, but they have now gone out of use.

### Althesin (Alphadione, Alphathesin)

Althesin is a mixture of two steroids, alphaxalone (3$\alpha$-hydroxy-5$\alpha$-pregnane-11,20-dione) and alphadolone (3$\alpha$,21-dihydroxy-5$\alpha$-pregnane-11,20-dione). It is presented as a clear colourless isotonic solution of neutral pH containing alphaxalone 9 mg and alphadolone 3 mg in each ml, which also contains 20 per cent Cremophor El (polyoxyethylated castor oil) and sodium chloride. It can be diluted with any isotonic solution. Its animal pharmacology was described by Child and colleagues.[30]

It is a brief-acting intravenous anaesthetic agent which is usually non-irritant at the site of injection. Both components are bound to plasma protein to about 30–40 per cent. Following intravenous injection of 0·05 mg/kg in man sleep is induced in 30 seconds and lasts about 5–10 minutes, whilst after 0·075 mg/kg sleep continues for around 10–15 minutes. Surgical anaesthesia is present for about half this time and full clinical recovery usually occurs within 30 minutes. Residual impairment of brain function may last up to 6 hours,[28] however, so patients should not drive a car the same day. It appears from animal experiments that termination of its action is determined largely by rapid metabolism in the liver[31, 32] rather than redistribution. It should therefore not be given to patients with liver disease.

There is a fall of arterial blood pressure of 10–20 per cent due to peripheral vasodilatation, a fall in central venous pressure and an increase of 20 per cent in the pulse rate.[33, 34] Apnoea may occur, particularly if the injection of Althesin is rapid, and there is a 2–3 per cent incidence of muscle tremors which is reduced by analgesic premedication.[35] Coughing, hiccup and laryngospasm have all been described, usually in response to stimulation during too light a plane of anaesthesia. It causes a low incidence of post-anaesthetic vomiting.

No hormonal effects due to the compounds' steroid configuration have been reported. Oyama and associates[36] found that no change took place in the concentration of plasma cortisol, though it did rise at the beginning of surgery. The plasma thyroxine was decreased but there was no change in the free thyroxine index, which was raised by surgery. Mehta and Burton[37] studied the effect of Althesin on carbohydrate metabolism and showed that blood sugar rose slightly during minor surgery and more during abdominal surgery, whilst the plasma insulin and human growth hormone levels did not change. Plasma-free fatty acids increased after 15 minutes of anaesthesia and minor surgery. The hyperglycaemic response to Althesin was the same in diabetics as in non-diabetic subjects.

The most important complication associated with its use is severe bronchospasm and circulatory collapse, an anaphylactoid reaction[38, 39] requiring treatment with oxygen, subcutaneous adrenaline, antihistamines, corticosteroids and plasma expanders. These reactions are probably due to the Cremophor El and have been seen following the administration of propanidid, a solution which also contains this substance. Evidence on the subject is, however, conflicting and true hypersensitivity to the steroids concerned may be involved in some cases. The frequency of bronchospasm and/or anaphylactoid reactions with this drug has been variously reported as 1 in 11,000[40] to 1 in 900[41] and may depend in part upon the speed of injection. In spite of its useful properties, therefore, Althesin cannot be recommended as a replacement for the older induction agents except where they are contra-indicated. Althesin is sometimes used as a long-term sedative by intravenous infusion in intensive care.

### Etomidate

[R-l-ethyl-l-(α-methylbenzyl) imidazole-5-carboxylate.]

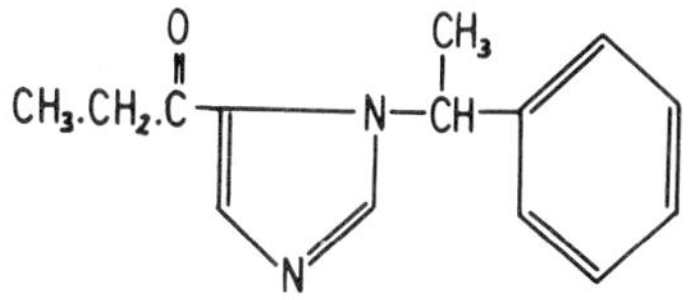


Etomidate is a water-soluble, non-barbiturate induction agent supplied as a solution of concentration 1·5 mg/ml containing propylene glycol. It has a rapid onset of anaesthetic action which coincides with the arm-brain circulation time, and within the dose range 0·1 to 0·4 mg/kg spontaneous wakening occurs in 7 to 14 min. On repeated administration there is little tendency to cumulation.[42] Anaesthesia with the larger doses is sometimes associated with apnoea of up to 45 sec duration and tachycardia of more than 20 beats per min increase.[43] There is an increase in muscle tone and a high incidence of involuntary movement[44] which can be decreased with opiates or diazepam premedication. The drug is without analgesic action.

Pain at the site of injection is common if the injection is made into a small vein but occurs in some patients when a large vein at the elbow is used. Carlos and Innerarity[45] reported that 20 per cent of their patients complained of burning pain even though the drug was administered by catheter inserted into an ante-cubital vein. This effect is independent of the drugs formulation.[46]

Early reports claimed that etomidate induction was free of the cardiovascular complications such as hypotension which are seen so often with established induction agents. More recent observations, however, indicate that such responses are more common than was previously thought.[47]

Recovery from anaesthesia is comparable with that after methohexitone and the drug has therefore been advocated particularly for outpatient work[44] and for bronchoscopy[48] or other brief operative procedures. The immediate post-anaesthetic period is, however, frequently complicated by nausea and vomiting so that adjuvant anti-emetic medication is needed.

Altogether the drug has no great advantage over other agents and it is recommended only if established agents are specifically contra-indicated. The drug has recently been implicated in adrenocortical failure occurring in patients receiving prolonged sedation in intensive care. It remains to be seen whether this is a genuine adverse drug reaction or rather a non-specific occurrence in seriously ill patients.

### Ketamine Hydrochloride (Ketalar)

2-(O-Chlorophenyl)-2-(Methylamino) cyclohexanone hydrochloride.

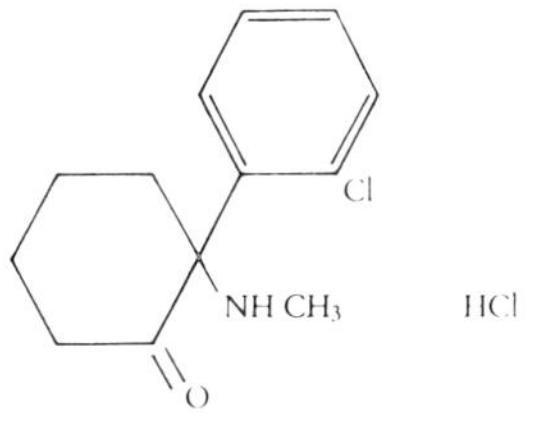


### Physical Properties

Ketamine hydrochloride is a white crystalline solid, soluble in water to a 20 per cent clear solution that is stable at room temperature. The base component is 86·7 per cent of the salt and the solution has a pH between 3·5 and 5·5. Benzethonium chloride is added as a preservative.

### Pharmacological Actions

Ketamine has unusual anaesthetic properties in that it produces unconsciousness with profound analgesia. For a brief initial period there may be a depression of respiration and a suppression of the pharyngo-laryngeal reflexes,[49] particularly after an intravenous injection. There is also an increase in systemic blood pressure and heart rate; originally this was believed to be due entirely to release of endogenous catecholamines, but other studies have suggested that ketamine produces a direct myocardial stimulant action combined with a peripheral effect.

Essentially, ketamine is a cataleptic analgesic and anaesthetic with hypnotic properties which are clearly distinguishable from the barbiturates. Electroencephalographic changes include the abolition of alpha waves and induction of theta activity. The short-lived depression of respiration and the pharyngolaryngeal reflexes are related to a high plasma concentration following intravenous administration.

### Metabolism

Ketamine undergoes N-demethylation and hydroxylation of the cyclohexanone ring with the formation of conjugates which are excreted in the urine. The unconjugated N-demethylated metabolite has only one-sixth the potency of ketamine and the unconjugated cyclohexanone derivative only one-tenth. Ketamine is relatively slowly distributed to the tissues and it has an elimination half-life of about 3 hours.[50] Analgesia is effected at circulating concentrations substantially lower than those which produce unconsciousness.

### Clinical Use

Ketamine was first introduced into clinical anaesthesia by Corssen and Domino in 1966.[51] Since that time it has been recommended for a wide variety of anaesthetic procedures. The principal advantage of this agent is that it produces satisfactory anaesthesia lasting from about 5 to 25 minutes with a relatively stable cardiovascular situation and the maintenance of a good airway. However, as already mentioned, both the circulation and respiration and the pharyngeal reflex can be affected during the first few minutes. The main disadvantage has been the recollection of unpleasant dreams by some of the patients during the recovery period. However, not all the dreams have been described as unpleasant yet some have been classified as nightmares. Various measures can be adopted to reduce the incidence of these dreams[52] and premedication with either hyoscine, droperidol or diazepam have been found useful. A quiet recovery room and minimal interference with the patient during this period can reduce the incidence of emergence phenomena.

Ketamine has a useful role for repeated anaesthetic procedures in small children, e.g. change of burns dressing. It is also an invaluable agent for the treatment of the trapped casualty or even for the Mass Casualty situation, so that it should always be available for the emergency and the induction of the shocked patient.[53] In regions where there is a dearth of anaesthetists then the satisfactory state of unconsciousness it can produce, with minimum training of the administrator, will be found useful for minor surgery but the lack of any muscular relaxation will limit this usefulness.

### Dosage

Intramuscularly: a dose of 10 mg/kg will usually produce 12 to 25 minutes of surgical anaesthesia.

Intravenously: 2·0 mg/kg will usually produce about 5 to 10 minutes of surgical anaesthesia.

*N.B.* It must be administered *SLOWLY* (i.e. over at least one minute) to reduce the incidence of respiratory depression.

Repeated dose: A half dose can be given when the patient shows the following signs.

(a) Movements in response to stimulation
(b) Nystagmus
(c) Phonation

### Contra-indications

Ketamine raises both the pulse rate and the systemic pressure. The studies of Tweed and his co-workers[54] have shown that ketamine has a direct stimulant action on the myocardium and peripheral vessels. The authors found that the myocardial minute oxygen consumption was increased and for this reason recommended that it should not be used in the presence of severe coronary or myocardial disease. Because it produces a marked rise in systemic and cerebrospinal fluid pressure, ketamine is contra-indicated in patients with hypertension, eclampsia, raised intra-ocular and intracranial pressure.

### Propanidid (Epontol)

This non-barbiturate, ultra-short-acting anaesthetic is a derivative of eugenol.

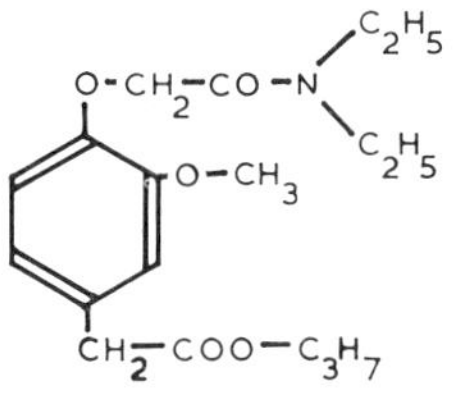


It is a pale yellow oil which, for clinical use, is dissolved in 20 per cent Cremophor El, a non-ionised, surface-active aqueous solution of ethoxylated castor oil, to give a 5 per cent solution of propanidid. This solution is highly viscous but it can be further diluted with an equal volume of physiological saline for easier administration.

It is rapidly metabolised to an anaesthetically inactive acid metabolite by enzymatic splitting of the ester bond, mainly in the liver but also in the blood by plasma-cholinesterase. This rapid breakdown determines the brief duration of anaesthesia.

When 5–6 mg/kg is administered intravenously over twenty seconds (the recommended rate) the unpremedicated patient is deeply asleep within about thirty seconds. 6 per cent of patients show involuntary muscular movements and 8 or 9 per cent a cough or hiccup. Awakening occurs in four to eight minutes and rational conversation is possible after a further two or three minutes.[55] There are no "hangover" effects but phlebitis occurs in 4 per cent, and as a large needle is used for the injection greater care than usual is necessary to prevent haematoma formation.

The blood pressure falls and the pulse rate rises in most patients.[56] The respiratory changes are characteristic,[57] the onset of anaesthesia being accompanied by a period of hyperventilation followed by apnoea which may last up to thirty seconds.

Propanidid prolongs the neuromuscular blocking effects of suxamethonium because of their common route of metabolism.[58]

The brevity of its effects means that to prolong anaesthesia either the dose of propanidid must be repeated or other agents administered rapidly to achieve a smooth transition. Premedication helps this but delays recovery. As with other induction agents containing Cremophor El, anaphylactoid reactions have been reported following propanidid. The drug is now seldom used.

**Diazepam (Valium, Diazemuls)** (see also Chapter 21)

Detailed description of the actions and uses of diazepam is inappropriate to a chapter devoted to intravenous anaesthesia, for diazepam should not be used clinically for this purpose. Intravenous doses of 10–20 mg provide light sedation with retention of pharyngeal reflexes and induce appropriate conditions for minor procedures such as endoscopy or dentistry, the resultant amnesia being such that the patient is unlikely to have unpleasant memories of the procedure itself. The drug can be used to induce anaesthesia, but doses of the order of 800 μg/kg are needed for a reliable "sleep dose",[59] there being wide variability in individual responsiveness. Furthermore, both onset and recovery are slow by comparison with other induction agents which greatly limits its usefulness. In its conventional organic solvent form with propylene glycol (Valium), the drug is painful on injection and the venous irritation it produces is followed by a high incidence of thrombosis. However, emulsion of diazepam in soya bean oil (Diazemuls) is almost always painless on injection and virtually free of thrombotic sequelae.[60]

**Midazolam (Dormicum)**, a water-soluble benzodiazepine derivative which is structurally related to diazepam, has similar properties, with a low incidence of pain on injection and subsequent thrombosis.[60] Like diazepam, there is wide inter-individual variability in the induction dose required and the onset of anaesthesia is slow.[61]

**Disoprofol (Diprivan)**

Disoprofol is 2,6-diisopropylphenol.

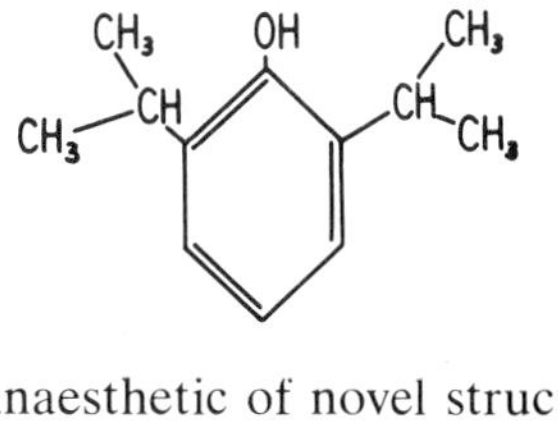


It is an anaesthetic of novel structure which has recently been introduced and is available as a 10 mg/ml solution in Cremophor El. It is equipotent with methohexitone and can be used in an induction dose of 2 mg/kg.[62] On injection it causes some pain due to venous irritation[63] but the onset of, and recovery from, anaesthesia are rapid. It causes transient hypotension and apnoea at higher dosage.

Assessment of the drug's true worth and place in anaesthetic practice is not possible so early after its introduction. Among the newer drugs, however, it looks promising.

### Minaxolone

Minaxolone is 11 $\alpha$-dimethylamino-2$\beta$-ethoxy-3$\alpha$-hydroxy-5$\alpha$-pregnan-20-one, a water-soluble derivative of alphadolone and alphaxolone, the components of Althesin. In limited clinical trials it has been shown not to cause venous irritation and to have a rapid onset of action, though accompanied by a high incidence of muscle movements.[64,65] By comparison with Althesin, recovery from anaesthesia is slow,[66] presumably because of the high water solubility. Though initially promising in some ways, this agent has now been withdrawn because of adverse effects on long-term toxicity testing in animals.

## REFERENCES


1. Price, H. L. (1975). General anesthetics: intravenous anesthetics. In: *The Pharmacological basis of Therapeutics*, 5th edit., p. 97. Ed. Goodman, L. S. and Gilman, A., New York: Macmillan.
2. Lundy, J. S. (1935). Intravenous anesthesia: preliminary report of the use of two new thiobarbiturates. *Proc. Mayo Clin.*, **10**, 536.
3. Ghonesin, M. M. and Korltila, K. (1977). Pharmacokinetics of intravenous anaesthetics: implications for clinical use. *Clin. Pharmacokin.*, **2**, 344.
4. Dundee, J. W. and Wyant, G. M. (1974). *Intravenous Anaesthesia*. Edinburgh: Churchill-Livingstone.
5. Whitwam, J. G. (1978). Adverse reactions to i.v. induction agents. *Brit. J. Anaesth.*, **50**, 677.
6. Beaven, M. A. (1981). Anaphylactoid reactions to anesthetic drugs. *Anesthesiology*, **55**, 3.
7. Toner, W., Howard, P. J., McGowan, W. A. W. and Dundee, J. W. (1980). Another look at acute tolerance to thiopentone. *Brit. J. Anaesth.*, **52**, 1005.
8. Wechsler, R. L., Dripps, R. D. and Kety, S. S. (1951). Blood flow and oxygen consumption of the human brain during anesthesia produced by thiopental. *Anesthesiology*, **12**, 308.
9. Fieldman, E. J., Ridley, R. W. and Wood, E. H. (1955). Hemodynamic studies during thiopental sodium and nitrous oxide anesthesia in humans. *Anesthesiology*, **16**, 473.
10. Brodie, B. B., Mark, L. C., Papper, E. M., Lief, P. A., Bernstein, E. and Rovenstine, E. A. (1950). The fate of thiopental in man and a method for its estimation in biological material. *J. Pharmacol. exp. Ther.*, **98**, 85.
11. Brodie, B. B., Bernstein, E. and Mark, L. C. (1952). The role of body fat in limiting the duration of action of thiopental. *J. Pharmacol. exp. Ther.*, **105**, 421.
12. Price, H. L. (1960). A dynamic concept of the distribution of thiopental in the human body. *Anesthesiology*, **21**, 40.
13. Morgan, D. J., Blackman, G. L., Paull, J. D. and Wolf, L. J. (1981). Pharmacokinetics and plasma binding of thiopental. I: Studies in surgical patients. *Anesthesiology*, **54**, 468.
14. Csögör, S. I. and Kerek, S. F. (1970). Enhancement of thiopentone anaesthesia by sulphafurazole. *Brit. J. Anaesth.*, **42**, 988.
15. Kaurinen, S., Eerola, M. and Ylitalo, P. (1980). Prolongation of thiopentone anaesthesia by probenecid. *Brit. J. Anaesth.*, **52**, 603.
16. Christensen, J. H., Andreasen, F. and Jansen, J. A. (1980). Pharmacokinetics of thiopentone in a group of young women and a group of young men. *Brit. J. Anaesth.*, **52**, 913.
17. Christensen, J. H., Andreasen, F. and Jansen, J. A. (1981). Influence of age and sex on the pharmacokinetics of thiopentone. *Brit. J. Anaesth.*, **53**, 1189.
18. Reiz, S., Balfors, E., Friedman, A., Haggmark, S. and Peter, T. (1981). Effects of thiopentone on cardiac performance, coronary hemodynamics and myocardial oxygen consumption in chronic ischaemic heart disease. *Acta anaesth. scand.*, **25**, 103.
19. Waters, D. J. (1966). Intra-arterial thiopentone. *Anaesthesia*, **21**, 346.
20. Taylor, C. and Stoelting, V. K. (1960). Methohexital sodium—a new ultrashort-acting barbiturate. *Anesthesiology*, **21**, 29.
21. Po, B. T., Watson, R. L. and Hansen, H. R. (1968). Arousal time following intravenous anesthetic agents, methohexital and thiopental: effect of doxapram hydrochloride. *Anaesth. Analg. Curr. Res.*, **47**, 446.
22. Kay, B. (1979). The measurement of occlusion pressure during anaesthesia. A comparison of the depression of respiratory drive by methohexitone and etomidate. *Anaesthesia*, **34**, 543.
23. Thornton, J. A. (1970). Methohexitone and its application in dental anaesthesia. *Brit. J. Anaesth.*, **42**, 255.
24. Male, C. G. and Allen, E. M. (1977). Methohexitone-induced convulsions in epileptics. *Anaesth. intens. Care*, **5**, 226.
25. Rowlands, D. J., Howitt, G., Logan, W. F. W. E., Clarke, A. D. and Jackson, P. W. (1967). Haemodynamic changes during methohexitone anaesthesia in patients with supraventricular arrhythmias. *Brit. J. Anaesth.*, **39**, 554.
26. Breimer, D. D. (1976). Pharmacokinetics of methohexitone following intravenous infusion in humans. *Brit. J. Anaesth.*, **48**, 643.
27. Coleman, J. and Green, R. A. (1960). Methohexital. A short acting barbiturate. *Anaesthesia*, **15**, 411.
28. Korttila, K., Linnoila, M. Ertama, P. and Häkkinen, S. (1975). Recovery and simulated driving after intravenous

anesthesia with thiopental, methohexital, propanidid or alphadione. *Anesthesiology*, **43**, 291.

29. Morgan, M., Holdcroft, A. and Whitwam, J. G. (1980). Comparison of thiopentone and methohexitone as induction agents for Caesarean section. *Anaesth. intens. Care*, **8**, 431.
30. Child, K. J., Currie, J. P., Davies, B., Dodds, M. G., Pearce, D. R. and Twissel, D. J. (1971). The pharmacological properties in animals of CT-1341, a new steroid anaesthetic agent. *Brit. J. Anaesth.*, **43**, 2.
31. Carson, I. W., Graham, J. and Dundee, J. W. (1975). Clinical studies of induction agents XLIII. Recovery from althesin, a comparative study with thiopentone and methohexitone. *Brit. J. Anaesth.*, **47**, 358.
32. Novelli, G. P., Marsili, M. and Lorenzi, P. (1975). Influence of liver metabolism on the actions of althesin and thiopentone. *Brit. J. Anaesth.*, **47**, 913.
33. Du Cailar, J. (1972). The effects in man of infusions of althesin with particular regard to the cardiovascular system. *Postgrad. med. J.*, **48** (suppl. 2), 72.
34. Savege, T. M., Foley, E. I., Ross, L. and Maxwell, M. P. (1972). A comparison of the cardiorespiratory effects during induction of anaesthesia of althesin with thiopentone and methohexitone. *Postgrad. med. J.*, **48** (suppl. 2), 66.
35. Dechene, J. P. (1976). Alphathesin, a new steroid anaesthetic agent. *Canad. Anaesth. Soc. J.*, **23**, 163.
36. Oyama, T., Maeda, A., Jin, J., Saltore, T. and Kudo, M. (1975). Effect of althesin (CT-1341) on thyroid adrenal function in man. *Brit. J. Anaesth.*, **47**, 837.
37. Mehta, S. and Burton, P. (1975). Effects of althesin anaesthesia and surgery on carbohydrate and fat metabolism in man. *Brit. J. Anaesth.*, **47**, 863.
38. Hester, J. B. (1973). Reaction to althesin. *Brit. J. Anaesth.*, **45**, 303.
39. Horton, J. N. (1973). Adverse reaction to althesin. *Anaesthesia*, **28**, 182.
40. Clarke, R. S. J., Dundee, J. W., Garrett, R. T., McArdle, G. K. and Sutton, J. A. (1975). Adverse reactions of intravenous anaesthetics; a survey of 100 reports. *Brit. J. Anaesth.*, **47**, 575.
41. Watt, J. M. (1975). Anaphylactic reactions after use of CT 1341 (Althesin). *Brit. med. J.*, **3**, 205.
42. Kay, B. (1976). A dose-response relationship for etomidate, with some observations on cumulation. *Brit. J. Anaesth.*, **48**, 213.
43. Holdcroft, A., Morgan, M. Whitwam, J. G. and Lumley, J. (1976). Effect of dose and premedication on induction complications with etomidate. *Brit. J. Anaesth.*, **48**, 199.
44. Miller, B. M., Hendry, J. G. B. and Lees, N. W. (1978). Etomidate and methohexitone. A comparative clinical study in out-patient anaesthesia. *Anaesthesia*, **33**, 450.
45. Carlos, R. and Innerarity, S. (1979). Effect of premedication on etomidate anaesthesia. *Brit. J. Anaesth.*, **51**, 1159.
46. Zacharias, M., Clarke, R. S. J., Dundee, J. W. and Johnston, S. B. (1978). Evaluation of three preparations of etomidate. *Brit. J. Anaesth.*, **50**, 925.
47. Criado, A., Maseda, J., Navarro, E., Escarpa, A. and Avello, F. (1980). Induction of anaesthesia with etomidate: haemodynamic study of 36 patients. *Brit. J. Anaesth.*, **52**, 803.
48. McIntosh, B. M. M., Lumley, J., Morgan, M. and Stradling, P. (1979). Methohexitone and etomidate for bronchoscopy. *Anaesthesia*, **34**, 239.
49. Taylor, P. A. and Towey, R. M. (1971). Depression of laryngeal reflexes during ketamine anaesthesia using a standard challenge technique. *Brit. J. Anaesth.*, **44**, 1163.
50. Clements, J. A. and Nimmo, W. S. (1981). Pharmacokinetics and analgesic effect of ketamine in man. *Brit. J. Anaesth.*, **53**, 27.
51. Corssen, G. and Domino, E. F. (1966). Dissociative anesthesia: further pharmacologic studies and first clinical experience with the phencyclidine derivative CI-581. *Anesth. Analg. Curr. Res.*, **45**, 29.
52. Johnstone, M. (1972). The prevention of ketamine dreams. *Anaesth. Intens. Care*, **1**, 70.
53. Bond, A. C. and Davies, C. K. (1974). Ketamine and pancuronium for the shocked patient. *Anaesthesia*, **29**, 59.
54. Tweed, W. A., Minuck, M. and Myrnia, D. (1972). Circulatory response to ketamine anesthesia. *Anesthesiology*, **37**, 613.
55. Wynands, J. E. and Burfoot, M. F. (1963). A clinical study of propanidid (F.B.A. 1420). *Canad. Anaesth. Soc. J.*, **12**, 587.
56. Johnstone, M. and Barron, P. T. (1968). The cardiovascular effects of propanidid. *Anaesthesia*, **23**, 180.
57. Harnik, E. (1964). A study of the biphasic ventilatory effects of propanidid. *Brit. J. Anaesth.*, **36**, 655.
58. Clarke, R. S. J., Dundee, J. W. and Hamilton, R. C. (1967). Interactions between induction agents and muscle relaxants. *Anaesthesia*, **22**, 235.
59. Brown, S. S. and Dundee, J. W. (1968). Clinical studies of induction agents. XXV: Diazepam. *Brit. J. Anaesth.*, **40**, 108.
60. Kawar, P. and Dundee, J. W. (1982). Frequency of pain on injection and venous sequelae following the i.v. administration of certain anaesthetics and sedatives. *Brit. J. Anaesth.*, **54**, 935.
61. Gamble, J. A. S., Kawar, P., Dundee, J. W., Moore, J. and Briggs, L. P. (1981). Evaluation of midazolam as an intravenous induction agent. *Anaesthesia*, **36**, 868.
62. Kay, B. and Stephenson, D. K. (1981). Dose-response relationship for disoprofol (ICI 35868; Diprivan). Comparison with methohexitone. *Anaesthesia*, **36**, 863.
63. Rogers, K. M., Dewar, K. M. S., McCubbin, T. D. and Spence, A. A. (1980). Preliminary experience with ICI 35868 as an i.v. induction agent: comparison with Althesin. *Brit. J. Anaesth.*, **52**, 807.
64. Mather, L. E., Seow, L. T., Gourlay, G. K., Roberts, J. G. and Cousins, M. J. (1981). Minaxolone, clinical effects and pharmacokinetics. Subanaesthetic infusion regimen. *Anaesthesia*, **36**, 586.
65. McNeill, R. G., Clarke, R. S. J., Dundee, J. W. and Briggs, L. P. (1981). Minaxolone: an evaluation with and without premedication. *Anaesthesia*, **36**, 592.
66. Sear, J. W., Prys-Roberts, C., Gray, A. J. G., Walsh, E. M., Curnow, J. S. H. and Dye, J. (1981). Infusions of minaxolone to supplement nitrous oxide-oxygen anaesthesia. A comparison with Althesin. *Brit. J. Anaesth.*, **53**, 339.

CHAPTER 20

# Sedative and Hypnotic Drugs



## Normal Sleep

Although sleep is a well-known phenomenon which is easy to define in broad terms, its scientific explanation is difficult. It is associated with a number of changes in body function: a reduction in awareness culminating in unconsciousness, progressive relaxation of body musculature, slight hypotension, bradycardia and reduction of the metabolic rate. The exact origin of sleep in the brain is not fully understood but probably arises in an integrated system involving ascending and descending pathways in the reticular formation, the cerebral cortex, intralaminary nuclei of the thalamus, caudate nucleus, posterior hypothalamus and anterior third of the pons. There appears to be no sleep centre as such, although electrical stimulation of certain parts of the reticular formation induces sleep in animals.

Different depths of sleep can be distinguished by the ease or difficulty with which the subject can be awakened and these have been correlated with electro-encephalographic changes. Five levels are distinguished: from A (drowsiness) to E (deep sleep). The deepest level occurs only for brief periods, usually early in the night. These types of sleep are referred to as orthodox or "slow wave" sleep. The normal person spends approximately one-quarter of the night in paradoxical or "rapid eye movement" (REM) sleep, this type being characterised by fast cortical electrical activity, greater reductions in skeletal muscle tone, rapid movement of the eyes and dreaming. The time spent in the various depths of sleep varies with age. In older people sleep is frequently broken by periods of wakefulness.[1]

### The Effects of Drugs on Sleep

Hypnotic and anaesthetic agents induce sleep

by mechanisms which are as yet poorly understood but which probably involve suppression of both cortical and subcortical activity. Progressive anaesthesia is associated with widespread inhibition, manifested by the absence of neuronal discharge. Electro-encephalographic patterns change with the depth of anaesthesia (see Chapter 27). During deep anaesthesia REM periods are absent, but in light anaesthesia they are often present and dreaming is common. The content of such dreams is usually highly emotional and often of a sexual nature, the latter being one reason why a chaperone is so essential when minor operations are being performed under solely gaseous anaesthetics.

The commonly employed hypnotic agents lessen the incidence and shorten the periods of REM sleep,[2] thus prolonging periods of orthodox sleep. With repeated administration recovery of REM sleep occurs, after which withdrawal of the drug precipitates massive compensatory increases of REM periods. Such observations probably explain why patients so often complain of sleeping badly the first night or two after stopping treatment with hypnotics and why so many become habituated to such drugs. Antidepressant drugs and narcotics usually have similar effects but major tranquillisers like phenothiazine derivatives may increase REM sleep and shorten the latent period before its onset. In elderly subjects hot drinks last thing at night tend to improve sleep,[3] an effect which is unlikely to be due entirely to suggestion.[4]

## SEDATIVES AND HYPNOTICS

Sedatives allay anxiety, while hypnotics induce sleep. Since most such drugs have different effects depending upon dosage, it is not possible to classify them too rigidly. For instance, most hypnotic drugs will merely produce sedation when administered in small enough doses.

In anaesthetic practice the principal use of hypnotic drugs is to ensure that the patient gets a satisfactory period of sleep the night before the operation, when anxiety about forthcoming anaesthesia and surgery may well result in insomnia. A routine prescription is, however, not advised and each case should be judged according to need.

### Factors Affecting the Response to Sedative Drugs

The response to a given dose of a sedative drug varies within wide limits which depend in the main on the state of the patient. When prescribing a sedative an appreciation must be made of the desired effect and of the condition of the patient—this is often difficult to assess accurately. A consideration of the following points will help.

**The effect of age.**—The elderly tend to be particularly sensitive to the action of sedative drugs. Quite small doses may produce unusually marked sedation but, more commonly, are liable to make patients noisy, confused and disorientated, particularly in strange surroundings like a hospital ward. So far as is possible, hypnotic agents should be avoided. If necessary, it is probably safest to give an alcoholic drink or a dose of chlormethiazole, which are less likely to cause problems than are other drugs such as benzodiazepines.

**The effect of body weight.**—Where precision of effect is required, the doses of drugs are best related to the weight of the patient, before making the necessary adjustments for the other factors. But here again allowance must be made, and the dose reduced for excess fat, or water—as in patients with ascites and oedema—or increased for patients who are unusually muscular.

**The effect of emotion.**—The state of reflex irritability depends mainly on the emotional condition of the patient. A placid individual needs less in the way of sedatives than one who is hyperexcitable.

**The effect of metabolic diseases.**—Where the basal metabolic rate is altered by a disease such as hyperthyroidism, the action of a given dose of sedative is likely to be less evident and of briefer duration than in a normal subject. Conversely where the metabolic rate is depressed the action of sedatives is profound and prolonged.

**The effect of previous medication with alcohol or narcotics.**—Long-continued use of these agents produces tolerance to the psychic effects of sedatives, and larger doses may be required. However, due to possible disturbances of metabolism already existing—particularly in the liver—sedatives may have a prolonged action and any depression of respiration and the circulation, which are the most important side-effects of these drugs, may be accentuated. In these circumstances a small dose given in plenty of time, so that the position can be reassessed and a further dose given if required, is the best policy.

**The effect of the presence of pain.**—Since drugs of this group have few if any analgesic properties, they should not be given to those who are in pain, because by removing the higher cortical functions they tend to allow the patient to over-react and produce restlessness. This may then be difficult to control with analgesics or narcotics without producing dangerous depression. The addition of a simple analgesic such as acetylsalicylic acid to a sedative will often make all the difference, and avoid the need for a narcotic. When long-acting sedatives are required pre-operatively it is important that they should be given early enough to allow most of their effect to wear off by the end of the operation, in order to avoid restlessness later.

**The general fitness of the patient.**—This is the most difficult factor to assess, especially for the inexperienced, and yet is the most vital because in those who are ill the margin of safety is narrow and the required dose may be extremely small. In all cases of doubt as to the fitness of the patient caution must be exercised. A dose which is thought to be too small is first given and when this has had time to act, which will vary with the drug and the route of administration, an assessment of the effect produced can be made and a further dose of the same or another drug added. Small repeated doses are safer than large doses at longer time-intervals. Patients who are ill frequently require very small quantities of a sedative to produce sleep, and these patients, who are least able to withstand any added insults, can all too easily have their respiration or circulation grossly depressed. It is often wiser not to use any pre-operative sedatives in the very ill, thus avoiding the risks of respiratory and circulatory failure.

### Classification of Sedative and Hypnotic Drugs

Five drugs, or groups of drugs, are in current clinical use:

1. Barbiturates
2. Benzodiazepines
3. Chloral derivatives
4. Chlormethiazole
5. Ethanol (ethyl alcohol)

The present tendency is to avoid the use of barbiturates because of their potential dangers, although many people believe that these drugs are more effective hypnotics than the presently favoured benzodiazepines. The choice of which drug to prescribe for pre-operative use is an individual one. Where patients are accustomed to the occasional or habitual use of a particular agent, then it is probably best to use the same one for this purpose although tolerance to the drug's pharmacological action may have developed.

Paraldehyde and bromethol (tribromethanol) have no justifiable place in modern therapeutics because of the dangers of toxicity, though the latter is still rarely used in the management of eclampsia.

Glutethimide (Doriden) is a structural analogue of thalidomide which has actions similar to those of barbiturates. Although once commonly used as a hypnotic agent, it is not now recommended.

For detailed exposition of the modes of action of hypnotics and sedatives, the reader should consult the review by Harvey.[5]

## BARBITURATES

Traditionally, barbiturates have been classified according to their duration of action, but this system, originally proposed on the basis of animal experiments, does not apply in man when they are used as hypnotics and administered orally. Indeed the duration of action of any one drug is conditioned by the patient's reaction to it rather than by its chemical structure. Although there are individual differences between many of the barbiturate drugs, all except the ultra short-acting ones, as typified by thiopentone, are discussed together in the following sections. Thiopentone and other similar drugs are discussed in greater detail in Chapter 19. The pharmacological actions of these drugs are as follows:

### Central Nervous System

All the sedative barbiturates produce a similar pattern of depression of the nervous system, the extent of which depends upon the level of excitability of the patient's nervous system and on the size of the dose administered.

The cerebral cortex and the reticular activating system are most sensitive to the barbiturates, the cerebellar, vestibular and spinal systems less so, and the medullary systems least of all. The circulatory and respiratory centres are affected by high concentrations but not the vomiting centre. Barbiturates are thought to work by increasing the effects of the inhibitory neurotransmitter gamma-aminobutyric acid (GABA), which produces widespread depression in the central nervous system. The exact mechanism involved, however, is unclear but may include inhibition of GABA uptake[6] which is normally responsible for inactivation of the transmitter.

**Hypnotic effect.**—This varies from mild impairment of performance of simple tasks to sleep. Depression of the cortex produces impairment of function and with high enough dosage sleep occurs in from twenty to sixty minutes. This sleep is usually dreamless. After awakening, depression of function can still be detected for some hours and the EEG does not return to normal for up to 48 hours. Following some of the barbiturates, these effects are felt by the patient as a "hangover".

**Effect on pain.**—In the presence of severe pain it is found that barbiturates may have an anti-analgesic action, making the patient restless and difficult to manage, as the control exercised by the higher centres is diminished. This is seen postoperatively in children who have had heavy premedication with barbiturates.

**Anticonvulsant effect.**—In anaesthetic doses all the sedative barbiturates are capable of inhibiting convulsions to some extent, such as those of tetanus, eclampsia, and epilepsy. Phenobarbitone has a specific anticonvulsant action not found in the others, which is clinically useful in treating epilepsy, particularly grand mal.

**Anaesthetic effect.**—If large enough doses of barbiturates are given, anaesthesia is produced, but there is no preliminary period of apparent stimulation and all the vital functions are depressed. The effect on respiration is particularly marked.

### Respiratory System

Barbiturates depress respiration by a direct action on the medullary respiratory centre. The depression is proportional to the dose of the barbiturate. The sedation and lessened muscular activity account for part of this fall in respiratory minute volume which is mainly brought about by a decreased tidal volume. Very large doses of barbiturates produce marked respiratory depression—indeed respiratory failure is the usual cause of death from barbiturate poisoning.

### Cardiovascular System

Ordinary oral hypnotic doses of the barbiturates have little effect on the circulation. The sedation they produce may cause a slight lowering of the blood pressure and/or pulse rate. Intravenous barbiturates may cause a fall in blood pressure due to depression of the vasomotor centre with consequent peripheral vasodilatation. Large doses of barbiturates affect directly the small blood vessels causing dilatation and increased capillary permeability.

### Alimentary Tract

Barbiturates decrease the tone and amplitude of contractions of the gastro-intestinal tract. The mechanism is probably a direct action on the smooth muscle or on the intrinsic ganglionic plexus. The gastric emptying time is little altered by hypnotic doses of the barbiturates but gastric secretion is depressed.

These findings are of little significance in clinical anaesthesia.

### Kidneys and Liver

Barbiturates produce no renal damage but anaesthetic doses do temporarily alter renal function.

The urine volume is decreased owing to increased tubular reabsorption of water produced by increased secretion of the pituitary antidiuretic hormone. Any hypotension produced by the barbiturate together with renal vasoconstriction leads to a decreased renal plasma flow and glomerular filtration rate. If the hypotension is prolonged, severe oliguria or anuria may occur. Therapeutic doses of the barbiturates have no effect on liver function. The liver is the most important organ for the destruction of the barbiturates, although other tissues such as kidney, brain and muscle also destroy the drug; therefore in cases of liver disease the action of barbiturates tends to be prolonged.

### Uterus

The uterus is relatively resistant to the depressant effects of barbiturates and hypnotic doses have not been found to depress uterine contractions in labour, although full anaesthetic doses may decrease the force and frequency of the uterine contractions. The barbiturates pass across the placental barrier easily and can produce marked respiratory depression in the fetus.

## Absorption, Metabolism and Excretion of Barbiturate Drugs

Barbiturates are readily absorbed from the intestine, the rate being slower for the longer-acting drugs. They are also easily absorbed from the rectum or from subcutaneous and intramuscular injection. Being lipid-soluble compounds, they are largely eliminated after biotransformation in the liver to oxidised and less lipid-soluble derivatives. The rate of biotransformation is slowest with the long-acting, more polar, derivatives such as barbitone and phenobarbitone, and fastest with the ultra-short-acting ones like thiopentone. Barbitone is consequently largely excreted unchanged, phenobarbitone is about 70 per cent metabolised and 30 per cent excreted unchanged, and butobarbitone about 90 per cent metabolised and 10 per cent excreted unchanged.

Rates of drug oxidation in the liver vary greatly from one individual to another, partly from inherent variability, and partly because barbiturates cause hepatic microsomal enzyme induction on repeated administration.[7] This accelerates their breakdown and causes tolerance to the drug's actions, making the individual relatively resistant to its effects. Cross-tolerance appears to occur with consumption of other cerebral depressant agents, notably alcohol, though this is often in the absence of enzyme induction. The mechanisms involved are obscure.

Barbiturates cause habituation, and a true addiction with withdrawal symptoms and signs including convulsions, particularly if they are repeatedly administered intravenously. Strong political moves have been made to ban these drugs from use as hypnotics or sedatives.

## Medium- and Long-acting Barbiturates

Individual compounds among the many available (Table 1) differ little in their pharmacological properties in that all are anticonvulsant, sedative and hypnotic according to dosage. For anticonvulsant activity, phenobarbitone (30 to 180 mg/day) is best for prophylaxis, though now largely superseded.

The disadvantages of the barbiturates are the "hangover" effect that follows the use of the longer-acting drugs, respiratory depression, and an occasional toxic skin rash.

As hypnotic agents there is little to choose between the many medium-acting drugs, amylobarbitone, butobarbitone, pentobarbitone, quinalbarbitone or the mixture Tuinal (amylobarbitone plus quinalbarbitone), all producing powerful sedation and hypnosis. Given to patients the evening before operation, any one of these drugs ensures a good night's sleep. Under the noisy conditions existing in many hospital wards, barbiturates are probably more effective than most of the alternatives presently available.

20/Table 1
Hypnotic and Anticonvulsant Barbiturates

| *Approved name* | *Proprietary and other names* |
|---|---|
| amylobarbitone | amobarbital, Amytal |
| butobarbitone | butobarbital, Soneryl |
| cyclobarbitone | cyclobarbital, Phanadorm, Rapidal |
| pentobarbitone | ethaminal, Napental, Nembutal |
| phenobarbitone* | phenobarbital, Gardenal, Luminal |
| quinalbarbitone | secobarbital, Seconal |

* Long-acting derivative.

Some of the proprietary names given apply to the sodium salts of these drugs which, being more soluble, are more rapidly absorbed from the gastro-intestinal tract.

Tuinal is a mixture of amylobarbitone and quinalbarbitone in equal parts.

## Barbiturate Poisoning

This may be chronic or acute. A regular daily dose of 200 mg of the powerful short-acting barbiturates can probably be taken without harm, but 800 mg per day will adversely affect performance, and after eight weeks withdrawal symptoms are likely. The average dose taken by the barbiturate addict is 1·5 g and unless this dose is exceeded severe intoxication is unusual. At any stage an overdose may be taken and then chronic poisoning becomes acute.

### Acute Barbiturate Poisoning

Acute barbiturate poisoning is less common now that barbiturates themselves are less frequently prescribed. The mortality rate of patients admitted to hospital with barbiturate poisoning is less than 2 per cent with expert treatment.[8]

**Symptoms and Signs.**—These reflect the degree of CNS depression. The patient may be merely lethargic with mild overdosage, inebriated in moderate overdose, or comatose in severe intoxication. Protective reflexes are impaired to an extent related to the depth of unconsciousness. Respiration is depressed: the minute volume is decreased but the rate may be slow or rapid. Occasionally Cheyne-Stokes respiration is seen. Hypoxia and respiratory acidosis develop.

The pupils may be constricted and react to light or show hypoxic paralytic dilatation. The blood pressure falls, mainly due to medullary vasomotor depression but also because of a direct effect on myocardial and smooth muscle. A tachycardia is present but tissue perfusion may be impaired producing a metabolic acidosis.

Urine output is decreased because of barbiturate induced vasopressin release and poor renal blood flow. Hypothermia occurs occasionally though its presence should suggest that a phenothiazine may also have been taken.

Death, when it occurs early, is usually due to respiratory depression and impaired laryngeal reflexes with aspiration of vomit, or to acute circulatory collapse. At a later stage bronchopneumonia, pulmonary oedema or renal failure may be responsible.

**Diagnosis.**—This depends in part on a knowledge of the circumstances in which the patient was found. Other causes of coma must be excluded. Frequently more than one drug, including alcohol, has been taken. Circumstantial evidence in the form of empty medicine bottles may be helpful. Specimens of blood, urine and stomach contents should be obtained for analysis; they may also be required for medico-legal reasons. Physical examination alone will not differentiate between the various CNS depressants.

### Management

Immediate care will depend upon an assessment of the level of consciousness and of respiratory and circulatory depression. In the fully conscious, gastric lavage may be beneficial; to be of value this should be performed soon after ingestion. Thereafter the patient is carefully observed for signs of any deepening CNS depression. In the semi-comatose and unconscious meticulous attention to the airway is essential. A patient with depressed pharyngolaryngeal reflexes should be intubated with a plastic cuffed endotracheal tube in order to isolate the respiratory tract. Certainly no attempt at gastric lavage should be made without this precaution. In borderline cases only an oropharyngeal airway may be tolerated; such patients should be turned from side to side with a slight head down tilt and oxygen administered by a face-mask. Equipment for tracheal intubation should be readily available. In severe intoxication arterial blood gas and pH estimations are valuable. Intermittent postive-pressure ventilation may be required and concomitant metabolic acidosis needs correcting. Regular chest radiography, electrolyte, creatinine and haematocrit estimations should be performed. Prolonged intubation may necessitate tracheostomy. Analeptics have no role in the management of acute barbiturate overdose.

Circulatory collapse is a major threat in severe cases. Intravenous fluids should be infused to maintain an adequate right atrial pressure which should be monitored by a central venous pressure cannula. Plasma, dextran and crystalloid solutions may be infused, but blood should only be given if there is evidence of coincidental blood loss. Myocardial (pump) failure as shown by an inadequate cardiac output in the face of a high filling pressure is best treated with a myocardial stimulant, e.g. isoprenaline or dopamine. Shubin and Weil[9] suggest digitalisation when diuresis does not occur with a high central venous pressure.

Hypothermia is probably best treated by passive means, and further heat loss should be avoided. Infections, especially of the respiratory tract, will require the appropriate antibiotic therapy. Corticosteroids used in the management of aspiration pneumonitis or cerebral oedema may deepen coma.

In severe intoxication methods of drug removal should be considered. These are:

(a) *Forced alkaline diuresis*

This requires normal renal function and careful, expert attention to water, electrolyte and acid-base balance. Osmotic or loop diuretics should be employed, in the presence of the high circulatory ADH, to obtain a diuresis of about 10 litres/day. Sodium bicarbonate infusion is used to produce an alkaline urine. Not all barbiturates are rapidly eliminated in this way. Renal excretion plays less part in the total elimination of those barbiturates with high protein binding and lipid solubility and whose main means of elimination is metabolic (e.g. pentobarbitone). However the elimination of longer-acting drugs such as phenobarbitone is greatly enhanced.

(b) *Haemodialysis*

This achieves rapid removal of all barbiturates. Less protein-bound drugs, e.g. long-acting barbiturates, are eliminated more quickly.

(c) *Peritoneal dialysis*

Peritoneal dialysis is far less effective than haemodialysis, and will not remove significant amounts of phenobarbitone.

## Benzodiazepines

Drugs of this class are now the commonest used hypnotic agents in clinical practice. Though they have sedative, anxiolytic and anticonvulsant and anaesthetic properties, they are usually classified as minor tranquillisers and are therefore dealt with elsewhere in this book. The reader is referred to Chapter 21.

## Chloral Hydrate ($CCl_3 . CH(OH)_2$) and its Derivatives

Chloral hydrate is a colourless non-deliquescent crystalline substance with a pungent odour and a strongly bitter taste. It is freely soluble in water.

**Pharmacological actions.**—Chloral hydrate is a sedative and hypnotic. In the usual dosage—0·7 to 2 g—sedation occurs in ten to fifteen minutes and is followed by sleep in about half an hour. The sleep is quiet and deep, but the patient can be easily aroused, and it lasts five to eight hours. Usually there are no after-effects and "hangover" is rarely seen. The EEG in resting man is depressed in a manner similar to that produced by the barbiturates, but in a less pronounced way.

Larger doses cause a prolonged and deeper sleep and may suppress pain. With doses of 6 g or more, complete anaesthesia may occur, and with it dangerous respiratory depression.

With the usual hypnotic doses respiration and blood pressure are depressed little more than in normal sleep. Cardiac depression is not seen with normal doses but does occur with large ones.

Chloral hydrate is rapidly absorbed from the gastro-intestinal tract but it is irritant to the stomach. It is mainly reduced to trichloroethanol, which is unpleasant to take and responsible for its hypnotic effect. Some of this substance is then inactivated by conjugation with glucuronic acid in the liver which is then excreted in the urine.

**Clinical use.**—Chloral hydrate is given in a dose of 0·3 to 2 g well diluted and with a suitable flavouring such as orange, to avoid gastric irritation and to mask the bitter taste. It is a non-cumulative, safe, and useful hypnotic and should be used more often than it is, especially when depression of respiration would be particularly dangerous.

Other preparations of chloral hydrate, its complexes or derivatives, are available. They have less gastric irritant effect and are therefore preferable for routine use, particularly in elderly patients. The most important of these are:

| *Approved name* | *Proprietary name* | *Tablet size* |
|---|---|---|
| dichloralphenazone | Welldorm | 0·15 g, 0·6 g |
| triclofos | Triclofos, Triclos | 0·5 g |

A syrup formulation of triclofos is available for paediatric use.

## Chlormethiazole Edisylate (Heminevrin)

Chlormethiazole has sedative, hypnotic and anticonvulsant properties. Adult doses of 1 to 2 g given orally or by intravenous infusion produce unconsciousness with a tachycardia but without other cardiovascular or respiratory changes.[10] It has been used to sedate elderly patients, though its repeated administration may cause dependence, and it is advocated for the management of drug- and alcohol-withdrawal states and for treatment of status epilepticus and eclampsia.

### Ethanol (Ethyl Alcohol) ($C_2H_5OH$)

Alcohol is a substance of more social than medical value, although a "nightcap" is a very useful hypnotic for the elderly. Its interest to the anaesthetist lies in its value for dealing with patients who are used to large quantities of it and who are therefore likely to be tolerant to the anaesthetic drugs. Alcohol was one of the first substances used to relieve pain: before 1847, spirits in large quantities were often given to patients prior to surgery. Although amnesia may well have been produced, the patients required to be restrained, since they were usually still in the so-called "excitement stage" of anaesthesia.

When a patient who is tolerant to alcohol has his normal quota withheld prior to anaesthesia, he way well be resistant. For such a person, the usual amount of alcohol, or even a little more—provided it can be given sufficiently far ahead to avoid the danger of aspiration from vomiting—may be helpful prior to anaesthesia. Induction of anaesthesia by intravenous ethanol has been reported but it is dangerous because of respiratory and circulatory depression.

## ANALEPTICS

Respiratory inadequacy has in the past been treated with a variety of analeptics, drugs which through their general nervous system stimulant properties activate medullary centres. They work either directly on the medulla or via chemoreceptor stimulation in the carotid body or both.

The management of underventilation, whether due to respiratory disease or to overdosage with cerebral depressant drugs, is, however, not greatly helped by the use of these agents. First, their ability to increase respiration is never very good but more importantly, particularly with the older agents, doses which are often only marginally greater than those needed for medullary stimulation activate cortical and other higher centres and produce convulsions. In practice, therefore, analeptic drugs are of little use and they should never be employed as substitutes for artificial ventilation if that is needed. In particular these drugs have no place in the management of drug poisoning.

Of the many agents used in the past, few are of more than historic interest. Ethamivan and nikethamide, both well-established drugs, and doxapram, which is the newest in the series, are discussed briefly below.

### Doxapram (Dopram, Stimulexin)

Doxapram [l-ethyl-4-(2-morpholinoethyl)-3,3-diphenyl-2-pyrrolidone] is a central nervous system stimulant. On intravenous administration it stimulates ventilation, increases cardiac output and work, and causes arousal from anaesthesia.[11] This stimulant phase is not followed by reactive hypoventilation. The ratio of convulsant to respiratory stimulant dose in animals is 70:1, that of nikethamide is 18:1.

The drug has a brief duration of action due to rapid inactivation in the liver and its ability to reverse drug-induced respiratory depression is therefore transient. Doses can be repeated hourly if necessary, or it may be given (well diluted) in an infusion.

Doxapram has been advocated as an adjunct to opiate analgesia for it does not reverse the analgesic effect[13] and by overcoming respiratory depression may allow more opiate to be given. Gawley and colleagues[14] showed that doxapram 1·8–2·0 mg/kg combined with morphine following upper abdominal surgery decreased cough and sputum production by comparison with morphine alone.

In the elderly and in patients with heart disease doxapram should be given cautiously, as ECG changes have been reported.

### Ethamivan. Vanillic Acid Diethylamide (Vandid, Clairvan)

Ethamivan is a central respiratory and circulatory stimulant. An intravenous dose of 0·6–2·0 mg per kg body weight will produce a rapid increase in the volume of respiration, followed in about a minute by an increase in respiratory and pulse rates with a moderate rise in blood pressure. All these effects are, however, of short duration—ten to fifteen minutes.

### Nikethamide (Coramine, Anacardone)

Nikethamide is a synthetic substance which

is made up as a 25 per cent solution. It stimulates respiration via the chemoreceptors of the carotid body and has a weak vasoconstrictor effect on the peripheral circulation. It has little, if any, effect on the myocardium unless large doses are given, when it raises the output slightly. The action of nikethamide is brief (10–15 minutes) and the dose is 1–2 ml of the 25 per cent solution given intravenously.

## REFERENCES


1. Březinová, V. (1975). The number and duration of the episodes of the various EEG stages of sleep in young and older people. *Electroenceph. clin. Neurophysiol.*, **39**, 273.
2. Oswald, I. (1968). Drugs and sleep. *Pharmacol. Rev.*, **20**, 305.
3. Březinová, V. and Oswald, I. (1972). Sleep after a bedtime beverage. *Brit. med. J.*, **2**, 431.
4. Adam, K., Adamson, L., Březinová, V. and Oswald, I. (1976). Do placebos alter sleep? *Brit. med. J.*, **1**, 195.
5. Harvey, S. C. (1980). Hypnotic and sedatives. In: *The Pharmacological Basis of Therapeutics*, 6th edit., p. 339. Ed. by A. G. Gilman, L. S. Goodman and A. Gilman. New York: Macmillan.
6. Sutton, I. and Simmonds, M. A. (1974). Effects of acute and chronic pentobarbitone on the $\gamma$-aminobutyric acid system in rat brain. *Biochem. Pharmacol.*, **23**, 1801.
7. Burns, J. J. and Conney, A. H. (1965). Enzyme stimulation and inhibition in the metabolism of drugs. *Proc. roy. Soc. Med.*, **58**, 955.
8. Clemmesen, C. and Nilsson, E. (1961). Therapeutic trends in the treatment of barbiturate poisoning. The Scandinavian method. *Clin. Pharmacol. Ther.*, **2**, 220.
9. Shubin, H. and Weil, M. H. (1971). Shock associated with barbiturate intoxication. *J. Amer. med. Ass.*, **215**, 263.
10. Wilson, J., Stephen, G. W. and Scott, D. B. (1969). A study of the cardiovascular effects of chlormethiazole. *Brit. J. Anaesth.*, **41**, 840.
11. Noe, F. E., Borrillo, N. and Greifensteen, F. E. (1965). Use of a new analeptic, doxapram hydrochloride, during general anaesthesia and recovery. *Anesth, Analg. Curr. Res.*, **44**, 206.
12. Winnie, A. P., Gladish, J. T., Angel, J. T., Ramamurthy, S. and Collins, V. J. (1971). Chemical respirogenesis II. Reversal of postoperative hypoxaemia with the "pharmacologic sigh". *Anesth. Analg. Curr. Res.*, **50**, 1043.
13. Dundee, J. W., Gupta, P. K. and Jones, C. J. (1973). Modification of the analgesic action of pethidine and morphine by three opiate antagonists, a respiratory stimulant (doxapram) and an analeptic (nikethamide); a study using an experimental pain stimulus in man. *Brit. J. Pharmacol.*, **48**, 326P.
14. Gawley, T. H., Dundee, J. W., Gupta, P. K. and Jones, C. J. (1976). Role of doxapram in reducing pulmonary complications after major surgery. *Brit. med. J.*, **1**, 122.

## CHAPTER 21

# Psychotropic Agents and Anti-Emetics



## ANTIHISTAMINES

Antihistamines are competitive antagonists of histamine. They are important because, apart from their value in treating conditions associated with the liberation of histamine, some of the compounds have useful side-effects.

To understand their value a knowledge of the pharmacological actions of histamine is essential.

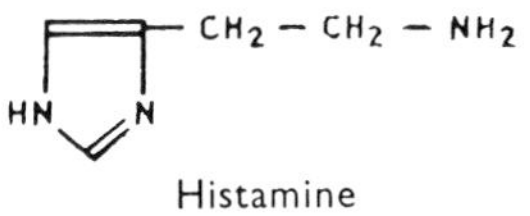


Histamine

**Actions of histamine.**—Histamine produces (1) *contraction of smooth muscle* which is most marked in the intestines, uterus and bronchioles; (2) *a fall of blood pressure* in man due to arteriolar and capillary dilatation with increased permeability and a flushed skin (essentially the same as the triple response of Lewis); (3) *increased glandular secretion*, particularly of the stomach, where it produces maximal stimulation to the secretion of hydrochloric acid—in fact histamine acid phosphate has been used as a test to find out how much hydrochloric acid the stomach can secrete. Histamine may also stimulate salivary, pancreatic and intestinal secretions. The headache, which occurs after the subcutaneous administration of histamine, is thought to be due to dilatation of the meningeal vasculature.

Research has shown that the actions of histamine are exerted on two populations of receptors, denoted $H_1$ and $H_2$, which can be distinguished by the actions of histamine analogues and of antagonists.[1] Smooth muscle and vascular effects are determined predominantly by $H_1$-receptors and are susceptible to blockade by $H_1$-antagonists. Gastric secretory effects are determined by $H_2$-receptors and are blocked by $H_2$-antagonists. There is, however, some overlap between the two and the hypotensive effect produced by histamine appears to involve both types.[2]

### $H_1$-antihistamines

Since the original work of Bovet and Staub,[3] many compounds have been synthesised and much comparative work done on their relative merits. A list of drugs in current use is given in Table 1. These compounds differ in potency and to some extent in their elimination characteristics, making some longer-acting than others, but there is no firm evidence of qualitative differences between them. Various animal tests have been used for quantitating the drugs' actions but to a certain extent the relationship of the potency of the different compounds varies with the tests used, and the correlation between the results in animals and those in man is uncertain.

21/Table 1
$H_1$-Antihistamines

| *Approved name* | *Proprietary name* |
|---|---|
| azatadine | Optimine |
| brompheniramine | Dimotane |
| chlorpheniramine | Piriton |
| clemastine | Tavegil |
| cyproheptadine | Periactin |
| dimethindene | Fenostil |
| dimethothiazine | Banistyl |
| diphenhydramine | Benadryl |
| diphenylpyraline | Histryl, Lergoban |
| mebhydrolin | Fabahistin |
| mepyramine | Anthisan |
| mequitazine | Primalan |
| phenindamine | Thephorin |
| pheniramine | Daneral |
| promethazine | Phenergan |
| terfenadine | Triludan |
| trimeprazine | Vallergan |
| triprolidine | Actidil, Pro-Actidil |

### Pharmacological Actions

The $H_1$-antihistmines show a variety of different pharmacological actions which can be summarised as follows:

1. *Antihistaminic action*.—The antagonistic action on bronchial and circulatory histamine receptors is competitive in type and depends therefore on the relative concentrations of histamine and antagonist present.

2. *Analgesia*.—Most derivatives have local analgesic properties, but it is doubtful if this is of any clinical importance.

3. *Central nervous system depression*.—Many of the antihistamines produce depression of the central nervous system which varies from an allaying of anxiety to intense drowsiness. For this reason promethazine, which produces the greatest depression, is given by mouth or injection as a pre-operative sedative and, in the form of an elixir, as a hypnotic for children. As premedication in small children, trimeprazine (Vallergan) elixir in a dose of 3–4 mg/kg is often used. The newly introduced drug terfenadine appears to have little or no sedative action.

4. *Synergism with analgesics and anaesthetics*.—Promethazine was used in anaesthesia by Laborit and Leger[4] in the hope that its antihistamine activity would avert certain forms of phlebitis which were thought to be due to anaphylaxis. It was found that promethazine was a powerful hypnotic and prolonged the action of the barbiturates and opiates. Summation of such hypnotic effects is to be expected with any drugs which have widespread central depressant actions. Promethazine, however, has some antanalgesic effect and this may give rise to dysphoric reactions in patients with pain unless adequate analgesia is also administered.

5. *Anti-emetic action*.—Many antihistamines have anti-emetic properties, largely due to their atropinic actions on the vomiting centre. They are of most benefit in motion sickness but the longer-acting drugs like promethazine have some beneficial effect against post-anaesthetic nausea and vomiting.

6. *Autonomic actions*.—Most antihistamines have atropine-like actions and dry salivary secretions. They show also mild alpha-adrenoceptor blocking properties and some show quinidine-like activity on the heart.

### Clinical Uses

The $H_1$-antihistamines are used in the treatment of urticaria and other allergic skin conditions, including drug sensitivity rashes, in the management of serum sickness, in hay fever, in vasomotor rhinitis and other diseases where there may be an allergic background. They are of little value in the treatment of asthma. Their use is recommended in Type 1 (anaphylactic) hypersensitivity reactions. But when these are severe, the mainstay of treatment is volume replacement, adrenaline and steroids.

### Side-effects

Drowsiness is common with most of these

drugs except phenindamine and terfenadine. Other side-effects which may occur are dizziness, headache, dry nose and mouth, with—more rarely—nausea and vomiting, intestinal colic and diarrhoea. The latter are seen most frequently with antazoline, mepyramine and tripelennamine, and can best be avoided by taking the drugs during or immediately after meals. If unpleasant side-effects are produced one of the other drugs should be used instead.

Promethazine in doses of 25 to 50 mg daily may produce ataxia and aching limbs. It is best administered at night because of the drowsiness produced. The other antihistamines are best administered throughout the day in repeated doses—triprolidine 2·5 mg, phenindamine 25–50 mg, diphenhydramine and tripelennamine 50 mg, mepyramine 100 mg. Gross overdosage produces widespread central nervous depression with convulsions, probably of hypoxic origin.

**Uses Associated with Anaesthesia**

Promethazine and trimeprazine have been used more in this context than the other true antihistamines because of their marked sedative properties which are unassociated with respiratory depression in clinical dosage. They can be used as a premedicant, to supplement anaesthesia during operation and postoperatively, and can be given intramuscularly or intravenously.

Promethazine (25–50 mg) with pethidine 50 or 100 mg and atropine 0·6 mg before operation produces a calm patient, sleepy but rousable, and with a normal blood pressure. Less thiopentone is required for the induction of anaesthesia than after premedication with morphine or papaveretum and hyoscine; there is a rapid return of reflexes post-operatively and a decreased need for post-operative analgesics for the first twelve hours, with less post-operative nausea and vomiting.

**$H_2$-antihistamines**

These drugs have an established place in the management of gastro-intestinal ulceration, reflux oesophagitis, gastric bleeding and peptic ulceration of the stomach and duodenum. Their effect results from antagonism of histamine at its $H_2$-receptor site which is responsible for gastric acid secretion. Administration of cimetidine (Tagamet) has been shown to promote healing of both gastric[5] and duodenal[6] ulcers and to reduce relapse rates with prolonged administration.

Following parenteral administration, the drug produces a reduction in gastric acid secretion which makes it potentially useful pre-operatively in situations where regurgitation of gastric contents is likely to occur. It cannot, however, neutralise the acid already in the stomach and therefore a time interval or some means of emptying the stomach is required for full effect.

A dose of 400 mg given orally between 1½ and 2½ hours prior to induction has been shown to reduce the volume of gastric secretions and reliably to raise the gastric pH above 2·5 in patients undergoing elective Caesarean section.[7] Some authorities, however, feel that a higher pH (> 3·5) should be aimed for to provide adequate prophylaxis against aspiration pneumonitis.[8] It must be stressed, moreover, that such treatment does not inhibit regurgitation nor obviate the need to prevent it occurring at the onset or during the course of anaesthesia. Rapid intravenous injection may cause hypotension which has been attributed to decreased peripheral resistance,[9] and there have been occasional reports of blood dyscrasias including thrombocytopenia and agranulocytosis. Otherwise, cimetidine appears comparatively devoid of serious side-effects and ranitidine, a newer $H_2$ antagonist appears similar in most respects.[10]

## PSYCHOTROPIC DRUGS

Various terms such as "tranquillisers" or "ataractics" have been loosely applied to a whole group of drugs which have only one property in common—namely an ability to produce "peace of mind". Yet this nebulous term makes it difficult or even impossible to measure or assess their efficacy with any real degree of accuracy, especially as they have little action on normal subjects. No general agreement has yet been reached on a satisfactory classification of this diverse group of drugs, largely because each one has so many actions that it is almost impossible to place them in a select compartment. The following groups of drugs are considered here:

(*a*) Major tranquillisers.
(*b*) Minor tranquillisers.
(*c*) Antidepressants.

The distinction between major and minor tranquillisers is that the former have widespread effects on the central and peripheral autonomic nervous systems and the ability to calm grossly disturbed psychotic patients. Minor tranquillisers have only restricted central action and in practice are useful only in mild anxiety and other reactive states.

## Major Tranquillisers

### Phenothiazine Derivatives

The phenothiazine nucleus has no antihistaminic action and little or no depressant effect upon the central nervous system; but derivatives of phenothiazine possess these as well as various other properties. Stemming from the work of Bovet and his colleagues in Paris very many have been synthesised. The first of the group to be used in medicine was promethazine, which has been discussed under the heading of antihistamine drugs, since it is one of the most powerful antihistaminics known. The addition of a chlorine atom to the nucleus and rearrangement of the side-chain of promethazine makes chlorpromazine, the most studied of the phenothiazine derivatives.

**Chlorpromazine** (Largactil, Thorazine).—2 - chloro - 10 - (3 - dimethyl - amino - n - propyl) phenothiazine hydrochloride.

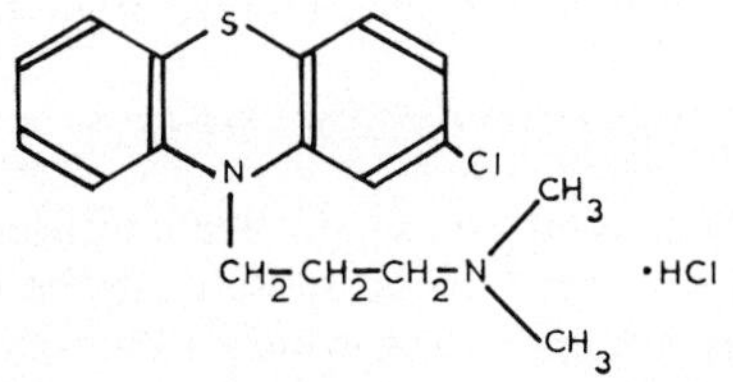


### Physical Properties

Chlorpromazine is a greyish-white crystalline powder with a slightly pungent odour. It is very soluble in water (1 g in 2·5 ml), a 5 per cent aqueous solution, having a pH of between 4 and 5. The powder and solution become discoloured in bright light.

### Pharmacological Actions

Chlorpromazine has slight antihistaminic activity but a profound action on the central nervous system and the peripheral circulation. It has so many actions on the central nervous system that it is very difficult to elucidate the different sites and mode of production of its effects. There is depression of hypothalmic function resulting in hypothermia, hypotension and a reduction in pituitary hormone secretion. Tranquillisation and general sedation also occur; all of these effects are thought to result from $\alpha$-adrenoceptor blockade in the relevant parts of the brain. Chlorpromazine is also a powerful anti-emetic and this activity together with the antipsychotic actions seen in schizophrenic patients probably results from antagonism of central dopamine receptors.

The mental effects noted in the conscious patient are drowsiness and loss of interest in the surroundings; euphoria sometimes occurs. If the drowsiness leads to sleep the patient can still be easily roused. The depressant action on the central nervous system lasts about eight hours after 0·7 mg/kg given intravenously in man.

The depressant actions of chlorpromazine are synergistic with those of other cerebral depressants, hypnotics, analgesics, alcohol and anaesthetics. Following chlorpromazine smaller quantities of general anaesthetics are needed to produce adequate anaesthesia. In the spinal cord, the drug reduces motor neurone activity with resultant muscular relaxation, an anticonvulsant effect, and potentiation of the competitive type of neuromuscular blocking drug.

**Autonomic nervous system.**—In the periphery, chlorpromazine produces innumerable effects which result from its actions as an $\alpha$-adrenoceptor and muscarinic cholinoceptor antagonist.

**Cardiovascular system.**—Chlorpromazine causes dilatation of peripheral blood vessels, particularly in the skin and splanchnic areas which results in hypotension, exaggerated by postural change and widespread heat loss from the skin. The normal vasoconstrictor response to hypovolaemia and shock is reduced with the result that operative blood loss causes an exaggerated fall in blood pressure which can be restored by fluid replacement.

**Respiratory system.**—Chlorpromazine has respiratory depressant effects, probably centrally mediated, which result in reductions of both tidal volume and respiratory rate.

**Hypothermic action.**—The drug has a powerful hypothermic effect as a result of several independent actions: suppression of the hypothalamic temperature regulating centres, reduction in spinal motor neurone activity (which abolishes shivering) and cutaneous vasodilatation.

**Anti-emetic action.**—Chlorpromazine is a powerful anti-emetic drug especially against vomiting produced by drugs and by radiation. It appears to act by depressing the chemoreceptor trigger zone.

**Fate in the body.**—Chlorpromazine, like the other phenothiazines, undergoes metabolic degradation by a number of pathways of which ring hydroxylation followed by conjugation and sulphoxide formation are the most important. These and several subsidiary pathways contribute to the formation of about 50 metabolites which appear in the urine and faeces. Some of these have modest biological activity but the extent to which their influence contributes to the action of the parent drug is unknown at present.

**Adverse effects.**—Treatment with chlorpromazine, as with other phenothiazines, commonly provokes unwanted responses. With single doses, the drug produces marked anticholinergic effects with resultant dry mouth and urinary retention. With repeated administration it can cause:

(*a*) abnormal involuntary movements including dystonia, Parkinsonism or tardive dyskinesia, due to dopamine antagonism in the basal ganglia;
(*b*) jaundice due to intrahepatic cholestasis from a delayed hypersensitivity reaction;
(*c*) contact dermatitis and light sensitivity resulting in a skin rash.

Such responses are, however, unlikely with use of the drug in anaesthetic practice except under exceptional circumstances.

### Clinical Uses

**Anaesthesia.**—Chlorpromazine is now little used in anaesthetic practice because of its numerous side-effects. It is, however, a constituent of Injectable Pethidine Compound B.P., a paediatric premedication; and chlorpromazine has been advocated in the technique of induced hypothermia because of its vasodilating action. It is also useful in the recovery period in situations where its combined actions of anti-emesis, sedation and peripheral vasodilatation may all be desirable. It potentiates the action of opiates and also of competitive neuromuscular blocking drugs.

**Administration.**—Concentrated solutions of chlorpromazine—and other phenothiazines—are irritant to the tissues, and must therefore be injected intra-muscularly. Intravenous injections should be limited to diluted solutions.

**Control of vomiting.**—Chlorpromazine is a powerful anti-emetic and has been used successfully in vomiting due to such varied causes as carcinomatosis, labyrinthitis, disulfiram (Antabuse) and alcohol, uraemia, nitrogen mustard, digitalis, hyperemesis gravidarum, acute gastritis and radiotherapy, as well as post-anaesthesia.

The doses used vary from 25 mg daily to 50 mg four times a day, but if vomiting is not controlled by two or three injections of 25 to 50 mg of chlorpromazine it is unwise to push the dosage because of the depression that is produced. A better alternative is to use another phenothiazine such as perphenazine (dose 5 mg).

**Psychiatry.**—Chlorpromazine has proved of value in the symptomatic control of most types of severe psychomotor excitement. Winkelman[11] summarised his results in 142 patients: "Chlorpromazine . . . is particularly outstanding in that it can reduce a severe anxiety, diminish phobias and obsessions, reverse or modify a paranoid psychosis, quieten manic or extremely agitated patients and make hostile, agitated senile patients quiet and easily manageable." Experimentally it antagonises the psychotomimetic effects of lysergide (LSD).

**Intractable pain.**—Because of its ability to increase the effectiveness of analgesics and its property of producing "pharmacological leucotomy"—a state where pain, although felt, does not distress the patient—chlorpromazine has found a place in the management of patients with intractable pain. Chlorpromazine has no analgesic properties, and therefore is of no value by itself, but in doses of 25 mg two or three times a day it is a useful adjuvant to the analgesics. It has been used extensively in the treatment of persistent hiccup.

### Other Phenothiazine Compounds

Many compounds based on the phenothiazine nucleus have been synthesised in an attempt to obtain more specificity without so many or dangerous side-effects and disadvantages. The structural grouping, approved and proprietary names of these derivatives are given in Table 2.

21/TABLE 2
SOME PHENOTHIAZINES AND RELATED DRUGS

| *Group* | *Approved name* | *Proprietary and other names* |
|---|---|---|
| *Dimethylamino-propyl side-chain* | chlorpromazine | Chloractil, Largactil, Thorazine |
| | promazine | Sparine |
| | trimeprazine | Alimemazine, Panectyl, Temaril, Vallergan |
| *Piperidine side-chain* | pericyazine | Neulactil, Propericiazine |
| | thioridazine | Melleril |
| *Piperazine side-chain* | fluphenazine | Modecate, Moditen, Moditen enanthate, Permitil, Prolixin |
| | perphenazine | Fentazin, Trilafon |
| | prochlorperazine | Compazine, Prochlorpemazine, Stemetil |
| | thiethylperazine | Torecan |
| | thiopropazate | Dartalan |
| | thioproperazine | Majeptil |
| | trifluoperazine | Stelazine |
| *Thioxanthines* | chlorprothixene | Taractan, Tarasan |
| | clopenthixol | Sordinol |
| | flupenthixol | Depixol |

Individual compounds in this vast collection differ from each other and from chlorpromazine itself only slightly in their properties. First, they differ in potency such that different doses are needed to produce equivalent effects. Secondly, they differ in anticholinergic activity, thioridazine being outstanding in its tendency to produce atropine-like side-effects. Thirdly, the piperidine and piperazine derivatives tend to produce antanalgesia, while the dimethylaminopropyl group tend to be analgesic.[12] Fourthly, the piperazine group have exaggerated antipsychotic properties and are more likely to produce extrapyramidal toxicity. The piperazine-substituted compounds also have preferential use as anti-emetics.

### Butyrophenone Derivatives

This group of drugs has actions which are essentially similar to those of the phenothiazines, particularly those with a piperazine side-chain (see above), although their structure is quite different. They show similar antipsychotic and anti-emetic properties and they are likely to produce extrapyramidal upsets. They do not appear to cause cross-sensitisation with phenothiazines and can safely be administered to patients who have developed jaundice after chlorpromazine.

They can cause hypotension because of both central and peripheral adrenergic blocking actions and the cerebral depressant actions summate with those of hynotics, narcotics, analgesics and other tranquillisers. Only three butyrophenones are in common use, benperidol (Anquil), droperidol (Droleptan) and haloperidol (Haldol, Serenace). All have powerful $\alpha$-adrenoceptor and dopamine receptor blocking activity and they induce mild sedation and tranquillisation. The very long half-life of haloperidol limits its use in anaesthetic practice. However, droperidol in combination with an opiate (usually fentanyl) is in common use for the production of *neuroleptanalgesia*. This combination, when used with nitrous oxide and oxygen, may form the basis for maintenance of general anaesthesia—either with or without the use of muscle relaxants. The technique is called *neuroleptanaesthesia* and the claimed advantages include avoidance of volatile inhalational agents, cardiostability, rapid awakening with return of protective reflexes, prolonged anti-emetic action (of the droperidol), and good postoperative analgesia. Droperidol should be used with care and in reduced dosage in the elderly as it may cause confusion. Also, as with all tranquillisers when given to patients in pain, it must be accompanied by adequate analgesia to avoid dysphoric reactions.

**Reserpine.**—This drug, an alkaloid of the plant *Rauwolfia serpentina*, was at one time in common use as a major tranquilliser, sedative and antihypertensive agent. Its clinical use has declined because of the intolerable side-effects of sedation, depression and diarrhoea and it is of historic interest only. Pharmacologically it depletes presynaptic stores of monoamines, which action is thought to be responsible for its widespread central and peripheral effects.

## MINOR TRANQUILLISERS

A number of mild cerebral depressant drugs have been used as sedatives and minor tranquillisers. Most of these, such as hydroxyzine, meprobamate, methylpentynol and tybamate, are largely of historic interest only. The most important of the minor tranquillisers in current use are the benzodiazepines.

### Benzodiazepines

Since their introduction into clinical practice in the early 1960s, a large number of compounds in this series has been introduced. Few real differences in pharmacological activity can be shown between them and their clinical use is dictated largely by their pharmacokinetic characteristics. Drugs with rapid disposal are more suited to hypnotic use, whilst those with slower disposal are used as tranquillisers and sedatives. The classification is complicated by the fact that many metabolites of the different benzodiazepines are themselves active and some are of very long duration of action. Moreover, several share with diazepam the same principal active metabolite which minimizes any differences there may be between the parent drugs. The derivatives which, at present, appear to have the most rapid disposal, absence of active metabolites and least clinical hangover are lormetazepam, temazepam and triazolam.

Those benzodiazepines with high lipid solubility are most suitable for parenteral use where a rapid effect is required as they will pass more quickly across the blood brain barrier (*cf.* lorazepam and diazepam). Low water solubility may cause problems with formulation of parenteral preparations and until recently this was the case with diazepam, which was only available in a propylene glycol formulation.

The following table lists some of the better known benzodiazepines together with details of their principal active metabolites or the absence of these. Half-lives of activity (T½ h.) are only relevant to (and only given for) those benzodiazepines without active metabolites.

**Diazepam** (Atensine, Valium).—7-Chloro-1,3-dihydro-1-methyl-5 phenyl-2H-1,4-benzodiazepin-2-one.

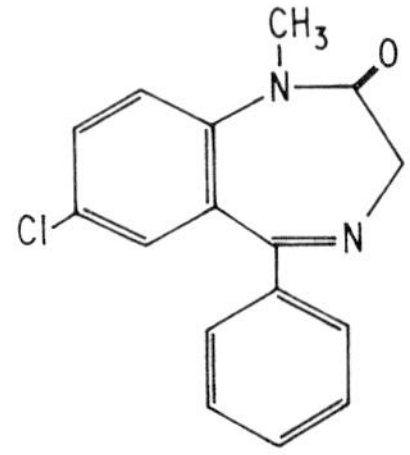


**Actions.**—Diazepam has general cerebral depressant properties, which make it suitable for use as anaesthetic, hypnotic, sedative or minor tranquilliser. At low dosage, it impairs concentration and the ability to perform skilled tasks. Larger doses produce amnesia, sleep or anaesthesia. Its depressant actions summate with those of all other cerebral depressant drugs, including anaesthetics. It has anticonvulsant activity,[13] probably supraspinal in ori-

21/TABLE 3
BENZODIAZEPINES

| *Approved name* | *Proprietary name* | *T½ h* | *Active metabolites* |
|---|---|---|---|
| chlordiazepoxide | Librium | | demethylchlordiazepoxide<br>demoxepam<br>desmethyldiazepam |
| diazepam | Valium, Atensine, Diazemuls, Evacalm, Sedapam, Solis, Tensium | | desmethyldiazepam |
| oxazepam | Serenid | 5–20 | none |
| chlorazepate | Tranxene | | desmethyldiazepam |
| lorazepam | Ativan | 10–15 | none |
| medazepam | Nobrium | | desmethyl medazepam<br>diazepam |
| temazepam | Normison | 8 | none |
| nitrazepam | Mogadon, Nitrados, Remnos, Somnite, Surem, Unisomnia | 18–28 | none |
| flurazepam | Dalmane | | desmethylflurazepam |

gin, which makes it a useful agent in the management of tetanus, severe pre-eclamptic toxaemia and status epilepticus. It depresses motor neurone activity in the spinal cord and can thereby have a useful effect in the management of muscle spasms in patients with cord lesions and multiple sclerosis. High doses markedly reduce the EEG voltage.

Used alone, large doses do not usually depress medullary respiratory and vasomotor centres, but in combination with other depressant agents severe respiratory and cardiovascular depression may result. Diazepam and other benzodiazepines are contra-indicated in patients with chronic obstructive airway disease who are dependent on hypoxic respiratory drive ("blue bloaters"), for these drugs inhibit such drive and may cause respiratory failure.

Diazepam is thought to exert its central effects by potentiation of the inhibitory transmitter gamma-aminobutyric acid (GABA), probably by competition, for a specific non-reactive binding site on the neurone.

**Absorption and fate.**—Diazepam is well absorbed when given by mouth and widely distributed in body tissues. It is broken down predominantly by oxidative metabolism in the liver, but this process is slow and at least two of the metabolites formed have marked pharmacological activity.[14] Thus much of the effect produced results from N-desmethyldiazepam (which has an elimination half-life of 100 hours) as well as from diazepam itself (with a half-life of 24 hours). Nitrazepam, having a somewhat shorter half-life (12–15 hours) is more suitable as a hypnotic agent than diazepam, though the difference is slight. On repeated administration diazepam accumulates in the body, and the effects of the drug and its metabolites take a long time to wear off. This is true also in cases of acute poisoning.

**Uses.**—Diazepam is at present one of the most commonly prescribed drugs in general and hospital practice. In mild anxiety states doses of 2 to 5 mg three times daily are used. In the management of agitated patients and in status epilepticus, as well as in premedication, larger doses may be needed.

However, the aforementioned problems of long half-life and active metabolites make diazepam unsuitable as a sole agent for induction or maintenance of general anaesthesia. It is used extensively in smaller intravenous doses (0·1–0·25 mg/kg) to sedate patients undergoing brief but unpleasant or painful procedures and, in this context, the production of a considerable degree of amnesia by the drug is considered an advantage. Diazepam is also being increasingly used orally as the sole premedicant in patients, where the analgesic and anticholinergic actions of traditional agents are not required. Furthermore, it is a commonly used adjunct to the induction of general anaesthesia when given intravenously. It reduces the requirement of induction agent and may thereby reduce the possible depressant effects on the circulation of barbiturates used alone. Also, reduction in reflex activity may aid smooth transition to maintenance agents. Diazepam is not water soluble and the traditional formulation in propylene glycol causes severe and prolonged thrombophlebitis if given into small peripheral veins. This problem has been largely overcome by a new formulation as a water-based emulsion (Diazemuls) which does not cause the same frequency or severity of reaction.

## ANTI-EMETICS

A proportion of patients undergoing anaesthesia and surgery suffer nausea and vomiting afterwards. This may be peripheral or central in origin, the latter arising either from stimulation of the chemoreceptor trigger zone or by activation of labyrinthine reflexes. Anti-emetic drugs act centrally either at the chemoreceptor trigger zone (CTZ) by antagonism of dopamine receptors or at the vomiting centre by antagonism of muscarinic cholinoceptors or histamine receptors or both. Additionally, metoclopramide (see below) accelerates gastric emptying which probably contributes to its anti-emetic action. Though anti-emetic drugs often reduce the incidence of postoperative nausea and vomiting, their accurate assessment is very difficult,[15] largely because the observations to be made are subjective and emotive. Clinical trials of potential drugs in this field require the strictest adherence to double-blind conditions.[16] The most useful drugs are anti-histamines and phenothiazines, some of which are indicated in Table 4.

Among these, the most active appear to be metoclopramide, perphenazine and prochlorperazine. All three are effective when adminis-

21/TABLE 4
ANTI-EMETICS

| *Approved name* | *Proprietary name* |
|---|---|
| betahistine | Serc |
| buclizine | Equivert |
| cinnarizine | Stugeron |
| cyclizine | Marzine, Valoid |
| dimenhydrinate | Dramamine, Gravol |
| droperidol | Droleptan |
| hyoscine | |
| meclozine | Ancoloxin |
| metoclopramide | Maxolon, Primperan |
| perphenazine | Fentazin, Trilafon |
| prochlorperazine | Stemetil, Vertigon |
| promethazine theoclate | Avomine |
| thiethylperazine | Torecan |
| trifluoperazine | Stelazine |

tered orally. In the postoperative phase, nausea and vomiting, especially that provoked by opiate analgesics, are best treated with one of these; the final choice being influenced by their differing degree of sedative side-effects and incidence of dyskinesias, especially in the elderly. When droperidol has been given during the anaesthetic, its powerful anti-emetic action usually lasts several hours into the recovery period.

### Metoclopramide (Maxolon)

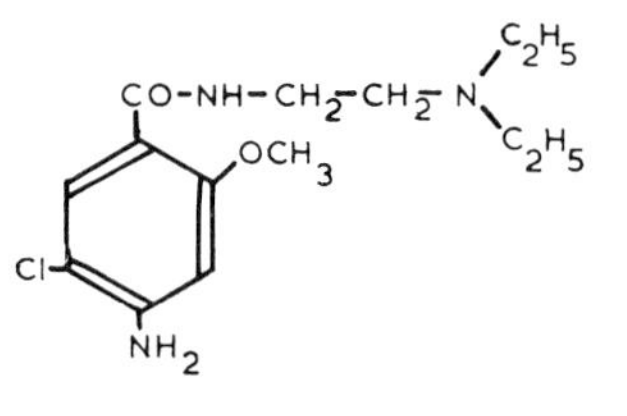


Metoclopramide is a dopamine antagonist which acts as an anti-emetic by blocking dopamine receptors in the chemoreceptor trigger zone. In doses of 10 mg t.d.s. it is non-tranquilising. It is not effective in vomiting of labyrinthine origin such as travel sickness, vertigo and Menière's disease. Handley[17] showed that metoclopramide (10 mg given at the end of the operation) was as effective as perphenazine 5 mg in preventing post-operative vomiting. Side-effects of prolonged administration of 60 mg per day include drowsiness, muscle dystonia, diarrhoea and headache. Oculogyric crisis is a rare but well documented side-effect of single dose *intravenous* administration.

Metoclopramide accelerates gastric emptying and has been advocated in the preparation of patients for obstetric anaesthesia. The degree of emptying obtained within a reasonable time is, however, small and no reliance should be placed on its action in this situation.

## ANTIDEPRESSANT DRUGS

### The Monoamine Oxidase Inhibitors (MAO inhibitors)

The commonly used drugs of this group are listed in Table 5. Their beneficial effect in the treatment of reactive depression is probably related to the accumulation of brain monoamines (5-hydroxytryptamine, dopamine and noradrenaline) which they cause. Inhibition of monoamine oxidase in the periphery causes sympathetic blockade and consequent hypotension, probably due to the formation of octopamine as a false transmitter at the sympathetic nerve ending. Among the various MAO inhibitors available, pargyline is occasionally used as an antihypertensive agent. Patients under treatment with MAO inhibitors are advised to avoid certain foodstuffs (cheese, Marmite and wines) and cold-cures which contain sympathomimetic amines, capable of producing exaggerated vasoconstriction and dangerous hypertension. Severe hypertensive episodes should be treated by $\alpha$-adrenoceptor blockade with phentolamine or chlorpromazine.

MAO inhibitors have inhibitory actions also on other enzyme systems, particularly those liver microsomal enzymes responsible for hydroxylation or oxidation of drugs such as barbiturates, alcohol, opiate narcotics, hyp-

21/TABLE 5
MONOAMINE OXIDASE INHIBITORS

| *Approved name* | *Proprietary name* |
|---|---|
| iproniazid | Marsilid |
| isocarboxazid | Marplan |
| phenelzine | Nardil |
| tranylcypromine | Parnate |
| tranylcypromine with trifluoperazine | Parstelin |

notics and tranquillisers. These drugs are thus potentiated and should be used only in small test doses to assess their effects. Pethidine should probably be avoided altogether, for on occasion hyperpyrexia, restlessness, unconsciousness, hypotension and death have followed its use.[18] If pethidine administration is essential, a small intramuscular test dose of 5 mg should be given followed by 10 mg and 20 mg at hourly intervals if no untoward effect on pulse, blood pressure, respiration or state of consciousness occurs. Thereafter the dose may be increased until normal dosage is achieved without complication. Such a procedure indicates that many patients respond normally.[19] It is mandatory, however, that other analgesics such as pentazocine, dihydrocodeine, or even morphine should be used before resorting to pethidine in view of the known sensitivity reaction.

The reason for the interaction between pethidine and monoamine oxidase inhibitors is not absolutely clear. In the resting state, amine neurotransmitters in the brain (noradrenaline; 5-hydroxytryptamine) are stored in granules at the nerve-ending. Any unstored transmitter is rapidly inactivated by the monoamine oxidase *enzyme* in the vicinity of the granules. On stimulation, the transmitter is released to act at the receptor. Thereafter some will be inactivated but the majority is *actively* taken up by the nerve-ending and re-stored in granules.

Pethidine and the tricyclic antidepressants tend to block the re-uptake process whilst the MAO inhibitors tend to build up the concentration of the neuro-transmitter. By this means the combination of an MAO inhibitor (permitting accumulation of transmitter in the nerve-ending) and pethidine (allowing accumulation near the receptor site) could lead to a severe reaction (convulsions, hypertension, etc.). In some animals, similar reactions occur, but not when morphine is substituted for pethidine. The finding that this sensitivity reaction is only rarely encountered in man remains a mystery.

There is no evidence that gaseous or volatile anaesthetic agents or neuro-muscular blockers are influenced by the administration of MAO inhibitors. The conduct of an anaesthetic may be made more difficult because of the combined hypotensive actions of the antidepressant and anaesthetic agents used. Elective operations under general anaesthesia are probably better postponed for one month, stopping MAO inhibitor treatment if the patient's psychiatric state permits. Stopping antidepressant treatment carries the risk that patients may make a suicidal attempt. This risk must be balanced against that of anaesthesia in the presence of the drugs.

### Tricyclic Antidepressants

Many compounds of this group are in common use for the treatment of depression, particularly of the endogenous or involutional type. The most important ones are listed in Table 6. These compounds have no inhibitory action against monoamine oxidase or other similar enzymes, their beneficial effect probably resulting from their action in preventing uptake of monoamines by nerve-endings.[20] Like the MAO inhibitors, they cause mild sympathetic blockade and consequent hypotension. They have also parasympathetic blocking (atropine-like) actions. The drugs are metabolised in the liver, partly by N-demethylation. Thus imipramine is converted into desipramine and amitriptyline into nortriptyline. Klerman and Cole[21] have reviewed the clinical pharmacology of this group of compounds.

In patients taking tricyclic antidepressant drugs dangerous potentiation of the cardiovas-

21/Table 6
Tricyclic and Related Antidepressants

| *Approved name* | *Proprietary and other Names* |
|---|---|
| amitriptyline | Domical, Elavil, Lentizol, Saroten, Tryptizol |
| amitriptyline with perphenazine | Triptafen |
| butriptyline | Evadyne |
| clomipramine | Anafranil |
| desipramine | Pertofran |
| dothiepin | Dosulepin, Prothiaden |
| doxepin | Adapin, Sinequan |
| imipramine | Berkomine, Janimine, Praminil, Tofranil |
| iprindole | Prondol |
| maprotiline | Ludiomil |
| mianserin | Bolvidon, Norval |
| nomifensine | Merital |
| nortriptyline | Allegron, Aventyl, Pamelor |
| protriptyline | Concordin, Vivactil |
| trazodone | Molipaxin |
| trimipramine | Surmontil |
| viloxazine | Vivalan |

cular effects of adrenaline and noradrenaline may occur, producing acute hypertension and dysrhythmias.[22] It is possible that some sudden deaths during local analgesia for dental treatment (where 1:80,000 adrenaline is commonly used) may have been caused by this interaction. Felypressin has been recommended as a safer alternative vasoconstrictor.

Overdosage with most of the drugs in this group entails a serious risk of tachydysrhythmias, due to combined atropine and indirect sympathomimetic actions, which are difficult to reverse. Some of the newer antidepressants which have somewhat different modes of action (e.g. maprotiline and mianserin) may prove less liable to induce this particular toxic effect. All tricyclic antidepressants have very large volumes of distribution. They can not, therefore, be removed by forced diuresis, by haemo- or peritoneal dialysis, or by haemofiltration. Acute overdosage should therefore be managed largely with cardiovascular and respiratory support.

## REFERENCES

1. Black, J. W., Duncan, W. A. M., Durant, G. J., Ganellin, C. R. and Parsons, M. E. (1972). Definition and antagonism of histamine $H_2$-receptors. *Nature (Lond.)*, **236**, 385.
2. Black, J. W., Owen, D. A. A. and Parsons, M. E. (1975). An analysis of the depressor responses to histamine in the cat and dog: involvement of both $H_1$- and $H_2$-receptors. *Brit. J. Pharmacol.*, **54**, 319.
3. Bovet, D. and Staub, A. M. (1937). Action protectrice des éthers phénoliques au cours de l'intoxication histaminique. *C.R. Soc. Biol. (Paris)*, **124**, 547.
4. Laborit, H. and Leger, L. (1950). Utilisation d'un antihistaminique de synthèse en therapeutique pré, per et post-opératoire. *Presse méd.*, **58**, 492.
5. Frost, F., Rahbek, I., Rune, S. J., Jensen, K. B., Gudmand-Høyer, E., Krag, E., Rask-Madsen, J., Wulff, H. R., Jensen, K. G., Højlund, M. and Nissen, V. R. (1977). Cimetidine in patients with gastric ulcer: a multicentre controlled trial. *Brit. med. J.*, **2**, 795.
6. Pounder, R. E., Williams, J. G., Milton-Thompson, G. J. and Misiewicz, J. J. (1975). 24-hour control of intragastric acidity by cimetidine in duodenal-ulcer patients. *Lancet*, **2**, 1069.
7. Johnston, J. R., McCaughey, W., Moore, J. and Dundee, J. W. (1982). Cimetidine as an oral antacid before elective Caesarean section. *Anaesthesia*, **37**, 26.
8. Crawford, J. Selwyn. (1981). Cimetidine in elective Caesarean section. *Anaesthesia*, **36**, 641.
9. Heining, M., Luthman, J., Groom, J. and Aps, C. (1983). Hypotension following cimetidine administration during cardiopulmonary bypass. *Anaesthesia*, **38**, 260.
10. Langman, M. T. S., Henry, D. A., Bell, G. D., Burnham, W. R. and Ogilvy, A. (1980). Cimetidine and ranitidine in duodenal ulcer. *Brit. med. J.*, **2**, 473.
11. Winkelman, N. W., Jnr. (1954). Chlorpromazine in the treatment of neuropsychiatric disorders. *J. Amer. med. Ass.*, **115**, 18.
12. Dundee, J. W., Love, W. J. and Moore, J. (1963). Alterations in response to somatic pain associated with anaesthesia. XV. Further studies with phenothiazine derivatives and similar drugs. *Brit. J. Anaesth.*, **35**, 597.
13. Randall, L. O., Heise, G. A., Schallek, W., Bagdon, R. E., Banziger, R., Boris, A., Moe, R. A. and Abrams, W. B. (1961). Pharmacological and clinical studies on Valium, a new psychotherapeutic agent of the benzodiazepine class. *Curr. ther. Res.*, **3**, 405.
14. Schwartz, M. A., Koechlim, B. A., Postma, E., Palmer, S. and Krol, G. (1965). Metabolism of diazepam in rat, dog and man. *J. Pharmacol. exp. Ther.*, **149**, 423.
15. Riding, J. E. (1963). The prevention of postoperative vomiting. *Brit. J. Anaesth.*, **35**, 180.
16. Purkis, I. E. and Ishii, M. (1963). The effectiveness of anti-emetic agents: comparison of the anti-emetic activity of trifluopromazine (Vesprin), perphenazine (Trilafon), and trifluoperazine (Stelazine) with that of dimenhydrinate (Gravol) in post-anaesthetic vomiting. *Canad. Anaesth. Soc. J.*, **10**, 539.
17. Handley, A. J. (1967). Metoclopramide in the prevention of post-operative nausea and vomiting. *Brit. J. clin. Pract.*, **21**, 460.
18. Perks, E. R. (1964). Monoamine oxidase inhibitors. *Anaesthesia*, **19**, 376.
19. Evans-Prosser, C. D. G. (1968). The use of pethidine and morphine in the presence of monoamine oxidase inhibitors. *Brit. J. Anaesth.*, **40**, 279.
20. Glowinski, J. and Axelrod, J. (1964). Inhibition of uptake of tritiated-noradrenaline in the intact rat brain by imipramine and structurally related compounds. *Nature (Lond.)*, **204**, 1318.
21. Klerman, G. L. and Cole, J. O. (1965). Clinical pharmacology of imipramine and related antidepressant compounds. *Pharmacol. Rev.*, **17**, 101.
22. Boakes, A. J. Laurence, D. R., Teoh, P. C., Barar, F. S. K., Benedikter, L. T. and Prichard, B. N. C. (1973). Interactions between sympathomimetic amines and antidepressant agents in man. *Brit. med. J.*, **1**, 311.

CHAPTER 22

# Neuromuscular Transmission

## History, Pharmacology and Physiology



### History

The history of the discovery of the South American arrow poison curare has been told many times by the early explorers of the New World. The fascination with the manner in which this extract of the bark of the creeper *Chondrodendron tomentosum* produced its lethal effect was masked in mystery and confusion. Clearly it killed when a small amount of the active compound contained on an arrow pierced the skin of an animal and yet, unlike most poisons, it did not render the animal unfit for consumption.

The early experiments of the Abbé Fontana,[1] using de la Condamine's sample of arrow poison established that contrary to earlier reports the fumes of curare were innocuous and that it was harmless if given by mouth. He demonstrated that it did not cause harm if applied topically but once it contaminated the blood of the animal it caused its death. In 1811–1812 Benjamin Brodie,[2,3] using the crude curare brought back to England by Charles Waterton, demonstrated that an animal poisoned by the drug could be kept alive by artificial ventilation. However, it remained for Claude Bernard (1856)[4] to demonstrate clearly that if curare was administered to frogs it caused paralysis without directly affecting the muscles' ability to contract if stimulated directly. He concluded from these lucid experiments that curare did not affect:

(*a*) the spinal cord
(*b*) the nerves or muscles directly
(*c*) the sensation

He also demonstrated that it was necessary for the poison to be given into the blood so that it could reach its site of action at the junction of the nerve and muscle.

In 1934 Dale and Feldberg[5] demonstrated that acetylcholine was produced by the stimulation of motor nerves and that this substance would cause contraction of muscles if injected close to the neuromuscular junction. When, in 1936, Dale, Feldberg and Vogt[6] showed that curare did not prevent the production of acetylcholine it became evident that the principal site of action of this drug was the acetylcholine receptor site, where it blocked the action of the neurotransmitter. This was confirmed by Eccles, Katz and Kuffler in 1941.[7] They demonstrated a progressive reduction in the electrical response at the motor end-plate on the muscle in the presence of increasing concentrations of curare.

In spite of this information curare remained a pharmacological curiosity until Richard Gill[8] brought back sufficient crude *Chondrodendron* to allow McIntyre[9] to extract sufficient purified drug (Intocostrin) in 1940 to permit its controlled use in patients. In 1942 Griffith and Johnson[10] in Montreal used 5 ml of this original preparation to supplement cyclopropane anaesthesia and to obtain adequate relaxation for an appendicectomy to be easily performed. Griffith and Johnson published the results of anaesthesia in 25 patients to whom Intocostrin had been administered in 1942 and with it heralded a new era of anaesthesia.

Once the use of curare became accepted as a means of producing muscle relaxation during anaesthesia the search started for alternative more specific agents. Harold King (1935)[11] in his original study of the crude curare extract in Henry Dale's laboratory suggested that the formula for the active compound was Fig. 1. This structure revealed 2 quaternary ammonium groups. The similarity of these quaternary ammonium groups with that of acetylcholine (Fig. 2) inspired the study of other bis-quaternary ammonium compounds. In their classic study of these compounds Paton and Zaimis (1949)[12] showed that where these two highly positively charged groups were separated by a 10 methyl chain, the maximum neuromuscular blocking effect was produced. However, this compound—decamethonium—had properties that differed from those of curare-like compounds. Zaimis (1953)[13] showed that instead of producing flaccid paralysis in chicks it produced tonic contraction and opisthotonus. Studies of the electrical changes produced at the end-plate when this drug was administered revealed that unlike curare it produced a depolarisation of the end-plate which was associated with the neuromuscular block.[14,15,16]

As a result of these experiments it became clear that neuromuscular block could be produced in two ways by neuromuscular blocking drugs either, like curare, by preventing the action of acetylcholine or, like decamethonium, by a depolarising action on the muscle end-plate.

Although recent work has questioned whether either of these activities is the only, or even the principal, cause of the neuromuscular block produced, they remain useful concepts on which to base our classification of the neuromuscular blocking drugs and our understanding of how they may produce their effects.

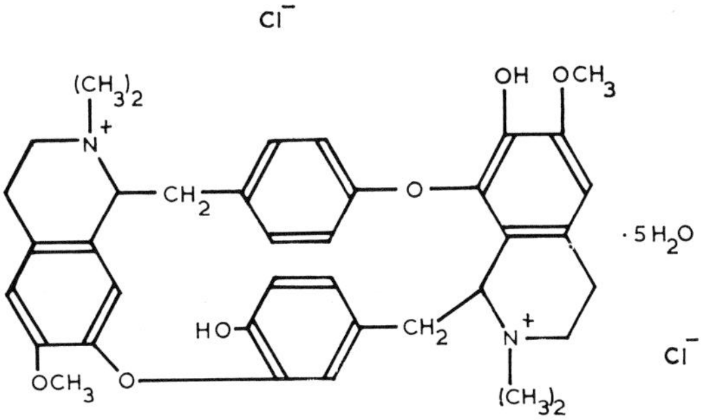


22/Fig. 1.—Structure of tubocurarine chloride (Suggested by King, 1935)

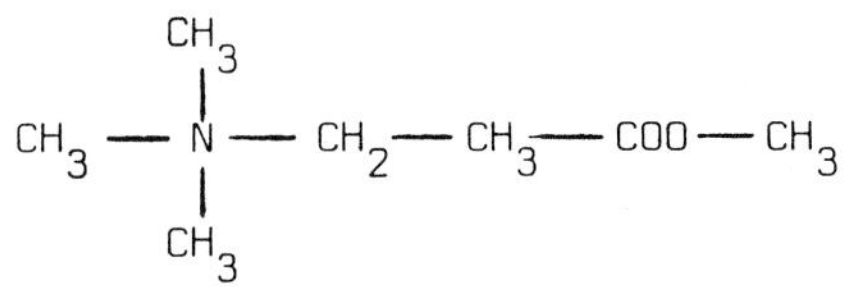


22/Fig. 2.—Acetylcholine

## NEUROMUSCULAR TRANSMISSION AND MUSCLE CONTRACTION

### Anatomy of Neuromuscular Junction

The synapse between the motor nerve and the muscle is termed the neuromuscular junction. As the motor nerve approaches the muscle it splits into many small fibres which innervate the muscle fibres. Muscles that perform fine intricate movements, like those of the hand and the eye, have relatively few muscle fibres innervated by each medullated nerve fibre whilst the postural muscles may have many hundreds of muscle fibres innervated by the same motor nerve fibre. Each of these motor units respond in an "all or none" manner to motor nerve stimulation, hence finely controlled gradation of response can only be achieved in those motor units containing relatively few muscle fibres.

Macroscopically, all the motor nerves pierce

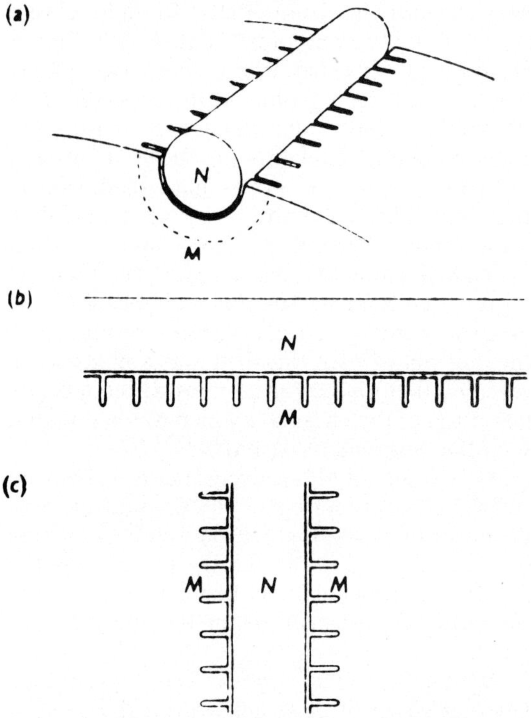


22/FIG. 3*a*.—Diagram of Neuromuscular Junction.
(*a*) Shows a small portion of the terminal axon branch N lying in a gutter formed by the surface of the muscle fibre M. The semicircular post-junctional folds are illustrated.
(*b*) Same in longitudinal section.
(*c*) Same in tangential section.
(Courtesy of Professor Sir Bernard Katz and the Editors of the *Journal of Physiology*)

the muscle epimysium at a point about midway between the origin and insertion, at the "motor point", before breaking up into the neurofibrils which innervate the muscle.

Each neurofibril loses its myelin sheath at the motor point and buries itself in a groove on the muscle fibre (Fig. 3*a* and *b*). However, it is anatomically separated from the muscle fibre by the synaptic cleft. The whole neuromuscular junction is surrounded by membrane which is closely adherent to the nerve, termed the Schwann cell membrane by Birks, Huxley and Katz[17] in their classical studies of the anatomy of this region. It is this membrane that separates the synaptic cleft from the extracellular fluid. More recent studies have elicited the specialised nature of this region in greater detail. The primary longitudinal groove in which the neurofibril lies is deeply furrowed by secondary clefts (Fig. 4*a* and *b*). Around the crest of each of these secondary clefts is a zone rich in cholinesterase.[18] In this cholinesterase-rich area at the orifice to the secondary clefts lie the cholinoreceptors. It is from the functionally discrete areas of the motor nerve directly opposite each of these crests that acetylcholine is discharged into the synaptic cleft.

Nicotinic cholinoreceptors, surrounding the

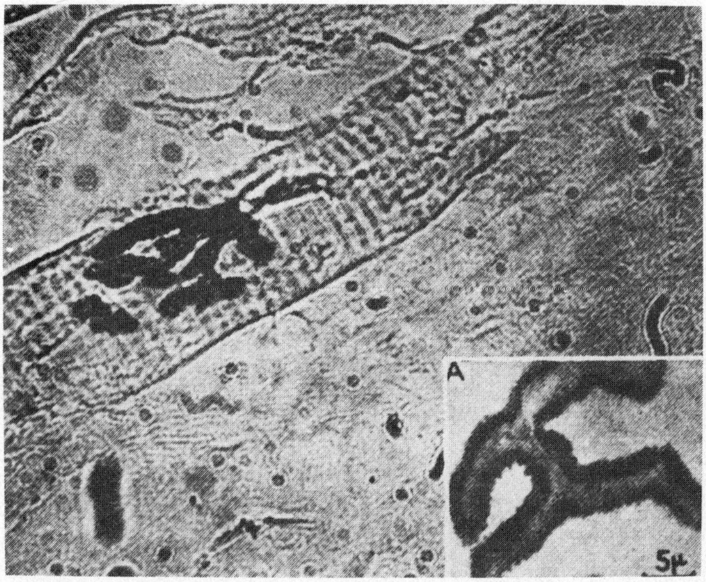


22/FIG. 3*b*.—Autoradiograph of the neuromuscular junction of the mouse showing its dimensions relative to that of the muscle innervated. Insert A is a magnification of the end-plate area. (Courtesy of Drs. Couteaux and Taxi and the editors and publishers of *Arch. Anat. Micros. Morph. Exp.*[48])

entrance to the sodium pore, have been demonstrated by Waser[19] using radioactive decamethonium. They are vulnerable to denervation and the specificity and localisation of the receptors is rapidly lost following section of the motor nerve.[20] There is a constant turnover of receptors—some disappearing whilst new ones develop. Following denervation the rate of new receptor synthesis continues at a slower rate. However, the receptors are not localised to the motor end-plate and become spread over the muscle surface causing denervation sensitivity of the whole muscle surface. New acetylcholine receptors can be produced by implanting a motor nerve under the perimysium and stimulating it so as to bombard the muscle with acetylcholine.

Two principal methods have been used to study the nicotinic receptors. In the method used by Tu[21] and Ceccarelli and Clementi[22] the receptor is labelled with $\alpha$ bungarotoxin and used to produce antibodies to cholinoreceptors of other species. The other method, pioneered by Waser and his co-workers,[19,23] used radioactive labelled drugs to identify and quantify the binding sites for curare-like drugs (Fig. 5) and agonist drugs such as decamethonium. With this method they demonstrated that it required 10–20 times as many molecules of decamethonium relative to curare to produce

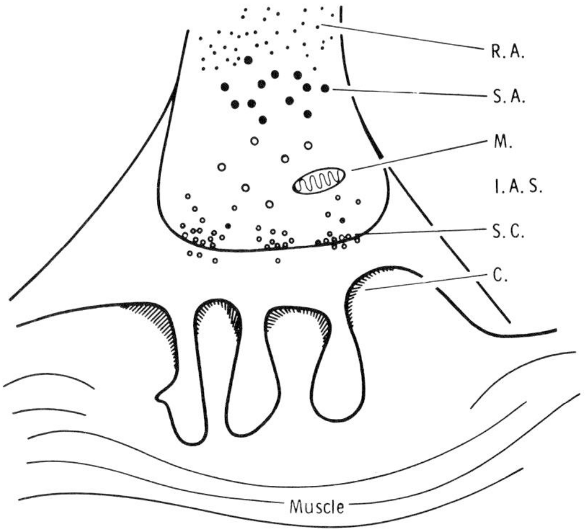


22/Fig. 4*a*.—Schematic representation of the neuromuscular junction.
R.A. = reserve acetylcholine
S.A. = storage acetylcholine
M. = mitochondria
I.A.S. = immediately available source of acetylcholine
S.C. = synaptic cleft
C. = cholinesterase around mouth of 2° cleft

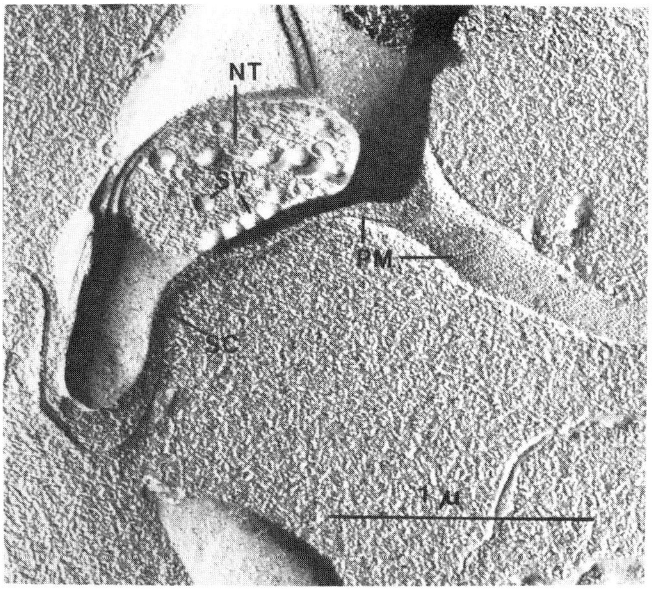


22/Fig. 4*b*.—Torpedo marmorata. Non-stimulated electroplax at 4°C. The synaptic vesicles (SV) are lined up along the synaptic cleft (SC). The post-synaptic membrane (PM) is densely covered with particles getting larger in the vicinity of the nerve terminal (NT). (Courtesy of Professor P. G. Waser and Dr. E. Schoenenberger and their publishers Excerpta Medica.[34])

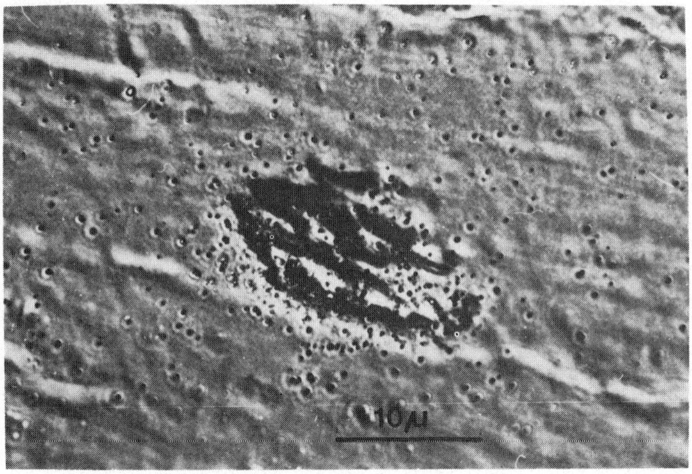


22/Fig. 5.—The distribution of cholinergic receptors at the neuromuscular end-plate of the mouse phrenic nerve diaphragm. Labelled with radioactive toxiferine. (Courtesy of Professor P. G. Waser and Dr. E. Schoenenberger and the publishers Excerpta Medica.[34])

neuromuscular block. This evidence that the receptors for curare-like drugs are separate from those for acetylcholine in the macromolecule of the receptor is supported by the observation that denervation caused a dispersion and loss of decamethonium receptors, whilst the curare receptors remained intact. Waser and associates[23] present a concept in which the curare receptors are associated with the molecules of cholinesterase that guard the mouth of the sodium pore whilst the acetylcholine receptors, where the radioactive decamethonium acts, are distributed immediately around this region (Fig. 6). This is similar to findings of workers using $\alpha$ bungarotoxin.[24] It was suggested by Nachmonsohn[25] that the reaction of acetylcholine with sufficient cholinergic receptors distorts the surface membrane opening the mouths of many sodium pores. This, in turn, allows the change in sodium conductance which is associated with depolarisation. Curare-like drugs act by attaching themselves to the receptors associated with cholinesterase at the mouth of the pore and act like a cork, blocking the sodium pore. Using isolated receptor substance, Patrick and co-workers[26] have demonstrated that conformational changes in the protein occur as the result of exposure to acetylcholine. Recent work by Colquhoun and Sheridan[27] suggests that drugs like gallamine are more active in the presence of a degree of acetylcholine-receptor activity, suggesting that they require some opening of the sodium channel before they bind to receptor sites. This

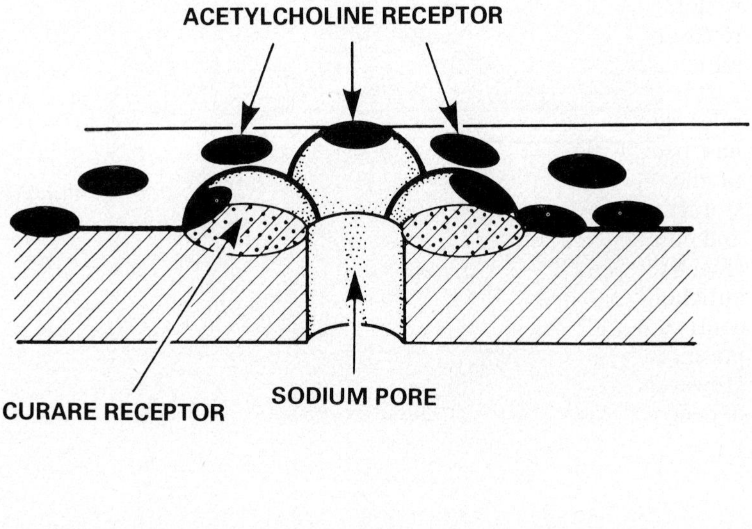


22/Fig. 6.—Cross-section of a sodium pore showing 3 of the 4 curare receptors which lie in close proximity to the mouth of the pore. Note also the surrounding acetylcholine receptors.

suggests that they act deeper in the sodium pore than toxiferine and tubocurare. Drugs which act by blocking the sodium channel itself are termed *channel blockers*. They are generally drug molecules of small size and characteristically the block they produce is greatest when sodium channels are opened by acetylcholine or other agonist drugs.

**Acetylcholine Formation and Release**

Acetylcholine is formed by the acetylation of choline within the nerve by a complex system of enzymes including acetyl CoA and acetyl transferase. The choline is transferred into the nerve from the extracellular fluid (ecf) by an active carrier system. This can be blocked by hemicholinium, which competes for the carrier.[28] Most of the choline comes from released acetylcholine but it is readily supplemented by the synthesis of new choline in the body.

Acetylcholine is "packaged" into vesicles before release from the nerve endings. Each of these vesicles contains between 4 or $5 \times 10^5$ molecules of acetylcholine and their random discharge from the motor nerve causes 1–2 mv depolarisation of the motor end-plate (postsynaptic membrane). This is the magnitude of change that might be caused by opening about 1500 sodium pores, but in order to cause a *propagated* action potential at least 20 to 30 times as many sodium channels must be opened. If 2 quanta are released simultaneously then the depolarisation is approximately doubled. The random leakage of quanta of acetylcholine causes the miniature end-plate potentials—MEPPs (Fig. 7). A study of the normal pattern of MEPPs reveals that the release of acetylcholine follows a random pattern suggesting that it is not restricted by the availability of readily releasable stores of neurotransmitter in healthy patients.

It is now appreciated that the formation and release of acetylcholine is quite complex. It has been suggested that acetylcholine exists in the motor nerve ending in three forms—storage acetylcholine; reserve acetylcholine; and immediately available acetylcholine[29,30] (Fig. 8). Studies in the presence of an anticholinesterase have demonstrated high concentrations of free acetylcholine in the axoplasm, in addition to that found in the vesicles. However, the importance of this finding really depends upon whether it is acetylcholine in transport to the vesicles or whether it is released from vesicles prior to motor activity. Only the immediately available acetylcholine represents acetylcholine that can be released immediately upon motor nerve stimulation. If reserve acetylcholine (which is already packaged in quanta) is not transferred to the immediately available

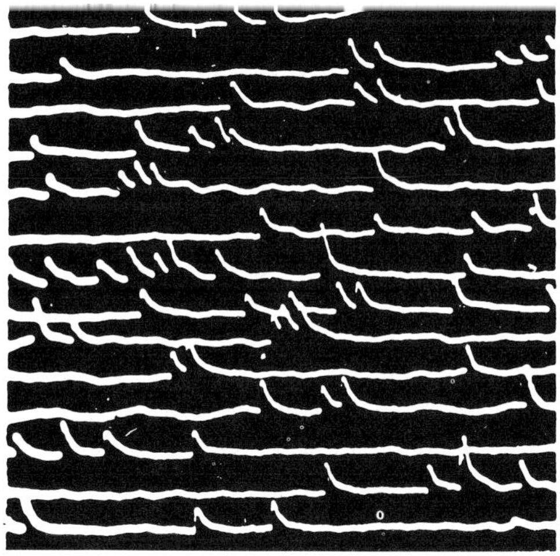

22/Fig. 7.—Miniature end-plate potentials of 1–2 mv occurring at random in a resting end-plate. (Courtesy of Dr. P. Fatt and Sir Bernard Katz, and the Cambridge University Press, publishers of the *Journal of Physiology*.[49])

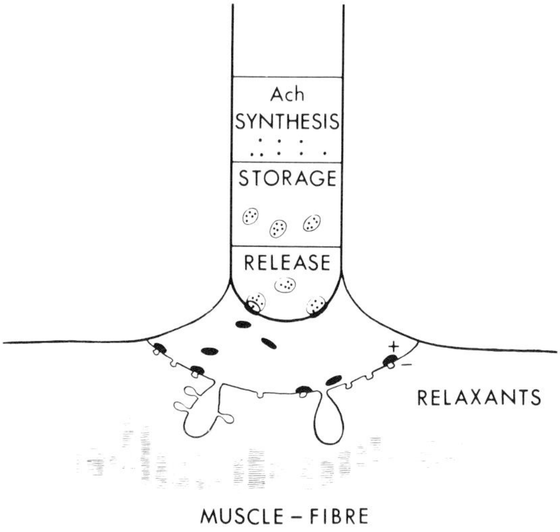


22/Fig. 8.—Diagram to show the three functional compartments at the nerve-ending. Note the packets or quanta of acetylcholine molecules in the storage region and their subsequent rupture on release.

source, then subsequent motor nerve stimulations will produce less and less effect. If the rate at which the transfer from the reserve pool keeps pace with the loss of immediately available acetylcholine, then twitch tension will be maintained. At slow rates of stimulation (between 1 and 10 Hz) the rate of formation of acetylcholine fails to match the loss of immediately available acetylcholine. This is revealed as a fade of successive twitch responses if the post-synaptic junction is partially curarised and in myasthenic patients. It is the basis of the train-of-four response test which, in the presence of residual curarisation, reveals a reduction in the first 4 or 5 twitch responses. It is also found in myasthenic patients when the motor nerve is stimulated at 2 Hz[31,32] (Fig. 9).

At faster rates of stimulation (over 20 Hz) acetylcholine itself reacts with cholinoreceptors on the motor nerve causing a feed-back effect by increasing the rate transfer of acetylcholine from the reserve pool to the immediately available pool.[33] This explains the *post-tetanic facilitation* found in curarised muscle as the increased formation of available acetylcholine produced during tetanic stimulation "overshoots" and causes the first few post-tetanic stimuli to a greater than normal outpouring of neurotransmitter.

With increasing attention upon possible pre-synaptic (motor nerve) sites of action of many drugs (previously thought to act only at the post-synaptic region) and the demonstration that drugs and physical effects, such as cold and nutritional states, can affect the rate of mobilisation and release of acetylcholine, details of this complex chain of events are assuming great importance.

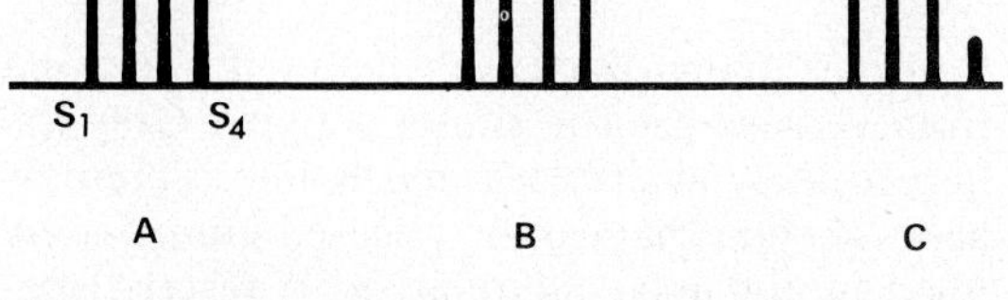

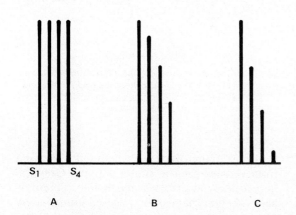


22/Fig. 9.—Train-of-four stimuli at 2 Hz. A—control; B—5 mg tubocurarine; C—12 mg tubocurarine.

Acetylcholine release is achieved by depolarisation of the motor nerve. This opens up channels in the presynaptic membrane through which calcium ions will pass. The essential role of calcium in this process is demonstrated by the inhibition of acetylcholine release that occurs in the absence of calcium from the extracellular fluid and by the presence of magnesium. Substances known to promote calcium transport across membranes, such as 4-amino pyridine, digitalis glycosides and guanidine, accelerate the rate of acetylcholine release, as does $\alpha$-adrenergic stimulation and phosphodiesterase inhibitors such as aminophylline. $\beta$-adrenergic drugs accelerate acetylcholine synthesis, possibly by activation of cyclic AMP, but do not affect the release process. It is possible that the cyclic AMP produces the energy necessary to concentrate acetylcholine in the vesicles.

What determines the precise locus of discharge is not obvious from electromicroscopy studies but the constancy of the position of discharge and its proximity to the receptor substance has been elegantly demonstrated using labelled acetylcholine.[34] High-resolution microscopy reveals a lattice in the presynaptic region within which the vesicles are released into the synaptic cleft.

### Hydrolysis of Acetylcholine

Acetylcholine is normally hydrolysed by cholinesterase at the post-synaptic membrane in a fraction of a millisecond. Of all the molecules of acetylcholine released the majority will be hydrolysed to choline which is then available for re-uptake by the motor nerve and re-synthesis to acetylcholine. It has been calculated that about half of the choline used in the synthesis of acetylcholine comes from this source. Some of the acetylcholine diffuses away from the receptor site to be hydrolysed in the bloodstream.

## THE PHYSIOLOGY OF NEUROMUSCULAR TRANSMISSION

### The Membrane Potential and Depolarisation

At rest there is a potential difference of about 90 mv across the post-synaptic membrane. This constitutes the resting membrane potential. This electro-motive force (emf) is the result of an excess of positively charged ions outside the cell relative to inside the cell. This uneven distribution of charged ions is principally due to the ease with which potassium ions permeate the membrane relative to sodium, so long as the sodium pores are closed. Because of the membrane's permeability to potassium ions, they will tend to pass out of the cell along their concentration gradient in the resting state (150 mmol inside the cell to about 5 mmol outside). As sodium cannot easily move in the opposite direction to counter this effect, there eventually will be an excess of positively charged ions outside the cell. When this occurs, and the electrostatic charge on the outside of the cell reaches a level at which it will inhibit the further migration of positively charged potassium ions—at this point equilibrium occurs, as the electrostatic force will balance the effect of the potassium concentrate gradient. It therefore follows that in the resting state the most important factor controlling the magnitude of the transmembrane potential is the potassium gradient across the cell membrane. This is explicit in the Gibbs Donnan law. For this reason changes in this potassium balance between the intracellular and extracellular concentrations cause alterations in the resting membrane potential as:

$$\text{emf} \propto \frac{[K^+]\text{ inside cell}}{[K^+]\text{ outside cell}}$$

As a result, a fall of extracellular potassium unaccompanied by a similar proportionate change in intracellular potassium will increase the transmembrane potential making it more difficult for acetylcholine to produce depolarisation. Because of this it will potentiate non-depolarising drugs. However, if both intracellular and extracellular potassium fall by a similar proportion, as commonly happens in chronic potassium depletion, such as accompanies ulcerative colitis, then the $K^+\text{I}/K^+\text{o}$ ratio will remain unchanged and the sensitivity to acetylcholine will be unaltered. However, in states of chronic potassium depletion relatively small shifts of potassium from inside to outside the cell (such as might occur with the administration of suxamethonium) could cause larger than usual changes in the resting membrane potential. As it is difficult to measure intracellular (or total body) potassium it is prudent to perform an ECG if the extracellular potassium is abnormal. Gross alterations in the transmembrane potential will usually be reflected in the ST segment of the ECG (see Chapter 12, p. 422).

When acetylcholine reacts with the post-synaptic receptors it produces an increase in sodium conductance by opening the sodium channels. For the 1–1·5 milliseconds during which the sodium pore is open about 12,000 cations enter the cell along the concentration and electrostatic gradient. As a result of this change in sodium conductance the transmembrane potential falls from −90 mV to zero, or +10 mV. This magnitude of change in the polarity of the membrane will normally trigger off a propagated action potential in the muscle fibre, causing muscle contraction to take place.

Towards the end of depolarisation $K^+$ conductance increases as $Na^+$ conductance falls back to its resting level and the excess of intracellular sodium is expelled by means of the sodium pump mechanism.

In 1953, Jenerick and Gerard[35] demonstrated that if the transmembrane potential was artificially reduced by a voltage clamp from −90 to −57 mV then the end-plate became refractory to acetylcholine propagated action potentials. This depolarisation is the basis of the type of block that is produced by suxamethonium and decamethonium[15,36] namely—a *depolarisation block*.

However, although depolarisation of this magnitude may occur when these agents are used it is now thought to be only a part of the cause of the neuromuscular block they produce.

### Margin of Safety

Most physiological processes in the body enjoy a large margin of safety against potential failure. This has also been found to occur in neuromuscular transmission. Although the synapse between the nerve and the muscle is the most vulnerable link in the initiation of muscle contraction, nevertheless it has been demonstrated that at least 70 per cent of the function has to be lost before neuromuscular failure occurs and that about 80 per cent of the activity has to be blocked by neuromuscular blocking drugs before the twitch response is affected[37, 38] (Fig. 10).

This finding is of great importance to anaesthetists for it implies that if one monitors neuromuscular block using the indirectly elected twitch response one cannot detect a block of less than 80 per cent of the receptors. If a tetanic stimulus is used then lesser degrees of receptor occupancy can be detected, but within the physiological range of tetanic activity 60 per cent or more receptor occupancy is necessary before this response is affected.[39]

### Sensitivity and Resistance

One can regard neuromuscular sensitivity as representing a shift in this response. Thus if the twitch response is depressed in the presence of only 50 per cent receptor occupancy then *sensitivity* to curare-like drugs will be present. This might be caused by potassium imbalance, decreased acetylcholine release or a myasthenic state. Conversely, if it required an even greater degree of receptor occupancy to reduce the twitch response then the patient would appear *resistant* to curare-like drugs.

## MUSCLE CONTRACTION

The process of muscle contraction starts by activation of the motor neurone in the spinal cord and then proceeds by rapid conduction of an action potential down the motor nerve by virtue of saltatory conduction. This wave of activity crosses the myoneural synapse with the assistance of the neurotransmitter acetylcholine. At the post-synaptic site it will cause depolarisation of the membrane causing the release of calcium, the excitation of the actin-myosin fibrils, and produce the muscle contraction essential for a life that is independent of its natural environment.

### Anatomy

The myofibrils that make up a muscle fibre are composed of sarcomeres. Each sarcomere contains thick and thin filaments alternating with each other (Fig. 11). The thick filaments are composed of myosin molecules each of which consists of a shaft from which "head" units are hinged (Fig. 12). The head units lie at an angle lateral to the shaft and extend from all surfaces of the main shaft of the thick filament. The direction of these head units

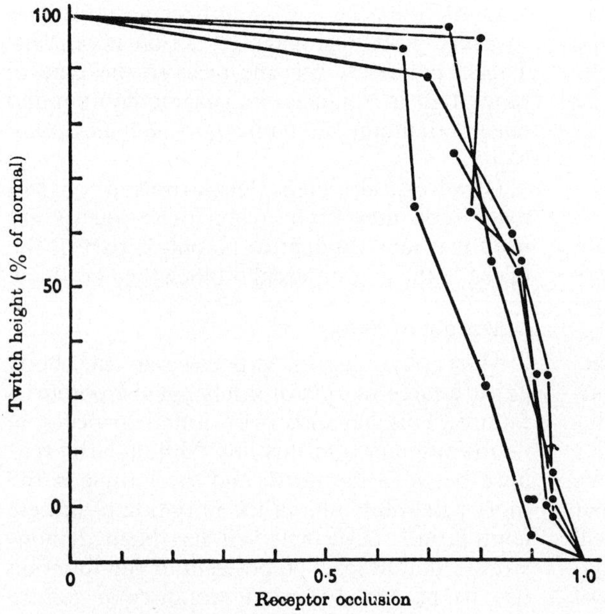


22/FIG. 10.—Receptor occupancy required to produce depression of twitch height. There is no depression of twitch response until over 70 per cent (0·7) receptors are occupied by curare. (Courtesy of Professor W. D. M. Paton and Dr. D. R. Waud (1967), and Cambridge University Press[38])

depends upon which end of the thick unit they lie.

The thin actin filaments, which interdigitate with the thick myosin filaments, spread out laterally from the central "Z line" and give striated muscle its striped appearance. The thin filaments are largely composed of two actin chains entwined in a double helix arrangement. Other protein elements, especially tropin and tropomysin are also found at regular intervals along the actin chain.[40]

The actin and myosin compose the contractile elements of muscle and they are controlled through the filament activation sites. These occur at regular intervals where the lateral heads of the myosin touch the actin helix.

The regulation of actin and myosin activity depends upon the sarcoplasmic reticulum. This is in the form of a complex tubule system composed of 3 main elements, the transverse tubules, the lateral cisterns and the longitudinal reticulum (Fig. 13*a* and *b*). The transverse tubules are contiguous with the surface membrane of the muscle fibre and penetrate and ramify deep into the muscle fibre from the surface. Although they do not directly open into the cisterns of the sarcoplasmic reticulum, they abut on to them. The lateral cisterns are themselves connected with each other by the longitudinal reticulum.

Each striated muscle fibre is composed of several hundred or more myofibrils containing actin and myosin chains and surrounded by the sarcoplasmic reticulum system, the whole being contained by the outer membrane—the sarcolemma.

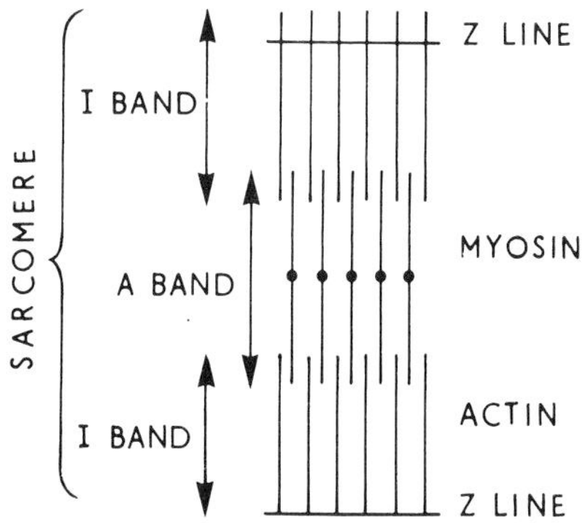


22/FIG. 11.—Diagram of a sarcomere showing the actin of the I band and the myosin of the A band.

**Activation of Contraction**

When a propagated action potential spreads over the surface of muscle fibre excitation, contraction coupling will occur. The electrical activity spreads out from the motor end-plate and down the open ends of the transverse tubules which are dispersed around the muscle fibre surface.[41] The depolarisation current produces its effect in the lateral cisterns adjacent to the tubules causing the sarcoplasmic reticulum to release calcium into the myofibril. In the resting state the sarcoplasmic reticulum sequestrates calcium, reducing the concentration in the myofibrils to sub-threshold levels. The passage of the depolarising potential into the transverse tubules and the subsequent release of this stored calcium activates muscle contraction.

The increased calcium concentration causes an interaction between the lateral heads of the

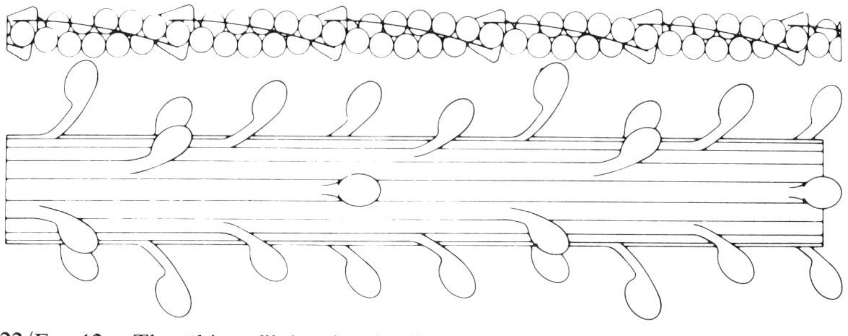

22/FIG. 12.—The "hinged" head units lie at angles to the myosin molecule and make contact with specific zones of the actin molecule. (With kind permission of Dr. G. Hooper and Eaton Laboratories.)

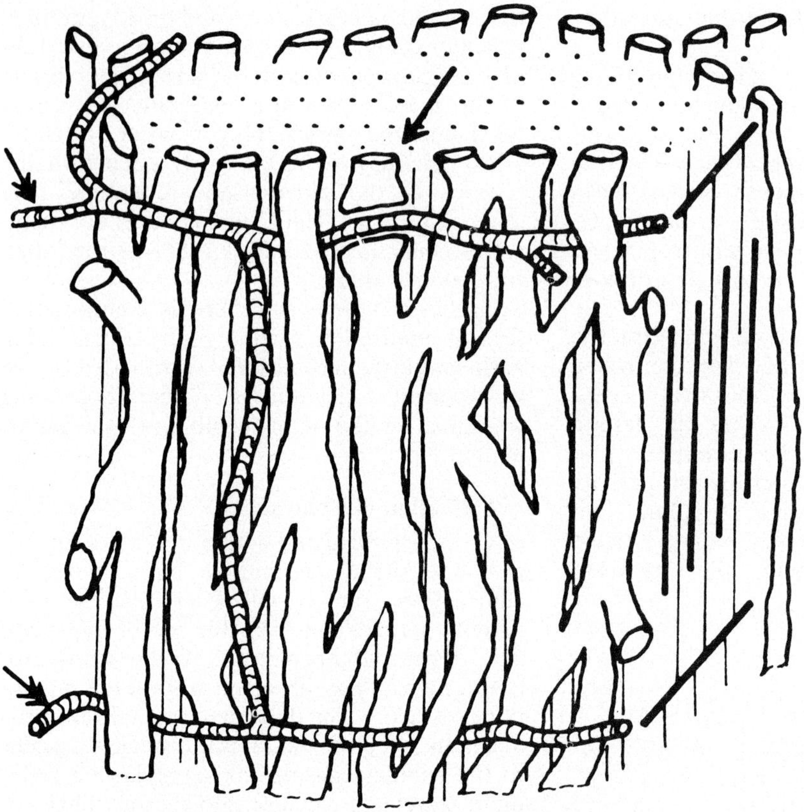

22/FIG. 13(*a*).—The sarcoplasmic reticulum of the myofibrils showing the transverse tubules (double arrow-head) and longitudinal reticulum (single arrow-head). (Courtesy of Dr. S. Page and the Editor of the *British Medical Bulletin*[50])

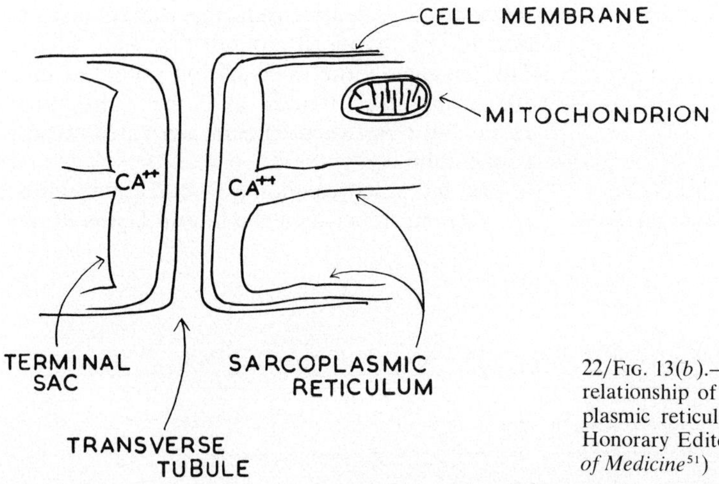


22/FIG. 13(*b*).—Diagram of muscle cell system showing relationship of terminal sac, transverse tubule and sarcoplasmic reticulum. (Courtesy of Dr. P. Furniss and the Honorary Editors of the *Proceedings of the Royal Society of Medicine*[51])

thick myosin filaments and the thin actin filaments with which they interdigitate. The protein molecules tropin and tropomyosin determine the actual sites of interaction. As a result of this action the thin filaments slide inwards over the thick filaments as the lateral heads of the myosin molecules pull on the thin actin filaments, causing a shortening of the muscle. If the muscle is stretched before contraction then there will be greater pull on the actin molecules and increased contraction results. The energy for this activity comes from the breakdown of ATP to ADP, a process encouraged by a local rise in calcium concentration.

If, however, the stretch is excessive then the actin molecules may be too far displaced from the lateral heads of the myosin to make contraction possible, as the linkage between the side heads of the myosin and the tropin on the actin filaments is disrupted. At this degree of stretch muscle contractibility fails.

To translate this action into muscular activity one has to bear in mind the basic all or none nature of the process. Each muscle fibre, indeed each motor unit, is only capable of one active contraction. To obtain gradation of muscle contraction requires a greater or lesser number of motor units to contract. To obtain altered speed of reaction one has to have changes in the rate of stimulation. This is, to some extent, determined by the nature of the motor neurone and muscle fibre since it has been demonstrated that some are intrinsically fast and others slow reactors. The slow twitch reactors have a longer lasting response, a greater resistance to fatigue and are metabolically more efficient. This is largely due to the nature of the myosin elements. This type of muscle fibre predominates in postural muscle.[42]

## INTERNUNCIAL NEURONE SYSTEM

The internuncial neurones are situated in the spinal cord between the anterior and posterior horns of the grey matter. Their function appears to be the co-ordination of impulses reaching the cord from many sources. This function allows the relaxation of one group of muscles when an opposing muscle group contracts during reflex and evoked activity. Thus they have connections with both sensory and motor fibres but are primarily influenced by impulses from the cerebellum. The role of the internuncial neurone system has been likened to a telephone exchange in that it relays impulses from various sources to the appropriate cell station. A single muscle movement can no longer be regarded merely as an impulse arising in the motor cortex and passing down the appropriate pathway via the anterior horn cell in the spinal cord to the muscle fibre. The muscles themselves have a complex system of signalling the degree of their contraction (see below) and the internuncial neurones play a role in regulating this movement and passing impulses to antagonistic muscles.

Clinically, the importance of the internuncial neurone system has increased since it has been found that certain drugs—notably mephenesin, diazepam and phenothiazines—can reduce or interrupt their activity and so lead to alterations in muscle tone. Nevertheless, the side-effects of mephenesin have made it unsuitable as an agent for producing muscular relaxation in clinical anaesthesia. Other members of the "tranquillising" series of drugs have been found to alter internuncial fibre activity and large doses of chlorpromazine and diazepam have been found to be effective, but their clinical value in this respect is largely limited to the treatment of tetanus.

### Muscle Spindles and the Small Fibre System

The motor pathway from the anterior horn cell down to the neuromuscular junction on the skeletal muscle fibre is now familiar to all (Fig. 14). Conduction along this route is rapid as the size of the fibre ($\alpha$ efferent) is large, i.e. 14 $\mu$m in diameter. Closer scrutiny of this nerve fibre reveals that besides these large fibres there are smaller ones—$\gamma$ efferent fibres measuring some 4 $\mu$m in diameter—which when traced peripherally are found to end in a special structure—the *muscle spindle* (Fig. 15).

The simple act of picking up a pencil from a table not only employs the motor pathway, but afferents reach the spinal cord from the sensory endings in the skin, joints and muscles. In fact, the muscle spindles are the sensory end-organ of the skeletal muscles and are responsible for signalling the degree of shortening of the whole muscle. In this way they can provide information so that only the exact amount of muscle activity required for the task is used. Histologically, the muscle spindle is an elongated and encapsulated structure which lies in parallel with the skeletal muscle fibres and shares its attachment. This latter point is of particular importance as its principal function is to signal the exact length of the skeletal fibre. Within the capsule small specialised (*intrafusal*) fibres can be recognised—the *nuclear bag* fibre and the *nuclear chain* fibre (Fig. 16*a* and *b*). Because the muscle spindle receives a motor innervation from the small efferent nerve fibres, contraction of the intrafusal fibres of the spindles sends a

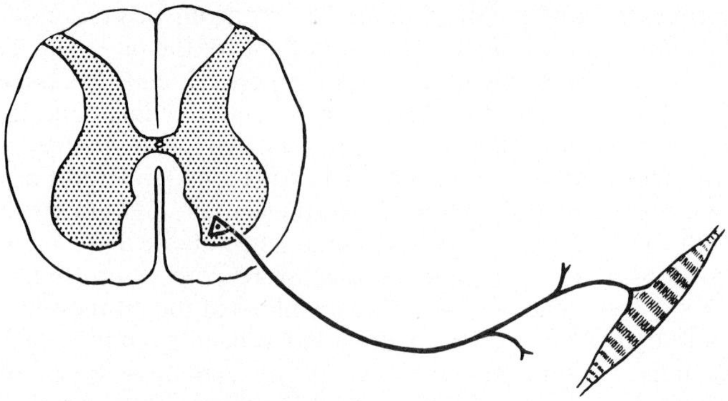

22/FIG. 14.—The motor pathway from the anterior horn cell to the neuromuscular junction.

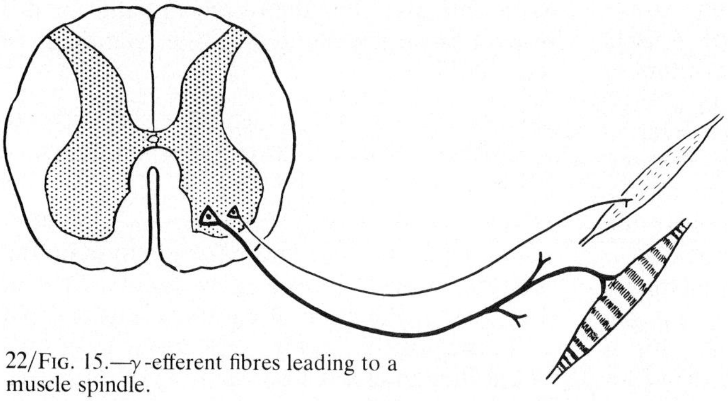

22/FIG. 15.—$\gamma$-efferent fibres leading to a muscle spindle.

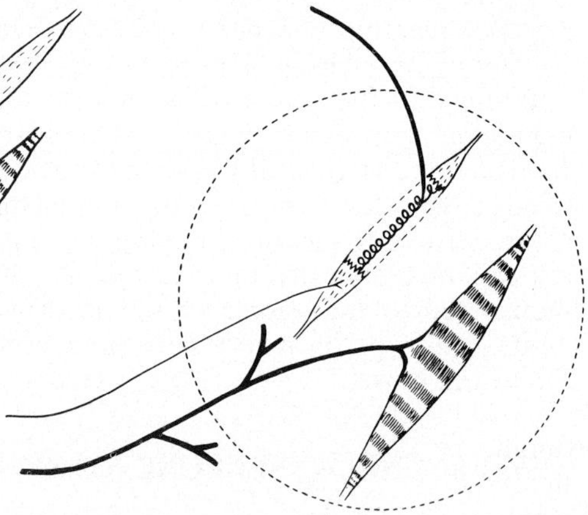

22/FIG. 16(*a*).—Intrafusal fibres.

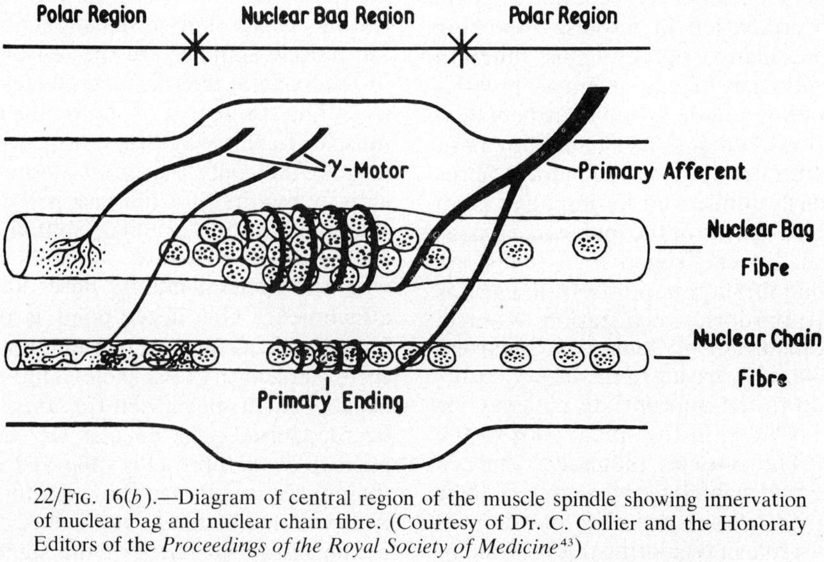


22/FIG. 16(*b*).—Diagram of central region of the muscle spindle showing innervation of nuclear bag and nuclear chain fibre. (Courtesy of Dr. C. Collier and the Honorary Editors of the *Proceedings of the Royal Society of Medicine*[43])

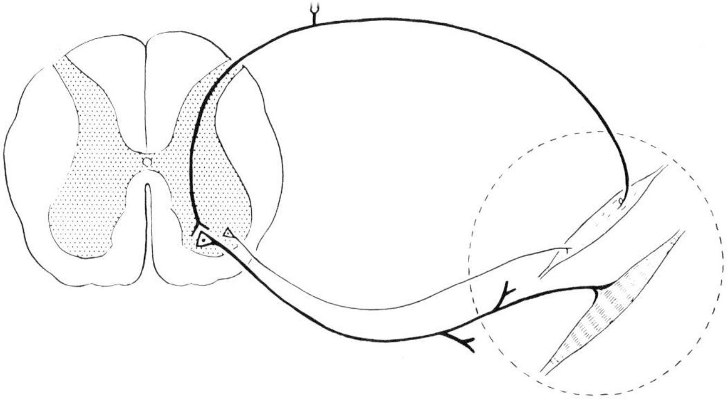

22/Fig. 17.—Connections of the muscle spindle.

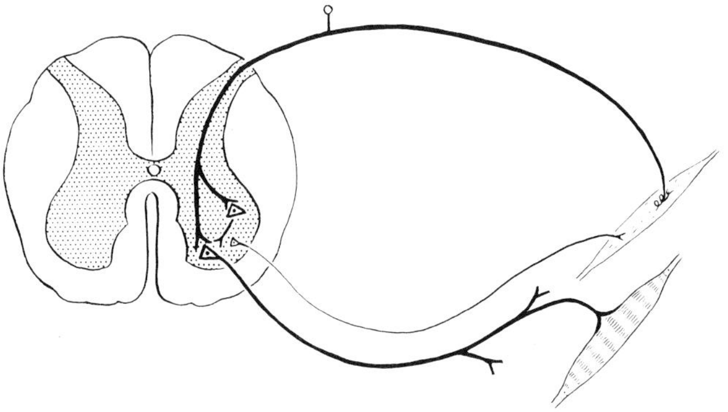

22/Fig. 18.—Small nerve fibre system.

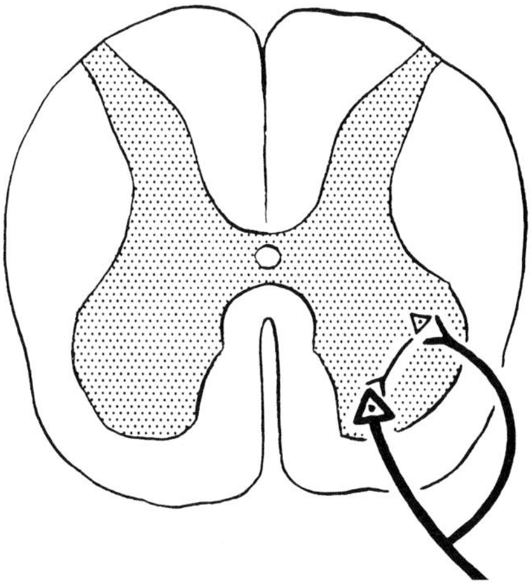

22/Fig. 19.—Renshaw cell.

stimulus back to the spinal cord along the large afferent sensory fibre. This fibre enters the spinal cord through the dorsal root and then traverses the grey matter, finally to synapse with the anterior horn cell of the corresponding muscle fibre (Fig. 17), or through an interneurone it may affect a motor nerve at a different spinal level (Fig. 18).

The small fibre system, therefore, consists of the gamma efferent fibre, the muscle spindle, and the large afferent fibre synapsing with the anterior horn cell of the motor unit. A servo-loop or feed-back mechanism is thus created which can either enhance or dampen the contraction of skeletal muscle according to the nature of the stimulus received.

Yet another feed-back loop has been described by Renshaw.[44] As the main motor nerve fibre courses through the white matter of the spinal cord a branch loops backwards to synapse with a cell in the anterior horn (Renshaw cell), and in turn this communicates with the large anterior horn cell again (Fig. 19).

Clinically the small fibre system has three important functions in relation to muscle activity:

(a) *Volitional effort* by modulating and damping the response of muscles to motor nerve activity results in a gradual regulation of muscle changes in muscle activity necessary for co-ordinated movements. The action of the various muscle relaxants on muscle spindle activity is difficult to study but the available evidence suggests that the interference with activity occurs simultaneously at both the intrafusal fibre of the muscle spindle and the neuromuscular junction. As a result there will be a loss of muscle tone, a loss of ability accurately to control volitional movements and a decrease in the nervous input into the reticular activating system and hence an indirect effect upon the brain.

Rack and Westbury[45] have shown that prolonged tetanic stimulation of the fibres of the muscle spindle in the cat can lead to damage to the mechanism (Fig. 16*b*). Both acetylcholine and suxamethonium are known to stimulate the motor and sensory nerve-endings on the muscle spindle. Collier[43] has suggested that the muscle pains of suxamethonium could be due to damage to the delicate muscle-spindle fibre rather than the tougher skeletal muscle fibre.

(b) *Reflex activity*.—The tone of the muscle spindles in resting muscle will set the level of stimulation required to produce a reflex response. This is demonstrated by the reinforcing effect of clasping the fingers upon the knee jerk reflex.[46]

(c) *Resting muscle-tone*.—Buller[47] has described muscle tone as the level of activity of the small fibre system. Increased muscle spindle activity is associated with a greater muscle tone.

## REFERENCES


1. Fontana, F. (1745). Memoire: sur le poison Americain appeler Ticunas et sur quelques autres poisons vegetaux. *Mem. de l'Acad. R. des Sciences*, p. 490.
2. Brodie, B. C. (1811). Experiments and observations on the different modes in which death is produced by certain vegetable poisons. *Phils. Trans. R. Soc. London*, 194.
3. Brodie, B. C. (1812). Further experiments with South American arrow poisons. *Phils. Trans. R. Soc. London*, 205.
4. Bernard, C. (1856). Leçons sur les effects des substances toxique et medicamentenses. English translation in *Survey of Anesthesiology*, 1961. Baltimore: Williams and Wilkins.
5. Dale, H. H. and Feldberg, W. (1934). Chemical transmission of the effects of nerve impulses. *Brit. med. J.*, **1**, 835.
6. Dale, H. H., Feldberg, W. and Vogt, M. (1936). Release of acetylcholine at voluntary motor nerve endings. *J. Physiol.* (*Lond.*), **86**, 353.
7. Eccles, J. C., Katz, B. and Kuffler, S. W. (1941). Nature of the end plate potential in curarised muscle. *J. Neurophysiol.*, **4**, 362.
8. Gill, R. (1940). *White Water and Black Magic*. New York: Henry Holt & Co.
9. McIntyre, A. R. (1959). Historical background. Early use and development of the muscle relaxants. *Anesthesiology*, **20**, 419.
10. Griffith, H. R. and Johnson, G. E. (1942). The use of curare in general anesthesia. *Anesthesiology*, **3**, 418.
11. King, H. (1935). Curare alkaloids. 1. Tubocurarine. *J. Chem. Soc.*, 1381.
12. Paton, W. D. M. and Zaimis, E. J. (1949). The pharmacological actions of the polymethylene bis methyl ammonium salts. *Brit. J. Pharmacol. & Chemother.* **4**, 381.
13. Zaimis, E. (1953). Motor end plate differences as a determining factor in the mode of action of neuromuscular blocking substances. *J. Physiol* (*Lond.*), **122**, 238.
14. Burns, B. D. and Paton, W. D. M. (1951). Depolarisation of the motor end-plate by decamethonium and acetylcholine. *J. Physiol.* (*Lond.*), **115**, 4.
15. del Castillo, J. and Katz, B. (1956). Interaction at the end plate receptors between different choline derivatives. *Proc. R. Soc. Lond.* (*Biol.*), **146**, 369.
16. Gissen, A. J. and Nastuk, W. L. (1970). Succinylcholine and decamethonium: comparison of depolarisation and desensitisation. *Anesthesiology*, **33**, 611.
17. Birks, R., Huxley, H. E. and Katz, B. (1960). The fine structure of the neuromuscular junction of the frog. *J. Physiol.* (*Lond.*), **150**, 134.
18. Davis, R. and Koelle, G. B. (1967). Electron microscopic localisation of acetylcholinesterase and non-specific cholinesterase at the neuromuscular junction by gold triocholine and gold thioactetic acid methods. *J. Cell. Biol.*, **34**, 157.
19. Waser, P. G. (1970). On receptors in the postsynaptic membrane of the motor endplate. *Ciba Foundation Symposium on Molecular Properties of Drug Receptors*, p. 59. Ed. Porter, R. and O'Connor, M. London: J. & A. Churchill.
20. Rohr-Hadorn, I. (1961). Beziehungen zwischen cholinergeschem und Acetylcholinesterase der Endplatte unter sucht wahrend der degeneration and regeneration des House Swerchfelles. *Helv. Physiol. Pharmacol. Acta*, **19**, 119.
21. Tu, A. T. (1977). Binding of neurotoxins to acetylcholine receptors. In: *Venous Chemistry and Molecular Biology*, Chap. 17, p. 240. New York: Wiley.
22. Ceccarelli, B. and Clementi, F. (Eds. (1979). Neurotoxins acting at post-synaptic sites. In: *Advances in Cytopharmacology*, Vol. 3, p. 141. New York: Raven Press.
23. Waser, P. G., Hofmann, A., Schaub, M. C., Hopff, W., Karis, J. H., Rosen, G. and Chang, A. (1972). Affinity labelling of cholinergic receptors with curarizing and depolarizing drugs. In: *Pharmacology Congress Reports* (San Francisco). Basel: Karger.
24. Rash, J. E., Hudson, C. S. and Ellisman, H. H. (1978). Ultrastructures of acetylcholine receptors at the mammalian neuromuscular junction. In: *Cell Membrane*

*Receptors for Drugs and Hormones*, p. 47. Eds. Straub and Bolis. New York: Raven Press.
25. Nachmonsohn, R. (1959). *Chemical and Molecular Basis of Nerve Activity*. New York: Academic Press.
26. Patrick, J., Valeur, B., Monneric, L. and Changeux, J. P. (1971). Changes in extrinsic fluorescence intensity of the electropax membrane during electrical excitation. *J. Mem. Biol.*, **5**, 102.
27. Colquhoun, D. and Sheridan, R. E. (1979). Modes of action of gallamine at the neuromuscular junction. *Brit. J. Pharmacol.*, **66**, 79.
28. Potter, L. T. (1968). Uptake of choline by nerve endings isolated from the rat cerebral cortex. In: *The Interaction of Drugs and Subcellular Components of Animal Cells*. Ed. Campbell. London: Churchill Livingstone.
29. Hebb, C. O. (1963). Formation, storage and liberation of acetylcholine. In: *Handbook of Pharmacological Experiments: Cholinesterase and Anticholinesterase*, p. 55. Ed. Eichler Farah and Koelle. Berlin: Springer.
30. Elmquist, D. and Quastel, D. M. J. (1965). A quantitative study of end-plate potentials in isolated human muscle. *Acta. Neurol. Scand.*, **45**, 257.
31. Ali, H. H., Utting, J. E. and Gray, G. T. (1971). Quantitative assessment of residual block (Part II). *Brit. J. Anaesth.*, **43**, 478.
32. Ali, H. H., Wilson, R. S., Savarese, J. J. and Kitz, R. J. (1975). The effect of tubocurarine on indirectly elicited train-of-four response and respiratory measurements in humans. *Brit. J. Anaesth.*, **47**, 570.
33. Bowman, W. C. and Webb, S. N. (1976). Tetanic fade during partial transmission failure produced by non-depolarising neuromuscular blocking drugs in the cat. *Clin. Exp. Pharmacol. Physiol.*, **3**, 545.
34. Waser, P. G. and Schoenberger, E. (1980). The structure and physiology of the cholinergic synapse. In: *Curares and Curarisation Proceedings XI*, p. 7. (International Meeting of Anesthesiology and Resuscitation, Paris.)
35. Jenerick, H. P. and Gerard, R. W. (1953). Membrane potential and threshold of single muscle fibre. *J. Cell Comp. Physiol.*, **42**, 79.
36. Jenden, D. J. (1955). The effect of drugs upon neuromuscular transmission in the guinea pig diaphragm. *J. Pharmacol. Exp. Ther.*, **114**, 3.
37. Waser, P. G. (1967). Receptor localisation by autoradiographic techniques. *Ann. N. Y. Acad. Sci.*, **144**, 737.
38. Paton, W. D. M. and Waud, D. R. (1967). The margin of safety of neuromuscular transmission. *J. Physiol. (Lond.)*, **191**, 59.
39. Waud, B. E. and Waud, D. R. (1971). The relation between tetanic fade and receptor occlusion in the presence of competitive neuromuscular block. *Anesthesiology*, **35**, 456.
40. Ebashi, S. and Endo, M. (1968). Calcium ion and muscle contraction. *Prog. Biophys. Chem.*, **18**, 125.
41. Adrian, R. N. (1969). Radial spread of contraction in frog muscle fibres. *J. Physiol. (Lond.)*., **204**, 231.
42. Buller, A. J., Eccles, J. C. and Eccles, R. M. (1960). Interactions between motoneurones and muscle in respect of their responses. *J. Physiol. (Lond.)*, **150**, 417.
43. Collier, C. (1975). Suxamethonium pains and fasciculations. *Proc. roy. Soc. Med.*, **68**, 105.
44. Renshaw, B. (1941). Influence of discharge of motoneurones upon excitation of neighboring motoneurones. *J. Neurophysiol.*, **4**, 167.
45. Rack, P. M. H. and Westbury, D. R. (1966). The effects of suxamethonium and acetylcholine on the behaviour of cat muscle spindles during dynamic stretching, and during fusimotor stimulation. *J. Physiol. (Lond.)*, **186**, 698.
46. Buller, A. J. and Dornhorst, A. C. (1957). Reinforcement of tendon reflexes. *Lancet*, **2**, 1261.
47. Buller, A. J. (1956). Muscle tone. *Physiotherapy*, **42**, 203.
48. Couteaux, R. and Taxi, J. (1952). Reserches histoetemiques sur la distribution des activitees cholinesterasiques au niveau de la synapse myoneurale. *Arch. Anat. micr. Morph. exp.*, **41**, 352.
49. Fatt, P. and Katz, B. (1952). Spontaneous subthreshold activity at motor nerve endings. *J. Physiol.*, **117**, 109.
50. Page, S. (1968). Structure of the sarcoplasmic reticulum in vertebrate muscle. *Brit. med. Bull*, **24**, 170.
51. Furniss, P. (1971). The etiology of malignant hyperpyrexia. *Proc. roy. Soc. Med.*, **64**, 216.

## FURTHER READING

Bowman, W. C. (1980). *Pharmacology of Neuromuscular Transmission*, Bristol: Wright.
Buller, A. J. (1981). Muscle Contraction. In: *Scientific Foundations of Anaesthesia*. Ed. Scurr and Feldman. London: Heinemann Med.
Feldman, S. A. (1979). *Muscle Relaxants*. Philadelphia: W. B. Saunders.

CHAPTER 23

# Neuromuscular Blocking Drugs



The observation of Buttle and Zaimis[1] that members of the bis-quaternary ammonium series of neuromuscular blocking agents caused opisthotonus and spasticity when injected into chicks whilst curare-like drugs caused a flaccid paralysis, confirmed that the new drugs produced a different type of block at the neuromuscular junction. This effect can also be verified by the action of these drugs *in vitro* on the cervical muscle of the chick. In addition, when studying the effect of the long-chain polymethylene series, a third phenomena was demonstrated—the occurrence initially of spastic paralysis followed by the development of flaccidity.

These three types of neuromuscular response correlate with depolarising block, non-depolarising block and Phase II or "dual" block (mixed block).

## NON-DEPOLARISATION BLOCK

### Pharmacodynamics of Non-depolarising Neuromuscular Block

The similarity between the parts of the structural formula of curare and that of the neurotransmitter acetylcholine, originally led to the "key in the lock" concept whereby the antagonist was envisaged as fitting into the receptor substance, preventing the access of acetylcholine.

The kinetic theory of action proposed in the competition theory envisaged the antagonist drug competing with acetylcholine for receptor sites (Fig. 1). This imposed a time course on the reaction

$$D + R \underset{K_2}{\overset{K_1}{\rightleftharpoons}} DR$$

$K_1$ = association rate
$K_2$ = dissociation rate

in which the rate of dissociation $K_2$ relative to the rate of association $K_1$ was termed the affinity constant. The classical means of studying this constant has in the past been by *in vitro* experiments where the log of the dose of agonist (usually carbachol) necessary to produce a progressive reversal of antagonist block has been plotted in the presence of increasing doses of non-depolarising blocker. This produces a series of parallel log dose-response curves from which the affinity, i.e. the amount of agonist required to neutralise the effect of given dose of antagonist, is calculated.

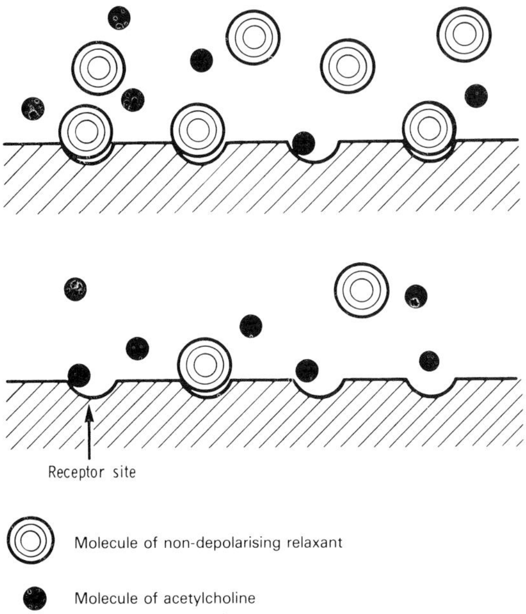


23/FIG. 1.—Competition theory of muscle relaxant action. *Upper figure:* the relatively high concentration of drug causes substantial receptor occupancy. *Lower figure:* as the concentration of drug falls, the receptors become available to acetylcholine. (With kind permission of Dr. S. A. Feldman and the publishers of *Muscle Relaxants*, W. B. Saunders.[2])

As long ago as 1959 Dermot Taylor[3] suggested that this was probably an inappropriate way of explaining the interaction of a drug as stable and long-acting as curare and a neurotransmitter which is as short-lived as acetylcholine. The theory has also been critically analysed by Wisliski and Benzakein.[4] In 1968 Gray and Ali[5] suggested that acetylcholine appeared to produce its action by "knocking off" curare from the receptor site rather than by direct competition. Evidence has been accumulating over the past 15 years to suggest that in the clinical situation the dissociation rate constant of all non-depolarising drugs is many times longer than its association rate and that it is dependent upon the chemical structure of the drug, rather than upon its physical properties. This strongly suggests that it is the result of physical-chemical interaction between drug and receptor rather than a simple process of competition. Armstrong and Lester[6] have demonstrated that the high concentration of drug retained in the synaptic cleft may prolong the dissociation of the drug-receptor complex twenty-fold relative to association in frog's muscle. However, this observation alone is insufficient to explain the differences in affinity found when various drugs are studied. This new theory is further strengthened by the suggestion that there are separate receptor sites for acetylcholine and curare-like drugs within the macromolecule of the receptor substance. It is difficult to envisage direct competition between two agents for different sites of activity.

Another reason for not accepting the competitive theory in clinical practice is the common experience that in the presence of a major degree of neuromuscular block[7] or a high plasma drug level[8–10] it is impossible to reverse a non-depolarising block by increasing the dose of agonist (neostigmine). This is in keeping with the concept presented by Feldman and Tyrrell[11] that non-depolarising block occurred when the drug occupied the receptor site and that it only dissociated slowly from the drug-receptor complex. In a series of experiments using the isolated-arm technique,* it has been

* *The isolated arm experiment* is carried out by injecting a dose of the drug under test (suitably diluted in 40 ml saline) into an indwelling needle on the dorsum of the hand. For example, 2 mg tubocurarine or 0·6 mg pancuronium or 8 mg gallamine diluted in 40 ml saline are rapidly injected whilst the arm is isolated from the general circulation by an

shown[2,12–14] that once receptor occupancy has been achieved, a reduction in plasma level of a non-depolarising drug to subclinical levels does not cause a rapid reversal of the block.

Although the blood level of the drug following release of the tourniquet is subparalytic, the recovery of the twitch response still takes from 14 to 40 minutes, depending upon the drug used. Under well-controlled conditions it can be demonstrated that, with shorter-acting drugs like vecuronium, gallamine and alcuronium, recovery is quicker than with the longer-acting drugs like pancuronium and tubocurarine (Table 1 and Fig. 2).

These figures are for the recovery index[15] which is the time for the twitch height to recover from 25 to 75 per cent of its control value, and are therefore less than half the time taken for complete recovery of the twitch response.

For recovery from 25 to 75 per cent of the control twitch response to occur about 5–10 per cent of the total receptor population has to be freed of the muscle relaxant and the displaced drug carried away from the receptor site. In these experiments the concentration gradient between receptor site and the blood is maximal and the blood flow through the arm is high as a result of the reactive hyperaemia following release of a tourniquet applied for 2–3 minutes. In spite of these favourable circumstances the spontaneous dissociation of drug from the receptor is a slow process even for the shortest-acting relaxants.

23/Table 1

Comparison of recovery times for a number of non-depolarising relaxants. Note that the most fat-soluble drug, vecuronium, has quickest spontaneous recovery rate.

| | | | |
|---|---|---|---|
| gallamine | 9·8 | ± | 1·3 min |
| pancuronium | 10·4 | ± | 1·4 min |
| tubocurarine | 12·8 | ± | 2·1 min |
| alcuronium | 9·6 | ± | 1·0 min |
| vecuronium | 6·8 | ± | 1·6 min |

The part played by acetylcholine in controlling the dissociation rate has also been studied.[4,5,10–12] Provided that the concentration of drug perfusing the neuromuscular junction is low, so that a satisfactory diffusion gradient exists between the end-plate and the blood, then

arterial tourniquet. The injected volume distends the veins, causing neuromuscular block. Once the block has been achieved, or at a preset time between 40 seconds and 2 minutes, the tourniquet is released, allowing blood from the general circulation containing no relaxant to perfuse the arm.

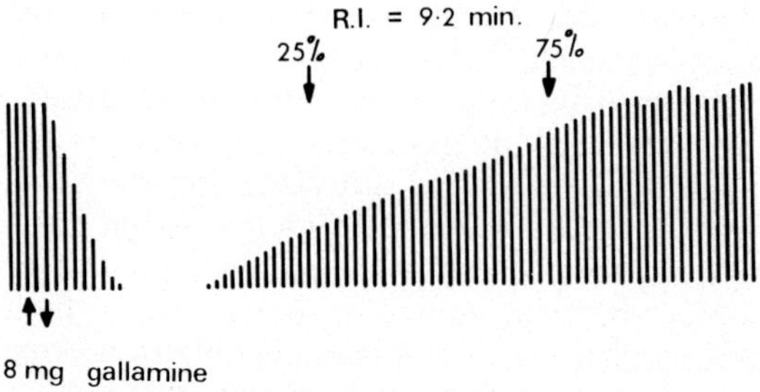


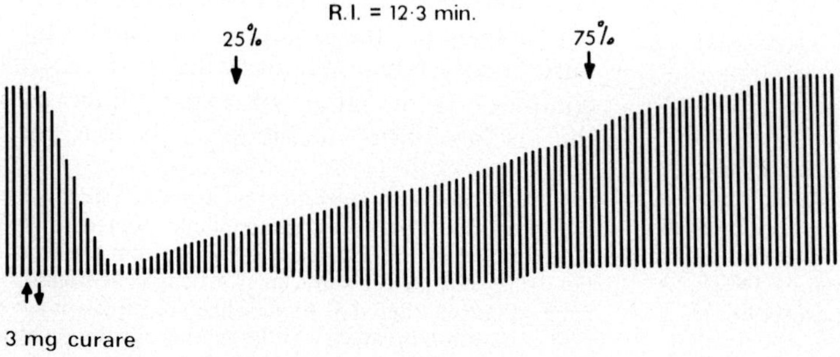


23/Fig. 2.—The isolated arm experiment.

*Upper trace:* recovery from gallamine paralysis in the absence of circulating gallamine. The recovery index (25–75 per cent recovery of twitch height) 9·2 min.

*Lower trace:* recovery from tubocurarine paralysis in absence of circulating curare. The recovery index (25–75 per cent of twitch height) 12·3 min.

acetylcholine will assist the dissociation of drug from the receptor. Small bursts of acetylcholine, such as are achieved by tetanic stimulus, will cause a small decurarising effect (Fig. 3). The same effect can be caused by other acetylcholine-like agents, including suxamethonium, (Fig. 4) and anticholinesterases. It is envisaged that the reaction of the agonist drug with the acetylcholine receptor produces sufficient molecular upheaval of the receptor area to cause the displacement of the non-depolarising drug, achieving reversal of the block.

If one accepts this concept, then studies using repeated bursts of acetylcholine or other agonist drugs will cause a much more rapid dissociation of the drug-receptor complex than occurs spontaneously in the clinical situation.

An alternative explanation was offered by Armstrong and Lester[6] to reconcile the kinetic theory of competition between acetylcholine and tubocurarine at a molecular level with the slow offset rate of tubocurarine found *in vivo* in the experiments of del Castillo and Katz and in their own frog-muscle preparation. They

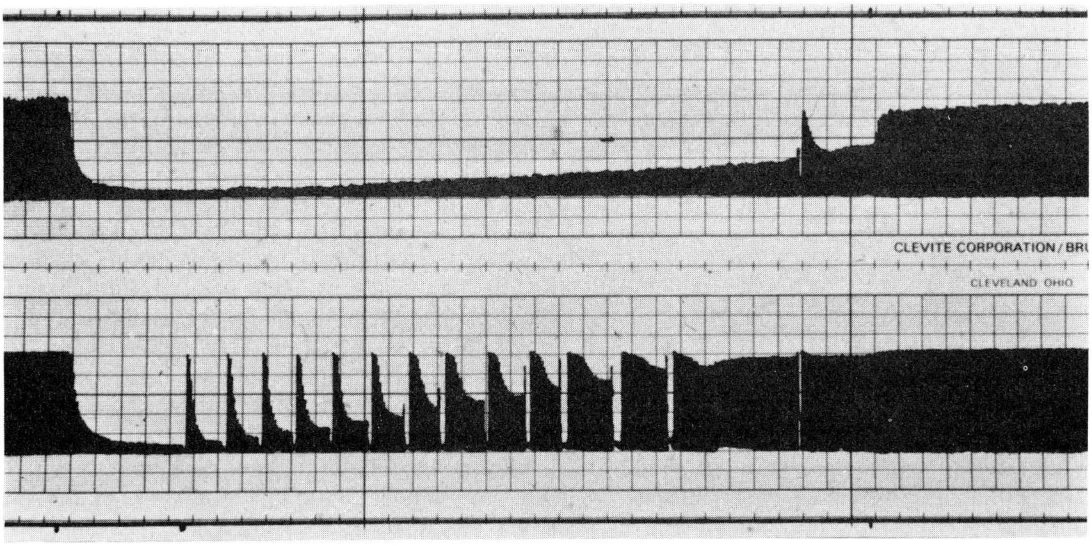


23/FIG. 3.—The decurarising effects of repeat small doses of acetylcholine (tetanic stimulation at 40 Hz) in the right arm (*lower trace*) compared with single-twitch stimulation in the left arm (*upper trace*) following systemic injection of 12 mg tubocurarine. (With the kind permission of Dr. S. A. Feldman and M. F. Tyrrell and the Honorary Editors of the *Proceedings of the Royal Society of Medicine*.[11])

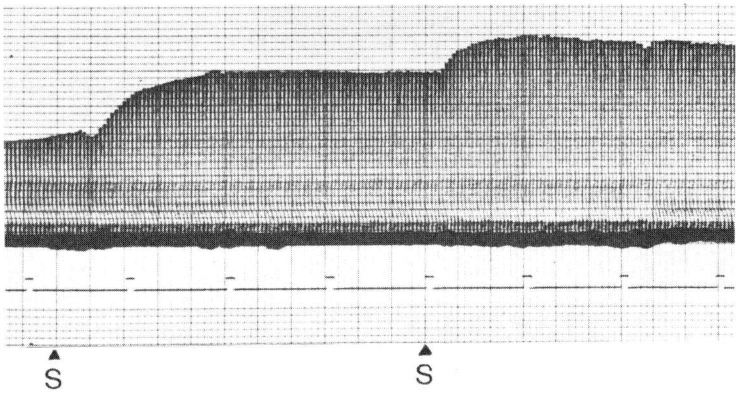


23/FIG. 4.—To illustrate the decurarising effect of small doses of suxamethonium upon partial curare block. S = 0·5 mg/kg suxamethonium.

proposed that *receptor binding* was not the crucial factor but rather the *diminished rate of diffusion* of tubocurarine molecules due to the high concentration of receptors locally confined within a synaptic membrane. This was termed *buffered diffusion*. This has given rise to a kinetic concept of an *access-limited biophase* in which the rate of access to, or egress from, a receptor area can be influenced by environmental factors. In this theory the amount of agonist and antagonist in the synaptic cleft is crucial. The arrival of an ionophoretic pulse of acetylcholine or a burst of tetanus will compete with antagonist for receptors. If there is more antagonist than available receptors, the concentration of free drug will rise sufficiently to produce a concentration gradient, allowing the drug to leave the biophase. In these circumstances it will appear to have been displaced by the acetylcholine. Armstrong and Lester demonstrated that when the amount of receptor substance is decreased by $\alpha$-cobra venom, acetylcholine more readily causes reversal of tubocurarine neuromuscular block.

### Characteristics of Non-Depolarising Block

Non-depolarising neuromuscular block is slower in onset than depolarising block and has a slower recovery time with all the drugs so far studied. Although onset time is affected by other factors such as muscle blood flow, the dose of drug administered, the size of the drug molecule and its lipophilicity, there appears to be an inevitable biophase delay before neuromuscular block occurs, which may reflect a slower penetration to a different site of action from that of the depolarising agents. Once a partial neuromuscular block is established, it demonstrates certain characteristics:

Fade on successive twitches in train-of-four response (see page 666).

With many drugs, i.e. tubocurarine, gallamine and alcuronium, tetanic fade is evident, although with pancuronium this may be less obvious.

Post-tetanic facilitation of the twitch response (see Fig. 12*a*).

Reversal by agonist drugs and by anticholinesterases (provided that the blood level of non-depolarising agent is sufficiently low to provide a concentration gradient for the drug to leave the receptor area).

In the chick and in the frog rectus muscle it causes flaccid paralysis.

## DEPOLARISATION BLOCK

### Characteristics of Depolarisation Block

Depolarising neuromuscular block is associated with a reduction of the transmembrane potential at the postsynaptic membrane. Originally this depolarisation was thought to explain totally the lack of response to motor nerve stimulation since it had been demonstrated that 40 to 50 mV depolarisation, produced physically by voltage clamp experiments or as a result of altering the extracellular potassium concentration, would cause inexcitability of the neuromuscular junction.[16] In recent years it has been appreciated that the duration of the neuromuscular block in mammals outlasts the depolarisation. Katz and Thesleff[17] suggested that this was due to a period of "desensitisation" that followed the depolarisation. During this phase the membrane potential is restored but the postsynaptic region remains inexcitable. Alternative explanations invoke a presynaptic effect of the drugs on the cholinoreceptors of the motor nerve terminal. This effect undoubtedly occurs, as antidromic firing of the nerve can be detected following administration of suxamethonium.[18] The importance of this prejunctional activity of the depolarising relaxants in the establishment of neuromuscular block is uncertain, as their principal presynaptic action appears to result in a facilitation of acetylcholine mobilisation and release. However evidence that they may produce a presynaptic block has been advanced by Galindo.[19]

The clinical characteristics of a depolarising block are its rapid onset and recovery and its association with muscle fasciculations. The fasciculations may be visible if a large dose of depolarising drug is given, or may be detected at lower doses using electromyography. They are nearly always obvious with suxamethonium but are only occasionally seen in patients following decamethonium. However, decamethonium produces marked fasciculations in most animals.

The response of a partial depolarisation block to tetanic stimulation varies but tetanic fade is seldom seen and tetanic contraction is well maintained. Post-tetanic facilitation does not occur unless an element of Phase II block is present. There is no fade on the train-of-four. Anticholinesterases and other agonist drugs will cause a potentiation of the block provided that a clinical Phase II block has not developed, in which case this effect is masked. By the time one comes to test the nature of the block in clinical practice it usually follows a prolonged effect of the depolarising drug. Due to the propensity with which a Phase II block occurs under these circumstances, pure depolarising characteristics are seldom elicited in clinical circumstances.

### Pharmacodynamics of Depolarising Neuromuscular Block

During their experiments using the isolated arm, Feldman and Tyrrell (1970)[11] and Feldman (1976)[12] found that the depolarising drug decamethonium ($C_{10}$) had a very short dissociation rate constant as the twitch response recovered rapidly once the plasma level was reduced by the release of the tourniquet and the drug washed out from the biophase (Fig. 5). This effect has been confirmed using suxamethonium. They suggested that depolarising drugs, unlike non-depolarising agents, do not bind to the receptor but associate and dissociate rapidly. As a result, their continuing relaxant activity in clinical use was dependent upon the plasma concentration of drug. Thus recovery from depolarising neuromuscular block depends on the rapidity with which the drug is washed out of the receptor area once the plasma level is lowered. This is in keeping with the findings of Churchill-Davidson and Richardson[20] that recovery from the effects of a small dose of decamethonium in volunteers was increased when the blood flow to the arm under study was increased.

Thus we have the concept of two types of neuromuscular block, one in which the receptor site is occupied by a drug that prevents the neurotransmitter fulfilling its function—non-depolarising block—and the other where the drug associates, produces an effect and then dissociates, but providing the plasma level is maintained it will then reassociate again causing a continuing agonist action. This is in keeping with Paton's rate theory of drug action.[21]

## PHASE II BLOCK

This effect was described by Churchill-Davidson and Richardson[20] in patients suffering from myasthenia gravis to whom decamethonium had been administered. A Phase II, "dual" or "mixed block" has since been observed as an almost inevitable concomitant of prolonged or excessive dosage with depolarising drugs.[22]

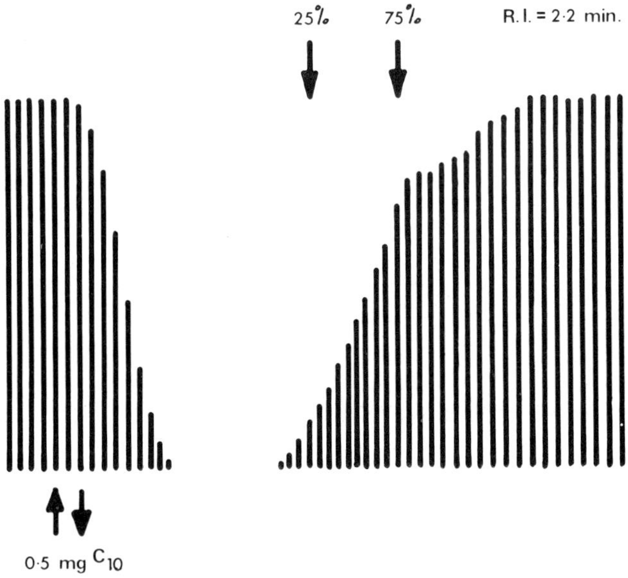

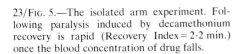

23/Fig. 5.—The isolated arm experiment. Following paralysis induced by decamethonium recovery is rapid (Recovery Index = 2·2 min.) once the blood concentration of drug falls.

Indeed it is probable that a subclinical Phase II effect occurs as an inevitable association of a depolarising drug block but only becomes overt when a sufficiently high proportion of receptors are affected. It is probable that this subclinical Phase II effect is the cause of the well documented tachyphylaxis that is seen with depolarising drugs. In myasthenia gravis there is a reduced "margin of safety" of neuromuscular transmission and as a result Phase II block occurs at an earlier stage than in normal patients.

The cause of Phase II block is unknown. Since it responds temporarily and partially to edrophonium and to neostigmine it clearly is not the same as desensitisation block as described by Katz and Thesleff.[7] Indeed many features of the block are indistinguishable from a non-depolarising block, except that it is seldom possible in well-established cases to reverse it successfully with neostigmine. This may be due to the presence of some residual depolarising agent, whose activity is potentiated at the same time as the non-depolarising effect of the Phase II block is antagonised. This possibility receives credance from the present concept of the duality of the receptors at the end-plate.

The historically classical test for the propensity of drugs to cause first a Phase I (depolarising block) followed by a Phase II block is to inject the agent into a chick, which will exhibit tonic contraction followed by flaccid paralysis.

## STRUCTURE ACTIVITY RELATIONSHIP

The similarity between the quaternary ammonium groups in the formula King described for tubocurarine in 1935[23] and the quaternary ammonium structure of acetylcholine led to the concept that this highly protonated grouping was essential for drugs that were active at the neuromuscular junction. This theory was confirmed by Paton and Zaimis's study of the bis-quaternary ammonium compounds in 1949.[24] By altering the number of methyl groups between the two positively charged quaternary groups, which by repelling each other kept the linear structure of the compound intact, they were able to demonstrate that when the distance between the quaternary ammonium moieties was 0·6–0·7 nm (6–7 Å) (i.e. 5 and 6 methyl molecules) the compounds were active as blockers of the sympathetic ganglia producing hypotension. When the chain was extended to ten methyl groups ($C_{10}$) neuromuscular block was produced. This led to the concept that the ideal distance between the 2 quaternary ammonium groups for neuromuscular block activity would be 1·2–1·4 nm (12–14 Å). The finding that certain neuromuscular blocking agents with only 1 quaternary ammonium ion such as *Erythrina Americana* were also effective neuromuscular blocking agents threw doubt upon this simple concept. Recently it has been demonstrated that the original King formula for curare which showed it as a bis-quaternary compound is erroneous at a physiological pH[25] (Fig. 6*a,b*) and that it is indeed a monoquaternary, monotertiary compound. It has also been shown that the presence of 2 quaternary ammonium groups is not an essential prerequisite for potent antagonist action at the neuromuscular junction. This has been confirmed by the introduction by Savage[26] of a monoquaternary steroid relaxant—vecuronium, whose potency is even greater than that of pancuronium. Even the original concept of the requirement of 2 onium groups and there-

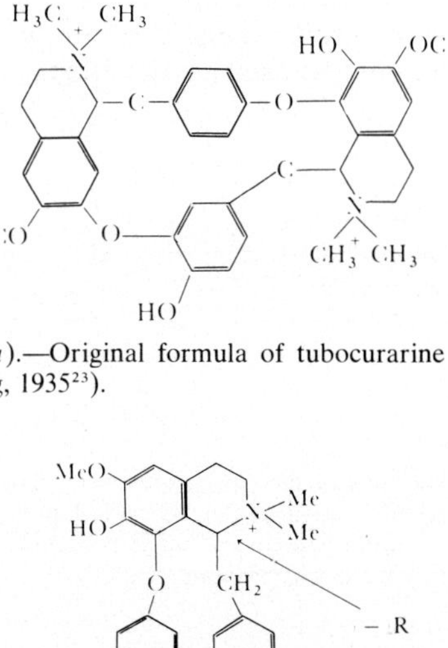


23/Fig. 6(*a*).—Original formula of tubocurarine chloride (after King, 1935[23]).

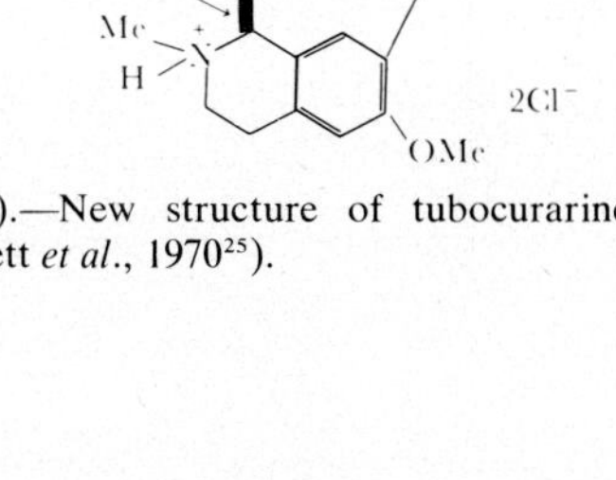


23/Fig. 6(*b*).—New structure of tubocurarine chloride (after Everett *et al.*, 1970[25]).

fore presumably the 2 onium receptors separated by 1·4 nm (14 Å) has had to be modified since the interonium distance of fazadinium is nearer 0·7 nm (7 Å) and that of pancuronium 1·0 nm (10 Å). Indeed it is easier to envisage the onium receptors as being in the four corners of squares whose sides are 0·7 nm (7 Å units). With this pattern the distance between opposing corners is about 1·0 nm (10 Å). Thus decamethonium with an interonium distance of 1·4 nm (14 Å) would span the sides of two squares (Fig. 7).

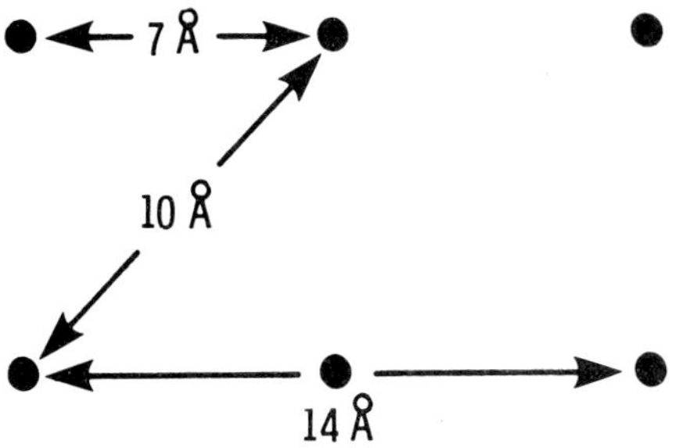


23/FIG. 7.—Possible arrangement of receptors at the myoneural junction.

The receptor is envisaged as having an onium receptor for the positively charged quaternary ammonium and an esteric receptor for the acetyl group or for esteric-like groupings.[27] It was by joining two acetylcholine-like groups onto the steroid androstane nucleus that Hewett and Savage[28] made pancuronium. However, the evidence for the necessity of an acetyl group in effecting the drug-receptor linkage in order to produce a curare-like action is by no means proven. It is possible to have potent neuromuscular blocking drugs, like the steroid relaxant chandonium, which do not possess acetyl or esteric groups; however, the loss of the 3 and 17 acetyl group from the steroid pancuronium molecule results in greatly diminished activity—indeed this is part of the metabolic pathway for the biotransformation of the drug.

## MONITORING NEUROMUSCULAR BLOCK

In order to detect the type of neuromuscular block present and to monitor the effect of any neuromuscular blocking agent two principal techniques are used:

1. Stimulation of a convenient motor nerve and watching (Fig. 8*a*,*b*,*c*) or recording (Fig. 9) the movement of the muscle innervated (indirect stimulation).
2. Stimulation of the motor nerve and recording the electrical activity of the corresponding group of muscle fibres of the muscle innervated. This is the compound electromyograph (Figs. 10–12).

Both techniques have their advocates and give similar but not identical results. Electromyography is especially suitable for neonates and for prolonged recording, but is more difficult to use in most clinical environments.

For comparative measurements to be made it is necessary to ensure supramaximal stimulation of the motor nerve and, if a pressure transducer is used, to ensure that a standard preload (stretch) is applied to the muscle studied.

In clinical practice neuromuscular transmission should be monitored whenever there is any doubt about the dose of drug which may be

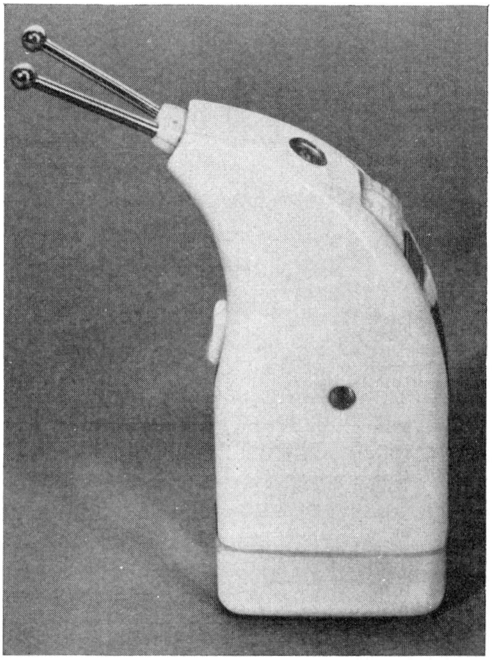

23/FIG.8(*a*).—A portable peripheral nerve stimulator. (Courtesy of the Editors and Publisher, J. B. Lippincott Company, of *Anesthesiology*.)

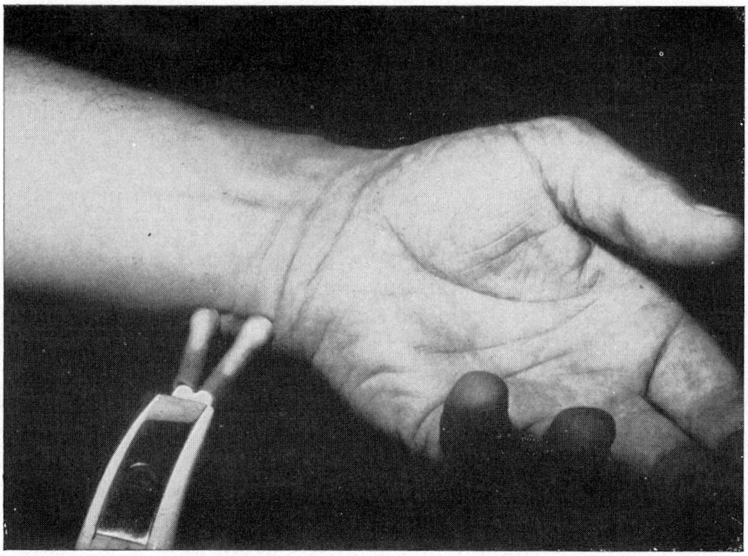

23/FIG. 8(*b*).—Method of applying the peripheral nerve stimulator to the ulnar nerve at the wrist. (Courtesy of The Editors and Publisher, J. B. Lippincott Company, of *Anesthesiology*.)

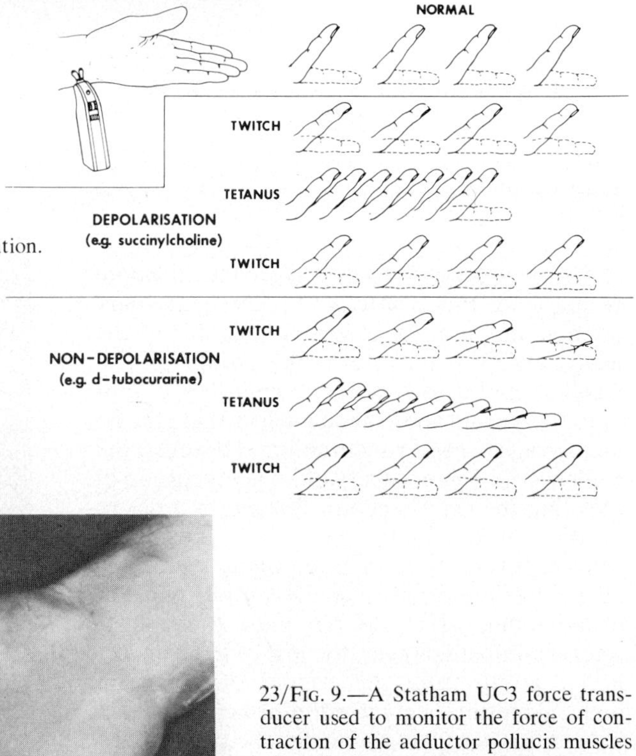


23/FIG. 8(*c*).—Finger movements with nerve stimulation.

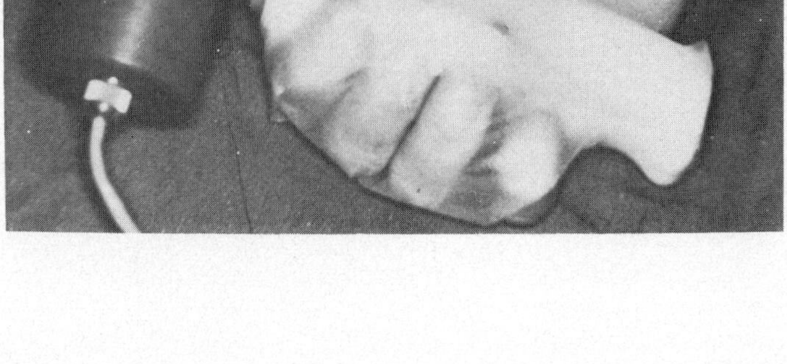

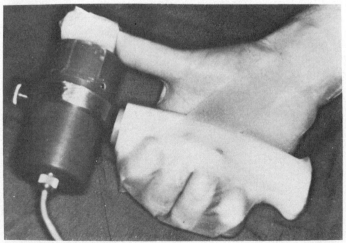

23/FIG. 9.—A Statham UC3 force transducer used to monitor the force of contraction of the adductor pollucis muscles when the ulnar nerve is stimulated.

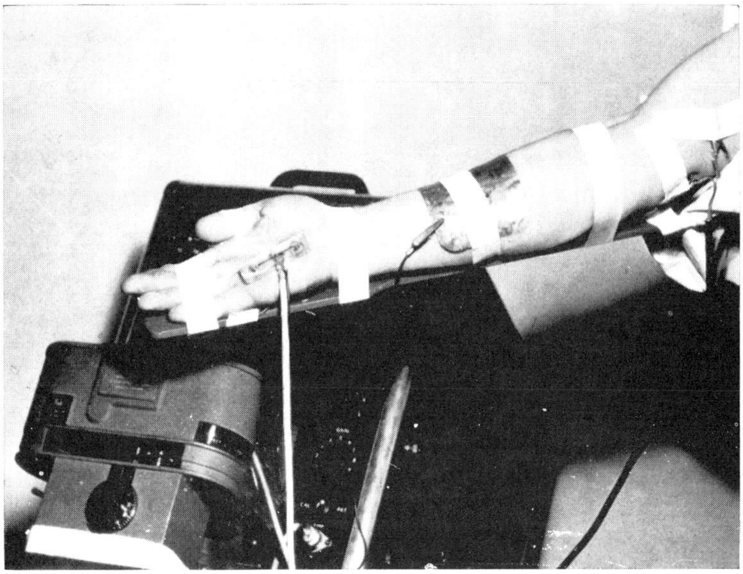

23/Fig. 10.—The electromyographic apparatus arranged for recording from the hypothenar muscles.

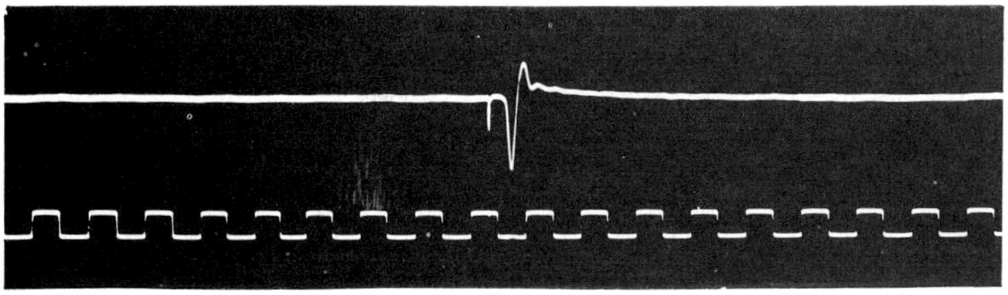

23/Fig. 11.—A normal action potential (twitch stimulus). The small downward depression before the origin of the complete action potential is the artefact caused by the electrical stimulus.

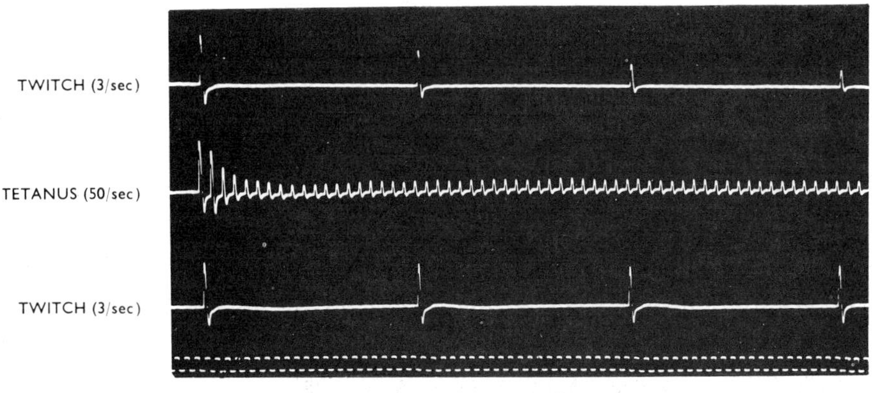


23/Fig. 12(*a*).—Non-depolarisation block.

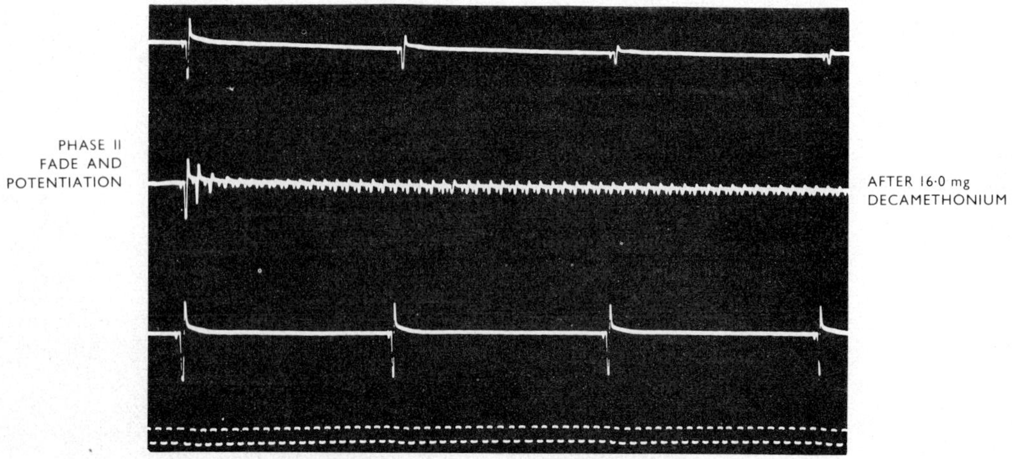


23/Fig. 12(*b*).—Phase II block showing fade of both twitch and tetanic responses together with post-tetanic potentiation after 16·0 mg decamethonium.

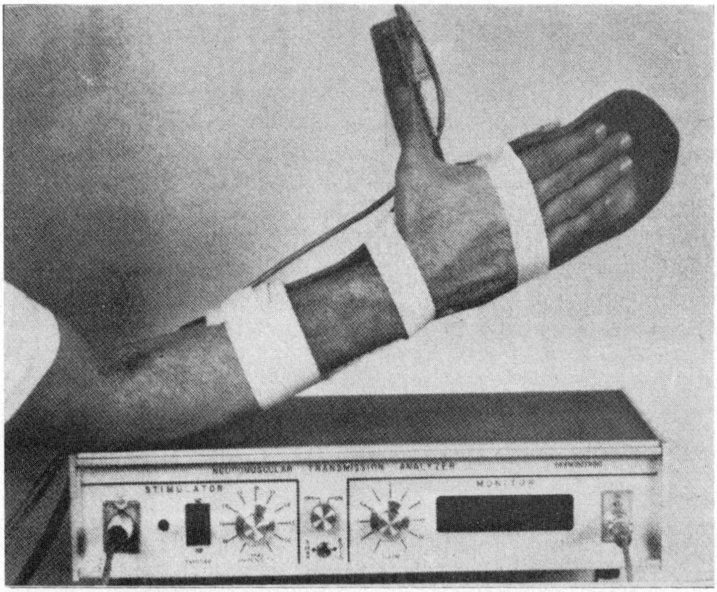


23/Fig. 13.—A view of the digital neuromuscular transmission analyser with the hand and forearm immobilised for recording from the thumb. (Courtesy of Drs. H. H. Ali, R. S. Wilson, J. J. Savarese and R. J. Kitz, and Macmillan Journals Ltd.[164])

required, such as in renal or liver disease, and when an unexpected or prolonged block has occurred. It is especially useful in the recovery room to ensure that complete and adequate reversal has been obtained before the patient is returned to his bed. Too often restlessness due to residual curarisation is misinterpreted as due to pain and a narcotic administered.[29,30] In these circumstances the result could be fatal. Special stimulators which automatically deliver four stimuli at 2 Hz, and demonstrate the ratio of the 4th to 1st twitch response, have been developed for this purpose.[31,32] (Fig. 13). With the introduction of drugs such as atracurium and vecuronium, which have a rapid offset time, it has become advisable to monitor neuromuscular conduction in order to administer the "top up" dose of drug before muscle relaxation has worn off.

## DEPOLARISING DRUGS

### Decamethonium

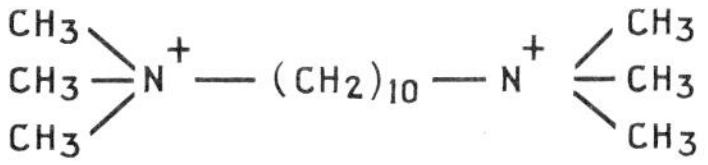


23/Fig. 14.—Decamethylene 1:10 bistrimethylammonium.

Decamethonium ($C_{10}$, Fig. 14) was introduced into anaesthesia by Organe, Paton and Zaimis in 1949.[33] Today this drug is now largely of historical and pharmacological interest. Although it does have its devotees who use it almost exclusively, most anaesthetists find that its disadvantages greatly outweigh its attractive features of rapid onset of action and the profound relaxation produced by a dose of 50 to 70 μg/kg. Its disadvantages are that it readily causes Phase II block in repeated doses; it cannot be reversed by antidotes; it is exclusively excreted by the kidneys and its action is therefore sometimes unduly prolonged. It may on occasions be associated with "scoline" type muscle pains and a shift of potassium ions from inside the cell to the e.c.f. in susceptible subjects. The tachyphylaxis described with decamethonium and typical of depolarising muscle relaxants[34] is probably a reflection of the progressive development of subclinical Phase II block.

### Suxamethonium

The neuromuscular blocking effect of suxamethonium (succinylcholine, Fig. 15) was described by Bovet and co-workers in 1949[35] and its effects in anaesthetised animals and man were described by Castillo and de Beer in 1950[36] and Thesleff in 1951.[37]

The rapid onset of the neuromuscular blocking action and the short duration of its effect render this drug unique. In spite of many disadvantages and some potentially lethal dangers, it remains the only drug presently available that will produce a rapid, complete neuromuscular block of about 5–10 minutes duration. The usual intravenous dose is between 1 mg/kg to 1·5 mg/kg.

### The Side-Effects of Suxamethonium

**Muscle pains.**—Between 20 and 50 per cent of patients receiving suxamethonium develop pains in the chest wall, upper abdomen, shoulders and back.[38] The severity of these pains vary but in extreme cases they can be debilitating, necessitating analgesics and bed rest for 2 or 3 days. Fortunately in the majority of patients it only presents as a mild ache. Although clinically there seems to be a relationship between the severity of muscle fasciculations and the occurrence of pains, this is by no means universally true.[39] Indeed it is possible to minimise or abolish the fasciculations by administering 10 mg of the drug 45 seconds to 60 seconds before the remainder of the drug is given.[40] However this "self taming" of the fasciculations, fails to affect significantly the incidence of pain. If prior to the administration of the suxamethonium a small dose of non-depolarising relaxant is administered such as 10–20 mg gallamine, 3 mg tubocurarine or 0·8 mg of pancuronium, this will significantly reduce the incidence of both the fasciculations and the pains.[41] Miller and Way,[42] in their very thorough study, suggested that for maximum effectiveness 3 minutes should elapse from the administration of the non-depolarising drug before giving the suxamethonium, but in the author's experience substantial mitigation of the pains can be achieved if suxamethonium is given 60 seconds after a small dose (8 mg) of gallamine. Although the use of larger doses of a non-depolarising drug before a depolarising agent can be criticised on the grounds that it complicates the neuromuscular pharmacology, its uneventful use in many thousands of anaesthetics supports the overall safety of this technique. Unfortunately, even when it is used, a few patients (5 to 7 per cent) will experience some muscle stiffness and discomfort. Prior treatment with a non-depolarising drug reduces the effectiveness of

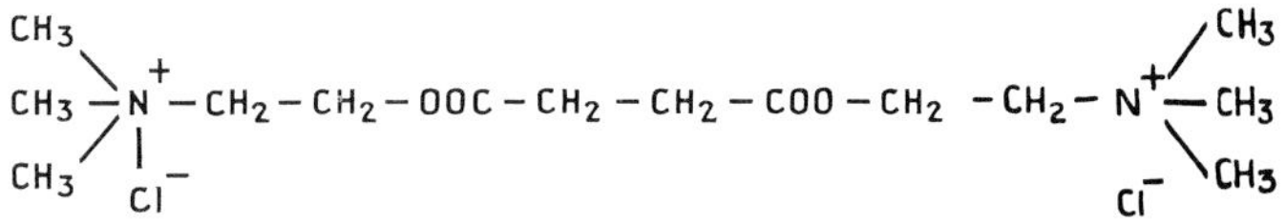


23/Fig. 15.—Suxamethonium chloride

the suxamethonium by about 30 per cent. If pancuronium is used to modify the suxamethonium pains, it may cause prolongation of the effect of the depolarising drug by virtue of its anticholinesterase properties.

Other factors that reduce the incidence and severity of the muscle pains include the use of a heavy premedication; the use of thiopentone as an induction agent in doses greater than 4 mg/kg; lignocaine,[43] diazepam and keeping the patient in bed for 24 hours following the operation. It follows that this side-effect is likely to be most troublesome following short anaesthetics in outpatients where early ambulation is essential and a minimal dose of hypnotic is used for induction. It is reasonable, therefore, to protect these patients by pretreatment with a non-depolarising relaxant unless it is specifically contra-indicated.

The cause of the muscle fasciculations after suxamethonium is now known. It is associated with presynaptic stimulation of the motor nerve and antidromic firing. Collier[39] proposed that it was associated with disturbance of the fusiform motor system whilst others have suggested it could be the result of rupture of muscle fibrils due to the unco-ordinated activity of the muscle. In support of this theory is the usual finding of a raised creatinine phosphokinase (CPK) level following suxamethonium, especially if fasciculations have been marked.[44]

In some otherwise normal patients, suxamethonium may cause spasms of certain groups of muscles (especially the masseters) whilst other muscles are flaccid. In many, but not all, patients with myotonia congenita, generalised muscle spasms may occur following suxamethonium injection.[45,46] Baraka and his colleagues[47] demonstrated that this effect could be modified by pretreatment with a small dose of tubocurarine. The association of muscle spasm with frank myoglobinuria leading to anuria has been reported.[48] However, Ryan, Kagan and Hyman[49] and Airaksinen and Tammisto[50] have found myoglobin in trace amounts in the urine of up to 30 per cent of patients who received suxamethonium.

Generalised muscle spasm has also been reported to follow the use of suxamethonium in patients with malignant hyperpyrexia, indeed Relton and his colleagues[51] suggested that it invariably occurred; however, other case reports have suggested that malignant hyperpyrexia might be provoked by suxamethonium without concomitant muscle spasms.[52]

### Effect of Suxamethonium on the Heart

The actylcholine-like action of suxamethonium on the heart[53] was confirmed by Goat in 1972.[54] She demonstrated that perfusing the isolated rabbit heart with an infusion containing suxamethonium produces an acetylcholine-like effect. This effect can be blocked by prior administration of a fully vagolytic dose of atropine.

A slowing of the heart rate is often observed on the administration of the first dose of suxamethonium to young children[55] although this effect is rarely seen in adults. However, if a second large dose is given to adults about 5 minutes after the first, then a severe bradycardia, and even a short period of cardiac arrest, may occur.[56] In clinical practice during a difficult intubation, this may have some practical importance. This response can be prevented or modified by large intravenous doses of atropine, producing vagal blockade, or by small doses of a non-depolarising drug. Atropine is capable of preventing the bradycardia and dysrhythmia of the repeated dose of suxamethonium, but only if it is present in sufficient concentration to produce some vagal blockade and tachycardia. When given intramuscularly one hour before induction of anaesthesia, it is seldom effective in preventing a bradycardia. However, if given in a dose of 0·01 mg/kg *intravenously* before a thiopentone, nitrous oxide and halothane anaesthetic, then it affords protection.[57] Thiopentone may play some role in reducing the incidence of bradycardia because the dose of atropine has to be increased to 0·015 mg/kg (given intravenously) if only nitrous oxide, oxygen and halothane are administered.[58] Glycopyrrolate is also effective in preventing the bradycardia and dysrhythmia of suxamethonium.[57] The precise mechanism of this action of suxamethonium is not known. Mathias and his colleagues[59] suggested that it might be reflex stimulation of the chemoreceptors in the great vessels, but in a recent study of tracheal muscle in the rabbit it was concluded that suxamethonium produced a direct stimulating action on the parasympathetic ganglia.

In clinical practice, if it is necessary to give a repeat dose of suxamethonium soon after the first, it is wise to precede this with either a small dose of a non-depolarising relaxant, or an intravenous dose of atropine sufficient to produce vagal blockade. Alternatively suxamethonium should be infused slowly so that the heart does not receive a bolus dose. The bradycardia of suxamethonium is not observed when it is administered by infusion.

Although suxamethonium has been incriminated as a cause of cardiac dysrhythmias, especially in digitalised patients, this has not been confirmed experimentally.[60] Indeed, Wong and his colleagues[61] produced evidence to suggest that the drug stabilised the myocardium against dysrhythmias induced by catecholamines.

### Potassium $K^+$ Ion Release

In the normal patient, the depolarisation caused by a paralytic dose of suxamethonium (1 mg/kg) will cause a rise in plasma $K^+$ of less than 0·5 mmol/l.[62] However, under certain circumstances the rise in plasma potassium due to the passage of potassium from inside the muscle cell during depolarisation is greatly in excess of this value. This is likely to occur following the effective denervation of the muscle and the resultant spread of acetylcholine-sensitive receptors away from the restricted end-plate region over the surface of the muscle. This loss of specifity of the receptor area can be demonstrated for up to 6 months following denervation. In clinical practice the "denervation response" is seen in the following circumstances:

*Massive burns* especially in children.[63–65]

*Massive muscle trauma.*[66,67]

*Lower motor neurone* lesions and denervation of motor nerves, Guillain-Barré syndrome, following spinal transection; acute spinal-cord compression, and rapid onset of demyelinating diseases of the motor nerves and other neuropathies.[68,69,70]

*Upper motor neurone lesions*, including cerebrovascular accidents, encephalitis and brain injury. Although the magnitude of the potassium response following suxamethonium is not as great as with lower motor neurone disease, nevertheless suxamethonium should not be given unless alternative techniques are inappropriate; if it is used it should always be preceded by a small dose of a non-depolarising drug.

*Abdominal infections.* A report by Kohlschutter, Baur and Roth,[71] suggests that in the presence of massive intra-abdominal infection large shifts of $K^+$ ion may occur, suggesting that suxamethonium may be contra-indicated in these patients unless alternative agents are considered to be more hazardous.

*Renal disease.* Although a suxamethonium-induced shift of potassium ions has been incriminated as the cause of sudden cardiac arrest in these patients,[72] Miller and his co-workers[73] failed to demonstrate a marked rise in plasma potassium in patients in renal failure following the administration of suxamethonium. It is possible that even the small potassium shift that invariably occurs when this drug is used may cause a serious effect on the membrane potential in patients, such as those suffering from renal failure, in whom a chronic potassium depletion often exists. Alternatively it is possible that some patients with renal disease may develop renal neuropathy of sufficient severity effectively to cause substantial muscle denervation. In any event it is better to avoid the use of suxamethonium in these patients whenever possible, especially if there is pre-existing ECG evidence of potassium imbalance.

### Raised Intra-ocular Pressure

The increase in intra-ocular pressure that follows the administration of suxamethonium lasts for an average of 6 minutes.[74] Although prior treatment with a non-depolarising relaxant usually modifies this response,[75,76] it cannot be relied upon to prevent the dangers of vitreous prolapse from an open eye wound.[77] It is therefore usually considered advisable to avoid the use of this drug in patients with penetrating injuries of the eye unless the use of alternative techniques carry a greater risk to the patient or to his eye. The cause of rise in intra-ocular pressure is believed to relate to the peculiar nature of the response of some of the extra-ocular muscles to acetylcholine-like drugs. Although most fibres respond with a brief contraction, others develop a slow *contracture* which produces a squeezing effect upon the globe and an increase in the intra-ocular pressure.

### Raised Intragastric Pressure

The rise to 12 cm $H_2O$ in intragastric pressure

that often follows the use of suxamethonium in adults[78] is probably of little significance provided that the oesophageal sphincter mechanism is intact, as it has been demonstrated that coincident with the rise in intragastric pressure there is a compensatory increase in oesophageal tone. This is confirmed by the overall safety of the use of suxamethonium for "crash induction" in patients with a potentially full stomach, provided that all other precautions are also taken to minimise the risk of regurgitation and inhalation of gastric contents.

### Malignant Hyperpyrexia

Suxamethonium, especially in patients anaesthetised with halothane, is often a triggering mechanism in this condition (see Chapter 26, p. 735).

### Anaphylactoid Response

Although suxamethonium causes only a modest release of histamine in most patients, cases of anaphylactoid reactions have been reported in sensitised individuals.[79]

### Phase II Block

The development of clinically demonstrable Phase II block will occur if the receptors are exposed to suxamethonium either in excess doses or for a prolonged time (see Fig. 12*b*).

### Suxamethonium and Plasma Cholinesterase

Suxamethonium is normally hydrolysed so rapidly to succinylmonocholine and then to choline by plasma cholinesterase that it is estimated that this process, together with rapid redistribution, results in only about 10–15 per cent of a given dose actually reaching the receptor area. Much of the succinylmonocholine (a very weak neuromuscular blocking drug) is hydrolysed to succinic acid and choline but substantial amounts may appear in the urine (Table 2). There are two ways in which this process can be impaired *in vivo*: (i) there can be a deficient blood content of plasma cholinesterase, or (ii) the plasma cholinesterase can be atypical, lacking the ability to hydrolyse suxamethonium.[80]

### Plasma Cholinesterase Deficiency

**Acquired factors** (Fig. 16) altering the level of the normal enzyme in man can be considered under three headings.

1. *Physiological.*—It has been demonstrated that low levels of plasma cholinesterase occur during pregnancy and the early puerperium,[81,82] and a number of cases of prolonged apnoea of mild duration following the use of suxamethonium have been reported.[83,84] The cause of the fluctuation in enzyme level is not known but could be related to changes in the oestrogen level, as women on the contraceptive pill have some reduction in their enzyme level.[85]

The level of plasma cholinesterase in the first six months of life is lower than the maternal but as clinically a resistance to suxamethonium has been recorded[86,87] it would not appear to be of great significance in clinical practice.

2. *Malnutrition.* — Plasma cholinesterase enzyme is formed in the liver and it follows that production of the enzyme will accompany any loss of hepatic function. In days gone by and before the introduction of more specific tests, the plasma cholinesterase blood level was used as a measure of hepatic function. Reduced levels, therefore, will be found in a large number of diseased states, but particular care in clinical practice must be exercised (in the dosage) when administering suxamethonium to patients with

23/TABLE 2
THE BREAKDOWN OF SUXAMETHONIUM

1st stage:

Suxamethonium —— (Rapid) / Plasma cholinesterase —— Succinylmonocholine + choline

2nd stage:

Succinylmonocholine —— (Slow) / Specific liver enzyme and Plasma cholinesterase —— Succinic acid + choline

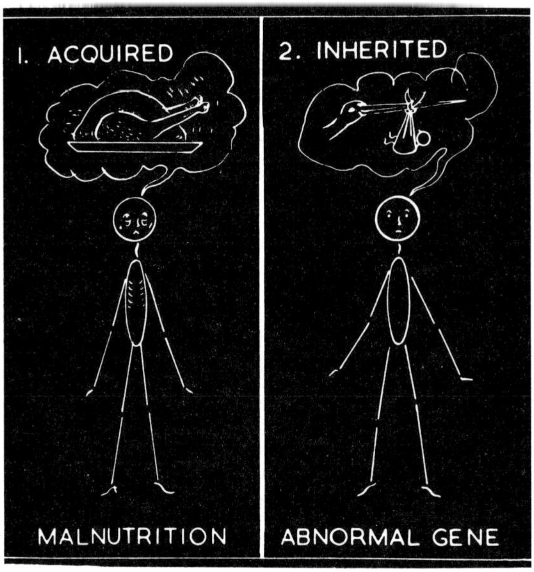


23/FIG. 16.—Illustration of the two causes of reduced plasma cholinesterase enzyme activity.

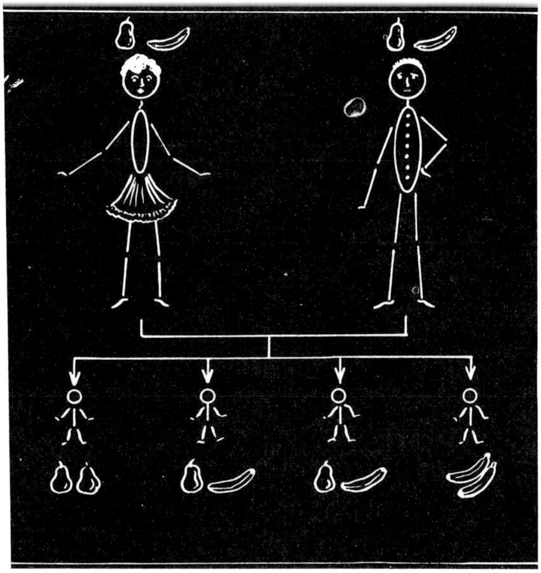

23/FIG 18.—Diagram of genetic response in the offspring when two heterozygotes marry.

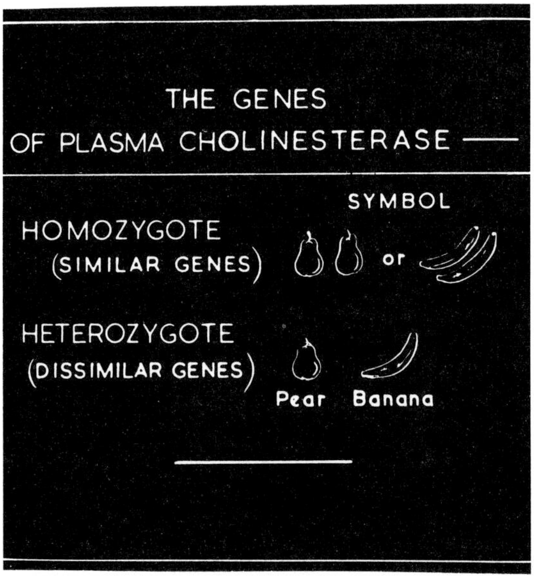


23/FIG. 17

terminal disorders (e.g. oesophageal obstruction).

3. *Drug interactions.*—Many drugs can reduce the level of the enzyme and the most potent of these are the anticholinesterase drugs including ecothiopate iodide.[88–90] Other interactions have been reported with e.g. phenothiazines,[91] cytotoxic agents,[92,93] ketamine,[94] trimetaphan,[95] pancuronium[96] and propanidid,[97] and the antibilharzial drug metrifonate.

**Genetic factors.** (Fig. 16).—Soon after the introduction of suxamethonium into clinical practice, numerous case reports appeared in the literature describing a prolonged paresis. The puzzle was resolved when Kalow and Davies[80] discovered in man that there were at least two types of plasma cholinesterase enzymes, a normal and an atypical one. Whilst the vast majority of the population possessed the normal or usual enzyme, rarely a patient was encountered who was either heterozygous (part normal and part atypical) or homozygous for the atypical gene. The way in which these combinations occur in the population is illustrated in Figs. 17 and 18. The frequency of each combination will clearly depend on the incidence of a particular gene in the population. Further studies have revealed that there are four principal genes associated with plasma cholinesterase; these are seen in Table 3, using the now accepted symbolic classification of Motulsky.[98]

The enzymes formed by variants of $E_1^a$ and $E_1^f$ have a qualitative difference from the usual ($E_1^u$) in that they have a reduced ability to hydrolyse suxamethonium.

23/Table 3
Classification of Genotypes of Plasma Cholinesterase

| *Genotype* | *Figure* | *Action* | *Reference* |
|---|---|---|---|
| Usual | $E_1^u$ | Normal hydrolysis | Kalow and Genest (1957)[99] |
| Atypical | $E_1^a$ | Dibucaine resistant | Kalow and Genest (1957)[99] |
| Fluoride | $E_1^f$ | Fluoride resistant | Harris and Whittaker (1961)[100] |
| Silent | $E_1^s$ | Complete lack of cholinesterase activity | Liddell et al. (1962)[101] |

*Determination of the genotype* is based on the differential inhibition of the enzyme by several substances such as dibucaine, fluoride, chloride and suxamethonium.

*Dibucaine test* examines the amount of inhibition of a particular plasma cholinesterase activity by dibucaine. If a specimen has a high usual (normal) enzyme content, then it will be inhibited to a large extent by dibucaine. This percentage inhibition can then be expressed as a number—the dibucaine number (Table 4).

23/Table 4
Dibucaine Number for Various Types of Sera

| | *Dibucaine Number* |
|---|---|
| $E_1^uE_1^u$ | 70–85 |
| $E_1^uE_1^a$, $E_1^uE_1^f$, $E_1^uE_1^s$ | 50–65 |
| $E_1^aE_1^a$, $E_1^fE_1^f$, $E_1^sE_1^s$ | 16–25 |
| $E_1^sE_1^s$ | 5–0 |

*Fluoride test* can similarly be performed and this will reveal a few instances where the samples may show a normal-looking dibucaine number yet an abnormally low fluoride number. Such a situation would be evident in the presence of $E_1^fE_1^f$ genotypes.

*Incidence of genotypes* will play an important part in the number of cases of prolonged response to suxamethonium that can be observed. If it is accepted that the enzyme formed from $E_1^uE_1^u$ genotypes can hydrolyse the clinical dose of suxamethonium in around four minutes, then the $E_1^uE_1^a$ and $E_1^uE_1^f$ genotypes would be expected to take 10–20 minutes to carry out the same task. It is only in the homozygotes $E_1^aE_1^a$, $E_1^fE_1^f$ and $E_1^sE_1^s$ that really prolonged periods of paresis can be anticipated. The number of times this prolonged paralysis will occur in the clinical situation will, therefore, depend on the estimation incidence of the various genotypes in the general population (Table 5).

23/Table 5
Incidence of Genotypes

| | |
|---|---|
| $E_1^uE_1^u$ | 94 per cent |
| $E_1^uE_1^a$ | 4 per cent |
| $E_1^uE_1^f$ | 0·4 per cent |
| $E_1^uE_1^s$ | 0·6 per cent |
| $E_1^aE_1^a$ | 0·04 per cent |
| $E_1^aE_1^f$ | 0·003 per cent |
| $E_1^aE_1^s$ | 0·01 per cent |
| $E_1^fE_1^f$ | 0·0003 per cent |
| $E_1^fE_1^s$ | 0·0005 per cent |
| $E_1^sE_1^s$ | 0·001 per cent |

Viby-Mogensen and Hanel[103] reported on a study of 225 patients by the Danish Cholinesterase Research Unit in Copenhagen, all of whom had experienced a prolonged apnoea after suxamethonium. Interestingly enough, 28·1 per cent of these apnoeas had normal plasma cholinesterase and were presumed due to other causes such as overventilation or central respiratory depression. In 6·2 per cent of patients there was a low plasma cholinesterase due to *acquired* factors. The incidence of the *genetic* factors in this sample together with the duration of apnoea are shown in Table 6.

23/Table 6
Incidence and related genotype together with duration of apnoea in 147 patients receiving suxamethonium.[103]

| *Genotype* | *No. of Cases* | *Duration of Apnoea (min)* | *Range* |
|---|---|---|---|
| $E_1^aE_1^a$ | 105 | 92 | 25–240 |
| $E_1^uE_1^a$ | 17 | 25 | 7–60 |
| $E_1^aE_1^s$ | 12 | 126 | 180–660 |
| $E_1^uE_1^s$ | 4 | 95 | |
| $E_1^sE_1^s$ | 3 | 170 | 240–360 |
| $E_1^aE_1^f$ | 4 | 38 | – |
| $E_1^uE_1^f$ | 2 | 18 | – |
| $E_1^fE_1^s$ | 1 | 35 | – |

A perusal of Table 6 reveals that the presence of one normal gene $E_1^u$ in the combination usually leads to a moderate duration of apnoea, whereas the presence of $E_1^s$ (particularly in homozygote form $E_1^sE_1^s$ or heterozygote $E_1^aE_1^s$) produced the largest periods of apnoea.

At the other extreme, Harris and his coworkers[104] described a $C_5$ variant as a rare variety of genetic disturbance which enables the holder to produce an extremely rapid hydrolysis of suxamethonium. Although no further studies appear to have been made, the presence of such a gene might help to explain the large dose of suxamethonium sometimes found necessary to produce complete paralysis.

**Administration**

Suxamethonium is usually administered intravenously, but it can be given intramuscularly or even by the subcutaneous route if the dose is sufficient. If either of the latter routes is used then there is a considerable delay in the onset of paresis and once established it lasts much longer than normal. An increase of at least 50 per cent in dose is required to produce paralysis by these routes. With the intravenous route the arrival in any group of muscle fibres is heralded by brief but visible twitches or fasciculations, and these are usually first observed in the eyebrow and eyelid muscles, passing later to the shoulder girdle and abdominal musculature, and finally to the hands and feet. Muscle fasciculations are more obvious in patients who are lightly anaesthetised.

**Dosage.**—The average single dose in man is 1 mg/kg, but when administered by continuous infusion as a 0·1 per cent solution a dose of 20–40 μg/kg/min will give relaxation of most skeletal musculature, but some assistance to respiration is required. Doses of 50–60 μg/kg/min and above usually result in complete respiratory paralysis. If total paralysis is produced by continuous infusion there is a considerable danger of administering an overdose, as there are no signs of muscle activity available. It is essential to monitor neuromuscular transmission continuously whenever an infusion of suxamethonium is used, as this will remove the risk of overdosage.

**Treatment of prolonged response to suxamethonium.**—The development of a Phase II block following prolonged exposure to suxamethonium presents the anaesthetist with a great temptation to try to expedite natural recovery by the administration of drugs. The dangers of this have been reviewed by Vickers[105] and Hunter.[106] Anti-cholinesterase agents may initially improve neuromuscular conduction but the results are seldom prolonged and unless the plasma level of drug is very low it will result in prolonging the action of suxamethonium in the depolarising phase. The use of cholase (purified human serum esterase) may effectively reduce the duration of the depolarising block,[107,108] but the shelf life of the enzyme is short. Many patients do not recover normal neuromuscular function after cholase, possibly due to the residual Phase II effect. Most anaesthetists are agreed that should there be a very prolonged effect from suxamethonium then the patient should be ventilated with 50 per cent nitrous oxide and oxygen until neuromuscular recovery occurs. Fluid infusions may assist recovery by increasing the distribution volume and promoting a diuresis and thus lowering the plasma concentration of drug.

Every patient who demonstrates a prolonged response to suxamethonium (over 30 min apnoea) should be investigated to determine if they have a reduction of plasma cholinesterase or an abnormal genotype. If an abnormal genotype is revealed then the immediate relatives of the patient should have their blood examined to determine the familial pattern. All patients with either the homozygous or heterozygous abnormality should carry warning cards to be given to the anaesthetist should an operation be necessary.

## NON-DEPOLARISING DRUGS

TUBOCURARINE (tubocurarine chloride)

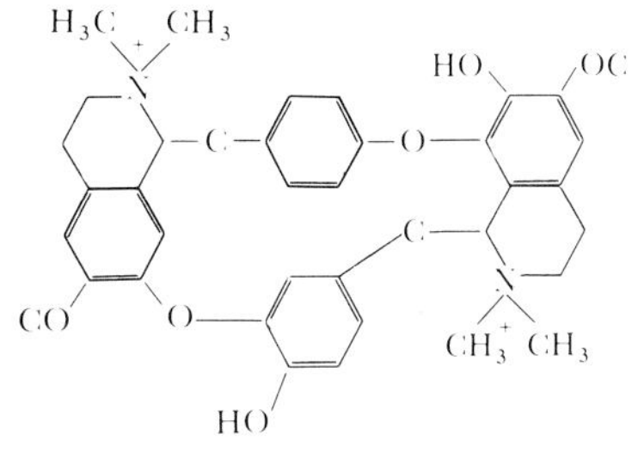


23/FIG. 19(*a*)—Original formula of tubocurarine chloride (after King, 1935).

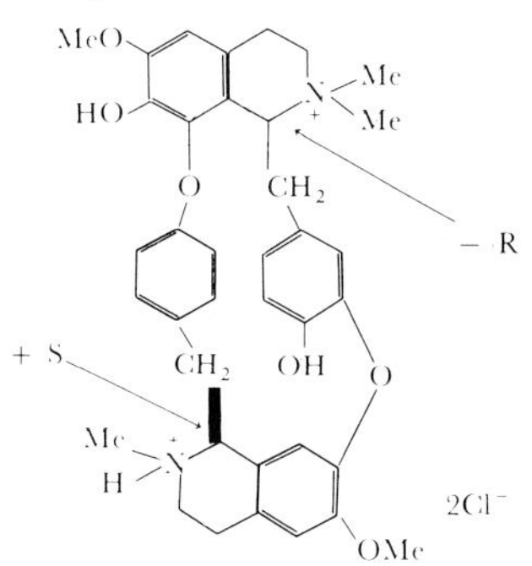


23/FIG. 19(*b*).—New structure of tubocurarine chloride (after Everett *et al.*, 1970).

This was the first neuromuscular blocking agent used in anaesthesia. Although originally described by King in 1935[23] (Fig. 19*a*) as a bisquaternary compound, it is now accepted as being a monoquaternary compound at physiological pH (Fig. 19*b*).

### Dose and Administration

To provide relaxation during anaesthesia, tubocurarine 0·2 to 0·4 mg/kg is administered intravenously. This provides a dose of about 20 to 35 mg to an average adult, in order to obtain good muscle relaxation for about 45 to 75 minutes. Depression of the adductor twitch response with this dose can be observed for up to 90 minutes. Although lesser doses will abolish the response of adductor muscles of the hands in lightly anaesthetised patients the abdominal relaxation produced is poor and the duration of good operative relaxation is shorter. Tubocurarine is a moderately cumulative drug; subsequent "top up" doses of 5 to 10 mg are usually adequate as a result. The duration of effect of each subsequent dose is usually slightly longer than the one preceding it.

### Excretion

Tubocurarine is normally largely excreted unchanged in the urine.[109] Miller and his co-workers[110] recovered 40 per cent of the drug unchanged from the urine in 24 hours in man. In the presence of reduced renal blood flow, Cohen and his colleagues[109] demonstrated that biliary excretion of the drug increased to provide a satisfactory alternative means of lowering the plasma level of drug, although under these conditions a modest prolongation of its action is usually evident.

### Non-Specific Effects

In addition to its action at the neuromuscular junction, tubocurarine has other non-specific effects, some of which may be deleterious in special circumstances.

**Histamine release.**—The drug causes more histamine release than any other available neuromuscular blocking agent and, although it has been the cause of anaphylactoid reactions,[111] this type of response is exceedingly rare even in atopic individuals. However, although the drug has been widely used in patients with asthma without adverse effect, it can produce severe bronchospasm and it should therefore be avoided in these patients.

**Hypotension.**—Tubocurarine is a weak ganglion-blocking drug. In susceptible patients it often produces a fall in systolic blood pressure of up to 20 per cent due to a decrease in peripheral resistance. Unless the dose of drug has been excessive or the patient hypovolaemic, the hypotension is usually of short duration compared with the duration of the muscle paralysis produced. The effect on the blood pressure is more pronounced in the presence of halothane. Although histamine release may contribute to the hypotension, and the hypotension has been demonstrated to be greatest in patients who release most histamine, it is little affected by the $H_1$ or $H_2$ blockers. Tachycardia, should it occur, is secondary to the hypotension. No effect on the cardiac vagus has been demonstrated with clinical doses of the drug. Johnson and his co-workers,[112] using volume pulse plethysmography studies, concluded that tubocurarine had a *direct* myocardial depressant action which was similar to that of verapamil, i.e. calcium ion ($Ca^{++}$) antagonism. This effect has not been confirmed by other workers.

### Clinical Use

Tubocurarine remains one of the safest and most predictable neuromuscular blocking agents available. Experience with this drug since 1946 has established its safety. It should be avoided in patients with a history of atopic reactions and in hypovolaemic patients. It should be used with caution in those patients in whom even a modest fall of peripheral resistance may endanger cardiac perfusion. Reversal of residual neuromuscular block at the end of the operation is usually easily accomplished with 30 μg/kg neostigmine (about 2·5 mg for an adult) administered intravenously mixed with atropine 1·2 mg (see Chapter 25, p 731). In the presence of an elevated plasma level greater than 1·0 μg/ml,[9,10] reversal by neostigmine will be incomplete. It is therefore essential to avoid administering large doses of tubocurarine shortly before the end of the operation. It is good clinical practice to test neuromuscular transmission with a peripheral nerve stimulator at the end of every anaesthetic in which a long-acting non-depolarising relaxant has been used, to ensure no residual paresis remains. The absence of any fade on twitch stimulation of the ulnar nerve at 2 Hz or the presence of the ability to sustain tetanic contraction both denote that neuromuscular transmission has returned to a satisfactory state.

### Dimethylcurare (Metacurine)*

This drug was originally synthesised by King in 1935[23] but due to difficulties in standardisation at that time, it was not widely used in anaesthesia until its pharmacological properties were re-investigated by Hughes and Chapple in 1976.[113]

Dimethylcurare is about half as potent as tubocurarine. It does not cause as much histamine release as the parent compound in clinical doses. Its main advantage over tubocurarine is that it causes less hypotension in a paralytic dose. Savarese and his colleagues[114] have demonstrated that doses greater than 40 μg/kg may cause fall in peripheral resistance. A major disadvantage of dimethylcurare is that it is almost entirely dependent upon renal excretion for elimination from the body and, as a result, its action is greatly prolonged in patients with poor renal function. It is very much more cumulative on repeated doses than tubocurarine.

### Pancuronium (Pavulon)

23/Fig. 20.

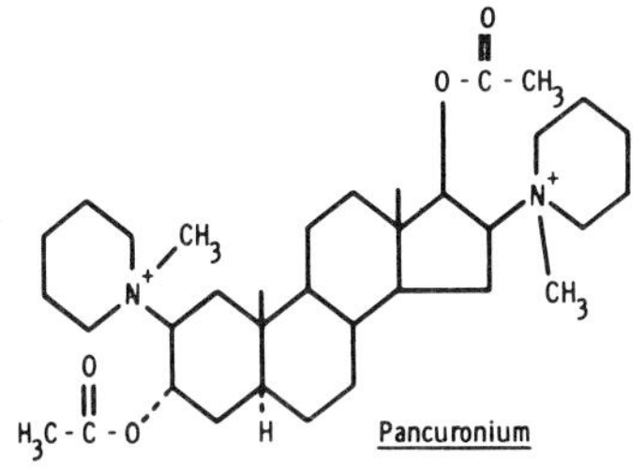


The addition of 2 acetylcholine-like groups onto the rigid steroid nucleus in the 2–3 and 16–17 positions produced this potent neuromuscular blocking drug. It was introduced into anaesthesia by Baird and Reid in 1967[115] and has found widespread acceptance as a safe, reliable agent in the subsequent years.

#### Dose and Administration

The drug is used intravenously in clinical practice in a dose of 60 to 100 μg/kg. Its rate of onset of action is slightly faster than tubocurarine,[116] and its duration of action is between 45 and 60 minutes. Pancuronium is a markedly cumulative drug. Because of this the "top up dose" should be between 5 to 10 per cent of the initial dose. It is advisable to time the last dose of pancuronium so that it is not less than 20 minutes before reversal of the block is attempted with neostigmine.

#### Excretion and metabolism

Pancuronium is principally excreted in the urine of animals and man.[117,118] Varying amounts of pancuronium are also recovered from the bile of patients, demonstrating the presence of an alternative hepatic pathway of excretion. Agoston and his co-authors in 1976[119] found from virtually zero to 30 per cent of the total dose of steroid could be recovered from the drainage T-tubes inserted into the bile ducts of patients following cholecystectomy. Up to 25 per cent of the biliary excretion is in the form of pancuronium metabolites, and a further 5 per cent of the injected dose, may appear as metabolites in the urine.[120] The principal metabolites are 17-hydroxy, 3-hydroxy and the 3–17 hydroxy compounds[117,118,121] (Fig. 21). The 3-hydroxy derivative, which is the first metabolite, has a potency of about one half of that of the parent compound, whereas the 17-hydroxy and 3–17 hydroxy compounds are very weak neuromuscular blocking agents.[120]

The considerable individual variation in the biliary excretion of pancuronium observed by Agoston and his colleagues[117] in patients after cholecystectomy may be explained by the observation of Somogyi and his co-workers[122] that in jaundiced patients the action of pancuronium was prolonged. This is probably due to the presence of bile salts which compete with steroid muscle relaxants for metabolic and excretory pathways.[123] Due to the limited biliary excretion and metabolism of pancuronium, its action is greatly prolonged in patients who are anephric or in whom the renal blood flow is decreased.

Although the prolongation of action is less dramatic than with gallamine, inability to reverse the action of pancuronium in patients with renal failure is common.[124–127] Clinical experience supports the findings of Miller and his colleagues[110] that tubocurarine is associated

* As tubocurarine is now considered to be a monoquaternary (as opposed to a bisquaternary) compound, because dimethylcurare has three extra methyl groups it should perhaps be more correctly termed *trimethylcurare*.

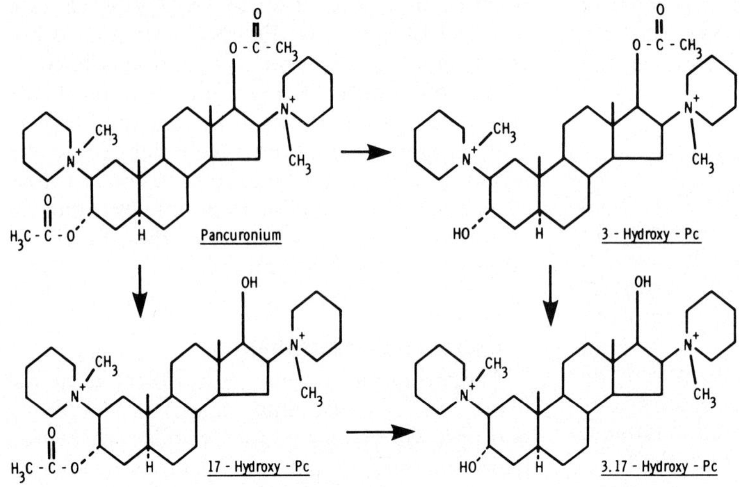


23/Fig. 21.—Metabolic breakdown of pancuronium.

with a lower incidence of incomplete reversal than pancuronium in patients with renal disease.

### Non-specific Effects

Pancuronium causes very little histamine release although allergic responses have been described.[128] It causes a mild transient depression on the plasma cholinesterase.

### Cardiovascular Effects

Pancuronium can cause tachycardia and increased peripheral resistance. Both of these effects are dose related. The chronotropic effect of pancuronium is principally due to an atropine-like action on the cardiac vagus.[113,129,130] This effect is always seen when the dose exceeds twice that required to paralyse the adducter twitch response, and can usually be demonstrated in non-atropinised patients at doses in excess of 80 μg/kg.

The increased peripheral resistance described following pancuronium[131] has been shown to be associated with an inhibition of the re-uptake of catecholamine by the heart muscle.[132,133] This effect is particularly likely to be of significance if the patient is lightly anaesthetised and the dose of pancuronium in excess of 120 μg/kg.

Because of its propensity to increase the rate and after-load of the heart, pancuronium in large doses may have serious disadvantages in patients with coronary artery insufficiency or myocardial failure.

### Clinical Use

Pancuronium is a popular muscular relaxant for intermediate duration operations. Although in modest doses it has little effect upon the heart, in the usual dose range of 8–10 mg in a fit adult it will produce an increase in cardiac work. It is a cumulative drug and its use should be avoided wherever possible in patients with jaundice and renal disease. Unless contra-indicated, its action should be reversed at the end of the operation by anticholinesterase.

## Alcuronium (Alloferin)

This compound is a derivative of C-toxiferine and was introduced into anaesthesia by Hugin and Kissling in 1961.[134]

### Dose and Administration

Alcuronium has about twice the potency of tubocurarine, requiring 10–15 mg i.v. for good abdominal relaxation in a 70-kg adult. Its duration of action in equiparalytic doses is rather shorter than that of pancuronium.

### Excretion

Alcuronium is largely excreted unchanged in the urine. Some drug may be excreted in the bile. Its duration of action is markedly prolonged in the absence of renal function.

### Non-specific Effects

Alcuronium causes little or no histamine release when injected intradermally or intravenously.

Although alcuronium may cause a fall in peripheral resistance,[131] this is seldom as marked as with tubocurarine. Tachycardia can follow its use in doses that are well in excess of those required to produce paralysis of the adductor muscles.

### Clinical Use

Alcuronium is a safe, reliable relaxant with few deleterious side-effects in modest clinical doses. It is usually easy to reverse with neostigmine except in anephric patients where a prolonged action may occur.[127]

It has been claimed that in equipotent doses alcuronium has a more rapid onset of action than tubocurarine, making it a more satisfactory drug for intubation.[135]

## Fazadinium Bromide (Fazadon)

Fazadinium is a yellow coloured azo pyridinium compound. In some animals it is rapidly hydrolysed by azo reductase enzymes in the liver (Fig. 23) causing a rapid fall in blood level and a non-cumulative, easily reversable neuromuscular block of short duration. Unfortunately, in the dog and in man there is relatively little metabolism of the drug, and the majority of fazadinium (70–80 per cent) is excreted in the urine.[136] As a result the drug is cumulative in man and produces a neuromuscular block of 30–50 minutes duration.

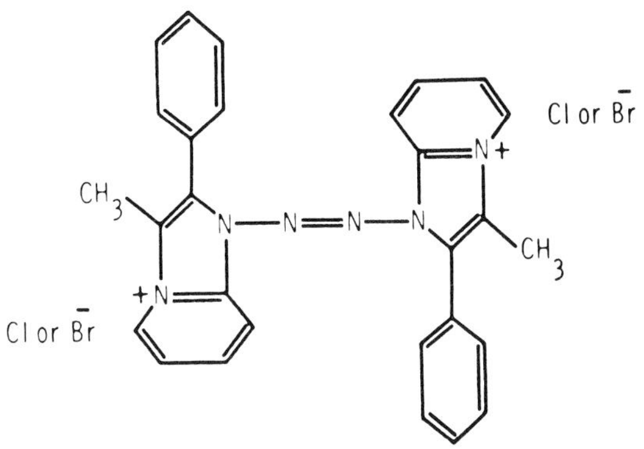


23/Fig. 22.—Fazadinium bromide.

**Dosage.**—The dose for neuromuscular block is about 1 mg/kg. However, for rapid intubation with this drug, 1·5 mg/kg is advised.

**Non-specific effects.**—Fazadinium causes vagolysis in a dose that produces only 80 per cent neuromuscular block.[113] It does not cause hypotension, although it may produce a fall in cardiac output when given during halothane anaesthesia.[137]

**Clinical uses.**—The only advantage of this drug over alternative agents is its ability to produce early relaxation of the vocal chords in doses that are 50 per cent above that required for neuromuscular block.

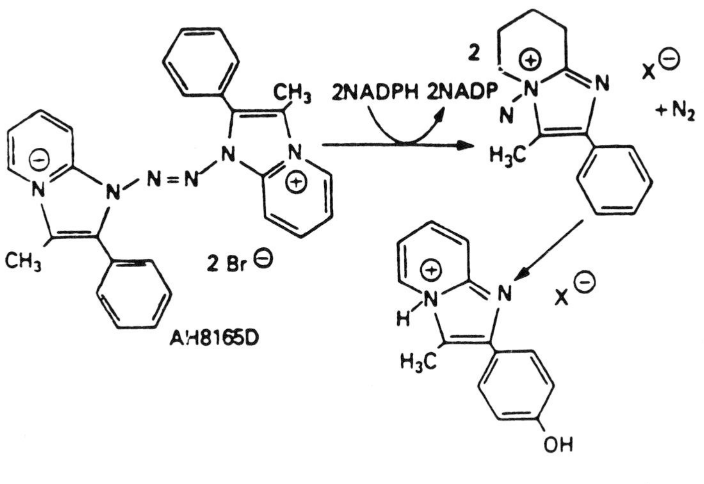


I

II

23/Fig. 23.—Hydrolysis of fazadinium by azo reductase in animals.

### Gallamine Triethiodide (Flaxedil)

#### History

Following the introduction of tubocurarine into clinical anaesthesia, pharmacologists throughout the world sought for synthetic drugs with a similar action. In 1947, Bovet[138] and his co-workers described the muscle relaxant properties of a synthetic product—gallamine triethiodide. The effects of this relaxant in man were first described by Huguenard and Boué (1948)[139] in France and by Mushin and his colleagues (1949)[140] in England.

#### Physical and Chemical Properties

Gallamine triethiodide is chemically tri-(β-diethylaminoethoxy)-benzene triethiodide with the following structural formula:

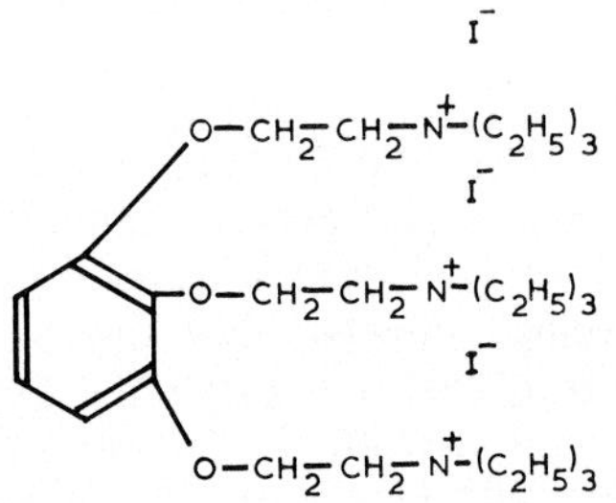


23/Fig. 24.—Structural formula of gallamine.

Ampoules of 80 mg (2 ml) and 120 mg (3 ml) are available. It is relatively stable and can be mixed with thiopentone.

#### Pharmacological Actions

**Mode of action.**—Gallamine triethiodide acts at the neuromuscular junction by non-depolarisation in a similar manner to tubocurarine.

**Cardiovascular system.**—Gallamine does not appear to have any direct action on the myocardium although it has been suggested that it reduces the incidence of cardiac dysrhythmias under cyclopropane anaesthesia.[141] It has a very marked vagal-blocking activity in the doses used in clinical anaesthesia and this factor is useful in combination with halothane, a drug which tends to stimulate this nerve. The action of gallamine on the parasympathetic system was not recognised in the early animal experiments using cats, but was described in man by Doughty and Wylie.[142] These authors noted that it occurred within 1–1½ minutes of an intravenous injection of the drug and was particularly marked in young people. The degree of tachycardia varied widely but, in over half the patients studied, showed an increase of 20–60 per cent over the control value. The rise in pulse rate is sometimes accompanied by an increase in the systemic blood pressure and cardiac output[143] The tachycardia can be abolished by both cyclopropane and halothane.

**Central nervous system.**—Like tubocurarine, there is no clear evidence available to suggest that gallamine has any action on the central nervous system in man. In animals, however, its intrathecal injection can lead to convulsions.

**Liver and kidneys.**—Gallamine has no direct action on either the liver or kidney. Indirectly, however, it has a weak inhibitory effect on the plasma cholinesterase produced by the liver.[144] Like tubocurarine it is excreted unchanged in the urine. Mushin and his colleagues[140] recovered 30 to 100 per cent of the original dose from the urine of rabbits in the two hours following its administration. Feldman and associates[145] found up to 82 per cent of the initial dose was excreted in the urine of dogs in 24 hours. It was demonstrated that in the absence of renal function there is no alternative mode of lowering the blood concentration of this drug.

A number of reports have appeared in the literature suggesting that a prolonged paresis may follow the use of gallamine in cases with poor renal function.[146–148] This is partly due to loss of redistribution sites in the kidney and also to the lack of alternative pathways of excretion for the drug[145] (Fig. 25).

Many case reports support the suggestion that the duration of action of gallamine triethiodide is prolonged in the absence of renal function.

It would appear unwise to use gallamine as the relaxant agent in the presence of poor renal function unless the total dose is less than 0·5 mg/kg.

**Histamine release.**—Courvoisier and Ducrot[151] failed to find any evidence of histamine release in dogs. Mushin and his colleagues,[140] working with the rat diaphragm preparation, found that gallamine liberated 1/5–1/2 the quantity of histamine as compared with tubocurarine.

**Uterus and placental barrier.**—There is no

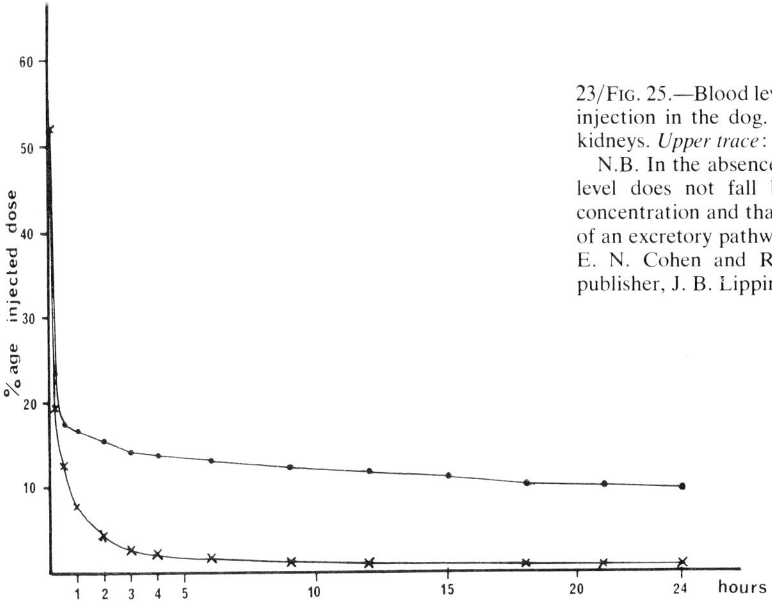

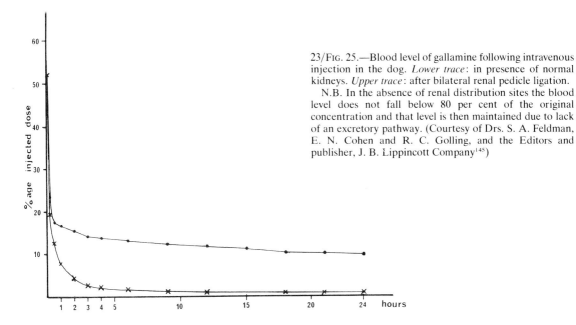

23/FIG. 25.—Blood level of gallamine following intravenous injection in the dog. *Lower trace*: in presence of normal kidneys. *Upper trace*: after bilateral renal pedicle ligation.

N.B. In the absence of renal distribution sites the blood level does not fall below 80 per cent of the original concentration and that level is then maintained due to lack of an excretory pathway. (Courtesy of Drs. S. A. Feldman, E. N. Cohen and R. C. Golling, and the Editors and publisher, J. B. Lippincott Company[145])

evidence available to suggest that gallamine influences the contractions of the pregnant uterus. Crawford[152] found direct evidence in patients undergoing forceps delivery or Caesarean section that gallamine crosses the placenta "in appreciable concentrations". Although he failed to notice any signs of paresis in the infants, gallamine was easily detectable in the cord serum. Nevertheless, Crawford was unable to find a simple relationship between the concentration of gallamine in the maternal and fetal bloods.

## Distribution

The distribution of gallamine throughout the body is illustrated in Fig. 26.

## Detoxication and Excretion

Gallamine is not detoxicated *in vivo* but is excreted unchanged in the urine. In the cat, 30–100 per cent of the total dose injected can be recovered from the urine within two hours.[140] In the dog, 82 per cent of the total dose can be

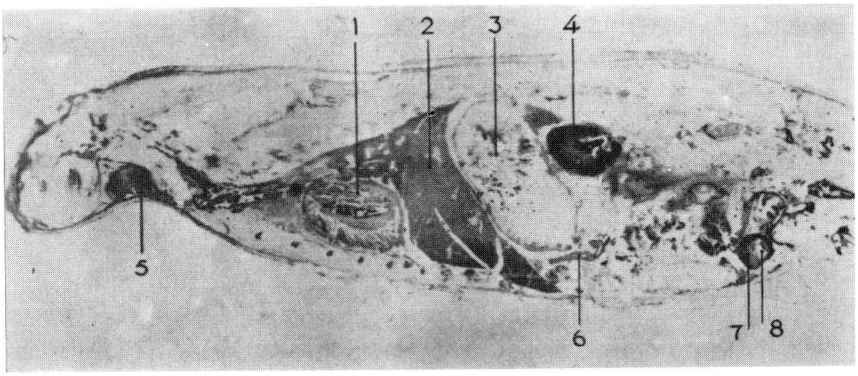


23/FIG.26.—Autoradiograph of rat sacrificed 15 minutes after intravenous injection of 2·4 mg/kg gallamine. 1, heart; 2, liver; 3, stomach; 4, kidney; 5, salivary gland; 6, intestine; 7, placenta; 8, fetus. (Courtesy of Drs. E. N. Cohen, N. Hood, R. C. Golling and the Editors and publisher, J. B. Lippincott Company[150]).

recovered from the urine in 24 hours, the majority being excreted in the first 5 hours.[145]

### Clinical use

Gallamine in a dosage of 1–1·5 mg/kg is an effective neuromuscular blocking agent. However, in view of its vagolytic action and the prolonged action in patients with poor renal function, it has few advantages over alternative agents.

### Vecuronium Bromide (Norcuron, Org NC45)

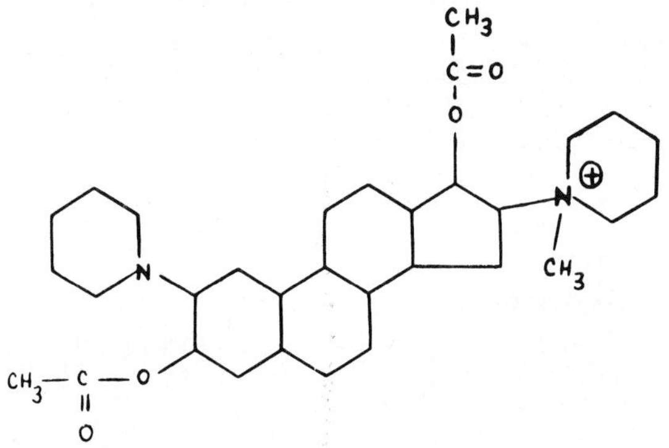

23/Fig. 27.—Structural formula of vecuronium bromide.

This agent was synthesised by Savage in 1979[26] and has been studied extensively in cats,[153] in the isolated arm of man,[14] and in man.[154–157]

Chemically the drug is the monoquaternary analogue of pancuronium. However, the stereoisometric relationship of the 3-acetyl group to the parent ring makes it structurally dissimilar. The loss of the quaternising methyl group on the molecule in the 2 position destabilises the 3 acetyl group. As a result, the solution has a short shelf-life and should be prepared in alkaline buffer solution shortly before use. The powder does not need to be kept refrigerated.

In spite of this monoquaternary structure, the drug appears to be more potent than pancuronium in man. The 90 per cent blocking dose (ED 90) of the adductor pollucis muscle is 0·03 mg/kg compared with 0·05 mg/kg for pancuronium. However, because of the brevity of its action, about 15–25 minutes (Fig. 28) when given in a dose that causes 95 per cent suppression of the twitch response, the relaxation produced by this dose is too short for most clinical purposes. It is more easily used in supraparalytic doses of 100 to 150 μg/kg. With this dose regime, 20 to 40 minutes of good surgical relaxation can be anticipated. Although it was initially claimed to be of rapid onset,

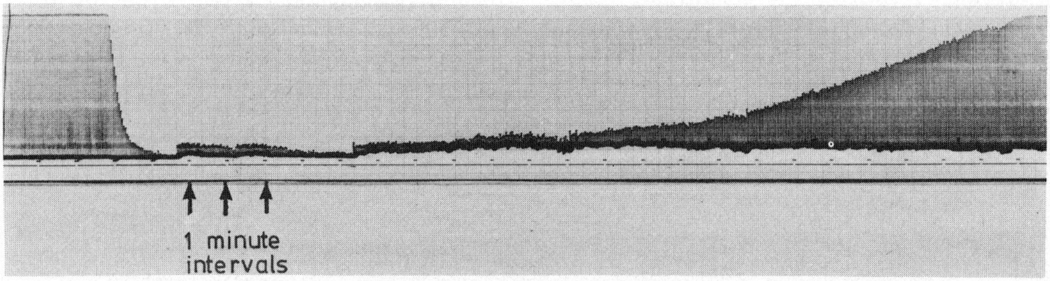


23/Fig. 28.—Recovery from vecuronium 0·04 mg/kg. Note rapid recovery 23 min. Time from 25 to 75% (RI) 5·2 min.

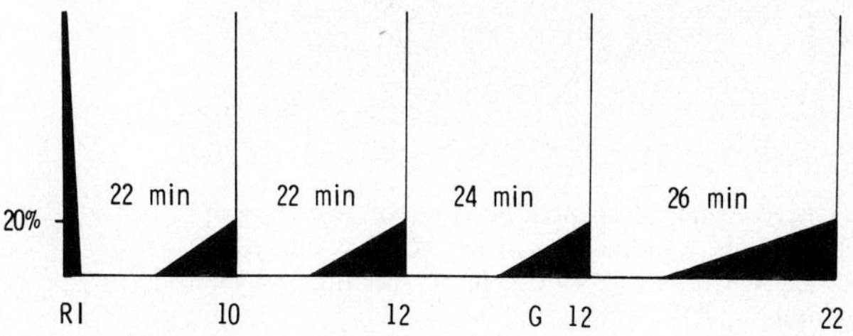


23/Fig. 29.—Diagrammatic representation of the adductor pollucis twitch response following repeated doses of vecuronium given at 20 per cent recovery of the twitch response. RI = recovery index (estimated time from 25 to 75 per cent recovery.) G = gentamicin 80 mg. i.v. causing prolongation of relaxant effect.

making it suitable for early endotracheal intubation, subsequent experience in 60 patients has demonstrated that doses of 150 μg/kg are required for consistently good intubating conditions within 2 minutes in lightly anaesthetised patients.[158] This has been confirmed in clinical practice.[165]

The principal advantages of this drug are its short duration of action in low doses, its lack of cumulative effect (Fig. 29) and its minimal cardiovascular side-effects in doses up to 20 times that required for paralysis.[159, 160, 166]

The duration of action of the drug is not affected by obstruction of hepatic blood flow or by occlusion of the renal arteries although, like pancuronium, its action is prolonged in jaundiced patients. The drug is rapidly cleared from the plasma, having a short $\alpha$ half-life compared to pancuronium. Its $\beta$ half-life, however, is similar to pancuronium. Present evidence from animal experiments suggests that biliary excretion may be an important alternative excretory pathway for this drug. Some workers have reported that up to 15 per cent of the drug appears as metabolites in the urine; however, this has not been confirmed in man. The drug has been used in anephric patients with only a minimal increase in the duration of the dose/response, causing an increase in the duration of block of about 10 per cent.[167]

Because of the lack of cumulative effects with this drug, it is possible to provide prolonged neuromuscular block by means of a continuous intravenous infusion and yet have a rapid reversal of action when the infusion is discontinued. This desirable characteristic increases the safety of a neuromuscular blocking agent as it allows a flexible duration of action and it ensures complete and safe reversibility of the drug even after many hours of relaxation. The lack of cardiovascular side-effects and the absence of histamine release make this the drug of choice for patients with autonomic and cardiac instability. Of all the neuromuscular blocking drugs available, vecuronium is the most specific for the neuromuscular junction, and therefore has the least side-effects. Because of this safety factor, it can be given in multiples of the ED 90 in order to prolong its clinical effect. Thus, in a 70 kg adult, 7 mg would be suitable for a 45-minute operation, 10 mg for an operation lasting 60 minutes, whilst 12–15 mg is likely to give 90 minutes of relaxation. Alternatively the drug can be administered in a dose of 0·1 mg/kg and the twitch response monitored. A 'top-up' dose of 0·02 mg/kg should be given when the first two twitches of the train-of-four are obvious. Failure to give the 'top-up' dose early enough produces uneven relaxation.

### ATRACURIUM (Tracrium)

This new drug (Fig. 30) whose pharmacological profile has been described by Hughes and Chapple[161] and Payne and Hughes[162] has many attractive properties. *In vitro* it is slowly hydrolysed by two separate reactions (1) Hofmann elimination* and (2) ester hydrolysis (Fig. 31). These processes have an *in vitro* half-life of 26 minutes when incubated with blood at pH 7·4.[168] The drug produces neuromuscular block of about 30–40 minutes in a fully paralytic dose of 0·5 mg/kg. Like vecuronium it is non-cumulative in repeated doses and has little effect on the cardiovascular system unless the dose is greater than 10 times that necessary to cause 90 per cent suppression of the adductor pollucis twitch response. The duration of action of atracurium is not prolonged by the absence of hepatic or renal pathways of excretion. Recent reports have suggested that owing to its rapid metabolism it may be the relaxant of choice for patients in renal failure.[163]

Unfortunately atracurium can cause the release of histamine. Although this is claimed to be less than that seen with tubocurarine, it is dose dependent and will produce flushing, bronchospasm and hypotension in a few sensitive individuals. As a result, it is recommended that a maximum dose of 0·5 mg/kg should be used. Some concern has been expressed about the tertiary amine derivative of the Hofmann degradation, as this compound will pass the blood-brain barrier and has analeptic properties in high concentrations. These concentrations are only likely to be achieved after prolonged use in anephric patients.

Atracurium is an attractive new drug which can be used as a single bolus for endoscopies

* The Hofmann elimination (degradation) is a pH sensitive splitting of quaternary ammonium into a tertiary state as a result of electron transfer. In this state the molecule of atracurium loses its neuromuscular blocking properties. The pH of atracurium in the ampoule is 3·5 and if kept at 5°C it is relatively stable. Once injected into blood at pH 7·4, Hofmann degeneration slowly occurs. It should not be mixed with thiopentone.

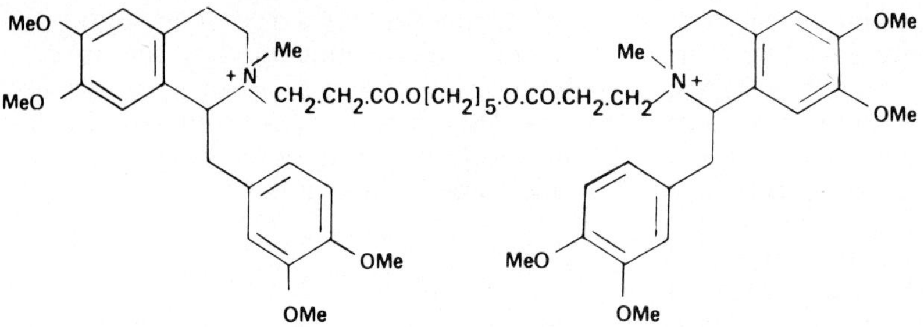


23/FIG. 30.—Structural formula of atracurium.

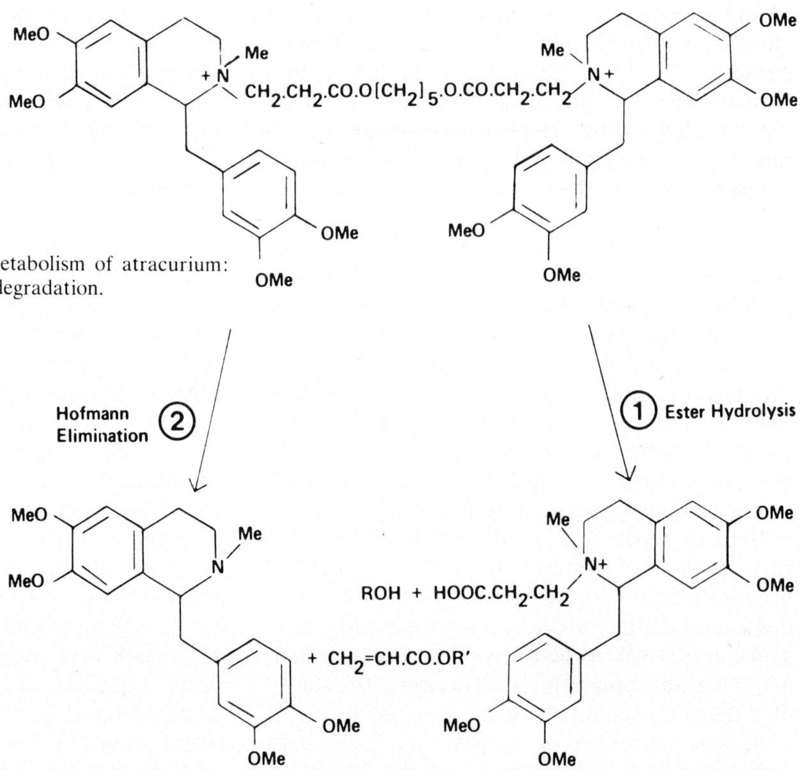


23/FIG. 31.—Two methods of metabolism of atracurium: 1. Ester hydrolysis. 2. Hofmann degradation.

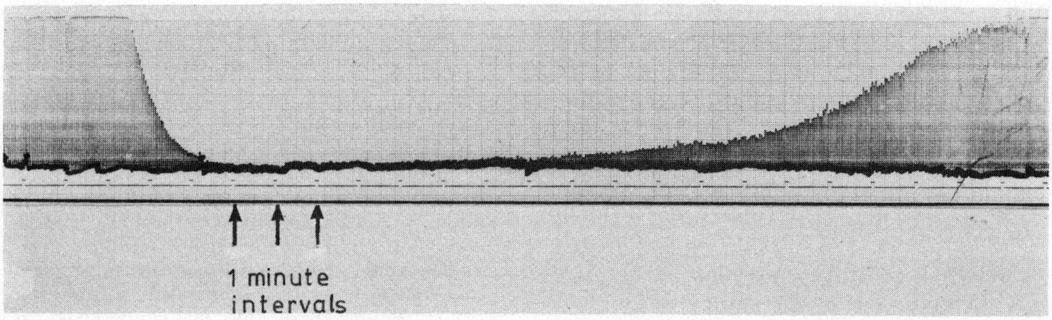


23/FIG. 32.—Recovery from atracurium 0·3 mg/kg. Note rapid rate of recovery 24 min. Time from 25 to 75% recovery (RI) 4 min.

(0·4 to 0·5 mg/kg) and short operations. It can be used as an infusion or in intermittent doses. Because of its rapid plasma clearance (short half-life) it is very predictable in use and 'top up' doses of 0·1 mg/kg are required every 10–15 min. Like vecuronium the rapid recovery from neuromuscular block causes uneven relaxation unless 'top-up' doses are given when the first two twitches of the train-of-four are obvious. It is claimed that intubation time is rapid with this drug. Under controlled conditions with light anaesthesia, the author has found 0·5 mg/kg produces good intubating conditions in 2 minutes, and this has been confirmed by Twohig, Ward and Corall.[169] Both atracurium and vecuronium are better drugs than other non-depolarising agents to give at the end of an operation when additional relaxation is required to close the abdomen.

### Pipecuronium (Arduan)

This aminosteroid (Fig. 33) has been synthesised and investigated in Hungary by Karparti and Biro[170] and Boros.[171] These workers suggest that pipecuronium is about 20 per cent more potent than pancuronium, the ED 95 dose being about 0·05 to 0·06 mg/kg. An investigation of the drug by Newton[172] confirmed this potency. The duration of action was found to be similar to that of pancuronium but without significant cardiovascular side-effects. The drug does appear to be cumulative on repeated doses when compared to vecuronium.

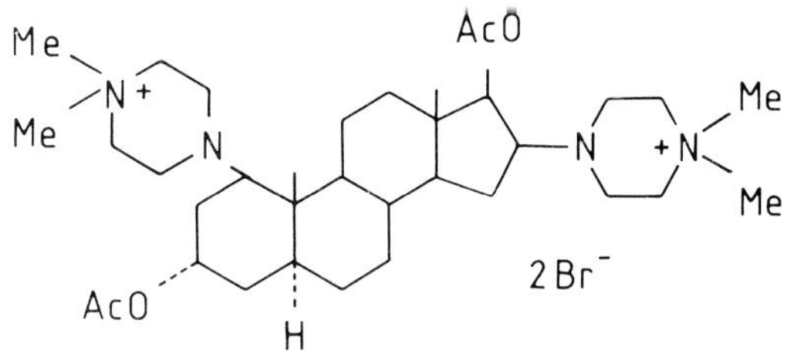

23/Fig. 33.—Pipecuronium bromide (Arduan.)

## REFERENCES


1. Buttle, G. A. M. and Zaimis, E. J. (1949). The action of decamethonium iodide in birds. *J. Pharm. (Lond.)*, **1**, 991.
2. Feldman, S. A. (1973). The relaxant-receptor reaction. In: *Muscle Relaxants*, p. 53. London: W. B. Saunders.
3. Taylor, D. B. (1959). The mechanism of action of muscle relaxants and their antagonists. *Anesthesiology*, **20**, 439.
4. Wisliski, L. and Benzakein, F. (1963). Post tetanic relief of neuromuscular block. *Arch. Int. Pharmacol.*, **142**, 23.
5. Gray, T. C. and Ali, H. (1968). In: *Progress in Anaesthesiology* (Proc. 4th World Congr. of Anaesthesiologists, London). Amsterdam: Excerpta Medica.
6. Armstrong, D. L. and Lester, H. A. (1979). The kinetics of tubocurarine action and restricted diffusion within the synaptic cleft. *J. Physiol. (Lond.)* **294**, 365.
7. Katz, R. L. and Katz, G. J. (1975). Clinical considerations in the use of the muscle relaxants. In: *Muscle Relaxants*. Ed. R. L. Katz. p. 330. Amsterdam: Excerpta Medica.
8. Baraka, A. (1967). Irreversible tubocurarine neuromuscular block in the human. *Brit. J. Anaesth.*, **39**, 891.
9. Baraka, A. (1977). Irreversible curarisation. *Anaesth. & Intensive Care*, **5**, 244.
10. Feldman, S. A. and Agoston, S. (1980). Failure of neostigmine to prevent tubocurarine neuromuscular block in the isolated arm. *Brit. J. Anaesth.*, **52**, 1199.
11. Feldman, S. A. and Tyrrell, M. F. (1970). A new theory of the termination of action of muscle relaxants. *Proc. roy. Soc. Med.*, **63**, 692.
12. Feldman, S. A. (1976). Affinity concept and the action of the muscle relaxants. *Acta anaesth. Belg.*, **27**, 89.
13. Agoston, S., Feldman, S. A. and Miller, R. D. (1979). Plasma concentrations of pancuronium and neuromuscular blockade after injection into the isolated arm, bolus injection and continuous infusion. *Anesthesiology*, **51**, 119.
14. Bencini, A., Agoston, S. and Ket, J. (1980). Use of human "isolated arm" preparation to indicate qualitative aspects of a new neuromuscular blocking agent ORG NC45. *Brit. J. Anaesth.*, **52**, 435.
15. Feldman, S. A. (1980). Clinical importance of affinity. *Abstract of the 7th World Congress of Anaesthesiologists, Hamburg*, p. 9. Amsterdam: Excerpta Medica.
16. Jenerick, H. P. and Gerard, R. W. (1953). Membrane potential and threshold of single muscle fibre. *J. cell. comp. Physiol.*, **42**, 79.
17. Katz, B. and Thesleff, S. (1957). A study of "desensitisation" produced by acetylcholine at the motor end plate. *J. Physiol. (Lond.)*, **138**, 63.
18. Standaert, F. G. and Adams, J. E. (1965). The actions of succinylcholine on the mammalian motor nerve terminal. *J. Pharmacol. exp. Ther.* **149**, 113.
19. Galindo, A. (1971). Depolarising neuromuscular block. *Pharmacol. exp. Ther.*, **178**, 339.
20. Churchill-Davidson, H. C. and Richardson, A. T. (1952). Decamethonium iodide (C10). Some observations using electromyography. *Proc. roy. Soc. Med.*, **45**, 179.
21. Paton, W. D. M. (1961). A theory of drug action based on the rate of drug-receptor combination. *Proc. roy. Soc. Biology*. **154**, 21.

22. Churchill-Davidson, H. C., Christie, T. M. and Wise, R. P. (1960). Dual neuromuscular block in man. *Brit. J. Anaesth.*, **31**, 290.
23. King, H. (1935). Curare alkaloids. I. Tubocurarine. *J. Chem. Soc.*, 1381.
24. Paton, W. D. M. and Zaimis, E. J. (1949). The pharmacological actions of polymethylene bis methylammonium salts. *Brit. J. Pharmacol. Chemother.* **4**, 381.
25. Everett, A. J., Lowe, L. A. and Wilkinson, S. (1970). Revision of the structure of (+) tubocurarine and (+) chondrocurarine. *Chem. Communications*, **16**, 1020.
26. Savage, D. S. (1979). Report to International Muscle Relaxant "Group" Meeting in Frieburg.
27. Kato, G. (1968). Nuclear magnetic resonance studies of functional transmitter-receptor substance. *Canad. Anaesth. Soc. J.*, **15**, 545.
28. Hewett, C. L. and Savage, D. S. (1968). Amino steroids (Part III) 2 and 3 amino 5 α-androstanes. *J. Chem. Soc. (C)*, 1134.
29. Viby-Mogensen, J. (1979). Residual curarisation in the recovery room. *Anesthesiology*, **50**, 528.
30. Feldman, S. A. (1980). La surveillance du bloc neuromusculaire. *Journees d'enseignement post-universitaire*, p. 337.
31. Crul, J. F., Severinghaus, J. W. and Booij, L. (1980). 7th World Congress of Anaesthesiologists—Poster session. In *Abstracts of Proceedings*, p. 539. Amsterdam: Excerpta Medica.
32. Viby-Mogensen, J. and Hanel, H. K. (1980). Demonstration Box 24. Poster session "Neuromuscular Blockade" (7th World Congr. Anaesthesiologists). In: *Abstracts of Proceedings*, p. 540. Amsterdam: Excerpta Medica.
33. Organe, G. S. W., Paton, W. D. M. and Zaimis, E. J. (1949). Bismethyl-ammonium diodide. *Lancet*, **1**, 21.
34. Organe, G. S. W. (1956). Some reflections on the muscle relaxants with special reference to decamethonium. *Canad. Anaesth. Soc. J.*, **3**, 5.
35. Bovet, D., Bovet-Nitti, F., Guarino, S., Longo, V. G. and Marotta, M. (1949). Proprieta farmacodinamiche di alcuni derivarti della succinilcolina dotatie di azione curarica. *R.C. 1st supp. Sanita*, **12**, 106.
36. Castillo, J. A. and de Beer, E. J. (1950). Neuromuscular blocking action of succinylcholine. *J. Pharmacol. exp. Ther.*, **97**, 458.
37. Thesleff, S. (1951). Pharmacologic and clinical experiments with succinylcholine iodide. *Nord. Med.*, **46**, 1045.
38. Churchill-Davidson, H. C. (1954). Suxamethonium (succinylcholine) and muscle pains. *Brit. med. J.*, **1**, 74.
39. Collier, C. (1975). Suxamethonium muscle pains and fasciculations. *Proc. roy. Soc. Med.*, **68**, 105.
40. Baraka, A. (1977). Self taming of succinylcholine-induced muscle fasciculations. *Anesthesiology*, **46**, 292.
41. Foster, C. A. (1960). Muscle pains that follow the administration of suxamethonium. *Brit. med. J.*, **2**, 25.
42. Miller, R. D. and Way, W. L. (1971). The interaction between succinylcholine and sub-paralysing doses of d-tubocurarine and gallamine in man. *Anesthesiology*, **35**, 567.
43. Haldia, K. N., Chatterji, S. and Kackar, G. N. (1974). Intravenous lignocaine for prevention of muscle pains after succinylcholine. *Anesth. Analg. (Clev.)*, **52**, 849.
44. Tammisto, T. and Airaksinen, M. (1966). Increase in creatinine-kinase activity in serum as sign of muscular injury, caused by intermittently administered suxamethonium during halothane anaesthesia. *Brit. J. Anaesth.* **38**, 510.
45. Kaufman, L. (1960). Anaesthesia in dystrophia myotonica. *Proc. roy. Soc. Med.* **62**, 1217.
46. Theil, R. E. (1967). The myotonic response to suxamethonium. *Brit. J. Anaesth.*, **39**, 815.
47. Baraka, A., Haddad, C. and Afifi, A. (1970). Control of succinylcholine induced myotonia by d-tubocurarine. *Anesthesiology*, **33**, 669.
48. Bennike, K. A. and Jarnum, S. (1964). Myoglobinuria with acute renal failure possibly induced by succinylcholine. A case report. *Brit. J. Anaesth.*, **36**, 730.
49. Ryan, F. J., Kagan, L. J. and Hyman, N. I. (1971). Myoglobinuria after a single dose of succinylcholine. *New Engl. J. Med.*, **285**, 824.
50. Airaksinen, M. M. and Tammisto (1966). Myoglobinuria after intermittent administration of succinylcholine during halothane anaesthesia. *Clin. Pharmacol. Ther.*, **7**, 583.
51. Relton, J. E. S., Creighton, R. E., Johnston, A. G., Pelton, D. A. and Conn, A. W. (1966). Hyperpyrexia associated with general anaesthesia in children. *Canad. Anaesth. Soc. J.*, **13**, 419.
52. Wilson, R. D., Dent, T. E., Traver, D. L., McCoy, N. R. and Allen, C. R. (1967). Malignant hyperpyrexia with anesthesia. *J. Amer. med. Ass.*, **202**, 183.
53. Purpura, D. P. and Grundfest, H. (1956). Blockade of cardial synapses by succinylcholine. *Science*, **124**, 319.
54. Goat, V. A. (1972). The actions of muscle relaxants on the cholinergic mechanisms in the heart. In: *Anaesthesia and Pharmaceutics*. Ed. Spierdijk and Feldman. University of Leiden Press.
55. Leigh, M. D., McCoy, D. D., Belton, M. K. and Lewis, G. B. (1957). Bradycardia following intravenous administration of succinylcholine chloride to infants and children. *Anesthesiology*, **18**, 698.
56. Mathias, J. A. and Evans-Prosser, C. D. G. (1970). An investigation into the site of action of suxamethonium on cardiac rhythm. *Progress in Anaesthesiology, 1968* (Proc. 4th World Congr. in Anaesthesiology). Amsterdam: Excerpta Medica.
57. Sorensen, O., Eriksen, S., Hommelgaard, P. and Viby-Mogensen, J. (1980). Thiopental–nitrous oxide–halothane anesthesia and repeated succinylcholine: comparison of preoperative glycopyrrolate and atropine administration. *Anesth. Analg. Curr. Res.*, **59**, 686.
58. Viby-Mogensen, J., Wisborg, K., Gabrielsen, J. and Spotoft, H. (1976). Halothane anaesthesia and suxamethonium. I. The significance of preoperative atropine administration. *Acta anaesth. Scand.*, **20**, 129.
59. Mathias, J. A., Evans-Prosser, C. D. G. and Churchill-Davidson, H. C. (1970). The role of the non-depolarising drugs in the prevention of suxamethonium bradycardia. *Brit. J. Anaesth.*, **42**, 609.
60. List, W. F. M. (1971). Succinylcholine induced cardiac arrhythmias. *Anesth. Analg. (Clev.)*, **50**, 361.
61. Wong, K. C., Whyte, S. R., Martin, W. E., Crawford, E. W. (1971). Antiarrhythmic effects of skeletal muscle relaxants. *Anesthesiology*, **34**, 458.
62. Paton, W. D. M. (1959). The effects of muscle relaxants other than muscular relaxation. *Anesthesiology*, **20** 453.
63. McCaughey, T. C. (1962). Hazards of anaesthesia for the burned child. *Canad. Anaesth. Soc. J.*, **9**, 220.
64. Bush, G. M. (1964). The use of muscle relaxants in burnt children. *Anaesthesia*, **19**, 231.

65. Tolmie, J. D., Joyce, T. H. and Mitchell, G. D. (1967). Succinylcholine danger in the burned patient. *Anesthesiology*, **28**, 467.
66. Birch, A. A., Mitchell, G. D., Playford, G. A. and Lang, C. A. (1969). Changes in serum potassium in response to succinylcholine following trauma. *J. Amer. med. Ass.* **210**, 490.
67. Mazze, R. I., Escue, H. M. and Houston, J. B. (1969). Hyperkalaemia and cardiovascular collapse following administration of succinylcholine to the traumatised patient. *Anesthesiology*, **31**, 540.
68. Stone, W. A., Beach, T. P. and Hamelberg, W. (1970). Succinylcholine danger in the spinal cord injured patient. *Anesthesiology*, **32**, 168.
69. Cooperman, L. H., Stobel, G. E. and Kennell, E. M. (1970). Massive hyperkalaemia after administration of succinylcholine. *Anesthesiology*, **32**, 164.
70. Tobey, R. E., Jacobsen, P. M., Kahle, C. T., Clubb, R. J. and Dean, N. A. (1972). The serum potassium response to muscle relaxants in neural injury. *Anesthesiology*, **37**, 332.
71. Kohlshutter, B., Baur, H. and Roth, F. (1976). Suxamethonium induced hyperkalaemia in patients with severe abdominal infection. *Brit. J. Anaesth.*, **48**, 557.
72. Roth, F. and Wuthrich, H. (1969). The clinical importance of hyperkalaemia following suxamethonium administration. *Brit. J. Anaesth.*, **41**, 311.
73. Miller, R. D., Way, W. L., Hamilton, W. K., Layzer, R. B. (1972). Succinylcholine induced hyperkalaemia in patients with renal failure. *Anesthesiology*, 36, 138.
74. Pandey, K., Badola, R. P. and Kumar, S. (1972). Time course of intraocular hypertension produced by suxamethonium. *Brit. J. Anaesth.*, **44**, 191.
75. Miller, R. D., Way, W. L. and Hickey, R. F. (1968). Inhibition of succinylcholine induced increased intraocular pressure by non-depolarising muscle relaxants. *Anesthesiology*, 29, 123.
76. Katz, R. L. and Eakins, K. E. (1969). The actions of neuromuscular blocking agents on extraocular muscle and intraocular pressure. *Proc. roy. Soc. Med.*, **62**, 1217.
77. Meyers, E. F., Krupin, T., Johnson, H. and Zink, H. (1978). Failure of non-depolarising neuromuscular blockers to inhibit succinylcholine-induced increased intraocular pressure. A controlled study. *Anesthesiology*, **48**, 149.
78. Miller, R. D. and Way, W. L. (1971). Inhibition of succinylcholine induced increased intragastric pressure by non-depolarising muscle relaxants and lidocaine. *Anesthesiology*, **34**, 185.
79. Mandappa, J. M., Chandrastetchava, D. N. and Nelvigi, R. G. (1975). Anaphylaxis to suxamethonium. *Brit. J. Anaesth.*, **47**, 523.
80. Kalow, W. and Davies, R. O. (1958). The activity of various esterase inhibitors towards atypical human serum cholinesterase. *Biochem. Pharmacol.*, **1**, 183.
81. Schnider, S. M. (1965). Serum cholinesterase activity during pregnancy, labour and puerperium. *Anesthesiology*, **26**, 335.
82. Oropollo, A. T. (1978). Abnormal pseudocholinesterase levels in a surgical population. *Anesthesiology*, **48**, 284.
83. Robertson, G. S. (1966). Serum cholinesterase deficiency. II: Pregnancy. *Brit. J. Anaesth.*, **38**, 361.
84. Wildsmith, J. A. W. (1972). Serum pseudocholinesterase, pregnancy and suxamethonium. *Anaesthesia*, **27**, 90.
85. Robertson, G. S. (1967). Serum proteins and cholinesterase changes in association with contraceptive pills. *Lancet*, **1**, 232.
86. Stead, A. L. (1955). The response of the newborn infant to muscle relaxants. *Brit. J. Anaesth.*, **27**, 124.
87. Cook, D. R. and Fischer, C. G. (1975). Neuromuscular blocking effects of succinylcholine in infants and children. *Anesthesiology*, **42**, 662.
88. McGavin, D. D. M. (1965). Depressed levels of serum pseudocholinesterase with ecothiopate iodide eye drops. *Lancet*, **2**, 272.
89. Pantuck, E. J. (1966). Ecothiopate iodide eye drops and prolonged response to suxamethonium. *Brit. J. Anaesth.*, **38**, 406.
90. Cavellero, R. J., Krumperman, L. W. and Kugler, F. (1968). Effect of echothiopate therapy on the metabolism of succinylcholine in man. *Anesth. Analg. Curr. Res.*, **47**, 570.
91. Hofstee, B. H. J. (1960). Mechanism of action of bivalent metal ions and of phenothiazine derivatives on serum cholinesterase. *J. Pharmacol. exp. Ther.*, **128**, 299.
92. Zsigmond, E. K. and Robins, G. (1972). The effect of a series of anticancer drugs on plasma cholinesterase activity. *Canad. Anaesth. Soc. J.*, **19**, 75.
93. Gurman, G. M. (1972). Prolonged apnoea after succinylcholine in a case treated with cytotoxics for cancer. *Anesth. Analg. Curr. Res.*, **51**, 761.
94. Schuh, F. T. (1975). Influence of ketamine on human plasma cholinesterase. *Brit. J. Anaesth.*, **47**, 1315.
95. Poulton, T. J., James, F. M. and Lockridge, O. (1979). Prolonged apnea following trimetaphan and succinylcholine. *Anesthesiology*, **50**, 54.
96. King, J. (1976). Inhibition of cholinesterase by pancuronium. *Brit. J. Anaesth.* **48**, 712.
97. Taussig, P. E., Stojak, H. E. and Bennett, N. R. (1979). *In vitro* interaction of propanidid and suxamethonium with pooled human plasma cholinesterase. *Brit. J. Anaesth.*, **51**, 181.
98. Motulsky, A. G. (1964). Progress in medical genetics. In: *Pharmacogenetics*. Ed. Steinberg and Bearn. New York and London: Grune and Stratton.
99. Kalow, W. and Genest, K. (1957). A method for the detection of atypical forms of human serum cholinesterase determination of dibucaine numbers. *Canad. J. Biochem.*, **35**, 339.
100. Harris, H. and Whittaker, M. (1961). Differential inhibition of human serum cholinesterase with fluoride; recognition of two new phenotypes. *Nature (Lond.)* **191**, 496.
101. Liddell, J., Lehman, M. and Silk, E. (1962). A silent pseudocholinesterase gene. *Nature (Lond.)*, **193**, 561.
102. Smith, S. E. (1976). Neuromuscular blocking drugs in man. In: *Handbook of Experimental Pharmacology*, New Series. Ed. G. V. R. Born, O. Eichler, A. Farah, H. Herken and A. D. Welch. (Vol. 42, Editor) E. Zaimis. Berlin: Springer Verlag.
103. Viby-Mogensen, J. and Hanel, H. K. (1978). Prolonged apnoea after suxamethonium. *Acta anaesth. Scand.*, **22**, 371.
104. Harris, H., Hopkinson, D. A., Robson, E. B. and Whittaker, M. (1963). Genetical studies on a new variant of serum cholinesterase detected by electrophoresis. *Ann. hum. Genet.*, **26**, 359.
105. Vickers M. D. A. (1963). The mismanagement of suxamethonium apnoea. *Brit. J. Anaesth.*, **35**, 260.

106. Hunter, A. R. (1966). Suxamethonium apnoea. *Anaesthesia*, **21**, 325.
107. Doenicke, A., Schmidinger, S. and Krumey, I. (1968). Suxamethonium and serum cholinesterase. Comparative studies in man *in vitro* and *in vivo* on the catabolism of suxamethonium. *Brit. J. Anaesth.*, **40**, 834.
108. Stovner, J. (1976). *Newer aspects of reversing neuromuscular block*. VI: World Congress of Anesthesiologists, Mexico.
109. Cohen, E. N., Brewer, N. H. and Smith, D. C. (1967). The metabolism and elimination of d-tubocurarine-$H^3$. *Anesthesiology*, **28**, 309.
110. Miller, R. D., Matteo, R. S., Benet, L. Z. and Sohn, Y. J. (1977). The pharmacokinetics of d-tubocurarine in man without renal failure. *J. Pharmacol. exp. Ther.*, **202**, 1.
111. Farmer, B. C. and Sivarajan, M. (1979). Anaphylactoid response to a small dose of d-tubocurarine. *Anesthesiology*, **51**, 358.
112. Johnson, M., Mahmoud, A. A. and Mrozinski, R. A. (1978). Cardiovascular effects of tubocurarine in man. *Anaesthesia*, **33**, 587.
113. Hughes, R. and Chapple, D. J. (1976). Effects of non-depolarising neuromuscular blocking agents on peripheral autonomic mechanisms in cats. *Brit. J. Anaesth.* **48**, 59.
114. Sávarese, J. J., Ali, H. H. and Antonio, R. P. (1977). The clinical pharmacology of metacurarine, dimethyltubocurarine revisited. *Anesthesiology*, **47**, 277.
115. Baird, W. L. M. and Reid, A. M. (1967). The neuromuscular blocking properties or a new steroid compound, pancuronium bromide. *Brit. J. Anaesth.*, **39**, 775.
116. Harrison, G. A. (1972). The cardiovasculur effects and some relaxant properties of four relaxants in patients about to undergo cardiac surgery. *Brit. J. Anaesth.* **44**, 485.
117. Agoston, S., Kersten, U. W. and Meijer, D. K. F. (1973). The fate of pancuronium bromide in the cat. *Acta anaesth. scand.*, **17**, 129.
118. Somogyi, A. A., Shanks, C. A. and Triggs, E. J. (1976). Clinical pharmacokinetics of pancuronium bromide. *Eur. J. Clin. Pharmacol.* **10**, 367.
119. Agoston, S., Vermeer, G. A., Kerstein, U. W. and Scaf, A. H. J. (1976). Renal and hepatic elimination of gallamine triethiodide in man. In *Disposition and Effects of Some Non-depolarising Neuromuscular Blocking Agents*. Thesis. Univ. of Groningen.
120. Miller, R. D., Agoston, S., Booij, L. H. D., Kersten, U. W., Crul, J. F. and Ham, J. (1978). The comparative potency and pharmacokinetics of pancuronium and its metabolites in anesthetised man. *J. Pharmacol. exp. Ther.*, **207**, 539.
121. Buzello, W. (1975). Der Stoffweschel von Pancuronium beim. *Menochem. Der Anaesthetist*, **24**, 13.
122. Somogyi, A. A., Shanks, C. A. and Triggs, E. J. (1977). Disposition kinetics of pancuronium bromide in patients with total biliary obstruction. *Brit. J. Anaesth.*, **49**, 1103.
123. Westra, P., Houwertjes, M. C., de Lange, A. R., Scaf, A. H. J., Hindricks, F. R. and Agoston, S. (1980). The effect of experimental cholestasis on muscle relaxants in cats. In: *Cholestasis and Muscle Relaxants* P. Westra, publ. University of Groningen Thesis.
124. Abrams, R. E. and Hornbein, T. F. (1975). Inability to reverse pancuronium blockade in a patient with renal failure and hepatic disease. *Anesthesiology*, **42**, 362.
125. McLeod, K., Watson, M. J. and Rawlings, M. D. (1975). Plasma concentrations of pancuronium bromide in patients with normal and impaired renal function. *Brit. J. Anaesth.*, **47**, 902.
126. Rouse, J. M., Galley, R. L. A. and Bevan, D. R. (1977). Prolonged curarisation following renal transplantation. *Anaesthesia*, **32**, 247.
127. Havill, J. H., Mee, A. D., Wallace, M. R., Chin, L. S. and Rothwell, R. P. (1978). Prolonged curarisation in the presence of renal impairment. *Anaesth. Intensive Care*, **6**, 234.
128. Heath, M. L. (1973). Bronchospasm in an asthmatic patient following pancuronium. *Anaesthesia*, **28**, 437.
129. Goat, V. A. and Feldman, S. A. (1972). The effect of non-depolarising muscle relaxants on cholinergic mechanisms in the isolated rabbit heart. *Anaesthesia*, **27**, 143.
130. Duke, P. C., Fung, J. and Gartner, J. (1975). The myocardial effects of pancuronium. *Canad. Anaesth. Soc. J.*, **22**, 680.
131. Coleman, A. J., Downing, J. W., Leary, W. P., Moyes, D. G. and Styles, M. (1972). The immediate cardiovascular effects of pancuronium, alcuronium and tubocurarine in man. *Anaesthesia*, **127**, 415.
132. Ivankovitch, A. D., Miletich, D. J., Albrecht, R. F. and Zahed, B. (1975). The effect of pancuronium on myocardial contraction and catecholamine metabolism. *J. Pharm. Pharmacol*, **27**, 837.
133. Salt, P. J., Barnes, P. K. and Conway, C. M. (1980). Inhibition of neuronal uptake of noradrenaline in the isolated perfused rat heart by pancuronium and its homologs ORG 6368, ORG 7268 and NC45. *Brit. J. Anaesth.*, **52**, 313.
134. Hugin, W. and Kissling, P. (1961). Preliminary reports on a new short-acting relaxant of the depolarisation-inhibiting type Ro4-38161. *Schweiz. med. Wschr.*, **91**, 455.
135. Lund, I. and Stovner, J. (1962). Experimental and clinical experiences with a new muscle relaxant, Ro. 4-3816 diallyl rev-toxiferine. *Acta anaesth. scand.*, **6**, 85.
136. Blogg, C. E., Savege, T. M., Simpson, J. C., Ross, L. A. and Simpson, B. R. (1973). A new muscle relaxant—AM.8165. *Proc. roy. Soc. Med.*, **66**, 1023.
137. Savage, T. M., Blogg, C. E. and Simpson, B. R. (1973). Initial experience with AH 8165D, a new rapidly acting muscle relaxant. *Anaesthesia*, **28**, 338.
138. Bovet, D., Depierre, F. and de Lestrange, Y. (1947). Proprietes curarisantes des ethers phenoliques a fonctions ammonium quaternaires. *C.R. Acad. Sci. (Paris)* **225**, 74.
139. Huguenard, P. and Boué, A. (1948). Un nouvel orthocurare francias de synthese le 3697 RP. *Rapport à la Soc. d'Anesthesie de Paris. Seance du 17.*
140. Mushin, W. W., Wien, R., Mason, D. F. J. and Langston, G. T. (1949). Curare-like actions of tri(dimethylamino-ethoxy)-benzine triethiodide. *Lancet*, **1**, 726.
141. Riker, W. F. and Wescoe, W. C. (1951). Pharmacology of Flaxodil with observations on certain analogs. *Ann. N. Y. Med. Sc.*, **54**, 373.
142. Doughty, A. G. and Wylie, N. D. (1951). An assessment of Flaxedil (gallamine triethiodide). *Proc. roy. Soc. Med.*, **44**, 375.
143. Kennedy, B. R. and Farman, J. V. (1968). Cardio-

vascular effects of gallamine triethiodide in man. *Brit. J. Anaesth.*, **40**, 773.

144. Vincent, D. and Parant, M. (1954). Action des alcoloides des curares sur les cholinesterases. *Bull. Soc. Chim. biol. (Paris)*, **36**, 405.

145. Feldman, S. A., Cohen, E. N. and Golling, R. C. (1969). The excretion of gallamine in the dog. *Anesthesiology*, **30**, 593.

146. Fairley, H. B. (1950). Prolonged intercostal paralysis due to a relaxant. *Brit. med. J.*, **2**, 986.

147. Montgomery, J. B. and Bennett-Jones, N. (1956). Gallamine triethiodide and renal disease. *Lancet*, **2**, 1243.

148. Feldman, S. A. and Levi, J. A. (1963). Prolonged paresis following gallamine. *Brit. J. Anaesth.*, **35**, 804.

149. Churchill-Davidson, H. C., Way, W. L. and de Jong, R. H. (1967). The muscle relaxants and renal excretion. *Anesthesiology*, **28**, 540.

150. Cohen, E. N., Hood, N. and Golling, R. (1968). Use of whole-body autoradiography for determination of uptake and distribution of labeled muscle relaxants in the rat. *Anesthesiology*, **29**, 987.

151. Courvoisier, S. and Ducrot, R. (1948). Sur l'effect histaminoide de la d-tubocurarine et des curares de synthese. *C. R. Soc. Biol. (Paris)*, **142**, 1209.

152. Crawford, J. S. (1956). Some aspects of obstetric anaesthesia. *Brit. J. Anaesth.* **28**, 146.

153. Durant, N. N., Marshall, I. G., Savage, D. S., Nelson, D. J., Sleigh, T. and Carlyle, I. C. (1979). The neuromuscular and autonomic blocking activities of pancuronium ORG NC45 and other pancuronium analogues in the cat. *J. Pharm. Pharmacol.*, **31**, 831.

154. Baird, W. L. M. and Herd, D. (1980). A new neuromuscular blocking drug ORG NC45, *Brit. J. Anaesth.*, **52**, 615.

155. Crul, J. F. and Booij, L. H. D. J. (1980). First clinical experiences with ORG NC45. *Brit. J. Anaesth.*, **52**, 595.

156. Krieg, N., Crul, J. F., Booij, L. H. D. J. (1980). Relative potency of ORG NC45, pancuronium, alcuronium and tubocurarine in anaesthetised man. *Brit. J. Anaesth.*, **52**, 783.

157. Savage, D. S. (1980). Mechanism of action of muscle relaxants and relationship between structure and activity. In *Curares and Curarisation*, p. 21. Amsterdam: Excerpta Medica.

158. Harrison, P. and Feldman, S. A. (1981). Intubating conditions with ORG NC45 (Norcuron). A preliminary study. *Anaesthesia*, **36**, 874.

159. Barnes, P. K. (1981). *Cardiovascular effects of ORG NC45 and pancuronium*. Presented to N.W. Soc. Anaesthetists. London.

160. Fahey, M. R., Morris, R. B., Miller, R. D., Sohn, Y. J., Cronnelly, R. and Gencarelli, P. (1981). Clinical pharmacology of ORG NC45 (Norcuron$^{TM}$). A new non-depolarizing muscle relaxant. *Anesthesiology*, **55**, 6.

161. Hughes, R. and Chapple, D. J. (1981). The pharmacology of Atracurium. A new competitive neuromuscular blocking agent. *Brit. J. Anaesth.*, **53**, 31.

162. Payne, J. P. and Hughes, R. (1981). Evaluation of atracurium in anaesthetised man. *Brit. J. Anaesth.*, **53**, 45.

163. Hunter, J. M., Jones, R. S., Utting, J. E. (1982). Use of the muscle relaxant atracurium in anephric patients: preliminary communication. *J. roy. Soc. Med.*, **75**, 336.

164. Ali, H. H., Wilson, R. S., Savarese, J. J. and Kitz, R. J. (1975). The effect of tubocurarine on indirectly elicited train-of-four muscle response and respiratory measurements in humans. *Brit. J. Anaesth.*, **47**, 570.

165. Kerr, J. W. and Baird, W. L. W. (1982). Clinical studies of ORG NC45. Comparison with pancuronium. *Brit. J. Anaesth.*, **54**, 1159.

166. Morris, R. B., Cahalan, M. K., Miller, R. D., Wilkinson, P. L., Quasha, A. L. and Robinson, S. L. (1983). The cardiovascular effects of vecuronium (ORG NC45) and pancuronium in patients undergoing coronary artery bypass grafting. *Anesthesiology*, **58**, 438.

167. Fahey, M. R., Morris, R. B., Miller, R. D., Nguyen, T. L., and Upton, R. A. (1981). Pharmacokinetics of ORG NC45 (Norcuron) in patients with and without renal failure. *Brit. J. Anaesth.*, **53**, 1049.

168. Marret, R. A., Thompson, C. N. and Webb, F. W. (1983). *In vitro* degeneration of atracurium in human plasma. *Brit. J. Anaesth.*, **55**, 61.

169. Twohig, M. M., Ward, S. and Corall, I. M. (1983). Conditions for tracheal intubation using atracurium compared with pancuronium. *Brit. J. Anaesth.*, **55**, 87S.

170. Karparti, E. and Biro, K. (1980). Pharmacological study of a new competitive neuromuscular blocking steroid: pipecuronium bromide. *Drug Research*, **30** (1), 346.

171. Boros, M. (1983). More information about pipecuronium; a new neuromuscular blocking agent. *Anesthesiology*, **58**, 108.

172. Newton, D. E. F., Richardson, E. J. and Agoston, S. (1982). Preliminary studies with pipecuronium bromide (Arduan). A new steroid muscle relaxant. *Brit. J. Anaesth.*, **54**, 789.

## FURTHER READING

Agoston, S. (1983). *Clinical experiences with Norcuron*. Amsterdam: Excerpta Medica.

Durant, N. (1982). Norcuron, a new non-depolarising neuromuscular blocking agent. *Seminars in Anaesthesia*, Vol. **1**, No. 1, page 47.

Lim, M. and Churchill-Davidson, H. C. (1981). Adverse effects of neuromuscular blocking drugs. In *Adverse Reactions of Anaesthetic Drugs*. Ed. J. A. Thornton. Ch. 4. Amsterdam: Excerpta Medica/Elsevier North-Holland Biomedical Press.

Viby-Mogensen, J. (1982). *Cholinesterase and succinylcholine*. Laegeforeningens forlag.

CHAPTER 24

# Factors Affecting Neuromuscular Block



## Pharmacokinetics

An appreciation of the drug receptor reaction—pharmacodynamics—allows us to understand some of the factors that determine how neuromuscular block is produced when a muscle-relaxant drug is administered to a patient. It will also explain why differing degrees of block may be produced when the same amount of drug is given to different patients, even though the plasma levels of drug may be similar. Clearly a patient with a reduced margin of safety for neuromuscular transmission will require less drug to achieve the same degree of block and it is this effect that underlies the different degree of sensitivity seen in the normal population.[1] However, in most normal people the most important factor in determining the *extent* of the neuromuscular block produced by a given dose of drug will be the number of molecules of the drug that penetrate the synaptic cleft following injection. In the absence of altered sensitivity, it is this peak concentration in the synaptic cleft, which parallels the plasma concentration obtained in the first few minutes following injection, that determines the *amount* of block produced. Figure 1 demonstrates that the effective neuromuscular blocking concentration of tubocurarine falls rapidly in the first few minutes after injection.

The *duration* of neuromuscular block is determined by the affinity of the drug for the receptor. However, other factors such as the rate of acetylcholine production and, more importantly, the ease with which the drug can leave the receptor area and diffuse away along a concentration gradient, will determine the duration of action in most clinical situations. The importance of the concentration gradient between the blood and the receptor was demonstrated by Agoston, Feldman and Miller.[2] By using three different techniques of administration of pancuronium they produced an approximately 3-fold variation in the concentration gradient between the receptor and the blood. At 50 per cent neuromuscular block, it will be observed that the blood levels ranged from 0·5 μg/ml to 0·14 μg/ml depending upon how

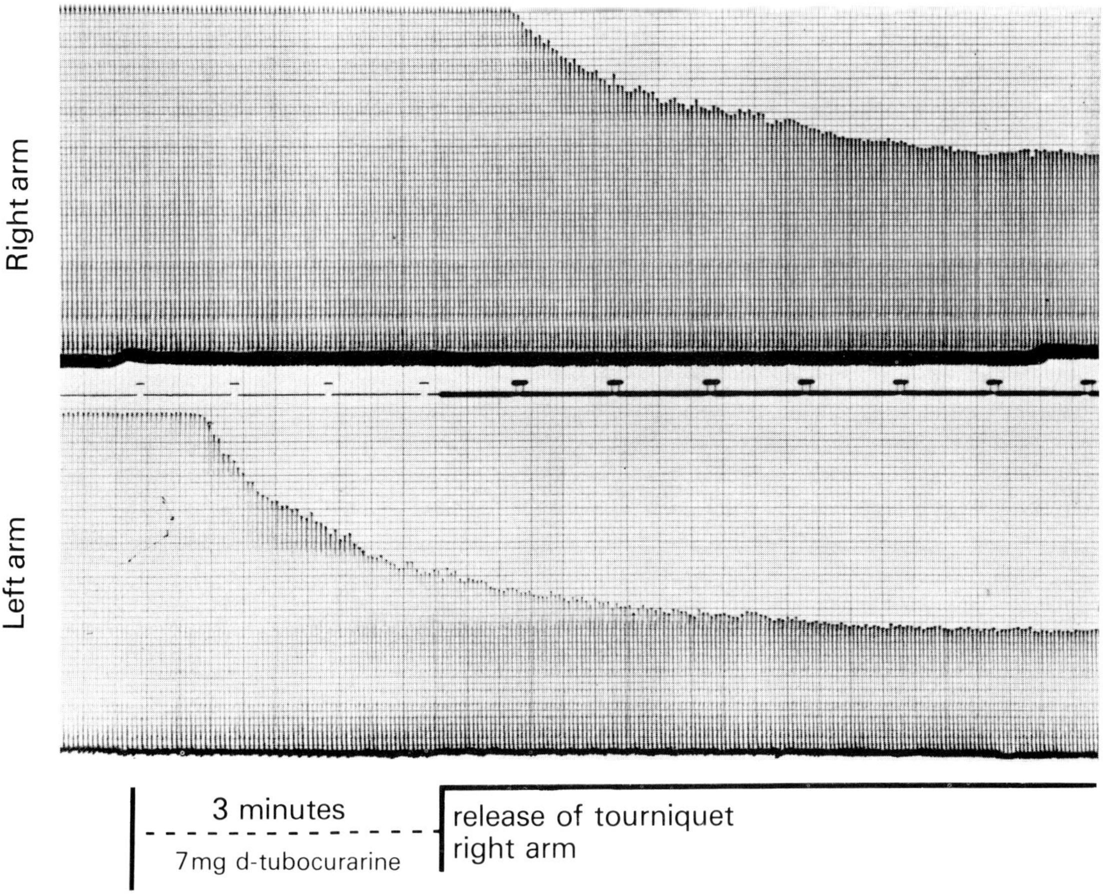


24/FIG. 1.—The effect of 7 mg of tubocurarine when injected systemically to compare twitch response in both hands. *Lower trace*: the blood flow is unimpeded, so the initial bolus leads to a high plasma concentration with resulting paralysis. *Upper trace*: the blood flow to the arm has been occluded (before the injection) for 3 minutes. Note the lesser degree of block when the tourniquet is released, due to the lowered concentration of tubocurarine in the plasma.

it had been produced. This resulted in a 4-fold increase in the time it took for the twitch to recover from 25 per cent to 75 per cent of its control height (Fig. 2). This demonstrates that although the plasma level of drug does not necessarily parallel the degree of block, it does play an important role in determining the blood receptor concentration gradient and so determining the rate of recovery from non-depolarising neuromuscular block in most clinical situations. Following neuromuscular block the receptor affinity of drug limits the recovery time (Fig. 3A). However, it can be shown that in similar fit individuals following a bolus injection of drug there is a good correlation between plasma level and the twitch height.[3–5] This correlates with Fig. 3B. Using a continuous infusion technique of drug administration where a state approaching equilibrum is achieved between the molecules of drug in the blood and receptor site, the blood level will control the amount of block produced.[6] This is represented by Fig. 3C. It is important therefore to understand those factors that control the blood level following the injection of a neuromuscular blocking agent in order to understand the factors controlling (a) the amount of block achieved and (b) the duration of its action. This is the study of pharmacokinetics.

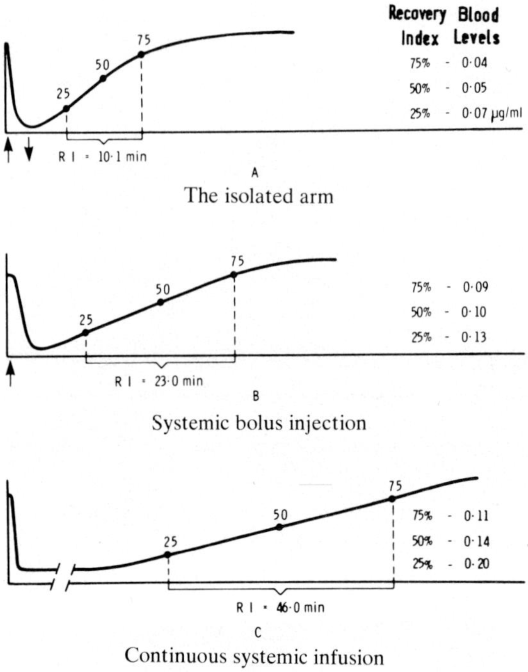


24/Fig. 2.—It will be observed that in the isolated arm experiment (A), the rapid fall in plasma concentration following release of the tourniquet results in a much quicker recovery, particularly when compared with the higher plasma concentration achieved with continuous systemic infusion (C). There is a three-fold difference in plasma levels of pancuronium at recovery to 50 per cent of the control twitch response. This corresponds with a four-fold variation in the Recovery Index (time for recovery of twitch response from 25–75 per cent). (Agoston *et al.*, 1979.[2])

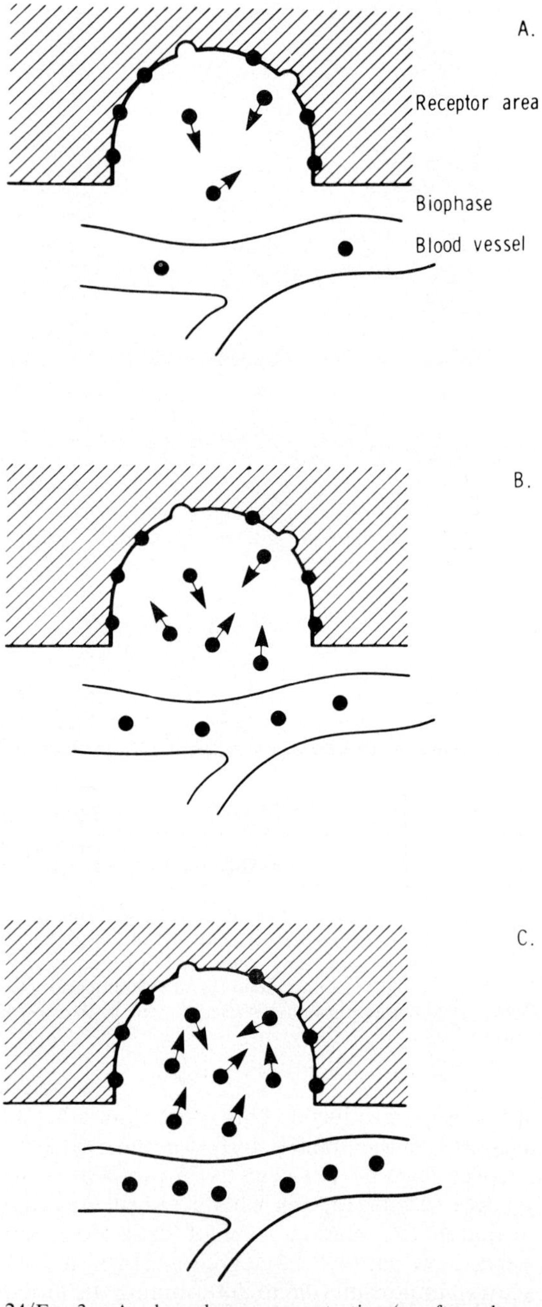


24/Fig. 3.—A – low plasma concentration (as after release of tourniquet in the isolated arm experiment); B – higher level following bolus injection; C – following a continuous infusion, very high plasma levels occur. Whilst pharmacodynamic forces remove pancuronium from the receptor, the blood concentration gradient determines the rate at which displaced molecules leave the receptor site and hence recovery from neuromuscular block. This explains the prolongation of the RI in the presence of high plasma levels.

**Distribution Volumes** (Fig. 4)

Once a drug is injected into the blood it will be rapidly distributed in the primary ($\alpha$) distribution volume. This distribution volume is about 4–7 litres in a 70 kg person; it is about twice the plasma volume but half the total e.c.f. volume. Although this volume does not correlate with any physiological volume, it does give a unit a measurement which allows us to compare one drug with another, or the effect of pathological circumstances upon different drugs. It is the effect of distribution in this volume that determines the peak plasma level of drug, which in turn affects the synaptic cleft concentration and hence the amount of neuromuscular block produced. Factors that increase the size of this compartment ($\alpha$ distribution volume) will lower the effective peak concen-

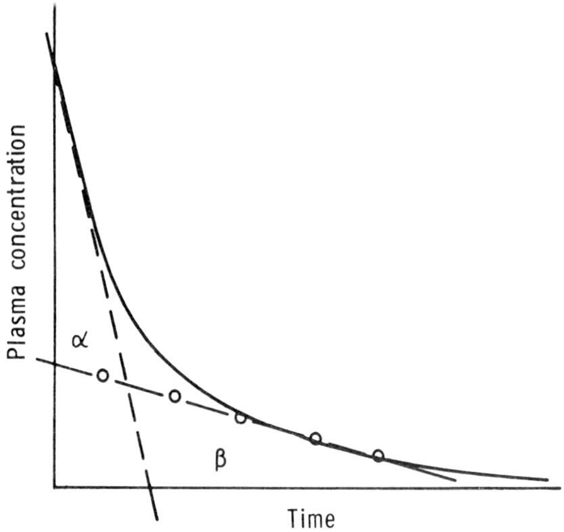


24/FIG. 4.—The $\alpha$ and $\beta$ distribution volumes can be derived from the plasma decay curve of a drug.

tration in the synaptic cleft and reduce the effectiveness of a given dose of drug. As the plasma concentration of drug is falling rapidly during the $\alpha$ phase—indeed its half-life (time to achieve a 50 per cent decrease in concentration) is about 3–4 minutes for most non-depolarising relaxants—anything that increases the muscle perfusion during this period will cause the neuromuscular junction to be exposed to a higher concentration of drug.

Redistribution from the primary ($\alpha$) distribution volume to the second, third and subsequent compartments starts once the drug has reached the blood, but due to the long time-constants for these processes they continue long after the $\alpha$ distribution phase has been completed. In theory, there are as many redistribution compartments as there are organs of the body, as the rate of drug uptake by each organ will depend upon its blood flow and the ability of that organ to sequestrate the drug.[7] In practice, it is usual to consider them as being of two main types: those with good perfusion and drug solubility, like muscle, liver and kidney, and those with poor perfusion and poor affinity, like fat (Fig. 5). Together they constitute the large ultimate non-active receptor volume into which the drug passes along a concentration gradient from the $\alpha$-volume. Metabolism (of some relaxants) and excretion of most muscle relaxants starts simultaneously with this redistribution process. These three factors determine the size of the $\beta$ distribution volume. Thus the size of the redistribution volume, together with metabolism and excretion, determine the rate at which the plasma level of drug falls and hence the concentration gradient between the receptor site and the plasma. This in turn has an important effect on controlling the rate of recovery from the neuromuscular block.

These useful pharmacokinetic concepts allow mathematical analysis and prediction of the effectiveness of given doses of drugs and the duration of recovery from their effects in a particular set of carefully controlled circumstances. However, it is important to realise that the distribution volumes do not represent actual body compartments nor any particular tissues of the body, and that physiological and pathological changes may affect them greatly. To extrapolate from formulae derived from the volumes calculated from this kind of analysis carried out under controlled circumstances, in order to determine the dose of drug required in patients in clinical practice, will inevitably lead to errors and dangers. It is more useful for the clinical anaesthetist to think in physiological and clinical terms when considering the factors affecting the *amount* of block that is likely to be produced following administration of a neu-

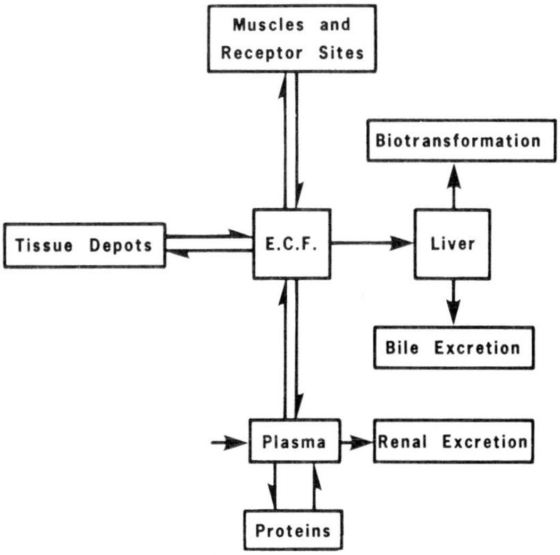


24/FIG. 5.—Redistribution of muscle relaxants occurs to sites with good perfusion, to tissue depots and sequestration to protein.

romuscular blocking agent, and the conditions which will affect the *duration* of its action.

## FACTORS AFFECTING AMOUNT OF BLOCK

As the plasma concentration will vary inversely with the size of the $\alpha$-distribution volume, factors altering the physical size of this compartment will affect the peak synaptic concentration of drug and hence the amount of block. Hydration, haemorrhage and factors affecting regional blood flow are important in this respect, as is plasma protein binding.

### Primary Distribution Volume

The most dramatic way to demonstrate the primary distribution volume for the muscle relaxants is by whole-body autoradiography. Cohen and colleagues[8] demonstrated that following administration of the drug it rapidly appeared in the highest concentration in the kidneys, although by virtue of its mass the largest amount has sequestrated in the liver and spleen (Fig. 6). This was similar for all the muscle relaxants studied (tubocurarine, gallamine and decamethonium). The redistribution shown by sacrificing the animal later than 5 minutes was mainly to the muscles. However, significant amounts of tubocurarine were found in the gut and salivary glands, and gallamine demonstrated an affinity for the mucopolysaccharide of cartilage.

These experiments emphasise the importance of the liver, the spleen and kidneys as rapid sequestration sites for neuromuscular blocking agents. Any reduction in blood flow to the kidneys reduces the distribution volume and so increases the amount of block produced by a given dose of drug. Similarly, provided the circulation to the organ is maintained, any increase in size of the liver or spleen will increase the distribution volume, lessening the effectiveness of a given dose of drug. This effect has been confirmed by Duvaldestin and his coworkers[9] who found that in patients with advanced liver disease the $\alpha$ distribution volume was greatly enlarged. As a result larger than normal doses of pancuronium were needed to achieve neuromuscular block, but the block lasted for a longer time. This is in keeping with the effects reported by Dundee and Gray[10] with tubocurarine.

### Plasma Protein Binding

In theory, the more drug sequestrated by plasma protein the less will be available for passage into the synaptic cleft. In practice the effect is to some extent offset by the ease with which the drug-protein complex dissociates as the blood level of drug falls.

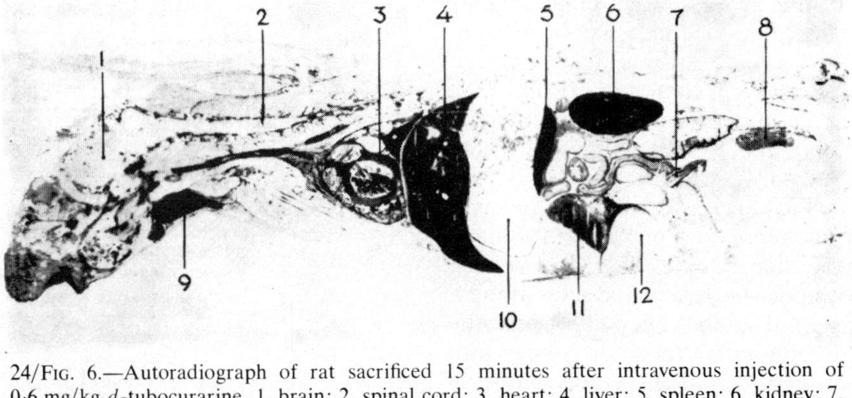


24/Fig. 6.—Autoradiograph of rat sacrificed 15 minutes after intravenous injection of 0·6 mg/kg *d*-tubocurarine. 1, brain; 2, spinal cord; 3, heart; 4, liver; 5, spleen; 6, kidney; 7, intestine; 8, bladder; 9, salivary gland; 10, stomach; 11, placenta; 12, fetus. (Courtesy of Drs. E. N. Cohen, N. Hood and R. Golling and the Editor and publisher of *Anesthesiology*, J. B. Lippincott Company[8].)

$$\text{Drug+protein} \underset{K_2}{\overset{K_1}{\rightleftharpoons}} \text{drug-protein complex}$$

$$K_2/K_1 = \text{affinity constant.}$$

If the affinity constant is low then the clinical effect of protein sequestration will be minimal.

There is little doubt that an increase in plasma protein does diminish the effectiveness of a given dose of many neuromuscular blocking drugs. Baraka and Gabaldi[11] showed a significant correlation between globulin levels and the dose of tubocurarine required. This effect was confirmed by Stovner *et al.*[12] Shanks and Penny[13] found that this correlation could only be demonstrated if small doses of tubocurarine were used—the larger the dose the less important this effect became. Although El Hakim and Baraka[14] postulated that the increase in gamma globulin associated with bilharzial cirrhosis was the cause of resistance to tubocurarine, the same effect has been demonstrated with pancuronium which is bound principally to plasma albumin. An alternative explanation, based upon the larger distribution volume observed in these patients due to their large liver or spleen, seems more appropriate. Alcuronium, gallamine and pancuronium,[15–17] and suxamethonium[18] have all been shown to bind to plasma albumin. There appears to be a correlation between the dose of alcuronium required to produce neuromuscular block and the plasma albumin content, the total plasma protein level and the packed cell volume.[19] Although it is generally accepted that 20–30 per cent of pancuronium can be bound to plasma proteins, figures for *in vitro* binding range as high as 70 per cent[17] depending upon the methodology used in the study. In clinical practice it is difficult to demonstrate a clinical effect from variations in dose requirements of pancuronium at different plasma protein levels within the physiological range. Similarly the effect of variations in plasma protein upon the action of suxamethonium are less obvious than the 70 per cent binding demonstrated by Dal Santo would suggest. Some of the explanation of these incongruities is no doubt due to the low affinity of the drug for protein and to the methods used to measure protein binding *in vitro* which do not accurately reflect the conditions *in vivo*.

## Blood Flow and Cardiac Output

In a series of experiments, it has been shown that the reactive hyperaemia produced by a few minutes ischaemia resulted in a more rapid onset and also a greater degree of block when tubocurarine was subsequently administered (Fig. 7). This observation confirms that of Churchill-Davidson and Richardson[20] using small doses of decamethonium. The importance of regional blood flow is too readily overlooked. Dehydration, haemorrhage and the release of catecholamines due to anxiety or pain will reduce profoundly the blood flow to organs classically regarded as being in the rapid distribution volume, including the kidney, the skin, the splanchnic area and the spleen, and may increase the blood flow to the muscles. Were this to occur it would result in an increase in the effectiveness of a given dose of drug. The influence of cardiac output is less easily determined. Cardiac output may alter four-fold between patients due to age, previous administration of thiopentone or hypnotic drugs, or due to diseases such as thyrotoxicosis and chronic anaemia. It might be anticipated that a reduction in circulation time might result in more loss of the drug from the rapid distribution compartment to tissues with a longer time constant for sequestration, so reducing the effectiveness of a bolus dose. Thus, giving the drug rapidly into a slow circulation might be analogous to giving the same dose of relaxant slowly into a fast circulation. However there is no experimental evidence to support this. In experiments in dogs in whom the cardiac output was altered four-fold by physical means, there is little difference in the amount of neuromuscular block produced by a given dose of pancuronium although the rate of onset of neuromuscular block is affected (Fig. 8).

## Age

Although sensitivity of the neonate to tubocurarine was first reported by Bush and Stead in 1962,[21] the extent of this effect has been the subject of controversy. Walts and Dillon[22] demonstrated that provided a dose based on surface area rather than body weight was used then the neonate was comparable to the adult in the requirement of more non-depolarising

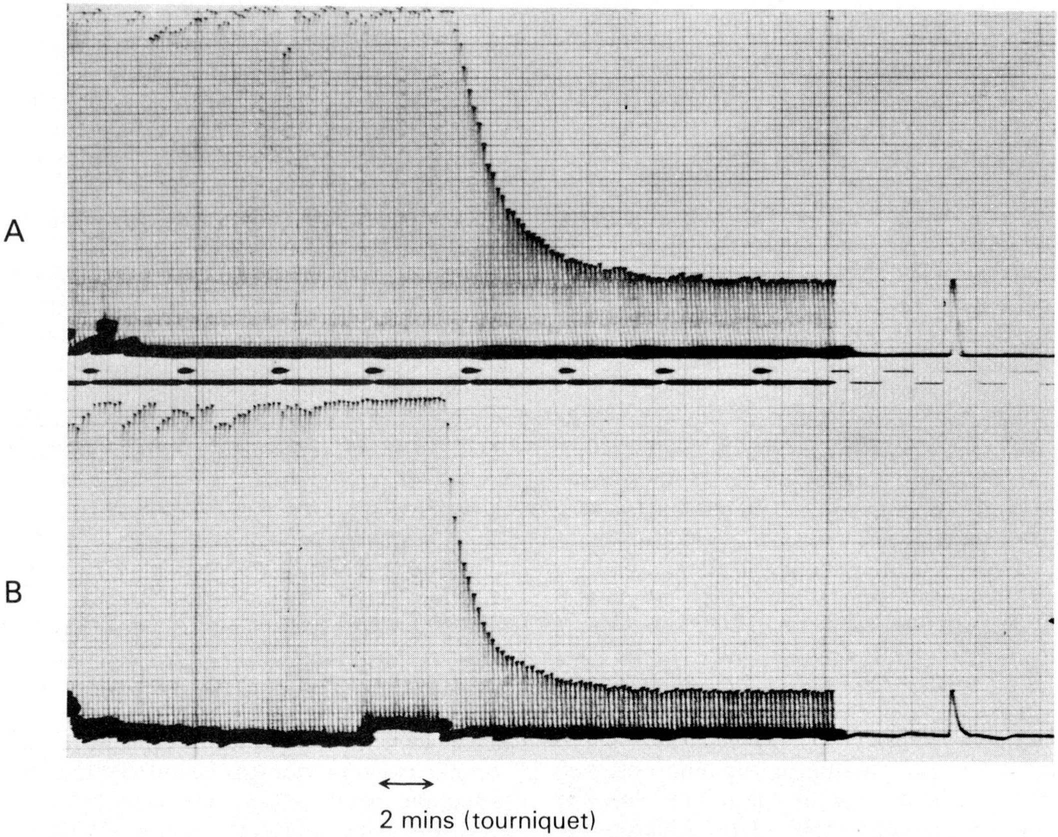


24/Fig. 7.—A. Right arm with normal perfusion. B. Left arm with blood supply occluded for two minutes prior to the injection of 10 mg tubocurarine. Note the block in the previously occluded arm (B) is more rapid in onset and greater in degree. This is due to the increased blood flow of the reactive hyperaemia.

drugs. As surface area accurately reflects the ECF volume it implies that provided the smaller distribution volume is taken into account the differences in neuromuscular sensitivity are minimal. Most paediatric anaesthetists, however, find that a reduced dose of non-depolarising relaxants is required in neonates. This effect is supported by the EMG findings suggesting that the neonate has a reduced margin of safety of neuromuscular transmission and will exhibit a post-tetanic depression of the twitch response which is similar to post-tetanic exhaustion of myasthenia gravis.[23,24] Neonates also have a resistance to depolarising agents and a propensity to develop Phase II block in a manner similar to patients with myasthenia gravis (Fig. 9).

It has been widely assumed that elderly patients require less muscle relaxant, due to their smaller ECF volume and lesser muscle bulk. However, in a study by McLeod *et al.*[25] it was demonstrated that the dose per kilogram of pancuronium required to produce neuromuscular block was approximately the same in all groups, although the effect lasted longer in the elderly, presumably due to less efficient excretion of the drug. However, in another study by Somogyi[26] no correlation between plasma clearance of pancuronium and the age of the patient was found.

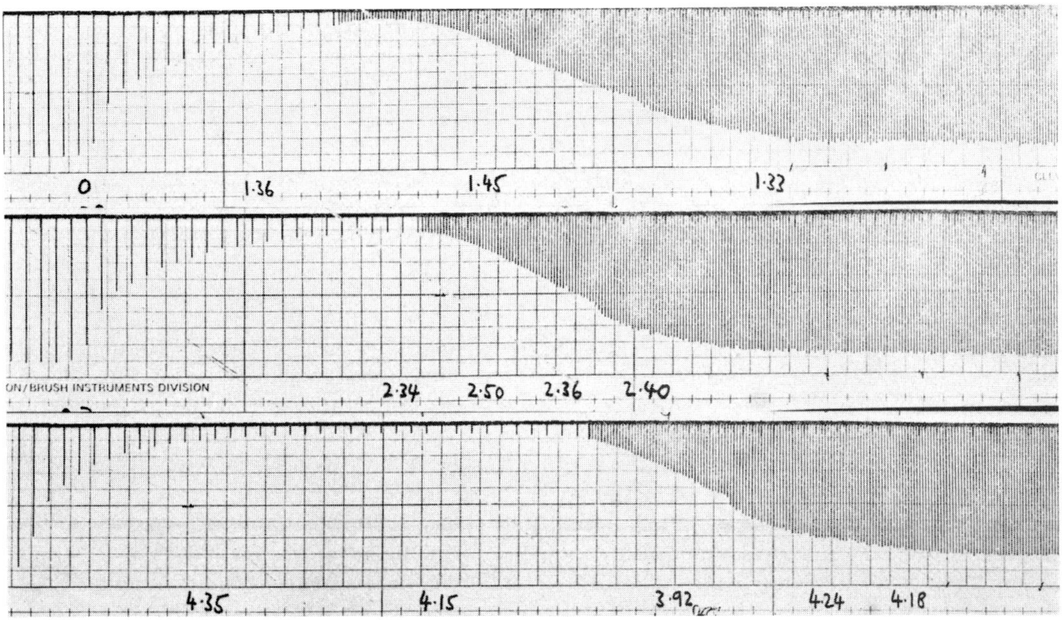


24/FIG. 8.—Effect of changes in cardiac output (volume in litres below trace) on rate of onset, amount of block and recovery from the same dose of pancuronium in a dog. *Upper trace* with lowest cardiac output (1·36 to 1·45 l/min). *Lower trace* with highest cardiac output (4·35 to 3·92 l/min). Onset of block (at fast paper speed) minimally faster at high outputs, whilst amount of block produced and recovery index unaffected by three-fold change in cardiac output.

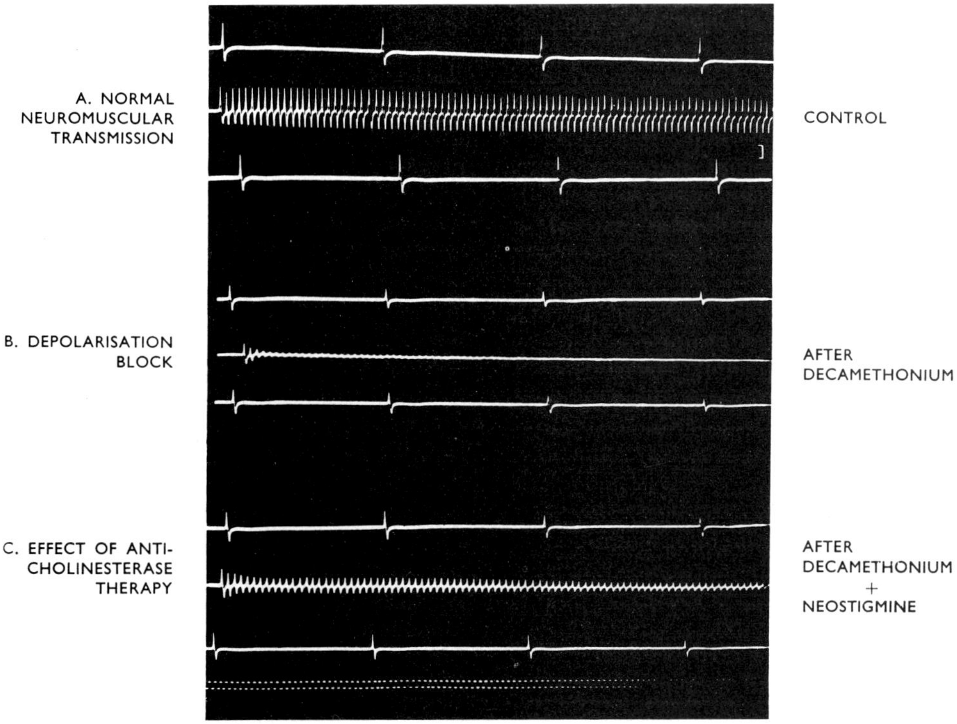


24/FIG. 9.—Signs of Phase II block following decamethonium in a neonate. (Courtesy of the Editors and publisher of *Anesthesiology*, J. B. Lippincott Company.)

### Carbon Dioxide and the pH of Blood

The results of studies on the effect of metabolic acidosis on the degree of block and rate of recovery of a non-depolarising neuromuscular block have been inconsistent. This may be a reflection on the method employed to produce the hydrogen ion charge, the animal chosen for study, or the degree of metabolic acidosis produced.

The most pronounced effect of pH change within the clinical range is upon the action of tubocurarine. There is universal agreement that respiratory acidosis in man potentiates the activity of this drug to a clinically meaningful extent, and most workers accept that a similar pH change produced by a combination of metabolic and respiratory acidosis has a similar effect. pH affects the action of suxamethonium in an opposite manner, potentiation occurring in alkalaemia and antagonism during acidaemia; however, the effect is less marked than with tubocurarine. The effect of acid-base changes in physiological range upon the action of the other relaxants including dimethyl curare, alcuronium, pancuronium and decamethonium appear to be small. Gallamine is mildly antagonised by acidaemia and potentiated by alkalaemia. Although in theory alkalaemia should increase the rate of Hofmann degradation of atracurium, *in vitro* studies suggest this would be unlikely to occur in the physiological range.

In clinical practice the only drug whose activity is sufficiently affected by pH changes in a clinical range to produce a noticeable effect is tubocurarine and the reason for this remains uncertain. Utting[27] found that the plasma level of tubocurarine varied with the pH of the blood during acidaemia, and this was confirmed in man by Baraka.[28] They ascribed this to a reduction in plasma protein binding at a lower pH. The change in binding, however, is small and does not account for the increased blockade observed. A more likely theory is that the change in pH can alter the binding of tubocurarine to the end-plate receptor.[29] An alternative theory suggested by Feldman[70] was based upon the new structure of tubocurarine proposed by Everett and his colleagues.[30] This new formula suggests that at a physiological pH tubocurarine is likely to be a monoquaternary monotertiary compound. In this state only about 75 per cent of the molecules are charged, whilst at a more acidic pH, ionisation will increase, causing a likely potentiation of the action of the drug.[31] Due to the increase in the charge density on the tertiary amine, tubocurarine will approach the activity of a bisquaternary compound. This will help to explain the unique potentiating effect of acidaemia upon the myoneural block produced by tubocurarine.

### Diseases and Drugs

Diseases that reduce the receptor population (such as myasthenia gravis) or the output of acetylcholine (such as the myasthenic syndrome and severe malnutrition) will cause a marked sensitivity to a non-depolarising muscle relaxant (see pp. 737 and 740).

Drugs such as the aminoglycosides, antibiotics, lithium carbonate, local anaesthetic agents, quinidine and hydrocortisone,[32,33] and the volatile anaesthetics all potentiate the action of the non-depolarising muscle relaxants. Different mechanisms are involved in these effects; thus the aminoglycoside antibiotics (see p. 722) and lithium carbonate[34,35] act by reducing transmitter release. The local anaesthetics[36–38] and quinidine are believed to act both by reducing acetylcholine release and by stabilising the postsynaptic membrane, and thus depressing the easy propogation of the action potential from the end-plate to the muscle.

The principal sites of action of volatile anaesthetics vary from one agent to another, but inevitably this is a combination of central nervous system depression and of spontaneously evoked neuronal discharge along the motor nerves.[39,40] There are other possible sites of action, such as the *prejunctional effect*, which is only seen at high concentrations,[41] an action on the *postsynaptic membrane*,[42–44] which is revealed when the margin of safety of neuromuscular transmission is reduced by the presence of a blocking agent[45] and, finally, the *direct effect* upon the muscle itself. The central action and the action upon the muscle contractile mechanisms are of minor clinical importance with most volatile agents in clinical concentrations. It was demonstrated that the major effect of the volatile agents was to increase the receptor sensitivity to the muscle relaxant drugs.[46] Further work showed that halothane did not depress renal blood flow in clinical concentrations and so interfere with the rate of excretion of tubocurarine.[6] Miller and his colleagues[47] found that both halothane and enflurane caused a significant effect upon the redistribution and excretion of pancuronium which could account for some of the increased activity seen when these drugs are administered to a patient, together with a volatile anaesthetic.

Clinically, all volatile anaesthetics potentiate both the amount of block produced by non-depolarising and depolarising relaxants and also the duration of action. This effect is most marked with the ethers, diethylether, enflurane and isoflurane, but it is also seen with halothane. The effect is related to the concentration of the inhalational agent used, and can be utilised to potentiate the action of these drugs under conditions when the total dose of drug needs to be minimised, as in patients with renal disease. It may also be helpful in assisting relaxation when the effect of a non-depolarising drug is wearing off and it is considered inappropriate to administer a supplementary dose.

### Burns

The increased dose requirement of non-depolarising relaxants in badly burned patients has been confirmed.[48] It was found that patients who had been burned some months previously demonstrated a marked tolerance to tubocurarine, and showed plasma levels of drug about six times that reported by Matteo and his colleagues[3] at 50 per cent block. The cause for this resistance is unknown. Although this may in part be explained by an increased binding capacity of the globulin fraction especially $\alpha$-aminoglycoprotein in burned patients blood,[49] it does not explain the magnitude of the different requirements found in these patients.

## FACTORS AFFECTING DURATION OF BLOCK

The duration of action of the neuromuscular blocking agents depends upon the rate of dissociation of the drug from the receptor site and the establishment of an adequate concentration gradient between the receptor and plasma to allow the displaced drug to leave the neuromuscular end-plate.

The rate of dissociation depends upon the chemical and physical properties of the drug and the rate of acetylcholine production. The establishment of a suitable concentration gradient to permit drug molecules to leave the receptor area is a function of redistribution of the drug to non-active acceptor sites in muscle, cartilage, fat and other tissues, as well as metabolism and excretion. The so-called $\beta$ distribution volume reflects the processes of redistribution, excretion and metabolism as a single conglomerate (see Fig. 3). It must be appreciated that this volume does not represent an anatomical or physiological entity as such but is merely a pharmacokinetically convenient expression covering many processes continuing at different rates and to a variable extent, according to the subject, the physiological state, physical conditions, the anaesthetic used and the drug studied.

### Redistribution of the Muscle Relaxants

The decay curve of the plasma concentration of the muscle relaxants indicates a slow but steady decline during the $\beta$ phase, which can be represented by simple mathematical models (if the processes of excretion, metabolism and redistribution are all lumped together). However, they do not yield useful information as to the rate at which the various components of redistribution occur, or the degree to which each tissue accepts the drug before an equilibrium state is achieved. In order to study redistribution quantitatively, recourse has to be made to studying the concentration of a drug in each organ over a period of time. Fleischli and Cohen,[50] using a radioactive drug, examined the redistribution of tubocurarine (Fig. 10) and demonstrated the differing time courses for the passage of drug into various tissues and their differing rates of removal from these sites, whilst renal and biliary excretion was also taking place. However, even the painstaking work of Cohen and his co-workers[8] could not cover all groups of tissues. They calculated that there was a considerable loss of drug from the organs studied, all of which had a relatively high blood flow into tissues that they did not study specifically, but which presumably constituted the low-blood-flow group with a high affinity for the drug—the so-called acceptor depots. It is the drug leaving tissue depot sites that is responsible for the long tail of the plasma concentration decay slope. However, if the tail of the $\beta$ decay curve occurs well below the plasma concentration required to effect neuromuscular

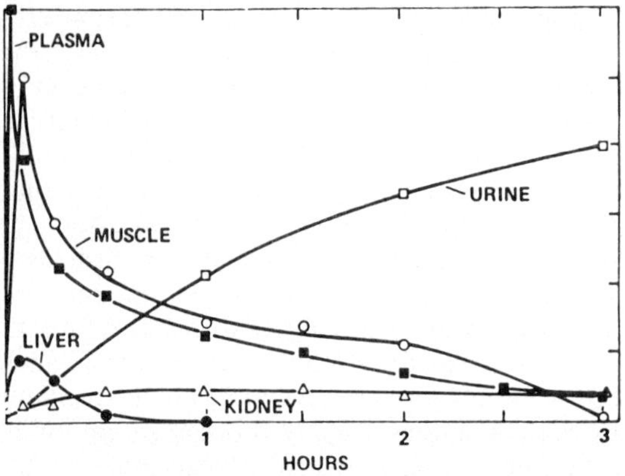


24/Fig. 10.—Redistribution of curare from the plasma during the first three hours. (With kind permission of Dr. G. Fleischli and Dr. E. N. Cohen and J. B. Lippincott Co., the publishers of *Anesthesiology*.[50])

block, it is unlikely to affect recovery from or reversal of a neuromuscular block.

### Renal Excretion

All the neuromuscular blocking agents are highly ionised, water-soluble compounds, and are therefore readily excreted by the kidney at a rate which is largely dependent upon the glomerular filtration rate and renal blood flow. During anaesthesia this is a variable quantity and it is this variation that contributes more than any other single factor to the individual differences in duration of action of the non-depolarising relaxants in present use, with the exception of atracurium, whose recovery time is very predictable. This is particularly obvious with drugs which rely solely upon the kidneys as the ultimate pathway for their excretion. This includes gallamine,[51,52] decamethonium and, to a large extent, dimethylcurarine (metacurarine). Alcuronium and fazadinium are largely excreted by the kidneys, whereas pancuronium and tubocurarine can be recovered to a variable extent from the bile. Pancuronium is excreted in amounts from 5 to 40 per cent in the bile as either the parent compound or one of the three metabolites (see page 695) and large amounts of tubocurarine can be recovered from the bile in dogs.[53] Of these two drugs with a capacity for alternate excretory pathways, it would appear that tubocurarine is more effectively excreted by the liver in patients with anuria, and so is preferred in conditions of renal failure.[54] Recently, Hunter and her colleagues[55] have described the use of atracurium in twenty anephric patients. This new, short-acting muscle relaxant is rapidly metabolised *in vivo* and no signs of residual curarisation were observed. They believe that atracurium is a suitable agent to use in the presence of renal failure. Suxamethonium, administered as an infusion or in a small dose potentiated by hexafluronium has also been advocated in renal failure.[56]

### Metabolism of Muscle Relaxants

The most important example of biotransformation as a means of reducing the blood drug concentration is the hydrolysis of suxamethonium to succinylmonocholine. In a normal patient, Kalow[57] estimated that only 10 per cent of an injected dose reacted with the receptors; the rest was hydrolysed. In these circumstances the distribution volume for suxamethonium would be so large that it is seldom considered as a separate entity.

Fazadinium was introduced as a muscle relaxant by Tyers[58] following the demonstration that certain azopyridines caused neuromuscular block. In most animals, fazadinium is hydrolysed by azoreductase in the presence of NADP (the active form of adenosine diphosphate nicotinamide) to the inactive monoquaternary compound. Unfortunately, this process does not appear to occur to a significant effect in the liver of man.

Pancuronium is metabolised in the liver to a varying extent up to 30 per cent. The reason for this variability is not obvious. The metabolites are principally excreted in the bile and for the most part they are weak relaxant compounds. As a result, the effect of hepatic biotransformation on the size of the distribution volume and the duration of action of pancuronium is unpredictable.

Newer muscle relaxants such as atracurium and the bulky esters, produced by Savarese and Wastila,[59] appear to depend largely on metabolism to lower the plasma level of drug and so allow early reversal of their neuromuscular blocking activities. The *in vitro* half-life of atracurium is 26 minutes, whilst some of the bulky esters are more rapidly hydrolysed than suxamethonium.

### Liver Disease

Duvaldestin and his co-workers[9] have demonstrated that liver disease increases the $\alpha$ distribution volume, necessitating more drug (pancuronium) to produce a given degree of block. It also decreases the $\beta$ volume. As a result, the duration of effect of a given dose of relaxant and especially the larger dose required to produce adequate block in these patients is increased. It seems likely that this is due to an increased blood flow to the enlarged liver and/or spleen, resulting in this being partially transferred from the second compartment to the first. However, it is possible that depression of renal excretion by a "hepatorenal" syndrome may contribute to the prolonged action of pancuronium. The importance of the liver as a redistribution site was well demonstrated by the experiments of Agoston and his colleagues in 1980.[60] The drug under study was injected directly into the portal vein of cats to demonstrate the "first-pass effect" and the liver was temporarily excluded from the general circulation by a reversible portacaval shunt. Working with the steroid series of relaxants, these workers were able to demonstrate the importance of hepatic uptake (first-pass effect) in the plasma clearance of ORG 6368 (17 acetoxy derivative of pancuronium). The neuromuscular block induced by pancuronium was greatly prolonged if the liver was excluded from the circulation. This demonstrated the importance of the liver as a redistribution site in lowering the plasma level of pancuronium.

## Effect of Jaundice

In 1977, Somogyi *et al.*[61] drew attention to the prolonged activity of pancuronium in jaundiced patients. This prolongation of the neuromuscular block by jaundice has been confirmed[62] even though renal excretion of the drug was not reduced. It has been further demonstrated[63] that this effect is due to a potentiation of the neuromuscular block by the bile salts, dehydrocholate and taurocholate. The effect can also be demonstrated with the steroidal relaxant vecuronium but is not found with gallamine, unless the level of taurocholate is very high (Fig. 11). It is probable that the explanation for this finding is that bile salts compete for certain microsomal enzyme systems or carrier mechanisms with the steroidal neuromuscular blocking agents.

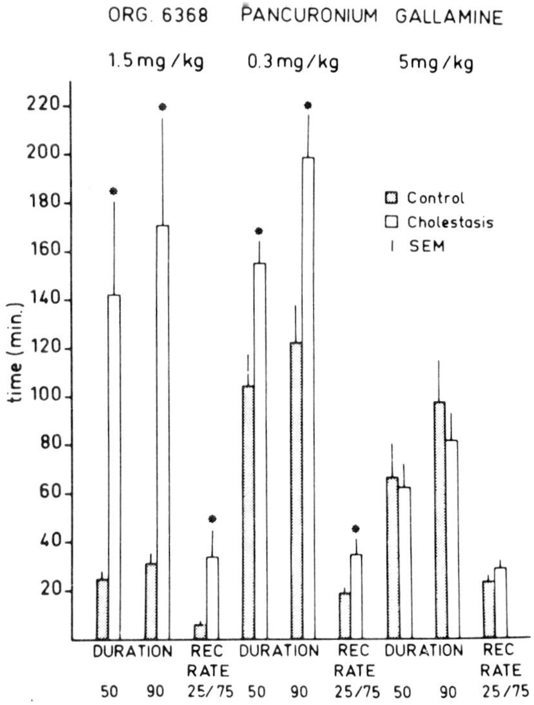


24/FIG. 11.—The effect of experimentally induced cholestasis upon the duration of action of the steroid relaxant ORG 6368, which has a high affinity for liver cells, and of pancuronium and gallamine. (Reproduced with kind permission of P. Westra, 1980.[63])

## Blood Flow

Churchill-Davidson and Richardson[20] demonstrated that the duration of action of decamethonium is reduced in conditions of high blood flow (Fig. 12). This finding is compatible with the concept of depolarising neuromuscular block as being associated with a low affinity.[64] Increasing the blood flow will increase the rate at which the drug is washed out of the receptor area. However, Feldman and Tyrrell suggested that non-depolarising relaxants have a high affinity for the receptor by virtue of the slow dissociation rate. In these circumstances alterations in blood flow would be expected to have less effect upon recovery time. This was confirmed[65] using a roller pump to produce an eight-fold change in blood flow to the limbs of the animal under study (Fig. 13). An absence of correlation between blood flow and recovery time from non-depolarising neuromuscular block was also demonstrated by Heneghan and his co-workers[66] using a xenon 133 washout technique to measure blood flow. This effect has been personally verified using conditions similar to that of Churchill-Davidson and Richardson,[20] by studying the recovery of adductor twitch response in the thumbs of the two hands of patients following surgical thoracic sympathectomy on one side.

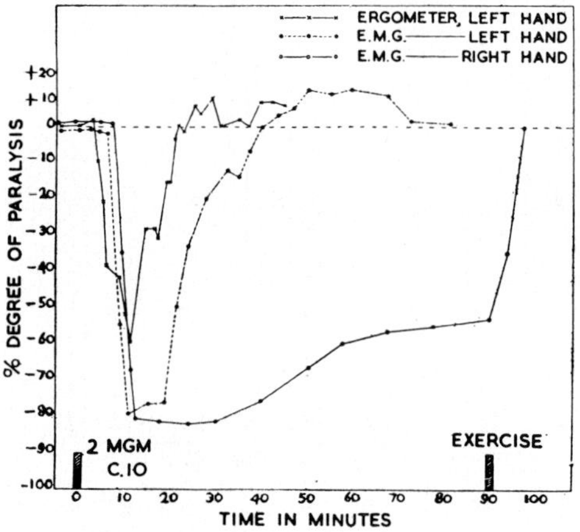


24/Fig. 12.—Comparison of the duration of paralysis from the administration of 2 mg of decamethonium in resting limb (right) and exercising limb (left). (Courtesy of the Honorary Editors of the *Proceedings of the Royal Society of Medicine*.)

## Other Factors

Physiological, pathological and drug induced changes in the rate of acetylcholine production or release will affect the duration of action of the muscle relaxants.

### Hypothermia

In recent years the findings of Holmes and associates,[67] Maclagen and Zaimis[68] and Cannard and Zaimis[69] that cooling reduced the effectiveness and duration of non-depolarising block, has been challenged,[70–76] and it is now generally accepted that hypothermia prolongs the duration of non-depolarising neuromuscular block.

In an elegant series of experiments, Thornton and his associates[75] controlled the temperature and blood flow of one hind limb of a dog, using an extracorporeal circuit containing a heat exchanger and a roller pump. They compared the response of directly stimulated muscle with indirect stimulation through the motor nerve in 10 dogs (Fig. 14*a*). They found that at about 30° C in the dogs a partial neuromuscular block occurred (Fig. 14*b*). This compares with a similar effect found by Feldman[70] in 5 patients

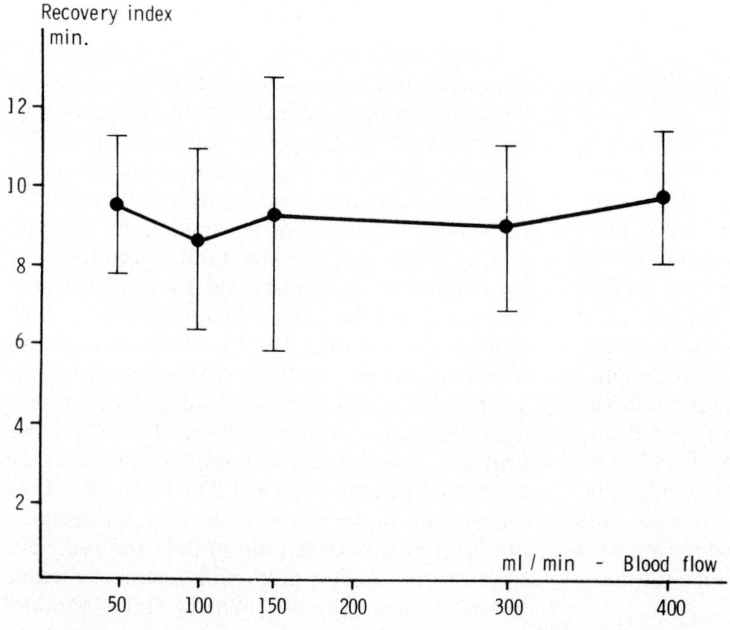


24/Fig. 13.—Alterations in blood flow on hind-limb of a dog paralysed with gallamine showing that an eight-fold increase in flow does *not* alter recovery index. (Courtesy of Drs. V. A. Goat, M. L. Yeung, C. Blakeney and S. A. Feldman, and Macmillan Journals Ltd.[65])

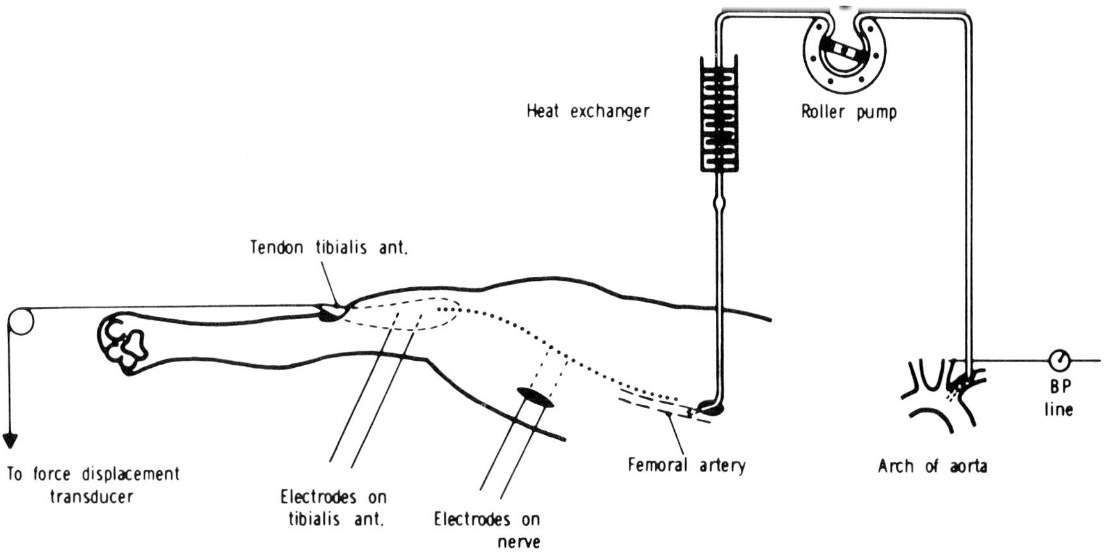


24/FIG. 14(*a*).—Experimental method used by Thornton *et al.*[75] to study effect of cold on neuromuscular conduction in dogs.

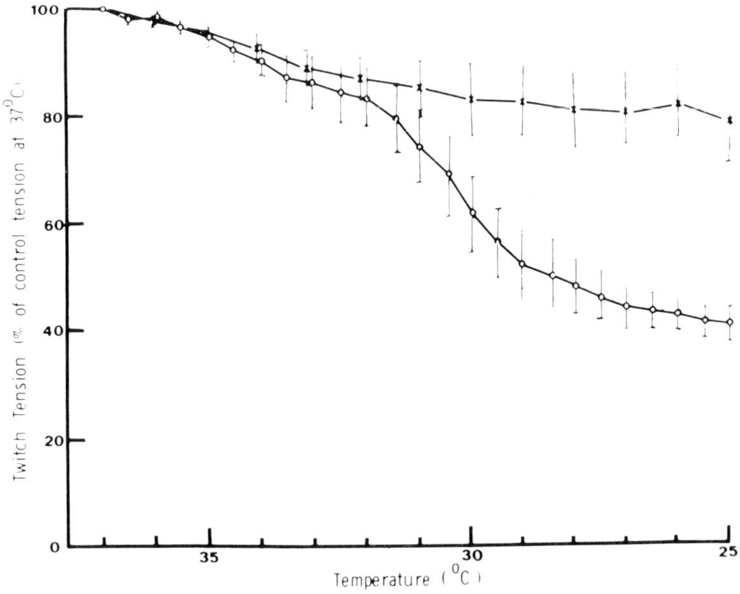


24/FIG. 14(*b*).—Effect of cooling upon the directly elicited twitch response (x) and the indirectly elicited twitch response (o) of dogs (n = 10). (Courtesy of Drs. R. J. Thornton, C. Blakeney and S. A. Feldman, and MacMillan Journals Ltd.[75])

studied during hypothermia (Fig. 15). The neuromuscular block, induced by cold, was reversed by rewarming and by anticholinesterase drugs such as edrophonium. Thornton and co-workers[75] concluded that in the cooling process, and at a specific temperature, there was a partial failure of acetylcholine release which varied from animal to animal. This occurred at lower temperatures in hibernating mammals.[77] As a result of the diminished acetylcholine output, there was a slower dissociation of non-depolarising neuromuscular blocking drugs from the receptor and a greatly prolonged action during hypothermia (Fig. 16). Ham and his co-work-

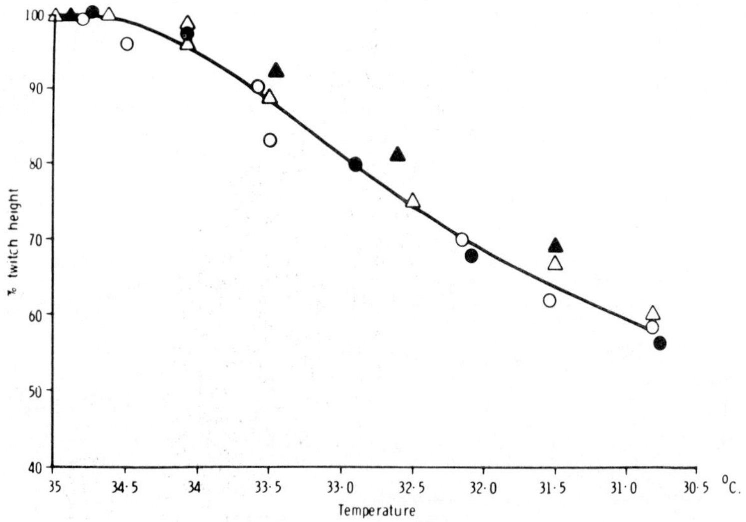


24/Fig. 15.—Effect of changes in muscle temperature upon the indirect twitch response of patients during hypothermia. (With kind permission of Dr. S. A. Feldman, and W. B. Saunders Ltd.[70])

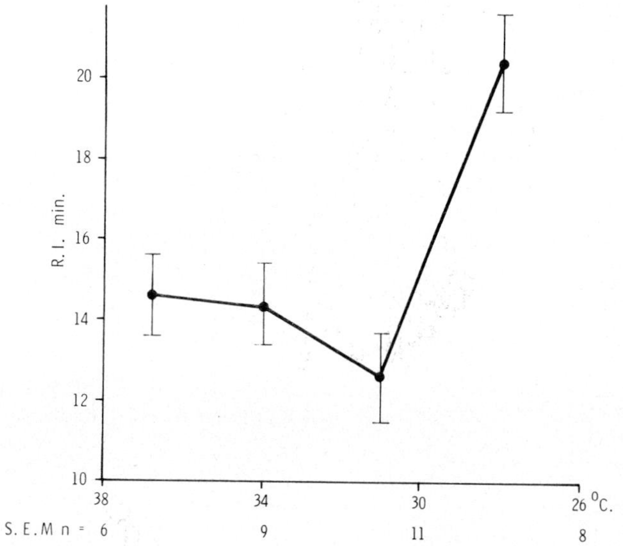


24/Fig. 16.—The effect of cold on the recovery index of gallamine in dogs, demonstrating the markedly prolonged duration of action of this drug below 30° C (Thornton *et al.*[75]).

ers[76] found an increased block produced by tubocurarine at lowered temperatures, as well as a prolonged activity. They attributed the prolongation of the block to a decrease in the renal blood flow during hypothermia as demonstrated by a reduced renal excretion of the drug. This mechanism would not explain the effect of hypothermia, demonstrated by Thornton and others in animals whose kidneys were normothermic and whose renal blood flow was unchanged by the experimental procedure.

In conclusion, from experimental observations, it would appear that hypothermia prolongs the action of the non-depolarising drugs. The mechanism for this action is probably related to a reduction in the production, or release, of acetylcholine at the nerve-ending and also to reduced cardiac output, with a falling liver and kidney blood flow.

## Antibiotics

The aminoglycoside antibiotics potentiate

the action of non-depolarising muscle relaxants by interfering with the transfer of calcium across the presynaptic membrane during depolarisation, and hence they reduce the quantal release of acetylcholine.[78,79] Prokic[80] reported the case-histories of 2 patients who were receiving streptomycin and who died after the administration of suxamethonium. However, the interaction of antibiotics with suxamethonium appears to be a rare occurrence. The potentiating potency of the antibiotics varies according to the chemical structure and the species in which it is tested. The response to treatment also differs. Polymyxin appears to be the most troublesome antibiotic followed by neomycin, streptomycin, gentamicin and kanamycin; all have weak actions and demonstrate their effect only in high doses. Lincomycin has a biphasic action, antagonising non-depolarising block in low concentrations but potentiating the block in high concentration.[81] The tetracylines also exhibit weak neuromuscular blocking effects at high concentrations.

The use of calcium salts to reverse the antibiotic effect has been recommended.[82–84] More recently Noble[85] reported successful reversal of gallamine block potentiated by kanamycin by the use of calcium gluconate. Singh and his colleagues[86] demonstrated the ability of high extracellular concentrations of calcium to antagonise the block caused by gentamicin in the phrenic-nerve diaphragm preparation. However, since the most that can be achieved by the administration of calcium is a more favourable concentration gradient for its entry into the motor nerve, it is less likely to be successful in correcting the basic defect than an agent such as 4-aminopyridine, which directly enhances conductance across the presynaptic membrane during depolarisation. The effectiveness of 4-aminopyridine in antagonising the effect of antibiotics has been demonstrated by Lee and his colleagues[87] both in experimental animals and in patients.

In view of the effect of the aminoglycoside antibiotics, their use should be carefully controlled to ensure that well under 1 g is given into a body cavity during anaesthetics that involve the administration of neuromuscular blocking agents. A prolongation of a non-depolarising block should be anticipated if an antibiotic such as gentamicin, in a dose greater than 40 mg, is given intravenously during the course of an anaesthetic.

### Pathological States

Pathological states, including the myasthenic syndrome (see page 740) and Addison's disease (or drug-induced adrenal suppression), will prolong the action of the non-depolarising muscle relaxants. Severe hypoxia and malnutrition may also increase the duration of action of relaxants by interfering with acetylcholine synthesis and release. Conditions causing reduced glomerular filtration (such as haemorrhagic shock or dehydration) will also prolong the action of muscle-relaxant drugs. In cases of impaired renal blood flow, an infusion of mannitol may increase renal excretion, but it does not increase the plasma clearance rate in normal patients.[88]

### Drugs

Drugs that reduce renal blood flow or glomerular filtration may be expected to increase the duration of action of non-depolarising muscle relaxants. It is possible that the prolonged action found after hypotension produced by ganglion-blocking drugs and nitroglycerine infusions are related to this effect, although a direct potentiation or presynaptic effect cannot be ruled out.[89–91]

Volatile anaesthetic agents not only potentiate the block produced by non-depolarising muscle relaxants, but they also prolong the block. Drugs that decrease the plasma cholinesterase levels, such as the antibilharzial drug metrifonate and certain cytotoxic drugs, will cause a prolonged response to suxamethonium. However, this is seldom of serious clinical significance.

Azathioprine (Imuran) has been found actually to antagonise neuromuscular blockade produced by non-depolarising relaxants. Dretchen and his colleagues[92] suggest that this is a result of a theophylline-like action, inhibiting the intracellular phosphodiesterase activity and leading to facilitation of calcium transport across the cell membrane.

## REFERENCES


1. Katz, R. L. and Katz, G. J. (1975). Clinical considerations in the use of muscle relaxants. In: *Muscle Relaxants, Monographs in Anesthesiology*. Ed. Katz. R. L. Amsterdam: Excerpta Medica.
2. Agoston, S., Feldman, S. A. and Miller, R. D. (1979). Plasma concentration and neuromuscular blockade after injection into the isolated arm, bolus injection and continuous infusion. *Anesthesiology*, **51**, 119.
3. Matteo, R. S., Spector, S. and Horowitz, P. E. (1974). Relation of serum d-tubocurarine concentration to neuromuscular blockade in man. *Anesthesiology*, **41**, 440.
4. Somogyi, A. A., Shanks, C. A. and Triggs, E. J. (1976). Clinical pharmacokinetics of pancuronium bromide. *Eur. J. clin. Pharmacol.*, **10**, 367.
5. Agoston, S., Crul, J. F. and Kersten, U. W. (1977). Relationship of the serum pancuronium to its neuromuscular activity in man. *Anesthesiology*, **47**, 17.
6. Stanski, D. R., Ham, J., Miller, R. D. and Sheiner, L. B. (1979). Pharmacokinetics and pharmacodynamics of d-tubocurarine during nitrous oxide—narcotic and halothane anaesthesia in man. *Anesthesiology*, **51**, 235.
7. Mather, L. E. (1980). Determination of drug action. *Anaesth. Intensive Care*, **8**, 233.
8. Cohen, E. N., Hood, N. and Golling, R. (1968). Use of whole body autoradiography for determination of uptake and distribution of labelled muscle relaxants in the rat. *Anesthesiology*, **29**, 987.
9. Duvaldestin, P., Agoston, S., Henzel, D., Kerstin, O. W. and Desmont, J. M. (1978). Pancuronium pharmacokinetics in patients with liver cirrhosis. *Brit. J. Anaesth.*, **50**, 1131.
10. Dundee, J. W. and Gray, T. C. (1953). Resistance to d-tubocurarine chloride in presence of liver damage. *Lancet*, **2**, 16.
11. Baraka, A. and Gabaldi, F. (1968). Correlation between tubocurarine requirements and plasma protein pattern. *Brit. J. Anaesth.*, **40**, 89.
12. Stovner, J., Theodorsen, L. and Bjelke, E. (1971). Sensitivity to tubocurarine and alcuronium with special reference to plasma protein pattern. *Brit. J. Anaesth.*, **43**, 385.
13. Shanks, C. A. and Penny, R. (1972). Plasma protein and dose requirements of tubocurarine. *Anaesth. Intensive Care*, **1**, 62.
14. El Hakim, M. S. and Baraka, A. (1963). d-tubocurarine in liver disease. *Kasrel Aini J. Surg.*, **4**, 99.
15. Stovner, J., Theodorsen, L. and Bjelke, E. (1971*b*). Sensitivity to gallamine and pancuronium with special reference to serum proteins. *Brit. J. Anaesth.*, **43**, 953.
16. Stovner, J., Theodorsen, L. and Bjelke, E. (1972). Sensitivity to dimethyltubocurarine and toxiferine with special reference to serum proteins. *Brit. J. Anaesth.*, **44**, 374.
17. Thompson, J. M. (1976). Pancuronium binding by serum proteins. *Anaesthesia*, **31**, 219.
18. Dal Santo (1968). Kinetics of distribution of radioactive labelled muscle relaxants. *Anesthesiology*, **29**, 435.
19. Yeung, M. L. (1976). Plasma proteins, packed cell volume and requirements for alcuronium. *Brit. J. Anaesth.*, **48**, 859.
20. Churchill-Davidson, H. C. and Richardson, A. T. (1952). Decamethonium iodide ($C_{10}$): some observations using electromyography. *Proc. roy. Soc. Med.*, **45**, 179.
21. Bush, G. M. and Stead, A. L. (1962). The use of tubocurarine in neonatal anaesthesia. *Brit. J. Anaesth.*, **34**, 721.
22. Walts, L. F. and Dillon, J. B. (1969). The response of newborns to succinylcholine and *d*-tubocurarine. *Anesthesiology*, **41**, 53.
23. Churchill-Davidson, H. C. and Wise, R. P. (1963). Neuromuscular block in the newborn infant. *Anesthesiology*, **24**, 271.
24. Churchill-Davidson, H. C. and Wise, R. P. (1964). The response of the newborn infant to muscle relaxants. *Canad. Anaesth. Soc. J.*, **11**, 1.
25. McLeod, K., Hull, C. J. and Watson, M. J. (1979). Effects of ageing on the pharmacokinetics of pancuronium. *Brit. J. Anaesth.*, **51**, 435.
26. Somogyi, A. (1980). Pancuronium plasma clearance and age. *Brit. J. Anaesth.*, **52**, 360.
27. Utting, J. (1963). pH as a factor influencing plasma concentration of *d*-tubocurarine. *Brit. J. Anaesth.*, **35**, 706.
28. Baraka, A. (1964). The influence of carbon dioxide on the neuromuscular block caused by tubocurarine in the human subject. *Brit. J. Anaesth.*, **36**, 272.
29. Maclagen, J. (1976). Competitive neuromuscular blocking drugs. In: *Neuromuscular Junction* p. 421. ed. E. Zaimis. Berlin: Springer Verlag.
30. Everett, A. J., Lowe, L. A. and Wilkinson, S. (1970). Revision of the structure of (+) tubocurarine chloride and (+) chandrocurarine. *Chem. Communications*, **16**, 1020.
31. Gibb, D. (1980). pKa value of neuromuscular blockers. *Anaesth. Intensive Care*, **8**, 380.
32. Torda, C. and Wolff, H. G. (1952). Effect of pituitary hormones cortisone and adrenalectomy on some aspects of neuromuscular function and acetylcholine synthesis. *Am. J. Physiol.*, **169**, 140.
33. Myers, E. F. (1977). Partial recovery from pancuronium neuromuscular blockade following hydrocortisone administration. *Anesthesiology*, **46**, 148.
34. Hill, G. E., Wong, K. C. and Hoges, H. R. (1977). Lithium carbonate and neuromuscular blocking agents. *Anesthesiology*, **46**, 122.
35. Borden, H., Clarke M. and Katz, H. (1974). The use of pancuronium bromide in patients receiving lithium carbonate. *Canad. Anaesth. Soc. J.*, **21**, 79.
36. Usubiaga, J. E. and Standaert, F. (1968). The effects of local anaesthetics on motor nerve terminals. *J. Pharmacol. exp. Ther.*, **159**, 353.
37. Kordas, M. (1970). The effect of procaine on neuromuscular transmission. *J. Physiol.*, **209**, 689.
38. Telivuo, L. and Katz, R. L. (1970). The effects of modern intravenous local anaesthetics on respiration during partial neuromuscular block in man. *Anaesthesia*, **25**, 30.
39. Barth, L. (1973). Paradoxical interaction between halothane and pancuronium. *Anaesthesia*, **28**, 5140.
40. Feldman, S. A. and Andrew, D. (1974). Paradoxical interaction between halothane and pancuronium. *Anaesthesia*, **29**, 100.

41. Kennedy, R. and Galindo, A. G. (1975). Neuromuscular transmission in a mammalian preparation during exposure to enflurane. *Anesthesiology*, **42**, 432.
42. Karis, J. H., Gissen, A. J. and Nastuk, W. L. (1967). The effect of volatile anesthetic agents on neuromuscular transmission. *Anesthesiology*, **28**, 128.
43. Katz, R. L. and Gissen, H. J. (1967). Neuromuscular and electromyographic effects of halothane and its interaction with d-tubocurarine in man. *Anesthesiology*, **28**, 564.
44. Epstein, R. A. and Jackson, S. M. (1970). The effect of depth of anesthesia on the neuromuscular refractory period of anesthetised man. *Anesthesiology*, **32**, 494.
45. Knight, C., Barnes, P. K. and Feldman, S. A. (1978). Interaction of halothane and pancuronium bromide. *Anaesthesia*, **33**, 139.
46. Miller, R. D., Crigne, M. and Eger, E. I. (1976). Duration of halothane and neuromuscular blockade with d-tubocurarine. *Anesthesiology*, **44**, 206.
47. Miller, R. D., Agoston, S., Vanderpol, F., Booij, L. H. D. J. and Crul, J. F. (1979). The effect of different anaesthetics on the pharmacokinetics and pharmacodynamics in the cat. *Acta. anaesth. Scand.*, **23**, 285.
48. Martyn, J. A. J., Szyfelbein, S. K., Alim, H., Matteo, R. S. and Savarese, J. J. (1980). Increased d-tubocurarine requirement following major thermal injury. *Anesthesiology*, **52**, 353.
49. Leibec, W. S., Martyn, J. A. J. and Millar, K. W. (1980). Increased d-tubocurarine plasma binding and clinical hyposensitivity following burns trauma. *Anesth Analg.*, **59**, 549.
50. Fleischli, G. and Cohen, E. N. (1966). An analog computer simulation for the distribution of d-tubocurarine. *Anesthesiology*, **27**, 64.
51. Feldman, S. A., Cohen, E. N. and Golling, R. C. (1969). The excretion of gallamine in the dog. *Anesthesiology*, **30**, 593.
52. Agoston, S., Vermeer, G. A., Kersten, U. and Scaf, A. H. J. (1976). Renal and hepatic elimination of gallamine triethiodide in man. In: *Disposition and Effects of Some Non-Depolarising Neuromuscular Blocking Agents*. Thesis. University of Groningen.
53. Cohen, E. N., Brewer, W. H. and Smith, D. (1967). The metabolism and elimination of *d*-tubocurarine[3] *Anesthesiology*, **28**, 309.
54. Miller, R. D., Matteo, R. S., Benet, L. Z. and Sohn, Y. J. (1977). The pharmacokinetics of *d*-tubocurarine in man without renal failure. *J. Pharmacol. exp. Ther.*, **202**, 1.
55. Hunter, J. M., Jones, R. S., Utting, J. E. (1982). Use of the muscle relaxant atracurium in anephric patients: preliminary communication. *J. roy. Soc. Med.*, **75**, 336.
56. Scaf, A. H. J. (1974). *Hexafluorenium*. Proefschrift, University of Groningen.
57. Kalow, W. (1959). The distribution, destruction and elimination of muscle relaxants. *Anesthesiology*, **20**, 505.
58. Tyers, M. B. (1975). Pharmacological studies on new, short-acting competitive neuromuscular blocking drugs. In: *Fazadon*. London: Duncan Flockhart.
59. Savarese, J. J. and Wastila (1979). BW444U. Intermediate duration non-depolarizing neuromuscular block—agent with significant lack of cardiovascular and autonomic effect. *Anesthesiology*, **51**, 279.
60. Agoston, S., Houwertjes, M. C. and Salt, P. J. (1980). A new method for studying the relationship between hepatic uptake of drugs and their pharmacodynamic effects in anaesthetised cats. *Brit. J. Pharmacol.*, **68**, 637.
61. Somogyi, A. A., Shanks, C. A. and Triggs, E. J. (1977). Disposition kinetics of pancuronium bromide in patients with total biliary obstruction. *Brit. J. Anaesth.*, **49**, 1103.
62. Vonk, R. J., Westra, P., Houwertjes, M. C. and Agoston, S. (1979). Prolongation by bile salts of the duration of action of a steroidal neuromuscular blocking agent. *Brit. J. Anaesth.*, **51**, 719.
63. Westra, P., Houwertjes, M. C., de Lange, A. R., Scaf, A. H. J., Hindricks, F. R. and Agoston, S. (1980). The effect of experimental cholestasis as muscle relaxants in cats. In: *Cholestasis and Muscle Relaxants*, by P. Westra. University of Groningen Thesis.
64. Feldman, S. A. and Tyrrell, M. F. (1970). A new theory of the termination of action of muscle relaxants. *Proc. roy. Soc. Med.*, **63**, 692.
65. Goat, V. A., Yeung, M. L., Blakeney, C. and Feldman, C. (1976). Effect of blood flow upon the activity of gallamine triethiodide. *Brit. J. Anaesth.*, **48**, 69.
66. Heneghan, C. P. M., Findley, I., Billbe, C. E. and Feldman, S. A. (1978). Muscle blood flow and the rate of recovery from pancuronium neuromuscular block in dogs. *Brit. J. Anaesth.*, **50**, 1105.
67. Holmes, P. E. B., Jenden, P. J. and Taylor, D. B. (1951). The analysis of the mode of action of curare on neuromuscular transmission, the effect of temperature changes. *J. Pharmacol. exp. Ther.*, **103**, 382.
68. Maclagen, J. and Zaimis, E. (1957). The effect of muscle temperature on twitch and tetanus in the cat. *J. Physiol. (Lond.)*, **137**, 89.
69. Cannard, T. H. and Zaimis, E. (1959). The effect of lowered muscle temperature on the action of neuromuscular blocking drugs in man. *J. Physiol.*, **149**, 112.
70. Feldman, S. A. (1973). Effect of blood flow, temperature and pH. In: *Muscle Relaxants, Major Problems in Anaesthesia*. London: W. B. Saunders.
71. Feldman, S. A. (1976). Hypothermia and neuromuscular transmission. Proc. VI World Congr. of Anaesthesiology, p. 27. Amsterdam: Excerpta Medica.
72. Feldman, S. A. (1979). Hypothermia and neuromuscular blockade. *Anesthesiology*, **51**, 369.
73. Feldman, S. A. (1979). Non-depolarizing neuromuscular block. In: *Muscle Relaxants, Major Problems in Anesthesia*, 2nd edition. Philadelphia: W. B. Saunders.
74. Foldes, F. F., Kuze, S. and Erdmann, K. A. (1974). The influence of temperature on the activity of neuromuscular blocking agents. In: *Abstracts of Scientific Papers*, p. 125. Annual Meeting Amer. Soc. Anesthesiologists.
75. Thornton, R. J., Blakeney, C. and Feldman, S. A. (1976). The effect of hypothermia on neuromuscular conduction in the dog. Anaesthetic Research Group. *Brit. J. Anaesth.*, **48**, 264.
76. Ham, J., Miller, R. D., Benet, L. Z., Matteo, R. S. and Roderick, L. L. (1978). The pharmacokinetics and pharmacodynamics of d-tubocurarine during hypothermia in the cat. *Anesthesiology*, **49**, 324.
77. South, F. E. (1961). The phrenic nerve diaphragm preparation in relation to temperature and hibernation. *Am. J. Physiol.*, **200**, 565.
78. Corrado, A. P., Rames, A. O. and de Escober, C. T. (1959). Neuromuscular blockade by neomycin potentiation by ether anaesthesia and d-tubocurarine and antagonism by calcium and prostigmine. *Arch. Int. Pharmacodyn. Ther.*, **120**, 380.

79. Torda, T. (1980). The nature of gentamicin induced neuromuscular block. *Brit. J. Anaesth.*, **52**, 325.
80. Prokic, C. (1976). Two deaths caused by drug combinations: muscle relaxants and intraperitoneal streptomycin as etiological agents. In: *VI World Congress of Anesthesiologists, Mexico City*. Amsterdam: Excerpta Medica.
81. Sokoll, M. D., Cronnelly, R. and Gergis, S. D. (1975). Neuromuscular blocking effects of lincomycin (Abstr.). *Pharmacologist*, **17**, 247.
82. Corrado, A. P. (1963). Respiratory depression due to antibiotics. Calcium in treatment. *Anesth. Analg.* (*Clev.*), **42**, 1.
83. Pandey, K., Kumer, S. and Badola, R. P. (1964). Neuromuscular blocking and hypotensive actions of streptomycin and their reversal. *Brit. J. Anaesth.*, **36**, 19.
84. Viljoen, J. F. (1968). Parenteral neomycin and muscle relaxants. Two case reports of interest. *Sth. Afr. Med. J.*, **40**, 968.
85. Noble, R. C. (1976). Respiratory insufficiency after intraperitoneal administration of kanamycin. Failure of calcium gluconate to reverse toxic effects. *South. med. J.*, **60**, 1218.
86. Singh, Y. N., Harvey, A. L. and Marshall, I. G. (1978). Antibiotic-induced paralysis of the mouse phrenic nerve hemidiaphragm preparation and reversibility by calcium and neostigmine. *Anesthesiology*, **48**, 418.
87. Lee, C. Y., de Silva, A. J. C. and Katz, R. L. (1978). Antagonism of polymixin $\beta$ induced neuromuscular and cardiovascular depression by 4-aminopyridine. *Brit. J. Anaesth.*, **50**, 1069.
88. Matteo, R. S., Nishitateno, K., Pua, E. K. and Spector, S. (1980). Pharmacokinetics of *d*-tubocurarine in man—effect of an osmotic diuretic on urinary excretion. *Anesthesiology*, **52**, 335.
89. Deacock, A. R. and Davies, T. D. W. (1958). The influence of certain ganglion blocking agents on neuromuscular transmission. *Brit. J. Anaesth.*, **30**, 217.
90. Wilson, S. L. (1976). Prolonged neuromuscular blockade associated with trimetaphan: a case report. *Anesth. Analg.* (*Cleve.*), **55**, 353.
91. Glissen, S. N., Eletr, A. A. and Lim, R. (1979). Prolongation of pancuronium-induced neuromuscular blockade by intravenous infusion of nitroglycerine. *Anesthesiology*, **51**, 47.
92. Dretchen, K. L., Morgenroth, V. H., Standaert, F. G. and Walts, L. F. (1976). Azathioprine—effect on neuromuscular transmission. *Anesthesiology*, **45**, 604.

CHAPTER 25

# Clinical use of Neuromuscular Blocking Drugs and Reversal Agents



The neuromuscular blocking agents are all exceedingly safe drugs. The ratio of the therapeutic dose to that producing serious side-effects in normal healthy individuals who are artificially ventilated is exceedingly high. The dangers that may accompany their use result either from a failure to appreciate the way in which some pre-existing disease in the patient may affect their activity, or the altered way in which the drug may act in the presence of certain pathological conditions. True allergic or anaphylactic responses to these drugs do occur but they are rare.[1]

## CLINICAL USE OF THE MUSCLE RELAXANTS

There remain certain areas of controversy in the use of the muscle relaxants, where claims that a certain view or particular technique is superior to another cannot be sustained. These will be briefly reviewed giving the author's personal preference. However, four fundamental facts must be borne in mind:

1. Every drug carries a potential mortality and morbidity which is generally greater with higher doses; therefore if muscle relaxation is not specifically indicated one must justify why a neuromuscular blocking agent should be used.

2. Muscle relaxants are not hypnotics, although they reduce the dose of analgesic or hypnotic required,[2] so paralysis must be accompanied by analgesia and hypnosis. Some of the reported side-effects of the muscle relaxants are at least in part due to the release of catecholamines during inadequate anaesthesia.

3. Whatever technique of drug administration is used, the aim should be to arrive at a situation where the blood concentration of drug is minimal at the time of reversal.

4. In an ideal world, the precise dose of muscle relaxant administered to each patient should be titrated against the neuromuscular block produced using a peripheral-nerve stimulator so that the clinician is fully cognisant of

the degree of block present at all stages of the operation.

### The Use of Suxamethonium for Intubation

The use of suxamethonium for endotracheal intubation, when it is to be followed by paralysis induced by a full dose of non-depolarising relaxant, exposes the patient to the hazard of two drugs with opposing actions, where it would be possible to use only one. The logic of this argument is unanswerable except in terms of utility – it is easier and quicker to intubate the trachea following suxamethonium than with a therapeutic dose of any non-depolarising drug. Provided that those patients in whom a side-effect of suxamethonium can be anticipated are avoided, the overall safety of the technique has been established by many hundreds of thousands of safe administrations. It is reasonable, therefore, to use suxamethonium for intubation in those patients in whom quick or perfect intubating conditions are desirable.

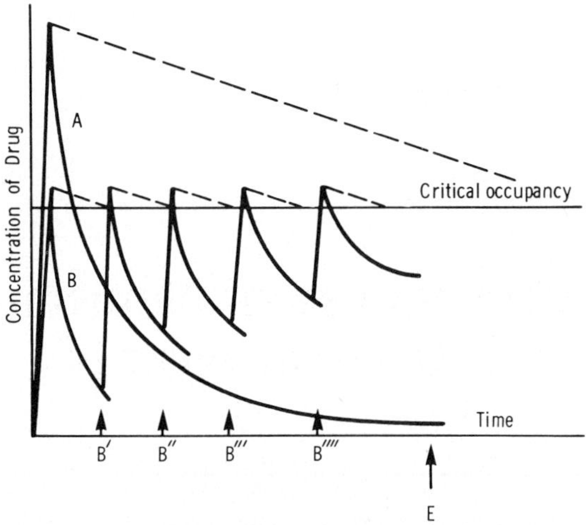


25/Fig. 1.—Predicted plasma concentrations following A, a large initial bolus of tubocurarine, and B, repeated, frequently administered "top up" doses. Note the higher concentration achieved by repeated small doses (B) as opposed to large bolus (A). E—End of operation. (Courtesy of Dr. S. A. Feldman, and W. B. Saunders Ltd.[3])

### The Dose Regime of Non-Depolarising Drugs

The advocacy by the "Liverpool School" of large initial doses of tubocurarine runs counter to that of the classical American authorities who have preferred the use of minimal doses frequently repeated. On theoretical grounds, Feldman[3] suggested that a large initial bolus dose of tubocurarine—although it produced the greatest incidence of side-effects—would also produce a lower plasma level of drug at the time of reversal than repeated "top-up doses" as the latter technique approached the continuous infusion state (Fig. 1). In an analysis of the two techniques, Sven[4] showed that although this is true for a single bolus injection of pancuronium, the drug is so cumulative that even a second dose mitigated most of the advantage and caused plasma levels almost as high as those produced by repeated injection (Fig. 2*a* and *b*). In a similar study, Ham and his colleagues[5] failed to demonstrate significantly different plasma levels between continuous infusion, intermittent injection and bolus injection but, as most of the patients in the latter group received "top-up" doses shortly before the comparison was made, a true comparison of plasma levels using the three techniques cannot be made.

The initial dose of neuromuscular blocker administered in Europe is often about 50 per cent greater than that used in America, where a lesser degree of surgical relaxation is accepted.

### Monitoring Neuromuscular Block

Continuous monitoring of neuromuscular block has its advocates.[6,7] The most convenient muscles for the anaesthetist to observe are the hand or the facial muscles, and a variety of suitable instruments are available. The hand muscles are particularly suitable, not only for access purposes, but also because there is evidence that they are affected earlier and recover later than the muscles of respiration.[8] Stimulation of the facial nerve and observation of the response of the facial muscles is useful, but care must be taken not to stimulate directly the muscle itself.

In clinical practice, a severe depression, or even abolition, of the twitch response of the adductor muscles may be necessary to produce ideal abdominal relaxation. For *lower* abdominal surgery, good relaxation can be obtained when only the first twitch of the train-of-four (i.e. less than 10 per cent) is visible, whilst for *upper* abdominal surgery it will often be necessary to suppress the whole of the train-of-four response. However, to prevent an overdose

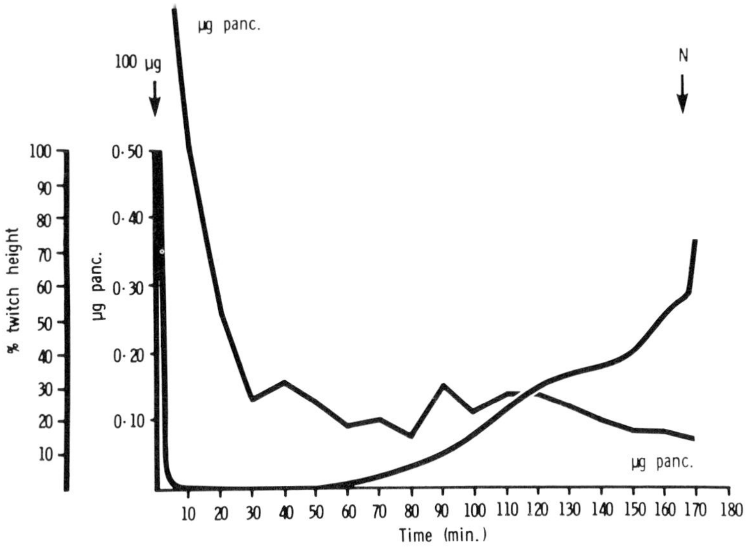


25/FIG. 2(*a*).—*Upper trace:* Plasma levels of pancuronium after single bolus of 100 μg/kg. *Lower trace:* Twitch response of hand muscles. N = neostigmine. (Personal communication, Sven, 1981.)

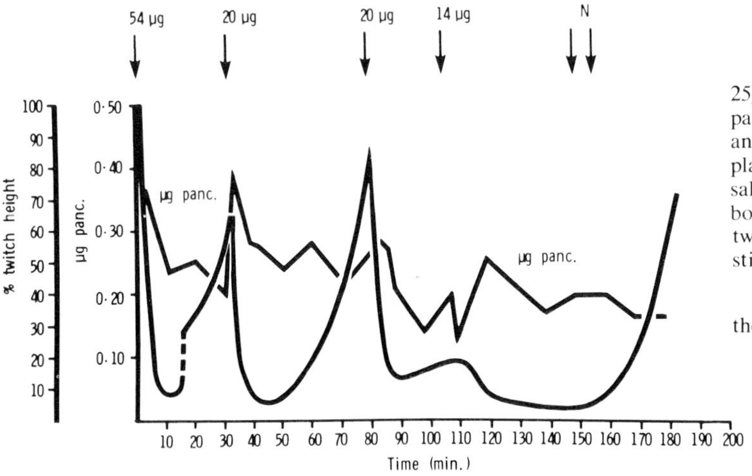


25/FIG. 2(*b*).—Plasma concentrations of pancuronium following 54 μg/kg bolus and repeated "top up" doses. Note the plasma concentration at the time of reversal was almost twice that following single bolus, whilst relaxation (*lower trace*, twitch response) was poor. N = Neostigmine.

In Figs. 2(*a*) and (*b*) ordinates denote the plasma concentration in μg/litre.

situation, some response to post-tetanic facilitation should always be maintained. Failure to obtain any post-tetanic facilitation represents a situation which is irreversible by neostigmine and the procedure recommended below should be followed.

In conditions of impaired renal function, hepatic disorders and in some long neurosurgical cases, it will be necessary to titrate carefully the dose of relaxant used, in order to achieve satisfactory surgical conditions with the minimum dose of relaxant. Possibly the most important use of monitoring is in the recovery room, where it is not uncommon for patients to exhibit restlessness due to residual paralysis.[9,10] This may be misinterpreted as due to pain and an analgesic administered unless the patient is tested for residual neuromuscular block.

### Treatment of Prolonged Paresis

It is probable that 95 per cent of patients in whom the neuromuscular block is inadequately reversed by 0·04 mg/kg of neostigmine have a plasma level of drug that prevents the establishment of an adequate concentration gradient for the drug to leave the receptor area. In these circumstances, it is pointless to continue administrating anticholinesterase drugs,[11] and the patient should be ventilated with an analgesic mixture of nitrous oxide and oxygen whilst steps are taken to reduce the plasma level by infusing fluid and electrolyte. If the urine secretion is adequate, mannitol may be given to improve diuresis. Once a good urine flow is established and the plasma level of drug reduced, it is usually possible to reverse the action of the relaxant drug.

### The Future

With the development of non-cumulative, shorter acting, non-depolarising relaxants without cardiovascular side-effects, it is possible that two equally acceptable forms of practice will develop. Either the dose of drug administered as an initial bolus will be adjusted so as to produce a suitable duration of action or alternatively the drug may be administered in the form of a constant infusion whose rate will be adjusted to abolish the twitch response of adductor muscles. The rate of flow may be increased to produce bursts of complete relaxation as and when it is demanded by the surgical procedure. With both techniques, the rapid recovery slope of the new relaxants such as atracurium and vecuronium make it desirable to monitor neuromuscular conduction so that the dose of drug can be adjusted in time to prevent reversal of the muscle relaxation.

## ANTICHOLINESTERASES AND THE REVERSAL AGENTS

Due to the inability to monitor less than 75 per cent receptor occlusion by non-depolarising relaxants, the use of neostigmine (with atropine) should always be considered before extubation of the patient. The dangers of neostigmine 0·04 mg/kg together with a fully vagolytic dose of atropine (1·0 mg–1·2 mg) are minimal in most patients, compared to the possible discomfort and the potential harmful effects of residual curarisation. It is not necessary to establish some degree of spontaneous breathing before neostigmine is administered, indeed, to do so deliberately may be harmful, as cardiac dysrhythmias are more common in the presence of a raised $Paco_2$.

### Anticholinesterases

As their name implies, all these compounds block the activity of both types of cholinesterase enzyme in varying degrees.

**Mode of action.**—The principal activity of anticholinesterase drugs is to depress the cholinesterase enzyme—both the plasma and true—thus permitting the local concentration of acetylcholine molecules to rise. There are, however, other effects of these drugs that must be mentioned. They are capable of acting in their own right to produce depolarisation if sufficiently large doses are used. This effect may be seen as a fibrillation of small muscles which may proceed to paresis in man if doses of more than 5·0 mg of neostigmine are given intravenously in the absence of any tubocurarine. The presence of even the smallest quantity of the latter drug will normally prevent this in clinical practice. These drugs may also have an action on the nerve-ending causing repetitive firing and increasing release of acetylcholine directly.[12] Indeed, there is considerable evidence to suggest that this facilitatory effect on acetylcholine mobilisation may be a major mode of action of the anticholinesterase drugs.[13,14]

Acetylcholine has a very widespread activity in the body, affecting not only peripheral autonomic ganglia, smooth muscle (including myocardium) and secretory glands, but also skeletal muscle. So various are these actions that they are usually sub-divided into two main groups. First, the *nicotine-like* activity accounting for the action at the neuromuscular junction and also at the autonomic ganglia. Secondly, the *muscarine-like* action which accounts for the effect on the myocardium, bowel, bladder, pupil, and secretory glands (Table 1).

Atropine sulphate opposes the muscarinic actions of acetylcholine and therefore is the drug of choice in the treatment of nerve-gas casualties where the most important lesion is usually spasm of the smooth muscle of the bronchioles. The anticholinesterases potentiate both the muscarinic and the nicotinic actions of acetylcholine. If, however, they are combined with a large dose of atropine (1–2 mg) then only the nicotinic action is revealed and the muscarinic side-effects are reduced or prevented. (For glycopyrronium, see p. 1144.)

Blaber and Bowman[15] have investigated the action of the anticholinesterase drugs and conclude that three distinct sites of activity can be illustrated. These are:

25/TABLE 1
ACTIONS OF ACETYLCHOLINE

| *Muscarinic effects* | *Nicotinic effects* |
|---|---|
| 1. Myocardium = bradycardia. | |
| 2. Gut = contraction. | |
| 3. Bronchioles = constriction. | 1. Autonomic ganglia stimulated. |
| 4. Pupil = contraction. | |
| 5. Salivary glands = mucus + +. | 2. Skeletal muscle stimulated. |
| 6. Sweat glands = stimulated. | |
| 7. Bladder = contracted. | |
| Opposed by atropine sulphate. | |

1. *Depression of acetylcholinesterase activity*.—This increases the amount of acetylcholine available at the motor end-plate.

2. *Action on the pre-junctional nerve-ending*.—The anticholinesterase drugs hasten the release of acetylcholine from the nerve-ending. Thus when high rates of nerve stimulation are used, the stores of acetylcholine are rapidly exhausted and neuromuscular transmission fails. However, these stores are sufficient for slow rates of nerve stimulation.

3. *Action on the post-junctional motor end-plate*.—This is one of simple depolarisation due to the presence of a greater quantity of acetylcholine for longer than the normal fraction of a millisecond.

**Neostigmine Methylsulphate (Prostigmin)**

This is a white crystalline powder, odourless and soluble in water. The formula is:

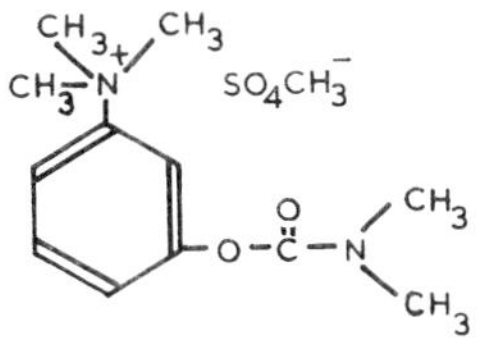


The fate of neostigmine in the body is interesting, for although a large proportion of the injected material can be accounted for by direct contact with the enzyme cholinesterase, most of the drug is excreted by glomerular filtration in the kidneys[30] and a similar proportion destroyed by the liver. When taken orally the gastro-intestinal tract appears to possess powerful destructive properties for neostigmine, as none survives long enough to reach the faeces, yet only one-thirtieth of the ingested material ever reaches the general circulation.[16] The plasma half-life of the drug is variously given as 30–50 minutes.

**Fasciculations.**—When neostigmine is given intravenously to a conscious subject, fasciculations may be seen or experienced by the individual. These are activations of motor units brought about partly by the accumulation of the packets or quanta of acetylcholine at the end-plate, but also by the direct action of the neostigmine on the motor nerve-ending causing repetitive firing with antidromic excitation of the motor unit.

*Clinical comment*.—Experience has shown that neostigmine in a dose of 40–45 μg/kg and atropine 20 μg/kg can be used with safety to reverse a non-depolarising block in man, and that neostigmine and atropine may be combined because the action of the atropine always precedes that of the neostigmine. In clinical practice a ratio of 1·0 mg of atropine sulphate to 2·5 mg neostigmine methylsulphate has been found satisfactory. The optimum time to administer this mixture is whilst the patient is still being hyperventilated and the carbon dioxide level of the blood is low. At least 5 min should be allowed for its effect to become obvious and improvement in neuromuscular conduction may occur for up to 10 min after its administration. It should, however, never be administered in the presence of a high concentration of halothane or cyclopropane.

Though almost every case that has received a paralysing dose of a non-depolarising drug will probably benefit from reversal of the neuromuscular block, it is now possible to demonstrate the degree of this block with a peripheral-nerve stimulator. If, for example, the hand muscles show adequate recovery of transmission (less than 20 per cent evidence of fade in the train-of-four stimulation and sustained contraction on tetanic stimulation) then it can safely be concluded that the respiratory muscles are no longer under the influence of the relaxant drug. Recovery of the respiratory muscles always precedes that of the peripheral hand muscles. The only exception to this rule is when a pathological state exists at the motor end-plate, e.g. myasthenia gravis.

In small children, cardiac cases, and severely ill patients it is advisable to titrate the exact dose of neostigmine and atropine required with the nerve stimulator. Also, in those patients who have received very large doses of a non-depolarising relaxant over a long period of time, it is often necessary to exceed a total dose of 2·5 mg of neostigmine and 1·0 mg of atropine. However, before further therapy is attempted it is important to verify with the stimulator that the signs of a non-depolarising neuromuscular block are still present.

If a dose of tubocurarine has been used which is much greater than the blocking dose (i.e. 100 per cent paralysis) then neostigmine will be unable to bring about complete reversal until the plasma level of relaxant has fallen below the critical threshold.[17] In clinical practice it is never advisable to exceed a total dose of 2·0 mg atropine and 5·0 mg neostigmine, as this is sufficient to depress all cholinesterase enzyme activity severely.

Though the combination of atropine and neostigmine is now considered safe it is perhaps wiser not to administer the mixture in the presence of a bradycardia. In such an instance atropine alone in dilute solution is sometimes used to raise the pulse rate to around 80 per minute before mixing the remainder of the atropine with 2·5 mg of neostigmine.

**Edrophonium Chloride (Tensilon)**

In a study of the quaternary ammonium compounds analogous to neostigmine the pharmacological activity of edrophonium was revealed. The compound is 3-hydroxy-phenyl-dimethylethylammonium chloride, a white, odourless and crystalline powder which is readily soluble in water but not in alkali.

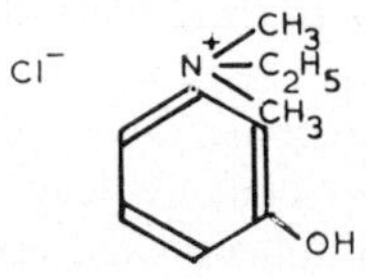


The mode of action of edrophonium has aroused considerable interest, since it was originally believed that it acted mainly by a direct action on the neuromuscular junction similar to that of acetylcholine. Its anticholinesterase activity was considered to be very weak.[18,19] Subsequently, however, Hobbiger[20] attacked this concept, and it is now generally accepted that the drug is an anticholinesterase and that the direct depolarising activity is secondary to its important prejunctional effect as a facilitator of acetylcholine mobilisation and release. Edrophonium is a weaker drug than neostigmine and a dose of 35 mg/70 kg has been found to be equipotent to neostigmine 3 mg/kg.[31] In this dosage it has a more rapid onset of action than neostigmine and its plasma level is sustained at an effective level for 20 min.[32] It has been recommended as a safe reversal to vecuronium neuromuscular block.[33–35] The muscarinic effects of edrophonium are less marked than with neostigmine and if the pulse rate is above 100/min, atropine may be omitted or only given if bradycardia ensues.

**Pyridostigmine (Mestinon).**—This compound (i.e. the dimethylcarbamic ester of 1-methyl-3-hydroxy-pyridinium bromide) is an analogue of neostigmine and was introduced into medicine for the treatment of cases of myasthenia gravis. Pyridostigmine has about one-quarter the potency of neostigmine so that 10 mg given intravenously are equivalent to 2·5 mg neostigmine by the same route, but the action of pyridostigmine on the myocardium and the bowel are far less marked.

Brown[21] investigated the use of this drug in anaesthesia and verified that the muscarinic side-effects are less than with an equivalent dose of neostigmine. He found, however, that about four minutes elapsed before the action at the neuromuscular junction became evident, and also that the drug was generally less reliable than neostigmine.

## Other Drugs Affecting Neuromuscular Function

**Galanthamine hydrobromide** (Nivalin).—This compound is an alkaloid which is extracted from the snowdrop bulb. It was widely used in Bulgaria as an antagonist to non-depolarising relaxants. Galanthamine has about one-tenth the anticholinesterase activity of neostigmine but the side-effects on heart rate and salivation are less.[22] The use of atropine is recommended.

**Germine acetate.**—Germine mono- and di-acetate are derivatives of the semi-synthetic ester alkaloids of the veratrum family. They are an interesting group of drugs because their principal site of action is on the muscle fibre itself. Germine diacetate is capable of improving neuromuscular transmission in the presence of both a depolarisation and a non-depolarisation block. This is achieved by converting a single muscle action potential into a brief period of tetanic firing by a direct effect on the fibre itself. However, it can have no effect at all if all neuromuscular transmission is blocked by complete paralysis. It would appear to be of possible value in the treatment of myasthenia gravis.

**Hexafluorenium.**—This is a drug with a variety of interesting actions. It achieved some notoriety in clinical anaesthesia when combined with suxamethonium because it prolonged the latter drug's action, reduced the dose required and therefore lessened the risk of Phase II block.[23] The main action is one of inhibition of plasma cholinesterase activity but it also has a specific action on the post-junctional membrane.[24] Apart from these actions, it also inhibits true cholinesterase and is a weak non-depolarising agent. It often causes disconcerting salivation in patients.

To those accustomed to using suxamethonium for short procedures and *d*-tubocurarine for long procedures, the value of combining hexafluorenium with suxamethonium has never seemed obvious. The combination lacked an adequate antidote. Added to this, there were reports of tachycardia, hypertension, cardiac dysrhythmias and fatal bronchospasm,[12] so it is hardly surprising that it failed to gain universal popularity.

**Tetrahydroaminacrine (THA).**—This drug has also been advocated for combination with suxamethonium. It is a weak anticholinesterase but a powerful direct stimulant of the respiratory centre.

**Quinidine.**—This agent potentiates the neuromuscular block of both the depolarising and the non-depolarising relaxants. In fact, the combination of quinidine and a muscle relaxant has resulted in a case of prolonged apnoea lasting six hours.[25] The most likely explanation of this enhancement of the activity of the muscle relaxants is that the cinchona alkaloids (like the local analgesic agents) depress the release of acetylcholine at the nerve-ending. However, Usubiaga[26] attacks this thesis and argues that the most likely explanation is a depressant action on the muscle fibre itself.

**4-Aminopyridine.**—This drug has been used to reverse the non-depolarising muscle relaxants at the end of operations, to reverse the effect of the amino-glycoside antibiotics at the myoneural junction[27] and to treat the Eaton-Lambert syndrome (myasthenic syndrome). The drug is not an anticholinesterase, but acts by increasing the rate of calcium transport across membranes, thereby increasing the rate of acetylcholine release and the force of muscle contraction.[28] It is believed to achieve this effect by prolonging the slow ingoing current, thereby allowing a greater calcium flux to take place. This results in an inotropic effect on cardiac as well as skeletal muscle, and also in a central nervous system stimulant action. Because of its action in promoting acetylcholine release, it has been used as a neostigmine synergist. If mixed with neostigmine, the dose of anticholinesterase required is greatly reduced.[36,37] As it crosses the blood brain barrier, it may cause convulsions in conscious patients.

### Clinical Comment on the Indications for the use of an Antidote to the Muscle Relaxants

Most anaesthetists today give an anticholinesterase drug at the end of all operations in which a non-depolarising muscle relaxant has been administered. This practice is usually commendable as it will lower the drug receptor occupancy to a safe level, but this can only be safely achieved if the blood level of the relaxant has been suitably reduced to a non-paralytic level. However, anticholinesterase therapy is not without complications and may cause disruption of intestinal anastomosis by promoting gut activity.[29] The more proximal the gut involved the more active is the resulting peristalsis caused by the neostigmine. But clinically all patients must be adequately reversed before artificial ventilation is discontinued and the trachea extubated.

## REFERENCES

1. Lim, M. and Churchill-Davidson, H. C. (1981). Adverse effects of neuromuscular blocking drugs. In: *Adverse Reactions to Anaesthetic Drugs*. Ed. J. A. Thornton. Amsterdam: Elsevier, North Holland Biomedical Press.

2. Forbes, A. R., Cohen, N. H. and Eger, E. I. (1979). Pancuronium reduces halothane requirements in man. *Anesthesiology*, **51**, S.1.

3. Feldman, S. A. (1973). The rational use of relaxants. In: *Muscle Relaxants*, p. 152. Philadelphia: W. B. Saunders Co.

4. Sven, J. (1979). Relationship between serum concentration and pharmacological effect on non-depolarizing muscle relaxants. In *Curares and Curarization*, p. 245. Post Graduate Course. XI International meeting of Anaesthesiology and Resuscitation, Paris. Amsterdam: Excerpta Medica.

5. Ham, J., Miller, R. D., Sheiner, L. B. and Matteo, R. S. (1979). Dosage-schedule independence of d-tubocurarine pharmacokinetics and pharmacodynamics and recovery of neuromuscular function. *Anesthesiology*, **50**, 528.

6. Churchill-Davidson, H. C. (1972). Neuromuscular blocking drugs. In: *A Practice of Anaesthesia*, 3rd edit. Ed. W. D. Wylie and H. C. Churchill-Davidson. London: Lloyd-Luke.

7. Katz, R. L. and Katz, G. (1975). Clinical considerations in the use of muscle relaxants. In: *Muscle Relaxants*. Ed. Katz. Amsterdam: Excerpta Medica.

8. Gerber, H. R., Johansen, S. H., Mortimer, J. T. and Yodlowski, E. (1977). Frequency sweep electromyogram and voluntary effort in volunteers after d-tubocurarine. *Anesthesiology*, **46**, 35.

9. Viby Mogensen, J., Jorgenson, B. C. and Ording, H. (1979). Residual curarization in the recovery room. *Anesthesiology*, 50, 528.

10. Feldman, S. A. (1980). La Surveillance du Bloc Neuromusculaire. *Journées d'Enseignement post-universaire*, p. 337. Paris: Librairie Arnette.

11. Feldman, S. A. and Agoston, S. (1980). Inability of neostigmine to prevent tubocurarine neuromuscular block. *Brit. J. Anaesth.*, **52**, 1199.

12. Katz, R. L. (1967). Neuromuscular effects of *d*-tubocurarine, edrophonium and neostigmine in man. *Anesthesiology*, **28**, 327.

13. Riker, W. F., Jr. (1960). Pharmacological considerations in a re-evaluation of the neuromuscular synapse. *Arch. Neurol. (Chic.)*, 3, 488.

14. Riker, W. F., Jr. and Standaert, F. G. (1966). The action of facilitory drugs on neuromuscular transmission. *Ann. N.Y. Acad. Sci.*, 135, 163.

15. Blaber, L. C. and Bowman, W. C. (1963). Studies on the repetitive discharges evoked in motor-nerve and skeletal muscle after injection of anti-cholinesterase drugs. *Brit. J. Pharmacol.*, **20**, 326.

16. Goldstein, A., Krayer, O., Root, M. A., Acheson, G. H. and Doherty, M. E. (1949). Plasma neostigmine levels and cholinesterase inhibition in dogs and myasthenic patients. *J. Pharmacol. exp. Ther.*, **96**, 56.

17. Baraka, A. (1967). Irreversible tubocurarine neuromuscular block in the human. *Brit. J. Anaesth.*, **39**, 891.

18. Randall, L. O. (1950). Anticurare action of phenolin quaternary ammonium salts. *J. Pharmacol. exp. Ther.*, **100**, 83.

19. Riker, W. F. Jr. and Wescoe, W. C. (1950). Studies on the inter-relationship of certain cholinergic compounds. V. The significance of the actions of the 3-hydroxy phenyltrimethylammonium ion on neuromuscular function. *J. Pharmacol. exp. Ther.*, **100**, 454.

20. Hobbiger, F. (1952). The mechanism of anticurare action of certain neostigmine analogues. *Brit. J. Pharmacol.*, **7**, 223.

21. Brown, A. K. (1954). Pyridostigmin. *Anaesthesia*, **9**, 92.

22. Wislicki, L. (1967). Nivalin (galanthamine hydrobromide), an additional decurarizing agent: some introductory observations. *Brit. J. Anaesth.*, **39**, 963.

23. Foldes, F. F., Hillmer, N. R., Molloy, R. E. and Monte, A. P. (1960). Potentiation of the neuromuscular effect of succinylcholine by hexafluorenium. *Anesthesiology*, **21**, 50.

24. Nastuk, W. L. and Karis, J. H. (1964). The blocking action of hexafluorenium on neuromuscular transmission and its interaction with succinylcholine. *J. Pharmacol. exp. Ther.*, **144**, 236.

25. Way, W. L., Katzung, B. G. and Larson, C. P. (1967). Recurarisation with quinidine. *J. Amer. med. Ass.*, **200**, 153.

26. Usubiaga, J. E. (1968). Potentiation of muscle relaxants by quinidine. *Anesthesiology*, **29**, 1068.

27. Lee, C., deSilva, A. J. C. and Katz, R. L. (1977). Reversal of Polymyxin B induced neuromuscular and cardiovascular depression by 4-aminopyridine. *Abstr. of Scientific Papers, ASA Meeting*, New Orleans, p. 445.

28. Illies, P. and Thesleff, S. (1978). 4-amino pyridine and evoked transmitter release from motor-nerve endings. *Brit. J. Pharmacol.*, **64**, 623.

29. Bell, C. M. A. and Lewis, C. B. (1968). Effect of neostigmine on integrity of iliorectal anastomosis. *Brit. med. J.*, **3**, 587.

30. Cronnelly, R., Stanski, D. R., Miller, R. D., Sheiner, L. B. and Sohn, Y. J. (1979). Renal failure and pharmacokinetics of neostigmine in anesthetised man. *Anesthesiology*, **51**, 222.

31. Cronnelly, R. (1983). Reversal agents after vecuronium and other competitive muscle relaxants. (Paper presented to the Muscle Relaxant Society, Geneva.) To be published.

32. Morris, R. B., Cronnelly, R., Miller, R. D., Stanski, D. R. and Fahey, M. R. (1981). Pharmacokinetics of edrophonium and neostigmine when antagonizing d-tubocurarine neuromuscular blockade in man. *Anesthesiology*, **54**, 399.

33. Foldes, F. F., Yun, H., Radnay, P. A., Badola, R. P., Kaplan, R. and Nagashima, H. (1981). Antagonism of the NM effect of ORG NC45 by edrophonium. *Anesthesiology*, **55**, A201.

34. Baird, W. L. M., Bowman, W. C. and Kerr, W. J. (1982). Some actions of ORG NC45 and of edrophonium in anaesthetised cats and man. *Brit. J. Anaesth.*, **54**, 375.

35. Cronnelly, R. and Morris, R. B. (1982). Antagonism of neuromuscular block. *Brit. J. Anaesth.*, **54**, 183.

36. Miller, R. D., Booij, L. H. D. J., Agoston, S. and Crul, J. F. (1979). 4-aminopyridine potentiates neostigmine and pyridostigmine in man. *Anesthesiology*, **50**, 416.

37. Booij, L. H. D. J., Van der Pol, F., Crul, J. F. and Miller, R. D. (1980). Antagonism of ORG NC45 neuromuscular blockade by neostigmine, pyridostigmine and 4-aminopyridine. *Anesth. Analg.*, **59**, 31.

CHAPTER 26

# Neurological Conditions and Anaesthesia



## MALIGNANT HYPERPYREXIA
(Hyperthermia)

Malignant hyperpyrexia is a rare condition in which genetically susceptible subjects exhibit an abnormal response to anaesthesia particularly, but not exclusively, if halothane or suxamethonium has been administered. The response causes a rapid increase in body temperature associated with profound metabolic acidosis usually associated with muscle rigidity. The syndrome carries a very high mortality in spite of symptomatic treatment unless this is established early and carried out vigorously. Specific and non-specific remedies are claimed to reduce the mortality of the condition.

Although there had been sporadic reports of hyperthermic response to anaesthesia for some years it was the report of Denborough and Lovell in 1960[1] noting the occurrence of the condition in susceptible members in one family, that provoked renewed interest in the disease. The occurrence of several cases in the Toronto area of Canada led Britt and associates[2] to describe the syndrome clearly and to point definitely to its being genetically linked. The present concept of the disease has been developed in a series of papers and on the two symposia published in 1973[3] and 1978.[4]

The task of elucidating the cause of this rare condition and the efficacy of the treatments proposed were made easier by the observation that certain strains of pigs (especially the Pietrain white Landrace pig) exhibited a similar phenomenon. This phenomenon has been known by pig breeders for many years and its genetic association recognised. It is triggered off by fear in the pigs, and if this occurs just before slaughter, it results in a particular jelly-like consistency of the muscles and a jelly-like exudate.[5] In 1966, Hall and his co-workers[6] demonstrated that suxamethonium and halothane induced a similar condition in those susceptible pigs and that it was associated with hyperthermia and the metabolic change associated with human malignant hyperpyrexia.

Halothane appears to be the most potent triggering agent for malignant hyperpyrexia in Landrace pigs[7–10] and susceptible patients.[11,12] Suxamethonium administration often accelerates or initiates the development of the syndrome.[10,11,13,14] In most patients, generalised muscle rigidity after the administration of suxamethonium is followed very shortly by a rapid increase in body temperature, profuse sweating, tachycardia and hyperventilation. However, some patients have not demonstrated generalised spasms. Donlon and his colleagues[15] described masseteric spasm as a warning sign of the development of this condition. Other muscle relaxants have been incriminated as causal agents, including tubocurarine in the presence of nitrous oxide.[16] However, in spite of one highly suggestive case report,[17] no proven case has been reported in which pancuronium has been used. Due to the difficulty of avoiding halothane-contaminated apparatus unless a predisposition to the disease is anticipated, it is possible that in those case reports, when the only volatile anaesthetic administered has been nitrous oxide, traces of halothane may have been received by the patient. Other agents that have been reported to trigger off malignant hyperpyrexia include the amide local anaesthetics (lignocaine), pethidine, ketamine, phencyclidine, monoamine oxidase inhibitors and tranquillisers.[18–21]

The pattern of inherited susceptibility to this syndrome suggests that it is transmitted as an autosomal dominant gene.[22,23] However, statistical analysis reveals fewer cases than would be expected on this basis, and this may be the result of generation skipping due to incomplete penetrance. Present opinion favours a multifactorial inheritance in the production of the fulminating condition.

Tests for susceptibility to the condition include the demonstration of a myopathy and *in vitro* muscle contractions when exposed to halothane.[24] Kalow and his colleagues[25] have demonstrated that caffeine, a known ATPase activator, will induce contractions. This forms a sensitive test for the presence of the syndrome.

Histological evidence of neurogenic disease and a die-back type of atrophy of muscle fibres has been reported. An increase in the plasma CPK (creatinine phosphokinase) is often, but by no means always, found in susceptible patients. It is always markedly increased after an actual attack of hyperpyrexia, presumably due to muscle breakdown.

### Diagnosis and Treatment

Patients should be questioned about relatives who have had anaesthetics. An unexplained death during anaesthesia should raise the possibility of the patient suffering from a predisposition to malignant hyperpyrexia. Dantrolene sodium offers a specific protection to patients but it is difficult to dissolve and an intravenous solution has only recently become available. As a prophylactic measure, dantrolene may be administered orally in a total dose of 5–7 mg/kg given in divided doses over 48 hours before the anaesthetic. In an established case during anaesthesia, a dose of 3–5 mg/kg i.v. is required. The intravenous solution has to be made up with sodium hydroxide to yield a pH of 9·5, and it should be administered along with mannitol to encourage diuresis. Extreme care must be taken to ensure that the solution does not extravasate outside the vein. Because of its high cost and the potentially dangerous nature of the solution, it should be used only in proven cases when the hyperpyrexia has not been controlled by conservative measures.

Less severe cases of hyperpyrexia should be treated symptomatically. The body temperature must be reduced as soon as possible, either by ice-bags, immersion in cold water, or even intraperitoneal and intravenous cooling, when considered practicable. The lactic acidaemia should be countered by an infusion of sodium bicarbonate. Intravenous procaine has been helpful in some cases.[14] Artificial hyperventilation with a high inspired oxygen is essential and the blood potassium must be monitored. If the muscle spasm is severe or myoglobinaemia present, then an infusion of mannitol should be given.

As evidence suggests that the greater the dose of triggering agent administered, the more severe the effect, so halothane or any other possible triggering agent should be discontinued. However, the patient must be kept sedated as there appears to be an association of sympatho-adrenal discharge and the severity of the symptoms. Indeed, some cases of sudden unexplained deaths not associated with anaesthesia may have occurred, triggered by an undue stress in susceptible patients due to the associated cardiomyopathy which sometimes occurs in such patients.[26]

### Mechanism of Malignant Hyperpyrexia

The importance of calcium in the activation of muscle contraction (see p. 669) and in the control of excitable tissues has led to the belief that susceptible patients suffer from a defect in the control mechanism of the calcium sequestrated in the sarcoplasmic reticulum and mitochondria. It has been demonstrated that the calcium-storage function of sarcoplasmic reticulum is *reduced* in susceptible subjects and pigs,[27] and this effect is exacerbated by high concentrations of halothane. It seems likely that the triggering event, following depolarisation of the muscle membrane or an altered permeability, produces an excessive and uncontrolled release of calcium into the transverse tubules, stimulating unco-ordinated and continued muscle activity. Dantrolene, which acts by blocking the passage of calcium into the terminal cisterns, mitigates this effect.

## MYASTHENIA GRAVIS

This disease, originally described in a young woman by Thomas Willis in 1684,[28] was re-described independently by Erb in 1879[29] and Goldflam in 1893.[30] It was given its name of myasthenia gravis pseudoparalytica by Jolly in 1895.[31]

### Pathological Changes

In early myasthenia gravis the motor end-plates are morphologically normal but as the condition becomes established, sprouting and branching of the terminal fibres is observed. The end-plates become elongated and show widening of the synaptic clefts and folds.[32] Infiltration with lymphorrhages is common. Atrophic end-plates are most frequently associated with neostigmine-resistant myasthenia gravis.

Two types of thymic enlargement have been described in patients with this disease. The commonest is simple hypertrophy of the gland in which lymphorrhages and germ centres are often seen. The second type is a tumour—a thymoma. This may be benign and encapsulated or it may be locally malignant within the thoracic cage. There is a close association between both thymic hyperplasia or tumour and the symptoms of myasthenia gravis, but their presence is by no means certain in every case.

### Clinical Features

(a) *Neonatal myasthenia* occurs in 1 out of 8 infants born to myasthenic mothers and a previous thymectomy performed on the mother is believed to reduce this incidence. The symptoms develop within three days of birth and the weakness persists for about six weeks after which it usually resolves. The condition responds well to the anticholinesterase drugs and may be related to circulating maternal antibodies.

(b) *Juvenile type*.—This condition occurs before the age of two years. It is usually confined to the bulbar musculature and consists of ptosis and ophthalmoplegia. It is usually mild or slowly progressive. In older children the pattern is similar to that found in the adult.

(c) *Adult type*.—Little can be added by modern physicians to the early description by Willis and others. Most cases occur in adults of either sex between the ages of 20 and 50, but it has been described in all the various age groups.

The onset of muscle fatigue is often so insidious that its significance may be missed by both doctor and patient. Occasionally it is precipitated by a severe illness or emotional disturbance. Fatigue of the eyelid muscles (on staring upwards) or of the limb girdle muscles (with elevation of the arms) are sometimes useful in eliciting the early signs of myasthenia. Though the bulbar muscles (i.e. eyelid, facial and swallowing) are the most commonly affected, the signs of disease can appear in any skeletal muscle throughout the body. Typically, the patient gives a history of fatigue increasing throughout the day with some recovery on awakening in the morning. In long-standing cases some wasting of the muscle fibres can be observed. The progress of the disease fluctuates but often reaches a certain level and then remains static for many years. In the early stages a remission may occur but these are rarely permanent. Abnormalities of thyroid function are present in a high proportion of patients with myasthenia gravis.

### Aetiology of Myasthenia Gravis

Until a few years ago, the aetiology of the disease was thought to be a primary disturbance of acetylcholine formation and release. This theory was based on the electromyographic findings of Desmedt[33] who demonstrated fade upon successive stimulation, post-tetanic facilitation (Fig. 1) and the classical occurrence of post-tetanic exhaustion. Elmquist and co-workers[34] were proponents of the *prejunctional* theory, as in 1964 they demonstrated a reduced incidence of miniature end-plate potentials in

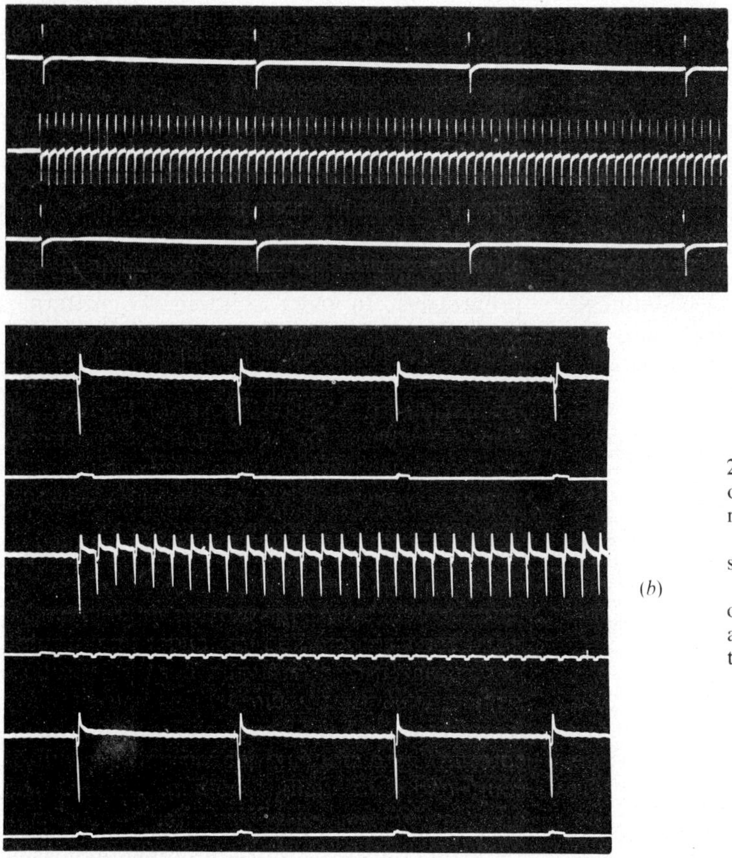

(*a*)

(*b*)

26/Fig. 1.—A comparison of the effects of electrical stimulation in a normal and myasthenic patient.
(*a*) Normal neuromuscular transmission.
(*b*) Myasthenia gravis. Note the "fade" of the twitch and tetanic response, and also the presence of post-tetanic facilitation.

myasthenic patients (Fig. 2). However, these and many other observations really demonstrated the reduced margin of safety of neuromuscular transmission that occurs in this disease and the close inter-relationship between prejunctional and postjunctional events. The realisation that the receptors are not static and permanent, but are part of a continuing turnover of postsynaptic structures, has allowed findings that were previously interpreted as due primarily to a motor nerve disease to be seen as secondary to a diminution in the receptor population caused by an increased receptor lysis, or a reduced replacement rate of the decaying receptors of the motor end-plate. The work of Fambrough and colleagues in 1973,[35] using $\alpha$-bungarotoxin to label postsynaptic receptors, demonstrated that they are greatly reduced in number in this disease. So the *postsynaptic* theory of the aetiology of myasthenia gravis began to receive support.

The shift towards accepting an alteration in receptor activity as the primary defect in this disease is in keeping with the aetiological changes seen in advanced disease, and also with the classical work of Churchill-Davidson and Richardson,[36] who demonstrated an altered response to decamethonium in these patients with a resistance to depolarising agents and a marked propensity to develop a Phase II block.

All the present evidence suggests that myasthenia gravis is an autoimmune disease in which the patient develops antibodies to acetylcholine receptors. This concept was first developed by Nastuk and colleagues[37] and Simpson[38] on the basis of the similarity of the disease with other autoimmune phenomena. The benefits resulting from the thymectomy and corticosteroid ther-

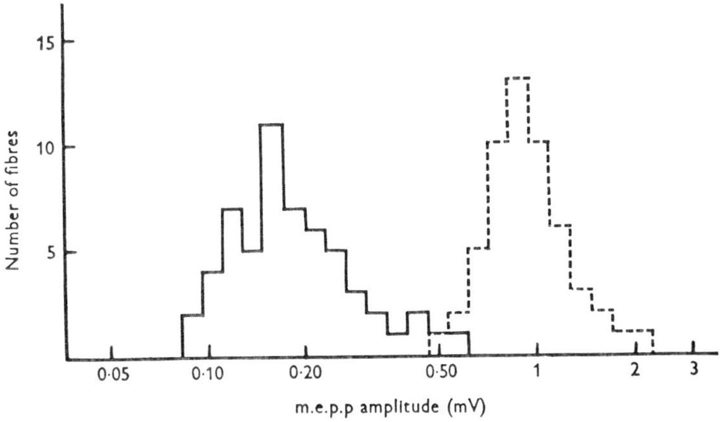


26/FIG. 2.—Distribution of mean miniature end-plate potential amplitudes from 57 myasthenic (solid line) and 54 normal (dotted line) human muscle fibres. All amplitudes corrected to a membrane potential of 85 mV. (Courtesy of Professor D. Elmquist, Drs. W. W. Hofman, J. Kugelburg and D. M. J. Quastel, and the Editors of the *Journal of Physiology*.[34])

apy, along with the occurrence of high levels of antibodies to muscle in some of these patients (especially those with thymomas), could be explained on this basis. Specific antibodies that bind to the receptor site—increasing the rate of turnover or actually causing their destruction—have now been demonstrated in 90 per cent of patients with myasthenia. The level of these antibodies correlates well with the severity of the disease.[39] The actual binding of antibody to receptors has been described in animals[40,41] and the passive, but shortlived transference of these receptor antibodies from man to animal, has been reported.[42]

### Treatment

The classical treatment of myasthenia gravis is based upon the observation of Mary Walker in 1934[43] that anticholinesterase drugs mitigated the effect of the disease. Many patients, especially those with ocular symptoms alone, are satisfactorily maintained on a mixture of atropine and either pyridostigmine, 60 to 240 mg or neostigmine 15 to 60 mg orally. This regime may be supplemented with other drugs such as ephedrine or guanidine hydrochloride. However, if this proves inadequate, then corticosteroid therapy is added, usually starting with relatively high doses of prednisone, which is then slowly reduced. In fulminating cases or in those developing resistance to anticholinesterase drugs, plasmapheresis may be used and immunosuppressive therapy given. Although successful in about 80 per cent of patients, the disadvantage of long-term therapy with Imuran, make it unattractive in young patients, except in life-threatening situations.

Thymectomy should be considered in all patients with troublesome symptoms not readily controlled by modest doses of anticholinesterase, and immunosuppressant therapy. It is less likely to be successful in elderly patients in whom little thymic tissue remains. The results of thymectomy are best in young patients (under 40 years) with high titre of receptor antibodies. In patients with thymomas, thymectomy is less effective in controlling the symptoms. Thymectomy is not indicated in juvenile (congenital) myasthenia, which appears to be a mixed pre- and postsynaptic phenomenon with a different aetiology from myasthenia gravis.

*Neonatal* myasthenia is a transient form of myasthenia gravis which appears in about 12 per cent of babies born to myasthenics. It is believed to be due to placental transfer from mother to baby of antibodies to acetylcholine receptors. The condition usually disappears within two months of birth.[44]

### Myasthenia and Anaesthesia

The anaesthetist may be called upon to assist in the diagnosis of myasthenia, in treating the patient by artificial ventilation during acute exacerbations, to anaesthetise the patient for surgery, including thymectomy or, more commonly, to provide conditions for general surgery in a myasthenic patient.

The *edrophonium test* remains the classical method of confirming the presence of the disease, although electromyographic or electromechanical evidence of the progressive fade of the twitch response on stimulation at rates of less than 10 Hz, is a strong indication of myoneural disease. The edrophonium test consists of administering 10 mg of the drug intravenously and recording the compound e.m.g. or the twitch response of the adductor muscles following stimulation of the ulnar nerve. An alternative technique is to use the isolated arm to determine if there is an abnormal sensitivity to 0·5 mg of tubocurarine in 40 ml of saline,[45] or resistance to 2 mg of decamethonium.[46]

Should a myasthenic patient require general anaesthesia, it is advisable to avoid the use of muscle relaxants. It is usually possible to intubate these patients at deeper levels of general anaesthesia, especially if the last dose of anticholinesterase before operation has been omitted. If a muscle relaxant is required, it is the author's preference to use 3 to 5 mg of tubocurarine and to avoid the depolarising drugs, to which the patients are often unduly resistant. Postoperative weakness remaining after the usual reversal doses of atropine and neostigmine is considered an indication for nasotracheal intubation and a trial of 24 hours of artificial ventilation. Following thymectomy, elective tracheostomy and artificial ventilation should be considered in the severely incapacitated patients, as the use of high doses of anticholinesterase, in the presence of muscle weakness and a sternotomy incision, predisposes to sputum retention and atelectasis. If the patient has been receiving corticosteroids pre-operatively, the dose should be suitably increased in the intra-operative and postoperative period.

## VON RECKLINGHAUSEN'S DISEASE

Although rarely a cause of any problem during anaesthesia, occasionally the neurofibromas may produce anatomical distortion, making intubation difficult. In a small proportion of patients with diffuse lesions, altered responses to suxamethonium have been reported[47] Baraka[48] reported a myasthenic response to non-depolarising drugs in a patient with this disease.

## CARCINOMATOUS NEUROPATHY

Henson and his colleagues[49] drew attention to the relationship between carcinoma (particularly of the bronchus) and a motor neuropathy. In most cases of advanced carcinoma the cachexia, anaemia and loss of weight are sufficient to produce severe peripheral weakness. However, in true carcinomatous neuropathy the fatiguability is out of all proportion to the severity of the disease. Microscopic examination discloses demyelination of nerve fibres and atrophy of muscle fibres. The response to anticholinesterase therapy is poor. The relationship of this condition to the myasthenic syndrome is not clear but carcinomatous neuropathy is much commoner than the myasthenic syndrome, and lacks the characteristic electromyographic "growth" of successive tetanic response which is so essential for diagnosis of the latter condition.

## MYASTHENIC SYNDROME

In recent years a number of cases have been described suggesting an association between a condition resembling myasthenia gravis and bronchial carcinoma. This relationship was first pointed out by Anderson and his associates[50] but it was not until four years later that Eaton and Lambert[51] detailed the specific condition which they termed "myasthenic syndrome".

Although superficially many of the features of the myasthenic syndrome resemble myasthenia gravis, a closer investigation has revealed a wide margin of differentiation. These have been fully described by Wise and Wylie[52] and are tabulated in Table 1.

The myasthenic syndrome is essentially a condition of peripheral muscle weakness developing in a patient with a bronchial carcinoma. This association is so common that the finding of the characteristic electromyographic response in the absence of obvious evidence of a neoplasm should be sufficient to stimulate an intensive search for its presence.

The specific electromyographic features are illustrated in Fig. 3.

They can be summarised as follows:

1. Low-voltage potential on twitch stimulation (Fig. 4).
2. The "fade" of successive responses on twitch stimulation.
3. The "growth" of successive responses on tetanic stimulation.
4. The presence of post-tetanic facilitation.

26/Table 1

| | *Myasthenia gravis* | *Myasthenic syndrome* |
|---|---|---|
| Sex | Twice as common in women. | Almost entirely men. |
| Age of onset | Commonly 20–40 years. | Commonly 50–70 years. |
| Presenting signs | Weakness of external ocular, bulbar and facial muscles. | Weakness and fatiguability of proximal limb muscles (legs > arms). |
| Other signs | Weakness of limbs, usually proximal, is a later sign (arms > legs). | Weakness of ocular and bulbar muscles is infrequent. |
| Other clinical features | Fatigue on activity. | Transient increase in strength on activity precedes fatigue. |
| | Muscle pains uncommon. | Muscle pains common. |
| | Tendon reflexes normal. | Tendon reflexes reduced or absent. |
| Response to muscle relaxants | Good response to neostigmine. | Poor response to neostigmine. |
| | Increased sensitivity to non-depolarising relaxants in clinically weak muscles. | Marked sensitivity to non-depolarising relaxants even in muscles relatively unaffected. |
| | Resistance to depolarising relaxants. | Sensitivity to depolarising relaxants. |
| Electromyographic features | Normal or slightly reduced amplitude of action potentials at slow rates of stimulation. | Very low voltage action potentials at slow rates of stimulation with fade. |
| | Fade of successive potentials especially on tetanic stimulation. | Marked growth of potentials on tetanic stimulation. |
| | Post-tetanic potentiation and post-tetanic exhaustion present. | Post-tetanic potentiation present. |
| Pathologic states | Thymoma in 25 per cent of patients. | Small-celled carcinoma of bronchus usually present. |
| | Motor end-plates abnormally elongated and distal nerves unusually branched. | Non-specific degenerative process of nerve fibres and end-plates. |
| Prognosis | Often good. | Rapid deterioration and death. |

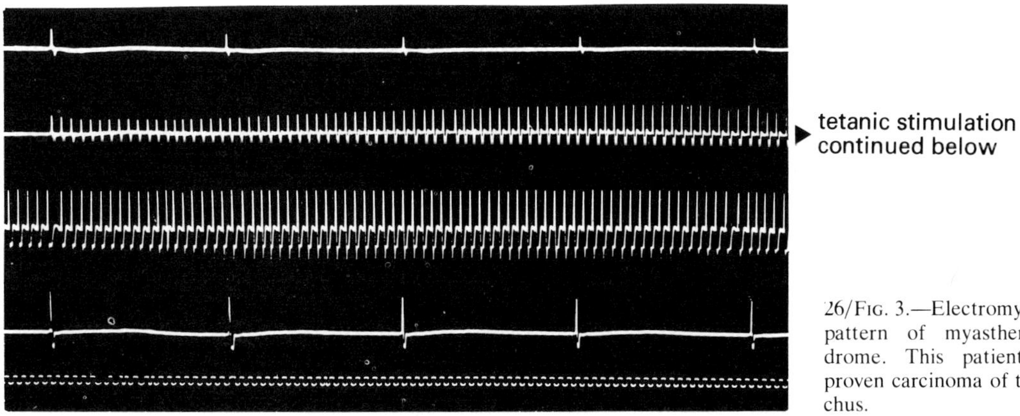


26/Fig. 3.—Electromyographic pattern of myasthenic syndrome. This patient has a proven carcinoma of the bronchus.

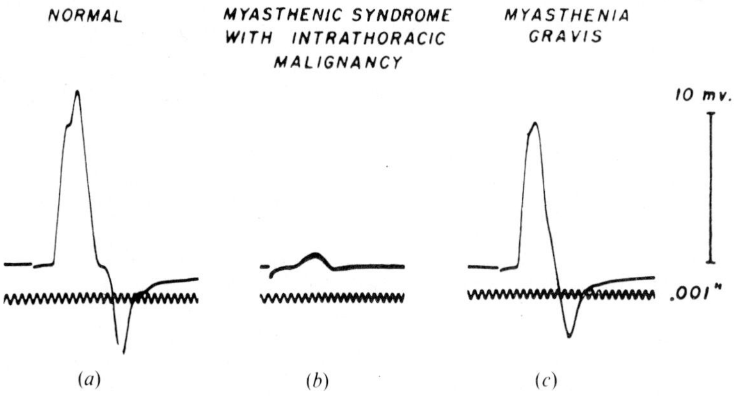


26/Fig. 4.—Illustrates the different height (i.e. voltage) of the action potential in response to a single twitch stimulus in (*a*) normal, (*b*) myasthenic syndrome, (*c*) myasthenia gravis. (Reproduced from a chapter in *Myasthenia Gravis*, courtesy of Dr. E. H. Lambert, and Charles C. Thomas, publisher.[54])

In a clinical assessment of the effect of relaxant drugs on patients with the myasthenic syndrome Wise[53] pointed out that these patients were highly sensitive to both the depolarising and the non-depolarising drugs. The presence of the peripheral weakness is always demonstrable in these cases if actually sought by the anaesthetist. However, if the patient has been confined to bed or is suffering from some incapacitating lesion then the presence of a myasthenic syndrome may be missed. The possible presence of this condition should always be borne in mind during the pre-operative examination of the patient for bronchoscopy under general anaesthesia or a thoracotomy for carcinoma of lung. If this condition is suspected, the diagnosis can easily be confirmed by electromyography. The use of all muscle relaxants is contra-indicated in the presence of the myasthenic syndrome. Improvement of neuromuscular conduction has been seen following the administration of 4-aminopyridine.

## DYSTROPHIA MYOTONICA

Dystrophia myotonica is a familial disease, usually occurring in adult life, characterised by muscle wasting, fatigue, and an inability to relax the muscles after a contraction (myotonia). The myotonia may precede the muscle wasting by many years or may occur independently. The condition is commonly associated with cataract, baldness and testicular atrophy and cardiomyopathy. Occasionally the anaesthetist may be privileged to diagnose the presence of myotonia when the patient "opens and squeezes" his hand before the induction of intravenous anaesthesia.

The abnormality in dystrophia myotonica is believed to be an increase in the sensitivity of the muscle fibre. Brown and Harvey[55] working with myotonic goats found that the myotonia persisted even after nerve-section and curarisation. Later Geschwind and Simpson[56] showed in man that neither tubocurarine nor decamethonium will abolish the myotonia. MacDermot,[57] however, has demonstrated histologically that not only is the muscle fibre itself involved but there is also a defect of the nerve-ending.

Kaufman[58] investigated the effect of anaesthetic drugs, including the relaxants and thiopentone, in patients with dystrophia myotonica. He observed that thiopentone did not influence neuromuscular transmission. The intense depression of respiration, therefore, that may follow the use of barbiturate or narcotic drugs is probably related to central depression of the respiratory centre in a patient with a limited respiratory reserve.

Both neostigmine and the depolarising drugs[59] may increase the degree of myotonia whereas tubocurarine will block neuromuscular transmission without necessarily overcoming the myotonia. Thiel[59] described a case in which the myotonic episodes were directly attributable to the action of suxamethonium.

Patients with dystrophia myotonica may also have some cardiac or endocrine dysfunction.

Regional analgesic techniques are well tolerated. The use of respiratory depressant drugs should be strictly limited. If general anaesthesia is required halothane (which is rapidly eliminated) is most useful.

## LOWER/UPPER MOTOR NEURONE DISEASES AND SUXAMETHONIUM

Any condition in which there has been a recent (4 days to 1 year) large loss of skeletal motor innervation, is a potential cause of a massive potassium shift from inside the cells into the extracellular fluid when suxamethonium is administered. This includes rapidly progressive demyelinating diseases and neuropathies, lower motor neurone disease, spinal-cord injuries and compression, upper motor neurone lesions and encephalitis. The possibility of an adverse reaction should preclude the use of suxamethonium in these situations, but if it is deemed essential to give a depolarising drug, it should be preceded by a small dose of a non-depolarising drug.

## FAMILIAL PERIODIC PARALYSIS

This is a hereditary condition characterised by recurrent attacks of flaccid paralysis. It is associated with an abnormality of potassium and is of two types:

(*a*) *Hypokalaemic form*.—The attacks of paresis are generally associated with a fall in the serum potassium concentration, but there is no critical level for the onset of muscular weakness. These attacks can be induced by the administration of glucose, insulin and epinephrine. During the paresis the muscles will no longer respond to electrical stimulation. Nevertheless, the volume of the muscle fibre increases, suggesting that not only potassium but water enters the fibre during the period of paralysis.

There is no data available on the response of these patients to anaesthetic drugs, but it is reasonable to assume that during an attack the patient will have an increased sensitivity to non-depolarising agents.

(*b*) *Hyperkalaemic form*.—This is a much rarer form of the condition and is associated with a high serum potassium, producing an intermittent depolarising type of neuromuscular block.

## PORPHYRIA

Porphyrins are tetrapyrrolic pigments produced mainly in the liver and bone marrow as intermediates in the synthesis of haem. The porphyrias are disorders of porphyrin metabolism, causing excessive production of porphyrins or their precursors, and are classified according to the major site of abnormal porphyrin production, the hepatic porphyrias being more common than the erythropoietic. The reader is referred to Goldberg and associates[60] for further details of the porphyrias in general; the only variety which will be mentioned here is acute intermittent porphyria.

### Acute Intermittent Porphyria

This is the commonest and most severe form of hepatic porphyria and usually presents in young adults. It is inherited as an autosomal dominant, but in 30 per cent of cases there is no family history. Typically there is an acute onset of colicky central abdominal pain with vomiting and constipation, although diarrhoea occurs in 10 per cent of cases. There is usually evidence of peripheral neuropathy which gives rise to paraesthesiae, numbness and cramp-like pains as well as weakness of limb and girdle muscles; weakness of trunk muscles is less common but can lead to respiratory embarrassment. The cardiovascular system is involved in about 70 per cent of attacks of acute intermittent porphyria; sinus tachycardia and hypertension are common and may be associated with left ventricular failure. It is important to remember that many of these patients present with psychiatric disturbances which include depression.

The diagnosis is confirmed initially by examination of the urine which turns dark on standing and has a very high porphobilinogen content (during an attack).*

A large number of drugs may precipitate or exacerbate an attack of acute porphyria. Barbiturates, especially thiopentone sodium, are most frequently involved and can produce severe porphyric neuropathy and coma. Other drugs, including those containing oestrogens,

* To test for porphobilinogen in the urine:
mix equal parts of fresh urine and Ehrlich's reagent;
red colour develops if porphobilinogen is present;
add 3 ml n-butanol, shake, allow to separate;
if red colour does not enter butanol (upper layer) it is porphobilinogen.

may precipitate an attack of the disease. If anaesthesia is needed for a patient suffering from porphyria, induction is best achieved with Althesin or an inhalational agent; there is no contra-indication to the use of opiate analgesics, diazepam or promazine and all these drugs may be needed in the treatment of an attack of porphyria itself. Most anaesthetists would be reluctant to use a local anaesthetic technique in a patient with (or at risk of) peripheral neuropathy.

## DERMATOMYOSITIS

Certain patients with this disease show a profound peripheral weakness, and in some this is associated with an improvement on the administration of an anticholinesterase drug. There is also a close relationship between carcinoma and dermatomyositis.

In an investigation of ten patients with dermatomyositis, Churchill-Davidson and Richardson (unpublished observations) found positive evidence of a myasthenic response (using decamethonium) in two: in one of these a neoplasm of bronchus was present. The muscle relaxants, therefore, must be used with caution when anaesthetising patients with dermatomyositis.

### Summary of Anaesthesia and Neurological Disease

In general, patients with some neurological impairment of muscle function are extremely susceptible to respiratory depressant or relaxant drugs; a fact which could safely be predicted, for in normal subjects the respiratory reserve is such that a considerable number of muscle fibres can be inactive yet the minute volume is well maintained. This is emphasised by the statement, "tidal volume is only 10 per cent of vital capacity in a normal patient," signifying that theoretically it is possible to lose 90 per cent of the fibre activity before diminished ventilation is apparent. In the presence of neurological disease the requirements for anaesthetic drugs are drastically reduced and the dose of any agent used should be selected accordingly.

## TETANUS

For a full discussion of this disease, see Chapter 10.

## REFERENCES


1. Denborough, M. A. and Lovell, R. R. H. (1960). Anaesthetic deaths in a family. *Lancet*, **2**, 45.
2. Britt, B. A., Locher, W. G. and Kalow, W. (1969). Hereditary aspects of malignant hyperthermia. *Canad. Anaesth. Soc. J.*, **16**, 89.
3. *International Symposium on Malignant Hyperthermia, 1973*. Ed. Gordon, Britt and Kalow. Springfield, Ill.: Charles C. Thomas.
4. *International Symposium on Malignant Hyperthermia, 1978*. Ed. Aldrete and Britt. New York: Grune and Stratton.
5. Briskey, E. J. (1964). Etiological status and associated studies of pale soft exudative porcine musculature. *Adv. Food Res.*, **13**, 89.
6. Hall, L. W., Woolf, N., Bradley, J. W. P. and Jolly, D. W. (1966). Unusual reaction to succinylcholine. *Brit. med. J.*, **2**, 1305.
7. Berman, M. C., Harrison, G. G. and Bull, A. C. (1970). Changes underlying halothane induced malignant hyperpyrexia in Landrace pigs. *Nature*, **225**, 653.
8. Hall, I. W., Trim, C. M. and Woolf, N. (1972). Further studies of porcine malignant hyperthermia. *Brit. med. J.*, **2**, 145.
9. Pan, T. H., Wollack, A. R. and De Marco, J. A. (1975). Malignant hyperthermia associated with enflurane anesthesia: a case report. *Anesth. Analg. (Clev.)*, **54**, 49.
10. Gronert, G. A., Milde, J. H. and Theye, R. A. (1976). Porcine malignant hyperthermia induced by halothane and succinylcholine, failure of treatment with procaine or procainamide *Anesthesiology*, **44**, 124.
11. Relton, J. E. S., Britt, B. A. and Steward, D. J. (1973). Malignant hyperpyrexia. *Brit. J. Anaesth.*, **45**, 269.
12. Britt, B. A., Endrenyi, L., Scott, E. and Frodis, W. (1980). Effect of temperature, time and fascicle size on the caffeine contraction test. *Canad. Anaesth. Soc. J.*, **27**, 1.
13. Britt, B. A., Kalow, W. and Gordon, A. (1973). Malignant hyperthermia; an investigation of 5 patients. *Canad. Anaesth. Soc. J.*, **20**, 431.
14. Noble, W. H., McKee, D. and Gates, B. (1973). Malignant hyperthermia with rigidity successfully treated with procainamide. *Anesthesiology*, **39**, 450.
15. Donlon, J. V., Newfield, P., Sreter, F. and Ryan, J. F. (1978). Implications of masseter spasm after succinylcholine. *Anesthesiology*, **49**, 298.
16. Ellis, F. R., Clarke, I. M. C. and Appleyard, T. N. (1974). Malignant hyperpyrexia induced by nitrous oxide and treated with dexamethasone. *Brit. med. J.*, **4**, 270.

17. Watson, P. M., Albin, M. S. and Smith, R. B. (1980). Malignant hyperthermia, a case report. *Anesth. Analg. Curr. Res.*, **59**, 220.
18. Stanley, B. and Pal, N. R. (1964). Fatal hyperpyrexia associated with phenelzine and imipramine. *Brit. med. J.*, **2**, 1011.
19. Kristo, I., Lewis, E. and Johnson, J. E. (1970). Severe hyperpyrexia due to tranylcypromine-amphetamine toxicity. *Ann. Intern. Med.*, **70**, 559.
20. Pollock, R. A. (1973). Prior drug intake malignant hyperthermia. In: *International Symposium on Malignant Hyperthermia, 1973* p. 179. Ed. Gordon, Britt and Kalow. Springfield, Ill.: Charles C. Thomas.
21. King, J., Barnett, P. S. and Kew, M. A. (1979). Drug induced hyperpyrexia: a case report. *S. Afr. med. J.*, **56**, 190.
22. Kalow, W. and Britt, B. A. (1973). Inheritance of malignant hyperthermia. In: *International Symposium on Malignant Hyperthermia*. Ed. Gordon, Britt and Kalow. p. 67. Springfield, Ill: Charles C. Thomas.
23. Kalow, W., Britt, B. A. and Chan, F. Y. (1979). Epidemiology and inheritance of malignant hyperthermia. *Int. Anesthesiol. Clin.*, **17**, 119.
24. Ellis, F. R., Cain, P. A. and Currie, S. (1978). Screening for malignant hyperpyrexia in susceptible patients. In: *2nd International Symposium on Malignant Hyperpyrexia*. New York: Grune and Stratton Inc.
25. Kalow, W., Britt, B. A. and Richter, A. (1977). The caffeine test of isolated human muscle in relation to malignant hyperthermia. *Canad. Anaesth. Soc. J.*, **24**, 678.
26. Wingard, D. W. (1974). Malignant hyperthermia, a human stress syndrome? *Lancet*, **4**, 1450.
27. Gronert, G. A., Heffron, J. J. A. and Taylor, S. R. (1979). Skeletal muscle sarcoplasmic reticulum in porcine malignant hyperthermia. *Eur. J. Pharmacol.*, **58**, 179.
28. Willis, T. (1684). *A Practice of Physick*, p. 167. London.
29. Erb, W. (1879). Ueber einen neuen, wahrscheinlich bulbären Symptomencomplex. *Arch. Psychiat. Nervenkr.*, **9**, 336.
30. Goldflam, S. (1893). Ueber einen scheinbar heilbaren bulbärparalytischen Symptomencomplex mit Betheiligung der Extremitäten. *Dtsch. Z. Nervenheilk.*, **4**, 312.
31. Jolly, F. (1895). Ueber Myasthenia gravis pseudoparalytica. *Berl. klin. Wschr.*, 32, 1.
32. Santa, T., Engel, A. G. and Lambert, E. H. (1972). Histiometric study of neuromuscular junction ultrastructure. *Neurology (Minneap.)*, **22**, 71.
33. Desmedt, J. E. (1961). Neuromuscular defect in myasthenia gravis. *Proceedings 2nd International Symposium on Myasthenia Gravis*. Ed. H. R. Viets. Springfield, Ill.: Charles C. Thomas.
34. Elmquist, D., Hofmann, W. W., Kugelberg, J. and Quastel, D. M. J. (1964). An electrophysiological investigation of neuromuscular transmission in myasthenia gravis. *J. Physiol. (Lond.)*, **174**, 417.
35. Fambrough, D. M., Drachman, D. B. and Satyamuri, S. (1973). Neuromuscular junction in myasthenia gravis: decreased acetylcholine receptors. *Science*, **182**, 293.
36. Churchill-Davidson, H. C. and Richardson, A. T. (1953). Neuromuscular transmission in myasthenia gravis. *J. Physiol. (Lond.)*, **122**, 252.
37. Nastuk, W. L., Plescia, O. J. and Osserman, K, E. (1959). Search for a neuromuscular blocking agent in the blood of patients with myasthenia gravis. *Amer. J. Med.*, **26**, 394.
38. Simpson, J. A. (1960). Myasthenia gravis. A new hypothesis. *Scot. med. J.*, **5**, 419.
39. Lindstrom, J. M., Seybold, M. E. and Lennon, V. A. (1976). Antibody to acetylcholine receptor in myasthenia gravis: clinical correlates and diagnostic value. *Neurology*, **26**, 1054.
40. Anwyl, R., Appel, S. M. and Narahashi, T. (1977). Myasthenia gravis serum reduces acetylcholine sensitivity in cultured rat myotubes. *Nature*, **26**, 262.
41. Kao, I. and Drachman, D. B. (1977). Myasthenic immunoglobulin accelerates receptor degradation. *Neurology*, **27**, 364.
42. Toyka, K. V., Drachman, D. B., Pestron, K. A. and Kao, I. (1975). Myasthenia gravis, passive transfer from man to mouse. *Science*, **190**, 397.
43. Walker, M. (1934). Treatment of myasthenia gravis with physostigmine. *Lancet*, **1**, 1200.
44. Scadding, G. K. and Havard, C. W. H. (1981). Pathogenesis and treatment of myasthenia gravis. *Brit. med. J.*, **283**, 1008.
45. Foldes, F. F. (1970). Regional intravenous neuromuscular block: a new diagnostic and experimental tool. In: *Progress in Anaesthesiology*, p. 425 (Proc. 4th World Congr. Anaesthesiol.). Amsterdam: Excerpta Medica.
46. Feldman, S. A. (1973). *Muscle Relaxants*. London: W. B. Saunders.
47. Yamashita, M., Matsuki, A. and Oyamei, T. (1977). Anaesthetic considerations in Von Recklinghausen's disease. *Anaesthesist*, **26**, 317.
48. Baraka, A. (1974). Myasthenic response to muscle relaxants in Von Recklinghausen's disease. *Brit. J. Anaesth.*, **46**, 701.
49. Henson, R. A., Russell, D. S. and Wilkinson, M. (1954). Carcinomatous neuropathy and myopathy. A clinical and pathological study. *Brain*, **77**, 82.
50. Anderson, H. J., Churchill-Davidson, H. C. and Richardson, A. T. (1953). Bronchial neoplasm with myasthenia. Prolonged apnoea after administration of succinylcholine. *Lancet*, **2**, 1291.
51. Eaton, L. M. and Lambert, E. H. (1957). Electromyography and electric stimulation of nerves in diseases of motor unit. Observations in myasthenic syndromes associated with malignant tumours. *J. Amer. med. Ass.*, **163**, 1117.
52. Wise, R. P., and Wylie, W. D. (1964). "The thymus gland. Its implications in clinical anesthetic practice." *Clinical Anesthesia: Anesthesia for Patients with Endocrine Disease*, Chapter II. Ed. M. T. Jenkins. Philadelphia: Davis & Co.
53. Wise, R. P. (1962). A myasthenic syndrome complicating bronchial carcinoma. *Anaesthesia*, **17**, 488.
54. Lambert, E. H., Rooke, E. D., Eaton, L. M. and Hodgson, C. H. (1961). Myasthenic syndrome occasionally associated with bronchial neoplasm: neurophysiologic studies. *Proceedings 2nd International Symposium on Myasthenia Gravis*, p. 368. Ed. H. R. Viets, Springfield, Ill.: Charles C. Thomas.
55. Brown, G. L. and Harvey, A. M. (1939). Congenital myotonia in the goat. *Brain*, **62**, 341.
56. Geschwind, N. and Simpson, J. A. (1955). Procaine amide in the treatment of myotonia. *Brain*, **78**, 81.
57. MacDermot, V. (1961). The histology of the neuromuscular junction in dystrophia myotonica. *Brain*, **84**, 75.

58. Kaufman, L. (1960). Anaesthesia in dystrophia myotonica—a review of the hazards of anaesthesia. *Proc. roy. Soc. Med.*, **53**, 183.
59. Thiel, R. E. (1967). The myotonic response to suxamethonium. *Brit. J. Anaesth.*, **39**, 815.
60. Goldberg, A., Beattie, A. and Campbell, B. (1975). The porphyrias and heavy metal intoxication. *Medicine (Balt.)*, Series 2, 600.

## FURTHER READING

Drachman, D. B., (1978). Myasthenia gravis—medical progress. *New Engl. J. Med.*, 136.

Gronert, G. A. (1980). Malignant hyperthermia. *Anesthesiology*, **53**, 395.

International Anesthesiology Clinics (1979). Ed. Britt. B.A. Boston: Little, Brown & Co.

International Symposium on Malignant Hyperthermia, 1973. Ed. Gordon, Britt and Kalow. Springfield, Illinois: Charles C. Thomas

International Symposium on Malignant Hyperthermia, 1978. Ed. Aldrete and Britt. New York: Grune and Stratton.

Scadding, G. K. and Havard, C. W. H. (1981). Regular Review. Pathogenesis and treatment of myasthenia gravis. *Brit. med. J.*, **283**, 1008.

Vickers, M. P. (1982). *Medicine for Anaesthetists*, 2nd edit. Oxford: Blackwell Scientific Publications.

CHAPTER 27

# Cerebral Circulation and Brain Metabolism



THE importance of the blood supply to the brain is well known and is emphasised by the frequency with which neurological damage is the factor limiting full recovery after an episode of circulatory arrest.

## ANATOMY

The arterial supply to the brain is derived from the internal carotid and vertebral arteries on each side, two-thirds of the supply coming from the carotid vessels. The left common carotid artery arises directly from the aorta, whereas the right is a branch of the innominate artery. The vertebral vessels arise from the subclavian artery on their respective sides and join together at the lower border of the pons to form the basilar artery. The circle of Willis (Fig. 1) is formed by anastomoses between the terminal branches of the basilar and two internal carotid arteries.

Kramer,[1] using a methylene blue technique, first suggested that the streams of blood passing to the circle of Willis do not normally mix but are distributed to sharply demarcated areas of brain on the same side, and work with cerebral angiography[2] has confirmed this. Flow across the anastomotic communications does occur though, and the importance of the circle of Willis was underlined by Brain[3] who stated "the purpose served by the circle of Willis is to guarantee that whatever the position of the head in relation to gravity and to the trunk, and however from one moment to another the relative flow through either carotid or vertebral artery may vary as a result, these variations are always compensated for distal to those vessels, and within the cranial cavity, by the freest possible anastomosis before the brain is reached." The efficiency of the circle of Willis in equalising pressures has been demonstrated in animal studies by Symon[4] who showed that complete occlusion of one internal carotid artery reduced pressure in both ipsilateral and contralateral middle cerebral arteries by about 14 per cent. Bilateral internal carotid occlusion caused a 50 per cent fall in middle cerebral artery pressure. Whilst in young subjects uni-

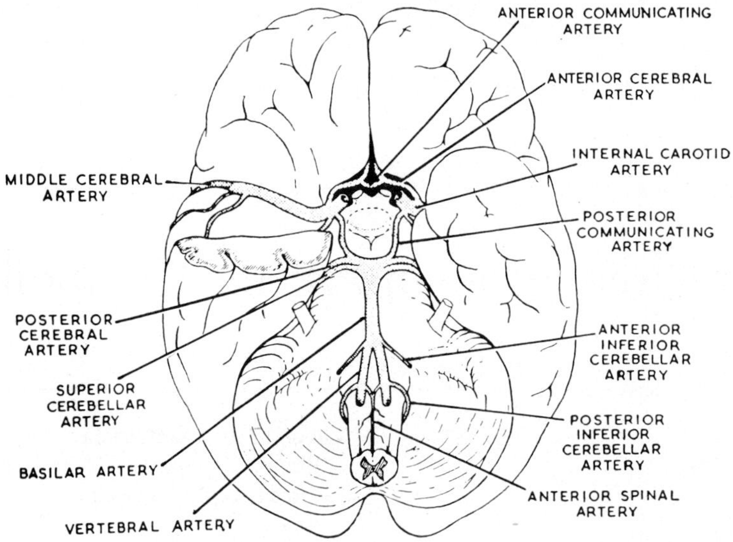


27/FIG. 1.—The circle of Willis.

lateral internal carotid occlusion does not affect total cerebral blood flow, a similar occlusion in the elderly often produces evidence of cerebral ischaemia. Individual anatomical variations, generalised arterial disease or acute reductions in systemic arterial pressure may all affect the efficiency of the circle of Willis.

Cerebral venous drainage, even in health, does not follow the unilateral pattern of the arterial supply.[5] About two-thirds of the blood in the superior jugular bulb comes from the ipsilateral side and there is also a small (approximately 3 per cent) extracerebral contribution at this level.[6] This may be important when a sample from one jugular bulb is taken as representative of the entire cerebral venous drainage. Kety and Schmidt[7] concluded that for most purposes, unilateral sampling is adequately representative, although Munck and Lassen[8] recommend bilateral sampling for greatest accuracy.

## MEASUREMENT OF CEREBRAL BLOOD FLOW

A variety of methods have been used for the study of cerebral blood flow in man.[9] The majority of these methods are based on the Fick principle, which states that the uptake or clearance of a suitable indicator from an organ is a function of the blood flow through that organ and the concentration gradient of indicator between blood supplying and draining the organ. The methods in general use diffusible indicators which are either inhaled or injected into the arterial supply to the brain.

**Inhalation techniques.**—The best known application of inhaled indicators to perfusion measurement is the Kety-Schmidt method of using nitrous oxide to measure cerebral blood flow.[7] A mixture of 15 per cent nitrous oxide and 21 per cent oxygen in nitrogen is inhaled for ten minutes whilst arterial and cerebral venous blood is sampled either intermittently or continuously. At the end of this time brain uptake is usually complete and is given by the product of the final cerebral venous indicator concentration and the blood-brain partition coefficient of nitrous oxide (which is approximately unity). Cerebral blood flow per unit weight of brain is obtained by dividing this uptake figure by the integrated arteriovenous nitrous oxide difference during the uptake period. Radioactive indicators such as $^{85}Kr$ and $^{133}Xe$ are nowadays more commonly employed than nitrous oxide, as standard counting techniques can be used to measure their blood concentration. The Kety-Schmidt method requires simultaneous sampling of arterial and jugular bulb blood. Such sampling allows concomitant measurement of cerebral oxygen metabolic rate. The method gives a measure of global cerebral blood flow with no indications of any regional variations in flow. If cerebral blood flow is low, equilibrium will be reached slowly, and inhalation may need to be continued for 15–30 minutes or arteriovenous difference extrapolated to infinite time. Lassen & Klee[10] suggested that under low-flow conditions measurements should be made during the washout period following inhalation of low concentrations of $^{85}$Kr.

**Inert gas injection techniques.**—When a bolus of $^{85}$Kr or $^{133}$Xe is injected into an internal carotid artery, entry of indicator into brain tissue and its subsequent washout will depend upon blood flow, diffusion and indicator solubility in blood and brain tissue. These indicators have very low blood solubilities and their pulmonary clearance will be virtually complete in one circulation time. Thus no effective arterial recirculation of indicator will occur. Radioactive xenon is the most commonly used indicator, as it has a relatively long half-life of 5·5 days and its activity can easily be recorded by external detectors placed over the head. Cerebral blood flow per unit weight of brain is determined from the peak height of the clearance curve, the area underneath it and the tissue blood partition coefficient of indicator.[11] Like the Kety-Schmidt method the use of injected indicators to measure cerebral blood flow represents an application of the Fick principle. The clearance curves obtained by this method can also be considered as the sum of two exponential curves, an initial fast component representing cortical flow and a slower component related to white matter flow. Use of multiple detectors allows regional blood flow to be assessed and instruments with up to 254 individual detectors have been described.[12]

**Other methods.**—Injected labelled microspheres and autoradiography following injection of diffusible tracers are methods which have been widely used in animal studies, but because of the need to sample brain tissue these methods are not applicable in man.

### Normal Values and Physiological Variation in Cerebral Blood Flow

Cerebral blood flow measured by the inhalation technique is 50–55 ml/100 g/minute in normal adults, indicating a total cerebral flow of approximately 750 ml/minute.[7] Similar cerebral blood flow values are given by the inert gas injection techniques. The flow rate is greater in the first decade of life, falling at puberty towards the adult values.[13] Most evidence suggests that cerebral blood flow tends to fall from middle age onwards.[14]

## FACTORS CONTROLLING CEREBRAL BLOOD FLOW

The Munro-Kellie doctrine of 1783 postulated that because the nearly incompressible brain is housed within a rigid cranium, the quantity of blood in the cerebral circulation will remain constant and flow through it will respond passively to changes in arterial pressure. In 1890, Roy and Sherrington[15] suggested that in addition to the effects of the systemic arterial pressure, the calibre of the cerebral vessels could vary in response to chemical changes in their environment, and it is now accepted that intrinsic regulation of the cerebrovascular resistance is the most important determinant of cerebral blood flow under normal conditions. The many factors which can influence cerebral blood flow do so either by altering the pressure gradient across the vessels, or by changing the resistance within them. The control of cerebral blood flow (CBF) can be considered in terms of the cerebral perfusion pressure, and the influence of chemical, metabolic and neurogenic factors on cerebral vascular resistance.

### 1. Cerebral Perfusion Pressure

In subjects with a normal intracranial pressure, cerebral perfusion pressure is the difference between mean arterial pressure (at the level of the head) and central venous or right atrial pressure. It is well known that CBF remains virtually constant when cerebral perfusion pressure is varied over a wide range. In normal subjects this autoregulation of CBF has a lower limit at a mean arterial pressure of about 60 mm Hg (8·0 kPa). Below this level CBF falls and the cerebral arteriovenous oxygen difference rises. Symptoms of cerebral ischaemia occur below a mean arterial pressure of about 40 mm Hg (5·3 kPa). The upper limit of autoregulation occurs at a mean arterial pressure of about 130 mm Hg (17·3 kPa). Outside the regulatory limits there is a passive relationship between CBF and perfusion pressure.

Blood flow autoregulation occurs in many body tissues and is not confined to the cerebral circulation. The most likely underlying mechanism is a stretch-induced myogenic response of arteriolar smooth muscle. The autoregulation of CBF is readily abolished by insults such as trauma, arterial hypoxaemia, hypercapnia and deep general anaesthesia.

Whilst an abrupt increase in arterial pressure above the upper limit of autoregulation will cause a considerable increase in CBF and may produce encephalopathic symptoms, chronic arterial hypertension is associated with a shift to the right of the autoregulation curve. The chronic hypertensive may be able to maintain a normal CBF with mean arterial pressures of 200 mm Hg (26·7 kPa) or more. An increase in the upper limit of autoregulation is associated with a nearly equal increase in the lower limit. Reduction of arterial pressure in a hypertensive subject will cause ischaemic symptoms at higher levels of arterial pressure than occurs in normotensive subjects. Adaptation of autoregulation to hypertension takes one or two months to become established. Effective antihypertensive therapy results in the autoregulatory limits returning towards the normal values.

In patients with raised intracranial pressure, cerebral perfusion pressure must be considered as the difference between mean arterial and intracranial pressures. Intracranial pressures below 50 cm $H_2O$ (4·9 kPa) do not reduce cerebral perfusion pressure below the lower limit of autoregulation and CBF is usually unaffected. Above this level of intracranial pressure marked falls in CBF will occur.

### 2. Chemical Factors Affecting Cerebral Blood Flow

Arterial carbon dioxide tension is the most important single factor controlling cerebral blood flow. Increasing arterial $CO_2$ tension increases flow whilst reduction in arterial $CO_2$ tension reduces cerebral blood flow. Harper[16] showed that in dogs cerebral blood flows changed by about 2·5 per cent for every 1 mm Hg (0·1 kPa) change in $Pco_2$, that sensitivity was greatest around the normal $Pco_2$ of 40 mm Hg (5·3 kPa), and that the relationship between $Pco_2$ and cerebral blood flow was virtually linear between 30 and 60 mm Hg (4–8 kPa). At $Pco_2$ levels over 150 mm Hg (20 kPa) no further increase in cerebral blood flow occurs, presumably because maximum cerebral vascular dilatation has then occurred. Similarly, cerebral blood flow reaches a level of about 45 per cent of normal at a $Pco_2$ of 15 mm Hg (2 kPa), and further reduction of $Pco_2$ does not cause a further decrease in flow. This limitation is probably due to local hypoxia, produced by vasoconstriction, exerting a local vasodilator effect which counters the effects of further hypocapnia.

Harper and Glass[17] showed that this response to $CO_2$ is diminished in the presence of hypotension and abolished when systemic blood pressure reaches 50 mm Hg (6·7 kPa). Similarly, Lennox and Gibbs[18] showed that the response of cerebral blood flow to carbon dioxide is diminished in the presence of arterial hypoxaemia.

Whilst acute changes in $CO_2$ tension cause the above changes, prolonged maintenance of arterial $CO_2$ at abnormal levels is associated with a return of cerebral blood flow to normal levels. After six to twelve hours of hyperventilation during acclimatisation to high altitude, Severinghaus and his colleagues[19] found cerebral blood flow to be unchanged from normal levels. Chronic hypercapnia, as seen in chronic respiratory failure, is usually associated with a normal cerebral blood flow.

The effect of carbon dioxide on cerebral blood flow is almost certainly due to a direct action on the smooth muscle of cerebral arterioles, mediated by local tissue pH changes.[20] If arterial carbon dioxide tension is kept constant marked changes in arterial pH produced by infusing acids or alkalis do not affect cerebral blood flow.[21] Thus the blood-brain barrier protects cerebral blood flow from the effects of metabolic acidosis and alkalosis.

The effects of changes in arterial oxygenation on cerebral blood flow are opposite to those produced by carbon dioxide. However, the cerebral circulation does not respond to $Pao_2$ changes around the normal value. When $Pao_2$ falls below 50 mm Hg (6·7 kPa) cerebral blood flow increases, and is doubled at a $Pao_2$ of about 30 mm Hg (4 kPa). The cerebral vasodilatation produced by hypoxia may be due to local tissue acidosis causing a fall in tissue pH and affecting smooth muscle of cerebral arterioles.[22]

Higher than normal oxygen tensions cause a

diminution in cerebral blood flow, 100 per cent oxygen inhalation reducing cerebral blood flow by 10 per cent, whilst a similar oxygen concentration at 2 atmospheres pressure causes a 20 per cent fall in cerebral blood flow. Whilst part of this response may be due to hypocapnia accompanying hyperoxia, oxygen also appears to have a direct constrictor effect on cerebral vessels. The fall in cerebral blood flow due to hyperoxia is not associated with fall in cerebral available oxygen.[23] Harper, McDowall and Ledingham[24] showed that cerebral vasoconstriction did not occur with hyperbaric oxygenation in dogs suffering from haemorrhagic hypotension, and Holbach and Gött[25] have shown a similar lack of effect of hyperbaric oxygenation on regional cerebral blood flow in areas of cerebral oedema following head injury.

### 3. Metabolic Regulation of Cerebral Blood Flow

In normal subjects the overall or global level of CBF is little different during sleep, resting wakefulness and with various types of brainwork. This constancy of CBF disguises changes that occur at regional levels due to brain activity. Thus Olesen[26] showed that during hand movement there was a 30 per cent increase in blood flow to the contralateral rolandic hand area. Extremes of overall brain activity seen in some diseases are associated with marked changes of CBF—high levels of CBF occur during epileptic seizures and CBF is reduced to low levels during coma. Marked reductions of CBF, paralleling metabolic activity, occur during deep levels of barbiturate and Althesin hypnosis. Little is known of the mechanisms that couple flow to metabolism.

### 4. Neurogenic Control of Cerebral Blood Flow

Although the cerebral vasculature is well supplied with both sympathetic and parasympathetic nerves, the cerebral circulation is less subject to autonomic control than other areas of the body. Maximal sympathetic stimulation decreases CBF by some 5–10 per cent,[27] and parasympathetic stimulation increases CBF by a comparable amount.[28]

It has been shown that sympathetic stimulation shifts the autoregulation curve to the right.[29] This implies that during states of acute arousal and effort the cerebral circulation can tolerate acute rises in blood pressure due to sympathetic activation, and may explain why lower levels of CBF are found during haemorrhagic hypotension (when sympathetic activity is high) than during pharmacologically induced hypotension of the same degree.

### Cerebral Blood Flow and Brain Tissue Acidosis

Inadequate brain perfusion leads rapidly to the production of an excess of lactic acids. As the cerebral vasculature is highly sensitive to brain tissue pH, brain lactic acidosis can have dire effects upon cerebral blood flow.

Brain tissue acidosis can be global, as occurs in patients resuscitated after circulatory arrest. It also develops in and around areas of focal ischaemia due to cerebrovascular disease, brain tumours or head injury. The major consequence of such acidosis on cerebral blood flow is an abolition of the normal autoregulation of CBF, resulting in a so-called "luxury perfusion syndrome".[20] Such luxury perfusion may imply an overall increase in CBF, but more often means that blood flow is in excess of metabolic demands.

When acidotic foci are present in the brain paradoxical flow responses can occur. A rise in $P_{CO_2}$ under these circumstances can lead to vasodilatation in vessels supplying the normal brain with blood supply to the damaged brain remaining passive. This will result in blood being diverted from the acidotic brain tissue—the so-called intracerebral steal syndrome. Conversely, during hypocapnia, as vessels supplying normal brain tissue constrict, so flow to the damaged area will increase—the inverse steal or Robin Hood syndrome.

## EFFECTS OF DRUGS ON THE CEREBRAL CIRCULATION

Care must be exercised in evaluating the effects of drugs on cerebral blood flow. Many drugs affect CBF by indirect mechanisms. CBF is increased by analeptic drugs which increase neuronal activity. Any drug which affects $P_{CO_2}$ will indirectly affect CBF. The CBF responses to drugs may be totally different in the diseased brain where CBF autoregulation is impaired.

Many agents which have marked effects on blood flow to other organs are without effect on cerebral blood flow. Thus noradrenaline, angiotensin, phenoxybenzamine and phentolamine do not affect CBF unless their effects on systemic pressure are so great that the normal limits of autoregulation are exceeded. Adrenaline does increase CBF, probably as a result of increased brain metabolism rather than any direct effect. Sodium nitroprusside increases CBF by a direct vasodilator effect on cerebral vessels, whilst trimetaphan and nitroglycerin are without direct effects on cerebral blood flow.

*Intravenous induction agents.*—Barbiturates can produce marked reductions in CBF (with parallel falls in cerebral oxygen uptake). Deep thiopentone anaesthesia can reduce CBF by up to 50 per cent. A similar cerebral vasoconstriction and fall in CBF is seen with Althesin. Both of these agents have been widely used to reduce intracranial hypertension. In contrast, ketamine produces pronounced cerebral vasodilatation and rises in CBF of 50 per cent or more.

*Inhalational anaesthetics.*—All gaseous and volatile anaesthetic agents increase cerebral blood flow. The increase in CBF is associated with a reduced cerebral oxygen uptake and an increase in cerebral venous oxygen content. Halothane has been the most widely studied agent and inspired concentrations of 1 per cent halothane have been shown to increase CBF by about 25 per cent.[30] Comparable effects on CBF have been demonstrated with methoxyflurane, trichloroethylene, enflurane and isoflurane. Low concentrations of cyclopropane may slightly reduce CBF,[31] but higher concentrations markedly increase CBF. In normal subjects nitrous oxide reduces cerebral oxygen uptake without affecting CBF—a state of relative overperfusion. In patients with intracranial disorders, nitrous oxide can markedly increase intracranial pressure due to cerebral vasodilatation.

As the use of inhalational anaesthetics during spontaneous breathing is commonly associated with a reduced ventilatory response to $CO_2$, the effects of these agents on CBF may be enhanced by hypercapnia. Conversely, Adams and his colleagues[32] have shown that the potentially dangerous effects of halothane on CBF and intracranial pressure can usually be abolished by the prior induction of a state of hypocapnia.

*Narcotic analgesics.*—These agents have little effect on CBF if $P_{CO_2}$ levels are controlled. In normal subjects during normocapnia morphine does not affect either CBF or cerebral autoregulation,[33] and similar effects have been shown for fentanyl.

*Muscle relaxants.*—Tubocurarine has been shown to increase CBF and cerebral blood flow in normal subjects.[34] These effects have been ascribed to histamine release and an increased pulsatile blood flow in the brain. Pancuronium is without an effect on CBF.

### General Anaesthetics and Intracranial Pressure

The inhalational anaesthetics (which raise cerebral blood flow by vasodilatation) lead to an increase in cerebral blood volume which, in turn, causes a rise in intracranial pressure. Usually the rises in CSF pressure are slight and readily controlled by hyperventilation. Large changes in intracranial pressure can occur in patients with space-occupying brain lesions.[35] Rapid fluctuations in cerebral blood volume can in these patients lead to dangerous pressure gradients being developed between different brain compartments. These effects of volatile anaesthetics can be reduced by a period of hyperventilation before their administration.[32,36]

## EFFECTS OF HYPOTHERMIA

Both cerebral blood flow and cerebral metabolic rate fall in dogs with decrease in body temperature.[37,38] Rosomoff[39] showed a diminution in cerebral blood flow in dogs of 6–7 per cent for each degree centigrade fall in temperature. At a temperature of 28° C, a fall in cerebral blood flow of 50 per cent was recorded and Kleinerman and Hopkins[38] reported that at temperatures between 22 and 27° C the reduction in cerebral blood flow exceeded the diminution of cerebral oxygen consumption. Albert and Fazekas[40] reported five cases of induced hypothermia in man; in two of these the diminution in cerebral blood flow exceeded the decrease in cerebral metabolic rate. However, Rosomoff and Holaday[37] reported a parallel reduction in both metabolic rate and blood flow in dogs cooled to 26° C and in clinical practice the technique is widely and successfully used to prevent cerebral damage during procedures which may jeopardise cerebral blood flow.

Hypothermia to a level of 30° C has been widely used in the past during neurosurgery, especially during carotid artery surgery. The complexity of inducing hypothermia and the complications of the technique have greatly reduced its popularity. Berntman and his colleagues[41] have shown that mild hypothermia (to 34° C) in rats afforded considerable protection against cerebral hypoxia and have suggested that a place for this technique may still exist in clinical practice.

## HYPERVENTILATION AND ANAESTHESIA

Hyperventilation raises the pain threshold in conscious volunteers and appears to reduce requirements for central depressant drugs during anaesthesia. It has been shown that hypocapnia does not alter anaesthetic requirements in man[42] and greater depth of anaesthesia during hyperventilation may be due to the higher alveolar tension of anaesthetic agent which develops when increased ventilation occurs at a constant inspired concentration.[43] There is conflicting evidence on the possible occurrence of cerebral hypoxia secondary to cerebral vasoconstriction and shift of the oxygen dissociation curve due to a low arterial carbon dioxide tension.[44–48] Many of these authors support the view that mild degrees of cerebral hypoxia can be produced by hyperventilation, but despite this theoretical disadvantage there is no clinical evidence that moderate hyperventilation of the anaesthetised patient to a $Pco_2$ of 30–35 mm Hg (4·0–4·7 kPa) produces cerebral damage and the benefits of controlled respiration, circulatory stability and minimal central depression, have made the technique widely popular. Harp and Wollman[49] have shown that normal man can tolerate hyperventilation to a $Pco_2$ of 20 mm Hg (2·7 kPa) for several hours with no impairment of cerebral metabolism. As has been already pointed out, abnormal blood flow responses can occur in and around ischaemic and acidotic areas of the brain.

### Value of Hyperventilation in Neurosurgery

Although it is sometimes claimed that hyperventilation can "shrink" the normal brain, Rosomoff[50] showed in dogs that hyperventilation does not reduce the volume of the brain tissue and that intracranial pressure is unaffected provided the carbon dioxide tension is normal before the onset of increased ventilation. The spontaneously breathing, anaesthetised patient is almost always hypoventilating to some extent so that controlled ventilation is likely to provide better and safer operating conditions. Similarly, in head injuries or patients with cerebral oedema, controlled ventilation with a guaranteed airway may be more satisfactory than possibly inadequate spontaneous respiration and an airway jeopardised by coma. Because of the factors associated with regional variations in cerebral blood flow hyperventilation may be of therapeutic value where localised areas of brain damage occur. By inducing an inverse steal syndrome blood flow to damaged areas will be increased and tissue damage may be minimised.[51]

## CEREBRAL METABOLISM

Measurement of overall cerebral metabolism depends upon the determination of cerebral arteriovenous differences and total cerebral blood flow. The venous sample is withdrawn from the superior jugular bulb in man, as this site provides blood which is almost exclusively representative of cerebral activity.

The cerebral metabolic oxygen rate ($CMRO_2$) is normally high (3–3·5 ml/100 g/min). Virtually all oxygen utilised by the brain is used to convert glucose aerobically to carbon dioxide and water. Under normal circumstances a small fraction of utilised glucose (about 5 per cent) is converted by anaerobic glycolysis to lactic acid. In hypoxia the electron transfer system necessary for aerobic metabolism cannot function and considerable increases in the level of anaerobic metabolism occur. Aerobic glucose oxidation provides 38 mol of APT per mol of glucose, whilst anaerobic metabolism of 1 mol of glucose only produces 2 mol of APT. Maximal anaerobic glycolysis yields only 2·5 per cent of the resting brain tissue energy requirements.[52]

Cerebral oxygen consumption is usually independent of cerebral blood flow, $CMRO_2$ being unaffected until cerebral blood flow has fallen to 60 per cent of its resting value. Available oxygen stores in the brain are so small that an uninterrupted circulatory supply is essential. Oxygen deprivation by total circulatory arrest causes loss of consciousness in 10 seconds.[53]

Hypoglycaemia, by reducing the amount of substrate, produces all degrees of functional disturbance progressing to coma, the degree of hypoglycaemia correlating well with the level of impairment.

Physiological variations of cerebral activity produce no change in the overall brain metabolic rate, but regional variations in both blood flow and metabolism do correlate with cerebral activity. Marked reductions in cerebral oxygen supply, as occur during severe hypocapnia with a $Pco_2$ of about 20 mm Hg (2·7 kPa), can produce brain tissue hypoxia as evidenced by EEG changes, alterations in critical flicker fusion frequency and reaction time, and metabolic abnormalities.[54–56]

Many drugs used during anaesthesia can markedly affect brain metabolism. Thiopentone in normal induction doses reduces $CMRO_2$ by about one-third, and deep thiopentone anaesthesia can result in a 50 per cent fall in $CMRO_2$, with a parallel fall in cerebral blood flow. Althesin has similar effects on $CMRO_2$ and CBF. The use of these agents to protect the ischaemic brain is discussed in the management of head injuries (p. 787). Ketamine increases both $CMRO_2$ and CBF. Most of the volatile anaesthetic agents reduce $CMRO_2$ whilst increasing CBF, though seizure activity induced by deep enflurane anaesthesia combined with hypocapnia results in a sudden increase in brain oxygen utilisation. Nitrous oxide and narcotic analgesics only minimally depress $CMRO_2$.

## THEORIES OF ANAESTHESIA

Anaesthesia may be defined as a progressive reversible depression of nervous tissue, or more simply as the controlled production of unconsciousness.

There is no simple theory explaining the production of the unconscious state. The many theories of anaesthesia which have been advanced depend either on physical properties of anaesthetics or the localisation of a site of action of anaesthetics.

### Physical Properties of Anaesthetics

A vast number of compounds have been shown to be capable of producing anaesthesia, and they lack any common chemical features. No theories have been advanced relating anaesthetic action to overall chemical structure. The anaesthetic agents in general use have however several common physical features. They are all substances of comparatively low molecular weight, chemically unreactive and unchanged. A fruitful source of theories of anaesthesia has been to correlate some physical property of anaesthetics with anaesthetic potency.

#### Lipid Solubility

Meyer and Overton were the first workers to correlate narcotic potency with lipid solubility, expressed as an oil-water partition coefficient.[57,58] There is general agreement that all anaesthetics are lipophylic, and the greater the lipid solubility the lower the concentration of anaesthetic required to produce its effects. It is more conventional to correlate potency with an oil/gas partition coefficient rather than differential solubility in oil and water. The minimum alveolar anaesthetic concentration (MAC) of any agent multiplied by its oil-gas partition coefficient tends towards a constant value of 140.[59] Lipid solubility does not lead to any explanation of how anaesthetics act but strongly suggests that they are acting in lipid regions of cells.

#### Water Solubility

The majority of anaesthetics are poorly soluble in water. Miller[60] and Pauling[61] independently showed that many anaesthetic molecules were capable of forming hydrates in the form of clathrates. In these compounds a cage of water molecules surrounds a central anaesthetic molecule. The presence of such "microcrystals" was believed to produce anaesthesia by affecting membrane permeability or altering the electrical properties of cells. Whilst there is a correlation between anaesthetic potency and hydrate dissociation pressure, it is a far poorer correlation than was originally thought. Moreover, whilst clathrates of many anaesthetic compounds can be formed, their formulation often requires extremes of pressure at body temperature.

#### Thermodynamic Activity

Ferguson[62] pointed out that many of the correlations invoked in theories of anaesthesia were concerned with partition of an anaesthetic between different phases. At equilibrium in such a partition the thermodynamic potential—

the partial molal free energy—will be the same in all phases. Ferguson showed that equipotent concentrations of anaesthetics had equal thermodynamic activities, assessed as the ratio of anaesthetic tension to saturated vapour tension. This finding, like that of lipid solubility, does not explain how anaesthetics act. It does explain why many different physical properties of anaesthetics can be to a greater or lesser extent correlated with narcotic potency.

### Protein Binding

Many proteins contain hydrophobic areas to which molecules of anaesthetic drugs can become attached by induced dipole bonding, and such binding may be involved in the mode of action of anaesthetics. Halsey, Brown & Richards[63] have shown that in the presence of anaesthetic agents protein structures can be reversibly altered.

### Membrane Permeability

Although many theories of narcotic action have invoked an effect on ion transport across cell membranes the evidence for such an effect is conflicting. Anaesthetics reversibly inhibit sodium and potassium transport *in vitro*, but higher concentrations of anaesthetics are required to produce this effect than those used clinically. Because of the likelihood that anaesthetics act at the cell membrane it has been suggested that their effects are due to actions on the sodium pores, which could be blocked by membrane swelling due to anaesthetics or to an effect of anaesthetics on membrane proteins.

### Pressure Reversal of Anaesthesia

High applied pressures can reverse the effects of many anaesthetics. Johnson & Flagler[64] showed that tadpoles anaesthetised with alcohol awoke if exposed to hydrostatic pressures of 50 atmospheres, and Smith and his colleagues[65] showed a similar effect of high gas pressures on mammals anaesthetised with volatile agents. Halsey & Wardley-Smith[66] showed that pressure reversal also applied to narcotics, tranquillisers and intravenous induction agents. These effects of raised pressure led to the "critical volume" hypothesis, which states that a critical hydrophobic molecular site was expanded by anaesthetics and restored to its previous state by raised pressure.[67,68] Halsey, Wardley-Smith & Green[69] have modified this theory to suggest that anaesthetics produce expansion of a number of sites with differing physical properties.

## ELECTROENCEPHALOGRAPHY

The electroencephalogram (EEG) is conveniently recorded from multiple symmetrically paired electrodes placed on the skull, although monitoring during anaesthesia is commonly performed with only two electrodes (frontal and occipital). A number of extraneous signals may interfere with the recording of these very small potentials (tens of microvolts only); excessive sweating, eye movements and contraction of scalp or limb muscles can all produce artefacts, and arterial or venous pulses, respiratory changes and the electrocardiogram can be superimposed on the EEG, particularly if the electrodes or earth lead are poorly applied or incorrectly sited. Proximity to other apparatus frequently causes interference and it may be necessary to perform the recording in a screened room.

### Normal Activity

A wide variety of patterns may be recorded from normal individuals and the following wave forms have been recognised.

*Delta waves*, 0·5–3·5 Hz, occur in infants and sleeping adults with an amplitude of about 100 microvolts. They are largest in the frontal lobes, symmetrical but asynchronous.

*Theta waves*, 4–7 Hz, occur in children with an amplitude of 50 microvolts and in adults with an amplitude of 10 microvolts. They are diffuse in children but become localised to the parietal and temporal regions in adults.

*Alpha waves*, 8–13 Hz, occur in infants with an amplitude of 20 microvolts, in children with an amplitude of 75 microvolts and in adults with an amplitude of 50 microvolts. These, like the theta rhythms, are diffuse in children but become localised to the parietal and occipital areas in adults. They are symmetrical and synchronous. The alpha waves are augmented by closing the eyes and during mental repose, and are reduced by visual and mental activity, sometimes to the extent of total removal or "blocking".

*Beta waves*, 14–15 Hz, of about 20 microvolts, usually occur in the fronto-central areas in children and are symmetrical and asynchronous.

*Gamma waves*, 26 or more Hz, usually have an amplitude of 10 microvolts and are rare in normal subjects.

**Some Abnormal Patterns**

It is very rare to obtain a record of a major convulsive seizure free from artefact but minor seizures are frequently well recorded, especially when a stimulus such as over-breathing is used (Fig. 2–*4*). Seizures produced in this way are often less severe than those usually suffered by the patient and are called "larval". About 50 per cent of people subject to "fits" have an "Abnormal" EEG record between attacks—that is they show patterns which are never seen in normal subjects (Fig. 2–*5*). Hysterical fits do not affect the EEG.

As the disturbances arise in differing parts of the brain, the pattern of the electroencephalogram will vary from lead to lead. A minor seizure pattern is characterised by "wave and spike" activity containing a very large component up to 1 millivolt at a frequency from 1·5 to 3·5 Hz (Fig. 2–*6*). The spike component lasts from 0·02 second up to 0·1 second. In organic diseases the relationship between the spike and wave varies from moment to moment.

The pattern of a major convulsion appears to be an all-or-none phenomenon and it is not much altered by drugs. The pattern depends on the site of onset and route of spread of the electrical disturbance but is symmetrical and synchronous when it is fully developed. It starts to alter thirty seconds or so before the onset of the convulsion is manifest, as shown by rhythms of 2–7 Hz which increase in amplitude and are most prominent in the pre-motor regions (Fig. 2–*7*). The tonic stage of the convulsion is characterised by the abrupt onset of spikes of moderate amplitude. The spikes then become "grouped" and there is a slow component at 1·5–3 Hz which bears a constant time relationship to the groups of spikes. Towards the end of the convulsion, the spikes occur only in synchronised groups on the crest of a rhythmic slow wave. The frequency of this wave slows to 1 Hz with no decline in amplitude, and then it suddenly ceases. After the convulsion there is random slow activity with an occasional spike which is followed by the gradual reappearance of the normal pattern.

**The Effect of Anaesthetic Drugs on the Electroencephalogram**

It is difficult to correlate the classical Guedel signs of anaesthesia with changes in the EEG and there is some variation in the changes which are produced by different anaesthetic agents. Sadove and his colleagues[70] state as a broad outline that the following changes occur. "When there is only slight mental impairment with mild analgesia and amnesia, low-voltage fast activity

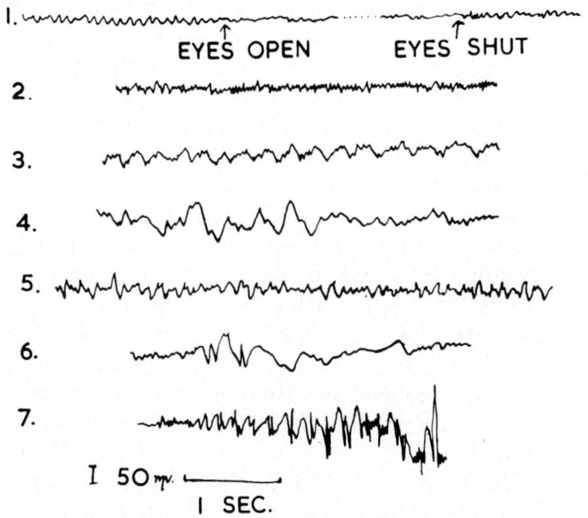


27/Fig. 2.—Some Electroencephalographic Patterns

1. Normal *alpha* rhythm showing effect of opening the eyes; 2. Normal fast activity; 3. Normal slow activity; 4. Slow activity in a child of 10 produced by hyperventilation; 5. Typical inter-seizure record; 6. Wave and spike activity; 7. Pre-convulsion trace.

is increased and the record resembles the normal 'attention' trace. With the onset of light anaesthesia, fast activity of high voltage predominates. Slowing of the electrical activity occurs with deepening of the anaesthetic, followed by brief periods of inactivity and finally, total electrical silence. The stage of brief periods of inactivity may be reached transitorily after a rapid intravenous induction."

Common sedatives (barbiturates, chloral hydrate and paraldehyde) can produce variable changes in the EEG but there is no correlation with the clinical effect of the drug. All sedatives producing sleep, even those used clinically as anticonvulsants, tend to activate seizure discharges in epileptic or predisposed persons.[71] Atropine, pethidine and morphine used in conventional doses produce no change in the EEG and curare likewise has no effect provided respiration is controlled.[72] Spinal anaesthesia produces no change in the EEG although coincidental sleep or sedation may have some effect on the record.

**Effects of Hypoxia**

Slowing of the wave frequency of the EEG is the most characteristic change associated with hypoxia, but cerebral venous oxygen tensions of 18 mm Hg (2·4 kPa) may be reached before there is any alteration of the record. An initial increase of frequency and amplitude lasting 1 to 2 seconds occurs sometimes with the onset of sudden and complete anoxia. By ten seconds there is slow cortical activity of 1 to 3 Hz which becomes slower and of greater amplitude. When it reaches 1 Hz the amplitude decreases so that by 18 to 20 seconds after complete anoxia, the EEG becomes a straight line. If hypoxia is rapidly relieved the EEG returns to normal in the reverse order, but changes may persist long after the oxygen tension has been restored to normal if the period of hypoxia was prolonged. Following a long period of hypoxia, a flat trace with superimposed low-voltage (5 microvolts), fast (50 Hz), spiky activity may occur.[73] This is known as "file pattern" and carries a poor prognosis.

It has been suggested that the EEG may be used to identify "cerebral death" in patients requiring support of cardiorespiratory function, and Hockaday and colleagues[74] were able to predict with considerable accuracy from the EEG whether anoxic damage following cardiac or respiratory arrest would prove fatal or non-fatal. However Haider and associates[75] have reported survival with complete normality in patients with a persistently flat EEG for many hours after barbiturate intoxication and it must therefore be realised that the EEG alone is insufficient evidence on which to decide whether supportive therapy should be continued or withdrawn from a patient with severe cerebral damage. Serial recordings, considered in conjunction with clinical assessment of the function of the central nervous and other systems and the aetiology of the condition, may be of some value in making these individual and difficult decisions.

**Effects of Hypercapnia**

Moderate increases in carbon dioxide tension (5 per cent inspired $CO_2$) cause an increase in frequency of cortical activity. Greater increases (more than 10 per cent $CO_2$) reverse this acceleration and slow waves appear.[70] High carbon dioxide tensions also potentiate the effects of barbiturates and other anaesthetic drugs.[76]

**Effects of Hypocapnia**

Voluntary hyperventilation in man produces high-voltage slow waves in the EEG which Brazier[77] concluded are due to the direct effect of a low $P_{CO_2}$ and are not secondary to hypoxia due to cerebral vasoconstriction. Holmberg[78] however found that voluntary hyperventilation with oxygen produced less alteration in brain potentials than voluntary hyperventilation with air, and Bollen[47] considered that the slow wave activity and accompanying analgesia of hyperventilation were indicative of mild cerebral hypoxia. The relevance of this clinical practice is discussed in the section on hyperventilation and anaesthesia.

**Effects of Hypotension**

The electroencephalographic pattern during hypotension depends not only on the level of blood pressure but also on the rate of fall to that level. At a rate of under 10 mm Hg (1·3 kPa)/minute, a fall of 100 mm Hg (13·3 kPa) in a hypertensive patient produced no electroencephalographic change,[86] whereas a rapid but smaller decrease in blood pressure can produce slow, high-amplitude waves or even temporary cessation of cortical activity

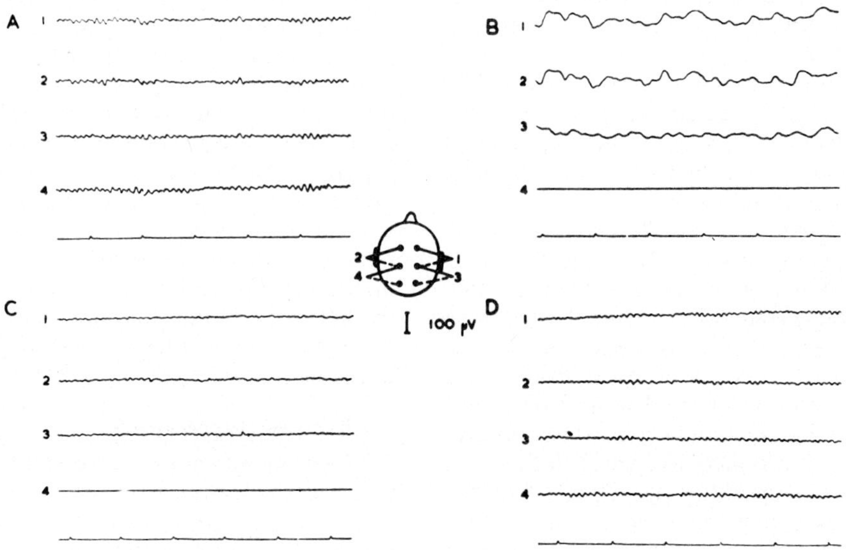


27/Fig. 3.—The Effects of Hypotension on the Electroencephalogram

EEG records of normal man, aged 38.
Time marker: 1 second intervals.
A—Normal resting rhythm of 9 Hz B.P. 130/80.
B—During acute fall of B.P. to unrecordable levels, after 100 mg C5 and 45 degrees foot-down tilt. Subject unconscious.
C—One minute after B, 10 degrees head-down. B.P. 40/? Consciousness returning.
D—Four minutes after C. B.P. 105/70. Conscious. Normal $\alpha$-rhythm.

(Courtesy of Professor P. R. Bromage and the Honorary Editors of the *Proceedings of the Royal Society of Medicine*[86])

(Fig. 3). These effects may be due to delay in the response of the cerebral blood vessels to sudden changes in blood pressure.

**Effects of Hypothermia**

Little change occurs in the EEG until the temperature has fallen to 35–31° C when some decrease in amplitude and frequency takes place. At 25° C the amplitude is further decreased and at 20° C there is no appreciable activity in either parietal or occipital regions, and only a very low-amplitude wave remains at 2 cycles per second in the frontal regions. Prolonged maintenance at low temperatures produces no further alterations. With rewarming the changes occur in the reverse order but at one or two degrees higher than on cooling and there are no permanent changes.[79]

The effect of circulatory arrest in the hypothermic patient is to produce a flat record but this appears more slowly than would be the case at normal temperatures. "File pattern" low-voltage fast activity may be seen in these circumstances, but it is not of grave significance.[80]

**Effects of Surgery and Cardiopulmonary Bypass**

Studies before and after major surgery show that in a high percentage of cases, changes are produced which generally last for two or three days but which can persist for up to two weeks.[70] During cardiopulmonary bypass, transitory slowing of the EEG may occur with the onset of perfusion, possibly due to differences in temperature, chemistry or drug content of the blood in the apparatus, but subsequently the EEG may be used to monitor the adequacy of cerebral perfusion.

### Interpretation of EEG Data

The availability of analogue and digital computers has led to many refinements in EEG presentation and interpretation. Sophisticated methods of power spectral analysis have been used to assess depth of anaesthesia from the EEG.[81] Simple methods of interpreting the EEG have also been investigated. The "Cerebral Function Monitor" described by Maynard, Prior and Scott[82] filters a single EEG signal to accept that portion with frequencies between 2 and 15 Hz. Branthwaite[83] has shown the value of this simple monitor in differentiating cerebral changes occurring during open heart surgery.

## TEMPERATURE REGULATION AND SWEATING

Man, like birds and other mammals, maintains a relatively constant body temperature over a wide range of climatic and environmental conditions. The deep body or "core" temperature is controlled within narrow limits whilst superficial tissues act as a variable insulator. Temperature control consists of a balance between heat production and heat transfer to the environment. The hypothalamus contains centres which respond to impulses from cutaneous cold and warm receptors. The hypothalamus also responds to local changes in blood temperature.

Heat is produced in the body mainly by metabolic activity. Heat production can be increased by increased muscle activity—shivering. Under most circumstances heat production is relatively constant and body temperature is controlled by variations in heat loss. Heat is lost by processes of conduction, convection, radiation and evaporation. Increasing skin blood flow is the primary mechanism by which heat loss is increased, the loss being mainly due to convection and radiation. Above a certain threshold the sweating rate markedly rises to increase heat loss by evaporation. The sweat glands are innervated by cholinergic sympathetic fibres. Sweating provoked by anxiety, anoxia and other non-thermal stimuli merely reflects increased sympathetic activity.

Current theories of temperature regulation suggest that the anterior hypothalamus acts as a biological thermostat with a built-in "set point".[84,85] Variations in this set point account for diurnal temperature variations, temperature changes during the menstrual cycle and changes during exercise. Fever is an example of a gross disturbance in the set point.

The anaesthetised patient tends to become poikilothermic. Depression of metabolism reduces heat production, whilst central depression and loss of vascular control impair the regulation of heat loss. Body temperature tends to fall, especially in children and when visceral cavities are opened. Alternatively, it should be remembered that atropine in children can block the activity of the sweat glands thereby sometimes leading to pyrexia in the presence of inflammatory conditions. A hot environment, theatre lights and impermeable drapes can cause an increase in body temperature. Unless central depression is profound this will produce sweating. Sweating during anaesthesia is more usually indicative of increased sympathetic activity due to too light an anaesthetic plane, hypoxia or hypercapnia. Extreme hyperpyrexia during general anaesthesia—malignant hyperthermia—is due to a massive increase in heat production, and is discussed in some detail in Chapter 26.

## DIAGNOSIS OF BRAIN DEATH

With the development of intensive care facilities throughout the world, it is a commonplace problem to have a deeply comatose patient whose life is maintained by a mechanical ventilator. The first formal definition of brain death was given by Mollaret & Goulon[87] who termed the condition "coma dépassé" or ultra coma. In 1968 a multidisciplinary committee under the chairmanship of H. K. Beecher published the Harvard Criteria[88] to guide practitioners on the diagnoses of brain death. The Conference of Medical Royal Colleges of the U.K. and their Faculties published the so-called "U.K. criteria" in 1976[89] and re-emphasized them in 1979[90] and these criteria have been embodied in the United Kingdom Health Department's code of practice[91] on the removal of cadaveric organs for transplantation. Jennett[92] has reviewed the changes in practice that have occurred in the diagnoses of brain death and shown that proper regard to the current criteria will never result in the incorrect positive diagnosis of brain death. The code of practice agreed by the Conference of Medical Royal Colleges and Faculties of the United Kingdom (1976)[89] is as follows (reproduced in part by kind permission of the Editor, *British Medical Journal*).

### Pre-conditions for considering diagnosis of brain death

All of the following should coexist.

1. *The patient is deeply comatose.*

(*a*) There should be no suspicion that this state is due to depressant drugs. Narcotics, hypnotics, and tranquillisers may have prolonged durations of action, particularly when some hypothermia exists. The benzodiazepines act cumulatively and their effects persist, and they are commonly used as anticonvulsants or to assist synchronisation with mechanical ventilators. It is therefore recommended that the drug history should be carefully reviewed and adequate intervals allowed for the persistence of drug effects to be excluded. This is of particular importance in patients whose primary cause of coma lies in the toxic effects of drugs followed by anoxic cerebral damage.

(*b*) Primary hypothermia as a cause of coma should have been excluded.

(*c*) Metabolic and endocrine disturbances that can cause or contribute to coma should have been excluded. Metabolic and endocrine factors contributing to the persistence of coma must be carefully assessed. There should be no profound abnormality of the serum electrolytes, acid base balance, or blood glucose concentrations.

2. *The patient is being maintained on a ventilator because spontaneous respiration had previously become inadequate or had ceased altogether.*

Relaxants (neuromuscular blocking agents) and other drugs should have been excluded as a cause of respiratory inadequacy or failure. Immobility, unresponsiveness, and lack of spontaneous respiration may be due to the use of neuromuscular blocking drugs, and the persistence of their effects should be excluded by eliciting spinal reflexes (flexion or stretch) or by showing adequate neuromuscular conduction with a conventional nerve stimulator. Equally, persistent effects of hypnotics and narcotics should be excluded as the cause of respiratory failure.

3. *There should be no doubt that the patient's condition is due to irremediable structural brain damage. The diagnosis of a disorder which can lead to brain death should have been fully established.*

It may be obvious within hours of a primary intracranial event such as severe head injury, spontaneous intracranial haemorrhage, or after neurosurgery that the condition is irremediable. But when a patient has suffered primarily from cardiac arrest, hypoxia, or severe circulatory insufficiency with an indefinite period of cerebral anoxia or is suspected of having cerebral air or fat embolism then it may take much longer to establish the diagnosis and to be confident of the prognosis. In some patients the primary condition may be a matter of doubt and a confident diagnosis may be reached only by continuous clinical observation and investigation.

### Tests for confirming brain death

*All brain-stem reflexes should be absent.*

(*a*) The pupils are fixed in diameter and do not respond to sharp changes in the intensity of incident light.

(*b*) There is no corneal reflex.

(*c*) The vestibulo-ocular reflexes are absent. These are absent when no eye movement occurs during or after the slow injection of 20 ml of ice-cold water into each external auditory meatus in turn, clear access to the tympanic membrane having been established by direct inspection. This test may be contra-indicated on one or other side by local trauma.

(*d*) No motor responses within the cranial nerve distribution can be elicited by adequate stimulation of any somatic area.

(*e*) There is no gag reflex response to bronchial stimulation by a suction catheter passed down the trachea.

(*f*) No respiratory movements occur when the patient is disconnected from the mechanical ventilator for long enough to ensure that the arterial carbon dioxide tension rises above the threshold for stimulating respiration—that is the $Pa{CO_2}$ must normally reach 50 mm Hg (6·7 kPa). This is best achieved by measuring the blood gases; if this facility is available the patient should be disconnected when the $Pa{CO_2}$

reaches 40–45 mm Hg (5·3–6·0 kPa) after administration of 5 per cent $CO_2$ in oxygen through the ventilator. This starting level has been chosen because patients may be moderately hypothermic (35° C to 37° C), flaccid, and with a depressed metabolic rate, so that $Pa{CO_2}$ rises only slowly in apnoea (about 2 mm Hg/min; 0·27 kPa/min). (Hypoxia during disconnection should be prevented by delivering oxygen at 6 l/min through a catheter into the trachea.)

If blood gas analysis is not available to measure the $Pa{CO_2}$ and $Pa{O_2}$ the alternative procedure is to supply the ventilator with pure oxygen for 10 minutes (preoxygenation), then with 5 per cent $CO_2$ in oxygen for five minutes, and to disconnect the ventilator for 10 minutes while delivering oxygen at 6 l/min by catheter into the trachea. This establishes diffusion oxygenation and ensures that during apnoea hypoxia will not occur even in 10 or more minutes of respiratory arrest. Schafer and Caronna[93] have shown that a 10-minute disconnection period will ensure a $Pa{CO_2}$ of 60 mm Hg (8 kPa), provided that the starting value exceeds 30 mm Hg (4 kPa).

Those patients with pre-existing chronic respiratory insufficiency, who may be unresponsive to raised levels of carbon dioxide and who normally exist on a hypoxic drive, are special cases and should be expertly investigated with careful blood gas monitoring.

### Other Considerations

*Repetition of testing.*—It is customary to repeat the tests to ensure that there has been no observer error. The interval between tests must depend on the primary condition and the clinical course of the disease. Some conditions in which it would be unnecessary to repeat tests since a prognosis of imminent brain death can be accepted as being obvious are listed under the third criteria for considering a diagnosis of brain death (see above). In some conditions the outcome is not so clear-cut and in these the tests should be repeated. The interval between tests depends on the progress of the patient and might be as long as 24 hours. This is a matter for medical judgment, and reception time must be related to the signs of improvement, stability, or deterioration that present themselves.

*Integrity of spinal reflexes.*—It is well established that spinal cord function can persist after insults that irretrievably destroy brain-stem function. Reflexes of spinal origin may persist or return after an initial absence in brain-dead patients.[94]

*Confirmatory investigations.*—It is now widely accepted that electro-encephalography is not necessary for diagnosing brain death.[95–100]

Indeed, this view was expressed from Harvard in 1969 by Beecher,[101] only a year after the original Harvard criteria were published. Electroencephalography has its principal value at earlier stages in the care of patients, when the original diagnosis is in doubt. When electroencephalography is used the strict criteria recommended by the Federation of EEG Societies[102, 103] must be followed. Other investigations such as cerebral angiography or cerebral blood flow measurements are not required for diagnosing brain death.

*Body temperature.*—The body temperature in these patients may be low because of depression of central temperature regulation by drugs or by brain-stem damage and it is recommended that it should be not less than 35° C before the diagnostic tests are carried out. A low-reading thermometer should be used.

*Specialist opinion and status of doctors concerned.*—Experienced clinicians in intensive care units, acute medical wards, and accident and emergency departments should not normally require specialist advice. Only when the primary diagnosis is in doubt is it necessary to consult with a neurologist or neurosurgeon. The decision to withdraw artificial support should be made after all the criteria presented above have been fulfilled and can be made by any one of the following combinations of doctors. (*a*) A consultant who is in charge of the case and one other doctor; (*b*) in the absence of a consultant, his deputy, who should have been registered for five years or more and who should have had adequate experience in the care of such cases, and one other doctor.

## REFERENCES


1. Kramer, S. (1912). On the function of the circle of Willis. *J. exp. Med.*, **15**, 348.
2. McDonald, D. A. and Potter, J. M. (1951). The distribution of blood to the brain. *J. Physiol.* (*Lond.*), **114**, 356.
3. Brain, R. (1957). Order and disorder in the cerebral circulation. (*Harvey Tercentenary Lecture*). *Lancet*, **2**, 857.
4. Symon, L. (1967). A comparative study of middle cerebral pressure in dogs and macaques. *J. Physiol.* (*Lond.*), **191**, 449.
5. Batson, O. V. (1944). Anatomical problems concerned in the study of cerebral blood flow. *Fed. Proc.*, **3**, 139.
6. Shenkin, H. A., Harmel, M. H. and Kety, S. S. (1948). Dynamic anatomy of the cerebral circulation. *Arch. Neurol. Psychiat.* (*Chic.*), **60**, 240.
7. Kety, S. S. and Schmidt. C. F. (1948). The nitrous oxide method for quantitative determination of cerebral blood flow in man: theory, procedure and normal values. *J. clin. Invest.*, **27**, 476.
8. Munck, O. and Lassen, N. A. (1957). Bilateral cerebral blood flow and oxygen consumption in man by use of Krypton 85. *Circulat. Res.*, **5**, 163.
9. Lassen, N. A. (1980). Cerebral and spinal cord blood flow. In *Anesthesia and Neurosurgery*, p. 1. Ed. J. E. Cottrell and H. Turndorf. St. Louis: C. V. Mosby Company.
10. Lassen, N. A. and Klee, A. (1965). Cerebral blood flow determined by saturation and desaturation with Krypton 85. *Circulat. Res.*, **16**, 26.
11. Lassen, N. A. and Ingvar, D. H. (1963). Regional cerebral blood flow measurement in man. *Arch. Neurol.* (*Chic.*), **9**, 615.
12. Sveinsdottir, E., Larsen, B., Rommer, P. and Lassen, N. A. (1977). A multidetector scintillation camera with 254 channels. *J. Nucl. Med.*, **18**, 168.
13. Kennedy, C. and Sokoloff, L. (1957). An adaptation of the nitrous oxide method to the study of the cerebral circulation in children; normal values for cerebral blood flow and cerebral metabolic rate in childhood. *J. clin. Invest.*, **36**, 1130.
14. Shenkin, H. A., Novak, P., Goluboff, B., Soffe, A. M. and Bortin, L. (1953). The effects of aging, arteriosclerosis and hypertension upon the cerebral circulation. *J. clin. Invest.*, **32**, 459.
15. Roy, C. S. and Sherington, C. S. (1890). On regulation of blood supply of brain. *J. Physiol.* (*Lond.*), **11**, 85.
16. Harper, A. M. (1965). Physiology of the cerebral blood flow. *Brit. J. Anaesth.*, **37**, 225.
17. Harper, A. M. and Glass, H. I. (1965). The effect of alterations in the arterial carbon dioxide tension on the blood flow through the cerebral cortex at normal and low arterial blood pressure. *J. Neurol. Neurosurg. Psychiat.*, **28**, 449.
18. Lennox, W. G. and Gibbs, E. L. (1932). The blood flow in the brain and the leg of man and the changes induced by alteration of blood gases. *J. clin. Invest.*, **11**, 1155.
19. Severinghaus, J. W., Chiodi, H., Eger, E. I. (II), Brandstater, B. and Hornbein, T. F. (1966). Cerebral blood flow in man at high altitude. *Circulat. Res.*, **19**, 274.
20. Lassen, N. A. (1966). The luxury perfusion syndrome and its possible relation to acute metabolic acidosis localised within the brain. *Lancet*, **2**, 1113.
21. Harper, A. M. and Bell, R. A. (1963). The effect of metabolic acidosis and alkalosis on the blood flow through the cerebral cortex. *J. Neurol. Neurosurg. Psychiat.*, **26**, 341.
22. Kogure, K., Scheinberg, P., Reinmuth, O. M., Fujishima, M. and Busto, B. (1970). Mechanisms of cerebral vasodilatation in hypoxia. *J. Appl. Physiol.*, **29**, 223.
23. Jacobson, I., Harper, A. M. and McDowall, D. G. (1963). Relationship between venous pressure and cortical blood flow. *Nature* (*Lond.*), **200**, 173.
24. Harper, A. M., McDowall, D. G. and Ledingham, I. (1965). The influence of hyperbaric oxygen on the blood flow and oxygen uptake of the cerebral cortex in hypovolaemic shock. *Proc. 2nd Internat. Conf. on Hyperbaric Oxygen*, Vol. 2.
25. Holbach, K. H. and Gött, U. (1970). Effects of hyperbaric oxygen therapy on neurosurgical patients. In: *Proc. 4th Internat. Congr. on Hyperbaric Medicine*. Washington D.C.: National Academy of Sciences.
26. Oleson, J. (1971). Contralateral focal increase of cerebral blood flow in man during arm work. *Brain*, **94**, 635.
27. Kobayashi, S., Waltz, A. G. and Rhoton, A. L. (1971). Effects of stimulation of cervical sympathetic nerves on cortical blood flow and vascular reactivity. *Neurology* (*Minneap.*)., **21**, 297.
28. Salanga, V. D. and Waltz, A. G. (1973). Regional cerebral blood flow during stimulation of tenth cranial nerve. *Stroke*, **4**, 213.
29. Fitch, W., Mackenzie, E. T. and Harper, A. M. (1975). Effects of decreasing arterial blood pressure on cerebral blood flow in the baboon: influence of the sympathetic nervous system. *Circ. Res.*, **37**, 550.
30. Christensen, M. S., Høedt-Rasmussen, K. and Lassen, N. A. (1967). Cerebral vasodilatation by halothane anaesthesia in man and its potentiation by hypotension and hypercapnia. *Br. J. Anaesth.*, **39**, 927.
31. Alexander, S. C., Colton, E. T., Smith, A. L. and Wollman, H. (1970). The effects of cyclopropane on cerebral and systemic carbohydrate metabolism. *Anesthesiology*, **32**, 236.
32. Adams, R. W., Gronert, G. A., Sundt, T. M. and Michenfelder, J. D. (1972). Halothane, hypocapnia and cerebrospinal fluid pressure in neurosurgery. *Anesthesiology*, **37**, 510.
33. Jobes, D. R., Kennell, E., Bitner, R., Swenson, E. and Wollman, H. (1975). Effects of morphine-nitrous oxide anesthesia on cerebral autoregulation. *Anesthesiology*, **42**, 30.
34. Tarkkanen, L., Laitinen, L. and Johansson, G. (1974). Effects of d-tubocurarine on intracranial pressure and thalamic electrical impedance. *Anesthesiology*, **40**, 247.
35. Jennett, W. B., Barker, J., Fitch, W. and McDowall, D. G. (1969). Effect of anaesthesia on intracranial pressure in patients with space-occupying lesions. *Lancet*, **1**, 61.
36. Misfeldt, B. B., Jörgensen, P. B. and Rishoj, M. (1975). The effect of nitrous oxide and halothane upon the intracranial pressure in hypocapnic patients with intracranial disorders. *Brit. J. Anaesth.*, **46**, 853.
37. Rosomoff, H. L. and Holaday, D. A. (1954). Cerebral blood flow and cerebral oxygen consumption during hypothermia. *Amer. J. Physiol.*, **179**, 85.
38. Kleinerman, G. and Hopkins, A. L. (1955). The effects

of hypothermia on cerebral blood flow and metabolism in dogs. *Fed. Proc.*, **14**, 410.
39. Rosomoff, H. L. (1956). Some effects of hypothermia on the normal and abnormal physiology of the nervous system. *Proc. roy. Soc. Med.*, **49**, 358.
40. Albert, F. N. and Fazekas, J. F. (1956). Cerebral haemodynamics and metabolism during induced hypothermia. *Curr. Res. Anesth.*, **35**, 381.
41. Berntman, L., Welsh, F. A. and Harp, J. R. (1981). Cerebral protective effects of low-grade hypothermia. *Anesthesiology*, **55**, 495.
42. Bridges, B. E. and Eger, E. I., II (1966). The effect of hypocapnia on the level of halothane anesthesia in man. *Anesthesiology*, **27**, 634.
43. Eger, E. I. (II), Saidman, L. J. and Brandstater, B. (1965). Minimum alveolar anesthetic concentration: a standard of anesthetic potency. *Anesthesiology*, **26**, 756.
44. Sugioka, K. and Davis, D. A. (1960). Hyperventilation with oxygen: a possible cause of cerebral hypoxia. *Anesthesiology*, **21**, 135.
45. Robinson, J. S. and Gray, T. D. (1961). Observations on the cerebral effects of passive hyperventilation. *Brit. J. Anaesth.*, **33**, 62.
46. Pierce, E. C., Lambertsen, C. J., Deutsch, S., Chase, P. E., Linde, H. W., Dripps, R. D. and Price, H. L. (1962). Cerebral circulation and metabolism during thiopental anesthesia and hyperventilation in man. *J. clin. Invest.*, **41**, 1664.
47. Bollen, A. R. (1962). The electroencephalogram in anaesthesia; some aspects of hyperventilation. *Brit. J. Anaesth.*, **34**, 890.
48. Wollman, H., Alexander, S. C., Cohen, P. J., Smith, T. C., Chase, P. E. and Van Der Molen, R. A. (1965). Cerebral circulation during general anesthesia and hyperventilation in man. *Anesthesiology*, **26**, 329.
49. Harp, J. R. and Wollman, H. (1973). Cerebral metabolic effects of hyperventilation and deliberate hypotension. *Br. J. Anaesth.*, **45**, 256.
50. Rosomoff, H. L. (1963). Distribution of intracranial contents with controlled hyperventilation: implications for neuro-anesthesia. *Anesthesiology*, **24**, 640.
51. Alexander, S. C. and Lassen, N. A. (1970). Cerebral circulatory response to acute brain disease. *Anesthesiology*, **32**, 60.
52. Harp, J. R. and Hagerdal, M. (1980). Brain oxygen consumption. In: *Anesthesia and Neurosurgery*, p. 28. Ed. J. E. Cottrell and H. Turndorf. St. Louis: C. V. Mosby Company.
53. Rossen, R., Kabat, H. and Anderson, J. P. (1943). Acute arrest of cerebral circulation in man. *Arch. Neurol. Psychiat.* (*Chic.*), **50**, 510.
54. Cohen, P. J., Alexander, S. C. and Smith, T. C. (1967). Effects of hypoxia and normocarbia on cerebral blood flow and metabolism in man. *J. Appl. Physiol.*, **23**, 183.
55. Smith, A. L. and Wollman, H. (1972). Cerebral blood flow and metabolism effects of anesthetic drugs and techniques. *Anesthesiology*, **36**, 378.
56. Wollman, S. B. and Orken, L. R. (1968). Postoperative human reaction time and hypocarbia during anaesthesia. *Brit. J. Anaesth.*, **40**, 920.
57. Meyer, H. H. (1899). Zur Theorie der Alkoholnarcose I mitt Welche Eigenschaft der Anesthetika bedingt ihre narkotische Wirkung? *Naunyn-Schmiedeberg's Arch. exp. Path. Pharmak.*, **42**, 109.
58. Overton, E. (1901). *Studien uber die Narkose*. Jena: Fischer.
59. Eger, E. I., Lundgren, C., Miller, S. L. and Stevens, W. C. (1969). Anesthetic potencies of sulphur hexafluoride, carbon tetrachloride, chloroform and Ethrane in dogs: correlation with the hydrate and lipid theories of anesthetic action. *Anesthesiology*, **30**, 129.
60. Miller, S. L. (1961). A theory of gaseous anesthetics. *Proc. nat. Acad. Sci.* (*Wash.*), **47**, 1515.
61. Pauling, L. (1961). A molecular theory of general anaesthesia. *Science*, **134**, 15.
62. Ferguson, J. (1939). The use of chemical potentials as indices of toxicity. *Proc. roy. Soc. B.*, **127**, 387.
63. Halsey, M. J., Brown, F. F. and Richards, P. E. (1978). Perturbations of model protein systems as a basis for the central and peripheral mechanisms of general anaesthesia. In: *Molecular Interactions and Activity in Proteins*, p. 123. (Ciba Foundation Symposium, No. 60). Amsterdam: Excerpta Medica.
64. Johnson, F. H. and Flagler, E. A. (1950). Hydrostatic pressure reversal of narcosis in tadpoles. *Science*, **112**, 91.
65. Smith, R. A., Winter, P. M., Halsey, M. J. and Eger, E. I. (1975). Helium pressure produces a non-linear antagonism of argon or nitrogen anesthesia in mice. *ASA Annual Meeting Scientific Abstracts*, 217.
66. Halsey, M. J. and Wardley-Smith, B. (1975). Pressure reversal of narcosis produced by anaesthetics, narcotics and tranquillizers. *Nature*, **257**, 811.
67. Lever, M. J., Miller, K. W., Paton, W. D. M. and Smith, E. B. (1971). Pressure reversal of anaesthesia. *Nature*, **231**, 368.
68. Miller, K. W., Paton, W. D. M., Smith, R. A. and Smith, E. B. (1973). The pressure reversal of general anaesthesia and the critical volume hypothesis. *Molecular Pharmacol.*, **9**, 131.
69. Halsey, M. J., Wardley-Smith, B. and Green, C. J. (1978). The pressure reversal of general anaesthesia: a multisite expansion hypothesis. *Br. J. Anaesth.*, **50**, 1091.
70. Sadove, M. S., Becka, D. and Gibbs, F. A. (1967). *Electroencephalography for Anesthesiologists and Surgeons*. Philadelphia: J. B. Lippincott Co.
71. Gibbs, F. A., Gibbs, E. L. and Fuster, B. (1947). Anterior temporal localisation of sleep-induced seizure discharges of the psychomotor type. *Trans. Amer. neurol. Ass.*, **72**, 180.
72. Kiersey, D. K., Bickford, R. G. and Faulconer, A., Jr. (1951). Electroencephalographic patterns produced by thiopentone sodium during surgical operations. Description and classification. *Brit. J. Anaesth.*, **23**, 141.
73. Gronquist, Y. K. J., Seldon, T. H. and Faulconer, J., Jr. (1952). Cerebral anoxia during anaesthesia. Prognostic significance of electroencephalographic changes. *Ann. Chir. Gynaec. Fenn.*, **41**, 149.
74. Hockaday, J. M., Potts, F., Epstein, E., Bonazzi, A. and Schwab, R. S. (1965). Electroencephalographic changes in acute cerebral anoxia from cardiac or respiratory arrest. *Electroenceph. clin. Neurophysiol.*, **18**, 575.
75. Haider, I., Oswald, I. and Matthew, H. (1968). EEG signs of death. *Brit. med. J.*, **3**, 314.
76. Clowes, G. H. A., Kretchmer, H. E., McBurney, R. W. and Simeone, F. A. (1953). Electroencephalogram in evaluation of effects of anaesthetic agents and carbon dioxide accumulation during surgery. *Ann. Surg.*, **138**, 558.
77. Brazier, M. A. B. (1943). The physiological effects of

carbon dioxide on the activity of the central nervous system in man. *Medicine* (*Baltimore*), **22**, 205.

78. Holmberg, G. (1953). The electroencephalogram during hypoxia and hyperventilation. *Electroenceph. clin. Neurophysiol.*, **5**, 371.
79. Wilson, S. M. (1957). Electro-encephalography in relation to anaesthesia. *Proc. roy. Soc. Med.*, **50**, 105.
80. Pearcy, W. C. and Virtue, R. W. (1959). The electroencephalogram in hypothermia and circulatory occlusion. *Anesthesiology*, **20**, 34.
81. Berezowskyj, J. L., McEwen, J. A., Anderson, G. B. and Jenkins, L. C. (1976). A study of anaesthesia depth by power spectral analysis of the electroencephalogram (EEG). *Canad. Anaesth. Soc. J.*, **23**, 1.
82. Maynard, D., Prior, P. F. and Scott, D. F. (1969). Device for continuous monitoring of cerebral activity in resuscitated patients. *Brit. med. J.*, **4**, 545.
83. Branthwaite, M. A. (1973). Factors affecting cerebral activity during open heart surgery. *Anaesthesia*, **28**, 619.
84. Benzinger, T. H. (1970). *Physiological and Behavioural Temperature Regulation*, p. 831. Edited by J. D. Hardy, A. P. Gagge and J. A. J. Stolwijk. Springfield, Ill.: Chas. C. Thomas.
85. Hammel, H. T. (1972). *Essays on Temperature Regulation*, p. 121. Edited by J. Bligh and R. Moore. Amsterdam: North-Holland.
86. Bromage, P. R. (1953). Some electro-encephalographic changes associated with induced vascular hypotension. *Proc. roy. Soc. Med.*, **46**, 919.
87. Mollaret, P. and Goulon, M. (1959). Coma dépassé. *Rev. Neurology*, **101**, 3.
88. Harvard (1968). Report of the Ad Hoc Committee of Harvard Medical School to examine the definition of brain death. Definition of irreversible coma. *J. Amer. med. Ass.*, **205**, 337.
89. Conference of Medical Royal Colleges and their Faculties of the U.K. (1976). Diagnosis of brain death. *Br. med. J.*, **2**, 1187.
90. Conference of Medical Royal Colleges and their Faculties of the U.K. (1979). Diagnosis of brain death. *Br. med. J.*, **1**, 322.
91. Health Departments of Great Britain and Northern Ireland (1979). The removal of cadaveric organs for transplantation: a code of practice. London: H.M.S.O.
92. Jennett, B. (1981). Brain death. *Br. J. Anaesth.*, **53**, 1111.
93. Schafer, J. A. and Caronna, J. J. (1978). Duration of apnea needed to confirm brain death. *Neurology*, **28**, 661.
94. Ivan, L. P. (1973). Spinal reflexes in cerebral death. *Neurology* (*Minneap.*), **23**, 650.
95. Walker, A. E. (1976). The neurosurgeon's responsibility for organ procurement. *J. Neurosurg.*, **44**, 1.
96. Mohandas, A. and Chou, S. N. (1971). Brain death. A clinical and pathological study. *J. Neurosurg.*, **35**, 211.
97. *Lancet* (1974). Brain damage and brain death, **1**, 341.
98. *British Medical Journal* (1975). Brain death. **1**, 356.
99. MacGillivray, B. (1973). The diagnosis of cerebral death. In: *Proc. 10th Congr. European Dialysis and Transplant Assn.* Ed. by J. F. Moorhead. London: Pitman Medical.
100. Chou, S. N. (1981). Brain death. *Lancet*, **1**, 282.
101. Beecher, H. K. (1969). After the "definition of irreversible coma". *New Engl. J. Med.*, **281**, 1070.
102. EEG Societies (1974). The International Federation of EEG Societies. Report. *Electroenceph. clin. Neurophysiol.*, **37**, 430.
103. EEG Societies (1975). The International Federation of EEG Societies. Report. *Electroenceph. clin. Neurophysiol.*, **38**, 536.

CHAPTER 28

# Neurological Anaesthesia



## CEREBROSPINAL FLUID

Anaesthesia for intracranial surgery involves above all other considerations a constant awareness of the intracranial pressure. All space-occupying lesions, including even small aneurysms, may interfere with cerebrospinal fluid circulation and absorption. Drugs and techniques used by the anaesthetist can by direct or indirect mechanisms cause catastrophic changes in cerebrospinal fluid pressure which threaten the viability of the brain.

### Formation of Cerebrospinal Fluid

Cerebrospinal fluid is secreted by the villous projections of the choroid plexuses in the lateral ventricles. It passes through the interventricular foramina into the third ventricle, cerebral aqueduct and fourth ventricle, and thence through the foramina of Magendie and Luschka into the subarachnoid space. The major portion passes upwards through the posterior fossa and over the surface of the cerebral hemispheres, whilst the remainder flows through the foramen magnum to surround the spinal cord. Absorption of cerebrospinal fluid occurs mainly through the arachnoid villi into the dural sinuses and spinal veins. A small amount passes out along the dural sheaths of cranial and spinal nerves to be absorbed into lymphatics. The volume of cerebrospinal fluid in adults is 100–150 ml, and with the subject in the lateral position this exerts a pressure of 50–150 mm (0·5–1·5 kPa) of cerebrospinal fluid.

### Raised Intracranial Pressure

The classical signs of raised intracranial pressure are headache, vomiting and papilloedema. Detectable papilloedema may take up to two weeks to develop. A dangerous rise in pressure occurring due to a supratentorial lesion is marked by drowsiness, clouding of consciousness, a loss of the ability to look upwards, and dilatation and loss of response to light, firstly of the pupil on the side of the lesion and finally of both pupils. Raised pressure in the posterior fossa causes bradycardia, bradypnoea and hypertension. Some drowsiness may be present. As pressure in the posterior fossa rises, medullary coning occurs, when the cerebellar tonsils are pushed down behind the cervical spinal cord through the foramen magnum, blocking this foramen and also the foramina of Magendie and Luschka. Increasing medullary pressure leads to respiratory failure. Developing medullary coning usually produces neck stiffness and head retraction.

Evidence of raised intracranial pressure may be seen on X-rays of the skull as enlargement of the pituitary fossa, erosion of the posterior clinoid processes, and in slowly developing cases a beaten silver appearance of the vault (Fig. 1). In children the sutures may be forced apart.

Diagnostic lumbar puncture, anaesthesia, posturing the patient, and neuroradiological and neurosurgical interference can all precipitate a medullary conus in a patient already suffering from severe hydrocephalus.

A knowledge of the presence and degree of hydrocephalus is of greater importance to the anaesthetist than a diagnosis of the specific disease, while an understanding of normal cerebrospinal fluid physiology, and the effects on it of anaesthetic drugs and procedures, is an essential prerequisite to the selection and administration of successful anaesthesia.

### Cerebral Perfusion Pressure

Because the cerebral venous sinuses have a pressure in them which approximates to the intracranial pressure,[1] blood flow through the brain is determined by the mean arterial to intracranial pressure gradient. This cerebral perfusion pressure is normally 80–90 mm Hg (10·5–12 kPa).[2] Work by McDowall and his colleagues[3] has drawn attention to the potentially damaging falls in cerebral perfusion pressure which can occur when volatile anaesthetic agents are given to patients with raised intracranial pressure. Such falls have been shown to occur when commonly used anaesthetic concentrations of halothane, trichloroethylene, enflur-

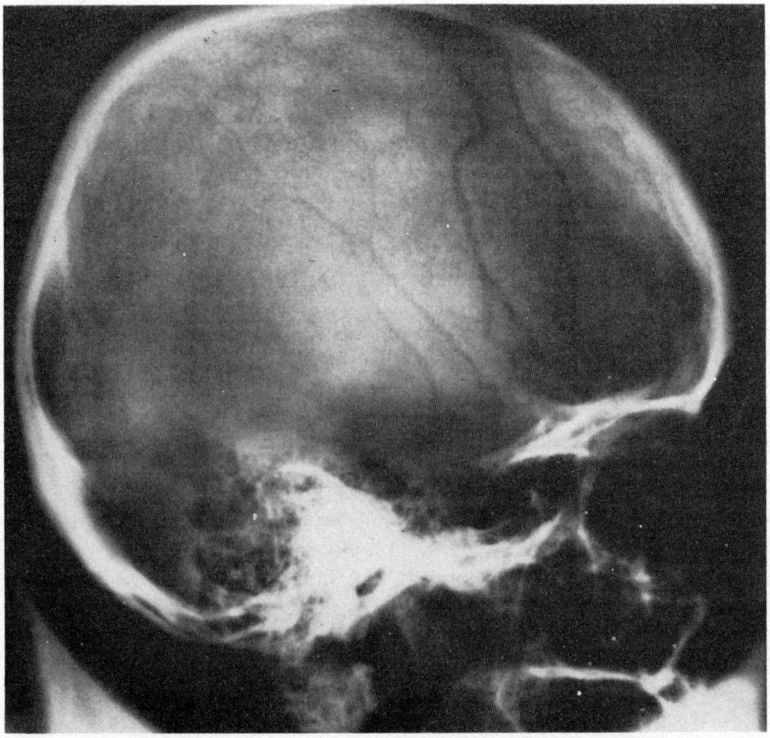

28/Fig. 1.—Raised intracranial pressure. Lateral skull radiograph of a 52-year-old woman with a malignant astrocytoma, showing a "smudged-out" appearance of the pituitary fossa typical of generalised raised intracranial pressure. (Courtesy of Dr. E. H. Burrows and The Wessex Neurological Centre.)

ane or isoflurane are administered.[2-6] All these agents cause an immediate but variable rise in cerebrospinal fluid pressure which is dose-dependent. The rise reaches a peak in 10 to 15 minutes and then declines. In the presence of an already raised intracranial pressure the rise caused by volatile anaesthetics may be very marked and intracranial pressure may continue to rise even after withdrawing the volatile agent. A high intracranial pressure, especially if associated with a reduced mean arterial pressure, may reduce cerebral perfusion pressure to near zero levels and cause hypoxic brain damage. The rise in cerebrospinal fluid pressure is due to increased cerebral blood flow and a raised cerebral blood volume and it is most evident when $Pco_2$ is either normal or raised. The practical importance of this is that when patients with raised intracranial pressure are to be anaesthetised, these agents should be avoided unless other measures to reduce intracranial pressure have been taken before they are exhibited. This is particularly applicable to investigations such as carotid angiography and in the management of patients having extracranial operations, usually for fractures, who also have recent head injuries. Relaxant drugs and moderate hyperventilation are to be preferred to spontaneous breathing and volatile agents.

## POSTURE

The posture of the patient has a pronounced effect on venous drainage. Unfortunately the ideal position for the anaesthetist is not always compatible with that needed by the surgeon, and although venous congestion may mitigate against a dry operation field, other more important factors sometimes decide the ultimate choice. Whenever possible the patient should be placed in a position so that venous drainage away from the operation site is encouraged, obstruction to major veins is avoided, and respiration is not impeded. There are four classical positions commonly used in neurosurgery—the supine, prone, lateral and sitting.

### 1. *Supine Position*

The supine position is used to approach the anterior fossa, and with the patient lying on his back and his head slightly raised and fixed in a special horseshoe rest, venous drainage and respiration are not embarrassed. The addition of a foot-down tilt is an advantage, but since it may lead to a very low pressure in the veins above the level of the heart there is a risk of air embolus occurring during the operation. This risk is at its highest when the sitting position is used.

### 2. *Prone Position*

The prone position is often used for laminectomies, and to approach the posterior fossa. It may lead to marked venous congestion, particularly if the operation area is dependent. Moreover, unless the patient is properly supported, undue abdominal compression may embarrass ventilation and obstruct the inferior vena cava. This last effect can seriously reduce blood pressure and also increase pressure in the vertebral veins. On the credit side, there is no risk of air embolus occurring.

The vertebral venous system consists of an extensive network of veins which drain into and communicate freely with the vena cavae.[7] Increased abdominal or thoracic pressure will be reflected in vertebral venous pressure and may reverse the normal direction of flow. Pearce[8] has shown that in patients in the prone position abdominal pressure sufficient to obstruct the inferior vena cava can cause caval pressure to rise by more than 30 cm of water (2·8 kPa), whilst even slight abdominal compression leads to a rapid increase in caval pressure of 3–4 cm of water (0·3–0·4 kPa). To produce minimal venous pressure Pearce recommended supporting the fully relaxed and ventilated patient so that the abdominal wall hangs free. A wedge-shaped pillow under the thorax with its broad edge just below the level of the acromion effectively maintains the patient in the correct position and gives reasonable freedom for diaphragmatic movement. Further help can be gained by raising the pelvis on supports. This position opens up the intervertebral spaces of the upper part of the spine but tends to close the lumbar intervertebral spaces. For this reason the jack-knife position with the patient flexed in the prone position over pillows or a "broken" operation table is often used for lumbar laminectomies, although respiratory embarrassment and venous congestion are more likely in this position.

3. ***Lateral Position***

Another approach to the problem of venous bleeding during laminectomy is to use the lateral position, which enables the patient to be postured with the back flexed. There is little, if any, venous engorgement in this position, provided the surgeon does not need excessive flexion to open up the intervertebral spaces. This can only be achieved by drawing up the thighs with full flexion at the hips, and results in some abdominal compression. The lateral position is also useful for posterior fossa surgery.

4. ***Sitting Position***

The sitting or upright position is undoubtedly the most effective method for producing an uncongested operating field for a cervical laminectomy or posterior fossa craniotomy. The patient is placed in a special chair with the head supported anteriorly in a cushioned horse-shoe. An alternative method is to place the patient supine on the operating table, but with the head well over the end and held forward and supported by a wire and caliper which is fixed to the head. The table is set with a pronounced foot-down tilt.

**Some Dangers of Posture**

Air embolus and severe hypotension are the two dangers associated with these upright positions, although any degree of anti-Trendelenburg tilt is conducive to such potential hazards.

**Air embolus.**—The incidence of air embolus is difficult to assess and published figures are not available, but it undoubtedly bears a relation to the competence of the surgeon. Furthermore, prompt diagnosis and treatment by both surgeon and anaesthetist sometimes prove surprisingly successful. In neurosurgical practice the quantity of air sucked into a vein may be comparatively small, but the site of entry may not be apparent at once. A tear in a venous sinus during the removal of bone is a likely site. Other vulnerable vessels are the suboccipital venous plexus and the mastoid emissaries.[9] Deep breathing or one or two deep respirations following a cough add to the hazard, as they increase the subatmospheric pressure which already exists in these veins. Hunter[10] considered that air embolism was very likely to occur when muscle relaxants and intermittent positive-pressure ventilation are used for a posterior fossa operation in the sitting position, and he considered the method unacceptable because effective ventilation, even without a negative phase, reduced the venous pressure above the heart to a dangerously low level. However, Millar[11] could find no evidence of a special danger of controlled ventilation during posterior fossa surgery. The risk of air embolism can be minimised by deliberately increasing venous pressure during the danger periods when the skull is being opened and closed, by intermittent compression of the jugular veins,[9] by providing an expiratory resistance,[12] or by use of a G-suit. The early signs of air embolism are an unexplained fall in blood pressure, a rise in pulse rate and (in the spontaneously breathing patient) the occurrence of a deep breath.[13] Useful simple adjuvants to diagnosis are an oesophageal stethoscope, electrocardiogram and a right atrial pressure line. Rapid diagnosis of early air embolus can be made using a Doppler ultrasonic detector,[14] end-tidal carbon dioxide analyser or pulmonary-artery pressure measurement. The Doppler detector is undoubtedly the most sensitive monitor of venous air embolism. Its high sensitivity leads to a relatively high incidence of false positive results. Moreover, it cannot be used to quantify the volume of air within the circulation. Sudden falls in end-tidal $CO_2$ (due to an increased alveolar dead-space) or rises in pulmonary artery pressure (due to increased pulmonary vascular resistance) are, in practice, reliable early indicators of venous air embolism.[15] At the first sign of air embolus, treatment must be immediately instituted. Ingress of more air into the circulation should be prevented either by identifying and closing the open vein or by flooding the operative site with saline. The patient should be given 100 per cent oxygen, for in the presence of nitrous oxide an air bubble in the circulation will increase in volume three or four-fold. Whilst in theory the patient should be placed flat and on his left side to minimise the danger of air entering the right ventricular outflow tract, it is rarely feasible to change posture rapidly during a neurosurgical procedure. If a right atrial catheter is in place air can be aspirated from the heart.[16] Large air emboli cause a marked reduction in cardiac output and vigorous cardiovascular supportive measures may be necessary.

**Hypotension.**—Adoption of the sitting position can impose a considerable disability on the circulatory system. This is most likely to occur in the thirty minutes after the patient has been placed in an upright position. The falls in blood pressure that occur in this position are usually due to impaired vasomotor stability produced by drugs given before and during anaesthesia. Although autoregulation maintains a normal cerebral blood flow in spite of falls in blood pressure there is a lower limit of arterial pressure below which this mechanism fails. It is unwise to allow the systolic pressure of a patient who has a normal circulation to fall below 70–80 mm Hg (9·3–10·7 kPa), and even this level may be unsafe in the presence of raised intracranial tension. To minimise falls in blood pressure the sitting position should be adopted gradually. Falls in blood pressure should initially be treated by a rapid infusion of bland fluid. If this is not effective a small dose of a pressor agent such as methoxamine (5–10 mg) may be necessary. Atropine may also be useful if bradycardia is present. The most effective form of therapy is to lower the patient to a more supine position. Some help towards the prevention of undue hypotension can be gained by firm bandaging of the legs from toes to groins, flexing the thighs and raising the legs[17] or by placing the lower part of the patient's body in a G-suit.[12]

The changes in the brain that can be caused by sub-oxygenation have been described elsewhere (see Chapter 29). Here it only needs to be stressed that specific histological changes in the cells are not visible if death takes place within 30 to 36 hours of the period of sub-oxygenation. Post-mortem diagnosis of the cause of sudden death in the operating theatre is rarely satisfactory, and depends far more upon clinical evidence of the sequence of events than upon abnormal pathology.

### Discussion

The choice between the upright and prone position usually depends upon the surgeon. Theoretically, better access to a particular part of the brain due to an uncongested and relatively bloodless operation wound enables delicate surgery to be performed with less risk of trauma to surrounding tissue. This is an important factor in neurosurgical work, where morbidity and mortality tend anyway to be high when the operation is in an area of the brain which abounds with vital functions. Yet there is insufficient practical evidence that the end results of series of similar operations differ greatly, if at all, when performed in either position by competent surgeons. For this reason it is as well to be certain that the complications specific to a particular position do not mar the ultimate result, and to select a posture which suits not only the surgeon but also the patient.

## ANAESTHESIA

The basis of good anaesthesia for neurosurgery has been well summarised by Bozza Marrubini[18] as a perfect airway, adequate ventilation, low venous pressure, a slack brain, minimal bleeding, the absence of coughing or straining and a rapid return to consciousness. Intracranial work does not require deep anaesthesia, and indeed the greatest and most frequent stimulus of an entire operation is usually the presence of an endotracheal tube in the trachea. The diathermy is an essential and constant part of neurosurgical technique, so that inflammable anaesthetic agents must not be used. Some surgeons may take upwards of six hours for an operation which is performed by others in under two. To satisfy these several requirements special techniques have been developed, but the differences between them only illustrate the importance that one anaesthetist attaches to some particular aspect of the problem and stress the value of the personal touch. There are few, if any, drugs or techniques which do not in some way adversely affect intracranial or intraspinal mechanics. Such factors can be minimised by careful selection and attention to detail.

### Local or General

No single drug or combination of drugs can be considered ideal in the circumstances of neurosurgical anaesthesia. Apart from the skin, fascia, temporal muscle, periosteum and bone of the skull, and certain parts of the basal dura where it is attached to bone, cranial surgery is carried out in an area which is entirely insensitive to pain. The nerves to the skin and fascia also supply the periosteum and bone. They pass through the fascia beneath the skin on a line encircling the skull and drawn approximately from the occipital protuberance to the eyebrows.[19] Thus, local subcutaneous infiltration with a solution of 1 per cent lignocaine produces satisfactory analgesia for burr holes and minor operations. If the incision impinges on the temporal muscle then a deeper infiltration must be made. In terms of pain relief this form of local analgesia is also effective for major craniotomies, and has the advantage of having no adverse effects on intracranial mechanics. Why, then, general anaesthesia?

**Local Analgesia**

Local analgesia leaves much to be desired in terms of sedation and comfort for the patient, and does nothing to aid the surgeon should the patient be unco-operative or unable to keep perfectly still. Although the mental state of many patients with intracranial disease is confused, the majority are conscious enough to dislike the discomforts of major surgery under local analgesia. The position on the operating table and the need to remain in it, and in a motionless state, for perhaps several hours are effective deterrents. There is a good deal of mental stress associated in the minds of many patients with an operation on the brain, and surgical manipulations in this area, even though painless, evoke indirect sensations, particularly during bone work. Stimulation of brain substance sometimes produces spontaneous motor or sensory activities for the patient, and though these may be valuable under certain circumstances as a guide to the localisation of the surgeon's work, they are unpleasant if repetitive or gross. A patient who is difficult to control because of his disease, or more simply because he or she is unco-operative, cannot be adequately sedated with complete safety, and certainly not as effectively as with a good general anaesthetic. Finally, the duration of action of all known local analgesic drugs is insufficient to cover the length of time that some surgeons take to complete certain operations.

General anaesthesia supplies an answer to all these disadvantages of local analgesia, but it does so at some slight cost. The dangers and disadvantages of general anaesthesia in the hands of inexperienced administrators must be appreciated before criticising those clinics where local methods of analgesia still find favour. So far as the operation of laminectomy is concerned, local infiltration analgesia is far from satisfactory, and either a more complete form, such as an epidural or spinal, must be used, or general anaesthesia preferred.

**General Anaesthesia**

**The airway.**—An absolute prerequisite of neurosurgical anaesthesia is that an adequate airway must be assured at all times. A non-kinkable armoured tube or a tube of the Oxford pattern provide satisfactory airway control during neurosurgery. If an Oxford tube is used a hole should be cut in its anterior wall near to the bevel or the bevel itself cut off to avoid obstruction of the outlet of the tube by the posterior tracheal wall during acute neck flexion. A curved or right-angled wide-bore connector must be firmly fixed to any tube used. Because access to the face may be impossible once surgery has started, the tube and its connectors must be firmly mounted and well fixed into position. In some neurosurgical procedures, especially posterior fossa explorations in children, there is a real danger of accidental endobronchial intubation occurring when the neck is acutely flexed. Hunter[9] recommends marking on the tube the distance from the mouth to the suprasternal notch, and not introducing the tube further than this distance.

**Premedication.**—The potential dangers of drugs which cause respiratory depression in patients with raised intracranial pressure are well known. Opiates and their analogues must be prescribed cautiously, if at all. Even when there is no apparent contra-indication to using such drugs pre-operatively, it must be remembered that their action may persist into the postoperative period. They may reduce reflex activity and the level of consciousness postoperatively, whilst pupillary effects may make assessment of the state of the patient difficult. Pre-operative sedation is an important factor in the preparation of patients for most forms of surgery, but for intracranial surgery this benefit may have to be foregone. In the positive absence of any evidence of raised intracranial pressure, tranquillisers such as diazepam may be used. These drugs have little cardiovascular or respiratory effects, and their anticonvulsant properties may be useful.[20,21] An adequate dose of atropine should be given about one hour before operation.

**Induction.**—Induction of anaesthesia must not be associated with hypoxia or hypercapnia. Drugs used during induction should have little effect on intracranial pressure and should neither stimulate nor depress cardiovascular function. After an initial period of pre-oxygenation and spontaneous hyperventilation, anaesthesia is induced by a slow intravenous injection of thiopentone, followed immediately by a muscle relaxant. Suxamethonium is the most widely used relaxant for intubation. Whilst fasciculations produced by this drug may raise intracranial pressure, pretreatment with a small dose of non-depolarising relaxant before induction minimises this problem. An alternative approach is to use pancuronium in a dose of 0·12 mg/kg. Loss of consciousness must be followed by controlled hyperventilation with oxygen, and intubation should not be attempted until full muscular relaxation has been obtained. The rise in blood pressure that commonly occurs during tracheal intubation may be dangerous in neurosurgical patients. It can be reduced by giving propranolol (0·04 mg/kg) before induction,[22] or an additional bolus dose of thiopentone can be given immediately before intubation.[23] Nitrous oxide should not be given until hyperventilation has been instituted for a few minutes.

**Maintenance.**—The majority of neurosurgical procedures are carried out during controlled ventilation. Adequate ventilation is important during anaesthesia for all forms of surgery, and is essential during neurosurgery. Carbon dioxide retention can play havoc with a neurosurgeon's operating field, whilst increased expiratory resistance due to obstruction, coughing or straining is even more disastrous. Raised venous pressure will increase intracranial pressure, as will oxygen lack and carbon dioxide retention.

Moderate hyperventilation to a $Pco_2$ of about 30 mm Hg (4 kPa) is widely practised in neurosurgical anaesthesia. This level of hyperventilation will usually assure adequate oxygenation, and result in a "slack" brain due to a reduced cerebral blood flow and intracranial pressure. Nitrous oxide/oxygen anaesthesia can be supplemented with intravenous narcotic drugs such as fentanyl. Small amounts of halothane (0·5 per cent) can be added if needed to prevent unwanted rises in blood pressure. The dangerous effects of inhalational anaesthetic agents on intracranial pressure are not evident if their use is preceded by the institution of hyperventilation.[24] Deep levels of anaesthesia are not necessary during neurosurgery, but inadequate depth of anaesthesia can result in rises in cerebral blood flow and intracranial pressure. Muscular relaxation can be provided by pancuronium or alcuronium. Tubocurarine is best avoided as there is some evidence that this drug may increase intracranial pressure.[25]

At one time all patients undergoing neurosurgery were allowed to breathe spontaneously. In many centres spontaneous ventilation is still used for patients undergoing posterior fossa surgery in the sitting position. A normal pattern of spontaneous breathing provides good evidence of the integrity of vital centres, and changes in the character of ventilation may warn of impending surgical danger. Many authorities believe that equally good indications of surgical invasion of the vital centres can be obtained by monitoring the circulation during controlled ventilation.[9] Campkin[26] has surveyed currently used methods of anaesthesia for infratentorial surgery in 37 neurosurgical units in the United Kingdom. Some 53 per cent of these institutions used the sitting position for posterior fossa surgery and just under half of these patients were allowed to breathe spontaneously.

### Reduction of Intracranial Pressure

The prevention of a rise in intracranial pressure (ICP) is a cardinal rule in safe neurosurgical anaesthesia. In this context controlled ventilation to a $Pco_2$ of about 30 mm Hg (4 kPa), the avoidance of venous congestion, and cautious use of volatile anaesthetic agents are all of importance. Occasionally intracranial pressure may rise to a dangerous level in spite of all precautions. Such rises may be due to the presence of a space-occupying lesion, or be related to brain oedema caused by severe hypoxia or trauma. In some patients ICP may be at a level which warrants its reduction before induction of anaesthesia. Reduction of ICP may be achieved by employing one or more of the following methods.

**Removal of CSF.**—The simplest method of removing CSF is by lumbar puncture followed, if necessary, by continuous drainage through a malleable needle.[27] The danger of this method is that it may precipitate medullary coning, especially if the raised ICP is not associated with a communicating hydrocephalus. Drainage by the lumbar route should be limited to a rate of less than 5 ml/min. Removal of large volumes of CSF by this route may produce arterial hypertension and cardiac dysrhythmias, and can be followed by a rebound increase in ICP.[28,29] CSF drainage is more safely performed by ventriculostomy, the ventricles being tapped either pre-operatively through burr holes, or at craniotomy.

**Hyperosmolar agents.**—Increases of plasma osmolality will cause a transfer of fluid from the brain to plasma. Many substances have been used in the past, including 50 per cent sucrose and fructose, hypertonic dextran and double- or quadruple-strength plasma. None of these agents was markedly efficient in shrinking a swollen brain.

*Urea.*—As a 30 per cent solution lyophilised in 10 per cent invert sugar was shown by Javid & Settlage[30] to have a useful dehydrating effect on the brain when given in doses of 1–1·5 g/kg body weight. Urea is a potent osmotic diuretic and has a more prolonged action than that of substances which merely increase plasma osmolality. Urea is contra-indicated in the presence of impaired renal function, and is a profound local irritant. Its major disadvantage is that it may cause a rebound rise in brain tension, due to a late diffusion of urea into brain substance, and a rise in brain osmolality.[31]

*Mannitol* has replaced urea for the purposes of cerebral dehydration. It also increases plasma osmolality to withdraw fluid from the brain, and acts as a potent diuretic. Rebound rises of ICP can occur but are less marked with mannitol than with urea and mannitol is much less irritant to tissues than urea. Mannitol is the drug of choice for the rapid reduction of ICP. It is used as a 20 or 25 per cent solution in doses of 0·5–1·5 g/kg body weight, and is given over 10–20 minutes. Its effects on ICP last for several hours.

*Glycerol* is a further useful agent for brain dehydration. It is given orally or intravenously as a 10 per cent solution in doses of 0·5–1 g/kg body weight. Rebound increases in ICP are rarer with glycerol than with mannitol, though such rebound can still occur.[32] Higher concentrations than this can cause haemolysis.[33] Glycerol is less widely used than mannitol for the urgent reduction of ICP, but has some advantages if long-term cerebral dehydration is required. As well as a lower incidence of rebound, glycerol has less diuretic effect and therefore is less likely to produce electrolyte derangements. As glycerol is metabolised it has some nutritional value and can be used (with caution) in the presence of reduced or absent renal function.

Osmotic dehydrating agents, as well as actively withdrawing fluid from the brain, reduce ICP by reducing the rate of CSF formation.[34] Large bolus doses of these agents can produce marked brain shrinkage and tearing of cortical veins and dural sinuses.[35] These agents, by increasing plasma volume and possibly by reducing blood viscosity, increase cerebral blood flow and may transiently increase ICP. If a raised ICP is due to a subdural or epidural haematoma, rapid reduction in ICP will remove the splinting effect of this raised pressure and may lead to further expansion of the haematoma.

**Systemic diuretics.**—Diuretics such as frusemide and ethacrynic acid have been widely employed for the reduction of ICP.[36,37] The reduction in ICP is produced partly by diuresis *per se*, and partly by a reduction in the rate of CSF formation. These agents have also been shown to reduce cerebral oedema by a direct effect.[38] Whilst the effects of diuretics on ICP are not as dramatic as those of mannitol, these drugs may occasionally have advantages over hyperosmolar agents when the increase in cerebral flow or increased plasma osmolality that these latter agents produce is thought to be undesirable.

**Steroids.**—Steroids, especially dexamethasone, are widely used to treat brain oedema associated with intracranial neoplasms. ICP falls due to a reduction in tumour bulk, and not due to any effect on CSF mechanics.

**Barbiturates.**—Bolus doses of thiopentone lower ICP by reducing cerebral blood flow. Long-term barbiturate therapy has been widely used for the control of intracranial hypertension due to head injury. Because of prolonged unconsciousness produced by large doses of barbiturates the use of these drugs to control ICP during neurosurgery is limited.

## Controlled Hypotension

There are few branches of surgery in which so strong a case can be made for induced hypotension, and in which the risks of the ancillary technique can be set against the advantages. At the outset, however, it is important to remember that most intracranial and spinal operations can be performed satisfactorily without it, provided due attention is paid to the essentials of good anaesthesia and posture. However, the presence of a tumour may cause congestion during surgery so that induced hypotension, by reducing swelling, may lessen the risks of some operations on the brain. Increased meningeal vascularity may lead to major haemorrhage during craniotomy which cannot be controlled until the skull is opened. Hypotension may reduce such blood loss to manageable levels. Minimal arterial bleeding with no venous ooze materially assists the surgeon to delineate the limits of the disease process and thus to remove it with less risk of damage to normal tissue. Control of haemorrhage may make possible operations which could not otherwise be attempted.[39] A raised intracranial pressure makes exposure at the operation site difficult, since the distended brain tends to bulge out when the dura is opened, and aggravates venous bleeding. A distended brain also necessitates considerable retraction which in turn leads to bruising of tissue. A marked reduction in arterial pressure will help to control these factors.

There are two situations in which hypotension during intracranial surgery may be particularly indicated. During the removal of vascular tumours such as meningiomata, reduction of systolic pressure to levels of 60–70 mm Hg (8·0–9·3 kPa) can be of great use. A more profound hypotension may be necessary during the control of aneurysms or angiomata to reduce the risk of vessel rupture. Hypotension during the removal of vascular tumours may have to be maintained for several hours. An adequate reduction of bleeding may be obtained by moderate hyperventilation and the use of low concentrations of halothane. Greater control of blood pressure can be obtained by the use of trimetaphan. This and other ganglion-blocking agents can produce a postoperative cycloplegia of several hours duration which may complicate neurological assessment. Hypotension necessary during aneurysmal surgery is best obtained by sodium nitroprusside[40] or nitroglycerin.[41]

The dangers of induced hypotension are well-recognised (see Chapter 12) and there are some problems associated with this technique of specific relevance to neurosurgical anaesthesia. Aserman[42] has described how hypotension produces a dough-like consistency of brain tissue, when it is easily compressed, slow to regain its normal conformity and equally slowly replenished with blood. In these circumstances pressure from a brain retractor may lead to "retractor anaemia." Aserman's advice that induced hypotension should only be used for those operations in which retraction is made on brain substance that is ultimately to be excised is however far too sweeping. If measures to keep brain bulk to a minimum are employed (which may necessitate ventricular tap) only minimum retraction is needed to expose even deep-seated lesions. A more important problem than retractor anaemia is the possibility of brain damage due to a low blood pressure. Abnormalities of the blood-brain barrier have been demonstrated after lowering mean arterial pressure of experimental animals to 30 mm Hg (4 kPa).[43] The loss of autoregulation which occurs at low arterial pressures may persist for some time after restoration of perfusing pressure. The cerebral circulation may be more vulnerable to the effects of hypotension during neurosurgery. With an open skull the siphon effect of the cerebral venous drainage in potentiating cerebral perfusion is lost.[9]

Trimetaphan camsylate, used as a 0·2 per cent solution, produces hypotension by ganglion blockade and possibly by histamine release and direct vasodilatation. At low levels of blood pressure trimetaphan may have direct cerebral toxic effects.[44] Tachyphylaxis is common during trimetaphan administration. Unlike more recently introduced hypotensive agents, trimetaphan does not increase intracranial pressure. Sodium nitroprusside is probably the most commonly used agent for controlled hypotension during neurosurgery. This agent directly dilates resistance vessels. Sodium nitroprusside is usually given as a 0·01 per cent solution in dextrose, and the solution must be protected from light. This drug allows rapid and precise control of blood pressure. As it increases cerebral blood flow its administration may result in a rise in ICP. *To prevent this danger the drug should not be administered until the dura has been opened*. Overdose with nitroprusside will result in cyanide toxicity. The dose should be limited to 1·5 mg/kg over 3 hours. Many methods of treating this cyanide toxicity have been suggested. Krapez and his colleagues[45] have recommended sodium thiosulphate (75 mg/kg) as an effective and safe antidote.

Nitroglycerin produces hypotension by an action on capacitance vessels. It is used as a 0·01 per cent solution, and in clinical practice its effects closely resemble those of nitroprusside. There are no toxic metabolic products of nitroglycerin. As with nitroprusside, this agent will increase cerebral blood flow, and can increase ICP.

## Hypothermia

Hypothermia leads to a fall in cerebral blood flow and cerebrospinal fluid pressure, and to a reduction in brain volume.[46, 47] Access to various parts of the brain is improved, and the surgeon can temporarily occlude a major end-artery. At rectal temperatures of about 30° C Burrows and his colleagues[48] have been able to clamp the middle cerebral artery for from 4½ to 12¾ minutes without evidence of permanent cerebral damage. The induction of hypothermia will lead to some fall in systemic blood pressure, but not necessarily to very much. The reduction in metabolism that the fall in temperature causes will, however, offer some protection against the potential dangers of induced hypotension. Hypothermia can also reduce or prevent cerebral oedema, which in some neurosurgical procedures is the ultimate factor leading to death. Induced hypothermia with surface cooling enjoyed considerable popularity during aneurysm surgery at a time when the usual surgical approach was temporarily to clip vessels feeding the aneurysm during approach to the sac, and the value of the technique in reducing problems of cerebral ischaemia was, under these circumstances, well proven. The current practice of a direct approach on the sac using an operating microscope, with an anaesthetic technique employing hypotension to a level sufficient to make the aneurysm lax, has effectively led to the abandonment of induced hypothermia during this form of neurosurgery. Even in 1971 McDowall,[49] in a survey of a large number of neurosurgical centres, found there was a general tendency to reduce the number of indications for the use of hypothermia.

Although hypothermia to about 30° C has been effectively abandoned in neurosurgical practice, Berntman and his colleagues[50] have shown that in rats a moderate level of hypothermia (34–35° C) gave good protection against the effects of global cerebral ischaemia. Such moderate hypothermia may have a place to play in the management of patients with severe head injuries.

## Monitoring During Neurosurgery

Neurosurgical procedures may be prolonged and are occasionally associated with considerable blood loss. Surgical manipulation of vital centres may endanger the patient's life; careful monitoring of cardiac and respiratory function is essential during these procedures.

*Cardiovascular system.*—An electrocardiogram is essential. Blood pressure may be monitored by indirect methods such as oscillotonometry, but the majority of neurosurgical anaesthetists insert an intra-arterial cannula for all but the briefest and most trivial of neurosurgical procedures. A radial or dorsalis pedis line also allows for intermittent sampling and blood gas estimation. An oesophageal stethoscope is useful. A central venous line should be inserted, especially for operations in the sitting position and in some institutions a pulmonary artery line is routinely inserted during neurosurgery. An ultrasonic transducer placed over the precordium will record any entry of air into the circulation.

*Respiratory system.*—Minute and tidal volume should be recorded. The character of the respiratory pattern is an important indicator of unimpaired medullary function in spontaneously breathing subjects during posterior-fossa surgery. Measurement of tidal carbon dioxide is a good indicator of the efficiency of ventilation, and will indicate the occurrence of venous air embolism.

*Other measurements.*—Oesophageal or rectal temperature should be measured and is especially important in children. Intracranial pressure monitoring is especially valuable in head-injured patients undergoing surgery.

## Posterior Fossa Surgery

Exploration of the posterior fossa is carried out for resection of space-occupying lesions and for aneurysm surgery. The commonest tumour found in this region is the acoustic neuroma.

Although benign in nature, the close proximity of this tumour to many cranial nerves and to the vital centres of the brain results in operative removal having a high morbidity and mortality.

As has been discussed above, posterior fossa surgery is often performed with the spontaneously breathing subject placed in the sitting position, with the attendant dangers of postural hypotension and air embolus. Surgical interference with the vital centres will produce changes in the arterial pressure, electrocardiogram and (in spontaneously breathing subjects) the respiratory pattern.

The specific postoperative complications of posterior fossa surgery relate almost entirely to brain-stem and cranial-nerve damage. Tenth-nerve damage may result in impaired swallowing and aspiration. Fifth, seventh and eighth nerve damage following surgery in the cerebellopontine angle may cause loss of the corneal reflex and lid closing, abnormal eye movements and hearing deficits. The most serious problems arise from oedema, haematoma or infarction of the brain stem and cerebellum. Patients suffering such damage will become unresponsive, with systemic hypertension, bradycardia and irregular respiration or apnoea. Such patients require urgent re-exploration to relieve pressure on the brain stem.

Systemic hypertension is common in the first postoperative day following posterior fossa surgery. Marked hypertension should be treated with nitroglycerin or nitroprusside because of the dangers of haematoma formation.

### Subarachnoid Haemorrhage

Three-quarters of all subarachnoid haemorrhages are due to rupture of an aneurysm of a large vessel in the floor of the cranium. Less frequently subarachnoid haemorrhage is due to intracranial angiomata or spreading haemorrhage from a burst atheromatous vessel in the brain. The distribution and incidence of the major groups of intracranial aneurysms is illustrated in Fig. 2.

Subarachnoid haemorrhage carries a high mortality. Repeat haemorrhage is common within 6 weeks of the original incident. Early surgery carries a high risk. Ruptured aneurysm is associated with a raised ICP which in part tamponades the bleeding vessel.[29] Re-bleeding may occur if ICP is lowered towards normal. Initial cerebral ischaemia in these patients is often followed by intense cerebral vasoconstriction. Pre-operatively, these patients are usually treated with epsilon-aminocaproic acid at a dose of 30–36 g/day in order to retard fibrinolysis.

At one time aneurysm surgery was commonly performed under hypothermia. Most neurosurgeons now prefer to carry out a careful dissection of the sac using an operating microscope, and induced hypotension is commonly employed in the normothermic patient. Mean systemic pressure should be reduced gradually to 50 mm Hg, when the sac will become lax and the danger of rupture during manipulation will be greatly reduced.

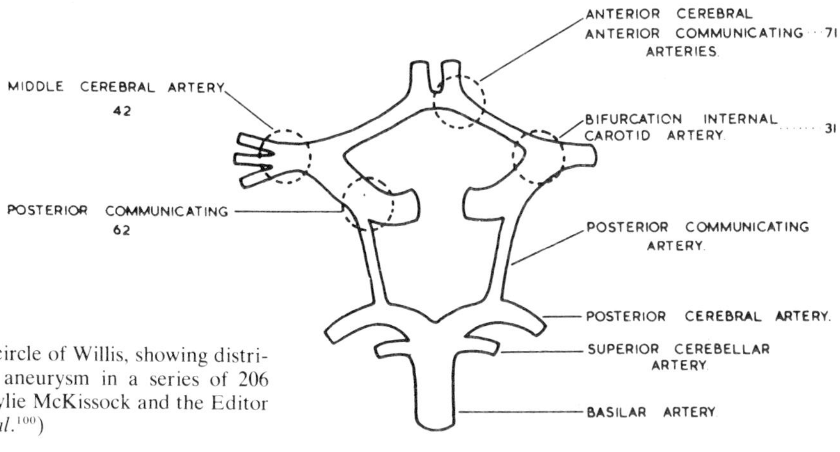


28/Fig. 2.—Diagram of the circle of Willis, showing distribution of major groups of aneurysm in a series of 206 patients. (Courtesy of Sir Wylie McKissock and the Editor of the *British Medical Journal*.[100])

### Stereotactic Operations

Localised lesions can be produced in the depths of the brain by thermocoagulation or by freezing with liquid nitrogen. Stereotaxis is the method by which the region to be treated is determined and localised. The technique is commonly used for making lesions of the globus pallidus in patients suffering from Parkinsonism. It is also valuable for the treatment of intractable pain and has recently been used for frontal leucotomy. Local analgesia will suffice but it is not always pleasant for the patient. When general anaesthesia is used it must be so chosen that at certain times during the operative procedure the patient will regain consciousness and co-operate fully with the surgeon. This is particularly important during the stage of stimulation when the area of the brain to be treated is being localised, and while the lesion is being made. Coleman and De Villiers[51] describe a technique for anaesthesia consisting simply of the continuous intravenous infusion of a 0·1 per cent solution of methohexitone. When tremor or abnormal movements are severe they also use small paretic doses of gallamine triethiodide to induce some reduction in muscle power. No premedication is used, and all sedative drugs are stopped for 24 hours before the operation. By stopping or slowing the drip it is possible to effect a rapid return of full consciousness, or, in an unduly apprehensive subject, produce a co-operative but sedated patient. An alternative technique is to make use of neuroleptanalgesia which provides sedation and suppression of mental and physical discomfort, but leaves the patient co-operative.[52] Because controlled lesions are best produced in the presence of tremor an alternative approach is to define the area to be treated under general anaesthesia, but delay the production of lesions until a later occasion and do this in a fully conscious patient.

### Cordotomy (Tractotomy) and Rhizotomy

Cordotomy is a gross but effective method of treating severe pain on either or both sides of the body. It is usually performed for those patients in whom neoplastic disease is the cause of the pain and in whom a reasonable expectation of life seems likely. A successful result enables more general treatment, such as that by opiates, to be stopped, or at least diminished. It is worth noting that patients who have been treated by large doses of opiates prior to a successful cordotomy do not always crave for these drugs when they are stopped. The therapy of genuine pain by large doses of opiates does not apparently invariably lead to addiction.

Cordotomy is always done at the cervical level so that the sense of touch is undisturbed, and a bilateral cut is rarely performed at the same operation, in order to avoid sphincter disturbances. If a bilateral cordotomy is needed then an interval of 6–8 weeks is usually allowed between the two. The approach is as for a laminectomy and the actual cord division is gross enough to be performed under general anaesthesia, although a more accurate assessment of the extent of section can be made if the patient is awake and co-operative. Simple infiltration is a not very successful method of ensuring good pain relief for laminectomy, though it can be used in combination with light enough anaesthesia to ensure sufficient return of consciousness at the crucial time. Segmental epidural analgesia will provide complete analgesia in the operation site without disturbing the area of pain and thus allowing adequate testing during the operation.[53]

Percutaneous electrical cordotomy is the coagulation of pain fibres in the anterior quadrant of the spinal cord by an electrode inserted through the second cervical intervertebral foramen. Originally described by Mullan and his colleagues[54] the technique has been popularised by Lipton.[55] As the active co-operation of the patient is essential, general anaesthesia is contra-indicated. Mehta[56] has suggested the use of phenoperidine and droperidol for this procedure.

Rhizotomy, or root section, is a precise method of treating pain which can be localised. With the exception of the cranial nerves, it is usual also to cut the nerve roots above and below the one supplying the affected segment, since there is an overlap in the sensory supply from the spinal nerves.

## NEUROSURGERY IN CHILDREN

Infants and small children may require neurosurgery for a variety of reasons, the commonest of which is probably the relief of congenital hydrocephalus. The other common reasons for paediatric neurosurgery are tumours such as astrocytomata and haemangioblastomata, and following severe head injury. Children with advanced intracranial tumours or head injuries may be in a critical state when they present for surgery, with a dangerously raised intracranial pressure. Management of these patients requires attention to all the basic demands of neurosurgical anaesthesia plus the problems particular to small and sick children. In general, best results are attained by anaesthesia with controlled ventilation. Premedication should consist of atropine 0·02 mg/kg, with a minimum dose of 0·2 mg. Anaesthesia is best induced with intravenous thiopentone. If no suitable vein can be found an inhalation induction may be needed. As soon as consciousness is lost an intravenous line is established. Suxamethonium (1 mg/kg) is used before intubation, and may be preceded by a small dose of thiopentone to limit any rise in intracranial tension that may result from intubation. Anaesthesia is continued after intubation with nitrous oxide and oxygen, tubocurarine (0·4 mg/kg) and controlled ventilation. Volatile anaesthetics are best avoided if intracranial tension is raised. Nitrous oxide can be supplemented with fentanyl in doses of up to 3 μg/kg. A minute volume in the order of 150 ml/kg/minute will usually produce a $Pco_2$ of 30–35 mm Hg (4–4·7 kPa). Severe brain-swelling during craniotomy may require mannitol (0·5–1 g/kg) for its control. At the end of the operation atropine (0·02 mg/kg) and neostigmine (0·05 mg/kg) are given to reverse the relaxant. During surgery monitoring of the cardiovascular and respiratory systems and of body temperature are important. A precordial or oesophageal stethoscope should be positioned before surgery commences, as should ECG leads. Accurate blood-pressure monitoring may require intra-arterial pressure measurements. A thermocouple or thermistor lead should be inserted in the oesophagus. Monitoring of tidal carbon dioxide concentration with a suitable infra-red analyser gives information on both respiration and cardiovascular function. Blood loss must be meticulously replaced as it occurs during surgery.

Anaesthetised infants are specially prone to hypothermia during surgery. A water blanket kept at 37° C or wrapping the infant in kitchen foil are useful methods to limit heat loss. Baum and Scopes[57] have described a polyester sheet, laminated on both surfaces with aluminium, as an effective "swaddler" during major paediatric surgery.

## POSTOPERATIVE CARE OF THE NEUROSURGICAL PATIENT

The immediate postoperative period is of considerable importance in neurosurgical practice. After cranial operations it may be difficult to distinguish between the effects of surgery and of anaesthesia—both may make common ground in the production of unconsciouness. In this respect anaesthesia can only be considered perfect when it ceases as soon as the surgeon completes the operation, for then the level of consciousness and the state of reflex activity are true guides to the condition of the patient. Unfortunately neither anaesthesia nor surgery is invariably perfect, and their combined or individual effects sometimes create problems which make the immediate postoperative period of considerable importance.

The sensitive intracranial mechanisms, already disturbed by the surgical procedure, may easily become unbalanced by apparently trivial complications of anaesthesia, and it is no exaggeration to suggest that a brief anoxic episode or a momentary rise in the level of carbon dioxide in the blood might even affect the patient's chance of survival. Either accentuates the element of cerebral oedema that follows all cerebral surgery. Oxygen should be given at this time for the first few hours and if there is any doubt about the adequacy of ventilation the endotracheal tube should be left in place and mechanical ventilation continued. Even successful surgery—successful that is, by the standard of removing a tumour completely—may be followed by nerve palsies, or more bizarre complications such as vasomotor collapse, hyperpyrexia, and respiratory disorders, all of which cause exceptional difficulties.

Thus the normal hazards of the postanaesthetic period and the special requirements of the neurosurgical patient are a strong indication for the provision of recovery room space next to the operating theatre, so that both anaesthetist and surgeon can be within sight and sound of the patient at this potentially critical time.

### Recovery from Neurosurgical Anaesthesia

It has been traditional that at the end of a neurosurgical procedure the patient should be awake and breathing spontaneously, so that the integrity of the nervous system can be tested. Difficulties can occur in attaining a smooth transition from anaesthesia to the awake state. Acute rises in intracranial pressure due to coughing or straining are as dangerous at the end of an operation as during the procedure. Secretions should be sucked out before any neuromuscular blockade is reversed and naloxone should be given to antagonise any narcotics that have been administered. Following major procedures when a possibility of brain-stem or cranial-nerve damage exists, where oedema may be expected, or when autoregulation may be impaired, it is much safer to continue to hyperventilate the patient in the postoperative period.

Seizure activity in the postoperative period must be rapidly brought under control, as the increase in systemic pressure and local increase in metabolic rate may lead to breakdown of the blood-brain barrier, and permanent neuronal damage. Diazepam (0·05–0·2 mg/kg), phenobarbitone (1–3 mg/kg), thiopentone (1–2 mg/kg) or phenytoin (10–20 mg/kg), all given intravenously and cautiously repeated when necessary, are effective drugs for seizure control.

## Routine Postoperative Care

The institution of continuous and skilled nursing care after surgery plays a vital part in the reduction of overall morbidity for many cranial operations. This is particularly so when cranial-nerve palsies are present, since the dangers associated with partial respiratory obstruction and tracheal aspiration are very real. All patients who have undergone major intracranial surgery are best treated postoperatively in a specialised neurological intensive care unit.

### Observation

The nurse must observe and record all essential clinical data at regular intervals—every ten minutes for the first hour or so. Pulse and respiration rates, blood pressure level, the level of consciousness, response to stimuli, fluid intake, drugs given and any other points likely to be of value must be written down. These observations are of paramount importance in assessing the progress of intracranial complications, while differentiation of the effects of anaesthesia from those of surgery is possible only if a record is available to show the general trend of events. Thus the earliest signs of reactionary haemorrhage may be the onset of sleep in a previously sleepy but conscious patient, or a rise in blood pressure in a semiconscious one.

### Posture

As soon as consciousness is regained, and provided the systolic blood pressure is over 100 mm Hg (13·3 kPa), patients who have had uncomplicated cranial operations should be brought to a sitting position. Even before this, if the danger of vomiting can be circumvented or appears unlikely—patients can be reflexly normal but cerebrally unconscious—it may be advisable to have the head raised on pillows. The prime object of posture at this early stage is to reduce the twin risks of cerebral oedema and reactionary haemorrhage. However, in the exceptional case it may be wiser to wait several hours before sitting the patient up at all. Occasions of this type occur after removal of a large tumour from the posterior fossa, when the adjacent compressed tissues cannot be expected to fill up the resulting hole straight away. In these circumstances a sudden change in posture could lead to marked movement of the brain stem, due to inadequate compensation for the change in blood pressure, and consequent disturbance of function.

Patients who have had a laminectomy are nursed flat for several days.

At a later stage in the postoperative period posture must also be adjusted to encourage lung drainage, and reduce incidence of ischaemic sores, particularly for those patients who remain semiconscious or suffer from respiratory dysfunctions.

Changes in posture are facilitated by nursing all neurosurgical patients in special beds designed to tilt or rise in various ways with minimal inconvenience to the patient or nursing staff.

### Sedation and Analgesia

Patients who have had cranial operations do not usually suffer from acute pain as a result of surgery. They are often restless and occasionally nauseated, particularly after operations in the posterior fossa, but rarely uncomfortable except from headache. The reason for this presumably lies in the insensitiveness of the structures involved, the skin being a notable exception, and the fact that movement of the patient is not, as in most other operative sites, reflected in increased tension in the wound. Laminectomy wounds, however, are very painful and usually require full doses of a potent analgesic such as an opiate or analogue. These agents are never necessary after cranial surgery, and indeed their potency, accentuated by the lack of acute pain, coupled with their well-known side-effects—particularly respiratory depression and pupillary contraction—contra-indicate their use.

The restlessness and headache can be adequately controlled by codeine phosphate in a dosage of from 32 to 65 mg, combined if necessary with phenobarbitone 100 to 200 mg and given intramuscularly. The effectiveness of codeine as an analgesic is open to doubt, but as a mild sedative without marked side-effects it is useful in these circumstances. Occasionally patients may be so seriously disturbed by the surgery as to become vociferous and in need of restraint. For these, paraldehyde intramuscularly (2–3 ml) is very effective.

**Intravenous Fluids**

There is still no general agreement about the exact distribution of water between the cells and the extracellular fluid in the brain. It is, however, agreed that cerebral oedema, unlike oedema in its more usual manifestations, is due to intracellular accumulation of water particularly in the white matter.[58] Equilibration of water between blood and brain is very rapid and occurs within a few minutes,[59] and it is extremely important not to overhydrate neurosurgical patients in the immediate postoperative period. Aqueous dextrose solutions should be avoided. Lactated Ringer's solution, with or without 5 per cent dextrose, may be used for maintenance fluid therapy.

Many patients are able to take fluids by mouth in a matter of hours and if the intravenous infusion has been left running it is very easy to give them more fluid than is desirable. It is wise to restrict the total fluid intake by all routes to 1½–2 litres on the day of operation and on the following day. Temporary diabetes insipidus is not uncommon after operations near the hypothalamus, and if a catheter has been passed can be recognised during operation by a sudden increase in urine volume—usually to between 7 and 12 ml/minute. In such cases dextrose/saline (4·3 per cent dextrose in 0·18 per cent saline) should be given 3-hourly in amounts equivalent to the previous 3-hourly urine volume if the patient is unable to drink. Treatment of diabetes insipidus with vasopressin (5–10 international units IM) may be necessary.

**Cerebral Oedema**

Apart from posture, the most effective method of reducing raised intracranial pressure is intravenous mannitol. Its use at induction is described on page 772. When used postoperatively, 500 ml of 10 per cent mannitol is given in the course of an hour and repeated 12-hourly. During this time the total fluid intake (including the volume of the mannitol solution) is restricted to 2 litres in 24 hours. Such a regime cannot usually be continued safely for more than 48 hours as it will cause progressive depletion of body water. This is indicated by a rise in serum sodium concentration which should not be allowed to exceed 155–160 mmol/l. Uncontrollable postoperative cerebral oedema may necessitate surgical decompression.

**Reactionary Haemorrhage**

Bleeding into the operation site leads to a rise in intracranial pressure which will be manifested by the signs already described, but specific localising signs, such as nerve palsies, which can be accounted for by the pressure of the accumulating blood clot, may also be present.

Treatment is essentially operative to remove the blood and stop the bleeding. Anaesthesia is often not required but an endotracheal tube should be passed, with the aid of a relaxant, and adequate ventilation ensured. Once the compression has been relieved, however, anaesthesia will be needed, since consciousness often rapidly returns.

Particular note must be taken of the quantity of blood lost when a craniotomy wound is reopened, and immediate replacement made should it appear necessary. Despite the constricted space in which the bleeding takes place, a surprisingly large quantity of blood can be lost while re-opening the wound, since such an emergency allows no time for meticulous haemostasis until after the clot has been evacuated. Circulatory collapse during reactionary haemorrhage or while re-opening is in part due to central factors, but undoubtedly owes something to blood loss. This simple fact must not be forgotten.

### Special Postoperative Care

Operations in the posterior fossa, particularly those for total extirpation of an acoustic neuroma, may be followed by cranial nerve palsies. Following removal of an acoustic tumour, a seventh-nerve palsy is not uncommon, but more dangerous in the immediate postoperative period are palsies of the glossopharyngeal and vagus nerves. These may be only temporary and incomplete, but while present, swallowing lacks co-ordination, and with laryngeal and glottic sensitivity diminished, normal feeding may lead to aspiration into the respiratory tract. For this reason it is a good plan to have a plastic tube of 4 to 6 mm diameter passed through the nose into the stomach before the operation is started. During the postoperative period all feeds should be given down this tube and great care taken to avoid vomiting or regurgitation, either of which may lead to aspiration. A suction apparatus should be next to the bed at all times. After 48 hours, a small quantity of water should be given to the patient by mouth to test whether swallowing is normal; if it is, the tube should be removed. When there is any likelihood of fifth-nerve damage, a tarsorrhaphy should be performed to protect the affected eye.

Patients who remain unconscious or semi-conscious for more than an hour or so after operation should be treated generally in a similar manner, and when they seem likely to remain in such a condition for several days—yet with a prospect of ultimate recovery—endotracheal intubation or a temporary tracheostomy must be considered. Certain complications—pulmonary aspiration lesions or inadequate ventilation—may be considered as indications for intubation or tracheostomy, but unconsciousness alone is not, provided competent nursing staff is available.

When gross aspiration of stomach contents into the lungs occurs during a bout of vomiting or regurgitation—a rare complication with adequate supervision and posturing—immediate bronchoscopy with lavage offers a reasonable prospect of removing the material and preventing infection. There are rarely, if ever, any other indications for bronchoscopy in the postoperative treatment of neurosurgical patients, or even for suction through an endotracheal tube. Simple pulmonary complications are best treated by posture and encouragement of normal drainage. If these fail, and the essential cause–such as unconsciousness or semi-consciousness—persists, then a tracheostomy enables efficient suction to be carried out simply and at regular intervals.

#### Respiratory Failure

This may be the terminal result of a rising intracranial pressure—in which case the essential treatment is that of the cause—of surgical interference, or of the direct effect of the disease process.

Operations on the cervical cord may be attended by bilateral phrenic paralysis, and although intercostal activity may be complete it is unlikely to be sufficient to maintain adequate ventilation, particularly during the immediate postoperative period. In cases of this type assisted or controlled respiration, preferably by a mechanical respirator, should be carried out, and a tracheostomy considered.

#### Vasomotor Failure

Hypotension is more often central than peripheral in origin. A peculiar type of circulatory collapse, characterised by a low blood pressure, with a slow pulse and dilated peripheral vessels, sometimes occurs after operations in the region of the fourth ventricle. The degree of hypotension is often sufficient to cause unconsciousness. Repeated intramuscular or intravenous doses of methoxamine, 5–10 mg, may be successful in restoring the blood pressure to normal, but more often than not the initial cause is incurable and the condition fatal.

#### Hyperpyrexia

So often in cranial surgery the postoperative complications are indicative of irreversible lesions in the brain itself, so that treatment, however effective in controlling the measurable signs or symptoms, only very rarely cures the cause. This is particularly true of severe hyperpyrexia, which is more often than not due to thrombosis in the region of the brain stem or thalamus. For such cases the production of hypothermia or the use of drugs such as chlorpromazine is unlikely to be successful—a more simple procedure, such as tepid sponging, is usually just as effective. If, however, the hyperpyrexia is likely to be due to cerebral oedema, then the more active measures may be found helpful.

### Pulmonary Oedema

Certain operations in the region of the midbrain, typically for tumours in the floor of the fourth ventricle, may be followed by pulmonary oedema. A rapid reduction in the circulating blood volume can be achieved with the use of diuretics (see Chapter 13). Intubation followed by positive-pressure respiration with a mechanical ventilator should be commenced if diuretics alone do not quickly control the situation.

## CAROTID ARTERY SURGERY

Carotid endarterectomy is frequently performed in subjects suffering from transient cerebral ischaemia due to carotid artery obstruction. The major problems arising during this procedure relate to the necessity of clamping the common, internal and external carotid arteries during removal of the atheromatous plaque and during arterial reconstruction. An additional problem lies in the fact that patients undergoing this procedure are usually elderly, hypertensive and suffering from generalised degenerative arterial disease. Whilst in normal subjects carotid flow may be unchanged by a 90 per cent reduction in the lumen of the artery, and in animals total occlusion of one carotid artery may only cause a 14 per cent decrease in pressure in the ipsilateral middle cerebral artery,[60] this maintenance of cerebral circulation depends upon collateral flow through the circle of Willis, and the common occurrence of abnormalities at this site makes it impossible to predict how an individual patient will tolerate carotid occlusion.

Many methods have been used to limit the dangers of cerebral ischaemia during carotid endarterectomy. These include the use of arterial bypass shunts, control of $Pco_2$, control of blood pressure, use of deep anaesthesia, heparinisation, hypothermia and hyperbaric oxygen.

**Bypass shunts.**—The use of a shunt between the common carotid artery and the distal internal carotid artery was described in 1972.[61,62] Although some surgeons claim that insertion of a shunt may cause internal damage and that its presence impedes the operator, the use of a bypass shunt during carotid artery surgery has become routine in most units.

**Control of $Pco_2$.**—Hypercapnia increases cerebral blood flow, and the use of deliberate hypercapnia (usually associated with induced hypertension) has been advocated during carotid artery surgery. Whilst any measure that increases cerebral blood flow would seem to be useful during such a procedure, there are objections to the use of hypercapnia. If hypercapnia affects cerebrovascular resistance on the side of the patent artery alone, an intracerebral "steal" can exist, decreasing perfusion on the side of the occlusion. Internal carotid artery occlusion pressure (the pressure in the cephalic portion of the internal carotid artery after clamping) has been shown to be lower during hypercapnia than during normo- or hypocapnia.[63] For these reasons, in most centres the use of hypercapnia is now avoided. Conversely, Michenfelder and Sundt[64] have shown in animal studies that hypocapnia could have an equally detrimental effect on cerebral metabolism. It would seem wise in patients undergoing this procedure to maintain $Pco_2$ close to the patient's normal resting level.

**Arterial blood pressure.**—In patients undergoing carotid endarterectomy, the brain may contain damaged areas in which circulatory autoregulation was already impaired. During surgery and occlusion, on theoretical grounds, deliberate hypertension may be of advantage, as normal parts of the brain would autoregulate blood flow whilst increased systemic pressure would benefit perfusion to those areas where occlusion had reduced local perfusion pressure below the autoregulatory limits. Some authorities[65] have recommended the use of systemic vasopressors to maintain a systolic pressure above 175 mm Hg (23·3 kPa). However, Fitch[66] has pointed out that deliberate hypertension will only influence compromised cerebral blood flow if a good collateral circulation exists, and where this is present the patient is less likely to suffer severe consequences of carotid occlusion at normal levels of blood pressure. It is generally agreed that hypotension of any degree should be avoided in these patients. Head pressure should be maintained at a "normal" level in relation to the patient's resting state.

**Deep anaesthesia.**—Marked depression of the central nervous system by anaesthesia reduces cerebral oxygen requirements and should confer some protection against the effects of carotid occlusion. Smith and his colleagues[67] showed that ligation of the middle cerebral and internal carotid arteries in dogs under deep halothane anaesthesia produced larger lesions than in animals under light halothane anaesthesia. They also showed that the same procedure in dogs given barbiturates rarely produced infarction. In clinical practice deep anaesthesia produced by any method is likely to be associated with depressed cardiac function, and a reduced cardiac output and cerebral perfusion pressure would vitiate any cerebral protective effects of anaesthesia.

**Heparinisation.**—Administration of heparin before carotid occlusion will improve carotid blood flow. Heparinisation alone has been advocated as the sole protection to the cerebral circulation during occlusion,[68] but most authorities now combine transient systemic heparinisation with a bypass shunt and other means of protecting the brain.

**Hypothermia.**—Surface cooling to a core temperature of 30° C considerably increases the time for which an internal carotid artery can safely be occluded. However, the deleterious effects that such hypothermia may produce in organs other than the brain have led to the virtual abandonment of its use.

**Hyperbaric oxygenation.**—This will increase cerebral oxygen delivery and, by constricting vessels in the normal parts of the brain, improve perfusion of those areas at risk.[69] The number of large, walk-in hyperbaric chambers in which this type of surgery can be performed is very limited.

**General considerations.**—Fitch[66] has summarised the principles of anaesthetic management of patients undergoing carotid artery surgery. His suggestions are for general anaesthesia at normothermia, supplemented by barbiturates, narcotics or low inspired levels of halothane, a normal or somewhat increased arterial oxygen tension, a normal carbon dioxide tension, a normal or slightly increased systemic blood pressure, the use of a bypass shunt and transient heparinisation instituted just before occlusion. Monitoring of the adequacy of cerebral perfusion is important during these procedures. A widely used measurement is that of stump pressure—that is, the pressure in the internal carotid artery distal to the occlusion. A stump pressure above 50 mm Hg (6·7 kPa) is taken to indicate adequate brain perfusion. The electroencephalogram is also of value during the procedure, and modern methods of processing the EEG to produce a compressed spectral array (CSA) or a density-modulated spectral analysis (DA) have diminished the problems of interpreting the large amount of data which the EEG can offer. The cerebral function monitor (CFM) is a less effective though simpler monitoring aid.

## NEURORADIOLOGICAL INVESTIGATIONS

Special neuroradiological investigations fall into four categories—air replacement of cerebrospinal fluid to outline the ventricular system, intraventricular or spinal subarachnoid of a radio-opaque dye to outline a tumour or other obstruction to the flow of CSF, angiography, and computerised axial tomography. It is possible to carry out all these investigations under local anaesthesia, with or without sedation, but because many of the procedures are unpleasant to the patient they are commonly performed under general anaesthesia. A co-operative patient is always essential if the procedure is to be performed without anaesthesia, and general anaesthesia is usually indicated in small children and in unco-operative adults.

General anaesthesia for neuroradiological procedures carries special risks to the patient by virtue of the various postures he will be required to adopt, and due to the effects of the underlying disease. The problems that the anaesthetist may encounter are identical to those met during neurosurgery itself, and the hazards are increased if these investigations are carried out in conditions which are less ideal than those usually available in the operating suite. During pre-operative assessment, the level of consciousness should be noted and clinical evidence of raised intracranial pressure should be carefully sought. If general anaesthesia is to be used, potent narcotic drugs should be avoided as premedicants for the same reasons as in neurosurgery. Atropine should be given pre-operatively, supplemented with oral diazepam if some sedation is needed. The principles of neuroradiological anaesthesia are identical to those of neurosurgical anaesthesia—to avoid all factors which may increase intracranial pressure.

**Air Encephalography**

This procedure consists of the incremental injection of air into the lumbar subarachnoid space. With the patient erect this air will rise, and will pass over the hemispheres outlining the brain sulci. By varying the position of the head air can be made to enter the ventricular system (Fig. 3). There has been a marked decrease in the number of air encephalograms performed since the introduction of computerised tomography. This investigation is still useful in detecting small suprasellar masses and small mass lesions in the cerebellopontine angle. The procedure is absolutely contra-indicated in the presence of a raised ICP as CSF removal may precipitate medullary coning. The procedure may be protracted in duration, requires many changes in posture, and air instillation usually causes severe headache. For these reasons the investigation is commonly carried out under general anaesthesia. Postural hypotension is a considerable problem during such anaesthesia. Either spontaneous or controlled ventilation may be used, but Campkin and Turner[70] have shown that hypotension is a greater problem in the spontaneously breathing anaesthetised patient. Better conditions are obtained if the procedure is carried out using controlled ventilation, and hypotension can be minimised by bandaging the legs. The problems associated with changes in the patient's posture have been reduced by the introduction of special rotatable chairs, into which the patient is firmly fitted. Following this investigation the patient should be nursed flat for 24 hours to reduce the problems of CSF leak and low-pressure headache. If nitrous oxide is administered to a patient in whom air is instilled into the subarachnoid space the volume of gas will increase as nitrous oxide diffuses into it.[71] Air encephalography during nitrous oxide anaesthesia is associated with a rise in ICP which is more marked if spontaneous respiration is used,[70, 72] but in the absence of previously raised ICP the rise is not significant. Whilst there are theoretical reasons for instilling nitrous oxide rather than air during the investigation, there is little evidence that this decreases the dangers of the procedure or reduces the severity or duration of postoperative headache,[73] and possibly because of the increased technical difficulty this approach has not been widely adopted.

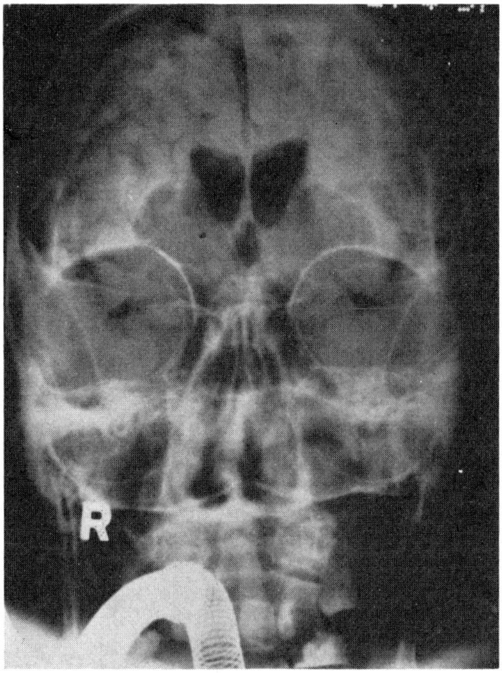


28/Fig. 3.—Normal air-encephalogram.

**Ventriculography**

This procedure consists of the injection of air or a radio-opaque contrast medium into the ventricular cavities via a burr hole. It is the investigation that should replace air encephalography in patients with a raised ICP. Ventriculography is often performed immediately preceding neurosurgery, and in any circumstances facilities for an immediate craniotomy should be available when this investigation is performed. The procedure is often performed under local anaesthesia. If general anaesthesia is required then it is safer to use controlled ventilation as for air encephalography. This is especially so if ICP is raised. As with air encephalography by the lumbar route, there is a danger of gas expansion and a rise in ICP if nitrous oxide is used as part of the anaesthetic technique. This is a lesser problem if oxygen is used as the contrast medium, or if liquid contrast medium is used.

### Cerebral Angiography

This entails the injection of contrast medium into an internal carotid artery to demonstrate the anterior and middle cerebral arteries and venous drainage from that side of the brain (Fig. 4, 5*a*, 5*b*, 6), or into the vertebral artery to visualise the circulation in the posterior fossa (Fig. 7). These investigations may be carried out by direct percutaneous puncture of the relevant vessels in the neck, or by retrograde catheterisation of the brachial, subclavian, or (most commonly) the femoral artery. Retrograde femoral artery catheterisation permits selective angiography and is less disturbing to the patient than direct puncture techniques. Cerebral angiography can be carried out using either local or general anaesthetic techniques. The advantages of general anaesthesia are improved patient comfort, immobility, and prevention of hypercapnia and hypoxaemia. An additional advantage of controlled hyperventilation is that it may lead to better quality angiograms. The slowing of the cerebral circulation produced by hypocapnia allows greater concentration of contrast medium,[74] and hypocapnic constriction of cerebral vessels improves radiological clarity.[75] By producing an intracerebral "steal" and diverting blood from normal to abnormal areas of brain, hyperventilation may improve the definition of cerebral tumours.[76] Complications of cerebral angiography relate mainly to the toxicity of the contrast medium used. With media such as meglumine iothalamate (Conray) severe hypotensive reactions are rare. Spasm produced by contrast medium is particularly dangerous in patients with a leaking aneurysm, where severe intracranial vascular spasm may already exist. After direct puncture of the carotid vessels pressure should be applied to the neck until the operator is certain that there is no leakage. Large haematomas may collect after carotid puncture and may compress the trachea to an extent that requires urgent intervention (Fig. 8).

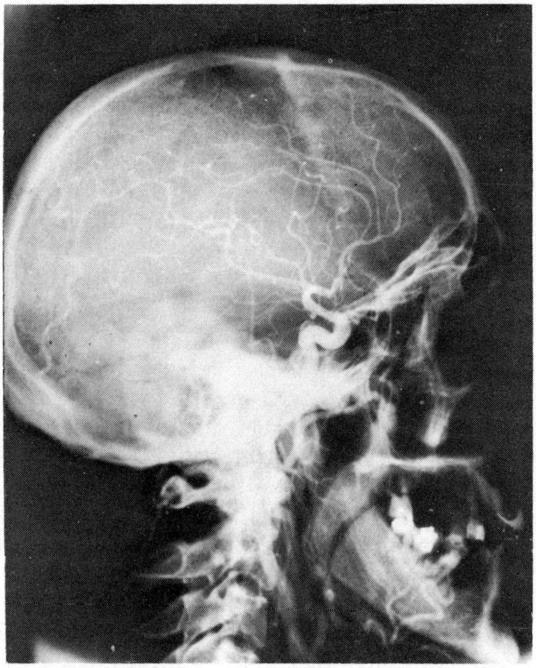

28/Fig. 4.—Normal carotid arterogram, lateral view.

Spinal cord angiography is performed by femoral artery catheterisation and selective retrograde catheterisation of the vertebral, intercostal or ileolumbar vessels. This investigation necessitates subtractive radiological techniques with a patient who is immobile and apnoeic during exposure, and is invariably carried out under general anaesthesia using IPPV.

### Computerised Axial Tomography

The introduction of computerised axial tomography (CAT or CT scanning) in 1973[77] has greatly enhanced the radiological investigation of intracranial disease. In this technique a well-collimated narrow x-ray beam is transmitted axially through the body from many angles of incidence. The transmitted photons are detected by solid state or gas detectors, and the system's computer builds up a picture of a slice of the body. During CAT scanning of the head the patient lies on an adjustable table with his head in the opening of the scanner's gantry. In the original equipment the head was placed in a latex cap surrounded by a plastic box containing water. Later generations of scanners have dispensed with the water interface. The procedure is non-invasive, but concomitant intravenous injection of a bolus of contrast

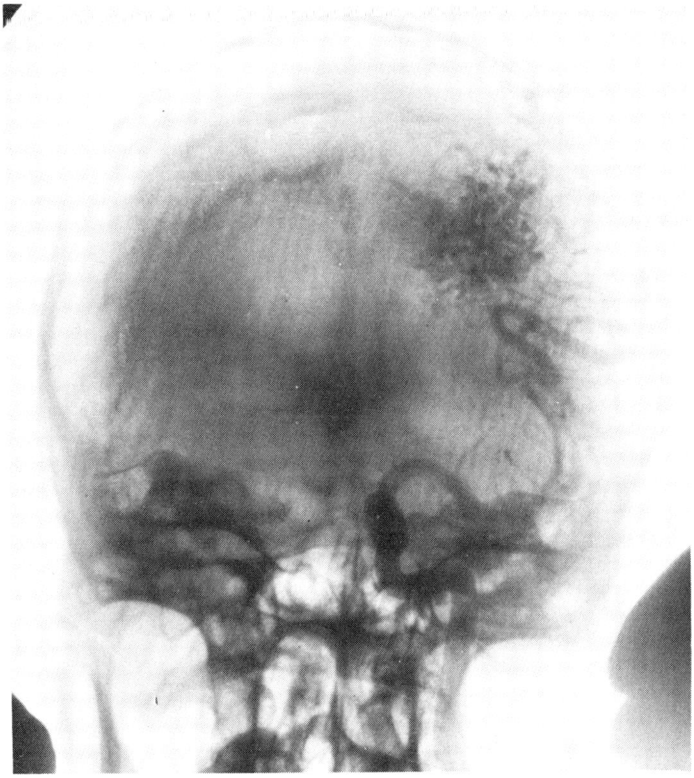

28/FIG. 5(*a*).—Carotid arteriogram—haemangioma (anteroposterior view).

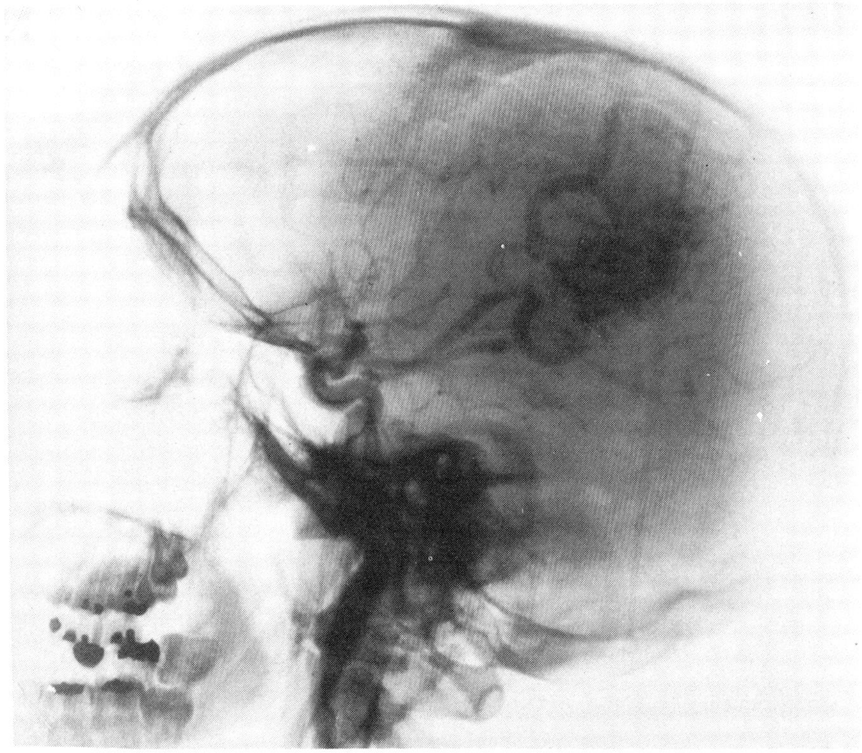

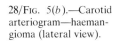

28/FIG. 5(*b*).—Carotid arteriogram—haemangioma (lateral view).

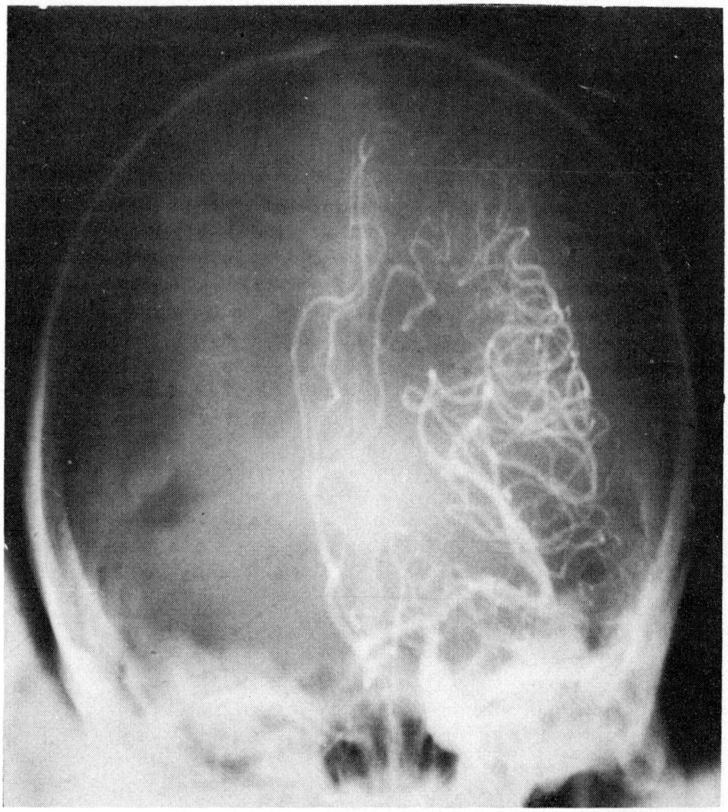

28/Fig. 6.—Subdural haematoma. Antero-posterior carotid arteriogram of a 60-year-old male with a severe head injury, showing lentiform avascular area over the cerebral hemisphere. (Courtesy of Dr. E. H. Burrows and the Wessex Neurological Centre).

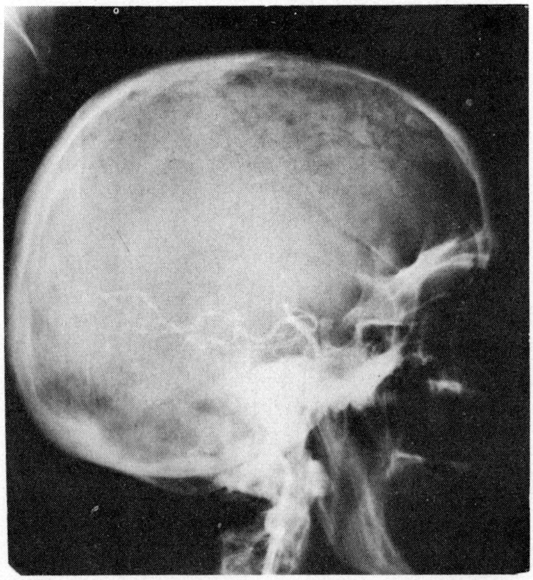

28/Fig. 7.—Normal vertebral arteriogram, lateral view.

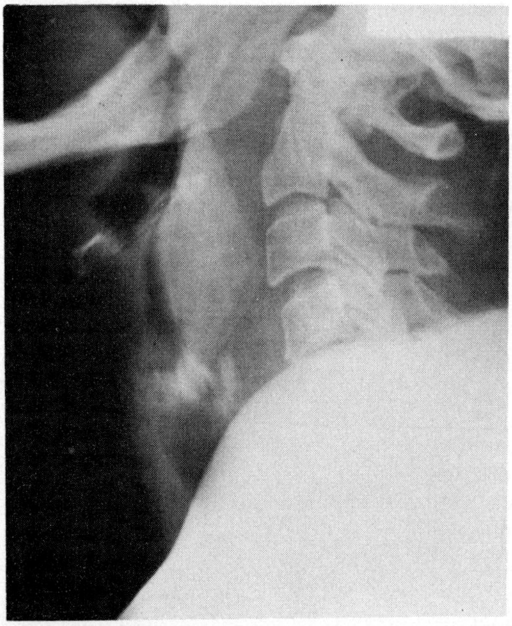

28/Fig. 8.—Haematoma causing tracheal obstruction following carotid arteriography. (Courtesy of the late Dr. Christine John).

agent is of great value in enhancing intracranial vascular lesions and masses. General anaesthesia is required where complete immobility cannot be guaranteed, and is therefore usually necessary in small children and in unco-operative adults. When general anaesthesia is indicated, the choice of technique should be governed by the general principles which apply to any neurosurgical anaesthetic.

## MANAGEMENT OF HEAD INJURIES
(see also Chapter 10)

Whilst large numbers of patients are admitted to hospital each year with head injuries, the majority of these have trivial injuries and suffer no long-term consequences. This section is devoted to the management of patients suffering severe head injury requiring urgent and skilled attention. Whilst severe head injury still carries a high mortality, it has become apparent in the last decade that aggressive therapy is worthwhile and can salvage a considerable proportion of these patients.[78, 79]

Brain damage due to head injury must be considered in terms of the primary biomechanical effects of forces applied to the skull at the time of injury, and secondary effects due to haemorrhage, oedema and infection. The ideal approach to the management of these patients is to ensure the best circumstances for recovery from the primary insult and to anticipate, and if possible prevent, secondary brain damage.[80] A major spur to the more optimistic approach to head injury has been the demonstration by Mitchell and Adams[81] that primary isolated brain-stem injury is a rare event.

### Assessment of Brain Damage

The Glasgow Coma Scale[82] is now widely used in many countries. It is based on assessment of three separate functions—eye opening, speech, and motor function (Table I). It has been shown that scaling in this system suffers little from observer error, and multicentre studies have shown good agreement between the initial score and the final outcome.[79]

All head injury patients require a detailed neurological examination to determine evidence of focal brain damage. The method of neurological assessment has been outlined by Teasdale.[80]

28/TABLE 1
GLASGOW COMA SCALE

| | |
|---|---|
| *Eye opening* | 4. Spontaneous |
| | 3. To speech |
| | 2. To pain |
| | 1. None |
| *Best verbal response* | 5. Orientated |
| | 4. Confused |
| | 3. Inappropriate |
| | 2. Incomprehensible |
| | 1. None |
| *Best motor response* | 6. Obeys commands |
| | 5. Localises pain |
| | 4. Withdraws |
| | 3. Flexes to pain |
| | 2. Extends to pain |
| | 1. None |

(After Teasdale and Jennett, 1974.[82])

### Initial Therapy

This should ideally be started at the site of the accident, and the primary concern is to secure an open airway and ensure adequate ventilation. Simple measures such as clearing the mouth of blood and vomit and turning the patient on to his side usually suffice. If not, endotracheal intubation should not be delayed. Muscle relaxants may be required to assist intubation if masseteric spasm is present, and cricoid pressure should be applied. Once the airway is secured a wide-bore nasogastric tube should be inserted. The degree of head injury may then be assessed and the patient must also be examined to determine the presence of associated injuries. An adequate airway, empty stomach and an effective circulation must be attained before the patient is moved from the accident room.

### Surgical Treatment

Surgical intervention may be necessary shortly on arrival in hospital or may be indicated during the course of therapy. Surgery is indicated for the treatment of compound depressed skull fractures and for the evacuation of epidural, subdural and large intracerebral haematomas, but has little place to play in the management of cerebral contusions or for the relief of a raised intracranial pressure *per se*. General anaesthesia for such surgery should follow all the precepts of neurosurgical anaesthesia as described above. Surgery is also often needed to treat concomitant non-cerebral injuries and here again the patient should be treated as if he were undergoing neurosurgery.

**Monitoring of intracranial pressure.**—Careful control of intracranial pressure and active treatment of intracranial hypertension has probably been the most important factor in the reduction of mortality following head injury. ICP can be monitored from the ventricular system. This requires insertion of a catheter into one or other lateral ventricle through a burr hole. Alternatively, ICP can be estimated from the extradural space by means of a transducer fixed into a burr hole. Better recordings are usually obtained by ventriculostomy, and with this method CSF can be removed for relief of high pressure, or acid-base status determination. Catheterisation of the ventricles may be difficult if the brain is distorted and with this method there is a possibility of brain infection. An extradural transducer is technically easy to insert. Care has to be taken that the transducer is coplanar with the dura (on the same plane) and does not indent it.[83]

The skull is a rigid and virtually closed box, and the pressure within it depends on the relative volumes of its contents—brain substance, CSF and blood. Initial expansion of brain substance due to a space-occupying lesion or brain oedema can be balanced by a displacement of CSF and venous blood, but as brain expansion increases this compensatory mechanism fails and pressure rises markedly. The well-known relationships between intracranial pressure and the volume of intracranial contents is shown in Fig. 9.

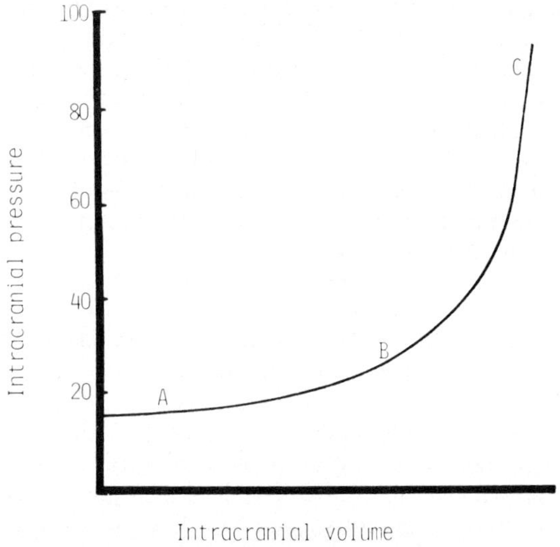


28/Fig. 9.—Diagrammatic relationship between intracranial volume and pressure. Point A represents a high compliance (low elastance) state. At point B compliance is beginning to fall and compensation starting to fail. At point C small rises in intracranial volume will cause large rises in intracranial pressure.

Normal intraventricular ICP varies from 5 to 15 mm Hg (0·7–2·0 kPa) (slightly higher levels being obtained by extradural measurements), and varies with both respiration and the heart beat. Patients who have suffered head injury *per se* may have a markedly raised ICP. They may also show abnormal waveforms. Lundberg[84] described the occurrence of A waves—plateau waves of 60–80 mm Hg (8·0–10·7 kPa) lasting for up to 20 mins—in patients in whom the limits of intracranial volume compensation were being approached. He also described B waves (occurring about once per minute) and C waves (up to 6/min). These are of lesser prognostic significance.

Because of the characteristics of the intracranial pressure-volume curve considerable attention has been paid to measurements of brain elastance (the inverse of compliance). The ventricular pressure response (VPR) is the pressure change produced by the bolus injection of 1 ml of fluid, which can be related to the steepness of the intracranial pressure volume curve.[85,86] VPR normally has a value of about 1·5 mm Hg (0·2 kPa). The combination of a low or normal ICP and a high VPR suggests a patient nearing the limits of volume compensation. Turner and McDowall[83] point out that each heart beat adds a volume of blood to the intracranial volume, and that increases in VPR are associated with an increased intracranial pulse pressure. The variation of pressures around mean ICP can indicate the degree of intracranial compression that exists.

**Treatment of raised ICP.**—An ICP greater than 20 mm Hg (2·7 kPa) should be regarded as an indication for intracranial hypotensive therapy. Many measures are available to reduce ICP. These include CSF removal, hyperosmolar agents, steroids, diuretics, hypothermia and controlled hyperventilation. Hyperventilation is almost invariably the first method of choice, and other methods are used if this fails to control ICP.

There has been considerable interest in recent

years in the use of large doses of barbiturates for protection of the ischaemic brain. There is considerable evidence that pretreatment of animals with barbiturates has a protective effect against induced ischaemia.[87–89] Various mechanisms of protection have been suggested, including reduction in cerebral oxygen requirements, increased activity of the hexose monophosphate shunt, reduction in cerebral oedema, and an antioxidant action in the control of free radical reactions initiated by hypoxia.[90–93] There is no good evidence that barbituates offer protection when given following cerebral insult. However, their use does markedly reduce ICP. Pentobarbitone in a loading dose of 5 mg/kg and then given at a rate of 1–5 mg/kg/hour can be used to maintain an ICP below 15 mm Hg (2·0 kPa) without pressure waves.[94] Care must be taken to preserve adequate cardiovascular function during this therapy. Thiopentone and Althesin have been similarly used in the control of raised ICP.

**Cerebral oedema.**—Cerebral oedema commonly occurs in severe head-injury cases, and is commonly treated with steroids. Whilst dexamethasone has a proven role in the reduction of cerebral oedema surrounding intracranial tumours, its efficiency when oedema is due to trauma is dubious. Faupel and his colleagues[95] have suggested that dexamethasone in these circumstances is only effective if given in high doses—1 to 1·5 mg/kg per day.

## ELECTROCONVULSIVE THERAPY

The precise mechanism by which the passage of an electric current through the brain should be able to bring about a therapeutic effect in cases of endogenous depression is still unknown. A simple explanation is that the current stimulates the mood centre in the hypothalamus, but in attempting to reach this innermost area of the brain it must also excite other centres such as the motor cortex. Before the introduction of anaesthesia and muscle paralysis into electroconvulsive therapy, the severity of the convulsions would put the patient at risk not only from compression fractures of the spine but from myocardial failure. An unmodified fit in a conscious subject comprises an immediate loss of consciousness with the passage of the electric current. This is followed by a tonic convulsion of about five seconds duration leading into a clonic convulsion with regular muscle movements lasting from about 10–50 seconds. Immediately after the passage of the current, signs of autonomic stimulation—"goose-pimples", dilatation of the pupil and flushing of the facial skin can be observed. Contraction of the jaw muscles is probably due to direct stimulation of the muscle fibres by the electric current as this takes place even in the completely paralysed patient. For this reason it is mandatory to protect the patient's teeth with some suitable mouth prop.

Cerletti and Bini[96] first described this method of treatment and since that time the clinical successes in many thousands of patients throughout the world bear witness to its value. The introduction of general anaesthesia and muscle paralysis has transformed the technique into one which can be conducted either as an out-patient or an in-patient with minimal risk. Mental depression increases in frequency with advancing age, so that a considerable number of patients will be encountered with hypertension and cardiac disease. Great care must therefore be used in selecting the sleep-dose of either thiopentone or methohexitone for each patient, but these doses need only be minimal as the passage of the electric current also produces unconsciousness.

In the majority of cases the electric current is applied to both temporal areas. In 1957, unilateral ECT to the non-dominant hemisphere was first proposed. It reduces the incidence and severity of memory disturbances associated with the bilateral technique,[97] but there is not general agreement that the therapeutic results are identical.

### Technique of General Anaesthesia

Sedative premedication is usually unnecessary but there is no objection to its use when specially indicated. A short-acting oral barbiturate is the most satisfactory method for such cases. To avoid the risk of vagal asystole, 0·5–1·0 mg of atropine sulphate should be given intravenously (either separately or mixed with the induction agent). Subcutaneous atropine in small doses given half an hour before treatment merely gives the patient an unpleasant dry-mouth feeling without influencing vagal activity.

Anaesthesia may be induced with any suitable intravenous induction agent. Thiopentone and methohexitone are the most widely used agents, but both propanidid and Althesin have been employed. Induction of anaesthesia is followed immediately by suxamethonium, 0·5–0·75 mg/kg. The doses of induction agent and suxamethonium and the patient's response to them are recorded so that any necessary adjustments may be made on subsequent occasions. Successful anaesthesia should allow slight twitching of the face and limbs, but little more. If no movements occur—because the dose of suxamethonium has been excessive—two signs may be useful as suggestive evidence of the successful passage of a current. The first is the presence of goose-flesh[98] and the second, dilatation of the pupils and their failure to react when inspected immediately after the stimulus.[99]

As soon as the patient is paralysed the lungs must be adequately inflated with oxygen. A mouth prop is then inserted to protect the teeth, and the electrodes applied. Great care must be used in selecting and fitting the mouth prop to protect the patient's own teeth. In rare instances it may be beneficial for the patient to retain a denture in position to give maximum support to his few remaining teeth.

Immediately after passage of the current the patient should again be gently ventilated with oxygen until adequate spontaneous respiration returns. The patient can then be turned on to his side and allowed to rest until fully conscious and orientated, when he can safely be allowed to return home, provided he is accompanied.

The return to consciousness is usually quiet if the patients have been properly selected for treatment, but unsuspected neurotics or hysterics may be difficult to control for a short period. The commonest complications are headache and retrograde amnesia.

## REFERENCES


1. Sosterholm, J. L. (1970). Reaction of the cerebral venous sinus system to acute intracranial hypertension. *J. Neurosurg.*, **32**, 652.
2. Fitch, W., Barker, J., McDowall, D. G. and Jennett, W. B. (1969). The effect of methoxyflurane on cerebrospinal fluid pressure in patients with and without intracranial space-occupying lesions. *Brit. J. Anaesth.*, **41**, 564.
3. McDowall, D. G., Barker, J. and Jennett, W. B. (1966). Cerebrospinal fluid pressure measurements during anaesthesia. *Anaesthesia*, **21**, 189.
4. Jennett, W. B., Barker, J., Fitch, W. and McDowall, D. G. (1969). Effect of anaesthesia on intracranial pressure in patients with space-occupying lesions. *Lancet*, **1**, 61.
5. Stullken, E. H., Milde, J. H., Michenfelder, J. D. and Tinker, J. H. (1977). The non-linear responses of cerebral metabolism to low concentrations of halothane, enflurane, isoflurane and thiopentone. *Anesthesiology*, **46**, 28.
6. Adams, R. W., Cuchiani, R. F., Gronert, G. A., Messick, J. M. and Michenfelder, J. D. (1981). Isoflurane and cerebrospinal fluid pressure in neurosurgical patients. *Anesthesiology*, **54**, 97.
7. Batson, O. V. (1940). The function of the vertebral veins and their role in the spread of metastases. *Ann Surg.*, **112**, 138.
8. Pearce, D. J. (1957). The role of posture in laminectomy. *Proc. roy. Soc. Med.*, **50**, 109.
9. Hunter, A. R. (1975). *Neurosurgical Anaesthesia*. Oxford: Blackwell Scientific Publications.
10. Hunter, A. R. (1960). Discussion on the value of controlled respiration in neurosurgery. *Proc. roy. Soc. Med.*, **53**, 365.
11. Millar, R. A. (1972). Neurosurgical anaesthesia in the sitting position. *Brit. J. Anaesth.*, **44**, 495.
12. Hewer, A. J. H. and Logue, V. (1962). Methods of increasing the safety of neuroanaesthesia in the sitting position. *Anaesthesia*, **17**, 476.
13. McComish, P. B. and Thompson, D. E. A. (1968). Respiratory disturbances in air embolism. *Anaesthesia*, **23**, 259.
14. Edmonds-Seal, J. and Maroon, J. C. (1969). Air embolism diagnosed with ultrasound. *Anaesthesia*, **24**, 438.
15. Paul, W. L. and Munson, E. S. (1981). Monitoring of end-tidal carbon dioxide to detect venous air embolism. *Brit. J. Anaesth.*, **53**, 313P.
16. Michenfelder, J. D., Terry, H. R., Daw, E. F. and Miller, R. H. (1966). Air embolism during neurosurgery, *Anesth. Analg. Curr. Res.*, **45**, 390.
17. Cheatle, C. A. and MacKenzie, R. M. (1953). Anaesthesia for cranial surgery in the sitting position. *Anaesthesia*, **8**, 182.
18. Bozza Marrubini, M. L. (1965). General anaesthesia for intracranial surgery. *Brit. J. Anaesth.*, **37**, 268.
19. Pitkin, G. P. (1953). *Conduction Anesthesia*, 2nd edit. Philadelphia: J. B. Lippincott Co.
20. Bozza Marrubini, M. L. and Tretola, L. (1965). Diazepam as a preoperative tranquillizer in neuro-anaesthesia. *Brit. J. Anaesth.*, **37**, 934.
21. Maekawa, T., Sakabe, T. and Takashiko, H. (1974). Diazepam blocks cerebral metabolic and circulatory responses to local anesthetic induced seizures. *Anesthesiology*, **41**, 389.
22. Greenbaum, R. (1976). General anaesthesia for neurosurgery. *Brit. J. Anaesth.*, **48**, 773.
23. Shapiro, H. M. (1975). Neurosurgical anesthesia. *Surg. Clin. North. Am.*, **55**, 913.
24. Adams, R. W., Gronert, G., Sundt, T. M. and Mich-

enfelder, J. (1972). Halothane hypocapnea and cerebrospinal fluid pressure in neurosurgery. *Anesthesiology* **37**, 510.
25. Tarkkanen, L., Laitinen, L. and Johannsen, G. (1974). Effects of d-tubocurarine on intracranial pressure and thalamic electrical impedance. *Anesthesiology*, **40**, 242.
26. Campkin, T. V. (1981). Posture and ventilation during posterior fossa and cervical operations: current practice in the United Kingdom. *Brit. J. Anaesth.*, **53**, 881.
27. Vourc'h, G. M. (1963). Continuous cerebral spinal fluid drainage by indwelling spinal catheter. *Brit. J. Anaesth.*, **35**, 118.
28. Barker, J. (1975). An anaesthetic technique for intracranial aneurysms. *Anaesthesia*, **30**, 557.
29. Nornes, H. and Magnaes, B. (1972). Supratentorial epidural pressure recorded during posterior fossa surgery. *J. Neurosurg.*, **35**, 541.
30. Javid. M. and Settlage, P. (1956). Effect of urea on cerebrospinal fluid pressure in human subjects. Preliminary report. *J. Amer. med. Ass.*, 160, 943.
31. Clark, K. and Einspruch, B. C. (1962). Osmotic rebound phenomena associated with agents used to lower intracranial pressure with emphasis on urea. *Arch. Neurol. (Chic).*, **6**, 414.
32. Guisado, R., Tourtelle, W. W., Arieff, A. I., Tomyasu, U., Mishra, S. K. and Scholtz, M. G. (1975). Rebound phenomenon complicating cerebral dehydration with glycerol. *J. Neurosurg.*, **42**, 226.
33. Hägnevik, K., Gordon, E., Lins, L. E., Wilhelmsson, S. and Forster, D. (1974). Glycerol-induced haemolysis with haemoglobinuria and acute renal failure. *Lancet*, **1**, 75.
34. Di Mattio, J., Hochwold, G. M. and Malhan, C. (1975). Effects of changes in serum osmolarity on bulk flow of fluid into cerebral ventricles and on brain water content. *Pflügers Arch. ges. Physiol.*, **359**, 253.
35. Marshall, S. and Hinman, F. (1962). Subdural haematoma following an administration of urea for diagnosis of hypertension. *JAMA.*, **182**, 813.
36. Miyazaki, Y., Suematsu, K. and Yamaura, J. (1969). Effects of ethacrinic acid on lowering of intracranial pressure. *Arzneimittelforschung*, **19**, 1961.
37. Wilkinson, H. A., Wepsie, J. G. and Austen, G. (1977). Diuretic synergy in the treatment of acute experimental cerebral edema. *J. Neurosurg.*, **34**, 203.
38. Reulen, H. J. (1976). Vasogenic brain oedema. *Brit. J. Anaesth.*, **48**, 741.
39. Anderson, S. and McKissock, W. (1953). Controlled hypotension with Arfonad in neurosurgery. *Lancet*, **2**, 754.
40. Siegel, P., Moraca, P. P. and Green, J. R. (1971). Sodium nitroprusside in the surgical treatment of cerebral aneurysms and arteriovenous malformations. *Brit. J. Anaesth.*, **43**, 790.
41. Fahmy, N. R. (1978). Nitroglycerin as a hypotensive drug during general anesthesia. *Anesthesiology*, **49**, 17.
42. Aserman, D. (1953). Controlled hypotension in neurosurgery with hexamethonium bromide and procaine amide. *Brit. med. J.*, **1**, 961.
43. Roth, D. A., Yanez, R., Andrew, N. W. and Mark, V. H. (1969). The combined effects of hyperventilation and hypotension on the blood-brain barrier. *Anesth. Analg. Curr. Res.*, **48**, 755.
44. Michenfelder, J. D. and Theye, R. A. (1977). Canine systemic and cerebral effects of hypotension induced by haemorrhage, trimetaphan, halothane, or nitroprusside. *Anesthesiology*, **46**, 188.
45. Krapez, J. R., Vesey, C. J., Adams, L. and Cole, P. V. (1981). Effects of cyanide antidotes used with sodium nitroprusside infusions, sodium thiosulphate and hydroxycobalamin given prophylactically to dogs. *Brit. J. Anaesth.*, **53**, 793.
46. Rosomoff, H. L. and Holaday, D. A. (1954). Cerebral blood flow and cerebral oxygen consumption during hypothermia. *Amer. J. Physiol.*, **179**, 85.
47. Rosomoff, H. L. and Gilbert, R. (1955). Brain volume and cerebrospinal fluid pressure during hypothermia. *Amer. J. Physiol.*, **183**, 19.
48. Burrows, M. Mc., Dundee, J. W., Francis, I. Ll., Lipton, S. and Sedzimir, C. B. (1956). Hypothermia for neurological operations. *Anaesthesia*, **11**, 4.
49. McDowall, D. G. (1971). The current usage of hypothermia in British neurosurgery. *Brit. J. Anaesth.*, **43**, 1084.
50. Berntman, L., Welsh, F. A. and Harp, J. R. (1981). Cerebral protective effects of low-grade hypothermia. *Anesthesiology*, **55**, 495.
51. Coleman, D. J. and De Villiers, J. C. (1964). Anaesthesia and stereotactic surgery. *Anaesthesia*, 19, 60.
52. Brown, A. S. (1964). Neuroleptanalgesia for the surgical treatment of Parkinsonism. *Anaesthesia*, **19**, 70.
53. Krumperman, L. W., Murtagh, F. and Wester, M. R. (1957). Epidural block anesthesia for cordotomy. *Anesthesiology*, **18**, 316.
54. Mullan, S., Harper, P. V., Hekmatpanah, J., Torres, H. and Dobbin, G. (1963). Percutaneous interruption of spinal pain tracts by means of Strontium 90 needle. *J. Neurosurg.*, **20**, 931.
55. Lipton, S. (1968). Percutaneous electrical cordotomy in relief of intractable pain. *Brit. med. J.*, **2**, 210.
56. Mehta, M. (1973). *Intractable Pain*, p. 229. London: W. B. Saunders Co.
57. Baum, J. D. and Scopes, J. W. (1968). The silver swaddler. *Lancet*, **1**, 672.
58. Aldridge, W. N. (1965). The pathology and chemistry of experimental oedema in the brain. *Proc. roy. Soc. Med.*, **58**, 599.
59. Bering, E. A. (1952). Water exchange of central nervous system and cerebrospinal fluid. *J. Neurosurg.*, **9**, 275.
60. Symon, L. (1967). A comparative study of middle cerebral artery pressure in dogs and macaques. *J. Physiol. (Lond.)*, **191**, 449.
61. Smellie, G. D. (1972). Surgery for occlusive vascular disease. In: *Scientific Foundations of Neurology*, p. 266. Eds: M. Critchley, J. O'Leary and W. B. Jennett. London: Heinemann.
62. Howe, J. R. and Kindt, G. W. (1974). Cerebral protection during carotid endarterectomy. *Stroke*, **5**, 340.
63. Boysen, G., Ladegaard-Pedersen, H. J., Henriksen, H., Olesen, J., Paulson, O. B. and Engell, H. C. (1971). The effects of $Pa_{CO_2}$ on regional cerebral blood flow and internal carotid artery pressure during carotid clamping. *Anesthesiology*, **35**, 286.
64. Michenfelder, J. D. and Sundt, T. M. (1973). The effect of $Pa_{CO_2}$ on the metabolism of ischaemic brain in squirrel monkeys. *Anesthesiology*, **38**, 445.
65. Sharbrough, F. W., Messick, J. M. and Sundt, T. M. (1973). Correlation of continuous electroencephalograms

with cerebral blood flow measurements during carotid endarterectomy. *Stroke*, **4**, 674.
66. Fitch, W. (1976). Anaesthesia for carotid artery surgery. *Brit. J. Anaesth.*, **48**, 791.
67. Smith, A. L., Hoff, J. T., Nielsen, S. L. and Larsen, C. P. (1975). Barbiturate protection against cerebral infarction. In: *Cerebral Circulation and Metabolism*, p. 347. Eds: T. W. Langfitt, L. C. McHenry, M. Reivich and H. Wollman. New York: Springer Verlag.
68. Kenyon, J. R., Thomas, A. B. W. and Goodwin, D. P. (1972). Heparin protection to the brain during carotid artery reconstruction. *Lancet*, **2**, 153.
69. Harper, A. M., Ledingham, I.McA. and McDowall, D. G. (1965). The influence of hyperbaric oxygen on blood flow and oxygen uptake of the cerebral cortex in hypovolaemic shock. In: *Hyperbaric Oxygenation*, p. 342. Ed: I.McA. Ledingham. Edinburgh: Livingstone.
70. Campkin, T. V. and Turner, J. M. (1972). Blood pressure and cerebrospinal fluid pressure studies during lumbar air encephalography. *Brit. J. Anaesth.*, **44**, 849.
71. Saidman, L. J. and Eger, E. I. (1965). Changes in cerebrospinal fluid pressure during pneumoencephalography under nitrous oxide anesthesia. *Anesthesiology*, **26**, 67.
72. Gordon, E. and Greitz, T. (1970). The effect of nitrous oxide on cerebrospinal fluid pressure during encephalography. *Brit. J. Anaesth.*, **42**, 2.
73. Wolfson, B., Siker, E. S. and Gray, G. H. (1970). Post-pneumoencephalography headache: a study of incidence and an attempt at therapy. *Anaesthesia*, **25**, 328.
74. Edmonds-Seal, J., Baulay, G. H. du and Bostock, T. (1967). The effect of intermittent positive pressure ventilation upon cerebral angiography: a preliminary study. *Brit. J. Radiol.*, **40**, 957.
75. Dallas, S. H. and Moxon, C. P. (1969). Controlled ventilation for cerebral angiography. *Brit. J. Anaesth.*, **41**, 597.
76. Samuel, J. R., Grange, R. and Hawkins, T. D. (1968). Anaesthetic technique for carotid angiography. *Anaesthesia*, **23**, 543.
77. Hounsfield, G. N. (1973). Computerised transverse axial scanning (tomography). I. Description of system. *Brit. J. Radiol.*, **46**, 1016.
78. Bruce, D. A., Raphaely, R. C., Goldberg, A. I., Zimmerman, R. A., Bilaniuk, L. T., Schut, L. and Kuhl, D. E. (1979). The pathophysiology, treatment and outcome following severe head injury in children. *Child Brain*, **5**, 174.
79. Jennett, B., Teasdale, G., Galbraith, S., Pickard, J., Grant, H., Braakman, R., Avezaat, C., Maas, A., Minderhoud, J., Vecht, C. J., Heiden, J., Small, R., Caton, W. and Kurse, T. (1977). Severe head injuries in three countries. *J. Neurol. Neurosurg. Psychiat.*, **40**, 291.
80. Teasdale, G. (1976). Assessment of head injuries. *Brit. J. Anaesth.*, **48**, 761.
81. Mitchell, D. E. and Adams, J. H. (1973). Primary focal impact damage to the brain stem in blunt head injuries. Does it exist? *Lancet*, **2**, 215.
82. Teasdale, G. and Jennett, B. (1974). Assessment of coma and impaired consciousness: a practical scale. *Lancet*, **2**, 81.
83. Turner, J. M. and McDowall, D. G. (1976). The measurement of intracranial pressure. *Brit. J. Anaesth.*, **48**, 735.
84. Lundberg, N. (1960). Continuous recording and control of ventricular fluid pressure in neurosurgical practice. *Acta Psychiat. scand.*, **36** (Suppl), 149.
85. Miller, J. D. (1975). Volume and pressure in the craniospinal axis. In: *Clinical Neurosurgery*, Vol. 22, p. 76. Ed: R. H. Wilkins. Baltimore: Williams & Wilkins Co.
86. Miller, J. D. (1976). Intracranial pressure-volume relationships in pathological conditions. *J. Neurosurg. Sci.*, **20**, 203.
87. Arnfred, I. and Secher, O. (1962). Anoxia and barbiturates—tolerance to anoxia in mice influenced by barbiturates. *Arch. int. Pharmacodyn.*, **139**, 67.
88. Michenfelder, J. D., Milde, J. H. and Sundt, T. M. (1976). Cerebral protection by barbiturate anesthesia: use after middle cerebral artery occlusion in java monkeys. *Arch Neurol.*, **33**, 345.
89. Yatsu, F. M., Diamond, I., Graziano, C. and Lindquist, P. (1972). Experimental brain ischemia: protection from irreversible damage with a rapid-acting barbiturate (methohexital). *Stroke*, **3**, 726.
90. Cohen, P. J. (1973). Effects of anesthetics on mitochondrial function. *Anesthesiology*, **39**, 153.
91. Flamm, E. S., Demopoulos, H. B., Seligman, M. L., Mitamura, J. A. and Ransohoff, J. (1979). Barbiturates and free radicals. In: *Neural Trauma*, p. 289. Eds. A. Popp and R. S. Bourne. New York: Raven Press.
92. Hakim, A. M. and Moss, G. (1976). Cerebral effects of barbiturates: shift from 'energy' to synthesis metabolism for cellular viability. *Surg. Forum*, **27**, 497.
93. Smith, A. L. (1977). Barbiturate protection in cerebral hypoxia. *Anesthesiology*, **47**, 285.
94. Bruce, D. A. (1980). Management of severe head injury. In: *Anesthesia and Neurosurgery*, p. 183. Eds: J. E. Cottrell and H. Turndorf. St. Louis: C. V. Mosby Co.
95. Faupel, G., Reulen, H. S., Miller, D. and Schurmann, K. (1976). Double-blind study on the effects of steroids on severe closed head injury. In: *Dynamics of Brain Edema*, p. 337. Eds: H. M. Poppins and W. Feindel. New York: Springer-Verlag.
96. Cerletti, V. and Bini, L. (1938). L'ettroshock. *Arch. gen. Neurol. Psichiat.*, **19**, 266.
97. Zinkin, S. and Birtchnell, J. (1968). Unilateral electroconvulsive therapy: its effect on memory and its therapeutic efficacy. *Brit. J. Psychiat.*, **14**, 973.
98. Edridge, A. (1952). Discussion on new muscle relaxants in electric convulsion therapy. *Proc. roy. Soc. Med.*, **45**, 869.
99. Thomas, E. and Honan, B. F. (1953). Electro-convulsive therapy. *Brit. med. J.*, **2**, 97.
100. McKissock, W. and Walsh, L. (1956). Subarachnoid haemorrhage due to intracranial aneurysms. *Brit. med. J.*, **2**, 559.

CHAPTER 29

# Neurological and Ophthalmic Complications of Anaesthesia



## Hypoxia and the Central Nervous System

Whatever the cause of hypoxia, the end results in the central nervous system appear to be the same, differing only in extent, which is in direct relation to the degree and duration of the period of sub-oxygenation. An acute anoxic episode caused by a period of cardiac arrest is dramatic enough to draw attention to any sequelae should the patient survive. Equally important are the equivalent degrees of acute hypoxia that can occur without cardiac arrest in some anaesthetic mishaps and certain disease states. Less obvious but just as potentially detrimental to the patient are the effects of prolonged but subacute hypoxia. Ancillary factors are the state of the brain prior to sub-oxygenation and repeated bouts of hypoxia. The normal brain will tolerate a moderate degree of oxygen lack for quite long periods without apparently being harmed, but the presence of disease, or even the ordinary changes associated with ageing, markedly increase its vulnerability. On the other hand, young babies have more resistance than adults. Repetitive bouts of moderate hypoxia may have cumulative effects, and once hypoxia of any degree has produced changes in the brain, loss of local circulatory autoregulation and disruption of the blood-brain barrier may lead to further brain damage. Ischaemic hypoxia is more dangerous than that associated with a normal flow of blood. It has been claimed that very low levels of cerebral blood flow produce more cerebral injury than no flow at all,[1] but more recent work has refuted this claim.[2]

### Clinical Picture

The clinical results of cerebral hypoxia are immensely variable, depending on the severity and duration of the episode. Transient hypoxia during anaesthesia and surgery may lead to a delayed recovery of consciousness, and no permanent sequelae, whilst circulatory arrest if not treated promptly will rapidly lead to brain death. Jennett[3] has described various levels of consciousness, varying from the totally alert state, through possible stages of clouded consciousness and drowsiness, to coma and brain death. Short of brain death a vegetative state may occur where there is no evidence of cortical function but retention of some brain-stem function.

### Physiopathology

Following arrest of the cerebral circulation, there is a brief period of reactive hyperaemia followed by a prolonged period of marked hypoperfusion.[4] Treatment directed at preventing the deleterious effects of this hypoperfusion may well improve the outcome. The lesions due to general brain anoxia are commonly widespread. Anaerobic metabolism and tissue acidosis leads to a loss of autoregulation in the affected areas, which can be focal or global. Increased blood flow and a damaged blood-brain barrier may lead to cerebral oedema, and can raise intracranial pressure and reduce cerebral perfusion pressure.

### Preventative Treatment

Hypoxia is generally regarded as being obvious in its clinical manifestations, but as Bedford[5,6] has shown there are innumerable occasions during and following anaesthesia and surgery when mild and insidious degrees of hypoxia may occur. Such occasions can be related to depressed cardiovascular function due to anaesthetic drugs or technique. Arterial oxygenation is known to be impaired during anaesthesia[7] and failure to enrich the inspired atmosphere with oxygen can lead to mild cerebral hypoxia. Virtually all patients subjected to anaesthesia and surgery undergo a period of postoperative hypoxaemia.[8,9] Whilst in itself of little consequence, moderate postoperative hypoxaemia occurring in a patient with a low haemoglobin and a reduced cardiac output may lower oxygen delivery to the brain to dangerous levels.

**Active treatment.**—The demonstration that aggressive treatment of severe head-injured patients improves the outcome has stimulated more active treatment of patients suffering cerebral hypoxia, and a less pessimistic view of the eventual prognosis. Many lines of treatment have been proposed, and a combination of several methods of treatment is often indicated. Current views on the treatment of established cerebral hypoxia relate to a limitation of the consequences of profound cerebral hypoperfusion, either by improving cerebral blood flow or by reducing cerebral metabolic requirements.

**Ventilation.**—Whether a patient should be allowed to breathe spontaneously or be artificially ventilated will depend on the degree of impairment of consciousness and on the adequacy of spontaneous ventilation. Oxygen enrichment of the inspired atmosphere is essential. Hypoventilation must be avoided at all costs, as hypercapnia will raise intracranial pressure and may increase the risk of cerebral oedema. Deliberate hyperventilation has been advocated in the treatment of cerebral hypoxia, but this form of therapy is less valuable in this state than in the patient who has suffered traumatic brain injury.

**Reduction of intracranial pressure.**—Any increase in intracranial pressure is likely to reduce cerebral blood flow. Mannitol given intravenously in a dose of 1 g/kg body weight is of proven value in reducing raised intracranial pressure. For long-term control of intracranial pressure glycerol may be given by a gastric tube in a dose of 1–2 g/kg body weight as a 50 per cent solution, and may be repeated 6 to 8 hourly.

**Steroids.**—Steroids, and especially dexamethasone, are well known to reduce cerebral oedema associated with brain tumours. There is little evidence of an advantageous effect of steroids when cerebral oedema and raised intracranial pressure are due to other causes. However, dexamethasone in an initial dose of 10 mg i.v. followed by 4 mg six-hourly is widely used in treating cerebral hypoxia, and whilst such therapy may not have proven good effects, it is unlikely to cause any harm.

**Hypothermia.**—Advantages claimed for the use of hypothermia include a decrease in cerebral blood flow, a corresponding reduction in cerebral oxygen requirement, decreased brain water and brain volume and a fall in intracranial pressure. Rosomoff[10] advocated lowering body temperature to 30–32° C for up to three weeks. The use of hypothermia to this degree has effectively been abandoned as the complexity and risks of severe hypothermia appear to outweigh any advantages.

**Barbiturates.**—There has been considerable enthusiasm for the use of barbiturates to protect the brain against ischaemia, stemming from the demonstration by Arnfred and Secher[11] that tolerance of mice to hypoxia was improved following barbiturate anaesthesia. Much of the work on the protective effects of barbiturates on the brain has been carried out in animal models, and there is little evidence of the clinical efficiency of this form of treatment. Pentobarbitone or thiopentone in an initial dose of 5 mg/kg followed by an infusion of 1–5 mg/hour causes a 50 per cent reduction in cerebral blood flow and cerebral oxygen requirements. Such therapy has a place in the management of severe head injuries, where its major role lies in the control of intracranial pressure. The evidence of the value of barbiturates in the clinical treatment of cerebral ischaemia is controversial and contradictory.[12,13] It has been suggested that barbiturates may protect the brain following hypoxia by scavenging "free radicals." The inner hydrophobic layer of all membranes contains unstable lipid side-chains. Free highly reactive molecules with a single electron in the outer shell form spontaneously in this layer and their formation may be propagated by hypoxia. This will lead to disturbed function of membrane-bound enzymes and eventual breakdown of the membrane barrier. Whilst there is *in vitro* evidence that barbiturates can prevent the initiation of free radical reactions and may be capable of diminishing these reactions once started, there is no evidence of such an effect during *in vivo* studies.[14]

The use of barbiturates for brain protection is now waning. They continue to have a place in the reduction of intracranial pressure, and in circumstances where it is desired to lower cerebral oxygen consumption abruptly. There is little agreement as to their place in treatment outside these two specific indications.

## Peripheral Nerve Palsies

Peripheral nerve palsies occurring during general anaesthesia are usually due to the effects, singly or combined, of pressure upon, or stretching of a nerve at some vulnerable point along its course. Occasionally such complications may result from the injection of an irritant substance into or near the nerve, or more simply from the trauma of a needle point. Evidence has accumulated to show that special conditions, such as induced hypothermia or hypotension, may themselves cause a neuropathy—while they will certainly aggravate any of the more common causes.

Stephens and Appleby[15] and Swan and his co-workers[16] describe the onset of nerve palsies following the use of hypothermia for cardiac operations. They were able to measure temperatures of 4° C in the gastrocnemius muscle of a patient who had a rectal temperature of 28° C. Exposure to cold in an ice water bath for periods of longer than thirty minutes led to peripheral nerve palsies in a number of patients.

In the assessment of any postoperative nerve palsy, a knowledge of the pre-operative neurological condition is of considerable importance. Not only is a diseased nerve more susceptible to trauma but the debilitating effects of both surgery and anaesthesia, even without any localised factor in the nerve itself, may accentuate pre-existing neurological disease. Diabetes mellitus, periarteritis nodosa and alcoholism are known predisposing causes.

### Compression and Stretching

**Brachial plexus palsy.**—A combination of factors is most commonly the cause of trouble. Clausen[17] described a case of brachial plexus palsy due to the effects of pressure alone, when a patient was maintained in the Trendelenburg position with inadequately padded shoulder supports. Presumably the supports were also badly positioned, because direct pressure upon the roots of the plexus is impossible if they are placed opposite the acromion processes.

The principal factors are weight bearing through the shoulder girdle in the Trendelenburg position, stretching of the plexus by moving the arm away from the side of the body, and abnormal relaxation of the muscles in this area. Weight bearing through the shoulder girdle leads to compression of the plexus between the first rib and the clavicle. When the arm is abducted from the side it is usually extended with some external rotation so that the plexus is put on the stretch. This may easily be accentuated to more than 90° by the unintentional and unnoticed movements of the surgeon, his assistants, or bystanders during the course of the operation. A further aggravating factor consists in placing the abducted arm at a lower horizontal level than the rest of the body.[18] This may occur if the arm drops away from the side of the body. Moreover the ill effects of this manoeuvre, which pushes the head of the humerus up into the already tightened plexus, are increased by raising the body still higher with a gall-bladder rest. The importance of the position of the arm, and hence of stretching as the principal cause of brachial plexus palsy, is illustrated by Kiloh's[19] description of four cases, all of which occurred during gall-bladder operations. Kiloh also stresses the fact that individual variations of anatomy and idiosyncrasy, such as cervical ribs, the size of the cervico-axillary canal, the shape of the first rib and the slope of the shoulder may all play a part sometimes in rendering the brachial plexus more vulnerable. Brachial plexus palsy as a result of faulty posturing during surgery was described long before relaxant drugs were introduced into anaesthetic practice, but there is little doubt that the extreme degrees of muscle relaxation they induce renders this complication much more likely in certain circumstances than with general anaesthesia alone.

### Compression

**Facial nerve palsy.**—The buccal branch of the facial nerve normally arises from the main stem in the substance of the parotid gland and emerges at the anterior edge of this gland to supply the lateral part of the orbicularis oris muscle. Occasionally this branch may arise more proximally and run superficial to the gland, in which case it is susceptible to pressure. Paresis of it may then be caused by compression when the jaw of an unconscious patient is held forward, or due to a firmly fitted head harness.

**Radial nerve palsy.**—The nerve is vulnerable as it winds round the mid-part of the inner surface of the humerus. In the lateral position—particularly with the arm placed away from the side of the body—it can easily be subjected to pressure.

**Ulnar nerve palsy.**—The ulnar nerve is unprotected as it passes superficially and inferior to the medial epicondyle of the humerus. Typically it may be compressed between the bone and the edge of the operating table should the arm not be placed close to the side of the body in the horizontal position. The surgeon, or his assistant, is likely to add further pressure during the operation as he stands up against the table. In 35 cases of ulnar nerve palsy reported by Cameron and Steward,[20] 34 followed general anaesthesia and one was associated with local anaesthesia.

**Common peroneal nerve palsy.**—This nerve, in a similar manner to the ulnar, may easily be compressed against the head of the fibula when the patient lies in the lateral position or from compression against the stirrups in the lithotomy position.

**Saphenous nerve.**—This nerve may be compressed against the stirrups on the medial side of the knee when the patient is in the lithotomy position.[21]

### Injection

**Median nerve palsy.**—The median nerve lies in close deep relationship to the basilic and median cubital veins at the medial side of the antecubital fossa. An extravenous injection of thiopentone in this area can easily reach the nerve. Pask and Robson[22] have drawn attention to the difficulty of appreciating the injection of very small quantities of fluid from a 10 ml syringe, and have shown that 0·2 ml of 1 per cent lignocaine can affect the median nerve significantly. Should the patient move after the needle of a syringe containing thiopentone has been successfully placed in the basilic vein, the point might easily advance sufficiently for some of the irritant fluid to reach the nerve.

**Lateral and median cutaneous nerves of the forearm.**—Either of these nerves may inadvertently come into contact with thiopentone solution should an attempted intravenous injection lead to some extravasation outside the vein, or the nerve itself be pricked.

**Radial nerve palsy.**—The radial vein, and its tributaries lying about 2·5–3·5 cm above the wrist on the radial side of the forearm, are popular not only for intravenous injection but also for intravenous infusion. Injudicious attempts at either of these procedures may lead to trauma of the radial nerve as it lies deep to but not far from the veins.

**Sciatic nerve palsy.**—Intramuscular injection into the buttock is always fraught with the potential hazard of traumatising the sciatic nerve, especially in infants. The upper and outer quadrant of the buttock should be used, but an alternative and safe site for injection is the anterolateral aspect of the mid-thigh.

### Prevention

General awareness of these dangers on the part of anaesthetists, surgeons, nurses, and all who care for unconscious patients is the best safeguard against their occurrence. Special precautions must be taken in particular instances where the risk of a certain posture must be accepted in the general interest of the patient. Thus it may be essential to use shoulder supports to maintain a patient in the Trendelenburg position, with the legs in the lithotomy position at the same time, during the operation of synchronous combined abdominoperineal resection of the rectum. In such an instance well-padded supports placed at the acromion processes are essential, and the arms should be placed by the side of the body. In all other inclined planes the body is more safely prevented from sliding by the use of a non-slip mattress (Fig. 1).[23]

If an arm is to be abducted from the body for the purpose of intravenous injections or infusions during an operation, it should be maintained at a higher horizontal plane from the body, and the use of a right-angle lock will help to ensure it is never fully abducted. In the "hands up" position, elevation of the upper arm 15 cm off the table prevents injury.[18]

### Treatment

This should consist of splinting to prevent deformities, and active exercises. Analgesics may be needed for a day or two after the onset of paresis.

### Prognosis

The greater the pressure and the longer it is applied, the more severe is the injury. Provided there is no pre-existing neurological disease the prognosis for peripheral nerve palsies of the types described is good. They may be slow to recover completely but the majority will clear within six months. The only notable exceptions are those due to hypothermia, which may take considerably longer. As a rule, power returns quickest in large muscles and more slowly in those concerned with fine movements. Thus patients who rely upon their fingers for everyday work and pleasure are more handicapped than manual workers.

The **neurological sequelae of spinal analgesia** are discussed in Chapter 32.

## Convulsions During Anaesthesia

Convulsions may occur during local or general anaesthesia. Those due to local anaesthetic drugs are discussed in Chapter 31. Convulsions during the administration of general anaesthesia have often, in the past, been associated with ether but are by no means limited to the use of this agent; indeed, accumulated experience suggests that they may be the result of a

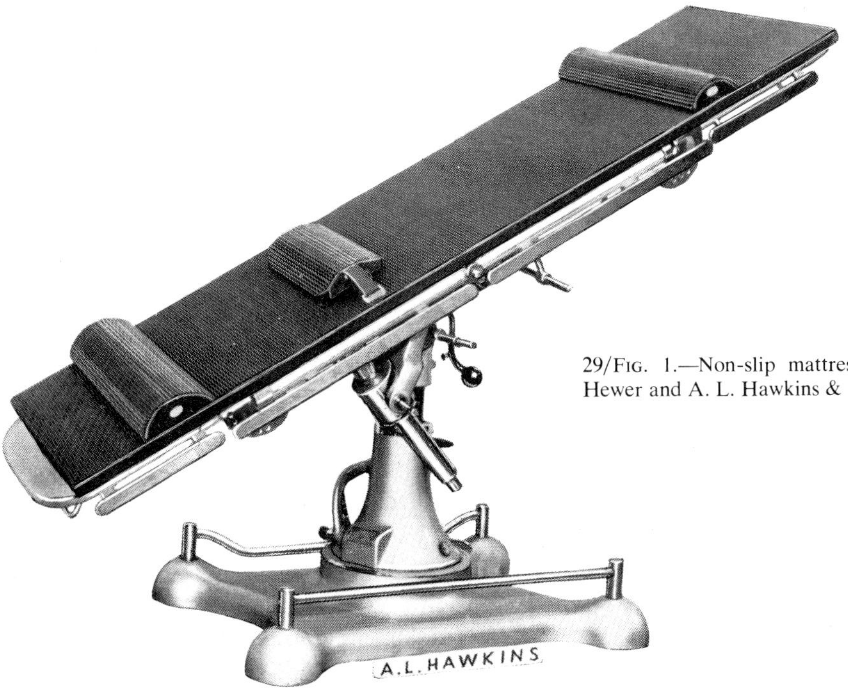


29/Fig. 1.—Non-slip mattress. (Courtesy of Dr. C. L. Hewer and A. L. Hawkins & Co. Ltd.)

combination of factors. These may be divided into three groups:

1. *Physical predisposition.* — Children undoubtedly have a greater propensity to convulse than adults, and this is presumably due to the lability of their central nervous systems. A fit may be induced in a true epileptic by various stimuli—such as hypoxia or hypercarbia—but the evidence for believing that all patients who convulse during general anaesthesia have an epileptic tendency is inconclusive.

2. *Disease.*—Sepsis with its associated high temperature and increased basal metabolism leads to some tissue hypoxia of the histotoxic type and frequently to dehydration. An excessively high body temperature may be produced by an overheated operating theatre or the injudicious use of surgical drapes on the patient.

3. *Anaesthesia.*—The contribution of anaesthesia lies primarily in its ability to accentuate the other factors. Hence excessive premedication with atropine raises the patient's temperature by increasing both metabolism and dehydration, while deep inhalational anaesthesia adds to the tissue hypoxia. Moreover, unless respiration is at least assisted at this stage, some carbon dioxide retention occurs. Convulsions in children following premedication with promethazine have been recorded[24] and an idiosyncratic reaction to the promethazine element has been postulated. Convulsions have also followed premedication in children with papaveretum and hyoscine[25] and the opiate held responsible. Increased seizure-like electroencephalographic activity is well known to occur during enflurane administration, and a few cases of frank seizure have been reported during use of this agent. The epileptogenic effects of enflurane are worsened in the presence of hypocarbia.

Malignant hyperthermia may be a cause of convulsions.[26] Its features and treatment are described elsewhere (Chapter 26).

Prevention of convulsions should consist of a reasoned appraisal of the risk in likely subjects, and the avoidance of all controllable and predisposing factors. The immediate treatment should be to ensure oxygenation and to control seizures. Either barbiturates or diazepam are effective for this purpose. Whilst administration of neuromuscular blocking agents and IPPV will control the outward manifestations of the seizure, electroencephalographic seizure activity continues. Further treatment consists in elimination of the cause of the convulsions, maintenance of a patent airway, full oxygenation and circulatory and respiratory support if hypotension or respiratory inadequacy occur.

## Ophthalmic Complications

Most ophthalmic complications follow direct trauma or the irritant effect of anaesthetic vapours, soda-lime dust, or sterilising solutions. Conjunctivitis, corneal abrasion and ulcers may also be caused in this fashion, and it is particularly important to ensure that the eyelids are closed, thus covering the eye at all times. In certain postures, such as the prone position in neurosurgery, and when the eyes are especially vulnerable, as in exophthalmos, it is a wise precaution temporarily to strap the eyelids together with adhesive plaster.[27] Indeed, in the latter case it is occasionally necessary to perform a tarsorrhaphy.

Less common complications affecting the eye as a result of anaesthesia and surgery are thrombosis of the central artery of the retina, acute glaucoma and pain in the region of the supra-orbital nerve. Thrombosis of the retinal artery, which causes blindness, is only likely to occur in those patients with pre-existing disease. Shock states, and excessive induced hypotension, could be a contributory cause. Postoperative blindness may also be part of a general syndrome caused by acute or subacute hypoxia. Ocular problems may follow cardiopulmonary bypass, varying from slight transient disturbances of visual acuity to total blindness.[28] Compression of the eye by an anaesthetic mask may cause indirect pressure on the central artery of the retina. If the patient suffers from arterial disease then ischaemic changes in the retina may be produced. Difficulties of accommodation are not uncommon immediately after anaesthesia and can usually be related to the varying effects of the drugs used—including pre- and postoperative medicants and relaxants—upon the ciliary and ocular muscles. Any agents which produce dilatation of the pupil and impede the circulation of the aqueous humour will accentuate a tendency towards glaucoma. Acute glaucoma, precipitated in a myopic patient, is a well-recognised postoperative complication, but its direct connection with either operation or anaesthetic is not always apparent. It has been suggested that the pressure of a face mask on the eye, and its subsequent release, is an important factor, but cases occur in which a mask has not been used. Certainly atropine and scopolamine should be used with caution for known cases of glaucoma, but the occasional acute case that occurs is more likely to be related to the general metabolic disturbance than to any single and specific factor.

Supra-orbital pain—a very rare complication—is almost certainly related to undue pressure in the area of the nerve.

The ocular complications of spinal analgesia are discussed in Chapter 32.

## REFERENCES


1. Hossmann, K. A. and Kleihues, P. (1973). Reversibility of ischemic brain damage. *Arch. Neurol.*, **29**, 375.
2. Steen, P. A., Michenfelder, J. D. and Milde, J. H. (1979). Incomplete versus complete cerebral ischaemia: improved outcome with a minimal blood flow. *Ann. Neurol.*, **6**, 389.
3. Jennett, B. (1980). Altered consciousness and coma. In: *Anesthesia and Neurosurgery*, p. 270. Eds: J. E. Cottrell and H. Turndorff. St Louis: C. V. Mosby Co.
4. Snyder, J. V., Nemoto, E. M. and Carroll, R. G. (1975). Global ischemia in dogs: intracranial pressures, brain blood flow and metabolism. *Stroke*, **6**, 21.
5. Bedford, P. D. (1955). Adverse cerebral effects of anaesthesia on old people. *Lancet*, **2**, 259.
6. Bedford, P. D. (1957). Cerebral damage from shock due to disease in aged people with special reference to cardiac infarction, pneumonia and severe diarrhoea. *Lancet*, **2**, 505.
7. Marshall, B. E. and Wyche, M. Q. (1972). Hypoxemia during and after anesthesia. *Anesthesiology*, **37**, 178.
8. Nunn, J. F. and Payne, J. P. (1962). Hypoxaemia after general anaesthesia. *Lancet* **2**, 631.
9. Conway, C. M. and Payne, J. P. (1963). Postoperative hypoxaemia and oxygen therapy. *Brit. med. J.*, **1**, 844.
10. Rosomoff, H. L. (1968). Cerebral oedema and brain swelling. *Acta anaesth. scand.*, Suppl. **29**, 75.
11. Arnfred, I. and Secher, O. (1962). Anoxia and barbiturates: tolerance to anoxia in mice influenced by barbiturates. *Arch. Int. Pharmacodyn.*, **139**, 67.
12. Bleyaert, A., Nemoto, E. M., Safar, P., Stezoski, W., Mickell, J. J., Moossy, J. and Rao, G. R. (1978). Thiopental amelioration of brain damage after global ischaemia in monkeys. *Anesthesiology*, **49**, 390.
13. Steen, P. A., Milde, J. H. and Michenfelder, J. D. (1979). No barbiturate protection in a dog model of complete cerebral ischemia. *Ann. Neurol.*, **5**, 343.
14. Steen, P. A. and Michenfelder, J. D. (1978). Cerebral protection with barbiturates: relation to anesthetic effect. *Stroke*, **9**, 140.
15. Stephens, J. and Appleby, S. (1956). Polyneuropathy following induced hypothermia. *Trans. Amer. neurol. Ass.*, p. 102 (80th Meeting, 1955).
16. Swan, H., Virtue, R., Blount, S. G., Jnr. and Kircher, L. T., Jnr. (1955). Hypothermia in surgery; analysis of 100 clinical cases. *Ann. Surg.*, **142**, 382.
17. Clausen, E. G. (1942). Post-operative ("anaesthetic") paralysis of brachial plexus; review of literature and report of nine cases. *Surgery*, **12**, 933.
18. Jackson, L. and Keats, A. S. (1965). Mechanism of brachial plexus palsy following anesthesia. *Anesthesiology*, **26**, 190.
19. Kiloh, L. G. (1950). Brachial plexus lesions after cholecystectomy. *Lancet*, **1**, 103.
20. Cameron, M. G. P. and Steward, O. J. (1975). Ulnar nerve injury associated with anaesthesia. *Canad. Anaesth. Soc. J.*, **22**, 253.
21. Schmidt, C. R. and Lincoln, J. R. (1966). Peripheral nerve injuries with anesthesia: a review and report of three cases. *Anesth. Analg. Curr. Res.*, **45**, 748.
22. Pask, E. A. and Robson, J. G. (1954). Injury to the median nerve. *Anaesthesia*, **9**, 94.
23. Hewer, C. L. (1953). Maintenance of the Trendelenburg position by skin friction. *Lancet*, **1**, 522.
24. Waterhouse, R. G. (1967). Epileptiform convulsions in children following premedication with Pamergan SP100. *Brit. J. Anaesth.*, **39**, 268.
25. Holmes, R. P. (1968). Convulsions following pre-operative medication. *Brit. J. Anaesth.*, **40**, 633.
26. Britt, B. A. and Gordon, R. A. (1969). Three cases of malignant hyperthermia with special consideration of management. *Canad. Anaesth. Soc. J.*, **16**, 99.
27. Snow, J. C., Kripke, B. J., Norton, M. L., Chandra, P. and Woodcombe, H. A. (1975). Corneal injuries during general anesthesia. *Anesth. Analg. Curr. Res.*, **54**, 465.
28. Taugher, P. J. (1976). Visual loss after cardiopulmonary bypass. *Am. J. Ophthal.*, **81**, 280.

CHAPTER 30

# Pain and the Analgesic Drugs



## PAIN

PAIN may serve a number of useful functions. It may be protective, defensive or diagnostic. The protective effect is most obvious in avoiding trauma; the burnt fingers of a patient with syringomyelia are evidence of this, while pressure sores which may occur in paraplegics are rare in poliomyelitis in which sensation is preserved. The defensive function is seen in the body's natural desire to immobilise an inflamed part or broken bone, which not only alleviates pain but also promotes healing. Angina pectoris may prevent the ischaemic myocardium from overexertion. Pain has an obviously diagnostic function in the acute abdomen, the onset of labour, and many other circumstances.

There are many conditions, however, such as carcinomatosis with bony metastases, where pain serves no useful function at all, and only makes a sad situation harder to bear.

Pain is one of the commonest symptoms to lead a patient to seek medical advice, and whatever the cause, it demands relief. To the general public, relieving pain is one of the most tangible roles the medical practitioner can play, and as such it merits our careful attention. Its importance was evinced by Sydenham in 1680: "Among the *remedies* which it has pleased Almighty God to give to man to relieve his sufferings, none is so universal and so efficacious as opium." The italics are mine.

The relief of pain during surgery is the *raison d'être* of anaesthesia. It is right that any expertise acquired in this field should be extended into the postoperative period, the labour ward and to the treatment of chronic pain.

## Neuroanatomy

### Pain Pathways[1,2]

Pain receptors appear to consist of peripheral plexuses of unmyelinated nerves, activated by high-intensity stimuli which may be thermal, mechanical, electrical or chemical (*vide infra*, Neuropharmacology). Pain is conducted along two types of fibres in the periphery, Aδ and C fibres. (For a classification of fibre types see Chapter 31, p. 835.) Aδ fibres are finely myelinated and relatively rapidly conducting (12–30 m/sec). They would appear to conduct the sharp pain produced by pinprick or electrical stimulation, as well as thermal stimuli, and are responsible for the withdrawal reflex. Aδ-conducted pain is felt quickly and is well localised.[3] C pain fibres are very fine non-myelinated fibres which conduct at a very slow rate of 2·3m/sec or less. Their threshold for stimulation is higher than that of Aδ fibres and they would appear to be responsible for more delayed and truly noxious burning or throbbing pain. There is, however, considerable overlap in the activation of Aδ and C fibres.

Peripheral sensory nerves have their cell bodies in the dorsal root ganglion, and the central projections of Aδ and C fibre neurones enter the dorsal horn in the lateral division of the dorsal root.

In the grey matter of the spinal cord, cell bodies are arranged in a series of laminae, some of which have classical names, but which are, more simply, given Roman numerals by Rexed,[4] starting with I at the tip of the dorsal horn. Aδ and C primary afferent fibres terminate principally in the marginal layer (lamina I) and the substantia gelatinosa (lamina II) (Fig. 1). Some of the neurones of lamina I which synapse with Aδ fibres, give off axons which ascend in the contralateral anterior columns without synapsing with neurones from deeper layers. The majority of pain fibres, however, synapse in the substantia gelatinosa with intermediate neurones which send projections to deeper layers, or with the dendrites of neurones whose cell bodies reside in deeper layers, principally in lamina V (Fig. 2).

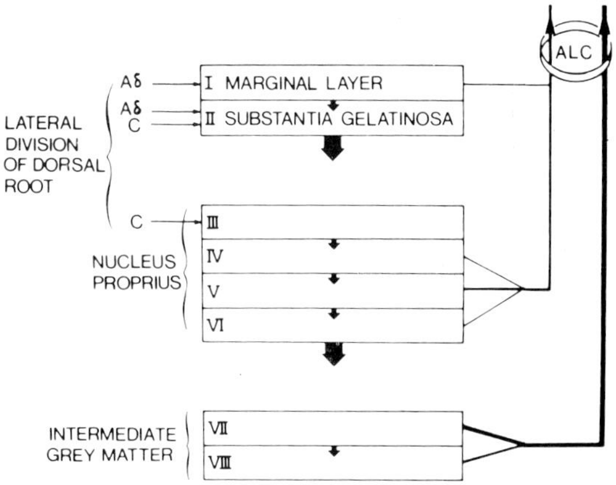


30/Fig. 1.—Diagram of the spinal cord grey matter. The laminae are numbered according to Rexed (Roman numerals). Cells in all laminae have axonal connections with deeper laminae. The main contribution for the spinothalamic tract is from lamina V, while a much larger number of pores from deeper laminae form the spinoreticular pathway. These two tracts ascend in the contralateral anterolateral column (ALC). (Courtesy of Bowsher (1978)[1] and the editor of *Anaesthesia*.)

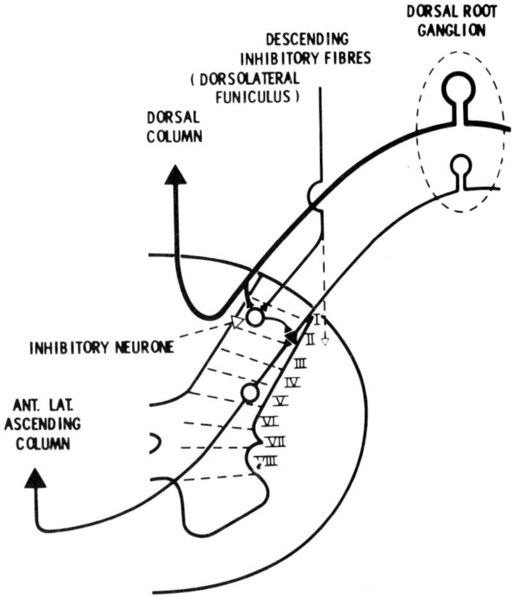


30/Fig. 2.—Diagram of the spinal cord showing pain pathways and connections.

The central projections from cell bodies in laminae IV, V and VI, with a contribution from lamina I, cross the midline in the anterior commissure to form the spinothalamic tract (Fig. 1) which ends in the thalamus, principally in the ventroposterior nucleus, sending a few fibres, *en route*, to the periaqueductal grey matter. The ventroposterior nucleus of the thalamus projects to the postcentral gyrus, the sensory cortex, where anatomical representation is reasonably precise.

Pain stimuli can also pass via interneurones to cell bodies in the intermediate grey matter (laminae VII and VIII), whose central projections also ascend in the contralateral anterolateral columns, forming the spinoreticular pathway. Pain impulses so transmitted in this multisynaptic pathway, pass via the reticular formation to be relayed non-specifically over a wide and poorly localised area of the cerebral cortex.

While it appears that the thalamus is involved in the experience of pain, the postcentral gyrus is necessary for its accurate localisation and the prefrontal cortex for the unpleasant affective reaction to it.

The existence of fast and slow neural pathways for pain conduction explains the occurrence of a double sensation of pain following a brief painful stimulus to the skin. The more distal the stimulus, the more distinctly can two successive peaks of pain be felt.

**Inhibitory pathways.**—There are various means by which pain transmission may be inhibited at spinal level (Fig. 2). They form part of a more modern and simplified explanation of the *gate theory* of Melzack and Wall.[166]

(i) *Large primary afferent fibres*, which mainly ascend in the dorsal columns and whose cell bodies lie in the dorsal root ganglion, send collaterals to synapse with and activate inhibitory interneurones in the dorsal horn. These in turn inhibit the release of transmitter along pain pathways. Thus stimulation of large $A\beta$ cutaneous afferents (for example by rubbing the part, or by transcutaneous nerve stimulation) may inhibit pain transmission.

(ii) *Inhibitory fibres*, which descend in the dorsolateral white funiculus and whose cell bodies lie in the medullary raphe nuclei, may also inhibit pain transmission, presumably by an action on the inhibitory interneurones. Activity in these descending inhibitory fibres may be provoked by stimulation of the cell bodies in the medulla directly, or of the periaqueductal grey matter.

(iii) *β-endorphin*, released into the third ventricle from long axons originating chiefly in the hypothalamus, is conveyed in the cerebrospinal fluid to the spinal cord where it may depress pain conduction in the substantia gelatinosa.

(iv) *Opiates* are also able to inhibit pain conduction in the cord either by activating descending inhibitory pathways or by a direct action on opiate receptors in the substantia gelatinosa (*vide infra*).

## Neurophysiology

The foregoing account of the anatomy of pain pathways is somewhat simplistic, and derived only by inference from much more complex results of neurophysiological and pharmacological experiments.[2,5,6]

While activity in sensory neurones may be excited in the periphery by thermoreceptor, nociceptor or mechanoreceptor stimulation, cell bodies in the posterior horn are responsive to different *intensities* of stimulation. Thus certain cells, found principally in lamina IV, respond only to a *low* intensity of stimulation, such as light touch; these are termed *low-threshold* or LT cells. They respond maximally to low-threshold stimuli and do not increase their firing rate with increased stimulus intensity. They are therefore incapable of conducting pain. Another type of cell, found principally in lamina V, responds over a wide range of stimulus intensities, the so-called *wide-dynamic-range* or WDR cells. Thus, in the periphery, mechanoreceptors which can respond over a wide range, including noxious stimuli, can excite a similarly variable response in WDR cells in lamina V. A third type of cell is responsive to stimuli only within the noxious range. Such cells are known as *high-threshold* or HT neurones, and are found mainly in lamina I. Thus volleys of activity provoked by $A\delta$ and C fibre stimulation in the periphery result in increased firing in HT and WDR cells in laminae I and V which is conducted up the anterolateral columns, principally in the spinothalamic tract. The spinothalamic tract receives contributions also from cells in laminae IV and VI, and is capable of conducting all types of afferent impulses; thus an individual without dorsal-column activity still possesses touch and position sense as well as appreciating pain.

## Neuropharmacology

**In the periphery.**—Prostaglandins of the E and I series sensitise pain receptors, and PGEs are believed to be involved in the amplification of pain in the inflammatory process. Several other autacoids such as bradykinin, acetylcholine, histamine and 5-hydroxytryptamine are known to produce intense pain on local injection and may also be involved in the mediation of natural pain.

**In the spinal cord and brain.**—Substance P, yet another peptide neurotransmitter, is present in the dorsal root ganglion and dorsal horn. Moreover Aδ and C fibre stimulation in the periphery results in release of substance P, which has itself been shown to excite 100 per cent of HT neurones in the spinal cord of cats, but only 14 per cent of LT units.[6] Substance P has now acquired an important role (long sought): that of principal pain transmitter in the cord.

**Inhibition of pain transmission.**—The neurochemistry of analgesia has been elucidated in recent years from studies of the behaviour of morphine and related drugs. It is now necessary to turn to opiate pharmacology in order to unfold the story.

Morphine administered systemically has been shown to depress the release of substance P in the substantia gelatinosa,[7] and to suppress the activity of lamina V neurones[8] and the responses to high-threshold noxious stimuli in dorsal-horn cells in the cord-transected cat.[9] Morphine also readily suppresses activity in ascending spinal axons evoked by C-fibre stimulation. Higher doses are necessary to suppress Aδ-evoked activity. All such opiate activities are reversed by naloxone.

### Opiate Receptors

It has long been apparent that opiates must act on receptors for three reasons:

(i) They exhibit stereospecificity
(ii) many possess high potency (for example, normorphine, etorphine, buprenorphine, fentanyl)
(iii) there exist competitive antagonists to their effects.

With the advance of highly selective radioligand binding techniques it became possible in the early 1970s to map opiate receptors in brain and spinal cord.[10,11] Opiates bind copiously to brain, but most binding sites possess relatively low affinity and are non-specific. A small proportion of the binding sites are highly selective and stereospecific, and possess high affinity only for active opiates. This affinity correlates closely with analgesic potency, suggesting that these binding sites are indeed opiate receptors.

Opiate receptors are widespread in brain stem and spinal cord.[11] They are found in areas associated with the emotions: the amygdala and the limbic system, in the area postrema,[12] associated with the stimulant effect upon the chemoreceptor trigger zone, and along the course of pain pathways in the medial thalamus, in the periaqueductal grey matter and in the substantia gelatinosa of the trigeminal nerve and spinal cord, and in the gastro-intestinal tract.

In accordance with the role of morphine in suppressing substance P release in the substantia gelatinosa, it would be anticipated that opiate receptors were on the substance P nerve terminals (Fig. 2). Nothing is ever quite so simple, however, and they would appear to be on closely associated interneurones.

Descending inhibitory neurones which activate the inhibitory interneurones (Fig. 2) are principally tryptaminergic (5HT-containing) while noradrenergic neurones are also involved.

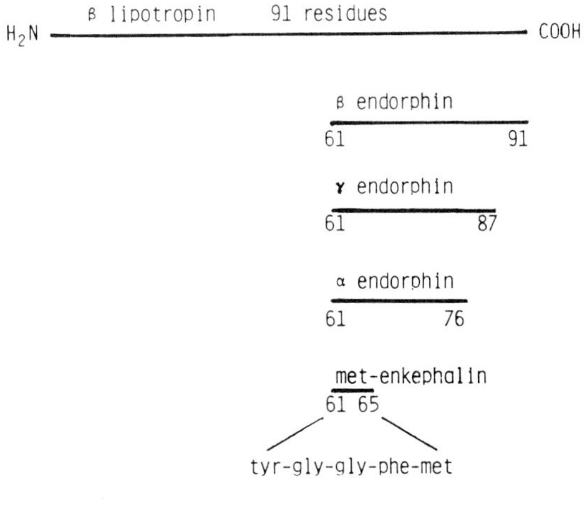


30/Fig. 3.

**Endogenous Opiates**

Knowledge of the existence of opiate receptors also stimulated a search for the endogenous opiate transmitter, since no known transmitter fulfilled this role. Aberdeen workers, using the guinea-pig ileum and the mouse vas deferens preparations in which opiates inhibit electrically induced activity, identified two related pentapeptides derived from pig brain which possessed potent, naloxone-reversed, opiate-like activity.[13] These they named *met-enkephalin* and *leu-enkephalin*, in which leucine is substituted for methionine (Fig. 3).

Longer peptides have been isolated, the endorphins, which also possess opiate-like activity, the principal one being termed β-endorphin. The various endorphins were found to form part of β-lipotropin, a pituitary hormone which induces fat metabolism, and which consists of 91 amino-acid residues. Sequence 61 to 91 is that of β-endorphin (Fig. 3), and 61 to 65 that of met-enkephalin. The residues 41 to 58 are those of β-melanotropin (MSH) concerned with skin pigmentation. It would appear therefore that β-lipotropin is the precursor of MSH and the endorphins, though not necessarily of the enkephalins which are more likely to be formed near their site of action. A giant pituitary prohormone, identified by Smythe, composed of about 200 amino-acid residues, contains those forming β-lipotropin and ACTH from different segments.

From Fig. 3 it would appear that opiate-like activity is dependent upon the sequence $H_2N$-tyr-gly-gly-phe-(61-64). This then is the activator sequence, while the remainder of the molecule is the specificity sequence, which addresses the molecule to a specific receptor.

The enkephalins have been found widely distributed in the brain stem and spinal cord of vertebrates, in general in nerve terminals closely associated with opiate receptors.[14] They are found in the globus pallidus, thalamus, periaqueductal grey matter, amygdala, dorsal horn (mainly the substantia gelatinosa) and intestine. Their half-life is extremely short, as befits neurotransmitters; they are rapidly inactivated by aminopeptidases.

Enkephalins are difficult to study because of their biological instability, but stable analogues of enkephalins are found to produce morphine-like effects, to inhibit substance P release in the substantia gelatinosa[7] and acetylcholine release in the brain.[15] Thus inhibitory neurones in the dorsal horn that are activated by descending inhibitory tryptaminergic fibres and collaterals from large sensory fibres (Fig. 2) are enkephalinergic.

β-endorphin is also widely distributed, but is found principally in the hypothalamus, whence it is passed via long axons to the third ventricle. It has a much longer half-life than the enkephalins, and is more suited to a hormonal rôle. It can therefore be assumed that after release into the cerebrospinal fluid, β-endorphin can act on opiate receptors in the brain stem and spinal cord.

β-endorphin appears to possess all the actions of morphine, producing analgesia, euphoria, behavioural effects and hyperglycaemia, and to be equipotent on all opiate receptors[16] (*vide infra*). Thus it can act as a neuromodulator, inhibiting release of acetylcholine and dopamine as well as substance P. But endorphins, unlike enkephalins, are found in the pituitary, and their primary role may well be in hormone regulation, promoting release of vasopressin (*cf* morphine), prolactin (reflecting *inhibition* of dopamine release) and growth hormone (relating to hyperglycaemia). The antidiuretic effect shared by β-endorphin and morphine may, in part, be independent of vasopressin release, since it has been demonstrated in rats devoid of this hormone.[17]

**Mechanisms of analgesia.**—There is good evidence that analgesia produced by electrical stimulation of the periaqueductal grey matter,[18] transcutaneous nerve stimulation, acupuncture (*vide infra*), nitrous oxide,[19,20] ketamine[21] and the placebo response[22] may all be associated with enkephalin or endorphin release, while generalised analgesic effects so produced can be reversed by naloxone.[19,23]

*Local* analgesia, such as may be produced by transcutaneous nerve stimulation[24] and of course by intraspinal opiates (*vide infra*), cannot so readily be reversed by *systemic* naloxone. Naloxone is a competitive antagonist and its effectiveness depends upon the relative concentrations of agonist and antagonist at the receptor. Local administration or release produces a massive local concentration, hard to achieve or to antagonise systemically.

**The mechanisms of acupuncture**[25] require more qualification. Mechanical and low-frequency (2–6 Hz) electroacupuncture releases β-endorphin into the cerebrospinal fluid and produces analgesia which is readily blocked by naloxone. High-frequency (200 Hz) acupuncture on the other hand is associated with met-enkephalin release. Descending tryptaminergic fibres may play a part in the analgesia so produced, since reducing brain 5HT inhibits the analgesic effect of high-frequency electro-acupuncture. Conventional doses of naloxone do not reverse this analgesia, which is in line with a *locally* mediated effect, from release of transmitter in close association with spinal cord receptors (Fig. 2).

Surprise has been expressed that cerebrospinal fluid levels of β-endorphin are very low in the presence of acute and chronic pain.[26] Surely this is precisely what would be expected in the *presence* of pain. The enkephalin/endorphin system is not tonically active along pain pathways, thus naloxone *per se* does not induce pain. It may however render pain-insensitive patients hypersensitive to pain,[27] as well as reversing the placebo response (*vide supra*). Arguments as to whether acupuncture, hypnotism, psychoprophylaxis or any other fringe methods of producing analgesia are better than the placebo, are entirely superfluous, since the placebo response is now so firmly rooted in explicable biochemistry. Placebo analgesia is inhibited by naloxone[22] even though the placebo responder is told when he receives the naloxone that it is an active analgesic!

### Classification of Opiate Receptors

While the enkephalins and β-endorphin would appear to be pure agonists, their potencies on all opiate receptors are not uniform.[16] Morphine-like drugs clearly vary in their agonist/antagonist profiles (see page 813) but this cannot explain certain qualitative differences in their effects. For example the partial agonists pentazocine and nalorphine produce dysphoria, which cannot be explained as the reverse of euphoria, as the pure antagonist naloxone does not produce dysphoria, nor does the partial agonist buprenorphine. To explain these and other anomalies it is necessary to postulate different types of opiate receptor. These have been classified by Martin[28] as

$\mu$ = supraspinal analgesia, euphoria, dependence
$\kappa$ = spinal analgesia, sedation
$\sigma$ = dysphoria

To this, the Kosterlitz classification would add $\delta$ receptors, to explain certain selective effects of leu-enkephalin.

It is now apparent from the effectiveness of $\mu$-agonists and the ineffectiveness of $\kappa$ agonists intraspinally,[29] that the spinal cord contains numerous $\mu$ receptors, but the distinction between $\mu$ and $\sigma$ remains relevant and valid clinically.

## Types of Pain

Pain may be classified according to its origin, that is somatic or visceral; according to its temporal nature, that is acute or chronic, continuous or intermittent; according to the nature of the sensation, that is aching, burning, stabbing, colicky; or, finally, according to its severity.

The origin of the pain can be further amplified as in Fig. 4.

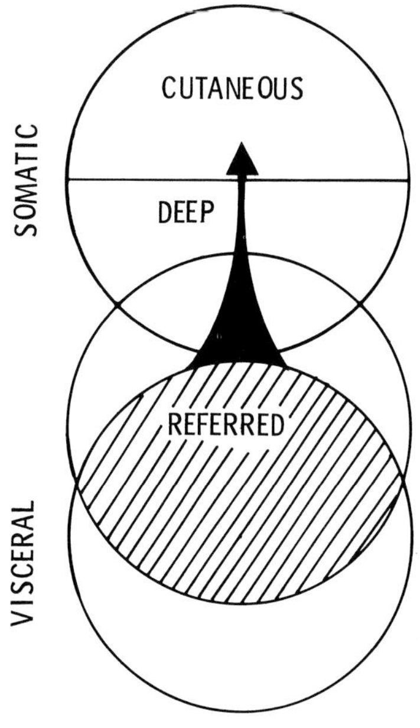


30/Fig. 4.

### Somatic Pain

*Superficial pain* is in general well-localised and much of the research on pain pathways and mechanisms (*vide supra*) relates to studies of superficial pain. Cutaneous sensation, including that to pinprick, can be related with reasonable reproducibility to the spinal segment concerned.

The cutaneous area supplied by a single posterior nerve root is termed a dermatome. Knowledge of these is important in determining the nerve roots that must be blocked when treating pain by epidural or spinal block, or when relieving persistent pain with alcohol, phenol or root section. A dermatome chart of the whole body is shown in Fig. 5, every spinal root being represented except C1. The dermatomes are in fact more extensive than those shown on such a chart as there is considerable overlap in the areas supplied by adjacent roots.

*Deep Pain*.—Pain impulses from joints, tendons, muscle and fascia arise in a network of fine fibres similar to those in the skin and travel by the same nervous pathways. The sensitivity of these tissues appears to vary with the richness of the innervation. Thus the low pain threshold of the periosteum is associated with dense innervation compared to the relatively insensitive and sparsely supplied fibrous muscle septa.[30]

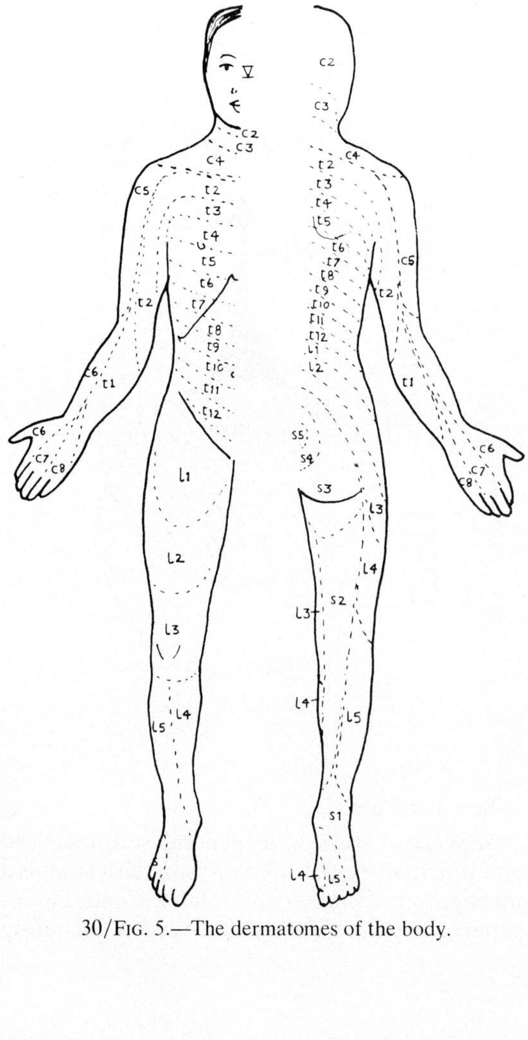

30/Fig. 5.—The dermatomes of the body.

The deep tissue area supplied by a single posterior nerve root is termed a sclerotome, which is not necessarily related to the overlying dermatome. As sclerotomes cannot be mapped as accurately as the dermatomes, it is often difficult to decide which roots are involved in patients with deep pain. For this reason the therapeutic blocking of spinal nerve roots to alleviate deep pain must be more extensive than that for superficial pain.

Deep pain usually has a dull aching character, and it may be accompanied by an unpleasant sickening sensation due to an autonomic response. It is poorly localised and tends to spread to other areas.

The occurrence of pain at some point distant from the site of stimulation is termed "referred pain" and it will be discussed in a later section. Although it is associated more commonly with visceral pain, it can occur with deep nonvisceral structures, as in the case of a diseased hip, when pain may be felt in the knee. Moreover, deep pain may be referred to the dermatome of the same posterior nerve root through which the impulses from the deep structures enter the spinal cord.

Deep pain endings can be stimulated by chemical substances or mechanical forces such as the stretching of muscle fibres. The receptors are especially sensitive in the presence of trauma or infection. Ischaemic muscle pain, as in intermittent claudication, and also the muscle pain provoked by excessive or sustained contractions, are probably due to stimulation of the nerve endings by various metabolic products. Sustained contraction is the likely cause of a large number of muscle pains, including many cases of backache and the neck stiffness associated with headaches. These may have an organic basis, as in meningitis, or may be due to the emotional tension accompanying an anxiety state.[31]

## Visceral Pain

This is transmitted mainly in the fibres which accompany sympathetic nerves, and so pass via the white rami communicantes to the posterior root ganglia, where the cell bodies are situated. The fibres essentially are components of spinal nerves utilising but not relaying in the sympathetic system. The modern tendency is to speak of them as autonomic or visceral afferents. Although the fibres connect with the spinothalamic tract, they are distributed more widely than somatic pain fibres within the cord. This explains why a more extensive cordotomy is generally required for visceral pain. The pain innervation of the viscera is shown in Fig. 6.

Not all visceral pain impulses travel with sympathetic nerves. Those from certain pelvic organs such as the bladder neck, prostate, uterine cervix and lower colon travel with the parasympathetic pelvic nerves to the cord. Also, some pain fibres from the trachea and oesophagus travel in the vagus nerve.

Visceral pain is caused by quite different stimuli from those which activate cutaneous receptors. It is possible, for example, to handle and even cut and burn viscera without producing pain, although mesenteric traction usually causes discomfort. Pain-producing stimuli include chemical irritants, as in peritonitis, sudden distension of organs and excessive contractions and spasms, especially when associated with changes in the blood supply. Normal activity of smooth muscle is painless except when the blood supply is impaired.

Compared with somatic pain, visceral pain is diffuse, less easily localised and often referred. It may be accompanied by either a rise or a fall in pulse and blood pressure, whereas these usually rise with somatic pain. Muscular rigidity and hyperaesthesia are commonly associated with visceral pain.

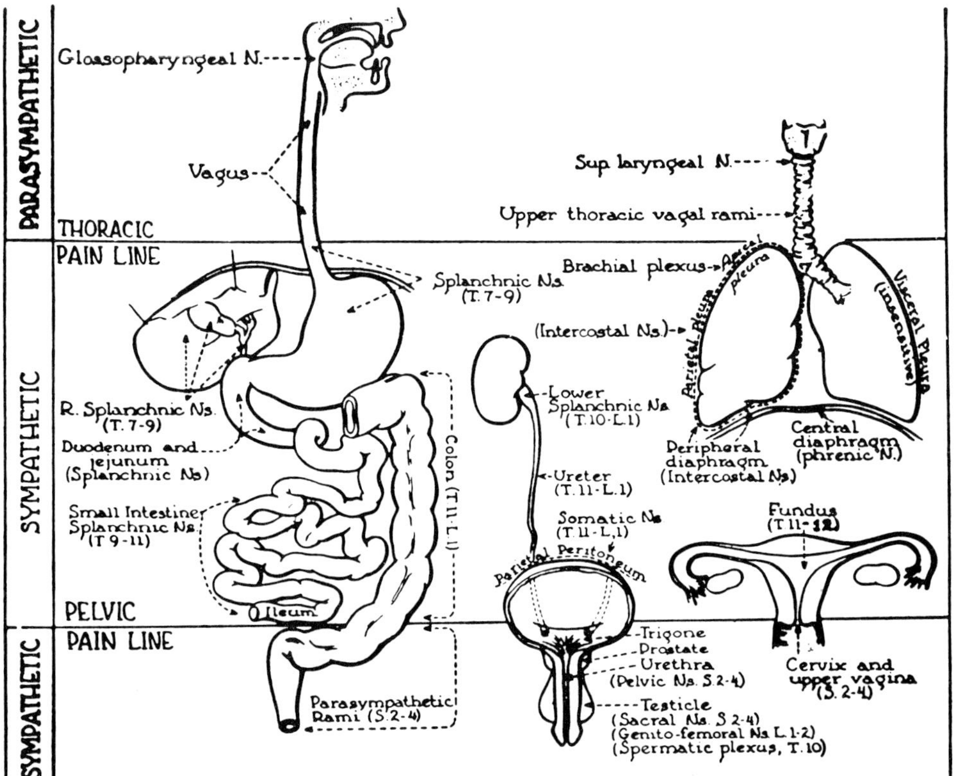


30/Fig. 6.—Pain innervation of the viscera (after Dr. J. C. White and by courtesy of the Williams and Wilkins Co.).

### Referred Pain

Deep pain, whether visceral or somatic in origin, may be felt in some part of the body other than the site of stimulation. Visceral pain tends to have a characteristic localisation for each organ, and is commonly referred to the dermatome of the spinal segment which the afferent fibres enter. The reference of cardiac pain to the left arm and diaphragmatic pain to the shoulder are well-known examples of this phenomenon. The whole of the relevant dermatome may not be involved; for example, pain from abdominal organs is usually felt anteriorly and not in the dorsal part of the segment. The neurophysiological basis of referred pain probably depends on the convergence of several cutaneous and visceral afferent fibres on the same secondary neurone at some point in the pain pathway. Although this may occur in the thalamus or cortex, it is known that the fibres in the spinothalamic tract are outnumbered by the pain fibres in the dorsal root, indicating a convergence of fibres at the spinal level.

### Psychogenic Pain

A psychogenic basis for pain can be inferred when no satisfactory organic cause for it can be found, and its distribution does not accord with a known anatomical pattern. The symptoms, which are a manifestation of a psychological disorder, are often described in a characteristic way. A feeling of pressure or of a tight band constricting the head are well-known examples of such a pain. Pains of psychological origin are usually continuous from day to day and involve more than one part of the body but they do not tend to disturb sleep.[32] The patients are prone to self-pity and have an easily aroused resentment, especially concerning previous treatment. The pain may enable the patient to escape some particular situation or duty and may be heralded by symptoms suggestive of an emotional disturbance.

Protracted organic pain frequently leads to exhaustion, while psychogenic pain is often preceded by a phase of exhaustion. Symptoms may occur at the site of previous trauma or infection, the pain persisting and growing in significance as it becomes the focus of the patient's preoccupation and apprehension. Sciatic pain from a prolapsed intervertebral disc may follow this pattern even when there is no question of impending litigation.

In severe cases psychotherapy may be as important as conventional pain-relieving measures. In any patient suffering from pain, both the somatic and the psychic aspects must be evaluated including the patient's personality and reaction to the present illness.

A strong psychogenic component to pain may be helped by the use of antidepressant drugs or ECT for endogenous depression, and psychotherapy and sedation in neurotic illnesses. There is no doubt that such patients can suffer as acutely as those with a clear-cut physical cause for their pain and are equally deserving of sympathy and compassion. The acceptance of pain at its face value and the institution of the appropriate treatment should be the underlying principle in cases of doubt, rather than the premature diagnosis of a psychogenic disorder.

It is important for the anaesthetist to realise that there is a psychological element to a greater or lesser extent in every patient, which can not only cause pain but can also increase its severity. Simple explanation and kindliness can do much to allay the anxiety of an apprehensive patient especially during a pre-operative ward visit.

## Assessment of Pain and Analgesic Drugs

Assessment of pain is extremely difficult because it is so entirely a subjective sensation. Nevertheless it is essential to have some means of measuring pain if one is to assess the value of analgesic drugs or techniques.

The *type* of pain (i.e. whether burning, aching, stabbing, whether acute or chronic and whether visceral, superficial, or musculoskeletal) must be assessed, in order to select the analgesic agents most suited to its treatment. For example, morphine-like drugs are indicated for aching, visceral pains; anti-inflammatory drugs for arthritic pains; only local anaesthesia can truly alleviate intermittent, sharp and stabbing pains. A potential addictive drug may be used for a short-lived severe pain, but should be avoided for chronic pain unless it is terminal.

The *intensity* of pain must be assessed in any analgesic clinical trial, as in many cases analgesia may only be partial. Methods of measuring pain intensity are described later.

Clinical trials of analgesic drugs and techniques are beset with difficulties, and anyone contemplating one should read at least some of the vast library that has been written on the subject of evaluating pain and analgesia[33–39] and should turn to the *Index Medicus* for recent publications.

The effects of analgesics may be tested on:

1. Experimental pain in animals and man;
2. Clinical pain.

*Experimental* pain has the value that the strength of the stimulus and hence the pain *threshold* and pain *tolerance*, can all be measured. *Clinical* pain, on the other hand, is at least real, it is generally more severe than experimental pain and more susceptible to systemically administered analgesic drugs.

### Experimental Pain in Animals

Techniques involving experimental pain generally measure the pain *threshold* and the effect on it of analgesic techniques. In animals a reflex response usually measures the end-point, and this appears to be related fairly satisfactorily to the pain threshold. The response to pin-prick by twitching of the skin in guinea-pigs can measure local anaesthetic activity. The use of heat (radiant heat causing rat tail-flicking[40] or causing rats and mice to jump from hot plates) has the advantage that the stimulus can be measured accurately, and the pain it produces is more susceptible to systemic analgesics.

Animals make better experimental subjects in this field than man because they are not subject to bias, and unlikely to be placebo reactors, and to them experimental pain is just as worrying as pathological pain.

### Experimental Pain in Man

Although experimental pain is useful for testing local anaesthetics in man (see Chapter 31) it is more difficult to devise experimental pain which is susceptible to systemic analgesic drugs in man. Moreover, nowadays, ethical considerations generally preclude giving potentially addictive agents to volunteers. However, unlike in animals, not only pain *threshold* but also pain tolerance and *intensity* can be assessed in man.

Pain may be produced by pressure on a bony surface, by radiant heat or a faradic current to the skin, or by exercising a limb rendered ischaemic with a sphygmomanometer, which can give predictable results with both classes of analgesic drugs.[41] In all these cases the stimulus *applied* can be measured (temperature, current, duration of exercise). The degree of pain *experienced* can then be assessed after various doses and various drugs.

The disadvantage of experimental pain in assessing systemic analgesics is that both mild analgesics and morphine-like drugs appear to have much less effect on it than on pathological pain. This may be because aspirin-like drugs depend in part for their analgesic effect upon an anti-inflammatory action, while morphine-like drugs are more effective against C-fibre transmitted pathological pain than against Aδ-fibre transmitted experimental pain. They are also more effective in stressful situations associated with clinical pain, in which activation of higher centres and descending inhibiting fibres may play a part.

Electrical stimulation of the tooth socket, however, produces severe pain which is often susceptible to systemic analgesia, and even to placebo.[23] The stimulus is best measured in terms of the electrical current passed, rather than the voltage.[39]

### Clinical Assessment

Clinical pain has the disadvantage that it waxes and wanes spontaneously and can only be evaluated subjectively.

A clinical trial of an analgesic should be limited to one particular field, for example: postoperative, obstetric, rheumatic or terminal pain. In theory, at least two dose levels of the test drug should be compared with a standard reference drug and a placebo, that is at least four treatments. In practice this usually results in the trial becoming too large, unless the duration of pain is long enough for complete cross-over of treatment groups (*vide infra*). A placebo is essential initially to ensure that the method of assessment is sufficiently sensitive to distinguish between the effect of the drug and the placebo response. But once the technique has been validated, a placebo can be omitted, if necessary, on ethical grounds. If the pain is of sufficient duration, a patient may act to an extent as his own control, that is to say he may receive in sequence two, three or more of the different treatments being studied. If pain is too brief or variable, patients must be randomly allocated into different treatment groups, or else be matched with others for age, sex, weight, degree of pain or disability, etc., for sequential analysis. With random allocation, groups must be checked at the end of the trial for comparability.

The possibility that a drug may have a different effect if given in a single dose or repeatedly should be remembered. It should be tested in the way that it is intended to be used. The timing and route of administration should be standardised as much as possible and doses given on a weight basis. The use of a double-blind technique need not preclude this.

**Evaluation of pain.**—The actual *assessment* is the most difficult part. A double-blind technique is essential as the assessment by both patient and observer is subjective and therefore open to bias. Occasionally objective methods, such as vital capacity and peak flow measurement after abdominal surgery, may reinforce evaluation of pain. Assessment should be sufficiently frequent to measure both peak effect and duration of the different treatments, otherwise variations in time course between treatments may falsify results. The patient may be asked to assess the pain as absent/slight/moderate or severe and the response to pain may be assessed by the observer as for example none/slight/marked or excessive. Fixed-interval scales as in the above example have now been superseded by the visual analogue scale, which has been found to be more sensitive, accurate and consistent.[38] By this technique the patient is shown a 10-cm line which he is told represents at one end "no pain at all" and at the other "pain as bad as he could possibly imagine", and is asked to mark the point on the line where his pain lies. This scale has the added advantage that, unlike the fixed-interval scale, the pain can be given a numerical value.

Finally, *side-effects* must be assessed. Appropriate signs such as vomiting, and alterations in blood pressure or respiration should be noted regularly. When seeking symptoms, the use of a check list is often advocated, but Huskisson and Wojtulewski[42] suggested that the incidence of side-effects may be more accurately recorded without a questionnaire, since the influence of suggestion is removed, and symptoms that might have been omitted from the check list are more likely to be volunteered.

Because the disease state may contribute to what appear to be side-effects, their incidence may be more accurately recorded in healthy volunteers, but such a technique would be acceptable only with non-addictive drugs.

## ANALGESIC DRUGS

Analgesic drugs relieve pain in doses which do not impair consciousness. Some drugs relieve pain by a direct effect on its cause: thus glyceryl trinitrate relieves anginal pain by reducing venous return and so reducing heart work; migraine may be relieved by ergotamine, which constricts meningeal vessels; colchicine relieves the pain of acute gout by virtue of an anti-inflammatory effect specific for this condition. None of these drugs is classed as an analgesic, since they affect rather the cause of the pain than its propagation. Anti-inflammatory analgesics, typified by aspirin, do, however, owe a variable but large component of their analgesic effect to a peripheral anti-inflammatory action.

Analgesics may be divided into two main groups:

1. Antipyretic and anti-inflammatory analgesics (prostaglandin synthesis inhibitors);
2. Narcotic analgesics: morphine and related drugs (drugs acting on opiate receptors).

### Prostaglandin Synthesis Inhibitors

These analgesics also possess either an antipyretic effect (e.g. paracetamol) or an anti-inflammatory effect (e.g. indomethacin), or both, as in the case of aspirin.

**Mode of action.**—Prostaglandins ($PGE_2$, $PGF_{2\alpha}$), prostacyclin (epoprostenol; $PGI_2$) and thromboxanes ($TXA_2$ and $TXB_2$) are all formed from the fatty-acid precursor arachidonic acid, via a series of unstable cyclic endoperoxides. It is the enzyme cyclo-oxygenase which catalyses the first step, that is the cyclising and oxygenating of arachidonic acid, which is inhibited by aspirin-like drugs. Synthesis of prostacyclin and thromboxanes as well as prostaglandins is therefore inhibited. Prostacyclin is found mainly in vascular endothelium and causes vasodilatation and diminished platelet adhesiveness. Thromboxanes on the other hand are vasoconstrictor and enhance platelet adhesiveness. Reduced synthesis of the latter results in the loss of platelet stickiness associated with aspirin.

It would appear that paracetamol affects only

the cyclo oxygenase within the central nervous system while anti-inflammatory drugs depress only the peripheral enzymes, and aspirin inhibits both.

These drugs are non-addictive and many are readily available across the counter. Many are incorporated in various BP and proprietary combination tablets, which may also contain other ingredients such as caffeine. The value of such mixtures probably lies simply in their additive effects. The cumulative self-administration over a few years of several kilograms of such combination tablets, principally those containing phenacetin, can cause renal papillary necrosis, an important cause of chronic renal failure.

**Aspirin (Acetylsalicylic Acid)**

This is the oldest and probably the most effective of the mild analgesics. It possesses analgesic, antipyretic and anti-inflammatory actions and although its analgesic effect is in part due to an action on the central nervous system, the peripheral anti-inflammatory action probably accounts for its remarkable effectiveness in relieving pain associated with inflammation. Although inferior to morphine and allied drugs in relieving visceral pain and that due to severe injury, it is superior in relieving headache, toothache, arthritic pain, dysmenorrhoea (probably because of the involvement of prostaglandins in uterine contraction) and that due to skin sepsis.

Aspirin has an antipyretic action mediated via the heat-regulating centre which is set at a lower level, so increasing the heat loss in febrile patients. This is achieved by cutaneous vasodilatation and sweating; aspirin is of especial value in relieving the aching pains associated with pyrexial illnesses such as influenza. When used at night, the antipyretic effect is a useful aid to inducing sleep in febrile patients. It has no effect upon the normal temperature, but since it is a metabolic stimulant it may cause hyperpyrexia in large or toxic doses, especially if there is absence of sweating, as there may be in dehydration and electrolyte depletion.

Aspirin has no effect on mood or consciousness, except when toxic doses cause severe pH and electrolyte disturbances, when coma ensues.

The only important side-effect of a normal dose of aspirin is gastric mucosal irritation with erosion and bleeding. This reaction depends upon a high concentration of non-ionised aspirin produced by stomach contents of a very low pH. Non-ionised aspirin is readily absorbed into the mucosal cells, whose interior pH is much higher. The aspirin will therefore ionise within the cells; it cannot easily diffuse out again once ionised, and so accumulates to produce concentrations which may cause a breach in the protective mucous coating of the stomach. Such an adverse reaction is more likely in the presence of a very low luminal pH, which explains the great differences in sensitivity between individuals. Its occurrence can be minimised by taking aspirin well crushed in a lot of water, with sodium bicarbonate, or as soluble aspirin.

Hypersensitivity occasionally occurs, producing skin rashes. The precipitation of asthma is probably not due to hypersensitivity to aspirin, but rather because excess leukotrienes are produced from arachidonic acid which is not being converted to prostaglandins. Leukotrienes may provoke bronchial muscle contraction, possibly in association with release of SRS-A.

Other adverse reactions to aspirin in general occur only after excessive dosage. It produces respiratory alkalosis due to direct stimulation of the respiratory centre, and metabolic acidosis due to uncoupling oxidative phosphorylation and disturbances of intermediary metabolism. Metabolic acidosis is especially prominent in children, and can occur when they are given large doses in the treatment of rheumatic fever.

Large doses may also prolong the prothrombin time, but the value of aspirin in preventing postoperative deep-vein thrombosis and other coagulative disorders is not yet established.

Symptoms of excessive doses typically are tinnitus and dizziness.

**Administration and dosage.**—Tablets contain 300 mg, and one to three tablets may be taken up to four times a day by adults. The dose commonly prescribed in adult rhematoid arthritis is 900 mg four-hourly (5 times a day). Aspirin soluble tablets BP, or Disprin, or one of many sustained-release or combined preparations (*vide infra*) may be preferred to reduce gastric irritation. An injectable form has been developed in combination with lysine for intramuscular injection.[43] Children should be given aspirin paediatric preparations, or Junior Aspirin tablets, which contain 75 mg of aspirin. The dose is approximately 10 mg/kg, three to four times a day. Aspirin is contra-indicated in the presence of peptic ulceration and bleeding disorders, and in those taking steroids (other than in rheumatoid arthritis) or oral anti-coagulants.

**Acute salicylate poisoning** represents about 15 per cent of all acute poisonings that are admitted to hospital,[44] and 45 per cent of analgesic poisoning.[45] The mortality in adults is 1–2 per cent, while in children it is around 7 per cent.

Direct stimulation of the respiratory centre leads initially to a respiratory alkalosis. This feature is not prominent in children. Metabolic stimulation leads to increased $CO_2$ production (which later overcomes the early reduction in $Paco_2$), increased $O_2$ demand, accumulation of fixed acids and hyperpyrexia from increased heat production. The consequent metabolic acidosis becomes increasingly severe with time, and may be marked from the start in children. Dehydration, because of sweating, hyperventilation and hyperpyrexia, is a prominent and serious complication. Consciousness is maintained unless the biochemical abnormality is severe. Ultimately, as in all forms of overdose, respiration is depressed.

**Treatment.**—Therapeutic measures include gastric lavage and intravenous fluid therapy to correct dehydration, electrolyte losses and acid-base disturbances. These changes can best be managed if repeated blood pH and $Pco_2$ or standard bicarbonate measurements are carried out. Intravenous sodium bicarbonate is especially valuable both to correct the metabolic acidosis and to alkalinise the urine, which promotes salicylate excretion. Diuretics are not usually indicated and may actually be harmful, especially in children, as they may add to the fluid and electrolyte disturbances; nor do they promote salicylate excretion.[167]

Rehydration is affected with 5 per cent dextrose solution with the addition of sodium bicarbonate and potassium chloride to correct acidosis and hypokalaemia. Sodium bicarbonate is indicated if the arterial blood pH is less than 7·5 and urinary pH less than 7·6. In severe intoxication accompanied by renal failure, haemodialysis is required, while in children in the presence of coma and hyperpyrexia, artificial ventilation may be indicated.

### Paracetamol (Acetaminophen USP, Panadol)

Paracetamol is an antipyretic analgesic which has no anti-inflammatory action. Many individuals find it to be a less effective analgesic than aspirin, but it is very popular and widely used, both by prescription and across the counter, owing to its freedom from side-effects in normal doses and lack of drug interactions. It does not cause gastric irritation or bleeding and may be taken with oral anticoagulants and steroids. There are thus no contra-indications to its use. Unlike aspirin it is of no value in the treatment of rheumatoid arthritis, though both aspirin and paracetamol may be used to treat post-operative pain once the worst is over and medication can be taken by mouth. Paracetamol tablets contain 0·5 g and two tablets may be taken four times a day.

The one serious disadvantage of paracetamol is its toxicity in acute overdose. It has become increasingly popular among those making suicide bids and now more than 1000 cases of paracetamol poisoning are admitted to hospital annually in England and Wales, of which at least 3 per cent die.[46] It is involved in 30 per cent of analgesic poisonings.[45] The major and notable danger of acute paracetamol overdose is hepatotoxicity, which may occur after as few as 12 to 14 tablets. This is caused by toxic products of intermediary metabolism, which accumulate in the liver when the normal metabolic pathways are saturated. After the overdose has been taken consciousness is not lost, and no effect is normally observed for the first few days, after which liver damage may become apparent and occasionally leads to hepatic coma and death. Treatment is extremely difficult and cannot be successful once severe liver damage has occurred. It is aimed at (i) limiting the absorption of paracetamol from the gastro-intestinal tract in the early stages with oral cholestyramine or activated charcoal, (ii) removing it from the blood by charcoal haemoperfusion, haemodialysis or diuresis, and (iii) reducing hepatotoxicity with steroids, or cysteamine, methionine or penicillamine.[47] Few of these procedures have proved to be of value, though the use of cysteamine, itself a rather toxic substance, appears to be very successful provided it is given within 10 hours of the ingestion of paracetamol.[48] Paracetamol overdose may also induce acute renal failure, either alone or in association with hepatic damage.[49]

### Phenacetin

Phenacetin used to be present in many compound analgesic tablets and was rarely used alone. Compound tablets containing phenacetin have now been withdrawn because of the danger of renal damage with continued use.

### Compound Analgesic Preparations

Numerous preparations are available which contain combinations of two or more analgesics and other odds and ends, and may include aspirin, paracetamol, codeine, dextropropoxyphene (*vide infra*) and other analgesics and caffeine. Their analgesic effects summate and in some instances preparations are formulated to reduce gastric irritation from aspirin. For example Safapryn contains paracetamol in the outer layer and aspirin in the core, while benorylate is a chemical combination of aspirin with paracetamol, which is only broken down after absorption. This preparation is in a liquid form and fairly well tolerated by many, though liable to give symptoms of aspirin toxicity.[50]

### Anti-inflammatory Agents

There is a large number of drugs of little use as analgesics except in the treatment of inflammatory conditions such as rheumatoid arthritis. All produce gastric irritation in proportion to their efficacy as anti-inflammatory agents. Phenylbutazone is one of the oldest and produces a surfeit of side-effects the most dangerous of which is hypersensitivity-type bone marrow depression. It may also produce rashes, diarrhoea and fluid retention. Indomethacin is now more commonly used, since hypersensitivity to it is rare. Other preparations include ibuprofen, ketoprofen, fenoprofen, alclofenac, mefenamic acid, flufenamic acid, oxyphenbutazone, naproxen, etc.

## Opiates

The term "opiate" used to refer only to the alkaloids of opium, the general term for any morphine-like drug being "narcotic analgesic." Because "narcotic" acquired a legalistic New York flavour, the term "opioid" was coined. This word, however, is somewhat dysphonic and frequently misspelt, and many now adopt the view that an opiate is correctly any drug which acts on opiate receptors.

This second group of analgesics includes a collection of drugs related to morphine either chemically or in their effects, or both.

They have certain chemical similarities, for example all are tertiary amines. They may be classified chemically into the following groups:

| | |
|---|---|
| 1. Natural alkaloids of opium (phenanthrene derivatives) | morphine<br>codeine |
| 2. Semi-synthetic derivatives: | diamorphine<br>dihydrocodeine<br>oxymorphone |
| Thebaine derivative: | buprenorphine |
| 3. Synthetic compounds: | |
| a. morphinans | levorphanol |
| b. benzmorphans | phenazocine<br>pentazocine |
| c. phenylpiperidine derivatives | pethidine<br>phenoperidine<br>fentanyl |
| d. diphenyl compounds | methadone<br>dextromoramide<br>dextropropoxyphene |

They vary in their agonist/antagonist profiles (see Chapter 18) and in their effects on different types of opiate receptor (see Classification of opiate receptors, page 805). Some, such as morphine and fentanyl, are effectively pure agonists at $\mu$ receptors, with a high efficacy—that is a high ceiling effect. They can combat severe pain and produce profound degrees of respiratory depression. Some, usually termed partial agonists or (perhaps less ambiguously) agonist/antagonists, also have some antagonist activity, which implies lower efficacy but a high affinity for receptors. Such drugs may also produce dysphoria by virtue of an agonist effect at $\sigma$ receptors (for example, pentazocine, nalorphine), or act only on $\mu$ receptors and so avoid this drawback (for example, buprenorphine). Some are weak agonists (for example, codeine, dextropropoxyphene or, somewhat stronger, methadone) without maximal efficacy, but because they lack high affinity for receptors, are devoid of antagonist activity. Naloxone, the pure antagonist, is quite without effect on receptors in its own right, but because of a high affinity for all opiate receptors, can reverse all the effects of the agonists. The predicted effects of these agonist/antagonist profiles on the log-dose/response curves of certain agents are shown in Fig. 7.

Morphine can be taken as the standard with which the others are compared. It produces a number of side-effects, which are possessed by the rest to a greater or lesser degree. They may induce drug dependence to an extent related to their euphoriant effect, and also, regrettably, to their agonist activity and consequently their efficacy as analgesics. The maximum respiratory depressant effect tends to be related to the maximum degree of analgesia of which each is capable; thus with codeine, maximum respiratory depression and analgesia are mild while with fentanyl, at the other end of the scale, both are profound. There is some variation in the sedative effect, but this may depend as much upon the individual as upon the drug. There is variation in absorption from the gastro-intestinal tract. Some, such as dextromoramide, diamorphine, and methadone, are well absorbed by mouth. Others, such as morphine, may be conjugated in the gut wall and little is absorbed unchanged. Those that are less well absorbed are more likely to produce constipation. Finally they vary in their duration of action, morphine, lasting about 4 hours, being intermediate in duration. The actions of morphine will be described first, and the remainder compared with it.

## Morphine

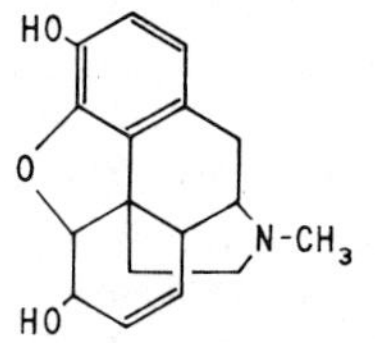


Morphine is the principal alkaloid contained in opium, of which it forms 10 per cent by weight. Opium is the dried powder derived from the milky exudate of the seed capsule of the poppy *Papaver somniferum*.

While the tertiary amine group confers on morphine the property of a weak base, the phenolic and alcoholic hydroxyl groups have weakly acidic properties and render the molecule very poorly lipophylic.

**Mode of action.**—Morphine produces its major effects on the central nervous system and the bowel. By virtue of an agonist effect on opiate receptors, it inhibits release of substance P along pain pathways[7] and in the gastro-intestinal tract,[51] and release of dopamine (probably in relation to the hormone-regulating role of $\beta$-endorphin) and acetylcholine[15] in the central nervous system.

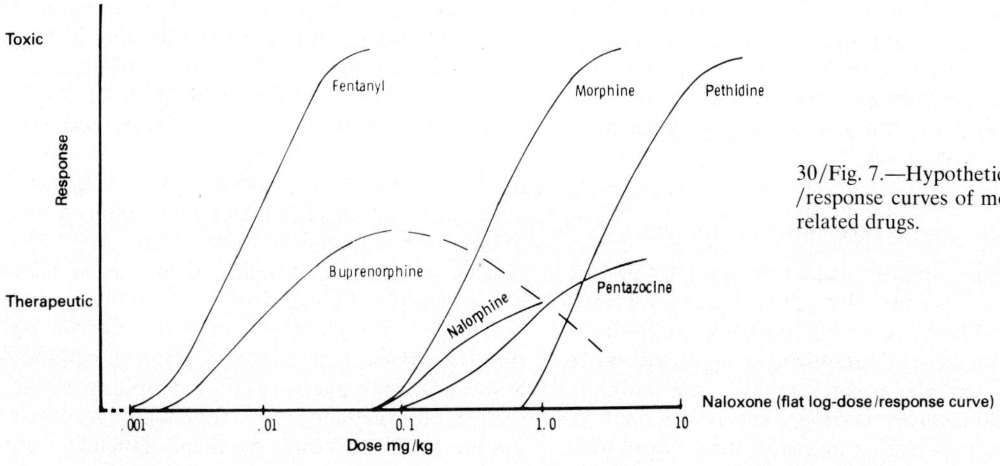


30/Fig. 7.—Hypothetical log-dose/response curves of morphine and related drugs.

The inhibition of transmitter release is a result of a reduction of cyclic AMP formation in opiate-sensitive neurones,[52] probably because of inhibition of adenylcyclase. Tolerance arises because such cells, continuously exposed to opiates, acquire a greater capacity to form cyclic AMP. Coffee is known to accentuate and, in overdose, to mimic opiate withdrawal, because by inhibiting brain phosphodiesterase it helps increase cyclic AMP levels in opiate-sensitive cells.

For an account of the neurophysiological effects of morphine *vide supra*, under inhibition of pain transmission, opiate receptors, endogenous opiates and mechanisms of analgesia (see p. 803 *et seq*.).

*Analgesia*.—It produces analgesia without impairing consciousness, although as the name narcotic implies it may induce drowsiness in many individuals. It is especially effective in combating dull, aching pain and less effective in sharp, intermittent pain.

*Mood*.—Morphine reduces worry, fear, hunger and fatigue and generally induces a drowsy and detached tranquillity. Accompanying this in most individuals is quite marked euphoria and associated with it a liability to produce dependence. While a very few individuals may be "hooked" after a single dose, physical dependence can be produced in all after a large number of doses. The sedative effect is species-dependent: cats and a few humans are stimulated by morphine.

*The respiratory centre* is depressed, leading to a reduction in the respiratory rate and minute volume. In therapeutic doses, the tidal volume is not necessarily decreased and may even be increased. The sensitivity of the respiratory centre to $CO_2$ is decreased and though the minute volume may appear to be within normal limits it will be found to be associated with a raised $Paco_2$. Respiratory depression is progressive with increasing doses and is the principal toxic effect of overdose, after which the respiratory rate may fall to three per minute. *Cough* is also markedly depressed.

*Other brain-stem effects*.—Morphine produces pin-point pupils because it stimulates the Edinger-Westphal nucleus—the parasympathetic nucleus of the oculomotor nerve. There is also stimulation of the chemoreceptor trigger zone, which appears to possess opiate receptors in series with dopamine receptors. Thus enkephalins, applied to the area postrema in the dog, induce emesis which is naloxone-reversible while that due to the dopamine agonist apomorphine is not,[12] and that due to morphine also can be inhibited by the dopamine antagonist metoclopramide. Vomiting is commoner in women than in men, and in ambulant than in resting patients. Morphine should only be given therefore to those confined to bed. The vasomotor centre is only slightly depressed, except in the presence of severe respiratory depression with brain-stem hypoxia.

*Cardiovascular system*.—Morphine releases histamine which may produce peripheral vasodilatation and a warm, itching skin. This property, coupled with mild vasomotor centre depression, may occasionally produce postural hypotension, and hypotension after haemorrhage. In the normal recumbent subject, blood pressure is not reduced by a standard intramuscular dose unless severe respiratory depression produces medullary hypoxia. Small (10 mg or less) intravenous doses may cause a slight fall in systolic blood pressure[53,54] and a dose-related fall in peripheral resistance.[55] Dilatation of capacitance vessels may contribute to the beneficial effect of morphine in acute left ventricular failure.

*Gastro-intestinal tract*.—Visceral muscle tone is increased, especially at the pyloric and ileocaecal sphincters. Furthermore, peristalsis throughout the gastro-intestinal tract is reduced, so causing delay in gastric emptying, and constipation. The muscle tone of the biliary ducts is increased and the sphincter of Oddi is contracted, effects which may aggravate the pain of biliary colic. The resultant increase in bile-duct pressure may be reversed by both atropine[56] and naloxone.[57]

*Hormonal effects*.—See under Endogenous opiates, page 804.

*Overdose*.—After an overdose of morphine the respiratory rate is extremely slow and the patient may become comatose, hypotensive and cyanosed. The respiratory depression, coupled with pin-point pupils, is usually diagnostic of narcotic overdose, though *in extremis* the pupils may dilate. A reduced tolerance to morphine is the most usual cause of such toxicity. Intense pain may antagonise the side-effects of morphine and the patient may require increasing doses of the drug. With a reduction in pain, tolerance is diminished and the patient may show signs of overdose. In acute coronary thrombosis such a collapse may be ascribed to the disease rather than to morphine, and similarly in the post-operative period surgical shock and blood loss may be incorrectly blamed. An addict becomes tolerant of narcotics, and may require vastly increasing doses. After a period of abstinence, sensitivity is restored, and if the addict then gives himself his previous dose, acute toxicity ensues.

Narcotic overdose should be treated with a narcotic antagonist (*vide infra*) as well as with the usual supportive measures.

*Absorption, distribution and fate.*—Morphine is poorly absorbed from the gastro-intestinal tract because it is poorly lipid-soluble and conjugated in the gut wall.[58] For reliable effect, therefore, it must be given by injection. When given intravenously, initially it is cleared fairly rapidly from the plasma and quite extensively taken up in the tissues having a distribution volume of 3·4 l/kg.[59] It crosses the blood-brain barrier extremely slowly in marked contrast to its more lipid-soluble derivative diamorphine.[60] After intravenous injection in dogs, the CSF concentration does not reach a peak for 15 to 30 minutes.[61] It has an elimination half-life of 1 to 2 hours, undergoing complete hepatic extraction and conjugation with glucuronic acid. In dogs, 66 per cent of a dose is excreted in 6 hours, glucuronides accounting for about 90 per cent.[61] Tolerance is not apparently related to enzyme induction.[168]

*Uses.*—The tranquillising effect of morphine makes it an excellent premedicant; moreover its analgesic property is a useful adjunct to anaesthesia. Probably its greatest value is in the treatment of severe pain due for example to myocardial infarction, injury, surgery and terminal cancer. It is little used in obstetrics, in which pethidine is the preferred narcotic in most centres. It is an effective cough suppressant, but other related drugs such as codeine or pholcodine, with more specific antitussive effects and less addiction liability, are to be preferred. It is sometimes used in the treatment of dyspnoea associated with acute left ventricular failure and pulmonary oedema, in which both the reduced respiratory drive and the cardiovascular effect described above are valuable. It may be used to facilitate controlled respiration, as depressing the respiratory centre may help to stop the patient fighting the ventilator when prolonged mechanical ventilation is required in intensive care. Finally, morphine is an excellent remedy for diarrhoea, for which purpose it is taken orally in kaolin and morphine mixture or in Chlorodyne, which cause minimal systemic effects. Its intraspinal use is discussed on page 823.

*Contra-indications and dangers.*—Narcotics should not be used in the control of chronic pain in non-terminal conditions, such as various musculoskeletal disorders, because the risk of producing dependence is too great. In such conditions aspirin, indomethacin or even steroids are to be preferred.

In subjects receiving morphine regularly the risk of addiction must be borne in mind. The onset of tolerance gives warning that addiction is developing. When satisfactory relief cannot be obtained with other analgesics the risk of addiction must be accepted, especially in the terminal stages of cancer when a fatal outcome is inevitable in a matter of months.

Narcotics should be avoided in acute asthmatic attacks and acute or chronic bronchitis and emphysema, not because of any effect upon the airways but because in such patients respiratory drive must be preserved, otherwise carbon dioxide narcosis may be precipitated. Obese and scoliotic patients may be quite disastrously sensitive to the respiratory depressant effects of even small doses of narcotics.

Morphine and all allied drugs are contra-indicated in head injury in the absence of controlled ventilation, because the $CO_2$ retention they produce causes cerebral vasodilatation and so increases the intracranial pressure. Exactly the same danger exists in eclampsia.

So long as the dose is administered on a body-weight basis, age makes little difference to narcotic sensitivity. Those with adrenocortical and thyroid deficiencies require reduced doses, which should probably also be used in renal failure, to avoid accumulation of conjugates. Patients with hepatic disease may require a reduced frequency of dosage, but hepatic disease does not always impair drug inactivation.

*Administration and dosage.*—The usual dose of morphine is 0·1–0·2 mg/kg, although more than this may be required in resistant individuals. It may be given 4-hourly by intramuscular or subcutaneous injection, though in the presence of severe vasoconstriction absorption from subcutaneous tissues may be very slow and small divided intravenous doses are preferred. Postoperatively, analgesia can be improved by the use of intravenous infusion.[62–64] One-ml ampoules may contain 10, 15, 20 or 30 mg of morphine sulphate. Morphine sulphate contains 75 per cent of anhydrous morphine base. Oral preparations are occasionally used, and recently controlled-release tablets have been introduced which are said to be of value in chronic pain when a very slow onset of action is immaterial. Plasma levels are just detectable in normal volunteers,[65] but oral preparations are in general singularly useless in the treatment of acute pain.[66]

**Papaveretum (Omnopon, Opoidine).**—This consists of all the water-soluble alkaloids of opium (morphine, codeine, papaverine, thebaine, narcotine, etc.) in the same proportions as they are in opium, and is standardised to contain 50 per cent of anhydrous morphine. The contribution of the other constituents to the overall effect of papaveretum is minimal. The adult dose of papaveretum is 10–20 mg, and that for a child 0·25 mg/kg. For premedication 10 mg of papaveretum combined with hyoscine gives good sedation for the average adult and a lower incidence of nausea and oversedation than when 20 mg of papaveretum is used. Papaveretum is useful for postoperative analgesia and may be preferred to morphine for intramuscular administration because it is cheaper.

**Nepenthe.**—Nepenthe is a liquid preparation of the opium alkaloids with added morphine such that one ml of nepenthe contains 8·4 mg of anhydrous morphine. It is thus *stronger* than the ordinary preparation of morphine sulphate 10 mg/ml and has no advantage over it for paediatric administration.

### Codeine

Codeine, or methyl morphine, is a homologue of morphine in which the $-OH$ group on the benzene ring is replaced with $-OCH_3$. It is therefore more lipid-soluble than morphine, and better absorbed by mouth.

The analgesic effect of codeine is weak and resides in part in the very small proportion of codeine which is converted to morphine in the liver. Codeine does not normally produce sedation, euphoria, addiction or marked respiratory depression, though it is an effective cough suppressant and usually causes constipation.

The analgesic dose of 60 mg of codeine phosphate serves no useful purpose for pain relief though it may help to suppress diarrhoea. 8–10 mg of codeine, present in various proprietary compound analgesic tablets, can have little analgesic effect. Codeine linctus, for cough suppression, contains 15 mg codeine phosphate per 5 ml dose.

### Diamorphine (Heroin)

Diamorphine is available legally in few western countries outside Great Britain but several differences from morphine make it valuable in certain fields of medicine.

In diamorphine, the two hydroxyl groups of morphine are replaced by acetyl ($CH_3COO-$) groups. This chemical alteration makes diamorphine more lipid-soluble, more readily and completely absorbed from the gastro-intestinal tract (until de-acetylated it cannot be conjugated) and more rapid in its passage across the blood-brain barrier.[60] It has a high ceiling for analgesia and produces less vomiting, constipation and sedation than morphine, but a very marked degree of euphoria. It is active as monoacetyl morphine and morphine to which it is broken down.

Its rapid onset of action and high-ceiling effect undoubtedly contribute to its worldwide popularity as a drug of abuse. However its oral effectiveness and relative freedom from side-effects make it of special value in the treatment of pain in terminal malignant disease, and in combination with cocaine it is of remarkable benefit. It is also used in a few centres in Great Britain for obstetric pain relief.

It is of similar potency to morphine.

### Dihydrocodeine (DF 118)

This is a semisynthetic derivative of codeine with superior analgesic activity. It is therefore an analgesic of intermediate activity producing little respiratory depression and dependence liability. Although useful for the latter reason in chronic pain, constipation can be a problem. It may be taken orally or by injection in a dose of 30–60 mg.

### Oxymorphone

This is a very potent morphine analogue with a high ceiling for analgesia and side-effects. It is little used clinically but its N-allyl derivative, naloxone (*vide infra*) is the first pure antagonist in therapeutic use.

**Buprenorphine (Temgesic)**

Buprenorphine is a highly lipid-soluble partial agonist, and slow dissociation from opiate receptors coupled with a long half-life, insure a long duration of action, depending upon the route of administration. If given by bolus intravenous injection intra-operatively, 0·3 mg has effects remarkably similar to low-dose fentanyl.[67] Unlike fentanyl, however, progressive increases in dose do not result in high-ceiling effects, but rather in antagonist effects,[68,69] resulting in a bell-shaped log dose/response curve (Fig. 7).

If given intramuscularly it is somewhat longer lasting than after intravenous administration, associated with more sustained plasma concentrations.[70] By the sublingual route (usefully non-invasive and bypassing the liver) 0·4 mg produces a slow and sustained rise in plasma concentration and a duration of action of 6–8 hours, significantly longer than that of 10 mg of morphine[71] or 20 mg of papaveretum,[72] though side-effects such as nausea and vomiting may be severe.[169,170] It increases intrabiliary pressure[73] and causes haemodynamic changes similar to morphine,[54] but 0·6 mg checks the rise in glucose and cortisol concentration that normally accompany major surgery.[74]

Its long duration of action when given sublingually makes it a useful analgesic for the postoperative period, but respiratory depression, though rare, is prolonged[171] and difficult to treat when it does occur. Naloxone, a drug of briefer duration of action anyway, has difficulty in counteracting the effects of buprenorphine, a partial agonist with remarkably high receptor affinity. For this reason, and also because it does not reverse analgesia, doxapram has been recommended to reverse respiratory depression due to buprenorphine.

**Levorphanol**

The properties of levorphanol are similar to those of phenazocine (*vide infra*) but because it is older it is less used nowadays. Its N-allyl derivative levallorphan, however, was used as an antagonist.

**Phenazocine (Narphen)**

Phenazocine is of similar efficacy as an analgesic to morphine, but is effective orally, produces less sedation, raises intrabiliary pressure less,[75] and has a longer duration of action. The incidence of other side-effects is similar. It is no longer available in injectable form and the oral dose is usually 5 mg.

**Pentazocine (Fortral)**

Pentazocine was first tested in animals as a narcotic antagonist but was found in man to be a partial agonist with useful analgesic activity. It was originally hoped that it would be as effective an analgesic as morphine but with less risk of addiction and severe respiratory depression. In practice it is intermediate in its efficacy as an analgesic: less effective than morphine and similar to dihydrocodeine. It also produces only slight respiratory depression and neither of these effects is augmented by increasing the dose. Hypertension rather than hypotension may be produced.[76] It produces little or no euphoria, but quite substantial dysphoria in a few individuals. Addiction is rare and typical physical dependence is not seen. It is less likely than morphine and pethidine to raise intrabiliary pressure.[56,75]

Its effects can be reversed by naloxone.

It is indicated in the treatment of chronic pain of intermediate severity when dependence must be avoided but it is generally less effective than "mild" analgesics for skeletal pain.[77] In obstetrics it produces less effective pain relief than pethidine, but fewer side-effects, and crosses the placenta less (see Chapter 41). It is of briefer duration than pethidine and less cumulative.

Because of its flat dose response curve, 20–60 mg may be equivalent to 10 mg of morphine by injection, while the oral dose is 25–100 mg. Because of its extremely brief duration it is rarely given with sufficient frequency, but is probably better never used at all.

**Pethidine (Meperidine USP, Demerol)**

The effects of pethidine are very similar to those of morphine, the principal difference being that both analgesia and side-effects are of quicker onset and briefer duration. The sedative and tranquillising effects are almost as good, and though the incidence of nausea, vomiting, dry mouth, hypotension and dizziness is transiently higher than after morphine, the duration of these side-effects is briefer.[78] Respiratory depression is as profound as with morphine, though of shorter duration. Indeed, significant respiratory depression has been demonstrated in volunteers in subanalgesic doses,[79] though pethidine cannot usefully suppress the cough reflex. Euphoria cannot be as reliably produced by pethidine as by morphine and diamorphine; nevertheless pethidine is widely abused.

Pethidine does not cause gastro-intestinal tract spasm as does morphine; it is less likely to produce constipation and cannot be used to treat diarrhoea. It has no spasmolytic action in therapeutic doses, and it increases intrabiliary pressure as markedly as does an equi-analgesic dose of morphine.[56] It does not produce meiosis. One serious disadvantage of pethidine is its dangerous interaction with monoamine oxidase inhibitors. Pethidine given to patients taking this type of antidepressant may produce coma, convulsions, hypertension, hyperpyrexia and occasionally hypotension and respiratory depression. The mechanism is probably an interaction occurring within the brain, where pethidine inhibits neuronal 5-HT re-uptake, an action not shared by most other opiates.[80] Although monoamine oxidase inhibitors may slightly retard the metabolism of all narcotics, they do not contra-indicate the cautious use of any except pethidine and dextromethorphan, a cough suppressant.

Pethidine is more lipid-soluble than morphine, possessing no polar hydroxyl groups. It cannot therefore be conjugated directly, but is fairly rapidly N-dealkylated and also hydroxylated in the liver. The first-pass clearance is about 50 per cent[81] and the principal initial metabolite, norpethidine, has convulsant properties. The distribution volume of pethidine itself is about 4 l/kg and the half-life 3–4 hours.[82]

Pethidine may be used for analgesia in all the situations in which morphine is used, though its duration of action is generally shorter, making it less suitable by intramuscular injection for postoperative pain. The important place it has in obstetric analgesia is hallowed by tradition. The effects it may have upon the fetus and neonate are far-reaching (see Chapter 41) but it is the preferred narcotic in this field because up to 300 mg can be given by midwives without medical prescription.

Pethidine is one-tenth as potent as morphine and the dose is 1·0–2·0 mg/kg. Though sometimes taken by mouth in 25 or 50 mg tablets, it has no merit by this route. If given intravenously, its onset of action is quicker than that of morphine, making it useful intra-operatively. It has also been given by this route postoperatively, either using a patient-demand system, or by a continuous infusion, whose rate must be reduced gradually for some hours to avoid accumulation.[83]

### Phenoperidine (Operidine) and Fentanyl (Sublimaze)

Both these agents are capable of producing profound analgesia and respiratory depression, and occasionally muscular rigidity, while delirium has been reported after fentanyl.[84] Phenoperidine is generally used when a prolonged action is required, for example, during controlled ventilation after major surgery. Fentanyl, on the other hand, is commonly used by bolus intravenous injection intra-operatively, though as a sole anaesthetic, even a high dose has been associated with awareness.[85] It causes a marked rise in intrabiliary pressure in guinea-pigs.[56] Both drugs are used in conjunction with butyrophenones during neuroleptanalgesia.

The dose of phenoperidine is 1–2 mg in an adult. Fentanyl may be given in a dose varying from 1–100 μg/kg. This is not because the log dose/response curve is any flatter than that of morphine, but rather because it is possible to produce a profound effect in terms of analgesia and respiratory depression with high-dose fentanyl without any undue disturbance of the circulation, because histamine release is negligible.[172] Hypotension has, however, been recorded with both agents when their use is associated with dramatic relief of pain. High-dose fentanyl greatly reduces the metabolic response to surgery, preventing the hyperglycaemia and increased cortisol levels which normally occur.[86,87] However, the risks of respiratory depression in the postoperative period[173] and of dangerous summation with other opiates given at this time are considerable after high intra-operative doses.

It should be stressed that the apparently brief action of fentanyl is *not* due to rapid elimination. Fentanyl is highly lipophilic and, therefore has a rapid onset of action after intravenous injection, but it dissociates rapidly from receptors and an enormous distribution volume insures rapid initial clearance of the drug from the circulation. It is concentrated in muscle, gastric lumen and all intracellular compartments and, consequently, plasma concentrations, having fallen, may rise again markedly with muscle movement[88] and gastric emptying.[89] Such resurgence into the circulation may be associated with delayed respiratory depression,[174] and Trudnowski[90] has suggested that antacid administration, by reducing fentanyl sequestration in the stomach, might enhance its safety. Because of fluctuations in fentanyl plasma concentrations after bolus administration, its elimination half-life is hard to measure and, certainly, extremely long. It has been found to be more than seven hours in post-cardiopulmonary bypass patients.[88] In order to achieve a constant plasma concentration in so extensively distributed a drug, it is necessary to make a 10- to 30-fold reduction in infusion rate over a few hours.[91,92]

**Methadone (Physeptone, Amidone)**

Methadone is similar to morphine in potency and in many of its actions but, in general, the onset and cessation of its effects are more gradual, its ceiling effect is lower and the total duration is much longer. Its half-life is one to three days.[93] It is effective orally, and sedation and constipation are less conspicuous. It is a powerful cough suppressant and may be taken in a linctus for severe intractable cough. It is useful orally in the treatment of severe chronic pain and is also used extensively in the treatment of heroin dependence. It can prevent withdrawal symptoms in an addict, while its own withdrawal symptoms are relatively gradual and mild. Despite a lower efficacy than morphine, methadone is devoid of antagonist properties because its affinity for opiate receptors is too low.

**Dextromoramide (Palfium)**

Dextromoramide is similar to morphine in most actions, but of briefer duration, less sedative and constipating, and as effective orally as parenterally. The adult dose is about 5 mg.

**Dextropropoxyphene (Propoxyphene USP)**

Propoxyphene is a mild analgesic, similar to codeine; the d-isomer possesses the analgesic activity. Dextropropoxyphene is present in Distalgesic tablets in a dose of 32·5 mg per tablet, in combination with 325 mg of paracetamol. The effect of 65 mg of dextropropoxyphene alone is better than that of placebo,[94] and there is no doubt that as Distalgesic it has become extremely popular in Great Britain in recent years. A proportion of its effectiveness may stem from the marked placebo effect of the coffin-shaped tablets. Overdose of Distalgesic can produce dangerous respiratory depression,[95] but the dose of paracetamol that is taken is rarely big enough to produce serious hepatic damage.[45]

## Tolerance and Dependence

Tolerance to all the effects of morphine-like drugs, with the possible exception of constipation, is readily acquired with continuous but not with intermittent use. Tolerance to the emetic effects occurs very quickly, while that to respiratory depression occurs more slowly but is present to an extent anyway in the presence of severe pain. Tolerance to the analgesic and euphoriant effects usually heralds the onset of dependence. Although on occasion almost any drug may induce psychological dependence, a narcotic agonist will always, after days or weeks of continuous administration, produce both psychological and physical dependence. On withdrawal, severe withdrawal symptoms result; these can be suppressed by the administration of another narcotic agonist. A partial agonist such as pentazocine cannot prevent withdrawal symptoms. If an addict is given a narcotic *antagonist*, withdrawal symptoms are precipitated. These typically consist of running eyes, nose and mouth, sweating, gooseflesh, anxiety, restlessness, dilated pupils, nausea, vomiting, and abdominal and muscle cramps. When methadone is substituted for heroin in the treatment of addiction, and then withdrawn, symptoms are mild and rarely worse than an influenza-like illness. For an explanation of tolerance, see page 815.

## Narcotic Antagonists

**Nalorphine (N-allylnormorphine: Lethidrone) and levallorphan (N-allylnorlevorphanol: Lorfan)** are partial agonists, with agonist effects on $\sigma$ receptors, thereby producing dysphoria. They have no place in clinical practice today.

**Naloxone (Narcan)**

Naloxone is the N-alkyl derivative of oxymorphone. It is a highly effective antagonist at all types of opiate receptors, and is devoid of agonist activity. When given alone therefore it produces neither analgesia nor respiratory depression and neither euphoria nor dysphoria. It blocks $\mu$, $\kappa$ and $\sigma$ receptors and therefore reverses all the effects of opiates. So selective is the action of naloxone on opiate receptors that it has been used to elucidate the role of enkephalins and endorphins in various processes, including nitrous oxide[19] and acupuncture[23] analgesia and numerous others[96] (see also page 804). Unlike the partial agonists nalorphine and levallorphan, it can reverse respiratory depression due to pentazocine overdose and is also useful in dextropropoxyphene (Distalgesic) poisoning.[97] It is less effective than doxapram in reversing respiratory depression due to the very high affinity of the partial agonist buprenorphine (see page 818).

It is probably best avoided during and after surgery in all but the most severe respiratory depression because, like levallorphan and nalorphine, it will also reverse the analgesia. In these situations doxapram may be preferred.[98] It is the agent of choice to reverse neonatal respiratory depression, in which it is harmless even if depression is not due to opiates. In view of this, and because the maximum neonatal effect of pethidine is observed 3–4 hours after maternal administration, naloxone should probably be given to all neonates whose mothers have received any opiates during labour. It should never be given to the mother before delivery, since she is not suffering from respiratory depression, nor is it desirable to sacrifice her analgesia.

Naloxone has rather a brief duration of action, particularly if given by intravenous bolus. The recommended adult dose by intravenous or other injection is 5–6 $\mu$g/kg, though if given intravenously such a dose may need to be repeated at intervals or given by infusion[175] until the effects of the narcotic have worn off. The recommended neonatal dose is 5–10 $\mu$g/kg, but this reverses the effects of pethidine for less than 30 minutes. If given intramuscularly to a neonate in a dose of 200 $\mu$g, however, naloxone has been found to reverse *all* the detrimental effects of pethidine (see page 1080) for at least 48 hours, with no ill effects.[99]

### Adjuncts to Analgesic Drugs

Many drugs have been used from time to time in combination with analgesics, in an attempt to potentiate the analgesia and alleviate the side-effects. Antihistamines such as cyclizine and promethazine, major tranquillisers (Chapter 21), and anticholinergics such as hyoscine, have all been used. All might be expected to combat nausea and vomiting, but enhance the respiratory depressant, sedative and hypotensive effects and constipation. Moreover promethazine has a mild anti-analgesic action,[100] and narcotic-induced emesis is not readily reversed by antihistamines, such as cyclizine or promethazine.[101] Dopamine antagonists are more effective and, in this context, metoclopramide is popular, since it may reduce emesis with fewer side-effects than the phenothiazine derivatives.

Postoperative analgesia due to papaveretum has been found to be prolonged by the addition of orphenadrine,[102] a skeletal muscle relaxant which has been used as an anti-acetylcholine agent in Parkinsonism. Physostigmine has been found to antagonise morphine-induced respiratory depression and somnolence but not analgesia,[103] although doxapram is now commonly used for this purpose.

## SPINAL OPIATES

In the following account the term "spinal" is used to describe intrathecal and epidural sites of administration collectively.

With the demonstration of opiate receptors in the spinal cord (see page 803) and of segmental analgesia from intrathecal opiates in rats[29, 104] clinicians soon began to explore the use of intrathecal[105] and epidural[106] opiates in medicine. A host of reports and a few clinical trials of their use in the treatment of postoperative, chronic and obstetric pain, followed.

**Site of Action**

The transmission of pain in the spinal cord can be inhibited by systemically administered morphine (see page 803, Inhibition of Pain

Transmission), the evidence suggesting a presynaptic inhibition of substance P release by an action on opiate receptors in the substantia gelatinosa. It is not surprising therefore that the analgesia produced by spinal administration should be profound, since using one tenth of the systemic dose the resulting local concentration can be expected to be about a hundredfold that produced by systemic administration. Spinal analgesia cannot be reversed by systemic naloxone, the relative concentration of the competitive antagonist being unfavourable. However intrathecal naloxone can not only reverse analgesia from spinal opiates, it also partly antagonises systemic morphine.[29] The production of analgesia in the lower part of the body exclusively is further evidence that the primary site of action is the cord rather than the brain. Such segmental analgesia has been demonstrated after intrathecal morphine in rats[104] and after epidural morphine in human volunteers[107] and patients.[108] Moreover, addiction is not supported by intrathecal morphine[109] suggesting low brain levels.

Neither analgesia nor side-effects is likely to result from systemic absorption of spinally-administered opiates. Intrathecal morphine is effective in a dose well below that required for systemic effects,[110,111] while analgesic effect generally correlates poorly with plasma concentration following epidural fentanyl,[112] pethidine[113,114] and morphine.[115] Side-effects (*vide infra*), when they occur, are often more pronounced than would be expected from systemic absorption. It is clear, however, that side-effects such as respiratory depression and emesis that are associated principally with the use of morphine, are produced by direct opiate action on the brain, probably attained via the cerebrospinal fluid or possibly, in the case of epidurals, via the vertebral venous plexuses.

It is easy to envisage how intrathecal opiates can gain access both to the substantia gelatinosa in the cord, and to the respiratory and vomiting centres via the cerebrospinal fluid. Epidurally-administered agents however are more distanced from the sites of action. They have two possible routes of access to the cord: one via cerebrospinal fluid, and the other via axonal transmission. Morphine, possessing a very poorly lipid-soluble molecule, has an extremely slow onset and prolonged action when given epidurally.[116] It penetrates dura and arachnoid very slowly, to remain for long hours in the cerebrospinal fluid. It appears therefore that prolonged effects and also a serious risk of side-effects are both strongly related to hydrophilicity. The much more lipid-soluble fentanyl may gain access to the cord either via cerebrospinal fluid or by axonal transmission. It has a rapid onset of analgesia, even when given epidurally, a more reliable but less prolonged effect than morphine, and has not been associated with serious side-effects,[117] since much less remains free in the cerebrospinal fluid.

### Effects of Spinal Opiates

Spinal opiate administration produces segmental analgesia (*vide supra* Site of Action) the extent and spread of which is dependent upon site of injection[118] and position, while the duration is generally longer than that produced by bupivacaine.[117,119–121] Yaksh and Rudy[29,104] showed that the potency and duration of analgesia of the $\mu$ agonists fentanyl, morphine, methadone and pethidine given intrathecally to rats, corresponded to the systemic properties and that the $\kappa$ and partial $\mu$ agonists pentazocine and cyclazocine were ineffective. In man opiates have been used successfully chiefly in the treatment of chronic pain, postoperative and obstetric pain. When pinprick analgesia is examined (principally A$\delta$ fibres) a reduction in "hurting pain" can be distinguished.[122] Touch and motor power are of course unaffected, as is sympathetic transmission[116,123,124] though a reduction in blood pressure may occur, associated with pain relief.[113,117]

Epidural morphine does not suppress the adrenocortical and hyperglycaemic responses to surgery, as does full epidural block with bupivacaine, but it does suppress the continued rise in cortisol in the postoperative period.[125,176]

### Adverse Effects

*Respiratory depression* has been reported in postoperative patients most frequently following intrathecal morphine,[126–130] but also occasionally following epidural morphine,[131] epidural pethidine[132,133] and a large dose of methadone.[134] It would appear to be a phenomenon particularly relevant to the postoperative period, and may be associated with the concurrent use of systemic opiates, anaesthetics and other depressant drugs.[135,177] Stanley[136] pointed out that if one tenth of the systemic dose were injected into the cerebrospinal fluid, this would represent a brain dose one hundred times that resulting from systemic administration. On occasion intrathecal doses many times larger than this have been used[137–139] subjecting the patient to considerable risk with no actual gain in terms of analgesia. In an attempt to prevent the passage of morphine into the cerebral ventricles, it has been combined with dextrose to form a hyperbaric solution given in the sitting position. There can be no logic in this, since respiratory depression may occur many hours after injection, and there is no reason why a simple mixture of morphine and dextrose should remain associated that long. Persistent use of the sitting position, however, does reduce respiratory depression.[178]

*Nausea and vomiting* occur very frequently following intrathecal morphine,[135] particularly in obstetric patients,[140,141] and have also been reported with epidural morphine[142,143] and epidural fentanyl given by infusion.[144,179] Single dose epidural fentanyl was however associated with lower incidence of vomiting than epidural bupivacaine.[117]

*Itching* is also a frequent complaint with intrathecal[140,141] and epidural[142] morphine in obstetrics. It may be nasal or generalised while regional itching has been reported in this field following epidural fentanyl.[117]

*Urinary retention* has been a feature of epidural[115,145,146] and intrathecal morphine[107,147] though it may be no more frequent than with intramuscular morphine following abdominal surgery.[180]

It would appear that systemic naloxone is able to reverse all the reported side-effects, even urinary retention, while leaving the analgesia intact, indicating that analgesia is the only direct spinal action of opiates.

*Long-term effects*.—No histological damage could be found in monkeys sacrificed 42 days after intrathecal morphine administration.[148] Epidural morphine has been given over many weeks to man, in the treatment of chronic pain, without any obvious detriment, with negligible side-effects and, even more remarkably, without the appearance of tolerance.[149–151] Transient tachyphylaxis may occur, when sensitivity may be restored to normal by the administration of local anaesthetic instead of opiate for a brief period.[181]

**Applications—Choice of Agent and Route of Administration**

**Morphine,** being very poorly lipid-soluble, has an extremely slow onset of action epidurally, rendering it useless by this route in obstetrics,[124,142,152–154] though often adequate for the postoperative period if given early enough.[115,119–121,145] It has also been used to treat ischaemic rest pain[155] and multiple fractured ribs,[156] a situation in which epidural bupivacaine may be associated with unacceptable hypotension.

Continuous epidural analgesia using morphine has certainly been very successful in the long-term treatment of chronic pain[150,151] and has even been used successfully in a totally implanted system.[149] Intrathecal morphine is quicker acting and more reliable than is epidural morphine, but fraught with side-effects (*vide supra*). For this reason it is really only suitable for patients who will be under close observation for 12–24 hours, and because of the remarkable and long-lasting analgesia it produces, it certainly has a place in open heart surgery[157] and has also been used successfully to treat the pain of myocardial infarction.[147] When used in obstetrics, a single dose may be expected to relieve pain throughout labour[140,141,182] though at the cost of a high incidence of itching and emesis, which nevertheless may be naloxone-reversible. By the intrathecal route, 1 mg or less of morphine may suffice, though more than this is frequently used. A duration of action of about 24 hours may be expected. Epidurally the dose used has been very variable, the mean initial dose being about 5 mg, and the duration about 12 hours. Standard ampoules of morphine sulphate contain preservative. Morphine for epidural and intrathecal use must therefore be specially prepared without any preservative. This stricture does not apply to other commercially available opiates mentioned here.

The addition of *adrenaline* to epidural morphine has not been found to prolong its action.[183]

**Pethidine,** being somewhat more lipid-soluble than morphine, is more reliable when given epidurally for postoperative pain[133] and in obstetrics.[158,184] It has to be used however in systemic-sized doses, and it has a duration of action in labour shorter than one might expect for a systemic dose,[185] though with of course more complete pain relief. Its epidural duration is not prolonged by the addition of adrenaline.[159] Such large doses may have a local anaesthetic effect if given epidurally[184] and moreover find their way in considerable concentration into the cerebrospinal fluid,[128] causing a significant risk of respiratory depression.[132, 133]

**Fentanyl** possessing much greater lipid solubility and also higher receptor affinity than pethidine is probably the safest and most reliable agent for producing epidural analgesia, albeit of short duration. It is particularly successful in obstetrics.[117, 160, 161] Side-effects are uncommon because high cerebrospinal fluid concentration is unlikely. A dose of 80–100 μg, diluted to 4–8 ml, produces analgesia for about 2·5 hours, slightly longer than bupivacaine.[117] As with local anaesthetics, analgesia lasts a little longer in the postoperative period[162, 163] than in labour. Fentanyl has also been used intrathecally in rats[29, 104] and man, but is less long-lasting than morphine by this as by the epidural route. There is likely to be systemic accumulation if it is given in repeated doses. Phenoperidine appears to have no advantage over fentanyl in terms of duration of epidural analgesia[164] and it is likely to be every bit as cumulative systemically.

**Diamorphine,** a lipid-soluble derivative of morphine, produces pain relief within a few minutes when given epidurally. Analgesia is longer lasting in the postoperative period than with intramuscular administration[186] or with epidural fentanyl,[163] though diamorphine is disappointing in the treatment of labour pain. Theoretically, as diamorphine is slowly hydrolysed to morphine in solution, there is a risk of respiratory depression from residual morphine in the cerebrospinal fluid. When used epidurally in a dose of 5 mg diluted to 8–10 ml with physiological saline however, no respiratory depression has been observed in several hundred patients in this hospital.

**Buprenorphine** is highly lipid soluble and has been reported to produce prolonged postoperative pain relief when added to a bupivacaine epidural. However, possibly because of its bell-shaped log dose/response curve on μ receptors its epidural action is inconsistent.

**Methadone** is also highly lipid soluble but has a rather low μ efficacy. It is not very efficient epidurally, and has to be given in doses appropriate for systemic use. Moreover it has a very long half-life and therefore systemic accumulation may well be sufficient to cause central depression.

**β-endorphin** itself has been used epidurally. It is lipid insoluble, and when used in the rather large dose of 3 mg it has a slow onset, a duration of analgesia of about 19 hours, and few side-effects.[165]

### The Ideal Spinal Opiate

It would appear that the ideal opiate for spinal use should have high μ-efficacy and be slowly dissociated from μ receptors to ensure long local action. It should have a short half-life so that once absorbed into the systemic circulation it is rapidly inactivated to minimise systemic accumulation. It should be lipid soluble to permit epidural use, since the lack of spinal headache and the use of an epidural catheter make this route preferable to the intrathecal in many circumstances. High lipid solubility also diminishes the risk of delayed respiratory depression resulting from the persistence of the drug in cerebrospinal fluid. A drug possessing all these properties may well become available in the future.

## REFERENCES


1. Bowsher, D. (1978). Pain pathways and mechanisms. *Anaesthesia*, **33**, 935.
2. Kitahata, L. M. and Collins, J. G. (1981). Spinal action of narcotic analgesics. *Anesthesiology*, **54**, 153.
3. Mayer, D. J. and Price, D. D. (1979). Neural mechanisms subserving pain in man. In: *Mechanisms of Pain and Analgesic Compounds*, p. 31. Ed. R. F. Beers and E. G. Bassett. New York: Raven Press.
4. Rexed, B. (1952). The cytoarchitectonic organisation of the spinal cord in the cat. *J. Comparative Neurol.*, **96**, 415.
5. Willis, W. D. (1979). Physiology of dorsal horn and spinal cord pathways related to pain. In: *Mechanism of Pain and Analgesic Compounds*. Ed. R. F. Beers and E. G. Bassett. New York: Raven Press.
6. Randic, M. and Miletic, V. (1977). Effect of substance P in cat dorsal horn neurones activated by noxious stimuli. *Brain Res.*, **128**, 164.
7. Jessell, T. M. and Iversen, L. L. (1977). Opiate analgesics inhibit substance P release from rat trigeminal nucleus. *Nature*, **268**, 549.
8. Dohi, S., Toyooka, H. and Kitahata, L. M. (1979).

Effects of morphine sulphate on dorsal horn neuronal responses to graded noxious thermal stimulation in the decerebrate cat. *Anesthesiology*, **51**, 408.
9. Yaksh, T. L. (1978). Inhibition by etorphine of the discharge of dorsal horn neurons: effects on the neuronal response to both high and low-threshold sensory input in the decerebrate spinal cat. *Exp. Neurol.*, **60**, 23.
10. Snyder, S. H. (1975). Opiate receptor in normal and drug altered brain function. *Nature*, **257**, 185.
11. Snyder, S. H. (1977). Opiate receptors and internal opiates. *Scientific American*, March, 44.
12. Bhargava, K. P., Dixit, K. S. and Gupta, Y. K. (1981). Enkephalin receptors in the emetic chemoreceptor trigger zone of the dog. *Brit. J. Pharmacol.*, **72**, 471.
13. Hughes, J., Smith, T. W., Kosterlitz, H. W., Fothergill, L. A., Morgan, B. A. and Morris, H. R. (1975). Identification of two related pentapeptides from the brain with potent opiate agonist activity. *Nature*, **258**, 577.
14. Goldstein, A. (1979). Endorphins and pain: a critical review. In: *Mechanisms of Pain and Analgesic Compounds*, p. 249. Ed. R. F. Beers, and E. G. Bassett. New York: Raven Press.
15. Jhamandas, K. and Sutak, M. (1980). Action of enkephalin analogues and morphine on brain acetylcholine release: differential reversal by naloxone and or opiate pentapeptide. *Brit. J. Pharmacol.*, **71**, 201.
16. Kosterlitz, H. W. (1979). Possible physiological significance of multiple endogenous opioid agonists. In: *Mechanisms of Pain and Analgesic Compounds*. Ed. R. F. Beers and E. G. Bassett. New York: Raven Press.
17. Huidobro-Toro, J. P. (1980). Antidiuretic effect of $\beta$-endorphin and morphine in Battleboro rates: development of tolerance and physical dependence after chronic morphine treatment. *Brit. J. Pharmacol.*, **71**, 51.
18. Akil, H., Richardson, D. E. and Hughes, J. (1978). Enkephalin-like material elevated in ventricular cerebrospinal fluid of pain patients after analgesic focal stimulation. *Science*, **201**, 463.
19. Yang, J. C., Clark, W. C. and Ngai, S. H. (1980). Antagonism of nitrous oxide analgesia by naloxone in man. *Anesthesiology*, **52**, 414.
20. Thomas, T. A., Fletcher, J. E. and Hill, R. G. (1980). Changes in $\beta$-endorphin concentrations during labour. *Anaesthesia*, **35**, 1129.
21. Lawrence, D. and Livingston, A. (1981). Opiate-like analgesic activity in general anaesthetics. *Brit. J. Pharmacol.*, **73**, 435.
22. Levine, J. D., Gordon, N. C. and Fields, H. L. (1978). The mechanism of placebo analgesia. *Lancet*, **2**, 654.
23. Mayer, D. J., Price, D. D. and Rafii, A. (1977). Antagonism of acupuncture analgesia in man by the narcotic antagonist naloxone. *Brain Res.*, **121**, 368.
24. Abram, S. E., Reynolds, A. C. and Cusick. J. F. (1981). Failure of naloxone to reverse analgesia from transcutaneous electrical stimulation in patients with chronic pain. *Anesth. Analg.*, **60**, 81.
25. Editorial (1981). How does acupuncture work. *Brit. med. J.*, **283**, 746.
26. Editorial (1981). Endorphins through the eye of a needle. *Lancet*, **1**, 480.
27. Stoelting, R. K. (1980). Opiate receptors and endorphins: their role in anesthesiology. *Anesth. Analg.*, **59**, 874.
28. Martin, W. R. (1979). History and development of mixed opioid agonists, partial agonists and antagonists. *Brit. J. clin. Pharmacol.*, **7**, 273.
29. Yaksh, T. L. and Rudy, T. A. (1977). Studies in the direct spinal action of narcotics in the production of analgesia in the rat. *J. Pharmacol. exp. Ther.*, **202**, 411.
30. Ruch, T. C. and Fulton, J. F. (1960). *Medical Physiology and Biophysics*. Philadelphia: W. B. Saunders Co.
31. Holmes, T. H. and Wolff, H. G. (1950). Life situations, emotions and backaches. *Res. nerv. Dis. Proc.*, **29**, 750.
32. Merskey, H. (1968). Psychological aspects of pain. *Postgrad. med. J.*, **44**, 297.
33. Beecher, H. K. (1957). The measurement of pain. *Pharmacol. Rev.*, **9**, 59.
34. Gruber, C. M. (1962). The design of experiments evaluating analgesics. *Anesthesiology*, 23, 711.
35. Fraser, H. F. and Harris, L. S. (1967). Narcotic and narcotic antagonist analgesics. *Ann. Rev. Pharmacol.*, **7**, 277.
36. Lasagna, L. (1964). Clinical evaluation of morphine and its substitutes as analgesics. *Pharmacol. Rev.*, **16**, 47.
37. Lasagna, L. (1970). Challenges in drug evaluation in man. *Ann. Rev. Pharmacol.*, **10**, 413.
38. Joyce, C. R. B., Zutshi, D. W., Hrubes, V. and Mason, R. M. (1975). Comparison of fixed interval and visual analogue scales for rating chronic pain. *Europ. J. clin. Pharmacol.*, **8**, 415.
39. Littlejohns, D. W. and Vere, D. W. (1981). The clinical assessment of analgesic drugs. *Brit. J. clin. Pharmacol.*, **11**, 319.
40. Bonnycastle, D. D. (1962). *The Assessment of Pain in Man and Animals* (Proc. Internat. Symp. held under auspices of UFAW, Middlesex Hosp. Med. School, 1961), p. 231. Ed. By C. A. Keele and R. Smith, Edinburgh: E. & S. Livingstone.
41. Parry, J. W. L. (1979). The evaluation of analgesic drugs – a case for experimental methods. *Anaesthesia*, **34**, 468.
42. Huskisson, E. C. and Wojtulewski, J. A. (1974). Measurement of side effects of drugs. *Brit. med. J.*, **2**, 698.
43. Korttila, K., Pentti, O. M. and Auvinen, J. (1980). Comparison of i.m. lysine acetylsalicylate and oxycodone in the treatment of pain after operation. *Brit. J. Anaesth.*, **52**, 613.
44. Matthew, H. and Lawson, A. A. H. (1970). *Treatment of Common Acute Poisonings*. Edinburgh: E. &. S. Livingstone.
45. The National Poisons Information Service Monitoring Group (1981). Analgesic poisoning: a multi-centre, prospective survey. *Human Toxicol.*, **1**, 7.
46. Douglas, A. P., Hamlyn, A. N. and James, O. (1976). Controlled trial of cysteamine in treatment of acute paracetamol (acetaminophen) poisoning. *Lancet*, **1**, 111.
47. Prestcott, L. F., Sutherland, G. R., Park, J. and Smith, I. J. (1976). Cysteamine, methionine and penicillamine in the treatment of paracetamol poisoning. *Lancet*, **2**, 109.
48. Prestcott, L. F., Newton, R. W., Swainson, C. P., Wright, N., Forrest, A. R. W. and Matthew, H. (1974). Successful treatment of severe paracetamol overdosage with cysteamine. *Lancet*, **1**, 588.
49. Cobden, I., Record, C. O., Ward, M. K. and Kerr, D. N. S. (1982). Paracetamol-induced acute renal failure in the absence of fulminant liver damage. *Brit. med. J.*, **284**, 21.

50. Aylward, M. (1973). Toxicity of benorylate (letter). *Brit. med. J.*, **2**, 118.
51. Gintzler, A. R. and Scalisi, J. A. (1982). Effects of opioids on non-cholinergic circulatory responses of the guinea-pig isolated ileum: inhibition of release of enteric substance P. *Brit. J. Pharmacol.*, **75**, 199.
52. Collier, H. O. (1979). Consequences of interaction between opioid molecule and specific receptor. In: *Mechanisms of Pain and Analgesic Compounds*, p. 339. Ed. R. F. Beers and E. G. Bassett. New York: Raven Press.
53. Rouby, J. J., Glaser, P., Simmoneau, G., Gory, G., Guesde, R. and Viars, P. (1979). Cardiovascular response to the I.V. administration of morphine in critically ill patients undergoing IPPV. *Brit. J. Anaesth*, **51**, 1071.
54. Scott, D. H. T., Arthur, G. R. and Scott, D. B. (1980). Haemodynamic changes following buprenorphine and morphine. *Anaesthesia*, **35**, 957.
55. Samuel, I. O., Morrison, J. D. and Dundee, J. W. (1980). Central haemodynamic and forearm vascular effects of morphine in patients after open heart surgery. *Brit. J. Anaesth.*, **52**, 1237.
56. Arguelles, J. E., Franatovic, Y., Romo-Salas, F. and Aldrete, J. A. (1979). Intrabiliary pressure changes produced by narcotic drugs and inhalational anesthetics in guinea pigs. *Anesth. Analg.*, **58**, 120.
57. Lang, D. W. and Pilon, R. N. (1980). Naloxone reversal of morphine-induced biliary colic. *Anesth. Analg.*, **59**, 619.
58. Brunk. S. F. and Delle, M. (1974). Morphine metabolism in man. *Clin. Pharmacol Ther.*, **16**, 51.
59. Murphy, M. R. and Hug, C. C. (1981). Pharmacokinetics of intravenous morphine in patients anesthestised with enflurane—nitrous oxide. *Anesthesiology*, **54**, 187.
60. Oldendorf, W. H., Hyman, S., Braun, L. and Oldendorf, S. Z. (1972). Blood-brain barrier: penetration of morphine, codeine, heroin and methadone after carotid injection. *Science*, **178**, 984.
61. Hug, C. C., Murphy, M. R., Rigel, E. P. and Olson, W. A. (1981). Pharmacokinetics of morphine injected intravenously into the anesthetised dog. *Anesthesiology*, **54**, 38.
62. Hug, C. C. (1980). Improving analgesic therapy (Editorial). *Anesthesiology*, **53**, 441.
63. Rutter, P. C., Murphy, F. and Dudley, H. A. F. (1980). Morphine: controlled trial of different methods of administration for postoperative pain relief. *Brit. med. J.*, **280**, 12.
64. Orr, I. A., Keenan, D. J. M. and Dundee, J. W. (1981). Improved pain relief after thoracotomy: use of cryoprobe and morphine infusion. *Brit. med. J.*, **283**, 945.
65. Leslie, S. T., Rhodes, A. and Black, F. M. (1980). Controlled release morphine sulphate tablets—a study in normal volunteers. *Brit. J. clin. Pharmacol.*, **9**, 531.
66. Hanks, G. W., Rose, N. M., Aherne, G. W., Piall, E. M., Fairfield, S. and Trueman, T. (1981). Controlled release morphine tablets. A double-blind trial in dental surgery patients. *Brit. J. Anaesth.*, **53**, 1259.
67. Kay, B. (1980). A double-blind comparison between fentanyl and buprenorphine in analgesic-supplemented anaesthesia. *Brit. J. Anaesth.*, **52**, 453.
68. Dum, J. E. and Herz, A. (1981). *In vivo* receptor binding of the opiate partial agonist, buprenorphine, correlated with its agonistic and antagonistic actions. *Brit. J. Pharmacol*, **74**, 627.
69. Rance, M. J. (1979). Animal and molecular pharmacology of mixed agonist-antagonist analgesic drugs. *Brit. J. clin. Pharmacol.*, **7**, 281.
70. Bullingham, R. E. S., McQuay, H. J., Dwyer, D., Allen, M. C. and Moore, R. A. (1981). Sublingual buprenorphine used postoperatively: clinical observations and preliminary pharmacokinetic analysis. *Brit. J. clin. Pharmacol.*, **12**, 117.
71. Edge, W. G., Cooper, G. M. and Morgan, M. (1979). Analgesic effects of sublingual buprenorphine. *Anaesthesia*, **34**, 463.
72. Fry, E. N. S. (1979). Relief of pain after surgery. A comparison of sublingual buprenorphine and intramuscular papaveretum. *Anaesthesia*, **34**, 549.
73. Tigerstedt, I., Turunen, M., Tammisto, T. and Hastbalka, J. (1981). The effect of buprenorphine and oxycodone on the intracholedochal passage pressure. *Acta anaesth. scand.*, **25**, 99.
74. McQuay, H. J., Bullingham, R. E. S., Paterson, G. M. C. and Moore, R. A. (1980). Clinical effects of buprenorphine during and after operation. *Brit. J. Anaesth.*, **52**, 1013.
75. Economou, G. and Ward-McQuaid, J. N. (1971). A cross-over comparison of the effect of morphine, pethidine, pentazocine and phenazocine on biliary pressure. *Gut*, **12**, 218.
76. Keats, A. S. and Telford. J. (1964). Studies of analgesic drugs VIII. A narcotic antagonist analgesic without psychotomimetic effects. *J. Pharmacol. exp. Ther.*, **143**, 157.
77. Huskisson, E. C. (1974). Simple analgesic for arthritis. *Brit. med. J.*, **4**, 196.
78. Dundee, J. W., Clarke, R. S. J. and Loan, W. B. (1965). A comparison of the sedative and toxic effects of morphine and pethidine. *Lancet*, **2**, 1262.
79. Rigg, J. R. A., Ilsley, A. H. and Vedig, A. E. (1981). Relationship of ventilatory depression to steady-state blood pethidine concentrations. *Brit. J. Anaesth.*, **53**, 613.
80. Gong, S. N. C. and Rogers, K. J. (1973). Role of brain monoamines in the fatal hyperthermia induced by pethidine or imipramine in rabbits, pretreated with a monoamine oxidase inhibitor. *Brit. J. Pharmacol.*, **48**, 12.
81. Moore, G. and Nation, R. (1976). Pharmacokinetics of meperidine in man. *Clin. Pharmacol. Ther.*, **19**, 246.
82. Koska, A. J., Kramer, W. G. Romagnoli, A., Keats, A. S. and Sabawala, P. B. (1981). Pharmacokinetics of high-dose meperidine in surgical patients. *Anesth. Analg.*, **60**, 8.
83. Austin, K. L., Stapleton, J. V. and Mather, L. E. (1981). Pethidine clearance during continuous intravenous infusions in postoperative patients. *Brit. J. clin. Pharmacol.*, **11**, 25.
84. Crawford, R. D. and Baskoff, J. D. (1980). Fentanyl-associated delirium in man. *Anesthesiology*, **53**, 168.
85. Hilgenberg, J. C. (1981). Intraoperative awareness during high-dose fentanyl—oxygen anesthesia. *Anesthesiology*, **54**, 341.
86. Cooper, G. M., Paterson, J. L., Ward, I. D. and Hall, G. M. (1981). Fentanyl and the metabolic response to gastric surgery. *Anaesthesia*, **36**, 667.
87. Walsh, E. S., Paterson, J. L., O'Riordan, J. B. A. and Hall, G. M. (1981). Effect of high dose fentanyl anesthesia on the metabolic and endocrine response to cardiac surgery. *Brit. J. Anaesth.*, **53**, 1155.
88. Bovill, J. G. and Sebel, P. S. (1980). Pharmacokinetics

of high dose fentanyl. A study in patients undergoing cardiac surgery. *Brit. J. Anaesth.*, **52**, 795.
89. Stoeckel, H., Hengstmann, J. H. and Schuttler, J. (1979). Pharmacokinetics of fentanyl as a possible explanation for recurrence of respiratory depression. *Brit. J. Anaesth.*, **51**, 741.
90. Trudnowski, R. J. (1981). Pharmacokinetics of fentanyl. *Brit. J. Anaesth.*, **53**, 439.
91. Hengstmann, J. H., Stoeckel, H. and Schuttler, J. (1980). Infusion model for fentanyl based on Pharmacokinetic analysis. *Brit. J. Anaesth.*, **52**, 1021.
92. Rigg, J. R. A., Wong, T. Y., Horsewood, P. and Hewson, J. R. (1981). Steady state plasma fentanyl in the rabbit. *Brit. J. Anaesth.*, **53**, 1337.
93. Berkowitz, B. A. (1976). The relationship of pharmacokinetics to pharmacological activity: morphine, methadone and naloxone. *Clin. Pharmacokinetics*, **1**, 219.
94. Wang, R. I. H. (1974). A controlled clinical comparison of the analgesic efficacy of ethoheptazine, propoxyphene and placebo. *Europ. J. clin. Pharmacol.*, **7**, 183.
95. Hunt, V. (1973). Treatment of dextropropoxyphene poisoning. *Brit. med. J.*, **1**, 554.
96. Baskin, D. S. and Hosobuchi, Y. (1981). Naloxone reversal of ischaemic neurological deficits in man. *Lancet*, **2**, 272.
97. Tarala, R. and Forrest, J. A. H. (1973). Treatment of dextropropoxyphene poisoning (letter). *Brit. med. J.*, **2**, 550.
98. Gairola, R. L., Gupta, P. K. and Pandley, K. (1980). Antagonists of morphine-induced respiratory depression. A study in postoperative patients. *Anaesthesia.*, **35**, 17.
99. Wiener, P. C., Hogg, M. I. J. and Rosen, M. (1977). Effects of naloxone on pethidine-induced neonatal depression. *Brit. med. J.*, **2**, 228.
100. Keats, A. S., Telford, J. and Kuroso, Y. (1961). "Potentiation" of meperidine by promethazine. *Anesthesiolgy*, **22**, 34.
101. Conner, J. T., Weldon Bellville, J., Wender, R. Wapner, S., Dorey, F. J. and Katz, R. L. (1977). Morphine and promethazine as intravenous premedicants. *Anesth. Analg.*, **56**, 801.
102. Fry, E. N. S. (1979). Postoperative analgesia using papaveretum and orphenadrine. A preliminary trial. *Anaesthesia*, **34**, 281.
103. Weinstock, M., Davidson J. T., Rosin, A. J. and Schnieden, H. (1982). Effect of physostigmine on morphine-induced postoperative pain and somnolence. *Brit. J. Anaesth.*, **54**, 429.
104. Yaksh, T. L. and Rudy, R. A. (1976). Analgesia mediated by a direct spinal action of narcotics. *Science*, **192**, 1357.
105. Wang, J. K., Nauss, L. A. and Thomas, J. E. (1979). Pain relief by intrathecally applied morphine in man. *Anesthesiology*, **50**, 149.
106. Behar, M., Magora, F., Olshwang, D. and Davidson, J. T. (1979). Epidural morphine in treatment of pain. *Lancet*, **1**, 527.
107. Torda, T. A., Pybus, D. A., Liberman, H., Clark, M. and Crawford, M. (1980). Experimental comparison of extradural and I.M. morphine. *Brit. J. Anaesth.*, 52, 939.
108. Prior, F. N. and Thyle, A. (1981). Epidural morphine (letter). *Anaesthesia*, **36**, 535.
109. Tung, A. S., Tenicela, R. and Winter, P. M. (1980). Opiate withdrawal syndrome following intrathecal administration of morphine. *Anesthesiology*, **53**, 340.
110. Chauvin, M., Samii, K., Schermann, J. M., Sandouk, P., Bourdon, R. and Viars, P. (1981). Plasma concentration of morphine after i.m. extradural and intrathecal administration. *Brit. J. Anaesth.*, **53**, 911.
111. Chauvin, M., Samii, K., Schermann, J. M., Sandouk, P., Bourdon, R. and Viars, P. (1981). Plasma morphine concentration after intrathecal administration of low doses of morphine. *Brit. J. Anaesth.*, **53**, 1065.
112. Wolfe, M. J. and Davies, G. K. (1980). Analgesic action of extradural fentanyl. *Brit. J. Anaesth.*, **52**, 357.
113. Cousins, M. J., Glynn, C. J., Wilson, P. R., Mather, L. E. and Graham, J. R. (1979). Aspects of epidural morphine (letter). *Lancet*, **2**, 584.
114. Glynn, C. J., Mather, L. E., Cousins, M. J., Graham, J. R. and Wilson, P. R. (1981). Peridural meperidine in humans: analgetic response, pharmacokinetics and transmission into CSF. *Anesthesiology*, **55**, 520.
115. Weddel, S. J. and Ritter, R. R. (1981). Serum levels following epidural administration of morphine and correlation with relief of post surgical pain. *Anesthesiology*, **54**, 210.
116. Bromage, P. R., Camporesi, E. and Chestnut, D. (1980). Epidural narcotics for postoperative analgesia. *Anesth. Analg.*, **59**, 473.
117. Justins, D., Francis, D. M., Houlton, P. G. and Reynolds, F. (1982). A controlled trial of epidural fentanyl in labour. *Brit. J. Anaesth.*, **54**, 409.
118. Asari, H., Inoue, K., Shibata, T. and Soga, T. (1981). Segmental effect of morphine injected into the epidural space in man. *Anesthesiology*, **54**, 75.
119. Chambers, W. A., Sinclair, C. J. and Scott, D. B. (1981). Extradural morphine for pain after surgery. *Brit. J. Anaesth.*, **53**, 921.
120. Graham, J. L., King, R. and McCaughey, W. (1980). Postoperative pain relief using epidural morphine. *Anaesthesia*, **35**, 158.
121. Shapiro, L-A., Hoffman, S., Jedeikin, R. and Kaplan, R. (1981). Single-injection epidural anaesthesia with bupivacaine and morphine for prostatectomy. *Anesth. Analg.*, **60**, 818.
122. Dirksen, R. and Nijhuis, G. M. M. (1980). Epidural opiate and perioperative analgesia. *Acta anaesth. scand.*, **24**, 367.
123. Cousins, M. J., Mather, L. E., Glynn, C. J. Wilson, P. R. and Graham, J. R. (1979). Selective spinal analgesia (letter). *Lancet*, **1**, 1141.
124. Writer, W. D. R., James, F. M. and Wheeler, A. S. (1981). Double blind comparison of morphine and bupivacaine for continuous epidural analgesia in labor. *Anesthesiology*, **54**, 215.
125. Christensen, P., Brandt, M. R., Nem, J. and Kehlet, H. (1982). Influence of extradural morphine on the adrenocortical and hyperglycaemic response to surgery. *Brit. J. Anaesth.*, **54**, 23.
126. Jones, R. D. M. and Jones, J. G. (1980). Intrathecal morphine: naloxone reverses respiratory depression but not analgesia. *Brit. med. J.*, **281**, 645.
127. Gjessing, J. and Tomlin, P. J. (1981). Postoperative pain control with intrathecal morphine. *Anaesthesia*, **36**, 268.
128. Glynn, C. J., Mather, L. E., Cousins, M. J., Wilson, P. R. and Graham, J. R. (1979). Spinal narcotics and respiratory depression (letter). *Lancet*, **2**, 356.
129. Davies, G. K., Tolhurst-Cleaver, C. L. and James, T.

L. (1980). Respiratory depression after intrathecal narcotics. *Anaesthesia*, **35**, 1080.

130. Sidi, A., Davidson, J. T., Behar, M. and Olshwang, D. (1981). Spinal narcotics and central nervous system depression. *Anaesthesia*, **36**, 1044.
131. Christensen, V. (1980). Respiratory depression after extradural morphine (letter). *Brit. J. Anaesth.*, **52**, 841.
132. Scott, D. B. and McClure, J. (1979). Selective epidural analgesia. *Lancet*, **1**, 1410.
133. Rutter, D. V., Skewes, D. G. and Morgan, M. (1981). Extradural opioids for postoperative analgesia. A double blind comparison of pethidine, fentanyl and morphine. *Brit. J. Anaesth.*, **53**, 915.
134. Welch, D. B. and Hrynaszkiewicz, A. (1981). Postoperative analgesia using epidural methadone. Administration by the lumbar route for thoracic pain relief. *Anaesthesia*, **36**, 1051.
135. Barron, D. W. and Strong, J. E. (1981). Postoperative analgesia in major orthopaedic surgery. Epidural and intrathecal opiates. *Anaesthesia*, **36**, 937.
136. Stanley, T. H. (1980). Intrathecal opiates, a potent tool to be used with caution (letter). *Anesthesiology*, **53**, 523.
137. Liolios, A. and Andersen, F. H. (1979). Selective spinal analgesia (letter). *Lancet*, **2**, 357.
138. Samii, K., Feret, J., Harari, A. and Viars, P. (1979). Selective spinal analgesia. *Lancet*, **1**, 1142.
139. Samii, K., Chauvin, M. and Viars, P. (1981). Postoperative spinal analgesia with morphine. *Brit. J. Anaesth.*, **53**, 817.
140. Scott, P. V., Bowen, F. E., Cartwright, P., Mohan Rao, B. C., Deeley, D., Wotherspoon, H. G. and Sumrein, I. M. A. (1980). Intrathecal morphine as sole analgesic during labour. *Brit. med. J.*, **281**, 351.
141. Baraka, A., Noueihid, R. and Hajj, S. (1981). Intrathecal injection of morphine for obstetric analgesia. *Anesthesiology*, **54**, 136.
142. Booker, P. D., Wilkes, R. G., Bryson, T. H. L. and Beddard, J. (1980). Obstetric pain relief using epidural morphine. *Anaesthesia*, **35**, 377.
143. Magora, F., Olshwang, D., Eimerl, D., Shorr, J., Katzenelson, R., Cotev, S. and Davidson, J. T. (1980). Observations on extradural morphine analgesia in various pain conditions. *Brit. J. Anaesth.*, **52**, 247.
144. Bailey, P. W. and Smith, B. E. (1980). Continuous epidural infusion of fentanyl for postoperative analgesia. *Anaesthesia*, **35**, 1002.
145. Reiz, S., Ahlin, J., Ahrenfeldt, B., Andersson, M. and Andersson, S. (1981). Epidural morphine for postoperative pain relief. *Acta anaesth. scand.*, **25**, 111.
146. Bapat, A. R., Kshirsagar, N. A. and Bapat, R. D. (1979). Aspects of epidural morphine (letter). *Lancet*, **2**, 584.
147. Pasqualucci, V., Moricca, G. and Solinas, P. (1981). Intrathecal morphine for the control of the pain of myocardial infarction (letter). *Anaesthesia*, **36**, 68.
148. Abouleish, E., Barmada, M. A., Nemoto, E. M., Tung, A. and Winter, P. (1981). Acute and chronic effects of intrathecal morphine in monkeys. *Brit. J. Anaesth.*, **53**, 1027.
149. Coombs, D. W., Saunders, R. L., Gaylor, M. S., Pageau, M. G., Leith, M. G. and Schaiberger, C. (1981). Continuous epidural analgesia via implanted morphine reservoir (letter). *Lancet*, **2**, 425.
150. Wishart, J. M. (1981). Epidural morphine at home (letter). *Canad. Anaesth. Soc. J.*, **28**, 492.
151. Zenz, M., Schappler-Scheele, B., Neuhaus, R., Piepenbrock, S., Hilfrich, J. (1981). Long-term peridural morphine analgesia in cancer pain. *Lancet*, **1**, 91.
152. Chayen, M. S., Rudick, V. and Borvine, A. (1980). Pain control with epidural injection of morphine. *Anesthesiology*, **53**, 338.
153. Crawford, J. S. (1981). Experiences with epidural morphine in obstetrics. *Anaesthesia*, **36**, 207.
154. Husemeyer, R. P., O'Connor, M. C. and Davenport, H. T. (1980). Failure of epidural morphine to relieve pain in labour. *Anaesthesia*, **35**, 161.
155. Layfield, D. J., Lemberger, R. J., Hopkinson, B. R. and Makin, G. S. (1981). Epidural morphine for ischaemic rest pain. *Brit. med. J.*, **282**, 697.
156. Johnson, J. R. and McCaughey, W. (1980). Epidural morphine. A method of management of multiple fractured ribs. *Anaesthesia*, **35**, 155.
157. Mathews, E. T. and Abrams, L. D. (1980). Intrathecal morphine in open heart surgery. *Lancet*, **2**, 543.
158. Perriss, B. W. (1980). Epidural pethidine in labour. A study of dose requirements. *Anaesthesia*, **35**, 380.
159. Perriss, B. W. and Malins, A. F. (1981). Pain relief in labour using epidural pethidine with adrenaline. *Anaesthesia*, **36**, 631.
160. Carrie, L. E. S., O'Sullivan, G. M. and Seegobin, R. (1981). Epidural fentanyl in labour. *Anaesthesia*, **36**, 965.
161. Francis, D. M., Justins, D. and Reynolds, F. (1981). Obstetric pain relief using epidural narcotic agents. *Anaesthesia*, **36**, 69.
162. Wolfe, M. J. and Nicholas, A. D. G. (1979). Selective epidural analgesia. *Lancet*, **2**, 150.
163. Houlton, P. G. and Reynolds, F. (1981). Epidural diamorphine and fentanyl for postoperative pain. *Anaesthesia*, **36**, 1144.
164. Perriss, B. W. (1979). Epidural opiates in labour. *Lancet*, **2**, 422.
165. Oyama, T., Fukushi, S. and Jin, T. (1982). Epidural $\beta$-endorphin in treatment of pain. *Canad. Anaesth. Soc. J.*, **29**, 24.
166. Melzack, R. and Wall, P. D. (1965). Pain mechanisms: a new theory. *Science*, **150**, 971.
167. Prescott, L. F., Balali-Mood, M., Critchley, J. A. J. H., Johnstone, A. F. and Proudfoot, A. T. (1982). Diuresis or urinary alkalinisation for salicylate poisoning. *Brit. med. J.*, **285**, 1383.
168. Sawe, J., Svensson, J. O. and Rane, A. (1983). Morphine metabolism in cancer patients in increasing oral doses—no evidence for autoinduction or dose dependence. *Brit. J. clin. Pharmacol.*, **16**, 85.
169. Kjaer, M., Henriksen, H. and Knudsen, J. (1982). A comparative study of intramuscular buprenorphine and morphine in the treatment of chronic pain of malignant origin. *Brit. J. clin. Pharmacol.*, **13**, 487.
170. Ellis, R., Haines, D., Shah, R., Cotton, B. R. and Smith, G. (1982). Pain relief after abdominal surgery—a comparison of i.m. morphine, sublingual buprenorphine and self-administered i.v. pethidine. *Brit. J. Anaesth.*, **54**, 421.
171. Cook, P. J., James, I. M., Hobbs, K. E. F. and Browne, D. R. G. (1982). Controlled comparison of i.m. morphine and buprenorphine for analgesia after abdominal surgery. *Brit. J. Anaesth.*, **54**, 285.
172. Rosow, C. E., Moss, J., Philbin, D. M. and Savarese,

J. J. (1982). Histamine release during morphine and fentanyl anaesthesia. *Anesthesiology*, **56**, 93.

173. Freye, E., Hartung, E. and Kaliebe, S. (1983). Prevention of late fentanyl-induced respiratory depression after the injection of opiate antagonists naltrexone and S-20682: comparison with naloxone. *Brit. J. Anaesth.*, **55**, 71.
174. Stoeckel, H., Schüttler, J., Magnussen, H. and Hengstmann, J. H. (1982). Plasma fentanyl concentrations and the occurrence of respiratory depression in volunteers. *Brit. J. Anaesth.*, **54**, 1087.
175. Gourlay, G. K. and Coulthard, K. (1983). The role of naloxone infusions in the treatment of overdose of long half-life narcotic agonists: application to normethadone. *Brit. J. clin. Pharmacol.*, **15**, 269.
176. Cowen, M. J., Bullingham, R. E. S., Paterson, G. M. C., McQuay, H. J., Turner, M., Allen, M. C. and Moore, A. (1982). A controlled comparison of the effects of extradural diamorphine and bupivacaine on plasma glucose and plasma cortisol in postoperative patients. *Anesth. Analg.*, **61**, 15.
177. Gustafsson, L. L., Schildt, B. and Jacobsen, K. (1982). Adverse effects of extradural and intrathecal opiates: report of a nationwide survey in Sweden. *Brit. J. Anaesth.*, **54**, 479.
178. McCaughey, W. and Graham, J. L. (1982). The respiratory depression of epidural morphine. Time course and effect of posture. *Anaesthesia*, **37**, 990.
179. Welchew, E. A. and Thornton, J. A. (1982). Continuous thoracic epidural fentanyl. A comparison of epidural fentanyl with intramuscular papaveretum for postoperative pain. *Anaesthesia*, **37**, 309.
180. Petersen, T. K., Husted, S. E., Rybro, L., Schurizek, B. A. and Wernberg, M. (1982). Urinary retention during i.m. and extradural morphine analgesia. *Brit. J. Anaesth.*, **54**, 1175.
181. McCoy, D. D. and Miller, M. G. (1982). Epidural morphine in a terminally ill patient. (Letter). *Anesthesiology*, **57**, 427.
182. Bonnardot, J. P., Maillet, M., Colan, J. C., Millot, F. and Deligne, P. (1982). Maternal and fetal concentration of morphine after intrathecal administration during labour. *Brit. J. Anaesth.*, **54**, 487.
183. Youngstrom, P. C., Cowan, R. I., Sutheimer, C., Eastwood, D. W. and Yu, J. C. M. (1982). Pain relief and plasma concentrations from epidural and intramuscular morphine in post-Cesarean patients. *Anesthesiology*, **57**, 404.
184. Husemeyer, R. P., Cummings, A. J., Rosankiewicz, J. R. and Davenport, H. T. (1962). A study of pethidine kinetics and analgesia in women in labour following intravenous, intramuscular and epidural administration. *Brit. J. clin. Pharmacol.*, **13**, 171.
185. Skjöldebrand, A., Garle, M., Gustafsson, L. L., Johansson, H., Lunell, N. O. and Rane, A. (1982). Extradural pethidine with and without adrenaline during labour: wide variation in effect. *Brit. J. Anaesth.*, **54**, 415.
186. Jacobson, L., Phillips, P. D., Hull, C. J. and Conacher, I. D. (1983). Extradural versus intramuscular diamorphine. A controlled study of analgesic and adverse effects in the postoperative period. *Anaesthesia*, **38**, 10.

CHAPTER 31

# The Pharmacology of Local Anaesthetic Drugs



A LOCAL anaesthetic drug reversibly blocks nerve conduction beyond the point of application, when applied locally in the appropriate concentration. Many drugs have local anaesthetic properties, notably quinidine-like antidysrhythmic drugs, antihistamines and tricyclic antidepressants, but this chapter refers only to those drugs used primarily for local anaesthesia.

## HISTORY

For many centuries the inhabitants of the highlands of Peru and Bolivia chewed the leaves of the indigenous shrub *Erythroxylum coca* for the sake of their effects of diminishing fatigue and appetite. These effects are due primarily to the principal alkaloid, cocaine. Numbing of the oral mucosa was, of course, merely regarded as a side-effect; it was not until the second half of the nineteenth century that the possible nature of the active substances contained in the plant roused the interest of scientific investigators in Europe. Cocaine was first isolated in 1860 by Neimann, who noted its local anaesthetic effect. It was over a generation, however, before this discovery was exploited. In the 1880s Sigmund Freud studied the physiological effects of cocaine and used it to treat morphine addiction, thereby producing the first cocaine addict in Europe. While Freud was away visiting his fiancée in 1884, a colleague, Karl Köller, introduced cocaine as a local anaesthetic for the eye at an ophthalmological congress, with immediate success. Freud was of course destined to become famous in other ways and so could afford to be magnanimous towards his colleague. Thereafter the field of local anaesthesia expanded quickly to include infiltration, nerve block and, later, spinal anaesthesia. Very soon the high systemic toxicity and addictive properties of cocaine stimulated the search for less toxic synthetic substitutes. A number of synthetic local anaesthetics emerged during this period, of which procaine, introduced by Einhorn in 1905, was the most important. It proved to be less toxic than cocaine, but somewhat unreliable and with a short duration of action. Numerous related compounds with few advantages over procaine emerged in the years that followed, but the major advance of the period was probably the production of cinchocaine in Germany in the late 1920s. The next milestone was the introduction of lignocaine in the 1940's: the forerunner of a new generation of chemically related and greatly improved local anaesthetics.

## Chemistry

The local anaesthetics in current use have a basic formula (Table 1).

Individual formulae are as shown in Fig. 1.

All modern local anaesthetics are amides. Esters are unstable in solution and cannot be autoclaved. Lignocaine, prilocaine, mepivacaine, bupivacaine and etidocaine all share a common basic structure that is sometimes termed aminoacyl amide.

The hydrophilic group in prilocaine is a secondary amine; the rest listed in Fig.1 are tertiary amines. The amine group confers on the molecule the property of a weak base (or proton acceptor) which can combine with an acid to form a water-soluble salt. This salt ionises in solution and is usually stable.

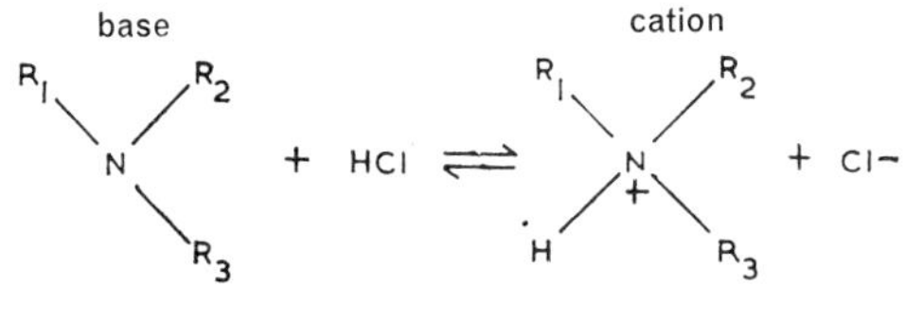


The non-ionised form of the molecule (the base) is lipid-soluble and consequently can penetrate tissue barriers. The proportions of the two forms of the molecule present in solution depend upon the $pK_a$ of the molecule (see Chapter 18) and on the pH of the environment, and can be calculated from the Henderson-Hasselbalch equation. The $pK_a$ values of the modern local anaesthetics are around 8 (see Table 4). At pH 7·4 a basic drug with $pK_a$ of 7·86 such as lignocaine is 25 per cent non-ionised, whereas for a drug with a $pK_a$ of the order of 9 such as procaine only 2·5 per cent is present in this form. At physiological pH, therefore, and at equal total concentrations, the concentration of lignocaine base is ten times that of procaine base. This factor contributes to the greatly enhanced penetrative power of lignocaine over procaine.

A local anaesthetic for injection is presented as a salt—usually the hydrochloride. The resulting solution is acidic, as the salt is derived from a strong acid and a weak base. The pH of a plain solution ranges from 4·4 for etidocaine to 6·3 for lignocaine.[1] In a more alkaline solution basic drugs are less soluble.

## Nerve Conduction

A nerve fibre consists of a central semi-fluid core, the axoplasm, enclosed in a tube, the cell membrane. The cell membrane is built up of a bimolecular lipid palisade, interspersed with large protein molecules. Each fibre of a peripheral nerve is enclosed in a tube of neurilemma, from which it is separated by the myelin sheath, except at the nodes of Ranvier. The myelin sheath, an insulating layer, is absent—or nearly so—in non-medullated nerves. Nerve fibres so encased are collected in bundles within the *endoneurium*. The *perineurium* surrounds a collection of bundles, and the *epineurium* encloses a whole nerve. There is therefore a substantial barrier between a local anaesthetic injected into the extracellular compartment and its site of action at the nerve cell membrane.

During nerve conduction, changes occur in

31/Table 1

| | | | | |
|---|---|---|---|---|
| Aromatic lipophilic group | — | Intermediate chain (ester: —COO— or amide—NH.CO—) | — | hydrophilic group 2ary or 3ary amine. |

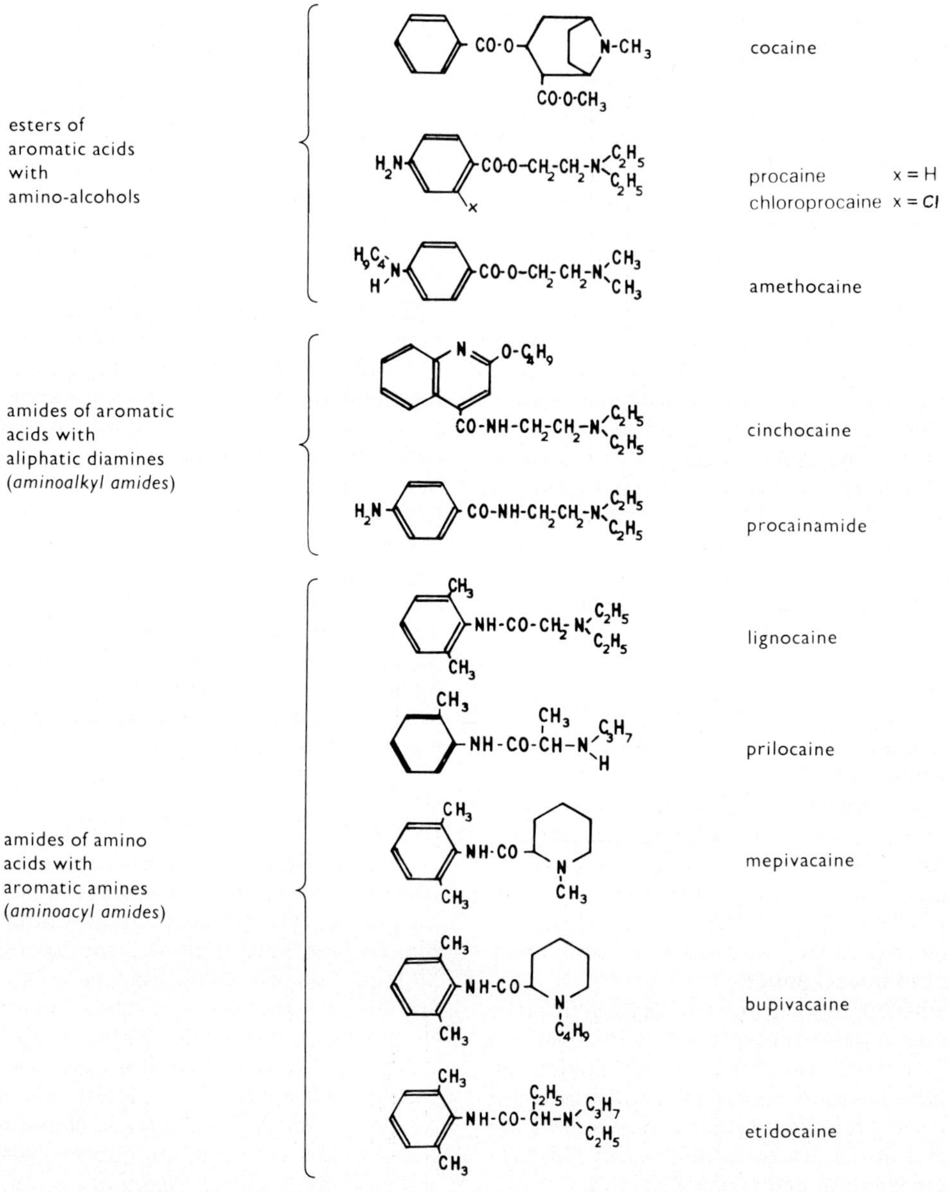


31/FIG. 1.—The structural formulae of local anaesthetic drugs. Procainamide is included here, although used only as an anti-dysrhythmic, because it is mentioned in this chapter.

the cell membrane. In the *resting state* there is a potential difference across the cell membrane, inside negative, due to a higher concentration of sodium ions outside than in. The cell membrane is relatively impermeable to sodium ions whose gradient is maintained by the sodium pump.

*Depolarisation phase.*—When a nerve is stimulated, partial depolarisation of the membrane is accompanied by a release of calcium ions and leads to a large transient increase in permeability to sodium ions which therefore enter the fibre, resulting in massive depolarisation. Thus, the threshold required to produce the action potential is exceeded, with consequent propagation of the nerve impulse.

During the *neutralisation phase*, potassium ions pass out of the fibre to restore electrical neutrality.

In the *restoration phase* sodium ions return to the outside and potassium ions re-enter the fibre.

In myelinated nerves these changes take place only at the nodes of Ranvier, giving rise to saltatory conduction of the nerve impulse.

## The Action of Local Anaesthetics on the Cell Membrane

The primary action of a local anaesthetic is on the cell membrane of the axon, on which it produces electrical stabilisation. The large transient increase in permeability to sodium ions, necessary for propagation of the impulse, is prevented, thus the resting potential is maintained and depolarisation in response to stimulation is inhibited. Initially the threshold for electrical excitation is raised, the rate of rise of the action potential reduced, and conduction slowed; eventually propagation of the impulse fails.

Classical local anaesthetics block sodium conductance, probably by a dual action on the cell membrane:

(1) They act directly on receptors within the sodium channels.

(2) They produce non-specific membrane expansion.

(1) **Action on receptors within the sodium channels.**—This action accounts for about 90 per cent of the nerve blocking effect of lignocaine and appears to be shared by both quaternary analogues of lignocaine[2] and by amine local anaesthetics acting in the cationic form (see below—active form of the local anaesthetic molecule). Quaternary derivatives of lignocaine, being fully ionised, cannot penetrate the cell membrane, and produce nerve block only if applied to its inner surface. The work of Hille[3] suggests that the receptor is *within* the sodium channel and while a polar quaternary compound can reach it only via the hydrophilic pathway, that is the axoplasmic opening of the sodium channel, an amine local anaesthetic can gain access either via the lipophilic pathway directly across the lipid membrane, or via the axoplasmic opening.[4]

(2) **Membrane expansion.**[5,6]—This is a non-specific action in contrast to a more specific drug-receptor interaction, and is analogous to the electrical stabilisation produced by a number of non-polar, purely lipid-soluble substances such as non-ionised barbiturates, general anaesthetics and benzocaine.

The production of nerve conduction blockade is associated with about a 3·5 per cent expansion of membrane volume; the actual volume of the anaesthetic occupying the membrane, however, is only about 0·3 per cent or less. The equivalent figures for general anaesthesia are a volume expansion of the membrane of 0·6 per cent compared with the volume of the anaesthetic of about 0·02 per cent. Since the volume occupied by the anaesthetic only accounts for about 10 per cent of this membrane expansion, a number of mechanisms have been suggested to account for the further 90 per cent. The most likely explanation is that there is an unfolding of membrane protein, together with a disordering of the lipid component of the cell membrane,[6] with consequent obstruction of the sodium channels. Displacement of membrane-bound calcium ions may also be involved; calcium is known to condense lipid layers and local anaesthetics to displace it. This mechanism may account for the major part of the effect of benzocaine and procaine, whose active form appears to be the uncharged base, but only the lesser part of the effect of lignocaine.[2] Nevertheless, pressure has been shown partially to reverse nerve block by lignocaine, though not by procaine.[7]

## The Active Form of the Local Anaesthetic Molecule

In order to act, a local anaesthetic must first penetrate the surrounding tissues and the nerve sheath. Only the uncharged form, therefore, can gain access to the cell membrane. Partitioning of local anaesthetic into tissues can be favoured by the addition of sodium bicarbonate, which by lowering the pH delays release of the drug into the circulation.[8]

According to the evidence of Ritchie *et al.*,[9] however, the cation is responsible for most of the nerve blocking effect. This they demonstrated in the following way. They suspended intact and desheathed nerves in bath fluids of different pH values and added different concentrations of lignocaine. They showed that while a high pH favoured block by lignocaine of an intact nerve, in a desheathed preparation the optimum pH for the action of lignocaine was neutral. Thus, where little or no penetration was required the lowest effective concentration was one which contained a predominance of the cationic form of the drug.

*Carbonated local anaesthetics.*—Research on carbonated local anaesthetics[10] provides further evidence that the cation is the active form of the local anaesthetic molecule and that it acts on the interior of the cell membrane. A number of factors may contribute to the enhanced effect of lignocaine carbonate over lignocaine hydrochloride:

(i) the pH of the solution is higher than that of the hydrochloride, thereby increasing the concentration of uncharged base available for penetration.

(ii) $CO_2$ is released and diffuses to the interior of the cell more rapidly than the local anaesthetic. Within the axon it lowers the pH thereby increasing the ionisation of the local anaesthetic. This has a two-fold effect:
(a) the concentration of base is reduced, so increasing its gradient for diffusion into the cell, a phenomenon known as diffusion trapping:
(b) the release of cation enhances the nerve blocking activity (*vide supra*).

(iii) $CO_2$ itself has some nerve blocking effect on desheathed preparations.

Clinically, carbonated lignocaine and prilocaine have both been shown to be superior to the hydrochlorides for epidural block in speed of onset, reduction in the incidence of missed segments and increased incidence of motor block,[11] though some workers find only a more intense[12] and more widespread[13] block.

*Tachyphylaxis* may be less evident with lignocaine carbonate than hydrochloride. Successive injections of the hydrochloride may lower the local pH, thus lignocaine becomes more ionised and less can penetrate to the site of action.[14] The carbonate, however, is a less acid salt. The advantages of carbonated *bupivacaine* are less clear.[15] Certainly, tachyphylaxis is rarely evident with the usual salt, bupivacaine hydrochloride, and other differences between the two salts in practice are negligible.[16]

## Potency and Duration of Action

Among local anaesthetics high potency and long duration of action tend to be directly related while the action of an individual drug can, to a certain extent, be prolonged by increasing the concentration and the dose.

In any one homologous series, for example in the mepivacaine-bupivacaine series, increasing the length of the side-chain on the amine nitrogen increases potency, but beyond $C_4$ tissue irritancy becomes too high and aqueous solubility too low for usefulness.

High potency is associated with high lipid solubility because this property facilitates solution in and passage across the cell membrane. The production of vasoconstriction by the drug will also tend to enhance and prolong its effect, while a vasodilator action will tend to accelerate its removal from the site of action.

Rapid biotransformation cannot shorten the action of amide local anaesthetics, which are only metabolised in the liver, while even the effect of pseudocholinesterase on procaine is negligible in the tissues.

The relationship between potency and toxicity is discussed below under Systemic Toxicity.

Some physicochemical properties mentioned are listed for individual local anaesthetics in Table 4 (p. 845).

## Sensitivity of Different Fibre Types

All types of nerve fibres are affected by local anaesthetics, but within any one fibre type (see Table 2) there is a tendency for small, slower-conducting fibres to be more readily blocked than large, fast-conducting fibres.[17]

Between fibre types, however, these rules do not hold good. It is well established that myelinated preganglionic B fibres which have a faster conduction time are about three times more sensitive to local anaesthetics than the slower non-myelinated postganglionic C fibres. In fact there is both experimental and clinical evidence that preganglionic fibres[18–20] are the most sensitive of all: vasodilatation, with consequent hypotension if sufficiently widespread, is a well-recognised early sequel to epidural, spinal or paravertebral block, which can all affect white

31/TABLE 2

| *Fibre Type* | *Function* *Sensory* | *Motor* | *Fibre Diameter* *μm* | *Conduction Speed* *m/sec* |
|---|---|---|---|---|
| A α | proprioception | somatic | 12–20 | 70–120 |
| β | touch, pressure | | 5–12 | 30–70 |
| γ | | muscle spindle | 3–6 | 15–30 |
| δ | pain, temperature | | 2–5 | 12–30 |
| B | | preganglionic | <3 | 3–15 |
| C | pain, reflex | post-ganglionic | 0·3–1·3 | 0·5–2·3 |

rami communicantes of the sympathetic chain. Gissen and colleagues[21] found that A fibres were more sensitive than B and C to a variety of local anaesthetics while Rosenberg and associates[20] found them the most resistant (Fig. 2). Data from laboratory experiments conducted at room temperature, as were those of Gissen, must be interpreted with care, because nerve blocking effects are highly temperature-dependent[22] and myelinated fibres most affected by cooling.[23] While large A fibres are certainly the most resistant to local anaesthetics, it is probable that Aδ fibres, subserving pain and temperature sensation, are more sensitive than C pain fibres, although more rapidly conducting.[24,25,185] Pathological pain (conducted by C fibres) such as that produced by impending uterine rupture or placental separation, may occasionally break through an epidural block which is relieving the physiological pain of labour: the "epidural sieve".[26] The greater sensitivity of A δ than C fibres to local anaesthetic block could perhaps go some way to explain this phenomenon. Sensory Aα fibres appear to be more sensitive to blockade than motor Aα fibres, although of the same conduction velocity. This may be because sensory fibres conduct at a higher *frequency*.[17] It has been suggested that this selectivity for sensory fibres exhibited by bupivacaine and lignocaine is a function of frequency-dependent block—a property not shared by etidocaine and amethocaine.[27] However, *all* local anaesthetics block sensory more rapidly than motor fibres clinically (Fig. 3), and show similar selectivity for different fibre types (Fig. 2). The varying ability of different agents to produce motor block would appear to be related largely to their epidural use (Fig. 3) and may be dependent upon the site at which each agent produces conduction block when applied epidurally.[28] Thus bupivacaine, the most selective for sensory fibres on epidural use, produces profound motor block on peripheral, intravenous regional[29] and intrathecal[30,31] administration. At other sites, the relative sensitivities of different fibre types may be dependent upon their placing within a nerve bundle.[32]

In summary the order of sensitivity to blockade appears to be (starting from the most sensitive): preganglionic, pain and temperature, touch, proprioception and motor fibres.

## PHARMACOLOGICAL EFFECTS

The effects produced by local anaesthetics may be:

(a) *local:* nerve blockade and a direct effect on smooth muscle (see below: vascular smooth muscle);

(b) *regional:* loss of pain and temperature sensation, touch, motor power, and vasomotor tone, in the region supplied by the nerves blocked;

(c) *systemic:* effects occurring as a result of systemic absorption, or intravenous administration. The production of nerve blockade requires a concentration many times higher than any that occurs systemically.[33] Lethal doses of lignocaine, for example, would be necessary to block sensory nerve endings systemically.[34] Thus the so-called analgesic properties of a procaine infusion are due to central sedation and not to any peripheral nerve blocking action. The chief systemic effects of local anaesthetics are on the heart and the central nervous system, and are probably produced by the same

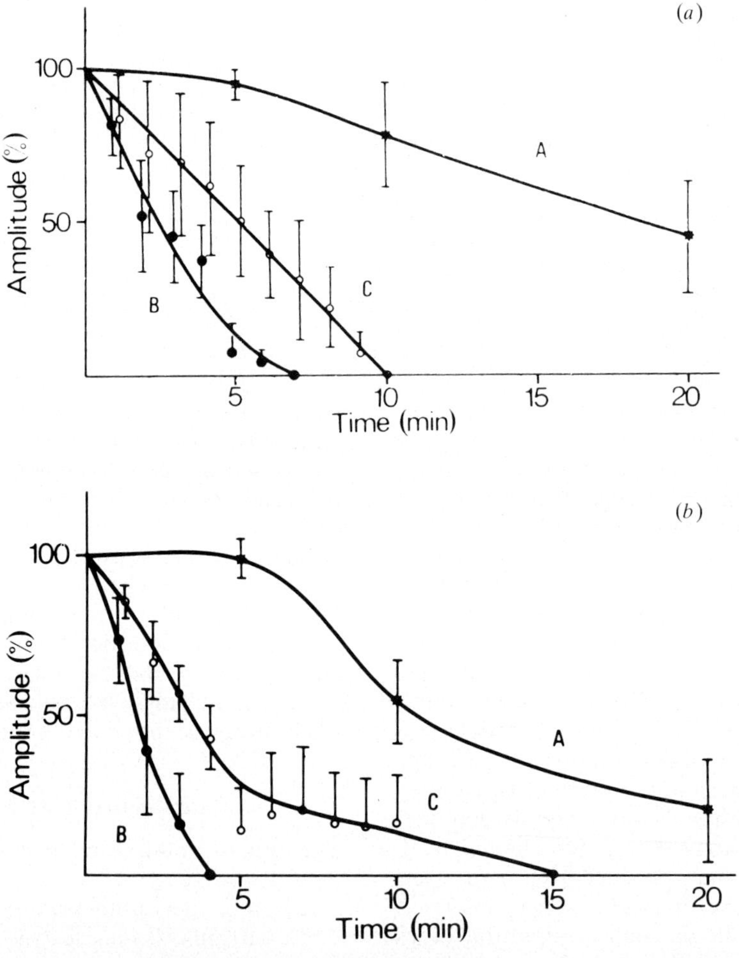


31/FIG. 2.—The effect of bupivacaine 200 μmol litre$^{-1}$ (*a*), and of 2-chloroprocaine 300 μmol litre$^{-1}$ (*b*), on the action potential amplitude in A, B and C fibres. 100% = control. Means ± SEM of at least three experiments. (Courtesy of Drs. P. H. Rosenberg, E. Heinomen, S. E. Jansson and J. Gripenberg, and the publishers of the *British Journal of Anaesthesia*, Macmillan Journals Ltd.[20])

action as is nerve blockade, that is by membrane stabilisation.

### Cardiovascular System

**The heart.**—Lignocaine and procaine have a stabilising effect on the cell membrane of cardiac tissue. They tend to depress automaticity in abnormal or damaged fibres and thereby suppress cardiac dysrhythmias. Procaine and procainamide also have quinidine-like effects; they prolong the action potential duration thus increasing the effective refractory period of cardiac cells, slowing conduction and so desynchronising ventricular contraction with a consequent depressant effect on myocardial contractility. Experimentally, all local anaesthetics appear to reduce cardiac sensitivity to adrenaline[35] and to produce dose-related depression of conduction and contractility.[36] Lignocaine, however, appears not to possess classical quinidine-like action and is remarkably non-cardiotoxic when used clinically. Its use as an antidysrhythmic is discussed on page 847.

Gross overdose of the longer-acting local anaesthetics bupivacaine and etidocaine has reputedly, on occasion, been associated with

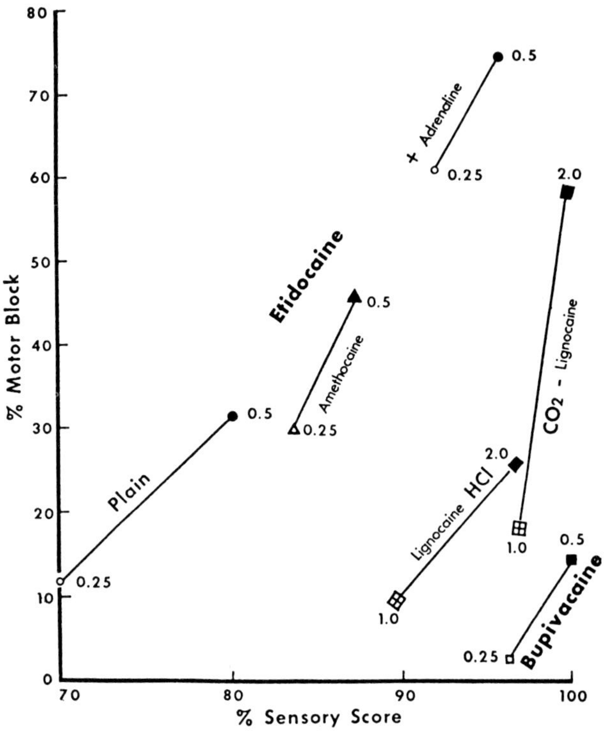


31/FIG. 3.—Comparison of average scores for motor and sensory blockade during epidural analgesia in obstetric patients. (Courtesy of Dr. P. R. Bromage and the Editor and publisher, Macmillan Journals Ltd., of the *British Journal of Anaesthesia*.[161])

ventricular tachycardia,[37] fibrillation[38] and cardiac arrest.[39] There is good evidence, however, that cardiac toxicity does not occur in subconvulsive doses,[40, 41] or in the absence of severe electrolyte disturbance,[42] or respiratory or metabolic acidosis.[41, 43] Asphyxia has been shown to increase lignocaine toxicity in baboon fetuses.[44]

**Vascular smooth muscle.**—The effects local anaesthetics may have on vascular smooth muscle cause some confusion[45] since they may be local, regional or systemic. The *local* effects vary. While procaine is undoubtedly vasodilator and cocaine vasoconstrictor (due to its sympathetic potentiating effect), vasomotor effects among modern local anaesthetics vary depending upon the nature of the drug and upon its concentration.[46] Vasoconstriction is more frequent at lower concentrations and vasodilatation at higher (see Fig. 4).[47, 48] Åberg[49] suggested that vasoconstriction and vasodilatation were associated with stimulation and inhibition respectively of tissue-bound $Ca^{++}$ release. Among the drugs in general use mepivacaine appears most likely to produce vasoconstriction at clinical concentrations, then prilocaine, lignocaine, and bupivacaine in that order. Of these drugs all but lignocaine exist as two stereoisomers, and the ability to produce vasoconstriction appears to be vested in one of the isomers,[50] though in the case of mepivacaine, both isomers have some vasoconstrictor power.[51] The *regional* effect is simply vasodilatation in the area supplied by blocked sympathetic nerves. *Systemic* effects may be produced in a variety of ways, reflexly and because of central nervous system involvement, but not as a result of any direct action on blood vessels outlined above, because the ambient concentration would be too low. Effects on the circulation of subconvulsive doses of modern local anaesthetics are variable but minimal, while large doses may produce circulatory collapse as a result of medullary depression and of convulsions causing respiratory impairment,[52] rather than because of any direct effect on the circulation.

**Central Nervous System**

The concept of local anaesthetics as central nervous system stimulants should be eschewed. It dates from the last century when cocaine was

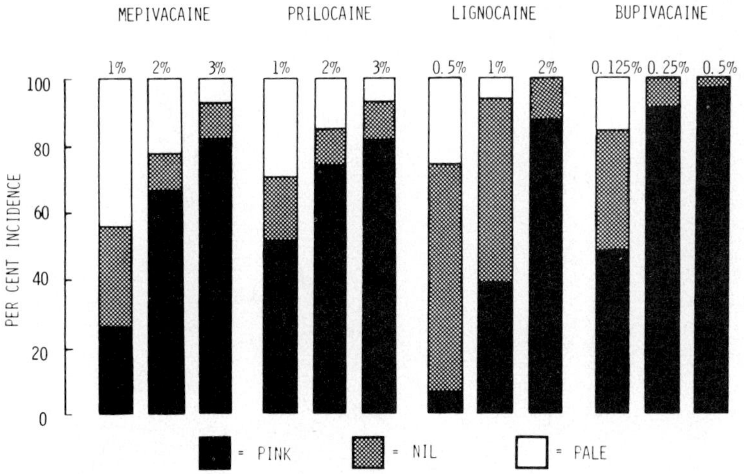


31/FIG. 4.—Local colour changes after intradermal injections of local anaesthetics in volunteers. Mepivacaine and prilocaine, n = 27; lignocaine and bupivacaine, n = 31. (Data from Reynolds *et al.*, 1976;[46] Aps and Reynolds, 1976.[47])

the only local anaesthetic. Cocaine has undoubted stimulant effects which are unrelated to its local anaesthetic action. The synthetic agents produce sedation and lightheadedness, while sometimes anxiety and restlessness occur, in which case inhibitory neurones have proved more susceptible than excitatory ones to depression, a situation not unfamiliar with alcohol. With more marked toxicity the patient may notice a numb tongue, circumoral pins and needles, twitching and visual disturbances. Severe toxicity proceeds to convulsions and coma with respiratory and cardiac depression,[53] as a result of medullary depression. Cardiac disturbances are compounded by convulsion-associated hypoxia (*vide supra*). Even with cocaine overdose, respiratory depression may be the cause of death.[54] Convulsions and unconsciousness may occur unheralded in severe intoxication of rapid onset. Treatment of intoxication is covered under Systemic Toxicity (p. 840).

Both lignocaine and procaine have been used by intravenous infusion primarily to produce central sedation at systemic concentrations which produce no elevation of the pain threshold[55] or nerve conduction block.[33] The sedative effect of lignocaine absorbed after epidural administration, for example, is well recognised.

**Autonomic nervous system.**—Cocaine, by inhibiting catecholamine uptake, has an undoubted sympathetic potentiating effect. Other local anaesthetics would appear not to block noradrenaline uptake.[56] Experimentally, local anaesthetics possess a weak blocking action on cholinergic[57,58] and adrenergic[59] receptors. The former may account for a bronchodilator effect.[60,61] *Ganglia:* local anaesthetics are not ganglion blockers in clinical doses and any apparent block produced locally at extremely high concentrations is probably due to a stabilising action on the nerve terminals.

**Neuromuscular junction.**—Local anaesthetics can certainly block motor nerves if present in sufficient concentration, and the presynaptic blocking effect that has been observed under experimental conditions with high concentrations of procaine again simply reflects a membrane stabilising action.

**Hypersensitivity.**—This implies an abnormal antigen-antibody response, and not an exaggerated normal response, correctly termed *supersensitivity*. The term has also been misused to describe adverse reactions due to accidental intravenous injection and frank overdose, while the lay public frequently claim "sensitivity" to the local anaesthetic when they have suffered a classical faint or a typical adrenaline reaction. It appears that dentists encounter true hypersensitivity to modern local anaesthetics, though rarely, more frequently than do anaesthetists, probably because of the much larger number of patients given dental local anaesthesia. Hypersensitivity to a local anaesthetic is more frequent in atopic individuals and may be manifested as local oedema initially, as generalised urticaria, or as angioneurotic oedema with or without lymphadenopathy. Dermatitis may be encountered as a delayed reaction to skin applications and as contact dermatitis in dentists. Anaphylaxis appears less common than atopic reactions.

Hypersensitivity to procaine and other ester derivatives of benzoic acid is not uncommon. There is likely to be cross sensitivity within the ester group of drugs and with *p*-aminobenzoic acid, widely used as a sunscreen, and *p*-hydroxybenzoic acid and its derivatives (paraben, methylparaben) which are preservatives and may be incorporated into amide local anaesthetic preparations. All these benzoic acid esters are relatively highly antigenic whereas the amide local anaesthetics are not, though true hypersensitivity to lignocaine[62–64] and bupivacaine[65] has been reported.

### Distribution and Fate

**Absorption.**—A dose of local anaesthetic must eventually be absorbed virtually entirely into the systemic circulation. The rate of absorption depends on several factors. The lipid solubility of the agent determines the proportion remaining in the aqueous phase available for rapid removal by the blood, and the proportion taken up by the tissues and therefore only slowly released into the systemic circulation (see also sections on Chemistry and Mode of Action). The vascularity of the tissues influences removal and can be altered by the local anaesthetic itself and by adrenaline (see below). Absorption of some local anaesthetics from mucosal surfaces such as the trachea[66] or an inflamed urethra, can give rise to plasma concentrations akin to those produced by direct intravenous injection. Absorption from the gastro-intestinal tract does occur, and for procainamide which is mainly excreted unchanged, oral antidysrhythmic therapy can be successful,[67] but for lignocaine, of which 70 per cent may be metabolised in a single passage through the liver, this route is ineffective.

**Distribution.**—In the plasma, local anaesthetics are bound to plasma proteins (principally to $\alpha_1$-acid glycoprotein) to an extent partly related to their potency and lipid solubility (see Table 4). A small proportion related to *free* concentration enters red cells. The cell/plasma ratio may therefore be reduced by enzyme induction which can increase the glycoprotein fractions in plasma.[68] Local anaesthetics are rapidly removed from the blood by the tissues. In general, distribution is so rapid that most of the drug has disappeared from the circulation before mixing in the blood is complete. Full equilibration with the tissues, however, may take many hours. Local anaesthetics readily cross lipid membranes such as cell membranes, the blood-brain barrier and the placenta (Chapter 41) and become more concentrated in tissues than in the blood. The distribution volume of lignocaine, for example, is about 2½ l/kg but varies widely between individuals.[69]

**Metabolism.**—Local anaesthetics are metabolised to more water-soluble compounds, which are therefore less concentrated in tissues and more rapidly excreted than the parent drugs. Amide local anaesthetics are metabolised in the liver, while most esters may also be hydrolysed in the plasma. In the liver, several pathways are involved. *N-dealkylation* of the tertiary amine has been shown to take place in a number of local anaesthetics[70] producing a more water-soluble secondary amine, and in the case of lignocaine for example, rendering it more susceptible to amide hydrolysis[71] as is the more rapidly metabolised secondary amine prilocaine.[72] *Hydroxylation* of the aromatic nucleus is believed to occur in the case of lignocaine, mepivacaine and bupivacaine,[73] to produce a compound which can be conjugated and so become solely water-soluble. Owing to its wide use as an antidysrhythmic, the breakdown of lignocaine has been most extensively studied. As much as 70 per cent may be broken down during a single passage through the liver, this high first-pass clearance yielding mainly the N-dealkylated product monoethylglycine xylidine, itself a moderately toxic and effective antidysrhythmic. The high clearance rate of lignocaine is markedly reduced in the presence of low cardiac output[69] and hence by halothane.[74] Amino*alkyl* amides (cinchocaine and procainamide) are metabolised much more slowly than amino*acyl* amides (lignocaine etc.—see Chemistry) and a much larger proportion is consequently excreted unchanged.[75]

In the plasma, procaine is rapidly hydrolysed by pseudocholinesterase, but at a rate which is saturable[75] and therefore subject to competition with suxamethonium. Amethocaine is hydrolysed at about a fifth the rate of procaine, while plasma cholinesterase appears unable to break down cocaine.[75]

**Excretion.**—With the exception of cinchocaine and procainamide, only a small fraction of the dose of a local anaesthetic is excreted unchanged in the urine. The water-soluble metabolites are readily excreted, but a lipid-soluble local anaesthetic base, once filtered in the glomerulus, can be re-absorbed in the renal tubule. In an acid urine it becomes highly ionised, tubular reabsorption is inhibited and renal clearance is high. However, with the high tissue uptake of the unchanged drug, renal excretion does not play a major role, even when the urine is acid.

## Systemic Toxicity

**Manifestations.**—Local anaesthetic toxicity affects mainly the central nervous system. Subconvulsive doses are unlikely to cause circulatory depression except through medullary depression or biochemical disturbances (see pp. 836–838).

**Drug factors.**—The toxicity of many drugs such as barbiturates which act systemically, is dose-related and merely an extension of the therapeutic action. Such need not be the case with drugs which act locally and whose toxic effects depend upon systemic absorption. Not surprisingly, the potency of a local anaesthetic is directly related to its acute intravenous toxicity,[76,77] that is when absorption is bypassed and the effect is so rapid that distribution and elimination cannot mitigate it. When a drug is used to produce local anaesthesia, the occurrence of systemic effects depends not upon the acute toxicity (since the dosage will be related to this) but upon the speed of absorption and elimination (see Distribution and Fate, p. 839). As the rate of metabolism of a local anaesthetic cannot affect its duration of action or potency, but can affect its *chronic* toxicity especially during repeated administration, a drug with a favourable ratio between duration of action and speed of elimination has an advantage.

**Other factors.**—There is evidence that the occurrence of toxicity is not necessarily related to the concentration of solution injected[78] as has been suggested, but rather to the total dose.[79] The speed of epidural injection similarly appears not to affect systemic absorption, although if the drug is injected intravascularly, rapid injection is more likely to result in serious toxicity. Clearly the site of injection and its vascularity will affect the speed of absorption[80] as will the addition of a vasoconstrictor. Although overdose is rightly feared in the very young and the very old, they are probably no more sensitive to a given plasma level than are other patients. Anoxia and acid-base disturbances lower the threshold both to CNS[81] and to cardiac toxicity (see p. 837).

The commonest cause of systemic toxicity is probably inadvertent intravascular administration, while rapid absorption from an inflamed urethra was a common cause of death from local anaesthesia before this hazard was realised.[82] Moreover, some disasters have been due to gross overdosage[37,83] (for example when unnecessarily high concentrations are used by surgeons for infiltration). Widespread field blocks and excessive surface application of local anaesthetics, sources of trouble in the past, should always be avoided, and a single dose of a local anaesthetic should never cause toxicity. The principal danger of true intoxication from a correctly administered local anaesthetic probably lies in its continuous or repeated administration. For this purpose the long duration of bupivacaine and the rapid elimination of etidocaine offer clear advantages.

An attempt has been made to suggest maximum safe doses of the various local anaesthetics in Table 4 (p. 845).

**Prevention.**—Toxicity, due to inadvertent intravascular injection, can be avoided by careful aspiration before injection and, most importantly, by *slow* injection with careful attention to the patient's symptoms. Toxicity from other routes of administration should be avoided by careful planning of procedures such that toxic doses are not used. Premedication with diazepam[84] or a barbiturate offers no licence to use excessive doses.

**Treatment.**—If signs of minor central nervous system toxicity occur, administration of the local anaesthetic should be discontinued. In the case of an intravenous infusion, simply stopping it may be sufficient treatment. In more severe cases and after local administration (when absorption cannot be stopped) oxygen should be given. In many cases correcting the cerebral hypoxia by this means may be all that is necessary. With full convulsions, artificial ventilation must be maintained with oxygen via an endotracheal tube if necessary. Where some form of drug treatment is necessary, neuromuscular blocking drugs alone have been advocated,[85] avoiding anticonvulsants in a condition with so large a component of cerebral depression. It can be argued, however, that the brain must be protected from prolonged electrical discharges, which enormously increase its oxygen requirement. Intravenous diazepam has been advocated[86] but thiopentone is probably as effective and is certainly quicker in onset, easier to monitor, and less prone to hangover[53] and less damaging to veins. Convulsions resulting from inadvertent intravascular injection should not be treated with anticonvulsants since they are likely to cease spontaneously before an anticonvulsant can take effect and leave the patient unnecessarily anaesthetised.

## VASOCONSTRICTORS

### Adrenaline (Epinephrine)

**Use.**—Adrenaline, by virtue of its $\alpha$-stimulant action, is used with a local anaesthetic to prolong its action and delay absorption into the systemic circulation, thereby it is hoped, reducing the incidence of systemic toxicity. When procaine and even lignocaine were among the few safe local anaesthetics the use of adrenaline for anything but the shortest procedures was justified. It increased the duration of action of lignocaine quite considerably, and when prolonged blockade was required it reduced the number of repeat doses needed and delayed the onset of chronic toxicity and tachyphylaxis. Its effects on the long-acting drug bupivacaine, and on prilocaine, are less marked, although it may prolong the action of etidocaine (see under individual local anaesthetics). By delaying and reducing peak absorption it may diminish the toxicity of big doses, even if local anaesthesia is not prolonged. It is more valuable in highly vascular areas such as the intercostal space and pelvic floor than in the less vascular epidural space, while in dentistry some form of vasoconstrictor is essential with most agents. In other fields, however, its dangers may outweigh its usefulness (*vide infra*), while in vascular areas it greatly increases the danger from accidental intravenous injection. Moreover, its inclusion in commercially available preparations necessitates the addition of antioxidants such as sodium metabisulphite and ascorbic acid, which in the quantities used in the United States, reduce the pH to less than 4·0.[1,87] In Britain, bupivacaine with adrenaline for example, contains fewer additives than in the United States and has a pH normally above 4·5.

For general puposes, adrenaline should not be used with local anaesthetic solutions in a concentration higher than 5 $\mu$g/ml (1:200,000), while in some cases an even lower concentration may be sufficient. In dentistry, however, adrenaline 12·5 $\mu$g/ml (1:80,000) is still frequently used, though in this situation of course the total dose is small.

*Systemic effects.*—Although adrenaline may reduce the systemic absorption of a local anaesthetic, toxicity usually occurs because of accidental intravenous injection. In this situation, adrenaline is more dangerous than the local anaesthetic itself. In clinical practice, were the entire dose of local anaesthetic containing say 100–150$\mu$g of adrenaline to be inadvertently given intravenously, one might expect marked tachycardia, palpitations, anxiety and sweating of brief duration. Such a dose, however, absorbed slowly after a correctly placed block, would have minimal systemic effects in the normal patient, with possibly some redistribution of blood to areas rich in $\beta$-receptors, such as skeletal muscle. Indeed Corall and associates[88] found the addition of 5 $\mu$g/ml of adrenaline to bupivacaine for obstetric epidurals to have no significant cardiovascular effects, though it may reduce uterine blood flow in sheep.[89] In patients taking certain antihypertensive drugs (because of denervation supersensitivity) and especially tricyclic antidepressants,[90] and in those with thyrotoxicosis, the systemic effects of adrenaline may be dangerously potentiated. In these situations adrenaline is contraindicated.

*Local effects.*—The local $\alpha$-vasoconstrictor effects of adrenaline may be dangerous in certain situations. It increases the likelihood of anterior spinal artery syndrome, a rare complication of epidural analgesia. If used for digital block it may produce gangrene. If given into a restricted area such as the dermis it may produce tissue anoxia because it also increases local oxygen consumption.[91]

### Noradrenaline (Norepinephrine)

Noradrenaline is a less potent $\alpha$-receptor stimulant than adrenaline, thus if used for local anaesthesia a higher concentration is required. It has been used in dentistry in concentrations of 20 or 40 μg/ml (1:50,000 or 1:25,000) and has given rise to dangerous hypertension.[92] Tricyclic anti-depressants may cause a 4- to 8-fold potentiation of its pressor effects.[90] It is contra-indicated in all those patients in whom adrenaline is contra-indicated, and in hypertension. There are thus no indications for its use in this field.

### Felypressin

Felypressin (Octapressin) is a synthetic polypeptide related to vasopressin. It is a vasoconstrictor that may be used as a substitute for adrenaline in local anaesthesia. It is used with prilocaine in dentistry in which it is more effective in prolonging the action of prilocaine than is adrenaline.[93] Its systemic toxicity is less than that of adrenaline[94] and used in dentistry it produces no cardiovascular changes, where adrenaline 12·5 μg/ml is likely to produce tachycardia.[95]

## Desirable Properties

There can be no such thing as the ideal local anaesthetic drug because different circumstances require different properties. However, certain characteristics are usually desirable. The first is good penetration. This tends to promote rapid onset of action, to eliminate patchy anaesthesia and to make topical application effective if this is required. A local anaesthetic should not produce local irritation, and systemic side-effects should be minimal. A safe therapeutic ratio is always necessary and not hard to achieve if the local anaesthetic is to be used in a single dose for most techniques in current use. In the past, paravertebral and intercostal block for tuberculosis surgery, for example, sometimes necessitated dangerously large doses. In the techniques commonly used at present, such as epidural blockade, it is relatively easy to keep within safe limits of dosage.

For the production of prolonged local anaesthesia many more properties are required. A long duration of action becomes an advantage for both convenience and safety, and it should be unnecessary to add adrenaline to achieve this. Tachyphylaxis should not occur and slow absorption but rapid elimination of the drug will tend to improve its therapeutic ratio (see discussion on Systemic Toxicity). Reversibility of action is stipulated by definition.

A local anaesthetic solution should be able to withstand repeated autoclaving and minor pH changes and should be stable in light and air.

## Assessment

Most local anaesthetics are fairly satisfactory drugs and improvements gained in the manufacture of new drugs are likely only to be marginal. Therefore careful assessment of a new drug is mandatory if it is to be adopted in preference to a well-tried agent. Local anaesthetics lend themselves to fairly accurate assessment as it is easier to measure their effects objectively than it is those of systemic analgesics.

Before the first clinical trials of a new drug take place, extensive preliminary investigations in both animals and man will have established a number of facts. It behoves the clinician about to embark on a clinical study to acquaint himself with the relevant literature.

### Laboratory Investigations in Animals and Man

Animal studies can be used to compare the acute and cumulative toxicity of drugs by various routes of administration (subcutaneous, intramuscular, intravenous, etc.) and to make a rough assessment of latency, potency and duration of action. The inhibition of the corneal reflex in the rabbit is used to measure surface anaesthetic activity. Inhibition of reaction to pinprick after intra-cutaneous injection in the guinea-pig can test infiltration analgesia. Conduction anaesthesia may be tested by sciatic nerve block in guinea-pig or frog, or by mouse tail root infiltration measuring inhibition of the pain reflex. In man a series of intradermal injections of different concentrations of the new drug, together with a standard drug and a blank (physiological saline) can be given in the forearm. A quantitative assessment of analgesia to pinprick can be made by counting the number of standard pinpricks that are felt as sharp out of a total of, say, five per intradermal weal, at regular intervals. This method can be used to compare the duration of action and vasoactivity of different preparations.[46,47,51,96,97]

Given a source of willing or needy volunteers,

other experimental tests may be carried out in man, such as bilateral ulnar nerve[98] or brachial plexus block,[99] one arm being used as control. Latency, potency, duration and penetration (patchy anaesthesia) of sensory and motor blockade may be tested.

Plasma concentrations which are associated with mild toxic symptoms, can be estimated during slow intravenous infusion in fit volunteers.[100]

### Clinical Trials[101, 102]

In the light of the information so obtained, clinical studies may now be planned and these should attempt to establish potency, latency, penetration, duration and potential toxicity in clinical practice. It is generally considered advisable to use a new drug initially in a pilot trial without the use of a control or double blind technique. In this way approximate potency may be confirmed and any major inadequacy detected. Having established feasibility, carefully planned and controlled double blind trials must be carried out (see Table 3) testing the agent against a standard drug such as lignocaine but not, of course, against a placebo. At this stage the help of an experienced organiser of clinical trials is valuable. The problem is simplified if a single type of local block is studied and the technique and rate of administration are standardised. When possible there should be a single operator and a single observer, to avoid minor variations in techniques of administration and assessment. Many hidden variables may arise, thus absolutely no comparisons between drugs can be made from a trial such as was published as recently as 1980, in which one agent was studied in one centre, and two others in another *continent*![103] A range of concentrations of the drug under scrutiny should be used and the volume of solution injected kept constant (which is, of course, essential for a double blind procedure). If a vasoconstrictor is used, its concentration should be constant in all the test solutions. If its concentration varies, then the nature and concentration of the local anaesthetic it accompanies should be constant. Where possible, a subject should act as his own control—for example, when a bilateral block is required. During continuous epidural anaesthesia, different solutions may be compared sequentially. Otherwise, patients should be selected randomly for the different treatments, the series should be as large and as homogenous as possible, and parity of age, sex, etc., in the several groups should be checked at the end of the series.

*Assessment of analgesia.*—Both artificial and natural pain should be used. Local anaesthesia lends itself better to testing with artificial pain than does systemic analgesia. Analgesia to pinprick is usually clear-cut, and can be used to measure onset, duration and spread, including patchy analgesia. The mean surface area involved in the block (e.g. the number of segments involved in the case of spinal or epidural analgesia) in each group is plotted graphically against the mean duration of action (Fig. 5). This supplies a visual means of instant comparison of two or more agents, showing the spread and completeness of analgesia and the onset and duration of action of each drug.

*Natural pain* should also be measured using a visual analogue scale: a 10 cm line with *no* graduations or labelling on it, except at one end "No pain at all" and at the other "pain as bad as you can possibly imagine". Pain can thereby be evaluated numerically. Natural pain, because of its variability, cannot be used to compare different solutions sequentially.

In addition to loss of pain, a numerical estimate of motor power and the incidence of hypotension, and other side-effects should be noted. As many data as possible should be recorded in each subject of a clinical trial, and measurements made at the same and sufficiently frequent time intervals.

31/TABLE 3
PLANNING A CLINICAL TRIAL

1. Search the literature.
2. Employ a double-blind technique using:
    reference drug (e.g. lignocaine)
    two or more concentrations of new drug
    patient as his own control where possible.
3. Standardise conditions:
    subjects
    route of administration
    technique of administration.
4. Standardise assessment of:
    artificial pain
    natural pain
    operating conditions
    side-effects
   and investigate potency, latency, spread and duration of action of the drug.
5. Evaluate results statistically where appropriate.

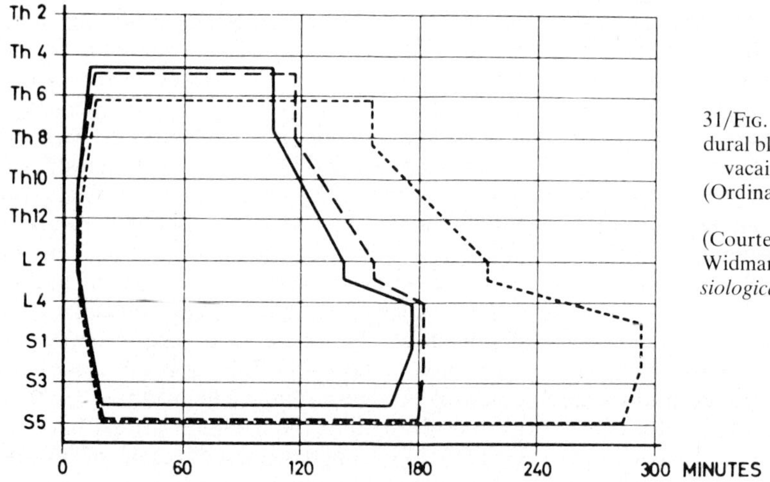


31/Fig. 5.—The extent and duration of epidural blockade using prilocaine (——), mepivacaine (– – –) and bupivacaine (- - - -). (Ordinate—dermatomes. Abscissa—duration.) (Courtesy of Dr. L. Ekblom and Dr. B. Widman and the Editors of *Acta Anaesthesiologica Scandinavica.*[104])

**Assessment of toxicity.**—After the correct administration of a single dose of a local anaesthetic by any accepted route, the incidence of systemic toxicity should be nil. It is nevertheless essential to judge the margin of safety that may be expected from a drug in any given situation, as for instance with a large dose, repeated injection after failed block, or for prolonged analgesia. Such assessment should not be made by trial and error as often happened in the past. It may be judged by measuring plasma concentrations of the local anaesthetic which occur in clinical practice in different situations and comparing these with the plasma concentration which gives rise to signs of systemic toxicity during experimental intravenous infusion in volunteers.

Complete testing of a local anaesthetic may take a long time if this regime is followed. For many years local anaesthesia was regarded as a safe alternative to general anaesthesia for surgery in the sick, and only reports of increasing numbers of deaths gave the lie to this idea. Now, with better techniques, safer drugs and a better understanding of their behaviour, local anaesthesia should be very much safer than it was in the past.

## INDIVIDUAL LOCAL ANAESTHETIC DRUGS

The number of drugs that have been marketed as local anaesthetics is legion, and only products in current use by anaesthetists, or those of historical importance, are included here. They are presented in chronological order. Numerical data are often misleading, because they may have been calculated from experiments under varying conditions by different workers. However, in Table 4, an attempt has been made to supply such as enable some quantitative comparison of different local anaesthetics. The pharmacological actions of the various drugs are covered mainly in earlier sections. The ensuing text deals principally with usage.

### Cocaine

This drug is now little used owing to its toxic and addictive properties. In addition to its nerve-blocking action it enhances the effect of sympathetic stimulation and of catecholamines.

Sympathetic activity is normally terminated because the transmitter, noradrenaline, is removed from the region of the receptor by its re-uptake into sympathetic nerve endings. Cocaine inhibits this re-uptake process and therefore allows accumulation of transmitter at the receptor site. The marked difference between the effects of cocaine and of other local anaesthetics is largely a reflection of this property. Cocaine is not a markedly potent or long-acting local anaesthetic and its therapeutic ratio in clinical use is substantially lower than that of

31/TABLE 4
PHYSICOCHEMICAL AND TOXICOLOGICAL DATA

| | *pKa* | *Protein binding at clinical Concentrations* | *Partition Coefficients Heptane/ buffer* | *Partition Coefficients Oleyl Alcohol/ buffer* | *Anaesthetic Concentration Relative to Lignocaine†* | *Maximum* Safe Dose* | *$LD_{50}$ mg/kg mice and rats IV* | *$LD_{50}$ mg/kg mice and rats SC* |
|---|---|---|---|---|---|---|---|---|
| COCAINE | 8·4 | | | | 2·0 | ?2 mg/kg | 17·5 | |
| PROCAINE | 9·0 | 35% | | 0·6 | 3·0 | 10 mg/kg | 55 | 370–630 |
| CINCHOCAINE | 8·5 | | | 530 | 0·1 | 0·4 mg/kg | 2·5–4·7 | |
| AMETHOCAINE | 8·4 | | | 80 | 0·25 | 1·0 mg/kg | 4·3–8·0 | 32–62 |
| LIGNOCAINE | 7·86 | 60–75% | 2·9 | 25–30 | 1·0 | 6 mg/kg | 15–38 | 300–400 |
| MEPIVACAINE | 7·7 | 75% | 0·8 | 10–17 | 1·0 | 6 mg/kg | 27–40 | 260–270 |
| PRILOCAINE | 7·9 | 55% | 0·4 | 11 | 1·0 | 8 mg/kg | 18–62 | 600–900 |
| BUPIVACAINE | 8·1 | 90–97% | 28 | 212–890 | 0·25 | 2 mg/kg | 7·8 | 83 |
| ETIDOCAINE | 7·7 | 94–97% | 142 | >1000 | 0·4 | 4 mg/kg | 5·8–7·2 | 89–102 |

From: Luduena *et al.*,[76] Truant and Takman,[105] Henn,[106] Sawinski and Rapp,[107] af Ekenstam,[108] Henn and Brattsand,[109] Tucker,[110] Messrs. Astra Pharmaceuticals, *Merck Index*, Reynolds (personal observation) IV = intravenous; SC = subcutaneous.

† These figures are only approximate. Relative potencies vary with site and especially with nerve fibre type.
* There is no single maximum safe dose for an individual local anaesthetic. The figures suggested here relate to plain solutions given by single shot into a non-vascular area such as the epidural space. These doses may often have been exceeded with impunity when adrenaline is added, while smaller doses of plain solutions may be toxic in vascular areas. If the doses were injected rapidly intravenously, severe toxicity might be expected.

the more modern drugs. It is active as a surface anaesthetic and the vasoconstriction it produces may delay its systemic absorption and, furthermore, has made it popular for ear, nose and throat work.

Although first used for eye surgery, the dangers of precipitating glaucoma and of causing corneal damage make it unsuitable in this field.

**Central nervous system effects.**—Cocaine, unlike modern local anaesthetics, has a stimulant effect like that of amphetamine, even in low doses. It produces excitement, euphoria and garrulousness and is prone to abuse. Medullary stimulation may cause hypertension, increased respiratory rate and vomiting. Body temperature may rise. In severe intoxication, coma, convulsions and medullary depression usually precede death.

**Cardiovascular system.**—Because of vasoconstriction and a sympathomimetic effect on the heart, the arterial pressure is initially raised by cocaine. Ventricular fibrillation may cause sudden death without premonitory signs of severe intoxication.

**Use.**—As a local anaesthetic, cocaine should be used only for surface application, if at all. A 10 per cent solution is used for endotracheal spraying and other surface application to the nose and throat, while some ENT surgeons use 20 per cent cocaine paste in the nose. Fortunately it appears to be fairly slowly absorbed in this form, though an element of risk in its use is undeniable.

For systemic use, it makes the perfect partner for heroin in the Brompton mixture for the terminally ill patient. It offsets the sedative effect of heroin, while the euphoriant properties summate most satisfactorily.

### PROCAINE AND PROCAINAMIDE

Procaine is a local anaesthetic of short duration and poor penetrative powers. These properties stem from its vasodilator activity and relatively high $pK_a$, which renders it highly ionised at physiological pH. It is therefore rapidly absorbed into the circulation when injected, and is inactive as a surface anaesthetic. It is less potent than lignocaine, and carries a lower incidence of successful nerve blockade. Its duration is about half that of lignocaine, but can be greatly prolonged by the addition of adrenaline.

Procaine, once in the circulation, is hydrolysed by pseudocholinesterase in the plasma and liver to *p*-aminobenzoic acid and diethylaminoethanol. It is therefore effectively of low toxicity. Several drug interactions, however, are possible:

1. Procaine may prolong the effect of suxamethonium by competing with it for the same enzyme.
2. One product of hydrolysis, *p*-aminobenzoic acid, is a potent inhibitor of the bacteriostatic effects of sulphonamides, as well as being allergenic.
3. Diethylaminoethanol potentiates the effect of digitalis and therefore might precipitate intoxication in patients on digitalis-type drugs.
4. Anti-cholinesterase drugs may increase the toxicity of procaine.

It has been stated that procaine should not be given to patients with myasthenia gravis. A reason for this is that such patients are likely to be taking anticholinesterase drugs, rather than because of any enhancement by procaine of neuromuscular blockade. Neither procaine nor any other local anaesthetic should be regarded as a ganglionic or neuromuscular blocker in therapeutic doses.

**Cardiovascular system.**—Procaine was early found to be an effective antidysrhythmic drug, but procainamide soon replaced it as it is less likely to produce central nervous system toxicity and because it is not broken down by pseudocholinesterase, it has a more prolonged cardiac effect. Both drugs have an antidysrhythmic effect like that of quinidine (see under Pharmacological effects, p. 836). Because conduction is readily depressed, a wide QRS complex may herald ventricular extrasystoles and fibrillation. Asynchronous contraction of the ventricle may be associated with a fall in cardiac output.

**Use.**—There are now no indications for the use of procaine as a local anaesthetic. It is too brief for most purposes and though perfectly satisfactory for local infiltration prior to setting up an intravenous infusion, for example, it has no specific clinical advantage over more modern drugs. As may be expected from its poor lipid solubility, it is singularly unreliable for epidural use.[111]

### Cinchocaine (Dibucaine, Nupercaine)

Cinchocaine is the most potent and toxic local anaesthetic that has been used medically. Its importance lies in the pride of place it has held over many years for spinal anaesthesia for which purpose its toxicity is of no moment. For some time three solutions of cinchocaine were made for this purpose: light (1:1,500 or 0·06 per cent), isotonic (1:200 or 0·5 per cent) and heavy (1:200 or 0·5 per cent in 6 per cent glucose). The light spinal technique, involving a subarachnoid injection of a large volume of dilute solution, was reputedly associated with chronic adhesive arachnoiditis and other serious neurological sequelae, and should not be used. Now only the heavy technique is employed for which purpose cinchocaine is generally longer-acting than other agents.[112,113]

*Other uses of cinchocaine.*—Under its USP name, dibucaine, this drug is used in the detection of atypical pseudocholinesterase (see Chapter 23).

### Amethocaine (Tetracaine, Decicaine, Pontocaine)

Amethocaine is a potent, long-acting local anaesthetic, and is a very effective surface anaesthetic. It is used in a 0·5 per cent concentration in the eye, and a 1 to 2 per cent solution for application to mucous membranes. Amethocaine hydrochloride for injection is usually presented as a dry powder and has been added to lignocaine solution to prolong the action of the latter in nerve blocks and epidural anaesthesia. It has also been used alone, in a 0·25 per cent or occasionally a 0·5 per cent concentration, 15—20 ml, for epidural anaesthesia, with or without adrenaline, when its duration of action is similar to that of bupivacaine. It appears that 0·5 per cent is no more effective or long-acting than 0·25 per cent.[114]

Amethocaine may also be used for spinal anaesthesia. Isobaric and hyperbaric solutions, concentrations of 0·5 and 0·75 per cent and volumes of 1–3 ml, have been employed.[115–117] The lower doses may be unreliable and certainly produce a smaller incidence of satisfactory analgesia than equal doses of bupivacaine,[118] though motor block is often profound and prolonged.[113] The larger doses of isobaric amethocaine may last up to six hours.[116]

## Lignocaine (Lidocaine, Xylocaine)

Lignocaine was synthesised in 1943 in Sweden, by Löfgren of AB Astra, and it was introduced into clinical practice in 1948. It has numerous advantages over many of its predecessors, and has been popular ever since.

Lignocaine is a local anaesthetic of moderate potency and duration, but of good penetrative powers and rapid onset of action. It is effective by all routes of administration and its advent was partly responsible for the increased popularity of epidural anaesthesia, because its excellent penetration renders blockade by this method highly successful.

It sometimes causes local vasodilatation. Adrenaline prolongs the action of lignocaine and also reduces its rate of systemic absorption. Thus the duration of action epidurally is about ¾–1 hour, prolonged up to 2½ hours with adrenaline. With repeated injection, tachyphylaxis often occurs; indeed it may occasionally be practically impossible to produce analgesia after some hours. Adrenaline can reduce but not abolish this feature.

The carbonate of lignocaine has remarkable penetrative powers, a rapid onset of action, a high incidence of motor block[119] and a reduced incidence of missed segments[120] when used for epidural anaesthesia (see also p. 834).

Lignocaine is very effective as a surface anaesthetic. Absorption from mucosal surfaces, however, is rapid and may give rise to high blood levels unless the dose is carefully controlled. For this reason, laryngo-pharyngeal and laryngeal spraying may be preferred to tracheal spraying for intubation, since they are as effective and lower plasma lignocaine levels result.[121]

Absorption from the inflamed urethra can take place at a rate equivalent to intravenous injection.

**Cardiovascular system** (see general section, p. 836).—Lignocaine is a useful drug in the treatment of cardiac dysrhythmias. It stabilises the membrane of damaged and excitable cells, tending to suppress ectopic foci. In therapeutic doses it causes no consistent rate change, and does not depress conduction in Purkinje tissue.[122] Widening of the QRS complex is not seen and there is usually no apparent myocardial depression. Even an improvement in cardiac output and blood pressure has been observed when it is used in the treatment of cardiac dysrhythmias.[123] It is less useful than quinidine or procainamide in the treatment of supraventricular dysrhythmias, in which the myocardial depressant action of the two latter drugs is often of little importance. The great value of lignocaine, however, is in the acute treatment of ventricular dysrhythmias, after myocardial infarction or cardiac surgery. Its lack of depressant effect in the myocardium is valuable in these circumstances. Toxicity affects the central nervous system producing sedation initially which, with an intravenous infusion, should give ample warning of more serious sequelae. Toxic effects are more likely in the presence of hepatic under-perfusion,[124] such as may accompany a reduced cardiac output.

**Dosage.**—A concentration of lignocaine hydrochloride of 0·25–0·5 per cent is used for infiltration. If extensive block is required 0·25 per cent with adrenaline should be used. Up to 40 ml of 0·5 per cent lignocaine without adrenaline is usually used for intravenous regional analgesia. 1 per cent lignocaine suffices for most nerve blocks. A concentration of 2 per cent, with adrenaline 12·5 μg/ml (1:80,000) is popular in dentistry. Concentrations of 1·2–2 per cent are used for epidural analgesia, sometimes with the addition of adrenaline 5 μg/ml (1:200,000). For surface application lignocaine may be used in solution as a liquid (4 per cent) for spraying or application on wool pledgets, or in a lubricating gel for the urethra (2 per cent) or on instruments, endotracheal tubes and oropharyngeal airways (4 per cent).

In the treatment of cardiac dysrhythmias, 1 mg/kg is usually given as a bolus dose intravenously, followed by an infusion of 1–2 mg/minute. Such a regime gives rise to a short-lived high blood concentration initially, followed by one which may be too low to be effective for 4–6 hours. Therefore infusion should be rapid at first (e.g. 4 mg/minute for 20 minutes) then gradually slowed down to 1 mg/min as the tissues begin to take up lignocaine less rapidly. Such an infusion continued at a steady rate for days is liable to give rise to systemic toxicity. A low infusion rate, and caution throughout, should be used in the presence of a low cardiac output and after cardiac surgery.[69]

The safe dose limit for lignocaine has been much disputed. After the publication by Deacock and Simpson[82] of a series of fatalities from lignocaine, the upper safe dose ascribed to it was 200 mg plain and 500 mg with adrenaline. However, this decision failed to take into account differences in weight of patients and different absorption rates from various sites of injection. The maximum safe dose in man is probably about 6 mg/kg—possibly less than this for plain solutions in vascular areas—while more than this has often been given with impunity with adrenaline into less vascular areas. Toxic symptoms may occur at plasma levels of 3 to 5 μg/ml (12·8–21·4 μmol/l)[125,126] yet such levels are not uncommonly produced after a single-shot epidural block.[79,127]

### Chloroprocaine (Nesacaine)

This agent, the 2-chloro derivative of procaine, was introduced into clinical medicine in the 1950s and has become increasingly popular in the USA since that time, though it has never been marketed in the United Kingdom.

It is a much more effective local anaesthetic than procaine, producing reliable nerve block by all routes, with good penetrative power. It has a rapid onset of action[128–130] which has made it popular for epidural analgesia in obstetrics, particularly when last minute blockade is practised. Its duration of action is very brief, however, with unpleasantly abrupt return of pain in labour,[128,130] usually within an hour. The incidence of motor block and hypotension tends to be higher than with bupivacaine. The abrupt offset of action has led to its combination with bupivacaine; however, it tends to abbreviate the action of bupivacaine;[131] this response has been shown in the rat to be related to the low pH of the mixture.[132]

Chloroprocaine is hydrolysed in plasma exceedingly rapidly, at a rate four times that of procaine itself, making its systemic toxicity remarkably low. Hydrolysis is, however, inhibited by the presence in the plasma of the amide local anaesthetics bupivacaine and etidocaine.[133]

Recent years have seen many reports of prolonged blockade and neurotoxicity associated with the epidural administration of chloroprocaine. Such complications appear to be dose-related and usually follow inadvertent subarachnoid injection of larger volumes.[134] It has been suggested that the formulation of chloroprocaine which is currently available in the United States and which is of low pH, might contribute to such neurotoxicity,[134] the cerebrospinal fluid having negligible buffering capacity in the face of large volumes.[135] There is evidence, however, for direct neurotoxicity[136] which is not produced by low pH alone[137] though osmotic disturbance produced by displacement of cerebrospinal fluid by large volumes of chloroprocaine solution may contribute.[138] Intrathecal chloroprocaine has been associated with subpial necrosis in dogs[137] and chronic adhesive arachnoiditis in man.[139]

Such risks, whether they be related to altered drug formulation or to error of technique, are generally deemed to outweigh the small advantage conferred by a rapid onset of action—which can usually be achieved by administering a local anaesthetic somewhat sooner!

### Mepivacaine (Carbocaine, Scandicaine)

Mepivacaine was synthesised by Bo af Ekenstam of AB Bofors in Sweden,[140] as one of a large homologous series. Mepicavaine is similar to lignocaine in local anaesthetic potency and speed of onset; it has good penetrative powers and a slightly longer duration of action. It produces vasoconstriction more readily than lignocaine[141] and prilocaine,[46] but its duration of action is increased by adrenaline. It has been used for all types of blockade, in doses and concentrations akin to those of lignocaine, and like lignocaine has caused death when used in excessive dosage.[83] The toxic plasma level may be slightly higher than that of lignocaine,[142] but as mepivacaine is cleared relatively slowly,[143] such toxic concentrations are readily produced by repeated doses. For long-continued use it is certainly less safe than bupivacaine. It has nevertheless been used extensively in obstetrics in the United States, with reports of fetal intoxication during caudal epidurals, accidental fetal injections and paracervical blocks. Whether any of these troubles can be directly laid at the door of mepivacaine remains debatable, but during caudal and lumbar epidural block there is no doubt that mepivacaine gives rise to relatively higher fetal blood concentrations than do other local anaesthetics that have been measured.[100,144,145]

Mepivacaine has undoubted value in dentistry. Unlike lignocaine, it has an acceptable success rate when used without adrenaline and a duration of dental anaesthesia of about 20 minutes[146,147] which is prolonged to 30–40 minutes by the addition of adrenaline.

Cartridges of 3 per cent plain solution for dental use and heavy solutions for spinal anaesthesia are rather mistakenly marketed in Great Britain under the confusing and inappropriate trade name of Chlorocain.

### Prilocaine (Citanest, Propitocaine, L67)

Prilocaine emerged in 1960, shortly after mepivacaine, from the same stable as lignocaine—AB Astra—having been synthesised some years previously by Löfgren.

Its potency and speed of onset as a local anaesthetic are similar to, or very slightly less than, those of lignocaine and its penetrative powers good. It can be used for all types of blockade, in concentrations similar to those of lignocaine. It is a moderate vasoconstrictor; its vasoactivity is intermediate between that of mepivacaine and lignocaine.[46] When used epidurally it may produce a higher incidence of motor block than does lignocaine and a slightly longer duration of action. After the addition of adrenaline its duration is only slightly prolonged, and is equal to that of lignocaine with adrenaline.[148]

It is used in dentistry in a 3 per cent solution. Its somewhat brief action can be more effectively prolonged by felypressin than by adrenaline.[93] It may be recommended in this field with felypressin (as Citanest with Octapressin) when a long duration of dental block is required in patients taking tricyclic antidepressants in whom adrenaline is contra-indicated.

The administration of prilocaine gives rise to much lower plasma concentrations than does an equal dose of lignocaine[78] or mepivacaine.[143] This is in part accounted for by more rapid metabolism and possibly also by greater tissue uptake[149] because it is less protein-bound than the other agents. It is only about two-thirds as toxic as lignocaine after a single dose, and considerably less cumulative.

Although it may be relatively unlikely to cause central nervous system toxicity, one product of its rapid metabolism, *o*-toluidine, induces methaemoglobinaemia. This is a dose-related phenomenon; when 600 mg of prilocaine have been given, the methaemoglobin level, normally about 1 per cent, may rise to 5 per cent or more. Levels greater than 10 per cent were observed in mothers and their babies after delivery, when prilocaine was used for epidural analgesia.[150] The maximum methaemoglobin concentration is normally seen four to six hours after prilocaine administration and declines to normal in about 24 hours. Methaemoglobinaemia can be treated successfully in this situation with methylene blue, 1 mg/kg. Nevertheless, its occurrence may contra-indicate prilocaine in many situations, though a slight, transient rise in methaemoglobin level is harmless to most people.

### Bupivacaine (Marcain, Marcaine, LAC 43)

Bupivacaine is one of the homologous series synthesised by Bo af Ekenstam to which mepivacaine belongs. First reports of its use were made in 1963.[151] Bupivacaine is three to four times as potent as lignocaine, and considerably longer lasting. Its speed of onset is sometimes found to be marginally slower than that of lignocaine and mepivacaine. It has been used for all manner of blocks when prolonged analgesia is required.

Bupivacaine crosses the placenta but little. For an account of its unique value in obstetrics, see Chapter 41.

It is used extensively for *lumbar epidural blockade*, particularly when prolonged analgesia is required. When given by intermittent injection, tachyphylaxis is much less common than with lignocaine, and safe and effective analgesia can usually be provided indefinitely. For pain relief in labour, a dose of about 30 mg provides analgesia for around two hours, and a low incidence of motor block (see Fig. 3). Analgesia in the postoperative period usually lasts four hours or so, while caudal administration may produce perineal analgesia for eight hours or more.

Concentrations of 0·125–0·5 per cent of bupivacaine may be used for epidural analgesia. A concentration of 0·125 per cent has a quite unacceptably high failure rate and brief duration of action, despite the addition of adrenaline.[152,153] Even 0·25 per cent has been found by some workers to fail to give complete blockade occasionally, while 0·5 per cent bupivacaine invariably achieves successful analgesia. Others have found 0·25 per cent satisfactory and the lack of motor blockade advantageous.[154] The lower concentrations are more satisfactory for continuous infusion.[155,156] Adrenaline 2·5–5·0 μg/ml (1:400,000–1:200,000) is sometimes added, though it is of little value and introduces an added risk. For surgery, 0·75 per cent bupivacaine may be used provided only limited spread is required. If a large number of segments must be blocked, it is difficult to keep within the maximum safe dose with this high concentration.

Bupivacaine has also become increasingly popular for spinal anaesthesia using either a hyperbaric solution containing 5–8 per cent dextrose or the commercial plain solution, which is slightly hypobaric.[31] Concentrations of 0·4, 0·5 and 0·75 per cent and volumes of 1–4 ml have been used,[157–159] though more than 15 mg is probably excessive.[160] Analgesia is generally good[118] and motor block profound.[30] Though maximum block may be slow to develop,[162] analgesia may persist in lower segments for more than four hours. For intravenous regional anaesthesia, a concentration of 0·2 per cent bupivacaine and a maximum dose of 1·5 mg/kg, produce good analgesia[163,164] which outlasts cuff deflation.[165] Problems associated with this procedure are related both to failures of technique and to the use of this somewhat excessive dosage, but bupivacaine is no longer recommended for this purpose.

Clinically occurring blood levels of bupivacaine are usually well below those likely to produce toxic symptoms[142] and it is a less cumulative drug than lignocaine or mepivacaine. For a single-shot epidural, the maximum safe dose is about 2 mg/kg. To provide prolonged analgesia, if 25–30 mg 2-hourly suffices, this dose rate can probably be given almost indefinitely. Geerinckx and associates[166] found bupivacaine not to accumulate in obstetric patients when 0·125 per cent was used. Reynolds, Hargrove and Wyman[167] showed that if 50 mg doses were repeated every 2–3 hours, a maximum dose without adrenaline of 320 mg and with adrenaline of about 500 mg, could probably be given with safety.

A few isolated cases of prolonged blockade have been noted following epidural bupivacaine,[168] but these have always recovered and it is doubtful if the incidence is any higher than with other agents, in view of the extensive use of bupivacaine in obstetrics.

### Etidocaine (Duranest)

Etidocaine is Astra's most recent addition to the field of local anaesthetic drugs. It has been used for ulnar nerve block,[169] axillary plexus block[170] and intercostal nerve block,[171] but principally for epidural block,[172,173] for induction of labour,[174] delivery,[175] pain relief in labour,[176,177] surgery[178] and postoperative pain relief.[179]

It is generally used in concentrations double those of bupivacaine, because it is less potent than bupivacaine in producing sensory block and also less reliable,[175,178,180] though more potent for motor block (see Fig. 2). Its onset of action is sometimes quicker than that of bupivacaine.[180] Although longer acting than lignocaine, its duration of action is less than that of bupivacaine. If adrenaline is added, duration of sensory blockade is only slightly briefer than that of bupivacaine, although motor block may occasionally be more prolonged.[181]

Etidocaine has been recommended when prolonged epidural blockade is required for surgery, in which the high degree of motor blockade is an advantage. For this purpose 20 ml of 1 per cent etidocaine with adrenaline 5 μg/ml (1:200,000) may be given, and should last 2–5 hours, though sensory block is not always adequate.[180] A 1·5 per cent solution may not necessarily be more satisfactory.[171] For obstetric pain relief it is less suitable than bupivacaine (although it crosses the placenta but little) because no concentration can produce reliable sensory block without an unacceptably high incidence of motor block.

Etidocaine is more rapidly eliminated than bupivacaine,[182] and less toxic after equal single doses. Thus for a single dose the therapeutic ratios of the two drugs are similar.[183] For continuous use, as etidocaine has to be given at double the dose of bupivacaine, and at a greater frequency unless adrenaline is added, it may have as great a cumulative tendency.[184] Accumulation, however, is not likely to be dangerous with either drug.

## REFERENCES


1. Moore, D. C. (1981). The pH of local anesthetic solutions. *Anesth. Analg.* **60**, 833.
2. Ritchie, J. M. (1975). Mechanism of action of local anaesthetic agents and biotoxins. *Brit. J. Anaesth.*, **47**, 191.
3. Hille, B. (1977). Local anesthetics: hydrophilic and hydrophobic pathways for the drug-receptor reaction. *J. Gen. Physiol.*, **69**, 497.
4. Narahashi, T., Frazier, D. T. and Yamada, M. (1970). The site of action and active form of local anesthetics I. Theory and pH experiments with tertiary compounds. *J. Pharmacol. exp. Ther.*, **171**, 32.
5. Seeman, P. (1972). The membrane actions of anesthetics and tranquillizers. *Pharmacol. Rev.*, **24**, 583.
6. Seeman, P. (1977). Anesthetics and pressure reversal of anesthesia. Expansion and recompression of membrane proteins, lipids and water. *Anesthesiology*, **47**, 1.
7. Kendig, J. J. and Cohen, E. N. (1977). Pressure antagonism to nerve conduction block by anesthetic agents. *Anesthesiology*, **47**, 6.
8. Donchin, Y., Ramu, A., Olshwang, D., Neiman, Z. and Magora, F. (1980). Effect of sodium bicarbonate on the kinetics of bupivacaine in i.v. regional anaesthesia in dogs. *Brit. J. Anaesth.*, **52**, 969.
9. Ritchie, J. M., Ritchie, B. and Greengard, P. (1965). The effect of the nerve sheath on the action of local anesthetics. *J. Pharmacol. exp. Ther.*, **150**, 160.
10. Catchlove, R. F. H. (1972). The influence of $CO_2$ and pH on local anesthetic action. *J. Pharmacol. exp. Ther.*, **181**, 298.
11. Bromage, P. R., Burfoot, M. F., Crowell, D. E. and Truant, A. P. (1967). Quality of epidural blockade III: carbonated local anaesthetic solutions. *Brit. J. Anaesth.*, **39**, 197.
12. Martin, R., Lamarche, Y. and Tétreault, L. (1981). Comparison of the clinical effectiveness of lidocaine hydrocarbonate and lidocaine hydrochloride with and without epinephrine in epidural anaesthesia. *Canad. Anaesth. Soc. J.*, **28**, 217.
13. McClure, J. H. and Scott, D. B. (1981). Comparison of bupivacaine hydrochloride and carbonated bupivacaine in brachial plexus block by the interscalene technique. *Brit. J. Anaesth.*, **53**, 523.
14. Tucker, G. T. and Mather, L. E. (1975). Pharmacokinetics of local anaesthetic agents. *Brit. J. Anaesth.*, **47**, 213.
15. Atkinson, R. E. and Nicholas, A. D. G. (1976). A comparison of bupivacaine hydrochloride and bupivacaine carbonate during labour. *Communication to the Obstetric Anaesthetists Association.*
16. Brown, D. T., Morison, D. H., Covino, B. C. and Scott, D. B. (1980). Comparison of carbonated bupivacaine and bupivacaine hydrochloride for extradural anaesthesia. *Brit. J. Anaesth.*, **52**, 419.
17. Franz, D. N. and Perry, R. S. (1974). Mechanisms for differential block among single myelinated and non-myelinated axons by procaine. *J. Physiol.* (*Lond.*), **236**, 193.
18. Heavner, J. E. and De Jong, R. H. (1974). Lidocaine blocking concentrations for B- and C-nerve fibers. *Anesthesiology*, **40**, 228.
19. Scurlock, J. E., Heavner, J. E. and de Jong, R. H. (1975). Differential B and C fibre block by an amide and ester-linked local anaesthetic. *Brit. J. Anaesth.*, **47**, 1135.
20. Rosenberg, P. H., Heinonen, E., Jansson, S. E. and Gripenberg, J. (1980). Differential nerve block by bupivacaine and 2-chloroprocaine. An experimental study. *Brit. J. Anaesth.*, **52**, 1183.
21. Gissen, A. J., Covino, B. G. and Gregus, J. (1980). Differential sensitivities of mammalian nerve fibers to local anesthetic agents. *Anesthesiology*, **53**, 467.
22. Rosenberg, P. H. and Heavner, J. E. (1980). Temperature-dependent nerve-blocking action of lidocaine and halothane. *Acta anaesth. Scand.*, **24**, 314.
23. de Jong, R. H. (1980). Differential nerve block by local anesthetics (Editorial). *Anesthesiology*, **53**, 443.
24. Strichartz, G. (1976). Review article: Molecular mechanisms of nerve block by local anesthetics. *Anesthesiology*, **45**, 421.
25. Nathan, P. W. and Sears, T. A. (1961). Some factors concerned in differential nerve block by local anaesthetics. *J. Physiol.* (*Lond.*), **157**, 565.
26. Crawford, J. S. (1976). The epidural sieve and MBC (minimum blocking concentrations) an hypothesis. *Anaesthesia*, **31**, 1277.
27. Scurlock, J. E., Meymaris, E. and Gregus, J. (1978). The clinical character of local anesthetics: a function of frequency-dependent conduction block. *Acta anaesth. Scand.*, **22**, 601.
28. Cusick, J. F., Myklebust, J. B. and Abram, S. E. (1980). Differential neural effects of epidural anesthetics. *Anesthesiology*, **53**, 299.
29. Magora, F., Stern, L. and Magora, A. (1980). Motor nerve conduction in intravenous regional anaesthesia with bupivacaine hydrochloride. *Brit. J. Anaesth.*, **52**, 1123.
30. Chambers, W. A., Edstrom, H. H. and Scott, D. B. (1981). Effect of baricity in spinal anaesthesia with bupivacaine. *Brit. J. Anaesth.*, **53**, 279.
31. Tuominen, M., Kalso, E., Rosenberg, P. H. (1982). Effects of posture on the spread of spinal anaesthesia with isotonic 0·75 per cent or 0·5 per cent bupivacaine. *Brit. J. Anaesth.*, **54**, 313.
32. Winnie, A. P., Lavallee, D. A., Sosa, B. P. and Masud, K. Z. (1977). Clinical pharmacokinetics of local anaesthetics. *Canad. Anaesth. Soc. J.*, **24**, 252.
33. Heavner, J. E. (1978). Conduction block by lignocaine and bupivacaine: neonate v. adult. *Brit. J. Anaesth.*, **50**, 1079P.
34. Haegerstam, G. (1979). Effect of i.v. administration of lignocaine and tetrodotoxin on sensory units in the tooth of the cat. *Brit. J. Anaesth.*, **51**, 487.
35. Chapin, J. C., Kushins, L. G., Munson, E. S. and Schick, L. M. (1980). Lidocaine, bupivacaine, etidocaine and epinephrine-induced arrhythmias during halothane anesthesia in dogs. *Anesthesiology*, **52**, 23.
36. Block, A. B. and Covino, B. G. (1981). Effect of local anaesthetic agents on cardiac conduction and contractility. *Regional Anesthesia*, **6**, 55.
37. Davis, D. L. and de Jong, R. H. (1982). Successful resuscitation following massive bupivacaine overdose. *Anesth. Analg.*, **61**, 62.
38. Prentiss, J. E. (1979). Cardiac arrest following caudal anesthesia. *Anesthesiology*, **50**, 51.
39. Albright, G. A. (1979). Cardiac arrest following

regional anesthesia with etidocaine or bupivacaine. *Anesthesiology*, **51**, 285.
40. Liu, P., Feldman, H. S. and Covino, B. G. (1981). Comparative CNS and cardiovascular toxicity of various local anesthetic agents. *Anesthesiology*, **55**, A156.
41. de Jong, R. H., Ronfield, R. A. and de Rosa, R. A. (1982). Cardiovascular effects of convulsant and supraconvulsant doses of amide local anesthetics. *Anesth. Analg.*, **61**, 3.
42. Avery, P., Redon, D., Schaenzer, G. and Rusy, B. (1981). Cerebral and cardiac toxicity of bupivacaine in the presence of normokalemia versus hyperkalemia. *Anesthesiology*, **55**, A164.
43. Moore, D. C., Thompson, G. E. and Crawford, R. D. (1982). Long-acting local anesthetic drugs and convulsions with hypoxia and acidosis. *Anesthesiology*, **56**, 230.
44. Morishima, H. O. and Covino, B. G. (1981). Toxicity and distribution of lidocaine in nonasphyxiated and asphyxiated baboon fetuses. *Anesthesiology*, **54**, 182.
45. Blair, M. R. (1975). Cardiovascular pharmacology of local anaesthetics. *Brit. J. Anaesth.*, **47**, S 247.
46. Reynolds, F., Bryson, T. H. L. and Nicholas, A. D. G. (1976). Intradermal study of a new local anaesthetic agent: aptocaine. *Brit. J. Anaesth.*, **48**, 347.
47. Aps, C. and Reynolds, F. (1976). The effect of concentration on the vasoactivity of bupivacaine and lignocaine. *Brit. J. Anaesth.*, **48**, 1171.
48. Altura, B. M. and Lassoff, S. (1981). Perivascular action of the local anaesthetic, lidocaine, on pial terminal arterioles: direct observations on the microcirculation. *Brit. J. Pharmacol.*, **73**, 577.
49. Åberg, G. (1972). Myogenic action of local anaesthetics on smooth muscle; role of $Ca^{++}$ and cyclic AMP. *Acta pharmacol. (Kbh.)*, **31**, Suppl. 1, 46.
50. Luduena, F. P. (1969). Duration of local anesthesia. *Ann. Rev. Pharmacol.*, **9**, 503.
51. Fairley, J. W. and Reynolds, F. (1981). An intradermal study of the local anaesthetic and vascular effects of the isomers of mepivacaine. *Brit. J. Anaesth.*, **53**, 1211.
52. Moore, D. C., Crawford, R. D. and Scurlock, J. E. (1980). Severe hypoxia and acidosis following local anesthetic-induced convulsions. *Anesthesiology*, **53**, 259.
53. Scott, D. B. (1981). Toxicity caused by local anaesthetic drugs (Editorial) *Brit. J. Anaesth.*, **53**, 553.
54. Weti, C. V., Wright, F. K. (1979). Death caused by cocaine use. *J. Amer. med. Ass.*, **241**, 2519.
55. Rowlingson, J. C. Difazio, C. A., Foster, J. and Carron, H. (1980). Lidocaine as an analgesic for experimental pain. *Anesthesiology*, **52**, 20.
56. Åberg, G., Morck, E. and Waldeck, B. (1973). Studies on the effects of some local anaesthetics on the uptake of $^3H$-1-noradrenaline into vascular and cardiac tissues *in vitro*. *Acta pharmacol. (Kbh.)*, **33**, 476.
57. Taylor, W. J., Wolf, A. and Young, J. M. (1980). The interaction of amine local anaesthetics with muscarinic receptors. *Brit. J. Pharmacol.*, **71**, 327.
58. Downes, H. and Loehning, R. W. (1979). An anticholinergic effect of hexylcaine on airway smooth muscle. *Anesthesiology*, **50**, 221.
59. Fleisch, J. H. and Titus, E. (1973). Effect of local anesthetics on pharmacologic receptor systems of smooth muscle. *J. Pharmacol. exp. Therap.*, **186**, 44.
60. Gal, T. J. (1980). Airway responses in normal subjects following topical anesthesia with ultrasonic aerosols of 4 per cent lidocaine. *Anesth. Analg.*, **59**, 123.
61. Downes, H., Gerber, N. and Hirshan, C. A. (1980). Intravenous lignocaine in reflux and allergic bronchoconstriction. *Brit. J. Anaesth.*, **52**, 873.
62. Waldman, H. B. and Binkley, G. (1967). Lignocaine hypersensitivity: report of a case. *J. Amer. dent. Ass.*, **74**, 747.
63. Eyre, J. and Nally, F. F. (1971). Nasal test of hypersensitivity—including a positive reaction to lignocaine. *Lancet*, **2**, 264.
64. Walker, R. T. (1971). Hypersensitivity reaction to local anaesthetic. *Brit. dent. J.*, **130**, 2.
65. Brown, D. T., Beamish, D. and Wildsmith, J. A. W. (1981). Allergic reaction to an amide local anaesthetic. *Brit. J. Anaesth.*, **53**, 435.
66. Rosenberg, P. H., Heinonen, J. and Takasaki, M. (1980). Lidocaine concentration in blood after topical anaesthesia of the upper respiratory tract. *Acta anaesth. scand.*, **24**, 125.
67. Koch-Weser, J. and Klein, S. W. (1971). Procainamide dosage schedules, plasma concentrations, and clinical effects. *J. Amer. med. Ass.*, **215**, 1454.
68. Routledge, P. A., Stargel, W. W., Finn, A. L., Barchowsky, A. and Shand, D. G. (1981). Lignocaine disposition in blood in epilepsy. *Brit. J. clin. Pharmacol.*, **12**, 663.
69. Aps, C., Bell, J. A., Jenkins, B. S., Poole-Wilson, P. A. and Reynolds, F. (1976). Logical approach to lignocaine therapy. *Brit. med. J.*, **1**, 13.
70. Reynolds, F. (1971). Metabolism and excretion of bupivacaine in man—a comparison with mepivacaine. *Brit. J. Anaesth.*, **43**, 33.
71. Hollunger, G. (1960). On the metabolism of Lidocaine II. The biotransformation of Lidocaine. *Acta pharmacol. (Kbh.)*, **17**, 365.
72. Geddes, I. C. (1965). Studies of the metabolism of Citanest $C^{14}$. *Acta anaesth. scand.*, Suppl. **16**, 37.
73. Boyes, R. N. (1975). A review of the metabolism of amide local anaesthetic agents. *Brit. J. Anaesth.*, **47**, 225.
74. Difazio, C. A. (1975). Biotransformation of lidocaine. In: *Biotransformation of Local Anesthetics, Adjuvants, and Adjunct Agents*, p. 21. Ed. by dal Santo, G. Boston: Little Brown & Co. *Internat. Anesthesiol. Clinics*, **13**, no. 4.
75. de Jong, R. H. (1975). Biotransformation of local anesthetics: general concepts. *Internat. Anesthesiol. Clinics*, **13**, no. 4, 1.
76. Luduena, F. P., Hoppe, J. O. and Borland, J. K. (1958). A statistical evaluation of the relationships among local anesthetic activity, irritancy and systemic toxicity. *J. Pharmacol. exp. Ther.*, **123**, 269.
77. Munson, E. S., Tucker, W. K., Ausinsch, B. and Malagodi, M. H. (1975). Etidocaine, bupivacaine and lidocaine seizure thresholds in monkeys. *Anesthesiology*, **42**, 471.
78. Scott, D. B., Jebson, P. J. R., Braid, D. P., Örtengren, B. and Frisch, P. (1972). Factors affecting plasma levels of lignocaine and prilocaine. *Brit. J. Anaesth.*, **44**, 1040.
79. Braid, D. P. and Scott, D. B. (1966). Dosage of lignocaine in epidural block in relation to toxicity. *Brit. J. Anaesth.*, **38**, 596.
80. de Jong, R. H. and Bonin, J. D. (1980). Local anesthetics: injection route alters relative toxicity of bupivacaine. *Anesth. Analg.*, **59**, 925.
81. Englesson, S. and Matousek, M. (1975). Central ner-

vous system effects of local anaesthetic agents. *Brit. J. Anaesth.*, **47**, 241.

82. Deacock, A. R. and Simpson, W. T. (1964). Fatal reactions to lignocaine. *Anaesthesia*, **19**, 217.
83. Sunshine, I. and Fike, W. W. (1964). Value of thin layer chromatography in two fatal cases of intoxication due to lidocaine and mepivacaine. *New Engl. J. Med.*, **271**, 487.
84. Moore, D. C., Balfour, D. I. and Fitzgibbons, D. (1979). Convulsive arterial plasma levels of bupivacaine and the response to diazepam therapy. *Anesthesiology*, **50**, 454.
85. Moore, D. C. and Bridenbaugh, L. D. (1960). Oxygen: the antidote for systemic toxic reactions from local anesthetic drugs. *J. Amer. med. Ass.*, **174**, 842.
86. Ausinsch, B., Malagodi, M. H. and Munson, E. S. (1976). Diazepam in the prophylaxis of lignocaine seizures. *Brit. J. Anaesth.*, **48**, 309.
87. McLeskey, C. H. (1980). pH of local anesthetic solutions (letter). *Anesth. Analg.*, **59**, 892.
88. Corall, I. M., Broadfield, J. B., Knights, K. M., Nicholson, J. R. and Strunin, L. (1975). Cardiovascular effects of extradural analgesia in labour: comparison of bupivacaine with lignocaine. *Brit. J. Anaesth.*, **47**, 1297.
89. Wallis, K. L., Shnider, S. M., Hicks, J. S. and Spivey, H. T. (1976). Epidural anesthesia in the normotensive pregnant ewe. *Anesthesiology*, **44**, 481.
90. Boakes, A. J., Laurence, D. R., Teoh, P. C., Barar, F. S. K., Benedikter, L. T. and Prichard, B. N. C. (1973). Interactions between sympathomimetic amines and antidepressant agents in man. *Brit. med. J.*, **1**, 311.
91. Klingenström, P. and Westermark, L. (1964). Local tissue oxygen tension after adrenaline, noradrenaline and Octapressin in local anaesthesia. *Acta anaesth. scand.*, **8**, 261.
92. Boakes, A. J. Laurence, D. R., Lovel, K. W., O'Neil, R. and Verrill, P. J. (1972). Adverse reactions to local anaesthetic/vasoconstrictor preparations. A study of the cardiovascular responses to Xylestesin and Hostacain with noradrenaline. *Brit. dent. J.*, **133**, 137.
93. Goldman, V. and Evers, H. (1969). Prilocaine-felipressin: a new combination for dental analgesia. *Dent. Practit. dent. Rec.*, **19**, 225.
94. Akerman, B. (1969). Effects of felypressin (Octapressin) on the acute toxicity of local anaesthetics. *Acta pharmacol. (Kbh.)*, **27**, 318.
95. Aellig, W. H., Laurence, D. R., O'Neil, R. and Verrill, P. J. (1970). Cardiac effects of adrenaline and felypressin as vasoconstrictors in local anaesthesia for oral surgery under diazepam sedation. *Brit. J. Anaesth.*, **42**, 174.
96. Aps, C. and Reynolds, F. (1978). An intradermal study of the local anaesthetic and vascular effects of the isomers of bupivacaine. *Brit. J. clin. Pharmacol.*, **6**, 63.
97. Morgan, M. and Russell, W. J. (1975). An investigation in man into the relative potency of lignocaine, bupivacaine and etidocaine. *Brit. J. Anaesth.*, **47**, 586.
98. Löfström, J. B. (1975). Ulnar nerve blockade for the evaluation of local anaesthetic agents. *Brit. J. Anaesth.*, **47**, 297.
99. Wencker, K. H., Nolte, H. and Fruhstorfer, H. (1975). Brachial plexus blockade for evaluation of local anaesthetic agents. *Brit. J. Anaesth.*, **47**, 301.
100. Reynolds, F. (1971). A comparison of the potential toxicity of bupivacaine, lignocaine, and mepivacaine during epidural blockade for surgery. *Brit. J. Anaesth.*, **43**, 567.
101. Bonica, J. J. (1957). Clinical investigation of local anesthetics. *Anesthesiology*, **18**, 110.
102. Covino, B. G. and Bush, D. F. (1975). Clinical evaluation of local anaesthetic agents. *Brit. J. Anaesth.*, **47**, 289.
103. Scott, D. B., McClure, J. H., Giasi, R. M., Seo, J. and Covino, B. G. (1980). Effects of concentrations of local anaesthetic drugs in extradural block. *Brit. J. Anaesth.*, **52**, 1033.
104. Ekblom, L. and Widman, B. (1966). A comparison of the properties of LAC 43, prilocaine and mepivacaine in extradural anaesthesia. *Acta anaesth. scand.*, Suppl. **21**, 33.
105. Truant, A. P. and Takman, B. (1959). Differential physical-chemical and neuropharmacologic properties of local anesthetic agents. *Anesth. Analg. Curr. Res.*, **38**, 478.
106. Henn, F. (1960). Determination of toxicological and pharmacological properties of Carbocaine, lidocaine and procaine by means of simultaneous experiments. *Acta anaesth. scand.*, **4**, 125.
107. Sawinski, V. J. and Rapp, G. W. (1963). Interaction of human serum proteins with local anesthetic agents, *J. dent. Res.*, **42**, 1429.
108. Ekenstam, B. af (1966). The effect of the structural variation on the local analgesic properties of the most commonly used groups of substances. *Acta anaesth. scand.*, Suppl., **25**, 10.
109. Henn, F. and Brattsand, R. (1966). Some pharmacological and toxicological properties of a new long-acting local analgesic, LAC-43 (Marcaine), in comparison with mepivacaine and tetracaine. *Acta anaesth. scand.*, Suppl. **21**, 9.
110. Tucker, G. T. (1975). Plasma binding and disposition of local anesthetics. *Internat. Anesthesiol. Clinics*, **13**, no. 4, 33.
111. Hunton, J. (1979). The use of procaine hydrochloride as a continuous lumbar epidural technique in labour. *Anaesthesia*, **34**, 274.
112. Fisher, A. and Bryce-Smith, R. (1971). Spinal analgesic agents: a comparison of cinchocaine, lignocaine and prilocaine. *Anaesthesia*, **26**, 324.
113. Rocco, A., Wark, J., Concepcion, M., Francis, D. and Covino, B. (1981). A controlled study of dibucaine and tetracaine in spinal anesthesia. *Anesthesiology*, **55**, A141.
114. Bromage, P. R. (1969). A comparison of bupivacaine and tetracaine in epidural analgesia for surgery. *Canad. Anaesth. Soc. J.*, **16**, 37.
115. Levin, E., Muravchick, S., Gold, M. I. (1981). Isobaric tetracaine, spinal anaesthesia and the lithotomy position. *Anesth. Analg.*, **60**, 810.
116. Brown, D. T., Wildsmith, J. A., Covino, B. G. and Scott, D. B. (1980). Effect of baricity on spinal anaesthesia with amethocaine. *Brit. J. Anaesth.*, **52**, 589.
117. Wildsmith, J. A. W., McClure, J. H., Brown, D. T. and Scott, D. B. (1981). Effects of posture on the spread of isobaric and hyperbaric amethocaine. *Brit. J. Anaesth.*, **52**, 273.
118. Moore, D. C. (1980). Spinal anaesthesia—bupivacaine compared with tetracaine. *Anesth. Analg.*, **59**, 743.
119. Bromage, P. R. and Gertel, M. (1970). An evaluation of two new local anaesthetics for major conduction blockade. *Canad. Anaesth. Soc. J.*, **17**, 557.
120. Bromage, P. R. (1972). Unblocked segments in epidural analgesia for relief of pain in labour. *Brit. J. Anaesth.*, **44**, 676.

121. Curran, J., Hamilton, C. and Taylor, T. (1975). Topical analgesia before tracheal intubation. *Anaesthesia*, **30**, 765.
122. Bigger, J. T. and Heissenbuttel, R. H. (1969). The use of procaine amide and lidocaine in the treatment of cardiac arrhythmias, *Progr. cardiovasc. Dis.*, **11**, 515.
123. Harrison, D. C., Sprouse, J. H. and Morrow, A. G. (1963). Antiarrhythmic properties of lidocaine and procaine amide: clinical and physiologic studies of their cardiovascular effects in man. *Circulation*, **28**, 486.
124. Prestcott, L. F., Adjepon-Yamoah, K. K. and Talbot, R. G. (1976). Impaired lignocaine metabolism in patients with myocardial infarction and cardiac failure. *Brit. med. J.*, **1**, 939.
125. Jewitt, D. E., Kishon, Y. and Thomas, M. (1968). Lignocaine in the management of arrhythmias after acute myocardial infarction. *Lancet*, **1**, 266.
126. Foldes, F. F., Molloy, R., McNall, P. G. and Koukal, L. R. (1960). Comparison of toxicity in intravenously given local anesthetic agents in man. *J. Amer. med. Ass.*, **172**, 1493.
127. Braid, D. P. and Scott, D. B. (1965). The systemic absorption of local analgesic drugs. *Brit. J. Anaesth.*, **37**, 394.
128. Allen, P. R. and Johnson, R. W. (1979). Extradural analgesia in labour. A comparison of 2-chloroprocaine hydrochloride and bupivacaine hydrochloride. *Anaesthesia*, **34**, 839.
129. James, F. M., Dewan, D. M., Floyd, H. M., Wheeler, A. S., Grant, W. M., Rhyne, L. and Westmoreland, R. T. (1980). Chloroprocaine vs. bupivacaine for lumbar epidural analgesia for elective cesarian section. *Anesthesiology*, **52**, 488.
130. Johnson, R. W. (1979). Editorial: Chloroprocaine. *Anaesthesia*, **34**, 837.
131. Corke, B. C., Carlson, G. and Dettbarn, W. D. (1981). The interaction of 2-chloroprocaine and bupivacaine. *Anesthesiology*, **55**, A162.
132. Galindo, A. and Witcher, T. (1980). Mixtures of local anesthetics: bupivacaine-chloroprocaine. *Anesth. Analg.*, **59**, 683.
133. Lalka, D., Vicuna, N., Burrow, S. R., Jones, D. J., Ludden, T. M., Haegele, K. D. and McNay, J. L. (1978). Bupivacaine and other amide local anesthetics inhibit the hydrolysis of chloroprocaine by human serum. *Anesth. Analg.*, **57**, 534.
134. Moore, D. C., Spierdijk, J. Van Kleef, J. D., Coleman, R. L. and Love, G. F. (1982). Chloroprocaine neurotoxicity: four additional cases. *Anesth. Analg.*, **61**, 155.
135. Covino, B. G., Marx, G. F., Finster, M. and Zsigmond, E. K. (1980). Prolonged sensory/motor deficits following inadvertent spinal anesthesia. *Anesth. Analg.*, **59**, 399.
136. Flowerdew, R. M. M. (1981). Chloroprocaine (letter). *Anaesthesia*, **36**, 535.
137. Ravindran, R. S., Turner, M. S. and Muller, J. (1982). Neurological effects of subarachnoid administration of 2-chloroprocaine—E, bupivacaine and low pH normal saline in dogs. *Anesth. Analg.*, **61**, 279.
138. Ravindran, R. S., Bond, V. K., Tasch, M. D., Gupta, C. D. and Luerssen, T. G. (1980). Prolonged neural blockade following regional analgesia with 2-chloroprocaine. *Anesth. Analg.*, **59**, 447.
139. Reisner, L. S., Hochman, B. N. and Plumer, M. H. (1980). Persistent neurologic deficit and adhesive arachnoiditis following intrathecal 2-chloroprocaine injection. *Anesth. Analg.*, **59**, 452.
140. Ekenstam, B. af, Egnér, B., Ulfendahl, H. R., Dhunér, K. G. and Aljelund, O. (1956). Trials with carbocaine: a new local anaesthetic drug. *Brit. J. Anaesth.*, **28**, 503.
141. Rochemont, W. Du M. De, and Hensel, H. (1960). Messung der Hautdurchblutung am Meschen bei Einwirkung verschiedener Lokalanaesthetica. *Naunyn-Schmiedeberg's Arch. exp. Path. Pharmak.*, **239**, 464.
142. Jorfeldt, L., Löfström, B., Pernow, B., Persson, B., Wahren, J. and Widman, B. (1968). The effect of local anaesthetics on the central circulation and respiration in man and dog. *Acta anaesth. scand.*, **12**, 153.
143. Arthur, G. R., Scott, D. H. T., Boyes, R. N. and Scott, D. B. (1979). Pharmacokinetic and clinical pharmacological studies with mepivacaine and prilocaine. *Brit. J. Anaesth.*, **51**, 481.
144. Morishima, H. O., Daniel, S. S., Finster, M., Poppers, P. J. and James, L. S. (1966). Transmission of mepivacaine across the human placenta. *Anesthesiology*, **27**, 147.
145. Moore, D. C., Bridenbaugh, L. D., Bagdi, P. A. and Bridenbaugh, P. O. (1968). Accumulation of mepivacaine hydrochloride during caudal block. *Anesthesiology*, **29**, 585.
146. Mumford, J. M. and Gray, T. C. (1957). Dental trial of Carbocaine—a new local anaesthetic. *Brit. J. Anaesth.*, **29**, 210.
147. Mumford, J. M. and Geddes, I. C. (1961). Trial of Carbocaine in conservative dentistry. *Brit. dent. J.*, **110**, 92.
148. Bromage, P. R. (1965). A comparison of the hydrochloride salts of lignocaine and prilocaine for epidural analgesia. *Brit. J. Anaesth.*, **37**, 753.
149. Eriksson, E. (1966). Prilocaine: an experimental study in man of a new local anaesthetic with special regards to efficiency, toxicity and excretion. *Acta chir. scand.*, Suppl. **358**.
150. Arens, J. F. and Carrera, A. E. (1970). Methemoglobin levels following peridural anesthesia with prilocaine for vaginal deliveries. *Anesth. Analg. Curr. Res.*, **49**, 219.
151. Telivuo, L. (1963). A new long-acting local anaesthetic solution for pain relief after thoracotomy. *Ann. Chir. Gynaec. Fenn.*, **52**, 513.
152. Bleyaert, A., Soetens, M. Vaes, L., Van Steenberge, A. L. and Van Der Donck, A. (1979). Bupivacaine, 0·125 per cent, in obstetric epidural analgesia: experience in three thousand cases. *Anesthesiology*, **51**, 435.
153. Stainthorp, S. F., Bradshaw, E. G., Challen, P. D. and Tobias, M. A. (1978). 0·125 per cent bupivacaine for obstetric analgesia? *Anaesthesia*, **33**, 3.
154. Duthie, A. M., Wyman, J. B. and Lewis, G. A. (1968). Bupivicaine in labour. Its use in lumbar extradural analgesia. *Anaesthesia*, **23**, 20.
155. Evans, K. R. L. and Carrie, L. E. S. (1979). Continuous epidural infusion of bupivacaine in labour: a simple method. *Anaesthesia*, **34**, 310.
156. Ross, R. A., Clarke, J. E., Armitage, E. N. (1980). Postoperative pain prevention by continuous epidural infusion. A study of the clinical effects and plasma concentrations obtained. *Anaesthesia*, **35**, 663.
157. Goodison, R. R., Josyala, A. (1979). Agents for spinal analgesia. Hyperbaric bupivacaine. *Anaesthesia*, **34**, 375.
158. Nightingale, P. J. and Marstrand, T. (1981). Subarachnoid anaesthesia with bupivacaine for orthopaedic procedures in the elderly. *Brit. J. Anaesth.*, **53**, 369.

159. Sundnes, K. O., Vaageness, P., Skretting, P., Lind, B. and Edstrom, H. H. (1982). Spinal analgesia with hyperbaric bupivacaine: effects of volume and solution. *Brit. J. Anaesth.*, **54**, 69.
160. Chambers, W. A., Littlewood, D. G., Edstrom, H. H., Scott, D. B. (1982). Spinal anaesthesia with hyperbaric bupivacine: effects of concentration and volume administered. *Brit. J. Anaesth.*, **54**, 75.
161. Bromage, P. R. (1975). Mechanism of action of extradural analgesia. *Brit. J. Anaesth.*, **47**, S 199.
162. Cameron, A. E., Arnold, R. W., Ghoris, M. W. and Jamieson, V. (1981). Spinal analgesia using bupivacaine 0·5 per cent plain. Variation in the extent of the block with patient age. *Anaesthesia*, **36**, 318.
163. Ware, R. J. (1975). Intravenous regional analgesia using bupivacaine. *Anaesthesia*, **30**, 817.
164. Ware, R. J. (1979). Intravenous regional analgesia using bupivacaine: a double blind comparison with lignocaine. *Anaesthesia*, **34**, 231.
165. Magora, F., Stern, L., Zylber-Katz, E., Olshwang, D., Donchin, Y. and Magora, A. (1980). Prolonged effect of bupivacaine hydrochloride after cuff release in i.v. regional anaesthesia. *Brit. J. Anaesth.*, **52**, 1131.
166. Geerinckx, K., Vanderick, G. G., Van Steenberge, A. L., Bouche, R. and De Muylder, E. (1974). Bupivacaine 0·125 per cent in epidural block analgesia during childbirth: maternal and foetal plasma concentrations. *Brit. J. Anaesth.*, **46**, 937.
167. Reynolds, F., Hargrove, R. L. and Wyman, J. B. (1973). Maternal and foetal plasma concentrations of bupivacaine after epidural block. *Brit. J. Anaesth.*, **45**, 1049.
168. Guerden, C., Buley, R. and Downing, J. W. (1977). Delayed recovery after epidural block in labour. A report of four cases. *Anaesthesia*, **32**, 773.
169. Radtke, H., Nolte, H., Fruhstorfer, H. and Zenz, M. (1975). A comparative study between etidocaine and bupivacaine in ulnar nerve block. *Acta anaesth. scand.*, Suppl. **60**, 17.
170. Hollmen, A. and Mononen, P. (1975). Axillary plexus block with etidocaine. *Acta anaesth. scand.*, Suppl. **60**, 25.
171. Bridenbaugh, P. O., Tucker, G. T., Moore, D. C., Bridenbaugh, L. D. and Thompson, G. (1973). Etidocaine: clinical evaluation for intercostal nerve block and lumbar epidural block. *Anesth. Analg. Curr. Res.*, **52**, 407.
172. Niesel, H. C. and Munch, I. (1975). Experience with etidocaine and bupivacaine in epidural analgesia. *Acta anaesth. scand.*, Suppl. **60**, 60.
173. Gitschmann, J. and Nolte, H. (1975). Comparative study with etidocaine and bupivacaine in epidural block. *Acta anaesth. scand.*, Suppl. **60**, 55.
174. Phillips, G. (1975). A double blind trial of bupivacaine (Marcain) and etidocaine (Duranest) in extradural block for surgical induction of labour. *Brit. J. Anaesth.*, **47**, 1307.
175. Moore, D. C., Bridenbaugh, P. O., Bridenbaugh, L. D., Thompson, G. E., Balfour, R. I. and Lysons, D. F. (1975). Bupivacaine compared with etidocaine for vaginal delivery. *Anesth. Analg. Curr. Res.*, **54**, 250.
176. Poppers, P., Covino, B. and Boyes, N. (1975). Epidural block with etidocaine for labour and delivery. *Acta anaesth. scand.*, Suppl. **60**, 89.
177. Wilson, J. (1975). A double-blind comparison of single doses of etidocaine 1 per cent and bupivacaine 0·5 per cent during continuous lumbar epidural block in obstetrics. *Acta anaesth. scand.*, Suppl. **60**, 97.
178. Moore, D. C., Bridenbaugh, P. O., Bridenbaugh, L. D., Thompson, G. E., Balfour, R. I. and Lysons, D. F. (1974). A double-blind study of bupivacaine and etidocaine for epidural (peridural) block. *Anesth. Analg. Curr. Res.*, **53**, 690.
179. Abdel-Salam, A. and Scott, B. (1975). Bupivacaine and etidocaine in epidural block for post-operative relief of pain. *Acta anaesth. scand.*, Suppl. **60**, 80.
180. Datta, S. D., Corke, B. C., Alper, M. H., Brown, W. U., Ostheimer, G. W. and Weiss, J. B. (1980). Epidural anaesthesia for cesarian section: a comparison of bupivacaine, chloroprocaine and etidocaine. *Anesthesiology*, **52**, 48.
181. Buckley, F. P., Littlewood, D. G., Covino, B. G. and Scott, D. B. (1978). Effects of adrenaline and the concentration of solution on extradural block with etidocaine. *Brit. J. Anaesth.*, **50**, 171.
182. Scott, D. B., Jebson, P. J. R. and Boyes, R. N. (1973). Pharmacokinetic study of the local anaesthetics bupivacaine (Marcain) and etidocaine (Duranest) in man. *Brit. J. Anaesth.*, **45**, 1010.
183. Munson, E. S. Tucker, W. K., Ausinsch, B. and Malagodi, M. H. (1975). Etidocaine, bupivacaine and lidocaine seizure thresholds in monkeys. *Anesthesiology*, **42**, 471.
184. Poppers, P. J. (1975). Evaluation of local anaesthetic agents for regional anaesthesia in obstetrics. *Brit. J. Anaesth.*, **47**, 322.
185. Rosenberg, P. H. and Heinonen, E. (1983). Differential sensitivity of A and C nerve fibres to long-acting amide local anaesthetics. *Brit. J. Anesth.*, **55**, 163.

CHAPTER 32

# Spinal and Epidural Block



## History

Spinal anaesthesia was initially produced inadvertently by Corning in 1885, and first used deliberately by Bier in 1898. In 1901 the French investigators Sicard[1] and Cathelin[2] described epidural injections through the sacral hiatus. By 1920 the technique had become popular and Zweifel[3] was able to analyse the incidence of fatalities encountered in 4,200 caudal epidural blocks recorded in the literature. Although the interspinous approach to the epidural space had also been demonstrated at the beginning of the century, Poges (1921)[4] was the first to describe the practical application of lumbar epidural anaesthesia. Later Dogliotti (1931–33)[5–7] in Italy popularised the technique, followed by other clinical exponents: Hess (1934),[8] Odom (1936)[9] and Harger and associates (1941)[10] in the USA, and Gutierrez (1939)[11] in South America.

The next important development was the adaptation of Tuohy's (1945)[12] catheter technique—devised for continuous spinal anaesthesia—to epidural anaesthesia, by Curbello (1949).[13]

Epidural blockade has increased steadily in popularity in the second half of this century, firstly with the decline in popularity of spinals because of possible serious neurological sequelae, and secondly with the advent of improved local anaesthetics such as bupivacaine.

## Anatomy

### The Vertebrae

The vertebral column is made up of 33 vertebrae: 7 cervical, 12 thoracic, 5 lumbar, 5 sacral, and 4 coccygeal. A typical vertebra is composed of the following parts (Fig. 1):

1. *The Body*, which is weight-bearing and separated from adjoining vertebral bodies by the intervertebral disc.
2. *The Vertebral Arch*, composed of pedicles and laminae which surround and protect the spinal cord and its coverings.
3. *The Transverse and Spinous Processes*, which give attachment to ligaments and to muscles acting on the vertebral column.
4. *The Superior and Inferior Articular Processes*.

Each pedicle is grooved, especially on the lower surface. These grooves are termed the superior and inferior vertebral notches, and together make up the intervertebral foramen for the passage of the spinal nerve. The transverse process arises at the junction of the pedicle and the lamina.

The posterior surface of the vertebral bodies together with the vertebral arches, intervertebral discs and the connecting ligaments collectively form the vertebral canal containing the spinal cord and its investing membranes. Deficiencies occur in the lateral and posterior walls of the vertebral canal, the former being the intervertebral foramen, while posteriorly is situated the interlaminar foramen. This foramen is bounded above and below by adjacent laminae, and at the sides by the inner aspect of the articular processes. In extension the interlaminar foramen is small, particularly in the thoracic region, but it enlarges in flexion and provides access for a spinal or epidural needle.

The spines of the thoracic vertebrae slope steeply downwards (Fig. 2), those of T5–8 are almost vertical. In consequence their tips lie at the level of the body of the vertebra below. The spines of T1 and 2 and of T11 and 12 are almost horizontal, while those of T3 and 4, and of T9 and 10 are somewhat oblique.

*The lumbar vertebrae*, five in number, have large and massive kidney-shaped bodies

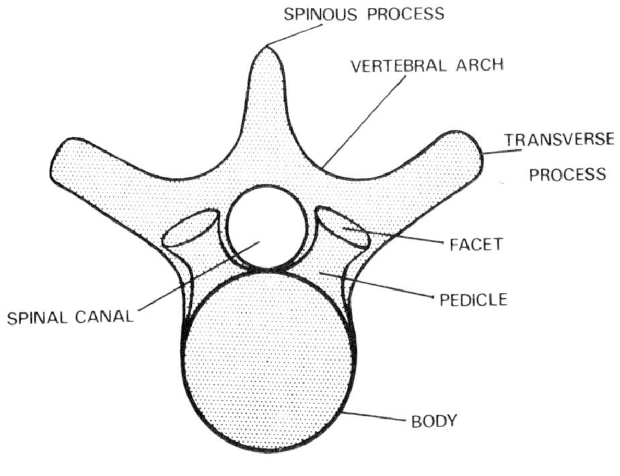


32/Fig. 1.—Diagram of a typical vertebra showing its components.

because of their weight-bearing function. They are distinguished from cervical vertebrae by having no foramen in the transverse process and from thoracic by having no articular facets for ribs on the vertebral bodies. The bodies are slightly taller anteriorly than posteriorly, producing the lumbar curve. The pedicles are directed backwards and laterally, as in the cervical region. The superior intervertebral notch is small and the inferior large. The laminae are thick and sloping, as in the thoracic region, and the spinal canal is triangular. The spine is hatchet-shaped and projects backwards nearly horizontally (Fig. 3).

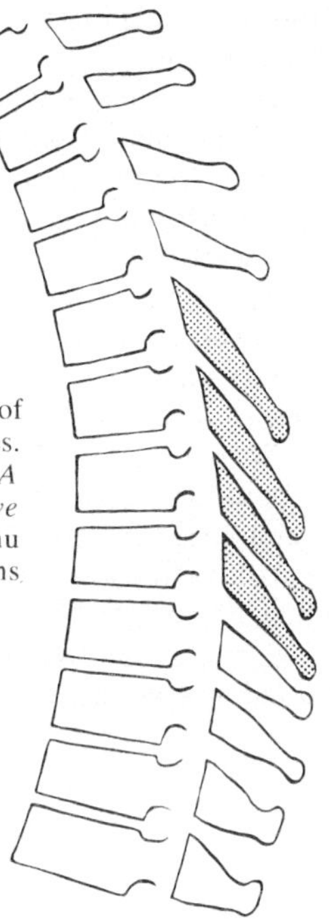

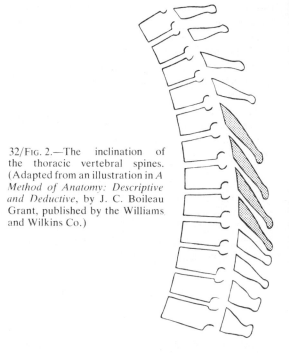

32/Fig. 2.—The inclination of the thoracic vertebral spines. (Adapted from an illustration in *A Method of Anatomy: Descriptive and Deductive*, by J. C. Boileau Grant, published by the Williams and Wilkins Co.)

### Important Ligaments of the Vertebral Column

It is essential for the anaesthetist to have an accurate knowledge of those ligaments in the spine through which the spinal or epidural needle passes. The different sensations of resistance that these ligaments impart to the advancing needle can with practice be appreciated by the operator and are an invaluable aid to successful technique.

The vertebrae are held together by a series of overlapping ligaments which not only bind together the vertebral column but assist in protecting the spinal cord (Figs. 4 and 5).

*The anterior and posterior longitudinal ligaments* bound the bodies of the vertebrae in front and behind, running from axis (C2) to sacrum.

*The ligamentum flavum* is of considerable importance to the anaesthetist. It is composed entirely of yellow elastic fibres, which account for its name. It runs from the anterior and inferior aspects of the lamina above to the posterior and superior aspect of the lamina below. Laterally it blends with the capsule of the facet joint and medially with the interspinous ligament, or with its fellow of the opposite side[14] (Fig 5). The ligamenta flava comprise over half of the posterior wall of the vertebral canal, the bony laminae accounting for the remainder. The ligament is thinnest in the cervical region and thickest in the lumbar region, where powerful stresses and strains have to be countered. Functionally, these ligaments are muscle sparers, assisting in straightening up after bending, and in maintaining the erect posture.

*Interspinous ligaments* connect adjoining spi-

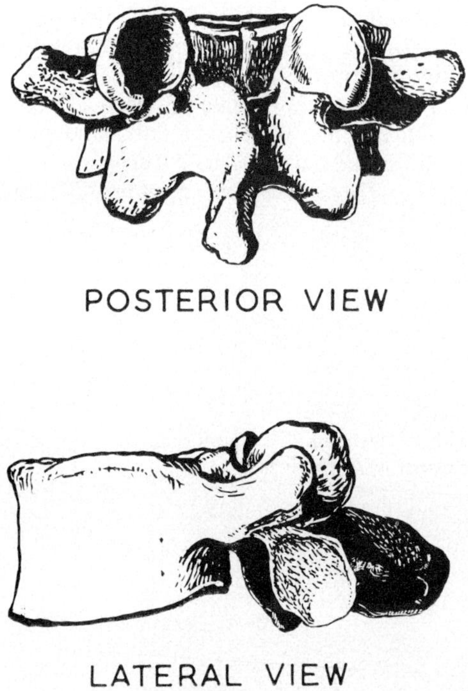


32/Fig. 3.—A lumbar vertebra.

nous processes from their tips to their roots (Fig. 4 and 5). They fuse with the supraspinous ligament posteriorly and with the ligamentum flavum anteriorly. In the lumbar region they are wide and dense.

*The supraspinous ligament* is a continuation of the ligamentum nuchae and joins together the tips of the spinous processes from the seventh cervical vertebra to the sacrum. It increases in thickness from above downwards and is thickest and widest in the lumbar region.

**The intervertebral discs** are responsible for a quarter of the length of the spinal column, and, functionally, are shock absorbers placed between the vertebral bodies. They are thicker in the cervical and lumbar regions, where they allow greater mobility, than in the thoracic region. Each disc consists of a peripheral fibrous portion—the annulus fibrosus—and a gelatinous central part—the nucleus pulposus—which accommodates itself to changes in shape during movement between the vertebra. If a lumbar-puncture needle is accidentally pushed too far through the subarachnoid space and into the annulus, the nucleus pulposus may prolapse and cause sciatica.

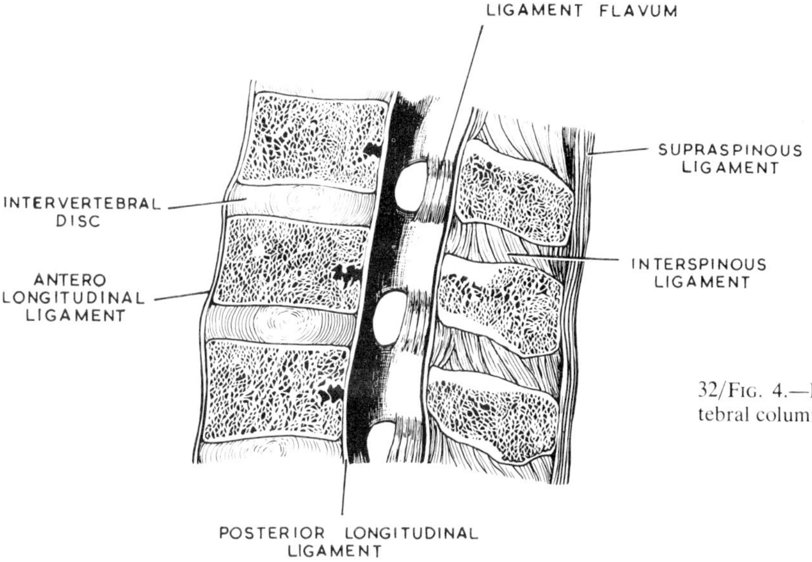


32/FIG. 4.—Important ligaments of the vertebral column.

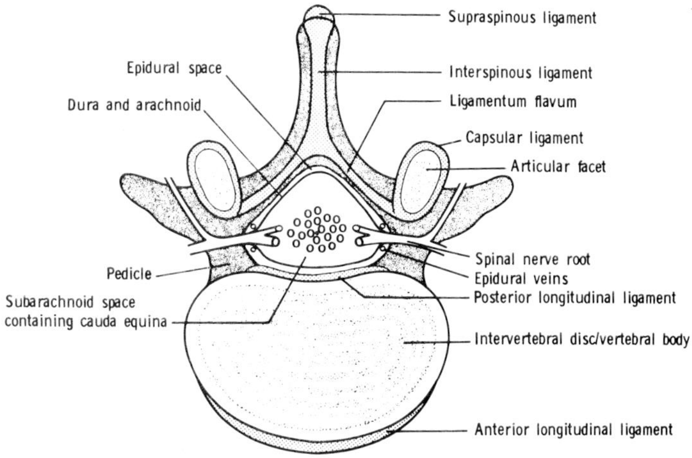


32/FIG. 5.—Diagrammatic transverse section through the vertebral column in the mid-thoracic region.

### The Spinal Cord and its Coverings

The spinal cord, a direct continuation of the medulla oblongata, begins at the upper border of the atlas and ends, in the adult, usually at the lower border of the 1st lumbar vertebra, being 42–45 cm in length. It may on occasion extend to the second or even more rarely to the 3rd lumbar vertebra. In the newborn child the cord ends at the 3rd lumbar vertebra, and in fetal life the cord extends the entire length of the vertebral canal and the spinal nerves run horizontally. As the vertebral column elongates with growth, the spinal cord does not keep pace and the nerve roots assume an increasingly oblique and downward direction towards their foramina of exit. Consequently, below the 1st lumbar vertebra the canal is occupied by a leash of lumbar, sacral and coccygeal nerve roots, termed the cauda equina (Fig. 5). The difference between the cord level of a given spinal root and the vertebral level must be remembered when blocking spinal nerve roots with small volumes of neurolytic agents, otherwise destruction of nerve roots below the desired levels will result (Fig. 6).

From the lower end of the spinal cord extends a thread-like structure known as the filum terminale interna, which ends with the dura and the arachnoid mater at the level of the second sacral vertebra (Fig. 6). It pierces the dura and arachnoid and is continued below this level as the filum terminale externa, eventually blending with the periosteum on the back of the coccyx.

The 31 spinal nerves emerge from the spinal cord in pairs, 8 cervical, 12 thoracic, 5 lumbar, 5 sacral, and one pair of coccygeal nerves. The spinal nerves are composed of the anterior and posterior roots, which unite in the intervertebral foramina to form the spinal nerve trunks. The cord has two enlargements, cervical and lumbar, corresponding to the nerve supply of the upper and lower limbs. The cervical enlargement extends from C3 to T2 and the lumbar enlargement from T9–12.

**The blood supply** of the spinal cord is somewhat tenuous, so that hypotension, local vasoconstriction, thrombosis or aortic clamping may lead to cord ischaemia. Such a mechanism may explain the occasional neurological disaster following spinal or epidural analgesia.

There are one or two posterior spinal arteries

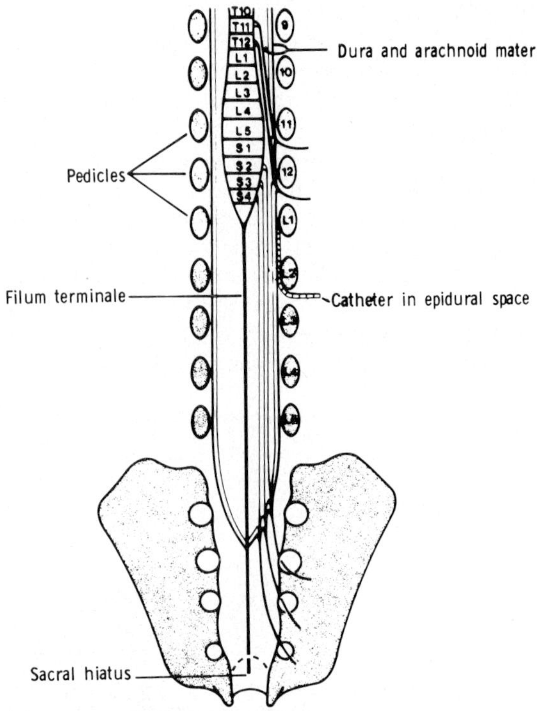


32/Fig. 6.—Diagrammatic longitudinal section through the lower end of the vertebral column. Artistic licence shows an epidural catheter entering the epidural space laterally instead of in the midline. For clarity, only a few spinal nerve roots are shown: those concerned with pain in labour. The spinal cord is seen to end at L1 and the dural sac at S2.

on each side arising from the posterior inferior cerebellar arteries at the base of the brain. They supply part of the posterior horns and posterior columns of the spinal cord and are replenished by numerous segmental arteries, the posterior radicular arteries.

There is a single anterior spinal artery lying on front of the anterior median fissure in the pia mater. It arises at the level of the foramen magnum by the union of a small branch from each vertebral artery and passes down the whole length of the spinal cord. Reinforcements for the anterior spinal artery are relatively few and irregular, many of the anterior radicular arteries petering out in the nerve roots. There are commonly two or three which join the anterior spinal artery in the cervical and upper thoracic regions, but only one, the Radicularis magna artery (or artery of Adamkiewicz) which is unilateral, supplying the lumbar enlargement

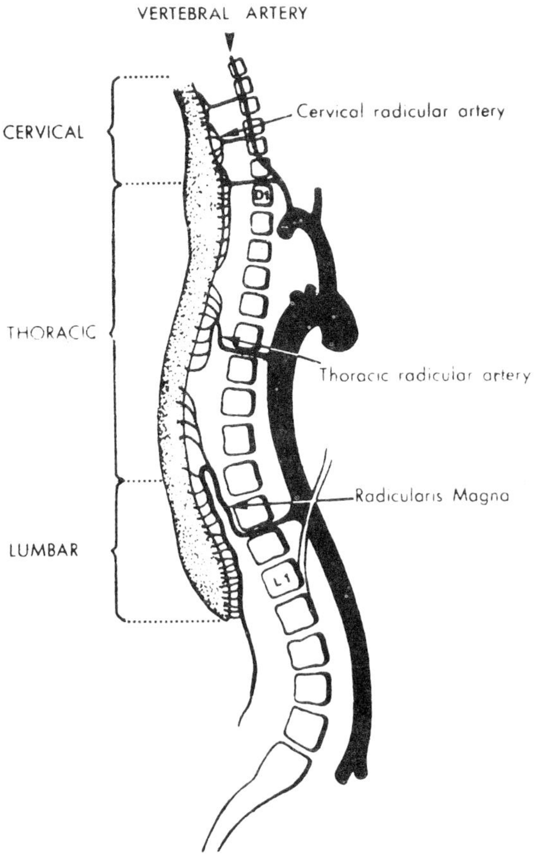


32/FIG. 7.—Blood supply of the spinal cord showing one arrangement of radicular vessels which feed the anterior spinal artery. (Courtesy of Little, Brown and Company, publishers of *International Anesthesiology Clinics*. From a paper by the late J. Usubiaga.[15])

(Fig. 7). The anterior and posterior spinal arteries do not anastomose with each other so that there are three distinct vascular areas within the cord, two posterior and one anterior (see Fig. 13, p. 887). The anterior spinal artery supplies the anterior and lateral columns and most of the grey matter of the cord. Thrombosis of this vessel causes the anterior spinal artery syndrome in which there is paraplegia without loss of posterior-column sensation (joint position, touch and vibration sense).

The spinal veins comprise anterior and posterior plexuses which drain through the intervertebral foramina into the vertebral, azygos and lumbar veins.

The spinal cord is enveloped by three membranes: dura, arachnoid, and pia mater, which are direct continuations of those surrounding the brain.

**The dura mater.**—In the cranial cavity the dura is arranged in two layers, periosteal and investing, which are firmly adherent except where they split to enclose venous sinuses. The outer periosteal layer is the periosteum of the inner surface of the skull bones and, in the spine, acts as the periosteum lining the spinal canal. The inner or investing layer is continued from the cranium into the spinal canal but is firmly adherent to the margins of the foramen magnum where it blends with the outer or periosteal layer. Between the spinal dura and the periosteum lining the spinal canal is the epidural space. Hence solutions deposited correctly in the spinal epidural space cannot enter the cranial cavity or produce nerve block higher than the 1st cervical nerves. In the spine the dura is loosely attached by fibrous strands to the posterior longitudinal ligament anchoring it in place anteriorly, and to the vertebral arch posteriorly.

The anterior and posterior nerve roots issuing from the spinal cord pierce the dura and carry tubular prolongations (dural cuffs) which blend with the perineurium of the mixed spinal nerve (Figs. 5 and 6).

The dura and arachnoid end as a tube usually at the 2nd sacral vertebra, so that cerebrospinal fluid is not found below this level. The dura ends by giving an investment to the filum terminale externa which blends eventually with the periosteum on the back of the coccyx.

**The arachnoid mater** is the middle of the three investing membranes covering the brain and spinal cord and is closely applied to the dura mater. The spinal arachnoid is a continuation of the cerebral arachnoid. The subarachnoid space contains the cerebrospinal fluid, and is divided by an incomplete midline septum along the dorsal suface of the cord. The subdural space between the dura and the arachnoid is a capillary interface containing a little serous fluid.

**The pia mater.**—In the vertebral canal the pia is closely applied to the spinal cord and extends into the anterior median fissure. The blood vessels going to the brain and spinal cord lie in the subarachnoid space before piercing the pia. They carry with them into the brain and spinal cord a sleeve of meninges derived from the pia mater.

### The Epidural Space

This is a potential space within the bony cavity of the spinal canal and outside the dural sac. It is bounded anteriorly by the bodies of the vertebrae and the posterior longitudinal ligaments, and posteriorly by the vertebral arches and the ligamenta flava. Superiorly it is closed by the fusion of dura and periosteum at the foramen magnum, and inferiorly by the sacrococcygeal ligament at the sacral hiatus. It communicates via the intervertebral foramina with the paravertebral spaces. Fibrous strands anchoring the dura posteriorly partly divide the epidural space in the midline, so that injected fluid frequently distends the space laterally rather than in the midline.[16]

The epidural space is always said to contain fat, but since the dural sac virtually fills the bony spinal canal (Fig. 5), this usually amounts to no more than a thin, transparent film of areolar tissue. The 31 pairs of spinal nerves with their dural cuffs traverse the space on their way to the intravertebral foramina, the lower ones travelling at an increasingly oblique angle (Fig. 6).

The venous plexuses of the vertebral canal lie in the epidural space (see Fig. 5). These veins receive tributaries from the adjacent bony structures and the spinal cord. They form a network running vertically within the epidural space, and can be subdivided into a pair of anterior venous plexuses which lie on either side of the posterior longitudinal ligament into which the basivertebral veins empty, and a posterior venous plexus. These veins, although divided into anatomical groups, all interconnect and form a series of horizontal segmental anastomoses. They connect with the intervertebral veins which pass out through the intervertebral foramina and so communicate with the vertebral, ascending cervical, deep cervical, intercostal, iliolumbar and lateral sacral veins. These veins have no valves and afford a connection between the pelvic veins below with the intracranial veins above. The epidural veins become distended during coughing and straining and also when the inferior vena cava is obstructed by large abdominal tumours, or in late pregnancy.

### The Paravertebral Space

The paravertebral spaces in the thoracic region lie between the heads of the ribs, and because they are in direct contact with the pleura they are subject to the same fluctuations as occur in intrathoracic pressure. The negative intrathoracic pressure is thus conducted via the paravertebral spaces to the thoracic epidural space and to a diminishing extent to the cervical and lumbar regions. The fat in the epidural space surrounds the intercostal nerves as they pass through the intervertebral foramina and so is in direct continuity with the fat in the paravertebral space.

## Cerebrospinal Fluid

Cerebrospinal fluid (CSF) is a clear colourless liquid with a pH of 7·4 and a light opalescence due to the presence of globulin. The average volume in the adult is about 135 ml, of which 35 ml is within the ventricles, 25 ml in the cerebral subarachnoid space and 75 ml in the spinal subarachnoid space.[17] It is secreted by the choroid plexus at a rate of 0·3–0·4 ml/min.

The normal protein content of CSF is 20 mg per cent (mg/dl) with equal albumin and globulin fractions, and glucose 2·5–4·4 mmol/l (45–80 mg per cent). After spinal block there is a rise in both the albumin and globulin content: the albumin level rises until about the 18th day, when it is nearly double the normal level.

Cerebrospinal fluid pressure in health varies between 70–180 mm $H_2O$ (0·7–1·8 kPa) in the lateral position to 375–550 mm $H_2O$ (3·7–5·4 kPa) in the vertical position. This pressure is transmitted to the epidural space[18] and any injection into the epidural space increases the pressure which is in turn transmitted to the cerebrospinal fluid. A conscious patient will occasionally notice a sensation of dizziness during the performance of epidural block; this can be attributed to a transient rise in CSF pressure.

An important factor determining the spread of drugs in the subarachnoid space is the specific gravity of the solution compared with that of the CSF. The specific gravity of CSF at body temperature referred to water at 4° C is 1·0003, that is its density is 1·0003 g/ml. Its specific gravity compared to water at the *same* temperature (a more meaningful value with little temperature dependence) is 1·007.[19] The specific gravity of 10 per cent dextrose, such as is commonly included in the so-called heavy or hyperbaric solutions (page 868), is 1·034 and that of amethocaine 0·5 per cent in 5 per cent dextrose is 1·02. These solutions are thus denser than cerebrospinal fluid at 37° and considerably more so when first injected at room temperature (see Fig. 8).

### The Effects of Spinal and Epidural Block

**Action of local anaesthetics.**—Local anaesthetics introduced into the subarachnoid or the epidural space block nerve conduction to an extent determined by the concentration and volume injected, the sensitivity of different fibre types (see page 834) and by the drug employed. Although all agents tend to block preganglionic B fibres most readily, then pain fibres, touch, proprioception and motor fibres, in that order, when injected epidurally there is a difference in their selectivity for sensory fibres. It has been found experimentally[20] that while bupivacaine given epidurally has a selective effect on the dorsal root, etidocaine appears rather to depress conduction in spinal-cord white matter. Clinically, epidural bupivacaine can produce analgesia without motor impairment, while etidocaine cannot. Given intrathecally, however, even bupivacaine will almost always produce motor as well as sensory block. After both types of block, however, muscle relaxation is a feature, muscle tone being reduced by loss of the afferent side of the reflex arc, even in the presence of good voluntary power.

Epidural local anaesthesia produces regional effects, the distribution and extent of which are determined by the site and volume of the injection, but in which lower segments may be spared. With spinal anaesthesia, however, it is much harder to produce sparing of the sacral

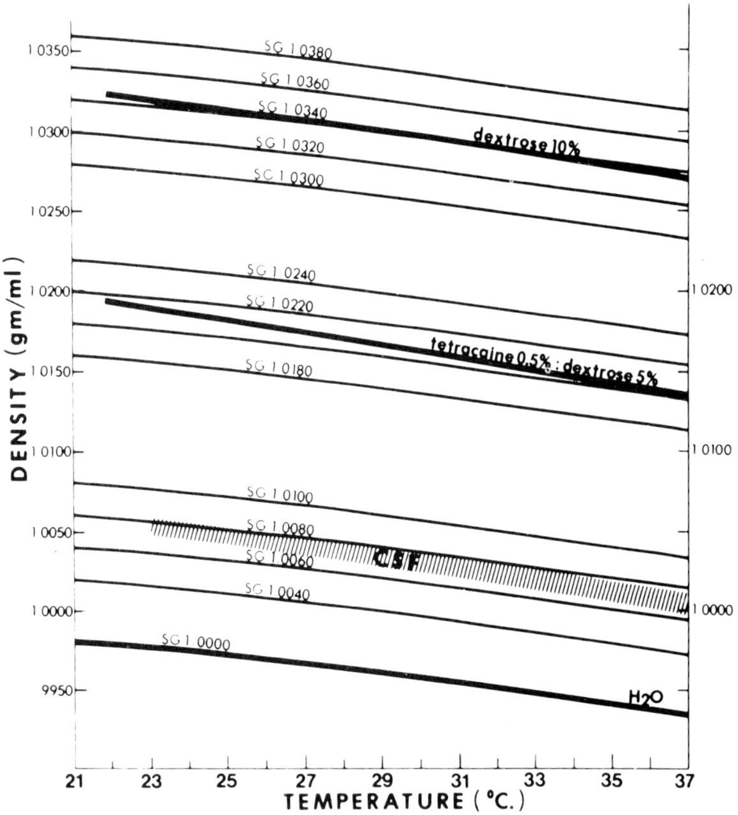

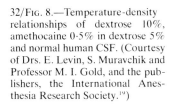

32/Fig. 8.—Temperature-density relationships of dextrose 10%, amethocaine 0·5% in dextrose 5% and normal human CSF. (Courtesy of Drs. E. Levin, S. Muravchik and Professor M. I. Gold, and the publishers, the International Anesthesia Research Society.[19])

segments. The factors determining the spread and degree of spinal and epidural block are dealt with later in the separate sections.

Local anaesthetics injected into the epidural space may gain access to their site of action by diffusing through the dural cuffs into the roots round which they are injected, by passing into the paravertebral spaces, or by diffusing into the cerebrospinal fluid. Though cerebrospinal fluid concentrations compatible with spinal anaesthesia may be noted following epidurals, the character of the block does not resemble that of spinal anaesthesia. Blockade, by passage into the cerebrospinal fluid after lumbar epidural administration, would result in preferential block of the sacral roots (see Fig. 6), while an asymmetric block would be extremely rare. Such is by no means the case. Clinical features suggest that epidural local anaesthetics block the roots near the site of injection, though experimentally conduction may be depressed at distant sites within the cord[20] and neuraxial spread of local anaesthetic is certainly likely to occur.

Intrathecally, local anaesthetics can block nerve conduction at about one tenth of the dose required epidurally. There is ready access to dorsal and ventral roots, which lie bare in the CSF at their point of entry into, or emergence from, the cord, unprotected by dural sleeves or any surrounding glial tissue.

### Cardiovascular Effects

The preganglionic sympathetic fibres arise in the spinal cord between T1 and L2 and travel in the corresponding anterior roots across the subarachnoid and epidural spaces. Sympathetic blockade leads to dilatation of both resistance and capacitance vessels in the region supplied by the blocked nerves. If this is extensive, a fall in peripheral vascular resistance will result together with a posture-dependent fall in cardiac output. The fall in blood pressure accompanying spinal and epidural anaesthesia depends upon the blockade, therefore, of a substantial number of thoracic segments. Sympathetic block extends somewhat higher than sensory block because B fibres are more sensitive than Aδ and C fibres to local anaesthetics. There is no difference between spinal and epidural block in this respect, though with epidurals, hypotension is usually of slower onset and can be minimised by preloading and by the use of small volumes of higher concentration of local anaesthetic in preference to bigger volumes of lower concentration.[21]

In the presence of sympathetic blockade in the lower part of the body, compensatory vasoconstriction in the upper part can help to maintain the total peripheral resistance. Provided that this reflex is not inhibited, for example by general anaesthesia, and that posture is such as to promote venous return, hypotension in the normovolaemic intact individual can be minimal. If blockade extends above the level of T5, it becomes progressively more difficult to compensate for the haemodynamic changes, and blood pressure will be markedly reduced.

The baroreceptors in the carotid sinus and aortic arch normally respond to a fall in blood pressure by producing a compensatory tachycardia (Marey's law) through vagal afferent and efferent pathways. Most patients under spinal or epidural anaesthesia, however, exhibit bradycardia and it would appear that the Bainbridge reflex predominates. Thus, in spinal or epidural anaesthesia, venous pooling in the periphery reduces stimulation of the volume receptors thereby diminishing activity of the cardiac sympathetic nerves. The result is vagal preponderance and a *slowing* of the heart rate. Block of the cardiac sympathetic nerves by either high spinal or epidural block may also be an additional factor causing bradycardia. Regional vasodilatation may have beneficial effects. The blood flow to the legs[22] and the splanchnic bed[23] are increased, which may confer a considerable advantage compared to general anaesthesia. Thus the incidence of deep-vein thrombosis after hip surgery is significantly reduced by spinal anaesthesia.[24,25] Epidural block as high as T1, however, has been shown to reduce blood flow to vital organs in rhesus monkeys,[26] not surprisingly, since such a high block is likely to be associated with a considerable fall in cardiac output.

Epidural blockade has been used to reduce bleeding during difficult abdominal surgery such as pancreatic and bile-duct operations,[27] for prostatectomy and in total hip replacement,[28] though hypotension should never be such as to jeopardise brain or cord blood supply in elderly, potentially atherosclerotic patients.

After preloading the circulation with crystalloid solution, epidural blockade of sufficient extent to provide analgesia in labour increases the maternal placental blood supply,[29] while blockade sufficient for Caesarean section has no detrimental effect,[30] unless there is hypotension or if preloading is omitted.

### Respiratory Effects

Correctly placed and conducted spinal and epidural blockade should not depress respiration because of motor block. With a high spinal anaesthetic intercostal nerves may become progressively blocked, but the phrenic nerve (C3, 4 and 5) should only be affected if gross errors of dosage or technique have occurred. The concentration of local anaesthetic in cerebrospinal fluid is normally too low, because of dilution and uptake by nerves, to block motor fibres at such a height.

Respiratory depression following lumbar epidural block is usually a result of inadvertent intrathecal injection of a full epidural dose. In this case, medullary depression is normally the cause of both respiratory and cardiovascular collapse, combined with coma. Occasionally a massive *epidural* block occurs in response to a correctly placed injection, in which case hypotension and respiratory paralysis may occur without coma. *High* epidurals, that is thoracic and even cervical injections, are occasionally given deliberately and, as would be expected, result in impaired respiratory function.[31]

When lumbar epidurals and spinals are used with care for surgery in high-risk and elderly patients, they are associated with a lower incidence of peri-operative morbidity and postoperative hypoxia than in general anaesthesia.[32, 33]

Because of its superior ability to relieve pain, epidural analgesia is associated with a reduction in respiratory alkalosis in labour. More importantly, metabolic acidosis is greatly reduced in mother and fetus.[34, 35]

**Bronchial muscles.**—Blockade of thoracic sympathetic fibres would not be expected to induce bronchospasm since, in this area, sympathetic tone is normally absent. With high epidural and spinal block there is in fact some increase in dead space, apparently associated with bronchodilatation, which could be secondary to hypotension or to reduced pulmonary blood volume.

**Management of respiratory depression.**—Hypoxia, whether from paralysis of respiratory muscle, from medullary depression, or secondary to convulsions, must always be treated immediately by the administration of oxygen and by intubation and controlled ventilation if necessary.

### Metabolic and Hormonal Effects

Recent interest has centred on the stress response to surgery and how it is modified by anaesthesia and analgesia. Major surgery under general anaesthesia alone can result in a marked rise in blood sugar, cortisol and catecholamines, with further increases postoperatively. It is clear that spinal and epidural blockade, if sufficiently high and prolonged, can minimise or even prevent these changes.[36–41] Moreover epidural anaesthesia has been shown to inhibit the stress-induced rise in renin and aldosterone release and the potassium loss[42] and postoperative negative nitrogen balance[43] associated with hysterectomy and the antidiuretic hormone hypersecretion which accompanies total hip replacement under general anaesthesia.[44]

### Gastro-intestinal Effects

The sympathetic blockade which accompanies spinal and epidural anaesthesia results in a contracted bowel with relaxed sphincters. In the absence of vagal block, there may be an increase in peristalsis and in intraluminal pressure which could be undesirable in the presence of intestinal obstruction. Because certain bowel afferents travel in the vagus, handling the viscera may cause considerable discomfort, nausea and hiccup in the conscious patient. A separate vagal block may therefore be advisable in upper abdominal surgery. The spleen and liver may be enlarged under spinal and epidural blockade.

## Techniques

### Preparation of the Patient

The anaesthetist should always visit a patient for whom spinal or epidural anaesthesia is planned, in order that he may examine the spine for any points of difficulty, and, if general anaesthesia is not also to be used, explain to the patient some important details. A few words about flexion of the spine and lying still during the procedure (particularly important for epidural anaesthesia) are of great assistance in securing the patient's co-operation at the time of injection. The psychological background to local anaesthesia cannot be over-emphasised. In units where operations are performed regularly under local anaesthesia, preparation begins in the out-patient department and continues in the ward, so that by the time the patient arrives in the theatre, most of his fears should have been allayed.

**Premedication.**—Local anaesthesia may be selected either because the patient wishes to remain alert, or because general anaesthesia carries a special hazard in the high risk patient or the fetus *in utero*. In any of these cases, heavy premedication would defeat the object. There are, however, some instances in which local anaesthesia is used by tradition or for surgical reasons, in which case sedative premedication is indicated. The choice must be suited to the patient and the circumstances. Diazepam has been advocated as it is said to increase the convulsive threshold to local anaesthetics. However, it is unthinkable that it should be used as a licence to overdose patients, in whom toxic doses of drugs and accidental intravenous injections should be avoided at all costs.

During surgery, needless and frivolous chat is unsuitable, while the patient should be included in any general conversation. It goes without saying that gasps must be avoided and panics concealed, while an atmosphere of calm and order should prevail.

**Intravenous infusion.**—A large-bore intravenous catheter must always be introduced prior to spinal or epidural blockade for the maintenance of blood pressure by fluid load, or if necessary by vasopressors. Also blood loss during surgery is ill-tolerated as the normal responses to haemorrhage are absent, and blood lost should be relaced *pari passu*.

**Monitoring the blood pressure.**—The blood pressure should be recorded every 5–10 minutes, but there is a considerable difference of opinion as to the extent to which it should be allowed to fall before corrective measures are taken. In a patient lying horizontal during spinal or epidural anaesthesia the tissues usually remain well perfused despite a low blood pressure, and coronary circulation is adequate for the reduced work level of the heart. A systolic pressure of 60 mm Hg (8·0 kPa) or less is dangerously low, and immediate measures should be taken to raise it. For previously normotensive subjects a systolic pressure of 80 mm Hg (10·7 kPa) is satisfactory but it needs to be monitored carefully so as to detect at once any further drop. In hypertensive patients, the systolic pressure should be maintained at more than half the original level, in order to maintain the blood supply to the central nervous system. In conscious patients, restlessness due to the accompanying cerebral hypoxia may be a sign of hypotension, but may be mistaken for incomplete analgesia. Should the anaesthetist fail to recognise the true cause of restlessness, he may be tempted to use sedation; such treatment may easily be fatal in the circumstances. When the systolic pressure falls below 80 mm Hg (10.7 kPa) in conscious patients, a vasovagal attack may be triggered, leading to profound hypotension with accompanying bradycardia, nausea and vomiting.[45] In anaesthetised patients the hypotension is usually well tolerated, provided the block does not reach the upper thoracic segments and so cause bradycardia. It is important to maintain the blood pressure in elderly patients who may have associated cerebrovascular and coronary atheroma, if cerebral or myocardial damage from hypotension is to be avoided.

Should severe arterial hypotension develop during spinal or epidural blockade, the oxygen concentration of the inspired mixture should be increased and the legs raised, if possible, to increase the venous return. The supine hypotensive syndrome caused by compression of the inferior vena cava by a tumour such as the gravid uterus, can be relieved by tilting the patient on to one side. When hypotension is associated with bradycardia, it can be effectively treated in most cases by giving small doses of atropine (0·2 mg) intravenously until the pulse is raised to a more normal rate. The most rational and effective treatment of severe hypotension is the rapid infusion of fluids intravenously, using compound sodium lactate (Hartmann's) solution. The rapid infusion of 500–1000 ml will fill the enlarged vascular bed produced by the spinal or epidural block and so raise the blood pressure to an acceptable level. Alternatively, colloid solutions may be used (see page 884).

The role of *vasopressors* in the management of hypotension is controversial. If despite a fall in blood pressure the patient remains pink, well perfused, has a good capillary circulation, constricted pupils and a palpable peripheral pulse, such as the superficial temporal, then he is unlikely to be in immediate danger. The use of vasopressors will raise the pressure but the benefit that results is difficult to evaluate as the vasoconstriction may reduce tissue perfusion and so accentuate the tissue hypoxia and metabolic acidosis. Vasopressors stimulate alpha and beta adrenoceptors to a varying degree, increasing arteriolar tone and the force of cardiac contraction respectively. The anaesthetist should restrict himself to ephedrine which has both $\alpha$ and $\beta$ actions, while pure $\alpha$-stimulants such as phenylephrine and methoxamine may be dangerous because they commonly cause reflex cardiac depression and tissue underperfusion. Vasopressors should only be used if the blood pressure remains low despite the other measures previously described. Particular care must be taken to guard against a sudden fall in blood pressure when the patient's posture is altered especially from the lithotomy position.

**General anaesthesia.**—Ideally, spinal and epidural blocks should be used as alternatives to general anaesthesia to avoid subjecting the patient to the risks of both procedures. However, there may be occasions when, with care, they are usefully combined.

Spinal or epidural blocks may be used as an adjunct to general anaesthesia to provide good operating conditions and hypotension in a patient who then needs only light general anaesthesia. They are particularly useful to provide effective postoperative analgesia without respiratory depression in relatively unfit patients who nevertheless require general anaesthesia for surgery.

In upper abdominal surgery it may be difficult to avoid undesirable vagal reflexes when handling and pulling on viscera. The patients may experience severe nausea and discomfort in the absence of general anaesthesia. Where both types of anaesthesia are combined electively, it is best for humane reasons to administer general before local anesthesia, but there are occasions when general anaesthesia has to be used to overcome an imperfect block.

The type of general anaesthesia employed will depend upon the patient, the surgery and, of course, the anaesthetist.

**Positioning the patient.**—The spine should be flexed as much as possible in order to widen the interspinous spaces. Even in flexion the spines of the lumbar vertebrae are considerably taller than the spaces (Fig. 4). The patient should normally adopt the left lateral position for right-handed operators, with the knees up and the chin down. The coronal plane of hips and shoulders should be as nearly as possible vertical so that the median plane is horizontal. Even so the midline can be difficult to identify in the presence of obesity, in which case the slumped sitting position may be helpful in the conscious patient.

**Sterility** is of vital importance, since infection introduced from without is a dangerous but completely avoidable complication of spinal and epidural block.

The anaesthetist should scrub up as for a surgical operation, and wear a sterile gown and gloves. Microbiological advice fluctuates as to the need for cap and mask. Most anaesthetists, however, would agree that, particularly as talking (and not least teaching) is necessary during the procedure, they would feel more assured of avoiding droplet contamination of equipment by the use of a mask.

As much as possible of the necessary equipment should be contained in a sterile pack. This should include sterile towels for covering the trolley top and one for the patient, a Sise introducer and a drawing-up needle, swabs, swab-holding forceps, a gallipot for skin-cleansing solutions and, for epidural blocks, an epidural needle and glass syringes, if required. Such may be prepared locally and sterilised by autoclaving, in which case disposable items, such as a small needle, plastic syringes, spinal needle or epidural cannula and filter must be added after opening the pack. Disposable spinal and epidural packs, which have been sterilised by gamma radiation, are now available commercially and commonly contain the necessary plastic items. These are very suitable for occasional use but are much more expensive than locally produced packs where large numbers are needed. Ampoules for spinal and epidural use should be sterile outside as well as in, so that they can be handled by the operator who can then inspect ampoule and contents closely. If sterile ampoules are not available, because of the danger of contamination on opening, the contents should be drawn up through a bacterial filter. Such a procedure may be necessary for heavy spinal solutions because heat sterilisation occasionally causes charing of dextrose.

The patient's back should be cleaned widely using 2 per cent iodine paint or some other coloured antiseptic, and sterile towels draped appropriately. Where bony landmarks are difficult to palpate, it can help to have the patient's hips and shoulders unobscured so that bearings are not lost.

### Spinal Anaesthesia

**Lumbar puncture** is generally carried out no higher than the 3/4 or 4/5 interspace, in order to avoid the danger of damaging the spinal cord. In the conscious patient, initial infiltration of the skin and subcutaneous tissues with local anaesthetic may be valuable to help the patient to keep still for lumbar puncture, particularly if a Sise introducer is used.

**Needles.**—Nowadays disposable spinal needles are generally used. The incidence of spinal headache is of course related to the size of needle used, and is least with a 25 or 26-gauge needle. Such a fine needle must be inserted via a Sise introducer (Fig. 9) or through a 20-gauge needle inserted as far as the epidural space.[46] Although CSF may not flow spontaneously through some 25-gauge needles, depending on the smoothness of the bore,[135] it can be gently aspirated.

An introducer offers an additional advantage in that it is used to pierce the epidermis so that no part of the spinal needle touches the skin. This reduces the infection hazard and the danger of carrying a piece of skin into deeper layers.

**The approach.**—In the midline approach, the needle is angled very slightly cephalad and passes through skin, subcutaneous tissue, supraspinous and interspinous ligaments, ligamentum flavum, dura and arachnoid, to enter the subarachnoid space. It is easier to find the interlaminar foramen (page 857) using the midline approach, but in the elderly the supraspinous and interspinous ligaments may be calcified, the adjacent spines even appearing fused on occasion, making introduction of the fine spinal needle extremely difficult. For such patients, the *lateral* approach may be advisable. In this case, the needle passes through skin and subcutaneous tissue, lumbar aponeurosis and lumbar muscles before reaching the ligamentum flavum. Little resistance is therefore experienced until this point. By this approach, however, it is easier to miss the interlaminar foramen and meet instead any part of the bony ring surrounding it, that is lamina, root of the spinous process or facet joint. Increasing the flexion of the spine opens up the interlaminar foramen, so improving access.

#### Solutions

The local anaesthetic solution is diluted by cerebrospinal fluid and therefore its original concentration is of less moment than the actual mass of drug injected. Spread is also determined by the specific gravity of the solution injected relative to that of cerebrospinal fluid: the so called baricity. This property is related to the mass of solute, and is not the same as tonicity, which depends upon the number of particles in the solution. For a brief discussion of the specific gravity of the cerebrospinal fluid see page 862. Hyperbaric solutions are rendered so by the addition of 10 per cent dextrose; simple solutions marketed for epidural use are commonly referred to as isobaric, yet they may, in practice, actually be slightly hypobaric, as for example, is 0·5 per cent Marcain plain.

*Hyperbaric solutions* contain from 5–9.5 per cent dextrose. They can be relied upon to move vertically downwards in the cerebrospinal fluid and will, therefore, block the sacral roots if the

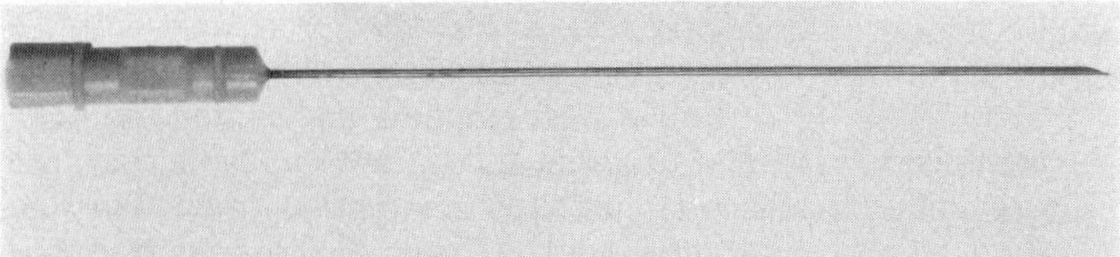

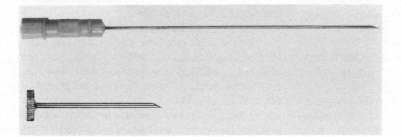

32/Fig. 9(*a*).—A disposable spinal needle with stilette in position.

32/Fig. 9(*b*).—A Sise introducer.

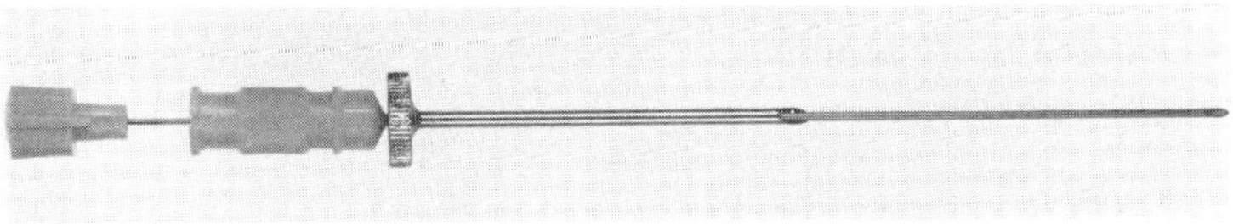

32/FIG 9(c).—The spinal needle can be passed down a Sise introducer.

32/FIG. 9(d).—A graduated epidural catheter (Portex) with bacterial filter attached. A graduated Tuohy needle showing stilette and side-facing hole.

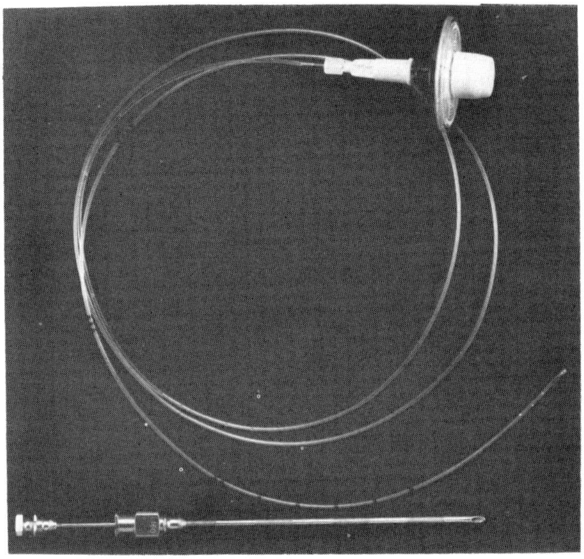

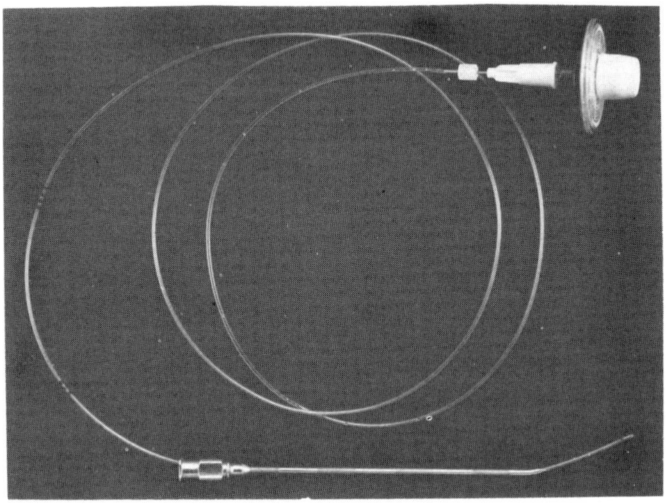

32/FIG. 9(e).—The catheter will pass down the needle which will deflect it to pass into the epidural space.

32/FIG. 9(f).—A caudal needle.

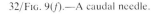

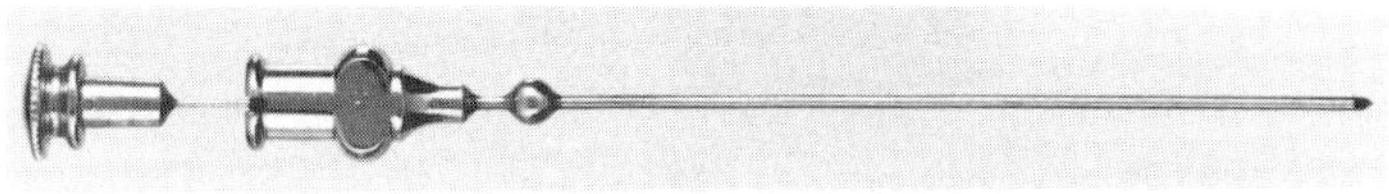

patient is sitting up and the dependent side in the lateral position. They will pass cephalad to the midpoint of the thoracic curve in the supine position and in this position produce a more consistently high block than hypobaric or isobaric solutions (Fig. 10).[47,48]

*Isobaric solutions* do not move under the influence of gravity in the cerebrospinal fluid. Spread of solution, and consequently the height of the block, is not influenced by the position of the patient[49] and is somewhat unpredictable.[47] Isobaric solutions are generally made by diluting local anaesthetic with physiological saline.

*Hypobaric solutions* move vertically upwards in the cerebrospinal fluid. The original light spinal technique involved using large volumes of dilute cinchocaine solution (1:1,500 or 0·06 per cent) and was sometimes associated with serious neurological disturbance. Consequently it has fallen into disuse. Currently, however, slightly hypobaric solutions, for example a 1 per cent solution of amethocaine diluted with an equal volume of water or commercial 0·5 per cent bupivacaine plain, may be used for spinal anaesthesia. Here the concentration of local anaesthetic is similar to that in heavy solutions, so the volume used is also similar. Thus the risks apparently attendant on the displacement of cerebrospinal fluid by large volumes of a foreign solution are avoided. Though the height of analgesia may be somewhat erratic (Fig. 10),[50] there is clearly a tendency for these solutions to rise in the subarachnoid space.[51]

### Drugs

*Cinchocaine* (dibucaine USP) is available in a 0·5 per cent solution in 6 per cent glucose ("heavy Nupercaine"). It has a specific gravity of 1·024 at 37° C and produces analgesia lasting 2–5 hours.

*Amethocaine* (tetracaine USP) hydrochloride 1 per cent or crystals may be mixed with 10 per cent glucose, physiological saline or distilled water to produce 0·5 per cent hyper-, iso- or hypobaric solutions respectively.[47] The hyperbaric solution has a specific gravity of 1·02 at 37.[19] The dose of amethocaine given intrathecally is 5–15 mg and the duration 4–6 hours.[49]

*Mepivacaine* hydrochloride is available for spinal use as a 4 per cent solution with 9·5 per cent dextrose. Its duration of action is considerably briefer than that of the other drugs mentioned here.

*Bupivacaine* hydrochloride (Marcain) has been increasing in popularity for spinal use recently, both as a hyperbaric solution in 8 per cent dextrose and as the commercial plain solution. Concentrations of 0·5 and 0·75 per cent have been used. The 0·5 per cent plain solution used in the U.K. is mildly hypobaric. The intrathecal dose is 7·5–15 mg. More than this is sometimes used but may produce exces-

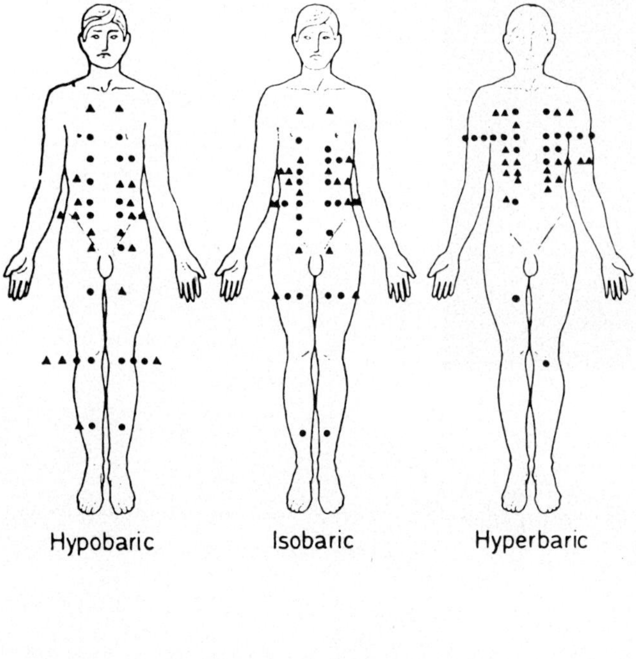


32/FIG. 10.—Height of analgesia 15 minutes after intrathecal injection of amethocaine in individuals given 10 mg(●) and 15 mg (▲). (Courtesy of Drs. D. T. Brown, J. A. W. Wildsmith, B. G. Covino and D. B. Scott, and the editor and publishers of the *British Journal of Anaesthesia*, Macmillan Journals Ltd.[47])

sive spread[52] and a high incidence of hypotension.[53] It has been found to be more effective than equal doses of amethocaine,[54] though motor block is less. The duration of analgesia is similar.

*Adrenaline* has, rather surprisingly, been used in spinal anaesthesia, though it must increase the risk of anterior spinal artery syndrome and cord ischaemia, particularly if there is concomitant hypotension. It may prolong blockade due to amethocaine[54] though it has little effect with bupivacaine.[55] In view of the increased risk, the intrathecal use of adrenaline, or indeed of other vasoconstrictors, would appear to be unjustified.

### Fate of Local Anaesthetics in the Subarachnoid Space

Following the injection of a local anaesthetic into the subarachnoid space, the concentration falls rapidly. The initial steep fall is due to mixing with cerebrospinal fluid and subsequently to absorption into nerve roots and spinal cord. It is during this period that spinal analgesia is said to become "fixed".

The later, more gradual, decrease in concentration reflects the removal of the drug by vascular absorption both from the cerebrospinal fluid and from the nervous tissue. There is a continuing slow uptake of local anaesthetic by the tissues, which have a higher affinity than cerebrospinal fluid for the more lipid-soluble drugs, and which also have a better blood supply. Bulk flow of cerebrospinal fluid into the venous sinuses via arachnoid villi may also contribute to a small extent to clearance of local anaesthetic as may, in an even smaller proportion, lymphatic drainage.

### Factors Controlling the Extent and Duration of Spinal Anaesthesia

1. *Specific gravity of the solution.*—Of the many factors which influence the spread of solutions in the cerebrospinal fluid, baricity is the most important[47] (Fig. 10). Only in the lithotomy position does baricity have little influence on the resultant block.[56]

2. *Position of the patient during and immediately after injection.*—The spread of hyperbaric solution is reliably determined by the position of the patient. Thus in the supine position, a hyperbaric solution may be relied upon to pass cephalad to the vertically lowest point of the thoracic curve and produce a relatively high spinal. In the sitting position it passes caudad to block sacral roots, while a unilateral block may be obtained by keeping the patient in the lateral position. When a unilateral block is desired for a hip or leg that is painful, however, use of a hypobaric solution will enable the patient to be positioned painful side uppermost. The sitting position encourages spread of hypobaric solutions.[137]

3. *Volume and concentration of solution.*—Most investigators have found the height of spinal block to be slightly dependent upon the volume of solution injected[57,138] and certainly upon the total mass of drug.[51,52] Increasing the dose certainly prolongs the blockade[47] while the greater the spread of a given dose of local anaesthetic, the briefer its duration of effect.[51] Thus, if spread is increased by baricity and posture, the effect is curtailed.

4. *Barbotage.*—The term is derived from the French *barboter*—to puddle, or to mix. The word "barbotage" was coined by Le Filliotre, and the technique was popularised in spinal anaesthesia by Labat. The basis of the technique is to leave the injecting syringe attached to the spinal needle and make repeated aspirations and injections, thus mixing and dispersing the original dose of local anaesthetic. The spread of a given dose of local anaesthetic can be increased by barbotage, which is now little used, however, since it has been shown to give rise to histological nerve damage.

5. *Site of injection.*—It is of course possible to use any spinal interspace for the introduction of a local anaesthetic, but in order to avoid possible damage to the spinal cord it is safer to restrict lumbar puncture to the L3–4 or L4–5 interspaces, other variables being then responsible for the ultimate height of the block.

### Applications and Dose Requirements

*Hyperbaric technique.*—Following injection into the cerebrospinal fluid, local anaesthetic is taken up into nerve tissue and disappears fairly rapidly. The position of the patient in the first few minutes is therefore crucial. A very useful technique for anorectal and bladder-neck operations such as transurethral prostatectomy, is to inject 1 ml of a heavy solution at the L4–5 interspace, with the patient sitting up. For operations about the anus where only the 4th and 5th sacral roots require to be blocked,

0·6 ml of solution is sufficient. The patient should be kept sitting up for five minutes after the injection while the heavy solution sinks rapidly to the bottom of the dural sac, blocking the necessary sacral nerves. There is little or no fall in blood pressure, so that a vasopressor is very seldom required.

For lower abdominal operations, 1·5–2 ml of solution is injected at the L3–4 interspace. Immediately after the injection the patient is turned on his back. The heavy solution then spreads under the influence of gravity up the thoracic segments. While in the average patient in the lateral position the vertebral column is more or less horizontal, in some women it may incline downwards towards the head because of the width of the pelvis relative to the shoulders, and in some men towards the coccyx because of the width of the shoulder relative to the pelvis. Thus the solution may spread in the wrong direction until the patient is rolled supine and tipped into the correct position. It is therefore best when using a heavy solution for an upper abdominal operation in a man, to tip the table until it is obvious that the vertebral column inclines towards the head. With the spine exactly horizontal the solution may not run high enough when injected at L3–4, the apex of the lumbar curve, and may tend to spread down towards the coccyx when the patient is rolled on to his back.

For upper abdominal operations where analgesia to the 4th or 5th thoracic segment is required, 2–3 ml of solution are injected with the patient head-down. As before, the solution spreads by gravity, and any excess of unfixed drug pools in the hollow of the thoracic curve, opposite the 4th and 5th nerve roots.

In planning the height to which analgesia is required for a particular operation it is useful to remember the following segmental levels:

| | |
|---|---|
| Nipple line | T4–5 |
| Xiphisternum | T6 |
| Umbilicus | T10 |
| Groin | L1 |
| Perineum | S2–4 |

For upper abdominal operations, anaesthesia must be sufficient not only to reach T7, but also to include the splanchnic nerves (greater splanchnic nerve T4, 5, 6, 7, 8), since an incomplete block of these makes surgical handling of the omentum and mesentery uncomfortable for a conscious patient. Moreover, it is advisable to combine the spinal block with para-oesophageal block of the vagus.

A point frequently not appreciated about lower abdominal operations such as abdomino-perineal resection of the rectum is that while the incision may not extend to the costal margin, nevertheless anaesthesia up to this region is needed since the surgeon requires to push the lower abdominal contents into the upper abdomen and may want to palpate the liver.

Dose requirements using isobaric and near-isobaric solutions are similar to those for hyperbaric techniques, but the posture must be varied accordingly.

### Lumbar Epidural Block

Preparation and positioning of the patient are described for both spinal and epidural block on p. 865 *et seq*. More skill is required for epidural than for spinal blockade, since the whole technique must be directed towards *avoiding* a lumbar puncture. For this reason the patient should be in the sitting position only when absolutely necessary, because the increase in cerebrospinal-fluid pressure so produced increases the likelihood of dural puncture. Absolute quiet and stillness must be ensured while an epidural is being inserted, so that the patient does not move, laugh or cry and so that the operator is not distracted.

The L2/3, 3/4 or 4/5 interspace may be used, the choice depending largely on the destination of the block. For abdominal and groin operations, using the L2/3 space minimises dosage requirements, while lower spaces may be suitable for lower leg, pelvic and perineal surgery. In a patient who has difficulty in flexing the spine or who possesses a marked lumbar lordosis the approach may be easier in a higher rather than a lower space. The thoracic approach to the epidural space is occasionally used by the skilled operator to provide analgesia in the upper abdomen and thorax.

The use of a large 16–18 gauge Tuohy needle makes prior local anaesthesia mandatory in the conscious patient. A skin bleb should be raised and subcutaneous layers infiltrated with about 2 ml of local anaesthetic solution. A Sise introducer is then used to remove a small core of skin which otherwise impedes the smooth passage of the Tuohy needle.

**Needles.**—A Tuohy needle is used for epidural blockade (Fig. 9). This needle nowadays always possesses a Huber point which is curved and rather blunt. The curve assists the passage of an epidural catheter round the corner into the epidural space. Both the curve and the bluntness reduce the risk of dural puncture. A 16- to 18-gauge needle is commonly used. The large calibre allows passage of an epidural catheter and also makes it easier to detect entry into the epidural space, particularly using the loss-of-resistance technique (*vide infra*). The Tuohy needle should be graduated in centimetres so that the depth of the epidural space can be assessed, then, using a graduated epidural catheter it is possible to measure the length of catheter in the epidural space.

**The approach,** as with spinal anaesthesia, may be midline or lateral, and the direction similar to that used for lumbar puncture. In the *midline* approach the resistance to advance of the Tuohy needle, and to injection of fluid down it, is considerable once the tip enters the supraspinous ligament. Painful sensation from this point is minimal, and with care it is possible to ensure entry into the epidural space in the midline. In the *lateral* approach sacrospinalis muscle offers only doughy resistance, and strong resistance to advance is not met until the needle hits either lamina or ligamentum flavum. Since the depth of the epidural space varies in the adult from 2·5 to >8 cm it is impossible to ensure by this approach that the needle enters the epidural space in the midline. Thus the risk of traumatic damage of nerve roots or epidural veins by the needle is increased using the lateral approach but, as with spinal anaesthesia, it may be a useful technique when the interspinous spaces are narrowed. In the lateral approach, the needle is angled towards the midline, and if bony rather than ligamenous resistance is met the needle tip is angled cephalad until it meets the ligamentum flavum.

### Methods of Identifying the Epidural Space

**Loss of resistance.**—There is almost complete resistance to injection of fluid through the epidural needle as it is advanced through the interspinous ligament and ligamentum flavum. As the needle tip emerges from the ligamentum flavum and enters the epidural space, the resistance to injection disappears dramatically.

Thus, using the midline approach, the Tuohy needle with its stilette in place is inserted until its tip is held firmly by the interspinous ligament. At all times the side hole of the Tuohy needle should be facing cephaled, to minimise trauma to the dura once the epidural space is entered. Then the stilette is removed and a large, fluid-filled syringe attached. Many operators use a 10 or 20-ml glass syringe whose plunger moves freely within the barrel. Provided it does not leak, this is the best tool to elicit the loss-of-resistance sign. Such syringes must be carefully maintained and sterilised completely clean with barrel and plunger separately wrapped. If such syringes are in short supply a 10 ml plastic syringe may be used, but the loss of resistance is less clear because of the friction of the plunger, though with experience this tool is perfectly reliable, and possibly more consistent in its behaviour than a glass syringe.

If the syringe is filled with *physiological saline*, the Tuohy needle may then be advanced solely by pressure on the *plunger* of the syringe. Thus, when the epidural space is entered and injection of fluid becomes possible, the movement of the barrel, and hence of the needle, is halted automatically. At this point, minimal saline should be injected so that little drips back when detaching the syringe, thereby avoiding confusion with cerebrospinal fluid. While advancing the needle towards the epidural space by pressure on the plunger with the dominant hand, the operator's non-dominant hand, it's dorsum braced against the patient's back, steadies the Tuohy needle and acts as a brake to sudden movement by increasing the inertia of the system.

The needle tip should approach the epidural space with the hole pointing cephalad. This minimises the angle at which the needle-tip encroaches on the dura, thereby reducing the chance of dural puncture. On entering the epidural space, the needle tip and the saline which is injected both help to push the dura away and so create an actual space. Once in the space, the needle should be moved as little as possible to avoid traumatising the dura.

If during the approach to the epidural space the needle tip strays out of the midline, a boggy and indefinite loss of resistance may be encountered. This is a source of trouble to the beginner, who must be taught constantly to check that the needle remains in the midline and precisely in the sagittal plane. It is important to notice that the needle is at right angles to the line of the patient's hips and shoulders, rather than parallel to the floor.

If the syringe is filled with *air*, this can give a very convincing loss-of-resistance sign, which is clearly differentiated from that encountered when the needle tip strays from the midline. Pressure on the plunger compresses the air within, but on releasing pressure the plunger bounces out again when the needle is in the ligament, subcutaneous tissue *or* muscle. Bounce is not elicited when the needle tip is in the epidural or subarachnoid space, or in a blood vessel. Moreover, when loss of resistance is encountered, if the epidural space has been entered, *no* fluid will drip back from the needle and no confusion is created. However, using loss of resistance to air, the needle cannot be advanced by pressure on the syringe plunger alone. The needle must be advanced step by step rather than in a continuous fashion, pausing to elicit bounce every millimetre or so. This method is slower and more prone to accidental dural puncture.[139] Also, should the needle tip enter a vein, apparently a not infrequent occurrence,[140] physiological saline would be harmless, whereas an air embolism is perhaps less so. Air is indubitably a foreign substance in this situation and excessive amounts will, of course, produce interstitial emphysema.[58]

Once the epidural space has been entered with the needle, the operator sucks gently down it to ensure that no cerebrospinal fluid or blood can be aspirated, and then injects air to establish the absence of bounce. Air passes in as if into the room.

At this point, either the local anaesthetic may be injected directly in the single-shot technique, or a catheter may be passed. Easy passage of the catheter is added confirmation that the epidural space has been entered, though twinges in one hip or leg suggest that the catheter is deviating to one side.

Mechanical aids to the loss-of-resistance sign, such as Macintosh's needle with spring-loaded stilette, Ilke's spring-loaded syringe, or Macintosh's balloon, are probably best avoided, since they may fail. Using a simple syringe, on the other hand, it is easy to check that the plunger flows freely, and failure is in the hands of the operator alone. Moreover, the simpler technique concentrates the attention of the anaesthetist on the feel of the ligaments the whole time, while visual and mechanical aids tend merely to be a distraction.

**The negative-pressure sign.**—A negative pressure can be detected in 50–80 per cent of cases on first entering the epidural space. It has been demonstrated in a number of ways.

*The hanging-drop sign*.–This is a very simple technique first described by Gutierrez.[59] The epidural needle is placed in the interspinous ligament, and a drop of fluid deposited on the hub; as the needle enters the epidural space the drop is sucked in.

*Odom's indicator*.–Odom[9] described a similar device to that of Gutierrez, the drop of fluid being contained in a small glass capillary tube attached to the needle. As the epidural space is entered. there is a movement inwards of the fluid: in some cases it disappears entirely. The Odom's indicator was later modified in a number of ways so as to increase its reliability.[60] On the whole, these modifications made the procedure so elaborate as to be far too time-consuming for routine use.

Three explanations have been put forward to account for this negative pressure:

(i) The first theory is that negative pressure is transmitted from the pleural cavity, via the thoracic paravertebral spaces, to the epidural space. Accordingly, it would be expected that negative pressure would be most marked in the thoracic region, and less so caudally. However, Dawkins[61] stated that in his own experience of 1,176 cases using Odom's indicator, he detected a negative pressure more frequently in the lumbar than in the thoracic region. There is thus no good evidence in favour of this theory.

(ii) The second theory is that negative pressure is created by flexion of the spine, so expanding the volume of the vertebral canal and consequently that of the epidural space. This may be a contributing factor.

(iii) The third theory is that the negative pressure is simply created by indenting the dura with the needle point. There is ample evidence to suppose that this is so.[62] Negative pressure is obliterated once fluid is injected, and indeed the epidural pressure may rise to as high as

30 cm of water during an epidural injection.[63]

Changes in both cerebrospinal fluid[18] and intra-abdominal[64] pressure are readily transmitted to the epidural space.

The negative-pressure sign has the advantage that it can be used with the lateral approach to the epidural space, since it does not depend on the continuity of ligaments to block the needle point as is the case with the loss-of-resistance sign. It has also been advocated for thoracic epidurals, where the thinner ligaments may make loss of resistance less easy to detect. However, Dawkins[61] detected a negative pressure in only 52 per cent of thoracic epidurals. Nevertheless, he later[65] advocated Brooks'[66] modification of Odom's indicator as the most satisfactory device for identifying the thoracic epidural space.

### The Single-Shot Epidural Injection

Only when the epidural space has been identified with certainty should any injection of anaesthetic solution be made. Few epidurals are instituted for surgery these days using the single shot-technique, and for pain relief it is rarely appropriate. It is a pity to go to the trouble of using epidural anaesthesia for surgery while denying the patient the option of repeat injections down the catheter for postoperative analgesia. If an epidural catheter is to be passed, then all injections of local anaesthetic should be made down it.

Nevertheless, there may be occasions when a short period of analgesia is required and direct injection down the Tuohy needle is indicated. A *test dose*, generally advocated to detect intrathecal or intravascular placement, is clearly inappropriate in this situation. It is obviously undesirable to have a patient with a Tuohy needle sticking in his back for 5 minutes, and there can be no guarantee that it is in the same place at the end of five minutes as it was when the test dose was injected. Moreover, the gush of cerebrospinal fluid which flows from an intrathecal Tuohy needle is quite unmistakable. Very occasionally, cerebrospinal fluid does not flow spontaneously from a needle whose tip, it appears, is at least partially within the subarachnoid space. It may be that a flap of dura covers the hole. In these cases, gentle aspiration may yield cerebrospinal fluid, and will also reveal intravascular placement of the needle. It is therefore a valuable part of the routine procedure. Injection down a needle with so large a bore as the Tuohy should be quite without resistance when the hole is correctly placed. Thus for a single shot epidural, the entire dose is injected down the needle at once, but the injection must be made slowly. Should any local anaesthetic solution pass directly into a vein, slow injection gives the patient time to report giddiness or light headedness, and the injection can be stopped before convulsions supervene.

Once the injection is complete, the needle is removed, the hole sprayed with Nobecutane and covered, and the patient positioned to assist the spread of solution towards the roots requiring blockade.

For drugs, dosage and posture, see below page 877.

### Continuous Epidural Blockade

Although the use of an epidural catheter is associated with a higher incidence of unilateral or asymmetrical blocks than is the single-shot technique, it is generally preferred because it so greatly enhances the versatility of the block and the duration of effect.

It is a matter of routine that before inserting the Tuohy needle, the catheter should be passed down it to confirm that it readily emerges from the tip. In the United Kingdom the Portex epidural catheter is generally used, and the 16G will pass down a 16G Tuohy needle. A graduated catheter (Fig. 9) should be used so that the length of catheter in the epidural space can be calculated. A detachable mount enables the operator to remove the Tuohy needle after insertion of the catheter.

Once the Tuohy needle is in the epidural space and its position has been checked using loss of resistance to saline, then air and gentle aspiration, the catheter is passed down, directing it, usually cephalad, with the side hole of the needle. The catheter tip emerges from the needle usually as the 10 cm mark is disappearing into the hub. Resistance may be felt at this point. If resistance to the passage of the catheter is felt beyond this point, it should *never be withdrawn, neither should it be forced onwards.* Withdrawal of the catheter once it has emerged may cause the end to be sheared off and remain in the epidural space.

*Causes of Obstruction to Passage of the Catheter*

(i) If insertion of the catheter produces pain or tingling in one hip or leg, it is abutting against a nerve root, and forcing its passage may cause root damage.

(ii) The catheter tip may be impinging on an epidural vein and forcing it may cause bloody tap, epidural haematoma or intravascular injection.

(iii) The catheter tip may be up against the dura and pushing too hard may cause it to penetrate the subarachnoid space.

(iv) The needle tip may not be in the epidural space at all.

A catheter entering the epidural space in the midline will generally pass freely, and should be inserted gently and no further than the 15 cm mark (at the needle hub). If resistance is encountered well before this, the needle may be carefully rotated through 90° (away from the twinges, should they occur). If this does not enable the catheter to pass, increasing spinal flexion may do the trick. Otherwise the Tuohy needle should be removed carefully while feeding the catheter through it. If, after the needle is out, calculation suggests that 2 cm or more of catheter remains in the epidural space, then all is well. If less, then the Tuohy needle should be reinserted, redoubling the efforts to keep it in the midline. If the catheter is well in, then it should be withdrawn until not more than 4 cm lies in the epidural space. Catheters may run for short distances in the epidural space and then double back on themselves or pass out through an intervertebral foramen. There has even been one report of a catheter tying itself in a knot in the epidural space.[67] The tendency of an epidural catheter to curl up at the site of introduction limits an important theoretical advantage of the catheter technique. It is tempting to assume that a catheter can be threaded to a predetermined level cephalad or caudad to the centre of the segments to be blocked, thus eliminating blockade of unnecessary segments and reducing dosage when the lumbar route is used. Bridenbaugh and associates[68] showed convincingly that it is well-nigh impossible to thread a catheter up the lumbar epidural space as it almost always curls up at the site of introduction. In their hands, only about 12 per cent of catheters could be threaded up to the desired levels. The tendency for a catheter to pass to one side in the epidural space increases the likelihood of an asymmetrical or unilateral block which, if resistant to treatment, may necessitate re-insertion of the catheter.

With the catheter correctly positioned, it should be anchored in place with Nobecutane by an assistant. While the operator remains in sterile garb, he detaches the mount and removes the Tuohy needle from the catheter (taking care not to pull the catheter out of the space), replaces the mount and aspirates down it gently. This manoeuvre should produce cerebrospinal fluid if the catheter has entered the subarachnoid space, particularly if a catheter with multiple eye holes rather than one with a single hole is used. There are reports, however, of total spinal anaesthesia resulting from attempted epidural injection, following negative aspiration.[69–71] It is possible that attempts at aspiration may be too hasty or that during aspiration the single hole may be temporarily obstructed by adjacent structures.

Aspiration will also reveal intravascular placement. If blood is aspirated, the catheter should be withdrawn a short distance. If the flow of blood is not readily stopped, the catheter should be inserted in an adjacent space.

Aspiration down the catheter is essential but not one hundred per cent reliable and does not, therefore, obviate the need for a test dose when using a catheter.

Next the operator attaches a bacterial filter to the mount and fixes the catheter to the patient's back before removing sterile garb. The catheter should be looped round near the skin to reduce the possibility of dislodging it from the epidural space. The area near the skin entry should be covered with a sterile dressing which, together with a length of catheter, is strapped securely to the patient's back. For abdominal operations, the catheter should be brought up over the patient's shoulder and the filter taped in front. The filter opening is kept covered between epidural injections, using the cap provided with the catheter.

**The test dose** of 2–3 ml of local anaesthetic solution is used to detect subarachnoid placement of the catheter, since a dose insufficient for epidural blockade may be expected to produce an effect if injected intrathecally; to wit, onset of analgesia and some degree of motor block can be expected to occur within 2 minutes.[72] If a full epidural dose were given intrathecally, however, it would produce a total spinal (see page 886), which is a serious complication. However, a test dose, like aspiration down the catheter, is not infallible, probably because the signs of spinal block are overlooked, and total spinal anaesthesia has been reported following an apparently ineffective test dose.[69–71] There is a school of thought which states that because a test dose may apparently fail occasionally, it should not be used, lest delay in analgesia cause distress to the patient.[73] This is not really a logical reason for omitting the test dose, though admittedly in a carefully conducted epidural service, total spinal *should* be vanishingly rare. In practice, the compromise measure is to allow an interval of time between test and main dose which is inversely proportional to the patient's pain!

A test dose of a local anaesthetic solution containing *adrenaline* has been advocated[72] to detect intravascular placement of the catheter which, in this case, would result in palpitations and tachycardia of rapid onset. Such a test fails of course if the patient is taking $\beta$-adrenoceptor-blocking drugs,[74] while the full dose containing adrenaline will, in such a patient produce dangerous hypertension due to unopposed $\alpha$ stimulation. Most workers consider that it is not justifiable to introduce the risks of adrenaline for the purpose of test-dosing alone, simply to guard against the rare event that catheter-aspiration yields a false negative for intravascular placement.

**Test dosing for repeat injections** is even more controversial. Examples can be quoted when injection down a catheter has produced epidural blockade, only to produce spinal block after a subsequent dose,[75] implying that an epidural catheter may with time migrate into the subarachnoid space. This is unlikely if there is minimal manipulation of the Tuohy needle in the space and *gentle* insertion of the catheter, thereby avoiding any trauma to the dura.

However, a test dose prior to each and every top-up dose has been advocated. Scott[73] pointed out, however, that if one really considers catheter migration to be a serious possibility, it is inadvisable to allow midwives, for example, to top-up, since one cannot expect them to judge whether a test dose has yielded a positive result. One must balance the very remote, though serious, possibility of a total spinal against keeping every patient waiting 5 minutes at every top-up. Paradoxically, since the anaesthetist is present for the first dose and can readily treat a total spinal, it can be argued that a test dose is more important for later injections during his absence. In the UK, however, test doses prior to top-up are the exception rather than the rule, though there can be no absolute contra-indication to their use.

**Drugs and Doses for Epidural Block**

Before the advent of bupivacaine, lignocaine hydrochloride 1·2–2·0 per cent (commonly 1·5 per cent) was used, together with adrenaline 5 μg/ml or amethocaine (50–100 mg) where appropriate to prolong its effect. The first dose of lignocaine might last 1–1½ hours with some prolongation from adrenaline, but with subsequent doses tachyphylaxis would occur, and it was impossible to maintain continuous analgesia without ultimately producing serious systemic toxicity.[76] Nowadays, bupivacaine hydrochloride is more commonly used, though it is occasionally combined with lignocaine initially, in an attempt to accelerate the onset of analgesia, though the evidence for this is variable. Duration of analgesia is longest with bupivacaine alone, while motor block is maximal using an equipotent mixture of the two drugs.[77] There is no advantage in terms of toxicity from using mixtures.[78]

For surgery, bupivacaine is used in a 0·5 or 0·75 per cent solution, which lasts more than 2 hours. Lower concentrations may be used for analgesia, easily avoiding motor block. A concentration of 0·25 per cent is usually satisfactory, though the duration and reliability of 0·125 per cent are not usually acceptable.[79] For postoperative analgesia a dose of bupivacaine generally lasts about 4 hours, though in labour 2 hours is the norm. In general, using a lower concentration necessitates a larger volume and the consequent increase in spread may result in a higher incidence of hypotension[21] (Fig. 11). Larger volumes, however, reduce patchy anaesthesia.

Amethocaine 0·5 per cent has also been used, though is it more toxic than bupivacaine, carries a higher incidence of motor block and, being an ester, is less stable in solution. Etidocaine is effective in about double the concentration of bupivacaine; it is no more toxic, produces much more motor block and is shorter in duration unless combined with adrenaline.

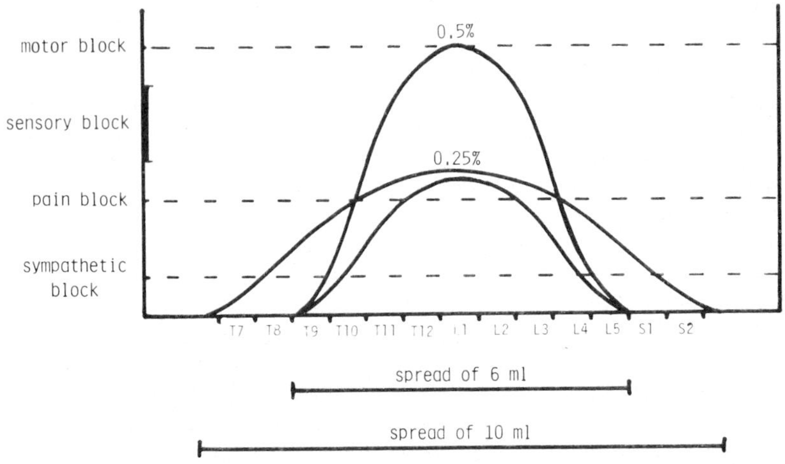


32/Fig. 11.—Theoretical relationship between spread of different volumes of bupivacaine in the epidural space and the thresholds for blockade of different fibre types. To produce adequate analgesia with 0·25% bupivacaine necessitates a larger volume and hence more widespread sympathetic block than is the case with 0·5%. (Courtesy of Dr. F. Reynolds, and Lloyd-Luke (Medical Books) Ltd.[21])

Extent of blockade in the epidural space is determined by dosage, though individual requirements vary for a number of reasons (see Factors Controlling the Spread of Epidural Block). In general, 20–30 ml of solution are required for abdominal surgery, but it should be borne in mind that the upper safe dose limit for bupivacaine is 2 mg/kg, that is 0·4 ml/kg of a 0·5 per cent solution. Constraints are somewhat greater for the other agents mentioned here. Upper abdominal surgery will require either a maximal volume given with the patient head down, or a thoracic approach to the epidural space. For lower abdominal and pelvic surgery combined, about half the dose may need to be given with the patient somewhat sitting up, and the remainder with the patient head down. Perineal surgery requires about 15 ml given in the sitting position and leg and groin surgery requires 15–20 ml horizontal.

For *analgesia*, low concentrations of local anaesthetics are effective. For analgesia after surgery in the lower abdomen, 8–10 ml of 0·25 per cent bupivacaine normally gives good analgesia for about 4 hours. Such a dose may be repeated indefinitely without any risk of systemic toxicity. There may, however, be minor degrees of motor block and some risk of circulatory instability, and such a technique would be unsuitable for upper abdominal or thoracic analgesia producing a high incidence of hypotension.[141]

Postoperative pain has been treated using a *continuous epidural infusion*[81, 82, 86] to avoid transient hypotension, supposedly associated with bolus injections. Bupivacaine 0·125–0·375 per cent has been used at infusion rates of 10–20 ml/hr. Dose requirements are generally greater by infusion than by bolus[21] however, while with higher concentrations it is hard to avoid progressive motor block and significant systemic accumulation.

**Fate of Local Anaesthetics in the Epidural Space**

Local anaesthetic solution injected into the epidural space can pass out of the intervertebral foramina to an extent depending on how completely these foramina are occluded by nerve roots and accompanying vessels. With age, skeletal changes tend to restrict the available gaps and therefore more effectively confine the solution to the epidural space, increasing spread and effectiveness (see Factors Controlling the Spread of Epidural Block).

Local anaesthetics also diffuse across dura and arachnoid into the cerebrospinal fluid. Though appreciable concentrations of drug can be measured in the CSF, it is unlikely that epidurals work entirely by intrathecal block, since the distribution of the two modes of block is different. Epidurals work segmentally at the roots nearest to the injection site, and readily spare the sacral roots. This would be impossible if intrathecal block were an important factor in epidural analgesia (Fig. 6).

It would appear, therefore, that local anaesthetics penetrate dural cuffs to block nerve roots in the vicinity. They may also pass by axonal transmission to block conduction within the spinal cord.[20]

Whatever the immediate destination of epidurally administered local anaesthetics, they must ultimately be absorbed into the bloodstream. Absorption of local anaesthetics into the circulation takes place more rapidly from the epidural than from the subarachnoid space.[83] The speed with which they are absorbed depends upon local vascularity, which may be influenced by injected adrenaline, and by drug characteristics which are discussed in Chapter 31.

**Factors Controlling the Spread of Epidural Block**

1. *Volume and concentration of local anaesthetic* (vide supra).

2. *Posture.*—Despite the slightly hypobaric nature of 0·5 per cent bupivacaine (Marcain plain) in relation to the cerebrospinal fluid, this solution, in common with other local anaesthetic preparations, tends to fall in the epidural space, though not as reliably as hyperbaric solutions given intrathecally. It is apparent that tilting can usually determine caudal and cephalad spread, while the lateral position produces a block which is significantly higher on the dependent side[84] and can be used to help overcome unilateral block. In most subjects, it is possible to induce sacral spread of local anaesthetic solution with the aid of the sitting position, though it may also be necessary to use a low space and/or a large volume. Sitting bolt upright may *discourage* caudal spread[142] possibly because the dural sac plugs the vertebral canal. For procedures involving both abdomen (thoracic roots) and pelvis or perineum (sacral roots), the semi-sitting position followed by a fully recumbent position may be used in an attempt to minimise the effect on the legs from blockade of all the intervening lumbar roots, though in practice it is impossible to eliminate lumbar effects in these circumstances.

Though fat has a lower specific gravity than aqueous local anaesthetic solutions, the thin film in the epidural space is unlikely to be sufficient to account for such positive geotropism. However, gravity *has* been shown to have a more marked effect on epidural spread in the obese than in normal subjects[85] and an increase in epidural fat in the obese could account for this difference.

3. *Lumbar interspace.*—The dermatomes of the anterior abdominal wall are *thoracic*, therefore even for lower abdominal surgery or analgesia, a higher lumber interspace is preferable. The L2/3 space is generally the most popular, being slightly safer than L1/2 because of the lumbosacral bulge in the cord (Fig. 6, p. 860). A lower approach than L2/3 for obstetric analgesia for example renders standard volumes of solution ineffective[86] and has too much effect on the legs.

For upper abdominal surgery, very large volumes that may border on the toxic, are necessary if given by the lumbar root. The thoracic approach greatly reduces dose requirement and unnecessary lumbar block. For lower leg and perineal block, the lower lumbar interspaces are suitable.

4. *Patient age.* Bromage[87] showed clearly that dose requirement per spinal segment dropped steadily from the age of 20 years onwards. Recently other workers[88] were not able to show this graded response, but confirmed that dose requirement was indeed less in patients over 40 than in those under 40 years of age. *Arteriosclerosis* has also been implicated[89] as a cause of excessive epidural spread. However, such a finding could be coincidental and purely age-associated. Osteoarthritis with increased closure of the intervertebral foramina in the aged may be a more important factor.[90]

5. *Pregnancy and intra-abdominal tumours.* In the presence of inferior vena caval compression from the gravid uterus or a large tumour, the venous return from the lower part of the body may be diverted to the vertebral and epidural venous plexuses. It is postulated that distension of the epidural veins will cause excessive epidural spread of local anaesthesia. However, Grundy and co-workers[91] found no increase in the number of segments blocked by a given dose of local anaesthetic in pregnant compared to non-pregnant women. True, pregnant women are much more sensitive to the *hypotensive* effect of vasodilatation, and pain relief in labour can be produced by very small volumes of solution because very few segments have to be blocked.

6. *Patient height and weight.*—Obesity does not increase the dose requirement for local anaesthetics epidurally, indeed it may even

reduce it.[92] Height, of course, increases dose requirement, as can be seen in the young age group,[87] though in an all-adult population the effect may be hard to detect as it tends to be swamped by the other factors. Certainly, determining dose requirement for obstetric analgesia on the grounds of patient height gives satisfactory results.

7. *Nerve-root size.*—The S1 root, outstandingly the thickest, can be notoriously resistant to block by the epidural route.[93] Analgesia in the S1 dermatome has a prolonged latency and frequently a shorter duration than the surrounding areas.

8. *Previous epidural block* is *not* associated with impaired spread of solution or unblocked segments, although previous epidural haematoma might be.[94]

## Indications for Spinal and Epidural Block

**Obstetric analgesia.**—By far the greatest number of epidurals are given in the UK for pain relief in labour. This is discussed in Chapter 39.

**Surgery.**—Local may be preferred to general anaesthesia when expert anaesthetists are in short supply, on the grounds that it is safer to have a conscious (albeit sympathetically-blocked) patient than an unconscious one in the hands of less highly trained staff.

Unfitness for general anaesthesia is occasionally an indication for spinal or epidural, but it must be remembered that the circulation can be rendered dangerously labile. Moreover, patients with heart or chest disease are rarely comfortably lying flat for surgery.

For Caesarean section, the fetus fares better under epidural than under general anaesthesia, provided the blood pressure is maintained (see Chapter 41), while for this, as for other operations, patients may prefer to be awake.

There is good evidence that elderly patients having total hip replacements and other hip surgery, fare better after spinal or epidural than after general anaesthesia. Postoperative hypoxaemia and disorientation are less evident[32] and deep-vein thrombosis less frequent.[24,25]

Epidural is sometimes used concurrently with general anaesthesia to reduce bleeding, particularly in repeat surgery, and for postoperative analgesia.

### Postoperative Analgesia

By using a continuous epidural technique, effective analgesia can be provided for the first 48 hours after operation. The patient is able to cough, expectorate and carry out breathing exercises unhampered by wound pain. The method is particularly indicated for patients with chronic bronchitis and emphysema. For analgesia after upper abdominal and thoracic surgery, however, the dose of local anaesthetic may have to be so large as to produce marked hypotension and leg weakness. The use of a mid-thoracic intervertebral space makes small volumes of solution effective and can reduce the incidence of hypotension, and improve vital capacity. Bromage[95] reported on the use of this technique to provide early ambulation after major abdominal procedures. For success, the technique must provide a narrow band of analgesia sufficient to cover the wound area, and leave the lower limbs unaffected.

The technique is exacting and unsuitable for routine use except where the facilities of a postoperative recovery ward or intensive care unit are available. Recently, opiates rather than local anaesthetics have been used by the lumbar and thoracic routes, thereby avoiding the associated hypotensive problems. This is discussed in Chapter 30.

**Crush injury of the chest.**—Continuous epidural analgesia with local anaesthetics or opiates is increasingly used in the treatment of chest injuries. The complete relief from pain that it affords reduces paradoxical respiration and allows the patient to clear the lower airways by coughing freely. Patients with moderate or severe chest injuries usually require tracheostomy and intermittent positive-pressure ventilation, but epidural analgesia with opiates may still be useful, though the extensive block needed would very likely be followed by marked hypotension if local anaesthetics were used. Epidural analgesia is worth considering, especially when the bony injury is limited to the lower part of the thoracic cage and also to help wean the patient off the ventilator after a period of intermittent positive-pressure ventilation.

**Intractable pain.**—This is discussed in Chapter 33.

**Lumbar-disc lesions.**—The use of epidural analgesia for the relief of sciatic pain was reported many years ago.[96,97] Cyriax[98] advocated it as the conservative treatment of choice for those patients who have a low lumbar disc lesion causing nerve-root pressure with neurological signs in the affected leg. Coomes,[99] from a comparison of the results of treatment by epidural injection with those from rest in bed, reinforced this view.

**Peripheral vascular disease.**—Preganglionic sympathetic (B) fibres are readily blocked by concentrations of local anaesthetic less than those required for sensory block. A single epidural injection is a convenient way of assessing the likely effects of a subsequent sympathectomy and saves the discomfort of blocking the sympathetic ganglia by several paravertebral injections. The prompt treatment by this technique may save a limb endangered by arterial embolism or traumatic injuries, as it will open up the collateral vessels that are in spasm. A white leg of pregnancy may also respond. Here the deep-vein thrombosis is thought to produce a reflex spasm of the small veins and arterioles, resulting in hypoxia and transudation of fluid from the capillaries into the tissue, where it increases the oedema further by pressing on the lymphatics. An early sympathetic block may break the vicious circle, but it usually has to be repeated or maintained over several days for successful treatment.

**Visceral pain.**—The severe pain of acute pancreatitis and the agonising pain of dissecting aneurysm of the aorta can be successfully relieved by continuous epidural analgesia.

## Caudal Epidural Anaesthesia

### Anatomy of the Sacrum, Sacral Canal and Hiatus

The sacrum represents the fusion of 5 sacral vertebrae. Variations of this fusion are common and have an important bearing on the failure rate of caudal epidural anaesthesia.

The sacrum is triangular in shape; the apex, below, articulates with the coccyx, while the base, above, has median and lateral portions. The median part represents the body of the 1st sacral vertebra and articulates with the corresponding surface of the body of the 5th lumbar vertebra. The lateral portions, known as the alae, represent fused costal and transverse elements.

The anterior surface is concave and ridged at the sites of fusion between the five sacral vertebrae. Lateral to the ridges are the large anterior sacral foramina through which the anterior primary rami of the first four sacral nerves pass. Local anaesthetic solutions injected into the sacral epidural space can pass freely through these foramina, and this is a factor in the unpredictable height to which caudal anaesthesia may extend.

The posterior surface has greater interest for the anaesthetist (Fig. 12). It is convex, and in the midline runs a bony ridge, the median sacral crest, with three or four rudimentary spinous processes. The sacral hiatus is a deficiency of the posterior wall resulting from failure of fusion of the laminae of the 5th sacral vertebra, and is triangular in shape, with its apex at the spine of the 4th sacral vertebra. In surface marking it normally forms an approximately equilateral triangle with the two posterior superior iliac spines. The lateral margins of the space each bear a prominence—the sacral cornu—which represent the inferior articular processes of the 5th sacral vertebra. The base of the hiatus is the superior surface of the coccyx. The posterior sacrococcygeal membrane, which in elderly subjects may be ossified, is attached to the bony margin and fills in the hiatus. In some cases the apex of the hiatus is the 3rd sacral spine, due to the absence of the 3rd and 4th laminae, and occasionally the whole of the bony posterior wall is deficient. When the laminae of the 5th sacral vertebra are present, the hiatus may be very small—with a diameter as narrow as 2 mm—making the introduction of a caudal needle almost impossible.

There are four pairs of posterior sacral foramina corresponding with the anterior ones. The sacral canal (Fig. 6) is triangular and contains a continuation of the epidural space, and the dural sac, which usually terminates at the lower border of the second sacral vertebra, though occasionally it extends below this point. The epidural space contains the sacral and coccygeal nerve roots and filum terminale, and a continuation of the epidural venous plexus. Fibrous bands may be present in the sacral epidural space dividing it into loculi which prevent the spread of solutions, and these may account for occasional incomplete anaesthesia.

### Needles

A malleable steel needle (Fig. 9) has been

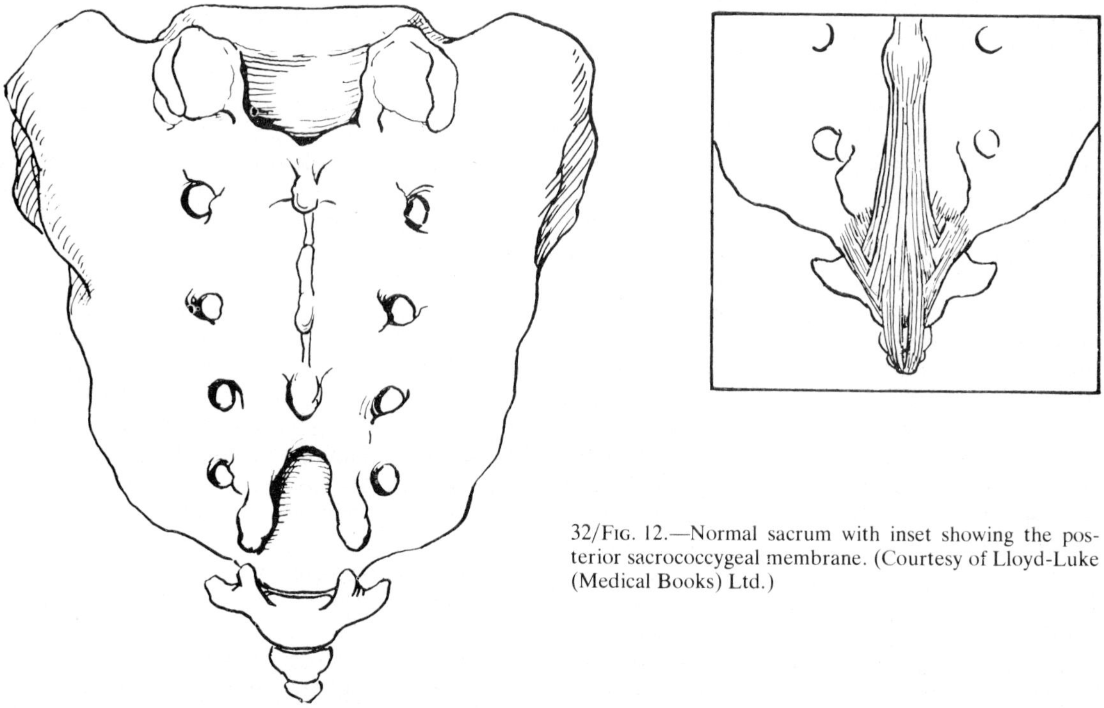

32/Fig. 12.—Normal sacrum with inset showing the posterior sacrococcygeal membrane. (Courtesy of Lloyd-Luke (Medical Books) Ltd.)

used as this will adapt itself to the curve of the sacrum and will not break. Such needles used occasionally to come apart where the hub joins the shaft, and for this reason there was near the hub a small round enlargement which ensured that a portion of shaft always stuck out of the skin. The length of the shaft, between point and enlargement, should be between 2 and 3 inches (5 and 7·5 cm). As with spinal epidural anaesthesia, a wider-bore needle gives a better feel of the structures it passes through, while a short bevel at the point minimises the risk of puncturing the dura. Nowadays many operators use an ordinary disposable hypodermic needle.

### Technique

The patient can be either prone or in the left lateral position. For obstetric patients the latter position is the more convenient. A scrupulous aseptic technique (see page 867) must be observed.

The sacral hiatus is identified by feeling for the sacral cornua with the tip of the index finger; a skin weal of local anaesthetic solution is then raised over it, using a fine needle. In obese patients it is difficult to feel, and in others it may be smaller than normal. When in difficulty, Galley[100] recommended identifying the tip of the coccyx and placing the tip of the index finger over this with the rest of the finger in the intergluteal fold. The hiatus should then coincide in position with the proximal interphalangeal joint. The caudal needle is passed through the skin weal to pierce the sacrococcygeal membrane at right angles to the skin surface. The hub of the needle is then depressed until it is almost in the intergluteal fold parallel to the skin over the sacrum. The needle is then pushed cephalad into the sacral canal, taking care that the point does not ascend any higher than a line joining the posterior superior iliac spines at which level the subarachnoid space begins.

Aspiration tests for blood and CSF are made. A drop or so of blood is no contra-indication to proceeding with the injection, but if CSF is aspirated the block must be abandoned or converted to spinal anaesthesia. Free bleeding from the needle hub means that an epidural vein has been pierced and the needle should be withdrawn for 0·5 cm. A test dose is then injected—say 5 ml of solution—and if the patient can move his toes at the end of 5 minutes the needle can be assumed to be safely in the epidural space and the main dose is injected.

In spite of careful technique the needle may pass into sites other than the epidural space: it may miss the sacrococcygeal membrane and pass dorsal to the sacrum. If this is suspected it can be tested for by injecting a few ml of air and palpating the skin over the tip of the needle for crepitus. The main danger is if the needle slips past the base of the coccyx into the rectum, or even pierces the fetal skull. Marked resistance to injection, with complaint of backache, suggests the needle point has run beneath the periosteal layer of the sacral canal, and this can be corrected by slightly withdrawing the needle. When the needle is correctly placed in the epidural space the solution should run freely without any sensation of resistance, as with lumbar epidural injection. Any feeling of resistance suggests that the needle is not correctly placed.

**Drugs.**—Local anaesthetic solutions appropriate for lumbar epidurals may be used, and though larger volumes are necessary to attain the same *height* of block, the resulting perineal analgesia can be very prolonged.

**Dosage.**—The level of anaesthesia depends on the volume of solution injected and the position of the patient. About 20–30 ml of solution are required for blocks up to L4–5 for operations on the anus, perineum or vagina. About 40 ml of solution plus a slight Trendelenburg position will give a block up to the umbilicus, but such a large dose risks toxic reactions.

### Indications for Caudal Epidural Blockade

**Surgical operations.**—The main value of this route is for the production of anaesthesia of the sacral nerves for such procedures as cystoscopy, anal operations and circumcision, and gynaecological operations on the vulva and vagina. In obese patients for whom a local block is likely to provide better operating conditions in these regions than is a general anaesthetic, the sacral approach to the epidural space may be technically difficult. In such cases it may be easier to perform a lumbar epidural block, with the patient sitting up to allow the local anaesthetic solution to diffuse down into the sacral canal.

**Postoperative analgesia.**—Caudals are frequently given in conjunction with general anaesthesia, because a single shot can provide prolonged postoperative analgesia. This is valuable for anal operations and particularly so for circumcision in children.[101]

**Obstetric analgesia.**—See Chapter 39.

## Contra-indications to Spinal and Epidural Block

The contra-indications to any form of injected local anaesthesia, be it spinal, epidural or simple nerve block, are the same, to wit: clotting defect and local sepsis.

It is never safe to put a needle into the tissues of a patient with a clotting deficiency, whether it be congenital or acquired as a result of intercurrent disease. It has been found, however, that the risk of a carefully inserted epidural may not be great in patients on well-controlled anticoagulant treatment.[143]

Sepsis in the skin in the vicinity of the injection is an obvious contra-indication but, bacteraemia and serious focal sepsis—a collection of pus anywhere in the body—can give rise to a metastatic abscess at the site of a foreign body or a haematoma in the epidural space.

Continuous techniques using an indwelling catheter are inappropriate for use intrathecally or caudally, in the former case because the danger of introducing infection into the cerebrospinal fluid is so great, and in the latter case because of the nearness of the decidedly contaminated anal region.[102]

Laminectomy is no contra-indication to spinal anaesthesia.[103,104] Adhesions between ligamentum flavum and dura may obliterate the epidural space, but epidurals are generally inserted well above the usual site for laminectomy, and so in practice laminectomy does not normally contra-indicate epidural blockade either.

In spina bifida it is usually possible to find an interspinous space above the spinal defect, to enable epidural loss of resistance to be detected.

Previous epidural analgesia does not normally impair spread of local anaesthetic in the epidural space, though theoretically a previous epidural blood patch might do.

## Complications of Spinal and Epidural Block

Not all complications are common to both techniques but as there is some overlap they are combined here to avoid repetition.

### Hypotension

Vasodilatation is a predictable, and occasionally a *desirable* feature of blockade involving nerve roots above L2. Serious hypotension is commonly provoked by a high block of *rapid* onset, because spread of effect may outstrip adequate cardiovascular compensation and fluid preloading. Hypotension therefore may appear a more prominent feature of spinal than epidural blockade, and of blockade with an agent of rapid onset, such as chloroprocaine,[105] not because of any differential neural effects by different techniques or drugs. Conversely, its incidence can be reduced when an extensive epidural is required, by giving the full dose in multiple small increments.[106] The physiology of hypotension and its management are discussed earlier (pp. 864 and 866). Hypotension is minimised by adequate fluid loading which, for spinal anaesthesia and for a rapid-acting local anaesthetic, must be given early. A litre or two of Hartmann's solution is commonly recommended, though colloid solutions such as 5 per cent albumin[107] and polygeline (Haemaccel)[108] are effective in reducing hypotension at lower volumes than is crystalloid solution. However, because colloids are more expensive and carry a slightly increased risk of allergic reaction, crystalloid is generally preferred for routine prophylaxis against hypotension.

### Complications Associated with Dural Puncture

It is often stated that a high incidence of inadvertent dural puncture is inevitable when epidurals are inserted by inexperienced operators. Doughty[109] has shown that even with a new trainee once a fortnight, it is possible to reduce the dural puncture rate to 0·4 per cent. He states that a high frequency of inadvertent dural puncture suggests a poor technique and a low standard of teaching and supervision.[110] Successful techniques involve the loss-of-resistance sign, using a saline-filled rather than an air-filled syringe,[139] and steady advance of the needle with pressure on the syringe plunger, the non-dominant hand creating a high-inertia system by acting as a brake to sudden advance (see page 873).

Dural penetration by the epidural catheter does occasionally occur, but minimal manipulation of the needle within the epidural space and gentle advancement of the catheter greatly reduce this risk.

**Headache.**—There is considerable evidence that most post-spinal headaches are due to a low CSF pressure consequent upon seepage of CSF through the dural puncture hole. Headache can also result from aseptic meningeal irritation or it may herald the onset of infective meningitis, but this should be infinitely rare. Typical post-spinal headache comes on within an hour or two of the anaesthesia. It is not, however, generally appreciated that its onset may be delayed for some days, and may last for weeks or even months.

Headache from the continued leakage of cerebrospinal fluid through a hole in the dura has certain well-defined characteristics. It is different from any other previously experienced and is made worse by sitting up and relieved by lying down or by abdominal compression. Pain may spread across the whole frontal area or be localised behind the eyeballs or in the nuchal region. In the latter case it is often accompanied by a stiff neck, typical of meningeal irritation. Nausea and vomiting not uncommonly accompany the headache and the patient may find difficulty in focusing his eyes. Tinnitus and deafness may occur, and are explicable on the basis of a low CSF pressure resulting in a fall in intra-labyrinthine pressure.

With a cerebrospinal fluid pressure of about 150 mm of water, fluid will continue to leak after lumbar puncture until the dural hole becomes sealed, and it is theoretically possible to lose up to 240 ml in a day. However, in post-spinal headaches the pressure is below 50 mm of water. Anything which is likely to increase the leak through the dura may increase the incidence of headache. Thus, spinal headache is commoner in obstetric patients in whom the cerebrospinal fluid pressure is raised during contractions, and in whom bearing down is believed to exacerbate the leak. However, Ravindran and his colleagues,[111] using a 22-gauge spinal needle, recorded an incidence of headache of 10 per cent in parturients who did not bear down, compared with 9 per cent in those who did. Reduction in the size of the dural hole by the use of a fine spinal needle significantly reduces the incidence of spinal headache. Dripps and Vandam[112] showed from their series that with a 16-gauge needle the incidence of headache was 24 per cent while with a 24-gauge needle it fell to 6 per cent. The latter is the smallest size needle which can, in practice, be used without the aid of an introducer but, using a 25- or 26-gauge needle, headache is even rarer.

Headache is no commoner following a correctly conducted epidural block than it is in an equivalent population not given an epidural.[113] Headache following accidental dural puncture with a Tuohy needle is both more frequent and more intractable than that with a finer spinal needle.

**Prophylaxis and treatment.**—The incidence of spinal headache can be minimised by the use of a ~~fine spinal~~ needle and also, it is said, by using the lateral approach to the subarachnoid space.[114] After lumbar puncture it is customary to keep the patient horizontal for 24 hours; however, this period of time is insufficient if a wide-bore (18 gauge) needle is used,[115] and particularly for obstetric patients, in whom complete bed rest for 72 hours may be required for repair of the punctured hole. The leak can be reduced by maintaining the prone position and by avoiding coughing and straining at stool.

In most cases, by such simple measures, a headache can be avoided completely. Should it occur, conservative measures should be continued and the patient should be given aspirin or paracetamol and encouraged to drink large volumes. An epidural injection or infusion of saline or Hartmann's solution has been recommended, but relief may be only temporary, especially when a wide-bore needle has done the damage.[116] When headache persists, an *epidural blood patch* may be considered. Its success rate in the treatment of CSF leak from a wide-bore needle is considerably higher than epidural saline,[116,117] a firm clot sealing the hole with remarkable effect. However, it frequently produces mild backache, neckache and paraesthesiae, and the introduction of infection by such a means would be disastrous, so it is a procedure which should only be used for severe refractory spinal headache.

Two sterile-gowned and gloved operators are required, one to carry out the epidural and the other to collect the patient's own blood with a sterile, anticoagulant-free syringe at the same time. A volume of 10 ml of blood is commonly used, though 20 ml has been recommended.[118] This procedure requires skill and care and is not to be undertaken lightly. Reynolds and his associates[119] reported a case of a patient who had been given 6 blood patches for a post-myelogram headache. Severe root compression necessitated neurosurgery at which a *subdural* (epiarachnoid) haematoma was revealed.

**Other sequelae of dural puncture.**—A low-pressure headache should always be taken seriously, as death has been reported from continued CSF leakage. In one case[120] in which a spinal headache was ignored, post-mortem revealed herniation of the uncus against the tentorium cerebellae. In another, a continuous subarachnoid block had been administered to an obstetric patient after accidental dural puncture.[121] Following 40 days of persistent headache, death resulted from bilateral temporal subdural haematoma. Indeed, subdural haematoma has been reported on several occasions following spinal block.[122]

Such disasters are obviously rare, however, and the patient should always be reassured, while any sign of persistent CSF leak, whether headache or frank cutaneous leakage,[123] should be treated conscientiously by whatever means are found necessary, until it is cured.

*Sixth cranial nerve palsy.*—Although paralysis of several cranial nerves has occasionally been reported (possibly as a result of excessive spread of local anaesthetic) the sixth nerve is most commonly affected because in its long, tortuous course it is susceptible to damage from low CSF pressure. Low pressure is assumed to result in descent of the medulla and pons and to cause stretching of the nerve—since it is anchored between its position in the cavernous sinus and origin from the pons—as it passes over the apex of the petrous temporal bone. Together with the low-pressure headache, there may be dizziness and photophobia, followed by double vision from impaired action of the external rectus muscle. The incidence can of course be reduced by using a fine spinal needle, and prophylaxis is exactly the same as for spinal headache.

The treatment of the lesion is to cover the affected eye to eliminate diplopia and prevent nausea. Spontaneous recovery can be expected in 50 per cent of cases in about a month, but muscle exercises and fusion training may help. Any surgical correction should be postponed for two years, as spontaneous recovery has been known to be delayed for as long as this.

*Accidental total spinal block.*—Should the entire epidural dose of local anaesthetic be unwittingly placed intrathecally, total spinal block will result. The patient may notice rising anaesthesia and difficulty in breathing, then become unconscious, severely hypotensive and apnoeic. The appearance resembles that of death. Immediate treatment is to intubate and ventilate with oxygen, and support the circulation by infusing fluid and administering ephedrine. Once the situation is stabilised, whatever procedure was intended should be carried out, as operating conditions are usually ideal. Provided hypotension has not been allowed to persist for too long, recovery normally takes place in two hours or more and is usually complete. However, whether because of hypotension, or because of some ill-defined irritant effect associated with the injection of a large volume of foreign fluid into the subarachnoid space, inadvertent intrathecal anaesthesia does appear to be associated with occasional prolonged neurological disturbance (*vide infra*).

Epidural analgesia for labour is commonly provided quite safely via an interspace adjacent to an inadvertent dural puncture. However, if more extensive blockade is required as, for example, for Caesarean section, the risk of producing a total spinal is considerable and there is good evidence that epidural block for Caesarean section should not be given following a dural puncture.[124]

*Respiratory failure.*—Respiratory failure is the great risk of high spinal anaesthesia whether deliberate or inadvertent. During the critical first few minutes of spinal anaesthesia when the solution is being "fixed" the anaesthetist should be constantly on the watch for signs of it. These signs are the progressive failure of intercostal respiration, with increasing diaphragmatic activity, reduction of the voice to a whisper, dilatation of the alae nasae, the use of the unparalysed accessory muscles of respiration, and a tracheal tug. The anaesthetist must be prepared to clear the airway, intubate, ventilate the lungs with 100 per cent oxygen, and restore the blood pressure by a combination of posture, intravenous fluids, atropine and possibly vasopressor drugs. The restoration of blood pressure is the primary physiological consideration, since most cases of apnoea during spinal block are due to hypotension rather than spread of the drug to the brain stem. Should the apnoea be due to phrenic paralysis, the same treatment is needed. Speed is vital in treatment as cardiac arrest rapidly follows respiratory arrest in cases of ischaemic medullary paralysis.

### Trauma

**Backache.**—This is caused by damage to the supraspinous and interspinous ligaments and the ligamentum flavum through which the spinal or epidural needle passes. With the fine spinal needles in use today, backache is very uncommon, but it is the commonest post-analgesia complication of epidural anaesthesia, though usually amounting to little more than mild local tenderness.

Damage to an intervertebral disc may occasionally follow lumbar puncture, particularly in childhood. It is possible that the flexion of the spine needed during lumbar puncture increases the pressure in the discs, causing them to bulge into the spinal canal. Backache associated with musculoskeletal and sacro-iliac strain is common in the puerperium, and if the patient has received an epidural, this is sometimes blamed. However, it is as common in patients who have *not* received epidurals as in those who have.[113]

**Haematoma.**—Injury to the epidural plexus of vessels causes "bloody tap". Bleeding can be severe enough to result in the formation of an epidural haematoma, and if blood reaches the subarachnoid space, signs of meningeal irritation will follow. Damage to the epidural vessels is more likely to occur with an epidural catheter technique than with a needle.[125] A clotting defect should be considered a contra-indication to epidural block, since the resulting epidural haematoma may be so large as to produce cord compression and neurological damage which may be permanent. An epidural haematoma can act as a nidus for infection if a bacteraemia occurs.

**Root damage.**—Damage to the nerve roots in the epidural space can occur if the needle is deviated laterally, and will be associated with pain in the appropriate distribution. Occasionally this produces an area of cutaneous paraesthesiae or numbness, which gradually recovers.

Root damage within the subarachnoid space, however, is more serious and may cause neurolysis with permanent neurological damage.

Theoretically a lumbar puncture could damage an unusually long cord, particularly in a child.

### Infection

**Meningitis** is completely preventable if a rigidly aseptic technique is used. A meningitic reaction may follow dural puncture, or injection of irritant solutions into the cerebrospinal fluid. Aseptic meningo-encephalitis has been reported as a coincidental sequel to epidural block in obstetrics.[126] Fever, backache and neckache are the features, and laminectomy is not indicated.

**Epidural abscess** again should not occur as a result of infection introduced from without. However, metastatic blood-borne infection may occur, particularly in an epidural haematoma, originating from some other focal source.[15] Localising signs are a feature and laminectomy is urgently required to evacuate the abscess and avoid permanent neurological sequelae from cord compression.

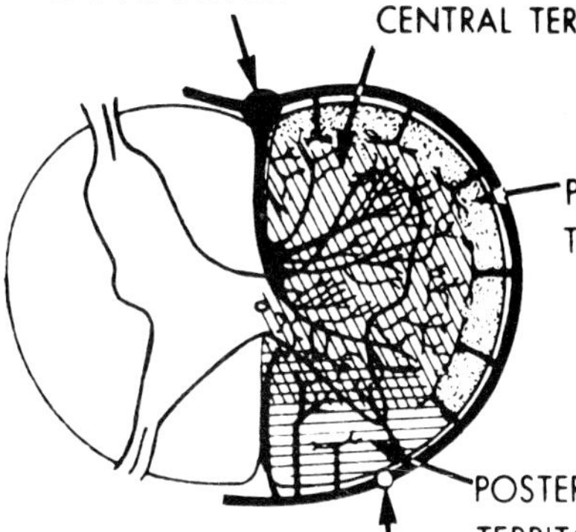

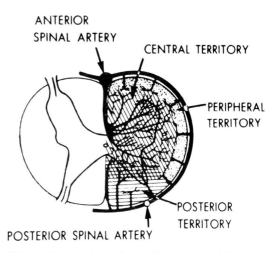

32/FIG. 13.—Blood supply of the spinal cord in cross-section showing the areas of distribution of anterior and posterior spinal arteries. (Courtesy of Little, Brown and Company, publishers of *International Anesthesiology Clinics*. From a paper by the late J. Usubiaga.[15])

### Ischaemic Damage

The blood supply of the spinal cord is always precarious (see page 860). It is jeopardised by any space-occupying lesion in the vertebral canal, such as epidural haematoma or abscess, or a neoplasm, any of which can cause compression of the functional end arteries, as well as compression of the cord itself, or of the roots. A prolonged period of hypotension, particularly when there is pre-existing arterial disease involving the aorta or radicular arteries, may cause functional ischaemia, or even obliteration of the anterior spinal artery, which supplies a large part of the cord (see Fig. 13). The *anterior spinal artery syndrome* is a predominantly motor disturbance, with sometimes loss of sphincter control and also occasionally of sensation. Hypotension from any cause may predispose to cord ischaemia but the factor which makes ischaemia a particular hazard of spinal or epidural blockade is the inclusion of adrenaline in the local anaesthetic solution.[127,128] Adrenaline produces localised vasoconstriction which, if coupled with systemic hypotension, is dangerous, particularly in eclamptic or arteriosclerotic subjects injected intrathecally or even epidurally.[129]

Other factors which may predispose to cord ischaemia are pressure from surgery on structures in the posterior abdominal wall, and possibly also an increase in venous pressure resulting from positive-pressure ventilation.

Profound hypotension from high or total spinal or epidural block, as from any cause, may also of course impair the cerebral circulation and cause brain damage, again particularly in patients with cerebral atherosclerosis.

### Chemical Irritation

A number of substances have been associated with definite nerve damage or irritation when injected into the epidural or subarachnoid space, namely detergents and antiseptics, alcohol, phenol, penicillin, preservatives, hypertonic saline, ammonium sulphate, potassium salts, propylene glycol, collodion and heavy metals.[15] Pain is commonly experienced on injection of an irritant substance and should lead the operator to abandon the administration at once, and check the nature of the solution injected. Moreover, if analgesia does *not* follow, this suggests that a local anaesthetic has *not* been injected.

Local anaesthetics generally cause reversible impairment of nerve function without histological damage, but abnormally large amounts in contact with nerves for a long time occasionally cause prolonged neurological sequelae. Thus the light spinal technique has been largely abandoned because it is believed that large volumes of solution, in displacing cerebrospinal fluid which is the normal environment for nerve roots, may be harmful. Permanent neurological sequelae have been reported in cases in which a large dose of local anaesthetic, destined for the epidural space, has accidentally been injected intrathecally.[130] In this case, profound hypotension may of course contribute to resultant neurological damage, though pH changes and electrolyte and osmotic disturbances may also be involved (see Chapter 31).

### Neurological Sequelae of Spinal and Epidural Block

Permanent neurological damage from correctly conducted spinal and epidural blocks in fit patients are vanishingly rare. It is impossible to quote an actual incidence, since the frequency of the problem will depend upon the skill and care of the operators. Thus large series are reported in which no permanent problems arise,[131] and in other cases there are crops of catastrophes all of which may be said to be avoidable.

Aetiologies of neurological damage are numerous. Horner's syndrome[144] presumably arises because of selective high block of sympathetic fibres. Sixth-nerve palsy may be caused by CSF leak; cord or root compression may result from epidural haematoma in the anticoagulated patient, or from epidural abscess. Direct needle trauma may cause root damage, temporary if epidural, permanent if intrathecal. Cord ischaemia may arise, most commonly in arteriosclerotic patients, following hypotension, particularly if adrenaline-containing solutions are used. Adhesive arachnoiditis may follow injection of contaminated local anaesthetic solutions, mistaken injection of irritant solutions, or accidental intrathecal injections of full epidural doses of local anaesthetics. Infection, possibly viral, has also been suggested.

The result may be transient or permanent palsy, paraplegia or cauda equina syndrome. The latter is characterised by retention or incontinence of urine and faeces, loss of perineal sensation and loss of sexual function.

Many causes of neurological deficit following spinals and epidurals are, however, purely fortuitous. Obstetric palsies may be attributed wrongly to epidural blockade. Thus the lithotomy position and stirrup pressure may produce perineal-nerve palsies, while the lateral cutaneous nerve of the thigh may be compressed as it emerges from the inguinal ligament. Pressure from the baby's head or rotation forceps may damage the lumbosacral trunk as it crosses the pelvic brim, and finally Keilland's rotation forceps may also be associated with postpartum bladder disturbance.[113]

Paraplegia following epidural analgesia has been reported in a number of patients in whom various anatomical abnormalities were believed to be the principal cause. For example, one patient had developmental laminar stenosis,[132] and two others, in whom haematomata apparently caused transient neurological damage, were found to have narrow spinal canals.[133,145] A fourth had an extradural spinal tumour.[134] Other cases of neurological damage following general anaesthesia[146] and aortic surgery[147] might well have been wrongly attributed to spinal or epidural blocks if they had been given. Thus, unless each case is carefully investigated, regional block may take the rap where actually it is only an unassociated or at worst a precipitating factor.

Aside from such chance and unconnected catastrophes, it is appropriate to approach epidural and possibly even spinal anaesthesia with the view that, by exercising due skill and care, and by correct selection of patients, permanent neurological damage can be avoided.

## REFERENCES

1. Sicard, A. (1901). Les injections médicamenteuses extradural par voie sacrococcygienne. *C. R. Soc. Biol. (Paris)*, **53**, 396.
2. Cathelin, F. (1901). Une nouvelle voie d'injection rachidienne. Méthode des injections épidurales par le procédé du canal sacré. Applications á l'homme. *C. R. Soc. Biol. (Paris)*, **53**, 452.
3. Zweifel, E. (1920). Die Todesfälle bei Sakrolanästhesie. *Zbl Gynäk.*, **44**, 140.
4. Poges, F. (1921). Anaesthesia metamerica. *Rev. Sanid. milit. argent.*, **11**, 351.
5. Dogliotti, A. M. (1931). Eine neue Methode der regionares Anästhesia: "Die peridurale segmentäre Anästhesia". *Zbl. Chir.*, **58**, 3141.

6. Dogliotti, A. M. (1932). Un nuovo metodo di anestesia tronculare: la rachianestesia peridurale segmentaria. *Arch. ital. Chir.*, **38**, 797.
7. Dogliotti, A. M. (1933). A new method of block anesthesia; segmental peridural spinal anesthesia. *Amer. J. Surg.*, **20**, 107.
8. Hess, E. (1934). Epidural anesthesia in urology. *J. Urol. (Baltimore)*, **31**, 621.
9. Odom, C. B. (1936). Epidural anesthesia. *Amer. J. Surg.*, **34**, 547.
10. Harger, J. R., Christofferson, E. A. and Stokes, A. J. (1941). Peridural anesthesia: a consideration of 1,000 cases. *Amer. J. Surg.*, **42**, 25.
11. Gutierrez, A. (1939). *Anestesia extradural*. Buenos Aires.
12. Tuohy, E. B. (1945). Continuous spinal anesthesia: a new method utilising a urethral catheter. *Surg. Clin. N. Amer.*, **25**, 834.
13. Curbello, M. M. (1949). Continuous peridural segmental anesthesia by means of a urethral catheter. *Curr. Res. Anesth.*, **28**, 12.
14. Doughty, A. (1980). The "impossible" epidural. In: *Epidural Analgesia in Obstetrics: a Second Symposium*. London: Lloyd-Luke (Medical Books).
15. Usubiaga, J. E. (1975). Neurological complications following epidural anesthesia. *Internat. Anesthesiol. Clinics*, **13**, 1.
16. Husemeyer, R. P. and White, D. C. (1980). Topography of the lumbar epidural space: a study in cadavers using injected polyester resin. *Anaesthesia*, **35**, 7.
17. O'Connell, J. E. (1970). Cerebrospinal fluid mechanics. *Proc. roy. Soc. Med.*, **63**, 507.
18. Shah, J. L. (1981). Influence of cerebrospinal fluid on epidural pressure. *Anaesthesia*, **36**, 627.
19. Levin, E., Muravchick, S. and Gold, M. (1981). Density of normal human cerebrospinal fluid and tetracaine solutions. *Anesth. Analg.*, **60**, 814.
20. Cusick, J. F., Myklebust, J. B. and Abram, S. E. (1980). Differential neural effects of epidural anesthetics. *Anesthesiology*, **53**, 299.
21. Reynolds, F. (1980). Optimum concentration and dosage: theoretical considerations. In: *Epidural Analgesia in Obstetrics: A Second Symposium*, p. 109. Ed. A. Doughty. London: Lloyd-Luke (Medical Books).
22. Modig, J., Malmber, G. P. and Karlström, G. (1981). Effect of epidural versus general anaesthesia on calf blood flow. *Acta anaesth. scand.*, **24**, 305.
23. Aitkenhead, A. R., Gilmour, D. G., Hothersall, A. P. and Ledingham, I. McA (1980). Effects of subarachnoid spinal nerve block and arterial $PCO_2$ on colon blood flow in the dog. *Brit. J. Anaesth.*, **52**, 1071.
24. Davis, F. M., Quince, M. and Laurenson, V. G. (1980). Deep vein thrombosis and anaesthetic technique in emergency hip surgery. *Brit. med. J.*, **2**, 1528.
25. Thorburn, J., Louden, J. R. and Vallance, R. (1980). Spinal and general anaesthesia in total hip replacement: frequency of deep vein thrombosis. *Brit. J. Anaesth.* **52**, 1117.
26. Sivarajan, M., Amory, D. W. and Lindbloom, L. E. (1976). Systemic and regional blood flow during epidural anesthesia without epinephrine in the rhesus monkey. *Anesthesiology*, **45**, 300.
27. Howat, D. D. C. (1977). Anaesthesia for biliary and pancreatic surgery. *Proc. roy. Soc. Med.*, **70**, 152.
28. Chin, S. P., Abou-Madi, M. N., Eurin, B., Witvoët, J. and Montagne, J. (1982). Blood loss in total hip replacement: extradural v phenoperidine analgesia. *Brit. J. Anaesth.*, **54**, 491.
29. Hollmen, A. I., Jouppila, R., Jouppila, P., Koivula, A. and Vierola, H. (1982). Effect of extradural analgesia using bupivacaine and 2-chloroprocaine on intervillous blood flow during normal labour. *Brit. J. Anaesth.*, **54**, 837.
30. Huovinen, K., Lehtovirta, P., Forss, M., Kivalo, I. and Teramo, K. (1979). Changes in placental intervillous blood flow measured by the $^{133}$Xenon method during lumbar epidural block for elective Caesarean section. *Acta anaesth. scand.*, **23**, 529.
31. Takasaki, M. and Takahash, T. (1980). Respiratory function during cervical and thoracic extradural analgesia in patients with normal lungs. *Brit. J. Anaesth.*, **52**, 1271.
32. Hole, A., Terjesen, T. and Breivik, H. (1980). Epidural versus general anaesthesia for total hip arthroplasty in elderly patients. *Acta anaesth. scand.*, **24**, 279.
33. McKenzie, P. J., Wishart, H. Y., Dewar, K. M. S., Gray, I. and Smith, G. (1980). Comparison of the effects of spinal anaesthesia and general anaesthesia on postoperative oxygenation and perioperative mortality. *Brit. J. Anaesth.*, **52**, 49.
34. Thalme, B., Belfrage, P. and Raabe, N. (1974). Lumbar epidural analgesia in labour. I. Acid-base balance and clinical condition of mother, fetus and newborn child. *Acta obstet. gynec. scand.*, **53**, 27.
35. Pearson, J. F. and Davies, P. (1974). The effect of continuous lumbar epidural analgesia upon fetal acid-base status during the second stage of labour. *J. Obstet. Gynaec. Brit. Cwlth.*, **81**, 975.
36. Brandt, M. R., Kehlet, H., Skovsted, L. and Hansen, J. M. (1976). Rapid decrease in plasma triiodothyronine during surgery and epidural analgesia independent of afferent neurogenic stimuli and of cortisol. *Lancet*, **2**, 1333.
37. Romano, E. and Gullo, A. (1980). Hypoglycaemic coma following epidural analgesia. *Anaesthesia*, **35**, 1084.
38. Rem, J., Møller, I. W., Brandt, M. R. and Kehlet, H. (1981). Influence of epidural analgesia on postoperative changes in various serum enzyme patterns and serum bilirubin. *Acta anaesth. scand.*, **25**, 142.
39. Namba, Y., Smith, J. B., Fox, G. S. and Challis, J. R. G. (1980). Plasma cortisol concentrations during Caesarean section. *Brit. J. Anaesth.*, **52**, 1027.
40. Traynor, C., Paterson, J. L., Ward, I. D., Morgan, M. and Hall, G. M. (1982). Effects of extradural analgesia and vagal blockade on the metabolic and endocrine response to upper abdominal surgery. *Brit. J. Anaesth.*, **54**, 319.
41. Pflug, A. E. and Halter, J. B. (1981). Effect of spinal anesthesia on adrenergic tone and the neuroendocrine responses to surgical stress in humans. *Anesthesiology*, **55**, 120.
42. Brandt, M. R., Ølgaard, K. and Kehlet, H. (1979). Epidural analgesia inhibits the renin and aldosterone response to surgery. *Acta anaesth. scand.*, **23**, 267.
43. Brandt, M. R., Fernandes, A., Mordhorst, R. and Kehlet, H. (1978). Epidural analgesia improves postoperative nitrogen balance. *Brit. med. J.*, **1**, 1106.
44. Bonnet, F., Harari, A., Thibonnier, M. and Viars, D. (1982). Suppression of antidiuretic hormone hypersecretion during surgery by extradural anaesthesia. *Brit. J. Anaesth.*, **54**, 29.

45. Scott, D. B. (1975). Management of extradural block during surgery. *Brit. J. Anaesth.*, **47**, 271.
46. Slattery, P. J., Rosen, M. and Rees, G. A. D. (1980). An aid to identification of the subarachnoid space with a twenty-five gauge needle (letter). *Anaesthesia*, **35**, 391.
47. Brown, D. T., Wildsmith, J. A., Covino, B. G. and Scott, D. B. (1980). Effect of baricity on spinal anaesthesia with amethocaine. *Brit. J. Anaesth.*, **52**, 589.
48. Chambers, W. A., Edstrom, H. H. and Scott, D. B. (1981). Effect of baricity on spinal anaesthesia with bupivacaine. *Brit. J. Anaesth.*, **53**, 279.
49. Wildsmith, J. A. W., McClure, J. H., Brown, D. T. and Scott, D. B. (1981). Effects of posture on the spread of isobaric and hyperbaric amethocaine. *Brit. J. Anaesth.*, **53**, 273.
50. Cameron, A. E., Arnold, R. W., Ghoris, M. W. and Jamieson, V. (1981). Spinal analgesia using bupivacaine 0·5% plain. Variation in the extent of the block with patient age. *Anaesthesia*, **36**, 318.
51. Tuominen, M., Kalso, E. and Rosenberg, P. H. (1982). Effects of posture on the spread of spinal anaesthesia with isobaric 0·75% or 0·5% bupivacaine. *Brit. J. Anaesth.*, **54**, 313.
52. Chambers, W. A., Littlewood, D. G., Edstrom, H. H. and Scott, D. B. (1982). Spinal anaesthesia with hyperbaric bupivacaine: effects of concentration and volume administered. *Brit. J. Anaesth.*, **54**, 75.
53. Nightingale, P. J. and Marstrand, T. (1981). Subarachnoid anaesthesia with bupivacaine for orthopaedic procedures in the elderly. *Brit. J. Anaesth.*, **53**, 369.
54. Moore, D. C. (1980). Spinal anesthesia: bupivacaine compared with tetracaine. *Anesth. Analg.*, **59**, 743.
55. Chambers, W. A., Littlewood, D. G. and Scott, D. B. (1982). Spinal anesthesia with hyperbaric bupivacaine: effect of added vasoconstrictors. *Anesth. Analg.*, **61**, 49.
56. Levin, E., Muravchick, S. and Gold, M. I. (1981). Isobaric tetracaine spinal anesthesia and the lithotomy position. *Anesth. Analg.*, **60**, 810.
57. Sundnes, K. O., Vaagenes, P., Skretting, P., Lind, B. and Edstrom, H. H. (1982). Spinal analgesia with hyperbaric bupivacaine: effects of volume and solution. *Brit. J. Anaesth.*, **54**, 69.
58. Laman, E. N. and McLeskey, C. H. (1978). Supraclavicular subcutaneous emphysema following lumbar epidural anesthesia. *Anesthesiology*, **48**, 219.
59. Gutierrez, A. (1933). Valor de la aspiracion liquida in el espacio peridural en la anestesia peridural. *Rev. Cirug. (B. Aires)*, **12**, 225.
60. Dawkins, C. J. M. (1969). An analysis of the complications of extradural and caudal block. *Anaesthesia*, **24**, 554.
61. Dawkins, C. J. M. (1963). The identification of the epidural space. A critical analysis of the various methods employed. *Anaesthesia*, **18**, 66.
62. Aitkenhead, A. R., Hothersall, A. P., Gilmour, D. G. and Ledingham, I. McA. (1979). Dural dimpling in the dog. *Anaesthesia*, **34**, 14.
63. Husemeyer, R. P. and White, D. C. (1980). Lumbar extradural injection pressures in pregnant women, an investigation of relationships between rate of injection, injection pressures and extent of analgesia. *Brit. J. Anaesth.*, **52**, 55.
64. Messih, M. N. A. (1981). Epidural space pressures during pregnancy. *Anaesthesia*, **36**, 775.
65. Dawkins, C. J. M. and Steel, G. C. (1971). Thoracic extradural (epidural) block for upper abdominal surgery. *Anaesthesia*, **26**, 41.
66. Brooks, W. (1957). An epidural indicator. *Anaesthesia*, **12**, 227.
67. Nash, T. G. and Openshaw, D. J. (1968). Unusual complication of epidural anaesthesia (C). *Brit. med. J.*, **2**, 700.
68. Bridenbaugh, L. D., Moore, D. C., Bagdi, P. and Bridenbaugh, P. O. (1968). The position of plastic tubing in continuous-block techniques. An X-ray study of 552 patients. *Anesthesiology*, **29**, 1047.
69. Ravindran, R. S., Bond, V. K., Tasch, M. D., Gupta, C. D. and Luerssen, T. G. (1980). Prolonged neural blockade following regional analgesia with 2-chloroprocaine. *Anesth. Analg.*, **59**, 447.
70. Reisner, L. S., Hochman, B. N. and Plumer, M. H. (1980). Persistent neurologic deficit and adhesive arachnoiditis following intrathecal 2-chloroprocaine injection. *Anesth. Analg.*, **59**, 452.
71. Moore, D. C., Spierdijk, J., Van Kleef, J. D., Coleman, R. L. and Love, G. F. (1982). Chloroprocaine neurotoxicity: four additional cases. *Anesth. Analg.*, **61**, 155.
72. Moore, D. C. and Batra, M. S. (1981). The components of an effective test dose prior to epidural block. *Anesthesiology*, **55**, 693.
73. Scott, D. B. (1978). Test doses in extradural analgesia (letter). *Brit. J. Anaesth.*, **50**, 307.
74. Soni, V., Peeters, C. and Covino, B. (1981). Value and limitations of test dose prior to epidural anesthesia. *Regional Anesthesia.*, **6**, 23.
75. Galloon, S. (1978). Test doses in extradural analgesia (letter). *Brit. J. Anaesth.*, **50**, 304.
76. Reynolds, F. and Taylor, G. (1970). Maternal and neonatal blood concentrations of bupivacaine. A comparison with lignocaine during continuous extradural analgesia. *Anaesthesia*, **25**, 14.
77. Seow, L. T., Lips, F. J., Cousins, M. J. and Mather, L. E. (1982). Lidocaine and bupivacaine mixtures for epidural blockade. *Anesthesiology*, **56**, 177.
78. deJong, R. H. and Bonin, J. D. (1981). Mixtures of local anesthetics are no more toxic than the parent drugs. *Anesthesiology*, **54**, 177.
79. Stainthorp, S. F., Bradshaw, E. G., Challen, P. D. and Tobias, M. A. (1978). 0·125% bupivacaine for obstetric analgesia? *Anaesthesia*, **33**, 3.
80. Gjessing, J. and Tomlin, P. (1979). Patterns of postoperative pain. A study of the use of continuous epidural analgesia in the postoperative period. *Anaesthesia*, **34**, 624.
81. Evans, K. R. L. and Carrie, L. E. S. (1979). Continuous epidural infusion of bupivacaine in labour: a simple method. *Anaesthesia*, **34**, 310.
82. Ross, R. A., Clarke, J. E. and Armitage, E. N. (1980). Postoperative pain prevention by continuous epidural infusion. A study of the clinical effects and plasma concentrations obtained. *Anaesthesia*, **35**, 663.
83. Giasi, R. M., D'Agostino, E. and Covino, B. G. (1979). Absorption of lidocaine following subarachnoid and epidural administration. *Anesth. Analg.*, **58**, 360.
84. Grundy, E. M. and Nageswara, L. (1978). Epidural anesthesia and the lateral position. *Anesth. Analg.*, **57**, 95.
85. Hodgkinson, R. and Husain, F. J. (1981). Obesity, gravity and spread of epidural anesthesia. *Anesth. Analg.*, **60**, 421.

86. Rolbin, S. H., Cole, A. F. D., Hew, E. M. and Virgint, S. (1981). Effect of lateral position and volume on the spread of epidural anaesthesia in the parturient. *Canad. Anaesth. Soc. J.*, **28**, 431.
87. Bromage, P. R. (1969). Ageing and epidural dose requirements. *Brit. J. Anaesth.*, **41**, 1016.
88. Park, W. Y., Massengale, M., Kim, S. I., Poon, K. C. and MacNamara, T. E. (1980). Age and the spread of local anesthetic solutions in the epidural space. *Anesth. Analg.*, **59**, 768.
89. Bromage, P. R. (1962). Exaggerated spread of epidural analgesia in arteriosclerotic patients. Dosage in relation to biological and chronological ageing. *Brit. med. J.*, **2**, 1634.
90. Sharrock, N. E. (1977). Lack of exaggerated spread of epidural anesthesia in patients with arteriosclerosis. *Anesthesiology*, **47**, 307.
91. Grundy, E. M., Zamora, A. M. and Winnie, A. P. (1978). Comparison of spread of epidural anesthesia in pregnant and non-pregnant women. *Anesth. Analg.*, **51**, 544.
92. Hodgkinson, R. and Husain, F. (1980). Obesity and the cephalad spread of analgesia following epidural administration of bupivacaine for Cesarean section. *Anesth. Analg.*, **59**, 89.
93. de Campo, T., Macias-Loza, M., Cohen, H. and Galindo, A. (1980). Lumbar epidural anaesthesia and sensory profiles in term pregnant patients. *Canad. Anaesth. Soc. J.*, **27**, 272.
94. Bray, M. C. and Carrie, L. E. S. (1978). Unblocked segments in obstetric epidural blocks. The influence of previous regional block on obstetric patients receiving lumbar epidural analgesia during labour. *Anaesthesia*, **33**, 232.
95. Bromage, P. R. (1967). Extradural analgesia for pain relief. *Brit. J. Anaesth.*, **39**, 721.
96. Evans, W. (1936). Intrasacral epidural injection in the treatment of sciatica. *Lancet*, **2**, 1225.
97. Kelman, H. (1944). Epidural injection therapy for sciatic pain. *Amer. J. Surg.*, **64**, 183.
98. Cyriax, J. H. (1957). *Textbook of Orthopaedic Medicine*, 3rd edit. London: Cassell & Co.
99. Coomes, E. N. (1961). A comparison between epidural anaesthesia and bed rest in sciatica. *Brit. med. J.*, **1**, 20.
100. Galley, A. H. (1949). Continuous caudal analgesia in obstetrics. *Anaesthesia*, **4**, 154.
101. Lunn, J. N. (1979). Postoperative analgesia after circumcision. *Anaesthesia*, **34**, 552.
102. Abouleish, E., Orig, T. and Amortegui, A. J. (1980). Bacteriological comparison between epidural and caudal techniques. *Anesthesiology*, **53**, 511.
103. Abouleish, E. (1977). *Pain Control in Obstetrics*. Philadelphia: J. B. Lippincott Co.
104. Berkowitz, S. and Gold, M. (1980). Spinal anesthesia for surgery in patients with previous lumbar laminectomy. *Anesth. Analg.*, **59**, 881.
105. Datta, S. D., Corke, B. C., Alper, M. H., Brown, W. U., Ostheimer, G. W. and Weiss, J. B. (1980). Epidural anesthesia for Cesarean section: a comparison of bupivacaine, chloroprocaine and etidocaine. *Anesthesiology*, **52**, 48.
106. Crawford, J. W. (1980). Experiences with lumbar extradural analgesia for Caesarean section. *Brit. J. Anaesth.*, **52**, 821.
107. Mathru, M., Rao, T. L. K., Kartha, R. K., Shanmugham, M. and Jacobs, H. K. (1980). Intravenous albumin administration for prevention of spinal hypotension during Cesarean section. *Anesth. Analg.*, **59**, 655.
108. Hallworth, D., Jellicoe, J. A. and Wilkes, R. G. (1982). Hypotension during epidural anaesthesia for Caesarean section. A comparison of intravenous loading with crystalloid and colloid solutions. *Anaesthesia*, **37**, 53.
109. Doughty, A. (1978). Epidural analgesia in labour: the past, the present and the future. *J. roy. Soc. Med.*, **71**, 879.
110. Doughty, A. (1979). Inadvertent dural puncture—an avoidable accident. *Anaesthesia*, **34**, 116.
111. Ravindran, R. S., Viegas, O. J., Tasch, M. D., Cline, P. J., Deaton, R. L. and Brown, T. R. (1981). Bearing down at the time of delivery and the incidence of spinal headache in parturients. *Anesth. Analg.*, **60**, 524.
112. Dripps, R. D. and Vandam, L. D. (1951). Hazards of lumbar puncture. *J. Amer. med. Ass.*, **147**, 1118.
113. Grove, L. H. (1973). Backache, headache and bladder dysfunction after delivery. *Brit. J. Anaesth.*, **45**, 1147.
114. Marx, G. F. (1981). Maternal complications of regional analgesia. *Regional Anesthesia*, **6**, 104.
115. Carbaat, P. A. T. and Van Crevel, H. (1981). Lumbar puncture headache: controlled study on the preventive effect of 24 hours' bed rest. *Lancet*, **2**, 1133.
116. Bart, A. J. and Scott Wheeler, A. (1978). Comparison of epidural saline placement and epidural blood placement in the treatment of post-lumbar-puncture headache. *Anesthesiology*, **48**, 221.
117. Ostheimer, G. W., Palahniuk, R. J. and Shnider, S. M. (1974). Epidural blood patch for post-lumbar puncture headache. *Anesthesiology*, **41**, 307.
118. Crawford, J. S. (1980). Experiences with epidural blood patch. *Anaesthesia*, **35**, 513.
119. Reynolds, A. F., Hameroff, S. R., Blitt, C. D. and Roberts, W. L. (1980). Spinal subdural epiarachnoid hematoma: a complication of a novel epidural blood patch technique. *Anesth. Analg.*, **59**, 702.
120. Eerola, M., Kaukinen, L. and Kaukinen, S. (1981). Fatal brain lesion following spinal anesthesia. Report of a case. *Acta anaesth. scand.*, **25**, 115.
121. Edelman, J. D. and Wingard, D. W. (1980). Subdural hematomas after lumbar dural puncture. *Anesthesiology*, **52**, 166.
122. Newrick, P. and Read, D. (1982). Subdural haematoma as a complication of spinal anaesthetic. *Brit. med. J.*, **285**, 341.
123. Jawalekar, S. R. and Marx, G. F. (1981). Cutaneous cerebrospinal fluid leakage following attempted extradural block. *Anesthesiology*, **54**, 348.
124. Hodgkinson, R. (1981). Total spinal block after epidural injection into an interspace adjacent to an inadvertent dural perforation. *Anesthesiology*, **55**, 593.
125. Verniquet, A. J. W. (1980). Vessel puncture with epidural catheters. Experience in obstetric patients. *Anaesthesia*, **35**, 660.
126. Neumark, J., Feichtinger, W. and Gassner, A. (1980). Epidural block in obstetrics followed by aseptic meningoencephalitis. *Anesthesiology*, **52**, 518.
127. Urquhart-Hay (1969). Paraplegia following epidural analgesia. *Anaesthesia*, **24**, 461.
128. Harrison, P. D. (1975). Paraplegia following epidural analgesia. *Anaesthesia*, **30**, 778.
129. Bromage, P. R. (1978). *Epidural Analgesia*. Philadelphia: W. B. Saunders Co.

130. Kane, R. E. (1981). Neurologic deficits following epidural or spinal anesthesia. *Anesth. Analg.*, **60**, 150.
131. Gordh, T. (1969). In: *Illustrated Handbook on Local Anaesthesia*. Ed. Eriksson, E. Copenhagen: Munksgaard.
132. Chaudhari, L. S., Kop, B. P. and Dhruva, A. J. (1978). Paraplegia and epidural analgesia. *Anaesthesia*, **33**, 722.
133. Ballin, N. C. (1981). Paraplegia following epidural analgesia. *Anaesthesia*, **36**, 952.
134. Hirlekar, G. (1980). Paraplegia after epidural analgesia associated with an extradural spinal tumour. *Anaesthesia*, **35**, 363.
135. Messahel, F. M., Robinson, J. S. and Mathews, E. T. (1983). Factors affecting cerebrospinal fluid flow in two spinal needles. *Brit. J. Anaesth.*, **55**, 169.
136. Russell, I. F. (1983). Spinal anaesthesia for Caesarean section. The use of 0·5% bupivacaine. *Brit. J. Anaesth.*, **55**, 309.
137. Kalso, E., Tuominen, M. and Rosenberg, P. H. (1982). Effect of posture and some CSF characteristics on spinal anaesthesia with isobaric 0·5% bupivacaine. *Brit. J. Anaesth.*, **54**, 1179.
138. McClure, J. H., Brown, D. T. and Wildsmith, J. A. W. (1982). Effect of injected volume and speed of injection on the spread of spinal anaesthesia with isobaric amethocaine. *Brit. J. Anaesth.*, **54**, 917.
139. Macdonald, R. (1983). Dr. Doughty's technique for the location of the epidural space (letter). *Anaesthesia*, **38**, 71.
140. Naulty, J. S., Ostheimer, G. W., Datta, S., Knapp, R. and Weiss, J. B. (1982). Incidence of venous air embolism during epidural catheter insertion. *Anesthesiology*, **57**, 410.
141. Conacher, I. D., Paes, M. L., Jacobson, L., Phillips, P. D. and Heaviside, D. W. (1983). Epidural analgesia following thoracic surgery. A review of two years' experience. *Anaesthesia*, **38**, 546.
142. Merry, A. F., Cross, J. A., Mayadeo, S. V. and Wild, C. J. (1983). Posture and the spread of intradural analgesia in labour. *Brit. J. Anaesth.*, **55**, 303.
143. Odoom, J. A. and Sih, I. L. (1983). Epidural analgesia and anticoagulant therapy. Experience with one thousand cases of continuous epidurals. *Anaesthesia*, **38**, 254.
144. Clayton, K. C. (1983). The incidence of Horner's syndrome during lumbar extradural for elective Caesarean section and provision of analgesia during labour. *Anaesthesia*, **38**, 583.
145. Newman, B. (1983). Postnatal paraparesis following epidural analgesia and forceps delivery. *Anaesthesia*, **38**, 350.
146. Schreiner, E. J., Lipson, S. F., Bromage, P. R. and Camporesi, E. M. (1983). Neurological complications following general anaesthesia. Three cases of major paralysis. *Anaesthesia*, **38**, 226.
147. Costello, T. G. and Fisher, A. (1983). Neurological complications following aortic surgery. Case reports and review of the literature. *Anaesthesia*, **38**, 230.

CHAPTER 33

# Pain Clinic and Operative Nerve Blocks



The present chapter is concerned with the practical management of pain by the anaesthetist and particularly with the symptomatic relief of chronic intractable pain. The last may be due to incurable malignant disease or to some condition such as post-herpetic neuralgia which does not immediately threaten the patient's life.

The various methods of relieving pain will be discussed with particular emphasis on nerve blocking procedures both in the context of pain clinic work and in operative and postoperative pain management.

## PRE-OPERATIVE PAIN

A patient suffering from some painful condition and awaiting surgery should receive the appropriate treatment, whether this necessitates morphine, some less potent analgesic, or merely sedation, rest and reassurance. In the immediate pre-operative period premedication affords the necessary pain relief and sedation, especially if morphine is used. Pain in the acute surgical emergency presents a more difficult problem. Analgesics should be withheld until a diagnosis has been reached and the course of action determined. Pain then having served its warning purpose, it is justifiable to relieve it with an opiate, given intravenously if necessary. Caution must be adopted in the elderly, toxic or shocked patient as a full therapeutic dose of morphine may cause collapse.

Patients in pain from acute trauma need and derive great benefit from morphine. A poor peripheral circulation from vasoconstriction may severely limit the absorption of drugs given by subcutaneous or intra-muscular injection. The optimal dose of morphine can be given much more safely and rapidly by incremental intravenous injections until the desired effect is achieved. A period of 10 minutes should elapse between each injection so that the full effect of each dose can be assessed. Patients in severe pain often need larger doses of narcotics than usual and the pain seems to antagonise the depressant effects of these drugs, although great care must be taken in elderly and severely shocked patients because of the possibility of circulatory and respiratory depression.

## POSTOPERATIVE PAIN

The incidence of postoperative pain varies with the individual patient, but is largely governed by the site and nature of the operation. Upper abdominal and intrathoracic operations cause most pain and distress and are associated with an increased incidence of pulmonary complications. Postoperative hypoxaemia, which is also directly related to pain[1] can persist up to five days and is more pronounced after upper abdominal surgery.[2] In a study on the incidence of postoperative pain after general surgical procedures, Parkhouse and his co-workers[3] found that during the first 48 hours postoperatively, the greatest number of analgesic injections was required by patients after gastric surgery. Much less pain occurs after operations on the head and neck, the extremities, and on the superficial tissues.

Pain may arise from the skin, tendons, bones, muscles or viscera, but from the functional viewpoint may be divided into the dull, aching pain which persists at rest and the severe, sharp pain produced by movement or coughing. The former pain is readily relieved by morphine but the sharp, severe pain which is caused by the contraction of recently incised or injured muscle is much more difficult to relieve. Fear and anxiety may aggravate postoperative suffering by causing rigid muscle contractions in an attempt to splint the operative site. This leads to a self-perpetuating cycle of increased pain, fear, and muscle spasm.

### Analgesics

The powerful effect of the placebo response must always be borne in mind when prescribing drugs for the relief of postoperative pain. Morphine sulphate in a dose of 10 mg has long been established as the standard drug for this purpose, despite its unpleasant side-effects, especially nausea and vomiting. The powerful narcotic analgesics are normally only required for the first 48 hours after surgery when the pain is most severe. Papaveretum is preferred by many clinicians because of a belief in its superiority as regards the incidence of side-effects. A dose of 20 mg is equivalent to 13·3 mg of morphine sulphate. In the immediate postoperative period, while the patient is still under the close supervision of the anaesthetist in the recovery room, it is often advantageous to give small incremental doses of these drugs intravenously until the desired degree of analgesia has been achieved. Anaesthetic techniques which include the use of intravenous analgesic drugs will postpone the need for postoperative analgesics and will reduce the total quantity required. The technique of neuroleptanaesthesia is often followed by a long period of postoperative analgesia and sedation. For patients who are intolerant of morphine, pethidine is probably the most widely used alternative drug, and indeed is used as the routine postoperative analgesic by many anaesthetists. The dose of pethidine is 100 mg and as its duration of action is shorter than that of morphine it may have to be given more frequently. Promethazine in a dose of 25–50 mg is frequently combined with pethidine both pre- and postoperatively. It affords increased sedation and reduces the incidence of nausea and vomiting. Promethazine is one of the drugs which have been described as having an antanalgesic effect—see below.[4] However, the increased sedation provided by the promethazine does appear to reduce the need for postoperative analgesics.

Increasing the dosage of analgesics enhances the severity of the side-effects but does not always produce more pain relief. The danger of addiction from the use of potent narcotic drugs in the relief of postoperative pain is small and is no reason for withholding their use. Nevertheless, non-addicting drugs should be substituted as soon as possible. If a series of painful operations is planned, the risk of dependence is increased, and for long-term pain therapy it may be useful to employ a drug such as pentazocine which has a low addictive potential.

The careful use of these pain-relieving drugs in the postoperative period will enable the patient to cough more effectively and to move more freely around the bed. Physiotherapy and breathing exercises should be timed to take place when the analgesia is at its maximum. Such a regime provides a safeguard against respiratory complications and thrombosis. The need of each patient for these drugs must be based on an assessment of his physical and mental state and the nature of the operation. Postoperative sedation must not be routine for all surgical patients as there is a considerable variation in prescribed therapeutic requirements.

Morphine and allied drugs, although relieving postoperative pain while the patient is lying quietly in bed, are unfortunately not as effective when the patient is coughing vigorously.[5] The use of larger or more frequent doses of these drugs in an attempt to improve the analgesia can lead to a highly dangerous situation. Respiratory and circulatory depression together with immobility, increased drowsiness and lack of co-operation may contribute materially to postoperative morbidity. In these circumstances such drugs, instead of preventing, may contribute to the development of respiratory and thrombotic complications. Morphine antagonists have been used to prevent these dangers and have been discussed in the previous chapter. Other side-effects which may cause problems include nausea, vomiting and dysphoria, particularly if the dose is increased. It is often necessary to give an anti-emetic on a regular basis to combat nausea and vomiting.

Pentazocine (Fortral), which is a narcotic antagonist, is less effective and has a shorter duration of action than pethidine. Although there is little risk of it causing addiction or respiratory depression, it may be associated with nausea, vomiting, sedation and dizziness and is unlikely to replace morphine and pethidine for postoperative pain relief.

Buprenorphine (Temgesic) in a dose of 0·3–0·6 mg by injection is another potent analgesic having antagonistic properties. It has a wide safety margin with little risk of causing respiratory depression. In the unlikely event of this complication occurring, naloxone may be only partially effective and it may be necessary to use doxapram to stimulate respiration. Nausea, vomiting, dizziness and drowsiness are possible side-effects but its long duration of action makes it a useful drug when nursing cover is limited. It is also available as a sublingual tablet (0·2 mg). Two tablets dissolved under the tongue may give up to 8-hours analgesia.

Not all patients require potent analgesics to relieve their pain after major surgical operations. Milder analgesics such as dihydrocodeine, pentazocine, aspirin, paracetamol and Distalgesic* are extremely useful and may be given freely during the first few days. The long term use of Distalgesic may be associated with abuse potential. Even patients who require morphine initially after operation can usually revert to simple remedies after the first 48 hours. Aspirin, if it is tolerated, is also very useful in relieving the stiffness and discomfort in back and limbs due to the unaccustomed and awkward positions which patients are forced to assume.

Children do not require the same scale of post-operative analgesia as an adult, perhaps because they have less fear of pain. Aspirin is often sufficient for children post-operatively. For severe pain, children may be given morphine (0·1–0·2 mg/kg), pethidine (1–2 mg/kg) or papaveretum (0·2–0·3 mg/kg), or codeine phosphate (1 mg/kg).

### Antanalgesia

Antanalgesia is the term applied to the action which certain drugs appear to have of lowering the pain threshold. This effect was first described by Clutton-Brock[6] and is manifest even if an analgesic has been administered previously. Further observations were made by Dundee[7]

* Dextropropoxyphene hydrochloride 32·5 mg and paracetamol 325 mg.

who found that small doses of thiopentone produced a transient fall in the pain threshold of patients premedicated with 100 mg of pethidine. Antanalgesia is in fact experimental confirmation of the clinical observations that sedatives and hypnotics, like phenothiazines and barbiturates, do not relieve pain unless administered in a dose which is large enough to produce unconsciousness. Smaller doses tend to produce an exaggerated response to pain and are clearly ineffective in relieving postoperative pain.

The postoperative restlessness which occurs so frequently in children who have been premedicated with barbiturates is almost certainly due to persistence of this antanalgesic effect. It is seen typically after painful operations like tonsillectomy and emphasises the advantages of an opiate as premedication or as part of the anaesthetic technique. Moreover, thiopentone which has been used for induction of anaesthesia, may exert an antanalgesic effect in the postoperative period. Low blood levels of thiopentone may persist for long periods and contribute to post-operative pain and restlessness. This effect may necessitate the use of larger doses of analgesics than would otherwise be required.

### Local Anaesthetic Techniques

(*a*) **Intercostal block.** — Post-operative somatic pain in the chest or abdomen can be controlled effectively by blocking the intercostal nerves innervating the area of the incision and including one nerve above and below the appropriate dermatomes. Bilateral injections have to be performed for midline incisions but for subcostal incisions only one side has to be blocked. It is most effective for superficial pain, but it does not block pain fibres from the viscera or peritoneum, thus deep pain may persist but it does enable the patient to cough more effectively. The need for repeated multiple injections is the main disadvantage and it carries the risk of pneumothorax but, unlike extradural block, the fall in arterial blood pressure is minimal, as the block is distal to the sympathetic outflow. Bonica[8] provided analgesia by repeating the injections daily for two to four days. The effect lasted for six to ten hours and the patients were able to breathe deeply and cough more effectively. Bridenbaugh and colleagues[9] found the technique compared favourably to the opiates in the management of upper abdominal and thoracic cases. The cryoprobe has also been used to produce long-lasting pain relief by blocking the intercostal nerves at the end of a thoracotomy under direct vision or by the external approach.[10]

(*b*) **Paravertebral block.** — Postoperative analgesia can be produced in any region of the body, except the head, by means of paravertebral block. Unlike intercostal block, it has the advantage of blocking all pain fibres (including those from the viscera) except for those in the vagus. It carries the risk of more severe complications including intrathecal injection, pneumothorax and hypotension.

(*c*) **Epidural block.**—A number of reports have stressed the superiority of epidural anaesthesia over other techniques for relieving postoperative pain.[8,11,12] Intermittent injections are given through an indwelling catheter. The complete pain relief which results from this block permits more effective coughing, better ventilation and increased mobility. After upper abdominal surgery the vital capacity is reduced to 25–30 per cent of the normal figure and to about 50 per cent after lower abdominal operations. This reduction in vital capacity is probably due to reflex muscle spasm because it is not augmented when the pain is relieved with morphine.[11] After epidural blockade there is a significant increase in vital capacity, which returns on average to 85 per cent of the preoperative level. Spence and associates[13] also found an improvement in respiratory function with epidural blockade following upper abdominal surgery, but it is not as great as might be expected, as other factors apart from pain cause respiratory difficulty in the postoperative period[14,15]

For the adequate relief of pain in upper abdominal surgery the block should extend as high as the 4th–5th thoracic segments. To minimise the risk of postural hypotension from sympathetic blockade, the thoracic approach to the epidural space is recommended,[16] so that the tip of the catheter lies at the level of the thoracic roots to be blocked. This enables small volumes (4–6 ml) of local anaesthetic to be used, plain bupivacaine having replaced lignocaine as the agent of choice. Bromage[17] suggested that the incidence of unblocked segments can be reduced by using carbonated local anaesthetics. The epidural technique affords excellent analgesia but requires special skill and training, strict asepsis and careful observation of the patient. There is always the risk of a total spinal anaesthetic developing after a top-up injection, which could have grave consequences if it had been undertaken by a nurse and the complication was not immediately diagnosed and treated. It is unsuitable for routine use at the present time because of the lack of adequate resources in most hospitals, but is of great value in selected patients with respiratory disease.

### Intrathecal and Epidural Narcotics

The use of narcotic analgesics injected intrathecally or epidurally for postoperative pain relief is discussed later in this chapter (p. 926). It has the advantage that small doses of these drugs can be introduced near the receptors in the dorsal horns. However, the possibility of the delayed development of severe respiratory depression is a limiting factor in the general use of this interesting new technique. At the present time it should be restricted to patients who are being closely monitored in intensive care units.

### Inhalational Techniques

The inhalation of known concentrations of volatile anaesthetic agents or nitrous oxide may be used to relieve postoperative pain and also for procedures such as changing dressings.[5] Nitrous oxide/oxygen mixtures are of value when narcotic analgesics are contra-indicated or when the analgesia they afford is inadequate, and in patients who are already receiving oxygen therapy.[18] Because of the risk of leucopenia, nitrous oxide can only be administered for 24 hours.

Entonox, the premixed 50 per cent mixture of nitrous oxide and oxygen, is freely available in hospitals in the United Kingdom but if inhaled undiluted for prolonged periods it leads to somnolence, and if used in the immediate postoperative period it results in a continuation of the state of anaesthesia with immobility and lack of co-operation.

If Entonox is substituted for oxygen therapy in upper abdominal cases, it is possible to achieve some analgesia without cerebral depression because of the air-dilution that occurs if it is administered by an MC or Edinburgh type oxygen mask. These will provide 10–25 per cent nitrous oxide in 25–35 per cent oxygen depending on gas flow.[19,20] The technique of deep breaths may help to cover movement, wound-dressing or post-operative physiotherapy. The contamination of the atmosphere with possible deleterious effects on staff working in the vicinity will restrict the use of nitrous oxide for this purpose.

### Discussion

There is usually a progressive reduction in the intensity of postoperative pain and after 48 hours narcotics are no longer required. Pain is the dominant factor in the production of post-operative chest complications and the effective relief of pain after surgery is not merely aimed at making the patient more comfortable, but is of vital importance in reducing the incidence and morbidity of such sequelae.

Morphine, papaveretum and pethidine have all been widely used in the relief of postoperative pain. They have the possible disadvantage of causing nausea and vomiting as a side-effect. Other analgesics such as phenazocine, methadone, levorphanol have a lower incidence of side-effects, are longer lasting and orally effective but have not gained wide acceptance in clinical practice. Most patients at present do not receive adequate postoperative pain relief, often being given only 2–4 analgesic injections in the first 48 hours. It has a low priority in nursing procedures and tends to be delegated to junior medical and nursing staff who do not have time to administer and supervise closely an effective analgesic regime. Many patients are reluctant to ask for analgesic injections and nurses often fail to recognise that the patient is in severe pain. The current development of techniques to supply self-administered potent analgesics by injection using an "on demand" system with an in-built safety mechanism to prevent overdose, is an interesting attempt to overcome this problem.

## CHRONIC PAIN

Severe intractable pain often presents a most difficult therapeutic problem. Many of the methods which are available for the symptomatic relief of pain are outside the sphere of the anaesthetist and are mentioned here only for the sake of completeness. These measures would include physiotherapy, psychotherapy, hormone therapy for hormone-dependent tumours, chemotherapy (including regional perfusion techniques), radiotherapy, surgery including palliative removal of tumours, amputation of painful useless limbs, adrenalectomy and hypophysectomy for bone secondaries from carcinoma of the breast, cordotomy, leucotomy, rhizotomy, and thalamotomy.

## PAIN CLINICS

In recent years, anaesthetists have taken an active role in the establishment and management of clinics for the relief of chronic pain. Because persistent pain may be due to many causes, its alleviation involves the use of a variety of techniques such as radiotherapy, pharmacology, neurosurgery, psychology, nerve blocking and chemical or physical neurolysis. Such a clinic will, therefore, ideally require the expertise of a number of different specialists, and this multidisciplinary approach has evolved in the larger regional centres,[21,22] where the availability of sophisticated equipment enables all types of cases to be treated.

Many pain clinics do not conform to this pattern and are run on a more modest basis, usually by an anaesthetist, who, by informal discussion with colleagues in other disciplines, is able to ensure that an accurate diagnosis is reached in each patient, and the appropriate scheme of treatment instituted.

Patients attending a clinic are referred by a specialist, either from the same or another hospital, or by a general practitioner. Many anaesthetists running a pain clinic adopt the policy of a "closed" referral system and only accept patients who have been seen and assessed by another specialist in the same hospital. The role of the anaesthetist in this field in Great Britain has been discussed by Swerdlow and his colleagues.[23] They consider that diagnostic or therapeutic nerve blocking will be used in about half the patients attending a pain clinic. Many nerve blocks, including the use of neurolytic agents, can be carried out during the clinic, but the more complex procedures requiring the use of the image intensifier and full operating theatre facilities are time consuming and are perhaps better carried out at a separate session. Some patients are able to go home after an appropriate period of recovery, but in-patient facilities are required for certain techniques, especially the intrathecal injection of neurolytic agents, and for the more technically demanding procedures of percutaneous cordotomy and chemical pituitary ablation. The anaesthetist is at a disadvantage in not having hospital beds of his own, but access to in-patient facilities can usually be arranged through the clinician referring the patient. The most satisfactory scheme is for the pain relief unit to have autonomous control of beds. This has been achieved with many of the larger units, as the value of this service has been increasingly appreciated within the hospital. Moreover, the observation and assessment of patients with long-standing chronic pain problems is often best achieved by admission to such an in-patient unit.[24]

The management of intractable pain due to malignant disease has always been an important aspect of pain clinic work, but it is the experience of those working in this field over the past decade that an increasing proportion of patients referred have chronic pain of non-malignant origin. The commonest causes of persistent pain are shown in Table 1. This change in emphasis is reflected in the wider range of techniques available, so enabling a broader spectrum of painful conditions to be treated than was possible in the past.

In addition to the extensive use of conventional nerve blocking techniques, there has been an upsurge in physical and electrical methods for interrupting pain pathways. These include the use of radio-frequency lesions, both for cordotomy and for suitable peripheral nerves, as well as cryo-analgesics, which produce a temporary block of transmission for 8–10 weeks. Transcutaneous nerve stimulation, vibration, percussion and acupuncture, illustrate the emphasis now being placed on techniques which utilise the stimulation of the large pain inhibitory nerve fibres and the possible release of endogenous opiates such as encephalin and endomorphan.[25,26]

All patients with chronic pain will have been taking analgesic drugs at some time and often over long periods, but without any discernible improvement in their symptoms. The prescribing and supervision of a suitable analgesic regime is an important aspect of pain clinic work in patients who are either unsuitable for a nerve block or other techniques, or who have failed to obtain adequate relief. The use of tranquillisers, the phenothiazine group of drugs, antidepressants and anticonvulsants such as carbamazepine, can often lead to a considerable degree of relief in refractory pain problems.

Pain clinic work involves the continuing clinical care of patients who, in addition to a physical disability, often have difficult emotional and psychological problems. Close liaison with the general practitioner regarding their treatment is essential. At times it may be necessary to involve the medical social worker or arrange home nursing care. Their management is often very difficult and demanding. Disappointments are not infrequent and relief is often partial or of short duration, but perseverance is rewarded with a worthwhile alleviation of suffering. A multidisciplinary approach, taking into account the possibility of referral to another specialist should more suitable alternative treatment seem necessary, and the use of all the supportive treatment available, are relevant in the current concept of the running of a pain clinic. The extension of the anaesthetist's interest into this field is a significant and important trend in modern anaesthetic practice.

### Pain From Malignancy

Pain due to malignancy is characterised by being constant, always at the same site and, over a period of time, increasing in extent and severity. The patient is never free of pain and it is usually described as being aching and boring in type. There are often acute exacerbations which can last for several hours. As the pain becomes more severe, sleep is disturbed, the patient waking up as the effect of the analgesic tablets wears off. The pain can be controlled by simple analgesics for a surprisingly long time provided a full dosage is given and at frequent enough intervals to maintain a constant action. One of the most striking features seen in a patient with inadequately controlled cancer pain is the progressive demoralisation that occurs over a period of time, leading to a state of total preoccupation with their symptoms to the exclusion of all other aspects of life.[27] Thus, he neglects his appearance, family, previous interests and presents an overall impression of suffering and withdrawal. This picture is also seen in patients with prolonged ischaemic limb pain and in causalgia.

When the patient is in severe pain but in good physical condition with a reasonable long-life expectancy, cordotomy, either by the open or the percutaneous technique should be considered. If this procedure is unavailable or contra-indicated, intrathecal neurolysis is an excellent method for relieving pain in the limb or trunk, and coeliac plexus block for upper abdominal malignancy. When the pain from inoperable cancer is severe and cannot be controlled by other means, narcotic analgesics should be administered in a dose and frequency adequate to relieve it. The use of these drugs under these circumstances, should in no way be inhibited by the fear of addiction.

### Non-Malignant Pain

Examples of chronic pain due to non-malignant causes are set out in Table 1. Despite complaining of severe and persistent pain, these patients do not show the signs of demoralisation and suffering seen in those with malignant disease. For example, patients with post-herpetic neuralgia maintain an interest in their hobbies and families and their state of nutrition is not impaired, despite constant protestations of the severity of their pain and of their need for stronger drugs. There are often periods when pain is absent and the remorseless advance in severity and extent that is seen in malignancy, does not occur. These patients often sleep surprisingly well and there is no constant waking

33/Table 1
Causes of Persistent Pain

| | |
|---|---|
| Malignant disease | Carcinoma<br>Sarcoma<br>Lymphoma |
| Post-traumatic | Postoperative scars<br>Neuroma<br>Amputation stump |
| Neuralgias | Trigeminal<br>Intercostal<br>Atypical facial<br>Post-herpetic |
| Nerve entrapment | |
| Spasticity and painful muscle spasms | |
| Musculo-skeletal | Disc protrusion<br>Facet joints<br>Osteoarthritis |
| Reflex sympathetic dystrophy | Causalgia<br>Sudeck's atrophy |
| Ischaemic limb disease | |
| Central | Headache<br>Thalamic |
| Psychogenic | |

pattern. In patients with chronic pain and normal life expectancy, narcotic analgesics should not be used because of the risk of addiction.

Many patients, whose pain is organic in origin, do have considerable emotional disturbance, manifesting itself in anxiety and depression. Again, some patients whose pain, although organic in origin, is neither disabling or severe, can become chronic complainers.[23] Such people should not be subjected to destructive procedures in an attempt to modify the pain impulses or placed on increasing drug therapy. The patient's condition should not be made worse if the treatment fails.

Referral for psychiatric help will be required in those patients in whom pain is a symptom of an underlying mental illness, or when pain of organic origin becomes dominated by psychiatric symptoms.

### Drug Therapy

For mild or moderate pain, simple analgesics which can be given orally and administered frequently are remarkably effective. Aspirin in one or other of its forms is widely used, especially for musculo-skeletal pain, and because of its anti-inflammatory action it is particularly useful in the rheumatic disorders. Aspirin interferes with prostaglandin synthesis and has a predominantly peripheral action. It has the disadvantage that it can cause gastric irritation and even haemorrhage in susceptible patients. Indomethacin and phenylbutazone are less effective than the salycilates for non-inflammatory pain, but their anti-pyretic and anti-inflammatory action are more pronounced so their long-term use is confined to the rheumatoid disorders, ankylosing spondylitis and similar conditions.

Paracetamol has no anti-inflammatory effect but, apart from this, is as effective as aspirin and has fewer side-effects. An overdose can produce fatal liver damage. Compound tablets, in which paracetamol is combined with codeine or d-propoxyphene (Distalgesic) or aspirin with codeine, are effective and widely used as mild analgesics.

If these drugs become ineffective, more potent ones can be prescribed. These would include dihydrocodeine tartrate (DF118), diflunisal (Dolobid), pentazocine (Fortral), buprenorphine (Temgesic) and mefenamic acid (Ponstan). For patients with malignant conditions who require still stronger drugs, recourse must be made to the narcotic analgesics which, because of their abuse potential, can be addictive. The following drugs are suitable for ambulant patients: dextromoramide (Palfium), methadone (Physeptone), levorphanol (Dromoran) and phenazocine (Narphen). These drugs are more potent than morphine when given by the oral route.[28] Dextromoramide, with a duration of action of only 1–2 hours, is useful if breakthrough pain occurs. Levorphanol and phenazocine have a longer duration of action and can be given at intervals of 6 hours. Methadone, because of its long half-life, gives good background control of pain if administered twice daily and can be given over long periods, enabling the patient to remain socially active. Oxycodone (Proladone) given as a suppository is useful for prolonged pain relief, especially during the night. Buprenorphine (Temgesic) is a powerful agonist-antagonist narcotic drug with a duration of activity of up to 8 hours. Because of its antagonistic properties, it may cause mild withdrawal symptoms in narcotic addicts. A sublingual preparation containing 0·2 mg buprenorphine is a useful drug for persistent severe pain before resorting to narcotics.

The non-ambulant patient in an advanced stage of malignant disease often requires morphine or heroin to control his increasingly severe pain. Because of the drowsiness and mental clouding which accompany the use of large doses of morphine, careful judgment is required as to when it is introduced, as most families will want the patient to remain alert and socially active as long as possible. Depression to the state of semi-consciousness is only acceptable in the terminal stages.

The absorption of morphine by mouth is unreliable and 60 mg is required to produce the analgesia equivalent to 10 mg given parenterally. Heroin (diacetylmorphine) when given by mouth is 2–3 times as potent as morphine as its increased lipoid solubility enables it to cross the blood-brain barrier more quickly.[28] Its pharmacological action is mainly due to its hydrolysis to morphine.

The euphoriant effect of cocaine and alcohol may be beneficial in the later stages of painful malignant disease and is given in combination with morphine or heroin. One popular preparation is the Brompton cocktail containing:

| | |
|---|---|
| Morphine sulphate | 15 mg |
| Cocaine | 10 mg |
| Gin | 1·5 ml |
| Water to | 5 ml |

The parenteral administration of heroin and morphine may be required when pain becomes very severe or oral medication is impossible.

Tolerance develops after narcotic analgesics have been used for two to three weeks, as will be demonstrated by a reduction in the duration and effectiveness of the analgesic effect. This will necessitate an increase in the dosage and frequency of administration. This effect is related to physical dependence and addiction but it should never be an inhibiting factor in controlling severe intractable pain due to malignant disease.

In practice, addiction is not a common problem in these patients and, if the neural pathway can be interrupted by a neurolytic block, the dose of narcotic can be rapidly reduced without withdrawal symptoms developing.

It is important to make a distinction between patients with a reduced life-expectancy and those with a normal one. Narcotics should never be withheld from patients with malignant disease and a life-expectancy of one to two years if analgesics are the most effective way of relieving their pain. However, in patients with chronic pain, who have a normal life-expectancy, the use of narcotic analgesics is contraindicated and treatment should be restricted to analgesics with a low potential for physical dependence. When analgesics are prescribed orally, they must be taken regularly so that, after allowing time for absorption, each subsequent dose produces its effect before the pain returns. There is considerable individual variation in the reaction to narcotics, particularly with regard to side-effects and it is by trial and error that the most suitable drug can be found for each patient.

Side-effects are not uncommon with the use of narcotics. These include nausea, vomiting, dysphoria and constipation so that anti-emetics, such as prochlorperazine (Stemetil), and suitable aperients will need to be given. The phenothiazines are often used in combination with the narcotics. Drugs, such as chlorpromazine, enhance the analgesic and sedative effects, combat nausea and help to reduce agitation. Some of the phenothiazines, such as promethazine, have an antanalgesic effect and are thus less suitable.

Depression and anxiety are common in patients with chronic pain. Tranquillisers and benzodiazepines, such as diazepam (Valium), are very effective for combating anxiety and helping the patient to sleep.

Depression is treated effectively by the tricyclic compounds, especially amitriptyline (Tryptizol) which has a sedative and anxiolytic action, as well as being an antidepressant. It must be explained to the patient that symptomatic relief may take 2–3 weeks. A single dose of 50 mg at night is often effective. A combination of amitriptyline and perphenazine (Triptafen) is also a useful drug when anxiety and depression are present in patients with chronic pain.

**Monoamine oxidase inhibitors** are the most effective antidepressant drugs available and also have analgesic properties, and can be used with striking success in certain selected patients with intractable pain from conditions such as post-herpetic neuralgia and intercostal neuralgia, when depression is the most prominent clinical feature. These patients have a meticulous obsessional type of personality and their lives become dominated by, and revolve around, their continuous pain. The most effective and popular of the monoamine oxidase inhibitors is phenelzine (Nardil) but it takes a month for the maximal elevation of mood and amelioration of symptoms to be obtained. The antidepressant effect is achieved by the accumulation of noradrenaline and other amines in the brain. Care must be taken to avoid tyramine-containing foods (cheese, yeast-extract, etc.) as this substance will no longer be inactivated in the gut by monoamine oxidase. Patients receiving monoamine oxidase inhibitors may also be sensitive to the analgesics—particularly pethidine.

Androgens and oestrogens are useful in the management of patients with hormone-dependent tumours while steroids are of value in carcinoma of the breast and leukaemia. Carbamazepine (Tegretol) is an anticonvulsant drug which has a membrane-threshold stabilising effect on the spinal nucleus of the trigeminal nerve, and thus depresses synaptic transmission. It is of considerable value in controlling the pain of trigeminal neuralgia, the initial dose of 100 mg being increased until a satisfactory clinical response is obtained. The blood count should be checked during the early stages of treatment as blood dyscrasias have been reported.

## TECHNIQUES FOR THE RELIEF OF PAIN

### Local Infiltration

One of the simplest ways of managing intractable pain is to inject 0·5 per cent lignocaine or 0·25 per cent bupivacaine into the painful tissues. In addition to relieving pain locally, this technique may also cause the disappearance of referred pain, muscle spasm and vasomotor disturbances at some distance from the site of injection. Furthermore this secondary relief frequently lasts for a considerable time after the block has worn off. It has been postulated that in certain myofascial disorders "trigger areas" act as a source of constant irritation and set up a vicious circle of impulses which produce the referred pain and other disturbances mentioned above. Local infiltration interrupts this vicious circle and may afford permanent relief of symptoms. Melzack and associates[29] have described a correlation between trigger points and acupuncture points for pain. Moreover, histological examination of trigger points which have been biopsied demonstrate destruction and degeneration of muscle fibres and fatty infiltration.[30] This technique is widely used for a variety of disorders such as sprains and strains, painful undisplaced fractures, low back pain, bursitis, tendinitis, arthritis, muscle disorders including myalgia, contusions, torticollis, muscle contractions and "fibrositis". Nowadays injections of corticosteroids are frequently given for these disorders, either by itself or in combination with a local anaesthetic. Painful scars following surgery and reflex dystrophies may also be treated successfully by local infiltration. It is often necessary to repeat the infiltration several times at intervals of three days to a week. The period of relief usually increases progressively after each injection.

### Injection of Somatic Nerves

The injection of a local anaesthetic into a peripheral nerve, or its immediate vicinity, will cause complete analgesia in the area supplied by the nerve for a period of about one hour to 3 hours depending on the drug used. In addition to its use in providing analgesia for surgery, it also has an important application for diagnostic purposes and for treating intractable pain. Like local infiltration, pain relief in the distribution of the nerve may persist long after the local anaesthetic has ceased to act and cutaneous sensation has returned. Post-herpetic neuralgia may be relieved by carrying out a paravertebral block on the appropriate spinal somatic nerve. Repeated nerve blocks may achieve long-lasting relief in this condition, particularly in patients with a short history of neuralgia. The mechanism by which prolonged relief is afforded in this way is not understood, but it has been suggested that nerve blocks may break up the vicious circle of pain by interrupting the reflexes which initiate or maintain the painful state.

From the gate theory of Melzack and Wall,[31,32] it could be postulated that local anaesthetic blocks reduce the sensory input bombarding the T-cells in the spinal cord so that it is below the critical level at which they are triggered to transmit pain impulses. The self-perpetuating activity in the neuron loops is also blocked, resulting in prolonged pain relief. Increased movements of muscles in the affected part provoke additional input of impulses in the large sensory fibres, so helping to close the gate and maintain pain relief.

Diagnostic nerve blocks are used for a variety of conditions such as reflex sympathetic dystrophies, peripheral vascular disease, nerve entrapment syndromes and neuralgias. As well as demonstrating the relief that can be anticipated by interrupting the transmission of impulses in that particular nerve, it enables the patient to experience the side-effects such as numbness that could follow permanent destruction of the nerve. As explained above, prolonged relief of chronic pain by a local anesthetic block may have a valuable therapeutic role in that repeated injections may result in abolition of the pain. The accuracy of nerve blocking can be improved by using an insulated needle and electrical stimulation with a peripheral nerve stimulator. The needle is insulated throughout its length, except at its tip and its correct placement adjacent to the nerve is indicated by twitching when a suitable current at 2 Hz is applied, while sensory stimulation occurs at about 50–100 Hz. The closer the tip of the needle to the nerve, the smaller the current needed to produce a response. The increased accuracy achieved by this technique is especially useful when it is proposed to destroy the nerve with a neurolytic solution.

It is not proposed to describe all the nerve blocks that may be practised. The following list merely sets out examples of conditions in which nerve blocks may be usefully employed. For a full description of the different blocks the reader is referred to Bonica's *Management of Pain*,[8] Moore's *Regional Block*,[33] Eriksson's *Illustrated Handbook in Local Anaesthesia*[34] and *Neural Blockade*[35] edited by Cousins and Bridenbaugh. The use of nerve blocks in the management of chronic pain is well discussed in Mehta's *Intractable Pain*.[36]

**Neurolytic Agents—Alcohol and Phenol**

By injecting agents which destroy nerve fibres, it is possible to obtain prolonged and even permanent pain relief. This technique is used in patients with severe intractable pain due to malignant disease or occasionally in conditions like post-herpetic neuralgia which have failed to respond to simpler measures.

Alcohol has been widely used as a neurolytic agent. Bonica[8] concluded that with concentrations below 50 per cent only sensory fibres are involved. After an alcohol block the maximum analgesic effect is not apparent for several days. Regeneration of the fibres occurs in time unless the nerve cells are destroyed as well. If superficial nerves are injected, sloughing of the overlying skin may occur. Alcoholic neuritis is a serious complication of this technique and is due to failure to place the alcohol in exactly the right place. This leads to incomplete destruction of the somatic nerve and causes an intense burning pain which may be worse than the original.

In recent years aqueous solutions of phenol (6 per cent) have been used as an alternative to alcohol. It seems to have little effect on tissues adjacent to the nerve and is more effective in blocking sympathetic fibres than somatic fibres. Phenol appears to diffuse less readily than alcohol. It used to be thought that these neurolytic agents destroyed the smaller fibres preferentially before the larger ones but it now seems that alcohol and phenol produce a patchy destruction of all sizes of fibres wherever contact with them occurs. The effect achieved is a quantitative reduction in the barrage of impulses emanating from the painful area rather than any specific qualitative change in the input. Lipton[27] has reported that a long-lasting block of accessible nerves, such as the intercostal, can be achieved by injecting in succession, 2 per cent benzocaine in arachis oil and then twice the volume of 6 per cent urethrane, down the same needle, so that mixing of these solutions occurs in the tissues. After injection of neurolytic solutions, a small volume of air or saline must be injected through the needle as it is withdrawn to prevent tracking of the solution to adjacent nerves or subcutaneous tissues. Deep nerve blocks should not be carried out in patients being treated with anticoagulant drugs because of the risk of extensive haematomata developing.

**Trigeminal nerve.**—Block of the Gasserian ganglion with a local anaesthetic only relieves trigeminal neuralgia for a few hours, but it is an aid to the differential diagnosis of this condition and also allows patients to experience the anaesthesia of the face which would follow permanent relief with alcohol injection or surgery. This is performed in patients who have failed to respond to medical treatment with drugs such as carbamazepine (Tegretol). Phenol may be used as an alternative to alcohol. Very small quantities are injected at a time, the aim being to abolish sensation to pin prick, yet retain light touch. The needle is introduced 3 cm lateral to the corner of the mouth at the medial border of the masseter muscle and passed through the soft tissues of the face to the foramen ovale at the base of the skull. X-rays are used to facilitate the procedure. The use of neurolytic solutions has largely been replaced by radiofrequency heat coagulation, using an insulated needle.[37] Its position is carefully localised to the desired divisions of the nerve according to the response to an initial stimulating current. If possible, a little sensation is left in the face.

If pain is limited to the distribution of one of the branches of the trigeminal nerve, then the individual branch can be blocked by the appropriate technique. The supra-orbital and supratrochlear branches of the 1st division, the maxillary nerve in the pterygo-palatine fossa or its infra-orbital branch and the mandibular division after its emergence from the foramen ovale, can all be blocked by local anaesthetics or neurolytic solutions. Such procedures are particularly useful in patients with pain due to malignant disease or post-herpetic neuralgia. The pain of a fractured jaw can be relieved with a superior alveolar or mandibular block.

**Supra-orbital and supratrochlear nerves.**—The supra-orbital nerve divides into two branches which cross the upper border of the orbit about 2·5 cm from the midline, near the supra-orbital notch. The nerve is injected directly after palpating it at the site of exit and eliciting paraesthesiae with the needle.

The supratrochlear nerve is injected at the root of the nose between the superior and medial borders of the orbit, paraesthesiae having first been obtained. The branches of these nerves can also be readily blocked by raising a weal of local anaesthetic above and along the whole length of the eyebrow.

**Infra-orbital nerve.**—This nerve, which is the continuation of the maxillary nerve, emerges from the maxilla through the infra-orbital foramen. This is situated about 1 cm below the midpoint of the lower border of the orbit. The nerve can usually be palpated at this point and is injected by inserting a needle 1 cm below and slightly medial to the foramen and directing it upwards and outwards towards the infra-orbital canal where paraesthesiae will usually be produced. Because of the risk of spread along the infra-orbital canal into the orbit, neurolytic solution, if used, must be injected slowly and in very small increments.

**Inferior dental nerve.**—This nerve enters the mandible in the inner aspect of the ramus, halfway between the anterior and posterior borders. The mandibular foramen lies 1 cm above the occlusal surface of the third molar teeth and local anaesthetic injected at this point will anaesthetise the teeth in half the lower jaw and the skin over the mental region.

**Mandibular nerve.**—This nerve can be blocked as it leaves the skull through the foramen ovale. A needle is inserted at right angles to the skin over the middle of the mandibular notch, between the coronoid and condyloid processes and immediately below the zygomatic arch. The nerve lies at a depth of 3–4 cm and when encountered by the needle, produces paraesthesiae like an electric shock over the mandible, lower teeth and lip. 5 ml of local anaesthetic are then injected or 1 ml of alcohol if a permanent block is required. If the needle strikes the lateral pterygoid plate, it is sited too far anterior and by redirecting it slightly posteriorly and deeper (0·5 cm), it will usually cause paraesthesiae.

**Glossopharyngeal nerve.**—It is sometimes necessary to block this nerve in patients with severe pain due to extensive malignant disease of the oropharynx. The nerve is injected at the base of the skull in the region of the jugular foramen but blockade may involve adjacent nerves such as the vagus, accessory and hypoglossal to which it is closely related.

### Cervical Plexus Block

The anterior branches of the cervical nerves can be blocked by a lateral approach as they lie in the sulci of the transverse processes. The patient lies in the supine position with his head turned away from the side to be blocked.

The tip of the mastoid process is marked together with the transverse process of the sixth cervical vertebra (Chassaignac's tubercle) which lies opposite the cricoid cartilage. This is the most prominent and easily palpable of the transverse processes. A line is drawn between these two points. The second cervical transverse process lies 1·5 cm below the mastoid process and 0·75 cm posterior to the line previously drawn. Likewise the transverse processes of C3, C4 and C5 are palpated and marked, each lying about 1·5 cm below the one above.

A needle is inserted perpendicularly through the skin and directed in a slightly caudad direction on to the transverse process at a depth of about 3 cm. The point of the needle lies in the sulcus adjacent to the nerve and paraesthesiae are usually obtained. Care must be taken to avoid puncturing the dura which can happen if the needle slips along the transverse process and through the intervertebral foramen. When the needles are correctly sited, 5 ml of local anaesthetic are injected, preceded by careful aspiration because of the risk of injection into the vertebral artery and other large vessels. This block can be used for operations on the thyroid and also for pain due to trauma, malignancy, neuralgia and osteo-arthritis.

If, as in malignancy, a chemical neurolytic block is indicated, it is preceded by an initial block with 1 to 1·5 ml of local anaesthetic to each nerve as a diagnostic test, paraesthesiae having first been elicited. This is followed by 1·0 to 1·5 ml of alcohol or 10 per cent phenol in glycerine.

Complications include hoarseness due to involvement of the recurrent laryngeal nerve, phrenic nerve block and cervical sympathetic block and subarachnoid injection.

### Brachial Plexus Block

The brachial plexus arises from cervical roots 5, 6, 7 and 8 and the greater part of thoracic 1. It may also receive some supply from cervical 4. Brachial plexus block is useful for fractures, dislocations, and skin and muscle injuries of the forearm and hand, and—provided it is complete—will suffice for the reduction of a dislocated shoulder. It also provides anaesthesia of the skin over the outer side of the upper arm, but not of the superior part of the inner side which is supplied by thoracic 2. Should anaesthesia of the latter be required, the block must be combined with an intradermal and subcutaneous infiltration of local anaesthetic solution in the form of a ring around the top of the upper arm.

**Supraclavicular technique.**—The simplest technique for injection of the plexus is to approach it by the supraclavicular route as described by Macintosh and Mushin.[38] Lignocaine 1 per cent should be used and adrenaline may be added (on the basis of 0·5 ml of adrenaline 1:1,000 to each 100 ml of local anaesthetic solution) if anaesthesia lasting more than 45 to 60 minutes is required. For prolonged operations 0·5 per cent bupivacaine gives good results. The patient lies in the dorsal position with a pillow under his shoulders and his head turned away from the side to be injected. The affected arm must be by his side and the shoulder lowered so that the subclavian artery can be easily palpated above the clavicle. A skin weal is raised 1 cm above the midpoint of the clavicle just lateral to the area where the subclavian artery can be felt, and avoiding the external jugular vein. A 5 cm (2 inch) 22-gauge needle is then introduced through the skin weal at an angle of about 80° in a backward, inward and downward direction towards the upper surface of the first rib over which the plexus runs (Fig. 1). While inserting the needle with one hand, it is helpful to push the subclavian artery medially with the first two fingers of the other, thus avoiding the risk of arterial puncture. Paraesthesia in the hand or forearm will most likely be felt by the patient as the point of the needle enters the plexus; at this stage 30 ml of local anaesthetic should be injected. If no paraesthesia is elicited, then the point of the needle must be advanced until it touches the upper surface of the first rib and local anaesthetic solution injected as it is withdrawn towards the skin. Repeated injections made in this manner, and with the needle point gradually moved along the upper surface of the first rib towards the subclavian artery, will block the plexus.

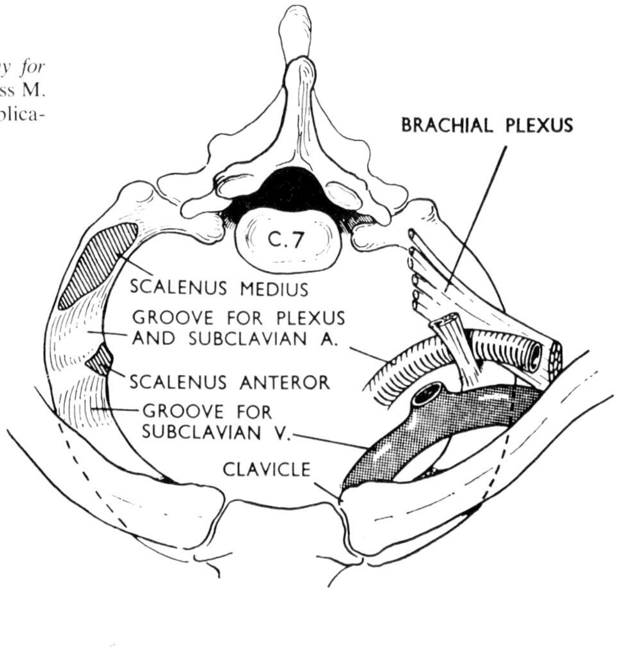


33/Fig. 1.—The first rib. (Reproduced from *Anatomy for the Anaesthetist* courtesy of Professor H. Ellis and Miss M. McLarty, and the publishers, Blackwell Scientific Publications.)

Puncture of the subclavian artery is not harmful provided local anaesthetic solution is not injected, but pressure should be temporarily applied to the vessel after removal of the needle to prevent the formation of a haematoma. The pleural cavity may also be entered if the direction of insertion of the needle is wrong, and this may be suspected if the patient begins to cough during the procedure. A pneumothorax may develop slowly and, even if the initial chest x-ray is normal, the patient should be kept in hospital under observation for 24 hours.

**Axillary technique.**—The axillary approach to the brachial plexus has gained in popularity in recent years. Using it, the success rate is equal to that by the supraclavicular route, and the complications of pneumothorax and phrenic paralysis are completely avoided. It is therefore particularly valuable when a bilateral block of the plexus is needed. It does not, however, produce analgesia of the shoulder. If this is required, the supraclavicular route must be used. The musculocutaneous nerve, which supplies the radial side of the forearm, is sometimes missed with this technique, because it leaves the sheath high up in the axilla, proximal to the point of injection.

The arm is abducted at a right angle from the body and the axillary artery palpated. The highest point in the axilla at which pulsation can be felt is the site for injection of local anaesthetic solution through a short, fine needle of 24 SW gauge. Such a needle lessens the risk of damage to the divisions of the plexus in the axillary sheath, and makes a haematoma unlikely should the axillary artery or vein be accidentally punctured. A finger is placed over the axillary artery, and after raising a skin weal the needle is advanced to one side of the artery until a definite and sudden "give" is experienced as the needle passes through the fascial wall of the axillary sheath. After aspiration, 15–20 ml of 1 per cent lignocaine are injected. The needle is then withdrawn as far as the subcutaneous tissues and then reinserted on the other side of the axillary artery where a further 15–20 ml of 1 per cent lignocaine are injected. The axillary sheath is effectively filled by 40 ml of solution and failure or partial block can follow the use of too small a volume of solution. In order to prevent the distal spread of the local anaesthetic solution and force it upwards into the axilla, it is advisable to apply a tourniquet to the upper arm immediately below the axilla. This should remain in place for about ten minutes.

### Intravenous Regional Anaesthesia

Holmes[39] has described a useful method of producing analgesia of either an arm or leg by a modification of Bier's[40] original intravenous analgesia technique.

**Technique.**—A butterfly needle or plastic intravenous cannula is placed in a suitable vein towards the extremity of the limb. The limb is then elevated and an Esmarch bandage applied from the fingers or toes proximally to reach a sphygmomanometer cuff on the upper arm or leg. This is now blown up to a level at least 50 mm Hg above the patient's systolic blood pressure, the Esmarch bandage is removed, and a solution of 0·5 per cent lignocaine is injected intravenously through the indwelling needle. Bupivacaine* (1·5 mg/kg of 0·5 per cent) diluted to 0·2 per cent with normal saline has proved satisfactory;[41] to achieve the recommended concentration of 0·2 per cent, each 10 ml of 0·5 per cent bupivacaine plain will require 15 ml of normal saline solution. Prilocaine in a concentration of 0·5 per cent is considered the drug of choice because of its rapid metabolism and low systemic toxicity.[42] The maximum adult dose of prilocaine for a 70 kg individual is 400 mg (5 mg/kg) i.e. 80 ml of 0·5 per cent solution. Smaller amounts and weaker concentrations directly proportional to body weight are indicated for children and debilitated patients. About 40 ml of solution are required for an adult arm and up to 70 ml for an adult leg. The onset of anaesthesia is rapid and accompanied by paraesthesia and a feeling of warmth in the limb. Muscular paralysis occurs. The technique can usually be carried out successfully without an Esmarch bandage provided the limb is elevated long enough to allow some drainage of blood. The sphygmomanometer must be kept above the level of the systolic blood pressure until the operation is completed. Holmes suggests that if this is uncomfortable for the patient, a second cuff should be used below it on the

* The Committee on the Safety of Medicines has recommended (October, 1983) that bupivacaine (Marcain) should not be used for intravenous regional anaesthesia, because it appears that toxic reactions, including cardiac arrest, are more likely to occur and are more difficult to treat when bupivacaine is used rather than lignocaine or prilocaine.

analgesic part of the limb, and the original cuff removed. The use of a double-ballooned sphygmomanometer cuff has been advocated as a refinement of this technique.[43] Intravenous regional anaesthesia is well suited for operations on the hand and forearm and also for the foot and lower part of the leg. It is contra-indicated in patients with known hypersensitivity to local anaesthetics, in patients with neurological or peripheral vascular disease and in sickle-cell syndrome.

The manner in which local anaesthesia and muscle paralysis are produced by this technique is not clear, but sensation and muscle power return within a matter of minutes after release of the sphygmomanometer cuff. The mode of action is probably on the large nerve trunks in the region of the elbow where the median and ulnar nerves lie close together. It has been suggested that the large venous channels which surround these nerves provide access for the drug to the vascular channels in the core of the nerves.[44]

At the end of the operation, at least 15 minutes should have elapsed since giving the injection of local anaesthetic before deflating the cuff, because of the increased risk of toxic reactions after short periods of circulatory occlusion. Some workers believe that the risk of toxic reactions to the local anaesthetic released into the circulation at the end of the procedure can be reduced by intermittent release, that is deflating the tourniquet for only a few seconds at a time on several occasions. The pharmacokinetic aspects of intravenous regional anaesthesia have been described in a study by Tucker and Boas.[45] This showed that after cuff release the peak plasma levels of lignocaine were 20 to 80 per cent lower than when the same dose of lignocaine was given by direct intravenous injection. The peak levels achieved were inversely proportional to the total time the tourniquet was applied and tended to be lower when the same dose was given by 0·5 per cent rather than 1·0 per cent solution. The release of the lignocaine into the circulation was noted to be biphasic, with an initial fast release of about 30 per cent of the dose, the remainder appearing by a gradual wash-out. 50 per cent of the dose of lignocaine can remain in the arm 30 minutes after release of the cuff, so it is possible to re-establish anaesthesia within 10–30 minutes of the initial deflation of the tourniquet by reinflating and injecting half of the original dose of the drug.

### Digital Nerve Block

The digital nerves to a finger or toe can be blocked by infiltration of local anaesthetic solutions on either side of the base of the proximal phalanx. Lignocaine, 0·5 per cent, should be used, but without the addition of adrenaline in case marked vasoconstriction of the digital vessels should lead to gangrene.

### Blocks for Abdominal Operations

Paravertebral and intercostal blocks for abdominal surgery are now rarely used. This is directly due to improvements in general anaesthesia, and, where a strong indication for local anaesthesia exists, to the many advantages of epidural or spinal block. However, the combination of intercostal blocks with coeliac plexus block provides excellent conditions for upper abdominal surgery and it is usually augmented with light general anaesthesia to cover any deficiencies in anaesthesia of the upper abdominal viscera. It requires up to sixteen separate injections and also carries the risk of an accidental pneumothorax or toxic reactions to the local anaesthetic. The block of the sympathetic fibres which results from the coeliac plexus injection causes a reduction in the size of the bowel and also a tendency for the blood pressure to fall but this is not usually so profound as that associated with a high spinal anaesthetic. It necessitates the infusion of an adequate volume of fluids and blood during surgery and, possibly, the injection of vasopressors such as metaraminol (Aramine) or ephedrine.

A local nerve block technique may be useful in a very aged or poor-risk patient with a strangulated hernia to avoid hazards of regurgitation and vomiting under general anaesthesia.

### Intercostal Block

Upper abdominal operations require bilateral intercostal block of the 6th to the 12th segments and lower abdominal operations the 7th to the 12th segments. Angle intercostal block is undertaken 7 cm from the midline of the back. At this point the rib is free from the cover of the sacrospinalis muscles and is easily palpable. The patient is placed in the lateral position with the scapula of the side to be blocked drawn as far as possible away from the midline. For a bilateral block it is easier to have the patient in the prone position. The lower border of the rib is palpated and a skin weal raised. The skin overlying the rib is drawn upwards and a 5 cm needle is passed down to the lower border of rib. Having made contact with bone, the needle is angulated so that the tip is pointing in a slight upward direction and then the needle is slowly moved down on the rib until it slips under its lower edge. The needle must not be allowed to advance to a depth greater than 3 mm from the lower border of the rib, where its position is fixed. After aspiration, 5 ml of 1 per cent lignocaine with adrenaline are injected while the needle is advanced and withdrawn 1–2 mm, to ensure that some of the injected solution is deposited in the correct plane between the internal intercostal muscles and the intercostales intimi (Fig. 2). The most important complication of intercostal nerve block is a pneumothorax caused by the needle advancing too far and puncturing the lung. A tension pneumothorax may ensue and as these blocks are often performed in poor-risk patients the whole value may be lost by this complication. Lignocaine 1 per cent with adrenaline produces satisfactory anaesthesia for up to two hours. For operations of longer duration bupivacaine 0·5 per cent should be used. If multiple intercostal blocks are being undertaken for abdominal surgery, it may be necessary to reduce the concentration of local anaesthetic used in order to avoid exceeding the permitted maximum dose.

### Paravertebral Somatic Nerve Block

The mixed spinal nerves formed by the fusion of the dorsal (sensory) and ventral (motor) roots can be blocked in the paravertebral space as they emerge from the intervertebral foramina. The cephalad aspect of the spinous process of the lumbar vertebrae is at the level of its own transverse process and these are the two bony landmarks that it is necessary to identify in order to block the corresponding lumbar nerve. In the thoracic region, because of the obliquity of the spines, the transverse process is at the level of the cephalad edge of the spinous process of the vertebra above, although the lower two thoracic spines are not angled so acutely. The patient lies in the prone position over a pillow to flatten out the lumbar curve. Skin weals are raised 3–4 cm from the midline opposite the cephalad aspect of the spinous processes. A 10–12 cm needle is inserted through each weal perpendicular to the skin and advanced until contact is made with the transverse process. This approach can be made much more easily if x-ray screening facilities are available. A rubber skin marker on the needle is positioned 3 cm from the skin in the

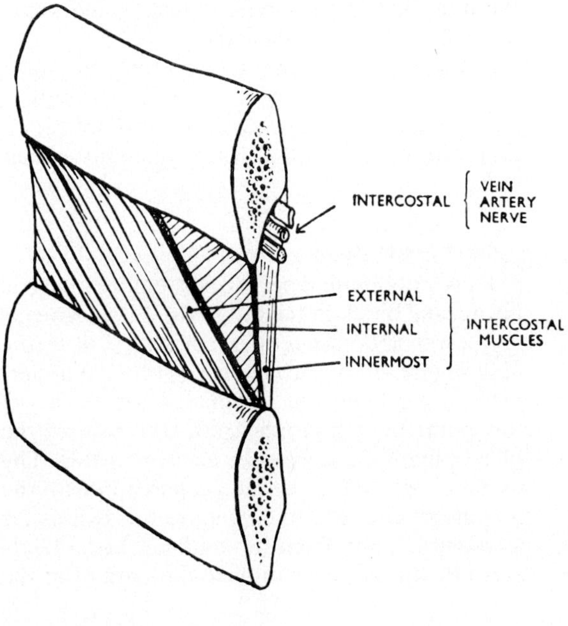


33/FIG. 2.—The intercostal space. (Reproduced from *Anatomy for the Anaesthetist* courtesy of Professor H. Ellis and Miss M. McLarty, and the publishers, Blackwell Scientific Publications.)

lumbar region and 2 cm in the thoracic region. The needle is withdrawn and directed slightly caudally so that it slips over the lower border of the transverse process and is then advanced into the paravertebral space until the marker reaches the skin. The needle often touches the spinal nerve producing paraesthesia but whether or not this occurs, after a preliminary aspiration to exclude blood or CSF, 10 ml of local anaesthetic are injected into the paravertebral space.

This block is useful for diagnostic and therapeutic pain relief in the dermatomes supplied by these nerves and also to provide anaesthesia of the lower abdomen in combination with intercostal blocks. Lumbar somatic block cannot provide complete anaesthesia of the leg because of the sacral fibres carried by the sciatic nerve.

Paravertebral block of the lumbar nerves is often performed for conditions such as post-herpetic neuralgia, disc protrusion and malignancy. The ilio-hypogastric and ilio-inguinal nerves often give rise to intractable pain from entrapment in the abdominal wall or in scars following hernia operation. Repeated blocks with bupivacaine will sometimes relieve the pain in such cases, although if this is only of short duration, it may be necessary to repeat the procedure with 6 per cent phenol. This may have the undesirable complication of motor weakness.

Thoracic and renal operations are occasionally followed by pain and tenderness which are distributed segmentally and usually appear shortly after the wound has well healed. The aetiology of this post-operative neuralgia is uncertain but may well be due to the involvement of segmental nerves in scar tissue. Intercostal or paravertebral block, repeated at intervals, may prove helpful in such cases. Local anaesthetics may suffice for this procedure but sometimes it is necessary to use 6 per cent aqueous phenol or cryoanalgesia for the intercostal nerves.

A paravertebral block may help control the pain of fractured ribs, vertebrae or sternum. The acute pain and disability of the early stages are relieved and mobility encouraged.

### Local Block for Herniorrhaphy

This can be very useful for a strangulated hernia in an aged or otherwise poor-risk patient.

A single epidural injection will do just as well in many cases, but in some circumstances it may be particularly desirable to avoid a fall in blood pressure or the risk of dural puncture in, for example, a severe bronchitic where repeated coughing may lead to severe post-spinal headache.

An iliac crest block of the twelfth thoracic, the ilio-inguinal and ilio-hypogastric nerves (Fig. 3), as they lie between the transverse abdominis and internal oblique muscles, is performed as follows. A skin weal is raised 2·5 cm from the iliac crest along a line joining the anterior superior spine to the umbilicus. A needle is then passed through this to strike the inner surface of the ilium just below the crest. Ten ml of 1 per cent lignocaine solution are deposited as the needle is slowly withdrawn. The injection is then repeated with the needle reinserted at a slightly steeper angle. The contents of the inguinal canal are catered for by a separate injection into the neck of the peritoneal sac 2 cm above the mid-inguinal point. The needle is inserted perpendicularly until it pierces the aponeurosis of the external oblique, and the needle then advanced a further 2–3 cm through the extra-peritoneal fat in this region. Ten ml of solution are deposited at this depth and a further 10 ml as the needle is withdrawn over 2 cm.[46] This ensures block of the neck of the peritoneal sac and the genital branch of the genito-femoral nerve. The block is then completed by a subcutaneous infiltration of the line of the surgical incision.

### Discussion

It is difficult to define precisely the place of regional analgesia for abdominal surgery. Some points have already been touched on in the general description of the blocks. Undoubtedly, in the whole field of regional analgesia, its use for abdominal surgery has suffered the greatest decline. Several factors contribute to this. The techniques are exacting for anaesthetist and patient, and are time-consuming. A considerable element of anxiety always exists for the whole surgical team when the patient is conscious. Anyone familiar with a patient nauseated and hiccupping from traction on upper abdominal viscera appreciates what the difficulties are. When a "light general anaesthetic" is given as well, conditions are certainly much improved, but if a light general anaesthetic can be given, why not a relaxant and controlled

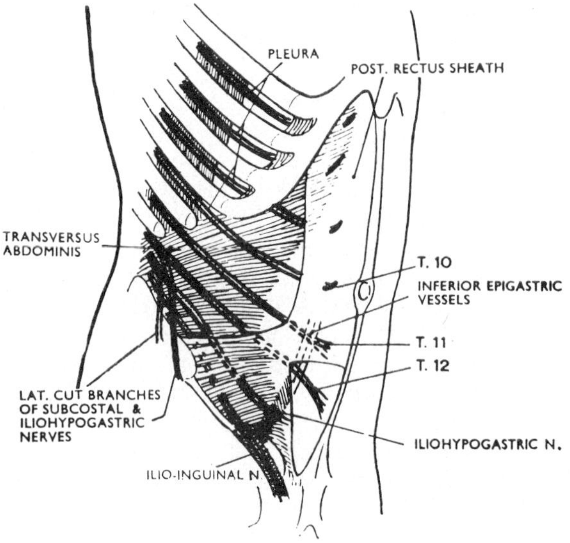


33/Fig. 3.—The lower intercostal, subcostal and first lumbar nerves. (Reproduced from *Anatomy for the Anaesthetist* courtesy of Professor H. Ellis and Miss M. McLarty, and the publishers, Blackwell Scientific Publications.)

respiration? A specific contra-indication to a relaxant may be present, for example an anatomical abnormality which prevents intubation, or, in some types of patient, the risk of an abnormal response to the relaxant.

Some patients with abdominal disease, such as poor-risk prostatectomies, can be managed by a combination of regional and spinal anaesthesia—rectus sheath block and saddle block spinal. This is a valuable method, since the blocks are technically easy to do and such a technique avoids the fall of blood pressure that is a concomitant of either spinal or epidural anaesthesia sufficient to cover the whole operation field itself.

Much depends on individual circumstances. In abstract discussion it is often easy to decide the ideal anaesthetic management of a patient, but surgical preferences play a part, as does the skill of the anaesthetist in regional anaesthesia. Present-day general anaesthesia has the supreme advantage of speed, and is a hundred per cent effective. Oxygenation, so important in the ill patient, and carbon dioxide elimination can often be best assured by controlled respiration using a high oxygen percentage in the gas mixture. All these factors must be assessed by the individual anaesthetist in the circumstances in which he finds himself.

## Application of Techniques

**Regional hip blockade.**—Blocking the obturator nerve and the nerve to quadratus femoris has been advocated for relieving pain in chronic osteo-arthritis of the hip joint and blocking them will afford pain relief in about 60 per cent of patients. This procedure is also useful in spastic conditions.

**Obturator block.**—This nerve is blocked as it lies in the obturator canal on the inferior surface of the pubic ramus. With the leg slightly abducted, an 18-gauge spinal needle is inserted vertically into the skin midway between the pubic tubercle and femoral artery, about 2 cm below the inguinal ligament. Having made contact with the superior ramus, the needle is withdrawn slightly and after turning the hub down through approximately 90°, the point is manoeuvred laterally and slightly cephalad so that it enters the obturator canal. The needle lies almost parallel with the shaft of the femur and it is advanced 3–5 cm into the canal which often produces paraesthesiae on the inner aspect of the thigh. After careful aspiration, 10 ml of local anaesthetic are injected. It may be helpful to use the image intensifier for this block. Adductor spasm due to spasticity can be relieved by blocking the obturator nerve with 6 per cent aqueous phenol using a nerve stimulator to localise the nerve.

**Block of the nerve to quadratus femoris.**—The patient is placed in the prone position with the leg externally rotated and a line is drawn between the posterior superior iliac spine and the sacrococcygeal joint. A mark is made on this line at the junction of its middle and lower thirds. A skin weal is raised at a point 5 cm posterior to the greater trochanter of the femur, level with the lower end of the sacrum. A 15-cm needle is inserted through the weal at an angle of 45° to the horizonal and directed towards the previously determined point on the line until it strikes bone. The needle is worked medially on the posterior surface of the ischium for about 1 cm so that it lies close to the sciatic nerve and the nerve to the quadratus femoris. 20 ml of local anaesthetic are injected which, in diffusing along the surface of the bone, will block both nerves and so produce numbness and motor weakness for several hours. Gentle manipulation and assisted mobility should be carried out in order to enhance the benefit of the nerve blocks.

**Post-herpetic neuralgia.**—Repeated nerve blocks with a local anaesthetic are disappointing in the relief of this condition. Good results can be obtained if the sympathetic chain supplying the affected part of the body is blocked with a local anaesthetic on a number of occasions, provided the treatment is carried out within three months of the onset of the pain. The pain and hyperaesthesia associated with post-herpetic neuralgia can sometimes be relieved by injecting the affected area subcutaneously with a mixture of local anaesthetic and methylprednisolone.

**Myofascial pain syndrome.**—This is a term used to describe a syndrome in which a 'trigger point' acts as a focus for a self-perpetuating cycle of pain, muscle spasm and stiffness. It may be related to a traumatic incident and occurs most frequently in the shoulder girdle and low back. The vicious circle of pain and muscle spasm can be broken and the symptoms relieved by injecting the trigger point with a local anaesthetic.

**Lateral femoral cutaneous nerve neuralgia** (Meralgia paraesthetica).—Pain, numbness and paraesthesiae in the distribution of the lateral femoral cutaneous nerve in the antero-lateral aspect of the thigh is often associated with obesity and prolonged pressure from belts, but may be due to entrapment of the nerve as it passes through the inguinal ligament or fascia lata of the thigh. Repeated blocks of the lateral femoral cutaneous nerve as it runs adjacent to the anterior superior iliac spine with local anaesthetics and possibly steroids, will often afford long-lasting relief of the pain, but sometimes surgical division of the nerve is necessary.

**Abdominal wall pain due to nerve entrapment.**—A little-known cause of long-standing abdominal pain is that due to entrapment of the intercostal nerves as they emerge from the rectus sheath.[47,48] The pain is sharp or burning in character and may persist for a long time with only occasional remission. The patient is usually a woman and the diagnosis can be made by getting her to tense her abdominal muscles by raising her head and shoulders off the pillow and palpating with one finger along the lateral border of the rectus sheath, where a localised very tender area will be discovered at the site of entrapment.

The diagnosis can be confirmed by injecting the affected nerve with local anaesthetic at the site of maximum tenderness, the needle being inserted through the lateral part of the rectus sheath and the solution injected as it is withdrawn. The addition of steroids to the local anaesthetic will enhance the period of relief but often two or three injections of 2–3 ml of 6 per cent aqueous phenol are required for prolonged improvement. If this treatment fails, surgical division of the nerve may be required.

## SYMPATHETIC NERVOUS SYSTEM

### Injection of Autonomic Nerves or Ganglia

There are many painful conditions in which the nerve impulses are carried by sympathetic pathways and in consequence sympathetic nerve blocks are among the most frequent that the anaesthetist is called upon to perform.

As the somatic nerves are separated from the sympathetic chain and ganglia, it is possible to block the latter without affecting motor or sensory somatic pathways. If a sympathetic block with local anaesthetic is beneficial, a permanent effect can be produced using a neurolytic solution with no impairment of sensory or motor function. A successful sympathetic block with local anaesthetic is followed by a rise in temperature, a feeling of warmth and an improvement in colour of the affected part, an increase in pulsation, dilatation of the veins, abolition of sweating as demonstrated by the starch-iodine or cobalt blue test, and the absence of changes in skin resistance, as shown by the sympatho-galvanic response when the skin is pinched. Sympathetically determined pain is relieved and there may be a demonstrable improvement in movement or function of the limb.

There are three different levels at which the sympathetic nervous system can be blocked: cervicothoracic (stellate ganglion), coeliac plexus and lumbar ganglia.

## Techniques of Sympathetic Blockade

### Stellate Ganglion Block

The cervical sympathetic chain normally consists of three ganglia, called the superior, middle, and inferior, according to their position in the neck, which are connected and through which the sympathetic supply to the upper limb, the neck, and the head is transmitted. A branch also runs to the cardiac plexus of nerves. The inferior cervical ganglion is frequently joined with that from the first thoracic nerve and is then known as the stellate ganglion. Sometimes the second thoracic ganglion is also included and occasionally either the fifth or sixth cervical ganglion, or both, are also incorporated, in which case the middle cervical ganglion is correspondingly smaller or absent.

The stellate ganglion is situated on the anterior surface of the neck of the first rib behind the subclavian artery and origin of the vertebral artery above, and the dome of the pleura below.

**Technique.**—The anterior approach to the ganglion is satisfactory in practice. The patient lies supine with the head fully extended at the atlanto-occipital joint. The point of insertion of the needle is determined by measuring two-finger's breadth (3·5 cm) lateral to the jugular notch of the sternum and then a similar distance above the clavicle. The skin weal, which is raised in this position, should lie on the medial border of the sternomastoid muscle and over the transverse process of the seventh cervical vertebra. As a further check, the prominent tubercle (Chassaignac's) of the sixth cervical vertebra can be palpated behind the lateral border of the sternomastoid muscle. The cricoid cartilage also lies at the level of the sixth cervical vertebra so the skin weal should lie on a plane about 1·3 cm below these landmarks. The sternomastoid muscle and the carotid sheath are retracted laterally by two fingers of the left hand which press backward and laterally while a fine 5–8 cm needle is inserted at right angles to the skin until it comes in contact with the bone of the seventh cervical transverse process. The needle passes between the sternomastoid muscle and common carotid artery on one side and the trachea and oesophagus on the other. If the needle is now withdrawn a few millimeters, its point will lie in the tissue plane anterior to the fascia which covers the prevertebral muscle and in which the sympathetic fibres run.[49] After aspiration for blood and cerebrospinal fluid, 10 ml of 1 per cent lignocaine or 0·5 per cent bupivacaine should be injected and this will diffuse up and down the fascial plane blocking the sympathetic ganglia from C2 to T4. The patient should not cough, talk or move while the injection is being carried out.

The signs of a successful block have been recapitulated by Macintosh and Mushin.[38] They are enophthalmos, ptosis, myosis (the original triad of Horner's syndrome), unilateral blockage of the nose due to congestion of the nasal mucosa, absence of sweating and flushing of the skin due to vasodilatation in the head and neck vessels and those in the arm, all of which occur on the side of the block.

**Indications.**—Stellate ganglion block may be of diagnostic and prognostic value in the treatment of Raynaud's disease of the upper limb and in scleroderma. It is also useful in assessing a phantom limb, and as an emergency measure in the treatment of accidental intra-arterial injection of thiopentone, arterial injuries, crushing injuries and embolism of the upper extremity. It is of value in the so-called post-traumatic syndrome and Sudeck's atrophy, when pain, swelling and vasomotor disturbances are present. A recent indication for stellate ganglion block is to produce vasodilatation in the vessels of the arm and so make the surgery easier when an arteriovenous fistula is being created to enable haemodialysis to be undertaken in patients with renal failure. It is worth a trial in the treatment of severe angina at rest, and if successful may be repeated with a neurolytic agent such as phenol. Successful block does not produce dilatation of cerebral vessels, and its value for patients with Menière's disease, cerebral thrombosis or embolism has not been proven.

**Complications.**—Intravascular and subarachnoid injections are dangerous and not necessarily excluded by a negative aspiration test. It is important that the needle, during its insertion, should not meet any appreciable resistance until it makes contact with bone. Traversing the prevertebral fascia or the ligaments joining the transverse processes could result in the needle piercing the vertebral artery or the dural cuff inside the cervical nerve sulci. Spinal anaesthesia could follow subarachnoid injection of local anaesthetic. Recurrent nerve paralysis or partial brachial plexus block may also occur but are not serious. Osteitis of the transverse process is a rare complication and may be due to the needle traversing the oesophagus.

### Chemical Stellate Ganglion Block

This technique is rarely used because of the risk of damaging adjacent somatic nerves such as the recurrent laryngeal or the pleura. Surgical sympathectomy is preferred if it is desired to produce a permanent effect.

In the rare case where surgery is contraindicated, and a neurolytic block is required, the technique is carried out as described above, but a marker is placed on the needle to indicate the depth of the fascial plane where the ganglion is located. The needle is then reinserted so that at the marked depth, its tip is 1 cm below the original position. If a small test dose of lignocaine (1·5 ml) produces a Horner's syndrome, it can be assumed that the tip of the needle is adjacent to the ganglion and 1 to 2 ml of 6 per cent aqueous phenol or 10 per cent phenol in Conray dye can then be slowly injected.

### Lumbar Sympathetic Block

The lumbar sympathetic chain runs on the anterolateral aspect of the lumbar vertebrae, lying in a groove between vertebral bodies and the attachment of the psoas major. It lies in a fascial compartment limited by the vertebrae, the psoas sheath and retroperitoneal fascia.

**Technique.**—To perform a lumbar sympathetic block, the patient lies in the lateral position with the side to be injected upwards. The gap between the iliac crest and costal margin is increased by lying the patient over a pillow. The skin of the lumbar region is prepared and the lumbar spines identified, the highest point of the iliac crest coinciding with the space between the L4 and L5 spines. Subcutaneous weals are raised about 8 cm lateral to the spinous processes of the L2 and L4 vertebrae. A 19-gauge needle 12–15 cm long, with a rubber marker is inserted at the L2 level and directed 45° in a cephalad direction until it reaches the transverse process of the vertebra above. The marker is then pushed down to the skin and the needle withdrawn. The position of the marker is now altered so that it is twice the original distance from the skin to the transverse process and, in the average patient, this should now indicate the distance from skin to the anterolateral aspect of the body of the vertebra. In obese patients, this distance should be reduced slightly and, in thin patients, increased slightly.

The needle is then reinserted through the weal at right angles to the sagittal plane and directed slightly medially between the transverse processes until the tip strikes the lateral side of the vertebral body. If necessary, the position of the needle is readjusted until the marker is almost touching the skin with the needle tip in contact with the vertebral body and the bevel facing medially. The needle should then be close to the sympathetic chain. A second needle is inserted in a similar manner opposite the L4 vertebra with the marker set to the same skin-to-vertebra distance as determined for the first needle. After aspirating, to exclude blood and CSF, 15 ml of 0·25 bupivacaine is injected through each needle. X-ray screening facilitates the performance of this block and the initial injection of a small volume of contrast medium (Conroy 280) will confirm spread along the anterolateral aspect of the lumbar vertebrae.

A simpler one-shot technique has been described by Bryce-Smith.[50] A weal is raised 5 cm from the mid-line opposite the L3 spine and a 12-cm needle is aimed medially at an angle of 70° to the skin surface so as to strike the body of the vertebra on its lateral aspect. 15 to 20 ml of local anaesthetic are injected which tracks forwards beneath the tendinous arch, bridging the sides of the vertebrae to reach the sympathetic chain. This technique is often accompanied by a somatic block so it is not suitable for the diagnostic investigation of pain syndromes.

**Indications.**—Lumbar sympathetic blocks with local anaesthetic are useful in the investigation of patients with circulatory insufficiency in the legs producing rest pain, intermittent claudication and incipient gangrene. It is also of value in Buerger's disease and arterial embolus.

A number of pain syndromes benefit from lumbar sympathetic blocks, including renal colic, post-traumatic syndrome, causalgia, Sudeck's atrophy, phantom limb pain and amputation stump pain. It may also be useful in patients with severe chilblains, hyperhidrosis, erythromelalgia and acrocyanosis.

**Complications.**—A fall of blood pressure may occur in elderly patients with severe arterial disease, necessitating an intravenous infusion. Subarachnoid puncture may occur if the needle is directed too medially and enters the intervertebral foramen.

Paraesthesiae may occur during insertion of the needle due to it impinging on a lumbar nerve root. Puncture of a major vessel or bleeding into the psoas sheath may occur. The latter may cause pain in the groin or thigh. Anticoagulant therapy is a contra-indication to lumbar sympathetic block because of the risk of a large retroperitoneal haematoma developing.

### Chemical Lumbar Sympathectomy

**Indications.**—The injection of aqueous phenol solution into the lumbar sympathetic chain produces an effect equivalent to surgical sympathectomy and is an invaluable technique when surgery is contra-indicated. As the patients requiring this procedure tend to be elderly with a high incidence of pulmonary and ischaemic heart disease, submitting them to surgical sympathectomy could carry an appreciable mortality and morbidity rate. There is the added advantage of a much shorter stay in hospital or even the possibility of performing the block on an out-patient basis. The effective duration of the phenol block of about six months is similar to surgical sympathectomy and, after this period, it can be repeated if necessary. After the procedure, the limb becomes warm as a result of dilatation of the smaller blood vessels, ischaemic pain is often relieved and sweating is abolished.

The technique has proved of considerable value in rest pain and ischaemic ulcers, incipient gangrene – prior to amputation to aid healing of skin flaps – intermittent claudication, Raynaud's disease, reflex sympathetic dystrophy and in conditions such as hyperhidrosis, phantom limb pain and that due to Paget's disease (osteitis deformans).[51]

**Technique.**—To facilitate a more accurate approach to the sympathetic chain, which lies on the anterolateral aspect of the lumbar vertebral bodies, Reid and his co-workers[51] advocate that the needles are introduced more laterally than in the conventional technique for lumbar sympathetic block using local anaesthetics. Needles inserted too near the midline are unable to negotiate the curve of the vertebral bodies to reach the sympathetic chain and success of the block depends on the volume of local anaesthetic (10 ml) injected. Such large volumes of neurolytic solutions are contra-indicated due to the risk of untoward damage caused by extensive spread.

The success of this modified technique is further enhanced by the use of the X-ray image intensifier. The patient is positioned with the side for injection uppermost lying over a pillow and skin weals are raised 10–12 cm from the midline, opposite the bases of the 2nd, 3rd and 4th lumbar spinous processes. 19-gauge, 15-cm needles are directed medially to the side of the vertebral body through each weal and then withdrawn and re-directed more laterally under image intensifier control, until in the lateral view (Fig. 4*a*) the tip of the needle is almost level with the anterior aspect of the vertebral body. The needle traverses the psoas muscle and a feeling of resistance is felt as the tip pierces the psoas fascia, at which point it is very close to the sympathetic chain. On screening (Fig. 4*a* and *b*) in the antero-posterior plane the tips of the needles should be just within the lateral borders of the vertebrae and the needles should not move with respiration.

After careful aspiration to exclude puncture of a blood vessel, the subarachoid space or renal pelvis, about 0·25 ml of Conray 280 is injected at each site to confirm the linear spread of the dye along the antero-medial aspect of the psoas fascia. Lateral spread over the psoas is to be avoided as this may predispose to involvement of the genito-femoral nerve. Localised accumulation of contrast medium indicates injection into muscle or fascia.

2–3 ml of 6·5 per cent aqueous phenol is injected through each needle in increments of 0·5 ml. As an alternative to phenol, 2–3 ml of absolute alcohol can be used. Another neurolytic solution which can be employed is 7–10

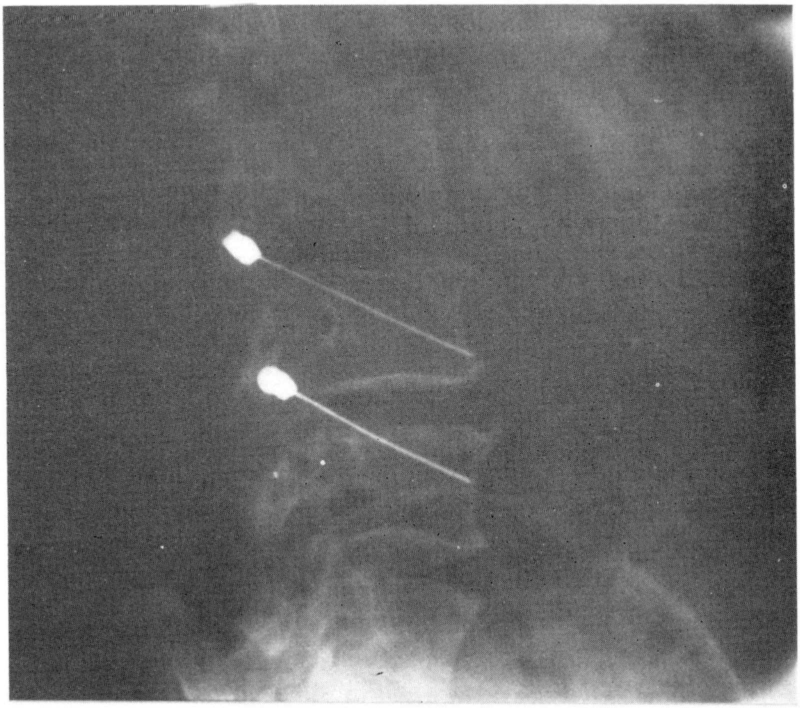

(*a*)

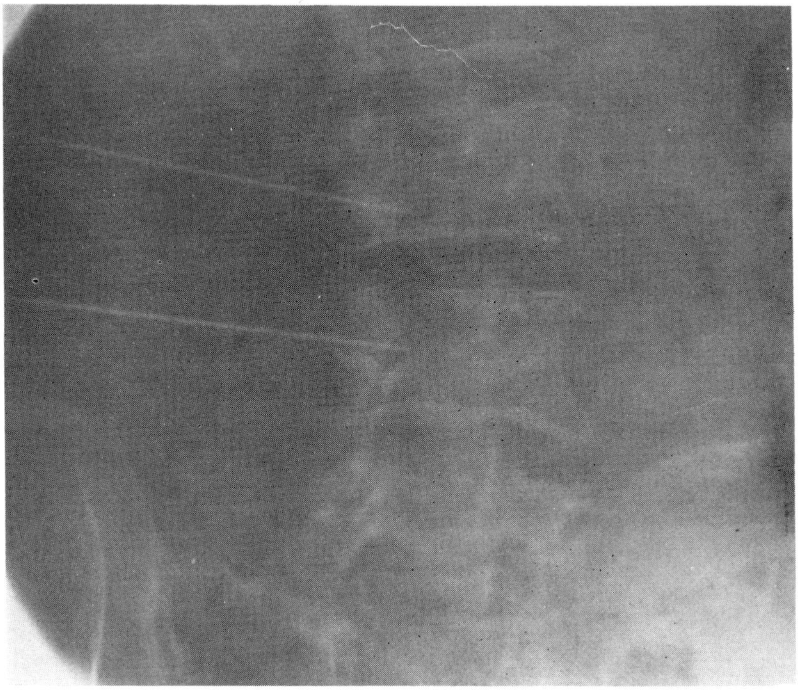

(*b*)

33/FIG. 4.—Chemical lumbar sympathetic block. (*a*) Lateral view; (*b*) antero-posterior view.

per cent phenol dissolved in Conray 280 contrast medium which, being visible on the image intensifier, obviates the need for the initial injection of dye.

Following the injection of the neurolytic solution and prior to removing the needles, 1 ml of air is injected at each level to prevent the phenol flowing along the needle tracks on to the somatic nerve roots, with the attendant risk of producing a neuritis.

Keeping the patient on the same side for about 10 minutes helps to localise the effect of the phenol to the sympathetic chain and stops it spreading laterally on to the genito-femoral nerve or posteriorly towards the somatic nerve roots. The blood pressure should be monitored for about one hour after the block. Preliminary injection of local anaesthetic is not used, unless a local block is performed the previous day, as it merely dilutes the effect of the phenol solution.

**Complications.**—The only common complication is a temporary neuritis in the groin or thigh, due to spread of the solution on to the first lumbar nerve root, producing burning pain and hyperaesthesia in the distribution of the genito-femoral nerve. This complication is also seen after surgical sympathectomy and the symptoms usually resolve after 2–3 months. Serious complications, such as paraplegia due to subarachnoid injection, are avoided by a meticulous technique, the use of the image intensifier and the initial injection of a radio-opaque dye.

**Coeliac Plexus Block**

The autonomic fibres innervating the upper abdominal viscera can be interrupted with a coeliac plexus block. Bridenbaugh and his co-workers[52] described the use of bilateral coeliac plexus block with 40 to 50 ml of 50 per cent alcohol in 41 patients with intractable pain from advanced carcinoma of the stomach, pancreas, gall bladder or liver. All these patients, with one exception, were rendered free from pain for periods varying from six weeks to one year. The block is carried out with the patient in the prone position with a pillow under the abdomen. Marks are made at the inferior edge of the 12th thoracic spine and at the lower border of each 12th rib at a distance of 7 cm from the lumbar spine (Fig. 5). Lines are drawn between these three marks to form a triangle. The coeliac plexus lies at the level of the upper part of the body of the 1st lumbar vertebra, which coincides with the tip of the 12th thoracic spine. A 12-cm (20-gauge) needle is inserted through the mark at the lower border of the 12th rib at an angle of 45 degrees to the skin, and advanced medially and upwards in the direction indicated by the side of the triangle marked on the patient's back. The depth at which the needle makes contact with the body of the 1st lumbar vertebra is noted and a marker is set 1·5 cm from the skin surface. After withdrawing the needle, it is reinserted at a slightly steeper angle until it just slips off the body of the vertebra. After advancing the needle a further 1·5 cm, its tip

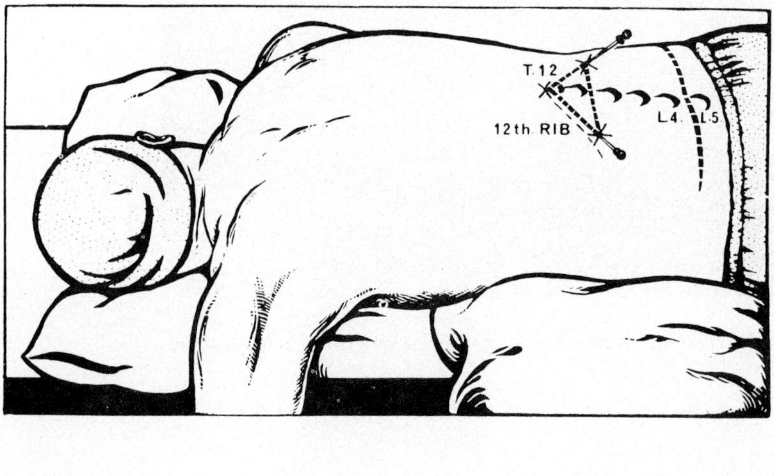


33/Fig. 5.—Coeliac plexus block. The position of the patient and skin markings for needle entries. (Redrawn from originals in *Regional Block*, courtesy of D. C. Moore and the publishers Charles C. Thomas).

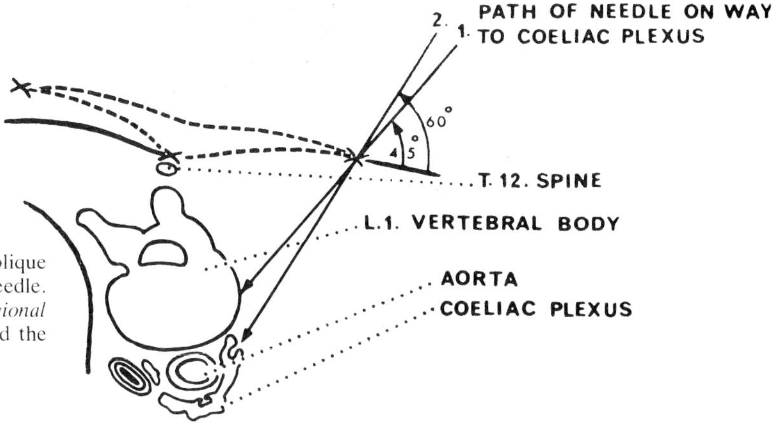

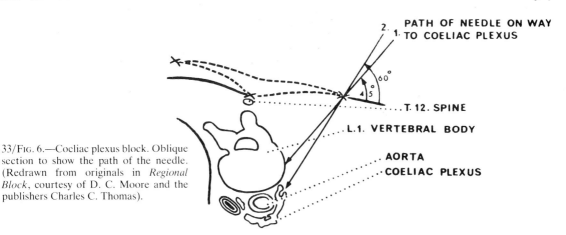

33/Fig. 6.—Coeliac plexus block. Oblique section to show the path of the needle. (Redrawn from originals in *Regional Block*, courtesy of D. C. Moore and the publishers Charles C. Thomas).

should lie adjacent to the coeliac plexus (Fig. 6). The distance to the plexus from the skin is between 7 and 10 cm. After a negative aspiration test, 15–25 ml of local anaesthetic is injected. These authors used 0·1 per cent tetracaine (Pontocaine) hydrochloride solution with 1 in 250,000 adrenaline, but 0·5 per cent lignocaine with 1 in 250,000 adrenaline or 0·25 per cent bupivacaine may be used as an alternative. There should be no resistance to the injection of this solution. The other side is similarly blocked and this should produce pain relief for up to eight hours. If the block is successful it is repeated the following day using 50 per cent alcohol. Alcohol is metabolised readily in the body and is preferred to phenol for this particular block because of the large volume of solution required.

Ideally the position of the needles should be checked with the image intensifier. On the antero-posterior view, the tips should be just within the lateral border of the first lumbar vertebra and, on lateral screening, they should lie 0·5 to 1 cm in front of the anterior surface of the vertebral body. The aorta, inferior vena cava and lumbar vessels all lie close to the needle points and, after careful aspiration to exclude accidental intravascular puncture, 0·5 to 1 ml of Conray 280 is injected. The dye should spread freely up and down the antero-lateral aspect of the vertebrae on x-ray screening.

Initially 1 ml of alcohol is injected to exclude somatic nerve paraesthesia. If the patient complains of a feeling of pressure resembling "a kick in the solar plexus" and of being unable to get his breath, the needle is correctly sited.

Bridenbaugh recommended that 25 ml of 50 per cent alcohol should be injected in each side, but a dose of 15 ml appears to produce effective and long-lasting pain relief.

A burning sensation lasting about one minute follows the injection of the alcohol. To prevent alcohol affecting the 1st lumbar nerve during withdrawal of the needle, the latter should be cleared by injecting 1·0 ml of air. The maximum effect from this block is not apparent for several days. Postural hypotension due to widespread interruption of vasomotor fibres may be a problem for a few days, especially in arterio-sclerotic subjects. This may be prevented by wrapping the legs in elastic stockings and applying an abdominal binder before the patient gets out of bed. Gorbity and Leavens[53] have modified this technique by introducing Teflon catheters under x-ray control onto the ganglia, using a trial of local analgesia before proceeding with 50 per cent alcohol. The development of paraplegia following a coeliac plexus block with 6 per cent aqueous phenol has been described by Galizia and Lahiri.[54] It was postulated that this complication was due to vascular ischaemia of the spinal cord from involvement of a lumbar artery.

This is a very effective block for relieving the pain of upper abdominal malignancy and has a high success rate. It has also been used for a similar purpose in patients with chronic pancreatitis, but owing to the interruption of the sympathetic supply to the pelvis, it may result in failure of ejaculation and, for this reason, may not be acceptable to the patient.

A combination of intercostal and coeliac plexus blocks with local anaesthetic produces good conditions for upper abdominal surgery, but carries the risk of hypotension.

**Intravenous Regional Sympathetic Block**

This is similar in concept to the Bier block using local anaesthetic but, in this incidence, intravenous guanethidine is used to produce a prolonged sympathetic block of a limb.[55–57]

After inserting a butterfly needle into a vein on the dorsum of the hand or foot, the limb is exsanguinated by elevation and then a tourniquet is inflated to 50 to 100 mm Hg above systolic blood pressure. A solution containing 10 mg guanethidinc plus 500 units of heparin in 25 ml of saline for the arm, or 20 mg guanethidine, plus 1000 units heparin in 50 ml of saline for the leg, is injected into the venous system via the butterfly needle. The tourniquet remains inflated for 10–15 minutes and is then released and reinflated several times to slow the release of any unfixed guanethidine into the circulation. The blood pressure is checked to exclude any fall resulting from this cause. The guanethidine is thought to bind to the sympathetic nerve endings, depleting the noradrenaline and producing a sympathetic block which can last a week or more. This is a useful alternative to sympathetic blocks with local anaesthetics in patients with reflex sympathetic dystrophies or causalgia.

## SYMPATHETIC BLOCKS IN PAIN RELIEF

In addition to the indications described in the section relating to the individual blocks, there are a number of other clinical conditions in with sympathetic blocks may be beneficial.

**Vascular disorders.**—An injury adjacent to a large vessel causes intense vasospasm which, if unrelieved, may progress to gangrene. Lesser degrees of vasospasm, whether due to trauma or vascular disease, are a frequent cause of pain. Disorders such as embolism, thrombophlebitis, Raynaud's disease, dissecting aneurysms and thromboangiitis obliterans all cause pain by vasospasm which may be relieved by the appropriate sympathetic block. The stellate ganglion may be blocked for disorders of the upper limb. It has been advocated to relieve the vascular spasm caused by the intra-arterial injection of thiopentone and also spasm after angiography. For circulatory disturbances of the lower limb a lumbar sympathetic block is indicated. When it is desired to interrupt both the somatic and the sympathetic pathways a paravertebral block of the spinal nerves can be carried out.

**Reflex sympathetic dystrophies (causalgic states).**—This term is applied to a group of conditions all exhibiting a similar symptomatology.[58] This consists of pain, hyperaesthesia, vasomotor disturbances and trophic changes. These conditions may be conveniently classified as follow:

1. *Major reflex dystrophies*
   (*a*) Causalgia—following peripheral nerve lesions.
   (*b*) Phantom limb pain.
   (*c*) Central pain—e.g. thalamic syndrome.
2. *Minor reflex dystrophies*

This group includes many conditions such as the shoulder–hand syndrome (Steinbocker), post-traumatic dystrophy, Sudeck's atrophy, post-traumatic oedema and the post-frostbite syndrome.

It is believed that in all these conditions a reflex disorder involving the sympathetic nervous system is initiated by local damage which acts as a chronic irritative lesion bombarding the spinal cord with a stream of afferent impulses. Conditions like Sudeck's atrophy and post-traumatic dystrophy follow injuries such as Pott's or Colles' fractures or contusion of a joint. The patient complains of a diffuse burning pain, often associated with cyanosis and sweating of the skin and decalcification of the bones. These syndromes may take eighteen months to two years to resolve but a lumbar sympathetic or stellate ganglion block usually affords complete but temporary relief of the pain and vasomotor disturbances. Repeated blocks at weekly intervals on four to six occasions often result in a complete resolution of these distressing disabilities. Intravenous regional sympathetic injection is useful in patients who do not get prolonged relief after stellate or lumbar blocks.

**Causalgia** is a distinct syndrome which develops after a peripheral nerve injury. It consists of a burning pain of varying severity which is exacerbated by minor stimuli, dryness, heat, or emotional disturbances, and often relieved by sympathectomy. Doupe and his co-workers[59] put forward a theory that causalgia is due to fibre interaction or artificial synapses developing at the site of nerve injury. This results in efferent sympathetic impulses being short-circuited at the site of trauma and stimulating sensory afferent fibres, whence they return to the spinal cord and are eventually interpreted in the thalamus as pain. At the same time impulses from the artificial synapse can also travel peripherally, causing the release of bradykinin.[60] The sensitisation of the peripheral nerve endings induced by this process causes the normal or damaged neurons to over-react and transmit impulses to the spinal cord that are interpreted in the central nervous system as a distal burning pain. In any particular patient one or other of these processes may predominate but both are abolished by sympathectomy. Repeated sympathetic blocks with local anaesthetic or the intravenous regional technique should be tried but if the beneficial effect is not prolonged, then it may be necessary to proceed to surgical or chemical sympathectomy.

**Cardiac pain.**—Cardiac pain impulses travel via sympathetic fibres through the middle and inferior cervical cardiac nerves and the thoracic cardiac nerves, to reach the upper four or five thoracic sympathetic ganglia and the corresponding posterior spinal nerve roots. Nowadays most cases of angina can be satisfactorily controlled with beta-blocking drugs but in special circumstances the sympathetic pathways may be interrupted and pain relieved by stellate ganglion block or paravertebral block of the upper four or five thoracic spinal nerves although the high risk of a pneumothorax in a seriously ill patient may well be unacceptable. A left-sided stellate ganglion block is usually sufficient to achieve relief, otherwise the right side must be blocked as well.

Severe incapacitating angina occasionally requires surgical interruption of the pain pathways either by posterior rhizotomy or thoracic ganglionectomy, but nowadays coronary artery bypass grafting together with drug therapy, has eliminated the need for these procedures.

**Cancer pain.**—Sympathetic pathways are implicated in many cases of cancer pain and sympathetic nerve blocks are often effective in relieving a large component of the pain associated with inoperable or recurrent malignant disease. Advanced carcinoma of the breast is often complicated by an uncomfortable oedematous arm and a severe burning pain in the shoulder and brachial plexus. To achieve complete pain relief by injection techniques, it is often necessary to interrupt the somatic pathways with a subarachnoid alcohol or phenol block and the sympathetic pathways with a stellate ganglion block.

The value of coeliac plexus block in patients with upper abdominal cancer has already been stressed. It may also be worth trying in patients with cancer of the uterus, bladder or prostate when there has been incomplete relief after a subarachnoid phenol block of somatic nerves. In such cases, tumour invasion may have spread to involve blood vessels and visceral sympathetic fibres. Blocking these fibres at the lumbar and lower thoracic cord, or even the lumbar chain itself, may be less effective than coeliac plexus block because of the additional effect of interrupting vagal fibres which occurs with the latter technique.

## Intrathecal Injections

The intrathecal route provides an excellent way of relieving intractable pain, especially that associated with incurable malignant disease. It enables neurolytic agents to be accurately placed so as to denervate localised areas of the body.

### Alcohol

The use of intrathecal alcohol in the management of intractable pain was first introduced by Dogliotti in 1931[61] and it has since become a widely used and valuable technique. Alcohol is a tissue poison which may cause necrosis if injected into subcutaneous tissues. When injected into the intrathecal space, it acts as a neurolytic agent, destroying nerve fibres wherever it comes into contact with them until it is diluted by the cerebrospinal fluid. Absolute alcohol has a lower specific gravity (0·806) than cerebrospinal fluid (1·007), so that when it is slowly injected intrathecally it acts as a hypobaric solution and forms a layer on top of the cerebrospinal fluid. By careful positioning of the patient it is possible to limit the spread of the alcohol so that it only bathes those dorsal roots whose ganglia it is desired to block. Subarachnoid alcohol block may cause serious complications, so it is obligatory to pay the most careful attention to details of technique and selection of patients.

**Selection and assessment of patients.**—Because of the risk of complications, this technique is usually reserved for the mangement of intractable pain in patients with incurable malignant disease. It may at times be justifiable in non-malignant conditions, such as severe long-standing sciatica in a patient considered unfit for laminectomy or patients with nerve root irritation due to arthritis, ankylosing spondylitis or fractured vertebrae. A careful history is taken from the patient, particular note being made of the duration, site and character of the pain. It is important to enquire if the patient has any disturbance of bladder or rectal function, as it would probably be aggravated by a block for pelvic or leg pain.

At the clinical examination detailed attention is paid to the nervous system and a note is made of any existing motor or sensory loss, muscle wasting, or alterations in the tendon reflexes. It is important to distinguish between difficulty in walking due to the aggravation of pain and that due to motor weakness.

The distribution of the pain should be plotted on a body dermatome chart. This serves as a guide to the nerve roots that need blocking but it is not accurate for pain arising in sclerotome structures such as bones, ligaments and muscles. Sympathetic pathways may also be implicated in carcinoma pain, particularly when viscera are involved.

The nature of the proposed treatment must be frankly discussed with the patient. A hopefully optimistic attitude should be adopted rather than a guarantee of success, and the need for a series rather than a single block must be stressed, otherwise the patient may be discouraged if the initial injection does not afford dramatic pain relief. The patient must be warned of possible complications such as numbness, weakness in the legs, and urinary retention. The low incidence of these complications must be pointed out, because if too pessimistic a picture is painted the patient may refuse treatment. In the more hopeless case, and especially if the patient is already partially incontinent, less emphasis should be placed on the risk of complications, although they should be fully discussed with a close relative and the reason for the treatment explained.

Most patients require more than one injection for complete relief, especially when the pain originates from a wide area. The response to the initial injection enables the anaesthetist to determine whether his assessment of the involved segments and site of block was correct.

**Technique.**—It is preferable to carry out the block on an operating table as it enables the patient to be positioned more accurately, but it can be carried out in the patient's bed with appropriately placed pillows. Morphine may be necessary beforehand to enable the patient to lie in the required position, but it is an advantage if the patient has some pain and is able to describe sensory changes and so confirm the level of the block.

The patient lies in the lateral position with the painful side uppermost. The body is angulated by breaking the table so as to produce a scoliosis with the maximum curve corresponding to the site of the block. Both the head and legs should be lower than the point of injection. The patient is rolled forward 45 degrees into the semi-prone position so that the sensory posterior roots lie uppermost. Subarachnoid tap is made under strict aseptic conditions, the site of puncture depending on the roots involved. Bonica[8] argued that it is better to deposit the alcohol at the point of emergence of the affected roots from the spinal cord. The spatial separation of the anterior and posterior roots is at a maximum at this point and, moreover, the expanded origin of the rootlets from the cord is thought to render them more susceptible to the action of the alcohol (Fig. 7). Blocking the roots at their exits through the intervertebral foramina carries an added risk of involving the anterior roots.

In carrying out the block an allowance must be made for the origin of the spinal nerves from the cord being above the level of the corresponding vertebra. It can be calculated as follows:

*Cervical region:*
Spinal cord segments are one vertebra above the corresponding vertebra.

*Upper thoracic region:*
Spinal cord segments are two vertebrae above the corresponding vertebra.

*Lower thoracic region:*
Spinal cord segments are three vertebrae above the corresponding vertebra.
L 1 segment is opposite T 10 spine.

Using this technique it is unnecessary to

33/FIG. 7.—Intrathecal alcohol block. Diagram of lower thoracic cord region showing method of blocking dorsal roots as they emerge from the spinal cord (see text).

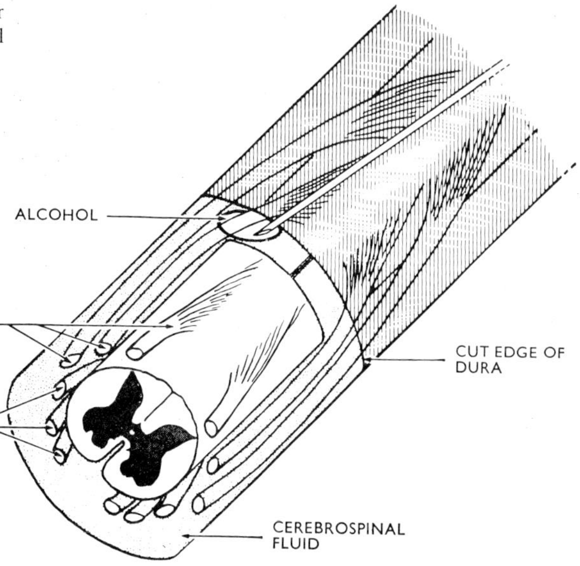

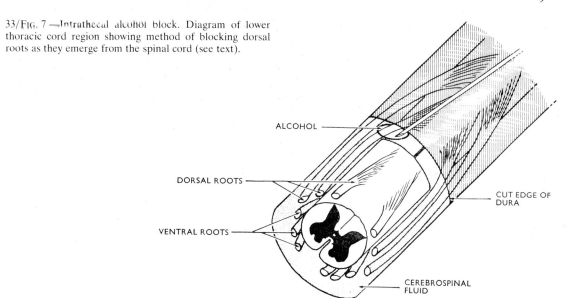

perform blocks below the L1–2 interspace. The exact segment being blocked becomes apparent during the injection and any necessary adjustment in the level can then be made. Great care must be exercised when inserting the needle in the cervical or thoracic regions, owing to the risk of entering the spinal cord. As the epidural space is approached the stilette is withdrawn and, while slowly advancing the needle, either the hanging drop or the loss of resistance test is used to demonstrate entry into this space. The needle is then very slowly advanced for a further 2 to 3 mm until its tip just enters the subarachnoid space.

The low pressure in the subarachnoid space may prevent the free flow of cerebrospinal fluid from the hub of the needle during a cervical tap. It is advisable therefore, to exert continuous suction with a syringe at this level so that the flow of fluid is immediately detected. It is important to position the patient with a slight head-down tilt to avoid spread of the alcohol to the medulla.

Absolute alcohol from a glass ampoule, the outside of which has been sterilised by autoclaving, is used and up to 0·5 ml is injected as an initial dose. The injection is made very slowly at a rate of about 0·1 ml per minute in order to localise the effect of the alcohol. The use of a 1 ml syringe facilitates this procedure. Burning paraesthesiae are experienced by the patient and ideally these should be located in the centre of the painful area. By testing sensory and motor functions the extent of the block can be assessed. In the absence of motor impairment, further small increments of alcohol may be injected, but as a general routine not more than 1 ml should be injected at any one segment. If the paraesthesiae do not coincide with the painful area it may be possible, by tilting the table slightly in the appropriate direction, to float the hypobaric solution on to the involved nerve roots. If the disparity is more than one dermatome, it is preferable to change the position of the needle.

When pain arises from a wide area two or more needles should be inserted at different levels and small volumes of alcohol injected through each needle, rather than trying to produce an extensive block through one. In such cases, and especially when the pain arises from both sides, it may be preferable to carry out these blocks at intervals of a few days. After the injection the patient should lie in the same position for about 20 minutes to avoid spread of the alcohol and to enable it to be "fixed" to the correct nerve roots.

This technique is unsuitable for out-patients owing to the risks which attend any intrathecal technique.

**Clinical effects and results.**—An initial injection of 0·5 ml of alcohol affords some pain relief but in patients with severe pain the block may have to be repeated, usually with a larger dose and perhaps in a different position. The maximum relief may be delayed as long as five days after the injection and a decision about a further block should be postponed until then. The larger the volume of alcohol injected, the greater the risk of side-effects. The precise dose in any individual patient can only be decided by a careful consideration of all the relevant factors, such as the severity and extent of the pain, and the willingness to accept the risk of side-effects. If the bladder sphincter is already paralysed, it may be permissible to use larger doses than usual. Incontinence is much more difficult to manage as a long-term problem in a woman than in a man.

Following the injection, a neurological examination will reveal a loss or diminution in sensation, especially to pin pricks and light touch. Tendon reflexes on the affected side are often absent and there may be a slight degree of motor weakness. These signs tend to disappear within a short time but areas of analgesia may persist for long periods. Some patients find this particularly distressing and complain vehemently. The results claimed by various authors are approximately 50 per cent good, 30 per cent fair and 20 per cent poor.[62]

The duration of pain relief ranges from six weeks to many months and even a year. The average duration is about three months, and if the pain does recur a further block can be carried out. Not all suitable patients are relieved by an intrathecal alcohol block.

**Complications.**—Some side-effects, such as headache and meningismus, are common to both spinal anaesthesia and subarachnoid alcohol block. The following complications are related to the neurolytic action of alcohol.

*Motor paralysis.*—This is due to involvement of the anterior roots and is more liable to occur when large volumes of alcohol are injected into the lumbar and lower cervical region. It may also result from bad positioning of the patient.

*Bladder paralysis.*—The injection of large volumes of alcohol into the lumbar region predisposes to this complication, which is due to involvement of the efferent parasympathetic fibres in the anterior sacral roots. These travel mainly in the second sacral nerve. Interrupting the sensory autonomic fibres, with consequent loss of bladder sensation, may lead to retention with overflow. Disturbance of bladder function occurs in about 5–10 per cent of cases but the incidence can be reduced by careful attention to technique. Spontaneous improvement usually occurs within a period of weeks or months.

*Rectal incontinence.*—The aetiology of this complication is the same as bladder paralysis but the incidence is less.

*Cutaneous analgesia.*—Areas of analgesia may persist for weeks and even months. It is particularly liable to occur when the block has been performed for a non-malignant condition in an otherwise healthy person.

*Adhesive pachymeningitis.*—Alcohol causes histological changes far beyond the point of injection, indicating that it diffuses widely in the subarachnoid space.

*Transverse myelitis and cauda equina syndrome.*—The risk of injecting alcohol into the cord can be avoided by ensuring that there is a free flow of cerebrospinal fluid before making the injection.

### Phenol in Glycerine

Alcohol has the disadvantage of diffusing extensively in the subarachnoid space. This rapid diffusion, together with the difficulties of accurately controlling the flow of a hypobaric solution, have led to the search for alternative agents. Maher[63,64] described a technique for using intrathecal phenol in glycerine to alleviate the pain of incurable cancer. Aqueous phenol is a caustic substance, but when dissolved in glycerine it only diffuses slowly from solution to affect the nerve roots over which it is flowing. Being a hyperbaric solution (Sp. G. glycerine 1·25: Sp. G. cerebrospinal fluid 1·007) it falls downwards in the subarachnoid space and is easier to control than alcohol. Maher concluded that 5 per cent phenol in glycerine is the optimal concentration to use as it will abolish pain without affecting other forms of sensation or disturbing motor function. These unwanted effects may result from the use of stronger solutions, while weaker solutions do not afford long-lasting relief. For patients unrelieved with phenol alone a phenol-silver nitrate solution can be used (silver nitrate 0·6 mg per ml of 4 per cent phenol in glycerine).[65] This is a more potent agent than phenol by itself but it may cause a meningeal reaction. With improvement in techniques, the need for this solution has decreased. Myodil (iophendylate) may also be used as a vehicle for phenol but it tends to protect the nerve roots and the phenol has to be used in a higher concentration (7 to 10 per cent) in order to achieve results comparable with 5 per cent phenol in glycerine.

In many centres phenol in glycerine has replaced alcohol as the agent of choice in the relief of intractable pain by intrathecal injections.

**Effect of phenol on the nervous system.**—The belief that intrathecal phenol has a selective action on the small unmyelinated fibres of the posterior roots is no longer tenable, as a result of a study by Smith.[66] She carried out post-mortem studies on the nervous systems of patients who had received intrathecal injections of phenol and also on a control series of spinal cords from patients with malignant disease who had not been given this treatment. The effect of phenol in Myodil on healthy nervous tissue was investigated in cats by means of electrophysiological and histological studies carried out on nerve roots which had been exposed by laminectomy.[67] These investigators concluded that initially intrathecal phenol affects a large number of fibres of many roots, acting as a local anaesthetic. This effect comes on in 50 seconds and lasts about 20 minutes. Some fibres recover completely but others subsequently degenerate, depending on the concentration and duration of application of the phenol. It was concluded that phenol in glycerine or Myodil did not affect the spinal cord or posterior root ganglia but acted on the nerve roots, causing indiscriminate degeneration of all fibres, irrespective of their size, wherever it came into contact with them. Although the anterior roots were affected to some extent, the site of action of the solution was predominantly on the posterior roots between the ganglia and the spinal cord. A striking feature in the injected patients was a marked degeneration of nerve fibres in the posterior columns of the spinal cord, secondary to the action of the phenol on the posterior roots. There was no suggestion of any marked meningeal reaction or direct damage to the cord. From these studies it was concluded that the effect of phenol in relieving chronic pain is not achieved by selectively destroying a particular type of nerve fibre (i.e. C fibres) because painful stimuli such as pricking and burning are still appreciated. The explanation is a quantitative rather than a qualitative one, depending on the destruction of a sufficient number of nerve fibres from the affected part of the body. This reduction in the sensory input and the lessening of the opportunity for summation between the opposing large and small fibre systems fits in with the Gate Control Theory of pain of Melzack and Wall (see Chapter 30).

**Technique.**—The selection of patients and the mapping out of the pain distribution on dermatome charts to determine the nerve roots that require blocking has already been discussed in the section on alcohol subarachnoid block. The needle should be inserted as near as possible to the vertebral outlets of the nerve roots it is desired to block with the phenol. A single injection of 1 ml of phenol in glycerine will usually block three nerve roots. Some patients require more than one injection and additional blocks are carried out at intervals of five days until all pain has been eradicated. With extensive bilateral pain it may be necessary to repeat the injections on three or four occasions.

Although Maher advocates carrying out this treatment at the bedside, the use of an operating table makes it easier to position the patient accurately and to control the flow of the solution after injection. With the patient lying on the painful side, subarachnoid puncture is performed with a 21-gauge needle, care being taken to ensure there is a free flow of cerebrospinal fluid. The needle is withdrawn to the edge of the subarachnoid space so that CSF is only just flowing. This reduces the possibility of the injected phenol affecting the more centrally placed roots in the cauda equina, with a consequent risk to bladder or bowel control. Rotating the patient posteriorly to an angle of about 30° with the vertical helps to localise the effect of the phenol to the posterior roots. With the bevel of the needle directed downwards, an initial dose of 0·3 ml of 5 per cent phenol in glycerine is slowly injected. If the needle is correctly sited, the relief of pain is immediate, and is accompanied by a sensation of warmth and paraesthesiae in the distribution of the affected roots. If these sensory symptoms do not coincide precisely with the painful area, the table may be tilted so that the solution flows on to the appropriate nerve roots. Incremental doses each of 0·3 ml are given at intervals of 5 minutes until the desired effect has been achieved. The "end-point" for stopping the injections is determined by testing sensation immediately before each injection. The object is to diminish or abolish sensation to pin-pricks compared with the other side while leaving light touch unaffected.

The patient is kept lying still in the position of the injection for thirty minutes afterwards in order to fix the phenol to the required roots. To minimise the risk of post-lumbar puncture headache, the patient is nursed lying flat in bed for 24 hours.

Details of technique and a guide as to the volume of solution required in each region of the vertebral column are set out below. Most patients suitable for an intrathecal phenol block have pain in the lower part of the body and, in consequence, most injections are carried out in the lumbar or lower thoracic regions. X-ray monitoring with a preliminary injection of a contrast medium (Myodil) to assess how the phenol in glycerine will flow within the subarachnoid space, is often used as part of this technique and is essential for cervical and upper thoracic nerve roots.

**Sacral region.**—A common cause of intractable pain in the perineum and bottom of the coccyx is a recurrence of carcinoma, following an abdominoperineal excision of the rectum. The problem is to transfer the phenol in glycerine from the site of injection to the lowest sacral and coccygeal roots with minimal involvement of the intervening sacral roots (S2, 3 and 4) which supply the bladder. The technique described by Maher and Mehta[68] is to perform a lumbar puncture in the exact midline at the L5-S1 space in the lateral position. Having withdrawn the needle to the edge of the subarachnoid space, 0·75 ml of 5 per cent phenol in glycerine is slowly injected. The needle is then withdrawn and the patient gradually turned on to his back, care being taken to avoid undue displacement of the phenol solution. After a minute's pause, the patient is slowly and carefully raised to the sitting position, so getting the phenol to flow along the posterior wall of the sacrum and pool at the bottom of the subarachnoid space. The patient leans forward on to pillows and stays sitting in this position for half-an-hour.

For pain involving the upper sacral roots, subarachnoid puncture is made at the L4–5 or L5–S1 space with the patient lying on the painful side and a 15°–20° head up tilt. 0·5 ml of phenol in glycerine is injected and allowed to flow slowly over the affected roots. If bladder control is normal prior to treatment, no disturbance should occur after blocking the sacral roots unilaterally.

**Lumbar region.**—After a successful lumbar tap, the needle is withdrawn to the edge of the theca so that the injected phenol does not cross the nerve roots which are descending centrally in the cauda equina and emerging at a lower level. The average volume of solution required for this region is 1 ml and it is given in increments of 0·3 ml as described above. At times as little as 0·5 ml of solution is enough to produce the desired effect. If necessary, the table is tilted slightly to localise the effect of the phenol to the appropriate nerve roots. The occurrence of sensory symptoms in the upper leg after the initial injection indicates that the needle has been inserted too far towards the unaffected side, allowing the phenol to trickle over all the roots of the cauda equina. Unless the injection is abandoned the patient may have difficulty in controlling his bladder.

**Dorsal region.**—Great care must be exercised in carrying out a subarachnoid tap in this region, particularly in the upper and mid-thoracic segments because of the obliquity of the spinous processes, the small size of the spinal canal and the risk of inadvertently transfixing the spinal cord. A short-bevelled needle is inserted initially into the epidural space, which may be recognised by the loss of resistance or hanging drop techniques. The needle is then advanced a millimetre at a time until cerebrospinal fluid just begins to flow. In view of the difficulty of performing a subarachnoid tap in the mid-dorsal region, pain at this level can be relieved by inserting a needle at the D9–10 interspace and by using a head-down tilt, allowing the neurolytic solution to flow in a cephalad direction to the affected nerve roots.[68] X-ray screening should be used in this procedure and to facilitate this, 1 ml of 7·5 per cent phenol in Myodil is injected followed by further increments of this solution or 5 per cent phenol in glycerine up to a total of 3 ml, until the desired pain relief has been achieved. Care must be taken to avoid the neurolytic solution ascending on to the brain stem by reducing the tilt once the desired level of analgesia has been achieved.

**Cervical region.**—Because of the danger of

phenol flowing into the cranium the patient must be positioned with a head-up tilt of 30° to 40°. The technique adopted is the same as in the thoracic region but as the spinal canal is narrow the needle must be inserted exactly in the midline. The results of intrathecal phenol are not so good in the cervical as in other regions, because the solution tends to flow away very quickly and also the cervical nerve roots are much shorter and hence the length available for absorption is less. The flow of a small volume of contrast medium is monitored by x-ray screening before injecting the phenol in glycerine. Maher considers that subdural injections give better results in this area. The technique is to introduce a spinal needle via the C6/7 interspace into the epidural space and then, by gentle pressure and rotation, the point is advanced into the subdural space. If the needle inadvertently enters the subarachnoid space, it is gradually withdrawn until the flow of CSF ceases. Reinserting the stilette helps to widen the subdural space prior to injecting 0·25 ml of 7·5 per cent phenol in Myodil. A honeycomb appearance on the x-ray, caused by the Myodil travelling down round the nerve roots, confirms the correct siting of the injection.[64] Further increments of the same solution or 5 per cent phenol in glycerine are injected up to a total of 3 ml until pain relief is obtained. The neurolytic solution will extend upwards against gravity to block the upper cervical nerve roots.

**Preparation of solutions.**—Phenol in Myodil must be prepared immediately before use. The outside of the Myodil ampoule cannot be sterilised by heat. The contents are drawn up and injected into a sterile ampoule containing phenol crystals.

**Factors influencing results of treatment.**—Most of the pain caused by cancer is of a constant, unremitting nature. It is carried by the small C fibres and can be eradicated by intrathecal phenol injections. A second type of pain, termed incident pain by Maher, is due to a sudden event such as a fracture or the collapse of a vertebra. This pain is not amenable to treatment by phenol, but as it is evoked by movement it can be relieved by complete rest.

Phenol has both a temporary and a permanent blocking effect.[69] When injected intrathecally it acts as a local anaesthetic, relieving all pain within a period of 50 seconds. Recovery takes place gradually after about 20 minutes but a varying number of pain fibres remain permanently damaged, so accounting for the relief of the constant pain in malignancy. Because of this dual effect phenol, unlike alcohol, destroys nerve fibres without causing pain.

Severe pain dominates a patient's whole existence, and if it cannot be relieved by analgesics it may materially shorten his life. Treatment of pain must not be an ordeal for these patients, as the majority have already endured operations and radiotherapy and many do not want anything further done. Good results can only be achieved if patients are referred early for treatment, preferably within two or three months of the pain becoming established. If it is longstanding and has been present for two or three years, the results are bound to be disappointing. Growth of tumour around the nerve roots may have a sheltering effect by preventing the phenol gaining access to them. Successful relief of pain in one part of the body frequently reveals pain in adjacent or more distant regions, which hitherto had been overshadowed by the patient's principal pain.

Long-lasting or even permanent relief can be anticipated if the patient is still pain-free three days after the phenol injection. Failure to obtain relief may be due to too few injections being given to cover adequately all the nerve roots innervating the painful area, or to the needle being inserted at the wrong place.

The return of pain after a period of relief may be due to the spread of tumour to another area or to the occurrence of incident pain.

**Results.**—The results of treatment depend largely upon the selection of patients and the other factors discussed above. Maher[65] reported complete relief in 61 (75 per cent) out of 81 cases when intrathecal phenol was used below the level of T 3. Other workers have not achieved such a high success rate. Gordon and Goel[70] used this technique on 37 patients and reported complete relief in 51 per cent and moderate to good relief in a further 30 per cent of patients. Nathan[71] reported that 77 per cent of patients obtained relief after cordotomy compared with 54 per cent after phenol injections, but that after phenol motor function in the legs was less affected and the incidence of sphincter trouble was only 12 per cent.

**Complications.**—The possible complications of this technique are the same as those described in the section on subarachnoid alcohol block.

The risk of interfering with the control of bladder or bowel function must always be borne in mind, but by using a meticulous technique the incidence can be kept down to about 5 per cent if the block is unilateral. Temporary difficulty with micturition may occur necessitating the use of an indwelling catheter for a few days or a week.

**Intrathecal phenol in the relief of spasticity.**—Intrathecal phenol, using either glycerine or Myodil as a solvent, has a most useful application in the relief of spasticity and the pain associated with flexor spasms.[72] 7·5 per cent–10 per cent phenol in Myodil is a suitable solution to use for these patients.

**Intrathecal Chlorocresol**

Maher[73] suggested using a 2 per cent solution of chlorocresol in glycerine as an alternative to phenol. Chlorocresol appears to have a delayed effect compared with phenol in glycerine and there are no immediate sensory changes or paraesthesiae. Fewer nerve roots are affected, so that a second injection may be required after three weeks. The higher proportion of success obtained with chlorocresol may be due to the diffusion affecting a greater length of nerve root. Swerdlow[74] concluded that intrathecal chlorocresol is marginally more effective than phenol, but the complication rate is higher.

For rectal, coccygeal and sacrosciatic pain the suggested dose of the solution is 0·5 ml; for the upper lumbar segments 0·75 ml; and for the thoracic segments 1·0 ml. This technique appears to be a more effective way of relieving the pain associated with carcinoma of the lung, especially that from a Pancoast tumour.

## Epidural Injection

The success achieved with intrathecal phenol solution has led to the use of this solution for epidural block in patients with pain due to malignant disease. By performing an epidural block with phenol at the T 12–L 1 space it is possible to interrupt sympathetic fibres and hence relieve cancer pain, particularly when it is due to involvement of viscera or blood vessels. Patients with perineal pain due to a carcinoma of the rectum are not always adequately relieved by a somatic block with intrathecal phenol. By performing an epidural block with phenol in glycerine at T 12–L 1 space, such cases can often be rendered pain-free. Doughty[75] suggested a dose of 5 ml of 5 per cent phenol in glycerine. If necessary the injection can be repeated after a few days using 7·5 ml of 7½ per cent or even 10 per cent phenol in glycerine. This block is especially effective in relieving the spasms of burning pain and tenesmus associated with advanced carcinoma of the rectum.

An epidural block may be preferred to an intrathecal one in the cervical or upper thoracic regions for patients with incurable malignant disease, but compared with subarachnoid injections, the technique is less precise in localising the solution to the affected nerve root. Moreover, because of the large doses of neurolytic agent used in the epidural approach, accidental dural puncture, if unrecognised, may lead to extensive neurological damage. Following a test dose of 0·2 ml of 7–10 per cent phenol in glycerine, Swerdlow[74] has advocated that 2 ml of the solution is injected into the epidural space for each nerve root to be blocked for intractable malignant pain above D6.

**Epidural injections for sciatica.**—The injection of local anaesthetic into the epidural space has been used successfully in the last decade in the treatment of sciatica, and the results of a large series have been described by Swerdlow and Sayle Creer.[76] In the lumbar approach for this condition, 10 ml of 1 per cent lignocaine or 0·25 per cent bupivacaine are injected. Many clinicians prefer the caudal approach to the epidural space using up to 30 ml of 0·5 per cent lignocaine. The injection is repeated at weekly or fortnightly intervals. Over half of the patients with subacute pain are helped by this treatment.

## Intrathecal and Epidural Narcotics

The discovery of opiate receptors in the dorsal horn of the spinal cord led to the idea that the subarachnoid injection of small doses of opiates could provide segmental analgesia by direct action at these sites.[77] Wang and associates[78] reported that intrathecal morphine in a dose of 0·5 to 1·0 mg was able to produce up to 24 hours relief in patients with severe intractable pain from pelvic malignancy. Other narcotics were shown to have similar effects and also that comparable results could be achieved by injecting morphine into the epidural space.[79] Using low dose morphine (2–3 mg) in 10 ml of 10 per cent dextrose by epidural injection, Magora and colleagues[80] reported good pain relief lasting 8 hours in 56 per cent of patients, especially after surgery and trauma and in patients with advanced peripheral vascular disease.

When pethidine (Demerol) 100 mg in 10 ml of physiological saline was used epidurally, there was a rapid transfer of the drug to the CSF which coincided with the onset of pain relief.[81] This technique gave good relief of severe postoperative pain for 6 hours, but was sometimes associated with transient hypotension and hypercarbia. Fentanyl (Sublimaze) in a dose of 0·1 mg diluted in normal saline has also been used epidurally for effective postoperative pain relief[82] and because of its high lipid solubility, insignificant concentrations appear in the plasma.[83]

Diamorphine in a dose of 2·5–5·0 mg diluted with saline is a more suitable agent for epidural injection than morphine because it is more lipophilic, but although longer acting it is overall less effective and reliable than fentanyl. These drugs may gain access to the receptor sites by axonal spread, as is thought to happen with local anaesthetics after epidural injection.

Morphine has a low lipid solubility and although effective intrathecally, it may persist in the CSF for long periods with the consequent possibility of delayed respiratory depression. If morphine is employed, it is imperative to use special preparations which do not contain preservative as these could possibly have a neurolytic effect or cause arachnoiditis, especially if injected intrathecally.

These techniques appear to have applications in the relief of pain in the postoperative period, in labour, in peripheral ischaemia and for easing intractable pain in terminal cancer.

The advantages, over the use of local anaesthetics, are that there are no detectable motor or sensory changes apart from analgesia and moreover the troublesome effects of autonomic blockade are avoided. As the effects of opiates on the gut are lessened, there should be a lower incidence of postoperative ileus.

A serious complication is the risk of severe respiratory depression which, in the case of intrathecal morphine, may be delayed for many hours.[84,85] This complication is presumably due to the narcotic in the CSF reaching the brain stem by a process of passive diffusion and so depressing the respiratory centre. This respiratory depression can be reversed by intravenous naloxone, although the analgesia persists. Further episodes of respiratory arrest may occur for up to 24 hours after the initial injection of morphine and require further doses of naloxone. This serious and delayed complication is the main limiting factor in the application of these interesting new developments and their place in clinical practice is not yet established.

## Percutaneous Electrical Cordotomy

Anterolateral cordotomy is the most satisfactory technique for the long-term relief of intractable pain due to malignancy, but it involves a major operation, with a variable mortality and morbidity, in patients who may be a poor operative risk.

The development of the technique of percutaneous electrical cordotomy[86–89] has been an important advance in this field, as it affords satisfactory pain relief in patients who may be too ill to submit to open surgical cordotomy. Most patients undergoing this procedure can leave hospital within a few days and may well submit to this type of cordotomy when major surgery would be rejected.

The technique used by Lipton[89] is to insert a spinal needle laterally, under x-ray control, between the first and second cervical vertebrae into the subarachnoid space. The aim of the technique is to place the point of the needle in front of the dentate ligament (ligamentum denticulum) (see Fig. 8) which is identified by injecting a mixture of CSF and iophendylate injection BP. This emulsion sinks down on to the ligament, which is recognised as a line on the lateral x-ray. An electrode, which is insulated apart from its terminal 2 mm, is introduced through the needle and inserted into the anterolateral column of the cord, the depth of penetration being assessed from an anteroposterior film. During insertion of the needle, impedence (electrical resistance) measurements are made to assess the position of the needle point. While the exposed tip is lying in the cerebrospinal fluid, the resistance falls to a lower level (200 ohm). It rises as the needle begins to enter the cord and when the conducting tip is no longer in contact with the CSF but entirely within the cord, it rises to 800 ohm. This is taken as the end point and prevents the needle penetrating too deeply.

If the tip of the electrode is situated too far posteriorly and is lying in the motor tract,

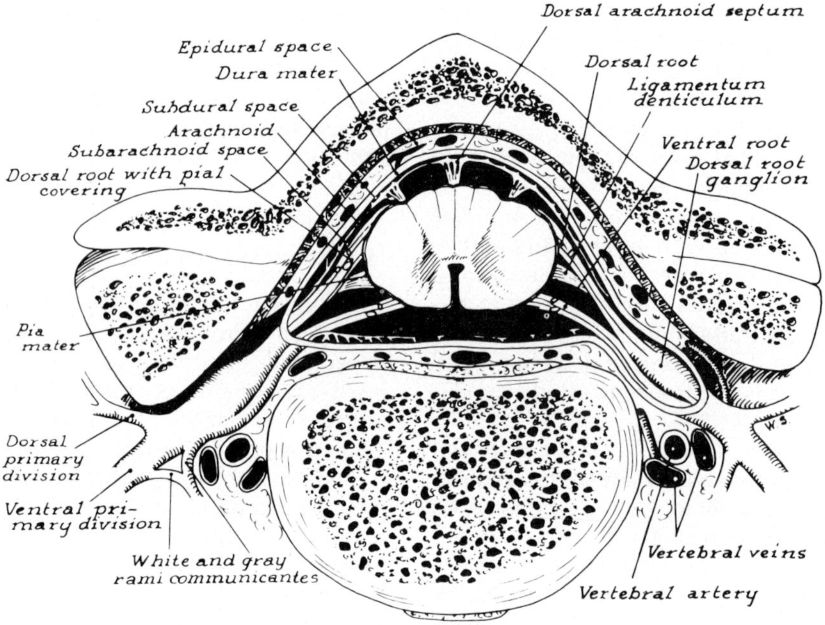


33/FIG. 8.—Cross-section of spinal cord in the spinal canal showing its meningeal coverings and the manner of exit of the spinal nerves (after Rauber). (From *Functional Neuroanatomy* courtesy of the editor, N. B. Everett and publishers, Lea and Febiger)

stimulation of the cord by passing a current through the electrode at 2 Hz, causes movement of the limbs or body of the same side (ipsilateral). Movement of the neck of the same side indicates that the electrode tip is placed too far anteriorly and is in the anterior horn cells. With correct positioning there is no movement but there may be paraesthesiae on the opposite (contralateral) side when stimulated at 100 Hz. The anterolateral tract is then coagulated by a radio frequency current to produce analgesia in the contralateral side. With accurate placement of the electrode this analgesia can be localised to one quadrant of the body (body and arm or body and leg). Coagulation is continued until there is loss of sensation to pinprick over the painful area, together with a few segments above and below. This technique gives good results for unilateral pain up to the C5 dermatome. Above this level the pain fibres ascend three or four segments before crossing to the anterolateral quadrant on the opposite side and so a lesion at C1–2 space will only produce analgesia up to C5.

In fifty-two patients Lipton achieved effective pain relief in 67 per cent and partial relief in 13 per cent.

**Complications.**—Percutaneous electrical cordotomy is relatively free from side-effects, although retention of urine may occur, especially after bilateral cordotomy. Headache is an almost invariable occurrence, while hyperalgesia and transient weakness may develop occasionally.

Respiratory embarrassment is a hazard of high cervical cordotomy and Mullan and Hosobuchi[90] reported nine fatalities in 400 cases due to this complication. It occurs because fibres descending from the medullary centre to the respiratory muscles lie very close to the lateral spinothalamic tract and are damaged by the cordotomy. These patients are able to maintain adequate ventilation while they are awake but during sleep respiration becomes ineffective and may require assistance. Six of Mullan and Hosobuchi's patients died during their sleep.

This hazard exists when bilateral cordotomies

are undertaken in the anterior quadrants of the cord and when unilateral lesions are produced in patients with impaired pulmonary function. Caution must be exercised in such cases as well as care and skill in localising the cordotomy to that part of the anterolateral column which is not essential for respiration.

In order to avoid this complication Lin and co-workers[88] described an anterior approach to the lower cervical cord for percutaneous cordotomy. The spinal needle is inserted below the origin of the phrenic nerve between the carotid sheath and the oesophagus and trachea. Under x-ray control the needle traverses an intervertebral disc and enters the anterolateral quadrant of the cord. Analgesia is produced by inserting an electrode and applying radio frequency current. Using this technique these authors claim it is possible to produce segmental analgesia in the thoracic and lumbar regions, sparing the sacral segments and so having a lower incidence of bladder complications. The upper cervical approach, however, probably gives better pain relief.

### Alcohol Injection of the Pituitary

Hormone ablation techniques such as orchidectomy, adrenalectomy and hypophysectomy are well-established procedures which may produce dramatic pain relief in patients with advanced hormone-dependent malignant tumours and may occasionally result in striking regression in the disease.

Moricca used chemical hypophysectomy for pain relief in patients with advanced hormone-dependent tumours, such as carcinoma of the breast, and this technique has been extended for pain relief in patients with any form of advanced carcinoma.[91,92] Moricca[91] considered that hormonal control exists to some degree in all malignant tumours.

This procedure is carried out using an image intensifier to control the position of a 15 cm trocar and cannula which is inserted through the nose and into the sphenoidal sinus. The trocar is then advanced in the midline through the bone at the base of the pituitary fossa into the pituitary gland itself just inferior to the posterior clinoid process. Having confirmed the position by injecting a radio-opaque dye, up to 1 ml of absolute alcohol is injected in increments while the pupillary size and light reflex are carefully monitored.

Lipton and associates[93] reported that 40 per cent of patients had complete pain relief for varying periods following this procedure and 30 per cent obtained partial relief. The injection can be repeated if the pain recurs.

The mechanism by which pain is relieved in non-hormone dependent tumours is uncertain but, in addition to the endocrine changes produced by this injection, it is possible that central pain transmission is affected by retrograde spread of the alcohol to the hypothalamus. The complications which have been reported with this technique include diabetes insipidus, meningeal irritation, diplopia, hemianopia, ptosis and CSF rhinorrhoea.

### Cryoanalgesia

The use of extreme cold to produce prolonged interruption of conduction in peripheral nerves is another physical method used in the management of chronic pain.[94] It is a direct development of the well recognised numbing effect of severe cold and the ability to perform painless amputations of limbs by refrigeration anaesthesia. There is less fibrous tissue reaction than after other destructive procedures and a lower incidence of neuralgia than with chemical agents such as alcohol and phenol, which can produce incomplete destruction of nerves. Cryoanalgesia does not result in neuroma formation. There is total functional loss in peripheral nerves after a cryolesion, due to a second degree nerve injury, based on Sunderland's[95] classification. Wallerian degeneration with axonal disintegration occurs, but the epineurium and perineurium remain intact so that nerve regeneration and recovery occurs after a period of weeks, depending on the rate and the distance of axonal regrowth that is required.

The maintenance of extreme cold by the absorption of heat from the tissues, is based on the Joule-Thomson effect. This occurs when the refrigerant gas, either nitrous oxide or carbon dioxide at about 45–60 kgf/cm$^2$ expands and cools to about $-75°$ C to $-70°$ C as it flows through a small nozzle. The inner surface of the tip of the cryoprobe is cooled by the gas and in turn heat is absorbed from the surrounding tissues. A suitable apparatus is the Lloyd Spembly Neurostat which incorporates a thermocouple in the cryoprobe so that the temperature at the tip can be monitored. It is important to place the probe within a few millimetres of the nerve to ensure that the latter is included in the ice ball and so suffers a cold injury. To help achieve accurate positioning it is possible to stimulate through the cryoprobe and so elicit the patient's pain when it is adjacent to the nerve. The duration of relief after producing a cryolesion is between 2 weeks and 5 months.[96] In patients with chronic pain, it may not produce permanent relief, but it is particularly useful in post-traumatic and postoperative pain. Blocking the intercostal nerves at the end of a thoracotomy under direct vision or by the external approach, significantly reduces the need for narcotic analgesics.[10] It can also be used for fractured ribs or intercostal neuralgia. Cryoanalgesia may be contra-indicated with mixed nerves because of the loss of motor function that occurs. This technique has also been used successfully in treating patients with intractable perineal pain, especially from pelvic cancer and coccydynia.[97] The cryoprobe was inserted into the sacral canal through the sacral hiatus and lesions were produced bilaterally on the posterior primary rami of the lower three sacral nerve roots. The best results were achieved in patients who received repeated and prolonged freeze applications.

The cryoprobe should not be used in the paravertebral space in the dural cuff region because of the risk of the lesion spreading to involve the spinal cord, by causing thrombosis of its main thoraco-lumbar feeder artery and so producing spinal cord ischaemia. It is also important to allow sufficient time for the tissues to thaw fully before the cryoprobe is withdrawn, otherwise nerves and blood vessels which may still be adhering to it could be accidentally torn.

A further problem with percutaneous use is that retrograde freezing along the cryoprobe may cause localised full-thickness destruction of the skin. This may be prevented by trickling hot water over the entry site of the probe during the freeze cycle.

## Electrical Neuromodulation

The use of electrical stimulation to produce pain relief by modifying the input of noxious stimuli to the central nervous system is based on the Gate Control Theory of Melzack and Wall. It is postulated that it is the small fibres which are transmitting impulses evoked by noxious stimuli and pain is produced if these gain access to higher centres in the central nervous system. By stimulating the large fibres electrically, it is believed that there will be suppression of small fibre activity, thus preventing the onward transmission of noxious impulses so that pain is no longer felt. It has also been suggested that the beneficial effects of electrical neuromodulation could be due to the production of endogenous morphine-like substances, as high levels of encephalins have been found in the cerebrospinal fluid following stimulation of brain electrodes for pain relief.[98]

### Transcutaneous Electrical Nerve Stimulation

Such stimulation is via a small portable battery-powered device which usually has a square wave pulse with controls for varying the pulse width, frequency and power. Various types of electrodes are available, some being similar to those used for the electrocardiogram, but the most satisfactory one, the flexible carbon type, are held in place by adhesive tape after application of electrode jelly to the skin. The best position for the electrodes is found by trial and error, the aim being to stimulate through the painful area. Each of the controls is adjusted in turn so that a tingling, pleasant sensation is produced. Initially, three periods of stimulation a day are tried, each lasting about an hour, but patients vary in their requirements and each person has to find the optimum regime for his own needs.

The conditions which might benefit from this treatment include postoperative scar pain, phantom limb pain, post-herpetic neuralgia and low-back pain. This is a useful method of pain relief which is non-invasive, devoid of risk and worth trying in patients with chronic pain which has a cutaneous element and it can produce significant analgesia.[99] There is probably a placebo response present,[100] and the percentage of patients gaining relief is comparable to that achieved in placebo reactors.

### Dorsal Column Stimulation

Stimulation of the large diameter afferent fibres in the dorsal columns of the spinal cord has also been used for pain relief.[101] Electrodes can be implanted surgically inside the dura or epidural electrodes can be inserted for test stimulation. The wires from the electrodes run to a subcutaneous receiver to which the electrical stimulation is transmitted. Despite the initial enthusiasm, this technique has not been adopted widely and, although of some value in carefully selected patients, it is used as a last resort.

### Denervation of the Posterior Vertebral (Facet) Joints

Chronic back pain is commonly due to prolapsed intervertebral discs causing nerve root compression or irritation. Pain can also arise from structures supplied by the posterior primary rami of the spinal nerves and, in particular, from the capsule and articular surfaces of the facet joints as a result of postural abnormalities, degeneration or collapse of the discs or bony structures or repeated trauma. There are seldom any abnormal neurological signs in such patients and straight leg raising is usually unaffected.

As a diagnostic measure, the lower lumbar facet joints can be injected with local anaesthetic. This is performed using the image intensifier, with the patient lying prone, but tilted slightly towards the side being injected in order to visualise the joint spaces in the vertical plane. After infiltration with local anaesthetic, a 22 swg disposable spinal needle is inserted vertically, under x-ray control, into the joint space, which is then injected with 1–2 ml of 0·5 per cent bupivacaine. The addition of 10 mg of methylprednisolone acetate (Depo-medrone) may prolong the duration of pain relief. The injections are usually performed bilaterally at the L3–4, L4–5 and L5–S1 joints, depending on the clinical findings. Pain relief, which may be long lasting, is an indication for denervating the joints.[102]

The posterior primary ramus passes dorsally and runs in a groove at the junction of the superior articular process and transverse process of the vertebra. It divides into a lateral and medial branch, the latter supplying the facet joint and the structures on its medial side. It continues downwards to supply the upper part of the capsule of the facet joint below. Each facet joint is thus supplied by two posterior primary rami, the one at its own level and the one arising from the spinal nerve above. In order to denervate the two lowest facet joints (L4–5 and L5–S1), it is therefore necessary to produce radiofrequency heat coagulation of the posterior primary rami of L3,4 and 5. The technique has been described by Mehta and Sluijter.[103]

With the patient sedated and lying face down, the tissues down to the transverse processes are infiltrated with local anaesthetic. Using x-ray screening, a needle, which is insulated apart from its terminal 4 mm, is inserted on to the junction of the upper border of the transverse process and the body of the vertebra. It is then moved slightly caudally, dorsally, and medially into the groove between the transverse process and the superior articular process of the facet joint where the posterior primary ramus is running.

Thermocoagulation of the nerve is carried out by a radio-frequency current, the temperature of the tip of the needle being maintained at 80° C for 60 seconds. The needle is repositioned so that it lies on the capsule of the facet joint itself and a second lesion is produced at this site. The procedure is repeated over the transverse processes at all three levels (L4, 5 and S1) and on the other side if this is clinically indicated. A machine suitable for this purpose is manufactured by Radionics Inc. of Massachusetts, USA. In selected patients this technique provides effective pain relief, particularly in those who have had no previous back surgery. Up to 60 per cent of patients in this group may benefit but the figure is lower in patients who have already had surgical intervention.

### Phantom Limb Pain

After amputation of a limb, the illusion that a phantom limb is still present is not uncommon, but is usually transient. Approximately 30 per cent of patients, however, suffer phantom limb pain which may develop immediately after amputation or be delayed for some time. It must be distinguished from stump pain which is due to irritation of cut nerves or pressure on a terminal neuroma, or between bone and a poorly fitting prosthesis.

Percussing the sensitive neuroma with a firm object or infiltration with local anaesthetic may afford relief. Resection of the neuroma is often followed by the growth of a new one but refashioning of the stump may be effective in relieving symptoms.

Phantom limb pain may be intermittent or continuous and may be provoked by peripheral stimuli or emotional factors. The pain is often described as a tingling, burning or cramping sensation and, occasionally, is severe, persistent and incapacitating. It occurs more commonly in patients who had pre-existing pain in the limb or if the amputation is delayed for a long period after injury.

Active treatment should be started as soon as possible, including repeated sympathetic blocks with local anaesthetics. If the latter are successful, then phenol sympathetic block should be considered in order to provide prolonged relief. Repeated injections of local anaesthetics into the stump or paravertebral blocks of the nerves supplying the limb may afford temporary relief, the duration of which may increase with each successive injection.

Vibration therapy, or the injection of hypertonic saline into the interspinous ligaments or into the stump itself may also have beneficial effects. Transcutaneous nerve stimulation has also been used successfully and psychological methods including relaxation techniques may be of value.

### Post-Herpetic Neuralgia

Herpes zoster is due to an acute infection of the posterior root ganglia with the varicella zoster virus, which has been lying dormant until falling immunity causes it to become reactivated. It usually occurs in older people and involves one to three nerves. The pain and cutaneous lesions along the segmental distribution of the involved nerves usually subside after 3–4 weeks. In some patients, however, the pain and scarring persist as post-herpetic neuralgia, the incidence of which increases markedly with age. The pain is persistent, demoralising, burning in character and often accompanied by marked hyperaesthesia, which is exacerbated by clothes or the slightest touch over the affected area. There is a tendency for the large sensory nerve fibres to be damaged or destroyed rather than the small unmyelinated fibres, so producing an imbalance in the sensory input to the spinal cord. In accordance with the Gate Control Theory, the preponderance of unmodulated small fibre activity would favour the production of pain sensation. Although many treatments have been advocated, there is no reliable method of relieving this distressing and debilitating condition once it has become established. Painting the eruption with idoxuridine during the acute phase has been advocated as a prophylactic measure to reduce the incidence of neuralgia.[98] Repeated sympathetic blocks with local anaesthetics are well worth trying during the early stages (first 3 months) and it has been claimed that this method of treatment also reduces the occurrence of post-herpetic neuralgia.[104] In the thoracic region, this will necessitate repeated paravertebral blocks of the involved nerves or, preferably, an indwelling epidural catheter for several days. The pain tends to improve slowly but the time scale for this is measured in years. A wide variety of treatments have been advocated and the earlier they are implemented the better the result.

Analgesics may give some relief but on no account should addictive narcotic drugs be prescribed. The combination of tricyclic antidepressants such as amitriptyline and phenothiazine may, on occasions, be helpful. The subcutaneous injection of up to 30 ml of 0·5 per cent marcaine, with or without the addition of 40–80 mg of methylprednisolone below the scarred and hyperaesthetic skin, may be beneficial on some patients. Repeated local anaesthetic blocks of the nerves supplying the affected area are also worth trying. Other methods of treatment which can be used include carbamazepine, cold sprays, vibration and percussion therapy, and transcutaneous nerve stimulation, the latter being very effective in some patients.[105]

## Neuroleptics and Neuroleptanalgesia

(see Chapter 21, p. 654).

## REFERENCES

1. Spence, A. A. and Alexander, J. I. (1971). Mechanisms of postoperative hypoxaemia. *Proc. roy. Soc. Med.*, **65**, 12.
2. Alexander, J. I., Spence, A. A., Parikh, R. K. and Stuart, B. (1973). The role of airway closure in postoperative hypoxaemia: *Brit. J. Anaesth.*, **45**, 34.

3. Parkhouse, J., Lambrechts, W. and Simpson, B. R. J. (1961). The incidence of postoperative pain. *Brit. J. Anaesth.*, **33**, 345.
4. Moore, J. and Dundee, J. W. (1961). Promethazine. Its influence on the course of thiopentone and methohexital anaesthesia. *Anaesthesia*, **16**, 61.
5. Simpson, B. R. J. and Parkhouse, J. (1961). The problem of postoperative pain. *Brit. J. Anaesth.*, **33**, 336.
6. Clutton-Brock, J. (1960). Some pain threshold studies with particular reference to thiopentone. *Anaesthesia*, **15**, 71.
7. Dundee, J. W. (1960). Alterations in response to somatic pain associated with anaesthesia. II. The effect of thiopentone and pentobarbitone. *Brit. J. Anaesth.*, **32**, 407.
8. Bonica, J. J. (1953). *The Management of Pain*. Philadelphia: Lea & Febiger.
9. Bridenbaugh, P. O., Dupen, S. L., Moore, D. C., Bridenbaugh, L. D. and Thompson, G. E. (1973). Postoperative intercostal nerve block analgesia versus narcotic analgesia. *Anesth. Analg. Curr. Res.*, **52**, 81.
10. Glynn, C. J., Lloyd, J. W. and Barnard, J. D. W. (1980). Cryoanalgesia in the management of pain after thoracotomy. *Thorax*, **35**, 325.
11. Simpson, B. R., Parkhouse, J., Marshall, R. and Lambrechts, W. (1961). Extradural analgesia and the prevention of postoperative respiratory complications. *Brit. J. Anaesth.*, **33**, 628.
12. Bromage, P. R. (1967). Extradural analgesia for pain relief. *Brit. J. Anaesth.*, **39**, 721.
13. Spence, A. A., Smith, G., Harris, R. (1970). The influence of postoperative analgesia and operative procedure on postoperative lung function: a comparison of morphine with extradural block. *Anaesthesia*, **25**, 126.
14. Spence, A. A. and Smith, G. (1971). Post-operative analgesia and lung function: a comparison of morphine with extradural block. *Brit. J. Anaesth.*, **43**, 144.
15. Wahba, W. M., Don, H. F. and Craig, D. B. (1975). Postoperative epidural analgesia: effects on lung volumes. *Canad. Anaesth. Soc. J.*, **22**, 519.
16. Wallace, P. G. M. and Norris, W. (1975). The management of postoperative pain. *Brit. J. Anaesth.*, **47**, 113.
17. Bromage, P. R. (1972). Unblocked segments in epidural analgesia for relief of pain in labour. *Brit. J. Anaesth.*, **44**, 676.
18. Parbrook, G. D. (1967). Techniques of inhalational analgesia in the postoperative period. *Brit. J. Anaesth.*, **39**, 730.
19. Parbrook, G. D. (1967). Comparison of trichloroethylene and nitrous oxide as analgesics. *Brit. J. Anaesth.*, **39**, 86.
20. Parbrook, G. D. (1972). Entonox for postoperative analgesia. *Proc. roy. Soc. Med.*, **65**, 8.
21. Bonica, J. J. and Block, R. G. (1974). The management of a pain clinic. In: *Relief of Intractable Pain*, 1st edit., Vol. 1, p. 116. (Monographs in Anesthesiology), ed. by M. Swerdlow. Amsterdam: Excerpta Medica.
22. Mushin, W. W., Swerdlow, M., Lipton, S. and Mehta, M. D. (1977). The pain centre. *Practitioner*, **218**, 439.
23. Swerdlow, M., Mehta, M. D. and Lipton, S. (1978). The role of the anaesthetist in chronic pain management. *Anaesthesia*, **33**, 250.
24. Lloyd, J. W. (1980). The anaesthetist and the pain clinic. *Brit. med. J.*, **281**, 432.
25. Pomerany, B. (1977). Brain opiates at work on acupuncture. *New Scientist*, **73**, 12.
26. Sjohund, B., Terenius, L. and Eriksson, M. (1977). Increased cerebrospinal fluid levels of endorphins after electroacupuncture. *Acta Physiol. Scand.*, **100**, 382.
27. Lipton, S. (1979). In: *The Control of Chronic Pain*. London: Edward Arnold.
28. Williams, N. E. (1977). In: *Persistent Pain: Modern Methods of Treatment*, p. 241. Ed. Lipton, S. London: Academic Press.
29. Melzack, R., Stillwell, D. M. and Fox, E. J. (1977). Trigger points and acupuncture points for pain: correlation and implications. *Pain*, **3**, 3.
30. Kraus, H. (1973). Trigger points. *N.Y. St. J. Med.*, **73**, 1310.
31. Melzack, R. and Wall, P. D. (1965). Pain mechanisms: a new theory. *Science*, **150**, 971.
32. Melzack, R. and Wall, P. D. (1968). Gate control theory of pain. In: *Pain* (Proc. Internat. Symp. organised by the Lab. of Psychophysiol., Faculty of Sciences, Paris, 1967), p. 11. Ed. by A. Soulairac, A. Cahn and J. Charpentier, New York: Academic Press.
33. Moore, D. C. (1979). *Regional Block. A handbook for use in the clinical practice of medicine and surgery*, 4th edit. Springfield, Ill.: Charles C. Thomas.
34. Eriksson, E. (1979). *Illustrated Handbook of Local Anaesthesia*, 2nd edit. London: Lloyd-Luke.
35. Cousins, M. J. and Bridenbaugh, P. O. (1980). *Neural Blockade*. Philadelphia: J. B. Lippincott Co.
36. Mehta, M. (1973). In: *Intractable Pain*. London: W. B. Saunders Co.
37. Sweet, W. T. and Wepsic, J. G. (1974). Controlled thermocoagulation of trigeminal ganglion and rootlets for differential destruction of pain fibres. *J. Neurosurg.*, **40**, 143.
38. Macintosh, R. R. and Mushin, W. W. (1954). *Local Analgesia: Brachial Plexus*, 3rd edit. Edinburgh: E. & S. Livingstone.
39. Holmes, C. McK. (1963). Intravenous regional analgesia. A useful method of producing analgesia of the limbs. *Lancet*, **1**, 245.
40. Bier, A. (1908). Ueber einen neuen Weg Localanasthesie an der Gliedmasse zu erzeugen. *Verh, dtsch. Ges. Chir.*, **37**, 204 (Part II).
41. Ware, R. J. (1975). Intravenous regional anaesthesia using bupivacaine. *Anaesthesia*, **30**, 817.
42. Thorn-Alquist, A. M. (1979). Chapter in *Illustrated Handbook of Local Anaesthesia*, 2nd edit. Ed. Eriksson, E. London: Lloyd-Luke.
43. Hoyle, J. R. (1964). Tourniquet for intravenous regional analgesia. *Anaesthesia*, **19**, 294.
44. Holmes, C. M. (1980). In: *Neural Blockade*, p. 352. Ed. Cousins, M. J. and Bridenbaugh, P. O., Philadelphia: J. B. Lippincott Co.
45. Tucker, G. T. and Boas, R. A. (1971). Pharmacokinetic aspects of intravenous regional anaesthesia. *Anesthesiology*, **34**, 538.
46. Macintosh, R. R. and Bryce-Smith, R. (1953). *Local Analgesia: Abdominal Surgery*. Edinburgh: E. & S. Livingstone.
47. Mehta, M. and Ranger, I. (1971). Persistent abdominal pain. Treatment by nerve block. *Anaesthesia*, **26**, 330.
48. Applegate, W. V. (1972). Abdominal cutaneous nerve entrapment syndrome. *Surgery*, **71**, 118.
49. Macintosh, R. R. and Ostlere, M. (1955). *Local Analgesia: Head and Neck*. Edinburgh: E. & S. Livingstone.

50. Bryce-Smith, R. (1951). Injection of the lumbar sympathetic chain. *Anaesthesia*, **6**, 150.
51. Reid, W., Kennedy, Watt, J. and Gray, T. G. (1970). Phenol injection of the sympathetic chain. *Brit. J. Surg.*, **57**, 45.
52. Bridenbaugh, L. D., Moore, D. C. and Campbell, D. D. (1964). Management of upper abdominal cancer. *J. Amer. med. Ass.*, **190**, 877.
53. Gorbitz, C. and Leavens, M. E. (1971). Alcohol block of the coeliac plexus for control of upper abdominal pain caused by cancer and pancreatitis. *J. Neurosurg.*, **34**, 575.
54. Galizia, E. J. and Lahiri, S. K. (1974). Paraplegia following coeliac plexus block with phenol. *Brit. J. Anaesth.*, **46**, 539.
55. Hannington-Kiff, J. G. (1974). Intravenous regional sympathetic block with guanethidine. *Lancet*, **1**, 1019.
56. Hannington-Kiff, J. G. (1977). Relief of Sudeck's atrophy by regional intravenous guanethidine. *Lancet*, **1**, 1132.
57. Hannington-Kiff, J. G. (1979). Relief of causalgia in limbs by regional intravenous guanethidine. *Brit. med. J.*, **2**, 367.
58. Sternscheim, M. J., Myers, S. J., Frewin, D. B. and Downey, J. A. (1975). Causalgia. *Arch. Phys. Med. Rehab.*, **56**, 58.
59. Doupe, J., Cullen, G. H. and Chance, G. Q. (1944). Post-traumatic pain and the causalgic syndrome. *J. Neurol. Neurosurg. Psychiat.*, **7**, 33.
60. Bergan, J. J. and Conn, J. (1968). Sympathectomy for pain relief. *Med. Clin. N. Amer.*, **52**, 147.
61. Dogliotti, A. M. (1931). Traitement des syndromes douloureux de la périphérie par l'alcoolisation sub-arachnoidienne des racines postérieures à leur émergence de la moelle épinière. *Presse méd.*, **39**, 1249.
62. Dwyer, B. and Gibb, D. (1980). In: *Neural Blockade*, p. 639. Ed. Cousins, M. J. and Bridenbaugh, P. O. Philadelphia: J. B. Lippincott, Co.
63. Maher, R. M. (1955). Relief of pain in incurable cancer. *Lancet*, **1**, 18.
64. Maher, R. M. (1957). Neurone selection in relief of pain. Further experiences with intrathecal injections. *Lancet*, **1**, 16.
65. Maher, R. M. (1960). Further experiences with intrathecal and subdural phenol. Observations on two forms of pain. *Lancet*, **1**, 895.
66. Smith, M. C. (1964). Histological findings following intrathecal injections of phenol solutions for relief of pain. *Brit. J. Anaesth.*, **36**, 387.
67. Nathan, P. W., Sears, T. A. and Smith, M. C. (1965). Effects of phenol solutions on the nerve roots of the cat: an electrophysiological and histological study. *J. neurol. Sci.*, **2**, 7.
68. Maher, R. and Mehta, M. (1977). In: *Persistent Pain: Modern Methods of Treatment*, Vol. 1, p. 72. Ed. Lipton, S. London: Academic Press.
69. Nathan, P. W. and Sears, T. A. (1960). Effects of phenol on nervous conduction. *J. Physiol.* (*Lond.*), **150**, 565.
70. Gordon, R. A. and Goel, S. B. (1963). Intrathecal phenol block in treatment of intractable pain of malignant disease. *Canad. Anaesth. Soc. J.*, **10**, 357.
71. Nathan, P. W. (1967). Some aspects of the cancer problem. *Brit. med. J.*, **1**, 168.
72. Nathan, P. W. (1959). Intrathecal phenol to relieve spasticity in paraplegia. *Lancet*, **2**, 1099.
73. Maher, R. M. (1963). Intrathecal chlorocresol (parachlormetacresol) in the treatment of pain in cancer. *Lancet*, **1**, 965.
74. Swerdlow, M. (1973). Intrathecal chlorocresol. *Anaesthesia*, **28**, 297.
75. Doughty, A. G. (1964). Personal communication.
76. Swerdlow, M. and Sayle Creer, W. (1970). A study of extradural medication in the relief of the lumbosciatic syndrome. *Anaesthesia*, **25**, 341.
77. Yaksh, T. L. and Rudy, T. A. (1976). Analgesia mediated by a direct final action of narcotics. *Science*, **192**, 1357.
78. Wang, J. K., Nauss, L. A. and Thomas, J. E. (1979). Pain relief by intrathecally applied morphine in man. *Anesthesiology*, **50**, 149.
79. Behar, M., Magora, F., Olshwang, D. and Davidson, J. T. (1979). Epidural morphine in treatment of pain. *Lancet*, **1**, 527.
80. Magora, F., Olshwang, D., Eimerl, D., Shorr, J., Katzenelson, R., Cotev, S. and Davidson, J. T. (1980). Observations in extradural morphine analgesia in various pain conditions. *Brit. J. Anaesth.*, **52**, 247.
81. Cousins, M. J., Mather, L. E., Glynn, C. J., Wilson, P. R. and Graham, J. R. (1979). Selective spinal analgesia. *Lancet*, **1**, 1141.
82. Wolfe, M. J. and Nicholas, A. D. G. (1979). Selective epidural analgesia. *Lancet*, **2**, 150.
83. Wolfe, M. J. and Davies, G. K. (1980). Analgesic action of extradural fentanyl (Letter). *Brit. J. Anaesth.*, **52**, 357.
84. Glynn, C. J., Mather, L. E., Cousins, M. J., Wilson, P. R. and Graham, J. R. (1979). Spinal narcotics and respiratory depression. *Lancet*, **2**, 356.
85. Davies, G. K., Tolhurst-Cleaver, C. L. and James, T. L. (1980). Respiratory depression after intrathecal narcotics. *Anaesthesia*, **35**, 1080.
86. Mullan, S., Hekmatpanah, J., Dobben, G. and Beckman, F. (1965). Percutaneous, intramedullary cordotomy utilizing the unipolar anodal electrolytic lesion. *J. Neurosurg.*, **22**, 548.
87. Rosomoff, H. L., Carroll, F., Brown, J. and Sheptak, P. (1965). Percutaneous radiofrequency cervical cordotomy: technique. *J. Neurosurg.*, **23**, 639.
88. Lin, P. M., Gildenberg, P. L. and Polakoff, P. P. (1966). An anterior approach to percutaneous lower cervical cordotomy. *J. Neurosurg.*, **25**, 553.
89. Lipton, S. (1968). Percutaneous electrical cordotomy in relief of intractable pain. *Brit. med. J.*, **2**, 210.
90. Mullan, S. and Hosobuchi. Y. (1968). Respiratory hazards of high cervical percutaneous cordotomy. *J. Neurosurg.*, **28**, 291.
91. Moricca, G. (1976). Neuro-adenolysis for diffuse unbearable cancer pain. In: *Advances in Pain Research and Therapy*, Vol 1, p. 863, Ed. J. Bonica, and D. Albe-Fessard. New York: Raven Press.
92. Tindall, G. T., Nixon, D. W., Christy, J. H. and Neill, J. D. (1977). Pain relief in metastatic carcinoma other than breast and prostate gland following transphenoidal hypophysectomy. *J. Neurosurg.*, **47**, 659.
93. Lipton, S., Miles, J. B., Williams, N. and Bark-Jones, M. (1978). Pituitary injection of alcohol for widespread cancer pain. *Pain*, **5**, 73.
94. Lloyd, J. W., Barnard, J. D. W. and Glynn, C. J. (1976). Cryoanalgesia. A new approach to pain relief. *Lancet*, **2**, 932.

95. Sunderland, S. (1978). *Nerves and Nerve Injuries*, 2nd edit., p. 131. Edinburgh: Churchill-Livingstone.
96. Barnard, J. D. W., Lloyd, J. W. and Glynn, C. J. (1978). Cryosurgery in the management of intractable facial pain. *Brit. J. Oral Surg.*, **16**, 135.
97. Evans, P. J. D., Lloyd, J. W. and Jack, T. M. (1981). Cryoanalgesia for intractable perineal pain. *J. Roy. Soc. Med.*, **74**, 804.
98. Lipton, S. (1979). In: *Relief of Pain in Clinical Practice*. Oxford: Blackwell Scientific Ltd.
99. Long, D. M. (1976). Cutaneous afferent stimulation for the relief of pain. *Progr. Neurol. Surg.*, **7**, 35.
100. Thorsteinsson, G., Stonnington, H. H., Stillwell, G. K. and Elveback, L. R. (1978). The placebo effect of transcutaneous electrical stimulation. *Pain*, **5**, 31.
101. Shealy, C. N. (1975). Dorsal column stimulation. *Surgic. Neurol.*, **4**, 142.
102. Shealy, C. N. (1975). Percutaneous radiofrequency denervation of spinal facets in treatment for chronic back pain and sciatica. *J. Neurosurg.*, **43**, 448.
103. Mehta, M. and Sluijter, M. E. (1979). The treatment of chronic back pain. A preliminary survey of the effect of radiofrequency denervation of the posterior vertebral joints. *Anaesthesia*, **34**, 768.
104. Colding, A. (1969). The effect of regional sympathetic blocks in the treatment of herpes zoster. *Acta anaesth. scand.*, **13**, 113.
105. Nathan, P. W. and Wall, P. D. (1974). Treatment of post-herpetic neuralgia by prolonged electrical stimulation. *Brit. med. J.*, **3**, 645.

*Section Four*

# THE METABOLIC, DIGESTIVE AND EXCRETORY SYSTEMS

CHAPTER 34

# Anaesthesia and the Gastro-intestinal Tract



## The Oesophagus

The oesophagus, which is about 25 cm long in the adult, extends from the cricopharyngeal sphincter at the level of the sixth cervical vertebra to the gastro-oesophageal junction. It is surrounded by an outer layer of longitudinal muscle with an inner, circular layer. Around the upper third of the oesophagus the latter muscle is striated while the lower part consists of smooth muscle. There is a sphincter at the pharyngo-oesophageal junction and another at the oesophago-gastric junction. The upper sphincter is 1–2 cm in length and is composed of striated circular muscle fibres of the crico-pharyngeus muscle and the circular fibres of the upper oesophagus. It is in a state of tonic contraction with a resting pressure of 15–60 cm of water thus preventing air entering the oesophagus from the pharynx under normal circumstances. The lower oesophageal sphincter (LOS) is a band of circular muscle surrounding the lower end of the oesophagus. It is approximately 3 cm in length and has a resting pressure of 10–15 cm of water.

The nerve supply to the oesophagus is both extrinsic and intrinsic. The former is derived from parasympathetic fibres from the vagi with sympathetic fibres from the superior and inferior cervical, and fourth and fifth thoracic, sympathetic ganglia. Stimulation of the parasympathetic fibres tends to increase the activity of the intestinal smooth muscle while stimulation of the sympathetic fibres tend to decrease the activity and cause contraction of the sphincters. The intrinsic nerve supply includes the myenteric nerve plexus of Auerbach, which lies between the outer longitudinal and the middle circular layers of muscle, and the submucosal plexus of Meissner which lies between the circular layer and the mucosa.

In the normal person a short segment of the lower oesophageal sphincter lies above the diaphragm, the remainder lying within the abdominal cavity. It used to be thought that the part of the sphincter below the diaphragm played an important part in preventing regurgitation, as the increased intra-abdominal pressure would increase the tone in that part of the sphincter lying below the diaphragm. However, Cohen and Harris[1] showed that displacement of the oesophago-gastric sphincter into the thoracic cavity in patients with a hiatus hernia did not necessarily result in reflux. The latter only occurred if the normal muscular tone of the sphincter was significantly reduced. There are a number of other factors that may play a small part in the prevention of reflux of gastric contents into the oesophagus. These include not only the intra-abdominal segment of the oesophagus but also the gastro-oesophageal angle, the diaphragmatic crura and the phreno-oesophageal ligament. However, by far the most important factor is the LOS.

The sphincteric pressure is affected not only by the intrinsic nerve plexus, but is also increased by gastrin released by the mucosa of the gastric antrum in response to the presence of acid. LOS pressure is also increased by alpha-adrenergic agents, acetylcholine, serotonin, histamine and pancreatic polypeptide, and decreased by beta-adrenergic agents, secretin, glucagon and dopamine.[2] Atropine and narcotics also tend to lower LOS pressure, while metoclopramide produces a marked increase.

*Abnormalities*.—While the LOS plays the predominant role in preventing reflux, in those patients in which the pressure is abnormally low, the other factors mentioned above may play a greater role as, for example, in hiatus hernia. In pregnancy, some 30–50 per cent of women have symptoms of heartburn. They have a reduced LOS pressure which returns to normal after the pregnancy and has been shown to correlate closely with the levels of oestrogen and progesterone during pregnancy.[3] The occurrence of reflux depends on an increase in intragastric pressure greater than the increase in LOS pressure and, under normal circumstances, these rise synchronously.[1] However, the presence of a grossly distended stomach and an abnormal LOS response, the presence of a nasogastric tube, or distension of the oesophagus by attempted inflation of the lungs against a closed glottis may all precipitate reflux. The cricopharyngeal sphincter will resist pressures of 100 cm water from below but will open with a positive pressure from above of only 15–25 cm water.[4]

*Posture*.—Although changes in position from supine to foot-down or to head-down produce alterations in intragastric pressure, they do not in a normal, unanaesthetised person, affect the proper functioning of the gastro-oesophageal junction. The effects of the position of a patient during the induction of anaesthesia and paralysis must be considered in relation to the action of the drugs administered at the time, and to the possible responses of that patient. All that can be said with any degree of objectivity is as follows: a steep foot-down tilt prevents the passive flow of fluid towards the oropharynx once paralysis is complete, but it renders tracheal aspiration probable should gastric or oesophageal contents reach the oropharynx by any other means, either before or during the onset of paralysis. A foot-down tilt lowers intragastric pressure, and enhances any adverse effects that the drugs used may have on the patient's circulation. A steep head-down tilt raises intragastric pressure and encourages the passive flow of fluid towards the oropharynx, but makes tracheal aspiration improbable in the presence of total paralysis. The supine, horizontal position combines in some measure the disadvantages of the two positions described, while the lateral position (left or right), used with a head-down tilt, assists fluid to drain away from the area of the glottis.

## Gastric Emptying

The time that the stomach takes to empty after a meal is very variable, even in a normal person. It is influenced principally by the following factors: the type of food eaten (protein leaves more slowly than carbohydrate, while fat is slowest of all), the quantity and the osmotic pressure and, finally, the motility of the stomach. Vagotomy will slow the rate of emptying, as will fear, while excitement increases the rate. There are a number of hormones which will delay gastric emptying.[5]

The more fluid the meal, the quicker it leaves the stomach, so that a slow emptying time is usually associated with food such as meat which contains proteins and can only slowly be rendered fluid or semi-fluid. Large quantities need a long time, and if the meal follows soon after a previous one, a full duodenum may delay stomach emptying.

Hypertonic solutions are delayed in the stomach until they are rendered more nearly isotonic. A marked prolongation of emptying time has been demonstrated by Hunt and his colleagues[6] who added sucrose in varying concentrations up to 25 per cent to a standard test meal.

King[7] demonstrated the influence of some of these factors by comparing a group of fasting but healthy young adults with a series of patients (diabetic and non-diabetic), none of whom had any clinical or radiological evidence of delay in stomach emptying. A volume of 200 ml of fluid containing 50 g of glucose and a little phenol red was given to the young adults. Gastric aspiration was then performed at intervals of 15 minutes up to 2 hours. On average the meal was diluted to about twice the volume, but after two hours an average of 46 ml of fluid containing 0·3 g of glucose remained. Similar solutions, but containing no phenol red, were given to twenty patients two hours before operation and gastric aspiration performed just before anaesthesia was due to be induced. These patients were prepared in the normal manner and premedicated. In ten of them volumes ranging from 100 to 265 ml (average 146 ml) and containing 2–10·2 g of glucose were removed from the stomach, thus demonstrating the influence of such factors as anxiety and premedication upon gastric function.

An easily digested meal will have left the stomach of a normal person in from one and a half to three hours, whereas a more solid one may take as long as four hours. Water, on the other hand, will pass into the duodenum almost as quickly as it is drunk. The introduction of metoclopramide has added a new dimension to gastric emptying. This agent has been shown to increase the rate at which the stomach empties, and also to increase intestinal motility.[8]

It is worth remembering that "There ain't no such thing as an empty stomach,"[9] since normal seretions are continuously produced—up to approximately 50 ml per hour—unless stimulated by food, by the presence of a gastric tube, or by emotion. Gastric secretions contain, amongst other things, about 0·5 per cent free hydrochloric acid.

**Discussion.**—The interplay of fear, disease and drugs on gastric emptying must at all times be present in the mind of an anaesthetist. Normality in this respect is so variable that the potential risk of even a small quantity of gastric secretion entering the respiratory tract must always be borne in mind when a patient's normal protective reflexes are depressed or abolished.

Silent regurgitation of gastric contents has been reported to occur in 25–70 per cent of patients having general anaesthesia, with as many as 76 per cent having tracheal aspiration.[10] Even in intubated patients, silent regurgitation has been reported in 14·5 per cent.[11] The type of cuff on the endotracheal tube plays a significant part in the prevention of aspiration.[12]

## SICKNESS

The syndrome of nausea, retching and vomiting is known as sickness, and each part of it can be distinguished as a separate entity.[13] Nausea is the subjective sensation of the desire to vomit but without any attempt at expulsive movements. It is frequently accompanied by such objective signs as the secretion of saliva, sweating and an increase in pulse rate, and variations in the rate, depth and regularity of respiration. Retching and vomiting, both active expulsive mechanisms, are differentiated by the results of the process, the latter always producing some gastric contents, the former nothing. The mechanism consists of a series of movements designed to squeeze the relaxed stomach between the descending diaphragm and contracting abdominal muscles. The gastro-oesophageal junction and the cricopharyngeal sphincter are open and the oropharynx is enlarged, the palate raised and the larynx held forward with the glottis closed. The act of vomiting is controlled by the vomiting centre situated near the respiratory centre in the medulla.

**Discussion.**—A knowledge of these mechanisms is important to the anaesthetist, particularly when dealing with patients who are likely to have fluid or food in either the oesophagus or stomach when anaesthesia is essential. The cricopharyngeal sphincter is affected both by anaesthetic drugs and muscle relaxants, becoming progressively incompetent as anaesthesia deepens or muscle paresis increases. A fully relaxed sphincter aids the surgeon during oesophagoscopy. Any degree of relaxation, should the position favour it or the intrathoracic pressure be high, may allow fluid retained in the oesophagus to flow or be forced into the pharynx. Pulmonary inflation with high pressures or coughing may cause oesophageal reflux of this type under anaesthesia. The use of suxamethonium is associated with a rise in intragastric pressure in some patients. There is no evidence to suggest that suxamethonium has a direct effect on the smooth muscle of the stomach, whilst a direct relationship between the rise in intragastric pressure (due to an increase in intra-abdominal pressure) and abdominal muscle tone has been shown.[14] Quite remarkable pressures can be applied directly to the stomach when it is full of air or fluid without evidence of reflux into the oesophagus in normal patients. During anaesthesia, provided the active processes of retching or vomiting are entirely suppressed and the gastro-oesophageal valve is not made incompetent, stomach contents will not enter the oesophagus in normal patients, even when postural changes, which would normally aid their movement, are taking place. Should a patient, however, be able to bring into action any part of the active mechanism of vomiting, then aspiration of stomach or oesophageal contents into the respiratory tract is always a potential danger due to the depressant effect of the anaesthetic or relaxant drugs upon laryngeal activity.

The syndrome of sickness may be initiated centrally by the effects of drugs or of hypoxia, or by stimulation of afferents throughout the body. Typically, these impulses arise from the stomach or other parts of the gastro-intestinal tract, and during light anaesthesia they may be started by surgical manipulation or by the anaesthetist inserting an airway or trying to introduce an irritant vapour too quickly. Afferent impulses can arise from almost any part of the body, and an important source is in the vestibular apparatus of the labyrinth.

## Preparation for Anaesthesia

Patients for elective operations should be prepared for anaesthesia—local or general—by pre-operative starvation for five hours. The last meal taken prior to this period should be light, preferably containing very little protein, and small in quantity. When the patient is to be anaesthetised as an out-patient, these instructions must be carefully explained, and it may be advisable to emphasise them by enlarging upon the unpleasantness, and perhaps even upon the danger, of sickness if they are not observed. Children need special care since they are unlikely to co-operate. The danger of hypoglycaemia in this group must always be remembered.[15] When they are out-patients it is safest to give the parent or responsible person written instructions so that no doubt can exist, and to stress that starvation includes both food and fluid. Out-patient operations are best performed in the early morning.

Unless the patient is known to have been prepared in the manner described, it must be assumed that the stomach is not empty and all non-urgent operations must be postponed until it is. An exception may be made for relatively minor operations which can be easily performed with local analgesia. If an operation is delayed, the physical condition and mental state of the patient must be taken into account when estimating how long to wait for normal emptying to be completed.

A surprisingly large number of factors can be responsible for the presence of material in the oesophagus or stomach of a patient presented for anaesthesia. The anaesthetist must be aware of these possibilities, which are listed in Table 1.[16]

## Preparation for Emergency Operations

It is possible to differentiate surgical emergencies into those which are true and will tolerate no delay in their treatment, or at the very most a short period for essential preparation, and those which are relative in their acuteness and can safely be delayed while the essential points of normal preparation are carried out. The final decision upon the time for operation can only be taken by the surgeon, but part of the responsibility for adequate preparation must fall upon the anaesthetist. The importance of this division of emergency cases lies in the increased safety that goes with adequate preparation before anaesthesia and operation—and furthermore in the greater comfort for the patient. In the true emergency, when there is any doubt about the oesophagus or stomach being empty, steps must be taken to drain them.

In most patients—92 out of the 110 patients investigated by Edwards and his colleagues[17]—the material is likely to be liquid, so that a small-bore stomach tube is helpful. A 6-gauge (4 mm) tube or a Ryle's tube (4 mm) which has not become flabby from repeated boiling, will cause little discomfort to the patient and enable

34/TABLE 1
CONDITIONS IN WHICH THE STOMACH MAY NOT BE EMPTY

| | |
|---|---|
| Material in the oesophagus | Oesophageal obstruction or pouch.<br>Pyothorax with oesophageal fistula. |
| Material introduced into the stomach from above | Food and drink given, i.e. lack of pre-operative "preparation".<br>Fluids given for medical reasons, e.g. to diabetics, or stomach washouts not completely removed.<br>Swallowed blood. Bleeding from nose, mouth or pharynx, due to accident or operation. |
| Material introduced into the stomach from below | Intestinal obstruction.<br>Ileus. |
| Material from the stomach itself | Normal or hypersecretion.<br>Bleeding from ulcer, neoplasm, or site of operation. |
| Prolonged emptying time of the stomach | A. Pyloric obstruction (including congenital pyloric obstruction).<br>B. Dilatation of the stomach.<br>C. Reflex I. Emotional states. Pain. Parturition. Shock. Accidents—e.g. cuts, fractures, burns.<br>II. Peritoneal irritation, e.g. perforated ulcer, twisted ovarian tumour.<br>D. Abdominal distension, e.g. large tumours, pregnancy at term. Gross ascites.<br>E. Severe illness. Toxaemia. Near-moribund patients.<br>F. Drugs. Morphia, papaveretum, pethidine, scopolamine, atropine. Most anaesthetic agents. |

Several causes are often present together, e.g. a patient brought to the theatre for resuture of a "burst abdomen" may be in poor general condition and may have taken food or fluids just before the incident. There will be shock, emotional disturbance, and peritoneal irritation, and morphine may have been given.

a lot of information to be gleaned about the stomach contents. Moreover, the surgeon may well require such a tube for the post-operative period. A double-lumen tube (the Salem Sump, Fig. 1) is largely replacing the old single-lumen tube in popularity. It is plastic and disposable and allows fluid to be instilled down the narrow bore whilst suction drainage can be applied to the larger lumen. Ideally these tubes are passed through the nose whilst the patient is still conscious and can aid the process with their swallowing reflex. However, these tubes can be passed satisfactorily in the anaesthetised patient particularly if the plastic tube is stiffened by keeping in a refrigerator prior to use.

Patients with early acute appendicitis and women in labour are often treated as exceptions to the general rule for gastric lavage—the former because nausea, vomiting and then a period of anorexia are typical of the disease, so that the patient is usually presented for anaesthesia with an empty stomach. If the inflammation has progressed to peritonitis, however, there may be some ileus, when full precautions must be taken. Obstetric patients are considered in greater detail in Chapter 40.

Even after apparently successful preparation, an anaesthetic technique must be chosen so as to lessen any risk of aspiration into the respiratory tract should any material remain in the oesophagus or stomach.

Whenever it is proposed to induce anaesthesia

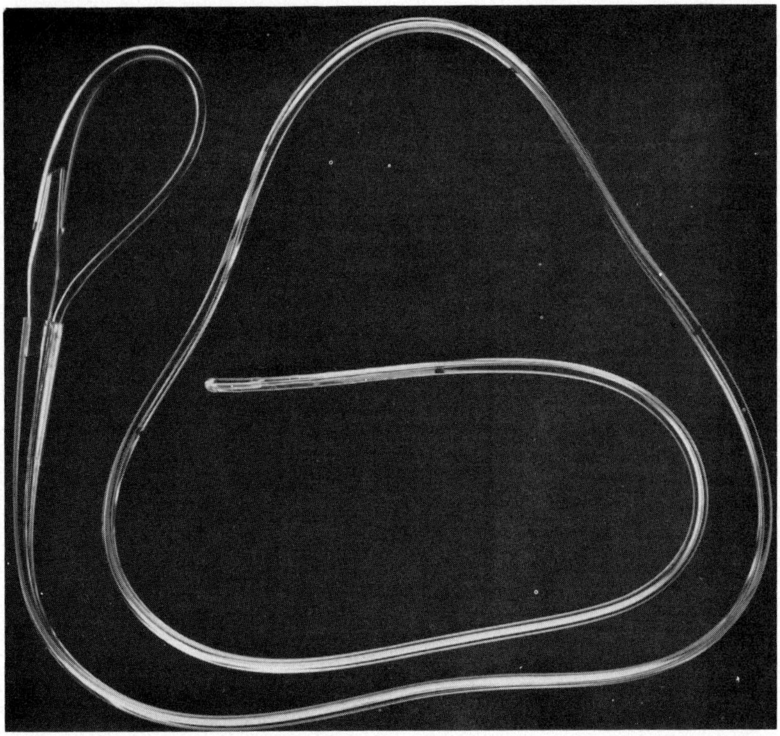

34/FIG. 1.—Salem sump tube.

with the risk of vomiting or regurgitation present, the essential apparatus must be checked beforehand. This must include an efficient suction apparatus. The patient should be induced on the operating table or a trolley which can rapidly be tilted head-down.

### General Anaesthesia

Safety during general anaesthesia for these cases can only be assured by a cuffed endotracheal tube. The most critical period is that between the loss of the patient's protective pharyngeal reflexes and the inflation of the cuff of the endotracheal tube in the trachea. It is this interval that must be kept to an absolute minimum. Pre-oxygenation with 100 per cent oxygen with a well-fitting face mask for 3 minutes is mandatory, and an open vein must be available. In a patient with a stable cardiovascular system, induction may be carried out with an intravenous agent followed by suxamethonium. Cricoid pressure should be applied immediately prior to induction of anaesthesia, by a competent assistant who has been told exactly what is required. All too often pressure is applied too late and released before the endotracheal cuff has been inflated.

In the very sick even a small dose of an intravenous inducing agent may be considered unsafe and an inhalational technique may be advisable. The use of cyclopropane and oxygen can be invaluable under these circumstances. In some centres this situation is considered a suitable justification for an awake intubation, whilst in others, ketamine has been recommended for the induction of anaesthesia. Once anaesthesia has been achieved suxamethonium may be given intravenously and intubation carried out. In all cases the dose of suxamethonium given must be adequate to produce complete paralysis, because attempts to intubate a partially paralysed patient will greatly increase not only the risk of regurgitation but also of active vomiting. If cricoid pressure is being carried out, the latter may result in oesophageal rupture.[18] Muravchick and associates,[14] using electromyography of the abdominal muscles, found a rise of intragastric pressure associated with fasciculations. They recommend that an anaesthetic induction sequence for patients with full stomachs should include pre-treatment with a non-depolarising muscle relaxant and generous doses of both thiopentone and suxamethonium.

The position of the patient at the time of induction will depend on the technique that has been chosen. Cricoid pressure which compresses the oesophagus between the back of the cricoid cartilage and the anterior surface of the body of the sixth cervical vertebra is best applied with the patient supine and horizontal. If competent assistance is not available, induction and intubation are best carried out with the patient head down in the *left* lateral position. Induction may be achieved with either of the two methods already described. The advantages of this position are: firstly, should any regurgitation occur tracheal soiling will not result. It is well known that position *per se* does not affect the intersphincteric pressure of the cardio-oesophageal junction; secondly, the tongue will fall to the side of the mouth allowing easy insertion of the laryngoscope blade with a clear view of the cords. Thirdly, in the pregnant patient compression of the inferior vena cava is prevented.

**Discussion**

The most important aspect of the management of a patient with a potentially full stomach is the awareness of the dangers. These include the realisation that despite the passage of a tube into the stomach, irrespective of the bore, both liquid and solid material may still be present within the stomach, and that the presence of a tube in the oesophagus at the time of induction is more likely to result in regurgitation from incompetence of the lower oesophageal junction and failure of cricoid pressure to be fully effective.

The attempts to minimise the effects of inhaled matter have centred not only on *mechanical emptying*, but also on *reduction of the acidity* of gastric contents and the increase of LOS pressure. The use of antacids to neutralise gastric acid is based on the belief that it is of critical importance for the gastric pH to be above 2·5, thus preventing a severe reaction within the lungs.[19] However, values greater than this have resulted in pulmonary complications, and a lower limit of pH 3·5 has been suggested.[2] While the special problems surrounding the obstetric patient will be considered in greater detail in Chapter 40, the general effects of antacids are of interest. Each contains stabilisers and preservatives which may contribute to the pulmonary lesion if inhaled, as may the alkalinity of the fluid, if complete mixing with the gastric contents has not occurred.[20] In the past, magnesium trisilicate has been recommended, but it has been suggested that because it is particulate, these very particles can cause pulmonary irritation. To this end, a non-particulate alkali such as sodium citrate might prove safer.[21]

The use of *cimetidine* and *ranitidine*, specific H-2 receptor antagonists which depress gastric acid production, have been advocated.[22] The drugs do not alter the volume of gastric content or the acidity of fluid already present and will only have a significant effect on gastric pH some 45 minutes after intravenous injection.[23] An intravenous dose of 200 mg, given one hour before induction for emergency surgery, produced a pH of gastric contents in excess of 2·5 in 80 per cent of patients. Howe and associates[24] demonstrated that cimetidine crosses the placental barrier, but they did not observe any untoward effects on either the fetus or newborn.

Much interest has been evoked in the consideration of drugs that will alter the LOS pressure and therefore the risk of regurgitation of gastric contents. The basic factors that alter the competence of the gastro-oesophageal junction have already been noted with the LOS pressure being of paramount importance. Drugs used in anaesthesia which alter this pressure are of significance. Atropine is known to decrease LOS pressure within 5 minutes of intravenous injection for a period of 60 minutes. This drug is still used extensively in routine premedication[25] to overcome the vagal effects of laryngoscopy and intubation, despite the fact that the response to the latter is sympathetic rather than parasympathetic.[26] Other drugs which decrease LOS pressure include hyoscine and glycopyrrolate.[27,28] Pethidine and morphine also decrease the pressure as do promethazine and droperidol. While metoclopramide markedly increases LOS pressure, it will not always overcome the effects of atropine or pethidine.[29] However, despite antacids and cricoid pressure, fatal aspiration can still occur,[30] and an awareness of this is absolutely vital.

**Treatment of Vomiting or Regurgitation Occurring during Anaesthesia**

If stomach or oesophageal contents enter the pharynx when the trachea is unprotected, urgent treatment is necessary. The patient must be quickly tilted into the head-down position, if not already in it, the obstructing material aspirated to clear the airway, and oxygen given. Priority for oxygen or suction will depend upon the particular state of affairs—obviously it will be a waste of time giving oxygen if the airway is completely blocked. Nevertheless, when the patient is breathing, and there is some sort of airway, it may be wiser to oxygenate first, with intermittent or continuous suction beneath the mask when possible, rather than risk death from anoxia. An oral airway will be a help if the jaw is relaxed. Attempts to intubate the patient before oxygenation, can be helpful only when the obstruction cannot be relieved by other methods or when the trouble arises in a paralysed patient. Attempted intubation in the presence of laryngeal spasm aggravates the situation; deliberate paralysis at this stage runs the risk of death before intubation and oxygenation can be completed, but may be the only step left.

Tracheal toilet down a bronchoscope may be necessary but should only be considered after the emergency treatment has been carried out, and the patient restored to a state in which the procedure can be justified. As an immediate measure it is very dangerous; an endotracheal tube is quite adequate for suction. As soon as the patient improves, bronchoscopy should be considered if it seems likely that material has been aspirated. Obvious food or fluid should be removed by suction and, if the fluid portion is considerable, 20 to 30 ml saline should be squirted into the bronchi and, if possible, sucked back again, repeating the procedure two or three times in an endeavour to neutralise or dilute any hydrochloric acid that may remain. Critics of this technique will point out that additional fluid may wash inhaled substances further down the bronchial tree and also increase the risk of infection. Lavage with large volumes of fluid is strongly contra-indicated.

The main lines of treatment of aspiration pneumonia have been reviewed by Broe and his associates[31] and are summarised in the following list:

1. Aspiration of particulate matter
2. Endotracheal suction
3. Pulmonary lavage
   Frequent installation of 5–10 ml of sterile saline
4. Steroids in large doses for 2–3 days
5. Albumin (IV)
   This is based on the concept that the basic injury in aspiration pneumonia is to the pulmonary capillary, with a marked increase in permeability, leading to extravasation of large volumes of extracellular fluid. Albumin, in theory, is believed to increase osmotic pressure in the capillary and reduce this extravasation. Cautious administration of 12·5 to 25 g of albumin every 4–6 hours with CVP monitoring has been recommended.
6. Positive-Pressure Ventilation (IPPV)
7. Positive End-Expiratory Pressure (PEEP)
   Excessive levels of PEEP elevate pulmonary arterial pressure leading to an increase in intra-alveolar oedema. Only minimum amounts of PEEP (sufficient to achieve adequate arterial oxygenation) should be used.

When possible the proposed operation should be postponed if the patient has suffered a long period of hypoxia or has aspirated material into the lungs.

**Local Anaesthesia**

Many emergency operations can be performed under local anaesthesia, and those on the extremities often lend themselves well to nerve-block procedures. Operations upon, or within, the abdomen can be performed under more extensive blocks, such as epidural anaesthesia, and the risk of the dangers associated wth a full stomach can usually be circumvented, but other dangers and considerations must be assessed. Other factors besides the risk of aspiration alone—a bad chest, for example—may suggest a local technique, but provided precautions are taken, general anaesthesia matches up to local anaesthesia in safety and is most often preferred by the patient and the surgeon.

Intubation of the trachea with a cuffed endotracheal tube may be undertaken with local anaesthesia and, once effected, general anaesthesia can be induced with safety. But this, like other local anaesthetic techniques in the presence of a full stomach, does not guarantee that vomiting or regurgitation will not occur, so that the risk of tracheal aspiration persists until intubation is accomplished.

### Postoperative Care

The risk of aspiration returns at the termination of the operation when the endotracheal tube is removed and the nasogastric tube aspirated. For this reason the tube must be left in place until the patient has been turned on the side and placed head down. This position should be maintained until the patient is fully conscious and the pharyngeal reflexes are active. All patients must be carefully observed during the period of recovery preferably in an area specifically designated for this purpose, with highly trained staff who will recognise any deleterious change in the patients' condition.

## Some Anaesthetic Considerations for Intraperitoneal Operations

It is not proposed to consider every operative procedure that can be performed on the gastro-intestinal tract or abdominal viscera, nor the differing types of general or local anaesthesia that have been employed for them from time to time.

### Muscle Relaxation

In no other part of the body is muscle relaxation more important for the surgeon. Inadequate relaxation not only hampers the surgeon's work but, in the long run, harms the patient. An important fundamental principle of anaesthesia is the provision of adequate reflex suppression in advance of surgical stimulation. Depression of sensory or motor reflexes before their threshold is lowered, besides enabling suitable conditions to be maintained with smaller quantities of drugs than would otherwise be the case, tends to prevent the end-results of those repetitive and harmful surgical manipulations, such as forceful pulling and retracting, which are made necessary by poor operating conditions.

The muscle relaxants have a special part to play in this area of the body. When the simple spinal reflex is broken completely by motor paralysis, severe depression and chemical disturbance from potent anaesthetic drugs in order to facilitate surgical access becomes unnecessary. This is particularly important for major and prolonged operations, and the control of respiration that of necessity follows, leads to a quiet and helpful operation site. Inflammable agents can be avoided and the surgeon enabled to use the diathermy with safety. Although similar principles apply for restricted or short procedures, such as appendicectomy, less importance need be attached to the value of the muscle relaxants.

### The Operative Incision

Some incisions are more helpful to the anaesthetist than others. Generally, the surgical incision chosen is that which offers the most convenient approach to the site of the disease, but in doubtful cases a less direct approach may be necessary. Paramedian and midline incisions sometimes result in quite extensive retraction to enable the surgeon to reach laterally placed organs, and this despite complete relaxation. Oblique incisions, such as that of Kocher for operations on the biliary system, avoid this. They are more comfortable for the patient in the postoperative period than longitudinal incisions, but because the muscles are cut across they are liable to be followed by a higher incidence of incisional hernia. The difficulties of access that may be associated with a small incision must not be confused with inadequate anaesthetic conditions.

### The Effects of Major Surgery

A number of procedures—most of which cannot be avoided even when well-accepted standards of anaesthesia are practised—may lead to some degree of peripheral circulatory depression, irrespective of obvious haemorrhage. Manipulating and freeing from the posterior abdominal wall a large carcinoma of the caecum or an extensive length of bowel affected with ulcerative colitis, common bile duct surgery, and operations in the region of the coeliac plexus, are typical examples. Although some patients sweat a little or show variations in pulse rate, blood pressure and capillary refill time, the majority usually have little discernible reaction to an operation, yet, *in all*, fundamental, but normally reversible, changes occur. Many of these changes can be objectively recorded. Alterations in peripheral blood flow, in the distribution and elimination of electrolytes and the output of endocrine glands have all been measured at one time or another. The results are of little immediate value to the clinical anaesthetist who must strive from more simple and constantly observable data to maintain or improve the state of his patient.

All potent anaesthetic agents tend to increase circulatory depression *pari passu* with the depth of anaesthesia obtained. Light anaesthesia ensures that the normal compensatory mechanisms remain essentially intact, yet it must be adequate to suppress noxious stimuli, or an attempt made to prevent these by using special techniques such as local blocks, or drugs with more or less specific properties.

**Anaesthesia**

The choice of technique will depend on the state of the patient, the length and type of the operation and the surgical requirements. In general, elective surgery for abdominal procedures may be carried out with inducton using thiopentone, intubation with either suxamethonium or a non-depolarising muscle relaxant followed by maintenance with nitrous oxide-oxygen analgesic sequence and intermittent positive-pressure ventilation. The choice of muscle relaxant for intubation will depend on the problems that are anticipated with the passage of the endotracheal tube. The aphorism that a patient should never be paralysed unless he can be ventilated must not be forgotten.[32] However, the introduction of pancuronium, which has a comparatively rapid onset of action, has resulted in its frequent use for intubation when required for elective surgery of long duration. It obviates not only the misery of postoperative muscle pains associated with suxamethonium but may also be of use in conditions associated with abnormal serum potassium levels. The hope that pretreatment with pancuronium would decrease these post-operative muscle pains has not been substantiated,[33] although both gallamine and tubocurarine have been shown to diminish them.[34, 35] However, in emergency situations (where there is a vital necessity to insert a cuffed endotracheal tube rapidly) suxamethonium still remains the agent of choice. Factors such as those discussed in the previous section, which suggest a deterioration in the patient's condition, demand special attention but there is no unanimity as to their treatment, other than to ensure that replacement of blood loss is adequate. In this respect, all estimates must allow for internal loss from the circulation—transfusion still remains the best method of combating incipient circulatory failure. With regard to cholecystectomy, two points are worth bearing in mind. Firstly, the assistant retracting the liver may, as he becomes more tired, allow the retractor to rest on and thus obstruct the inferior vena cava with a consequent sharp fall in cardiac output and systemic pressure, and secondly, traction on the vagal fibres in the hepatic region may cause a marked bradycardia. This will respond to atropine. The choice and necessity for supplementation of the nitrous oxide-oxygen anaesthetic will depend on the premedication and response of the patient. Incremental doses of narcotic agents, for example pethidine, omnopon and fentanyl, are frequently used. Fluid replacement should be given as required.

**Intestinal obstruction.**—An ageing population with a high incidence of chronic pulmonary and circulatory disease, and the associated disorders of fluid and electrolyte balances that result from the obstruction, account for some of the problems of anaesthesia. Vomiting, regurgitation and distended bowels present practical difficulties. It is probably no coincidence that this type of patient has been largely associated with prolonged periods of apnoea following the use of non-depolarising relaxants, intermittent positive-pressure respiration and antidotes. The increasing sensitivity of the elderly to pancuronium, probably as a result of dimishing renal function, may well be a contributory factor.[36] The use of suxamethonium,[37] rather than a non-depolarising agent, enables complete relaxation of the abdominal musculature to be produced without the special risk of prolonged apnoea, or side-effects upon the circulation. However, if the procedure is a particularly lengthy one the problems of a Phase II block in association with large doses of suxamethonium must always be remembered. Seriously ill patients often require only very small doses of a non-depolarising relaxant to produce excellent abdominal-muscle relaxation. The correct dose for each situation can only be ascertained by careful titration using a peripheral-nerve stimulator before the commencement of surgery. Provided an overdose is not administered and other factors such as anuria, metabolic acidosis, etc. are not present, then the neuromuscular block is readily reversible.

### Obesity

The problems associated with the anaesthetic management of the overweight patient essentially involve all physiological systems. During the past years surgical treatment has been added to the list of methods of attempting to correct obesity, and thus the anaesthetist has been faced with the many difficulties associated with its management.

Obese patients are more prone to a number of diseases including gall-stones, hiatus hernia, osteoarthritis, varicose veins, fractures, prolapse, diabetes with associated arterial disease and renal calculi.[38] They also have a mortality rate some 2–3 times that of a normal patient even for comparatively minor surgery, for example appendicitis.

The surgical procedures that may be undertaken include apronectomy and intestinal bypass. The latter may involve a number of different techniques, the most common of which is currently the production of a blind loop of small intestine which results when the proximal 14 inches of jejunum are anastomosed to the last 4 inches of the terminal ilium. This is the 14/4 operation described by Payne and DeWind.[39]

In considering the anaesthetic management of the obese surgical patient, the respiratory and circulatory systems are of particular importance. Many of the patients cannot lie down because of the decreased inspiratory capacity that ensues. It is known that the functional residual capacity is decreased and the closing capacity increased in the obese,[40] and with the addition of anaesthesia in the supine position, the alveolar arterial oxygen tension gradient will be increased even further. While pre-operative physiotherapy and breathing exercises are of benefit, the great danger is of hypostatic pneumonia postoperatively. The lung compliance is decreased by the cuirass of fat surrounding the chest. The Pickwickian syndrome associated with hypoventilation and a raised carbon dioxide tension is less common than originally believed.[41]

Obesity is associated with an increase in cardiac output, hypertension and cardiomegaly with a strong correlation with sudden death.[42]

The explanation of this increase in cardiac output (essentially stroke volume as the heart rate remains constant) is probably not due so much to the cuirass effect of the fat on the chest wall as to the overall increased body mass of fat. In fact, it has been estimated that 13·5 kg of fat contain five miles of blood vessels.[43]

The anaesthetic management of the obese patient requiring surgery will necessitate a full clinical, biochemical and radiological assessment. Blood gas analysis and pre-operative lung function studies are particularly important. Evidence of existing cardiac disease must be sought.

Induction may be hindered by the absence of suitable veins, although a small indwelling needle can usually be inserted on the ventral aspect of the wrist. Pre-oxygenation should be carried out prior to induction because inflation of the lungs may be difficult and a coincidental hiatus hernia is common. Thiopentone followed by intubation using suxamethonium may be used. As intubation is often technically difficult, a laryngoscope with a long blade and a stilette for introduction of the tube should always be available.

Maintenance of anaesthesia essentially requires a technique that will allow rapid return of consciousness at the end of the operation while permitting full relaxation of the abdominal muscles during the procedure. Pancuronium with small incremental doses of narcotic analgesic (e.g. pethidine or fentanyl) has been found to be satisfactory. There is, however, no evidence to commend any specific technique as mandatory. In a randomised, prospective clinical study using fentanyl, enflurane or halothane, there was no difference in awakening time or recovery time in morbidly obese subjects.[44] The addition of intra-operative PEEP had been shown to be of no advantage,[45] the emphasis being on IPPV with large tidal volumes. The inspired oxygen concentration should not be less than 40 per cent.

Postoperatively the important considerations include oxygen therapy with blood gas determinations to ensure adequate ventilation. The patient should be sat up as soon as possible and chest physiotherapy commenced. Wound infections are more common and the incidence of deep venous thrombosis is twice that found in the normal patient. Postoperative pain must be adequately treated. Vaughan and Wise[46] have shown that the postoperative arterial oxygen tension is lower in those patients in whom surgery is carried out through a vertical incision rather than a transverse one; the former resulting in prolonged shallow respiration as a consequence of pain, with resultant patchy pulmonary atelectasis.

## Postoperative Sickness

Postoperative sickness is generally no more than a temporary, but unpleasant, malady for the patient. Occasionally in severe cases it can be incapacitating, leading to serious disturbance of fluid and electrolyte balance, and to a considerable strain on some operation wounds.

### Incidence

This is so dependent upon the differing circumstances of individual series that quoted figures must be considered in relation to the type of premedication, anaesthesia, and operation, as well as to many other factors, if they are to have any practical meaning. Thus Knapp and Beecher[13] using a standard anaesthetic sequence of nitrous oxide, oxygen and ether for many different operations, had an incidence of sickness of all kinds as high as 82 per cent, whereas Dent and his associates[47] showed an incidence of only 27·2 per cent with a series of 2,000 patients undergoing all types of surgery with many anaesthetic sequences and, in a comparable investigation, Burtles and Peckett[48] had a total incidence of 32 per cent.

In a more recent study on possible remedies, Korttila and his associates[49] quote an incidence of nausea and vomiting between 50 and 70 per cent after balanced general anaesthesia, depending on whether pethidine (meperidine) or morphine is used in the premedication. So, despite the changes in the agents used for general anaesthesia, the incidence of postoperative nausea and also vomiting remains distressingly high.

### Aetiology

A multitude of factors may play a part in the production of postoperative sickness, but the anaesthetic agents themselves are of greatest importance. Thus, the effects of ether and chloroform are well known, and no inhalational agent—not even nitrous oxide—can be exonerated. Gold[50] showed that in a series of some 1,200 gynaecological patients, those induced with thiopentone and maintained with halothane or cyclopropane had a significantly lower incidence of postoperative vomiting than those induced and maintained with cyclopropane or halothane. Some patients are very easily upset, and a history of vomiting after a previous anaesthetic should always be an indication for special care and perhaps the use of precautionary measures of treatment. Females are notoriously more susceptible to this complication than males. Sensitivity to the emetic effects of opiates and related analogues is a very real problem for some patients, while others are undoubtedly psychologically attuned to the attitude that all anaesthetics make them sick. The technique of anaesthesia is also of some importance, since hypoxia and carbon dioxide retention predispose to sickness, as does inflation of the stomach with air!

The site and type of operation have always been considered to play some part in the aetiology of postoperative sickness, but Knapp and Beecher[13] found no evidence that intraperitoneal operations are more likely to produce this complication than non-abdominal cases. There is, however, no doubt that operations on or in the region of the semi-circular canals can produce sickness, particularly following movement, for a period of days afterwards.

Sickness is sometimes induced by the early or too liberal use of sweetened fluid in the immediate postoperative period.

### Treatment

Carefully selected and administered anaesthesia, including both pre- and postoperative medication, will limit both the incidence and severity of sickness. Specific anti-emetics can be used routinely to prevent sickness or more selectively to treat the severer cases, but since none of the powerful anti-emetics is without side-effects, their routine use can only be justified if these other actions are thought to be reasonable and acceptable in the circumstances.

Drugs of the phenothiazine and associated groups are the most effective anti-emetics. A specific effect on the vomiting centre in the medulla is claimed for them, while their general sedative action also plays a part. Prevention of sickness is most usefully attempted by combining the chosen drug with the premedication, and then administering further doses at 3- to 4-hourly intervals in the postoperative period. Alternatively, they can be used as the main component of premedication instead of an opiate or one of its analogues, and only combined with atropine or scopolamine. Yet another way is to give a dose intramuscularly just before the patient leaves the operating theatre, and then to repeat the dose at intervals during the next 24 hours. All these methods will tend to prolong the period of unconsciouness or semi-consciousness which follows general anaesthesia, while the selective effect on the respiratory-tract reflexes and autonomic ganglia may increase the hazards of the immediate postoperative period. It is therefore probably safer, and not much less effective, to use them when indicated in the postoperative period and only after the initial recovery of consciousness—though even then the induced hypotension is not without its dangers. Occasional patients who are known to have a severe sickness after anaesthesia might be counted as the exceptions and treated more thoroughly.

The principal drugs used as anti-emetics are promethazine (25–50 mg), metoclopramide (10 mg) and perphenazine (5 mg). Lind and Breivik,[51] following a clinical trial, concluded that metoclopramide was superior to perphenazine. More recently, domperidone was claimed to be an effective anti-emetic,[52] but later studies have shown that it is only effective if given intravenously and also only lasts for a short period. However, it is claimed that it will counteract the decrease in the lower oesophageal pressure brought about by atropine.[53] Metoclopramide is also believed to have an action at this site. Korttila and his associates[49] in a comparative study of domperidone (5 mg), metoclopramide (10 mg) and droperidol (1·25 mg) found that the latter drug was significantly more effective than either of the other two agents. Nevertheless, patients given droperidol tended to sleep longer. These authors concluded that anti-emetics acting principally on increasing gastric motility (i.e. domperidone and metoclopramide) might be less effective after atropine and opiates than a drug such as droperidol with a principal central effect.

Other compounds have their advocates for the prevention and treatment of postoperative sickness. Dimenhydrinate (Dramamine) and promethazine-8-chlorotheophyllinate (Avomine) are best used for cases of motion sickness typified in the postoperative period after operations on or near the labyrinth. The dose is from 25 to 50 mg. They are not of great use for other types of sickness. Prochlorperazine (Stemetil, 12·5 mg i.m.) is widely used after aural surgery.

The relative mildness of much postoperative sickness suggests that some of the old-fashioned remedies may still have their place in treatment. Moreover, even the special drugs fail to control sickness in some patients, so that less specific and homely, but none the less practical, procedures may be helpful. Sips of cold water to which a little bicarbonate or iodide has been added are often beneficial.

A small-bore tube (Ryle's or similar type of 4 mm diameter) for gastric suction is often a useful ancillary in the treatment of severe cases, and can also be helpful if used prophylactically in cases known to be liable to this complication. Occasionally, especially in episodes following operations upon children, intravenous replacement of fluid, food and electrolytes may be an essential part of treatment.

No case of persistent or severe postoperative vomiting should be treated by routine therapy until a surgical cause has been excluded.

## REFERENCES


1. Cohen, S. and Harris, L. D. (1971). Does hiatus hernia affect competence of the gastro-oesophageal sphincter? *New Engl. J. Med.*, **284**, 1053.
2. Cohen, S. (1979). Motor disorders of the esophagus. *New Engl. J. Med.*, **301**, 184.
3. Van Thiel, D. H., Gavaler, J. S., Stremple, J. (1976). Lower esophageal sphincter pressure in women using sequential oral contraceptives. *Gastroenterology*, **71**, 232.
4. Brooks, F. (1978). Applied anatomy and physiology of the oesophagus. In *Gastroenterology* Vol. 1, p. 113. Edited by H. I. Bockus. Philadelphia: W. B. Saunders Co.
5. Ganong, W. F. (1981). *Review of Medical Physiology*, p. 381. California: Lange Publications.
6. Hunt, J. N., Macdonald, I. and Spurrell, W. R. (1951). The gastric response to pectin meals of high osmotic pressure. *J. Physiol. (Lond.)*, **115**, 185.
7. King, R. C. (1957). The control of diabetes mellitus in surgical patients. *Anaesthesia*, **12**, 30.
8. Eisner, M. (1971). Effect of metoclopramide in gastro-intestinal motility in man: a manometric study. *Amer. J. dig. Dis.*, **16**, 409.
9. Hohmann, J. E. (1979). Routine gastric aspiration. *Anesthesiology*, **50**, 170.

10. Weiss, W. A. (1950). Regurgitation aspiration of gastric contents during inhalational anesthesia. *Anesthesiology*, **11**, 102.
11. Turndorf, H., Rodis, I. D., Clark, I. S. (1974). "Silent" regurgitation during general anesthesia. *Anesth. Analg. (Cleve.)*, **53**, 700.
12. Bernhard, W. N., Cottrell, J. E., Sivakumaran, C., Patel, K., Yost, L. and Turndorf, H. (1979). Adjustment of intracuff pressure to prevent aspiration. *Anesthesiology*, **50**, 363.
13. Knapp, M. R. and Beecher, H. K. (1956). Postanesthetic nausea, vomiting and retching. Evaluation of the antiemetic drugs dimenhydrinate (Dramamine), chlorpromazine, and pentobarbital sodium. *J. Amer. med. Ass.*, **160**, 376.
14. Muravchick, S., Burkett, L. and Gold, M. I. (1981). Succinylcholine-induced fasciculations and intragastric pressure during induction of anesthesia. *Anesthesiology*, **55**, 180.
15. Editorial (1974). Hypoglycaemia and personality. *Brit. med. J.*, **2**, 134.
16. Morton, H. J. V. and Wylie, W. D. (1951). Anaesthetic deaths due to regurgitation or vomiting. *Anaesthesia*, **6**, 190.
17. Edwards, G., Morton, H. J. V., Pask, E. A. and Wylie, W. D. (1956). Deaths associated with anaesthesia. A report on 1,000 cases. *Anaesthesia*, **11**, 194.
18. Sellick, B. A. (1961). Cricoid pressure to control regurgitation of stomach contents during induction of anaesthesia. *Lancet*, **2**, 204.
19. Bannister, W. K. and Sattilaro, A. J. (1962). Vomiting and aspiration during anesthesia. *Anesthesiology*, **23**, 251.
20. Gibbs, C. P., Schwartz, M. D., Wynne, J. W., Hood, C. I. and Kuck, E. J. (1979). Antacid pulmonary aspiration in the dog. *Anesthesiology*, **51**, 380.
21. Moir, D. D. (1981). Anaesthesia for obstetrics. *Hospital Update*, **7**, 1091.
22. Husemeyer, R. P., Davenport, H. T. and Rajesekaran, T. (1978). Cimetidine as a single oral dose for prophylaxis against Mendelson's syndrome. *Anaesthesia*, **33**, 775.
23. Dobb, G., Jordan, M. J. and Williams, J. G. (1979). Cimetidine in the prevention of the pulmonary acid aspiration (Mendelson's) syndrome. *Brit. J. Anaesth.*, **51**, 967.
24. Howe, J. P., McGowan, W. A. W., Moore, J., McCaughey, W. and Dundee, J. W. (1981). The placental transfer of cimetidine. *Anaesthesia*, **36**, 371.
25. Mirakhur, R. K., Clarke, R. S. J., Dundee, J. W. and McDonald, J. R. (1978). Anticholinergic drugs in anaesthesia. A survey of their present position. *Anaesthesia*, **33**, 133.
26. Prys-Roberts, C., Greene, L. T., Meloche, R. and Foex, P. (1971). Studies of anaesthesia in relation to hypertension. II: Haemodynamic consequences of induction and endotracheal intubation. *Brit. J. Anaesth.*, **43**, 521.
27. Brock-Utne, J. G., Rubin, J., Welman, S., Dimopoulos, G. E., Moshal, M. G. and Downing, J. W. (1978). The effect of glycopyrrolate (Robinul) on the lower oesophageal sphincter. *Canad. Anaesth. Soc. J.*, **25**, 144.
28. Wilson, S. L., Mantona, N. R. and Halverson, J. D. (1981). Effects of atropine, glycopyrrolate and cimetidine on gastric secretions in morbidly obese patients. *Anesth. Analg. Curr. Res.*, **60**, 37.
29. Hey, V. M. F., Ostick, D. G., Mazumder, J. K. and Lord, W. D., (1981). Pethidine, metoclopramide and the gastro-oesophageal sphincter. *Anaesthesia*, **36**, 173.
30. Whittington, R. M., Robinson, J. S. and Thompson, J. M. (1979). Fatal aspiration (Mendelson's) syndrome despite antacids and cricoid pressure. *Lancet*, **2**, 228.
31. Broe, P. J., Toung, T. J. K. and Cameron, J. L. (1980). Aspiration pneumonia. *Surgical Clinics of North America.*, **60**, 1551.
32. Greene, N. M. (1976). Familiarity as a basis for the practice of anesthesiology. *Anesthesiology*, **44**, 101.
33. Brodsky, J. B., Brock-Utne, J. G. and Samuels, S. I. (1979). Pancuronium and post-succinylcholine myalgias. *Anesthesiology*, **51**, 259.
34. White, D. C. (1962). Obervations on the preventon of muscle pains after suxamethonium. *Brit. J. Anaesth.*, **34**, 332.
35. Lamoreaux, L. F., and Urbach, K. F. (1960). Incidence and prevention of muscle pain following the administration of succinylcholine. *Anesthesiology*, **21**, 394.
36. McLeod, K., Hull, C. J. and Watson, M. J. (1979). Effects of ageing on the pharmacology of pancuronium. *Brit. J. Anaesth.*, **51**, 435.
37. Morton, H. J. V. (1957). Intestinal obstruction and anaesthesia. *Brit. med. J.*, **2**, 224.
38. Bliss, B. P. (1973). The surgical management of obesity. *Brit. J. hosp. Med.*, **10**, 19.
39. Payne, J. H. and DeWind, L. T. (1969). Surgical treatment of obesity. *Amer. J. Surg.*, **118**, 141.
40. Fisher, A., Waterhouse, T. D. and Adams, A. P. (1975). Obesity: its relation to anaesthesia. *Anaesthesia*, **30**, 633.
41. Farebrother, M. J. B. and McHardy, G. J. R. (1974). Respiratory complications of obesity. *Brit. med. J.*, **3**, 469.
42. Kannel, W. B., LeBauer, E. J., Dawber, T. R. and McNamara, P. M. (1967). Relation of body weight to development of coronary heart disease: the Framingham Study. *Circulation*, **35**, 734.
43. Smart, G. A. (1956). In: *Price's Textbook of the Practice of Medicine*, 9th edit., p. 450. Ed. D. Hunter. London: Oxford Med. Publishers.
44. Cork, R. C., Vaughan, R. W. and Bentley, D. M. (1981). General anesthesia for morbidly obese patients—an examination of postoperative outcomes. *Anesthesiology*, **54**, 310.
45. Salem, M. R., Dala, F. Y., Zygmunt, M. P., Mathrubhutham, M. and Jacobs, H. K. (1978). Does PEEP improve intraoperative arterial oxygenation in grossly obese patients? *Anesthesiology*, **48**, 280.
46. Vaughan, R. W. and Wise, L. (1975). Choice of abdominal operative incision in the obese patient: a study using blood gas measurements. *Ann. Surg.*, **181**, 829.
47. Dent, S. J., Ramachandra, V. and Stephen, C. R. (1955). Post-operative vomiting: incidence, analysis and therapeutic measures in 3,000 patients. *Anesthesiology*, **16**, 564.
48. Burtles, R. and Peckett, B. W. (1957). Postoperative vomiting. Some factors affecting its incidence. *Brit. J. Anaesth.*, **29**, 114.
49. Korttila, K., Kauste, A. and Auvinen, J. (1979). Comparison of domperidone, droperidol and metoclopramide in the prevention and treatment of nausea and vomiting after general anaesthesia. *Anesth. Analg. Curr. Res.*, **58**, 396.
50. Gold, M. I. (1969). Post-anaesthetic vomiting in the recovery room. *Brit. J. Anaesth.*, **41**, 143.

51. Lind, B. and Breivik, H. (1970). Metoclopramide and perphenazine in the prevention of postoperative nausea and vomiting. *Brit. J. Anaesth.*, **42**, 614.
52. Fragen, R. J. and Caldwell, N. (1978). A new benzimidazole anti-emetic, domperidone, for the treatment of post-operative nausea and vomiting. *Anesthesiology*, **49**, 289.
53. Brock-Utne, G. (1980). Domperidone antagonises the relaxant effect of atropine on the lower oesophageal sphincter. *Anesth. Analg. Curr. Res.*, **59**, 921.

## FURTHER READING

Eralam, R. (1975). *Clinical Tests of Oesophageal Function*. London: Crosby Lockwood Staples.

CHAPTER 35

# Anaesthesia and the Liver



## ANATOMY

THE liver, which is the largest glandular organ of the body, lies below the right costal margin under the diaphragm. In the adult the liver constitutes approximately one-fortieth of the body weight, ranging between 1000 and 1500 g, and is divided imperfectly into two lobes—a large right and a small left one. Neither of these two lobes is derived exclusively from the right and left hepatic buds of the embryo nor do they receive their blood supply solely from one or other of the two hepatic arteries. On the inferior and posterior surface between the right and left lobes are two smaller lobes—the caudate and the quadrate. The falciform ligament consists of two layers of peritoneum which are closely united until they reach the upper surface of the liver, where they part company to cover the peritoneal surface of the right and left lobe. This ligament joins the liver to the diaphragm and the anterior abdominal wall. In its free edge stretching from the umbilicus to the lower border of the liver is the ligamentum teres containing small para-umbilical veins. At its upper end the two layers of the falciform ligament separate widely to expose a small triangular area–the bare area of the liver. The right fold of the ligament joins the upper layer of the coronary ligament and the left fold sweeps away to become continuous with the anterior layer of the left triangular ligament.

The porta hepatis is found on the inferior surface of the liver, lying between the quadrate lobe in front and a process of the caudate lobe behind. This structure is important because it consists of a deep fissure containing most of the essential structures of the liver. Viewed from below these structures, from right to left, are the common hepatic duct, which gives off a branch—the cystic duct—leading to the neck of the gall bladder, the bile duct, the portal vein and finally the hepatic artery with a plexus of hepatic nerves.

The minute structure of the liver comprises a whole mass of neatly arranged lobules. Each lobule consists of numerous cells arranged in columns which radiate from around a central vein. Irregular blood vessels or sinusoids can be found between the columns of cells. The blood supply to these lobules comes from the hepatic artery and the portal vein. Both these vessels, soon after entering the porta hepatis, divide into right and left branches. Each branch then undergoes dichotomy many thousands of times to supply all the lobules. The hepatic artery, which arises from the coeliac axis, brings fresh oxygenated blood for the liver cells almost directly from the aorta, whereas the portal vein carries all ingested material in the venous blood from the gastro-intestinal tract and spleen. These two vascular supplies are carried throughout the liver on the periphery of the lobules. Small branches are given off from both vessels which encircle the lobule as the interlobular plexus and from these plexuses small capillary-like vessels (sometimes described as sinusoids) run between the column of cells of the lobule and finally drain into the vein in the centre of the lobule—the central vein. All the central veins join up to form the hepatic veins which finally drain into the inferior vena cava.

The nerve supply of the liver—the hepatic plexus—consists of non-medullated fibres from the sympathetic ganglia of $T_7$ and $T_{10}$ which synapse in the coeliac axis, with fibres from both vagi and the right phrenic nerve. The nerves ramify around the vessels and bile ducts and finally terminate in the liver cells.

## Physiology

The blood flow to the liver is about 1,500 ml per minute. Of this total, about 80 per cent (1,200 ml) reaches the liver through the portal vein and the remaining 20 per cent (300 ml) passes along the hepatic artery. However, the blood in the hepatic artery is about 95 per cent saturated with oxygen whereas that in the portal vein is around 85 per cent.

It has been estimated that the liver normally requires about 60 ml of oxygen per minute, of which about 17 ml are supplied by the hepatic artery and the remainder by the portal vein. The total amount of oxygen available to the liver cells can be reduced by a number of conditions:

1. Anaesthesia, due to:
   (*a*) reduced hepatic blood flow
   (*b*) reduced arterial oxygen saturation through pulmonary shunting
2. Lowered cardiac output as in shock, haemorrhage or hypotension
3. Inhalation of a low inspired concentration of oxygen
4. Hypermetabolic states, e.g. pyrexia
5. Hepatotoxic substances
6. Obstruction of the portal vein or hepatic artery
7. Portal hypertension, with extensive extrahepatic collateral circulation or internal portal hepatic venous shunts and arterio-venous hepatic shunts.

It is clear therefore that, as the cells surrounding the central lobular vein are the last to receive nourishment, they are the first to suffer from any deprivation. With toxic substances one might expect the cells surrounding the hepatic artery to receive the worst damage, but it is liver toxins which cause the hepatic cells to swell, and it is their swelling which further interferes with the blood supply of the central cells and causes them to suffer the worst damage.

## Functions of the Liver

**General metabolism.**—Ingested carbohydrates are broken down in the intestine and the resulting monosaccharides are absorbed and stored in the liver in the form of glycogen (glycogenesis). The breakdown of glycogen (glycogenolysis) is through the Embden-Meyerhof pathway to pyruvic acid and then via the citric acid cycle to carbon dioxide and water. Any excess glucose not converted to glycogen may be converted to fatty acids.

Fats pass from the depots throughout the body to the liver and are broken down, almost as fast as they arrive, into glycerol and fatty acids under the influence of the enzyme liver lipase.

The end-products of protein digestion are amino acids which play such an important part in cellular structure. The "amino acid pool" is composed not only of the fresh supplies from the gut, but also from the continual breakdown and rebuilding of the tissues. The amino acids number about twenty and each protein molecule is a composite group of most of them. Of these eight are essential amino acids which the body cannot make, and to ensure survival they must form part of a normal diet. About one half of the body protein synthesis and resynthesis takes place in the liver and it is here that the surplus amino acids undergo oxidative deamination. In this process the amine group ($NH_2$) is released as ammonia ($NH_3$); the latter substance is either excreted as urea or is used again for building other amino acids. The remainder of the molecule (the non-nitrogenous part) is broken down to produce energy for the general metabolism.

The amino acid methionine is of special interest because it is concerned in the synthesis of choline; it generously donates three methyl groups to ethanolamine to form choline, and this may then become acetylated in the presence of the enzyme choline acetylase to form the essential substance of neuromuscular transmission—acetylcholine. Another of methionine's important functions is to supply a methyl group to noradrenaline to synthesise adrenaline.

**Storage.**—Fats, protein and glycogen and likewise certain vitamins—such as vitamin B, which plays such an important part in pernicious anaemia—are all stored in the liver.

**Production and destruction.**—Amongst its tasks the liver synthesises plasma proteins, prothrombin, fibrinogen and heparin. In early life it plays an important part in red blood cell formation and later becomes one of the principal places where the breakdown products of old red blood corpuscles are dealt with.

**Formation of the bile secretion.**—This is carried out in the liver.

**Detoxication of drugs.**—The liver is able to remove many foreign substances by oxidation. For example pethidine is removed in this manner and therefore liver function is important in any assessment of drug activity. Barbiturates in common with many other drugs metabolised in the liver have the ability to stimulate the microenzyme systems within the hepatic cells. The effect of this "enzyme induction" results in an increase in the amount of enzyme present in the cells, with the result that repeated doses of the same drug are metabolised with increasing speed and in consequence have a decreasing effect.The enzymes stimulated by a particular drug are not specific to that drug and may thus increase the rate of metabolism of other drugs given at the same time. For example the alcoholic patient will tolerate barbiturates very well. However, once the liver begins to fail such a patient becomes extremely sensitive to barbiturates, particularly the short-acting group, because there is insufficient functioning hepatic tissue to metabolise them.

## Liver Function Tests

In attempting to assess the functional state of the liver a number of points must be remembered. Because the liver carries out such diverse functions, a great variety of biochemical tests have been used to assess the overall state of the organ, and many of these may be normal in the presence of liver disease, while factors other than liver disease may cause abnormal results.

### Serum Bilirubin Estimations

Bilirubin is formed mainly from the breakdown of the haem part of the haemoglobin molecule. This occurs in the reticulo-endothelial cells of the liver and spleen. The unconjugated bilirubin (which is carried in the plasma bound to albumin) is taken up by the liver cells which convert it from a fat-soluble to a water-soluble form by conjugating it with glucuronic acid. Unconjugated bilirubin is not normally present in the urine, but in patients with conjugated bile in the plasma some will pass through the glomerulus and appear in the urine, giving it a dark colour.

The Van den Bergh reaction determines the conjugated level of bilirubin [normal value 0·2 mg/100 ml (3·4 μmol/l) or less] and by the addition of methyl alcohol also the total concentration of the serum bilirubin, that is the sum of the conjugated and unconjugated bilirubin [normal value 0·8 mg/100 ml (13·7 μmol/l) or less].

### Bromsulphthalein Test

This dye, consisting of phenol and tetrabromphthalein disodium sulphonate, is taken up by the liver cells and excreted unchanged in the bile. The test, which is now rarely used, is based upon a study of the concentration remaining in the blood after the intravenous injection of this dye and is expressed as a percentage of the control value. The patient is given 5 mg/kg body weight of 5 per cent bromsulphthalein intravenously, and if normal, should have 0 to 3 per cent of it left in the blood after forty-five minutes. In patients with hypoalbuminaemia a normal result may be found even in the presence of liver disease. This is in consequence of an inverse relationship that exists between the rate of removal from the plasma of bromsulphthalein and plasma albumin concentration.[1]

**Serum Enzyme Tests**

The multiplicity of tests for liver function is evidence of the complexity of processes carried out by this organ and the inadequacy, in consequence, of a single test to give an overall picture of the state of the liver. Enzymes are present in most of the cells of the major organs throughout the body and the serum of the blood contains a steady level of each, because there is a constant small breakdown of cells. However, if an organ such as the heart or liver suddenly undergoes an ischaemic episode, then cellular breakdown will increase precipitously and this will be reflected in a dramatic elevation of the serum level of the corresponding enzymes. Similarly, if obstruction to the biliary tract occurs, the enzymes normally excreted by this route will spill into the blood stream with a marked increase in serum levels. For this reason these enzyme tests play an important role in distinguishing jaundice due to hepatic cellular damage and that following early obstruction of the common bile duct.

The enzymes in question include transaminases, dehydrogenases and phosphatases.

**The transaminases.**—Transamination is a chemical reaction in which an amino group of an amino acid replaces the keto group of another acid to form a new amino acid, with the enzyme for this process being a transaminase. There are two principal hepatic transaminases:

1. *Aspartate aminotransferase (glutamic oxaloacetic transaminase).*—This is present in large quantities in the liver, heart, kidney and skeletal muscle. High serum values for this enzyme are found in both hepatocellular necrosis and myocardial infarction. Normal serum value 5 to 17 International units/dl.*

2. *Alanine aminotransferase (glutamic pyruvic transaminase).*—This is also present in many organs but there is relatively less in the liver cells as compared with the heart and skeletal muscle. Normal serum value 4 to 13 International units/dl.[2]

* There is a wide variation in the normal range quoted by different laboratories. This is because each uses its own technique, and there are no generally agreed standards for temperature, pH or buffering solutions. Though there are International units, there is no International technique.

In severe liver disease, such as acute hepatitis, the level of these enzymes in the serum may rise to 800 International units/dl or more, whilst in the presence of simple obstructive jaundice the level is usually in the region of 50 to 100 International units/dl.

**The dehydrogenases.**—These enzymes catalyse an oxidation-reduction reaction in the presence of a coenzyme which serves as a hydrogen donor or acceptor.

The principal enzymes of this group include lactic dehydrogenase (LDH) and isocitric dehydrogenase (ICD). The former is a relatively insensitive index of hepatocellular injury, although the serum level may be greatly raised in association with hepatic neoplasms. In the latter case raised levels are found in hepatic damage, but normal values occur in the presence of myocardial infarction.[2]

Normal values for LDH are up to 500 International units/dl. This figure is considerably raised in infective or toxic hepatitis but is usually within normal limits in early obstructive jaundice.

**The phosphatases.**—The serum alkaline phosphatase is also useful in helping to diagnose the cause of jaundice, as a low figure in King Armstrong units (0–15 units/dl) suggest either a normal response or the presence of inflammation of the liver cells. A high figure (35 or more units/dl), on the other hand, signifies an obstruction to the flow of bile. Serum gamma-glutamyl transpeptidase (GGT) which is found in the liver and other tissues, may be increased in both biliary and liver cell disease. Alcohol and drugs, for example barbiturates, may also increase enzyme activity. Normal values are 6–28 units in males and 4–18 units in females. Increases are also found in alcoholics from microsomal enzyme induction, and drugs, for example phenobarbitone, may produce the same effect. Other phosphatases that may be affected by liver disease include serum glucose 6-phosphatase and serum 5-nucleotidase.

**Pseudo (Plasma) Cholinesterase Test**

Pseudocholinesterases are responsible for the breakdown of acetylcholine and also suxamethonium. These esterases are believed to be formed mainly in the liver, and in the presence of damage to this organ, or of starvation, low values may be expected. Nevertheless, a low pseudocholinesterase level may be present in otherwise healthy subjects and this is one of the first points that comes to mind if a prolonged apnoea follows suxamethonium. It must be assumed, therefore, that there are other causes of a low pseudocholinesterase reading besides liver damage; and it is known that merely altering the protein intake in the diet is rapidly reflected in the level of the esterase in the blood.

Other diagnostic procedures for assessing liver function include needle biopsy and hepatic scanning using a gamma-emitting isotope.

### Jaundice and its Differential Diagnosis

The cause of the yellow tinge in the skin, so characteristic of jaundice, is an increase in the concentration of bilirubin in the blood. This may occur for a variety of reasons:

(*a*) **Haemolytic jaundice** is due to an excessive destruction of red blood cells with the consequent accumulation of large quantities of unconjugated bilirubin, which is formed so fast that the liver cells are simply unable to remove it quickly enough, so that the concentration in the blood rises. This type of jaundice most commonly occurs after the transfusion of incompatible blood or the injection of haemolytic drugs and sera. It also occurs in association with a number of hereditary defects of the red cell membrane (e.g. hereditary spherocytosis) or its haemoglobin content (sickle-cell anaemia).

(*b*) **Hepatic jaundice.**—This results from failure of the liver cell to conjugate the bilirubin and excrete it into the biliary system. This may be the direct result of toxic damage to the cell (e.g. drugs). The cells surrounding the central part of the lobule are the most susceptible to damage because they are supplied with the lowest saturation of oxygen and are thus the first to suffer. Damage to these central cells often introduces an element of "obstruction" into this type of jaundice. Alternatively, there are a number of comparatively rare conditions, often familial, in which there is an abnormality of bilirubin conjugation (e.g. Gilbert's syndrome).

(*c*) **Obstructive jaundice** signifies some form of blockage in the biliary system preventing the outflow of bile. A rare type of this condition occurs in the newborn where the congenital abnormality is some failure in the cannulation of the bile duct system. More commonly it is seen in adults as an acquired condition following obstruction of the common bile duct by a stone or by carcinoma of the head of the pancreas.

Bilirubin being the essential cause of jaundice, a description of its formation and fate is important in any attempt to differentiate between the various types of jaundice described above.

Normally the red blood cells are broken down by the reticulo-endothelial system. The globin portion of the molecule is split off and returns to the metabolic protein pool. The haem is then broken down to iron and porphyrin. The iron is carried to the bone marrow where it is used again for further haemoglobin synthesis. The porphyrin is broken down to bilirubin and carried in the blood bound to albumin which is insoluble in water and cannot pass into the urine. A rise in red cell destruction, therefore, will lead to a corresponding rise in the protein-bound bilirubin. On reaching the liver the latter is conjugated with glucuronic acid to form the water-soluble bilirubin glucuronide which passes from the liver cell down the bile duct to the intestines where it is acted upon by bacteria and forms urobilinogen. Some of this is then reabsorbed and passes into the blood stream, but about half passes on down to join the faeces and in contact with air it becomes oxidised to form urobilin. Of that part of urobilinogen that is reabsorbed, some returns to the liver to complete the cycle, whilst the rest passes to the kidney and is excreted in the urine. Ultimately it is likewise oxidised in the presence of air to form urobilin.

In haemolytic jaundice the total quantity of protein-bound bilirubin is greatly increased. The liver cells just cannot manage to deal with the huge quantities that are reaching them and a rise in concentration is inevitable. The urine does not contain any bilirubin because the bilirubin in the blood is insoluble in water. The concentration of urinary urobilinogen is increased. In obstructive jaundice the water-soluble bilirubin cannot be excreted down the bile duct into the intestine and it overflows from the liver cell back into the blood stream. The concentration of the serum water-soluble bilirubin rises and it appears in the urine. As no urobilinogen is able to be formed in the intestine the stools are pale and the urine contains no urobilinogen. In hepatic jaundice which has resulted from toxic damage to the liver the biochemical picture is more confused, giving usually an initial obstructive type picture with a haemolytic element superimposed a little later. Assessment of liver function tests will show evidence of hepatic cell damage.

## Liver Blood Flow

The splanchnic vascular system supplies all the blood passing to the intestines from which it finally drains into the portal system and is carried to the liver. The liver blood flow, however, receives another contribution from the hepatic artery so that variations in the splanchnic flow and in that of the hepatic artery are reflected in the final amount of blood which passes through the liver.

### Measurement of Liver Blood Flow

This is a complex procedure based on the extraction of bromsulphthalein by the liver cells.[3] This technique has been adapted for use in anaesthetised patients by Shackman and his associates.[4] The conscious patient is first screened and a radio-opaque catheter is passed under vision up an arm vein via the superior vena cava into the inferior vena cava and from there into a branch of the right hepatic vein. This provides samples of portal blood *after* it has passed through the liver. Bromsulphthalein is injected intravenously, first as an initial primary dose and then as a continuous infusion of a 3 per cent solution in saline at an average of about 1·4 ml/minute. Once stabilisation has been reached the concentration in a peripheral artery is taken to equal that in the blood reaching the liver cells. A comparison between this concentration and that in the hepatic vein will reveal a relative drop due to the extraction by the liver cells. Since the arteriovenous difference can also be determined for similar samples, the actual amount of blood flowing through the liver can be calculated. Caesar and his colleagues[5] have described a technique using indocyanine green in order to measure the splanchnic blood flow. Other substances which have also been used include galactose and ethanol.

### Flow in the Conscious State

Measurements made on conscious subjects suggest that the average liver blood flow is about 1·25 to 1·5 litres per minute. As the normal cardiac output for a patient at rest is about 5 litres/minute this means that about 25 per cent of this output passes to the liver. Under certain conditions, however, the liver has to sacrifice some of this flow in order to protect the homeostatic mechanism, maintain the systolic pressure, and ensure a blood supply to the most "vital" centres. Haemorrhage, congestive heart failure and severe exercise are amongst these causes.

### Flow in the Anaesthetised Patient

The induction and maintenance of general anaesthesia is sufficient to produce a drop of up to 50 per cent in the amount of blood flowing through the liver.[6] As the average flow in the conscious patient is about 1500 ml/min it follows that the onset of anaesthesia reduces this flow to around half (750 ml/min). Deeper planes of anaesthesia produce an even greater fall. Price and his colleagues[7] used indocyanine green to measure the splanchnic blood flow during anaesthesia in a group of volunteers who were not undergoing surgery. When cyclopropane was the anaesthetic used, the liver blood flow was significantly reduced by splanchnic vasoconstriction. If, at this point, a small dose of hexamethonium (i.e. one insufficient to lower the blood pressure yet capable of some ganglion blockade) was also given, then both the hepatic and the splanchnic flow could be returned to normal. On the basis of these findings the authors concluded that the reduced liver blood flow of cyclopropane anaesthesia is probably secondary to increased sympathetic activity in the splanchnic vascular bed.

In contrast, halothane anaesthesia produces a fall in liver blood flow *without* altering the splanchnic vascular tone. In this case the fall in hepatic blood flow parallels the decrease in cardiac output.[8] The latter has been shown to vary with arterial carbon dioxide tension[9] and Juhl and Einer-Jensen[10] have shown that as a consequence of this response hypercapnia may lessen the fall in hepatic blood flow and hypocapnia increase it.

In other words, a rise in arterial $P_{CO_2}$ leads to an increase in cardiac output which, in view of the unaltered splanchnic tone, will lead to an increase in liver blood flow. Conversely, a fall in arterial $P_{CO_2}$ leads to a reduction in cardiac output and a diminution of hepatic blood flow.

Methoxyflurane anaesthesia causes an even more marked reduction in splanchnic blood flow than either halothane or cyclopropane.[11] This seems to result from an increase in splanchnic resistance and decreased mean arterial pressure. Epstein and associates[12] found that general anaesthesia, using thiopentone, nitrous oxide, oxygen and succinylcholine, with intermittent positive-pressure ventilation and maintenance of normal arterial carbon dioxide tension, altered splanchnic blood flow very little. Cowan and colleagues[13] have measured hepatic blood flow under conditions of routine general anaesthesia and they state: "Studies in man using hepatic vein catheters have shown that blood flow through the liver falls significantly after induction with various anaesthetic agents, but returns to pre-anaesthetic levels during the subsequent abdominal surgery. This fall, which is greater with trichloroethylene than with halothane, may be large enough in some patients to contribute to postoperative liver dysfunction." Their results suggest that though *induction* of anaesthesia can cause a sharp fall in hepatic blood flow, the *trauma* of surgery could be responsible for a rapid return to normal levels in the lightly anaesthetised patient. However, these results were not confirmed by Gelman.[14] He estimated hepatic blood flow (EHBF) using radioactive colloidal gold. Patients were anaesthetised with either halothane or enflurane and showed a reduction in EHBF of about 15 per cent. Surgery reduced the flow further and the degree increased with the extent of the surgical trauma, being some 80 per cent of the initial value during minor surgical procedures but falling to about 45 per cent in patients undergoing partial gastrectomy or cholecystectomy.

Any reduction in hepatic blood flow must be considered in the light of the tremendous increase in flow that takes place in the skin and muscle vessels at the same time. As there is no compensatory increase in the cardiac output in most forms of anaesthesia, it follows that the liver—ably helped by the kidney—is the source of this extra amount of blood passing to the periphery. In fact, active vasoconstriction may take place. There is no evidence to suggest that this reorganisation of the blood flow is in any way beneficial to the patient, and certainly it is extemely troublesome for the surgeon.

**Flow during Autonomic Blockade**

The effects of autonomic blockade depend in part on the technique by which it is produced. Kennedy and associates[15] have shown in conscious volunteers that epidural anaesthesia (to the level of $T_5$) using lignocaine solutions containing adrenaline, results in an initial fall in splanchnic vascular resistance, while the hepatic blood flow decreased by about 25 per cent 30 minutes after $T_5$ anaesthesia had been achieved and then slowly returned to normal. When plain lignocaine was used, the splanchnic vascular resistance rose significantly with a rapid fall in hepatic blood flow also of about 25 per cent, which gradually returned to normal. The difference in effect between the two solutions used may depend on a splanchnic vasodilator action of adrenaline.[16]

In high spinal anaesthesia hepatic blood flow decreased by an amount similar to that with epidural anaesthesia. However, the splanchnic vascular resistance did not alter significantly, the decrease in flow being associated with a fall in mean arterial pressure.[17] It would thus appear that the high serum levels of lignocaine that are found in epidural anaesthesia when adrenaline is not used may have specific action on splanchnic vasculature.

Ganglionic blockade does not cause any change in splanchnic vascular resistance, but a fall in flow proportional to the fall in mean arterial pressure.[18]

**Flow during Hypotension associated with Vasoconstriction**

This follows oligaemia from severe blood loss. The splanchnic bed attempts to compensate for this alteration in the haemodynamics by vasoconstriction which, in turn, results in a drop in the portal flow. When the systemic pressure falls the flow through the hepatic artery also drops. Thus the combination of vasoconstriction in the splanchnic bed with hypotension—as occurs after severe haemorrhage—may lead to a serious depletion of liver blood flow.

**Flow during Hypothermia**

Hypothermia causes both a fall in blood pressure and a reduction in liver blood flow, but it has the great advantage that in this case the metabolism (oxygen requirements) of the hepatic cells are reduced *pari passu* with the fall in temperature and blood pressure. There is little evidence to suggest that the liver cells suffer any damage from hypothermia alone, but if a period of cardiac arrest is also included then severe congestion of the liver cells may result from temporary occlusion of the inferior vena cava.

**Flow and Vasoconstrictor Drugs**

The administration of such drugs may reduce the liver blood flow. While the local action of adrenaline on the liver is one of vasoconstriction, the effects of a raised systemic blood pressure and splanchnic vasodilatation predominate, and the result is that hepatic blood flow increases. Noradrenaline, on the other hand, is such a powerful vasoconstrictor that the liver flow usually shows a slight fall despite the rise in systemic pressure. Cases of damage to the liver cells following the infusion of noradrenaline have been reported. Other vasopressors, like methylamphetamine, which stimulate cardiac output, increase the hepatic flow.

## Anaesthesia and the Hepatic Cells

Most anaesthetic drugs can be classed as protoplasmic poisons of lesser or greater degree, which is why they figure prominently in any study of liver function. As has already been mentioned, the liver cells surrounding the central lobular vein are working with a low oxygen saturation; it is hardly surprising, therefore, that they are the first to suffer damage if the saturation falls even lower. This, if coupled with the action of any anaesthetic drug used, may be sufficient to produce signs of liver damage. In essence the two causes—hypoxia and drugs—are inseparable and complementary.

Hypoxia may be the result not only of a fall in the oxygen content of the hepatic blood but also of a fall in the absolute amount of blood arriving at the liver in a given time. While the oxygen consumption of the liver may decrease during general and regional anaesthesia, the splanchnic blood flow is reduced to a greater degree.[19] Price and colleagues[20] examined the effects of cyclopropane and halothane anaesthesia to see if this disproportionate reduction in oxygen requirement and splanchnic blood flow caused any evidence of hepatic cell anoxia, but found none. However, as Cooperman[18] pointed out, the problem remains of applying this data, obtained in general from fit, healthy young volunteers, to the ill and aged patient undergoing surgery.

One added factor that is often not considered is the effect on splanchnic circulation of surgical trauma and stimulation which occurs during intra-abdominal surgery. Torrance[21] showed that hepatic blood flow could fall markedly as a result of even the most minor surgical manoeuvre such as manipulation of the peritoneum, and it is not difficult to see how hypoxia of the centrilobular cells of the liver could arise. It seems surprising that hepatic dysfunction does not occur more commonly after intra-abdominal surgery.

Sherlock[2] has divided therapeutic agents that may effect the liver into two broad groups, the predictable and the unpredictable.

In the *predictable* group are included drugs that interfere with bilirubin metabolism and those with a direct hepatotoxic effect. The hepatic effects of drugs in this group can be reproduced in animals. Novobiocin is an example of a substance that interferes with the conjugation of bilirubin, and this may be of particular relevance in the neonate, while carbon tetrachloride produces a direct dose-dependent action on the liver. Large doses of intravenous tetracycline are also directly hepatotoxic.

In the *unpredictable* group only a small number of those receiving the drug concerned will be affected. The incidence is unrelated to the dose though it is more common after multiple exposures suggesting a sensitivity reaction. Furthermore, the liver lesion cannot be reproduced in animals. This hypersensitivity type of reaction is either hepatitic, being indistinguishable from viral hepatitis (for example, isoniazid), or cholestatic, with obstruction to the excretion of bilirubin as may be seen with the phenothiazine group of drugs. For the past twenty years much interest has been centred on the effects of the inhalational anaesthetic agents, particularly halothane. An association between its use and hepatitis prompted the National Halothane Study[22] and the subsequent literature on this topic has been as profuse as it has been inconclusive. While Sherlock in 1978[23] stated that "the case against halothane *seems* to be proved", by 1980, Deinstag[24] noted that "despite vitriolic controversy over the existence of halothane-induced hepatitis, a consensus has been reached that it *is* a distinct although rare syndrome".

The difficulties surrounding clarification of the condition have arisen firstly from its rarity, with a quoted incidence of between 1 in 6000 and 1 in 110,000,[25] secondly from the lack of specificity of the pathological changes, and thirdly from the difficulty in reproducing the condition in animal models.

The mechanisms by which halothane causes hepatic damage are by no means clear and include both the allergic and the hepatotoxic theories. While the former postulates a direct hypersensitivity reaction to halothane, the latter is believed to be the consequence of the biotransformation of halothane to reactive intermediates which are responsible for the hepatic damage.[26] (See also Chapter 6, p. 198.)

The clinical syndrome presents as fever, usually with rigors, which develops more than 7 days (range 8–13) after halothane anaesthesia. Associated malaise and non-specific gastrointestinal symptoms including right upper abdominal pain may also occur. The fever may appear between one to twelve days postoperatively after repeated exposure to halothane. Jaundice appears rapidly after the pyrexia. The white blood count is usually normal but the eosinophil count may fall to zero.[27] Hepatic reactions have also been reported with methoxyflurane[28] and enflurane.[29]

**Comment**

Where does this leave the practising clinician who wishes to use halothane? Certainly, the advice that unexplained jaundice or delayed pyrexia after a previous halothane administration should be a contra-indication to further use,[23] would appear to be generally accepted. If biotransformation to reactive metabolites is a causal factor, what may increase this process? Hypoxia and certain enzyme-inducing agents have been shown to increase the rate.[30] Thus there is a theoretical risk in a second halothane anaesthetic to patients who are fat, elderly, likely to have enzyme induction, are stressed with other reactive metabolites (e.g. radiotherapy), or are having an operation which may reduce hepatic blood flow significantly.[31,32] However, it must not be forgotten that the risk of using an alternative but unfamiliar anaesthetic technique may be greater.

**The muscle relaxants and liver damage.**— The exact relationship between tubocurarine and the metabolism of the liver is still obscure. Dundee and Gray[33] drew attention to the observation that patients with liver dysfunction required more tubocurarine to produce complete muscular paralysis than was normally required in similar healthy subjects. This has also been noted in patients given pancuronium.[34] Investigation of patients with total biliary obstruction[35] showed that plasma clearance of pancuronium was less than half the normal value with a corresponding increase in neuromuscular blockade of almost twice normal. Some 11 per cent of pancuronium is normally excreted in bile.[36] A similar finding was also observed by Duvaldestin and colleagues[37] in patients with cirrhosis, but they found that the total apparent volume in which the pancuronium was distributed was increased by 50 per cent. Westra and associates[38] also found prolongation of the action of pancuronium with extrahepatic cholestasis from decreased clearance from the liver. They reconfirmed that the action of gallamine is not affected by hepatic disease and suggested its use in such circumstances. While Thompson[39] has shown that pancuronium is bound by serum proteins, particularly the gammaglobulin fraction, a decrease in plasma protein binding may be one of the factors giving rise to an enlarged volume of distribution in patients with extrahepatic cholestasis.[38]

As a result of these findings, it would appear that an *increase* in the volume of distribution of pancuronium would lead to a diminished effect. However, due to the *decrease* in hepatic elimination, the reverse is the case and the overall effect is increased. Great care, therefore, must be taken with incremental doses and the necessity for their use should be carefully monitored with a nerve stimulator.

## Acute Liver Failure in Relation to Anaesthesia and Surgery

In clinical anaesthesia liver damage may result from a number of different causes, the most important of which is probably a period of severe hypotension occurring during or immediately after major surgery. The extent of the hepatic changes will depend on the degree and duration of the hypotension.

The onset of postoperative jaundice may be due to a number of other causes which may be subdivided into those producing increased serum levels of unconjugated bilirubin, impaired hepatocellular function and extra-hepatic obstruction.[40]

The increase in serum bilirubin may be the result of blood transfusion. One unit of 14-day-old stored blood may contain 250 mg of bilirubin which is the normal daily production. Jaundice after massive transfusions of blood, for example after cardiac surgery, is generally of the order of 10 per cent. The reabsorption of massive haematomata may also result in postoperative jaundice.

Hepatocellular damage may result from drugs that have been administered either pre- or intra-operatively, from sepsis, or from pre-existing liver disease, for example, anicteric hepatitis. Extrahepatic biliary obstruction may arise from bile duct injury during surgery or postoperative cholecystitis.

One of the important associations with hepatocellular failure is renal failure which occurs even in the presence of previously normal renal function. It is common in two groups of patients: those with biliary obstruction and those with hepatic cirrhosis, usually severe. If the obstruction is relieved or the cirrhosis treated by transplantation, the renal function rapidly recovers. The exact cause is not known, although it has been suggested that the high level of circulating endotoxins found in both conditions may be responsible.[41] Similarly, the failure of the liver to remove various vasoactive substances would also explain the changes that occur. These include an alteration in renal cortical perfusion[42] in conjunction with a reduction in effective renal blood flow.[43] The exact aetiology of this phenomenon is not known.

The symptoms and signs of hepatic failure are rather vague and indefinite at first but gradually become more obvious. At the start the patient complains of lassitude, malaise, anorexia and headache. Vomiting and pyrexia are often prominent. At about the third day vomiting is persistent and at the end of a week jaundice may be present. This heralds the final stages when the mental state becomes confused, with periods of delirium, and finally drifts into coma and death.

### Treatment

The management of hepatic failure[2] is essentially supportive with treatment of the biochemical abnormalities that occur. Great care must be taken to see that nothing is given that might increase the degree of failure or coma that may be present. If sedation is essential, diazepam is probably the drug of choice.[44] Great care should be taken, since this drug is metabolised by the liver and has a half-life of two days. The serum albumin level has been shown to be a useful index for the prediction of the effect of intravenous diazepam, and therefore a low level would suggest the possibility of marked sensitivity. Essentially protein intake is stopped and intestinal absorption of protein minimised by oral neomycin in order to prevent or decrease the encephalopathy. Hypoglycaemia is treated with i.v. 50 per cent glucose if the blood sugar falls below 100 mg/100 ml (5·6 mmol/l). Electrolytic disorders, particularly hyponatraemia, must be corrected and renal failure may necessitate dialysis. Bleeding tendencies and anaemia may require vitamin K, fresh frozen plasma and fresh blood. In general, the complications of corticosteroid therapy outweigh the benefits. Finally, temporary hepatic support either by exchange transfusion, cross-circulation or extracorporeal liver perfusion may be necessary.

## Hepatic Disease and Anaesthesia

The pre-operative assessment of liver function is important, but often neglected.[45] Of particular importance is an attempt to estimate the metabolic ability of the liver, and this is best achieved by measurements of serum albumin and the prothrombin ratio.

When considering anaesthetic drugs, the reserves of the liver are so great that unless the patient is rapidly approaching hepatic failure, there are few agents that cannot be used in small dosage. Two factors must, however, always be kept in mind: first, the extent to which any particular agent depends upon liver function for its breakdown and removal from the body, and secondly, the effect of the agent, and indeed of the anaesthetic and surgical procedure as a whole, on liver function.

In practice, minor surgical procedures in the presence of hepatic disease are best performed under local anaesthesia. It must be borne in mind that amide local anaesthetic drugs are metabolised in the liver. Thus with single-dose spinal and epidural anaesthesia the low doses used cannot lead to a toxic concentration. However, if these drugs are infused (or given continuously) then the presence of severe hepatic dysfunction (with delayed metabolism) can rapidly lead to a toxic concentration accumulating in the plasma. Similarly, the barbiturates, the opiates, and the phenothiazines must only be used in small quantities (if at all) as they primarily rely on the hepatic cells for their metabolism or conjugation.

If general anaesthesia is mandatory then a light level in association with full muscular paralysis is the method of choice, as the volatile agent and relaxant can be excreted unchanged. In selecting a particular anaesthetic agent or technique in the patient with hepatic disease, it should be remembered that the cardiac output, the hepatic blood flow and the oxygen saturation are probably more important factors than the effect of a particular agent on liver function. For extensive operations in association with severe liver disease particular problems arise from the dangers of hypoxaemia and myocardial depression. The patients concerned tend to have a hyperdynamic circulation with a high cardiac output and depressed total peripheral resistance.[46] A high inspired oxygen concentration is essential throughout the procedure if desaturation is to be avoided. Both systemic and pulmonary shunting of blood occur which contributes to the hypoxaemia. The pulmonary shunting in liver disease is particularly important, being associated with a marked increase in ventilation/perfusion imbalance.[47]

In view of the greater risk of renal failure in patients with obstructive jaundice or cirrhosis, the use of 10 per cent mannitol to maintain adequate urinary output is advisable; the mannitol should be given immediately before and during surgery and, again, in the postoperative period if required.

**Hepatitis**

The outbreak of hepatitis, particularly in dialysis and transplant units, has become a recognised hazard in recent years. The aetiology is in almost all cases one of two viral agents known as Virus A and Virus B. Hepatitis A and B, which results from infection with the respective virus, produce two distinguishable clinical diseases, the differences between which are summarised in Table 1. The pathology of the two diseases is essentially the same, with acute inflammation of the entire liver. In hepatitis B, antibodies are produced against an antigen that was initially found in an Australian aborigine.[48] This antigen was initially called *Australia antigen* but has now been redesignated as *Hepatitis B* antigen (HBAg.). It is found in 83 per cent of sera tested within 12 days of the onset of symptoms of type B hepatitis and has usually been cleared by 3–4 weeks.[2]

It is hepatitis B rather than A that is of importance to the anaesthetist.[49] It may be transmitted in the blood or secretions of a patient who may either have acute hepatitis clinically or be a symptom-free carrier. It is the latter group that are the great danger. It is not possible at the present time to test blood from every patient for the presence of hepatitis B

35/Table 1
Viral Hepatitis in Man

| | Hepatitis A | Hepatitis B |
|---|---|---|
| Synonym | Infectious hepatitis | Serum hepatitis |
| HB antigen in serum | Negative | Positive |
| Transmission | Faecal-oral<br>By food or water | Parenteral transfer or close physical contact<br>Blood and blood products |
| Incubation period | 3–5 weeks (mean 28 days) | More variable, generally longer |
| Presumed infective particle | 27 nm, enterovirus-like RNA (probably) | 44 nm, double-shelled virion (Dane particle) DNA |
| Found mainly in | Faeces | Blood |
| Small laboratory animal | None | None |
| Cell culture technique | None | None |

antigen. There are, however, "certain categories of patient who should be regarded with suspicion, treated with respect, and tested without fail",[49] and these are shown in Table 2.

35/TABLE 2
PATIENTS UNDER SUSPICION AS HEPATITIS B CARRIERS

(1) All patients with liver diseases however acute or chronic.
(2) Patients undergoing haemodialysis, or who have had a renal transplant.
(3) All patients with leukaemia, reticuloses, polyarteritis nodosa or polymyositis.
(4) Patients being treated with radiotherapy or immunosuppressive drugs.
(5) Immigrants or visitors from countries with a high background of carriers.
(6) Persons who have been transfused in, or recently returned from, countries with a high background incidence (namely tropical and sub-tropical areas and Greenland).
(7) Patients who have received blood or a blood product in the last 6 months, or who have been transfused with blood or blood products from paid blood donors.
(8) Inmates of prisons or institutions for the mentally defective.
(9) Drug addicts, prostitutes, and homosexuals.
(10) The tattooed.
N.B. This list should not be regarded as complete.

(Tables 1 and 2 courtesy of Professor A. P. Waterson, and Macmillan Journals Ltd.[49])

In patients who are hepatitis B antigen-positive or in whom time does not allow screening tests to be carried out, full precautions must be taken from the time the patient leaves the ward. All staff entering theatre should be gowned, gloved and masked, preferably in disposable material that can be incinerated after the operation. The anaesthetist must take particular care to see that contamination does not arise from blood spilt at the time when intravenous infusions are set up, or from syringes and needles that have been used. The practical details of the management of hepatitis B antigen-positive patients who require surgery has recently been fully reviewed by Waterson.[49]

There is no specific treatment for hepatitis B infections. A trial of a vaccine has produced encouraging results for the future.[50] For those who have been contaminated to an extent which is likely to result in the disease, a preparation of concentrated specific hepatitis B antigen antiserum should be given as soon as possible and at any rate within 48 hours, a further injection being given at 28 days.[51]

## LIVER TRANSPLANTATION

The first successful orthoptic liver transplant was carried out in 1963 by Thomas Starzl in Denver and, since that time, more than 200 livers have been grafted, with the longest survival time being 10 years after transplantation.[52] The indications for this operation have been summarised by Williams[53] as a primary hepatoma (without extrahepatic metastases), advanced cirrhosis without a severe bleeding tendency in patients under the age of 60, and inoperable biliary atresia in children over the age of 1 year.

The selection and preparation of a patient for liver transplantation is an extremely important and difficult task. Sherlock[54] has described the problems in detail, which in summary include general investigations with emphasis on assessment of liver function; methods of determining the hepatic vasculature and anatomy of the biliary system; tissue compatibility tests and control of hepatocellular failure.

The difficulties associated with anaesthesia have been discussed by Samuel[55] and Farman and associates.[56] The latter report their experiences in a series of 27 orthoptic liver allografts. In summary they emphasise the effect of hepatic dysfunction on drug metabolism and conclude that a conventional technique using nitrous oxide, oxygen and pancuronium is best. Two particular problems arise: firstly, the rapid loss of blood that may occur in the initial stages of the operation, and secondly, the fall of cardiac output that results from clamping of the inferior vena cava. Both may be corrected by blood transfusion. The donor liver, which is cooled immediately after removal and may be kept for up to ten hours stored in ice, releases cold acid perfusate which is rich in potassium. The effects of the latter on the myocardium can be reversed by intravenous calcium chloride, while sodium bicarbonate will reverse the acidosis. In the postoperative period it is essential that good oxygenation is maintained and repeated examinations made for biochemical abnormalities.

## REFERENCES


1. Grauz, H. and Schmid, R. (1971). Reciprocal relation between plasma albumin level and hepatic sulfobromophthalein removal. *New Engl. J. Med.*, **284**, 1403.
2. Sherlock, S. (1975). *Diseases of the Liver and Biliary System*, 5th edit. Oxford: Blackwell Scientific Publications.
3. Bradley, S. E., Inglefinger, F. J., Bradley, G. P. and Curry, J. J. (1945). The estimation of hepatic blood flow in man. *J. clin. Invest.*, **24**, 890.
4. Shackman, R., Graber, I. G. and Melrose, D. G. (1953). Liver blood flow and general anaesthesia. *Clin. Sci.*, **12**, 307.
5. Caesar, J., Shaldon, S., Chiandussi, L., Guevara, L. and Sherlock, S. (1961). The use of indocyanine green in the measurement of hepatic blood flow and as a test of hepatic function. *Clin. Sci.*, **21**, 43.
6. Thorshauge, C. (1970). Hepatic blood flow during anaesthesia. *Acta anaesth. scand.*, Suppl. **37**, 205.
7. Price, H. L., Deutsch, S., Cooperman, L., Clement, A. J. and Epstein, R. M. (1965). Splanchnic circulation during cyclopropane anesthesia in normal man. *Anesthesiology*, **26**, 312.
8. Ahlgren, I., Aronsen, K.-F., Ericsson, B. and Fajgelj, A. (1967). Hepatic blood flow during different depths of halothane anaesthesia in the dog. *Acta anaesth. scand.*, **11**, 91.
9. Prys-Roberts, C., Kelman, G. R., Greenbaum, R., Kain, M. L. and Bay, J. (1968). Hemodynamics and alveolar-arterial $Po_2$ differences at varying $Paco_2$ in anesthetized man. *J. appl. Physiol.*, **25**, 80.
10. Juhl, B. and Einer-Jensen, N. (1974). Hepatic blood flow and cardiac output during halothane anesthesia: an animal study. *Acta anaesth. scand.*, **18**, 114.
11. Price, H. L. and Pauca, A. L. (1969). Effects of anesthesia on the peripheral circulation. *Clin. Anesth.*, **3**, 674.
12. Epstein, R. M., Wheeler, H. O., Frumin, M. J., Habif, D. V., Papper, E. M. and Bradley, S. E. (1961). The effect of hypercapnia on estimated hepatic blood flow, circulating splanchnic blood volume, and hepatic sulfobromophthalein clearance during general anesthesia in man. *J. clin. Invest.*, **40**, 592.
13. Cowan, R. E., Jackson, B. T. and Thompson, R. P. H. (1975). The effects of various anaesthetics and abdominal surgery on liver blood flow in man. *Gut*, **16**, 839.
14. Gelman, S. I. (1976). Disturbances in hepatic blood flow during anesthesia and surgery. *Arch. Surg.*, **3**, 881.
15. Kennedy, W. F., Everett, G. B., Cobb, L. A. and Allen, G. D. (1971). Simultaneous systemic and hepatic hemodynamic measurements during high peridural anesthesia in normal man. *Anesth. Analg. Curr. Res.*, **50**, 1069.
16. Bearn, A. G., Billing, B. and Sherlock, S. (1951). The effect of adrenaline and nor-adrenaline on hepatic blood flow and splanchnic carbohydrate metabolism in man. *J. Physiol. (Lond.)*, **115**, 430.
17. Kennedy, W. F., Everett, G. B., Cobb, L. A. and Allen, G. D. (1970). Simultaneous systemic and hepatic hemodynamic measurements during high spinal anesthesia in normal man. *Anesth. Analg. Curr. Res.*, **49**, 1016.
18. Cooperman, L. H. (1972). Effects of anaesthetics on the splanchnic circulation. *Brit. J. Anaesth.*, **44**, 967.
19. Cooperman, L. H., Warden, J. C. and Price, H. L. (1968). Splanchnic circulation during nitrous oxide anesthesia and hypocarbia in normal man. *Anesthesiology*, **29**, 254.
20. Price, H. L., Deutsch, S., Davidson, I. A., Clement, A. J., Behar, M. G. and Epstein, R. M. (1966). Can general anesthetics produce splanchnic visceral hypoxia by reducing regional blood flow? *Anesthesiology*, **27**, 24.
21. Torrance, H. B. (1957). Liver blood flow during operations on the upper abdomen. *J. roy. Coll. Surg. Edinb.*, **2**, 216.
22. National Halothane Study (Summary). (1966). *J. Amer. med. Ass.*, **197**, 775.
23. Sherlock, S. (1978). Halothane heptitis. *Lancet*, **2**, 364.
24. Deinstag, J. L. (1980). Halothane hepatitis: allergy or idiosyncrasy? *New Eng. J. Med.*, **3**, 102.
25. Strunin, L. (1979). Liver dysfunction after repeated anaesthesia. *Brit. J. Anaesth.*, **51**, 1097.
26. Brown, B. B. (1981). Pharmacogenetics and the halothane hepatitis mystery. *Anesthesiology*, **55**, 93.
27. Sherlock, S. (1981). *Diseases of the Liver and Biliary System*, 6th edit. Oxford: Blackwell Scientific Publications.
28. Katz, S. (1970). Hepatic coma associated with methoxyflurane anesthesia. *Amer. J. dig. Dis.*, **15**, 733.
29. Denlinger, J. K., Lecky, J. H. and Nahrwold, H. L. (1974). Hepatocellular dysfunction without jaundice after enflurane anesthesia. *Anesthesiology*, **41**, 86.
30. McLain, G. E., Sipes, I. G. and Brown, B. R. (1979). An animal model of halothane hepatotoxicity: roles of enzyme induction and hypoxia. *Anesthesiology*, **51**, 321.
31. Editorial (1980). The liver and halothane—again. *Brit. med. J.*, **2**, 1197.
32. Editorial (1980). Immunization against hepatitis B. *Brit. med. J.*, **2**, 1585.
33. Dundee, J. W. and Gray, T. C. (1953). Resistance to *d*-tubocurarine chloride in the presence of liver damage. *Lancet*, **2**, 16.
34. Ward, M. E., Adu-Gyamfi, Y. and Strunin, L. (1975). Althesin and pancuronium in chronic liver disease. *Brit. J. Anaesth.*, **47**, 1199.
35. Somogyi, A. A., Shanks, C. A. and Triggs, E. J. (1977). Disposition kinetics of pancuronium bromide in patients with total biliary obstruction. *Brit. J. Anaesth.*, **49**, 1103.
36. Agoston, S., Vermeer, G. A., Kersten, U. W. and Meijer, D. K. E. (1973). The fate of pancuronium bromide in man. *Acta anaesth. scand.*, **17**, 267.
37. Duvaldestin, P., Agoston, S., Henzel, U., Kersten, U. W. and Desmonts, J. M. (1978). Pancuronium pharmakokinetics in patients with liver cirrhosis. *Brit. J. Anaesth.*, **50**, 1131.
38. Westra, P., Vermeer, G. A., de Lange, A. R., Scaf, H. J., Meijer, D. K. F. and Wesseling, H. (1981). Hepatic and renal disposition of pancuronium and gallamine in patients with extrahepatic cholestasis. *Brit. J. Anaesth.*, **53**, 331.
39. Thompson, T. M. (1976). Pancuronium binding of serum proteins. *Anaesthesia*, **31**, 219.
40. LaMont, J. T. and Isselbacher, K. D. (1973). Postoperative jaundice. *New Engl. J. Med.*, **288**, 305.
41. Wilkinson, S. P., Moodie, H., Stamatakis, J. D., Kakkar, V. V. and Williams, R. (1976). Endotoxaemia and

renal failure in cirrhosis and obstructive jaundice. *Brit. med. J.*, **2**, 1415.
42. Kew, M. C., Brunt, P. W., Varma, R. R., Hourigan, K. J., Williams, R. and Sherlock, S. (1971). Renal and intrarenal blood-flow in cirrhosis of the liver. *Lancet*, **2**, 504.
43. Lieberman, F. L. (1970). Functional renal failure in cirrhosis. *Gastroenterology*, **58**, 108.
44. Branch, R. A., Morgan, M. H., James, J. and Read, A. E. (1976). Intravenous administration of diazepam in patients with chronic liver disease. *Gut*, **17**, 975.
45. Strunin, L. (1978). Preoperative assessment of the patient with liver dysfunction. *Brit. J. Anaesth.*, **50**, 25.
46. Kaplan, J. A., Bitner, R. L. and Dripps, R. D. (1971). Hypoxia, hyperdynamic circulation, and the hazards of general anesthesia in patients with hepatic cirrhosis. *Anesthesiology*, **35**, 427.
47. Ruff, F. (1971). Regional lung function in patients with hepatic cirrhosis. *J. clin. Invest.*, **50**, 2403.
48. Blumberg, B. S., Alter, H. J. and Visnich, S. (1965). A "new" antigen in leukemia sera. *J. Amer. med. Ass.*, **191**, 541.
49. Waterson, A. P. (1976). Hepatitis B as a hazard in anaesthetic practice. *Brit. J. Anaesth.*, **48**, 21.
50. Szmuness, W., Stevens, C. E., Harley, E. J., Zang, E. A., Oleszko, W. R., William, D. C. Sadovsky, R., Morrison, J. M., and Kellner, A. (1980). Hepatitis B Vaccine: Demonstration of efficacy in a controlled clinical trial in a high-risk population in the United States. *New Engl. J. Med.*, **303**, 833.
51. Editorial (1980). Hepatitis B virus infections among surgeons. *Lancet*, **2**, 300.
52. Starzl, T. E., Koep, L. J., Halgrimson, C. G., Hood, J., Schroter, G. P. J., Porter, K. A. and Weil, III, R. (1979). Fifteen years of clinical liver transplantation. *Gastroenterology*, **77**, 375.
53. Williams, R. (1970). Transplantation of the liver in man. *Brit. med. J.*, **1**, 585.
54. Sherlock, S. (1972). Selection and preparation of the patient for liver transplantation. In: *Anaesthesia in Organ Transplantation*, p. 32. Basel: Karger.
55. Samuel, J. R. (1972). Anaesthesia for liver transplantation. In: *Anaesthesia in Organ Transplantation*. Basel: Karger.
56. Farman, J. V., Lines, J. G., Williams, R., Evans, D. B., Samuel, J. R., Mason, S. A., Ashby, B. S. and Calne, R. Y. (1974). Liver transplantation in man. *Anaesthesia*, **29**, 17.

CHAPTER 36

# Anaesthesia and the Kidney



## ANATOMY

The two kidneys lie retroperitoneally in the abdomen on either side of the vertebral column. Each normally weighs between 120 and 170 g and measures 12×7×3 cm. In the cadaver the upper and lower poles are at the level of the twelfth thoracic and third lumbar vertebrae respectively. The right kidney may lie slightly lower than the left due to the mass of the liver. During normal inspiration each kidney moves up and down over a distance of one vertebral body.

The anterior surface of each kidney bears important relationships to many intra-abdominal structures, the upper pole is closely attached to the adrenal gland, and the renal vessels and ureter join the hilum at its medial border. The kidney itself is covered in a fibrous capsule which may easily be removed, exposing a layer of smooth muscle fibres beneath. A cross-section of the kidney reveals the outer cortical and the inner medullary substance.

### Vascular System

The main renal arteries pass directly from the abdominal aorta to the kidneys. After giving off small branches to the capsule and pelvis, each main artery then enters the hilum and divides into five segmental arteries which in turn divide into interlobar arteries as they run through the renal medulla towards the cortex.

Each of the segmental arteries is an end artery, which means that it does not anastomose with its neighbouring artery, and if one should become occluded the segment of the kidney which it supplies will become infarcted. On reaching the point of junction between medulla and cortex at the base of the pyramids each interlobar artery divides into two, and in a T-shaped fashion each branch runs at right angles to the parent stem between cortex and medulla. These vessels give off important branches, the interlobular arteries. These run through the cortex giving off a large number of branches which pass directly to the glomeruli (the afferent glomerular arterioles) and finally terminate as perforating arteries which supply the surface of the kidney. Although the renal veins follow the same course as the arteries the larger veins anastomose freely through the arcuate veins.

### Urinary System

Each individual renal tubule and its glomerulus is called a nephron and each adult kidney has approximately 1½ million of these structures. The glomerulus consists of a mass of capillary vessels surrounded by the blind end of an expanded renal tubule called Bowman's capsule. This apparatus is concerned with the filtering of substances from the blood stream. Bowman's capsule leads to the proximal convoluted tubule, down the descending limb of the loop of Henle and bends sharply back as the ascending limb to become the distal convoluted tubule which finally drains into the collecting tubule. The function of this tubular system is both selective reabsorption and excretion so that the material that finally reaches the ureters is urine.

At the point where the distal tubule begins, it lies close to the arterioles which enter and leave its own glomerulus and is modified histologically being known as the macula densa. The area formed by these cells, the arterioles and the few cells lying between these structures is called the juxtaglomerular apparatus from which renin is secreted.

### Nerve Supply

The kidney has a sympathetic supply which is derived from the 12th thoracic to the 2nd lumbar segments of the spinal cord. The adrenergic fibres enter the renal substance along the renal arteries and are predominantly vasoconstrictor in action being distributed to the afferent and efferent glomerular arteries. Nerve fibres have also been shown to terminate close to the cells of the juxtaglomerular apparatus. Cholinergic fibres have also been found in the kidney but their exact function is not known.

## Physiology

Under normal resting conditions about 20–25 per cent of the total cardiac output passes through the renal circulation each minute. In other words, the two kidneys between them receive a blood flow of 1,100–1,200 ml/minute. Approximately half of this total consists of plasma and the rest is made up of cells. Although the distribution of blood flow to the glomeruli in different parts of the cortex may alter, there do not appear to be any arteriovenous shunts present. However, not all the blood which enters the interlobular arteries in the cortex passes to the glomeruli, since these arteries may emerge on the surface of the kidney and anastomose with the capsular vessels. In the glomerular capillaries the arterial pressure, which is probably some 10–20 mm Hg (1·3–2·6 kPa) below the systemic pressure, tends to drive the fluid across the glomerular membrane, being opposed by the osmotic pull of the proteins in the blood and the hydrostatic pressure in Bowman's capsule. Thus of the original total of about 1000 ml of blood that enters the kidneys every minute, about 1/10th or 100 ml is filtered off and passed down the tubules. At this point the selective reabsorption mechanism plays a major role and almost all the fluid content passes back into the circulation again. Of each 100 ml of fluid entering the tubules, 99 ml is reabsorbed. Put in another way, this means that 1 ml of urine is formed from every 1,000 ml of blood that goes to the kidneys.

### Glomerular Filtration

The glomerular membrane is permeable to both fluid and electrolytes, but not to protein or cells. In fact a small amount of protein does pass through even in the normal kidney but is reabsorbed in the proximal tubules. The driving force across this membrane is called the effective filtration pressure (EFP) and is calculated as the glomerular capillary pressure minus the sum of the osmotic pressure of the plasma proteins and the hydrostatic pressure in Bowman's capsule. In man this value has been estimated to be about 20 mm Hg (2·7 kPa).[1] The fraction that passes across the glomerular membrane is normally about one-sixth of the renal plasma flow or one-tenth of the renal blood flow.

Thus:

If the renal blood flow is . . . . 1,200 ml/min,
and the renal plasma flow is . . . . 750 ml/min,
the total reaching the tubules
is one-sixth of 750 ml/min, i.e. . . 125 ml/min.

There are a number of factors which influence the EFP, which include the systemic blood pressure, alterations in the osmotic pressure of the plasma proteins and increase in the pressure within Bowman's capsule resulting from obstruction in the tubules lower down the nephron. While the kidney is able to maintain the glomerular capillary pressure at a constant level over a wide range of systemic pressures, it is very vulnerable if the latter falls markedly. Clinically, it is known that in cases of severe hypotension during or immediately after surgery renal excretion ceases altogether, and this may be associated with signs of renal damage in the postoperative period.

In renal disease there is a close relationship between the severity of the damage and the number of functioning glomeruli, so that any further damage by anaesthetic agents or the like becomes of prime importance. The glomerular membrane itself is particularly susceptible to damage by hypoxia, ischaemia and drugs. Normally, molecules with a weight of 69,000 or more cannot pass through the membrane, while those of lower weight pass through with increasing ease as their size diminishes. For example, albumin, with a molecular weight of 69,000 is essentially impermeable to the membrane while, if present, free haemoglobin with a molecular weight of 68,000 passes through in appreciable quantities. Ischaemia of the glomerulus destroys this semi-permeability, hence the value of albumin in the urine as a guide to renal damage.

**Tests of glomerular filtration.**—In normal circumstances the glomeruli filter the plasma contents without showing any favours. Substances with large molecules pass across more slowly than those with small ones. The glomerular filtration rate is described as the amount of fluid passing from the capillaries in the glomerular tuft into the lumen every minute.

Precise measurements of GFR are not usually carried out because of the technical difficulties of the methods available, but reasonably accurate values may be obtained by determination of the "clearance" of a substance from the plasma. If a substance is completely filtered into Bowman's capsule from the glomerular capillaries and is neither absorbed nor excreted during its passage through the renal tubules then the volume of plasma which initially held the amount of substance excreted will be equal to the GFR.

The calculation is made from the following equation:

$$\frac{\text{Concentration of substance in urine} \times \text{volume of urine}}{\text{Concentration of substance in plasma}} = \text{clearance in ml/min}$$

1. *Inulin clearance.*—The most accurate method of assessing glomerular filtration rate is by the use of inulin, as this substance is filtered unchanged by the glomeruli but is not reabsorbed by the tubules. Despite this, such measurements are usually reserved for estimations requiring great accuracy, as the continuous infusion of inulin and the repeated blood sampling make this method unsuitable for routine clinical testing.

2. *Creatinine clearance.*—As creatinine is a normal constituent of the blood which is filtered rapidly by the glomeruli yet is not reabsorbed in the tubules, it has become a popular means of assessing glomerular function. Unfortunately a very small quantity is secreted by the tubules, but this can be taken into account in the final assessment. Fortunately the blood level of creatinine remains remarkably constant, so that a long period of study can be contemplated, yet it is only necessary to measure the blood level once during this period. The concentration of creatinine is determined colorimetrically, based on the intensity of the orange colour produced in the sample by alkaline sodium picrate.

*Details of test.*—The patient first empties his bladder thoroughly and this specimen is discarded. A 24-hour save of all urine passed is then commenced. Creatinine in the blood and in the urine is known, together with the total volume of urine passed during the period, hence the total quantity of glomerular filtrate can be calculated.

Although the creatinine clearance test is not quite as accurate as that with inulin (see below), its simplicity makes it much more convenient in routine clinical practice, and even with advanced renal disease the differences between inulin and creatinine clearances are not of clinical importance.

The normal value in an adult patient of the creatinine clearance (i.e. glomerular filtration rate) is approximately 120 ml/minute.

There is a wide variation of about ± 15 ml/minute, and as the age of the patient increases so the glomerular filtration rate declines steadily until by the time the age of 90 or over is reached, the rate has fallen by approximately 50 per cent to 60 ml/minute.

3. *Urea clearance*.—Like creatinine, urea is a normal constituent of the blood and therefore it is easy to measure the clearance simply by determining its blood and urine concentrations and measuring the total volume of urine passed. Since some of the urea entering the tubules is reabsorbed into the circulation, an allowance must be made for this, and if the glomerular filtration rate is 120 ml/minute, then the urea clearance is 60 per cent of 120, or 75 ml/minute. Furthermore, the urea clearance is very dependent on the rate of urine flow and when the flow drops below 2 ml/minute the inaccuracies are considerable. Then a figure can only be calculated with the use of a complex formula, and is sometimes referred to as the *standard urea clearance*, but in clinical practice it is rarely used. Under normal conditions of the test, the fluid intake of the patient is so adjusted that the total quantity of urine passed exceeds 2 ml/minute. The result may then be termed a *maximal* urea clearance. Although once popular this test is now very seldom used, having been replaced by creatinine clearance or radioisotope studies.

4. $^{51}$*Cr-EDTA*.—A number of substances have been introduced which have radioactive markers. Initially these included labelled forms of inulin, but these tended to be expensive and relatively unstable. The most widely used alternative is $^{51}$Cr-EDTA (ethylene diaminetetracetate) which is readily available and can be stored satisfactorily.[2] This is filtered and passes through the renal tubule in exactly the same way as inulin. The usual calculation may be applied either by using a constant intravenous infusion or a single-shot technique in which the fall of plasma concentration of the gamma-emitting isotope, during a 2-hour period, is determined.

5. *Blood urea and creatinine levels*.—As both urea and creatinine clearance values are useful methods of assessing glomerular filtration rates, so the level of these substances in the blood gives some indication of renal function.

The normal blood values are:
Urea 15·0–40·0 mg per cent (2·5–6·7 mmol/l)
Creatinine 0·7–1·5 mg per cent (62–132 μmol/l).

A rise in blood urea is a relatively late sign of renal damage. Unfortunately, as both urea and creatinine are produced in the body, their concentrations in the blood can be altered by other factors. For example the effect of high- and low-protein diets can be seen in Fig. 1. As GFR decreases the blood urea rises quite slowly and even a fall of 50 per cent in GFR will only result in a blood urea of 30 mg/100 ml (5 mmol/l) if a low-protein diet is being eaten; and this value is within the normal range for the population. Serum creatinine concentrations are less affected by dietary protein, being in general proportional to the muscle mass, so that a slightly raised serum level in a patient with a very small muscle mass may mask a severely decreased GFR.

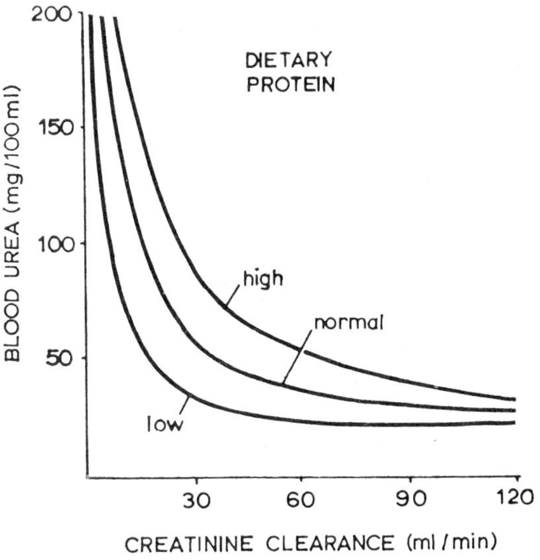


36/Fig. 1.—Schema of the relationship between glomerular rate (creatinine clearance) and the blood urea at varying levels of protein intake. (Courtesy of Professor H. E. de Wardener, author of *The Kidney*, published by Churchill Livingstone.[3])

6. *Proteinuria*.—The presence of significant quantities of protein in the urine denotes the presence of glomerular or tubular damage. Normally about 10–20 mg per cent of protein passes across the glomerular membrane, but almost the entire quantity is reabsorbed by the tubules. The method of detection of protein in the urine depends either on simple precipitation by boiling, or by flocculation with 25 per cent salicyl sulphonic acid.

### Salicyl Sulphonic Acid Test

*Trace* of precipitate—approximately equivalent to a concentration of 0·2 g protein/litre

*Heavy* precipitate—approximately equivalent to a concentration of 5·0 g protein/litre.

The significance of a positive result to this test is influenced by the dilution of the urine. Thus a positive response in a very concentrated urine is of less importance than the same result in a dilute one. Macroscopic blood or pus will be responsible for some precipitate, and care should be taken to avoid this error. Albustix is a convenient way of demonstrating urinary protein, although it will not show the presence of Bence Jones protein.

The exact type of proteins excreted is sometimes of significance in diagnosis of the underlying renal disease. Thus electrophoretic separation can be used to distinguish between albumin and globulin. In acute nephritis both protein types are excreted in the same proportions as in the plasma, whereas in myelomatosis a protein of low molecular weight (22,000) may appear with albuminuria.[3]

7. *Blood cells and casts.*—Small amounts of blood cells (red and white) and hyaline casts may be found in the urine of normal subjects. Nevertheless if a 4-hour save of urine is taken and the phosphates in it precipitated by glacial acetic acid then, when the resultant fluid has been centrifuged, the number of cells recognised microscopically in a counting chamber can be determined:

Normal urine contains 50,000 cells, with a range of 0–200,000 white cells per hour.

Abnormal urine contains over 200,000 white cells per hour,[3] and the rate of excretion of red cells is approximately the same.

The only casts that are of any clinical importance are the blood and granular types, and both these denote renal damage.

### Tubular Reabsorption

The constituents of the contents of Bowman's capsule are a direct ultrafiltrate of plasma. But although this liquid starts out on its journey through the tubular system resembling plasma, by the time it reaches the end it bears no relation to it at all. On its way down, enormous quantities of water and certain electrolytes are reabsorbed. This process is selective, so that the kidney tubules play an important part in controlling the electrolyte balance of the body. For example, for every 100 litres of water that enters the tubules less than 1 litre reaches the urine. Reabsorption may be either an active process requiring energy, or a passive process which depends on diffusion along a concentration gradient. A single substance may be reabsorbed by both processes in different parts of the nephron. Substances which are actively absorbed include calcium, amino acids and uric acid. There are specific mechanisms controlling the reabsorption of salts and water. In the latter case the water content of the body is controlled through the antidiuretic hormone of the posterior pituitary, and it is well known that nearly all anaesthetic drugs stimulate the release of this substance. Adrenal corticoid excretion controls sodium and chloride levels, and again this would appear to be slightly stimulated by anaesthetic drugs.

### Tubular Secretion

The secretion of substances into the tubular lumen may also be either active or passive. In man active secretion appears to be limited to a number of steroid metabolites, while potassium and urea are examples of passive secretion.

**Tests of tubular function.**—As the role of the tubules is largely one of selective reabsorption, most of the tests are based on the concentration of solids in the urine. Similarly, as the primary function of the tubules is to withdraw most of the water from its lumen, the ability to pass a concentrated or dilute urine under different conditions can be used as a gauge of tubular activity.

(i) *Urine concentration test.*—The specific gravity of the urine can be measured with a hydrometer. Normally, the range lies between 1003–1030 depending on the fluid intake. In diabetes, when large quantities of glucose are reaching the urine, the specific gravity is high, whereas tubular damage leads to a very dilute urine.

The ability of the kidney to concentrate urine may be studied in two ways: (*a*) complete abstinence from fluids for a 24-hour period has been used. This method is extremely unpleasant for the patient. A normal kidney should produce one specimen during this period with a specific gravity of 1,020 or more. (*b*) An intramuscular injection of pitressin tannate (5 mg) in oil is found to be a much more satisfactory alternative because it does not interfere with the patient's normal fluid intake. The action of the pitressin is to inhibit diuresis, so again a 24-hour urine save is instituted. The patient is allowed to eat and drink in a normal manner. One sample during this period should have a specific gravity of 1,020 or more if normal tubular function is present.

(ii) *Urine dilution test*.—For this test the patient consumes a known quantity of water (1 litre) and the ability of the kidney to excrete most of this intake is then studied. First the bladder is emptied and the contents discarded in the usual manner. Samples are then taken hourly for the next four hours. Normally at least 750 ml out of the 1 litre drunk by the patient should be recovered in the urine, and the specific gravity will be less than 1,004 in at least one specimen. Smoking and extreme emotion, however, may limit the diuresis.

Other methods used to study tubular function are more complex and involve the measurement of sodium, potassium, calcium, phosphate, and ammonium excretion.

### Measurement of Renal Blood Flow (RBF)

The renal blood flow is the total quantity of blood passing to both kidneys each minute. In order to measure this amount of blood, it is necessary to find a substance which is completely removed from the plasma during a single passage through the glomerular tuft, yet is neither reabsorbed nor excreted by the tubules. Then the plasma flow can be measured, and from this the blood flow to the kidney can be calculated. Diodrast and para-amino-hippuric acid (PAH) nearly fulfil these criteria, but PAH is technically easier to use. In fact only 90 per cent of it passes across the membrane and the remaining 10 per cent recirculates. Nevertheless, allowances can be made for this fraction in the final calculation. The exact proportion of PAH removed by a normal kidney has been confirmed in patients by simultaneous sampling of the concentration in the renal artery and vein during a steady infusion. Theoretically, if this substance was completely removed the concentration in the renal vein would be nil. In practice it was found that a small percentage (10 per cent) eluded filtration. Thus, measurements using PAH give an estimation of the "effective" renal plasma flow (ERPF) and this is converted to the true renal plasma flow by multiplying the results obtained by 1·1.

Measurement of renal plasma flow is made by first giving the patient a priming dose of PAH, followed by an infusion of it given at a rate which just compensates for its loss in the urine. In these circumstances the concentration of PAH in the peripheral venous plasma is essentially the same as that in the arterial plasma of the glomerular capillaries, so that venous samples may be used in the estimation. Thus:

$$\text{PAH clearance} \times 1{\cdot}1 = \text{Renal plasma flow in ml/minute.}$$

The plasma flow can be converted to blood flow if the value for the haematocrit is known:

$$\text{RBF} = 1{,}100\text{–}1{,}200 \text{ ml/minute.}$$

In renal disease the extraction of PAH may well be lower than the normal value of 90 per cent, and unless the renal vein is catheterised at the same time an accurate value for RBF cannot be calculated. More commonly $^{125}$I-Hippuran and $^{131}$I-Hippuran are now used instead of PAH. A single shot of the substance is given and the rate at which it disappears from the plasma measured. It is usual to estimate ERPF and GFR simultaneously using $^{131}$I-Hippuran and $^{51}$Cr-EDTA.

### Renal Blood Flow in the Conscious Patient

In normal circumstances the flow through the renal vessels does not vary widely. This constancy is maintained largely by alteration in the calibre of the renal arterioles. The kidney has its own regulating mechanism which ensures that it receives as adequate a supply of blood as possible despite variations in the systemic pressure. The range of mean systemic pressures over which autoregulation acts has been shown to be 70–200 mm Hg (9·3–26·7 kPa) in the dog. There are many factors which can reduce the renal blood flow in a conscious patient, and prominent amongst them are haemorrhage, fainting, asphyxia and cardiac failure.

The mechanism by which these various conditions reduce the renal blood flow is not the same in each case.

(*a*) *In hypovolaemia*, as is evidenced by haemorrhage, the mechanism is complex. In man there is a profound fall in renal blood flow and glomerular filtration. This fall is out of all proportion to the drop in blood pressure and is caused by severe renal vasoconstriction. One of the principal features of this condition is that even if the patient is thoroughly transfused and the blood volume and pressure returned to normal levels, the vasoconstriction does not wear off for several hours.[4]

The cause of this vasoconstriction has been thoroughly investigated and is now believed to be one of two factors—one nervous, the other humoral. Following severe haemorrhage with renal ischaemia, transfusion will slowly reverse the vasoconstriction if it is given within the first four hours. During this period the vasoconstriction is believed to be nervous in origin.

After four hours of renal ischaemia produced by hypotension the vasoconstriction may take many days to pass off even after suitable transfusion therapy; alternatively it may be irreversible. This persistent vasoconstriction is thought to be humoral in origin. Various substances have been suggested, and the most likely is renin.[5]

(*b*) *In the faint reaction*, there is essentially a slowing of the heart rate with marked peripheral vasodilatation. The cardiac output falls and the renal blood flow is reduced.

(*c*) *A high concentration of carbon dioxide or a low oxygen tension* in the blood reaching the kidneys causes the renal vessels to constrict. The latter response is induced reflexly through the sympathetic nervous system from stimulation of the carotid chemoreceptors, and is markedly increased if the hypoxia is associated with a fall in systemic blood pressure, which will also stimulate the carotid baroreceptors.[6]

(*d*) *In denervation*, as in autonomic block due to spinal analgesia or to the use of ganglion-blocking drugs, the renal vessels are dilated and the renal flow closely follows any changes in the systemic blood pressure. If the pressure remains unchanged the renal flow will do likewise; if it falls, so will the flow through the kidney. The decrease in GFR is parallel to the fall in mean arterial pressure. The ERPF falls slightly less than the GFR, suggesting that the decrease in renal vascular resistance is greater in the post-glomerular capillary bed.[7]

## Renal Blood Flow in the Anaesthetised Patient

### Effect of Anaesthesia

It would appear that all general anaesthetic agents commonly employed cause a decrease in renal blood flow to a greater or lesser extent. The degree of depression of the flow will depend upon the depth of anaesthesia. Thus, under very light anaesthesia the flow will be about 800 ml/minute (*cf* conscious = 1,200 ml/minute), but under deep anaesthesia it falls to 200 ml/minute or even less. So fine and rapid is this change in flow in relation to alterations in the depth of anesthesia with both ether and cyclopropane, that the renal blood flow could easily be used as an accurate sign of anaesthetic depth. During a long operation with a constant level of anaesthesia the flow remains unaltered, and as soon as the anaesthetic is withdrawn the blood flow starts to return to normal. Thus in lightly anaesthetised patients the fall will be moderate, while in those in whom the alpha-blocking agents (for example, droperidol) are used in conjunction with a balanced anaesthetic technique no significant alteration in renal blood flow may occur.[8]

The mechanism of this reduction in flow has been studied in animals[9] using ether and cyclopropane. Dogs were anaesthetised by a continuous intravenous infusion of pentobarbitone sodium, which produces little change in the renal circulation. The kidney was then perfused with a constant volume pump. The inhalation of ether and cyclopropane resulted in a pronounced and sustained rise in the perfusion pressure. Since this effect no longer occurred after denervation of the kidney it was concluded that the fall in blood flow was due to neurogenic vasoconstriction. Halothane, like most other general anaesthetic agents, brings about a fall in renal blood flow in premedicated patients.[10] However, at comparable depths of anaesthesia the reduction with cyclopropane and ether is greater than that with halothane. This could be explained on the basis that halothane produces less catecholamine excretion (leading to renal vasoconstriction) than either ether or cyclopropane.

Methoxyflurane produces a decrease in renal blood flow (RBF) by two different mechanisms. Firstly it modifies autoregulation so that RBF is directly dependent on the systemic pressure, and secondly it depresses RBF by a separate mechanism which is pressure independent.[11]

### Effect of Surgery

Habif and his co-workers[12] have shown that most operative procedures do not produce any change in the renal circulation. de Wardener[13] has confirmed these findings, but referred to one case where severe traction upon the large bowel had produced temporary vasoconstriction. Since there is considerable difficulty in obtaining adequate data on patients undergoing major surgery, it would at present seem advisable to conclude that major surgical stimulation—particularly under very light anaesthesia—may lead to depression of renal blood flow.

### Effect of Ganglion-blocking Drugs

Since the introduction of the hypotensive technique many authors have strongly condemned this method of reducing bleeding during surgery, on the grounds that it leads to increased damage to the kidney. It is difficult to gather, from a simple comparative study of patients under anaesthesia with and without hypotension, whether any renal damage occurs. Hampton and Little[14] stated that the incidence of renal complications following the use of hypotensive drugs during anaesthesia was no greater than in a comparable control series. Evans and Enderby[15] in a similar study based upon fluid excretion, proteinuria and the appearance of casts and red cells in the urine found, in a small series of 50 patients, that although the incidence of damage was slightly greater in the hypotensive group it was statistically insignificant. Miles and his colleagues[16] produced valuable evidence by measuring the renal blood flow and glomerular filtration rate of patients undergoing hypotensive anaesthesia without surgery. They used pentamethonium bromide and found, in a series of 10 patients, that although the systemic pressure fell by an average of 34 per cent, the average fall in the renal blood flow was only 5 per cent. In one of their cases the mean blood pressure fell below 40 mm Hg (5·3 kPa) yet the renal blood flow—though depressed—was still greater than they had found under deep anaesthesia in the absence of ganglion-blocking drugs.

From these observations it is concluded that renal vasodilatation must occur in the presence of hypotensive anaesthesia due to ganglion-blocking drugs. The experimental evidence available suggests that as the systemic pressure falls, so the renal vessels dilate to keep an almost steady flow of blood. On this basis it can be said that the normal kidney does not suffer damage from relatively short periods of hypotensive anaesthesia. It must be emphasised, however, that no data are available for very long periods of hypotension or the pathological kidney.

Moyer and McConn,[17] in a group of anaesthetised patients receiving pentamethonium, hexamethonium, and trimetaphan, were unable to confirm these results obtained by Miles and his colleagues.[16] In their patients the fall in blood pressure was followed by a reduction in the renal blood flow and the glomerular filtration rate in both normal and hypertensive patients. Associated with the fall in glomerular filtration rate was a marked reduction in the excretion of water and sodium. This was so great that they emphasised the dangers of overloading such a patient with fluids. Wakim,[18] using a flow meter inserted into the renal vein of dogs, also found a fall in their renal blood flow during hypotension with hexamethonium.

This evidence completely contradicts that of Miles and his colleagues,[16] but on close scrutiny of the figures the actual reduction in blood flow is not very great. Most significant of all, little or no mention is made by Moyer and McConn[17] of steps taken to prevent any fluctuation in depth of anaesthesia or to prevent a rise in the carbon dioxide tension of the blood. Since the smallest change in anaesthetic depth or carbon dioxide tension is sufficient to produce marked changes in the renal blood flow, variations in either of these measurements may account for the fundamental differences in these results.

### Effect of Haemorrhage

On purely theoretical grounds it might be reasoned that the renal vessels would constrict in the presence of increasing blood loss. de Wardener and his associates[19] have shown that this is not the case. In the anaesthetised subject the renal vessels dilate as the systemic pressure falls, so that they maintain an even flow of blood to the renal tissue despite the obvious paucity of flow in other parts of the body.

In their study these investigators measured the cardiac output, right atrial pressure, forearm blood flow, systemic pressure, heart rate, glomerular filtration and renal blood flow in a series of patients under light anaesthesia. The anaesthetic agents used were ether and cyclopropane. Haemorrhage was produced by venesection in amounts varying from 800–1,500 ml at a rate of 70–200 ml/minute. In the whole group the average fall in the estimated blood volume was 23 per cent. The only frequent change that they observed was a small reduction in renal flow during the actual venesection, but this rapidly returned to the previous level after the bleeding was completed. In twelve out of their fourteen patients venesection produced no *significant* change in the renal blood flow. In the two remaining patients the blood pressure fell to such a low level (below 40 mm Hg; 5·3 kPa) that the flow of urine ceased. When it started again the data available suggested, however, that the renal blood flow had continued during the period of anuria and that this flow had been reduced far less than would have been expected. The severe hypotension and bradycardia that occurred in these two patients was corrected immediately by rapid transfusion.

There are two important facts that emerge from this work on haemorrhage in the anaesthetised patient. First, the normal kidney does not apparently suffer acute ischaemia from severe hypotension under anaesthesia, and any reduction in flow that may occur can quickly be restored by transfusion therapy. Secondly, it is possible for the normal anaesthetised patient to lose up to 25–30 per cent of his total circulating blood volume without showing any significant changes in blood pressure or heart rate. This finding is of particular importance in any discussion upon the aetiology of postoperative renal failure.

In man, complete renal ischaemia lasting longer than 30 minutes is usually followed by tubular damage, and such an event is most likely to occur during the removal of an aortic aneurysm. This damage can be largely prevented by hypothermia; periods of up to two hours of total occlusion with only minor signs of renal damage at a body temperature of 28° C have been reported.[20]

**Auto-regulating mechanism.**—In the conscious subject even a relatively small haemorrhage is followed by a vasovagal attack where the blood pressure falls, largely due to widespread dilatation of the muscle vessels. At the same time the renal vessels dilate.[21] Under anaesthesia, even after a relatively massive haemorrhage, the renal vessels still dilate, but now the muscle vessels are found to be constricted. It was originally thought that the renal dilatation that occurred on fainting might be part of a widespread neurogenic vasodilating mechanism. The finding that under anaesthesia the muscle vessels constrict whilst the renal vessels dilate supports, however, the concept that the kidney has its own auto-regulating mechanism which tends to maintain an even level of renal blood flow despite alterations in the cardiac output and systemic pressure. The presence of such an intrinsic mechanism has been confirmed in animals.[22] Phillips and his associates,[23] working with dogs, also commented upon the relative stability of the renal circulation after haemorrhage, and they stated "the kidneys appear now to be favoured at the expense of the other peripheral circulation". Severe renal vasoconstriction occurred, however, after 4 to 6 hours of oligaemia.

Therefore, on the basis of all this evidence, it seems improbable that a transient reduction in blood volume, as may occur during surgery, can be responsible for the ischaemic renal damage that occasionally follows operations. Nevertheless, it is important to stress that all these measurements were made upon people with good kidney function and these deductions certainly do not hold when severe renal disease is already present.

### Effect of Vasopressor Drugs

When hypotension develops during anaesthesia a vasopressor drug is often used to restore the systemic pressure to a normal level. Two assumptions are usually made when considering the injection of these drugs. First, that the low blood pressure is necessarily associated with a reduced flow to the vital organs, and secondly, that raising the blood pressure by pressor drugs will automatically improve the flow. When considering the kidney both these assumptions may be unwarranted.

In the conscious patient, raising the blood pressure either with adrenaline[24] or noradrenaline[25] is associated with a pronounced renal vasoconstriction and fall in renal blood flow.

In the anaesthetised patient, the action of adrenaline, noradrenaline and methylamphetamine upon the renal blood flow have been studied.[26] These pressor drugs were given to both a group of patients with a normal blood pressure and a group with induced hypotension produced by pentamethonium bromide. The effect of the drugs upon the renal vessels was essentially the same, whether a low blood pressure was present or not. Adrenaline and noradrenaline both produced a rise in blood pressure accompanied by a consistent fall in the renal blood flow. On the other hand, methylamphetamine led to a rise in blood pressure and an overall increase in renal blood flow. No information is available about the action of these drugs upon the renal circulation in cases of hypotension due to haemorrhage. Moyer and McConn[17] studied the effects of vasopressor drugs on a group of hypertensive patients. Their results showed an increase in renal flow when the blood pressure was raised by noradrenaline after an injection of pentamethonium.

Dopamine possesses a selective renal vasodilatory action and also has positive inotropic cardiac activity. It, therefore, might be considered the most suitable agent for use in the presence of poor renal perfusion (see p. 431). If, however, the latter was mainly due to reduced cardiac output, then isoprenaline (with its stronger inotropic action) might be preferable.

### Renal Failure in Relation to Anaesthesia and Surgery

Following major surgery it is commonplace to find traces of albumin, red cells and casts in the urine during the first three postoperative days. In fact, Evans and Enderby[15] found that 78 per cent of a small series of normal patients developed proteinuria on the day after operation and in 34 per cent this persisted for more than three days. Cases of severe renal damage are fortunately rare, but when they occur they are often attended by a fatal result. The clinical picture of postoperative renal damage may be classed as either mild or severe.

In the mild condition the patient passes a plentiful supply of water in the first few days after operation. If it were accurately measured a polyuria would be noticed. Around the 7th–10th day the patient becomes mentally difficult or drowsy, and it is this change in the patient's mental attitude that often draws attention to the underlying condition. A blood urea taken at this stage reveals a level of 250 mg (41·7 mmol/l) or more. In all probability these patients had underlying renal damage before operation and a careful history usually reveals that they had polyuria at the same time. This can most easily be ascertained by a history of rising in the night to pass water with the absence of any prostatic enlargement on examination.

The severe type is the commoner condition and usually oliguria or anuria are noticed on the first postoperative day. Anuria is exceptional. The blood urea shows a steadily rising value and the rate of this rise is often taken as an indication of the severity of the condition. Vomiting and diarrhoea are early signs, together with restlessness, a wandering mind, and severe headache. Insomnia may be a marked feature and in the later stages muscle twitches and cramps may occur.

#### Causative Factor

Many factors have been blamed in the past, but at the present time the general opinion favours a prolonged period of hypotension leading to renal ischaemia as the principal cause. Anaesthesia, surgery, and even haemorrhage hardly affect the normal kidney, but then it is rare for the patient with normal kidney function to suffer failure postoperatively. During major surgery, particularly on the heart, a period of severe hypotension may occur. The resulting hypoxia of the renal cells is believed to lead to damage which is only revealed during the postoperative period. In the immediate postoperative period, when consciousness has been regained, a low blood volume state—as occurs after blood loss—is the most likely cause of intense renal vasoconstriction. Experimental data have shown that it is possible for a patient under light anaesthesia to lose 25 per cent of his blood volume without obvious circulatory signs. When consciousness has been regained, however, a hypovolaemia of this extent may be sufficient to cause intense renal vasoconstriction while producing only a slight fall in blood pressure.

Under normal circumstances the renal blood flow in the conscious patient remains remarkably constant despite considerable fluctuations in the perfusion pressure. This intimate control is believed to be exerted through neural and hormonal influences as part of the homeostatic mechanism controlling the extracellular fluid volume. In severe haemorrhage there is an immediate increase in intrarenal vascular resistance, presumably due to vasoconstriction.[27] In turn, this leads to a decrease in renal blood flow, a fall in the amount of sodium and water excreted and possibly a reduction in glomerular filtration rate. These changes, which are at first reversible but eventually lead to tubular damage, are more severe in those patients with pre-existing renal disease.

The induction of general anaesthesia causes a fall in the renal blood flow which is roughly proportional to the depth of anaesthesia. The exact mechanism of renal ischaemia in the surgical patient is still not entirely clear but probably arises from the effects of anaesthesia on the renin-angiotensin system. The stimulation of renin release by anaesthetic agents would result in a decrease in renal blood flow mediated by angiotensin.[28] The most widely held view is that cellular damage takes place either during or immediately after a period of hypotension. On the re-establishment of a normal blood flow these cells either recover completely or their permeability is damaged so that they swell with oedema and partially or totally occlude the lumen of the tubule. This theory is the basis for the use of mannitol in the prophylactic treatment of suspected cases of renal damage. As mannitol is excreted virtually unchanged, it is presumed that a hypertonic solution not only tends to keep the lumen of the tubules patent but may also withdraw some of the water from the tubule cells, thus diminishing the effects of the oedema.[29]

Evidence to support the hypotensive theory of postoperative renal failure is mostly clinical. Certainly oliguria and anuria are very rare complications in patients undergoing routine minor surgery with general anaesthesia. Yet in major surgery—particularly in association with the extracorporeal circulation with a poor total perfusion—the signs of renal damage are frequently observed.

### Diagnosis

The first indication of renal damage in the postoperative period is oliguria. This is a term used to denote a total urinary output in twenty-four hours of less than 500 ml. Nevertheless, oliguria in the postoperative period is not always due to renal failure, for it is commonly brought about by dehydration. This form of renal failure is often referred to as "pre-renal" and if not treated will progress to true renal failure. If a patient's fluid intake by mouth is curtailed or abandoned for many hours before operation, yet the "insensible" loss of sweating, humidification and alimentary secretions continues, it is not surprising that dehydration rapidly occurs. The "insensible" loss is usually estimated at about 1 litre per 24 hours. To this must be added any haemorrhage at the time of operation together with the extrusion of fluid into the lumen of the bowel during surgical manipulations. If adequate precautions are not taken to maintain the circulating fluid volume by infusion then dehydration will result. This will lead to haemoconcentration with a raised haematocrit and haemoglobin level.

In attempting to differentiate between oliguria due to dehydration and that due to intrinsic renal failure, the determination of two ratios are of greatest value, namely the urine: plasma ratio of urea and osmolality.

In the dehydrated group a high urine: plasma osmolality ratio greater than 1·8–2·0 and a urine: plasma urea ratio greater than 20 are usually found, while in those patients with established renal failure values of these ratios are less than 1·15 and less than 10 respectively.[30] The distinction is not however cast-iron and between the two groups fall those with intermediate values who may well respond to the institution of a forced diuresis with either mannitol or diuretics. Contrast radiography may also be invaluable as it may show the presence of treatable extrarenal obstruction.

### Treatment

In patients with pre-renal failure any deficit in blood volume should be rapidly corrected. Metabolic acidosis, if present, should be corrected by administration of bicarbonate, because it increases renal vasoconstriction.[31]

If this fails to restore the renal output, a dopamine infusion should be initiated. The selective renovascular effects of this drug in low concentrations has become an invaluable asset. A starting dose of 2 μg/kg/min should be tried, and increased slowly if there is no improvement of renal output.

A patient with severe, acute postoperative renal failure rarely survives for more than ten days unless effective treatment is employed quickly. In the less severe type of case which responds fairly rapidly to therapy, the oliguria gives way to polyuria.

The basic principle, therefore, of any treatment of this condition is twofold. First, since the cells of the collecting tubules are damaged, the fluid intake of the patient must be kept as nearly as possible equal to the fluid output. This latter figure must take into account any insensible loss from sweating, vomiting and diarrhoea, besides any small amount of urine that is passed. Secondly, the diet must be so arranged that protein metabolism is kept as low as possible, because the waste products of nitrogen metabolism soon mount to toxic levels. In normal subjects it is known that a carbohydrate intake of 100 g depresses protein metabolism, and it is assumed that the same process takes place under the conditions of acute renal failure.

The present-day management of patients with early postoperative renal failure is based on a strict surveillance of body weight and the biochemical changes in both blood and urine.

**Preliminary measures.**—1. The *weight* of the patient is accurately determined, as this will give an indication of gain or loss of fluids in the future treatment.

2. *Biochemical data* are also obtained as a baseline for the effectiveness of the therapy. The measurements made are:

(*a*) Blood. Values for urea, creatinine, calcium, potassium, sodium, chloride and bicarbonate are obtained. The haematocrit is also measured.

(*b*) Urine. Values for urea, sodium and potassium are estimated.

3. *An indwelling catheter* is inserted into the bladder so that a close watch can be kept on the exact amount of urine that is excreted.

4. *Restriction of fluids*.—The vital importance of the water obtained from metabolism within the body must be remembered. This sum amounts to approximately 600 ml daily. The total fluid required for a perfect balance of fluid therapy is composed of the sum of fluid lost by "sensible" and "insensible" loss. The "sensible" loss is the fluid which leaves the body either as urine or vomit. The "insensible" is the amount of fluid used up in sweating, humidification of the air in the lungs, and secretions into the bowel lumen which are lost in the faeces, and is usually taken as 1 litre per day. Thus a patient's fluid requirements will be 400 ml of sugar solution which together with the 660 ml produced within the body will provide for the 1,000 ml lost from "insensible" sources. To this total intake must also be added exactly the amount lost through urinary excretion and vomit.

The basis for restricted fluid therapy in acute renal failure can be expressed in ml as in Table 1. In this way fluid intake and output can be finely balanced. However, a small steady weight loss of 200–500 g daily will occur when a balance has been achieved, presumably due to a loss of body proteins.

**Further measures.**—1. *Carbohydrate* in the form of laevulose is most commonly used because not only is the sugar more easily metabolised but it is also believed to be the least nauseating when given by mouth in high concentration. Normally 100 g of laevulose are added to 400 ml of water, and this can be taken orally. If vomiting occurs as a complication, then a sterile solution of fructose can be infused into a large vein. As high concentrations of sugar solutions produce a severe reaction with thrombosis in small veins, a subclavian vein catheter is often used. Nevertheless the oral route is preferable because of the risk of infected emboli from the use of intravenous catheters.

2. *Anabolic steroids* (i.e. testosterone) are given to reduce the breakdown of protein within the body.

3. *Antibiotics* and *anticoagulants* must only be used with caution as many tend to accumulate in the circulation if renal function is poor. For example, streptomycin is contra-indicated in such circumstances, as even small doses may lead to VIIIth cranial nerve damage. Similarly, the sulphonamides should not be used as they tend to form crystals in the renal tubules, thus increasing the renal damage. Use of the aminoglycoside, particularly gentamicin, has been found to be satisfactory. Blood levels of this

36/TABLE 1
RESTRICTED FLUID THERAPY

| | | | | |
|---|---|---|---|---|
| Insensible | | 400 ml of sugar solution | | |
| loss (1,000 ml) | | + 450 ml from tissue metabolism | } = | 600 ml from body metabolism |
| + | = | + 150 ml from carbohydrate metabolism | | |
| sensible loss | | + sensible loss (urine or vomit) | | |

and other antibiotics should be estimated to establish the correct serum levels.

Most of the long-acting anticoagulants (e.g. dicoumarin) tend to accumulate in the presence of renal failure, but heparin can be used with safety because it is detoxicated in the liver.

4. *Ion-exchange resins* can be used to control the serum potassium level which tends to rise steadily in the presence of acute renal failure. These resins are in powder form and can be given either orally or rectally. They act by accepting potassium and releasing sodium in exchange. Using Resonium 15 g four times a day, it is often possible to keep the serum potassium level between 3·5 and 4·0 mmol/l. Alternatively in an emergency, the administration of glucose (50 g) and insulin (15 units) tends to lower the serum potassium level by holding the electrolyte within the cell and also actively promoting its uptake by the cell.

Once this regime has been fully established it is then only necessary to observe closely the effects of this therapy. The future progress will reveal the extent and severity of the renal damage. If it is clear that restriction of fluids alone is not preventing a gradual deterioration in the patient's state then the question of dialysis must be considered.

*Indications for dialysis* are:

(*a*) Worsening of the clinical state of the patient—particularly the appearance of pre-uraemic features together with mental retardation
(*b*) Blood urea nitrogen (BUN) over 25–28 mmol/l(150–170 mg per cent) or a blood urea over 50 mmol/l (300 mg per cent)
(*c*) A rise in the serum potassium level over 7·0 mmol/l
(*d*) A fall in the plasma bicarbonate to 12 mmol/l) or below.

**Dialysis.**—There are two principal methods of removing the waste products of metabolism from the circulation in the presence of poor renal function.

(*a*) *Peritoneal dialysis* necessitates the introduction of a large volume of fluid of known composition into the peritoneal cavity. Those electrolytes and nitrogenous substances which are in excess in the circulation can then diffuse out into the fluid and so finally be removed. This technique requires an intraperitoneal catheter with numerous fine holes in the terminal 4 cm. The tubing is inserted under local analgesia about one-third of the way along a line drawn from the umbilicus to the pubic symphysis; 2·5 litres of either an isotonic (if the patient is not overloaded already with water) or hypertonic (if waterlogged) solution are run in and left *in situ* for about 40 minutes, after which it is all drained out again. Antibiotics and heparin are added to the solution to prevent infection and the formation of fibrin clots. The whole technique is simple and effective in mild or moderate cases. It can be repeated frequently without much trouble. The only disadvantage is that it removes the plasma proteins and also exposes the patient to the risk of infection.

(*b*) *Haemodialysis* is based on the principle of passing the blood through semi-permeable Cellophane tubing in its passage from an artery to a vein. The tubing or membrane is surrounded by a solution of known concentration so that during the passage of the blood the electrolytes and other waste products can diffuse out. Such an apparatus is often described as an "artificial kidney". The development of these machines has now progressed to a stage where it is perfectly feasible to keep a patient alive indefinitely without renal function provided his blood is dialysed at least twice weekly.

### Histological Findings in a Fatal Case of Postoperative Renal Failure

The glomerular membrane is less sensitive to hypoxia and ischaemia than is the tubular system, so that it is not surprising that the latter structures suffer most in cases of acute postoperative renal failure. The distal convoluted tubules show dilatation with flattening of the epithelium, and pigmented casts may be found in the lumen of these tubules, and also that of the loop of Henle and the collecting tubule.[32] Necrosis of the tubules is not a common finding in this condition, but the cells of the tubules show cellular infiltration and oedema. The anuria or oliguria is clearly not due to any damage to the glomerular apparatus but rather to alteration in the function of the tubules. Biopsy specimens have failed to confirm that swelling of the tubules occurs and blocks the flow of urine. The most acceptable explanation is that the tubules lose their semi-permeability and almost all the water passing down the lumen is reabsorbed.

## KIDNEY TRANSPLANTATION

For many years it has been established that in man tissues can easily be transferred from one region of the body to another, yet great difficulty is experienced if an attempt is made to transfer this same tissue to another person. This failure to accept the tissues of other human beings is due to the immune response. A significant advance in our knowledge of the mechanism of this response has been made by the contributions of Medawar[33] and Burnet,[34] both of whom were jointly awarded the Nobel Prize for Medicine in 1962. These authors demonstrated that the immune reaction is a protective mechanism possessed by every animal and is most easily illustrated as the inflammatory reponse to an invading organism or the allergic reaction to a foreign protein. Without this protection, man would have succumbed to the microbe many centuries ago.

The treatment of chronic renal failure by means of renal transplantation has now become a well-established practice, with well over 8300 transplants being recorded by the International Transplant Registry.[35] Analysis of the results has shown that the number of grafts functioning at the end of the first and third year for cadaveric kidneys was 53 per cent and 40 per cent while for kidneys taken from living related donors the number was 73 per cent and 58 per cent respectively.[36]

### The Immune Response

This is generated mainly by lymphoid tissue. It is most easily studied by observing the reaction to a homologous skin graft, though the same principle applies to transplanted organs such as the kidney. At first the new graft thrives, so that during the initial five days or so it become vascularised and pink with a really healthy appearance. On about the 5th to 7th day, the homograft takes on a discoloured appearance, and soon the evidence of necrosis begins to appear, until by the 12th day it is obviously dead. Pathological examination of the grafted region will reveal a lymphocytic reaction with also, but to a lesser degree, a proliferation of plasma cells. If a second attempt is now made to repeat the grafting process, then the time taken for the rejection phenomenon to reveal itself is even less.

It is clear, therefore, that the immune response is a fundamental law permitting the body to recognise self from non-self and involves two factors, cellular and humoral. The cellular factor is believed to be more important than the humoral one. The whole process is intimately linked with the lymphoid tissue throughout the body, and this system is known to be closely concerned with the production of antibodies. Burnet[37] has suggested that the probable role of the thymus gland is to organise the immune response and this takes place around the time of birth. Once achieved, the thymus no longer has a function to fulfil so that it atrophies and shrinks. In mice, if the thymus gland is removed soon after birth this immune response does not develop. Thus it is established that if a successful homologous tissue transplantation is to be achieved in man, it is vital to try and match the donor and recipient tissues as nearly as possible and also to suppress the immune response.

### Tissue Typing

The antigens (which are on the surface of grafted cells and are responsible for the immune response in patients receiving grafts) are called histocompatibility antigens. It is the immune response of the recipient against these antigens that results in the rejection of the tissue that has been grafted. In man the most important histocompatibility antigens are called the HL-A antigens and these are found in all nucleated cells of the body including leucocytes. Each person can carry up to 6 different HL-A antigens.

After initially confirming ABO compatibility, which is the first essential step, two general methods are used to determine the compatibility between the donor and the recipient of grafted tissue. The first involves the determination *in vitro* of the histocompatibility antigens in both donor and recipient and only if there are some antigens common to both are the tissues for grafting considered acceptable. In the second method donor and recipient tissues are mixed *in vivo* and observed for signs of incompatibility.

### Suppression of the Immune Response

Although there are numerous methods, the principal difficulty is to achieve a delicate balance between a lethal dose on the one hand and yet an adequate one on the other.

**Genetic compatibility.**—A number of successful kidney transplant operations have been reported between identical twins. Because of the genetic compatibility between these two beings, the immune response is not present. However, some of these patients have developed glomerulonephritis (the initial disease of the host) in the grafted kidney, but this complication is less likely to occur if the diseased kidney is removed first. The genetic relationship between children and parents and between siblings enhances the chance of successful transplantation in these groups.

**Current methods of treatment.**—1. *Corticosteroids*. These are usually given in the form of prednisone or prednisolone. Three general schemes are in current use. In the first, high doses are given from the time of transplantation and then gradually reduced until either signs of rejection occur or a maintenance level of 10–15 mg daily is reached.[38] Secondly, minimal steroid therapy is given until signs of rejection are seen, when the dosage is rapidly increased.[39] Thirdly, over and above a maintenance dose of steroids a large bolus of methyl prednisolone (10–30 mg/kg) is given as a single dose or on several occasions. This must be injected slowly as there have been reports of cardiac irregularities and even arrest.

2. *Azathioprine*. This is an antimetabolite which interferes with nucleic acid synthesis in the cell. It only becomes active after conversion in the liver to 6-mercaptopurine. Azathioprine and its metabolites are excreted by the kidney and the dosage is dependent on renal function, which is assessed by creatinine clearance. With normal renal function the dosage currently in use (3 mg/kg) does not depress bone-marrow function but the white-cell and platelet counts must be checked regularly. Treatment with azathioprine is usually continued indefinitely.

3. *Antilymphocytic globulin*. This is an antiserum produced in a foreign species against the recipient's lymphocytes. It inhibits cellular delayed-type sensitivity and will prevent or delay graft rejection. It is usually given at the time of transplantation.

4. *Cyclophosphamide*. This is an alkylating agent which may be used in place of azathioprine.

5. *Radiotherapy*. Local radiation of the graft with 150 rads on 3 occasions over a 4-day period has been used,[40] and this has replaced whole-body irradiation.

6. *Anticoagulants*. During the rejection period of a graft, it has been shown histologically that platelets and fibrin are deposited in the small renal vessels. Treatment of the recipient with heparin, oral anticoagulants and the platelet de-aggregating agent dipyridamole, has shown that these lesions can be prevented.[41]

### The Rejection Phenomenon

The success or failure of a graft to "take" is determined by histocompatibility factors which are inherited. For this reason it follows that the nearer the donor tissue is to that of the recipient the more likely is the grafting to be successful. Ideally, therefore, the most suitable donor tissue is that taken from an identical twin. Next comes a close family relationship such as the mother for her son. Finally, a donor of a compatible blood group with as many HL-A antigens as possible similar to those of the patient should be selected.

The rejection response is a very complicated process and the signs can first be observed at any time from a few days to even months after the grafting. Sometimes the process can be halted and even reversed by local irradiation or increasing the dose of drugs if the diagnosis is established sufficiently early.

**Diagnosis of the rejection response.**—The initial finding is deterioration of renal function with decreasing urine output, reduced urinary concentration of urea and sodium, and increased protein excretion. The creatinine clearance falls and the serum creatine and urea rise. The graft may swell and become tender and hypertension and pyrexia may occur. Urine examination may show an increased number of lymphocytes, and blood examination a leucocytosis, eosinophilia and a thrombocytopenia. Although a number of enzyme estimations may show evidence of an immunological reaction, clinical examination and simple laboratory tests are usually adequate to confirm that rejection is occurring.[42]

### Treatment

The most common method of treatment of the rejection episode is with large doses of methylprednisolone given intravenously.[43] 1–2 g of methylprednisolone are given twelve-hourly for 36 hours. In this dosage, the long-term side-effects of steroid therapy are not seen. Alternatively, either the oral steroid therapy or, less often, the dose of azathioprine may be increased.

## RENAL DISEASE AND ANAESTHESIA

Anaesthesia for patients with renal disease may be broadly divided into four categories:

1. Insertion of arteriovenous shunt or construction of an arteriovenous fistula
2. Nephrectomy related to transplantation
3. Kidney transplantation
4. Surgery unrelated to the coincidental renal disease.

The choice of anaesthetic agents is dependent on the degree of remaining renal function because it is necessary to limit the drugs to those in which the degree of reduction of renal excretion will not lead to prolonged action. If the drugs are metabolised to inactive substances before excretion no difficulties will arise from their use. The metabolism of the inhalational agents, with the exception of methoxyflurane, do not affect renal function. The latter has been shown to produce an impairment of renal concentrating power directly related to the total dose given and to the resulting serum levels of ionic fluoride which are formed from the metabolism of the methoxyflurane.[44] It has also been suggested that enflurane, which is also a fluorinated methylethyl ether, may also cause renal damage[45] and a case of renal failure following enflurane anaesthesia has been reported.[46]

The non-inhalational anaesthetic agents are essentially dependent on the kidney for their excretion either unchanged or as active or inactive end-products, and each drug must be considered on its own merits. In some instances the presence of renal failure may result in alternative metabolic pathways being used, for example an increased amount being excreted in the bile, as is found with tubocurarine.[47]

### General Considerations

In patients with advanced renal failure the major problems are those of uraemia, anaemia, hypertension, infection, and electrolyte disorders, especially hyperkalaemia. In those awaiting transplantation, uraemia can be satisfactorily treated by dialysis and most patients will have been attending a dialysis unit twice weekly, or more frequently in the acute stage. Dialysis will ensure normal fluid balance as well as correcting electrolyte disturbances and eliminating urea. Haemodialysis is performed through an arteriovenous shunt placed on the forearm or lower leg. The Scribner Teflon shunt has been widely used for this purpose, but recently the Cimino-Brescia shunt has become increasingly popular. This involves the establishment of a direct arteriovenous fistula between the radial artery and an adjacent vein by open operation. The marked dilatation of the veins in the forearm that results from this shunt enables frequent and easy access to be established with the circulation, using needles of sufficient calibre to carry the blood flow required for haemodialysis. Once a satisfactory shunt has been established, dialysis can be performed whenever required.

Almost all patients presenting for transplantation are severely anaemic, as the anaemia associated with uraemia is very resistant to treatment. The anaemia is caused, in part, by failure of the kidney to produce renal erythropoietic factor. This substance acts on a plasma globulin to produce erythropoietin which, in turn, stimulates red-cell production in the bone marrow.[48] The infusion of large volumes of blood carries a risk of precipitating pulmonary oedema. Blood is only added sparingly during dialysis, as the stimulus to the patient's own erythrocyte production would be thereby reduced and moreover, each transfusion carries the risk of introducing serum hepatitis, and infection is liable to spread rapidly in dialysis units.

Most patients will have a haemoglobin level in the region of 7 g/dl when they present for operation, a figure which would be regarded as totally unacceptable for other operative procedures. Nevertheless, patients undergoing renal transplantation survive surgery and anaesthesia remarkably well despite this severe degree of anaemia. Because of the frequency of infections during chronic renal failure many patients having renal transplants will be receiving antibiotic therapy. The potentiation of the action of non-depolarising muscle relaxants following the intraperitoneal administration of polymyxin, streptomycin and neomycin is well known. This phenomenon may also become manifest in patients with a low urinary output who are receiving certain antibiotics by injection, because their requirements for these drugs are considerably reduced.[49] Particular care should be taken with the aminoglycosides, tetracycline, polymyxins, colistin, and lincomycin.[50]

### Arteriovenous Shunts and Fistulae

While anaemia and some degree of uraemia will usually be present, the use of peritoneal dialysis and cation exchange resins should have resulted in the patient having normal electrolytes. The initial procedure that is usually carried out is the insertion of a Teflon/silastic shunt. At the same time or at a subsequent operation, a subcutaneous arteriovenous fistula is formed. It is necessary to insert the shunt first, because the fistula will take some weeks before it may be used satisfactorily.

### Renal Transplantation

With the exception of transplantation from a living (related) donor, this procedure is usually undertaken as an emergency. The donor kidney is removed from the cadaver as soon as possible after death has been certified. The warm ischaemic time—that is the time between the cessation of renal perfusion until the kidney has either been surface cooled or perfused with a cold solution at 4° C (for example Hartmann's solution), should ideally be less than thirty minutes. Although subsequent storage for up to 16 hours has been reported without severe tubular necrosis,[35] this should be kept to an absolute minimum. Tissue cross-matching between donor and intended recipient is carried out and, if satisfactory, blood is taken for full blood count, urea and electrolyte estimation and cross-matching.

### Bilateral Nephrectomy

This has been carried out after renal transplantation when the grafted kidney is functioning well. The problems are essentially the same as those for transplantation although the problem of renal excretion of drugs will be of less importance in the presence of an adequate renal output. The patient will still be receiving both steroids and immunosuppressive drugs, and the dosage of these should be increased over the period of surgery.

### Anaesthetic Management

Initial pre-operative examination of the patient is vital with particular emphasis to see if any signs of fluid overload are present. A full explanation of what may be expected postoperatively is essential, for the patient may understandably be extremely apprehensive. When time will allow a small premedicant dose of morphine 5–10 mg and scopolamine 0·2 mg can be given.

Either regional or general anaesthesia techniques may be suitable. In many instances regional anaesthesia may not appear acceptable to the patient, but a full explanation of what such a technique would involve, with adequate sedation (for example, oral diazepam), will usually result in the patient's agreement. For surgery involving the arms, brachial plexus block has been used. The problem of postoperative clotting of the arteriovenous fistula has resulted in the use of infiltration with local anaesthetic of the operative site and sympathetic blockade which, in the arm, is achieved by stellate ganglion block. The latter may be carried out with 10 ml of 0·5 per cent bupivacaine, because its length of action will ensure continued dilatation of the forearm vessels well into the postoperative period.

The long-term survival of most patients with chronic renal failure depends on access to the vascular system for dialysis for the rest of their lives. Anything that may damage vessels needed in the future for shunts and fistulae must be avoided at all costs. When it is necessary to set up an intravenous infusion, the ideal veins are those on the back of the hand, and care should be taken to see that no drugs that are known to cause thrombosis of small veins are given via this route. If there are no obvious veins in the hand, the insertion of a subclavian catheter under local anaesthesia, prior to induction, is probably the best alternative. If, in desperation, a forearm vein has to be used, it is worth asking the surgeon which vein is going to be the least valuable for access in the future.

When multiple procedures are being performed, or in very apprehensive patients, general anaesthesia will be required. Induction with thiopentone or methohexitone followed by maintenance with nitrous oxide, oxygen and minimal amounts of halothane has proved satisfactory. However, the latter may cause marked hypotension, and trichloroethylene or isoflurane may be used in such cases. As blood levels of thiopentone are altered by redistribution and tissue uptake[51] its length of action is unaffected by the degree of renal failure. The technique of intermittent thiopentone with a small supplementary dose of narcotic, even in the sickest patient, is extremely useful.

If it is necessary to intubate the patient, the dangers associated with the use of suxamethonium in patients with renal failure must be considered. It has been shown that injection of suxamethonium causes a small but statistically significant rise in serum potassium, and it has been suggested that this may be the cause of cardiac arrest in uraemic patients.[52,53] The maximum increase, in two separate studies, was 0·5 mmol/l[54] and 0·7 mmol/l,[55] and no difference was found between normal patients and those in renal failure. In Miller's series none of his patients with renal failure was uraemic although the highest serum potassium was 6·6 mmol/l. He concluded that suxamethonium is not contra-indicated in patients with renal failure in the absence of uraemia. Samuel and Powell[49] used suxamethonium without a problem for intubation in 97 patients for renal transplantation. Measurements of serum potassium and blood urea ranged between 3·0–7·2 mmol/l for potassium and 2·5–42·5 mmol/l (15–256 mg/100 ml) for urea. Serum cholinesterase levels are known to be reduced in chronic renal failure but this does not normally create any difficulties.[56]

Although the antigenic profile of the recipients awaiting transplant will already be on record it will take approximately two hours to determine for which recipient the donor kidney is suitable. In consequence it is likely that the acceptable recipient will have eaten recently and thus have a full stomach. Although attempts to empty the stomach by gastric aspiration have been advocated, the results are usually incomplete and the procedure both time-consuming and distressing to the patient. Because the time factor is critical in emergency transplantation, premedication with oral antacids alone (magnesium trisilicate 30 ml) has been recommended.[49] An alternative is to give metoclopramide 10 mg intravenously to hasten gastric emptying. For any subsequent doses of this drug given to patients in renal failure, the normal dose should be halved, since the clearance is greatly reduced.[57]

Immediately prior to *induction* oxygen should be given for at least 3 minutes. An open vein should be secured in the back of the hand. To save veins, the intravenous infusion that will be required during surgery may be inserted at this stage rather than using a small-gauge indwelling metal needle. In view of the potential danger of hyperkalaemia in patients with renal failure, no crystaloid solution given should contain potassium. This is an even greater danger in insulin-dependent diabetics who come to transplantation.[58] Great care must be taken of any fistula or shunt that is present, so the limb should be wrapped in cotton-wool, kept immobile and in extension. The blood-pressure cuff should be placed on another limb to minimise any chance of clotting in the shunt. ECG electrodes should be positioned on the chest.

The patient may be induced with a small dose of thiopentone or methohexitone mixed with a normal premedicant dose of atropine and followed by suxamethonium and rapid intubation. Cricoid pressure should be applied to prevent regurgitation of gastric contents. The potential hazards of using suxamethonium have already been discussed; in patients who have been adequately starved, intubation may be carried out using either tubocurarine or pancuronium. However, not only does the onset of laryngeal paralysis take longer to supervene but the large dose required for intubation increases the risk of administering an overdose. It is advisable, therefore, to titrate each patient with a peripheral-nerve stimulator (Chapter 23). In view of the high risk of infection in patients receiving corticosteroids and immunosuppressive drugs, all equipment used for intubation and ventilation should have been sterilised. Maintenance of anaesthesia with nitrous oxide/oxygen/tubocurarine and minimal doses of halothane has been reported by Samuel and Powell[49] in 100 patients. In six of these a small dose of either morphine or pethidine was added. They noted that halothane, when used as the main anaesthetic agent, could cause unpredictable hypotension in patients with potentially abnormal plasma volumes after dialysis. It would seem that halothane and tubocurarine can decrease renal blood flow.[59] As about 90 per cent of doses of morphine, pethidine and fentanyl are inactivated before excretion, these drugs may be used as the main agent for maintaining anaesthesia, with halothane being confined to the treatment of any acute hypertensive episodes that may occur.

While gallamine is contra-indicated because

it is excreted by the kidney in an active form, both tubocurarine and pancuronium have been used satisfactorily as neuromuscular blocking agents. The total dose should be kept to the minimum requirements because prolonged action has been reported with both agents. Incremental doses of suxamethonium have also been used satisfactorily for providing muscular relaxation during transplantation, and are particularly useful for children. A supplementary dose of atropine should be given to protect the heart against the effect of reflex bradycardia. Once anaesthesia has been established, the intravenous infusion in the hand can be set up if not already present, and a subclavian catheter inserted for measurement of central venous pressure. At this stage both corticosteroids and immunosuppressive drugs are usually given, the exact dosage depending on the renal unit concerned. The kidney is usually placed retroperitoneally in the pelvic cavity with anastomosis of the renal artery and vein to the iliac vessels. On completion of the anastomosis either diuretics or mannitol may be given. In kidney grafts that show signs of vascular spasm after release of the vascular clamps, any evidence of hypovolaemia, shown by central venous pressure measurement, should first be corrected. If there is no improvement, an infusion of dopamine 2 $\mu$g/kg/min should be started and will often reverse the spasm. The infusion is usually discontinued at the end of the operation provided any fluid deficit has been corrected. At the end of the operation non-depolarising muscle relaxants are reversed in the usual way with atropine and neostigmine. The ECG should be carefully observed during this period because dysrhythmias may occur which may lead to cardiac arrest particularly in patients with hyperkalaemia. Great care should be taken to see that no antibiotics with neuromuscular-blocking properties are given in the immediate postoperative period or the patient will rapidly become reparalysed. Postoperatively patients are transferred to a specialised unit and nursed in as near a sterile condition as possible.

## REFERENCES


1. Lambert, P. P., Gassee, J. P., Verniory, A. and Ficheroulle, P. (1971). Measurement of the glomerular filtration pressure from sieving data from macromolecules. *Pflügers Arch. ges. Physiol.*, **329**, 34.
2. Lingardh, G. (1972). Renal clearance investigations with 51 Cr-EDTA and 125 I-Hippuran. *Scand. J. Urol. Nephrol.*, **6**, 63.
3. de Wardener, H. E. (1973). *The Kidney. An outline of normal and abnormal structure and function.* 4th edit. London: Churchill Livingstone.
4. Lauson, H. D., Bradley, S. E. and Cournand, A. (1944). Renal circulation in shock. *J. clin. Invest.*, **23**, 381.
5. Wright, S. (1965). *Applied Physiology*, 10th edit. London: Oxford Univ. Press.
6. Pelletier, C. L. and Shepherd, J. T. (1975). Effect of hypoxia on vascular responses to the carotid baroflex. *Amer. J. Physiol.*, **228**, 331.
7. Kennedy, W. F., Sawyer, T. K., Gerbershagen, H. U., Everett, G. B., Cutler, R. E., Allen, G. D. and Bonica, J. J. (1970). Simultaneous systemic cardiovascular and renal hemodynamic measurements during high spinal anaesthesia in normal man. *Acta anaesth. scand.*, **14**, Suppl. 37, 163.
8. Gorman, H. M. and Craythorne, N. W. B. (1966). The effects of a new neuroleptanalgesic agent (Innovar) on renal function in man. *Acta anaesth. scand.*, Suppl. **24**, 111.
9. Miles, B. E. and de Wardener, H. E. (1952). Renal vasoconstriction produced by ether and cyclopropane anaesthesia. *J. Physiol. (Lond.)* **118**, 141.
10. Mazze, R. I., Schwartz, R. D., Slocum, H. C. and Kevin, G. B. (1963). Renal function during anesthesia and surgery. 1. The effects of halothane anesthesia. *Anesthesiology*, **4**, 279.
11. Leighton, K. M., Koth, B. and Wenkstein, B. M. (1973). Autoregulation of renal blood flow: alteration by methoxyflurane. *Canad. Anaesth. Soc. J.*, **20**, 173.
12. Habif, D. V., Papper, E. M., Fitzpatrick, H. F., Lowrance, P., Smythe, C. McC. and Bradley, S. E. (1951). The renal and hepatic blood flow, glomerular filtration rate and urinary output of electrolytes during cyclopropane, ether and thiopental anesthesia, operation and the immediate postoperative period. *Surgery*, **30**, 241.
13. de Wardener, H. E. (1955). Renal circulation during anaesthesia and surgery. *Anaesthesia*, **10**, 18.
14. Hampton, L. J. and Little, D. M. (1953). Complications associated with the use of "controlled hypotension" in anesthesia. *Arch. Surg.*, **67**, 549.
15. Evans, B. and Enderby, G. E. H. (1952). Controlled hypotension and its effect on renal function. *Lancet*, **1**, 1045.
16. Miles, B. E., de Wardener, H. E., Churchill-Davidson, H. C. and Wylie, W. D. (1952). The effect on the renal circulation of pentamethonium bromide during anaesthesia. *Clin. Sci.*, **11**, 73.
17. Moyer, J. H. and McConn, R. (1956). Renal hemodynamics in hypertensive patients following administration of pendiomide. *Anesthesiology*, **17**, 9.
18. Wakim, K. G. (1955). Certain cardiovasculorenal effects of hexamethonium. *Amer. Heart. J.*, **50**, 435.
19. de Wardener, H. E., Miles, B. E., Lee, G. de J.,

Churchill-Davidson, H. C., Wylie, W. D. and Sharpey-Schafer, E. P. (1953). Circulatory effects of haemorrhage during prolonged light anaesthesia in man. *Clin. Sci.*, **12**, 175.
20. Churchill-Davidson, H. C. (1955). Hypothermia. *Brit. J. Anaesth.*, **27**, 313.
21. de Wardener, H. E. and McSwiney, R. R. (1951). Renal haemodynamics in vasovagal fainting due to haemorrhage. *Clin. Sci.*, **10**, 209.
22. de Wardener, H. E. and Miles, B. E. (1952). The effect of haemorrhage on the circulatory autoregulation of the dog's kidney perfused *in situ*. *Clin. Sci.*, **11**, 267.
23. Phillips, R. A., Dole, V. P., Hamilton, P. B., Emerson, K., Jr., Archibald, R. M. and van Slyke, D. D. (1945). Shock and renal function *Amer. J. Physiol.*, **145**, 314.
24. Smith, H. W. (1943). *Lectures on the Kidney*. (Porter Lectures, Series IX, and the William Henry Walch Lectures.) Lawrence, Kan.: Univ, of Kansas Press.
25. Barnett, A. J., Blacket, R. B., Depoorter, A. E., Sanderson, P. H. and Wilson, G. M. (1950). The action of noradrenaline in man and its relation to phaeochromocytoma and hypertension. *Clin. Sci.*, **9**, 151.
26. Churchill-Davidson, H. C., Wylie, W. D., Miles, B. E. and de Wardener, H. E. (1951). The effects of adrenaline, noradrenaline and methedrine on the renal circulation during anaesthesia. *Lancet*, **2**, 803.
27. Parsons, F. M., Blagg, C. R. and Williams, R. E. (1963). Chemistry, therapy and hemodialysis of acute renal failure. *Biochem. Clin.*, No. **2**, p. 457.
28. Pettinger, W. A. (1978). Anesthetics and the renin-angiotensin-aldosterone axis. *Anesthesiology* **48**, 393.
29. Flores, J., Di Bona, G. F., Beck, C. H. and Leaf, A. (1972). The role of cell swelling in ischemic damage and the protective effect of hypertonic solute. *J. clin. Invest.*, **51**, 118.
30. Luke, R. G., Briggs, J. D., Allison, M. E. M. and Kennedy, A. C. (1970). Factors determining response to mannitol in acute renal failure. *Amer. J. med. Sci.*, **259**, 168.
31. Zimmerman, W. E. (1969). Metabolic disorders, renal and hepatic blood flow in shock and the effect of infusion fluids on parameters of acid-base balance. *Bibl. haemat. (Basel)*, **33**, 408.
32. Brun, C. and Munck, O. (1957). Lesions of the kidney in acute renal failure following shock. *Lancet*, **1**, 603.
33. Medawar, P. B. (1958). *The Immunology of Transplantation*, p. 144. (Harvey Lectures No. 52.) New York: Academic Press Inc.
34. Burnet, F. M. (1959). *The Clonal Selection Theory of Acquired Immunity*. (Abraham Flexner Lectures.) Nashville: Vanderbilt University Press.
35. Hulme, B. (1975). Medical aspects of renal transplantation. In: *Recent Advances in Renal Disease*, ed. Jones, N. F. London: Churchill Livingstone.
36. Gurland, H. J., Brunner, F. P., Dehn, H., Harlen, H., Parsons, F. M. and Scharer, K. (1973). Combined report on regular dialysis and transplantation in Europe. *Proc. Europ. dial. & transpl. Ass.*, **10**, 42.
37. Burnet, F. M. (1962). Role of the thymus and related organs in immunity. *Brit. med. J.*, **2**, 807.
38. Straffan, R. A., Hewitt, C. B., Kiser, W. S. Stewart, B. H., Nakamoto, S. and Kolff, W. J. (1966). Clinical experience with the use of 79 kidneys from cadavers for transplantation. *Surg. Gynec. Obstet.*, **123**, 483.
39. Mowbray, J. F., Cohen, S. L., Doak, P. B., Kenyon, J. R., Owen, K., Percival, A., Porter, K. A. and Peart, W. S. (1965). Human cadaveric renal transplantation: report of twenty cases. *Brit. med. J.*, **2**, 1387.
40. Hume, D. M., Magee, J. M., Kaufman, H. M., Rittenbury, M. S. and Prout, G. R. (1963). Renal homotransplantation in man in modified recipients. *Ann. Surg.*, **158**, 608.
41. Kincaid-Smith, P. (1969). Modification of vascular lesions of rejection in cadaveric renal allografts by dipyridamole and anticoagulants. *Lancet*, **2**, 920.
42. Merrill, J. P. (1971). Diagnosis and management of rejection in allografted kidneys. *Transplant Proc.*, **3**, 287.
43. Woods, J. E., Anderson, C. F., De Weerd, J. H., Johnson, J. H., Donadio, W. J., Leary, F. J. and Frohnert, P. P. (1973). High dosage intravenously administered methylprednisolone in renal transplantation: a preliminary report. *J. Amer. med. Ass.*, **223**, 896.
44. Cousins, M. J. and Mazze, R. I. (1973). Methoxyflurane nephrotoxity: a study of dose-response in man. *J. Amer. med. Ass.*, **225**, 1611.
45. Loehning, R. W. and Mazze, R. I. (1974). Possible nephrotoxicity from enflurane in a patient with severe renal disease. *Anesthesiology*, 40, 203.
46. Eichhorn, J. H., Hedley-White, M. D., Steinman, T. I., Kaufmann, J. L. and Laasberg, L. H. (1976). Renal failure after enflurane anesthesia. *Anesthesiology*, **45**, 557.
47. Cohen, E. N., Winslow Brewer, H. and Smith, D. (1967). The metabolism and elimination of *d*-tubocurarine $H^3$. *Anesthesiology*, **28**, 309.
48. Ganong, W. F. (1981). *Review of Medical Physiology*, 10th edit. Los Altos (California): Lange.
49. Samuel, J. R. and Powell, D. (1970). Renal transplantation. *Anaesthesia*, **25**, 165.
50. Pittinger, C. and Adamson, R. (1972). Antiobiotic blockade of neuromuscular function. *Ann. Rev. Pharmacol.*, **12**, 169.
51. Saidman, L. J. and Eger, E. L. (1966). The effect of thiopental metabolism on the duration of anaesthesia. *Anesthesiology*, **27**, 118.
52. Striker, T. W. and Morrow, A. G. (1968). Effect of succinylcholine on the level of serum potassium in man. *Anesthesiology*, **29**, 214.
53. Roth, F. and Wuthrich, H. (1969). The clinical importance of hyperkalaemia following suxamethonium administration. *Brit. J. Anaesth.*, **41**, 311.
54. Koide, M. and Waud, B. E. (1972). Serum potassium concentrations after succinylcholine in patients with renal failure. *Anesthesiology*, **36**, 142.
55. Miller, R. D., Way, W. L., Hamilton, W. K. and Layzer, R. B. (1972). Succinylcholine-induced hyperkalaemia in patients with renal failure. *Anesthesiology*, **36**, 138.
56. Ryan, D. W. (1977). Preoperative serum cholinesterase concentration in chronic renal failure. *Br. J. Anaesth.*, **49**, 945.
57. Bateman, D. N. and Gokal, R. (1980). Metoclopramide in renal failure. *Lancet*, **1**, 982.
58 Hirshman, C. A. and Edelstein, G. (1979). Intraoperative hyperkalemia and cardiac arrests during renal transplantation in an insulin-dependent diabetic. *Anesthesiology*, **51**, 161.

59. Deutsch, S., Bastron, R. D., Pierce, E. C. and Vandam, L. D. (1969). The effects of anaesthesia with thiopentone, nitrous oxide, narcotics and neuromuscular blocking drugs on renal function in normal man. *Brit. J. Anaesth.*, **41**, 807.

*Section Five*

# THE ENDOCRINE SYSTEM

CHAPTER 37

# Anaesthesia and the Endocrine Glands



THE endocrine system is both affected by anaesthesia and also influences the anaesthetic management of a patient with an endocrine disorder. It has long been recognised that the stress response can be initiated by the administration of a general anaesthetic. More recently, considerable efforts have been expended to suppress the stress response.[1] It remains unsettled whether the stress response is a necessary part of this physiological process.

Stanley and associates[2] were able to demonstrate that high doses of fentanyl were able to effect a considerable reduction in the cortisol response to cardiothoracic bypass. Their attempts at cortisol suppression must be viewed against the current policy regarding patients receiving corticosteroid therapy, when endogenous cortisol output may be suppressed and considerable emphasis is placed upon adequate cortisol cover for operative procedures. The observer may be excused if he sees an apparent conflict in the two viewpoints.

## THE THYROID GLAND

Surgery is undertaken on patients with thyroid disease, either because the gland is excessively enlarged or malignant, or because it is overactive and cannot be controlled by medical treatment. Surgery is also indicated in preference to medical treatment during pregnancy when antithyroid drugs may not be given for fear of causing cretinism in the developing fetus.

### Pre-operative Preparation

If the patient is not hyperthyroid, no particular preparation is necessary. If, however, the thyroid is overactive, every effort should be made to bring the excess activity under control, using antithyroid drugs such as carbimazole. It was formerly the practice to administer iodine in the form of Lugol's iodine, for a brief period immediately prior to surgery. This had two functions: firstly it inhibited thyroxine output temporarily and, secondly, it altered the physical consistency of the gland which could become friable under the influence of carbimazole.

The adequacy of medical treatment is monitored by measuring the serum thyroxine level. Occasionally, troublesome cardiac effects of thyrotoxicosis may be controlled with $\beta$-blocking drugs and the anaesthetist should be aware of this. A chest radiograph, including anteroposterior and lateral views of the neck and thoracic inlet should be available. An assessment may then be made of the degree of tracheal compression that may be present or of any thoracic extension of the goitre.

An ECG should be available as thyrotoxicosis may cause atrial fibrillation. A full blood count will reveal any substantial degree of bone marrow depression caused by carbimazole. Indirect laryngoscopy should be performed prior to surgery, so that normal function of the vocal cords may be recorded at that stage. This is largely a medico-legal precaution which may only be required in the unlikely event of a recurrent laryngeal nerve being damaged during the surgery.

### Positioning of the Patient

The patient lies supine on the operation table with a slight foot-down tilt of the table in order to minimise venous filling of the neck. The neck is extended by placing a firm pad between the shoulders and by further extension of the atlanto-occipital joint.

Great care must be taken to protect the eyes, particularly as the eyelids may not close due to exophthalmos. Soft pads should be placed over the closed eyes as inadvertent pressure may be exerted on the eye by an assistant. Some surgeons may require the superficial tissues of the neck to be infiltrated with a vasoconstrictor. If adrenaline is used, it should be diluted to 1:200,000 and the patient closely observed for myocardial hyperexcitability during the infiltration, especially if a halogenated anaesthetic agent is being administered.

The anaesthetic technique employed requires endotracheal intubation, but whether spontaneous or controlled ventilation is used is a matter of individual preference.

The thyroid gland is a very vascular organ and the vascularity may be increased following carbimazole treatment. It may, therefore, be considered prudent to provide some degree of hypotension to limit operative blood loss, though this is rarely great enough to warrant blood replacement. One difficulty occasionally encountered during the manipulative phase of the thyroidectomy, is the occurrence of acute changes in heart rate. This may be due to release into the circulation of thyroxine. If the tachycardia is troublesome or ectopic beats occur, then a $\beta$-adrenergic blocking agent such as propranalol 1–2 mg may be used intravenously.

### Postoperative Care

Occasionally problems are encountered which may, or may not, be anticipated. For instance, in patients where the enlarged thyroid gland has caused a significant degree of tracheal compression, when the gland is removed much of the structural support of the trachea is lost. This may lead to tracheal collapse following extubation. This is an uncommon complication but can be very difficult to treat. As an immediate measure, should the patient develop inspiratory stridor and increasing difficulty with breathing following extubation, the anaesthetist should re-intubate the trachea. The tube may have to be retained for a day or more.

Another cause of postoperative stridor is laryngeal and supralaryngeal oedema. This can be caused by a haematoma in the neck. The haematoma should be released as a matter of urgency and without general anaesthesia. A marked degree of glottic oedema can be present with only minimal symptoms, and it is an extremely hazardous procedure to embark upon general anaesthesia with paralysis of the respiratory muscles, as visualisation of the glottis may not be possible. Release of the haematoma will enable the oedema to disperse and improve respiratory exchange.

A later complication following thyroidectomy or, more precisely, parathyroidectomy, is tetany. This is due to either loss of the parathyroid glands along with the thyroid, or due to a temporary loss of parathormone production. Tetany is caused by a lowered ionised calcium level and is manifested by hyperexcitability of neuromuscular transmission or by frank spasms. The muscular spasms may be very severe and cause respiratory embarrassment. Treatment is with intravenous calcium chloride or gluconate and is urgently indicated when muscular spasms occur.

## MYXOEDEMA

Although surgery is not often undertaken for the treatment of myxoedema, anaesthesia may be necessary for a patient with the disease. It should be considered in patients known to have the disease or who require supportive therapy (thyroxine). In either case, the patient may be sufficiently unwell to have neglected his treatment and consequently become hypothyroid. In extreme instances, the patient will be in danger of developing myxoedematous coma.

Certain anaesthetic agents, for instance halothane and suxamethonium, exacerbate a pre-existing slow heart rate in a hypothyroid patient, and the cardiac output may fall dangerously. Another factor which must be taken into account in patients with myxoedema is the diminished metabolic rate in such patients and this will mean that drug metabolism is impaired. Many drugs, such as opiates, will have more prolonged and profound effects in these circumstances.

Myxodema should be suspected in a patient where recovery of consciousness is unduly delayed.

## PARATHYROID

The parathyroid glands, usually four in number, have an important physiological role in controlling the level of the serum ionised calcium. The hormone responsible is parathormone, and it maintains the serum calcium by mobilising calcium from bone, increasing calcium absorption from the gut and by increasing calcium reabsorption from the renal tubules. It also is reponsible for facilitating the loss of phosphate via the renal tubules, by lowering the tubular transport maximum (TmP) for phosphate with resulting phosphaturia.

Disturbances in parathyroid function occasionally present for surgical correction. They fall into two groups:

*Primary hyperparathyroidism.*—In this condition, excess production of parathormone usually results in an adenoma of one or more of the parathyroid glands.

*Secondary or tertiary hyperparathyroidism.*—In secondary hyperparathyroidism, there is clear evidence of an associated disease such as malabsorption disease, or chronic renal failure. In these conditions, the lowered serum calcium levels stimulate the secretion of parathormone which may lead to overproduction and adenoma formation, which is described as the tertiary state.

### Anaesthesia

It should be borne in mind that patients presenting for surgical removal of parathyroid adenoma may have severe bone disease or be in renal failure. The search for an adenoma may prove to be an extensive one and has been known to extend beyond the neck into the mediastinum. Methylene blue dye is usefully taken up by parathyroid tissue, and the parathyroid glands—usually a yellowish colour—are coloured blue by the dye. The dose of methylene blue is 75–100 mg in a 1 per cent solution. Conduct of the anaesthesia for parathyroidism is much as for thyroidectomy, but ionised calcium levels must be monitored in the post-operative periods when sudden falls may occur. Treatment is with calcium chloride or gluconate, intravenously.

## ADRENAL GLANDS

There are two in number and these are situated at the upper pole of each kidney. Sections of the gland reveal two distinct areas. An outer yellow cortex and an inner brown medulla. Histologically the cortex is composed of three layers: zona glomerulosa, zona fasiculata and zona reticularis.

It is thought that the mineral corticoids (aldosterone and deoxycortone) are produced in the cells of the zona glomerulosa, whilst the middle layer, i.e. zona fasciculata, secrete the glucocorticoids (cortisone and hydrocortisone), and the inner zona reticularis is responsible for the sex hormones.

Control of the secretions of adrenal cortical hormones is by the anterior pituitary hormone ACTH, although it seems that this has little influence on the secretion of aldosterone.

**Mineralocorticoids.**—Aldosterone levels are influenced by the release of renin. Renin is a peptide hormone released from the juxtaglomerular cells of the afferent arterioles in the kidney. It is released in response to alterations in the plasma volume. Renin, in turn, causes a polypeptide angiotensin I to be converted to angiotensin II. Angiotensin II promotes the release of aldosterone. As aldosterone controls the tubular reabsorption of sodium, and as angiotensin II is a vasoconstrictor, the system as a whole controls the blood volume.

**Glucocorticoids.**—These are principally concerned with carbohydrate and protein metabolism and by far the most important is cortisol (hydrocortisone).

**Sex hormones.**—There are a number of different hormones of this type secreted by the adrenals, some are androgenic and some oestrogenic. It is the removal of these hormones that is intended when bilateral adrenalectomy is performed for palliation of metastasising hormone-dependent tumours (e.g. breast).

**Glucocorticoid excess.**—Excessive production of glucocorticoid hormones leads to a condition known as Cushing's syndrome. This is characterised by truncal obesity, a red and moon-like face, hypertension, muscle wasting and osteoporosis. It may be the result of a primary adrenal disorder (e.g. adenoma of the adrenal gland) or of excessive ACTH secretion from the anterior pituitary gland (Cushing's disease). Occasionally the syndrome may be produced by ectopic ACTH-secreting tumours.

Laboratory diagnosis is directed towards firstly establishing the presence of glucocorticoid excess (by measurement of plasma or urinary levels—looking in particular for loss of diurnal rhythm in the plasma cortisol levels) and, secondly, differentiating between excess hormone production from primary adrenal disease and that from excessive ACTH production (using the dexamethasone suppression or metyrapone tests).

If an adrenal adenoma is demonstrated, surgical extirpation is indicated. Following surgery, the patient will have to be closely observed as normal adrenal activity may have been suppressed and acute Addisonian crisis may ensue.

**Primary aldosteronism (Conn's syndrome).**—This condition, with an elevated serum sodium, lowered potassium and hypertension, may occasionally present for surgery.

**Adrenocortical insufficiency (Addison's disease).**—Addison's disease may present as chronic, progressive tiredness, weakness, anorexia and skin pigmentation. The patient will be dehydrated and have low blood pressure. Occasionally, the patient will present *in extremis*, severely dehydrated and sodium depleted, with an elevated serum potassium which may be causing ECG changes. The condition is known as Addisonian crisis, and requires immediate saline infusion with cortisol. It may occur in a patient with Addison's disease who has developed a surgical condition making increased demands on the stress mechanism, or in a patient on long-term steroid therapy for a variety of conditions who inadvertently fails to receive his normal dosage (e.g. road traffic accident with head injury, or acute intestinal disorder causing vomiting).

### Anaesthesia for Patients Receiving Corticosteroid Therapy

The administration of steroids to a patient will lead, to a greater or lesser extent, to suppression of the endogenous excretion of cortisol. It now seems improbable that significant suppression will be present 2 months after the cessation of therapy. Current practice is still fairly conservative and most anaesthetists administer hydrocortisone 100 mg with premedication for all patients who have had a course of steroid therapy in the preceding six months.

Hydrocortisone is continued 6-hourly for 24 hours following major surgery. It should be noted that this dosage of hydrocortisone is considerably in excess of the maximum that can be excreted by the adrenals in the most severe stress. It is interesting that much effort is now being expended to suppress the stress response to routine surgery.[1]

## DIABETES MELLITUS

The main factor which controls the level of circulating insulin is the blood sugar. The principal function of insulin is to facilitate the uptake of glucose by peripheral tissues and to promote storage in the liver as glycogen. It can be demonstrated that the level of insulin rises almost concurrently with the ingestion of a carbohydrate meal.

Growth hormone has a stimulant effect on the cells of the islets of Langerhans leading to an increased insulin output and eventual exhaustion. The glucocorticoids also affect the level of the circulating blood sugar, principally by glycogenolysis (i.e. breaking down liver glycogen). The diagnosis of diabetes mellitus may be suspected in any patient with glycosuria, but is confirmed by the time-honoured oral glucose tolerance test. The fasting blood sugar should be less than 6·5 mmol/l; the peak level after the ingestion of 50 g glucose should not exceed 10 mmol/l, and by 2 hours, the level should have fallen below 7 mmol/l.

Patients with diabetes mellitus conveniently fall into two groups:

Type I: 'Juvenile onset'—Insulin dependent.

Type II: 'Mature onset'—Insulin independent.

In the former type, it is important to match the insulin requirements to the caloric requirement and this will be altered by the stress of the operation. In the latter, Type II, the usual increase in insulin output will not take place and severe hyperglycaemia may occur if the stress is great.

The anaesthetist will encounter diabetic patients quite frequently, as it is a fairly common disease with many aspects that require surgical treatment. Regardless of whether the disorder is related to the diabetic condition or not, the preparation of the patient will require the same careful attention. The aim of the management of the diabetic during anaesthesia must be to prevent the effects of insulin deficiency with consequent increased catabolism and electrolyte changes. In practice, this may be best achieved by the administration of insulin, glucose and electrolytes, and the careful avoidance of hyperglycaemia or hypoglycaemia.

### Practical Pre-anaesthetic Management

**Type I (Juvenile onset) diabetes.**—It is useful, practically, to distinguish between minor and major procedures. A minor procedure can be considered as one in which a patient may be reasonably expected to recover fully within a few hours and be able to resume normal oral intake of fluids and food. A major procedure is one where the patient is expected to require intravenous support for a few days postoperatively.

*Minor procedures*: A patient on long-acting insulin alone should be changed to twice-daily Actrapid insulin subcutaneously. Then, either the morning dose of insulin should be omitted and the patient starved, or the morning dose given and the blood sugar levels estimated before anaesthesia. Following recovery from anaesthesia, should the blood sugar be found to be normal or low, a dextrose infusion should be set up. It should be noted that during and following anaesthesia, a low blood sugar is more life-threatening in the short term than a temporarily raised blood sugar. There can be no reason for failing to check blood sugar levels as convenient diagnostic kits are readily available (Figs. 1 and 2). If the patient is controlled on a morning dose of Actrapid followed by a longer-acting insulin, the patient may be starved and the morning dose of Actrapid omitted altogether. The blood sugar level should then be checked and corrected with 5 per cent dextrose if necessary. Normal diet may be restored as soon as possible and the usual insulin requirements resumed.

*Major surgery*.—The diabetic patient should be admitted 2–3 days prior to the proposed operation and the insulin regime altered to twice daily Actrapid. The pre-operative management may be conducted in one of two ways, depending upon the availability of a syringe pump. If a syringe pump is available, insulin may be given by slow intravenous injection. An intravenous infusion of 5 per cent dextrose is

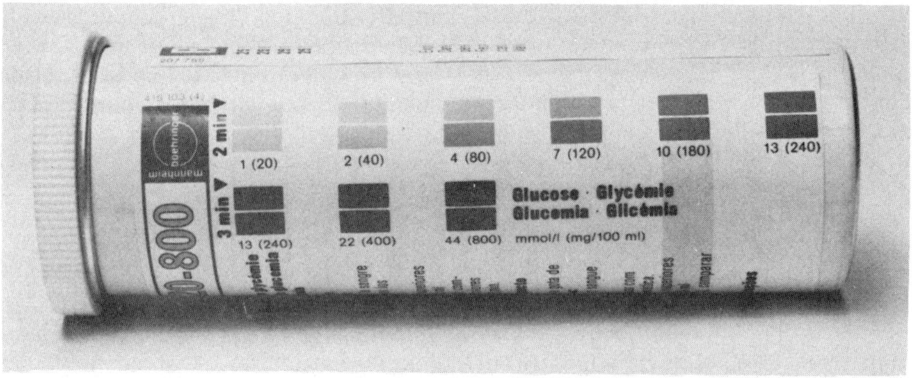


37/FIG. 1.—BM Stix. Two-tone colour comparison sticks, giving reasonably accurate blood sugar estimations.

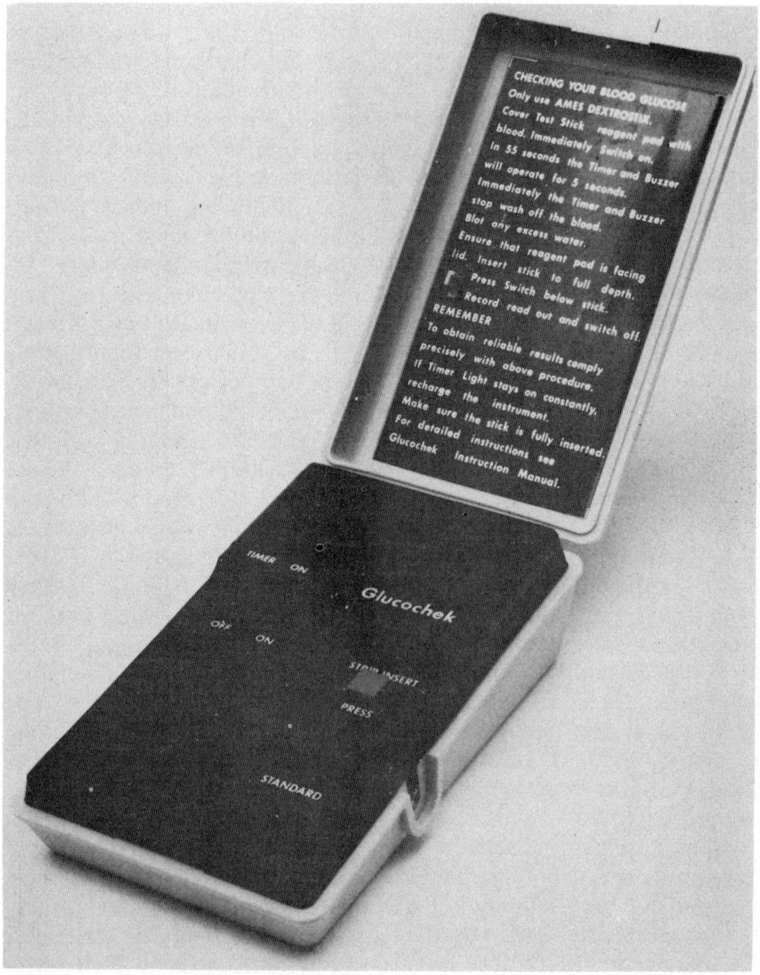


37/FIG. 2(*a*).—Glucochek apparatus and user chart.

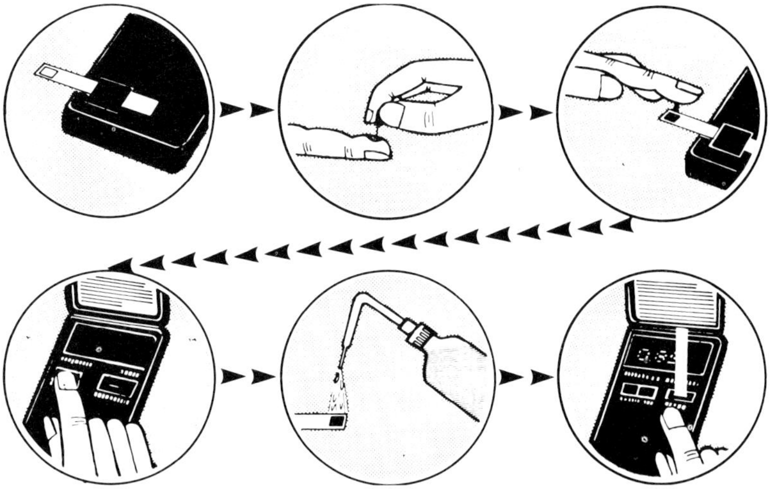
Clip a fresh test stick under the holder on the front of the case with the reagent strip outwards and facing up.
Prick a finger and obtain a drop of blood sufficiently large to cover the reagent area of the stick.
Transfer blood from the finger to the reagent strip of the test stick, ensuring the whole area is covered.
Immediately switch on GLUCOCHEK. The "On" light will glow. Glucochek has a built-in timer which begins timing on switching on.
After 55 seconds the timer will start to buzz and will light the "Timer" lamp. This gives a warning that the timing period is nearly up. After a further 5 seconds the buzzer will stop and the light will go out. Immediately wash the blood off the test stick and blot it with tissue.
Insert the test stick in the carrier, with the reagent area towards the top of the instrument, making sure it goes right in, and press the button nearby. The blood glucose value will be shown on the display. The reading will be held until the display is switched off.

37/Fig. 2(*b*).—Automated colorimetric estimations of blood sugar using Dextrostix.

set up and a solution of insulin (Actrapid) prepared as follows:

48 ml 0·9% sodium chloride
2 ml human albumin
50 units Actrapid insulin
} (1 unit of insulin/ml)

The albumin prevents the insulin from becoming adsorbed onto the plastic surface of the syringe and tubing. The tubing from the insulin syringe is connected into the infusion and the pump run at a rate appropriate to the blood sugar level. If human albumin is not readily available in small amounts, a convenient alternative may be prepared by allowing 10 ml of the patient's heparinised blood to stand, and withdrawing 3–5 ml of the supernatant plasma, which contains albumin.

An example of such a regime is given in Table 1.

The blood sugar levels should be checked hourly and the injection rate of insulin adjusted accordingly. Alternatively, should there not be a syringe pump available, the following regime may be followed.

37/Table 1

| *Blood Sugar Level* | *Injection Rate of Insulin* (1 unit/ml) |
|---|---|
| *mmol/l* | *ml/hr* |
| >20 | 6 |
| 15–20 | 5 |
| 10–15 | 4 |
| 8–10 | 2 |
| 6–8 | 1·5 |
| 5–6 | 1 |
| 2–5 | 0·5 |
| <2 | STOP (increase dextrose infusion rate) |

An infusion is prepared as follows:

5% dextrose 1000 ml
13 mmol potassium chloride
15 units Actrapid insulin
5 ml human albumin

The drip rate is set at 1 drop every two seconds (approximately 1 litre 8-hourly).

A sliding scale is suggested for different

strengths of insulin infusions against different levels of blood sugar (Table 2). This is a disadvantage of the regime, as varied strengths of insulin infusion have to be prepared.

37/TABLE 2

| *Blood Sugar Level* | *Insulin Content of Infusion* |
|---|---|
| 5 mmol/litre | 5 units Actrapid/litre |
| 5–10 mmol/litre | 15 units Actrapid/litre |
| 10 mmol/litre | 20 units Actrapid/litre |
| 20 mmol/litre | 25 units Actrapid/litre |

**Duration of action of insulin.**—Numerous compounds of insulin are now available and the particular one selected will be based on the duration of action required (Table 3).

**Emergency Anaesthesia for Diabetic Patients**

Should a surgical emergency arise in a diabetic patient, it is very important that the attendant anaesthestist ensures that the diabetic control of the patient is fully attended to before surgery is embarked upon.

It is quite likely that the diabetic control has been disturbed in a surgical emergency. Either the patient has not been receiving regular insulin or the metabolic demands have increased due to fever or increased catabolism. In both instances, the diabetic condition may have deteriorated markedly and it is therefore incumbent upon the anaesthetist to ensure adequate hydration, restoration of the acid/base balance, correction of any gross electrolyte disturbance

37/TABLE 3
DURATION OF ACTION OF INSULIN COMPOUNDS

| *Conventional Type* | *Duration of Action* | *Highly Purified Type* | |
|---|---|---|---|
| Soluble | Short 4–6 hours | Neutral | Actrapid |
| Neutral | | | Led Neutral |
| Globin Insulin Zinc Suspension | Intermediate 15–18 hours | Biphasic | Rapitard |
| | | | Semitard |
| | | Isophane | Hypurin |
| Isophane | | | Initard |
| | | | Insulatard |
| | | | Mixtard |
| | | | Neuphane |
| Insulin Zinc Supension (Lente) | Long 24 hours | Insulin Zinc Suspension (Mixed) | Hypurin (Lente) |
| Insulin Zinc Suspension (Crystalline) Ultralente | | | Lentard MC |
| | | | Montard MC |
| | | | Neulente |
| Protamine Zince Insulin | | Insulin Zinc Suspension Crystalline | Ultratard MC |

(particularly potassium) and the adequate administration of insulin.

**Intravenous fluids.**—The choice of intravenous fluids for replacement in diabetic ketoacidosis is either physiological saline (0·9 per cent) or dextrose (5 per cent). The use of Hartmann's solution (lactated Ringer) has been shown to cause rises in blood sugar levels due to conversion of lactate to glucose.[3]

If an electrolyte solution is preferred, Ringer's solution would seem a suitable choice.

**Type II (Non-insulin dependent: mature onset diabetes).**—This type of diabetes mellitus is associated with high blood insulin levels. It is unlikely to develop to ketoacidosis and it is usually treated either by restriction of caloric intake or with oral hypoglycaemic agents (sulphonylurea or diguanides).

*Minor procedures.*—It is suggested that patients with Type II diabetes treated with diet alone should not be prepared in any particular way, but that blood sugar levels should be checked before and after surgery.

Patients who are treated with diguanides should have that treatment stopped or altered to sulphonylureas pre-operatively.

Patients being treated with sulphonylureas should not be given treatment on the day of operation. As this group of drugs has a prolonged duration of action, it is likely that the previous day's therapy may be active on the day of operation when the patient is being starved prior to surgery. It is prudent, therefore, to check the blood sugar pre-operatively and should it be normal or low, an infusion of 5 per cent dextrose should be set up.

*Major procedures.*—It is preferable that such patients anticipating major surgical operations should be stabilised on insulin 2–3 days pre-operatively. Patients should be on at least twice daily insulin (e.g. Actrapid and Isophane). On the day of operation, the patients should be prepared in exactly the same way as Type I diabetic patients, either with dextrose and insulin pumps, or with dextrose, potassium and insulin infusions—with the insulin concentration related to the blood sugar levels.

**Total Pancreatectomy**

Following the procedure for total pancreatectomy, there is often insufficient islets of Langerhans' tissue remaining to provide adequate blood sugar control and the patient will develop diabetes. This can happen early in the postoperative period and the patient will require insulin. Therefore, all patients should have blood sugar levels monitored following pancreatectomy.

As a guide to insulin requirement, about 0·1 units of Actrapid/kg body weight/hour, is a suitable base-line dosage and will enable a more accurate dose range to be assessed according to the blood sugar response.

## THE APUD CONCEPT

This achronym is given to a series of cells widely distributed in the body with a common cytochemical property. The achronym is derived from the initial letters of the functions:

AMINE PRECURSOR, UPTAKE and DECARBOXYLATION

The grouping together of these cells under a common heading is useful in that it enables a widely different group of conditions, caused by tumours of these cells, to be considered as a whole.

The cells are embryologically derived from neuro-ectoderm. They then divide into two groups:

1. Central Group, which form
   - Hypothalamus
   - Pituitary
   - Pineal
2. Peripheral Group which form
   - Sympathetic nervous system
   - Adrenal medulla
   - Gut
   - Thyroid ('C' cells)
   - Pancreas, including gastrin and islet cells
   - Carotid body
   - Skin
   - Lungs

Tumours arising from any of these cells are termed "Apudomas". It is not intended to provide an exhaustive list of all the possible variations here, but to account for some of the more usual ones:

**Glucagonoma.**—These can cause skin erythematous rashes and diabetes mellitus.

**Insulinoma** ($\beta$-cell tumours).—Patients suffer from periodic attacks of hypoglycaemia, which may lead to bizarre behaviour and often, mistakenly, leads to a psychiatric diagnosis.

**Gastrinoma** (Zollinger-Ellison syndrome).—These pancreatic tumours cause hyperchlorhydria with recurrent and intractable peptic ulceration.

**Neuroblastoma.**—These tumours usually occur in childhood and mature into ganglioblastomas, which are discovered in later life. Some neuroblastomas secrete catecholamines or VIP (vasoactive intestinal polypeptide). They behave occasionally in a similar manner to phaeochromocytomas when handled during excision (see below).

**Vipoma.**—These are tumours of the Apud series which secrete principally VIP. They cause a syndrome which is characterised by marked weight loss, diarrhoea, hypokalaemia and achlorhydria. The patients complain of intestinal colic and flushing attacks which are not unlike those associated with carcinoid tumours (see below). The tumours are usually located in the pancreas, but occasionally may be encountered as ganglio neuroblastomas anywhere along the neural crest distribution.

## Phaeochromocytoma

Although this is a relatively rarc cause of hypertension, it does hold some special problems for the anaesthetist.

As has been described earlier, these tumours arise from the neural crest tissue and are generally situated within the adrenal medulla, although not necessarily so. They are usually benign but can be malignant.

**Clinical symptoms and signs.**—The classical picture is of paroxysmal hypertension, but this may take the form of a sustained high blood pressure with intermittent episodes when it rises even higher. In an attack, apart from having a very high blood pressure, the patient will complain of sweating, palpitations and headache. Occasionally the symptomology may be unusual and the presence of phaeochromocytoma may only be suspected at operations for some incidental disease, when the blood pressure becomes markedly unstable. When undiscovered, the presence of a phaeochromocytoma eventually leads to a permanently high blood pressure which makes the disease difficult to differentiate from essential hypertension on clinical grounds.

### Diagnosis

*Provocative tests.*—Certain substances can provoke the release of catecholamines from a phaeochromocytoma and form the basis of provocative tests. Histamine (25–50 mg), glucagon (0·5–1·0 mg) or tyramine (0·1–0·5 mg) will produce substantial rises in blood pressure (>60 mm Hg). However, the tests are unreliable and possibly dangerous. It is wise to have an $\alpha$-adrenergic blocking agent (such as phentolamine) at hand if a provocative test is to be performed, in order to prevent excessive rises in blood pressure.

*Urinary VMA (Vanillylmandelic acid).*—24-hour urinary collections for estimation of catecholamine degradation products such as VMA are useful tests for phaeochromocytomas.

*Plasma catecholamines.*—The plasma catecholamine levels are invariably raised in patients with a phaeochromocytoma.[4] Normal range is below 1000 ng/l whilst patients with phaeochromocytoma usually have levels in excess of 2000 ng/l. Once the possibility of a tumour has

37/Table 4
Drugs Used in Treatment

| *Name* | *Type of Drug* | *Comment* |
|---|---|---|
| phenoxybenzamine | $\alpha$-blocker | Long acting, cumulative |
| phentolamine | $\alpha$-blocker | Short action. Rapid onset |
| prazosin | $\alpha$-blocker | 1st dose marked effect |
| propranolol | $\beta$-blocker | May have little action on BP. May raise BP if used alone |
| labetalol | $\alpha$ & $\beta$-blocker | Little effect. May raise BP |
| sodium nitroprusside | vasodilatation | Useful in pre-operative control. Limited dose |
| $\alpha$-methyl tyrosine | substrate inhibitor | Useful in pre-operative control. Drug of choice. |

been confirmed, it is necessary to localise the tumour and aortic angiography will thus be indicated. Angiographic localisation can occasionally precipitate a hypertensive crisis and caution must be exercised if pharmacological control has not been secured at this stage.

### Pre-operative Preparation

The principle of pre-operative treatment is based upon the severity of the disease, because over-enthusiastic treatment can cause postoperative problems as the half-life of circulating catecholamines is only of the order of 3 minutes. Complete adrenergic blockade will persist postoperatively when circulating catecholamine levels will be dramatically reduced. Adrenergic blockade may cause profound cardiovascular collapse under such conditions. Pre-operative use of $\alpha$-adrenergic blocking agents is thus restricted to patients with sustained hypertension or who are subject to frequent hypertensive attacks. $\beta$-blocking drugs should always be given in association with $\alpha$-blockers due to the high incidence of cardiac dysrhythmias. $\beta$-blocking drugs should not be given alone as they are liable to cause a rise in blood pressure.

*$\alpha$-Methyl p-tyrosine* blocks the first step in the synthesis of catecholamines (by inhibiting tyrosine hydroxylase) and has proved to be extremely effective in securing pre-operative control, but there may be postoperative problems similar to those following $\alpha$-adrenergic blockade.

### Anaesthetic Management

The overall principle of anaesthetic management for the excision of phaeochromocytoma is to prevent undue rises or falls in blood pressure and to prevent the occurrence of cardiac dysrhythmias caused by circulating catecholamines. It was formerly believed that there was a considerable change in the blood volume following excision of the phaeochromocytoma due to the loss of vasoconstrictive effect of catecholamines. When Levenson and his colleagues[5] measured pre-operative and postoperative blood volumes in cases of phaeochromocytoma, they were unable to demonstrate significant changes. Nevertheless, the concept persists and the anaesthetist may well find considerable changes in right atrial filling pressures following tumour excision.

It is therefore incumbent upon the anaesthetist to have available the means of measuring central venous pressure and, preferably, the ability to measure arterial pressure directly by intra-arterial manometry. The cardiac rhythm must be directly observed with an ECG monitor.

Many anaesthetic techniques have been described for operative excision: neuroleptanaesthesia has been advocated,[6] whilst halothane and muscle relaxant techniques are advocated by Sever, Roberts and Snell.[4]

Control of the blood pressure during the procedure may be achieved by intermittent use of sodium nitroprusside or phentolamine. Dysrythmias may be treated by the use of intravenous propranolol or practolol.

The central venous pressure is maintained with the administration of blood, plasma or crystalloid. It is recommended that 1–2 litres of fluid are infused prior to clamping the vessels on the tumour. In severe cases of postoperative vascular collapse, it may be necessary to employ a noradrenaline infusion until catecholamine production is restored.

The choice of muscle relaxants at present appears to be between tubocurarine, which can cause a mild ganglion blockade, or pancuronium, which can enhance the cardiac output and heart rate. This latter effect may not be desirable in a patient who is already hypertensive.

## Carcinoid Tumours

These tumours, again cytologically classified in the APUD series, arise from the enterochromaffin cells of the gut. They secrete a variety of vaso-active peptides, the precise agent depending upon the site in which the tumours arise.

The tumours that arise in mid- and hindgut secrete predominantly 5-hydroxytryptophan, kallikrein and possibly E-prostaglandin. Those of the foregut (e.g. stomach and lungs) secrete 5-hydroxytryptophan and histamine.

The clinical features of the condition are of flushing attacks, diarrhoea, abdominal pain, bronchospasm and the presence of cardiac valvular lesions on the right side of the heart. With carcinoid tumours of the gut, systemic symptoms are not marked unless there are hepatic metastases. This is because the primary growths secrete the vaso-active peptides into the portal circulation and, initially, the liver is able rapidly to detoxicate the substances, nullifying the systemic effects. However, when secondary growths of the liver start to secrete, the full clinical picture is seen. Pulmonary carcinoids will produce systemic symptoms at an early stage.

It is thought that the flushing attacks are caused by the formation of bradykinin as a result of the action of kallikrein in the blood stream. It is possible that E-prostaglandin, also secreted by carcinoid tumours, may cause vascular flushing.

If the tumour is producing histamine (gastric carcinoids in particular), then attacks of bronchospasm may occur and may pose a problem during anaesthesia.

### Anaesthetic Management

Unless the clinical picture has fully emerged pre-operatively, the unsuspecting anaesthetist may be precipitated into the management of these cases during an otherwise straightforward laparotomy. Occasionally it is the bizarre response of the patient to the handling of an abdominal mass that gives a clue as to the nature of the tumour. The commonest symptom is that of wide cardiovascular variations, with blood pressure rising or falling unpredictably. Bronchospasm can be a rare occurrence.

*Drugs.*—Flushing attacks occurring pre-operatively may be controlled with steroids. The hypertensive episodes that can manifest themselves during surgery may be controlled with methotrimeprazine.

Aprotonin is an inhibitor of the peptide kallikrein and may prove useful in an attack. Other agents that have been used with partial success are streptozocin and methysergide. $H_1$ and $H_2$ (histamine) receptor blockade may help to alleviate some of the symptoms and this may be achieved by the administration of chlorpheniramine and cimetidine.

Codeine phosphate may be useful in controlling excessive intestinal activity and diarrhoea.

## REFERENCES

1. Hall, G. M. (1980). Fentanyl and the metabolic response to surgery. *Brit. J. Anaesth.*, **52**, 561.
2. Stanley, T. H., Berman, L., Green, O., Robertson, D. H. and Roizen, L. (1979). Fentanyl-oxygen anaesthesia for coronary artery surgery: plasma catecholamines and cortisol responses. *Anesthesiolgy*, **51**, S139.
3. Alberti, K. G. M. M. and Thomas, D. J. B. (1979). The management of diabetes during surgery. *Brit. J. Anaesth.*, **51**, 693.
4. Sever, P. S., Roberts, J. C., Snell, M. E. (1980). Phaeochromocytoma. *Clin. in Endocrinol. & Metabolism*, **9** 543.
5. Levenson, J. A., Safar, M. E., London, G. M. and Simon, A. (1980). Haemodynamics in patients with phaeochromocytoma. *Clin. Sci.*, **58**, 349.
6. Desmonts, J. M., Le Honelleur, J., Redmond, P. and Duvaldestin, P. (1977). Anaesthetic management in patients with phaeochromocytoma. *Brit. J. Anaesth.*, **49**, 991.

*Section Six*

# THE REPRODUCTIVE SYSTEM

CHAPTER 38

# Physiological Changes of Pregnancy and Labour



THE average duration of a human pregnancy is 280 days calculated from the first day of the last menstrual period, and during this time the uterus alone increases in weight from 30 g to 1000 g. As a result of the hormonal and mechanical influences, major physiological adjustments occur to meet the increasing metabolic demands of the uterus, placenta and fetus.

## Haematological Changes (Fig. 1 and Table 1)

**Maternal blood volume** increases by approximately 40 per cent but plasma volume increases more than red cell volume, so that the dilutional effect may apparently reduce haemoglobin concentrations. Prophylactic iron therapy during pregnancy can largely prevent this so-called *physiological* anaemia. The mean plasma volume towards the end of pregnancy is almost 4 litres.[2] It was previously held that the maximum dilutional effect occurred at 34 weeks of pregnancy, but this incorrect assumption was probably the result of aortocaval compression (see p. 1007). These haematological changes facilitate gas exchange with the fetus and minimise the effects of blood loss at delivery.

**Plasma protein** concentration falls during

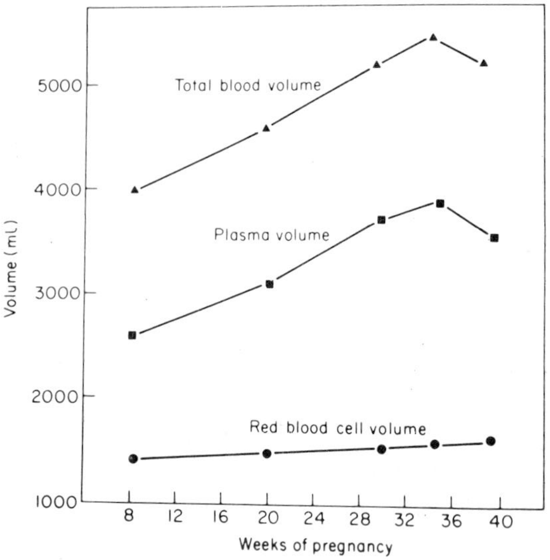


38/Fig. 1.—Changes in plasma volume, red cell volume and total blood volume during pregnancy. The late falls are probably the result of supine caval occlusion. (Courtesy of Dr. D. D. Moir and the publishers, Baillière Tindall.[1])

38/Table 1
Haematological Changes During Pregnancy

| | | |
|---|---|---|
| Blood volume | | +40% |
| Plasma volume | | +45% |
| Red cell volume | | +20% |
| White cell count | | ↑↑ |
| Haematocrit | | −16% |
| Plasma proteins: | Albumin | −20% |
| | $\alpha_1\alpha_2,\beta$ Globulin | ↑ |
| | $\gamma$ Globulin | ↓ |
| | Fibrinogen | +60% |
| Erythrocyte sedimentation rate | | ↑↑ |
| Clotting factors VII, VIII, IX, X | | ↑ |
| Plasma cholinesterase | | ↓ |

pregnancy mainly due to a 25 per cent reduction in plasma albumin concentration. $\alpha_1$, $\alpha_2$ and $\beta$ globulin concentrations rise progressively during pregnancy, $\gamma$ globulin concentration falls slightly, whilst a substantial increase in fibrinogen concentrations may produce ESR readings as high as 50–80 mm in the first hour. The overall albumin:globulin ratio decreases from 1·5 to 1·0. The alterations in plasma protein concentrations may affect the pharmacokinetics of drugs administered during pregnancy and in general drugs exhibit increased protein binding. Significant changes in plasma protein concentrations occur in pre-eclampsia.[3]

**Plasma cholinesterase** is reduced in pregnancy although it is doubtful if this reduction is of clinical significance when suxamethonium is used.[4,5] Interestingly the incidence of muscle pain following suxamethonium is reduced in pregnancy.[6]

**Coagulation.**—The rise in plasma fibrinogen is accompanied by increases in factors VII, VIII, IX and X during pregnancy. Platelet count and platelet adhesiveness probably remain unchanged although the overall effect is one of hypercoagulability, and this may be related to the production of deep venous thrombosis as well as being implicated in the aetiology of pre-eclampsia and disseminated intravascular coagulation.

**Cardiovascular Changes** (Fig. 2 and Table 2)

The circulatory changes that occur are designed to serve two functions,

(i) to maintain normal uteroplacental circulation;
(ii) to facilitate the exchange of oxygen, carbon dioxide, nutrients and waste products between mother and fetus.

**Anatomy.**—The myocardium hypertrophies, whilst the elevated diaphragm displaces the heart upwards, laterally and forwards and rotates it to a more transverse position.

**Chest x-ray** demonstrates these anatomical changes.

**ECG.**—General left axis deviation secondary to the anatomical shift in position is commonly accompanied by flattened T waves or Q waves in lead III, as well as innocent depression of the ST segments. Sinus tachycardia, premature contractions and bouts of paroxysmal atrial tachycardia are more common in pregnancy.

**Heart rate** averages 80–90 per minute by term.

**Blood pressure.**—Systolic pressure changes only slightly but diastolic pressure decreases considerably in mid-pregnancy, then rises again during the third trimester. In normal labour, systolic pressure rises 5–10 mm Hg (0·7–1·3 kPa) during first-stage contractions, but may increase by 30 mm Hg (4·0 kPa) during second-stage contractions despite the large reduction in venous return produced by the Valsalva manoeuvre effect of bearing down efforts by the mother.

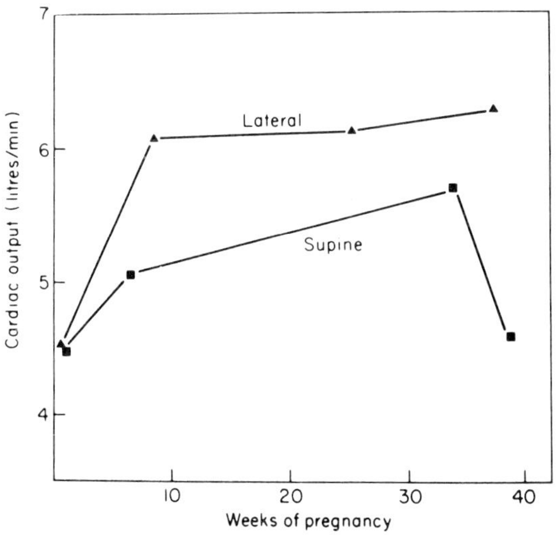


38/FIG. 2.—Changes in cardiac output during pregnancy. (Courtesy of Dr. D. D. Moir and the publishers, Baillière Tindall.[1])

38/TABLE 2

| | |
|---|---|
| Heart rate | +15% |
| Stroke volume | +30% |
| Cardiac output | +40% |
| Peripheral vascular resistance | −15% |
| Systolic pressure | −0 to 5 mm Hg (−0 to 0·7 kPa) |
| Diastolic pressure | −10 to 20 mm Hg (−1·3 to 2·7 kPa) (mid pregnancy) |
| Central venous pressure | unchanged |

Cardiovascular changes during pregnancy. During second-stage contractions accompanied by maternal expulsive efforts, very large increases may occur in systolic blood pressure and CVP.

**Venous pressure.**—Central venous pressure is generally normal during pregnancy unless measured with the mother supine, when substantial increases are recorded (see below). Pressure in lower-limb venous systems is greatly increased during pregnancy and even more so in the supine position. Expulsive efforts in the second stage will produce enormous rises in CVP, which are superimposed upon the smaller rises in pressure accompanying contractions throughout labour. Up to 300 ml of blood is expelled from the uteroplacental circulation during the contraction. Ergometrine injected during the third stage will produce a prolonged elevation of the CVP.[7]

**Peripheral resistance** is reduced in pregnancy and sympathetic blockade produced by regional anaesthesia may cause further reductions.

**Cardiac output** rises substantially in early pregnancy and this elevation is sustained until delivery. The rise is accomplished by an increase in both heart rate and stroke volume. The large arteriovenous shunt across the placenta increases venous return.

The view that cardiac output rose until 32 weeks of pregnancy and thereafter declined has been shown to be incorrect. This erroneous conclusion was reached after measurement in the supine position, when caval occlusion produced profound reductions in venous return. The influence of position upon the haemodynamics of pregnancy is of fundamental importance and must be understood by everyone who deals with pregnant women, be they anaesthetist, obstetrician or midwife.

**Aortocaval compression.**—Compression of the inferior vena cava upon the vertebral bodies by the pregnant uterus when the mother lies supine obstructs venous return (Figs. 3*a*,*b*). Compensatory mechanisms act to increase peripheral vascular resistance and heart rate and may maintain normal brachial artery pressure, whilst collateral venous channels assure an adequate venous return (see Fig. 4). The mother seldom experiences any symptoms, and this is called *concealed caval occlusion*.

However, six per cent of unanaesthetised mothers experience hypotension and bradycardia when lying supine, and cardiac output may fall by 50 per cent. This is *revealed caval occlusion* and the result is termed the *supine hypotensive syndrome* (see Fig. 5). Symptoms such as dizziness, nausea, anxiety and restlessness accompany the hypotension.

The aorta is also compressed by the uterus when the woman lies supine and this results in decreased femoral artery pressures. There are no compensatory mechanisms to counter this effect. Seventy-seven per cent of women show decreased brachial and/or femoral pressures after 5 minutes lying supine. The decrease in femoral pressures may be noted as early as the 19th week of pregnancy but the decreased brachial pressures only after 28 weeks.[9]

Aortocaval compression has damaging effects

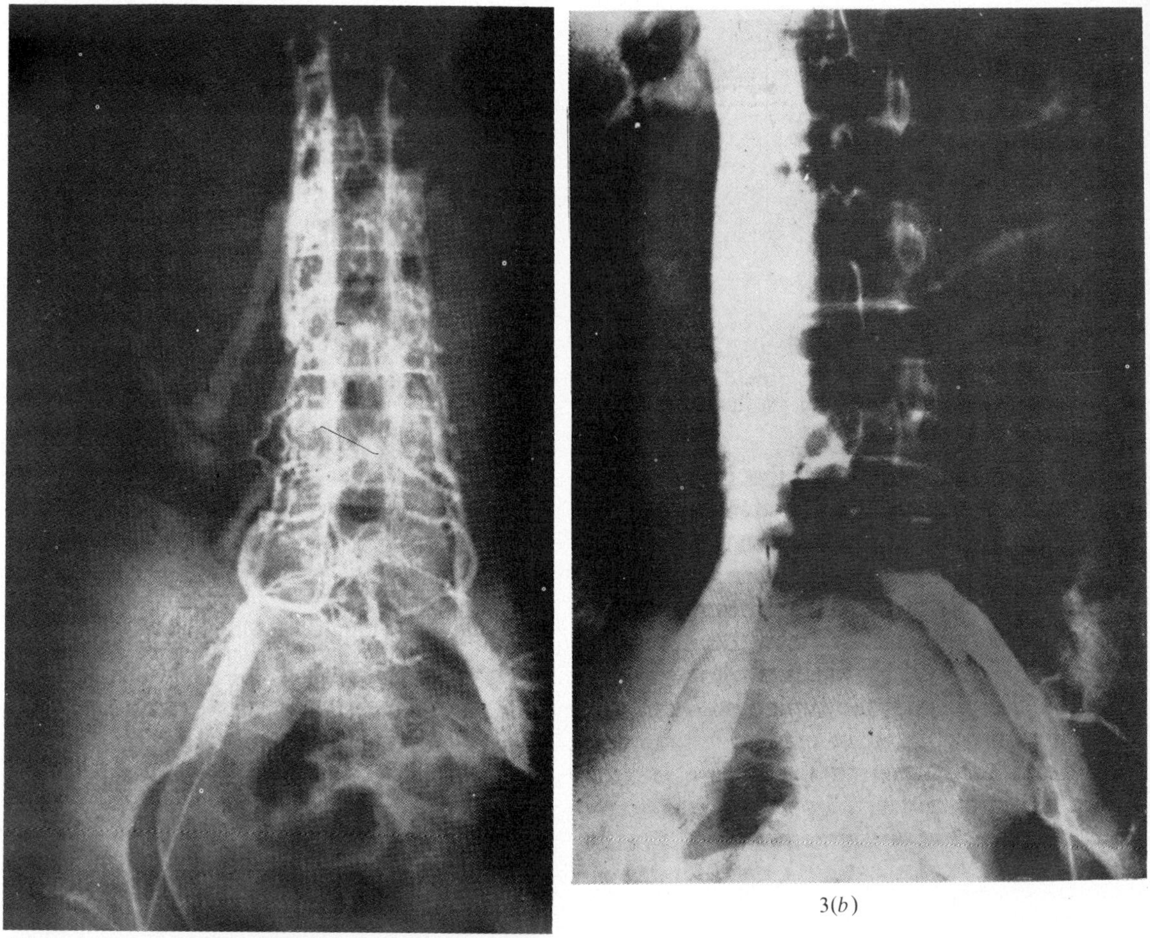

3(*b*)

3(*a*)

38/Fig. 3(*a*).—Inferior vena cavogram in the supine position immediately before caesarean section. Little or no dye enters the inferior vena cava, traversing instead the collateral circulation through the paravertebral veins.

38/Fig. 3(*b*).—The same patient immediately following delivery. Virtually all the dye now travels up the inferior vena cava. (Fig. 38/3*a* and *b*, courtesy of Professor M. G. Kerr, Dr. D. B. Scott and Dr. E. Samuel, and the Editor of the *British Medical Journal*.)

far beyond the revealed fall in maternal blood pressure. The reduction in uteroplacental blood flow produced by the decreased cardiac output, the aortic compression and the increased sympathetic tone results in fetal hypoxia and acidosis.[10] Transient abnormalities of the fetal heart rate occur in 56 per cent of supine patients compared with only 10 per cent of those with lateral uterine displacement and, importantly, only 50 per cent of these fetal heart rate changes are associated with overt or revealed maternal hypotension.[11] Intervillous blood flow decreases by 20 per cent in the supine compared to a patient with 45° left lateral tilt.[12] Fetal pH is lower if the mother is supine during the second stage, and effective pelvic tilt will counter this.[13] There may be a strong argument for delivering patients in the lateral rather than the lithotomy position.

Uterine contractions are less efficient in the supine position,[14] and maternal $Pa_{O_2}$ decreases by 13 mm Hg (1·7 kPa).[15] The caval obstruction

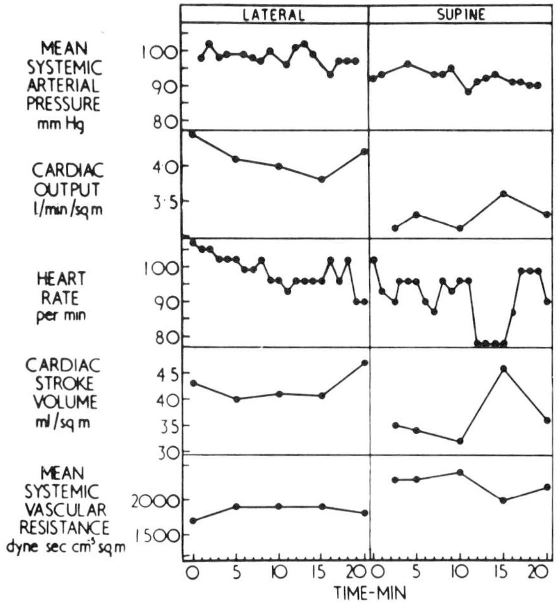


38/Fig. 4.—Concealed caval occlusion. The patient was symptom-free in the supine posture, but with a reduced cardiac output and an increased peripheral resistance. (Courtesy of Dr. D. B. Scott and John Sherratt and Son Ltd., publishers of the *British Journal of Anaesthesia.*[8])

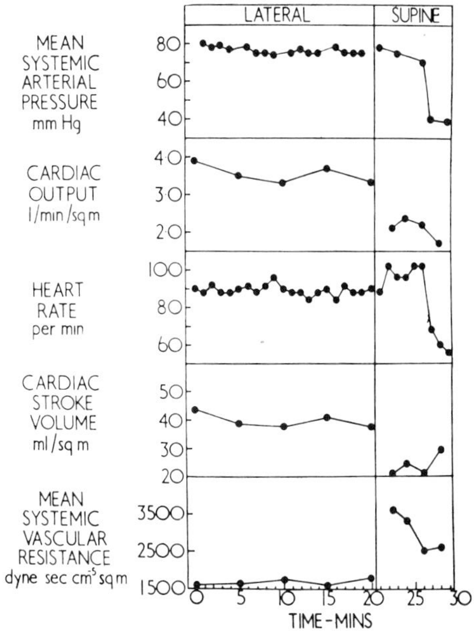


38/Fig. 5.—Revealed caval occlusion. Patient exhibiting the typical supine hypotensive syndrome. There was an immediate fall in cardiac output in the supine position but the arterial pressure was temporarily maintained by a rise in peripheral resistance. Then a sudden bradycardia occurred accompanied by fainting and hypotension. (Courtesy of Drs. M. M. Lees, D. B. Scott, M. G. Kerr and S. H. Taylor, and Blackwell Scientific Publications, publishers of *Clinical Science*.)

diverts blood flow to the vertebral venous plexus, producing a relative decrease in the volume of the epidural space, and this has been suggested as a partial explanation of the reduced dose requirements needed for epidural blockade in pregnancy.

When a uterine contraction occurs in a woman lying supine there is a further reduction in pelvic perfusion and pulse pressure in the legs as the compressive effect of the uterus on the vertebral bodies is enhanced. This is called the Poseiro effect.[16]

Aortocaval compression is one of the prime factors which renders cardiopulmonary resuscitation of late pregnant women very difficult, and uterine displacement should precede urgent delivery as essential steps in the management of cardiac arrest.[17]

The problems of aortocaval compression will be grossly aggravated following the sympathetic blockade produced by epidural and subarachnoid anaesthesia, so strict avoidance of the supine position and an adequate intravenous fluid preload are essential parts of the anaesthetic technique.

Aortocaval compression, whether or not a regional nerve block exists, can almost always be prevented by a complete avoidance of the unmodified supine position after about 30 weeks of pregnancy (Fig. 6). *The complete lateral position is preferable*. Maternal and fetal biochemistry is usually better in the left position, whilst hypotension may still be apparent in the right position, although sometimes the reverse is true.[18] Excessive flexion of the spine around a gravid uterus in the lateral position may result in severe inferior vena caval obstruction, and if this is evident, then the sitting position should be chosen for the insertion of an epidural catheter (see Fig. 7).

When the complete lateral position is not practical, then lateral uterine displacement, usually to the left, should be achieved by placing a wedge under the appropriate buttock to tilt the pelvis or by tilting the whole operating table. There are also mechanical devices which

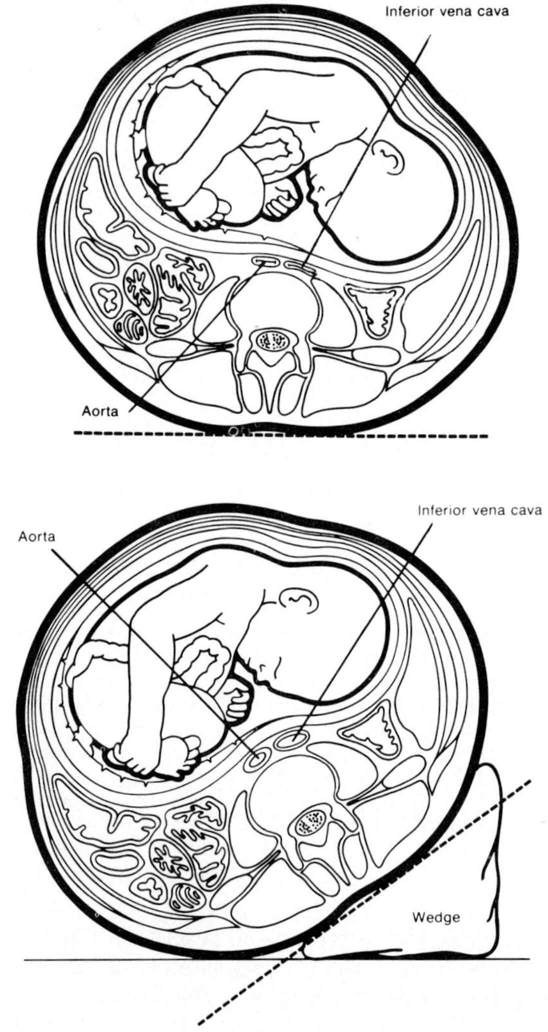


38/Fig. 6.—Aortocaval compression relieved following lateral uterine displacement achieved with a wedge under the right buttock. (Courtesy of Gerald W. Ostheimer and Breon Laboratories, Inc., U.S.A.[20])

38/Table 3
Respiratory Changes During Pregnancy

| | |
|---|---|
| *Dynamics* | |
| Tidal volume | +40% |
| Respiratory rate | +15% |
| Minute ventilation | +50% |
| Alveolar ventilation | +70% |
| Airway resistance | −36% |
| Total pulmonary resistance | −50% |
| Total compliance | −30% |
| Dead space | unchanged |
| *Volumes* | |
| Vital capacity | unchanged |
| Total lung capacity | −5% |
| Inspiratory lung capacity | +5% |
| Functional residual capacity | −20% |
| Expiratory reserve volume | −20% |
| Residual volume | −20% |
| Closing volume | unchanged |
| *Arterial Gases* | |
| $Pao_2$ | +10 mm Hg (1·3 kPa) |
| $Paco_2$ | −10 mm Hg (−1·3 kPa) |
| pH | no change |
| *Oxygen Consumption* | +20% |

have been especially designed to produce uterine displacement.

**Respiratory Changes** (Table 3)

**Anatomy.**—The diaphragm is elevated about 4 cm, although this shift is effectively compensated for by an increase in both anteroposterior and transverse diameters of the thoracic cavity as hormone-induced relaxation occurs in the costal ligaments.

Capillary engorgement occurs throughout the respiratory tract, resulting in, amongst other things, an increase in the incidence of nose bleeds especially following procedures such as nasal intubation.

**Function.**—Tidal volume and respiratory rate increase, and by term alveolar ventilation rises to 70 per cent above non-pregnant levels. Residual volume and functional residual capacity are such that airway closure may occur during normal tidal ventilation in one-third of pregnant women.[19] Dyspnoea may occur in about 60 per cent of normal pregnant women, although the reason for this is unknown.

Because of the increased oxygen consumption, the increased pulmonary ventilation and the decreased functional residual capacity, the pregnant woman is much more sensitive to the effects of apnoea, and the $Pao_2$ will fall by a mean of 139 mm Hg (18·5 kPa) after one minute of apnoea, compared with a mean fall of 58 mm Hg (7·7 kPa) in the non-pregnant following pre-oxygenation.[21]

Conversely, hyperventilation, whether the result of unrelieved pain or of the effects of mechanical ventilation, can quickly lower the

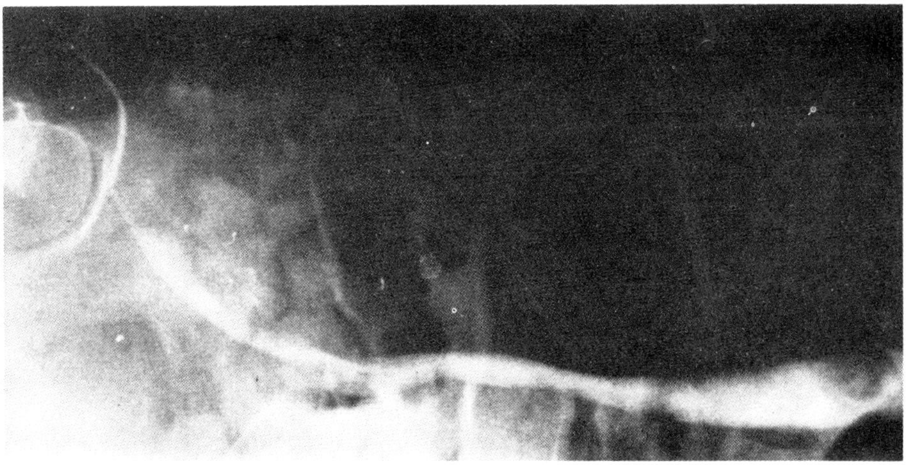

38/FIG. 7.—Cavogram (lateral view) of pregnant patient lying on her side. Despite the lateral posture a long segment of the inferior vena cava is seen to be partially compressed. (Courtesy of Professor M. G. Kerr, Dr. D. B. Scott and Dr. E. Samuel, and the Editor of the *British Medical Journal*.)

$Paco_2$ such that the hypocarbia and respiratory alkalosis produce a reduction in uteroplacental blood flow and impairment of maternal-fetal gas exchange.

Apparatus designed to provide inhalational analgesia during labour must be capable of accurate performance when subjected to high minute volumes and peak inspiratory flow rates.

### Changes in Gastro-intestinal Functions

**Gastric emptying** takes place at widely varying rates during labour and it may be considerably delayed particularly following the administration of opiates.[22] Gastric emptying times are only slightly prolonged if no analgesia or an epidural block is provided during labour.[23] Metoclopramide will speed gastric emptying in early labour, but is unable to reverse the effects of opiate drugs.

**Lower oesophageal sphincter tone,** and the resultant barrier pressure which prevents gastro-oesophageal reflux, are both usually increased during pregnancy, but sphincter tone may be reduced. It is this loss of tone, and not the rise in intra-abdominal pressure which is given as the main reason for the high incidence of heartburn occurring during pregnancy.[24] In addition, the displacement of the diaphragm by the enlarging uterus may disturb the gastro-oesophageal angle, which normally creates a valvular effect to aid the lower oesophageal sphincter in preventing regurgitation. As many as 70 per cent of women experience some symptoms of oesophageal reflux during pregnancy.[25] Heartburn must be regarded as a warning signal suggesting that an increased risk of regurgitation will exist during anaesthesia. Many of the drugs given during labour will influence lower oesophageal sphincter tone. The opiates, atropine, hyoscine, glycopyrrolate and diazepam will all lower sphincter tone and thus decrease the barrier pressure preventing regurgitation.[26] Metoclopramide, which effectively increases sphincter tone in non-pregnant patients does not consistently reverse the effect of the previously mentioned drugs, nor will metoclopramide reliably increase sphincter tone when no other drugs have been given. When metoclopramide and atropine are given together, the atropine effect predominates. Alkaline stomach contents will increase sphincter tone but the presence of a stomach tube will lower tone and increase the likelihood of regurgitation, which means that the removal of such tubes is mandatory before anaesthesia is induced.

**Intragastric pressure** is considerably increased in the last weeks of pregnancy and this increase is further exaggerated by the lithotomy or Trendelenburg position. At most times, this increase in intragastric pressure which tends to produce regurgitation, is opposed by a concurrent increase in the barrier pressure (or lower oesophageal sphincter opening pressure) so that the risk of reflux of stomach contents into the oesophagus during pregnancy is actually reduced. Patients who experience heartburn exhibit a considerably reduced barrier pressure.

Suxamethonium produces a rise in intragastric pressure during the fasciculations, but this rise is opposed by a greater rise in lower oesophageal sphincter tone, which causes a slight increase in the pressure gradient and creates no increased risk of regurgitation.[27]

**Gastric-acid secretion** is reduced during most of pregnancy, but increased gastric secretion results in enhanced acid production during the last few weeks of pregnancy.[28]

### Changes in Renal Function

Renal blood flow and glomerular filtration rate are increased by up to 80 per cent in early pregnancy and are maintained throughout. Suggestions of a reduction in these rates in the third trimester were based on measurements made in the supine position (see Aortocaval compression). Glycosuria is frequently observed because of an intermittent failure of tubular reabsorption to deal with the increased glomerular filtration rate and this may confuse the diagnosis of gestational diabetes.

### Changes in Hepatic Function

The influence of various hormones upon hepatic enzyme activity is reflected in the variations of plasma protein and serum cholinesterase; binding of drugs to plasma proteins and the metabolism of drugs by the liver may both be affected.

## PHYSIOLOGY OF LABOUR

### Onset of Labour

The chain of events responsible for initiating the onset of labour remains a mystery. At a cellular level it is known that increased calcium ion concentrations within smooth muscle promotes uterine contractions. Reduction in intracellular calcium caused, for example, by cyclic AMP activity, promotes uterine relaxation.

Hormones, produced by the mother, placenta or fetus may be the initiating factors. Oxytocin released from the posterior pituitary gland is a potent uterine stimulant but is probably more important in the second stage of labour.[29] Fetal production of cortisol and oestrogen increases dramatically near term, and these hormones may stimulate prostaglandin synthesis and release progesterone which inhibits uterine activity. The concentration of progesterone falls gradually before the onset of labour and may block the action of prostaglandins on the myometrium until then.

The role of the prostaglandins would appear to be of central importance. Prostaglandins $E_2$ and $F_2\alpha$ initiate myometrial contractions, and the precursors of these hormones are stored in the fetal membranes during pregnancy before being released at the appropriate time by some unknown mechanism.

**Neural control of uterine activity** is of less importance in the onset and maintenance of contractions than hormonal influences. The myometrium possesses $\alpha$- and $\beta$-adrenergic receptors and some cholinergic receptors. $\alpha$-adrenergic stimulation enhances resting uterine tone and contraction strength, whereas $\beta$-stimulation, primarily through $\beta_2$ receptors, produces the opposite effect. Endogenous catecholamines released by the stimulus of pain, stress or fear may precipitate inco-ordinate uterine action and $\beta$-receptor stimulants are used to retard premature labour. The addition of adrenaline to local anaesthetic solutions used during labour has been claimed to reduce uterine activity for up to 60 min.[30]

### Normal Labour

The first stage of labour commences with the onset of regular uterine contractions and continues until the cervix is fully dilated, which usually takes 10–12 hours in primigravid labours and 6–8 hours in multigravid labours. The second stage commences with full dilatation of the cervix and ends with delivery of the fetus. Traditionally applied time limits for the duration of the second stage are probably inappropriate when applied to women who have received an epidural injection. The third stage of labour has been much shortened by the use of oxytocic drugs and lasts from the delivery of the fetus until the delivery of the placenta.

**The mechanism of normal labour** depends on the interaction of three basic factors which when acting together produce cervical dilatation, descent and rotation of the presenting part, and expulsion of the fetus into the outside world. Traditonally these have been described as the passages, the passenger and the powers.

The dimensions and shape of the female pelvis will determine the ease with which the fetus, of variable configuration, will pass through during labour, and as the fetal head descends through the pelvis in normal labour, the occiput, which initially lies in a transverse position, is rotated so that it comes to lie directly anterior. This rotation is encouraged by the shape of the pelvis and by the tone of the levator ani muscle which forms the pelvic floor. Absence of this muscle tone may delay rotation and descent of the fetal head, and this is frequently cited as the reason for the increased incidence of rotational forceps associated with epidural analgesia in many centres. With patience and careful monitoring, this increased need to use forceps may be avoidable.

Uterine contractions of varying frequency and strength are described as inco-ordinate and are associated with a slow rate of cervical dilatation. Pain and anxiety may aggravate this situation by increasing sympathetic tone and effective epidural analgesia is strongly indicated to restore a normal pattern of contraction.

During the second stage, maternal expulsive efforts utilising the diaphragm and the abdominal musculature aid the uterine contractions in delivering the fetus. Regional neural blockade prevents the involuntary triggering of these expulsive efforts by each contraction, though the mother can be encouraged to push voluntarily in concert with the contractions. Powerful motor block of the abdominal muscles will prevent even this pushing and will render assisted delivery obligatory.

### Assessment of the Progress of Labour (Fig. 8)

The rate of cervical dilatation and the descent of the presenting part indicates the progress of labour, and graphical representations of this (called partograms) facilitate the clinical assessment of the progress.[31] The rate of progress of any individual is charted alongside expected rates so that any aberrations may be diagnosed at an early stage. Undue prolongation of labour, especially if painful, is potentially harmful to the mother and fetus and may be caused by abnormalities in either the passage, passenger or the power. Gross abnormalities in either of the first two factors will produce obvious mechanical obstruction which may preclude vaginal delivery, but abnormalities in the powers are often more subtle and may be overcome by stimulation of the uterus with oxytocin. This has led to the modern concept of the active management of labour, particularly in the primigravida.[32] Delay in a multigravid labour will be more frequently due to a mechanical cause and not a deficiency in the powers.

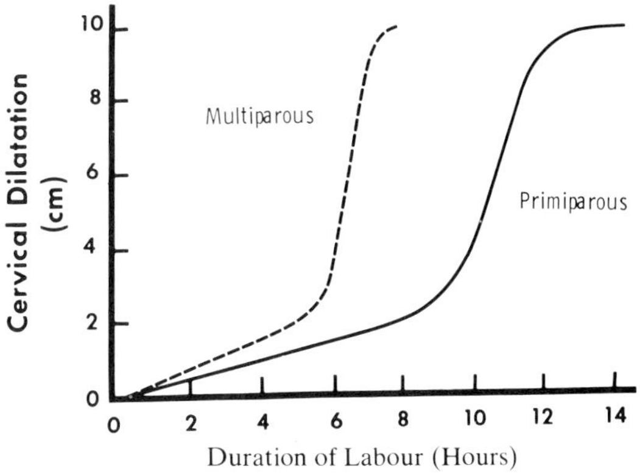


38/Fig. 8.—Partograms: graphical representations of normal progress in labour. (After Friedman, 1955, 1956.[33,34])

## SOME PATHOLOGICAL CONDITIONS OF PREGNANCY AND LABOUR

### Pre-eclamptic Toxaemia and Eclampsia

Pre-eclampsia is said to be present if two out of three signs – oedema, proteinuria and hypertension – are present in the second half of pregnancy. The diastolic blood pressure should be greater than 90 mm Hg (12·0 kPa) or have risen 20 mm Hg (2·7 kPa) above the pressure measured in early pregnancy. The differential diagnosis from other forms of hypertension in pregnancy is often very difficult. Eclampsia is a severe form of the disease characterised by gross hypertension and proteinuria compounded by the development of convulsions. Various immunological mechanisms have been suggested as possible causes, but the aetiology of the syndrome remains obscure.[35]

Oedema is a very common sign in pregnancy, found in up to 35 per cent of normotensive pregnant women, and even when accompanied by mild hypotension does not seem to be harmful to mother or fetus. The increased medical attention these symptoms attract may actually improve the perinatal outcome.[36]

The appearance of proteinuria is of much more ominous significance, particularly when early on in the pregnancy. The likelihood of eclampsia developing is increased with the attendant risks of convulsions or cerebrovascular accidents in the mother, and decreased placental blood flow causing growth retardation, hypoxia and death in the fetus.

Hypertensive disease occurs in up to 26 per cent of pregnancies and pre-eclampsia is the diagnosis made in 22 per cent.[37] Severe pre-eclampsia can be expected in 5 per cent of pregnancies, and hypertensive disorders directly caused 29 deaths during 1976–78. Cerebral haemorrhage was the commonest cause of death.[38]

Many pathophysiological changes accompany the signs. Plasma volume is reduced, blood viscosity increases and a relative polycythaemia develops. Capillary walls exhibit increased permeability. It is essential to appreciate that despite the oedema and hypertension, the circulation is grossly hypovolaemic and will show an exaggerated response to haemorrhage, hypotensive agents or extensive sympathetic blockade.

Intravascular coagulation occurs, although the initiating stimulus is obscure, and the concentration of fibrin degradation products rises sharply.[39] This potential disturbance of the microvasculature may explain the effects of pre-eclamptic toxaemia (PET) upon organs such as the placenta, lungs and kidneys. Ventilation perfusion abnormalities may occur in the lungs. If a severe coagulopathy develops, regional analgesic procedures may be contra-indicated.

Renal blood flow and glomerular filtration rate are reduced, even in the presence of oedema. Placental perfusion shows highly significant reduction in severe PET but the intervillous blood flow can be largely restored by an epidural block ($T_{10}$–$S_5$).

Laryngeal oedema has been reported as a potential complication of PET which may cause respiratory obstruction or create intubation difficulties.[40,41]

**Management.**—The delivery of the baby and placenta is the only certain cure, so treatment should be aimed at (i) controlling hypertension, (ii) preventing convulsions and (iii) ensuring rapid delivery by the safest route possible, which should include the liberal use of caesarean section. The significant reduction in perinatal mortality associated with PET justifies the modern aggressive management.[42]

Arterial pressure, ECG, urine output and composition and fetal heart rate and biochemistry must be intensively monitored. Frequent haematological and biochemical tests should be performed and should include urea and electrolytes, creatinine, plasma proteins, haemoglobin, haematocrit, coagulation screen and urine osmolality. Measurement of plasma colloid osmotic pressure may be very useful.

**Hypovolaemia** should be vigorously corrected using central venous pressure as a guide, and this is best achieved using salt-poor albumin, or plasma protein fraction to restore intravascular colloid pressure. The CVP has been shown to bear an inverse relationship to diastolic pressure and as CVP increases, blood pressure reduces and a diuresis occurs.[43]

**Hypertension** can be rapidly controlled with drugs such as diazoxide, hydralazine, sodium nitroprusside or nitroglycerin. Hydralazine 40 mg in 500 ml 5 per cent dextrose may be given at the rate of 2–20 mg/hour following a 20 mg bolus injection. Hydralazine is superior to sodium nitroprusside, despite the more rapid action of the latter, and it also increases utero-placental blood flow.[44] Sodium nitroprusside carries the potential risk of producing fetal cyanide toxicity. Nitroglycerin has fast onset and short duration of action, combined with rapid hepatic clearance so that quick, precise blood-pressure control is possible. The fetal affects of nitroglycerin are unknown.[45]

**Convulsions** can be prevented or controlled with diazepam or a 0·8 per cent infusion of chlormethiazole. Diazepam can be given as an infusion, 40 mg in 500 ml 5 per cent dextrose at 2–4 mg/hour, after a bolus injection of 10 mg.

Magnesium sulphate is commonly used in the USA. In the extreme case, muscle relaxation, intubation and IPPV may be necessary but this only prevents the external manifestations without suppressing the central neural hyperactivity. Eclamptic convulsions may occur after delivery in up to 50 per cent of cases (for further details see Hibbard[46] and Turner[47]).

**Pain relief** should be provided by epidural

block if there is no coagulopathy, although this technique must never be used primarily as a method for lowering blood pressure. Effective analgesia will reduce the blood pressure and prevent swings in arterial pressure during painful contractions, whilst producing a beneficial effect on the placental blood flow. Effective analgesia also facilitates early delivery which is the only certain cure for PET.

**Coagulation Disorders**

Coagulation mechanisms are usually enhanced and fibrinolytic activity reduced during pregnancy, but disruption of the clotting system may occur with increased fibrinolysis or intravascular coagulation (for details see also Chapter 17, p. 601), and also in conditions such as abruptio placentae, intra-uterine fetal death, septicaemia, or amniotic-fluid embolism.

**Abruptio placentae.**—Premature separation of a placenta situated in a normal position in the uterus is associated with severe haemorrhage, and 40 per cent of patients will develop hypofibrinogenaemia, probably as a result of excess consumption. Twenty per cent may exhibit severe coagulation deficiencies.

Such premature placental separation is often associated with hypertensive disorders, and if bleeding is concealed retroplacentally, central venous pressure may give the only true indications of the extent of blood loss.

Fetal mortality is very high and caesarean section may be indicated to gain control of the bleeding even after fetal death.[48] Fresh whole blood or fresh frozen plasma should be used in conjunction with expert coagulation screening. Renal failure may follow intravascular fibrin deposition, so vigorous therapy with mannitol is indicated if oliguria occurs.

**Septicaemia.**—Endotoxic shock following either septic abortion, or antepartum or postpartum infection, may be associated with disseminated intravascular coagulation.

**Intra-uterine fetal death.**—The depletion of coagulation factors does not become significant until 3–4 weeks after the fetus perishes, and the current availability of effective uterine stimulants usually circumvents the problem by ensuring early delivery. Regional analgesia is strongly indicated for this distressing condition but it would be wise to perform a coagulation screen test before inserting an epidural or subarachnoid block.

**Haemorrhage**

A normal vaginal delivery is accompanied by an average blood loss of 200 ml, increased by 150 ml if an episiotomy is performed. But blood loss may be considerably greater and, if in excess of 500 ml, is described as postpartum haemorrhage. Routine use of oxytocic drugs in the third stage limits blood loss.

Blood loss following forceps delivery or caesarean section is substantially reduced when epidural anaesthesia is provided rather than pudendal nerve block or general anaesthesia. Under general anaesthesia blood loss at forceps delivery or caesarean section averages 520 ml, and upwards of one litre respectively, but with an epidural block, these losses average only 270 ml for a forceps delivery while the loss at caesarean section is halved.[1]

The increased blood volume due to the autotransfusion from the empty, contracted uterus compensates for this loss, so that transfusion is not indicated unless clinical signs of hypovolaemia are apparent and usually only after the loss exceeds 1·2–1·5 litres.

Abnormal haemorrhage may be associated with coagulation disorders, placenta praevia, retained placenta, or following miscarriage. Twenty-six deaths were directly due to haemorrhage in the 1976–1978 period.[38]

The management of the coagulopathies has already been mentioned. The bleeding in the other conditions will usually stop only when the uterus is empty, so rapid delivery or curettage may be indicated before optimal resuscitation can be achieved.

**Amniotic Fluid Embolism**

Amniotic fluid embolism is a rare condition but possesses a very high mortality, such that the condition caused 11 maternal deaths in England and Wales (1976–1978).[38] Other causes of sudden collapse during labour or delivery are listed in Table 4.

The exact route by which the amniotic fluid penetrates the maternal circulation is uncertain, although probably powerful uterine contractions force the fluid into uterine venous sinuses through lacerations in the membranes.

Pulmonary vascular obstruction by the cells and debris in the fluid is considered a prime factor in the development of profound pulmonary and circulatory effects.[49] The disseminated

38/TABLE 4
CAUSES OF SUDDEN COLLAPSE DURING LABOUR OR DELIVERY.
The anaesthetist may be required to provide both resuscitation and urgent anaesthesia if necessary.

*Obstetric*
- Haemorrhage, with or without coagulopathy
- Acute uterine inversion
- Amniotic fluid embolus
- Endotoxic shock
- Acute adrenal haemorrhage

*Non-obstetric*
- Eclampsia
- Cerebrovascular accident
  - hypertensive disease of pregnancy
- Cardiovascular collapse
  - pre-existing cardiac disease
  - hypertensive disease
  - aortocaval compression
  - neural blockade
- Pulmonary embolus
  - clot or air
- Drug overdose or other adverse drug reaction
- Water intoxication or hyponatraemia
- Pulmonary acid aspiration

intravascular coagulopathy which almost invariably appears causes further mischief in the pulmonary circulation and often precipitates severe haemorrhage.

**Management** must include intensive circulatory and respiratory support whilst an attempt is being made to identify and treat the coagulopathy. Fresh blood should be used for volume replacement but the decision to administer fibrinogen, fibrinolysis inhibitors or heparin must be based on expert haematological advice. Vigorous treatment has resulted in survival, and a serine proteinase inhibitor, FOY, has been successfully used to treat the disseminated intravascular coagulation (DIC).[50]

## DRUGS USED IN LABOUR

There is an intimate pharmacological relationship between the myometrium and the muscle in the cardiovascular system, so that drugs used to stimulate or retard labour may also exert strong influences on the heart and vasculature, thereby creating anaesthetic problems.

### Drugs Used to Inhibit Uterine Activity

**$\beta$-Agonists.** — $\beta$-adrenergic stimulation *increases* intracellular cyclic AMP, which acts to reduce free calcium and thereby diminish myometrial contractility. $\beta$-sympathomimetic agents currently used to retard labour include salbutamol, ritodrine, terbutaline and isoxsuprine. These drugs are initially administered intravenously to control an acute episode of premature labour, then orally as prophylaxis, once the contractions have settled. Their efficacy in arresting premature labour remains controversial, whilst the side-effects of the drugs may be very severe.[51]

Cardiovascular effects of the drugs include hypotension following generalised vasodilatation, tachycardia, palpitations and increased cardiac irritability. Acute pulmonary oedema has been described following administration of $\beta$-agonist drugs in conjunction with corticosteroids given to induce fetal lung maturity.[52] Carbohydrate metabolism may be disrupted and these drugs must be used cautiously in diabetic patients.

Problems have been encountered when patients taking $\beta$-agonists present for general anaesthesia, and $\beta$-blockers may have to be employed to control tachycardia and increased cardiac output, but should only be given after the umbilical cord has been clamped.[53]

**Ethanol**, by suppressing the release of oxytocin from the posterior pituitary gland, may be used to control uterine contractions, though the effect of ethanol may be less marked than that of the $\beta$-agonist, whilst the side-effects may be quite unpleasant.

**Prostaglandin synthetase inhibitors** will suppress uterine activity, but animal experiments suggest that premature closure of the fetal ductus arteriosus may make these drugs unsuitable for use in premature labour.

### Drugs Used to Augment Uterine Activity

**Prostaglandins.**—The prostaglandins, of which only $PGE_2$ and $PGF_2\alpha$ are of importance in obstetrics, are a group of 20 carbon hydroxy fatty acids. They increase cyclic AMP, causing direct stimulation of smooth muscle, and indirect stimulation following increased oxytocin output from the pituitary. The endogenous prostaglandins are thought to play a key role in the spontaneous initiation of labour. When administered as an intravaginal pessary the prostaglandin will induce ripening of the cervix, often initiating labour and thus avoiding the need for a formal induction. Labours so induced have a high rate of spontaneous delivery and a diminished analgesic requirement.[54]

Intravenous administration of prostaglandins is as effective as Syntocinon in the artificial induction and maintenance of labour. However, nausea, vomiting or diarrhoea occur in many patients, and thrombophlebitis often develops at the site of i.v. administration.

Prostaglandins are also used to stimulate delivery after intra-uterine fetal death relatively early in pregnancy, when the uterus is less sensitive to the effects of oxytocin.

**Syntocinon** is used both to augment uterine activity during labour and during active management of the third stage following delivery. Syntocinon is a synthetic preparation of oxytocin which is normally used in preference to natural oxytocin. Given intravenously, oxytocin produces powerful uterine contractions along with a brief fall in blood pressure and peripheral resistance. This transient hypotension should not be a problem in a well-hydrated, tilted patient, but can be severe when oxytocin is given as a bolus during general anaesthesia with the patient supine.[55] As a general practice, oxytocin should be given as an infusion (e.g. 20 units in 500 ml of crystalloid solution) rather than in an intravenous bolus.

Syntocinon causes water retention and, if combined with large volumes of carrier fluid for prolonged intravenous administration during labour, water intoxication may result, manifesting as convulsions or sudden collapse. Haematological and electrolyte concentrations will confirm the diagnosis[56] The use of more concentrated solutions, accurately administered by infusion pump, will avoid this problem.

Over-enthusiastic intravenous administration of relatively hypotonic fluids throughout a prolonged labour, even without Syntocinon, may result in hyponatraemia in mother and neonate.

**Ergometrine** administration produces powerful uterine contractions, but is accompanied by sustained vascular spasm persisting for several hours, which results in increased peripheral resistance, systemic hypertension, increased central venous pressure and coronary artery vasoconstriction.[57] This may be very dangerous in patients with pre-existing disease of the cardiovascular system or pre-eclampsia, and could precipitate pulmonary oedema or a cerebrovascular accident. Ergometrine causes vomiting in up to 50 per cent of cases and this can be a most serious side-effect when procedures such as caesarean section are performed on an awake patient under an epidural block.

Oxytocin 10 units is as effective as ergometrine 0·5 mg in controlling bleeding when either is given intravenously after delivery.

**Syntometrine** is a combination which contains Syntocinon 5 units for every 0·5 mg of ergometrine, and this is the standard drug given intramuscularly after delivery in most obstetric units. The rapid onset of action of Syntocinon is reinforced by the more sustained action of ergometrine and blood loss is claimed to be reduced in the third stage of normal delivery when this combination is used.[58]

## REFERENCES


1. Moir, D. D. (1980). *Obstetric Anaesthesia and Analgesia*, 2nd edit. London: Baillière Tindall.
2. Hytten, F. F. and Leitch, I. (1971). *The Physiology of Human Pregnancy*, 2nd edit. Oxford: Blackwell.
3. Studd, J. W. W. (1975). The plasma proteins in pregnancy. Physiological adjustments in pregnancy. *Clin. in Obst. & Gynaecol.*, **2:2**, 285.
4. Shnider, S. M. (1965). Serum cholinesterase activity during pregnancy, labor and the puerperium. *Anaesthesiology*, **26**, 335.
5. Blitt, C. D., Petty, W. C., Alberternst, E. E. and Wright, B. J. (1977). Correlation of plasma cholinesterase activity and duration of action of succinylcholine during pregnancy. *Anesth. Analg.*, **56**, 78.
6. Datta, S., Crocker, J. S. and Alper, M. H. (1977). Muscle pain following administration of suxamethonium to pregnant and non-pregnant patients undergoing laparoscopic tubal ligation. *Brit. J. Anaesth.*, **49**, 625.
7. Williams, C. V., Johnson, A. and Ledward, R. (1974). A comparison of central venous pressure changes in the third stage of labour following oxytocic drugs and diazepam. *J. Obstet. Gynaec. Br. Cwlth.*, **81**, 596.
8. Scott, D. B. (1968). Inferior vena caval occlusion in late pregnancy and its importance in anaesthesia. *Brit. J. Anaesth.*, **40**, 120.
9. Marx, G. F., Husain, F. J. and Shiau, H. F. (1980). Brachial and femoral blood pressures during the prenatal period. *Am. J. Obstet. Gynecol.*, **136**, 11.
10. Willcourt, R. J., Paust, J. C. and Queenan, J. T. (1982). Changes in fetal $TcPo_2$ values occurring during labour in association with lumbar extradural analgesia. *Brit. J. Anaesth.*, **54**, 635.

11. Huovinen, K. and Teramo, K. (1979). Effect of maternal position on fetal heart rate during extradural analgesia. *Brit. J. Anaesth.*, **51**, 767.
12. Kauppila, A., Koskinen, M., Puolokka, J., Tuimala, R. and Kuikka, J. (1980). Decreased intervillous and unchanged myometrial blood flow in supine recumbency. *Obstet. Gynecol.*, **55**, 203.
13. Humphrey, M. D., Chang, A., Wood, E. C. and Hounslow, D. (1974). A decrease in fetal pH during the second stage of labour when conducted in the dorsal position. *J. Obstet. Gynaecol. Brit. Cwlth.*, **81**, 600.
14. Caldeyro-Barcia, R. (1960). Effect of position changes on the intensity and frequency of uterine contractions during labor. *Am. J. Obstet. Gynecol.*, **80**, 284.
15. Ang, C. K., Tan, T. H., Walters, W. A. W. and Wood, C. (1969). Postural influence on maternal capillary oxygen and carbon dioxide tension. *Brit. med. J.*, **4**, 20.
16. Poseiro, J. J. (1967). Compression of the aorta or iliac arteries by the contracting human uterus during labor. In: *Effects of Labor on Fetus and Newborn*. Ed. R. Caldeyro-Barcia. New York: Pergamon Press.
17. Marx. G. F. (1982). Cardiopulmonary resuscitation of late pregnant women. *Anesthesiology*, **56**, 156.
18. Buley, R. J. R., Downing, J. W., Brock-Utne, J. G. and Cuerden (1977). Right versus left lateral tilt for Caesarean section. *Brit. J. Anaesth.*, **49**, 1009.
19. Bevan, D. R., Holdcroft, A., Loh, L., MacGregor, W. G., O'Sullivan, J. C. and Sykes, M. K. (1974). Closing volume and pregnancy. *Brit. med. J.*, **1**, 13.
20. Ostheimer, G. W. (1980). *Regional Anesthesia Techniques in Obstetrics*. New York: Breon Laboratories, Inc.
21. Archer, G. W. and Marx, G. F. (1974). Arterial oxygen tension during apnoea in parturient women. *Brit. J. Anaesth.*, **46**, 358.
22. Nimmo, W. S., Littlewood, D. C., Scott, D. B. and Prestcott, L. F. (1978). Gastric emptying following hysterectomy with extradural analgesia. *Brit. J. Anaesth.*, **50**, 559.
23. Wilson, J. (1978). Gastric emptying time in labour, some recent findings and their clinical significance. *J. int. med. Res.*, **6**, Suppl. 1, 54.
24. Van Thiel, D. H., Gavaler, J. S., Joshi, S. N., Sara, R. K. and Strempe, J. (1977). Heartburn of pregnancy. *Gastroenterology*, **72**, 666.
25. Hart, D. M. (1978). Heartburn in pregnancy. *J. int. med. Res.*, **6**, Suppl. 1, 1.
26. Rubin, J., Brock-Utne, J. G., Dimopoulos, G. E., Downing, J. W. and Moshal, M. G. (1982). Flunitrazepam increases and diazepam decreases the lower oesophageal sphincter tone when administered intravenously. *Anaesth. Intens. Care*, **10**, 130.
27. Smith, G., Dalling, R. and Williams, T. I. R. (1978). Gastro-oesophageal pressure gradient changes produced by induction of anaesthesia and suxamethonium. *Brit. J. Anaesth.*, **50**, 1137.
28. Attia, R. R., Ebeid, A. M., Fischer, J. E. and Goudsouzian, N. G. (1982). Maternal fetal and placental gastrin concentrations. *Anaesthesia*, **37**, 18.
29. Bisset, G. W. (1976). Neurohypophyseal hormones. In: *Peptide Hormones*. Ed. by J. A. Parsons. London: MacMillan.
30. Jouppila, P., Jouppila, R., Kaar, K. and Merila, M. (1977). Fetal heart rate patterns and uterine activity after segmental epidural analgesia. *Brit. J. Obstet. Gynaec.*, **84**, 481.
31. Beazley, J. M. and Kurjak, A. (1972). Influence of a partograph on the active management of labour. *Lancet*, **2**, 348.
32. O'Driscoll, K., Jackson, R. J. A. and Gallagher, J. T. (1970). Active management of labour and cephalo-pelvic disproportion. *J. Obstet. Gynaec. Brit. Cwlth.*, **77**, 385.
33. Friedman, E. A. (1955). Primigravid labor: A graphicostatistical analysis. *Obstet. Gynecol.*, **6**, 567.
34. Friedman, E. A. (1956). Labor in multiparas: A graphico-statistical analysis. *Obstet. Gynecol.*, **8**, 691.
35. MacGillivray, I. (1981). Aetiology of pre-eclampsia. *Brit. J. Hosp. Med.*, **26**, 110.
36. Redman, C. W. G., Beilin, L. J., Bonnar, J. and Wilkinson, R. H. (1976). Plasma-urate measurements in predicting fetal deaths in hypertensive pregnancy. *Lancet*, **1**, 1370.
37. Chamberlain, G., Phillipp, E., Howlett, B. and Masters, K. (1978). *British Births, 1970*. Vol. 2: Obstetric Care. London: Heinemann.
38. Department of Health and Social Security (1982). *Report on Confidential Enquiries into Maternal Deaths in England and Wales*, 1976–1978. London: HMSO.
39. Howie, P. W. (1977). The haemostatic mechanisms in pre-eclampsia. (Hypertensive states in pregnancy.) *Clin. in Obst. & Gynaecol.*, **4:3**, 595.
40. Brock-Utne, J. G., Downing, J. W. and Seedat, F. (1977). Laryngeal oedema associated with pre-eclamptic toxaemia. *Anaesthesia*, **32**, 556.
41. Jouppila, R., Jouppila, P. and Hollmen, A. (1980). Laryngeal oedema as an obstetric anaesthesia complication. *Acta anaesth. scand.*, **24**, 97.
42. Tejani, S. N., Paydar, M., Tejani, N. A., Mann, L. I. and Weiss, R. R. (1977). Modern management of hypertensive disorders of pregnancy. *Obstet. Gynecol.*, **51**, 648.
43. Joyce, T. H., Debnath, K. S. and Baker, B. A. (1979). Pre-eclampsia – relationship to CVP and epidural analgesia. *Anesthesiology*, **51**, S297.
44. Ring, G., Krames, E., Shnider, S. M., Wallis, K. L. and Levinson, G. (1977). Comparison of nitroprusside and hydralazine in hypertensive pregnant ewes. *Obstet. Gynecol.*, **50**, 598.
45. Snyder, S. W., Wheeler, A. S. and James, F. M. (1979). Use of nitroglycerin to control severe hypertension of pregnancy during Cesarean section. *Anesthesiology*, **51**, 563.
46. Hibbard, B. M. and Rosen, M. (1977). The management of severe pre-eclampsia and eclampsia. *Brit. J. Anaesth.*, **49**, 3.
47. Turner, G. M. (1981). Management of pre-eclampsia and eclampsia. *Brit. J. Hosp. Med.*, **26**, 120.
48. Odendaal, J. H., Brink, S. and Steytler, J. G. (1978). Clinical and haematological problems associated with severe abruptio placenta. *S. Afr. Med. J.*, **54**, 476.
49. Morgan, M. (1979). Amniotic fluid embolism. *Anaesthesia*, **34**, 20.
50. Taenaka, N., Shimada, Y., Kawai, M., Yoshita, I. and Kosaki, G. (1980). Survival from DIC following amniotic fluid embolism. Successful treatment with a serine proteinase inhibitor – FOY. *Anaesthesia*, **36**, 389.
51. Editorial (1979). Drugs in threatened preterm labour. *Brit. med. J.*, **1**, 71.
52. Tinga, D. J. and Aarnoudse, J. G. (1979). Postpartum pulmonary oedema associated with preventive therapy for premature labour. *Lancet*, **1**, 1026.
53. Knight, R. J. (1977). Labour retarded with $\beta$-agonist

drugs. A therapeutic problem in emergency anaesthesia. *Anaesthesia*, **32**, 639.
54. Emburey, M. P. (1981). Prostaglandins in human reproduction. *Brit. med. J.*, **283**, 1563.
55. Weis, F. R. and Peak, J. (1974). Effects of oxytocin on blood pressure during anesthesia. *Anesthesiology*, **40**, 189.
56. Feeney, J. G. (1982). Water intoxication and oxytocin. *Brit. med. J.*, **285**, 243.
57. Johnstone, M. (1972). The cardiovascular effects of oxytocic drugs. *Brit. J. Anaesth.*, **44**, 826.
58. Docherty, P. W. and Hooper, M. (1981). Choice of an oxytocic agent for routine use at delivery. *J. Obstet. Gynaecol.*, **2**, 60.

## FURTHER READING

Moir, D. D. (1980). *Obstetric Anaesthesia and Analgesia*, 2nd edit. London: Baillière Tindall.

Whitfield, C. R. (1977). Medical disorders of pregnancy. *Clin. in Obst. & Gynaecol.*, **4:2**.

CHAPTER 39

# Relief of Pain in Labour



THE responsibility of the anaesthetist in obstetrics is arguably greater than in any other field of anaesthesia for the consequences of maternal or fetal death or incapacitation are of serious, long-term social and financial importance to both the family involved and to the community as a whole.

## PAIN IN LABOUR

### Pathways and Mechanisms

The description of peripheral pain pathways proposed by Cleland in 1933[1] has been modified by Bonica[2] and is fundamental to any consideration of obstetric analgesia.

**Pain in the first stage of labour.**—Uterine contractions cause stretching, tearing and distortion and possibly ischaemia of the uterine tissues, whilst simultaneous dilatation of the cervix and stretching of the lower uterine segment is occurring. The intensity of the pain increases progressively with the rising strength of the contractions and these painful stimuli are transmitted by A δ and C afferent fibres which accompany sympathetic pathways through the pelvic, inferior, middle and superior hypogastric plexuses, the lumbar sympathetic chain, the white rami of the spinal nerves T10, T11, T12 and L1 and the posterior roots of these nerves to reach the spinal cord (see Fig. 1). In early labour, only the nerve roots of T11 and T12 are involved, but as the intensity of contractions increases, T10 and L1 are recruited.[2]

Backache is a frequent complaint during labour and may be caused by one or other of two mechanisms. Pain originating in the uterus or cervix may be referred to the cutaneous branches of the posterior divisions of T10–L1 which migrate caudally for an appreciable distance before they innervate the skin overlying

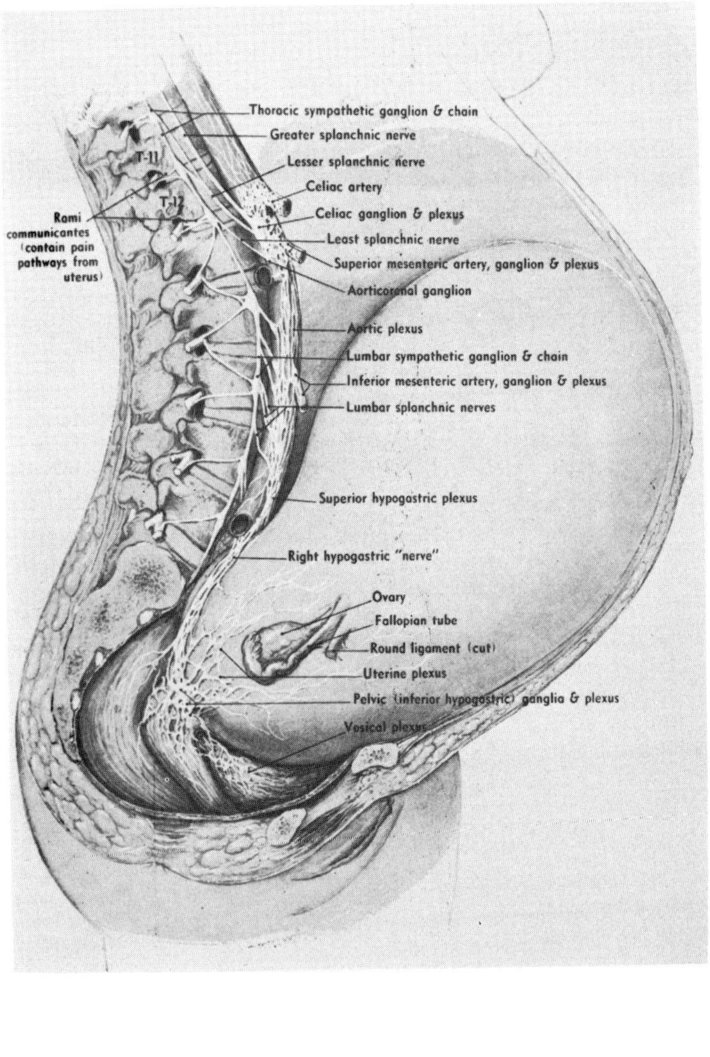


39/Fig. 1.—This anatomical view illustrates the pathways followed by pain fibres which originate in the uterus and cervix and reach the spinal cord at T10, 11, 12 and L1 segmental levels. The afferent fibres are not part of the autonomic system and merely accompany the sympathetic nerves. (Courtesy of J. J. Bonica and the publishers, F. A. Davis Company, Philadelphia.[3])

the vertebral column. The cutaneous branches of T11, for example, supply the skin overlying L3 and L4 vertebrae.[2] Pressure on peri-uterine tissues often, in association with fetal malposition or an unusual shape of sacrum, refer to the L5, S1 segments and are felt as very low back pain.

**Pain in the second stage of labour.**—The pain caused by distension of the pelvic structure and perineum following descent of the presenting part is added to the pain of uterine contractions although, once cervical dilatation is complete, the pain induced by contractions may become less intense. The uterine pain continues to be referred to T10–L1, while the pain produced by stretching or pressure exerted on intrapelvic structures, including the peritoneum, bladder, urethra and rectum is referred to sacral segments. Pressure on the roots of the lumbosacral plexus may manifest itself as pain felt low in the back or in the thighs. Pain produced by stretching the perineum is transmitted by the pudendal nerve (S2, 3, 4) and in part by the posterior cutaneous nerve of the thigh (S2, 3), the genito-femoral nerve (L1, 2) and the ilio-inguinal nerve (L1) (see Table 1).

*Clinical implications.*—During the first stage of labour, an epidural block limited to the T11, T12 segments at the beginning and later extending to involve T10 and L1 will usually be sufficient to provide excellent pain relief whilst avoiding neural blockade of sacral segments. Premature sacral blockade can result in the loss of the stimulating effect upon contractions of Ferguson's reflex and the loss of pelvic muscle tone, which aids the rotation of the presenting part.

Later in the first stage and during the early part of the second stage, pain is often experienced in lower lumbar and upper sacral segments; so the block will have to be extended if analgesia is to be guaranteed.

Complete block of the sacral segments need only be performed when perineal pain becomes worrisome and, by this stage, the block of thoracolumbar segments will hopefully be decaying to such an extent that abdominal muscle strength will be adequate to permit voluntary expulsive efforts by the mother.

### Consequences of Pain in Labour

Pain is a noxious and unpleasant stimulus

39/Table 1

Pain in Labour: Pathways and Mechanisms (after Crawford[5])

The pain produced by overdistension of the bladder is conducted via sympathetic pathways to T11, L1 and appears as suprapubic pain.

| *Site of Origin* | *Mechanism* | *Pathway* | *Site of Pain* |
|---|---|---|---|
| Uterus and cervix | Distortion, stretching, tearing of fibres | (i) Afferents which accompany sympathetic pathway to T10, T11, T12 and L1<br>(ii) Dorsal rami T10–L1 referred to cutaneous branches of posterior divisions | upper abdomen and groin<br>mid-back |
| Peri-uterine tissues<br>Lumbosacral region | Pressure often in association with fetal malposition or platypelloid pelvis | Lumbosacral plexus L5, S1 (? pelvic splanchnic nerves) | low-back, thigh |
| Bladder, urethra, rectum | Pressure by presenting part | S2, 3, 4 | referred to perineum and sacral area |
| Vagina | Distension, tearing | Somatic S2, 3, 4 | not referred |
| Perineum | Distension, tearing | Pudenal (S 2, 3, 4)<br>Genito-femoral (L1, 2)<br>Ileoinguinal L1<br>Posterior cutaneous Nerve of thigh, S2, 3 | not referred |

which produces fear and anxiety. It was once held that fear, ignorance and anxiety exacerbated the pain of labour, but it should be stressed that the converse may also be true.[4]

The maternal and fetal consequences of unrelieved pain in labour have been summarised in Fig. 2. Unrelieved stress in the pregnant baboon causes a reduction in uterine blood flow, fetal heart rate and fetal oxygenation which all return to normal when the stress is removed.[6,7]

Unrelieved stress in labour produces increased plasma cortisol and catecholamine concentrations and this may be responsible for the reduction in utero-placental blood flow[8,9] (see Figs 3 & 4). Effective pain relief reduces plasma noradrenaline,[10] prevents the rise during first and second stage of labour of 11-hydroxy-corticosteroid,[11] prevents metabolic acidosis developing by reducing the rate of rise of lactate, pyruvate and excess lactate levels,[12] and decreases maternal oxygen consumption by up to 14 per cent.[13] Effective epidural analgesia prevents the pain-induced hyperventilation and hypocapnia which can be severe enough in painful labour to produce tetany[14] and also reduces utero-placental blood flow by up to 25 per cent. The respiratory alkalosis further impairs feto-maternal gas exchange by shifting the oxyhaemoglobin dissociation curve to the left and fetal $Pa_{O_2}$ may fall by up to 23 per cent.[15]

## Methods of Pain Relief in Labour

There have been many approaches to the relief of pain in labour throughout history up to the present time. The possible sites of action of some of the currently available analgesic techniques are illustrated in Fig. 5. The requirements of a satisfactory analgesic technique in labour may be listed as follows (after Bromage, [16]):

1. Safety
2. Effective analgesia throughout painful periods of labour
3. No depressant effect on the maternal respiratory or cardiovascular system
4. No depressant effects on the progress of labour
5. No depressant effects on the baby before or after delivery
6. No unpleasant maternal side-effects
7. High technical success rate.

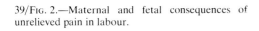

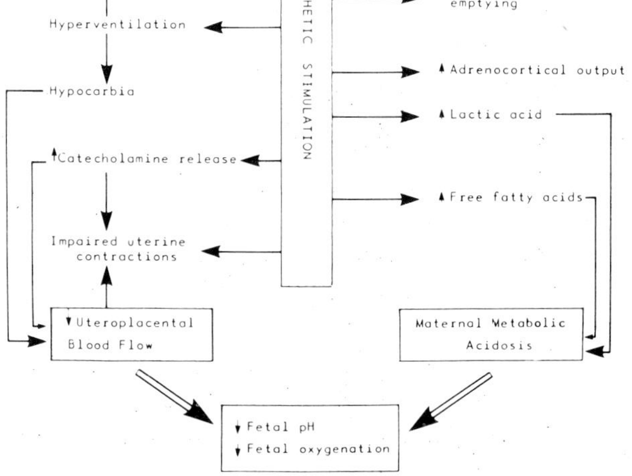

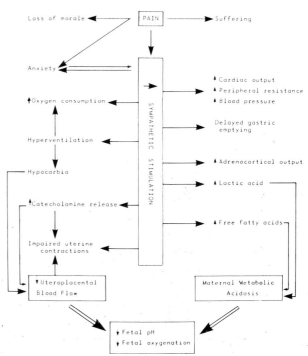


39/FIG. 2.—Maternal and fetal consequences of unrelieved pain in labour.

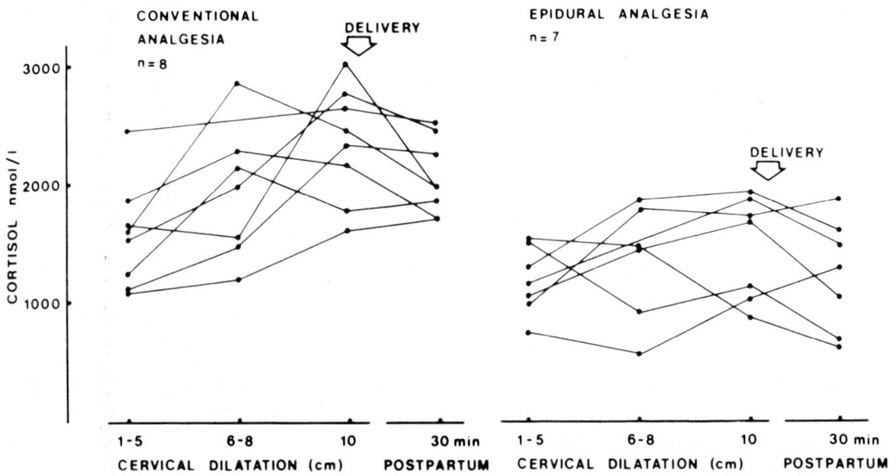


39/FIG. 3.—Effect of pain on plasma cortisol concentration during labour. *Left:* Patients receiving pethidine and Entonox. *Right:* Patients receiving continuous epidural analgesia. (Courtesy of Drs. Maltau, O. V. Eielsen and K. T. Stokke and the publishers C. V. Mosby Co.[8])

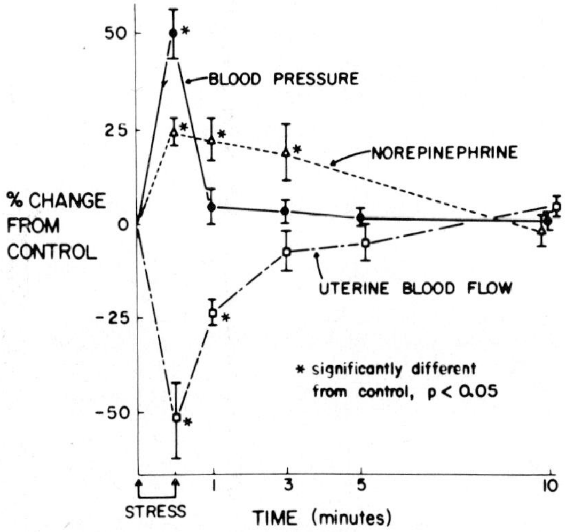

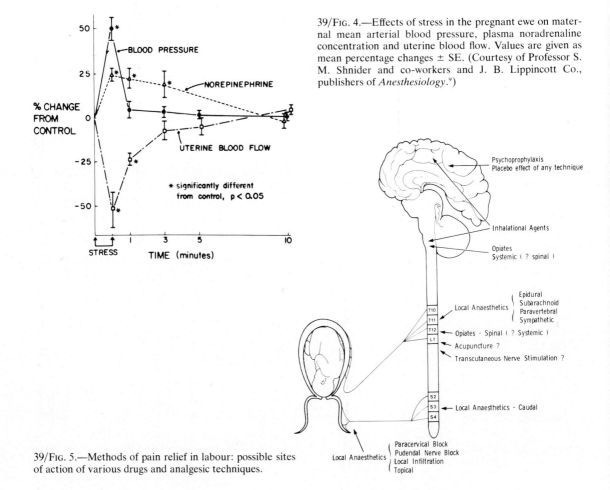


39/FIG. 4.—Effects of stress in the pregnant ewe on maternal mean arterial blood pressure, plasma noradrenaline concentration and uterine blood flow. Values are given as mean percentage changes ± SE. (Courtesy of Professor S. M. Shnider and co-workers and J. B. Lippincott Co., publishers of *Anesthesiology*.[9])

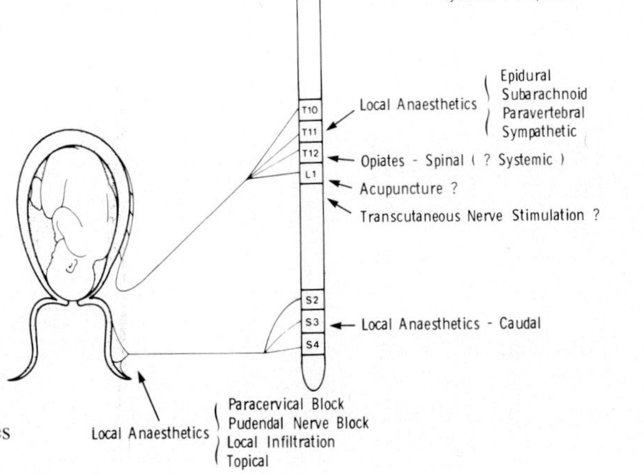


39/FIG. 5.—Methods of pain relief in labour: possible sites of action of various drugs and analgesic techniques.

Very few of the available techniques fulfil all of these criteria.

### Consequences of Pain Relief Techniques

Although the provision of adequate pain relief has physiological and psychological benefits for both mother and fetus, the analgesic techniques may exert other effects which may be quite undesirable. The psychoprophylactic and physical methods carry few risks, apart from the frequency with which a method fails to provide adequate analgesia. The use of drugs given systemically or by inhalation introduces potentially depressive drugs into the maternal and fetal circulations. The mother may experience clouding of consciousness, reduced co-operativeness and nausea and vomiting. She may find the intramuscular injections or the inhalation of a smelly vapour unpleasant. The infant may be severely depressed by these drugs, particularly the opiates.

Regional neural blockade involves considerable interference with the mother as intravenous and epidural cannulae are inserted, monitoring carried out and posture changed frequently. Potentially serious complications may follow incorrect application of these regional blocks and mother and infant may be placed in great peril.

These analgesic methods must be utilised with great care and skill to ensure that no harm is done.

## SYSTEMIC ANALGESICS

*Pethidine* alone or in combination with an inhalational agent has been the mainstay of obstetric analgesia for many years and this remains so in hospitals where full time obstetric anaesthetic services are unavailable.

The results of using pethidine in labour are often very disappointing. Intramuscular pethidine 100 mg or 150 mg was deemed satisfactory by only 22·4 per cent of women in the first stage of labour and in 47·7 per cent it gave no relief at all, meaning that 77·6 per cent had inadequate or no pain relief.[17] Other trials have demonstrated pethidine's serious shortcomings.[18]

Pethidine has a short duration of action and repeated doses will be necessary in a long labour although most recommendations hold that two doses only should be given. Maternal side-effects from pethidine are troublesome. Nausea and vomiting occur in 50 per cent of patients. Pethidine lacks the euphoric properties of morphine and patients complain of drowsiness and unpleasant dysphoric reactions.

Pethidine rapidly crosses the placenta and exerts both immediate and long-term effects on the fetus. There is immediate reduction in the extent of beat-to-beat variability in the fetal heart rate[19] and a fall in fetal pH and oxygenation. Administration of any of the opiate drugs during labour results in prolonging the time to spontaneous respiration of the neonate, lower Apgar scores, lower $Pa{O_2}$, increased $Pa{CO_2}$ (for up to 5 hours after birth), reduced respiratory minute volume and depressed neurobehavioural responses for up to 48 hours.[20] Maximum respiratory depression in the neonate occurs 2½ to 3½ hours after pethidine administration.

Intermittent intramuscular administration of an opiate takes no account of variations in the pharmacological behaviour of the drug in different patients, nor of the different plasma concentrations of the drug which each individual may require to produce analgesia. This concentration may vary considerably between individuals and has been defined as the minimum effective analgesic concentration.[21]

Patient-controlled analgesic systems have been developed in an attempt to balance some of these deficiencies. The Cardiff palliator responds to push button patient demands by delivering doses of 15–25 mg of pethidine at intervals of not less than 10 minutes, and this system can increase the proportion of patients achieving considerable relief to upwards of 43 per cent.[22,23]

*Morphine* is a powerful opiate with a longer duration of analgesic action compared to pethidine. It benefits from the ability to allay anxiety but frequently causes nausea and vomiting and is a potent depressor of neonatal respiration.

*Pentazocine* is a synthetic opiate with a partial agonist-antagonist profile. It is not a controlled drug in the UK and is approved for use by midwives. The incidence of nausea and vomiting is claimed to be less than with equianalgesic doses of pethidine and because it is only a partial agonist the respiratory depressant effect reaches a ceiling. In doses of 40–60 mg i.m. the analgesic effect is similar to pethidine and, after repeated doses of both drugs, the pentazocine produces less severe neonatal respiratory depression. This drug, however, may produce very unpleasant dysphoric reactions in the mother.

*Other opiates*.—Advances in the understanding of opiate receptor pharmacology may soon lead to the development of drugs with very specific analgesic activity without the attendant maternal and fetal side-effects.

*Ketamine* has been used to produce analgesia during labour. Doses in the region of 0·25 mg/kg reportedly produce effective analgesia without any adverse effect on uterine blood flow, uterine activity or neonatal status.[24, 25]

*Opiate antagonists*.—The opiate agonist-antagonist combinations such as Pethilorfan (pethidine and levallorphan) represent an illogical concept, were never effective and have no place in obstetrics.

When pure opiate antagonism is required, it is no longer necessary to use drugs such as nalorphine which possess partial agonist activity, as the pure opiate antagonist, naloxone, is now available. A dose of 200 μg i.m. is effective in reversing respiratory depression in the neonate and, in very urgent situations, 40 μg can be administered i.v. Infants given naloxone after suffering the effects of maternal opiate administration display a superior long-term neurobehavioural performance compared to infants who do not receive naloxone.[20] Despite this apparent long-term effect, naloxone produces only a very short-lived reversal of opiate-induced respiratory depression and signs of relapse must be watched for as the naloxone action abates.

## SYSTEMIC SEDATIVE AND ANXIOLYTIC DRUGS

Sedative, anxiolytic and hypnotic drugs are often advanced for use during labour but drugs of this class are very powerful, with a wide range of effects and a prolonged duration of action. Before administering one of these agents, medical staff should consider whether friendly reassurance and encouragement might be more effective, whether the presence of the husband would help, whether effective analgesia is what is required or whether there is some other simple way of avoiding the use of the drug. Adequate antenatal preparation will prevent the anxiety which is the result of fear and ignorance.[26]

Some suggested indications for the use of these drugs have included: to allay anxiety, to promote sleep in early labour, to aid in the treatment of hypertension (this indication is quite illogical), to prevent convulsions or to act as an anti-emetic. It is the last two indications which should provide for most use of these drugs.

Many of the drugs (e.g. promethazine) have an antanalgesic effect which, when combined with the sedative effect, may result in a mother who is actually less able to cope with her labour.

Drugs which might be considered are given below:

*Hypnotic* in early labour. Avoid the barbiturates. Chloral hydrate or perhaps nitrazepam may be suitable.

*Anxiolytic*.—Promazine (i.m. 50 mg) has enjoyed wide popularity in this role and has even been claimed to potentiate pethidine analgesia. Promazine, like most of the phenothiazines, is also an anti-emetic. Diazepam, in small doses of 5–10 mg, is often recommended to allay anxiety, but even small doses affect beat-to-beat variations in fetal heart rate and when more than 30 mg is given before delivery, the infant may exhibit the "floppy infant syndrome" which is characterised by hypotonia, hypothermia, lethargy, respiratory depression and poor feeding. The metabolites of diazepam persist in the infant's circulation for at least a week. Strong positive indications should exist before this drug is prescribed and it should not be given intramuscularly because absorption is very erratic and even slower than that following oral administration.

*Anticonvulsant*.—Diazepam and chlormethiazole are suitable drugs whilst in the USA magnesium sulphate is commonly used. Magnesium sulphate produces relaxation of skeletal muscles and does not alter the cerebral excitation, but care must be exercised if it is necessary to administer a muscle relaxant.

## INHALATIONAL ANALGESICS

Sub-anaesthetic concentrations of some of the inhalational anaesthetics produce marked analgesia and, provided that higher concentrations can be avoided, can be prescribed safely by midwives during labour. Nitrous oxide is almost always delivered premixed with oxygen from Entonox cylinders, while trichloroethylene and methoxyflurane require special draw-over vaporisers. These vaporisers should be robust and safe, capable of delivering the set concentration reliably and unaffected by changes in minute volume, peak flow or variations in room temperature.

The risk of overdose producing unconsciousness is a major drawback of the inhalational anaesthetic in labour. In analgesic concentrations, these drugs do not alter the progress of labour.

Many mothers object to the smell of the agent or to the use of a mask, and a mouthpiece has been used instead. Nausea and vomiting occur frequently and impaired consciousness may lead to confusion and lack of co-operation.

Success with this form of analgesia in labour depends on adequate instruction and supervision by the midwife, and on proper use by the mother, yet despite this, results are often poor. Comparisons between the different agents generally show little difference in analgesic efficiency.

**Entonox**

Nitrous oxide is almost always used as Entonox, premixed 50:50 with oxygen in a cylinder. The constituents normally remain mixed in the gaseous phase because of the Poynting effect, but after exposure to ambient temperatures below −6° C, the nitrous oxide may remain in the liquid phase allowing the oxygen to be exhausted first after which the cylinder will deliver only 100 per cent nitrous oxide. Certain guide-lines are laid down for the storage and handling of Entonox cylinders.[27]

Although a relatively lipid insoluble inhalational agent, nitrous oxide needs to be inhaled for 45 seconds before the maximum analgesic effect can be attained, so during the first stage, inhalation should be commenced at the first warning of a contraction and not delayed until pain appears. Once inhalation ceases, blood and alveolar concentrations decline rapidly and the analgesic effect is very short lived. Pain dominates the whole of a second stage contraction and no warning is perceived by the mother. Dependence should be placed on the regularity of second stage contractions, and inhalation commenced at least 30 seconds before the next expected contraction. When the mother is bearing down late in the second stage, she should quickly inhale 4 or 5 times from the machine, hold her breath and then push. The manoeuvre can be repeated if the analgesia wears off before the contraction is completed.

A continuous supply of nitrous oxide (e.g. 5 l/min) provided by nasal prongs or a catheter has been given between contractions and this will marginally increase the effectiveness of Entonox, although acceptance of the catheter by the mother is mixed.[28]

The analgesia provided by Entonox is inadequate for operative manoeuvres such as forceps delivery, episiotomy or manual removal of the placenta and will need to be supplemented by local or regional block. Up to 25 per cent of mothers find artificial rupture of the membranes an uncomfortable procedure and should at least be offered Entonox.

When used correctly, Entonox can be surprisingly effective, producing considerable relief in as many as 46–72 per cent of mothers.[17,23] Entonox is twice as effective as pethidine alone.

**Trichloroethylene**

Trichloroethylene is delivered in concentrations of 0·35 per cent or 0·5 per cent from either Tecota (Temperature Compensated Trilene Apparatus) or Emotril (Epstein, Macintosh, Oxford Trilene) inhalers. No cumbersome cylinders are required as with nitrous oxide. Trichloroethylene and methoxyflurane both have higher lipid solubilities than nitrous oxide and thus exhibit more prolonged uptake distribution and elimination phases. Trichloroethylene will not produce analgesia before 4 minutes after commencement of inhalation; however, the slow rate of elimination means that high blood and alveolar concentrations can be maintained and will thus provide a background level of analgesia which can be reinforced by further inhalation during each contraction. After two hours of intermittent use, considerable quantities of the drug may accumulate and the use of trichloroethylene should rarely be prolonged beyond this time if drowsiness, lack of co-operation and increased likelihood of fetal depression are to be avoided.

Trichloroethylene commonly causes nausea

and vomiting and its sweet smell may be unpleasant. Its use in labour is now uncommon.

**Methoxyflurane**

This potent anaesthetic is delivered in a concentration of 0·35 per cent from a Cardiff inhaler. These inhalers are painted bright green to distinguish them from Tecota inhalers which are grey. The analgesia produced by methoxyflurane persists into the period after inhalation ceases. Nausea and vomiting are uncommon and although inorganic fluoride concentrations are increased in both mother and infant, the risk of renal damage seems negligible as long as inhalation is restricted to low concentrations for limited periods.

**Other Inhalational Agents**

Enflurane 0·5 per cent has been claimed to produce satisfactory analgesia in 89 per cent of mothers during the second stage,[29] and isoflurane 0·2–0·7 per cent has also been used in labour.

## Psychoprophylaxis

Knowledge of what is going to happen during labour coupled with support and encouragement from the labour ward staff can greatly reduce maternal anxiety and reduce analgesic requirements. Methods which depend on very intensive antenatal preparation and the conduct of the labour in a defined manner are developed from time to time and often enjoy a period of great popularity.

The Lamaze method involves the use of breathing techniques, minimal analgesia, strictly limited operative intervention and the presence of the father. One trial suggested that it was beneficial to both mother and infant.[30]

The Leboyer method was regarded as having no advantage over a gentle conventional delivery in influencing infant and maternal outcome.[31]

It is virtually impossible to mount strictly controlled double blind trials to test such methods although it must never be forgotten that some women obviously benefit immensely from these psychoprophylactic techniques and many may feel much happier for having participated in such schemes, whatever the outcome. Only if harm is likely to come to the mother or child should discouragement be voiced.

The advocates of some of these methods occasionally believe in the efficacy of their techniques above all others and may, very unwisely, suggest to the mother that should the method fail in her own case it is a reflection of her own inadequacy and not due to any shortcomings in the procedure. This, of course, is most unfortunate. The anaesthetist should always be ready to provide support and effective analgesia if any particular mother is no longer able to cope with the pain. The main emphasis of these natural childbirth methods should be towards preparation and participation, and not towards withholding pain relief.[32]

## Other Methods of Analgesia

Many different methods and devices find brief favour as relievers of the pain of labour but most suffer from having a useful effect in only selected individuals and can never provide adequate analgesia for operative obstetrics. Sometimes complicated or cumbersome equipment is required and this may further reduce the attractiveness of a technique. Methods which have been recently used include white sound (audioanalgesia), abdominal decompression, acupuncture, hypnosis, transcutaneous nerve stimulation and electroanalgesia.

Reports of investigations testing such methods of analgesia must be examined very closely. Maternal expectations regarding pain relief in labour vary from country to country and trials must be stringently designed to take account of the many variables which may afflict pain relief investigations, particularly the placebo effect which can influence over 30 per cent of positive results when testing analgesic methods.

*Hypnosis* is very effective in a small proportion of patients but is not universally useful and is very time consuming both before and during labour.

*Acupuncture* does not seem to be of any use in labour.[33]

*Transcutaneous nerve stimulation (TNS)* has been shown to be a safe and useful addition to methods of pain relief available in the first stage, and is especially helpful for backache. Various investigations have reported up to 54 per cent of patients helped by TNS and that analgesic requirements are reduced in these patients.[34–36]

*Electroanalgesia* is an intriguing treatment

which requires the application of low intensity currents to frontal and mastoid regions. Electroanalgesia has been reported as being helpful to Russian women in labour.[37]

## REGIONAL ANALGESIA

Before employing any local or regional anaesthetic technique, the anaesthetist should satisfy himself that adequate equipment and drugs for resuscitation are immediately available and that the mother has an intravenous cannula in place. As a routine, a syringe of thiopentone and a syringe of suxamethonium should be drawn up daily and stored in a refrigerator so that the drugs are instantly available to treat untoward local anaesthetic reactions or to induce general anaesthesia. Figure 6 illustrates possible sites for regional nerve block in labour.

### Local Anaesthetics used in Obstetrics

**Ester-linked agents**

*2-Chloroprocaine* has been recommended for use in labour because the very short plasma half-life the drug possesses suggests that neonatal depression and cumulative toxicity are unlikely to be problems. The short duration of action may be considered a disadvantage if 2-chloroprocaine is used for continuous epidural analgesia. Doubts about potential neurological damage caused by the drug have rather restricted the adoption of 2-chloroprocaine outside the USA.

*Tetracaine* is the most commonly used agent for subarachnoid blocks in North America but is little used elsewhere.

*Cinchocaine* (Dibucaine) is popular in the UK for producing subarachnoid block.

**Amide-linked Agents**

The implications of maternal and fetal plasma concentrations and effects of these drugs are discussed elsewhere.

*Lignocaine* is used for many procedures although the frequent requirement to add adrenaline is regarded as a major disadvantage by some (see below). Lignocaine is less suitable for continuous epidural analgesia than bupivacaine because tachyphylaxis develops, but stronger concentrations (e.g. 1·5–2 per cent with adrenaline) are very useful for epidural anaesthesia for caesarean section.

*Prilocaine* has a very high fetal maternal ratio and fetal methaemoglobinaemia has been reported.

*Bupivacaine* is the agent of choice for epidural analgesia during labour and the 0·5–0·75 per cent solutions provide excellent anaesthesia for major obstetric operations.

*Etidocaine* possesses a rapid onset of action, produces excellent muscle relaxation and is a suitable agent for caesarean section anaesthesia, but quite unattractive for continuous epidural analgesia.

### Lumbar Epidural Analgesia

**Epidural Space in Pregnancy**

Alterations in the anatomy of the epidural

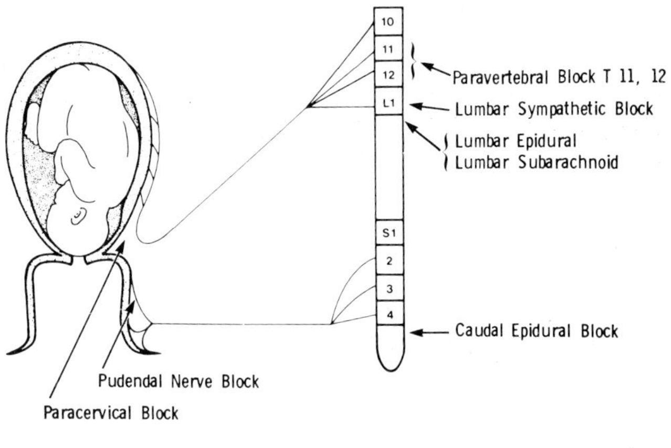


39/Fig. 6.—Regional analgesia: sites for suitable nerve blocks in labour.

and subarachnoid spaces are induced by pregnancy and labour and are commonly held to be responsible for the reduced local anaesthetic dose requirements of pregnant women, although it has been suggested that this decreased dose requirement is not apparent if caval occlusion is avoided.[38]

**Volume.**—Intermittent obstruction of the inferior vena cava by the enlarging uterus encourages venous drainage through alternative pathways and so the vertebral and azygous venous systems dilate. The epidural veins are part of the internal vertebral venous plexus and these veins become particularly engorged when the mother is supine or during uterine contractions. The enlarged veins act to reduce the internal volume of the epidural space into which local anaesthetic solutions are introduced. Thus the same volume will spread further than in the epidural space of a non-pregnant woman.

*Clinical significance:* Segmental dose requirements are generally reduced in pregnancy and labour.

**Pressures.**—In the non-pregnant subject, the pressure in the lumbar epidural space is normally −1 cm $H_2O$ whereas in early labour, between contractions, pressures in the lateral position average 1·63 cm $H_2O$ and rise to between 4–10 cm $H_2O$ by the end of the first stage. Assuming the supine position will increase epidural space pressure by up to 50 per cent, and this increase is proportional to the degree of inferior vena caval obstruction, uterine displacement will moderate the rise produced in this position.[39]

*Clinical significance:* the pressure in the epidural space is positive during labour so methods for identifying the space which depend on negative pressure should not be used.

During contractions, the reflex increase in abdominal muscle tone and the sudden efflux of blood from the contracting myometrium into the venous system contributes to a further rise in epidural space pressure of from 2–8 cm $H_2O$, even in the lateral position. Adequate epidural pain relief minimises the pressure rise produced during contractions.

The spread of local anaesthetic solution in the epidural space will be exaggerated during a contraction so injections should not be made at this time. Also the epidural veins will be greatly engorged and the risk of puncture by needle or catheter will be increased if either is inserted into the epidural space during a contraction.

## Some Technical Considerations During Labour

### Preliminaries

Antenatal classes should usually familiarise the mother with the concept of epidural analgesia but further explanation should always be offered before consent (at least verbal in the UK) is obtained. A brief history should search for any major contra-indications. Always remember that some time will elapse before the catheter is inserted and the local anaesthetic has taken effect, so if the mother is in pain, provide Entonox and stop the Syntocinon infusion to reduce the severity of the contractions and create a much more co-operative patient. Check fetal heart rate and maternal blood pressure and commence the intravenous fluid loading before positioning the patient for the epidural injection.

### Prehydration

An intravenous fluid load of 500–1000 ml of Hartmann's solution should be given to every mother and will reduce the incidence of fetal heart rate disturbance and maternal hypotension following the epidural.[40] Beware of giving too much fluid during labour, for impaired water excretion may eventually lead to maternal or fetal hyponatraemia. Albumin and various synthetic plasma volume expanders have been recommended, but expense and the risk of adverse reactions should preclude their general use. Specific indications may exist when hypotension must be avoided at all costs.

### Position of Patient

Adequate spinal flexion may be more difficult to achieve in the pregnant patient and opinions differ as to whether sitting or using the left lateral position is best. Moir[41] advocates the sitting position and this position is certainly very useful in the obese or in the patient with a difficult back, but most other authors recommend the left lateral position. Sitting may be quite uncomfortable when the patient is in strong labour.

### Approach to the Epidural Space

The midline approach between the lumbar spines is most commonly used but the paramedian approach is an alternative method enthusiastically recommended by some centres.[42,43] This approach is often very useful in the difficult back when the interspinous ligaments feel impenetrable.

### Identification of the Epidural Space

Methods which depend on a negative pressure in the epidural space must never be used (see above) and loss of resistance should be sought using a freely sliding syringe filled with air, or preferably saline. Some use a local anaesthetic solution. Should inadvertent dural puncture by the Tuohy needle occur, there will rarely be any doubt about whether the fluid gushing out is cerebrospinal fluid or injected saline.

### Insertion of Epidural Catheter

If labour is progressing rapidly or the pain is severe, then to save time, the first dose should be injected through the Tuohy needle before the catheter is inserted. A catheter should always be inserted once the anaesthetist has gone to the trouble of identifying the epidural space, even if delivery seems imminent because further analgesia may be required postpartum for a retained placenta or episiotomy repair.

The catheter should not be inserted during a contraction when the epidural veins are maximally engorged and care should be taken to ensure the catheter has not penetrated the dura. Continuous back flow down the catheter or a positive aspiration test may suggest this.

### Timing of Injections

Injections into the epidural space during labour should be made between contractions so as to avoid the risk of increased spread. That this risk exists at all is disputed.[44]

### Injections in the Lateral Position

Strict avoidance of the supine position, vital throughout labour, is imperative once an epidural block is established. Use of the complete lateral position and not just a lateral uterine tilt is still compatible with satisfactory epidural analgesia in labour. The dependent side will show earlier onset, increased spread and increased duration of sensory block, but this is of only minor clinical significance and can be simply overcome by regular turning from side to side within the first 10–15 minutes.[45–48]

### Segmental Block

The successful use of epidural blocks in labour depends greatly on restriction of the block to selected nerve roots, thus minimising the problems of hypotension, bladder impairment and motor weakness which result from indiscriminate blocks. The substantially reduced doses of local anaesthetic required also benefit mother and fetus.

In the early first stage of labour, T11, T12 segments need to be blocked and this is later extended to T10 and L1. Blockage of the sacral roots is required before delivery proceeds during the second stage. The reality is not always as simple as this but Fig. 7 illustrates those approaches to the provision of segmental blockade in labour and demonstrates why a third approach, the caudal, is unsatisfactory.

### Local Anaesthetic: Concentration and Dose

**Dose.**—It is widely accepted that epidural dose requirements are reduced by about one-third in pregnancy and that this reduction is a result of the distension of the internal vertebral venous plexus. The pump-like action of these swollen epidural veins which pulse and swell during uterine contractions may further enhance spread, though the reduced segmental dose requirement has been demonstrated to be already present by the first trimester.[49]

Recent work suggests that the uterine contractions may not affect spread[44] and others claim that the increased dose requirement is not present if aortocaval compression is avoided.[45] Obesity will further reduce epidural dose requirements and the anaesthetist must exercise caution with the obese pregnant patient.[50]

Whatever dose is chosen, or whenever doubt exists about a suitable dose, it is always wise to err on the side of caution. Adjustment of the block can be made with further doses if the mother complains of residual pain, or testing of sensory levels reveals an inadequate block.

The duration of action of all local anaesthetics is shorter in labour, perhaps because of the accelerating nature of the pain and the increased vascularity of the epidural space.[51]

**Concentration.**—The concentration of local anaesthetic should be chosen after consider-

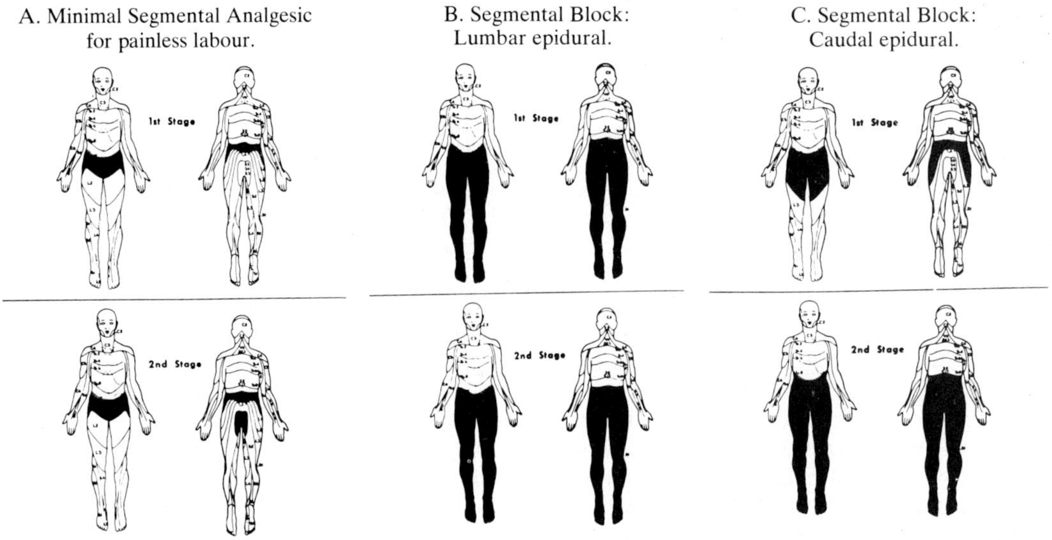


39/FIG. 7.—Segmental blockade produced by different regional techniques in labour. A. First stage: block $T_{11}$–$T_{12}$ (extended to $T_{10}$–$L_1$). Second stage: add $S_2$ (not illustrated here), $S_3$, $S_4$, $S_5$. This technique requires the least quantity of local anaesthetic and can be achieved with Cleland's double catheter technique (see p. 1041). B. Single lumbar catheter is a satisfactory compromise. C. Continuous caudal block is totally inappropriate for first stage pain relief. (Courtesy of Professor P. R. Bromage and the publishers, W. B. Saunders.[16])

ation of the present stage and likely duration and outcome of the labour, the need for muscular relaxation and the nature and severity of the pain. The desired effect should be secured with the lowest dose possible and standard regimes should be used to ensure staff familiarity with the technique. Results of research indicate that drug dosages and concentrations used successfully in one centre may fail when used elsewhere.

Bupivacaine is the agent of choice for continuous lumbar epidural analgesia because it is relatively safe and long-acting, produces acceptable motor block, has a low feto-maternal ratio and has minimal effects on neonatal neurobehavioural tests.

Concentrations of bupivacaine are available from 0·125 per cent to 0·75 per cent and increasing concentration produces increased frequency and duration of adequate analgesia, greater motor block, faster onset and wider segmental spread.[52] Reduction in the degree of motor block may result in an increased incidence of spontaneous delivery as abdominal and pelvic muscle tone is maintained, although the incidence of rotational forceps is the same whether 0·25 per cent or 0·5 per cent solution is used. After 5 top-ups of either solution, the degrees of motor block are indistinguishable.[53]

The use of the 0·125 per cent solution is strongly advocated by some who claim very high success rates with minimal or no motor block, using an initial mean dose of 13±2 mg and a mean total dose of 55±20 mg.[54] However, other groups have reported significantly higher failure rates using the 0·125 per cent solution when compared with the 0·25 per cent or 0·5 per cent, but they have also noted that when the 0·125 per cent is effective, then these patients also require a significantly smaller total amount of drug during the labour.[55] Failure of epidural analgesia must be very carefully defined, for many women who remain aware of their contractions are actually pleased to have some sense of "being in labour" and, despite often minor discomfort, are in no way failures. Bromage[16] states that high volumes of low concentration local anaesthetic will not produce excessive spread because spread is determined by the mass of local anaesthetic injected, not the volume. This may not always be apparent in practice.

Other authors prefer to opt for a middle course and recommend 0·25–0·375 per cent solutions for use in normal labour.[41] The potent 0·75 per cent solution should be reserved to produce analgesia for operative obstetrics.

Recommended volumes for a first dose might range from 15–20 ml of 0·125 per cent to 5–10 ml of 0·5 per cent. Table 2 details a scheme which is used with great success at St. Thomas' Hospital, although it would be quite reasonable to substitute 0·25 per cent solution for all the top-ups.[5,56]

*Other local anaesthetics* should rarely be required if bupivacaine is available. Lignocaine is used as a test dose by some because the more rapid onset might aid in identification of an intrathecal block; carbonated lignocaine has been claimed to be more effective with troublesome blocks, and 2-chloroprocaine enjoys some popularity because of the rapid onset of action.

**Adrenaline.**—The addition of adrenaline to local anaesthetic solutions is recommended to reduce systemic absorption, to prolong the action and intensify sensory and motor block. Trials have shown this to be true with lignocaine 2 per cent, bupivacaine 0·25 per cent and 0·5 per cent.[52] However, the effect on small repeated doses of bupivacaine is negligible and bupivacaine also has low toxicity and an adequate duration for obstetrics without the need for adrenaline.[57] Enhanced motor block is rarely desirable in obstetrics.

Doses of adrenaline less than 50 μg do not affect intervillous blood flow[58] but may diminish uterine contractility for up to 60 minutes.[59] No advantage exists to justify the use of adrenaline in obstetric epidural injections.

39/Table 2

Lumbar Epidural Analgesia in Labour: A Suggested Scheme

1. Explanation, history, consent.
2. Maternal BP, cervical dilatation and state of labour, fetal heart rate and condition.
3. Position: left lateral, comfortable. Turn off Syntocinon: Entonox as necessary.
4. Intravenous Hartmann's solution 500–1000 ml.
5. Prepare equipment: strict sterility; check patency of catheter, and passage through Tuohy needle.
6. Insert catheter 2–3 cm, L2–L3 interspace. (Loss of resistance technique to locate space).
7. Test dose: Bupivacaine 0·5 per cent 3 ml; wait 5 minutes.
8. Full dose: Bupivacaine 0·5 per cent; to give total 5–8 ml.
9. Maintain lateral position; turn from side to side every 4–5 min; NEVER SUPINE.
10. Monitor: BP at 5-min intervals for 20–30 minutes
    Fetal heart rate
    Uterine contraction.
11. Assess segmental block after 30 minutes.
12. Top-up doses. According to height of original block.

| | |
|---|---|
| Abdominal pain: | Bupivacaine 0·5 per cent 3–6 ml recumbent; |
| Perineal pain, Sacral pain | Bupivacaine 0·25% 8–10 ml sitting. |

### Test Dose

Opinions differ as to whether a test dose should be given for an obstetric epidural block, not because of any wanton disregard for the patient's safety but because a test dose can so often produce unreliable results. Moore[60] has defined the components of an effective epidural test dose:

(i) dose of the local anaesthetic in 3 ml sufficient to produce rapid spinal block
(ii) 0·015 mg adrenaline to indicate intravascular injection
(iii) ECG and pulse rate monitor to indicate any changes.

An inadvertent intravascular injection of local anaesthetic without adrenaline may produce tingling of the tongue and a light-headed feeling. However, signs of inadvertent subarachnoid injection are less definite and less reliable, and a genuine positive result is infrequent. Reports of false negative results are common.[61] A compromise may be arrived at by using a test dose of a short-acting drug such as lignocaine 2 per cent before giving the therapeutic dose of bupivacaine.[51]

The incidence of vessel puncture by the epidural catheter has been stated to be as high as 9 per cent,[62] and the dangers of the catheter penetrating the dura after one or more successful epidural injections is well known. The problem of detecting delayed dural puncture by the catheter is difficult to overcome, especially when midwives administer top-up injections. A test dose could be given before every top-up, but the fallibility of a test dose has already been examined and also the signs of an intrathecal injection may be less apparent against the background of an already established block.

### Epidural Infusions

Continuous infusion techniques have been devised in an attempt to even out the fluctuations in pain relief which sometimes result from intermittent techniques. Short-acting drugs, such as 2-chloroprocaine and procaine would seem ideal for this style of administration, but bupivacaine has been successfully used in concentrations of 0·125 per cent—0·25 per cent. After an initial loading dose of up to 10 ml, an infusion of 6–10 ml per hour is administered using a paediatric drip set, an Intraflo device or an infusion pump. The patient should turn from one side to the other at least every 30 minutes and the head of the bed may be elevated to achieve sacral block in the second stage.

The technique is claimed to preserve maximum motor function with minimal sympathetic block although blood pressure must be continuously monitored. Bladder problems seem to occur frequently and there is a tendency for a larger dose of local anaesthetic to be given. The technique requires very careful supervision and may actually create more work for nursing and anaesthetic staff.[63–65]

### The Difficult Back

Anatomical abnormalities or disruption created by surgery on the lumbar spine may cause problems for the epidural anaesthetist. If the lumbar approach is too difficult or seems too hazardous, then a continuous caudal block may be indicated. A subarachnoid block may be simpler to perform, is less traumatic and will provide analgesia for the end of stage one and delivery.

### Care of the Patient

The anaesthetist should remain with the patient throughout the epidural induction period and thereafter should regularly ensure that adequate segmental blockade is being maintained with the top-up doses he or she has ordered.

The patient must never be allowed to lie supine without uterine displacement or lateral tilt. A full lateral position is preferred.

Monitoring should involve regular checks on the maternal blood pressure as well as continuous display of fetal heart rate and uterine contractions.

All women in labour should receive nothing to eat or drink and an antacid (mist magnesium trisilicate or 0·3 m sodium citrate, 15 ml) should be given every two hours. The likelihood of urinary retention occurring should be borne in mind.

#### Top-up doses

Delay in providing top-up injections is a potential cause of failure of epidural analgesia in labour. In most centres midwives, who are on the spot, administer top-ups but other units insist on the anaesthetist administering every top-up dose because of the risk of delayed intravascular or subarachnoid injection. If the midwife administers the top-up dose then a doctor, skilled in resuscitation, must be instantly available on the labour ward.

The Central Midwives Board for England and Wales has recommended the following safeguards for midwives who give top-up injections:

1. That the ultimate responsibility for such a technique should be clearly stated to rest with the doctor.
2. That written instructions as to the dose should be given by the doctor concerned.
3. That in all cases the dose given by the midwife should be checked by one other person.
4. That instruction should be given by the doctor as to the posture of the patient at the time of injection, observation of blood pressure etc., and measures to be taken in the event of any side-effect.
5. That the midwife should have been thoroughly instructed in the technique so that the doctor concerned is satisfied as to her ability.

Failure strictly to observe these criteria has resulted in tragedy.

**Delivery.**—Some obstetric units allow the epidural to wear off gradually during the late first, and early second stage so that full voluntary muscle power is available for maternal bearing down. If sensory loss persists, the second stage contractions may not be perceived by the mother and reflex bearing down will not result. However, the mother may compensate by making voluntary efforts when palpation of the abdomen reveals a contraction is occurring, so that it seems unnecessary to allow the analgesia to wane during the second stage. If maternal expulsive efforts are inadequate, then a lift out forceps may be indicated and, unlike mid-cavity forceps, this manoeuvre is said to be relatively innocuous for the infant.[66]

All mothers should be given high concentrations of oxygen for 5–20 minutes prior to delivery. An increase in maternal inspired oxygen concentration is reflected by an increase in fetal arterial oxygen tension within 50 seconds.[67] The administration of oxygen for short periods does not reduce uteroplacental blood flow and may be very beneficial to the neonate.[68]

Studious avoidance of the supine position and aortocaval compression should be carried right through until delivery. A wedge must be used even in the lithotomy position. The unmodified supine position in the second stage causes a progressive fall in fetal pH.[69]

**Contra-indications to Lumbar Epidural Analgesia**

*Absolute:* Patient refusal
Local infection
Coagulopathy or anticoagulant therapy
Hypovolaemia—haemorrhage or shock
Previous Caesarean section for contracted pelvis
Inadequate facilities or supervision.

*Relative:* Pre-existing neurological disease
Severe deformity of the spine.

**Indications: Lumbar Epidural Analgesia**

If adequate facilities and experienced staff are available, epidural analgesia should be available to any woman who requests pain relief and does not exhibit a specific contra-indication. The relief of pain in labour can be shown to be of physiological and psychological benefit to both mother and child. There are certain conditions in which the benefits of an epidural block are particularly marked. These include: pre-eclampsia, inco-ordinate uterine action, premature labour, maternal cardiovascular or respiratory disease and diabetes mellitus. Breech presentation and multiple pregnancy, once listed as contra-indications, are now regarded as positive indications for epidural analgesia.

**Maternal and Fetal Effects of Epidural Analgesia**

Many of the conclusions drawn from early research into the effects of epidural analgesia in obstetrics have been invalidated because no account was taken of aortocaval compression, which has subsequently been shown to exert a powerful influence on uterine performance, utero-placental blood flow, and fetal and infant well being. Serious hazards are still associated with the use of epidural blocks in labour and the technique demands faultless performance by skilled practitioners. Many of the alternative methods of obstetric analgesia may not be as efficient as epidural blockade but the risks are often considerably less in inexperienced hands. Bromage[16] says that perfection is the only practical and acceptable goal for the practice of epidural analgesia in obstetrics.

A summary of potential maternal and fetal problems is given in Table 3.

**Inadvertent Dural Puncture**

The incidence of dural puncture varies widely from centre to centre and decreases sharply as individual experience increases. An overall rate of 2–3 per cent could be expected in a training hospital, although much higher rates have been cited.[41]

Dural puncture with a 16–18G Tuohy needle will be immediately apparent even if a fluid-filled syringe has been used to locate the epidural space. Puncture by the much thinner catheter will be less apparent and Dextrostix or litmus paper may be necessary to differentiate CSF from the injected saline. Catheter puncture of the dura may occur after previously successful epidural injections have been given.[70]

If dural puncture by needle or catheter is not recognised and a dose of local anaesthetic is injected, a total spinal block is likely and will be characterised by a rapid loss of sensation and motor power, hypotension and eventually respiratory failure due to medullary depression. This is a very rare occurrence but the possibility of a total spinal block demands that expert personnel are immediately available. Maternal deaths have occurred as a result of inadvertent subarachnoid injection producing total spinal block.

Management of an inadvertent subarachnoid injection may require full respiratory and cardiovascular support for the duration of the local anaesthetic block. The threats of aortocaval compression and regurgitation of stomach contents complicates the management of these patients.

39/Table 3
Adverse Maternal and Fetal Effects of Epidural Analgesia

| | |
|---|---|
| **Maternal** | |
| Immediate | |
| (a) *Insertion*—needle or catheter | wrong place<br>penetrates blood vessel, dura, neural tissue<br>broken catheter |
| (b) *Injection* | subarachnoid<br>intravascular<br>adverse reaction to local anaesthetic |
| (c) *Neural blockade* | hypotension<br>motor block<br>bladder dysfunction<br>Horner's syndrome<br>? shivering |
| (d) *Inadequate analgesia* | total failure<br>partial failure |
| (e) *Progress of labour* | prolong labour<br>increase instrumental deliveries |
| Delayed | |
| (a) *Neurological* | |
| (b) *Headache* | Post-dural puncture |
| **Fetal** | |
| Immediate | |
| (a) *Direct effect of local anaesthetic* | |
| (b) *Indirect effects* | changes in uterine blood flow<br>maternal hypoxia<br>change in progress and outcome of labour |
| Delayed | |
| (a) *Condition at birth* | |
| (b) *Subsequent neurobehavioural testing* | |

## Management of Inadvertent Dural Puncture

1. **Immediate.**—Conversion may be made immediately to a subarachnoid block by injection down the Tuohy needle. Otherwise the needle should be removed and a catheter inserted in an adjacent space. The risks of large amounts of local anaesthetic penetrating the dural puncture hole are negligible. Alternatively, the whole procedure may be abandoned and resort made to alternative methods of analgesia.

An elective forceps delivery is recommended to avoid maternal pushing.

2. **Headache prophylaxis.**—The hole in the dura produced by a Tuohy needle allows a considerable leak of cerebrospinal fluid and this is thought to be responsible for the high incidence of headache following inadvertent dural puncture. The parturient may be even more susceptible to headache than the non-pregnant and 70–80 per cent will experience headache, 20 per cent being severe in nature.[71]

The headache may commence immediately but is more commonly delayed for up to 24 hours. The pain is usually occipital and is always postural, being relieved when the sufferer is recumbent.

### Suggested Prophylactic Measures

(a) Bed rest: prone, supine and lateral positions have been recommended.
(b) Hydration, intravenous or oral.
(c) Abdominal binder to raise epidural space pressure.
(d) Epidural injections. The injection of 40–60 ml of Hartmann's solution immediately after delivery may be given as a single treatment or followed with a gravity drip of 1–1·5 litres of Hartmann's solution into the epidural space over the next 24 hours. It has been suggested that this technique raises the pressure in the epidural space and prevents CSF leakage, but evidence to support this argument is slight and the advantages of these epidural injections unconvincing.
(e) If headache occurs and is not controlled by analgesics, proceed immediately to a blood patch injecting up to 20 ml of autologous blood. Results from this treatment are often dramatic and problems are very unusual.[72,73]

### Inadvertent Intravascular Injection

Intravascular injection of a full dose of bupivacaine may produce toxic concentrations in the blood sufficient to precipitate an adverse reaction, although it appears that bupivacaine has a wide safety margin and slow intravascular injection of epidural type doses may not precipitate convulsions.[51,74] Early signs of intravascular injection include numbness of the tongue and lips and euphoria and if these signs appear, local anaesthetic injection must be halted immediately.

The elimination half-life of the amide local anaesthetics is long enough for systemic accumulation to occur following frequent top-up, although this is unlikely to produce toxic levels.

The risks of inadvertent intravascular injection are minimal with careful aspiration prior to injection, use of a test dose containing adrenaline, and use of small doses of highly protein-bound, rapidly metabolised, agents.

### Cardiovascular Effects

The hypotension which follows an epidural block is a consequence of the loss of sympathetic vasomotor tone which reduces venous return. Caval occlusion in these circumstances may produce drastic reductions in cardiac output because the normal compensatory mechanisms are paralysed. The reduced cardiac output during epidural induced hypotension results in reductions in uteroplacental blood flow, uterine action and fetal oxygenation. An epidural block will not reduce uteroplacental blood flow if hypotension is avoided. Short periods of hypotension (less than 2 minutes) may result in increased fetal acidosis, but may be otherwise harmless.[75]

Hypotension is usually said to occur if blood pressure falls 20–30 mm Hg (2·7–4·0 kPa) below the pre-epidural level or systolic pressure drops below 100 mm Hg (13·3 kPa).

Hypotension can be prevented by giving an intravenous fluid preload and by avoiding caval compression. Should hypotension occur following an epidural further left uterine displacement should be performed or the full lateral position adopted. The left side is usually best for both displacement and turning, but occasionally the right side is preferred. Further crystalloid and, if indicated, colloid solution should be infused and if after 2 minutes no response has occurred, ephedrine should be given intravenously in 5 mg increments. Rarely will more than 30 mg be necessary. Crawford has had to resort to vasopressors in only 8 out of 17,000 epidurals administered during labour.[5] Oxygen should always be administered to the hypotensive mother and atropine given if bradycardia is present.

### Vasopressors

Vasopressors which depend on peripheral vasoconstriction to produce their effect will reduce uterine artery blood flow and an agent such as ephedrine, which has a positive inotropic effect on the heart, and does not greatly alter uterine blood flow, is to be preferred (see Fig. 8).

Ephedrine can be administered intramuscularly and intravenously or as an infusion (e.g. 50 mg ephedrine in 500 ml balanced salt solution) to be titrated against the blood pressure. Overdose can produce hypertension, and drug interaction with ergometrine may be dangerous.

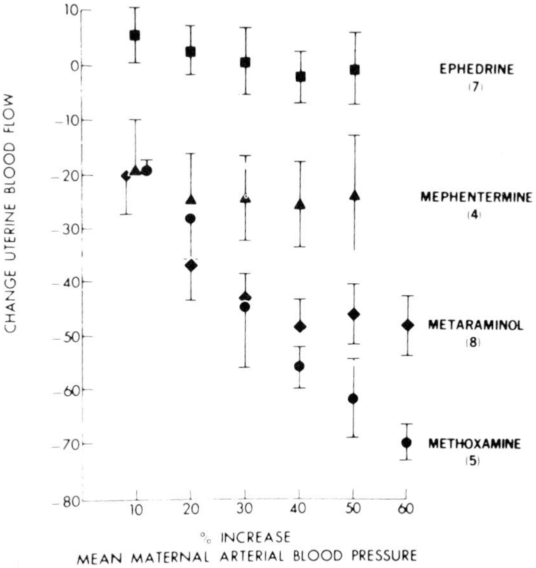


39/Fig. 8.—Influence of different vasopressors on uterine blood flow and mean maternal arterial blood pressure in the pregnant ewe. (Courtesy of D. H. Ralston, S. M. Shnider and A. A. deLorimer and the publishers, J. B. Lippincott Co.[76])

Prophylactic intramuscular ephedrine is not recommended before caesarean section under regional block,[77] but prompt administration of 10–30 mg i.v. at the first sign of falling blood pressure will help to prevent further falls and reduce the incidence of nausea and vomiting during these procedures.[78]

Dopamine has been used to control hypotension in labour and when given as an infusion of 2 $\mu$g/kg/min, blood pressure was easily controlled and neonatal status was no different from that following ephedrine administration.[79] However, dopamine probably reduces uterine placental blood flow so ephedrine should remain the vasopressor of choice.

**Effects on Labour and Delivery**

**First stage.**—The myometrium is not heavily dependent on motor innervation and is driven mainly by humoral stimulation so that even a high segmental block cannot influence this aspect of uterine control. Earlier studies which suggested that epidural blockade retarded labour took no account of the influence of aortocaval compression since normal uterine activity is very dependent on adequate myometrial perfusion and any decrease in flow quickly reduces uterine contractility.[80]

In the absence of hypotension or aortocaval compression, epidural analgesia may actually produce a slight but insignificant increase in uteroplacental blood flow and this increase is particularly marked in the presence of pre-eclamptic toxaemia (PET).[81]

Systemic absorption of epidurally administered drugs may result in direct drug effects on the myometrium. At low concentrations, most local anaesthetics have a net stimulating effect and act to increase contractility. High drug concentrations are necessary to depress myometrial activity and such high concentrations are unlikely in normal obstetric epidural practice.[82] No correlation can be demonstrated between uterine activity and plasma bupivacaine.[83]

Adrenaline added to local anaesthetic solutions seems not to affect uterine blood flow if the dose is less than 50 $\mu$g but can reduce uterine activity for up to 60 minutes after administration.[84, 85]

Painful inco-ordinate uterine contractions in the first stage of labour will revert to a more normal painfree pattern after an epidural block is established, perhaps as a result of suppressed catecholamine secretion.

If the perineum is anaesthetised in very early labour, contractions may cease. This is said to be due to the abolition of Ferguson's reflex. Carefully administered segmental block should avoid this problem and an oxytocin infusion will re-establish contractions if necessary.

So in the absence of hypotension or aortocaval compression, an epidural block will not alter the overall rate of progress of the first stage.[85, 86] The other point that needs to be made here is that epidural analgesia should be given when the pain demands it, and not delayed until some pre-determined degree of cervical dilatation is attained.

**Second stage.**—Epidural blockade can influence the progress of the second stage in several ways. Diagnosis of the commencement of the second stage is often delayed because the sensory blockade obtunds the desire to bear down. Relaxation of the pelvic floor muscles may delay rotation of the descending presenting part and weakness of abdominal muscles may impede the mother's expulsive efforts. Finally, the abolition of the reflex desire to bear down may further complicate matters, especially for the primigravida who may find difficulty in co-ordinating the forces necessary to expel the fetus by her own efforts.

The second stage of labour is almost certainly prolonged by epidural blockade but what is unclear is whether it follows that the proportion of assisted deliveries, particularly rotational forceps, should increase accordingly. A twenty-fold increase in rotational forceps has been reported when an epidural group is compared to a control group.[86]

A number of factors need to be examined. Firstly there is far from universal agreement as to the indications for forceps delivery and the wide variation between different obstetricians in the same hospital has been highlighted.[87]

Secondly, the use of segmental analgesia limited to T10–T12 during the first stage of labour should not be associated with an increase in malposition or instrumental delivery.[85]

Thirdly, the use of weaker concentrations of bupivacaine (0·125–0·25 per cent) will increase the proportion of spontaneous deliveries.[53, 88]

And finally, prolongation of the second stage beyond previously accepted limits has not been shown to be harmful to the infant so long as close fetal monitoring continues and aortocaval compression is avoided. Opinion is now strongly in favour of allowing the second stage to evolve slowly[5, 89] towards spontaneous delivery, thereby reducing the need for instrumental delivery which has been shown to be associated with significant immediate and long-term morbidity and mortality,[90, 91] Unnecessary bearing down should also be discouraged, for bearing down will reduce placental blood flow and fetal oxygenation[92] and is traumatic for the fetus.[93]

### Inadequate Analgesia

Epidural analgesia is satisfactory in over 80 per cent of mothers immediately, useful but incomplete in 15 per cent and unsatisfactory in 2–3 per cent. When compared to other methods of pain relief in labour, epidural blockade produces superior analgesia and comfort. There are, however, dissatisfied mothers and some of the possible causes of an inadequate block are listed below:

| | |
|---|---|
| A. Total failure | Catheter in wrong place<br>Given too late in labour. |
| B. Partial failure | Unilateral block<br>Missed segment<br>Inadequate dose or concentration<br>Low backache<br>Full bladder<br>Rectal pain<br>Pathological pain, e.g. uterine rupture<br>Failure to give top-ups. |

### Total Failure

If the labour is progressing rapidly, the block may never control the pain and a subarachnoid block may have been a more appropriate choice. If the epidural injection has absolutely no effect, the catheter is in the wrong place and should be re-inserted.

### Partial Failure

Many women wish to remain aware of their contractions whilst others will regard any sensory input as indicating failure.

*Unilateral block* may occur in up to 12 per cent of cases and follows the insertion of too much catheter or is a result of the mother being left lying on just one side. Very circumscribed unilateral analgesia may follow the paravertebral passage of a catheter. In any of these cases, the patient should be turned onto the painful side, the catheter slightly withdrawn and a further dose of local anaesthetic injected.

*Missed segments*.—Sometimes pain is felt during contractions in just one or two spinal segments, often confined to the groin. The explanation behind this phenomenon is uncertain but missed segments may occur in 6–14 per cent of cases and the pain is often quite severe. The L1 nerve root,[94] the S1 nerve root,[95] anterior placement of the catheter in the epidural space, or epidural space adhesions have all been invoked as possible sites or causes of the missed segment. Previous epidurals or spinal injections do not increase the likelihood of missed segments occurring.[96]

The incidence is much less if stronger concentrations of local anaesthetic are used initially and treatment should consist of catheter withdrawal if necessary, followed by a top-up of a stronger concentration solution given with the painful side down. The use of carbonated lignocaine has been claimed to reduce the incidence of missed segments although the evidence is contradictory.[97,98] Epidural injection of an opiate such as fentanyl 100 μg may sometimes solve the problem but a very low tolerance to re-inserting the catheter should prevail.

*Low backache*.—Backache may be referred via the posterior cutaneous branches of T10–L1 and originate in the uterus and peri-uterine tissues or may be related to pressure on the vertebral bodies and intra-pelvic structures. Backache is frequently associated with malpresentation or platypelloid pelvis and is sometimes very resistant to treatment. A top-up dose given with the patient sitting should be tried first. If pain persists, epidural fentanyl, a subcutaneous injection of local anaesthetic in the painful area or transcutaneous nerve stimulation could be used.

*Failure of top-up procedures*.—Even though 80–90 per cent of mothers are completely satisfied with the epidural, when interviewed after delivery only 46 per cent report a completely pain-free labour and list delay by the midwife in topping-up as the most common cause of failure.[99] The questions of appropriate dose, volume and concentration have been considered already as has the problem of pathological pain.

### Postpartum Problems

Women who have epidural or spinal blockade in labour sometimes experience an increased incidence of problems such as shivering, headache, nausea and vomiting, hypotension, backache and difficulties with micturition in the postpartum period.[100]

Uneventful labours conducted without any

form of regional analgesia may still result in postpartum headache, backache and disturbances of micturition, so the epidural should not attract the blame as a routine (see Table 4). From 14–23 per cent of women without an epidural will experience postpartum headache and the incidence of bladder disturbance is high following a forceps delivery irrespective of the method of anaesthesia.

The cause of the shivering which occurs before or after delivery is not known but 22 per cent of women without an epidural will shiver during labour so the suggestion that the epidural induced peripheral vasodilatation was somehow responsible cannot be wholly true. An immunological response to amniotic fluid or fetal cells entering the maternal circulation, or a transitory septicaemia are other suggested mechanisms. The incidence of shivering in women receiving epidural analgesia may range from 20–50 per cent.[101]

Up to 4 per cent of mothers may complain of feeling deprived of some essential experience, as of being denied participation in the birth process, if their labour is conducted with an epidural block.[102] It is interesting to note that women who reported intense levels of pain when questioned during labour, recall this pain as being of much diminished intensity when interviewed again after six months and may sometimes feel that the pain was insufficient to even justify the epidural block.

## Neurological Sequelae

Serious neurological sequelae due to properly conducted epidural analgesia in obstetrics are extremely rare. Transient minor neurological problems do occur more frequently. Postpartum neurological problems can be expected in 1:2000 to 1:3000 deliveries conducted without regional anaesthesia[106] and the causes may be spontaneous in nature, or iatrogenic.[16] Most common (1:400) are compression and injury of peripheral nerves (e.g. lumbosacral trunk, femoral nerve, common peroneal) by the fetal head against the pelvic brim (see Fig. 9) or by lithotomy poles. These lesions have well-defined sensory and motor deficits and are often termed obstetric palsies. Moderately common (1:6000) is spinal root compression from a prolapsed vertebral disc, while rare causes (1:15,000) of postpartum neurological deficits are caused by a haemangioma of the spinal cord or spontaneous epidural haematoma.

*Serious neurological problems* could be directly attributable to the epidural block in the following instances:

—Trauma to spinal cord or roots during insertion
—Wrong solution injected
—Spinal cord ischaemia due to prolonged hypotension
—Epidural abscess (occurs spontaneously)
—Epidural haematoma (occurs spontaneously).

*Horner's syndrome* is a less serious neurological finding which unaccountably appears during obstetric epidural blocks.[107]

*Delayed recovery*, taking up to 48 hours, has been reported after an otherwise uneventful labour and epidural block.[108] The problem of postdural puncture headache, and the convulsions which may follow intravascular injection have been discussed elsewhere.

39/TABLE 4
INCIDENCE (%) POSTPARTUM SEQUELAE OF VARIOUS ANALGESIC TECHNIQUES

| | Grove (1973)[103] No epidural n = 187 | Crawford (1972)[104] Epidural n = 923 | Moir & Davidson (1972)[97] No epidural n = 50 | Moir & Davidson (1972)[97] Epidural n = 50 | Moir *et al.* (1976)[105] Epidural n = 335 | Ostheimer (1981)[100] Pudendal Nerve Block n = 100 | Ostheimer (1981)[100] Spinal n = 500 | Ostheimer (1981)[100] Epidural n = 1000 |
|---|---|---|---|---|---|---|---|---|
| Headache | 23 | 19·4 | 10 | 18 (no dural punctures) | 9 | 0 | 2·0 | 6·1 |
| Backache | 37·5 | 45 | 32 | 22 | 15 | — | — | — |
| Bladder dysfunction | 18 | 25·8 | 20 | 34 | 34·3 | — | — | — |
| Shivering | — | — | — | — | — | 22·2 | 36·6 | 39·7 |
| Nausea | — | — | — | — | — | 3·3 | 10·0 | 17·3 |

Bladder dysfunction is much higher following forceps delivery than after spontaneous delivery

39/Fig. 9.—Obstetric palsy: the lumbosacral plexus is vulnerable to compression by the fetal head against the pelvic brim. (Courtesy of J. T. Cole and the publishers, C. V. Mosby Company.[106])

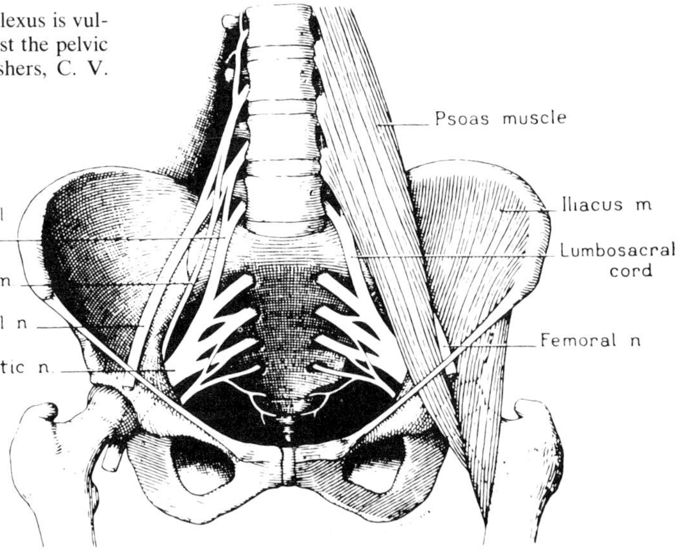


### Fetal Effects of Lumbar Epidural Analgesia

This matter is covered in detail in the chapter on the fetus, but it is important to note that the effects of the epidural may be exerted directly by the local anaesthetic drug or indirectly by the changes in uterine blood flow, changes in uterine contractility, and changes in the duration and mode of delivery. Figure 10 summarises these influences.

The supine position and resulting aortocaval compression are more important influences than the epidural itself and epidural blockade only produces falls in fetal oxygenation if hypotension is allowed to develop.[109] If mean arterial pressure remains below 70 mm Hg (9·3 kPa) for more than 3 minutes, then neonatal neurobehaviour will be impaired.

### Epidural Analgesia—Double Catheter Technique

Proposed by Cleland in 1952,[110] this technique requires insertion of two epidural catheters, one at T11 level to block T10–T12 segments during the first stage of labour, and a second caudal catheter to provide sacral block in the second stage.

The use of two catheters allows very precise control of segmental distribution using small doses of local anaesthetic. Only 4–5 ml of bupivacaine 0·5 per cent should need to be

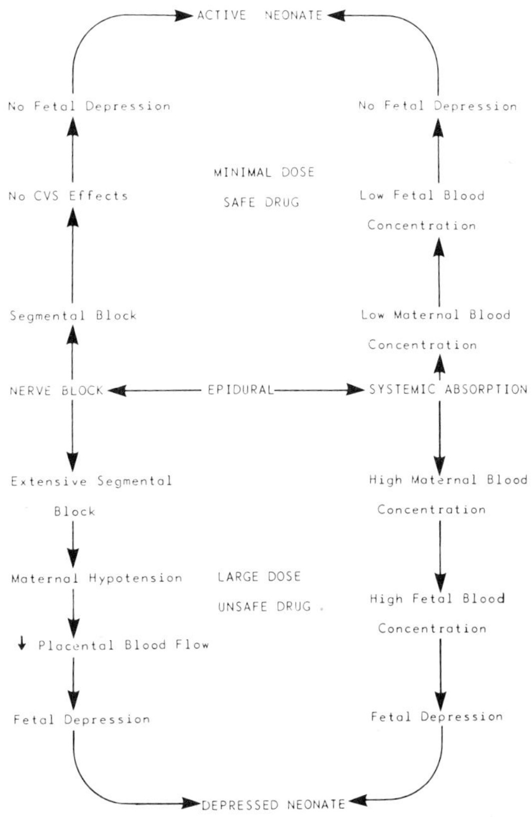


39/Fig. 10.—Summary of the influence of epidural analgesia on neonatal condition. (After Bromage, 1978.[16])

injected into either catheter, there is no need to position the mother to obtain perineal analgesia; maternal hypotension is less and the analgesia produced is very satisfactory.[111]

The double catheter technique is not widely used but may be especially indicated for the very sick mother with pre-eclampsia or heart disease.

### Caudal Epidural Analgesia

Once a very popular technique,[112] the caudal route has been overshadowed by the lumbar route. The major disadvantage of caudal analgesia is that it is non-selective and a block which reaches T10 will also block all lumbar and sacral segments. Larger doses of local anaesthetic are required and the risk of toxicity increased, yet the onset of an adequate block to T10 during the first stage is much slower than for the lumbar route. The overall success rate for the insertion of caudal block is lower than for lumbar blocks because the sacral hiatus demonstrates many anatomic variations, so that the lumbar injection is often technically easier and less painful. Pelvic muscle tone is not maintained during the first stage and rotation of the fetal head may be impaired so that the rate of forceps delivery is increased. The sacral area is potentially more infective than the lumbar region and the risks of dural puncture or intravascular injection are not avoided. Puncture of the rectum has occurred and, more seriously, of the fetal head.

However, the caudal route may be very useful, as part of the two catheter technique, or to provide perineal analgesia when delivery is imminent and lumbar injection is not practical. In a very distressed and restless patient a caudal block may be more rapidly and safely accomplished. The perineal analgesia and muscle relaxation which results is ideal for instrumental delivery. A subarachnoid block is probably simpler to perform and more certain to be effective and might be preferred in many of these indications.

### Paracervical Block

Injection of 8–10 ml of local anaesthetic into each fornix, blocks most of the afferent supply from the uterus and produces adequate first stage pain relief in 80 per cent of cases. However, fetal bradycardia occurs in 20–50 per cent of patients receiving a paracervical block and may be due to a decrease in placental blood flow resulting from uterine artery vasoconstriction, although direct local anaesthetic toxicity, on the fetus, may contribute. Lignocaine and etidocaine may actually relax the uterine artery. Bupivacaine causes constriction in the range of 5–25 $\mu$g/l but exerts inconsistent effects either side of this range.[113]

Fetal scalp blood pH and oxygenation remain reduced for a half hour following paracervical block and the likelihood of neonatal depression is increased.[114] Fetal deaths have been directly attributed to this procedure and paracervical block is contra-indicated in any circumstance where fetal wellbeing may be compromised.

### Lumbar Sympathetic Block

Block of the lumbar sympathetic chain is capable of producing reliable analgesia of long duration with a low incidence of side-effects during the first stage of labour. However, the procedure is technically difficult to perform, is generally more painful, cannot be used as a continuous technique and produces inadequate analgesia for delivery. This method might be useful if lumbar epidural block was contra-indicated for some reason.[115]

### Paravertebral Block

Paravertebral block has been used to block the nerves involved in the first stage of pain transmission after they leave the protection of the vertebral foramen. Considerable experience is required to perform these blocks and there is a risk of causing a pneumothorax.

## MIDWIVES

Instruction of midwives in the methods of pain relief available in labour is the responsibility of anaesthetists and, in the UK, it is a requirement of the Central Midwives Board that student midwives receive a certain number of lectures on the subject. Specific texts are available for midwives.

The anaesthetist's responsibility should not end with these lectures and he should teach midwives on the labour ward and thus make them more aware of what pain relief methods are available and the relative merits of each method. It is a great pity if the obstetric anaesthetist acts only as an epidural catheter insertion technician—he or she has much more to contribute to the labour ward.

## REFERENCES


1. Cleland, J. G. P. (1933). Paravertebral anesthesia in obstetrics. Experimental and clinical basis. *Surg. Gynecol. Obstet.*, **57**, 51.
2. Bonica, J. J. (1979). Peripheral mechanisms and pathways of parturition pain. *Brit. J. Anaesth.*, **51**, 3S.
3. Bonica, J. J. (1967). *Principles and Practice of Obstetric Analgesia and Anesthesia*. Philadelphia: F. A. Davis.
4. Dick-Read, G. (1959). *Childbirth Without Fear*, 2nd edit. New York: Harper and Row.
5. Crawford, J. S. (1982). *Obstetric Analgesia and Anaesthesia*. 1. Current Reviews in Obstetrics and Gynaecology. Edinburgh: Churchill Livingstone.
6. Morishima, H. O., Pederson, H. and Finster, M. (1978). Influence of maternal psychological stress on the fetus. *Am. J. Obstet. Gynecol.*, **131**, 286.
7. Morishima, H. O., Yeh, M. N. and James, L. S. (1979). Reduced uterine blood flow and fetal hypoxaemia with acute maternal stress: experimental observation in the pregnant baboon. *Am. J. Obstet. Gynecol.*, **134**, 270.
8. Maltau, J. M., Eielsen, O. V. and Stokke, K. T. (1979). Effect of stress during labour on the concentration of cortisol and estriol in maternal plasma. *Amer. J. Obstet. Gynecol.*, **134**, 681.
9. Shnider, S. M., Wright, R. G., Levinson, G., Roizen, M. F., Wallis, K. L., Rolbin, S. H. and Craft, J. B. (1979). Uterine blood flow and plasma norepinephrine changes during maternal stress in the pregnant ewe. *Anesthesiology*, **50**, 524.
10. Falconer, A. D. and Powles, A. B. (1982). Plasma noradrenaline levels during labour. Influence of elective lumbar epidural blockade. *Anaesthesia*, **37**, 416.
11. Buchanan, P. C., Milne, M. K. and Browning, M. C. K. (1973). The effect of continuous epidural blockade on plasma 11-hydroxycorticosteroid concentrations in labour. *J. Obstet. Gynaecol. Brit. Cwlth.*, **80**, 974.
12. Marx, G. F. and Greene, N. M. (1964). Maternal lactate, pyruvate and excess lactate production during labour and delivery. *Am. J. Obstet. Gynecol.*, **90**, 786.
13. Sanguol, F., Fox, G. S. and Houle, G. L. (1975). Effect of regional analgesia on maternal oxygen consumption during the first stage of labour. *Am. J. Obstet. Gynecol.*, **121**, 1080.
14. Argent, V. P. (1982). Treatment of severe tetany due to hyperventilation during labour with a mixture of nitrous oxide, oxygen and carbon dioxide. *Brit. med. J.*, **2**, 117.
15. Levinson, G., Shnider, S. M., de Lorimier, A. A. and Steffenson, J. L. (1974). Effects of maternal hyperventilation on uterine blood flow and fetal oxygenation and acid-base status. *Anesthesiology*, **40**, 340.
16. Bromage, P. R. (1978). *Epidural Analgesia*. Philadelphia: W. B. Saunders.
17. Holdcroft, A. and Morgan, M. (1974). An assessment of the analgesic effect in labour of pethidine and 50 per cent nitrous oxide in oxygen (Entonox). *J. Obstet. Gynaecol. Brit. Cwlth.*, **81**, 603.
18. Beazley, J. M., Leaver, E. P., Morewood, J. H. M. and Bircumshaw, J. (1967). Relief of pain in labour. *Lancet*, **1**, 1033.
19. Petrie, R. H., Yeh, S., Murata, Y., Paul, R. H., Hone, E. H., Barron, B. A. and Johnson, R. J. (1978). The effect of drugs on fetal heart rate variability. *Am. J. Obstet. Gynecol.*, **130**, 294.
20. Wiener, P. C., Hogg, M. I. and Rosen, M. (1979). Neonatal respiration, feeding and neurobehavioural state. Effects of intrapartum bupivacaine, pethidine and pethidine reversed by naloxone. *Anaesthesia*, **34**, 996.
21. Glynn, C. J. and Mather, L. E. (1982). Clinical pharmacokinetics applied to patients with intractable pain: studies with pethidine. *Pain*, **13**, 237.
22. Evans, J. W., Rosen, M., McCarthy, J. and Hogg, M. I. J. (1976). Apparatus for patient controlled administration of intravenous narcotics during labour. *Lancet*, **1**, 17.
23. Rosen, M. (1979). Systemic and inhalation analgesia. *Brit. J. Anaesth.*, **51**, Suppl. 1, 115.
24. Gallon, S. (1976). Ketamine for obstetric delivery. *Anesthesiology*, **44**, 522.
25. Hodgkinson, R., Marx, G., Kim, S. S. and Miclat, N. M. (1977). Neonatal neurobehavioural tests following vaginal delivery under ketamine, thiopental and extradural analgesia. *Anesth. Analg. Curr. Res.*, **56**, 548.
26. O'Driscoll, K. (1975). An obstetrician's view of pain. *Brit. J. Anaesth.*, **47**, 1053.
27. Cole, P. V., Crawford, J. S., Doughty, A. G., Epstein, H. G., Hill, I. D., Rollason, W. N. and Tunstall, M. E. (1970). Specifications and recommendations for nitrous oxide/oxygen apparatus to be used in obstetric analgesia. *Anaesthesia*, **25**, 317.
28. Arthurs, G. J. and Rosen, M. (1979). Self-administered intermittent nitrous oxide analgesia for labour. Enhancement of effect with continuous nasal inhalation of 50 per cent nitrous oxide (Entonox). *Anaesthesia*, **34**, 301.
29. Abboud, T. K., Shnider, S. M., Wright, R. G., Rolbin, S. H., Craft, J. B., Henriksen, E. A., Johnson, J., Jones, M. J., Hughes, S. C. and Levinson, G. (1981). Enflurane analgesia in obstetrics. *Anesth. Analg. Curr. Res.*, **60**, 133.
30. Hughey, M. J., McElin, T. W. and Young, T. (1978). Maternal and fetal outcome of Lamaze-prepared patients. *Obstet. Gynec.*, **51**, 643.
31. Nelson, M. N., Enkin, M. W., Saigal, S., Bennett, K. J., Milner, R. and Sackett, D. L. (1980). Randomised clinical trial of the Leboyer approach to childbirth. *New Eng. J. Med.*, **302**, 655.
32. Marx, G. F. (1981). Childbirth in the nineteen-eighties. *Regional Anesthesia*, **6**, 67.
33. Wallis, L., Shnider, S. M., Palahniuk, R. J. and Spivey, H. T. (1974). An evaluation of acupuncture analgesia in obstetrics. *Anesthesiology*, **41**, 596.
34. Stewart, P. (1979). Transcutaneous nerve stimulation as a method of analgesia in labour. *Anaesthesia*, **34**, 361.

35. Robson, J. F. (1979). Transcutaneous nerve stimulation for pain relief in labour. *Anaesthesia*, **34**, 357.
36. Miller-Jones, L. M. H. (1980). Transcutaneous nerve stimulation in labour. *Anaesthesia*, **35**, 372.
37. Persianinov, L. S. (1975). The use of electro-analgesia in obstetrics and gynecology. *Acta obstet. gynec. Scand.*, **54**, 373.
38. Grundy, E. M., Zamora, A. M. and Winnie, A. P. (1978). Comparison of spread of epidural anesthesia in pregnant and non-pregnant women. *Anesth. Analg. Curr. Res.*, **57**, 544.
39. Galbert, M. W. and Marx, G. F. (1974). Extradural pressures in the parturient patient. *Anesthesiology*, **40**, 499.
40. Collins, K. M., Bevan, D. R. and Beard, R. W. (1978). Fluid loading to reduce abnormalities of fetal heart rate and maternal hypotension during epidural analgesia in labour. *Brit. med. J.*, **2**, 1460.
41. Moir, D. D. (1980). *Obstetric Anaesthesia and Analgesia*, 2nd edit. London: Baillière Tindall.
42. Carrie, L. E. S. (1977). The paramedian approach to the epidural space. *Anaesthesia*, **32**, 670.
43. Abboud, T. K. (1981). An easy approach for difficult spinal anesthesia in the parturient. *Anesth. Analg. Curr. Res.*, **60**, 770.
44. Sivakumaran, C., Ramanathan, S., Chalon, J. and Turndorf, H. (1982). Uterine contractions and the spread of local anesthetic in the epidural space. *Anesth. Analg. Curr. Res.*, **61**, 127.
45. Grundy, E. M., Rao, L. and Winnie, A. P. (1978). Epidural anesthesia and the lateral position. *Anesth. Analg. Curr. Res.*, **57**, 95.
46. Husemeyer, R. P. and White, D. C. (1980). Lumbar extradural injection pressures in pregnant women. An investigation of relationships between rate of injection, injection pressures and extent of analgesia. *Brit. J. Anaesth.*, **52**, 55.
47. Rolbin, S. H., Cole, A. F. D., Hew, E. M. and Virgint, S. (1981). Effect of lateral position and volume on the spread of epidural anaesthesia in the parturient. *Canad. Anaesth. Soc. J.*, **28**, 431.
48. Apostolou, G. A., Zarmakoupis, P. K. and Mastrokostopoolos, G. T. (1981). Spread of epidural anesthesia and the lateral position. *Anesth. Analg. Curr. Res.*, **60**, 584.
49. Fagraeus, L., Urban, B. J., Groce, A. M. and Bromage, P. R. (1979). Spread of epidural analgesia in early pregnancy. *Anesthesiology*, **51**, S299.
50. Hodgkinson, R. and Husain, F. J. (1980). Obesity and the cephalad spread of analgesia following epidural administration of bupivacaine for Cesarean section. *Anesth. Analg. Curr. Res.*, **59**, 89.
51. Scott, D. B. (1977). Analgesia in labour. *Brit. J. Anaesth.*, **49**, 11.
52. Littlewood, D. G., Buckley, T., Covino, B. G., Scott, D. B. and Wilson, J. (1979). Comparative study of various local anaesthetic solutions in extradural block in labour. *Brit. J. Anaesth.*, **51**, Suppl. 1, 475.
53. Thorburn, J. and Moir, D. D. (1981). Extradural analgesia, the influence of volume and concentration of bupivacaine on the mode of delivery, analgesic efficacy and motor block. *Brit. J. Anaesth.*, **53**, 933.
54. Bleyaert, A., Soetens, M., Vaes, L., Van Steenberge, A. L., Van Dier Donck, A. (1979). Bupivacaine, 0·125 per cent, in obstetric epidural analgesia: experience in three thousand cases. *Anesthesiology*, **51**, 435.
55. Stainthorp, S. F., Bradshaw, E. G., Challen, T. D. and Tobia, S. M. H. (1978). 0·125 per cent bupivacaine for obstetric analgesia. *Anaesthesia*, **33**, 39.
56. Harley, N. F., Moir, B. J. and Brighten, P. W. (1978). The concentration of bupivacaine for obstetric analgesia. *Anaesthesia*, **33**, 648.
57. Reynolds, F. (1972). The influence of adrenaline on maternal and neonatal blood levels of local analgesic drugs. In: *Proceedings of the Symposium on Epidural Analgesia in Obstetrics*. Ed. A. Doughty, London: H. K. Lewis.
58. Albright, G. A., Jouppila, R., Hollmen, A. I., Jouppila, P., Vierola, H. and Koivula, A. (1981). Epinephrine does not alter human intervillous blood flow during epidural anesthesia. *Anesthesiology*, **54**, 131.
59. Jouppila, P., Jouppila, R., Kaar, K. and Merila, M. (1977). Fetal heart rate patterns and uterine activity after segmental epidural analgesia. *Brit. J. Obstet. Gynaecol.*, **84**, 481.
60. Moore, D. C. and Batra, M. S. (1981). The components of an effective test dose prior to epidural block. *Anesthesiology*, **55**, 693.
61. Soni, V., Peeters, C. and Covino, B. (1981). Value and limitations of test dose prior to epidural anesthesia. *Regional Anesthesia*, **6**, 23.
62. Verniquet, A. J. W. (1980). Vessel puncture with epidural catheter. Experience in obstetric patients. *Anaesthesia*, **35**, 660.
63. Evans, K. R. L. and Carrie, L. E. S. (1979). Continuous epidural infusion of bupivacaine in labour. A simple method. *Anaesthesia*, **34**, 310.
64. Davies, A. O. and Fettes, I. W. (1981). A simple safe method for continuous infusion epidural analgesia in obstetrics. *Canad. Anaesth. Soc. J.*, **28**, 484.
65. Taylor, H. J. C. (1982). Continuous infusion epidural analgesia. *Canad. Anaesth. Soc. J.*, **29**, 283.
66. Livnat, E. J., Fejcin, M., Scommegna, A., Bieniarz, J. and Burd, L. (1978). Neonatal acid-base balance in spontaneous and instrumental vaginal deliveries. *Obstet. Gynec.*, **52**, 549.
67. Myers, R. E., Strange, L., Joelson, I., Huzell, B. and Wussow, C. (1977). Effects upon the fetus of oxygen administration to the mother. *Acta Obstet. Gynecol. Scand.*, **56**, 195.
68. Ramanathan, S., Gandhi, S., Arismendy, J., Chalon, J. and Turndorf, H. (1982). Oxygen transfer from mother to fetus during Cesarean section under epidural anaesthesia. *Anesth. Analg. Curr. Res.*, **61**, 576.
69. Humphrey, M. D., Change, A., Wood, E. C. and Hounslow, D. (1974). A decrease in fetal pH during the second stage of labour when conducted in the dorsal position. *J. Obstet. Gynaecol. Brit. Cwlth.*, **81**, 600.
70. Philip, J. H. and Brown, W. U. (1976). Total spinal anesthesia late in the course of obstetric bupivacaine epidural block. *Anesthesiology*, **44**, 340.
71. Craft, J. B., Epstein, B. S. and Coakley, C. S. (1973). Prophylaxis of dural puncture headache with epidural saline. *Anesth. Analg. Curr. Res.*, **52**, 228.
72. Ostheimer, G. W., Palahniuk, R. J. and Shnider, S. M. (1974). Epidural blood patch for post-lumbar-puncture headache. *Anesthesiology*, **41**, 307.
73. Crawford, J. S. (1980). Experiences with epidural blood patch. *Anaesthesia*, **35**, 513.
74. Moore, D. C., Bridenbaugh, L. D., Thompson, G. E., Balfour, R. I. and Horton, W. G. (1978). Bupivacaine: a

review of 11,080 cases. *Anesth. Analg. Curr. Res.*, **57**, 42.
75. Corke, B. C., Datta, S., Ostheimer, G. W., Weiss, J. B. and Alper, M. H. (1982). Spinal anaesthesia for Caesarean section. The influence of hypotension on neonatal outcome. *Anaesthesia*, **37**, 658.
76. Ralston, D. H., Shnider, S. M. and de Lorimer, A. A. (1974). Effects of equipotent ephedrine, metaraminol, mephentermine and methoxamine on uterine blood flow in the pregnant ewe. *Anesthesiology*, **40**, 354.
77. Rolbin, S. H., Cole, A. F. D., Hew, E. M., Pollard, A. and Virgint, S. (1982). Prophylactic intramuscular ephedrine before epidural anaesthesia for Caesarean section: efficacy and actions on foetus and newborn. *Canad. Anaesth. Soc. J.*, **29**, 148, 152.
78. Datta, S., Alper, M. H., Ostheimer, G. W. and Weiss, J. B. (1982). Method of ephedrine administration and nausea and hypotension during spinal anesthesia for Caesarean section. *Anesthesiology*, **56**, 68.
79. Clark, R. B. and Brunner, J. A. (1980). Dopamine for the treatment of spinal hypotension during Caesarean section. *Anesthesiology*, **53**, 514.
80. Schellenberg, J. C. (1977). Uterine activity during lumbar epidural analgesia with bupivacaine. *Am. J. Obstet. Gynecol.*, **127**, 26.
81. Jouppila, R. (1982). Placental blood flow and obstetric anaesthesia. Proceedings of the Association of Paediatric Anaesthetists. *Anaesthesia*, **37**, 505.
82. Greiss, F. C., Still, J. G. and Anderson, S. G. (1976). Effects of local anesthetic agents on the uterine vasculatures and myometrium. *Am. J. Obstet. Gynecol.*, **124**, 889.
83. Tyack, A. J., Parsons, R. J., Millar, D. R. and Nicholas, A. D. G. (1973). Uterine activity and plasma bupivacaine levels after caudal epidural analgesia. *J. Obstet. Gynaecol. Brit. Cwlth.*, **80**, 896.
84. Jouppila, R., Jouppila, P., Hollmen, A. and Kuikka, J. (1978). Effect of segmental extradural analgesia on placental blood flow during normal labour. *Brit. J. Anaesth.*, **50**, 563.
85. Jouppila, R., Jouppila, P., Karinen, J. M. and Hollmen, A. (1979). Segmental epidural analgesia in labour: related to progress of labour, fetal malposition and instrumental delivery. *Acta Obstet. Gynaecol. Scand.*, **58**, 135.
86. Studd, J. W. W., Crawford, J. S., Doignan, N. M., Rowbotham, C. J. F. and Hughes, A. O. (1980). The effect of lumbar epidural analgesia on the rate of cervical dilatation and the outcome of labour of spontaneous onset. *Brit. J. Obstet. Gynaec.*, **87**, 1015.
87. Doughty, A. (1978). Epidural analgesia in labour. The past, the present and the future. *J. roy. Soc. Med.*, **71**, 879.
88. Phillips, J. C., Hochberg, C. J., Petrakis, J. K., Van Winkle, J. D. (1977). Epidural analgesia and its effects on the "normal" progress of labor. *Am. J. Obstet. Gynecol.*, **129**, 316.
89. Ralston, D. H. and Shnider, S. M. (1978). The fetal and neonatal effects of regional anesthesia in obstetrics. *Anesthesiology*, **48**, 34.
90. O'Driscoll, K., Meacher, D., Macdonald, D. and Geoghegan, F. (1981). Traumatic intracranial haemorrhage in first born infants and delivery with obstetric forceps. *Brit. J. Obstet. Gynecol.*, **88**, 577.
91. Friedman, E. A. (1981). The effect of lumbar epidural analgesia on the rate of cervical dilatation and the outcome of labour of spontaneous outset. *Brit. J. Obstet. Gynaec.*, **88**, 464.
92. Bassell, G. M., Humayun, S. G. and Marx, G. F. (1980). Maternal bearing down efforts—another fetal risk? *Obstet. Gynecol*, **56**, 39.
93. Maltau, J. M. and Egge, K. (1980). Epidural analgesia and perinatal retinal haemorrhages. *Acta anaesth. Scand.*, **24**, 99.
94. Crawford, J. W. (1980). The enigma of the missed segment. *Canad. Anaesth. Soc. J.*, **27**, 594.
95. De Campo, T., Macias-Loza, M., Cohen, H. and Galind, A. (1980). Lumbar epidural anaesthesia and sensory profiles in term, pregnancy patients. *Canad. Anaesth. Soc. J.*, **27**, 274.
96. Bray, M. C. and Carrie, L. E. S. (1978). Unblocked segments in obstetric epidural blocks. *Anaesthesia*, **33**, 232.
97. Moir, D. D. and Davidson, S. (1972). Postpartum complications of forceps delivery performed under epidural and pudendal nerve block. *Brit. J. Anaesth.*, **44**, 1197.
98. Bromage, P. R. (1972). Unblocked segments in epidural analgesia for relief of pain in labour. *Brit. J. Anaesth.*, **44**, 676.
99. Morgan, B. M., Rehor, S. and Lewis, P. J. (1980). Epidural analgesia for uneventful labour. *Anaesthesia*, **35**, 57.
100. Ostheimer, G. W. (1981). Neurobehavioral effects of local anesthesia and fetal resuscitation. *Regional Anesthesia*, **6**, 136.
101. Webb, P. J., James, F. M. and Wheeler, A. S. (1981). Shivering during epidural analgesia in women in labor. *Anesthesiology*, **55**, 706.
102. Billewicz Driemel, A. M. and Milne, M. D. (1976). Long term assessment of extradural analgesia for the relief of pain in labour. II. Sense of 'deprivation' after extradural analgesia in labour: relevant or not. *Brit. J. Anaesth.*, **48**, 139.
103. Grove, L. H. (1973). Backache, headache and bladder dysfunction after delivery. *Brit. J. Anaesth.*, **45**, 1147.
104. Crawford, J. S. (1972). Lumbar epidural block in labour: a clinical analysis. *Brit. J. Anaesth.*, **44**, 66.
105. Moir, D. D., Slater, P. J., Thorburn, J., McLaren, R. and Moodie, J. (1976). Epidural analgesia in obstetrics: a controlled trial of carbonated lignocaine and bupivacaine HCl solutions with and without adrenaline. *Brit. J. Anaesth.*, **48**, 129.
106. Cole, J. T. (1946). Maternal obstetric paralysis. *Am. J. Obstet. Gynecol.*, **52**, 372.
107. Carrie, L. E. S. and Mohan, J. (1976). Horner's syndrome following obstetric extradural block. *Brit. J. Anaesth.*, **48**, 611.
108. Cuerden, C., Buley, R. and Downing, J. W. (1977). Delayed recovery after epidural block in labour. A report of four cases. *Anaesthesia*, **32**, 773.
109. Willcourt, R. J., Paust, J. C. and Queenan, J. T. (1982). Changes in fetal $TcPo_2$ values occurring during labour in association with lumbar extradural analgesia. *Brit. J. Anaesth.*, **54**, 635.
110. Cleland, J. G. P. (1952). Continuous epidural and caudal block in obstetrics and surgery with postoperative analgesia. *Anesth. Analg. Curr. Res.*, **31**, 289.
111. Hollmen, A. (1979). Regional techniques of analgesia in labour. *Brit. J. Anaesth.*, **51**, 175.
112. Rubin, A. P. (1972). The choice between the lumbar

and the caudal route. In: *Proceedings of the Symposium on Epidural Analgesia in Obstetrics*. Ed. Doughty, A. London: H. K. Lewis.

113. Tuvemo, T. and Willdeck-Lund, G. (1982). Smooth muscle effects of lidocaine, prilocaine, bupivacaine and etidocaine on the human umbilical artery. *Acta anaesth. Scand.*, **26**, 104.

114. Baxi, L. V., Petrie, R. H. and James, L. S. (1979). Human fetal oxygenation following paracervical block. *Am. J. Obstet. Gynecol.*, **135**, 1109.

115. Meguiar, R. V. and Wheeler, A. S. (1978). Lumbar sympathetic block with bupivacaine: analgesia for labour. *Anesth. Analg. Curr. Res.*, **57**, 486.

## FURTHER READING

Bromage, P. R. (1978). *Epidural Analgesia*. Philadelphia: W. B. Saunders.

Moir, D. D. (1980). *Obstetric Anaesthesia and Analgesia*, 2nd edit. London: Baillière Tindall.

CHAPTER 40

# Anaesthesia for Obstetrics



## Maternal Mortality

In the triennium 1976–1978, there were 40 deaths associated with anaesthesia in England and Wales. Thirty deaths were directly due to anaesthesia and there were avoidable factors in 28. Emergency caesarean section was the operative procedure for which anaesthesia was given in 18 cases, but 3 women died during elective caesarean section.

Table 1 shows that the mortality rate per million maternities was 17·2 for deaths directly associated with anaesthesia and that this rate has actually risen. Alarmingly the percentage of true maternal deaths due to anaesthesia is the same for the two periods 1973–1975 and

40/TABLE 1
MATERNAL MORTALITY
Deaths associated with anaesthesia; estimated rates per million maternities and percentages of true maternal deaths, 1964–1978.[4]

| | 1964–66 | 1967–69 | 1970–72 | 1973–75 | 1976–78 |
|---|---|---|---|---|---|
| Number of deaths directly associated with anaesthesia | 50 | 50 | 37 | 31 | 30 |
| Rate per million maternities | 19·2 | 10·3 | 16·1 | 16·1 | 17·2 |
| Percentage of true maternal deaths due to anaesthesia | 8·7 | 10·9 | 10·4 | 13·2 | 13·2 |

1976–1978 and this is higher than in any of the previous three periods. Anaesthesia caused 16·6 per cent of true maternal deaths in Ireland in 1979[1] and general anaesthesia was listed as the greatest cause of maternal deaths over a twenty-year period at a specialist London obstetric hospital.[2]

### ANAESTHETIC CAUSES OF DEATH

**Inhalation of stomach contents** caused 14 deaths and most of these were the result of poor anaesthetic practice. Nine of the patients died of Mendelson's syndrome. Only 4 of these patients had apparently received routine antacid premedication. Cricoid pressure was either not applied or was applied casually or incorrectly in all of these cases. These figures confirm North American experiences where 50 per cent of anaesthetic-related maternal deaths are due to aspiration of vomitus.

**Difficulty with endotracheal intubation** was the cause of death in 16 patients. Unsuccessful attempts at intubation were followed by hypoxia and cardiac arrest. Cardiopulmonary resuscitation is very difficult in the pregnant woman at term.[3]

**Other causes** included misuse of drugs, accidents with apparatus and epidural analgesia. At least one death occurred when total spinal anaesthesia complicating an epidural block was incorrectly managed.

A number of conclusions about avoiding maternal mortality mave been drawn from these reports and are summarised below:

1. The anaesthetist, irrespective of status or training, must have skilled help.
2. Inexperienced anaesthetists should not have sole responsibility for obstetric anaesthesia.
3. Antacid therapy will not give total protection against Mendelson's syndrome.
4. Cricoid pressure must be applied correctly by a skilled assistant.
5. Failed intubation drills must be mastered by all obstetric anaesthetists.
6. Epidural analgesia during labour requires skilled supervision and an anaesthetist must be immediately available.
7. No matter how urgent the obstetric emergency, the anaesthetist must not neglect to monitor the condition of the anaesthetised patient.

## ACID ASPIRATION SYNDROME

In 1946, Mendelson[5] described 66 cases in which gastric contents had been regurgitated, and initiated the syndrome which now bears his name. Morbidity and mortality following aspiration depends on the volume, nature, acidity and distribution of the aspirated material. At least 62 per cent of patients may die following aspiration, the mortality being 40 per cent if only one lobe is involved and greater than 90 per cent if more than one lobe is involved. The mortality following aspiration is probably high because of the frequency with which large surface areas of the lung are involved.

Inhalation of gastric contents of sufficient volume or solidity will cause asphyxia. In other cases, the risk of serious pulmonary reaction increases progressively as the pH of the aspirate decreases to less than 2·5. Volumes as small as 25 ml of such acid fluid may be sufficient to cause widespread damage and it has been noted that 55 per cent of obstetric patients at term have more than 40 ml liquid gastric contents and in 40 per cent of patients, the pH is less than 2·5.[6] Aspiration of partially digested food is particularly damaging.[7]

Irrespective of the aetiological mechanism or agent responsible for injuring the alveolar-capillary substrates in the lungs, the pathophysiological consequences are similar and the clinical picture will fit into the *adult respiratory distress syndrome.*[8] Four phases have been described.[9]

Phase 1 Profound dyspnoea and tachypnoea
Bronchospasm is often present
Chest x-ray may be normal

Phase 2 (latent period)
Increasing cyanosis and hypoxaemia
Minor chest x-ray abnormalities

Phase 3 Respiratory failure; profound hypoxaemia, reduced compliance
Diffuse bilateral infiltrates

Phase 4 Hypoxaemia unresponsive to oxygen
Metabolic and respiratory acidosis.

**Diagnosis.**—Severe liquid aspiration may cause immediate collapse, but symptoms following aspiration of more moderate amounts may only become apparent 6–8 hours after the incident. Suction down an endotracheal tube which reveals bile-stained fluid is often diagnostic, while over the longer term, serial chest x-rays and arterial blood gas estimates will reveal progressive changes (Fig. 1).

### Management

A. Solid gastric contents require urgent removal by bronchoscopy.
B. Aspiration of liquid contents should be managed in the following way.[10]

1. Early diagnosis and appropriate management is essential in order to reduce mortality.
2. The ultimate degree of pulmonary destruction cannot be gauged at the time of aspiration.
3. Thorough endotracheal suction must be performed and the pH of the aspirate measured. Bronchial lavage is contra-indicated and is likely to aggravate the injury by removing or dispersing surfactant.
4. Intermittent positive-pressure ventilation with PEEP appears to be the one factor that can readily alter the prognosis.
5. Correction of blood volume and acid-base balance. Hypovolaemia is a prominent feature of pulmonary aspiration and central venous pressure or pulmonary-artery wedge pressures may be helpful to guide volume restoration. Over-enthusiastic infusion of crystalloid solution may encourage the formation of interstitial pulmonary oedema.
6. Steroids are not of proven value, but are often used.
7. Antibiotics should only be used when bacterial culture results are available.
8. Antispasmodics should only be used if bronchospasm is present.
9. Use of a membrane oxygenator may be indicated if $Pa_{O_2}$ continues to fall below 50 mm Hg (6·7 kPa) despite the above measures.

## Prevention of the Acid Aspiration Syndrome

### 1. Decreasing Gastric Fluid Volume

**Restriction of oral intake** during labour would seem an obvious precaution but this is only a recent innovation in many places. Intravenous infusions should be used to prevent dehydration and ketoacidosis in prolonged labour.

**Empty the stomach by physical means.**—The passage of a large-bore stomach tube may be used to empty the stomach but this is very uncomfortable for the patient and rarely achieves complete emptying, because of the separate pools of fluid which exist within the stomach. The tube must be withdrawn before general anaesthesia is induced.

**Empty the stomach by pharmacological means.**—Apomorphine has been used to promote vomiting. A slow intravenous injection of 1–3 mg of apomorphine diluted in water is given until vomiting occurs, this is followed by naloxone 0·4 mg which will suppress the vomiting, and atropine 1·0 mg or hyoscine 0·6 mg which will control the intense salivation.[11] Up to 75 per cent of stomach contents may be vomited, but the method is not reliable.

Deliberate emptying of the stomach should be employed if circumstances suggest that the patient is at increased risk of regurgitating. Metoclopramide hastens gastric emptying but this effect is not reliable in labour. Cimetidine will decrease gastric volume but the effect of the drug on gastric acid pH is of greater significance. Glycopyrronium (glycopyrrolate) and atropine can both decrease gastric acid secretions,[12], but this effect is very variable[13] and both these drugs produce a reduction in lower oesophageal sphincter tone; their place in obstetric anaesthesia has been questioned

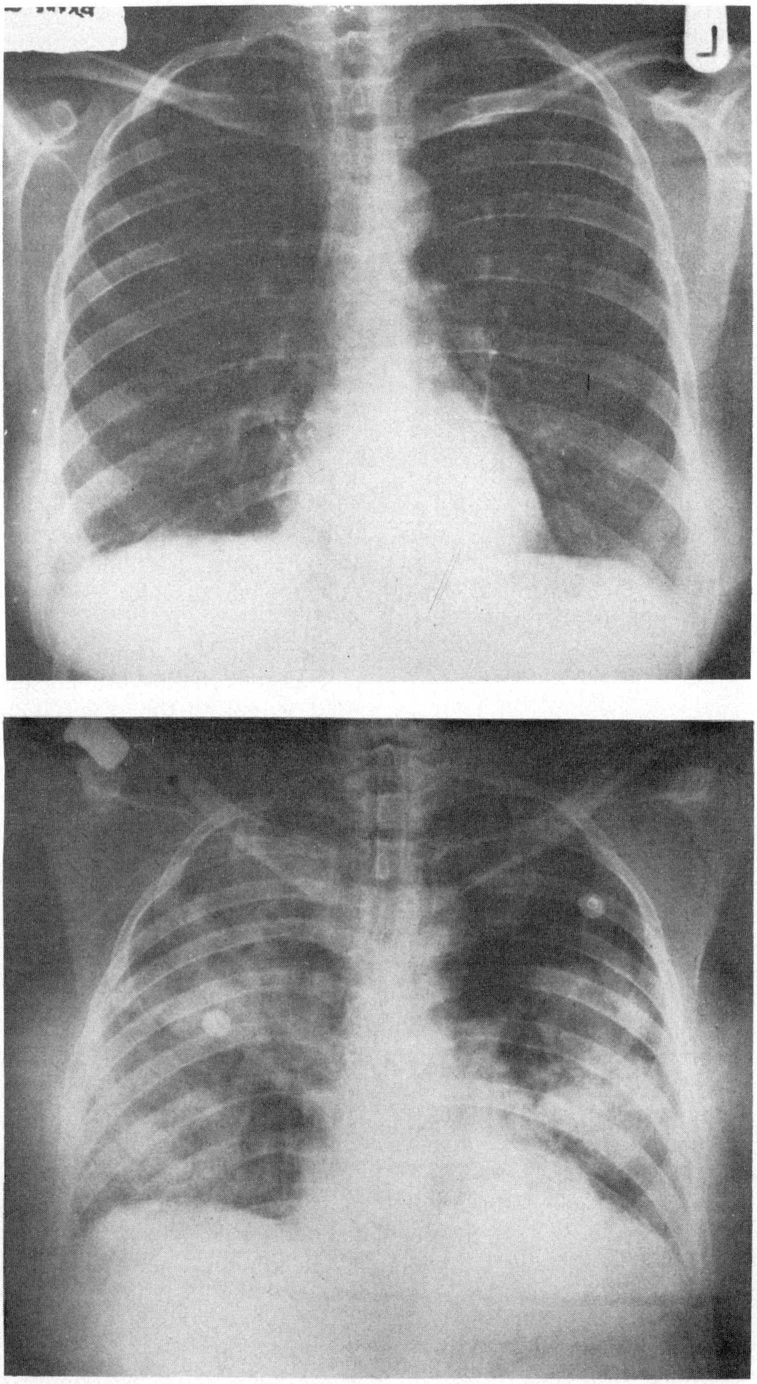

(a)

(b)

40/Fig. 1.—Obstetric aspiration syndrome: (a) before, (b) after. (Courtesy of Dr. G. C. Hanson and the Whipps Cross Hospital, London.)

40/Table 2
Approaches to the Problem of Acid Aspiration

*Decrease gastric fluid volume*
- Restrict intake
- Empty stomach:
  - physical
  - pharmacological
- Suppress gastric secretion

*Decrease gastric fluid acidity*
- Neutralise existing acid
- Elevevate pH, pharmacological

*Prevent regurgitation*
- Increase tone of lower oesophageal sphincter
- Avoid increase in intragastric pressure
- Induction in upright posture

*Prevent inhalation if regurgitation occurs*
- Cricoid pressure
- Induction in lateral position
- Powerful sucker available

*Avoid intubation difficulties*
- Careful patient assessment
- Skilled obstetric anaesthetist

*Avoid general anaesthesia*
- Regional anaesthesia

unless repeat doses of suxamethonium are being used or some other specific indication exists.[14]

## 2. Decreasing Gastric Fluid Acidity

**Antacids** will increase gastric fluid pH above 2·5 in over 80 per cent of cases, but alkalinisation may further delay gastric emptying although gastro-oesophageal sphincter tone is increased.[15] The antacids may produce significant pulmonary damage if aspirated and deaths have been reported following aspiration of gastric fluids containing antacids. The routine use of antacids does not seem to have influenced the maternal mortality figures,[16] and animal experiments suggest that aspiration of antacid-gastric acid mixtures, or even of particulate antacid solutions alone will produce more severe lung pathology than following aspiration of acid alone.[17,18] It may be the particulate nature of the antacids that is responsible for the pulmonary damage, and suspensions containing aluminium hydroxide seem to be most potent in this respect.

Cohen[16] questions the wisdom of giving repeatedly any fluid to a patient in labour with delayed gastric emptying, especially when the substance may actually stimulate acid secretion or further delay gastric emptying.

Despite all these apparent disadvantages, there are many reports of survival, with little or no pulmonary damage following aspiration of antacid-containing gastric fluid.[19]

A non-particulate antacid such as sodium citrate may be the solution of choice in obstetrics and will cause less pulmonary damage if aspirated.[20] Fifteen to thirty ml of the 0·3 molar solution should be given, chilled to make the taste more palatable.[21,22,23] Sodium citrate mixes more thoroughly with stomach contents compared to particulate antacids such as Mist Magnesium Trisilicate, and mixing is further improved by rotating the patient through 180° or even 360°.[24] Inadequate mixing of antacids with stomach contents may partially explain the inability of antacids to be uniformly effective, since the stomach is divided into right and left pockets by the vertebral column when the patient is supine or slightly tilted.

If sodium citrate is not available, mist magnesium trisilicate should be used:

*Mist Magnesium Trisilicate BPC*

| | |
|---|---|
| Magnesium trisilicate | 500 mg |
| Light magnesium carbonate | 500 mg |
| Sodium bicarbonate | 500 mg |
| Peppermint emulsion concentrate | 0·25 mg |
| Chloroform water, double strength | 5 ml |
| Water to | 10 ml |

Patients having a trial of labour should continue to receive antacid, 15 ml two-hourly, and everyone should receive 30 ml before general anaesthesia. Rotation should be encouraged, to promote mixing, and if the pre-operative dose is given on the ward, the transfer process from bed to trolley to operating table before induction will aid antacid distribution.

### Pharmacological Agents Used to Decrease Gastric Acidity

Histamine plays a major role in acid production by the parietal cells in the stomach and this action is mediated by histamine $H_2$ receptors, at which site $H_2$ antagonists such as cimetidine and ranitidine also act. Single doses of these antagonists produce unreliable results, but repeated doses of cimetidine, for example, can increase gastric pH to above 2·5 in 90–100 per cent of cases.[25] Cimetidine 400 mg stat, then

200 mg orally every two hours during labour, is an effective regimen but gastric pH may remain low for 90 minutes or so after the initial dose.[26] The concurrent administration of an antacid with cimetidine will inhibit the absorption of cimetidine, so that administration should be separated by one hour.[27]

Ranitidine is more potent, has a longer duration and produces fewer side-effects than cimetidine, and for elective operations a dose of 150 mg on the evening before and again on the morning of operation will decrease gastric-fluid volume and increase pH to safe levels in virtually every case.[28]

Glycopyrronium and atropine have been claimed to decrease gastric acidity,[29] but the effects are very inconsistent.[30]

### 3. Preventing Regurgitation

**Increase tone of lower oesophageal sphincter.**—Metoclopramide increases the tone of the lower oesophageal sphincter and since it is also an effective anti-emetic, routine intravenous administration before general anaesthesia can be recommended.[31,32] Alkalinisation of stomach contents will increase lower oesophageal sphincter tone, but many of the other drugs which might be used pre-operatively such as atropine, hyoscine, glycopyrronium and diazepam will actually reduce lower oesophageal sphincter tone and increase the likelihood of regurgitation.

**Avoid increases in intragastric pressure.**—The fasciculations produced by suxamethonium were thought to cause a rise in intragastric pressure, but recent work has shown that the pressure in the lower oesophageal sphincter increases by a greater amount than the intragastric pressure so that the risk of regurgitation is not increased.

Pretreatment with a small dose of tubocurarine or pancuronium to suppress the suxamethonium-induced fasciculation and thereby prevent the rise in intragastric pressure would seem to be an unnecessary procedure and anyway might be hazardous, since the paralysing dose of suxamethonium needs to be increased after the patient has received a pretreatment dose of a non-depolarising relaxant.[33]

**Induction in the upright position** has been suggested from time to time as a means of avoiding regurgitation, though this method cannot be recommended in obstetrics because of the added dangers of aortocaval compression in the sitting position, the often increased difficulty in inserting an endotracheal tube, and the certainty that should regurgitation occur, the stomach contents are sure to be inhaled.

### 4. Preventing Inhalation

**Cricoid pressure** is the single most important manoeuvre in the prevention of the acid aspiration syndrome, and must be applied correctly in every case, irrespective of any other precautions that may have been taken. The method was described by Sellick[34] and will effectively prevent regurgitation in the face of high rises in intragastric pressure. Regurgitation has been reported during application of cricoid pressure but if the cricoid pressure was being correctly applied, this is very difficult to understand.

Table 2 summarises the various approaches to the problem of regurgitation and aspiration and emphasises that reliance must never be placed on one precaution alone, but rather that every patient should receive as many different measures as are compatible and safe.

## ANAESTHESIA FOR OPERATIVE OBSTETRICS

The requirements of the ideal obstetric anaesthetic may be listed as follows (after Moir[31]).

1. Avoid pulmonary aspiration of stomach contents
2. Avoid neonatal respiratory depression
3. Avoid hypoxia and provide optimal fetal oxygenation
4. Avoid hypotension (including aortocaval compression) and maintain uteroplacental blood flow
5. Avoid uterine atony and consequent haemorrhage
6. Avoid maternal hyperventilation and hypocapnia
7. Provide satisfactory operating conditions, with muscular relaxation where necessary
8. Ensure unconsciousness throughout any general anaesthetic
9. Comply with the mother's wish to be awake or asleep at the time of delivery
10. Avoid depression of neonatal neurobehavioural responses.

## General Anaesthesia

General anaesthesia in obstetrics should always be performed by an experienced anaesthetist, with skilled assistance, and using a well-tried, methodical technique.

### Preparation – Patient

Unless the operation is an absolute emergency, then the anaesthetist should visit the patient to explain the anaesthetic procedure and to give as much reassurance as possible.

**Premedication** is rarely indicated. Crawford[35] has suggested that diazepam 5 mg may be helpful in allaying anxiety and reducing peri-operative awareness. However, other studies have stated that the benzodiazepines are unsatisfactory as pre-operative obstetric sedatives and that delirium may be an unwanted side-effect.[36] Diazepam also reduces lower oesophageal sphincter tone, thereby increasing the possibility of regurgitation.[37] For the same reason, the anticholinergic drugs should be avoided; also these drugs possess the unpleasant side-effect of producing a dry mouth. Pre-induction anxiety can be more simply allayed by a calm and confident atmosphere in the anaesthetic room than by having recourse to drugs. Always remember that these women are facing the prospect of a major operation and the arrival of a new baby, whilst many may be disappointed at being denied a normal vaginal delivery. All these mothers warrant gentle handling.

**Transport.**—All patients having caesarean section benefit by being in the lateral position for at least 30 minutes before anaesthesia is induced, so the journey to the operating theatre should be accomplished with the patient in this position, and certainly never with the patient in the unmodified supine position. Thirty minutes in the lateral position will decrease maternal metabolic acidosis and enhance fetal oxygenation.

**Regurgitation prophylaxis.**—The mother should receive a dose of 30 ml of 0·3 M sodium citrate before leaving the ward. If so desired, cimetidine or ranitidine, in an appropriate regime, can be ordered some time pre-operatively, although single doses of these histamine $H_2$ antagonists exert no reliable effect.

Artificial emptying of the stomach using apomorphine-induced vomiting or a large-bore stomach tube is still practised routinely in some centres, but many might prefer to reserve these measures for cases in whom regurgitation seems likely.

### Preparation – Anaesthetist

The anaesthetist should perform an obsessional "cockpit check" before every obstetric anaesthetic, whether it is to be a general or a regional procedure. He should ensure that the following items are present and function correctly:

1. Tilting table or bed
2. Powerful suction apparatus
3. High-flow oxygen; full reserve cylinders
4. Two working laryngoscopes
5. Malleable endotracheal tube introducers; Magill's forceps
6. Endotracheal tubes with connectors and working cuffs, sizes 7, 8 at least
7. Wedge or left uterine displacement apparatus
8. Drugs drawn up: induction agent, suxamethonium, non-depolarising relaxant, maintenance opiate, anticholinergic, metoclopramide, oxytocin
9. Intravenous equipment: infusion set up; crystalloid, plasma volume expanders and blood all immediately available
10. Assistant instructed in how to perform Sellick's manoeuvre
11. Calm and quiet in the anaesthetic room
12. Surgeon present before induction.

### Induction

**Position.**—The patient must never lie supine, and induction and intubation may be completed with the patient in a full lateral position, or with lateral tilt or left uterine displacement. The wedge or uterine displacement must be maintained until delivery, and some surgeons will now sit down to operate on the patient in the full lateral position. Whatever the circumstances or the indications for a general anaesthetic, no woman should ever be induced in the lithotomy position; her legs must always be taken out of the stirrups and, if necessary, held by someone in the theatre.

**Pre-oxygenation,** with an oxygen flow of 6–8 l/min, should be maintained for at least 3 minutes before induction. As a consequence of the increased oxygen consumption and altered lung volumes of pregnancy, one minute's apnoea in the parturient will result in a decrease of 139 mm Hg (18·5 kPa) in $Pao_2$, compared with 58 mm Hg (7·7 kPa) in the non-pregnant; thus pre-oxygenation and immediate re-oxygenation following intubation are vital.

**Metoclopramide.** 10 mg, given intravenously, will increase the tone of the lower oesophageal sphincter and sometimes will also encourage gastric emptying, although this effect is variable in labour. Time must be given for metoclopramide to take effect and it might be best given as the pre-oxygenation period commences.

**Anticholinergic agents,** either atropine, hyoscine, or glycopyrronium may be used to decrease salivation and reduce the likelihood of bradycardia, but these drugs will oppose the effects of metoclopramide and should be avoided.

**Cricoid pressure** should be applied before the injection of the induction agent, after the assistant has been satisfactorily instructed in the correct technique, and the mother has been warned.

**Induction agent.**—Thiopentone 4 mg/kg, methohexitone 1 mg/kg, etomidate, ketamine, Althesin and propanidid have all been tried as induction agents for caesarean section. Sodium thiopentone in a dose of 4 mg/kg produces a highly significant fall in intervillous blood flow, which is likely to be a reflection of the decreased cardiac output and splanchnic vasoconstriction caused by this drug.

Althesin has been associated with an increased incidence of metabolic acidosis and also carried an increased risk of producing an adverse drug reaction, the consequences of which may be totally unacceptable in obstetric anaesthesia. Etomidate has been described as resulting in infants with superior neonatal status and in a dose of 0·3 mg/kg may be indicated for the clinically ill fetus.[38]

Ketamine, in a dose of 1–2 mg/kg has been recommended as a routine induction agent but reports of unpleasant dreams may limit the usefulness of the drug.[39] Although ketamine may actually increase uterine-artery blood flow,[40] other reports show that neonates from mothers induced with ketamine may fare less well and exhibit depressed neurobehavioural responses. The use of ketamine is contra-indicated in any of the hypertensive diseases of pregnancy, including pre-eclampsia, but the drug may otherwise be useful, especially in the very ill or hypovolaemic patient.

**Muscle relaxant.**—Despite recommendations to the contrary, suxamethonium is the relaxant of choice for intubation in caesarean section. The risk of regurgitation is not increased by suxamethonium-induced fasciculations,[41] and comparisons with the speed of onset and quality of intubating conditions produced by other agents show suxamethonium to be the safest agent.[42,43]

Once intubation has been achieved, relaxation may be maintained using pancuronium, alcuronium or – especially in the hypertensive – tubocurarine. Suxamethonium drips, or the use of tacrine to prolong the duration of the suxamethonium injection, are now rarely used.

### Failed Intubation

Although failure to intubate a paralysed patient is a rare event, the difficulties, if encountered during obstetric anaesthesia, are compounded by the risks of maternal acid aspiration and by the need to ensure fetal well-being.

Every obstetric anaesthetist should have a clear plan of action prepared to cope with such an emergency. The decision to abandon repeated attempts at intubation must be made promptly before serious hypoxaemia develops or continued manipulation triggers coughing and regurgitation.

The classic failed intubation drill was detailed by Tunstall,[44] but consideration of each individual situation may dictate different management, depending primarily on the urgency of the indication for surgery.

If the obstetrician insists that immediate operation is imperative, three problems confront the anaesthetist.

(i) *To maintain oxygenation*, initially by gentle IPPV with mask and airway, then with spontaneous ventilation as the suxamethonium effect wears off.

(ii) *To minimise the risk of airway contamination.*—Cricoid pressure should be maintained and the patient turned head-down and on to the left side. Tunstall recommends passing a wide-bore stomach tube, but the passage of such a tube in a lightly anaesthetised patient may precipitate laryngospasm, vomiting and aspiration.

(iii) *To provide surgical anaesthesia* so that the operation can proceed as soon as possible. If oxygenation is being satisfactorily maintained, nitrous oxide and an inhalational agent should be added whilst the IPPV continues, so that when spontaneous respiration returns the patient will be anaesthetised. Often no choice of inhalational agent will be possible and although ether and methoxyflurane have been recommended as the agents of choice, it is more likely nowadays that halothane, enflurane or isoflurane will be available, and despite the uterine-relaxing properties of agents such as halothane and enflurane, the urgency of the situation may demand their use. Supplementation with small doses of thiopentone may allow lower concentrations of the inhalational agent to be used, or intravenous ketamine might be given to produce excellent surgical anaesthesia, thus allowing the administration of 100 per cent oxygen.

If the obstetrician declares that the operation should proceed as soon as safe anaesthesia can be provided, the patient should be allowed to wake up whilst oxygenation, cricoid pressure and the left lateral position are maintained. As soon as the mother is fully recovered and co-operative, the operation should proceed using a regional technique. A simple subarachnoid block will produce the most rapid anaesthesia whilst presenting the possibly compromised fetus with the lowest exposure to depressant drugs.

For an elective operation, a longer delay may be sensible until a more experienced anaesthetist and special intubation equipment is obtained or a planned regional technique is embarked upon. The safety of the regional techniques is very attractive.

The incidence of failed intubation may be reduced by adequate pre-operative assessment of every patient and by meticulous preparation of the anaesthetic equipment and drugs. Different laryngoscopes with long blades or special handles should be available along with a range of introducers for the endotracheal tube. If a semi-rigid suction catheter is used as an introducer, any fluid regurgitated during intubation can be immediately sucked out of the pharynx. The labouring patient with pre-eclampsia may develop laryngeal oedema, so a range of endotracheal tube sizes should be available for these patients.

**Awareness**

Awareness may be auditory or tactile and may or may not involve the appreciation of pain by the mother. The experience may be remembered as an unpleasant dream, or even not remembered at all postoperatively even though the patient was definitely conscious peri-operatively.[45] Up to 9 per cent of patients have reported that they were aware during the course of their operation, and this is important not only because these people are suffering unduly, but also because the increased stress of awareness may stimulate sympathetic tone, resulting in decreased uteroplacental blood flow at a crucial time.

The problem of awareness is not peculiar to obstetrics, but is more common during this form of anaesthesia because sedative and depressive drugs are avoided and high concentrations of oxygen are administered in the fetal interest before delivery. Once the umbilical cord has been clamped, powerful opiates and high concentrations of nitrous oxide can be employed.

Various methods aimed at reducing the incidence of awareness have been suggested. Premedicant drugs such as hyoscine and diazepam have been claimed to reduce maternal awareness but the use of these drugs may be objected to for other reasons.

Mark[46] recommends the use of thiopentone increments whilst administering 100 per cent oxygen up until delivery. The use of ketamine as an induction agent may reduce the incidence of awareness and an etomidate infusion has been investigated as another answer to the problem.

Tunstall[45] demonstrated a reduction in awareness by using 66 per cent nitrous oxide for the period from 2 to 5 minutes following induction, before reverting to a higher inspired oxygen tension prior to delivery.

The method which currently finds most to commend it involves the addition of a low concentration of inhalational agent to the inspired mixture before delivery, remembering always that the MAC for the potent inhalational agents is substantially reduced in pregnancy.[47] Halothane 0·3–0·5 per cent, enflurane 0·6 per cent, methoxyflurane 0·2 per cent and trichloroethylene 0·2 per cent have been added to oxygen/nitrous oxide mixtures producing thereby a very low incidence of awareness and often resulting in the birth of infants in superior condition.

Halothane and isoflurane up to 1·5 MAC will produce an increase in uterine artery blood flow but, at the same MAC, will cause pronounced uterine relaxation, so the inspired concentration must be kept below these levels if increased haemorrhage is to be avoided. At the concentrations previously recommended, these inhalational agents do not result in increased blood loss at caesarean section.

### Ventilation

Relative hyperventilation is commonly used in non-obstetric anaesthesia but is potentially harmful to the fetus in obstetric anaesthesia, and even moderate hyperventilation, which may produce a $Paco_2$ of 23 mm Hg (3·1 kPa) is associated with falling fetal $Pao_2$, increasing base deficit, lower Apgar score at one minute and a delayed time to spontaneous respiration.[48] More severe hyperventilation which, in the pregnant woman, may easily lower $Paco_2$ to below 17 mm Hg (2·3 kPa) is associated with increasing fetal acidosis.[49]

Mechanisms which might be responsible for this deleterious effect on the fetus include uterine artery vasoconstriction secondary to the maternal hypocarbia, umbilical artery vasoconstriction secondary to fetal alkalosis, altered haemodynamics produced by the IPPV causing decreased uterine blood flow, or finally, a shift to the left of the oxyhaemoglobin dissociation curve with the respiratory alkalosis making oxygen exchange with the fetus more difficult.

Whatever the exact mechanism, minute volumes in excess of 100–120 ml/kg/min should be avoided during general anaesthesia for caesarean section.[50] There is no advantage to be gained by adding $CO_2$ to the inspired gas mixture to compensate for hyperventilation when the same result can be achieved safely by simply adjusting the minute volume.

### Oxygen Concentration

Early work had suggested that maternal hyperoxygenation was harmful to the fetus and that increases in the maternal inspired oxygen percentage beyond 66 per cent failed to produce any improvement in fetal oxygenation. Recent work has shown that the highest fetal oxygen tensions are obtained with inspired maternal oxygen concentrations of 95–100 per cent and that maternal hyperoxia increases fetal oxygen stores and improves both maternal and fetal acid-base status.[51–53] No problems have been encountered from the theoretical possibility of early closure of the ductus arteriosus.

There is a current trend towards the use of high concentrations (up to 100 per cent) of oxygen with reliance on a volatile agent to prevent awareness prior to delivery, and without doubt the maternal $Pao_2$ should be maintained above 300 mm Hg (40 kPa). This can only be achieved with a minimum maternal inspired oxygen concentration of 66 per cent.

### Induction-Delivery Interval

During general anaesthesia, the concentration of nitrous oxide, volatile agent or intermittently administered intravenous agent will progressively rise in the fetal circulation and, if delivery is long delayed, the agents may cause neonatal depression.

The optimal induction delivery interval is 10–20 minutes but up to 30 minutes is satisfactory so long as a high inspired oxygen concentration is maintained and aortocaval compression is studiously avoided.

Unawareness of the effects of aortocaval compression in the supine anaesthetised woman may have been responsible for the very hazardous, rapid surgery which was sometimes advocated for caesarean section.

The so-called U.D. interval (time from uterine incision to delivery of infant) is, however, of greater significance, and after 90 seconds fetal asphyxia and acidosis begin to become apparent, probably as a result of partial placental separation, impaired placental blood flow and premature fetal respiratory efforts causing aspiration of liquor.

### Conduct of Anaesthesia after Delivery

Once the umbilical cord has been clamped, the gas flow should be adjusted to deliver 66 per cent nitrous oxide, and an opiate given intravenously in an appropriate dose. Too large an opiate dose should be avoided, otherwise sedation postoperatively may further delay maternal infant contact.

Very low concentrations of an inhalational agent may be continued after delivery to counter the risk of awareness, but caution should be exercised as these agents may oppose uterine

40/TABLE 3
GENERAL ANAESTHESIA FOR CAESAREAN SECTION: AN OUTLINE

1. Pre-operative visit and explanation.
2. Antacid—30 ml before transport to theatre.
3. Journey tilt—NEVER transport supine. Maintain left lateral tilt UNTIL delivery.
4. Pre-oxygenation 6–8 l/min.
5. Check maternal blood pressure, fetal heart rate.
6. Intravenous cannula (use local anaesthetic).
7. Intravenous metoclopramide 10 mg.
   After minimum 3 minutes pre-oxygenation.
8. Cricoid pressure (instruct assistant).
9. I.V. Sodium thiopentone 250–300 mg over 10–20 sec
   Suxamethonium 100–120 mg.
10. Intubate when relaxation complete.
11. Remove cricoid pressure ONLY when endotracheal tube cuff inflated.
12. Ventilation: $O_2$ 6 l/min plus $N_2O$ 3 l/min
    Avoid hyperventilation
    Add halothane 0·3–0·5 per cent; enflurane 0·5–0·75 per cent.
13. Pancuronium 5–7 mg when necessary.
14. After delivery: increase $N_2O$, reduce $O_2$
    I.V. opiate
    I.V. oxytocin 5–10 iu.
15. ? empty stomach.
16. Monitor blood loss.
17. Reverse muscle relaxation, extubate with patient on side, head down.

contraction and may also cause prolonged maternal drowsiness postoperatively.

**Blood loss** during caesarean section under general anaesthesia usually measures 700–1000 ml, but transfusion can often be delayed because the mother is protected by the increased blood volume of pregnancy and by the autotransfusion she receives from the utero-placental circulation once the baby has been delivered and the uterus has contracted.

**Emptying the stomach.**—It is often worthwhile passing a tube into the stomach during anaesthesia to remove by suction whatever fluid there might be, especially if pre-induction emptying had not been performed. This reduces the risk of regurgitation either following extubation or in recovery, for the risks are often just as great during this period as at induction. The patient should always be extubated lying head down and on her side, but this should only take place after the muscle relaxation has been fully reversed with neostigmine and atropine.

## REGIONAL ANAESTHESIA FOR OPERATIVE OBSTETRICS

The risk of regurgitation and aspiration of stomach contents, the likelihood of drug-induced neonatal depression and the other problems associated with general anaesthesia may be largely avoided by using regional anaesthesia techniques. Pudendal nerve block or low spinal block may be appropriate for a lift-out forceps delivery or episiotomy repair; spinal or epidural blockade to T10 creates very good conditions for removal of a retained placenta or a mid-cavity forceps, whereas higher segmental blockade is ideal for caesarean section.

Regional anaesthesia is not without risks, and complications such as inadvertent intravascular injection or unexpectedly high segmental block with cardiovascular collapse may be life-threatening. There should be no relaxation in the high standard of care and supervision which every pregnant woman should receive, irrespective of the method of anaesthesia.

### Pudendal Nerve Block

The pudendal nerve is derived from the anterior primary rami of the second, third and fourth sacral nerves and carries the sensory nerves from most of the perineum, vulva and lower two-thirds of the vagina, and the motor supply to the external anal sphincter and the perineal muscles. Bilateral pudendal nerve block is only suitable for operations involving the lower vagina and perineum and will not relieve the pain of uterine contractions nor of operations such as removal of a retained placenta. Even so, the method has an unacceptably low success rate in many cases and it has been suggested that mid-cavity forceps should always be performed using other techniques such as lumbar or caudal epidural or spinal block.[31] However, pudendal nerve block is usually performed by the obstetrician, and the substitution of alternative blocks will signal a large increase in anaesthetic workload.

**Transperineal pudendal nerve block.**—The pudendal nerve can be blocked behind the ischial spine before it enters the canal in the wall of the ischiorectal fossa. A skin weal is raised over the ischial tuberosity and through this a 10 cm needle is inserted. The fingers of the free hand are placed in the vagina and the needle is guided through the ischiorectal fossa until the point lies above and behind the ischial spine, where 10 ml of local anaesthetic are injected. The nerve must be blocked on both sides.

**Transvaginal pudendal nerve block.**—This technique is performed with a guarded needle, the tip of which is inserted just above and behind the ischial spine. Compared to the transperineal method, this approach is technically simpler, less painful, has a higher success rate and is less likely to result in damage to the fetus or rectum. The needle point is passed first through the vaginal mucous membrane and then through the sacrospinous ligament to lie in the vicinity of the pudendal nerve.

Local infiltration will be required to block branches of the posterior cutaneous nerve of the thigh, the inferior haemorrhoidal nerve and the ilio-inguinal and genitofemoral nerves.

## Lumbar Epidural Block for Caesarean Section

Profound neural blockade of 17 spinal segments is required to guarantee pain-free surgery, so the anaesthetic technique needs to be meticulous in the extreme. Particular attention must be paid to ensure that cardiovascular stability is maintained and aortocaval compression avoided so that uteroplacental perfusion remains adequate. Supplementary oxygen for the mother is also essential.

### Technical Points

The outline of a suitable scheme is given in Table 4.

40/Table 4
Epidural Anaesthesia for Caesarean Section: An Outline

1. Visit and full explanation pre-operatively.
2. Routine antacid—0·3 M sodium citrate 30 ml before theatre.
3. Journey tilt; NEVER supine; wedge or tilt until delivery.
4. Check equipment and drugs for general anaesthesia.
5. Oxygen, by mask, until delivery.
6. Check maternal BP, fetal heart rate.
7. Intravenous cannula: (local anaesthetic)
   Commence Hartmann's 1 litre during block,
   1 litre during surgery.
8. Insert epidural catheter.
9. First dose: bupivacaine 0·5 per cent 10–12 ml; sitting; wait 10 minutes.
10. Assess upper level of analgesia.
    Second dose: bupivacaine 0·5 per cent 1·5 ml per segment unblocked below T6 level. Patient recumbent; wedge or tilt.
    (Note: a single dose of bupivacaine 0·75% 14–16 ml recumbent, may be excellent)
11. Prevent hypotension throughout.
    Avoid supine position.
    Treat falling BP early: I.V. fluid—ephedrine 5–10 mg I.V.; repeat if necessary.
12. Commence operation when block adequate.
13. Oxytocin 5–10 iu at delivery.
14. Additional bupivacaine 0·5 per cent, up to 6 ml.
15. Treat nausea: perphenazine;
    boredom: husband or diazepam.
16. Postoperative analgesia: maintain epidural.

**Preparation.**—The patient requires from the anaesthetist a very full explanation of everything that is likely to happen during the operation; she must be starved and have received 30 ml of antacid, as is the case for caesarean section under general anaesthesia.

The anaesthetist must prepare the anaesthetic room for a general anaesthetic and be satisfied that drugs and equipment are available to convert rapidly to a general anaesthetic should it become necessary.

**Position.**—The supine position must be avoided on the journey to theatre and thereafter until the baby is born. A wedge under the buttock, lateral tilt of the operating table, or one of the uterine displacement devices should be used. Babies delivered by caesarean section under epidural anaesthesia, of mothers who lie supine throughout, have a lower pH, higher plasma bupivacaine concentration and generally poorer condition than babies of mothers in whom aortocaval compression is avoided.[54]

**Intravenous fluid preloading** is an essential part of the epidural technique and up to 2 litres of a crystalloid solution (e.g. Hartmann's solution) should be infused while the block is being established and as surgery commences. Haemaccel and albumin have been recommended in volumes of 10–15 ml/kg but are much more expensive than crystalloid solutions and carry the risk of producing an adverse drug reaction.[55,56]

Prophylactic administration of intravenous ephedrine is not indicated, but ephedrine in increments of 5–10 mg should be given at the first sign of an impending fall in blood pressure. This technique will prevent any major fall occurring.[57] Atropine should be given if bradycardia occurs.

**Insertion of the epidural catheter** may be

accomplished with the patient sitting or in the left lateral position, and as soon as the catheter is secured, the patient should receive the first dose sitting and remain in this position for 10 minutes.[58] This refinement has overcome the problems of unblocked sacral segments transmitting pain during incision, and of manipulation of the pelvic peritoneum over the lower uterine segment. After 10 minutes, the height of the block should be assessed using gentle needle pricks and with the patient recumbent, either wedged or in a full lateral position. Additional local anaesthetic is given to shift the upper limit of the block to T6. A block to T4 produces increased maternal comfort when compared to a T7 block and by giving prophylactic ephedrine 25 mg (i.m.), the authors of this trial detected no change in the incidence of hypotension or fetal problems that are associated with the higher block compared to the T7 block.

When using bupivacaine 0·5 per cent plain solution, the sitting dose should be 10–12 ml and, after 10 minutes, a dose of 1·5 ml should be given in the recumbent position for every unblocked segment below the T6 dermatome. The mean total volume is 23 ml (115 mg) of the 0·5 per cent solution.[58] A further dose of 6 ml may be given after delivery of the infant and this will ensure the mother reaches the recovery ward pain free.

The administration of the local anaesthetic in this divided fashion, one dose sitting and one dose recumbent, reduces the impact of the large dose on the cardiovascular system and allows time for more of the fluid preload to be infused.

**Timing.**—Establishing a satisfactory block for a caesarean section operation is time-consuming and this technique is not suitable for the solo anaesthetist with a busy operating list or for the emergency case when rapid delivery is indicated. Undue haste will disturb the mother and attempting to start the surgery before the block is fully effective is likely to jeopardise the whole procedure. Always allow from 30–45 minutes from when the patient arrives in the anaesthetic room to when she will be ready for the incision. The presence of an epidural cannula inserted during labour will, of course, simplify matters.

**Choice of drug.**—Bupivacaine 0·5 per cent plain generally produces very good results and is, at present, the most popular choice in the United Kingdom, although the 0·75 per cent solutions of bupivacaine and etidocaine 1 to 1·5 per cent produce blocks of more rapid onset with an increased quality of sensory and motor block.[59] Initial experiences using 14–16 ml of bupivacaine 0·75% given as a single dose in the left lateral wedged position have produced excellent results and this may well be the technique of choice. Lignocaine 1·5–2 per cent with adrenaline 1:200 000 is also a very satisfactory choice. The safety of bupivacaine is an attractive feature and doses of 30 to 40 ml of the 0·5 per cent solution have been used without apparent maternal or infant problems.[60,61]

**Delivery.**—The mother should breathe 100 per cent oxygen until the baby is delivered, although some centres use a nitrous oxide/oxygen mixture instead.

Oxytocin 5–10 iu given slowly after delivery may be supplemented, if necessary, by a slow infusion of a solution containing 20 iu oxytocin diluted in 500 ml of a carrier such as dextrose 5 per cent. Too rapid injection of an oxytocin bolus may produce transient hypotension during high epidural blockade. Ergometrine should not be given to the awake patient because of the high incidence of nausea and vomiting which would result.

After delivery of the infant and the initial pleasure at handling her new child, the mother may become bored or restless, for this part of the operation occupies the most time. The husband can act as a very useful distraction at this stage or, if really indicated, a sedative such as diazepam may be given.

**Surgical considerations.**—Rough handling of the uterus or the insertion of packs above the uterus may be perceived as discomfort or pain by the mother, or may precipitate vomiting, so great gentleness is required on the part of the surgeon.

**Blood loss** is usually halved compared to caesarean section performed under general anaesthesia.

**Postoperative pain** can be controlled by using the epidural cannula to administer local anaesthetics or if adequate supervision is available, epidural opiates.

### Advantages and Disadvantages

Not all patients are psychologically suited to having major abdominal surgery whilst they are awake and if a mother is reluctant, she must never be forced to accept an epidural instead of general anaesthesia. The procedure is very time-consuming and because of this is unsuitable for emergency caesarean section. Failure to produce adequate sacral block will result in patient discomfort when the uterus is incised and to avoid undue stimulation, the whole surgical technique must be one of gentleness. Mothers having caesarean section under epidural analgesia not surprisingly experience greater psychic stress during the procedure but this has not been demonstrated as being harmful to the fetus.[62]

Epidural anaesthesia for caesarean section substantially reduces the risk of aspiration of stomach contents, and also the blood loss at operation and, at the same time, will provide an excellent form of postoperative analgesia. The mother is not denied total participation in the birth of her child and maternal-infant bonding can be established immediately. Successful breast-feeding is more likely with neural blockade than following general anaesthesia.[63] An earlier return of appetite, and enhanced gastric emptying occur when the epidural group is compared to patients receiving narcotic analgesics.

When the fetus is in good condition preoperatively, neither general nor epidural anaesthesia that is well conducted, seem to confer any advantage on the biochemical status of the infant, nor does either method improve performance in neonatal neurobehavioural tests. However, the ill or compromised fetus definitely benefits from having caesarean section delivery performed under epidural anaesthesia.[64–66]

## Subarachnoid Block

Subarachnoid block is widely used in the USA to provide analgesia for operative delivery and caesarean section, and recent calls have been made for the technique to be used more widely in the United Kingdom.[31,67]

Subarachnoid block is very easy to perform, is guided by a definite end point, and enjoys a very high success rate in producing excellent analgesia of very rapid onset. Unlike a lumbar epidural block, an intrathecal injection is assured of blocking all the sacral nerve roots, thus overcoming one of the problems of epidural analgesia for caesarean section. Because of the very small doses of local anaesthetic, fetal effects are minimal and neonatal neurobehavioural testing is superior in a spinal anaesthetic group compared to other forms of anaesthesia.

However, the technique possesses a number of *disadvantages*, the impact of which can be minimised by careful attention to detail:

(i) *Hypotension* is said to be more common than with epidural block, although it is unlikely to be a problem with low spinal and saddle blocks. The strategies to avoid hypotension are similar to those used for epidural blocks in obstetrics. The high incidence of hypotension which complicates the use of midspinal blocks for caesarean section has prompted trials of prophylactic ephedrine and the use of colloid solutions to a greater degree than with epidurals.[55,56]

(ii) *Headache*.—The incidence of headache following subarachnoid block seems to vary widely from centre to centre but rates as high as 16 per cent have been reported.[67] By using 25-gauge spinal needles, this incidence should reduce to less than 1 per cent. It has also been suggested that by puncturing the dura laterally, thereby avoiding a midline approach, this complication has been reduced.[66]

It is often thought that an instrumental delivery is obligatory once a dural puncture has been performed, in order to avoid the risk of increased cerebrospinal-fluid pressure associated with maternal pushing. However, one study was unable to demonstrate any difference in the incidence of headaches between women who delivered after bearing down and those who had elective forceps following subarachnoid block.[68]

(iii) *Single-shot technique*.—Because only a single injection is made, inadequate blocks cannot be topped-up or adjusted as with an epidural catheter, and no use can be made of the block to provide postoperative analgesia.

### Technique

**Saddle block** will block S2-4 and is suitable for forceps lift-out or episiotomy repairs only. The block will not abolish the pain of uterine contractions nor of any operative manipulations.

40/TABLE 5
SUBARACHNOID BLOCK
Suggested doses for blocks in obstetrics.
Injections should be given over 5–10 seconds and timing commenced from then.

| *Technique & Block* | *Saddle* | *Block to T10* | *Block to T6* |
|---|---|---|---|
| Lumbar puncture | L 4, 5 | L 3, 4 | L 3, 4 |
| Position | Sitting for 1–3 min | Sitting for 5–15 sec | Lateral to supine, with wedge |
| *Drugs* | | | |
| lignocaine (hyperbaric) 5·0% | 15–20 mg | 30–50 mg | 50–75 mg |
| cinchocaine (hyperbaric) 0·5% | 3·0 mg | 4–5 mg | 6–9 mg |
| amethocaine (hyperbaric) 0·5% | 3·0 mg | 4–5 mg | 6–9 mg |
| Volume (approximately) | 0·6 ml | 0·8–1 ml (but may be as high as 1·5 ml) | 1·2–1·8 ml (but may be as high as 2·5 ml) |

The injection should be given slowly over 5–10 seconds and the patient should remain in a sitting position for 1–3 minutes (see Table 5).

**Low spinal block** will block to T10 and will block the pain of contractions as well as providing excellent analgesia for mid-cavity forceps, assisted breech delivery or manual removal of the placenta. Compared to a pudendal nerve block, the analgesia produced by a low spinal block is infinitely superior for the mother, the infant and the obstetrician.

Once the injection is completed, the patient should remain sitting for 5–15 seconds and then placed supine with a wedge in position before being placed into the lithotomy position.

**Mid-spinal block** will block from above T6 to S5 and is suitable for caesarean section. The injection should be inserted with the patient lying in the left lateral position and she should be immediately turned to lie supine with a wedge. A slight degree of head-down tilt may sometimes be desirable to spread the upper extent of the block.

### Local Infiltration for Caesarean Section

Where expert anaesthetic help is unavailable, caesarean section can be very readily performed using local infiltration and women who have had one such operation will willingly submit to a second caesarean section using the same form of anaesthesia. The technique is well described by Ranney,[69] who uses 60–100 ml of procaine 1 per cent plain, and by Gordh[70] using up to 100 ml of lignocaine 0·25 per cent with adrenaline 1:200,000.

### Postoperative Analgesia after Operative Obstetrics

Caesarean section, or other operative delivery, often leaves the mother in a great deal of pain postoperatively and the pain of the incision may be exaggerated by the discomfort of a urinary catheter, of sore breasts, or by feelings of disappointment if the mother was hoping for a vaginal delivery.

The need for analgesia must be weighed against the needs for the mother and baby to be alert and able to interact with each other as soon as possible, for this early bonding is said to be a vital determinant of future infant development. Systemic analgesics are often very sedative, so regional techniques are strongly indicated, bearing in mind that urinary retention and peripheral motor weakness may be undesirable results. Whenever an epidural catheter has been used during pre-operative labour, or for the actual operation, top-up doses of either local anaesthetic or opiates should be given postoperatively. Bupivacaine 0·125–0·25 per cent in modest doses of 5–10 ml may give satisfactory analgesia with minimal side-effects. The use of epidural opiates is fraught with hazard in inexperienced hands (see below).

## EMERGENCY OPERATIONS DURING LABOUR

When fetal or maternal survival demand an immediate operation, no time should be lost trying to perform a regional block and the anaesthetist must proceed immediately to general anaesthesia. For this reason, syringes of thiopentone and suxamethonium should be freshly drawn up every day and stored in a refrigerator on the labour ward so that these drugs are instantly available in an emergency. All the anaesthetic equipment needed for a major abdominal operation should also be stored and maintained in working condition on the labour ward.

Irrespective of the urgency of the operation, no patient must ever be induced whilst in the lithotomy position. The need to avoid aortocaval compression is nowhere more vital than in these situations where fetal wellbeing may be already compromised. Every general anaesthetic must be conducted using the full obstetric anaesthetic routine, since the risks of regurgitation do not alter with the indicaton for the operation. There is absolutely no place for the quickly administered inhalational anaesthetic in obstetrics.

If some delay is permissible, a subarachnoid block will produce the most rapid anaesthesia, providing a regional technique is thought justifiable.

As a guide-line, Davis[71] has related the degree of urgency of the caesarean section with the method of anaesthesia that would be appropriate. He feels that unless 30–45 minutes are available from the time the decision to operate is made until the time delivery is desirable, general anaesthesia is the only feasible anaesthetic. Between 30 and 45 minutes, subarachnoid block could be used; between 45 and 60 minutes, extension of an existing epidural; and only if 60–90 minutes is allowable between decision and delivery should a new epidural block be contemplated. In one hospital which practised a high rate of epidural caesarean section, 64 per cent of the administration of general anaesthesia was given because of time factors.[71]

Table 6 illustrates some of the factors associated with an increased likelihood of caesarean section. Early identification of these patients and of those likely to require assisted delivery (such as breech presentations) should enable the anaesthetist to establish a working epidural unhurriedly and early in labour. This will further reduce the need for urgent general anaesthetics on the labour ward.

### Operative Obstetrics

**General versus regional anaesthesia.**—The anaesthetist must not be lured into the sole advocacy of one or other technique for obstetric anaesthesia. The advantages to the mother and baby and the satisfaction gained by the anaesthetist is often greater with a regional procedure; but in many circumstances, general anaesthesia may be best for the baby, may be desired by the mother or may be more safely and easily performed by the anaesthetist, whilst leaving the obstetrician better able to deal with the problems facing him.

40/Table 6
Factors Associated with Increased Likelihood of Caesarean Section (from Davis, 1982[71]).

| | |
|---|---|
| Obstetric background | Short stature/large baby<br>Unfavourable cervix<br>Malpresentation<br>Multiple pregnancy<br>Primigravida over 30 |
| Developments during labour | More than 10 hours in labour<br>Slow dilatation of cervix<br>Failure of presenting part to descend<br>Failure of conventional methods of analgesia<br>Warning signs of impaired fetal wellbeing |

Although regional analgesia vastly reduces the risks of pulmonary acid aspiration, the consequences of cardiovascular collapse from poorly conducted epidural or spinal analgesia could alter the nature, but not the numbers, of maternal deaths.

## COMPLICATED OBSTETRICS

In many complicated obstetric situations, the survival of the mother or fetus may be in question and anaesthetic or analgesic techniques which reduce uteroplacental blood flow or depress neonatal respirations are totally inappropriate and must not be employed. Likewise, dangers of the supine position and aortocaval compression are nowhere more harmful. Regional techniques are generally the methods of choice.

### Breech Presentation

An anaesthetist should be present for every breech delivery and, if possible, an epidural block should be established early in labour. Epidural block provides both maximum analgesia and pelvic relaxation for the delivery of the after-coming head. If uterine relaxation is required suddenly, an amyl nitrate capsule can be crushed and inhaled from a Magill circuit, or two puffs taken from a salbutamol inhaler. There should never be a need for sudden, hazardous induction of general anaesthesia.

When breech-presentation labour is conducted with epidural analgesia, there is no increase in the duration of labour, the incidence of breech extraction is reduced and infant condition after birth is improved. Thus epidural analgesia is the method of choice.[72]

### Prematurity

These immature infants require special consideration for vaginal delivery. Descent of the head should be well controlled and achieved with minimal pushing, followed by gentle lift-out forceps delivery through a generous episiotomy. Epidural analgesia or a low spinal block will provide adequate conditions for the premature delivery and will also avoid the risks of neonatal depression in an immature infant following systemic analgesia.

### Multiple Gestation

A multiple delivery often combines the problems of prematurity and breech presentation with consideration for the well-being of the second twin. There is a well-recognised increase in morbidity and mortality associated with second twins, and this often follows a prolonged interval between the first and second deliveries. Epidural analgesia is now considered to be positively indicated and produces no prolongation of the first stage, no increase in the incidence of breech extraction, often a shorter interval between first and second twin delivery, and no adverse effect on neonatal morbidity or mortality. An adequate block allows prompt intervention to deliver either twin.[73,74]

The larger uterus will increase the likelihood of aortocaval compression. Quadruplets have been successfully delivered using epidural analgesia.

### Uterine Scar

If a scar exists in the uterus, following previous caesarean section or other uterine surgery, the question arises as to whether epidural analgesia during a subsequent labour will either increase the risk of the scar rupturing or cause delay in diagnosis once rupture has occurred. Opinion differs, but many now feel that epidural block does not increase the risk of rupture and that the main danger lies in overstimulation with oxytocin. Pain is a relatively infrequent sign of scar dihescence[75] and a selective epidural technique is thought unlikely to impede the appreciation of such pain as might occur. The pain will "get through" the epidural block.

Other signs of rupture, apart from pain, should be constantly sought. These signs include increasing heart rate, decreasing blood pressure, sudden cessation of contractions, fresh vaginal bleeding and alteration in the scar to palpation. In one series of 119 cases with uterine scars who had labour conducted under epidural analgesia, only two suffered rupture of the scar.[76]

A suggested scheme for providing epidural blockade for a "trial of the scar" is as follows:[77]

1. Minimal analgesia, e.g. bupivacaine 0·125 per cent, intermittent, not continuous.
2. Stringent monitoring, frequent abdominal examination, and urgent caesarean section if any doubt exists.
3. Avoid oxytocic drugs unless absolutely essential.
4. If uterine overactivity occurs, discontinue epidural block until normal activity is resumed.

### Pre-eclampsia

Epidural blockade is strongly indicated during labour and apart from providing pain relief, will often encourage an increase in uteroplacental and intervillous blood flows. The epidural block should never be used to lower the blood pressure; other pharmacological methods are indicated, but once the block is established, the blood pressure will fall and the swings of blood pressure with contractions will be minimised. Epidural blockade has no effect on maternal cardiac output in the pre-eclamptic patient.[78]

Anaesthesia for caesarean section is best provided by epidural blockade, although any tendency to hypotension must be carefully controlled.[79] General anaesthesia in the pre-eclamptic patient may present a number of problems. Induction and intubation are likely to precipitate large rises in blood pressure with the risk of pulmonary oedema or a cerebrovascular accident. It is recommended that hydralazine or nitroglycerine infusion be commenced before induction, to allow prompt control of any rises in blood pressure. Ketamine must not be used as an induction agent. Laryngeal oedema has been frequently described in association with pre-eclampsia and may cause difficulty with intubation.

If magnesium sulphate has been used in the pre-operative management of pre-eclampsia, then the dose of non-depolarising muscle relaxant should be cautiously titrated against the response to a peripheral-nerve stimulator.

### Maternal Heart Disease

The clinical details of each individual case will dictate any special anaesthetic consideration but in general the aim should be to minimise the wide fluctuations in heart rate and cardiac output that may be associated with the pain and stress of delivery. Intensive monitoring, including central venous pressure and pulmonary artery wedge pressure, should be employed where necessary.

Epidural analgesia is the method of choice for lesions such as mitral stenosis and incompetence, aortic incompetence and congenital heart disease with left-to-right shunts. Some other lesions such as aortic stenosis and cases with pulmonary hypertension may not tolerate the cardiovascular changes induced by an epidural block, although selective epidural block has been used in labour for a patient with pulmonary hypertension.[80] A parturient with a single ventricle obtained satisfactory analgesia during labour from two intrathecal injections of 1 mg of morphine.[81]

Regional analgesia will permit easy forceps delivery and avoid the potentially very harmful Valsalva effect produced by maternal pushing in the second stage.

The use of ergometrine should be avoided. For further details, see Gothard, 1978.[82]

### Diabetes Mellitus

Pregnancy and labour in a woman who suffers from insulin-dependent diabetes is a more hazardous affair than for the non-diabetic woman. The incidence of large babies is increased, unexplained stillbirths, premature labour and pre-eclampsia occur more commonly, and perinatal mortality may be as high as 9 per cent.[83]

Analgesia during labour should be provided with an epidural block to minimise any hormonal upset caused by pain and anxiety. Maternal blood sugar levels should be checked regularly and neonatal hypoglycaemia watched for after delivery.

Careful control of insulin dosage coupled with glucose infusion is necessary before caesarean section (see p. 995). General anaesthesia is suitable but epidural blockade provides excellent, stress-free operating conditions.

### Antepartum Haemorrhage

Patients with placenta praevia or abruptio placentae may present for examination under anaesthesia following antepartum haemorrhage, and this examination has to be conducted so that it can proceed rapidly to caesarean section if necessary. The situation may sometimes be very grave as a coagulopathy develops and complete volume replacement is often impossible to achieve before surgery has to be undertaken. Central venous pressure should be monitored in every case and regional anaesthesia should not be used in the face of severe hypovolaemia or a coagulopathy. General anaesthesia using a faultless obstetric anaesthetic technique is indicated and induction should be performed with very cautious doses of thiopentone or ketamine. Ketamine is much better tolerated by the hypovolaemic circulation.

### Acute Inversion of the Uterus

This may present as a sudden emergency on the labour ward following delivery and the patient will suffer severe shock, either haemorrhagic or neurogenic in origin. Rapid induction of general anaesthesia with relaxation of the uterus may be necessary.

### Retained Placenta

In the absence of an established epidural block, which will provide excellent conditions for the removal of a retained placenta, the choice of anaesthesia lies between a full obstetric general anaesthetic (modified because of the absence of a fetus), or a simple subarachnoid block, which will rapidly provide analgesia up to the T10 segmental level. If the patient is hypovolaemic, vigorous volume replacement is necessary and if hypovolaemia is severe, then regional block should be avoided in favour of a general anaesthetic. Uterine relaxation can be achieved during regional block by inhaling two puffs from a salbutamol inhaler, or by crushing an amyl nitrate capsule into a Magill circuit and breathing from a mask.

## Monitoring in Obstetrics

**Maternal** monitoring should be very intensive in many of these complicated obstetric situations.

**Central venous pressure** and, if necessary, pulmonary artery wedge pressures, can greatly assist the management of severe pre-eclampsia, maternal cardiac disease and any of the haemorrhagic conditions. A negative correlation exists between diastolic pressure and central venous pressure in the pre-eclamptic states.

**Arterial blood gas** measurement is very important in diagnosing the aetiology of maternal acidosis which often develops during prolonged or difficult labour. Lactacidaemia will result from excessive stress and should be treated with epidural analgesia, whereas ketoacidosis requires an infusion of intravenous dextrose.[84]

**Fetal monitoring** is detailed in Chapter 41.

### Epidural and Intrathecal Opiates in Obstetrics

The use of spinal opiates in obstetrics originally promised the following potential advantages:

1. Only small doses of opiate would be necessary, thereby avoiding the problems of maternal and neonatal depression from large systemic doses.
2. Effective regional analgesia without the problems of local anaesthetic block—hypotension, motor weakness and bladder disturbances.
3. Preservation of normal abdominal and pelvic muscle tone will aid rotation of the fetal head and allow the mother to push when necessary.

In reality, the results have been very variable and the role of the currently available opiates given spinally in obstetrics is still uncertain.

#### Analgesia During Labour

The effect produced by the spinal opiates is incapable of providing analgesia for operative obstetrics and in many cases supplementation with local anaesthetic has been necessary in the second stage of labour.

Best results have been obtained using morphine or $\beta$-endorphin given intrathecally. Intrathecal morphine in doses of 1–2 mg produces analgesia throughout the whole of the first stage in a high percentage of cases,[85,86] although the incidence of side-effects such as somnolence, nausea and vomiting, and severe pruritis is often very high.

Intrathecal $\beta$-endorphin produces analgesia in the range of 12–32 hours (mean 18 hours) with very few maternal side-effects and no neonatal depression. Unfortunately, the size of the molecule makes intrathecal injection necessary, and this, of course, creates all the problems associated with dural puncture. However, the results are said to show great promise[87]

Morphine possesses relatively poor lipid solubility so, not surprisingly, the epidural route is less favourable and, in fact, results of epidural morphine in obstetrics have been very poor.[88–92] Sometimes better results have been reported using pethidine in doses of 25–100 mg with or without adrenaline 1:200,000[93–94] and with fentanyl,[95] although the effects of these drugs is never as reliably reproducible as is the effect of a local anaesthetic epidural block.

The use of a highly soluble opiate such as fentanyl may be advantageous in very early labour when local anaesthetic block is undesirable, in some cases where motor and sympathetic block need to be specifically avoided, and in the supplementation of local anaesthetic blocks that are providing unsatisfactory analgesia. Epidural morphine was used successfully to provide analgesia for labour in a woman with a single ventricle.[81]

#### Postoperative Analgesia

The spinal opiates find much more satisfactory use in the treatment of postoperative pain. After caesarean section, epidural morphine 4 mg has produced analgesia with a mean duration of 22–27 hours in a number of trials.[96,97] The incidence of unwanted side-effects, particularly pruritus, was high. Epidural morphine in a dose of 2 mg was much less effective postoperatively.[98] Fentanyl, pethidine, methadone, diamorphine and phenoperidine have all been used postoperatively, with variable results.

Whenever a patient receives an epidural or intrathecal opiate injection, she may be in great danger of suffering delayed respiratory depression at any time in the ensuing 12 hours. The risk of this occurring is increased if other sedative or opiate drugs have been given to the patient, and the literature abounds with reports of respiratory arrests occurring in such cases. Great caution should be exercised in the use of these drugs, and constant supervision must be available for at least twelve hours after any spinal opiate injection. Respiratory depression can be readily treated with intravenous naloxone, but only if the patient is actually being observed at the time her respiration rate declines.

## REFERENCES


1. Breheny, F. and McCarthy, J. (1982). Maternal mortality. A review of maternal deaths over twenty years at the National Maternity Hospital, Dublin. *Anaesthesia*, **37**, 561.
2. Morgan, C. A. and Paull, J. (1980). Drugs in obstetric anaesthesia. *Anaesth. Intens. Care*, **8**, 278.
3. Marx, G. F. (1982). Cardiopulmonary resuscitation of late-pregnant women. *Anesthesiology*, **56**, 156.
4. Department of Health and Social Security (1982). *Report on Confidential Enquiries into Maternal Deaths in England and Wales, 1976–1978*. London: HMSO.
5. Mendelson, C. L. (1946). The aspiration of stomach contents into the lungs during obstetric anaesthesia. *Am. J. Obstet. Gynecol.*, **52**, 191.
6. Taylor, G. and Pryse-Davies, J. (1966). The prophylactic use of antacids in the prevention of acid pulmonary aspiration syndrome. *Lancet*, **1**, 288.
7. Schwartz, D. J., Wynne, J. W. and Gibbs, C. P. (1980). The pulmonary consequences of aspiration of gastric contents at pH values greater than 2·5. *Am. Rev. Respir. Dis.*, **121**, 119.
8. Fein, A. M., Goldberg, S. K., Lippmann, M. L., Fisher, F. and Morgan, L. (1982). Adult respiratory distress syndrome. *Brit. J. Anaesth.*, **54**, 723.
9. Gomez, A. C. (1968). Pulmonary insufficiency in non-thoracic trauma. *J. Trauma*, **8**, 656.
10. Hanson, G. C. (1978). The pulmonary aspiration syndrome. In: *The Medical Management of the Critically Ill*. Edited by G. C. Hanson and P. L. Wright. London: Academic Press.
11. Crawford, J. S. (1978). *Principles and Practice of Obstetric Anaesthesia*, 4th edit. Oxford: Blackwell.
12. Roper, R. E. and Salem, M. G. (1981). Effects of glycopyrrolate and atropine combined with antacid on gastric acidity. *Brit. J. Anaesth.*, **53**, 1277.
13. Manchikanti, L., Kraus, J. W. and Edds, S. P. (1982). Cimetidine and related drugs in anesthesia. *Anesth. Analg. Curr. Res.*, **61**, 595.
14. Cotton, B. R. and Smith, G. (1981). Comparison of the effects of atropine and glycopyrrolate on lower oesophageal sphincter pressure. *Brit. J. Anaesth.*, **53**, 875.
15. Gibbs, C. P., Spohr, L. and Schmidt, D. (1982). The effectiveness of sodium citrate as an antacid. *Anesthesiology*, **57**, 44.
16. Cohen, S. E. (1979). Aspiration syndromes in pregnancy. *Anesthesiology*, **51**, 375.
17. Gibbs, C. P., Schwartz, D. J., Wynne, J. W., Hood, C. I. and Kuck, E. J. (1979). Antacid pulmonary aspiration in the dog. *Anesthesiology*, **51**, 380.
18. Eyler, S. W., Cullen, B. F., Murphy, M. E. and Welch, W. D. (1982). Antacid aspiration in rabbits: a comparison of Mylonta and Bicitra. *Anesth. Analg. Curr. Res.*, **61**, 288.
19. Bassell, G. M. and Gatha, M. K. (1980). Pulmonary aspiration following antacid therapy (letter). *Anesthesiology*, **52**, 450.
20. Gibbs, C. P. and Wynne, J. W. (1980). Maternal mortality and anaesthesia (letter). *Brit. J. Anaesth.*, **52**, 842.
21. Dewan, D. M., Writer, W. D. R., Wheeler, A. S., James, F. M., Floyd, H. M., Bogard, T. D. and Rhyne, L. (1982). Sodium citrate premedication in elective Caesarean section patients. *Canad. Anaesth. Soc. J.*, **29**, 355.
22. Viegas, O. J., Ravindran, R. S. and Shumacker, C. A. (1981). Gastric fluid pH in patients receiving sodium citrate. *Anesth. Analg. Curr. Res.*, **60**, 521.
23. Wrobel, J., Koh, T. C. and Saunders, J. M. (1982). Sodium citrate: an alternative antacid for prophylaxis against aspiration pneumonitis. *Anesth. Intens. Care*, **10**, 116.
24. Holdsworth, J. D., Johnson, K., Mascall, G., Gwynne Roulston, R. and Tomlinson, P. A. (1980). Mixing of antacids with stomach contents. Another approach to the prevention of the acid aspiration (Mendelson's) syndrome. *Anaesthesia*, **35**, 641.
25. Coombs, D. W., Hooper, D. and Colton, T. (1979). Pre-anesthetic cimetidine alteration of gastric fluid volume and pH. *Anesth. Analg. Curr. Res.*, **58**, 183.
26. Dundee, J. W., Moore, J., Johnston, J. R. and McCaughey, W. (1981). Cimetidine and obstetric anaesthesia. *Lancet*, **2**, 252.
27. Steinberg, W. H., Lewis, J. H. and Katz, D. M. (1982). Antacids inhibit absorption of cimetidine. *New Engl. J. Med.*, **307**, 400.
28. Andrews, A. D., Brock-Utne, J. G. and Downing, J. W. (1982). Protection against pulmonary acid aspiration with ranitidine. A new histamine $H_2$ receptor antagonist. *Anaesthesia*, **37**, 22.
29. Baraka, A., Saab, M., Salem, M. R. and Winnie, A. P. (1977). Control of gastric acidity by glycopyrrolate premedication in the parturient. *Anesth. Analg. Curr. Res.*, **56**, 642.
30. Stoeling, R. K. (1978). Responses to atropine, glycopyrrolate and Riopan of gastric fluid pH and volume in adult patients. *Anesthesiology*, **48**, 367.
31. Moir, D. D. (1980). *Obstetric Anaesthesia and Analgesia*, 2nd edit. London: Baillière Tindall.
32. Hey, V. M. F., Ostick, D. G., Mazumder, J. K. and Lord, W. D. (1981). Pethidine, metoclopramide and the gastro-oesophageal sphincter. A study in healthy volunteers. *Anaesthesia*, **36**, 173.
33. Freund, F. G. and Rubin, A. D. (1972). The need for additional succinylcholine after d-tubocurarine. *Anesthesiology*, **36**, 185.
34. Sellick, R. A. (1961). Cricoid pressure to control regurgitation of stomach contents during induction of anaesthesia: preliminary communication. *Lancet*, **2**, 404.

35. Crawford, J. W. (1979). Premedication for elective Caesarean section. *Anaesthesia*, **34**, 874.
36. Ong, B. Y., Pickering, B. G., Palahniuk, R. J. and Cumming, M. (1982). Lorazepam and diazepam as adjuncts to epidural anaesthesia for Caesarean section. *Canad. Anaesth. Soc. J.*, **29**, 31.
37. Rubin, J., Brock-Utne, J. G., Dimopoulos, G. F., Downing, J. W. and Moshal, M. G. (1982). Flunitrazepam increases and diazepam decreases the lower oesophageal sphincter tone when administered intravenously. *Anaesth. Intens. Care*, **10**, 130.
38. Downing, J. W., Buley, R. J. R., Brock-Utne, J. G. and Houlton, P. C. (1979). Etomidate for induction of anaesthesia at Caesarean section: comparison with thiopentone. *Brit. J. Anaesth.*, **51**, 135.
39. Dich-Nielsen, J. and Holasek, J. (1982). Ketamine as induction agent for Caesarean section. *Acta anaesth. scand.*, **26**, 139.
40. Oats, J. N., Vasey, D. P. and Waldron, B. A. (1979). Effects of ketamine on the pregnant uterus. *Brit. J. Anaesth.*, **51**, 1163.
41. Smith, G., Dalling, R. and Williams, T. I. R. (1978). Gastro-oesophageal pressure gradient changes produced by induction of anaesthesia and suxamethonium. *Brit. J. Anaesth.*, **50**, 1137.
42. Corall, I. M., Ward, M. E., Page, J. and Strunin, L. (1977). Conditions for tracheal intubation following fazadinium and pancuronium. *Brit. J. Anaesth.*, **49**, 615.
43. Blackburn, C. L. and Morgan, M. (1978). Comparison of speed of onset of fazadinium, pancuronium, tubocurarine and suxamethonium. *Brit. J. Anaesth.*, **50**, 361.
44. Tunstall, M. E. (1976). Failed intubation drill. *Anaesthesia*, **31**, 850.
45. Tunstall, M. E. (1979). The reduction of amnesic wakefulness during Caesarean section. *Anaesthesia*, **34**, 316.
46. Mark, L. C. and Poppers, P. J. (1982). The dilemma of general anaesthesia for Caesarean section: adequate fetal oxygenation v. maternal awareness during operation. *Anesthesiology*, **56**, 405.
47. Palahniuk, R. J., Shnider, S. M. and Eger, E. I. (1974). Pregnancy decreases the requirements for inhaled anesthetic agents. *Anesthesiology*, **41**, 82.
48. Peng, A. T. C., Blancato, L. S. and Motoyama, E. K. (1972). Effect of maternal hypocapnia v. eucapnia on the foetus during Caesarean section. *Brit. J. Anaesth.*, **44**, 1173.
49. Moya, F., Morishima, H., Shnider, S. M. and James, L. S. (1965). Influence of maternal hyperventilation on the newborn infant. *Am. J. Obstet. Gynecol.*, **91**, 76.
50. Datta, S. and Alper, M. H. (1980). Anesthesia for Cesarean Section. *Anesthesiology*, **53**, 142.
51. Marx, G. F. and Mateo, C. V. (1971). Effects of different oxygen concentrations during general anaesthesia for elective Caesarean section. *Canad. Anaesth. Soc. J.*, **18**, 587.
52. Palahniuk, R. J., Scatliff, J., Biehl, D., Wiebe, H. and Sankaran, K. (1977). Maternal and neonatal effects of methoxyflurane, nitrous oxide and lumbar epidural analgesia for Caesarean section. *Canad. Anaesth. Soc. J.*, **24**, 586.
53. Ramanathan, S., Gandhi, S., Arismendy, J., Chalon, J. and Turndorf, H. (1982). Oxygen transfer from mother to fetus during Cesarean section under epidural anesthesia. *Anesth. Analg. Curr. Res.*, **61**, 576.
54. Datta, S., Alper, M. H., Ostheimer, G. W., Brown, W. U. and Weiss, J. B. (1979). Effects of maternal position on epidural anesthesia for Cesarean section, acid-base status and bupivacaine concentrations at delivery. *Anesthesiology*, **50**, 205.
55. Huovinen, K., Lehtovirta, P., Forss, M., Kivalo, I. and Teramo, K. (1979). Changes in placental intervillous blood flow measured by the $^{133}$Xenon method during lumbar epidural block for elective Caesarean section. *Acta anaesth. scand.*, **23**, 529.
56. Mathru, M., Rao, T. L. K. Kartha, R. K., Shanmugham, M. and Jacobs, K. H. (1980). Intravenous albumin administration for prevention of spinal hypotension during Cesarean section. *Anesth. Analg. Curr. Res.*, **59**, 655.
57. Datta, S., Alper, M. H., Ostheimer, G. W. and Weiss, J. B. (1982). Method of ephedrine administration and nausea and hypotension during spinal anesthesia for Cesarean section. *Anesthesiology*, **56**, 68.
58. Thorburn, J. and Moir, D. D. (1980). Epidural analgesia for elective Caesarean section. *Anaesthesia*, **35**, 3.
59. Sinclair, C. J. and Scott, D. B. (1982). Double-blind comparison of 0·75% bupivacaine and 1·5% etidocaine with and without epinephrine in epidural block. *Regional Anesthesia*, **7**, 77.
60. McGuiness, G. A., Merkow, A. J., Kennedy, R. L. and Erenberg, A. (1978). Epidural anaesthesia with bupivacaine for Cesarean section. *Anesthesiology*, **49**, 270.
61. Crawford, J. S. (1982). *Obstetric Analgesia and Anaesthesia*. 1. Current Reviews in Obstetrics and Gynaecology: Edinburgh: Churchill/Livingstone.
62. Kanto, J., Vinamaki, O., Gronroos, M., Lammintausta, R. and Liukko, P. (1981). Blood glucose, insulin, antidiuretic hormones and renin activity response during Caesarean section performed under general anaesthesia or epidural analgesia. *Acta anaesth. scand.*, **25**, 442.
63. Brownridge, P. and Jefferson, J. (1979). Central neural blockade and Cesarean section. II. Patient assessment of the procedures. *Anaesth. Intens. Care*, **7**, 163.
64. James, F. M., Crawford, J. S., Hopkinson, R., Davies, P. and Naiem, H. (1977). A comparison of general anaesthesia and lumbar epidural analgesia for elective Cesarean section. *Anesth. Analg. Curr. Res.*, **56**, 228.
65. Downing, J. W., Houlton, P. C. and Barclay, A. (1979). Extradural analgesia for Caesarean section: comparison with general anaesthesia. *Brit. J. Anaesth.*, **51**, 367.
66. Marx, G. F. (1980). Regional analgesia versus general anaesthesia for Caesarean section. *Anaesthesia*, **35**, 1126.
67. Crawford, J. S. (1979). Experience with spinal analgesia in a British obstetric unit. *Brit. J. Anaesth.*, **51**, 531.
68. Ravindran, R. S., Viegas, O. J., Tasch, M. D., Cline, P. J., Deaton, R. L. and Brown, T. R. (1981). Bearing down at the time of delivery and the incidence of spinal headache in parturients. *Anesth. Analg. Curr. Res.*, **60**, 524.
69. Ranney, B. and Stanage, W. F. (1975). Advantages of local anesthesia for Cesarean section. *Obstet. Gynecol.*, **45**, 163.
70. Gordh, T. (1979). Infiltration anaesthesia for caesarean section. In: *Illustrated Handbook in Local Anaesthesia*, 2nd edit. Edited by E. Eriksson. London: Lloyd-Luke.
71. Davis, A. G. (1982). Anaesthesia for Caesarean section. The potential for regional block. *Anaesthesia*, **37**, 748.
72. Breeson, A. J., Kovacs, G. T., Pickles, B. G. and Hill, J. G. (1978). Extradural analgesia: the preferred method

of analgesia for vaginal breech delivery. *Brit. J. Anaesth.*, **50**, 1227.
73. Crawford, J. S. (1975). An appraisal of lumbar epidural blockade in labour in patients with multiple pregnancy. *Brit. J. Obstet. Gynaec.*, **82**, 929.
74. Weekes, A. R. L., Cheridjian, V. E. and Mwanje, D. K. (1977). Lumbar epidural analgesia in labour in twin pregnancy. *Brit. med. J.*, **2**, 730.
75. Case, B. D., Corcoran, R., Jeffcoate, N. and Randle, G. H. (1971). Caesarean section and its place in modern obstetric practice. *J. Obstet. Gynaec. Brit. Cwlth.*, **78**, 203.
76. Carlsson, C., Nybell-Lindahl, G. and Ingemarsson, I. (1980). Extradural block in patients who have previously undergone Caesarean section. *Brit. J. Anaesth.*, **52**, 827.
77. Bromage, P. R. (1978). *Epidural Analgesia.* Philadelphia: W. B. Saunders.
78. Graham, C. and Goldstein, A. (1980). Epidural analgesia and cardiac output in severe pre-eclampsia. *Anaesthesia*, **35**, 709.
79. Hodgkinson, R., Husain, F. J. and Hayashi, R. H. (1980). Systemic and pulmonary blood pressure during Caesarean section in parturients with gestational hypertension. *Canad. Anaesth. Soc. J.*, **27**, 389.
80. Sørensen, M. B., Korshin, J. D., Fernandes, A. and Secher, O. (1982). The use of epidural analgesia for delivery in a patient with pulmonary hypertension. *Acta anaesth. scand.*, **26**, 180.
81. Ahmad, S., Hawes, D., Dooley, S., Faure, E. and Brunner, E. A. (1981). Intrathecal morphine in a parturient with a single ventricle. *Anesthesiology*, **54**, 515.
82. Gothard, J. W. W. (1978). Heart disease in pregnancy. *Anaesthesia*, **33**, 523.
83. Essex, N. L., Pyke, D. A., Watkins, P. J., Brudnell, J. M. and Gamsu, H. R. (1973). Diabetic pregnancy. *Brit. med. J.*, **4**, 89.
84. Marx, G. F., Desai, P. K. and Habib, N. S. (1980). Detection and differentiation of metabolic acidosis in parturients. *Anesth. Analg. Curr. Res.*, **59**, 929.
85. Scott, P. V., Bowen, F. E., Cartwright, P., Rao, B. C. M., Deeley, D., Wotherspoon, H. G. and Sumrein, I. M. A. (1980). Intrathecal morphine as sole analgesic during labour. *Brit. med. J.*, **281**, 351.
86. Baraka, A., Noveitrid, R. and Hajj, S. (1981). Intrathecal injection of morphine for obstetric analgesia. *Anesthesiology*, **54**, 136.
87. Oyama, T., Matsuki, A., Taneichi, T., Ling, N. and Guillemin, R. (1980). $\beta$ endorphin in obstetric analgesia. *Amer. J. Obstet. Gynecol.*, **137**, 613.
88. Bapat, A. R., Kshirsagar, N. A., and Bapat, R. D. (1979). Aspects of epidural morphine. *Lancet*, **2**, 584.
89. Booker, P. D., Bryson, T. H. L. and Beddard, J. (1980). Obstetric pain relief using epidural morphine. *Anaesthesia*, **35**, 377.
90. Writer, W. D. R., James, F. M. and Wheeler, A. S. (1981). Double-blind comparison of morphine and bupivacaine for continuous epidural analgesia in labor. *Anesthesiology*, **54**, 215.
91. Chayen, M. S., Rudick, V., Bervine, A. (1980). Pain control with epidural injection of morphine. *Anesthesiology*, **53**, 338.
92. Husemeyer, R. P., O'Connor, M. C. and Davenport, H. C. (1980). Failure of epidural morphine to relieve pain in labour. *Anaesthesia*, **35**, 161.
93. Perriss, B. W. (1980). Epidural pethidine in labour. A study of dose requirements. *Anaesthesia*, **35**, 380.
94. Perriss, B. W. and Malins, A. F. (1981). Pain relief in labour using epidural pethidine with adrenaline. *Anaesthesia*, **36**, 631.
95. Justins, D. M., Francis, D., Houlton, P. G. and Reynolds, F. (1982). A controlled trial of epidural fentanyl in labour. *Brit. J. Anaesth.*, **54**, 409.
96. Carmichael, F. J., Rolbin, S. H. and Hew, E. M. (1982). Epidural morphine for analgesia after Caesarean section. *Canad. Anaesth. Soc. J.*, **29**, 359.
97. Danielson, D. R., Coombs, D. W., Vageau, M. and Kippe, E. (1981). Epidural morphine for post-cesarean analgesia. *Anesthesiology*, **55**, A323.
98. Crawford, J. S. (1981). Experiences with epidural morphine in obstetrics. *Anaesthesia*, **36**, 207.

## FURTHER READING

Department of Health and Social Security (1982). *Report on Confidential Enquiries into Maternal Deaths in England and Wales, 1976–1978.* London: HMSO.

Datta, S. and Alper, M. H. (1980). Anesthesia for Cesarean section. *Anesthesiology*, **53**, 142.

Marx, G. F. and Hodgkinson, R. (1975). Anaesthesia in the presence of complications of pregnancy. Obstetric Analgesia and Anaesthesia. In: *Clinics in Obstetrics and Gynaecology*, **2:3**, 609.

CHAPTER 41

# The Fetus and Placenta



## THE PLACENTA

Fetal welfare depends upon good placental function for the supply of nutrients and oxygen and for the removal of waste products. The placenta performs for the fetus the function of gastro-intestinal tract, lung, liver, kidney and endocrine gland. The human placenta is of the villous type, consisting of multiple fetal villi which branch progressively throughout gestation, thereby increasing its surface area. It is also classified as haemomonochorial, indicating that at term only a single layer of fetal chorionic tissue (the syncytiotrophoblast) separates maternal blood from fetal capillary endothelium. Maternal blood in the intervillous spaces or placental sinuses is thus in direct contact with fetal chorionic villi. These chorionic villi are covered with a continuous layer, the syncytiotrophoblast, with isolated remnants of cytotrophoblast beneath it. The fetal capillaries lie in chorionic connective tissue. As gestation advances, the fetal capillaries come to fill the terminal villi, and the syncytiotrophoblast directly overlying fetal capillaries becomes thin and fused with the endothelium, forming vasculosyncytial membranes, areas specialised for rapid exchange by simple diffusion.

The syncytiotrophoblast is the active part of the placenta, performing several functions. (1) It produces placental hormones: chorionic gonadotrophin, placental lactogen, oestrogens, progesterone. (2) It produces enzymes for the active transport of certain essential requirements, and for the breakdown of a few pharmacologically active substances. (3) It has a brush border which can engulf macromolecules and plasma droplets (pinocytosis).

The placenta is supplied with maternal blood from the uterine vessels. The uterine blood supply is thus shared by the uterine muscle, the placenta and the fetus. Blood enters the maternal sinuses in jets from the open ends of the uterine spiral arteries. Two umbilical arteries, arising from the fetal internal iliac arteries, carry fetal blood via the umbilical cord to the placenta, and a single umbilical vein returns it to the fetus. Figure 1 shows the arrangement of the fetal circulation and its relationship to the maternal.

Substances may cross the placenta in several ways:

1. *By active transport processes*, which are available for the transport of such essential requirements as amino acids, vitamins, etc, enabling them to cross to the fetus against a concentration gradient. Such specialised processes involve the consumption of metabolic energy.
2. *By facilitated diffusion*, which transfers glucose, for example, down a concentration gradient but at a rate more rapid than simple physical laws would allow.
3. *By pinocytosis* or by leakage across porous defects.
4. *By simple diffusion*, which occurs only down a concentration gradient and is a purely passive process governed by physical laws. *Respiratory* gases and *drugs* used by anaesthetists cross the placenta mainly by passive diffusion.

The supply of nutrients is very sensitive to impaired placental function which, if it occurs chronically, will result in intra-uterine growth retardation. Acute and more severe impairment, however, produces fetal anoxia and acidosis and, if severe, results in brain damage and death. Labour and delivery present particular hazards to the fetus, and it is important that the anaesthetist understands how the procedures which he undertakes may affect the fetus. After discussing placental transfer in general, and that of respiratory gases and drugs in particular, this chapter includes a section on fetal monitoring and the diagnosis of fetal distress.

## PLACENTAL TRANSFER

The importance of placental transfer rate is as a measure of the amount of oxygen reaching the fetus in unit time, the amount of carbon dioxide and waste products that can be eliminated in unit time, and the dose of potentially harmful drug that is likely to reach the fetus.

Rate of transfer by diffusion depends upon:

1. *the permeability* of the placenta to the compound concerned, and
2. *the tension gradient* of diffusible substance. This in turn is affected by
3. *the relative affinities* of maternal and fetal blood for the substance, and
4. *the blood flows* on the two sides of the placenta;
5. *the area* available for placental exchange also affects the mass of transfer.

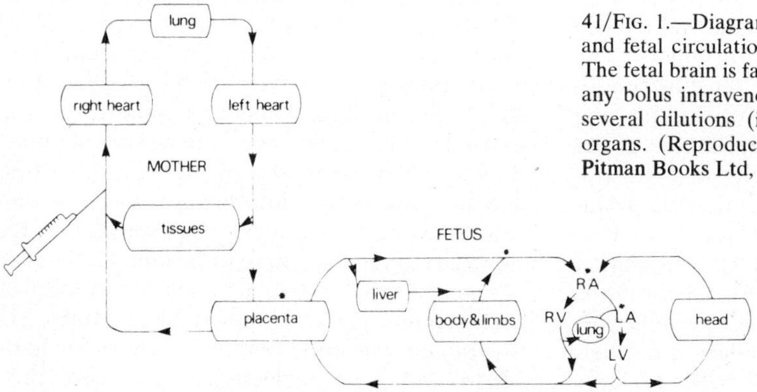


41/FIG. 1.—Diagrammatic representation of the maternal and fetal circulations and the relationship between them. The fetal brain is far removed from the maternal blood and any bolus intravenous injection to the mother undergoes several dilutions (indicated *) before reaching the fetal organs. (Reproduced from Reynolds (1979) courtesy of Pitman Books Ltd, London.[126])

The placental membrane, being covered by a continuous syncytial layer, behaves essentially as any lipid membrane where passive diffusion is concerned. Thus, small non-ionised water soluble molecules with molecular weights less than 100 (such as respiratory gases) diffuse readily across the placenta, while lipid soluble molecules can cross up to a molecular weight of 600–1000. Large water soluble and any ionised particles cross only very slowly. Such relatively poorly diffusible substances are said to be *permeability* dependent in their rate of transfer, which is little affected by blood flow. On the other hand, respiratory gases and lipid soluble drugs are very freely diffusible, readily equilibrate across the placenta, and are said to be *flow* dependent in their transfer rate, that is the amount crossing the placenta depends upon transport to and from that organ.

The *thickness* of the placental membrane affects the time taken to diffuse across it from one side to the other and therefore affects permeability of the less diffusible substances, particularly those which are only present in the circulation for a brief period, for example drugs given by bolus. For the flow-dependent transfer of readily diffusible substances however, particularly those continuously present in maternal blood, placental thickness serves only as a minor delaying factor, with a negligible effect on overall transfer rate once the substance of the placenta is effectively in equilibrium with maternal blood. This takes only a few seconds as at term most diffusion takes place across the ultra-thin vasculosyncytial membranes, presenting no barrier whatever. Theoretically diffusion may be slightly slower in early gestation, when the placental membrane is thicker.

## PLACENTAL TRANSFER OF RESPIRATORY GASES

### Permeability

Respiratory gases pass across the placenta by passive diffusion. The placenta does not impose any barrier to diffusion of such small molecules which therefore show *flow* dependence. A persistent tension gradient for oxygen and carbon dioxide exists across the placenta but appears to be due not so much to a barrier for diffusion as to a relatively inefficient multivillous flow pattern (*vide infra*) apparently producing mismatch.

### Tension Gradient and Relative Affinities

The oxygen and carbon dioxide tensions of maternal and fetal blood are given in Table 1.

An important factor which tends to preserve these concentration gradients and so enhance respiratory gas exchanges is the differences in

41/TABLE 1
OXYGEN AND CARBON DIOXIDE TENSIONS IN MATERNAL AND FETAL BLOOD

| | *Maternal* | *Fetal* | *Tension Gradient* |
|---|---|---|---|
| Oxygen | Arterial: 95 mm Hg<br>(12·7 kPa)<br>(96 per cent saturated)<br><br>Venous: 33 mm Hg<br>(4·4 kPa)<br>(51 per cent saturated) | UA: 15 mm Hg<br>(2·0 kPa)<br>(26 per cent saturated)<br><br>UV: 28 mm Hg<br>(3·7 kPa)<br>(64 per cent saturated) | 80 mm Hg<br>(10·7 kPa) |
| Carbon dioxide | Arterial: 33 mm Hg<br>(4·4 kPa)<br>Venous: 46 mm Hg<br>(5·6 kPa) | UA: 55 mm Hg<br>(7·3 kPa)<br>UV: 40 mm Hg<br>(5·3 kPa) | 22 mm Hg<br>(2·9 kPa) |

UA = umbilical artery, i.e. "venous" blood
UV = umbilical vein, i.e. "arterial" blood

affinities for oxygen and carbon dioxide between maternal and fetal blood.

**Carbon dioxide.**—The $CO_2$ dissociation curve is nearly linear and maternal and fetal $CO_2$ tensions are closely correlated over a wide range of values. Carbon dioxide is a highly diffusible gas and the difference in tension between fetal and maternal blood is usually remarkably constant, although Baillie[1] found that the gradient was considerably increased in the presence of perinatal asphyxia. The double Haldane effect (see Chapter 3), analogous to the double Bohr effect described below, promotes the passage of carbon dioxide from fetus to mother and allows passage of large volumes of carbon dioxide for relatively slight changes in tension.

**Oxygen.**—Many factors influence the partial pressure and content of oxygen in maternal and fetal blood. The simple effect of tension gradient is very much modified by the presence of haemoglobin and its effect on oxygen affinity on the two sides of the placenta.

(a) *The shape of the curve.*—An increase in maternal $Po_2$ beyond the flat upper part of the dissociation curve increases the maternal oxygen content relatively little, and therefore little additional oxygen becomes available to the fetus. Rorke and colleagues[2] showed that an increase in maternal $Po_2$ up to about 300 mm Hg (40 kPa) was accompanied by a related rise in fetal $Po_2$ but beyond this point no further increase in fetal $Po_2$ occurred.

(b) *Fetal haemoglobin* has a higher affinity for oxygen than does maternal haemoglobin, as is shown in Fig. 2. Thus at a tension of 22 mm Hg (2·9 kPa) maternal blood is only 38 per cent saturated with oxygen whereas fetal blood reaches a value of 75 per cent saturation. With the progress of pregnancy, adult haemoglobin begins to appear, so that the concentration of this type rises from 6 per cent at the twentieth week to just over 20 per cent at birth. After birth, fetal red cells, and with them fetal haemoglobin, begin to disappear, so that by the fourth month they can no longer be detected.

(c) *Increased fetal haemoglobin concentration.*—As pregnancy nears term the fetal packed cell volume (PCV) rises, while that of the mother is well below normal. At term the fetal haemoglobin concentration is 17–19 g per 100 ml (g/dl) blood, which may be almost double that in the mother.

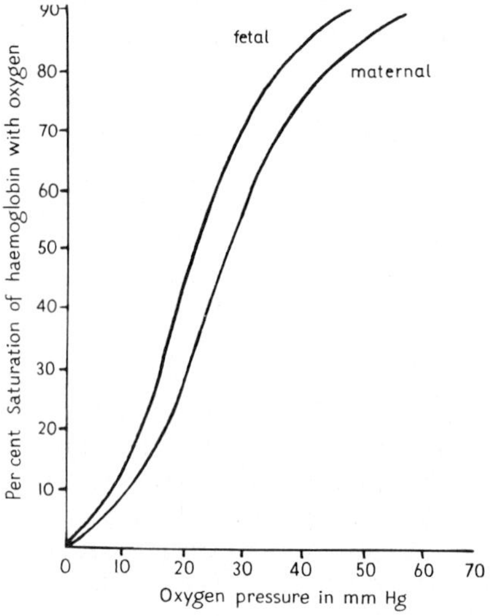


41/Fig. 2.—Oxygen Dissociation Curves of Human Infant at Birth (upper line) and Pregnant Woman (lower line).

Note the large difference in oxygen saturation of fetal and maternal blood at an oxygen pressure of 22 mm Hg (2·9 kPa). (Adaptation of a figure in *The Physiology of the Newborn Infant* by C. A. Smith, published by Blackwell Scientific Publications Ltd.)

(d) *The Bohr effect.*—The oxygen dissociation curves of fetal and adult haemoglobin are influenced by the acid-base state.

A double Bohr effect was described by Hauge.[3] The transfer of acids from the fetal blood into the maternal intervillous spaces causes the fetal pH to rise and increases the affinity of fetal blood to oxygen (Bohr shift to the left). At the same time the acids, passing to the maternal circulation, cause the maternal pH to fall, thereby reducing the affinity of maternal blood for oxygen (Bohr shift to the right), so further oxygen is released to the fetus.

The influence of the Bohr effect on fetal oxygen uptake has been demonstrated principally in sheep, in whom maternal hyperventilation with marked respiratory alkalosis caused hypoxia in the fetus, but when maternal carbon dioxide tension was restored, while hyperventilation continued, fetal oxygen content rose to its former value (see Fig. 3). When the duration of maternal hypocapnia was prolonged, a metabolic acidosis could be detected in the fetus.

There may be several causes for the observed fetal hypoxia: Levinson and associates[4] showed

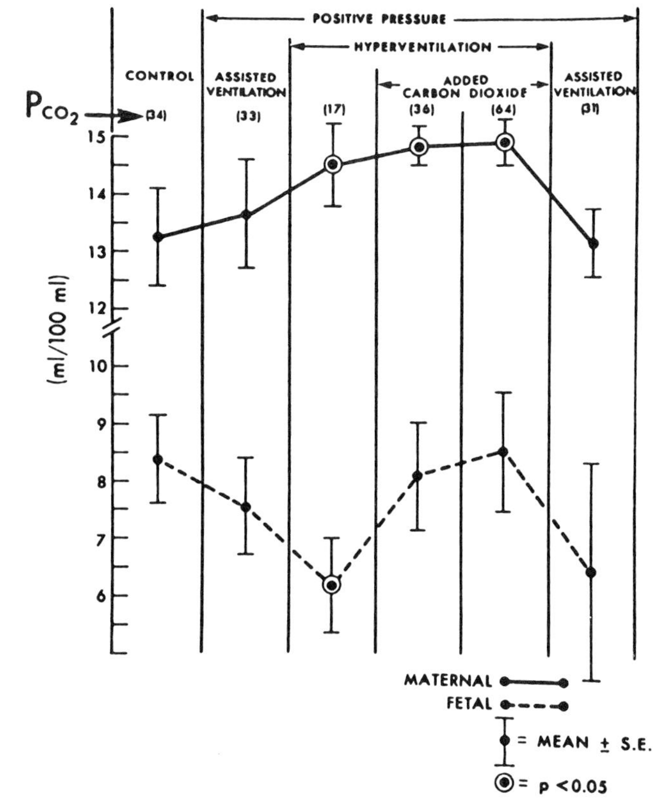


41/Fig. 3.—Changes from control values in mean maternal and fetal arterial oxygen content during five periods of positive-pressure ventilation. Mean maternal $Paco_2$ (mm Hg) during each period indicated at top of figure. (Courtesy of Drs. G. Levinson, S. M. Shnider, A. A. Lorimer and J. L. Steffenson and the Editor and publisher, J. B. Lippincott Company, of *Anesthesiology*.[4])

that uterine blood flow was reduced during periods of hyperventilation, even when the $Paco_2$ was kept within normal limits by added $CO_2$, but even when uterine blood flow was reduced by hyperventilation, the fetal oxygen content was only reduced during periods of maternal respiratory alkalosis. The best explanation for this phenomenon was therefore the Bohr effect.

Ralston and his co-workers[5] confirmed this hypothesis by showing that an infusion of sodium bicarbonate to produce a metabolic alkalosis in ewes did indeed cause a significant degree of fetal hypoxia.

### Maternal Placental Blood Flow

This factor is of paramount importance since, together with the maternal respiratory gases, it is capable of modification by the anaesthetist. The uterine blood flow is distributed to the uterine musculature and to the placenta. The respiratory gases available for exchange with the fetus are contained in that portion of the uterine flow destined for the placenta, allowing for the metabolism of the placenta itself (see Table 2). The placental metabolic oxygen consumption has been found to be between 1 and 2 ml $O_2$ per minute for an average 0·5 kg placenta.[6]

Placenta blood flow is largely passive and depends on:

i. The maternal cardiac output and blood pressure.
ii. The vasomotor tone of the uterine vessels.
iii. The state of uterine contraction.
iv. Pathological changes in the placenta.

i & ii. **Maternal cardiac output and blood pressure** and the **tone of the uterine blood vessels** may be influenced by a number of factors:

*Hypotension*, resulting from spinal or epidural

blockade may cause a fall in uterine blood flow,[7] fetal heart rate changes and minor degrees of neonatal acidosis.[8]

*Aortocaval occlusion* in mothers nursed or anaesthetised supine is the most important remediable cause of a fall in cardiac output and placental underperfusion which may occur in the absence of maternal hypotension.[9] Myometrial flow is less affected than placental blood flow, suggesting that only the former is capable of autoregulation. Aortocaval occlusion occurs in any mother at or near term but decompensation is especially likely during epidural block or general anaesthesia, causing overt supine hypotension. Datta and colleagues[10] showed that babies born by Caesarean section to mothers kept supine under epidural anaesthesia were more acidotic than those whose mothers did not lie supine.

*General anaesthesia* may be associated with a rise[11] or a fall in cardiac output; the latter is likely if halothane is used in any but low concentrations. A fall in cardiac output may not be accompanied by a fall in uterine flow, but *placental* flow is likely to be adversely affected. The work of Downing and his colleagues[12] however, suggests that enflurane need not have a detrimental effect on placental exchange. Levinson and associates[4] showed that both positive-pressure respiration and hyperventilation could reduce uterine blood flow, but that the effect on fetal oxygenation was more dependent on the maternal acid-base state than upon blood flow (*vide supra*).

*Epidural blockade* is free from ill effects upon the fetus unless it is associated with hypotension, when fetal bradycardia is likely. Hypotension, resulting from a block limited in extent to that required for pain relief in labour, is commonly due to decompensation in the presence of aortocaval occlusion and as such is readily remediable by left uterine displacement. Moreoever, the beneficial effects of fluid loading, in preventing disorders of the fetal heart pattern, have been well demonstrated.[13] Epidural blockade, in preventing reflex vasoconstriction in the region supplied by the blocked sympathetic outflow, could theoretically mitigate the detrimental effect of aortocaval occlusion on uterine blood flow. This beneficial effect however is likely to be offset by hypotension itself, occurring in the supine position.[14]

Actual changes in intervillous (placental) and myometrial flow have been measured in a variety of circumstances. In the presence of segmental epidural blockade for obstetric analgesia, both uterine[7] and intervillous[15,16] flow tend to rise, while after a more extensive block for Caesarean section, intervillous flow is more likely to fall,[17] though with adequate preloading of the circulation, any detriment to either maternal blood pressure or intervillous flow is usually eliminated.[18] Though relatively large doses of adrenaline have been shown to reduce uterine blood flow in sheep, a concentration of 5 $\mu$g/ml added to local anaesthetic for epidural blockade has been shown not to alter intervillous flow in humans.[19] This may be an effect of dose rather than a species difference.

Various different workers have shown, however, that epidural analgesia in labour improves both the maternal and fetal acid-base status, and that the metabolic acidosis that usually occurs progressively throughout labour is much reduced in both mother and baby.[20,21] Moreover if epidural analgesia replaces pethidine, the rise in $P_{CO_2}$ and fall in pH which may occur in the baby after delivery (even following small doses of pethidine) are avoided.[21]

*Maternal hyperventilation* may reduce uterine blood flow. Hyperventilation can reduce cardiac output and blood pressure and a reduced maternal $P_{CO_2}$ might theoretically produce uterine vasoconstriction. However, Levinson and coworkers[4] suggest that in fact the effect of hyperventilation in reducing placental flow is mechanical and, moreover, has little effect *per se* on fetal oxygenation. A significant reduction in fetal oxygenation occurs only in the presence of maternal alkalosis, and is probably the result of the Bohr effect (*vide supra*). Motoyama and colleagues[22] found that the production of very low maternal $P_{CO_2}$ levels in ewes reduced *umbilical* blood flow and significant maternal-fetal circulatory mismatch reduced oxygen transfer to the fetus. Prolonged maternal hyperventilation could lead to severe fetal hypoxia and metabolic acidosis. Provided maternal oxygenation remains constant, a maternal $Pa_{CO_2}$ of 30–34 mm Hg (4·0–4·5 kPa) is probably the optimum for fetal oxygenation[2] which falls only when the maternal $P_{CO_2}$ is well below this level.

However, the combination of maternal hypotension, associated with hyperventilation, diminished uterine blood flow, and the shift of the oxygen dissociation curve may all impair placental transfer of oxygen and produce fetal hypoxaemia. The implication of this observation upon clinical practice is that *excessive* artificial ventilation of a patient anaesthetised at or near term, will tend to restrict the oxygen supply to the fetus. It is most unlikely that apnoea in a baby born in such circumstances is due to a low arterial $CO_2$ level. A more probable cause is hypoxia, and appropriate resuscitative measures should be instituted.

*Maternal $PaO_2$.*—The importance of the maternal $Pao_2$ lies in the direct effect it has upon the oxygen tension gradient across the placenta, and its effect on placental perfusion is probably less important.

*Maternal bearing down*, although often essential in the second stage of labour, is a form of Valsalva manoeuvre which markedly reduces placental perfusion.[14]

*Vasopressor drugs.*—When a sympathomimetic drug with a predominantly $\alpha$-stimulant action, such as methoxamine, is used to raise the blood pressure, it is likely to reduce tissue perfusion both because of local vasoconstriction in areas where $\alpha$-receptors are numerous and also because of reflex cardio-depression.[23] The detrimental effect is prominent in the uterine vessels whose $\alpha$-receptors appear particularly sensitive.[24] A sympathomimetic agent with mixed $\alpha$ and $\beta$ effects, such as ephedrine, methylamphetamine and mephentermine, has a less detrimental effect on tissue perfusion and is to be preferred in obstetrics.[5] However, even a drug with mixed $\alpha$ and $\beta$ effects may cause uterine vasoconstriction. Thus it is clear that in obstetrics no vasopressor should be used until the patient has been turned on her side, the legs have been raised, and plasma expanders tried, and yet a dangerous degree of hypotension is still present; then only a mixed $\alpha$ and $\beta$ stimulant, such as ephedrine, should be used. In these circumstances it is highly likely to benefit placental perfusion.

iii. **Uterine contraction.**—While halogenated hydrocarbon anaesthetics tend to relax uterine muscle,[25–27] local anaesthetics have no such effect, though large doses may improve contractility.[28]

During strong uterine contractions the pressure in the maternal intervillous space rises, occluding the uterine veins and compressing the open ends of the spiral arteries. Placental flow is therefore greatly reduced, and the fetus uses the reserves of oxygen from the intervillous space. If placental function was previously borderline, the onset of labour will lead to fetal distress. Moreover, if labour is augmented with oxytocin, such is the requirement of the overworked myometrium that reactive hyperaemia in the muscle bed may steal from the placental blood supply to an extent that placental and fetal demands cannot be met. It is important that uterine overstimulation is not overlooked as a remediable cause of fetal distress.

iv. **Pathological changes in the maternal blood vessels** supplying the placenta, such as are associated with pre-eclampsia, may result in impaired placental blood supply and placental insufficiency leading to fetal hypoxia and acidosis.

### Fetal Placental Blood Flow

Fetal umbilical flow is proportional to the functional chorionic surface. It therefore increases with gestation and at term amounts to about half the fetal cardiac output. Fetal placental flow is passive and largely dependent upon the cardiac output, which is reflected in the fetal heart rate. Autoregulation of umbilical blood flow and its distribution are absent, but flow does vary with fetal activity. Cord compression is the one important cause of a reduced fetal placental flow, and if it produces villous oedema, may also serve to reduce intervillous flow past the important terminal villi.

### Maternal and Fetal Flow Matching

In various small animals, with labyrinthine placentae (e.g. the rabbit and guinea-pig), maternal and fetal placental flows tend to run in opposite directions—an efficient counter-current system. In the human, intervillous flow is mainly from the centre to the periphery of each lobule, while villous flow is running in all directions—a haphazard cross-current system with a lot of functional shunting. There is no local autoregulation apart from villous fibrosis beneath areas of fibrin deposition (*vide infra*). The system relies upon a superfluity of flows on both sides to ensure an exchange adequate for fetal welfare. Moreover, that fetal haemoglobin is operating on the steep part of its curve ensures that where oxygen is plentiful, extra supplies can be taken up. This means that the effect of mismatch, *per se*, on oxygen uptake is less severe than in the lungs.

### Area Available for Placental Exchange

The area available for placental exchange can be reduced by fibrin deposition on the maternal side, which is usually accompanied by fibrosis of the associated villi. Up to 30 per cent of the surface area of the placenta can be lost in this way without apparent harm to the fetus. This is distinct from the fetal detriment that may be associated with placental infarcts accounting for only 10 per cent of the placenta, because these represent serious impairment of the maternal supply line.

Placental separation is an obvious cause of an abrupt reduction in exchange area, and a clear threat to the fetus.

In the second stage of labour, with descent of the fetus, the uterine wall and consequently the placental bed retract. Descent of the head coupled with bearing down and a progressive maternal acidosis serve to make the second stage of labour a hazardous time for the fetus.

Table 2 summarises factors involved in oxygen transfer across the placenta in an ideal "normal" case.

## PLACENTAL TRANSFER OF DRUGS

The effects that drugs given to a woman in labour may have upon the fetus and neonate have increased in importance in recent years as graver dangers to the baby have diminished.

Drugs may affect the fetus either indirectly, by altering maternal physiology, or directly

41/Table 2
Summary of Oxygen Exchanges across Placenta

| | | | |
|---|---|---|---|
| Uterine arterial $O_2$ content (ml/100 ml) | 15·8 | 17·0 | Umbilical venous $O_2$ content (ml/100 ml) |
| Uterine venous $O_2$ content | 10·8 | 7·0 | Umbilical arterial $O_2$ content |
| $O_2$ released per 100 ml | 5·0 ml | 10·0 ml | Oxygen acquired per 100 ml |
| But uterine blood flow is 700 ml/min | | | But umbilical blood flow is 300 ml/min |
| $O_2$ availability for uterus, placenta and fetus (5·0 ml/100 ml × 700) | 35 ml/min | 30·0 ml/min | $O_2$ acquired *could* be (10 ml/100 ml × 300) |

*Assumptions*

| Maternal: | | Fetal: | |
|---|---|---|---|
| Hb | 12 g/100 ml (g/dl) | Hb | 19 g/100 ml (g/dl) |
| $PaO_2$ | 95 mm Hg (12·7 kPa) | $PvO_2$ | 28 mm Hg (3·7 kPa) |
| $SaO_2$ | 95 per cent | $SvO_2$ | 64 per cent |
| $PvO_2$ | 33 mm Hg (4·4 kPa) | $PaO_2$ | 15 mm Hg (2·0 kPa) |
| $SvO_2$ | 55 per cent | $SaO_2$ | 26 per cent |

(from nomograms of Hellegers and Schruefer, 1961)

$O_2$ *Balance Sheet*

| | | |
|---|---|---|
| Uterine $O_2$ availability | | 35 ml/min |
| Fetal $O_2$ requirement (at term) | 18 ml/min | |
| Uterine $O_2$ consumption | 15 ml/min | |
| Placental $O_2$ consumption | 1·5 ml/min | |
| Total debit | 34·5 | |
| Balance | | +0·5 ml/min |

after passage across the placenta. When assessing the direct effect, it is useful to understand the factors that influence the extent to which a drug may cross the placenta.

Where passive diffusion is concerned, the placenta appears to behave like any other lipid membrane, such as the blood-brain barrier. It is self-evident, therefore, that drugs which act upon the nervous system and can cross the blood-brain barrier are certain to be able to cross the placenta. Inhalational anaesthetics, highly diffusible lipid-soluble molecules, cross the placenta with ease. Weak acids such as barbiturates and weak bases such as narcotic analgesics and local anaesthetics all cross the placenta readily in the non-ionised state. Fully ionised drugs, such as neuromuscular blocking drugs and other quaternary ammonium compounds, which do not readily cross other lipid barriers in the body, diffuse across the placenta only very slowly. Large particles, such as macromolecules and even fetal cells, that cannot diffuse across lipid membranes, do cross the placenta to a small extent, either by pinocytosis or across hypothetical porous defects.

Both placental and drug characteristics influence the rate of passive diffusion.

### Placental Factors

(i) *The area of the membrane.*—The reduction in area available for exchange in the aging placenta could theoretically retard net drug transfer and so delay equilibration. In practice this factor is probably less important in the context of drug transfer than it is to the supply of metabolic requirements.

(ii) *Maternal and fetal blood flow.*—The flow arrangements in the human placenta (see p. 1075) mean that at best umbilical venous blood leaving the placenta comes into equilibrium with maternal venous blood leaving the placental bed, and not with the maternal arterial blood, as is the case in the more efficient countercurrent systems encountered in labyrinthine placentae.

Blood flow on either side of the membrane maintains the concentration gradient of any substance that is not in equilibrium across the placenta, and so promotes its passage. Maternal placental flow may be reduced by a number of mechanisms which are of vital importance in the transfer of respiratory gases (see p. 1073), but the only factor of note concerned in drug transfer is the effect that transient reduction in blood flow during uterine contraction may have upon transfer of a drug injected by intravenous bolus.

The fact that the rate of transfer of freely diffusible drugs is flow dependent, means that in the short term, in the presence of good placental function, a larger dose of drugs reaches the fetus. Thus in the elective caesarean section it is perhaps more important to keep the dose of general anaesthetic drugs to a minimum than it is in the emergency where labour and fetal distress both indicate reduced placental function.

(iii) *Placental enzymes.*—The placenta contains numerous enzymes and there is evidence of some drug metabolism, for example of barbiturates, within the placenta.[29] This facility, however, is readily saturated and probably has little protective effect on the fetus.

### Drug Characteristics

**Permeability** of drugs used by anaesthetists is principally determined by lipid solubility. The *concentration gradient* of diffusible drug determines its rate of transfer but the overall dose received by the fetus depends not only upon transfer rate but also upon the length of time the maternal concentration remains high. Only *free, non-ionised* drug is readily diffusible, thus high-protein binding and a high degree of ionisation can both reduce the effective concentration gradient. There is ample evidence that inhalation anaesthetics and induction agents, and local and systemic analgesic drugs, all possess molecular weights compatible with lipid diffusion and all cross the placenta very rapidly (*vide infra*) with no barrier to diffusion. Fully ionised drugs such as quaternary ammonium compounds, on the other hand, would be expected to cross at a very slow rate.

#### Relative Affinities

For local anaesthetic drugs and those acting upon the central nervous system, the umbilical venous-maternal plasma concentration ratio is not, beyond the first few minutes, directly related to sampling time, as it would be if the rate of transfer were slow. In fact, there is a persistent and fairly consistent apparent gradient for a given drug even in the presence of a

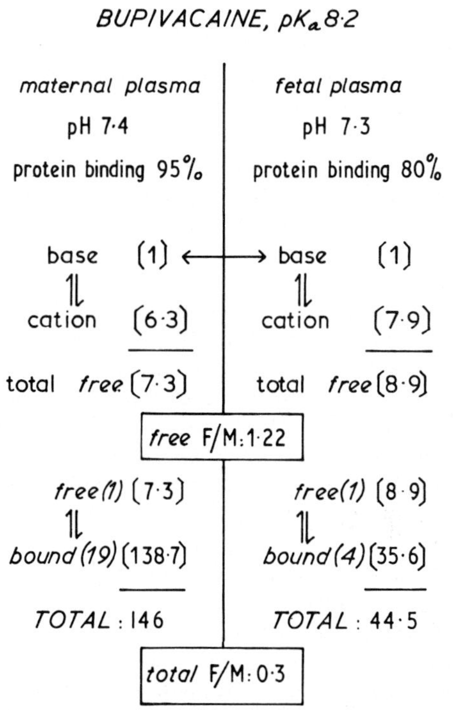


41/FIG. 4.—Transplacental distribution of a basic drug such as bupivacaine with a pKa of 8·2. At equilibrium the concentration of *unbound, non-ionised* drug (free base), the diffusible component, is equal in maternal and fetal plasma. The top half of the figure shows how the distribution of *free* (unbound) drug is determined by the pH gradient and the pKa, relative concentrations of cation and base having been calculated from the Henderson-Hasselbalch equation. The lower half of the figure shows how disparities in protein binding alter the final total concentration in mother and fetus.

A pH gradient of 0·1 between maternal and fetal plasma is in accord with the findings of Thalme *et al.*[21] Protein-binding figures are derived from Reynolds.[37] The figure for fetal plasma is higher than that reported by Tucker *et al.*[34] of 65 per cent. This percentage may be artificially low because it was measured at a concentration much higher than that found clinically. The same balance was demonstrated by Thomas *et al.*[35] who found a fetal-maternal ratio for bupivacaine of 0·24, and slightly lower fetal and maternal protein binding, demonstrating no gradient for free non-ionised bupivacaine.

relatively steady maternal concentration. In other words, something near equilibrium probably exists but the partition coefficient of the drug between the two compartments is not unity.

Two drug characteristics influence this steady state ratio:

(i) **pKa** (see p. 617).—This property determines the degree of ionisation at a given pH. There is normally a small pH gradient across the placenta; basic drugs are more ionised in the more acid fetus, while acidic drugs are more ionised in the mother. Only the non-ionised form diffuses across readily, and so the free concentration of a basic drug tends to be higher in the fetus (see Fig. 4), and that of an acidic drug higher in the mother. The stronger the base or acid, the more marked this disparity will be. A very weak acid or base—virtually non-ionised—would by contrast tend to have a fetal-maternal free concentration ratio near unity. More importantly, it has been shown that a fall in fetal pH, such as may accompany the supine position,[10] maternal diabetes[30] or fetal asphyxia from any cause,[31] or indeed as may be induced by lactic acid infusion in lambs[32] is accompanied by an increase in fetal-maternal ratio of the weak bases, lignocaine and bupivacaine.

(ii) **Protein binding.**—Disparity in protein binding between fetal and maternal plasma is probably the most important determinant of the equilibrium in fetal-maternal ratio (see Fig. 4). *In vitro* studies of the binding of a range of acidic drugs[33] and of local anaesthetics[34,35] suggest more extensive binding by maternal than by fetal plasma. At term there is a higher concentration of albumin in the umbilical cord than in the maternal circulation,[36] although $\alpha_1$ acid glycoprotein (which binds bases) is higher in the mother.

One can postulate, therefore, that unless maternal concentration of a drug is changing rapidly, there may actually be little or no gradient for *diffusible* (free, non-ionised) drugs between maternal and umbilical venous plasma. Drugs may continue to cross the placenta because of a gradient between maternal arterial and umbilical arterial plasma, accounting for a persistent gradient between umbilical artery and vein. High maternal protein binding, in that it slows placental transfer, does have the effect of reducing the total dose to the fetus of a drug given over the short term, as for example in labour.

### Other Factors Influencing the Placental Gradient

Any rapid rise or fall in maternal concentration of a drug is likely to recreate a gradient across the placenta. A rise may be produced by maternal inhalation or a bolus intravenous injection. The reverse occurs when stopping inhalation, because the fetus cannot exhale drugs as can the mother, or after a bolus when drug redistribution produces a more rapid fall in the maternal than in the fetal circulation.

The maternal rate of drug metabolism may exceed that of the fetus, especially for aromatic hydroxylation and conjugation processes, but the disparity may be less than one might suppose for the comparatively small load imposed by analgesic drugs. The fetus may be protected to some extent because a proportion of drug in umbilical venous blood is detoxicated in the liver before gaining access to the systemic circulation.

### Total Dose of Drug Received by the Fetus

The absolute concentration of a drug in fetal plasma and tissues is, of course, of greater importance to the infant's welfare than is the fetal-maternal ratio. As this concentration is a product of maternal concentration and fetal-maternal ratio, the extent to which a drug accumulates in the maternal circulation may be crucial for the baby. From the pharmacokinetic point of view, the fetus represents a very deep compartment in comparison with maternal tissues (see Fig. 1), therefore his own tissues become saturated only very slowly. The longer the time that the baby is exposed to high concentrations of a drug and its metabolites, the more nearly will fetal tissues become saturated with the substances, and the longer it will take the fetus to eliminate them. Thus Apgar scores, measured within minutes of birth, may fail to distinguish deleterious effects of cumulative depressant drugs which could better be detected by later neurobehavioural assessment.

## PLACENTAL TRANSFER OF INDIVIDUAL DRUGS

### Inhalational Anaesthetics

Inhalational anaesthetics diffuse rapidly across the placenta, and provided they are evenly distributed between cells and plasma (because of the difference between maternal and fetal haematocrits) one would expect the equilibrium whole blood fetal-maternal ratios to be near unity. Indeed, the solubility of inhalation agents in maternal and fetal blood is very similar; the greatest disparity has been observed with halothane, which is about 1·3 times as soluble in maternal as in fetal blood.[38]

Yet it has long been remarked that babies frequently emerge awake from anaesthetised mothers, a phenomenon contributing to the impression of a placental "barrier". The presence of a barrier is a misconception and the phenomenon is rather due to delay in equilibration of maternal blood with fetal brain (see Fig. 1). Stenger and his co-workers[39] who measured *uterine* venous concentrations of nitrous oxide at caesarean section, found them to be equal to umbilical venous at delivery, but only slowly to approach maternal *arterial* levels. The incidence of depressed neonates increased with duration of anaesthesia before delivery.

The much more soluble methoxyflurane equilibrates even more slowly than nitrous oxide. Maternal and fetal plasma concentrations of methoxyflurane have been measured during both analgesia and anaesthesia and in both cases, umbilical venous-maternal ratios were about 0·7 with evidence of continuing uptake after 15 minutes of anaesthesia. The neonatal methoxyflurane levels and incidence of depression were higher when methoxyflurane anaesthesia succeeded analgesia, than when analgesia or brief anaesthesia were given on their own.[40,41] In a study of enflurane anaesthesia for caesarean section, Wickström and colleagues[42] found umbilical venous concentrations to be 0·7 of maternal shortly after delivery. Levels in both individuals fell rapidly thereafter.

In a study of the distribution of radioactive halothane in maternal and fetal guinea-pig tissues, the concentration after 5 to 45 minutes was higher in all maternal than fetal tissues except the liver, in which fetal concentrations exceeded maternal.[43]

The likelihood of neonatal depression is clearly greater from anaesthetic than from analgesic doses of anaesthetics. Yet for such cumulative agents as trichloroethylene and methoxyflurane, long duration of analgesia may often be detrimental. Phillips and Macdonald[44] found lower Apgar scores in infants of mothers given trichloroethylene analgesia than in the control group, while nitrous oxide, a much less cumulative drug, had no such effect. The 50 per cent oxygen in Entonox may contribute an overall benefit. This is in contrast to the necessarily limited concentration of oxygen in nitrous oxide anaesthesia, which may be one factor in the detrimental effect of prolonged nitrous oxide anaesthesia.[45]

**Barbiturates**

Barbiturates are weak acids whose pKa values are near or above the physiological pH range. They are, therefore, largely non-ionised and pass readily across the placenta by lipid diffusion. Protein binding may be more extensive in maternal than in fetal plasma,[33] thus at equilibrium both free and total concentrations are higher in mother than in fetus. Bolus intravenous injection of the more highly lipid-soluble barbiturates produces early massive transfer and early peak fetal levels, with backwash occasionally producing levels transiently higher in fetus than mother. Cassano and associates[46] showed that thiopentone administered intravenously to mice produced peak fetal levels in 10 minutes whereas the much less lipid-soluble phenobarbitone did not reach a maximum in the fetus until 30 minutes. In a well-conducted study of thiopentone in women at caesarean section Heslop and colleagues[47] found umbilical venous to be approximately equal to maternal venous concentration at delivery, but the decline thereafter was much slower in neonates than in the mothers. Like nitrous oxide, thiopentone crosses the placenta freely but does not immediately put the baby to sleep because the placenta is not the fetal brain, and further dilutions take place (Fig. 1) before this organ is reached. Although within about a minute of bolus administration umbilical venous levels are probably falling, fetal tissue levels will continue to rise for perhaps 40 minutes.[48]

Finster and co-workers[49] found lower cord concentrations of thiopentone after vaginal delivery than after caesarean section and suggested that cord compression limits transfer.

Large doses of barbiturates given to women in labour are recognised to produce neonatal depression and have been found to delay the establishment of breast feeding by as much as two days.[50]

**Narcotic Analgesics**

Narcotic analgesic drugs, being amines, are bases and are more than 95 per cent ionised at physiological pH. Nevertheless the non-ionised fraction is of sufficient lipid solubility for rapid placental transfer by lipid diffusion. Shier and colleagues[51] gave pethidine intravenously over 3 minutes to pregnant ewes and found that umbilical venous exceeded maternal arterial concentrations within a minute of the end of infusion, and thereafter remained higher, which is compatible with the pH gradient effect and an element of backwash. Clinical studies have demonstrated fetal-maternal pethidine ratios of usually less than unity,[52,53] although always higher than those of pentazocine.[54–56] A fetal-maternal ratio of less than one can be accounted for by incomplete fetal-maternal equilibration, and indeed it has been found that[57,58] two-and-a-half hours may elapse before the fetal concentration exceeded that found in the mother. The more marked accumulation of pethidine than pentazocine in mothers results in neonatal pethidine levels many times higher than pentazocine. The half-life of pethidine in the neonate may be more than 20 hours—greatly in excess of that found in the mother.[57,59] Refstad and Lindbaek[60] found that neonatal respiratory depression was briefer following maternal analgesia with pentazocine than with pethidine. However, pentazocine usually produces less effective pain relief than pethidine, albeit with fewer side-effects.[61,62]

Pethidine has long been known to produce neonatal sedation with respiratory depression.[63] Even small doses impair the acid-base state,[21] suckling and other neurobehavioural responses.[64] The detrimental effect has been found to be dose related[65] and to be greatest when pethidine has been given 3 hours or more before delivery[66,67] and has been attributed to the accumulation of metabolites.[68,69] All adverse effects in the neonate are, however, readily reversed by the administration of naloxone[70] which must be given in an adequate dose (*200* μg) if reversal is not to be short-lived[71,72] (see also Chapter 30).

**Tranquillisers**

Although phenothiazines are used extensively in labour and, as weak bases, are certain to cross the placenta, few studies of their placental transfer have been made. Promazine crosses the placenta rapidly, but fetal levels have been found to be lower than maternal.[53] Chlorpromazine crosses the placenta readily but its conjugated metabolites (water soluble substances) do not, nor can the baby produce them.[73,74]

In contrast to the phenothiazines, diazepam, during its short period of popularity for routine obstetrics, was quite extensively studied. It is a very poorly ionised base and concentrations in the fetus are commonly greater than those in the mother[75–77] probably because of a more extensive fetal than maternal protein binding. The concentration in the fetal heart is high, an interesting finding in view of the depression of cardiac autonomic control with which diazepam is associated. It causes loss of beat-to-beat variation of fetal heart rate and, if given in doses of 30 mg or more, hypothermia and hypotonia in the neonate. Even the less lipid soluble lorazepam is found in equal concentrations in fetal and maternal plasma, when given a few hours or more before delivery.[78] Moreover, when used (surely erroneously) in the treatment of hypertension in pregnancy, it has been associated with reduction in Apgar scores, respiration, temperature and suckling in the neonate.[79] Adverse effects are likely to be prolonged since the neonate can conjugate lorazepam only very slowly.[80]

### Local Anaesthetics

Local anaesthetics are weak bases and all cross the placenta readily, but their equilibrium fetal-maternal ratios vary greatly. They range from about 0·3 for bupivacaine and etidocaine, 0·55 for lignocaine, 0·7 for mepivacaine to 1 for prilocaine.[81–87] These fetal-maternal ratios appear to be related to protein binding, the most highly bound yielding the lowest ratios. Tucker and associates,[34] Reynolds[37] and Thomas and colleagues[35] demonstrated more extensive binding of local anaesthetics to maternal than to fetal plasma proteins. Thomas and co-workers[35] found that there was actually no gradient for free non-ionised bupivacaine across the placenta. The effect of a high degree of maternal binding on the fetal-maternal ratio is explained in Fig. 4. More recently, however, Khunert and colleagues[82] suggested that low fetal-maternal ratios of bupivacaine were due not to high maternal binding but to fetal tissue uptake. Such an explanation *cannot* apply to low umbilical *venous*-maternal ratios, such as are consistently found by all workers.

Bupivacaine and etidocaine used epidurally yield low maternal concentrations, consequently neonatal concentrations are very much lower than those of lignocaine and mepivacaine: both markedly cumulative when used for continuous epidural analgesia in labour. Prilocaine, although producing low maternal levels is little used in obstetrics because of the danger of methaemoglobinaemia. Epidural chloroprocaine yields very low rapidly disappearing plasma concentrations in both mother and baby,[88] but its usefulness is limited by its characteristically brief and abrupt analgesia.

There is evidence that the neonate can eliminate lignocaine much as can the mother,[89–92] while the breakdown of mepivacaine,[91,93] bupivacaine[82,94] and possibly etidocaine also[95] is delayed.

Low Apgar scores associated with high plasma concentrations of local anaesthetics have been reported after prolonged epidural analgesia with lignocaine[96] and mepivacaine.[86] No such association has been reported with bupivacaine. In a trial without random allocation of patients, infants born of mothers who had received epidural analgesia with lignocaine or mepivacaine, had lower scores for muscle strength and tone.[97] The same workers found no such detrimental effect associated with bupivacaine,[98] though more recently in a detailed neurobehavioural scrutiny, suckling and muscle tone scores for bupivacaine were found to be lower than those for pethidine *plus* naloxone.[70] The authors stated that the effects were not such as could be detected in any routine paediatric examination and were probably therefore clinically unimportant. The same view was echoed by Abboud and associates,[99] while Rosenblatt and co-workers[100] detected some dose-related neonatal detriment, though an *increase* in muscle tone, with epidural bupivacaine, and Merkow and colleagues[101] detected no neurobehavioural deficit with bupivacaine, mepivacaine or chloroprocaine used in pudendal block.

### Neuromuscular Blocking Drugs

Neuromuscular blockers are all quaternary ammonium compounds, which are fully ionised, and therefore would be expected to diffuse across the placenta only very slowly. The delivery of a vigorous baby from a mother paralysed by a normal dose of a neuromuscular blocking drug provides familiar clinical evidence to support this theory. True neonatal neuromuscular blockade may occur only after prolonged and profound curarisation. A case was reported of a curarised baby born at 28 weeks' gestation to a mother who had been given 245 mg of tubocurarine in the treatment of status epilepticus.[102]

Studies of small doses of alcuronium, pancuronium, dimethyltubocurarine, fazadinium and suxamethonium suggest that a bolus injection may force small quantities of these drugs across the placenta, but that in such circumstances, equilibrium distribution between fetus and mother does not occur and paralysing levels are not reached in the fetus.[103–110] Umbilical venous : maternal venous ratios as high as 0·4 have been reported for pancuronium after 20 minutes anaesthesia,[107] but this compares a pre-mixed fetal level with a post-mixed maternal, and therefore does not represent anything approaching a clinically effective fetal dose.

Drabkova and colleagues[106] state that the placenta does not break down suxamethonium, and they showed that fetal monkey plasma broke down suxamethonium more slowly than maternal. They therefore suggest that large successive doses to the mother and the administration of anticholinesterase to the baby, might cause neonatal paralysis.

### Atropine and Neostigmine

Atropine, a weak base, crosses the placenta and, after intravenous injection to the mother causing a rapid rise in maternal heart rate, produces a slow rise in fetal heart rate.[111] The fetal-maternal ratio has been found to rise rapidly to about 93 per cent at 5 minutes,[112] and to equilibrate in about 10 minutes.[113] Neostigmine, which possesses a quaternary ammonium group, is unlikely to cross the placenta readily. Indeed, there is circumstantial evidence that it does not cross, since when given to the mother, it fails to reduce atropine tachycardia in the fetus.

## MANAGEMENT OF LABOUR AND ITS EFFECT ON THE BABY

An attempt will be made in this section to summarise the various ways in which analgesic and anaesthetic management and related factors can affect the welfare of fetus and neonate.

**Fluid loading** with crystalloid (Hartmann's solution or saline) or colloid solution tends to improve maternal placental blood flow following epidural blockade (p. 1074) and reduces the incidence of disordered fetal heart rhythms.[13] Fluid loading with watery solutions such as 5 per cent dextrose, however, can cause serious hyponatraemia in mother and baby,[114] the main component of which is water overload rather than sodium deficit. Very *little* water is required by the labouring mother, whose ability to excrete a water load is defective. Obstetricians and midwives, however, frequently feel constrained to treat ketonuria (an entirely predictable finding in the starving parturient) with dextrose, although a 5 per cent concentration offers little in the way of calories, whilst the administration of more than 20 g/h of dextrose has been found to be associated with neonatal hypoglycaemia, and may make fetal acidosis worse.[115] *The moral is probably to give only such amounts of 5 per cent dextrose as is necessary as a vehicle for an oxytocin infusion.*

### Epidural Analgesia and Anaesthesia

The effect on the neonate of placentally administered local anaesthetics that are currently used in obstetrics is clinically unimportant (see p. 1081). Provided hypotension is prevented, a selective epidural block such as is necessary for analgesia in labour, tends to improve placental blood flow and acid-base status in mother and baby. Epidural anaesthesia for caesarean section need not impair placental blood supply provided the maternal circulation is pre-loaded, and is associated with less neonatal depression than is general anaesthesia.[116] Moreover, the lack of maternal sedation, not to say coma, allows early all-important bonding.

Local anaesthetics do not depress uterine contractility[28] neither does epidural analgesia prolong the first stage of labour.[117] The second stage, however, is prolonged but the decline in fetal acid-base status is much slower,[118] making a long second stage relatively safe for the baby. Moreover, the incidence of serious retinal haemorrhage is reduced in neonates following vaginal delivery under epidural block[119] despite a longer second stage.

The population of mothers receiving epidural analgesia in labour usually includes most of the high risk and complicated cases, and one can expect that the majority of assisted vaginal deliveries of one sort and another will fall into this group. It is therefore quite irrelevant to ask whether epidurals *cause* abnormal deliveries, because the reverse is more often true.

In a large retrospective survey, despite this bias *against* epidural babies, the incidence of perinatal death was slightly, though not significantly, *lower* in the epidural group.[120]

### Pethidine and Adjuncts

The potentially harmful neonatal effects of maternal pethidine analgesia can be reversed by administering an adequate dose of naloxone to the baby. Sedative anti-emetics and benzodiazepines on the other hand have no antidotes. Moreover, in terms of early bonding of mother and baby, the direct effect of pethidine or any sedative drug on the neonate may be of little importance if the mother herself is somnolent, exhausted or amnesic.[121]

### General Anaesthesia

The greatest danger of general anaesthesia is, of course, respiratory obstruction or inhalation of stomach contents at induction, which put both mother and baby at risk. Once past this acute danger, the more prolonged the anaesthesia before delivery, the more harmful it is to the baby. Positional effects on the maternal circulation, positive-pressure hyperventilation and increasing fetal doses of all anaesthetic agents, may all contribute to neonatal depression.

Doses of inhalational agents, particularly those which are slowly eliminated from the body, should be kept to a minimum before delivery of the baby, though analgesic concentrations given over a short period are probably harmless to the fit neonate.

### The Effect of Labour Itself on the Baby

With each uterine contraction, maternal placental blood flow falls to a very low level, even though maternal arterial blood pressure rises. Thus the transfer of oxygen to the fetus falls with, and rises again after, each contraction. Labour is therefore a form of stress to the fetus which, if placental function is already compromised, for example because of maternal hypertension or partial placental separation, may lead to fetal asphyxia. The normal progress of the second stage of labour leads to a progressive diminution in the placental circulation, thus submitting the fetus to an increasing degree of hypoxia and acidosis.[20] In ordinary circumstances this is compatible with the birth of a living child. Unduly prolonged labour or continuous uterine hypertonus may lead to such a degree of fetal hypoxia as to cause permanent cerebral damage. This hazard can be compounded by the uncontrolled use of oxytocin particularly if the fetus is otherwise at risk.

### Signs of Fetal Distress

In labour, the fetus signals his distress in two ways; one by the appearance of fresh meconium in the liquor and the other by changes in the fetal heart pattern (see below) that can be detected by fetal monitoring. A measurement of pH on a fetal blood sample may be used to verify the diagnosis of fetal distress which cannot be made with certainty from the heart pattern alone. A fetal pH of less than 7·25 is a signal of asphyxia (*vide infra*) but fetal $Po_2$ measurement is less reliable.

## Fetal Monitoring

**Cardiotocography.**—The limitations of intermittent auscultation of the fetal heart are generally recognised and fetal welfare is better monitored by continuous recording of the fetal heart rate (FHR) and uterine contractions, the latter being essential in the interpretation of the data.

*The fetal heart rate* may be measured:

(i) using an ECG derived from a unipolar electrode applied to the presenting part. The second electrode is in contact with the maternal vagina. The cardiotachometer is triggered by the R wave of the ECG. This is an accurate and reliable method, provided the electrode is securely applied, but necessitates ruptured membranes and an accessible cervical os;

(ii) with an external monitoring transducer, using ultrasound. This is a non-invasive technique which can be used before the onset of labour, if the os is tightly closed, or for the second twin. It is less accurate than the ECG and often disturbed by movement of mother and baby, while certain changes in heart pattern may be difficult to interpret.

*Uterine contractions* may be recorded:

(i) using a pressure transducer within the uterine cavity. This can give an accurate measure of intra-uterine pressure but is invasive and not without risk, so it is rarely used;

(ii) using an external tocodynamometer,

applied over the uterine fundus. This provides a record of duration and frequency of uterine contractions but is not an accurate measure of their force, the height of the trace depending as much on the thinness of the abdominal wall.

Fetal heart rate patterns involve *baseline* changes, which occur independently of uterine contraction, and periodic changes, which are closely associated with them (Fig. 5).

### I. Patterns that are Rarely Associated with any Reduction in Fetal pH

*The "normal" pattern*, which is between 120 and 160 beats per minute, with no change in rate during contractions. There should be a short-term variation in heart rate (commonly termed beat-to-beat variation, though the periodicity is normally longer than this) of 5 or more beats per minute.

*Accelerations* taking place during uterine contractions signal a good reflex response on the part of the fetus, and are of excellent prognostic significance.

*A baseline bradycardia*, with good beat-to-beat variation but with no periodic decelerations, is not an adverse pattern and is rarely associated with a fetal pH below 7·25.

### II. Warning Patterns

*The Early deceleration* or Type I dip is a slowing in the fetal heart rate, the lowest point of which coincides with the peak of the contraction, the normal rate being restored when the uterus relaxes. The change is thought to be due to compression of the fetal head and is usually physiological and not of serious significance, if the pattern remains unaltered. However, it may herald more serious changes, such as variable or late deceleration, and slow recovery of the rate following uterine relaxation, or a dip of more than 40 beats/minute may be an early sign of fetal distress.

*A baseline tachycardia* is a fetal heart rate averaging more than 160 beats/minute. If it is not associated with loss of variability or decelerations, it does not normally herald fetal hypoxia, and is not reversed by administering oxygen to the mother. It may be associated with maternal pyrexia and ketosis, and the temperature and urine of the mother should be examined.

*Loss of baseline variability*, or a beat-to-beat variation of less than 5 beats/minute, may signal fetal hypoxia, or it may be a drug effect. It is commonly observed following maternal administration of diazepam and may be seen occasionally after other sedatives[122] and epidural blockade. If not associated with any of these, it should be treated as a sign of fetal distress requiring adjustment of the mother's position

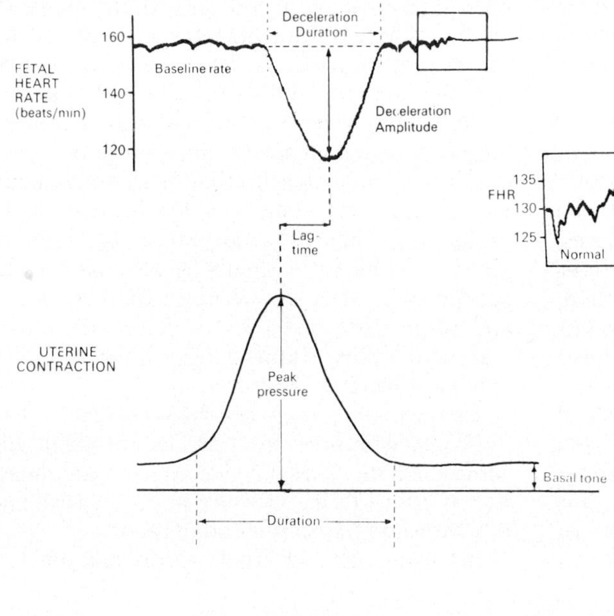


41/Fig. 5.—The cardiotocograph. (Courtesy of Professor R. W. Beard and Sonicaid Ltd., publishers of *Fetal Heart Patterns and Their Clinical Interpretation*.)

and possibly administration of oxygen and fetal blood sampling. It carries a serious prognosis if complicated by any other changes.

*Variable decelerations* involve slowing of the FHR persisting for unequal periods and irregularly co-ordinated with the uterine contractions. If prolonged and severe, they may be of serious significance but in the early stages are not associated with biochemical changes in the fetus. They should be taken as a warning of the possible development of the late deceleration pattern.

III. **Changes of Serious Prognostic Significance**

*Late decelerations* or type II dips involve a fall in fetal heart rate which is maximal *after* the peak of uterine contraction. This is thought to be due to fetal hypoxia following contractions and is normally taken as a sign of fetal distress though a reduced fetal pH is not always present. It is this time lag between uterine contraction peak and heart rate trough (see Fig. 5) that is significant, even if the rate stays above 120 beats/minute, though on the whole deeper dips are viewed more seriously.

Late deceleration patterns were observed by Thomas[123] in 8·4 per cent of labours but the fetal pH was less than 7·25 in only 41 per cent of these and the one-minute Apgar score was less than 7 in only 47 per cent. Epidural anaesthesia and the supine position were associated with late deceleration in 71 per cent of cases but in spite of this the fetal scalp pH and the 1-minute Apgar scores were identical in the epidural and non-epidural cases.

In the presence of late decelerations, the mother should be turned on her side, given oxygen and intravenous fluids and possibly a fetal blood sample should be taken. If conservative measures fail, and if there is fetal acidosis, urgent delivery is required.

*Complicated patterns.*—Combinations of baseline tachycardia, loss of beat-to-beat variation and decelerations may generally be taken to be of the worst prognostic significance and demand immediate action.

A ghastly fetal heart pattern may herald the second stage of labour and be due simply to compression of the baby's head. It may also be due to cord compression and shrinking of the placental site with descent of the head, in which case, delivery should be expedited.

Ideally, cardiotocography should be regarded only as a screening method of fetal monitoring. Without fetal blood sampling, cardiotocography may result in unnecessary operative deliveries.

**Fetal Blood Sampling**

The measurement of the pH of fetal blood has provided the most accurate and reliable means of assessing the condition of the fetus during labour.[124] If the fetus is deprived of oxygen its glycogen metabolism proceeds anaerobically to the formation of lactic acid rather than through the normal aerobic metabolic cycle via pyruvic acid to carbon dioxide and water. The accumulation of lactic acid in the fetal blood lowers its pH and results in metabolic acidosis. Thus a fall of the fetal blood pH can be an index of fetal asphyxia.

The mean range of variability of the fetal blood pH during labour is from 7·35 to 7·26. This should remain constant until shortly before delivery; then a fall in pH occurs due not only to the natural interruption of placental flow during the uterine contraction but also to an accumulation of lactic acid in the mother and fetus. In general a fall in fetal pH to below 7·25 would be considered abnormal and a fall in pH to 7·20 suggests that early delivery would be desirable.

Some caution is needed in the interpretation of these figures. An abnormally low pH value can be caused by errors of technique in collecting the sample from the fetal scalp, such as contamination with liquor, inadequate mixing of the sample or a delay of more than a few minutes before making the measurement. Ideally, the pH electrode should be sited within the labour ward area, not only to avoid delay in obtaining the result but also for the convenience of repeated tests, as clinical action on the basis of only one measurement may not be justified. Serial estimations at short intervals showing a steady fall in pH suggests the need to deliver the baby.

Before taking action on the basis of a low fetal pH it should be remembered that any degree of metabolic acidosis in the mother will be reflected in the fetus. For instance if the mother herself is dehydrated and ketotic, a pH of below 7·25 in her infant may not be as diagnostic of placental insufficiency as it would be if her own acid-base status had been normal.

The benefits derived from fetal blood sampling are shown by the reduction in the number of caesarean sections done for fetal distress at Queen Charlotte's Hospital from 86 cases in 1964/65 to 27 in 1966/67 after the advent of fetal blood sampling. It was unusual to perform the operation solely because of the clinical signs of fetal distress if the pH remained within normal limits.[125]

## REFERENCES


1. Baillie, P. (1970). Acid-base balance at birth. *Proc. roy. Soc. Med.*, **63**, 78.
2. Rorke, M. J., Davey, D. A. and du Toit, H. J. (1968). Foetal oxygenation during Caesarean section. *Anaesthesia*, **23**, 585.
3. Hauge, A. (1969). Gasvekslingen i placenta. *Nord. Med.*, **20**, 621.
4. Levinson, G., Shnider, S. M., Lorimer, A. A. and Steffenson, J. L. (1974). Effects of maternal hyperventilation on uterine blood flow and fetal oxygenation and acid-base status. *Anesthesiology*, **40**, 340.
5. Ralston, D. H., Shnider, S. M. and Lorimer, A. A. (1974). Uterine blood flow and fetal acid-base changes after bicarbonate administration to the pregnant ewe. *Anesthesiology*, **40**, 348.
6. Friedman, E. A., Little, W. A. and Sachtleben, M. R. (1962). Placental oxygen consumption *in vitro*. *Am. J. Obstet. Gynecol.*, **84**, 561.
7. Brotanek, V., Vasicka, A., Santiago, A. and Brotanek, J. D. A. (1973). The influence of epidural anesthesia on uterine blood flow. *Obstet. Gynec.*, **42**, 276.
8. Corke, B. C., Datta, S., Ostheimer, G. W., Weiss, J. B. and Alper, M. H. (1982). Spinal anaesthesia for Caesarean section. The influence of hypotension on neonatal outcome. *Anaesthesia*, **37**, 658.
9. Kauppila, A., Koskinen, M., Puolokka, J., Tuimala, R. and Kuikka, J. (1980). Decreased intervillous and unchanged myometrial blood flow in supine recumbency. *Obstet. Gynec.*, **55**, 203.
10. Datta, S., Alper, M. H., Ostheimer, G. W., Brown, W. U. and Weiss, J. B. (1979). Effects of maternal position on epidural anesthesia for Cesarean section, acid-base status, and bupivacaine concentrations at delivery. *Anesthesiology*, **50**, 205.
11. Newman, B. (1982). Cardiac output changes during Caesarean section. Measurement by transcutaneous aortovelography. *Anaesthesia*, **37**, 270.
12. Downing, J. W., Houlton, P. J. C., Brock-Utne, J. G. and Buley, R. J. R. (1978). The contrasting effects of enflurane on transplacental exchange after methohexitone and ketamine induction of anaesthesia for Caesarean section. *Anaesth. Intens. Care*, **6**, 239.
13. Collins, K. M., Bevan, D. R. and Beard, R. W. (1978). Fluid loading to reduce abnormalities of fetal heart rate and maternal hypotension during epidural analgesia in labour. *Brit. med. J.*, **277**, 1460.
14. Weaver, J. B., Pearson, J. F. and Rosen, M. (1975). Posture and epidural block in pregnant women at term. Effects on arterial blood pressure and limb blood flow. *Anaesthesia*, **30**, 752.
15. Jouppila, R., Jouppila, P., Hollmen, A. and Kuikka, J. (1978). Effect of segmental extradural analgesia on placental blood flow during normal labour. *Brit. J. Anaesth.*, **50**, 563.
16. Hollmen, A. I., Jouppila, R., Jouppila, P., Koivula, A. and Vierola, H. (1982). Effect of extradural analgesia using bupivacaine and 2-chloroprocaine on intervillous blood flow during normal labour. *Brit. J. Anaesth.*, **54**, 837.
17. Jouppila, R., Jouppila, P., Kuikka, J. and Hollmen, A. (1978). Placental blood flow during Caesarean section under lumbar extradural analgesia. *Brit. J. Anaesth.*, **50**, 275.
18. Huovinen, K., Lehtouirta, R., Forss, M., Kivalo, I. and Teramo, K. (1979). Changes in placental intervillous blood flow measured by the $^{133}$Xenon method during lumbar epidural block for elective Caesarean section. *Acta anaesth. scand.*, **23**, 529.
19. Albright, G. A., Jouppila, R., Hollmen, A. I., Jouppila, P., Vierola, H. and Koivula, A. (1981). Epinephrine does not alter human intervillous blood flow during epidural anesthesia. *Anesthesiology*, **54**, 131.
20. Pearson, J. F. and Davies, P. (1974). The effect of continuous lumbar epidural analgesia upon fetal acid-base status during the first stage of labour. *J. Obst. Gynaec. Brit. Cwlth.*, **81**, 971.
21. Thalme, B., Belfrage, P. and Raabe, N. (1974). Lumbar epidural analgesia in labour I. Acid-base balance and clinical condition of mother, fetus and newborn child. *Acta obstet. gynec. scand.*, **53**, 27.
22. Motoyama, E. K., Rivard, G., Acheson, F. and Cook, C. D. (1966). Adverse effect of maternal hyperventilation on the foetus. *Lancet*, **1**, 286.
23. Forrest, A. L., Lawson, J. I. M. and Otten, P. E. (1974). A non-invasive technique of comparing myocardial performance following epidural blockade and vasopressor therapy. *Brit. J. Anaesth.*, **46**, 662.
24. Wallis, K. L., Shnider, S. M., Hicks, J. S. and Spivey, H. T. (1976). Epidural anesthesia in the normotensive pregnant ewe: effects on uterine blood flow and fetal acid-base status. *Anesthesiology*, **44**, 481.
25. Naftalin, N. J., McKay, D. M., Phear, W. P. C. and Goldberg, A. H. (1977). The effect of halothane on pregnant and non-pregnant human myometrium. *Anesthesiology*, **46**, 15.
26. Munson, E. S., Maier, W. R. and Caton, D. (1969). Effects of halothane, cyclopropane and nitrous oxide on isolated human uterine muscle. *J. Obstet. Gynaecol. Brit. Cwlth.*, **76**, 27.
27. Munson, E. S. and Embro, W. J. (1977). Enflurane, isoflurane and halothane and isolated human uterine muscle. *Anesthesiology*, **46**, 11.
28. Willdeck-Lund, G. and Nilsson, B. A. (1979). The effect of local anaesthetic agents on the contractility of

human myometrium in late pregnancy. *Acta anaesth. scand.*, **23**, 78.

29. Kyegombe, D., Franklin, C. and Turner, P. (1973). Drug-metabolising enzymes in the human placenta, their induction and repression. *Lancet*, **1**, 405.
30. Datta, S., Brown, W. U., Ostheimer, G. W., Weiss, J. B. and Alper, M. H. (1981). Epidural anesthesia for Cesarean section in diabetic parturients: maternal and neonatal acid-base status and bupivacaine concentration. *Anesth. Analg.*, **60**, 574.
31. O'Brien, W. F., Cefalo, R. C., Grissom, M. P., Viera, S. F., Golden, S. M., Uddin, D. M. and Davies, S. E. (1982). The influence of asphyxia on fetal lidocaine toxicity. *Am. J. Obstet. Gynecol.*, **142**, 205.
32. Kennedy, R. L., Erenberg, A., Robillard, J. E., Merkow, A. and Turner, T. (1979). Effects of changes in maternal-fetal pH on the transplacental equilibrium of bupivacaine. *Anesthesiology*, **51**, 50.
33. Ehrnebo, M., Agurell, S., Jalling, B. and Boreus, L. O. (1971). Age differences in drug binding by plasma proteins: studies on human foetuses, neonates and adults. *Europ. J. clin. Pharmacol.*, **3**, 189–193.
34. Tucker, G. T., Boyes, R. N., Bridenbaugh, P. O. and Moore, D. C. (1970). Binding of anilide-type local anesthetics in human plasma: II Implications *in vivo*, with special reference to transplacental distribution. *Anesthesiology*, **33**, 304.
35. Thomas, J., Long, G., Moore, G. and Morgan, D. (1976). Plasma protein binding and placental transfer of bupivacaine. *Clin. Pharmacol. Ther.*, **19**, 426.
36. Mendenhall, H. W. (1970). Serum protein concentrations in pregnancy III. Analysis of maternal-cord serum pairs. *Amer. J. Obstet. Gynec.*, **106**, 718.
37. Reynolds, F. (1970). *Systemic toxicity of local analgesic drugs with special reference to bupivacaine.* M.D. thesis (Univ. of London).
38. Gibb, C. P., Munson, E. S. and Tham, M. K. (1975). Anesthetic solubility coefficients for maternal and fetal blood. *Anesthesiology*, **43**, 100.
39. Stenger, V. G., Blechner, J. N. and Prystowsky, H. (1969). A study of prolongation of obstetric anesthesia. *Am. J. Obstet. Gynecol.*, **103**, 901.
40. Clark, R. B., Cooper, J. O., Brown, W. E. and Greifenstein, F. E. (1970). The effect of methoxyflurane on the foetus. *Brit. J. Anaesth.*, **42**, 286.
41. Siker, E. S., Wolfson, B., Dubnansky, J. and Fitting, G. M. (1968). Placental transfer of methoxyflurane. *Brit. J. Anaesth.*, **40**, 588.
42. Wickström, I., Kjellmer, I., Kristianson, B. and Magno, R. (1980). Anaesthesia for Caesarean section—VII. Early effects on neonatal renal function of enflurane anesthesia for Cesarean section. *Acta anaesth. scand.*, **24**, 190.
43. Geddes, I. C., Brand, L., Finster, M. and Mark, L. (1972). Distribution of halothane-$^{82}$Br in maternal and foetal guinea-pig tissues. *Brit. J. Anaesth.*, **44**, 542.
44. Phillips, T. J. and Macdonald, R. R. (1971). Comparative effect of pethidine, trichloroethylene and Entonox on fetal and neonatal acid-base and $Po_2$. *Brit. med. J.*, **3**, 558.
45. Palahniuk, R. J., Scatliff, J., Biehl, D., Wiebe, H. and Sankaran, K. (1977). Maternal and neonatal effects of methoxyflurane, nitrous oxide and lumbar epidural anaesthesia for Caesarean section. *Canad. Anaesth. Soc. J.*, **24**, 586.
46. Cassano, G. B., Ghetti, B., Gliozzi, E. and Hansson, E. (1967). Autoradiographic distribution study of "short-acting" and "long-acting" barbiturates: $^{35}$S-thiopentone and $^{14}$C-phenobarbitone. *Brit. J. Anaesth.*, **39**, 11.
47. Heslop-Christensen, J., Andreasen, F. and Jansen, J. A. (1981). Pharmacokinetics of thiopentone in Caesarean section. *Acta anaesth. scand.*, **25**, 174.
48. Dawes, G. S. (1973). Theory of fetal drug equilibration. In: *Fetal Pharmacology*, ed. L. Boréus, New York: Raven Press.
49. Finster, M., Mark, L. C., Morishima, H. O., Moya, F., Perel, J. M., James. L. S. and Dayton, P. G. (1966). Plasma thiopental concentration in the newborn following delivery under thiopental-nitrous oxide anesthesia. *Am. J. Obstet. Gynecol.*, **95**, 621.
50. Brazelton, T. B. (1961). Psychophysiological reactions in the neonate II. Effect of maternal medication in the neonate and his behaviour. *J. Pediat.*, **58**, 513.
51. Shier, R. W., Sprague, A. D. and Dilts, P. V. (1973). Placental transfer of meperidine HCl. Part II. *Am. J. Obstet. Gynecol.*, **115**, 556.
52. Apgar, V., Burns, J. J., Brodie, B. B. and Papper, E. M. (1952). The transmission of meperidine across the human placenta. *Am. J. Obstet. Gynecol.*, **64**, 1368.
53. Crawford, J. S. and Rudofsky, S. (1965). Placental transmission and neonatal metabolism of promazine. *Brit. J. Anaesth.*, **37**, 303.
54. Beckett, A. H. and Taylor, J. F. (1967). Blood concentrations of pethidine and pentazocine in mother and infant at time of birth. *J. Pharm. Pharmacol.*, **19**, Suppl., 50.
55. Duncan, S. L. B., Ginsburg, J. and Morris, N. F. (1969). Comparison of pentazocine and pethidine in normal labor. *Am. J. Obstet. Gynecol.*, **105**, 197.
56. Moore, J., McNabb, T. G. and Glynn, J. P. (1973). The placental transfer of pentazocine and pethidine. *Brit. J. Anaesth.*, **45**, 798.
57. Caldwell, J., Wakile, L. A., Notarianni, L. J., Smith, R. L., Lieberman, B. A., Jeffs, J., Coy, Y. and Beard, R. W. (1977). Transplacental passage and neonatal elimination of pethidine given to mothers in childbirth. *Brit. J. clin. Pharmacol.*, **4**, 715P–716P.
58. Tomson, G., Garle, R. I. M., Thalme, B., Nisell, H., Nylund, L. and Rane, A. (1982). Maternal kinetics and transplacental passage of pethidine during labour. *Brit. J. clin. Pharmacol.*, **13**, 653.
59. Caldwell, J., Notarianni, L. J. and Smith, R. L. (1978). Impaired metabolism of pethidine in the human neonate. *Brit. J. clin. Pharmacol.*, **5**, 362P.
60. Refstad, S. O. and Lindbaek, E. (1980). Ventilatory depression of the newborn of women receiving pethidine or pentazocine. A double-blind comparative trial. *Brit. J. Anaesth.*, **52**, 265.
61. Moore, J., Carson, R. M. and Hunter, R. J. (1970). A comparison of the effects of pentazocine and pethidine administered during labour. *J. Obstet. Gynaec. Brit. Cwlth.*, **77**, 830.
62. Oliva, G. C., Marchetti, P., Di Maggio, A., Arduini, D., Mancuso, S. and Romanini, C. (1980). Effetti della Meperidina e della pentazocina sub feto e sull'attivita contrattile uterina. *Ann. Ost. Gin. Med. Perin.*, **CI**, 67.
63. Roberts, H., Kane, K. M., Percival, N., Snow, P. and Please, N. W. (1957). Effects of some analgesic drugs used in childbirth with special reference to variation in

respiratory minute volume of the newborn. *Lancet*, **1**, 128.
64. Brackbill, Y., Kane, J., Manniello, R. L. and Abramson, D. (1974). Obstetric meperidine usage and assessment of neonatal status. *Anesthesiology*, **40**, 116.
65. Belsey, E. M., Rosenblatt, D. B., Lieberman, B. A., Redshaw, M., Caldwell, J. Notarianni, L., Smith, R. L. and Beard, R. W. (1981). The influence of maternal analgesia on neonatal behaviour. I. Pethidine. *Brit. J. Obstet. Gynecol.*, **88**, 398.
66. Shnider, S. M. and Moya, F. (1964). Effects of meperidine on the newborn infant. *Am. J. Obstet. Gynecol.*, **89**, 1009.
67. Morrison, J. C., Wiser, W. L., Rosser, S. I., Gayden, J. O., Bucovaz, E. T., Whybrew, W. D. and Fish, S. A. (1973). Metabolites of meperidine related to fetal depression. *Am. J. Obstet. Gynecol.*, **115**, 1132.
68. Stephen, G. W. and Cooper, L. V. (1977). The role of analgesics in respiratory depression: a rabbit model. *Anaesthesia*, **32**, 324.
69. Morrison, J. C., Whybrew, W. D., Rosser, S. I., Bucovaz, E. T., Wiser, W. L. and Fish, S. A. (1976). Metabolites of meperidine in the fetal and maternal serum. *Am. J. Obstet. Gynecol.*, **126**, 997.
70. Wiener, P. C., Hogg, M. I. and Rosen, M. (1979). Neonatal respiration, feeding and neurobehavioural state. Effects of intrapartum bupivacaine, pethidine and pethidine reversed by naloxone. *Anaesthesia*, **34**, 996.
71. Wiener, P. C., Hogg, M. I. J. and Rosen, M. (1977). Effects of naloxone on pethidine-induced neonatal depression. *Brit. med. J.*, **2**, 228.
72. Moreland, T. A., Brice, J. E. H., Walker, C. H. M. and Parija, A. C. (1980). Naloxone pharmacokinetics in the newborn. *Brit. J. Clin. Pharmacol.*, **9**, 609.
73. O'Donoghue, S. E. F. (1971). Distribution of pethidine and chlorpromazine in maternal, foetal and neonatal biological fluids. *Nature (Lond.)*, **229**, 124.
74. Ullberg, S. (1973). Autoradiography in fetal pharmacology. In: *Fetal Pharmacology*. Ed. by L. Boreus. New York: Raven Press.
75. Idanpaan-Heikkila, J. E., Jouppila, P. I., Poulakka, J. O. and Vorne, M. S. (1971). Placental transfer and fetal metabolism of diazepam in early human pregnancy. *Am. J. Obstet. Gynecol.*, **109**, 1011.
76. Erkkola, R., Kangas, L. and Pekkarinen, A. (1973). The transfer of diazepam across the placenta during labour. *Acta obstet. gynec. scand.*, **52**, 167.
77. Mandelli, M., Morselli, P. L., Nordio, S., Pardi, G., Principi, N., Sereni, F. and Tognoni, G. (1975). Placental transfer of diazepam and its disposition in the newborn. *Clin. Pharmacol. Ther.*, **17**, 565.
78. McBride, R. J., Dundee, J. W., Moore, J., Toner, W. and Howard, P. J. (1979). A study of the plasma concentrations of lorazepam in mother and neonate. *Brit. J. Anaesth.*, **51**, 971.
79. Whitelaw, A. G. L., Cummings, A. J. and McFadyen, I. R. (1981). Effect of maternal lorazepam on the neonate. *Brit. med. J.*, **282**, 1106.
80. Cummings, A. J. and Whitelaw, A. G. L. (1981). A study of conjugation and drug elimination in the human neonate. *Brit. J. clin. Pharmacol.*, **12**, 511.
81. Reynolds, F. and Taylor, G. (1970). Maternal and neonatal concentrations of bupivacaine: a comparison with lignocaine during continuous extradural analgesia. *Anaesthesia*, **25**, 14.
82. Kuhnert, P. M., Kuhnert, B. R., Stitts, J. M. and Gross, T. L. (1981). The use of a selected ion monitoring technique to study the disposition of bupivacaine in mother, fetus and neonate following epidural anesthesia for Cesarean section. *Anesthesiology*, **55**, 611.
83. Poppers, P., Covino, B. and Boyes, N. (1975). Epidural block with etidocaine for labour and delivery. *Acta anaesth. scand.*, Suppl. 60, 89.
84. Lund, P. C., Cwik, J. C., Gannon, R. T. and Vassallo, H. G. (1977). Etidocaine for Caesarean section—effects on mother and baby. *Brit. J. Anaesth.*, **49**, 457.
85. Moore, D. C., Bridenbaugh, L. D., Bagdi, P. A. and Bridenbaugh, P. O. (1968). Accumulation of mepivacaine hydrochloride during caudal block. *Anesthesiology*, **29**, 585.
86. Morishima, H. O., Daniel, S. S., Finster, M., Poppers, P. J. and James, L. S. (1966). Transmission of mepivacaine hydrochloride (Carbocaine) across the human placenta. *Anesthesiology*, **27**, 147.
87. Epstein, B. S., Banerjee, S. G. and Coakley, C. S. (1968). Passage of lidocaine and prilocaine across the placenta. *Anesth. Analg. Curr. Res.*, **47**, 223.
88. Kuhnert, B. R., Kuhnert, P. M., Prochaska, A. L. and Gross, T. L. (1980). Plasma levels of 2-chloroprocaine in obstetric patients and their neonates after epidural anesthesia. *Anesthesiology*, **53**, 21.
89. Shnider, S. M. and Way, E. L. (1968). The kinetics of transfer of lidocaine (Xylocaine ®) across the human placenta. *Anesthesiology*, **29**, 944.
90. Blankenbaker, W. L., Difazio, C. A. and Berry, F. A. (1975). Lidocaine and its metabolites in the newborn *Anesthesiology*, **42**, 325.
91. Brown, W. U., Bell, G. C., Lurie, A. O., Weiss, J. B., Scanlon, J. W. and Alper, M. H. (1975). Newborn blood levels of lidocaine and mepivacaine in the first postnatal day following maternal epidural anesthesia. *Anesthesiology*, **42**, 698.
92. Aps, C., Bell, J. A., Jenkins, B. S., Poole-Wilson, P. A. and Reynolds, F. (1976). Logical approach to lignocaine therapy. *Brit. med. J.*, **1**, 13.
93. Meffin, P., Long, G. J. and Thomas, J. (1973). Clearance and metabolism of mepivacaine in the human neonate. *Clin. Pharmacol. Ther.*, **14**, 218.
94. Caldwell, J., Moffatt, J. R., Smith, R. L., Lieberman, B. A., Cawston, M. O. and Beard, R. W. (1976). Pharmacokinetics of bupivacaine administered epidurally during childbirth. *Brit. J. clin. Pharmacol.*, **3**, 956P.
95. Morgan, D., McQuillan, D. and Thomas, J. (1978). Pharmacokinetics and metabolism of the amide local anaesthetics in neonates. 11 etidocaine. *Europ. J. clin. Pharmacol.*, **13**, 365.
96. Shnider, S. M. and Way, E. L. (1968). Plasma levels of lidocaine (Xylocaine ®) in mother and newborn, following obstetrical conduction anesthesia. *Anesthesiology*, **29**, 951.
97. Scanlon, J. W., Brown, W. U., Weiss, J. B. and Alper, M. H. (1974). Neurobehavioural responses of newborn infants after maternal epidural anesthesia. *Anesthesiology*, **40**, 121.
98. Scanlon, J. W., Ostheimer, G. W., Lurie, A. O., Brown, W. U., Weiss, J. B. and Alper, M. H. (1976). Neurobehavioural responses and drug concentrations in newborns after maternal epidural anesthesia with bupivacaine. *Anesthesiology*, **45**, 400.
99. Abboud, T. K., Khoo, S. S., Miller, F., Doan, T. and

Henriksen, F. H. (1982). Maternal, fetal and neonatal responses after epidural anesthesia with bupivacaine, 2-chloroprocaine or lidocaine. *Anesth. Analg.*, **61**, 638.

100. Rosenblatt, D. B., Belsey, E. M., Lieberman, B. A., Redshaw, M., Caldwell, J., Notarianni, L., Smith, R. L. and Beard, R. W. (1981). The influence of maternal analgesia on neonatal behaviour: II. Epidural bupivacaine. *Brit. J. Obstet. Gynecol.*, **88**, 407.
101. Merkow, A. J., McGuinness, G. A., Erenberg, A. and Kennedy, R. L. (1980). The neonatal neurobehavioural effects of bupivacaine, mepivacaine and 2-chloroprocaine used for pudendal block. *Anesthesiology*, **52**, 309.
102. Older, P. O. and Harris, J. M. (1968). Placental transfer of tubocurarine. *Brit. J. Anaesth.*, **40**, 459.
103. Thomas, J., Climie, C. R. and Mather, L. E. (1969). The placental transfer of alcuronium. *Brit. J. Anaesth.*, **41**, 297.
104. Speirs, I. and Sim, A. W. (1972). The placental transfer of pancuronium bromide. *Brit. J. Anaesth.*, **44**, 370.
105. Kivalo, I. and Saarikoski, S. (1976). Placental transfer of $^{14}$C-dimethyltubocurarine during caesarean section. *Brit. J. Anaesth.*, **48**, 239.
106. Drabkova, J., Crul, J. F. and van der Kleijn, E. (1973). Placental transfer of $^{14}$C labelled succinylcholine in near-term Macaca Mulatta monkeys. *Brit. J. Anaesth.*, **45**, 1087.
107. Booth, P. N., Watson, M. J. and McLeod, K. (1977). Pancuronium and the placental barrier. *Anaesthesia*, **32**, 320.
108. Duvaldestin, P., Demetriou, M., Henzel, D. and Desmonts, J. M. (1978). The placental transfer of pancuronium and its pharmacokinetics during Caesarean section. *Acta anaesth. scand.*, **22**, 327.
109. Bertrand, J. C., Duvaldestin, P., Henzel, D. and Desmonts, J. M. (1980). Quantitative assessment of placental transfer of fazadinium in obstetric anaesthesia. *Acta anaesth. scand.*, **24**, 135.
110. Abouleish, E., Wingard, L. B., De La Vega, S. and Uy, N. (1980). Pancuronium in Caesarean section and its placental transfer. *Brit. J. Anaesth.*, **52**, 531.
111. Schifferli, P-Y. and Caldeyro-Barcia, R. (1973). Effects of atropine and beta-adrenergic drugs on the heart rate of the human fetus. In: *Fetal Pharmacology*, pp. 259–278. Ed. by L. Boreus. New York: Raven Press.
112. Kivalo, I. and Saarikoski, S. (1977). Placental transmission of atropine at full-term pregnancy. *Brit. J. Anaesth.*, **49**, 1017.
113. Kanto, J., Virtanen, R., Iisalo, E., Mäenpää, K. and Liukko, P. (1981). Placental transfer and pharmacokinetics of atropine after a single maternal intravenous and intramuscular administration. *Acta anaesth. scand.*, **25**, 85.
114. Tarnow-Mordi, W. O., Shaw, J. C. L., Liu, D., Gardner, D. A. and Flynn, F. V. (1981). Iatrogenic hyponatraemia of the newborn due to maternal fluid overload: a prospective study. *Brit. med. J.*, **283**, 639.
115. Mendiola, J., Grylack, L. J. and Scanlon, J. W. (1982). Effects of intrapartum maternal glucose infusion on the normal fetus and newborn. *Anesth. Analg.*, **61**, 32.
116. Brownridge, P. (1979). Extradural analgesia for Caesarean section (letter). *Brit. J. Anaesth.*, **51**, 1092.
117. Studd, J. W. W., Crawford, J. S., Duignan, N. M., Rowbotham, C. J. F. and Hughes, A. O. (1980). The effect of lumbar epidural analgesia upon cervimetric progress and the outcome of spontaneous labour. *Anaesthesia*, **35**, 419.
118. Pearson, J. F. and Davies, P. (1974). The effect of continuous lumbar epidural analgesia upon fetal acid-base status during the second stage of labour. *J. Obstet. Gynaec. Brit. Cwlth.*, **81**, 975.
119. Maltau, J. M. and Egge, K. (1980). Epidural analgesia and perinatal retinal haemorrhages. *Acta anaesth. scand.*, **24**, 99.
120. David, H. and Rosen, M. (1976). Perinatal mortality after epidural analgesia. *Anaesthesia*, **31**, 1054.
121. Dodson, M. E. and Chiswick, M. L. (1981). Anaesthetic drugs and maternal-infant bonding (letter). *Brit. J. Anaesth.*, **53**, 551.
122. Johnson, E. S. and Colley, P. S. (1980). Effects of nitrous oxide and fentanyl anaesthesia on fetal heart-rate variability intra- and post-operatively. *Anesthesiology*, **52**, 429.
123. Thomas, G. (1975). The aetiology, characteristics and diagnostic relevance of late deceleration patterns in routine obstetric practice. *Brit. J. Obstet. Gynaec.*, **82**, 126.
124. Saling, E. E. and Schneider, D. (1967). Biochemical supervision of the foetus during labour. *J. Obstet. Gynaec. Brit. Cwlth.*, **74**, 799.
125. Beard, R. W. and Morris, E. D. (1969). *Modern Trends in Obstetrics*, p. 298. London: Butterworths.
126. Reynolds, F. R. (1979). Transfer of drugs. In: *Placental Transfer*. ed. by G. V. P. Chamberlain and A. W. Wilkinson. London: Pitman Books.

CHAPTER 42

# Paediatric Anaesthesia



## Introduction

Specialised anaesthesia for paediatric patients is necessary for those below the age of about five years (or less than 20 kg body weight), though strictly speaking all patients below the age of 14 years are paediatric. Marked differences exist between infants and older children or adults, not only in their anatomy, but also in their physiology, handling of drugs, and other pathological processes. With many babies of 27 weeks' gestation surviving with weights as low as 600 g, the peculiarities of neonatal physiology may persist longer than the defined period.

Specialised centres have evolved for treating babies in the neonatal period (first 28 days of extrauterine life) with paediatric physicians, surgeons, anaesthetists and nursing staff trained in the care of this vulnerable group of patients.[1]

## CHANGES THAT TAKE PLACE AT BIRTH

### Cardiovascular System

In the fetal circulation oxygenated blood

coming from the placenta via the umbilical vein and ductus venosus passes through the liver and the very short inferior vena cava and as quickly as possible to the coronaries and developing brain. There is only minimal mixing with desaturated blood from the gut and lower limbs. This division of the vena cava into two streams is achieved by the ridge, termed the crista dividens. The superior margin of the foramen ovale (crista terminalis) guides the blood flow from the right to left atrium and so to the aorta via the left ventricle. Only 10 per cent of the right ventricular output flows through the lungs, the remainder bypasses the lungs by right-to-left shunting through the patent ductus arteriosus because the pulmonary vascular resistance is higher than the systemic (Fig. 1).

After clamping of the umbilical cord, right atrial pressure falls. At the same time the lungs become inflated and the pulmonary vascular resistance falls, allowing increased pulmonary blood flow. The change in right and left atrial pressures causes closure of the foramen ovale which usually seals in most cases. This represents the transitional circulation.

Physiological closure of the ductus arteriosus is completed within 10–15 hours by contraction of the smooth muscle at the end of the pulmonary artery, under the influence of increasing $Pa_{O_2}$ after the first breath. Anatomical closure is delayed for 2–3 weeks.[2] E prostaglandins relax ductal muscle and contraction will occur with inhibitors of prostaglandin synthesis such as indomethacin.[3]

The administration of prostaglandin E will maintain patency of the ductus in patients with pulmonary atresia until a systemic-pulmonary shunt can be created surgically. The neonatal circulation is labile and may revert to a transitional type with blood flowing right-to-left through a ductus arteriosus or patent foramen ovale. This state, caused by increased pulmonary vascular resistance in response to hypoxia, hypercapnia or acidaemia, is especially important in patients with hyaline membrane disease or congenital diaphragmatic hernia. The vicious circle of cyanosis, acidaemia, falling cardiac output and death, may be reversed by drugs such as tolazoline, which dilate the pulmonary vasculature.[4] The neonatal physiological shunt is in the order of 20 per cent (adult 7 per cent).

At birth the heart rate averages between 130 and 160 per minute, but gradually falls to around 100 by 5 years of age. Neonates have a mean systolic blood pressure of 80±16 mm Hg (10·7±2·1 kPa) and mean diastolic blood pressure of 46±16 mm Hg (6·1±2·1 kPa). Cardiac output falls from a level of 400–500 ml/kg per minute to 150–200 ml/kg per minute as fetal channels close during the first week of life. As the cardiac output falls, peripheral vasoconstriction must occur to produce the rise in blood pressure seen after birth.

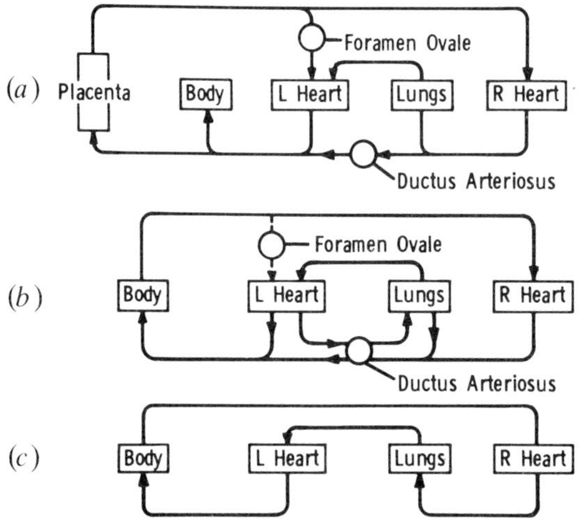


42/FIG. 1.—Diagram of (*a*) the fetal, (*b*) transitional and (*c*) adult circulations.

### Respiratory System

After 16 weeks of fetal life *in utero*, the total number of airways and blood vessels are present, though the number of alveoli are relatively few even at term.

From 24 weeks *in utero*, granules appear in the alveolar lining cells, from which surfactant develops. Lipoproteins which lower surface tension "*in vitro*" to less than 10–15 dyne/cm are called surfactants. Without surfactant to lower the surface tension in the fluid alveolar lining, once a fluid/air interface has developed, the lungs would be unable to retain gas within them and would be unstable. Surfactant deficiency is the most important factor in the development of hyaline membrane disease of the newborn.

The active constituents of surfactant are phospholipids, 85 per cent of which is lecithin and this appears in the amniotic fluid towards term. Gluck and his co-workers (1971)[5] showed that the terminal increase in lecithin in amniotic fluid is greater than that of sphingomyelin (another surface-active phospholipid). When the ratio of lecithin to sphingomyelin is above 2, the risk of hyaline membrane disease is low, but when the ratio is less than 1·5 the risk is high. Such investigations are obviously useful when premature induction of labour is being considered.

Glucocorticoids, when infused into the animal fetus, accelerate the production of surfactant and it is possible that the early presence of surfactant in "poorer risk" pregnancies is provoked by the steroids. The role of steroids in normal conditions is not clear, though infants who develop hyaline membrane disease have lower blood cortisols than infants who have no pulmonary disease.[6] Normal thyroid function is also necessary for surfactant development.[7]

Regular respiratory movements of the fluid-filled lungs can be detected in the fetus from an early gestational age. The movements increase in size and frequency as maturation of the fetus proceeds.[8] The periods of fetal breathing are increased in the presence of fetal hypercapnia and cease during hypoxia.[9] They can be detected by ultrasound, are present for up to 90 per cent of the time and are taken to be a sign of fetal wellbeing.

### The First Breath

Within one minute of clamping of the umbilical cord the neonate establishes and maintains a pattern of regular respiration. Many factors such as sound, touch, and temperature stimulate the first breath, but major factors appear to be a sudden resetting of the chemoreceptors and the effect of hypoxia. Sensory activity impinges on the reticular system, causing a resetting of the respiratory centre so that levels of oxygen and carbon dioxide tension, which before had no effect on respiration, now do so. The tension of oxygen in carotid blood rises at birth from 23 mm Hg (3·1 kPa) to more than 60 mm Hg (8·0 kPa) and the carbon dioxide level falls from 45 to 35 mm Hg (6·0–4·7 kPa).

The infant's first breath generates respiratory pressures exceeding 70 cm $H_2O$. Active expiration expels lung fluid and then progressively each respiratory cycle shows smaller pressure-volume loops with steadily decreasing effort for breathing (Fig. 2). A normal functional residual volume of 70–80 ml is established within 60 minutes of birth. Some of the reasons why respiratory failure is so common in infants can be seen in Table 1.

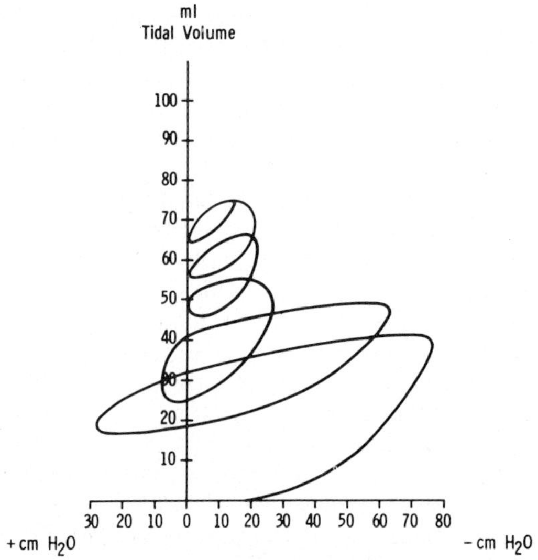


42/Fig. 2.—Pressure-volume loops of a neonate's first five breaths. Note the large negative and positive swings during the first two breaths, and the gradual increase in residual volume until the lungs are filled.

42/Table 1

Causes of Low Respiratory Reserve of the Infant

1. Higher dead-space : tidal volume ratio
2. Higher respiratory rate
3. Sole reliance on diaphragmatic function
4. Alveolar ventilation twice the adult (150 ml/kg)
5. Low lung compliance (6 ml/cm $H_2O$)
6. High total pulmonary resistance (25 cm $H_2O\ l^{-1}\ sec^{-1}$)
7. Large physiological shunt (20 per cent on day 1). Closing volume occurs within tidal breathing.

## THE SURGICAL NEONATE

A neonate loses weight from the time of birth, but generally the birth weight is regained in ten days. A normal child can be expected to double its birth weight in five months and by one year weighs three times the birth weight.

Haemoglobin falls rapidly from the level at birth of approximately 19g/dl and after a period of relative anaemia rises to adult levels.

42/TABLE 2
SOME AVERAGE VALUES FOR A NEONATE WEIGHING 3·4 kg

| | |
|---|---|
| Respiratory rate | 30–40/min |
| Tidal volume | 17 ml |
| Alveolar ventilation | 460 ml/min |
| Pulse rate | 120–160/min |
| Mean blood pressure | 65 mm Hg (8·7 kPa) |
| Haemoglobin concentration | 17–19 g/100 ml (g/dl) |
| Urinary output | 17–85 ml/kg/24h |
| Fluid requirement | 100–170 ml/kg/24h |

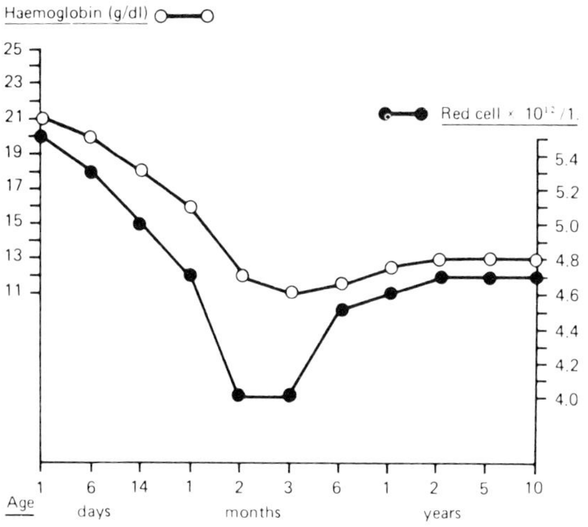


42/FIG. 3.—Changes in haemoglobin concentration and red-cell count in the first ten years of life. (Courtesy of Dr. H. T. Davenport and William Heinemann Medical Books.[10])

## Thermal Regulation

The neonate attempts to maintain core temperature at 37° C, but because of an initial low basal metabolic rate, large surface-to-weight ratio, immature sweat function, poor insulation, and an inability to move from an adverse thermal environment, this may not be successful. The newborn baby is very vulnerable to changes in environmental temperature, and low-birth-weight babies particularly so. Silverman and his associates[11] showed that a reduction in infant mortality of 40 per cent could be achieved if infants of less than 1·5 kg were nursed in ambient temperatures of 31·7° C rather than 28·9° C.

Superfical thermoreceptors exist, especially in the trigeminal distribution of the face, and a cold stimulus causes an increase in metabolic heat production from the hydrolysis of triglycerides in brown fat. This very vascular fat is situated in the upper part of the body and thermally lags the great thoraco-abdominal vessels. The ability to shiver is poorly developed. Metabolism of brown fat increases metabolic rate, cardiac output and oxygen consumption, so that any existing hypoxia is worsened.[12] The metabolic response to cold is greatly inhibited by general anaesthesia.

The ability to sweat is limited and starts only when the core temperature rises by 1° C.

The neutral thermal environment is that temperature in which the oxygen consumption of the baby is minimal, and this is approximately 31° C in a term baby and almost 36° C for a low-birth-weight baby. These are the temperature settings for incubators.

The neonate in the delivery room or operating theatre is very vulnerable to cold stress but some heat loss is inevitable. This is reduced by the use of aluminised plastic swaddlers, warm wrappings, aluminium foil to the limbs, a heated mattress and an overhead heater. The ambient temperature should be 24° C.

## Fluid Balance

The neonatal kidney is able to cope with the normal demands made on it, because 50 per cent of dietary protein is incorporated into new tissue. Because of a lower glomerular filtration rate per unit surface area, poor capacity to concentrate urine and no diuretic response to a water load, it is less well equipped to deal with the effects of dehydration, excess water and electrolyte load, trauma or acidosis.

Urine volume begins at about 25 ml/kg per day and rises to 100–120 ml/kg body weight per day by the end of the first week. 92 per cent of all healthy babies pass urine within 24 hours of birth. Insensible loss in normal babies is 25–30 ml/kg per day, but is much greater in premature babies and also if phototherapy* and overhead heaters are used.

Maintenance requirements for the full-term neonate are 20–40 ml/kg per day on the first day, increasing by 20 ml/kg per day up to

* Phototherapy is a technique using a wavelength of 425–475 nm to decompose bilirubin in peripheral vessels. It has greatly reduced the number of exchange transfusions necessary in neonates.

120 ml/kg per day. Some centres do not give maintenance fluids in the first 2–3 days of life unless abnormal losses occur. All maintenance fluids for neonates should include dextrose – 4 per cent with 0·18 per cent saline. If there is difficulty in maintaining a normal blood sugar, then 10 per cent dextrose in saline should be substituted.[13]

### Hepatic Function

Some aspects of liver function such as detoxication of drugs and carbohydrate metabolism are poorly developed at birth, but others such as synthesis of albumin and coagulation factors are relatively normal. By 6 weeks of age enzyme systems function at adult levels.

Because of low glycogen stores and hepatic immaturity, *hypoglycaemia*, defined as 1·6 mmol/1 (30 mg per cent) or less, in a *term* baby, is common. In *low-birth-weight* babies hypoglycaemia is below 1·1 mmol/1 (20 mg per cent). The possibility of hypoglycaemia must be anticipated, and four-hourly Dextrostix performed. The condition is usually without symptoms unless the level is very low, when apnoeic attacks or convulsions may occur. 10 per cent dextrose may be infused at a rate of 75–100 ml/kg per day. Hypothermia can also cause hypoglycaemia.

### Hypocalcaemia

This condition occurs commonly in the first 2 days of life in sick babies. Causative factors are immaturity of the parathyroids and high phosphate content of some milk formulae. Non-specific neurological signs such as irritability may lead to tetany or convulsions, and should be treated with an infusion of 2 per cent solution of calcium gluconate at 5 mg/kg per hour. Calcium should be given if the total calcium level falls below 1·5 mmol/l.

## NEONATAL RESUSCITATION

### Neonatal Asphyxia

Neonatal asphyxia may be due to a failure to breathe or an inability to expand the lungs. A failure to breathe may be due to respiratory-centre depression caused by intra-uterine hypoxia or by narcotic or anaesthetic drugs. The depressant action of opiates is well known but diazepam has also been shown to produce neonatal depression when given in large doses (in excess of 30 mg) to the mother in the 24 hours prior to delivery.[14] Asphyxia may also be caused by brain-stem injury due to cerebral haemorrhage. The lungs may not be able to expand if the infant is very premature or if the airway is obstructed by mucus or meconium.

After observing experimental animals subjected to birth asphyxia, Dawes[15] described neonatal asphyxia in two phases, i.e. primary apnoea and terminal apnoea.

The sequence of events (as observed in animals) is as follows. After an initial period of

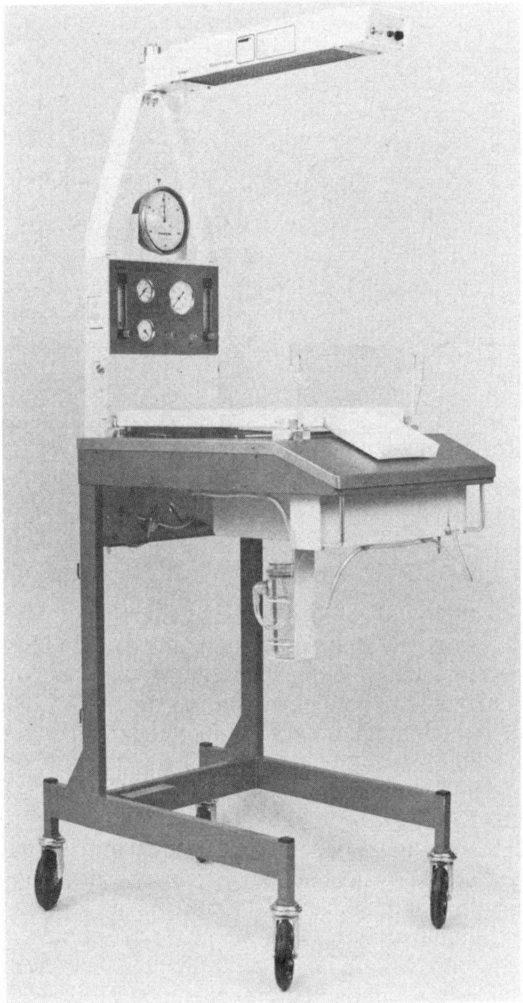

42/Fig. 4.—Neonatal resuscitation trolley (Vickers Medical Model 60 Resuscitaire; courtesy of Vickers Medical).

distressed attempts at breathing, a period of apnoea occurs (primary apnoea). This is followed, after an interval, by a series of gasps increasing in frequency, but diminishing in effectiveness until all activity ceases (terminal apnoea). Unless active measures are taken very quickly, the heart stops and the animal will be dead. There is every reason to believe that these observations apply equally to the human infant.

**Primary apnoea.**—An infant in this state makes active efforts to breathe at first, but is cyanosed and only responds weakly to external stimuli. The tone is weakly flexural, though the heart rate is usually over 100/min. The Apgar score is about 6.

Most cases of primary apnoea respond to routine care – clearing the nasopharyngeal mucus, and application of oxygen. "Lazy" babies often gasp actively if expansion of the lungs is initiated by application of positive pressure (e.g. by mask and inflating bag).

If the period of asphyxia has been prolonged or severe, the baby passes to a stage of terminal apnoea. It is important to recognise this state as urgent resuscitative measures are required to save the child.

**Terminal apnoea.**—At this stage the baby is white or pale and makes no attempt to breathe. There is no muscle tone and no response to external stimuli. The heart rate is below 100 and gradually becomes even slower. The Apgar score is less than 3.

### The Apgar Score

A more objective method of evaluating the state of a newborn infant is by means of scoring, using five signs noted sixty seconds after birth of the baby.[16,17] The signs are heart rate, respiratory effort, muscle tone, reflex irritability, and colour. Each sign is given a score of 0, 1 or 2. A total score of 10 shows that the infant is in the best possible condition. Active resuscitation is necessary below 5. Details of this Apgar score are given in Table 3.

A systematic approach to resuscitative intervention has been described by Gregory (1975)[18] and is summarised in Table 4.

In practice it is often difficult to distinguish between primary and terminal apnoea and little is lost, and a great deal gained, by early active treatment of apnoeic infants. *The infant should be intubated and given artificial ventilation. Resuscitation must not be delayed in an attempt to assess the Apgar score correctly.*

### Artificial Respiration

This must take place if there are no respiratory movements after one minute, or the heart rate is less than 100/min at any time. It is possible to ventilate the patient with a face

42/TABLE 3
THE APGAR SCORE

| *Sign* | *Score* | | |
|---|---|---|---|
| | 0 | 1 | 2 |
| Heart rate | absent | slow (below 100) | over 100 |
| Respiratory effort | absent | weak cry<br>hypoventilation | good strong cry |
| Muscle tone | limp | some flexion of extremities | well flexed |
| Reflex irritability (response of skin stimulation to feet) | no response | some motion | cry |
| Colour | blue<br>pale | body pink<br>extremities blue | completely pink |

42/Table 4

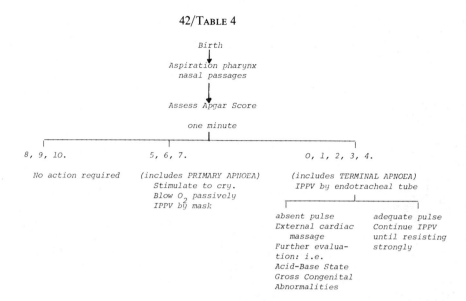

Birth
↓
Aspiration pharynx nasal passages
↓
Assess Apgar Score one minute

- **8, 9, 10.** No action required
- **5, 6, 7.** (includes PRIMARY APNOEA) Stimulate to cry. Blow $O_2$ passively IPPV by mask
- **0, 1, 2, 3, 4.** (includes TERMINAL APNOEA) IPPV by endotracheal tube
  - absent pulse: External cardiac massage. Further evaluation: i.e. Acid-Base State, Gross Congenital Abnormalities
  - adequate pulse: Continue IPPV until resisting strongly

mask,[19] but ventilation is most readily and efficiently achieved by endotracheal intubation.

The technique of intubation involves the use of the straight-bladed laryngoscope (e.g. Magill-Anderson (U.K.) or Flagg (U.S.A.) blade. The tip of the blade of the laryngoscope is advanced into the posterior pharynx or upper oesophagus. The blade is then slowly withdrawn whilst maintaining pressure on the tongue anteriorly. The larynx springs into view, whilst the epiglottis is retained anterior to the blade. A tube of size 12FG (equivalent to 2·5 mm internal diameter) will be suitable for most neonates, although a 10 FG (2·0 mm) may be necessary for a small baby. Cole-pattern shouldered tubes are traditionally used for this purpose.[20]

Hey[21] suggests that an inflation pressure of 30 cm $H_2O$, maintained for 1–2 seconds, is the best way of initially aerating the lungs, though slightly higher pressures may be needed in some babies. Excised lungs when inflated at autopsy tend to rupture at inflation pressures in excess of 30 cm $H_2O$, though in clinical practice pneumothorax is rare. Neonatal resuscitators are all fitted with relief valves to vent at 30 cm $H_2O$. After the initial breath, regular ventilation at pressures of 15–20 cm $H_2O$ should be given until normal regular spontaneous respiration begins.

If intravenous drugs are to be given, they may be injected into the umbilical vein, but prolonged cannulation of the umbilical vein may lead to thrombosis of the portal vein. Narcotic depression is best treated with naloxone 0·005–0·01 mg/kg.

**Cardiac Arrest or Severe Bradycardia** (<30/min)

In these circumstances, external cardiac massage must be instituted to maintain a cardiac output. The technique is slightly different to that used on the adult. Pressure is applied over the middle sternum as there is danger of causing damage to the liver by depression of the lower sternum. Pressure is applied with two fingers only or, alternatively, the upper thorax is held with both hands and pressure applied to the mid-sternum with both thumbs.

## PRE-OPERATIVE ASSESSMENT

A pre-operative visit to children of all ages by the anaesthetist is crucial. Children between the ages of 2 and 5 years are particularly prone to unreasonable fears and do not have the intellectual ability to rationalise these. Careful handling, an explanation of what will take place and that the sleep essential for a pain-free operation is only temporary, will usually calm these fears. Emotional upsets are fewer if the mother is admitted to hospital with the child.

A detailed history and physical examination, with emphasis on assessment of cardiovascular and respiratory function are important. Children frequently suffer from upper respiratory-tract infections and surgery should be delayed if the child has a nasal discharge, inflamed tonsils or ear-drums, or a fever. In the latter circumstances, the incidence of complications is high: for example, severe laryngeal spasm during anaesthesia, and pneumonia postoperatively. Upper respiratory-tract infection (URTI) may be the prodromal phase of one of the childhood exanthemata—notably chicken-pox and measles.

The anaesthetist will be alerted to possible intubation difficulties associated with conditions such as Still's disease or Pierre-Robin syndrome.

All children should be accurately weighed after admission and a haemoglobin estimation performed. All children over 3 months of age, originating from Africa or Mediterranean countries, who are likely to be carriers of sickle-cell disease should have a screening sickle test and haemoglobin electrophoresis if that is positive.

A nasogastric tube should be passed in any sick paediatric patient because gastric distension occurs readily, with acidosis and hypoxaemia as predisposing causes. Gastric distension may prejudice normal respiratory function and regurgitation is likely, with subsequent pulmonary aspiration.

Oral fluids are given until 4 hours prior to surgery. Starvation for longer periods is undesirable in paediatric practice as there may be a risk of hypoglycaemia developing before surgery.

### Premedication

The aim of premedication is to produce a calm, co-operative child; this is usually easy to achieve in a normal, well-prepared child, but more difficult in one needing repeated anaesthetics, or in the subnormal. Sedation must never be achieved at the expense of respiratory depression, and is contra-indicated in patients with respiratory insufficiency or obstruction, cleft palate surgery and neurosurgery. Much less sedation is required if the child has been carefully prepared.

Sedation may be administered orally, by intramuscular injection or rectally, though the latter is less used nowadays in the U.K. because the effect of such administration is likely to be unpredictable. Doses are based on the body weight of the child. Few children welcome injections, but the intramuscular route is the only way to ensure certainty of action of the drugs.

Sedative premedication is not used in the neonate, though atropine is indicated, as secretions in narrow airways may cause respiratory embarrassment (Table 5). Vagal tone is low in the neonate and in some centres atropine is given intravenously on induction of anaesthesia, and this is especially important if the anaesthetic technique involves the use of cyclopropane, suxamethonium or halothane. Hyoscine may cause cerebral excitation in the very young. If the baby is pyrexial and toxic, atropine should be used in a smaller dose, or even omitted, as the combination has been incriminated in the production of febrile convulsions.

42/Table 5
Dosage of Atropine for Premedication
(Intramuscular injection—1 hour pre-operatively)

| *Body Weight (kg)* | *Dosage (mg)* |
|---|---|
| Below 2·5 | 0·15 |
| 2·5–8 | 0·2 |
| 8–15 | 0·3 |
| 15–20 | 0·4 |
| Over 20 | 0·5 |

(Oral doses twice the above, 2 hours pre-operatively)

Vitamin $K_1$ 1·0 mg should be given to newborns pre-operatively by intramuscular injection. Vitamin K is relatively deficient at this age and the liver enzyme system synthesising prothrombin is immature.

After the age of 9–10 months sedative premedication is desirable, though younger children having repeated surgery or cardiac surgery should be considered as suitable.

### Children up to 15 kg

*Trimeprazine elixir forte B.P.* (Vallergan) contains 6 mg/ml and may be given in doses of 3 to 4 mg/kg orally 2 hours pre-operatively. This phenothiazine has antihistamine and anti-emetic properties in addition to its sedative effect.

*Injection pethidine compound.* Each ml contains pethidine 25 mg, promethazine 6·25 mg and chlorpromazine 6·25 mg. It may be given in doses of 0·06–0·08 ml/kg by intramuscular injection one hour pre-operatively, to a maximum of 1·5 ml. This mixture provides excellent sedation, analgesia and anti-emesis without respiratory depression or prolonged sedation.

*Diazepam syrup B.P.* (contains 1 mg in 2·5 ml) is suitable as a sedative for particularly anxious children, two hours before routine premedication. Doses of 0·4 mg/kg orally are usual.

**Over 15 kg body weight**

Papaveretum and hyoscine may be used in doses of 0·4 mg/kg and 0·008 mg/kg respectively by intramuscular injection one hour pre-operatively. This is the most satisfactory premedication in the majority of older children and is particularly well tolerated in patients with cyanotic congenital heart disease.

## ANAESTHETIC APPARATUS

Equipment for paediatric anaesthesia is specialised to provide low apparatus dead-space and minimal resistance to respiration. In addition it should be lightweight, safe to use, allow humidification of inspired gases and incorporate a scavenging system for expired gases.

The tidal volume of a neonate is approximately 20 ml with a physiological dead-space of one-third, so that alveolar ventilation amounts only to some 14 ml. Thus, the addition of only a few millilitres of apparatus dead-space represents a very large proportional increase.

**Face masks.**—Masks are not used in small babies for prolonged periods as they will usually require intubation. A good fit to the face is a more important consideration than a very low dead-space since the latter is reduced in practice by streaming effects of the fresh gas flow (FGF) within the mask. The Rendell-Baker and Soucek mask[22] with a nominal dead-space of 4 ml for the neonatal size may not make a good air seal on the face.

**Endotracheal tubes** (Figs. 6 and 7).—Tubes of the Magill type may be either disposable or rubber, and the latter, though possibly more irritant to the mucosa, are less liable to kinking and are easier to insert. Cuffed tubes are not used in children under the age of 10 years. See Table 6 for the approximate size based on the

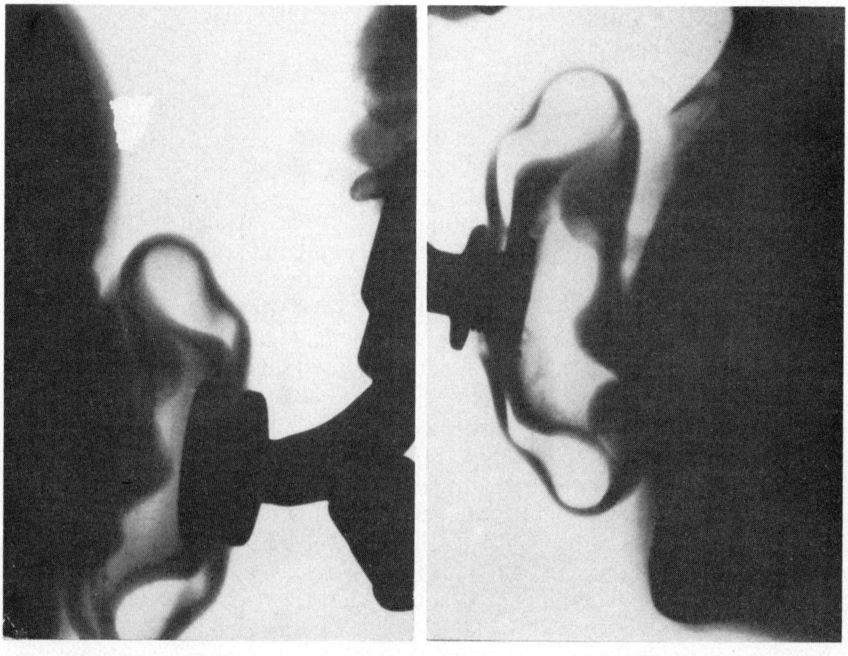

(*a*) (*b*)

42/Fig. 5.—X-ray pictures showing the difference in contour of the face of an infant (*a*) and a 4-year-old child (*b*). This illustrates the need for a special type of mask for the infant. (Courtesy of Dr. H. B. Sandiford.)

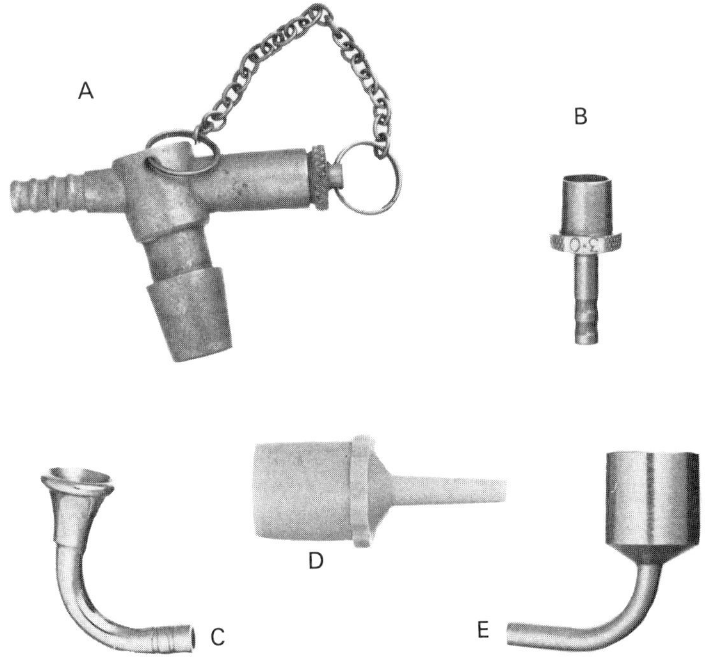


42/Fig. 6.—Endotracheal tube connectors suitable for paediatric use.
A. CARDIFF
B. OXFORD
C. MAGILL
D. PORTEX 15 mm
E. PENLON 15 mm
(With kind permission of Dr. D. J. Hatch and Dr. E. Sumner, and the publishers, Edward Arnold.[20])

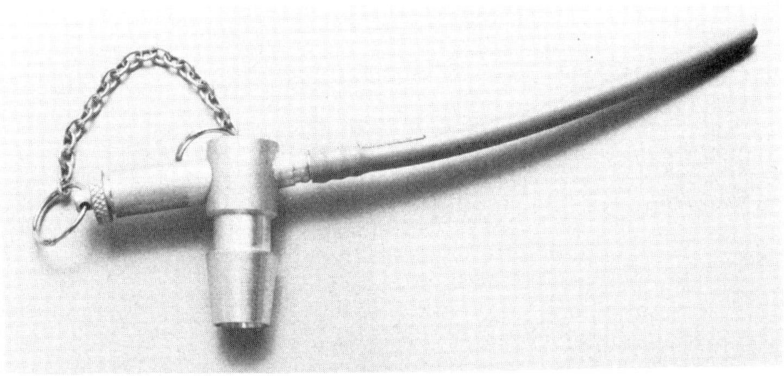

42/Fig. 7.—Plain Magill tube with Cardiff connector. (With kind permission of Dr. D. J. Hatch and Dr. E. Sumner, and the publishers, Edward Arnold.[20])

age of the child. Variations in the calibre of children's airways make it advisable to prepare tubes one size larger and smaller than the selected tube. The ideal tube, when in place has a small air leak around it, thus preventing damage to the rigid subglottic region, the cricoid ring, this being the narrowest part of a child's upper airway (see Table 6).

After intubation, auscultation of both lung fields is necessary to ensure that endobronchial intubation has not taken place.

Lightweight Cardiff connectors are very satisfactory for use with small tubes as fixation is

42/Table 6
Suggested Endotracheal Tube Sizes

| *Age* | *Internal diameter (mm)* |
|---|---|
| Up to 2 months | 2·5 and 3·0 |
| 3 to 5 months | 3·0 and 3·5 |
| 6 to 9 months | 3·5 and 4·0 |
| 10 months to 1 year | 4·0 and 4·5 |
| 2 to 4 years | 4·5 and 5·0 |
| 5 years | 5·0 and 5·5 |
| 6 to 7 years | 5·5 and 6·0 |
| 8 to 9 years | 6·0 and 6·5 |
| 10 years | 6·5 and 7·0 |
| 11 to 12 years | 7·0 and 7·5 |
| 13 to 14 years | 7·5 and 8·0 |

secure, suction is easy and they have a low resistance to airflow.

Oxford tubes have tapered outside diameter so that if too large a tube is used, the larynx is stretched as the tube is inserted. This may lead to oedema and post-extubation stridor.

Endobronchial tubes for paediatric anaesthesia are not manufactured. It is possible, however, to intubate one or other main bronchus by positioning correctly a long endotracheal tube. Provision must be made for the right upper lobe bronchus by cutting a hole in the side of the tube close to the tip.

### Anaesthetic Circuits

The anaesthetic circuit most commonly used for children under 5 years of age (20 kg bodyweight) in the U.K. and perhaps in the world, is the Ayre's T-piece with the Rees modification.

The circuit is ideal for either spontaneous breathing or controlled ventilation. To prevent dilution by air or rebreathing the capacity of the expiratory limb must be greater than the tidal volume of the patient, and the fresh gas flow (FGF) twice the minute volume of the patient.[23,24]

No rebreathing occurs unless the FGF falls below 200 ml $kg^{-1}$ $min^{-1}$ with spontaneous ventilation. With halothane anaesthesia rebreathing occurs sooner than with enflurane.[25]

The main advantages of the T-piece are its simplicity, low resistance and dead-space, and the ease of manual ventilation. Scavenging devices must be indirectly connected to the

42/Table 7
Suggested Lengths of Oral Endotracheal Tubes

| *Internal diameter (mm)* | *Length (cm)* |
|---|---|
| 2·5 and 3·0 | 8 to 9 |
| 3·5 | 9 to 10 |
| 4·0 | 10 to 11 |
| 4·5 | 11 to 12 |
| 5·0 | 12 to 13 |
| 5·5 | 13 to 14 |
| 6·0 | 14 to 15 |
| 6·5 | 15 to 16 |
| 7·0 | 16 to 17 |
| 7·5 | 17 to 18 |
| 8·0 | 18 to 19 |

42/Table 8
Fresh Gas Flow in a T-Piece to Prevent Rebreathing with Spontaneous Respiration

| *Body weight (kg)* | *Face mask (litres/min)* | *Endotracheal tube* (litres/min) |
|---|---|---|
| 5 | 8 | 6 |
| 10 | 8 | 6 |
| 15 | 10 | 7·5 |
| 20 | 12 | 9 |
| 25 | 14 | 10·5 |
| 30 | 14 | 10·5 |
| 35 | 15 | 11·5 |
| 40 | 16 | 12·0 |
| 45 | 17 | 12·5 |

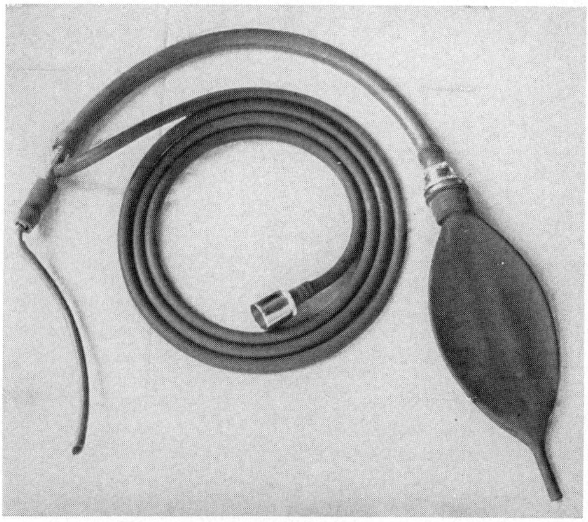

42/Fig. 8.—T-piece system for paediatric anaesthesia. (Courtesy of Dr. G. J. Rees.)

circuit to prevent any possibility of blockage to the expiratory flow.[26] A disadvantage is the absence of a pressure-relief valve in the circuit. It is also possible to reduce FGF during *manual ventilation* to avoid hypocapnia, though the flow should never be less than 3 l/min.

Bain and Spoerel[27] devised an alternative circuit using coaxial tubing, which may also be used in patients under 20 kg for spontaneous or controlled respiration with the same characteristics as the T-piece (Fig.9).

The circuit can be used with most standard ventilators including T-piece occluders (Sheffield or Loosco) or Nuffield.[29]

Non-rebreathing valves are used in paediatric anaesthesia but they tend to stick and introduce more resistance and dead-space. Circle absorption systems are popular in the U.S.A. and have light tubing, silicone-rubber valves, low gas flows with efficient humidification, warming and scavenging.

Manual ventilation is most satisfactory for small babies because changes in compliance or air leaks are easy to detect quickly, e.g. in repair of oesophageal atresia. In other situations the use of a mechanical ventilator may be preferable and simple T-piece occluders such as Loosco or Sheffield are ideal for use in the operating theatre.

The method of cycling involves the intermittent occlusion of the expiratory limb of a basic T-piece anaesthesia circuit.

In the Loosco, the rate is set electronically between 20 and 60 per min and the inspiratory: expiratory time ratio varies from 1:1 to 1:3. The ventilator normally works as a volume-constant device. The gas-flow rate required to produce a given minute volume is obtained using a nomogram which takes into account the volume of gas "lost" during the expiratory phase. PEEP may be applied to the expiratory limb of the ventilator, which can also be used as a pressure-constant device by incorporating a pressure-limiting relief valve.

The Sheffield ventilator is a similar device with an electronically-timed solenoid valve which occludes the expiratory limb (Fig. 10).

For children over 20 kg, adult circuits are suitable and for mechanical ventilation in the operating theatre the Manley ventilator is most satisfactory.

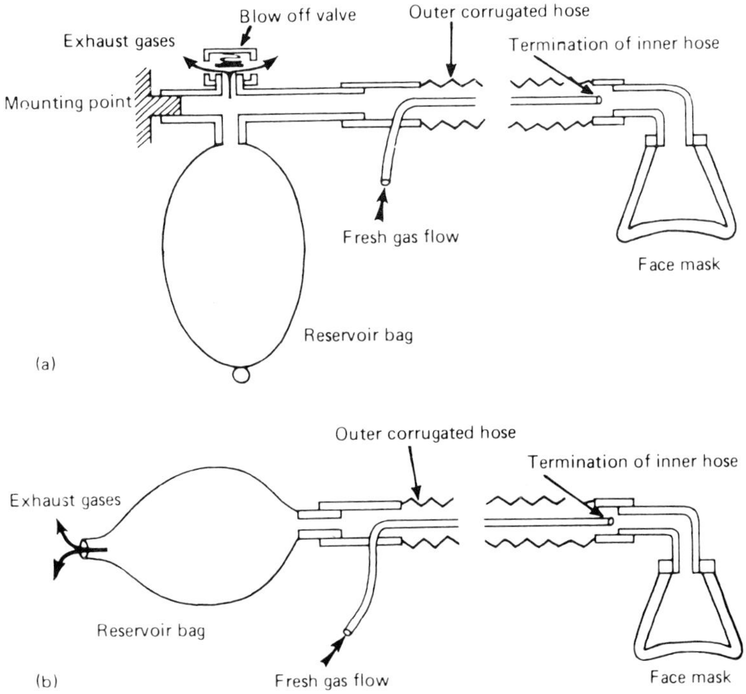


42/FIG. 9.—(a) The Bain circuit. (b) Paediatric modification of the Bain circuit. (Courtesy of Pitman Medical Ltd.[28])

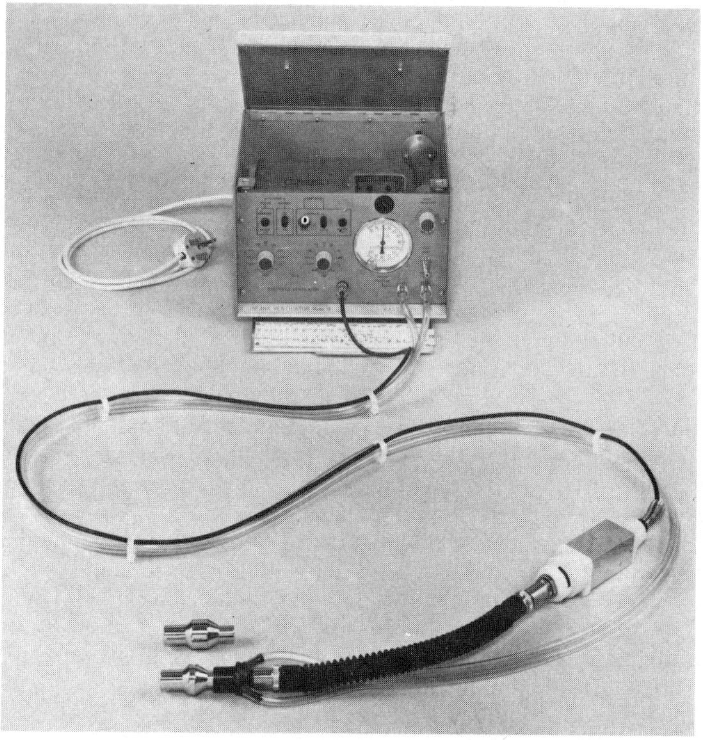

42/Fig. 10.—Sheffield ventilator. (Courtesy of H. G. East & Co. Ltd., Oxford.)

**Laryngoscopes**

For the first year of life, a straight-bladed instrument is preferable, because the larynx lies more anterior and is covered by a large, soft epiglottis inclined at an angle of 45° to the glottis – features which make visualisation with a curved blade more difficult.

## GENERAL PRINCIPLES OF ANAESTHESIA

**Induction of Anaesthesia**

The induction may be by inhalation or intravenous injection and the child may want to choose. Cyclopropane and oxygen, or nitrous-oxide/oxygen and halothane or enflurane are suitable agents for use in all children after the neonatal period. The heavy vapours are best directed by the hand over the patient's nose and mouth, the mask being connected only when the child is asleep. After application of the mask, it is an advantage to keep the T-piece bag taut, to maintain the FRC and to overcome any mild laryngeal obstruction which tends to occur during inhalational induction.

For intravenous induction 2·5 per cent thiopentone in doses of up of 4 mg/kg are the most satisfactory. Other drugs such as methohexitone, Althesin, etomidate and ketamine are also used, but all have disadvantages. Ketamine in particular has undesirable side-effects of emergence delirium, prolonged recovery and tendency to cause laryngeal spasm and, because it causes increase in cardiac output, should never be given to patients with cardiac outflow-tract obstruction.

In neonates, induction of anaesthesia takes place after intubation. After pre-oxygenation, the baby is firmly held by an assistant and laryngoscopy performed, then the larynx is intubated as the infant takes a breath. This manoeuvre is easily performed and overcomes the great problem of maintenance of the airway and oxygenation during inhalational anaesthesia in this age group. *Awake intubation* should be attempted in most babies under 21 days of life as the ease of intubation is related to muscular resistance, not to the age of the baby. The technique should be abandoned in favour of general anaesthesia if the muscular resistance is judged to be too great.

### Maintenance of Anaesthesia

Halothane is the most satisfactory agent for use in paediatric anaesthesia as it is rapidly absorbed and eliminated, with minimal cardiovascular effects, and gives excellent operating conditions. Enflurane has few advantages over halothane.[30] At the Hospital for Sick Children, Great Ormond Street, halothane is used in over 90 per cent of anaesthetics, and is the obvious choice for spontaneous breathing anaesthesia for surface operations which take up to one hour for the older child (over one year of age). In the National Halothane Study there was no report of jaundice ascribed to halothane under the age of 10 years. It is clear that the incidence of post-halothane jaundice, if it indeed occurs at all, is extremely low and many frequently repeated administrations are a tribute to the safety of halothane.[31,32]

Induction of anaesthesia is followed by the administration of a muscle relaxant, commonly suxamethonium 1 mg/kg intravenously if intubation is indicated.

Controlled ventilation after endotracheal intubation is the technique of choice for neonates and for most babies up to 5 kg body weight, even for minor procedures. Small babies are very sensitive to the respiratory depressant effects of inhalational anaesthesia, and controlled ventilation ensures adequate alveolar ventilation and maintenance of a normal residual lung volume. A rate of 30–40 a minute is used with pressures of 25–30 cm $H_2O$ with PEEP of 5 cm $H_2O$ to preserve the FRC with a fresh gas flow of 4 litres.

For babies over 5 kg body weight spontaneous breathing without intubation is possible if the surgery allows.

### The Muscle Relaxants

The relaxant drugs are discussed in Chapter 23, and are as suitable for paediatric anaesthesia as for adults.

The effects of suxamethonium are probably the same in the neonate as the adult and reports of decreased sensitivity in the former may relate to the larger extracellular fluid volume in which the drug is distributed. If repeated doses are to be administered, atropine premedication is mandatory.

The neonate is sensitive to non-depolarising muscle relaxants, which may be related to immaturity of the neuromuscular junction or to differences in bio-availability of the drug with dilution or binding by plasma proteins. Bennett and colleagues[33] showed that for the first 7 days of life 0·25 mg/kg tubocurarine is necessary for curarisation, from 7–14 days, 0·4 mg/kg, and 0·5 mg/kg thereafter. At birth pancuronium is 9 times as potent as tubocurarine, though this drops to 6 times by 28 days of life. Doses of pancuronium of 0·04 mg/kg are safest in babies of less than 7 days old.[34] In practice, tubocurarine is diluted to 0·5 mg/ml (0·25 mg/ml for prematures) and increments of 0·25 mg (0·125 mg) given to achieve satisfactory conditions. Tubocurarine has little cardiovascular effect in the young and is possibly the drug of choice. After the first two weeks of life, infants require similar doses to adults on a weight-for-weight basis. Atracurium, with its independence of renal and hepatic function, may be a logical drug to use for neonates.

At least 20 minutes should elapse between the last dose of tubocurarine and the end of surgery if full reversal is to be achieved. A mixture of atropine (0·025 mg/kg) and neostigmine (0·05 mg/kg) is given intravenously for reversal of residual curarisation.

### Supplements

Doses of halothane up to 0·5 per cent may supplement anaesthesia with controlled ventilation, and fentanyl in doses of up to 10 $\mu$g/kg are equally satisfactory. The latter drug should not be used in neonates unless mechanical ventilation is planned for the postoperative period.

### Monitoring

Careful, continuous monitoring of the clinical status of the patient is essential, and conventional adult methods of monitoring are readily applicable, with modification, to the small infant. The best methods of monitoring are those which increase the contact between anaesthetist and patient.[35] At least one peripheral pulse should be accessible, e.g. radial or

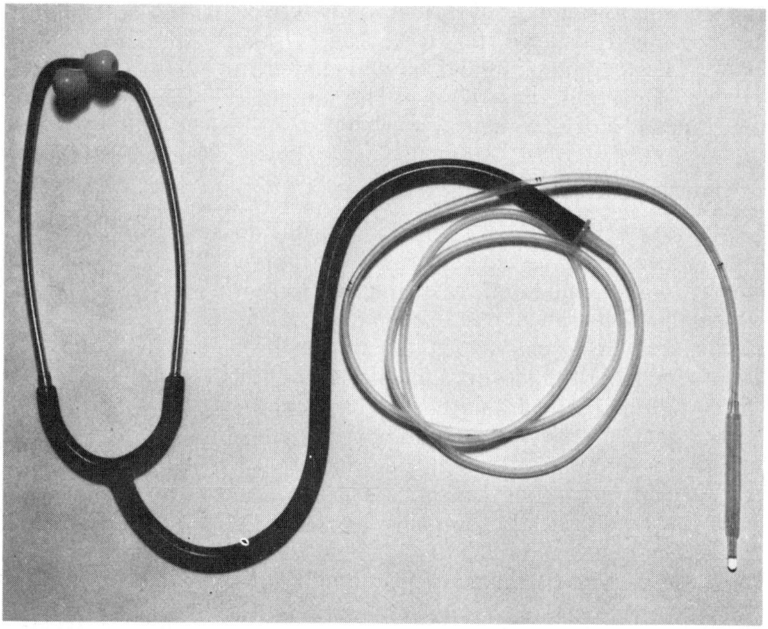

42/Fig. 11.—Oesophageal stethoscope.

axillary, and the use of a precordial or oesophageal stethoscope assists in monitoring heart rate, quality of heart sounds and pulmonary ventilation (Fig. 11).

The sphygmomanometer method of determining blood pressure in a small baby is difficult because of the inaudibility of the Korotkoff sounds, though it may be achieved very satisfactorily using an automatic device such us the Dinamap or Sentry. The width of the cuff must cover at least ⅔ of the upper arm and surround at least ¾ of the limb. ECG with a heart-rate counter is used on almost all patients. Direct monitoring of arterial and venous pressures is easily achieved after radial-arterial and internal-jugular venous cannulae have been placed. End-tidal $CO_2$ may be measured using a capnograph with a paediatric cuvette. At the moment transcutaneous $O_2$ and $CO_2$ tensions are rarely measured in the operating theatre, most electrodes being adversely affected by anaesthetic gases.

Temperature must always be measured during surgery on small babies because of the increased susceptibility of this age group to heat loss. Nasopharyngeal, oesophageal or rectal temperatures are easily measured. Temperature conservation may be achieved by wrapping the limps and head in aluminium foil and placing the child on a thermostatically controlled electrical or water blanket at 38–40° C.

**Fluid Replacement**

20 g, 22 g and 24 g cannulae exist for peripheral venous cannulation and suitable veins are to be found on the dorsum of the hand. Correct holding of the limb is essential for successful venepuncture and many anaesthetists prefer to perform the manoeuvre single handed, distending the vein by compressing the wrist between index and middle fingers of the left hand. Optimal venous distension and stretching of the overlying skin are more easily achieved this way.

Blood volume is very variable at birth and in the neonate ranges from 85–100 ml/kg. By one month it is 80 ml/kg and by 2 years 75 mg/kg. A blood loss of more than 10 per cent of the calculated blood volume (BV) should be replaced with colloidal solution. If the Hb level is in excess of 15 g/dl up to 20 per cent of the BV may be given as plasma, if available; if below 15 g/dl blood loss should be replaced with whole blood. Blood loss is estimated from both swab-weighing and the loss into a calibrated suction bottle. Small amounts of blood may be transfused from a syringe, using a standard giving set and a 3-way tap. Microfilters are necessary if massive transfusion is expected or if the patient has pulmonary vascular disease. Adequate warming of the blood is achieved if the tubing of a standard giving set is held in a thermostatically controlled water bath. Certain calibrated infusion sets do not have a filter proximal to the drip chamber and are only suitable for infusions of clear fluids.

Intra-operative maintenance fluids may be given as 4 per cent dextrose with 0·18 per cent saline at a rate of 5–6 ml $kg^{-1}$ $h^{-1}$. The adequacy of fluid replacement is judged most satisfactorily by monitoring heart rate, blood pressure, peripheral perfusion and urine output.

### Extubation

Neonates are extubated *completely awake* after spontaneous respiration has been judged to be fully adequate. The lungs are lightly distended using the T-piece bag so that the infant coughs as the tube is withdrawn. Older children may be extubated deeply anaesthetised. Extubation at an in-between stage must be avoided or severe laryngeal spasm may follow.

### Postoperative Analgesia

*Neonates do not need and should not be given opiate analgesic postoperatively*. Older children may be given papaveretum 0·25 mg/kg (Omnopon) 4-hourly intramuscularly, or codeine phosphate 1 mg/kg 4-hourly intramuscularly. Postoperative vomiting is unusual in childhood but, if it does occur, may be controlled with prochlorperazine B.P. (Stemetil) 0·2 mg/kg intramuscularly (maximum 12·5 mg).

## SPECIFIC SURGICAL CONDITIONS

### Congenital Diaphragmatic Hernia

In this condition, which occurs in 1 in 4000 live births, part of the abdominal contents herniate through an incompletely formed diaphragm, usually on the left. The degree of respiratory distress at birth is related mainly to the degree of associated pulmonary hypoplasia. After birth, the midgut fills with air, causing further distension in the chest and increasing respiratory and cardiovascular distress. The diagnosis should be suspected in any case of respiratory distress postpartum; there is also a small abdomen which is scaphoid in contour. The diagnosis is confirmed on chest x-ray. If gas is blown or swallowed into the stomach, the respiratory distress is increased. A large nasogastric tube must be passed to deflate the stomach within the chest. If ventilatory assistance is required this must be via an endotracheal tube. Mortality from this condition remains high and occurs in those patients with symptoms in the first six hours of life; up to 50 per cent of this group may survive.[36] Treatment is by immediate laparotomy, decompression of the chest, repair of the diaphragmatic defect and correction of the associated malrotation of the gut.

Postoperatively, all patients with symptoms in the first six hours of life should be mechanically ventilated, and weaned only after 48 hours of stability of gas exchange. Occurrence of transitional circulation is common in this condition and may be treated with the pulmonary vasodilator tolazoline.[4] Survival is in the region of 72 per cent if all cases are taken into account.

### Congenital Lobar Emphysema and Lung Cysts

These conditions, which may be a cause of serious respiratory distress in the newborn period, are due to congenital weakness of the bronchial cartilages and overdistension of a lobe of the lung. The distension causes both collapse of the surrounding normal lung and mediastinal shift.

Anaesthesia with endobronchial intubation has been described, but is unnecessary if care is taken with controlled manual ventilation to avoid further distending the lobe or cyst or even producing pneumothorax.

### Oesophageal Atresia with Tracheo-oesophageal Fistula

Oesophageal atresia, with or without fistula, occurs in 1 in 3000 live births, and should be suspected if hydramnios has been a complication of pregnancy. The infants are often of low birth-weight, and associated abnormalities commonly include other atresias and cardiac defects. The baby may present with respiratory difficulties, choking with feeds or drooling saliva. The abdomen may distend with gas if the fistula is in the common site (Fig. 12).

The diagnosis is confirmed if a nasogastric tube cannot be passed into the stomach.

The main risk to life comes from soiling of the lungs with saliva, gastric contents or contrast

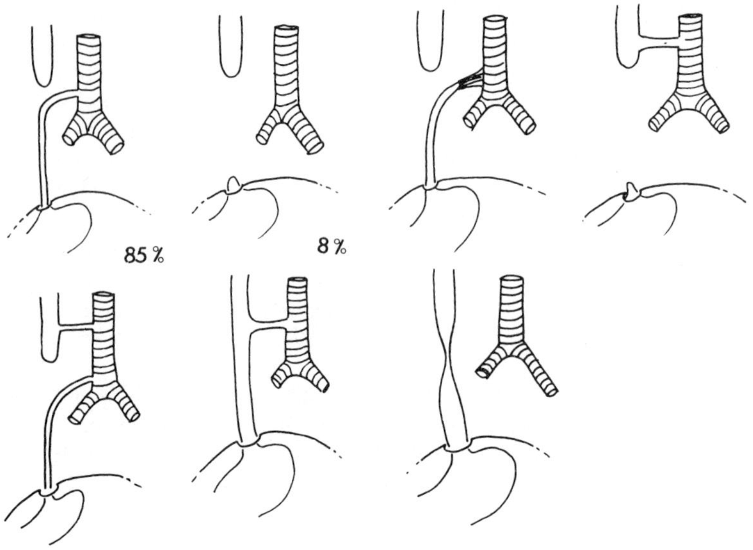


42/FIG. 12.—Varieties of tracheo-oesophageal fistulae or atresia. The incidence of the common types is also indicated.

medium (this should not be used). The blind upper pouch of the oesophagus should be kept continuously asiprated using a double lumen Replogle tube as soon as the diagnosis is made. Surgery may be delayed to allow antibiotics and physiotherapy to improve the lungs.

During anaesthesia gentle controlled manual ventilation is established at once and problems such as overdistension of the stomach during such ventilation are of theoretical interest only. Leaks of gas to the stomach are easily audible with a precordial stethoscope. The ventilation must be monitored very carefully during surgical dissection of the fistula. The thoracotomy is usually followed by formation of a gastrostomy for feeding.

Postoperatively, IPPV may be necessary if the baby has soiled lungs, low birth-weight with a tendency to apnoea, or has associated cardiac abnormalities.

### Intestinal Obstruction in the Neonate

The causes of intestinal obstruction in the neonate are many and some may only be diagnosed at laparotomy. The symptoms are vomiting and abdominal distension. The patient may need urgent surgery, but fluid replacement should begin at once and attempts made to correct deficits.

*Severe* dehydration should be urgently treated with blood or plasma in volumes up to 40 ml/kg. *Mild* dehydration of 5 per cent body-weight (loss of skin turgor, mildly depressed fontanelles) and *moderate* dehydration of 10 per cent body-weight (sunken eyes and fontanelles) are treated with 0·9 per cent NaCl or 4 per cent dextrose with 0·18 per cent saline. Half the estimated deficit is given in 6–8 hours. Metabolic acidosis should be treated using the formula mmol $HCO_3^-$ = base deficit × kg weight × 0·3. Potassium replacement starts when the urine output improves, at a rate not exceeding 3 mmol of $K^+$/kg per 24 hours at a concentration of 0·5 mmol $kg^{-1}$ $h^{-1}$. As the circulating blood volume increases, peripheral perfusion improves and peripheral temperature increases.

**Duodenal atresia.**—One-third of the patients with this condition also have Down's syndrome (mongolism). Plain abdominal x-ray shows a double gas bubble in the dilated stomach and proximal duodenum. If the obstruction is below the ampulla of Vater, vomiting is bile stained. Atresias or stenosis may also occur in the jejunum or ileum.

**Malrotation (volvulus).**—The failure of the midgut to be correctly fixed in normal rotation may cause obstruction by bands of peritoneum (Ladd's bands) from the caecum to the posterior abdominal wall. Volvulus with intestinal strangulation demands urgent surgery after infusion of plasma or blood to improve the circulating blood volume.

**Meconium ileus.**—This is the abdominal manifestation of fibrocystic disease in 10–15 per cent of patients with this condition. Obstruction is caused by inspissated meconium, and volvulus or perforation with peritonitis are common complications.

**Hirschsprung's disease.**—This disease is caused by lack of ganglia in the distal colon and rectum, causing a functional obstruction with increasing distension. Barium and manometric studies with rectal biopsy establish the diagnosis. Defunctioning colostomy is performed, followed at a later date by a formal "pull through" operation of the affected segment.

**Necrotising enterocolitis.**—This condition is characterised by abdominal distension with ileus, blood in the stools and a typical x-ray appearance of gas in the bowel wall. There is a very high mortality (up to 50 per cent) and this condition affects up to 8 per cent of babies in special-care units. Fifty per cent of the patients have a Gram-negative septicaemia and most have a history of birth asphyxia. Surgical intervention may be necessary if perforation occurs. Intravenous feeding, gentamicin and metronidazole are used in supportive therapy.

**Exomphalos and Gastroschisis.**—Exomphalos is a herniation of varying degree into the umbilical cord, and gastroschisis is a defect of the abdominal wall. There is often severe loss of fluid from exposed guts, and surgery involves repair of the abdominal wall. Compression of the contents frequently causes respiratory embarrassment so that mechanical ventilation is required postoperatively for all except the smallest defects.

### Anaesthetic Management of Intestinal Obstruction in the Neonate

A large nasogastric tube will keep the stomach decompressed and diminish the risk of aspiration of gastric contents. Awake intubation after pre-oxygenation is the preferred technique as this also minimises the risks of aspiration.

#### Pyloric Stenosis

This common malformation occurs in 1 in 400 live births, of which 85 per cent are male. Gross thickening of the pyloric smooth muscle, forming a hard tumour, causes obstruction to thicker feeds with increasing vomiting after the second week of life. The infant loses weight, becomes dehydrated and, with the loss of gastric acid, has a hypochloraemic alkalosis. Extremes of dehydration are not nowadays seen, but with prolonged vomiting the baby would eventually become acidotic with a falling cardiac output. The operation of pyloromyotomy is not an emergency, but is preceded by complete correction of fluid and electrolyte balance. 2 ml/kg 0·9 per cent NaCl raises the serum chloride by 1 mmol/l and surgery should not take place until the chloride is at least 90 mmol/l and the bicarbonate 24 mmol/l (up to 400 ml of 0·9 per cent NaCl may be necessary).

A large nasogastric tube is passed, the gastric residue drained off and 4-hourly washouts with saline performed until the aspirate is clear and odourless.

The patients are usually too old and lusty for awake intubation, and induction of anaesthesia should involve the use of cricoid pressure, which is as effective in infants as it is in adults. A technique using intermittent suxamethonium in doses of 5 mg is suitable for this procedure.

Oral feeding is usually re-established immediately after the patient has returned to the ward.

#### Intussusception

This commonly occurs between the ages of 6–18 months in previously healthy infants. Usually the ileum invaginates into the caecum, causing pain, vomiting, distension and bleeding. Fluid losses are always greater than expected and infusions of plasma or blood in volumes up to 40 ml/kg may be needed to restore the circulating blood volume.

## ANAESTHESIA FOR OTHER CONDITIONS

#### Hare-lip and Cleft Palate

The hare-lip deformity and anterior palatal deformity are usually corrected at the age of about 3 months, whereas the posterior palatal deficiency is repaired between the ages of 12 and 18 months.

The conditions are often associated with other abnormalities such as Pierre Robin syndrome (micrognathia), Treacher-Collins syndrome (hypoplasia of the first bronchial arch) and Klippel-Feil syndrome (fused cervical vertebrae), which may cause incipient or actual respiratory obstruction and make intubation very difficult indeed. Sedative premedication should be avoided and inhalational anaesthesia employed as for any case of respiratory obstruction. Suxamethonium for intubation may be given when it is established that ventilation with a face mask is possible. A preformed endotracheal tube such as Oxford (or a newer, disposable variety) is used, and a wad of gauze placed in the roof of the mouth will prevent the blade of the laryngoscope from slipping into the cleft. The surgeon inserts a mouth gag (e.g. Dott's) and care must be taken to check the patency of the tube after insertion of the gag as the latter may occlude the tube by pressing it onto the mandible. The pharynx must be packed to prevent aspiration of blood. An anaesthetic technique which ensures rapid recovery of pharyngeal reflexes should be selected. Blood should be cross-matched as the surgical loss may exceed 10 per cent of the total blood volume.

It is common practice to insert a strong suture in the tongue postoperatively to ease the maintenance of a clear airway. Codeine phosphate 1 mg/kg (i.m.) is satisfactory for postoperative analgesia.

### Choanal Atresia

This condition may cause respiratory obstruction if the posterior nares are blocked by bony or membranous walls. Immediate relief is obtained by fixing an oropharyngeal airway in the mouth until surgery takes place—this consists of transnasal or transpalatal puncture and dilatation.

### Induced Hypotension

This may be indicated for palatal surgery in the older child, but children are more resistant to hypotensive agents than adults. Trimetaphan (250 mg in 100 ml 5 per cent dextrose) or sodium nitroprusside are suitable agents. (The total dose of nitroprusside should not exceed 1–1·5 mg/kg.) A reflex tachycardia is controlled with increments of 0·1 mg propranolol. Careful control of the rate of administration of the drugs and their effect on the blood pressure is mandatory.

## Cardiac Surgery

Anaesthesia for cardiac surgery in childhood follows the same general principles as for adults (see Chapter 13), but is usually carried out for congenital heart disease, rather than acquired disease.

The incidence of major congenital heart disease is approximately 8 per 1000 live births, the commonest condition being ventricular septal defect (75 per cent of these close spontaneously). Lesions may be divided into three groups: those which cause *cardiac failure*—VSD, patent ductus arteriosus, aortic stenosis, and coarctation of the aorta; those causing *cyanosis*—pulmonary or tricuspid atresia, tetralogy of Fallot, and univentricular heart with pulmonary stenosis; and those which cause *failure and cyanosis*—transposition of the great vessels, truncus arteriosus, and total anomalous pulmonary venous drainage. Any of these may require urgent surgery.[37]

Cardiac catheterisation for neonates and infants is satisfactorily performed with sedation and local analgesia. Controlled ventilation may be required for the very sick. Non-invasive two-dimensional echocardiography has removed the need for catheterisation in many lesions and children come to surgery in an improved condition. Injections of hyperosmolar contrast medium initially may overload the circulation and the subsequent diuresis may dangerously reduce the circulating blood volume and cause severe haemoconcentration.

### Open Heart Surgery

Neonates do not tolerate cardiopulmonary bypass as well as older babies, nevertheless lesions such as critical aortic stenosis or total anomalous pulmonary venous drainage need urgent surgery. Preliminary surface cooling may be used to produce uniform cooling and to protect the brain in the event of cardiac arrest before bypass.[38] This technique may cause a higher incidence of postoperative renal failure and is becoming less popular.[39]

Opiate premedication is particularly well tolerated in the older cyanosed child.

During the rewarming period on bypass it is common practice to infuse sodium nitroprusside (3 mg/kg in 100 ml 5 per cent dextrose) to overcome vasoconstriction and thus improve the rewarming process and ensure a full peripheral circulation. Inotropic agents, if necessary, are similar to those used in adults. Dopamine is the drug of first choice[40] and if used in a dilution of 6 mg/kg in 100 ml 5 per cent dextrose, each microdrop is 1 $\mu g\ kg^{-1}\ min^{-1}$. If the infant requires severe fluid restriction, the concentration of such drugs may need to be increased.

Peripheral venous, arterial, and central venous lines are inserted percutaneously. The arterial line is put into a radial artery and one or two cannulae are inserted into the right internal jugular vein. Oesophageal, nasopharyngeal and rectal temperatures are monitored.

Patients with cyanotic congenital heart disease have a deficiency in clotting factors and platelet function, so that increased haemorrhage is likely in the post-bypass period. Fresh blood, fresh frozen plasma, platelet-rich plasma and vitamin $K_1$ should all be available for such patients.

Cold cardioplegic solutions containing potassium are used to produce asystole and minimise myocardial metabolic demands after aortic cross clamping.[41]

Particular care is necessary in anaesthetising those patients with balanced intracardiac shunts, e.g. tetralogy of Fallot or Eisenmenger's syndrome. With tetralogy of Fallot, *deep* anaesthesia causes peripheral vasodilatation and a relative increase in right-to-left shunting, whilst too *light* anaesthesia with tachycardia causes spasm of the infundibulum of the right ventricle. The former state is treated with adrenaline and the latter with a $\beta$-adrenergic blocking drug such as propranolol. A relaxant technique with narcotic supplementation (morphia, papaveretum or fentanyl) is suitable.

### Closed Heart Surgery

The main closed heart operations in childhood are ligation of patent ductus arteriosus, Blalock pulmonary to systemic shunt* and resection of coarctation of the aorta.

The infants may be very sick with cardiac failure and cyanosis, and in need of pre-operative respiratory and cardiac support.

**Patent ductus arteriosus.**—The incidence of PDA in preterm infants has doubled in the last decade and causes significant left-to-right shunting with cardiac failure in over 20 per cent of cases. Attempts to close the ductus using a prostaglandin synthetase inhibitor such as indomethacin often fail, and surgical closure is necessary.[42] Conversely, patency of the ductus is life-saving in patients with pulmonary atresia. Infusions of prostaglandin $E_2$ will ensure that the ductus remains open until a surgical shunt of the Blalock type can be created surgically. Some of the smaller babies are already being ventilated, and ligation of the ductus often allows the weaning process to begin.

In older children the operation is a simple affair and though blood should be standing by at the moment of ligation, transfusion is very rarely necessary. Standard anaesthesia for thoracotomy is employed.

**Pulmonary-systemic shunts.**—Severe cyanosis and polycythaemia are common in patients who require Blalock shunts. Small babies need direct arterial pressure monitoring using the radial artery on the opposite side to the shunt. Blood loss of up to 20 per cent of the blood volume is replaced with plasma to lower the haematocrit. If the baby is sick and postoperative mechanical ventilation is indicated, supplementation with fentanyl and intra-operative ventilation with 100 per cent $O_2$ after curarisation is a very satisfactory technique.

**Coarctation of the aorta.**—Infantile coarctation of the aorta is of the preductal type and is associated with very severe left ventricular failure and pulmonary oedema. Other anomalies may be present, such as VSD, which further increase the risks. Severe respiratory and cardiac failure are always present. Anaesthesia with halothane is very poorly tolerated. Arterial pressure monitoring by direct means is mandatory. Controlled ventilation with 100 per cent $O_2$ is advisable as even nitrous oxide may cause hypotension. Supplementation with fentanyl is usually well tolerated and doses of 10 $\mu$g/kg may be given after monitoring is established. Acidosis must be corrected, and an infusion of adrenaline ½–1 mg in 100 ml 5 per cent dextrose prepared for use if necessary. It may be necessary for the surgeons to reclamp the aorta several times before the clamp is finally removed. Postoperatively respiratory support is always needed for at least 48 hours.

### Neurosurgery

Neurosurgical anaesthesia in childhood follows the same general principles as for adults.

Neurosurgery in infancy usually involves operations for developmental anomalies in the spine and cranium or for hydrocephalus. Clo-

* The Blalock shunt consists of an anastomosis between the pulmonary artery and subclavian artery of the same side, to improve oxygenation in patients where total correction of a lesion is impossible or inappropriate.

sure of a myelomeningocele, in selected cases, is carried out within 24 hours of birth. 80 per cent of these babies have the Arnold-Chiari malformation* and also have hydrocephalus at birth or will develop the condition shortly afterwards. During intubation the baby's back is supported on a "head ring" to protect the lesion from pressure. The infant is positioned prone on pads supporting the chest and pelvis so that the abdomen remains free and obstruction of the inferior vena cava avoided. Controlled ventilation is especially necessary for neonates operated on in the prone position with pressure on the chest.

Occipital encephalocele may be associated with abnormalities of the cervical spine, micrognathia or cleft palate and such patients may be difficult to intubate.

A great deal of the neurosurgery in childhood is for the treatment of hydrocephalus associated with myelomeningocele or caused by aqueduct stenosis. Surgical treatment involves the implantation of a low-pressure valve system to drain CSF from the ventricle to the right atrium, pleural cavity or to the peritoneum. Controlled ventilation must be employed for neonates, but older babies and children may be allowed to breathe spontaneously, though controlled ventilation is essential for patients with raised intracranial pressure.

## POSTOPERATIVE CARE

### Fluid Requirements

Because of inappropriate antidiuretic hormone (ADH) secretion and fluid retention in the immediate postoperative phase, it is usual to restrict the volume of intravenous fluids to 40 ml/kg per day rising to 80 ml/kg per day by 7 days of age, when the urine output should have increased to 150 ml/kg per day.[43] Suitable solutions are 10 per cent dextrose with 0·18 per cent saline for babies with tendency to hypoglycaemia, or 4 per cent dextrose with 0·18 per cent saline for larger babies. In addition, the volume of gastric aspirate is replaced by normal saline intravenously. Supplementation with potassium (at a rate not exceeding 3 mmol/kg in 24 hours) is usual after the first postoperative day.

* The Arnold-Chiari malformation is a downward displacement of the pons and medulla, and protrusion of the cerebellar vermis through the foramen magnum, causing obstruction to the normal flow of CSF.

### Respiratory Support

Postoperatively many babies require respiratory support because of the poor respiratory reserve of the neonate, and severe hypoxaemia may occur as a result of an increase in the work of breathing or reduction in the lung $\dot{V}/\dot{Q}$. Intrapulmonary shunting may increase if the FRC is further reduced after abdominal or thoracic surgery. Other babies may suffer from pre-existing lung disease such as hyaline membrane disease or pneumonia.

The decision to provide respiratory support is always made on clinical grounds such as apnoeic attacks, respiratory rate over 60, signs of increasing work of breathing (nasal flaring, subcostal recession), increasing oxygen dependence, and failure to clear secretions. Such babies will be unable to maintain an arterial oxygen tension between 50 and 80 mm Hg (6·7 and 10·7 kPa) with increasing inspired oxygen concentrations, and the carbon dioxide tension will rise above 50 mm Hg (6·7 kPa).

The measurement of cutaneous oxygen and carbon dioxide tensions is increasingly satisfactory and is particularly helpful in very small babies where the risks of cicatricial retrolental fibroplasia and pulmonary oxygen toxicity are highest and from whom it may be difficult to obtain arterial blood for blood gas analysis.[44] A reasonable correlation exists between transcutaneous and arterial gas levels when the peripheral circulation is good. Significant discrepancy may occur in patients with poor tissue perfusion and with arterial oxygen tensions at the extremes of hypoxia and hyperoxia.

**Nasotracheal intubation.**—The nasal route is preferred for long-term intubation, as the tube may be fixed more securely and gives greater comfort and ease of nursing. Long-term intubation for respiratory support is a fully established technique.[45] In our series of over 4,000 babies and children over the past eight years in the Hospital for Sick Children, Great Ormond Street, there have been no serious complications, some babies having been intubated continuously for as long as eight months.

All the *complications* of the technique are avoidable:

1. *Dislodgement* is prevented by firm fix-

ation of the nasal tube, using a connector such as the Tunstall (Fig. 13).

2. *Blockage* of the tube is avoided by full humidification of the inspired gases, and endotracheal suction at least every 30 minutes.

3. *Subglottic stenosis*, potentially the most dangerous complication from pressure necrosis of the cricoid mucosa is avoided by the use of a biologically inert, loose-fitting tube, allowing an air leak at an airway pressure of 20 cm $H_2O$.

4. *Nasal ulcers* are avoided by careful nursing and regular changing of the tube from nostril to nostril every 10 days.

5. *Post-extubation stridor* occasionally occurs after short intubations (24–36 hours) and is treated with dexamethasone 0·25 mg/kg intravenously.

Tracheostomy is very rarely necessary for respiratory support, although, because handling, nursing and stimulating a growing baby are easier with a tracheostomy, it may be performed after 6–8 weeks.[47]

**Mechanical ventilation.**—Major criteria for the choice of a paediatric ventilator must be that the machine has the facility to deliver a low flow rate, is reliable, has an efficient humidifier and an accurate control of inspired oxygen concentration, possesses reliable alarm system, and is easy to sterilise between cases. Suitable machines include the Servo 900B (flow generator) and the Bourns BP 200 (pressure generator) both of which have important characteristics for mechanical ventilation of the neonate.[48] (Figs. 14 and 15)

Ventilator settings are initially chosen on clinical grounds, and blood gas measurement, which is essential for the management of patients on mechanical ventilation, is performed after a short time to confirm adequacy of ventilation. It is more satisfactory to paralyse small babies to be ventilated, though many patients are easily managed with small doses of morphine (0·2 mg/kg i.v.) or diazepam (0·2 mg/kg i.v.)

Small babies are very likely to develop a type of lung damage known as bronchopulmonary dysplasia, following mechanical ventilation. Factors associated with this progressive destruction of the lung architecture and function with fibrosis and cyst formation are: pulmonary hypoplasia, surfactant deficiency, the presence

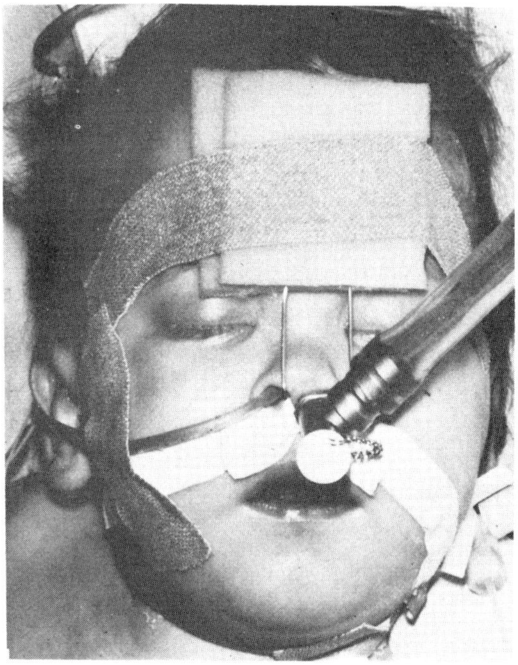

(*a*)

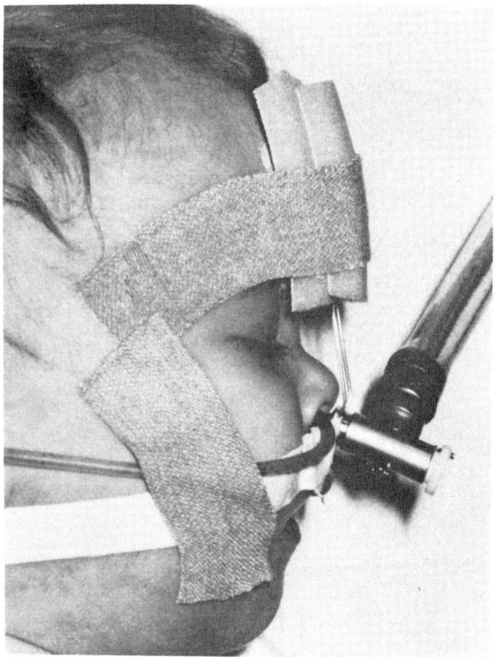

(*b*)

42/Fig. 13(*a*) and (*b*).—Fixation of tracheal tube with Tunstall connector. (Courtesy of Dr. M. Branthwaite, and Blackwell Scientific Publications.[46])

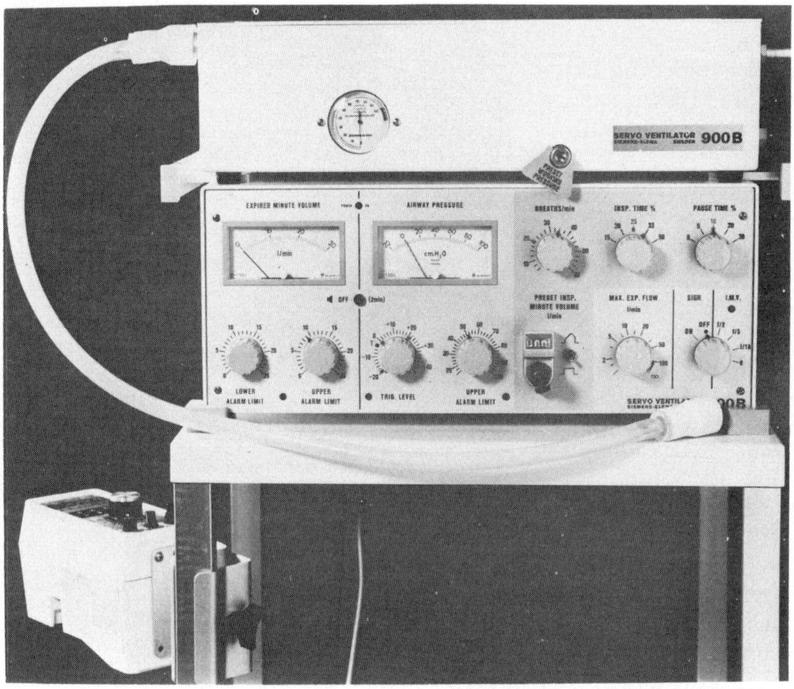


42/Fig. 14.—Servo ventilator 900B with intermittent mandatory ventilation.

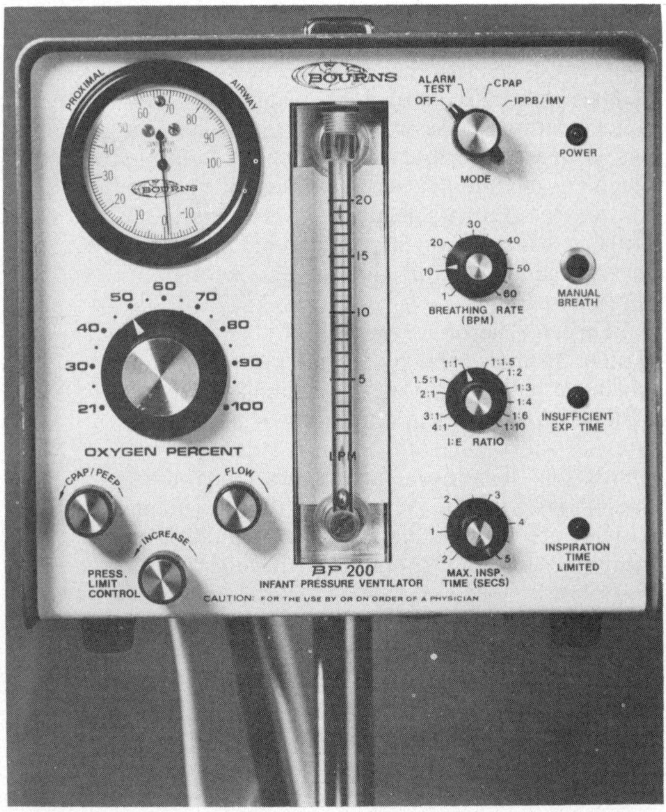


42/Fig. 15.—Bourns BP 200 ventilator.

of a left-to-right shunt (e.g. PDA) *high ventilatory pressures* (more than 30 cm $H_2O$), *high inspired oxygen concentrations* (over 60 per cent), chronic infection, and poor mucociliary function. The condition is progressive as increased $\dot{V}/\dot{Q}$ mismatching demands higher inspired oxygen concentrations and falling lung compliance needs even higher inflation pressures, unless the factors known to cause the bronchopulmonary dysplasia are minimised. However, recovery is then very slow.

Neonatal ventilators have a variety of facilities which help to minimise bronchopulmonary dysplasia.

The *ventilatory rate* is usually set at a level below which the infant would be breathing spontaneously, but the machine must have the capacity for high rates, as this is a way of increasing the minute ventilation without increasing the peak airway pressure. Work is proceeding on the use of high-frequency IPPV.[49] It is an advantage to have the facility to change the *cycling method* and *wave form*. A pressure generator produces a square wave of pressure which is an advantage in ventilating the very stiff lungs of hyaline membrane disease so that the alveoli are held distended, thus improving gas exchange and allowing the inspired oxygen concentration to be reduced. A pressure-limiting facility will also tend to minimise lung damage.

It is occasionally necessary to reverse the inspiratory:expiratory time ratio from 1:2 to 2:1, which often helps to improve gas exchange in hyaline membrane disease, though not necessarily in patients with other lung pathology.

The machine must have the ability to apply positive end expiratory pressure (PEEP), the term for Constant Distending Pressure (CDP) during IPPV. The effect of the CDP is to increase functional residual capacity in relation to closing volume, thus decreasing intrapulmonary shunting (alveolar recruitment) in diseased states of the lungs associated with fluid retention.

Early application of CDP to patients with hyaline membrane disease improves gas exchange and may decrease the severity of the disease by reducing surfactant consumption. The net effect of PEEP on tissue oxygenation depends on the degree to which the cardiac output is reduced by the technique. Levels of PEEP of up to 10 cm $H_2O$ are used.

The aim of maintenance ventilation is for peak inflation pressures of less than 30 cm $H_2O$ and as low an inspired oxygen concentration ($F_{IO_2}$) as possible, using the above techniques to establish an arterial $Pa_{O_2}$ of 60 to 80 mm Hg (8 to 10·7 kPa).

Infants of less than 36 weeks' gestation are at risk from retrolental fibroplasia associated with a high $Pa_{O_2}$. The safe level is not known but it is unwise to allow it to rise above 70 to 80 mm Hg (9·3 to 10·7 kPa) for any length of time.[50]

Weaning from the ventilator takes place after cardiovascular and biochemical stability has been achieved with inflation pressures of less than 25 cm $H_2O$, $Pa_{CO_2}$ of less than 50 mm Hg (6·7 kPa) and $Pa_{O_2}$ more than 80 mm Hg (10·7 kPa) at $F_{IO_2}$ 0·5 (i.e. the inspired oxygen concentration is 50 per cent).

Babies must never breathe through an endotracheal tube without CDP. Zero end expiratory pressure allows the small, stiff lungs to collapse progressively so the closing volume encroaches further into the functional residual capacity (FRC), with increased right-to-left intrapulmonary shunting and hypoxia. As lung volume falls, the airway resistance to gas flow rises, so that the work of breathing and oxygen consumption rise. With the endotracheal tube in place, the normal mechanism is lost whereby the glottis generates 2–3 cm $H_2O$ pressure in times of respiratory distress.

**CPAP.**—Constant positive airway pressure, constant distending pressure with spontaneous ventilation is now always used for weaning small babies from ventilators and for respiratory support in some patients who do not need ventilation. CPAP, by keeping small airways distended, reduces airway resistance and thus the work of breathing and also improves $\dot{V}/\dot{Q}$ characteristics. The technique was originally described by Gregory and his colleagues[51] using a tight-fitting headbox. This is rarely used nowadays and CPAP is better applied through a face mask, one nasal prong or an endotracheal tube.

CPAP may be applied using a modified T-piece (Fig. 16)[52] or Bain circuit, both of which rely on a fresh gas flow of three times the patient's minute volume. A CDP of 6–8 cm $H_2O$ is suitable to start with. Apnoea of prematurity responds to CPAP by activation of sensory stretch receptors in the chest wall.

Modern infant ventilators are fitted with integral CPAP circuits and most use *intermittent*

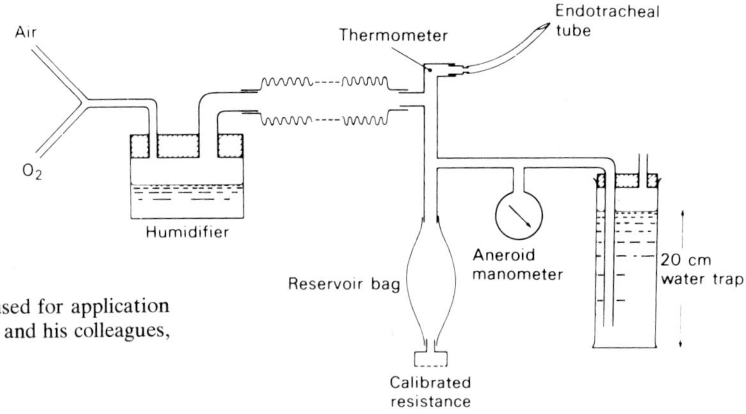


42/FIG. 16.—Modified T-piece circuit used for application of CPAP. (Courtesy of Dr. D. J. Hatch and his colleagues, and the Editor of the *Lancet*.[52])

*mandatory ventilation* (IMV). This facility allows the patient to breathe with CPAP between a preset number of mandatory breaths from the machine. As the patient progresses, the number of IMV breaths are gradually reduced. Systems which rely on a continuous fresh gas flow (Bourns) are better than where the flow is of the demand type (Servo).

**Mandatory minute ventilation** is a relatively new concept and available commercially in relatively few machines. The preset minute volume is available for the patient to breathe spontaneously if he is able to do so, but if he does not, the machine will ventilate him.

After extubation from 2 cm $H_2O$ CPAP, pulmonary atelectasis is common and repeated intubation for physiotherapy and suction may be necessary. Temporary support with CPAP via one nasal prong may be needed until the glottis recovers the ability to generate its own pressure.

*Bronchoscopy is never needed merely to remove secretions or to expand collapsed lobes.*

**Hyaline Membrane Disease** (HMD)

Significant advances have been made in the management of HMD (Idiopathic Respiratory Distress Syndrome) in recent years, so that it is no longer the principal cause of death in preterm infants.[53] The condition occurs in 1 per cent of all live births and 1 in 3 premature babies, being caused by deficiency of lung surfactant associated with prematurity. The severity is increased by interference with surfactant synthesis in type II alveolar cells by hypoxia or asphyxia in the neonatal period. The lungs are unable to maintain a functional residual capacity by failing to stabilise small air spaces at the end of expiration. $\dot{V}/\dot{Q}$ is mismatched, causing hypoxaemia and increased pulmonary vascular resistance (Fig. 17).

The clinical features are grunting respiration, tachypnoea, dyspnoea, cyanosis and tachycardia. The chest radiograph shows a typical "ground glass" uniform opacity in all lung fields with an air bronchogram. The tachypnoea with stiff lungs increases the work of breathing by up to ten times. Right-to-left shunts through a patent ductus or foramen ovale increase the arterial hypoxaemia, which in turn impairs myocardial function leading to metabolic acidosis.

Davies and his associates[55] showed one regimen for treatment of HMD (Table 9). Regular frequent clinical assessments with blood gas analysis are essential, and transcutaneous $Po_2$ monitoring is invaluable. Continuous gas monitoring is possible using an indwelling umbilical arterial cannula, but this carries a risk of serious thrombo-embolic problems if the cannula is left *in situ* for periods longer than 48 hours. Repeated samples may be taken from the radial arteries.

Careful respiratory support involves the use of constant distending pressure or mechanical ventilation with square-wave form and possibly using reversed inspiratory:expiratory time ratios (e.g. 2:1) and positive end-expiratory pressure.[56]

The very stiff lungs of HMD are especially prone to damage by high ventilatory pressures and inflation pressures should be limited

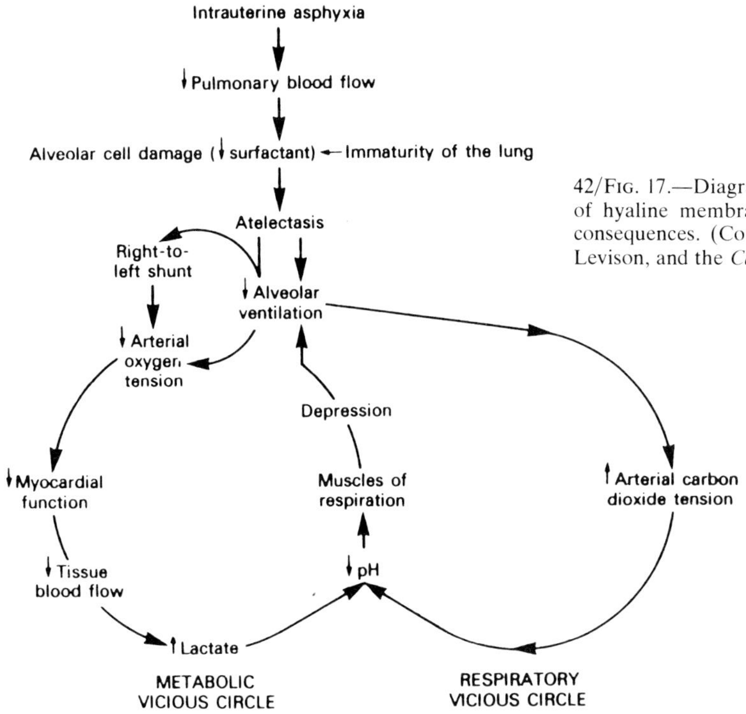


42/FIG. 17.—Diagrammatic representation of the aetiology of hyaline membrane disease and its pathophysiological consequences. (Courtesy of Dr. P. R. Swyer and Dr. H. Levison, and the *Canadian Medical Association Journal*.[54])

## 42/TABLE 9
## OXYGEN THERAPY IN RESPIRATORY DISTRESS

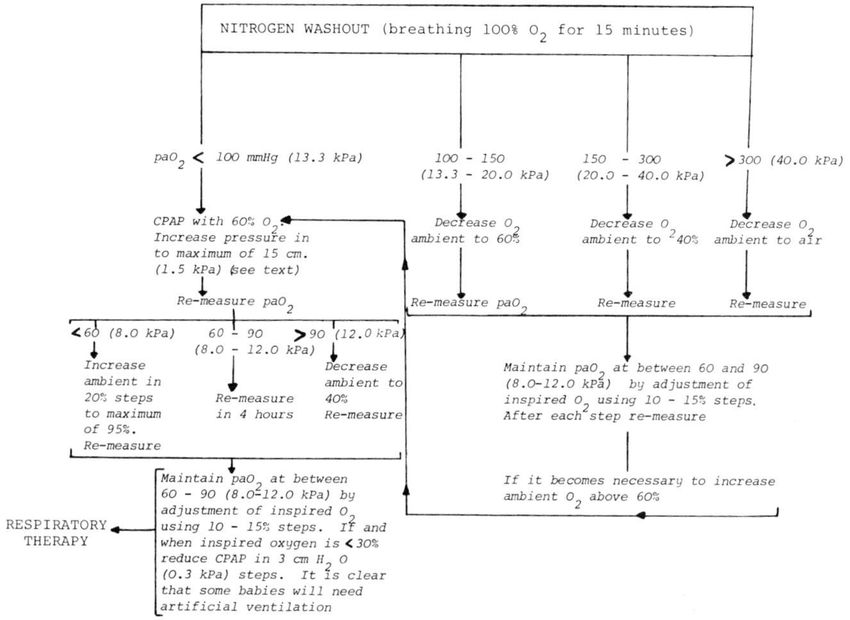

to 30 cm $H_2O$. Results are better if the patients are paralysed and ventilated using a square-wave form.[57] In the future it may be possible to replace the surfactant using an artificial preparation, as has been achieved experimentally.[58]

**Intravenous Hyperalimentation**

Parenteral nutrition is very frequently required in infants after major surgery, with necrotising enterocolitis, protracted diarrhoea, extreme prematurity or renal failure.

The technique requires very strict aseptic conditions and intensive nursing care. Some centres recommend that peripheral veins are used and the site changed every 24 hours. The inclusion of Intralipid in doses of 4 g fat/kg per day means that peripheral veins may be used for longer periods without the increased risks of infection and venous thrombosis as when central veins are used.

When central silastic catheters are used, they are tunnelled under the skin for a distance before entering the central vein, thus minimising infection. Catheters of the Broviac or Hickman type with a Teflon cuff are the most satisfactory. A bacterial filter is fitted into the system as close to the patient as possible, though Intralipid will not pass through such filters. A series of 3-way stopcocks is arranged so that solutions may be given in rotation, and all infusion tubing drip sets and solutions are changed every 24 hours.[59]

Regimens are available to maintain positive nitrogen balance and growth for many months at a rate of 0·42 MJ/kg (100 kcal/kg) per day.

*Vamin* with additional glucose is the most satisfactory amino-acid solution for use in infants at an infusion rate not exceeding 72 ml/kg per day.

*Intralipid* as 10 or 20 per cent is the usual fat solution used and is rapidly cleared from the plasma even in patients with mild liver dysfunction. The rate of administration is reduced if the serum remains thick.

*Monosaccharide* is usually given as dextrose 10 or 15 per cent. Fructose, though less dependent on insulin for its metabolism, causes an osmotic diuresis. Hypoglycaemia may occur during fructose administration.

*A multivitamin* infusion is given in a dose of 3 ml per day with the additions of folic acid 0·5 mg per day, vitamin K, 3 mg twice weekly, and vitamin $B_{12}$ 100 $\mu$g once each month. If intravenous feeding is continued for more than one week, biotin (part of vitamin B complex) 0·5 mg per day and choline chloride 150 mg must be given. Trace elements are provided by weekly infusions of plasma 10 ml/kg or, better,

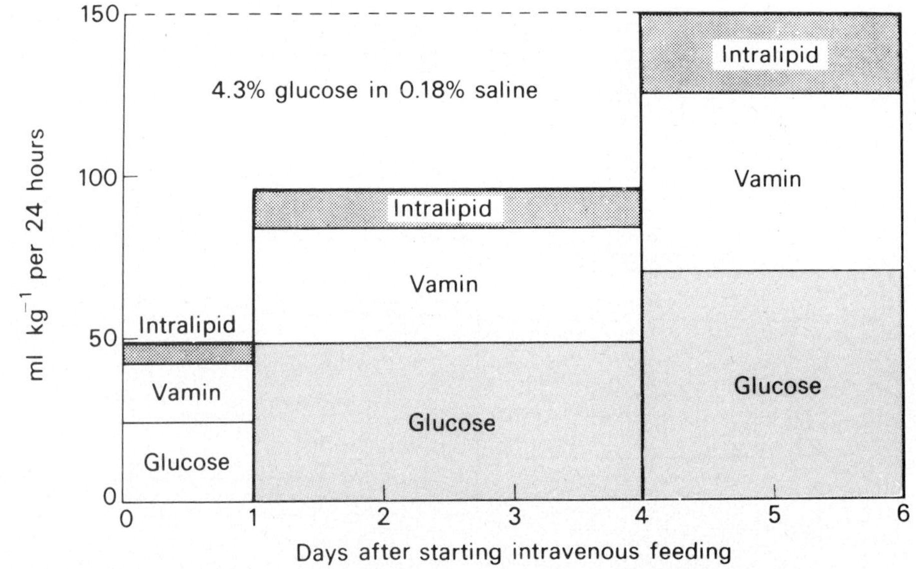


42/Fig. 18.—A technique for the introduction of infusates for complete intravenous feeding in infants. (Courtesy of Dr. J. Harries, and the *British Medical Journal*.[60])

by adding a proprietary mixture such as Ped-El to a Vamin amino-acid solution.

The volumes of each nutrient are increased daily, maximum volumes being achieved on the fourth day, if the clinical and biochemical state of the patient remains satisfactory (Fig. 18). Small volumes of each solution are given in a rotational system so that an even distribution of solutions is achieved during a 24-hour period.

All additives such as vitamins or electrolytes must be infused with the dextrose-saline and each electrolyte solution given separately or precipitation may occur with mixtures. The daily doses of calcium and potassium are spaced out to avoid the possibility of excess concentrations producing cardiac dysrhythmia.

If possible some oral feeding should continue during total intravenous feeding to maintain a continuous stimulant effect on the small-intestinal mucosa. Intravenous alimentation should not be abruptly withdrawn or hypoglycaemia (caused by the high levels of circulating insulin) may develop. Full oral feeding should be re-introduced over several days before the i.v. alimentation is withdrawn.

Complications of the technique are common and include septicaemia with *Candida albicans, Staphylococcus aureus* and *Escherichia coli.*

42/TABLE 10
A COMPLETE REGIMEN FOR THE PARENTERAL NUTRITION OF INFANTS

| | ml/kg/day | | |
|---|---|---|---|
| | Day 1 | Days 2–5 | 6th day on |
| Vamin 100 ml, Ped-El 12 ml | 20 | 35 | 50 |
| 10% dextrose 100 ml | 30 | 50 | 60 |
| 4% dextrose/saline 0·18% 100 ml, Multibionta 1 ml, $K_2HPO_4$ (17·42%) 3 ml, Folic acid 0·06 ml | 100 | 60 | 20 |
| Intralipid 20% | — | 10 | 20 |

Maximum volumes may be made up to 160 ml/kg/day using 5 per cent dextrose.

Topical antibiotics with nystatin at the point of skin entry of the catheter may reduce the incidence of infection. Central venous catheters must be removed if blood cultures are found to be positive. Phlebitis and venous obstruction are common, though the incidence is reduced by including Intralipid in the regimen.

Most of the amino-acid solutions contain high sodium concentrations and are markedly hyperosmolar, so that excess may cause oedema and cardiac failure.

## REFERENCES


1. Leader (1978). Paediatric Anaesthesia. *Brit. Med. J.*, **2**, 717.
2. Heymann, M. A. and Rudolph, A. M. (1975). Control of the ductus arteriosus. *Physiol. Rev.*, **55**, 62.
3. Kitterman, J. A. (1980). Patent ductus arteriosus: Current clinical status. *Arch. Dis. Childh.*, **55**, 106.
4. Sumner, E. and Frank, J. D. (1981). Tolazoline in the treatment of congenital diaphragmatic hernia. *Arch. Dis. Childh.*, **56**, 350.
5. Gluck, L., Kulovich, M. V., Bores, R. C., Brenner, P. H., Anderson, G. G. and Spellacy, W. N. (1971). Diagnosis of respiratory distress syndrome by amniocentesis. *Amer. J. Obstet. Gynec.*, **109**, 440.
6. Auld, P. A. M. (1976). Pulmonary transition from fetal life. In *Reviews in Perinatal Medicine*. Ed. E. M. Scarpelli and E. V. Cosmi. Baltimore: University Park Press.
7. Wu, B., Kikkawa, Y., Orzales, I. M., Motoyama, E. K., Kaibara, M., Zigas, C. J. and Cook, C. D. (1973). The effect of thyroxine on the maturation of fetal rabbit lungs. *Biol. Neonat. (Basel)*, **22**, 161.
8. Dawes, G. S., Fox, H. E. and Richards, R. T. (1972). Variations in asphyxial gasping with fetal age in lambs and guinea pigs. *Quart. J. Exp. Physiology*, **57**, 131.
9. Boddy, K., Dawes, G. S. and Robinson, J. S. (1974). In *Modern Perinatal Medicine*. Chicago: Year Book Medical Publishers.
10. Davenport, H. T. (1980). *Paediatric Anaesthesia*, 3rd edit. p. 16. London: Heinemann.
11. Silverman, W. A., Agate, F. J. and Fertic, J. W. (1963). A sequential trial of the non-thermal effect of atmospheric humidity on survival of newborn infants of low birth weight. *Pediatrics*, **31**, 719.
12. Hey, E. (1972). Thermal regulation in the newborn. *Brit. J. Hosp. Med.*, **5**, 51.
13. Bennett, E. J. (1975). Fluid balance in the newborn. *Anesthesiology*, **43**, 210.
14. Cree, J. E., Meyer, J., Hailey, D. (1973). Diazepam in labour: its metabolism and effect on the clinical condition and thermogenesis of the newborn. *Brit. Med. J.*, **4**, 251.
15. Dawes, G. S. (1968). *Fetal and Neonatal Physiology*. Chicago: Year Book Medical Publishers.
16. Apgar, V. (1953). Proposal for new method of evaluation of newborn infant. *Anesth. Analg. Curr. Res.*, **32**, 260.
17. Apgar, V., Holadam, D. A., James, L. S., Weisbrot, I. M. and Berrien, C. (1958). Evaluation of the newborn infant; second report. *J. Amer. Med. Ass.*, **168**, 1985.
18. Gregory, G. A. (1975). Resuscitation of the newborn. *Anesthesiology*, **43**, 225.
19. Mushin, W. W. (1967). A neonatal inflating bag. *Brit. Med. J.*, **1**, 416.
20. Hatch, D. J. and Sumner, E. (1981). Neonatal resusci-

tation. In *Neonatal Anaesthesia*. London: Edward Arnold.

21. Hey, E. N. (1977). Resuscitation at birth. *Brit. J. Anaesth.*, **49**, 25.
22. Rendell-Baker, L. and Soucek, D. H. (1962). New paediatric face-masks and anaesthetic equipment. *Brit. Med. J.*, **1**, 1960.
23. Ayre, P. (1956). The T-piece technique. *Brit. J. Anaesth.*, **28**, 520.
24. Willis, B. A., Pender, J. A. and Mapleson, W. W. (1975). Rebreathing in a T-piece. Volunteer and theoretical studies of the Jackson-Rees modification of the Ayre's T-piece during spontaneous respiration. *Brit. J. Anaesth.*, **47**, 1239.
25. Byrick, R. J. and Janssen, E. G. (1980). Respiratory wave form and rebreathing in T-piece circuits: A comparison of enflurane and halothane wave forms. *Anesthesiology*, **53**, 371.
26. Hatch, D. J., Miles, R. and Wagstaff, M. (1980). An anaesthetic scavenging system for adult and paediatric use. *Anaesthesia*, **35**, 496.
27. Bain, J. A. and Spoerel, W. E. (1972). A streamlined anaesthetic system. *Canad. Anaesth. Soc. J.*, **19**, 426.
28. Sumner, E. and Patrick, E. (1980). In *Preparation for Anaesthesia*. edited by A. J. Stevens. Tunbridge Wells: Pitman Medical.
29. Newton, N. I., Hillman, K. M. and Varley, J. G. (1981). Automatic ventilation with the Ayre's T-piece. A modification of the Nuffield Series 200 ventilator for neonatal and paediatric use. *Anaesthesia*, **36**, 22.
30. Steward, D. J. (1979). Manual of pediatric anesthesia. New York: Churchill Livingstone.
31. Solosko, D., Frissell, M. and Smith, R. B. (1972). 111 halothane anesthesias in a pediatric patient. A case report. *Anesth. Analg. Curr. Res.*, **51**, 706.
32. Carney, F. M. T. and van Dyke, R. A. (1972). Halothane hepatitis: a critical review. *Anesth. Analg. Curr. Res.*, **51**, 135.
33. Bennett, E. J., Ignacio, A., Patel, K., Grundy, E. M. and Salem, M. R. (1976). The use of d-tubocurarine in neonatal anaesthesia. *Brit. J. Anaesth.*, **34**, 721.
34. Nightingale, D. A. and Bush, G. H. (1973). A clinical comparison between tubocurarine and pancuronium in children. *Brit. J. Anaesth.*, **45**, 63.
35. Battersby, E. F. (1981). Monitoring during anesthesia for pediatric surgery. *Intern. Anesthesiol. Clin.*, **19**, 95.
36. Marshall, A. G. and Sumner, E. (1982). Improved prognosis in congenital diaphragmatic hernia: experience of 62 cases over 2-year period. *J. Roy. Soc. Med.*, **75**, 607.
37. Stark, J. (1980). Current status of cardiac surgery in early infancy. *Proceedings of the 8th European Congress of Cardiology, Paris, 1980*, p. 253, Basel: Karger.
38. Subramanian, S., Wagner, H., Vlad, P. and Lambert, E. (1971). Surface induced deep hypothermia in cardiac surgery. *J. Pediat. Surg.*, **6**, 612.
39. Radney, P. A. (Ed.) (1980). Anesthetic considerations for pediatric cardiac surgery. *Intern. Anesthesiol. Clin.*, **18**, 1–217.
40. Lang, P., Williams, R. G., Norwood, W. I. and Castaneda, A. R. (1980). The hemodynamic effects of dopamine in infants after corrective cardiac surgery. *J. Pediat.*, **96**, 630.
41. Buckberg, G. D. (1979). A proposed 'solution' to the cardioplegic controversy. *J. Thorac. Cardiovasc. Surg.*, **77**, 803.
42. Neuman, G. G. and Hansen, D. D. (1980). The anaesthetic management of preterm infants undergoing ligation of patent ductus arteriosus. *Canad. Anaesth. Soc. J.*, **27**, 248.
43. Rickham, P. P., Lister, J. and Irving, I. M. (1978). *Neonatal Surgery*, London: Butterworth.
44. Soueff, P. N. L., Morgan, A. K., Soutter, L. P., Reynolds, E. O. R. and Parker, D. (1978). Comparison of transcutaneous oxygen tension with arterial oxygen tension in newborn infants with severe respiratory illnesses. *Pediatrics*, **62**, 692.
45. Allen, T. H. and Steven, I. M. (1972). Prolonged nasotracheal intubation in infants and children. *Brit. J. Anaesth.*, **44**, 835.
46. Branthwaite, M. (1977). *Anaesthesia for Cardiac Surgery*, p. 162. Oxford: Blackwell Scientific Publications.
47. Aberdeen, E. (1965). Tracheostomy and tracheostomy care in infants. *Proc. Roy. Soc. Med.*, **58**, 900.
48. Reynolds, E. O. R. (1974). Pressure waveform and ventilator settings for mechanical ventilation in severe hyaline membrane disease. *Int. Anesthesiol. Clin.*, **12**, 259.
49. Kirby, R. R. (1980). High frequency positive pressure ventilation. What rôle in ventilatory insufficiency. *Anesthesiology*, **52**, 109.
50. James, L. S. and Lanman, J. T. (1976). Symposium: Retrolental fibroplasia. *Pediatrics*, **57**, Suppl. 591.
51. Gregory, G. A., Kitterman, J. A., Phibbs, R. H., Tooley, W. H. and Hamilton, W. K. (1971). Treatment of the idiopathic respiratory distress syndrome with continuous positive airway pressure. *New Engl. J. Med.*, **284**, 1333.
52. Hatch, D. J., Taylor, B. W., Glover, W. J., Cogswell, J. J., Battersby, E. F. and Kerr, A. A. (1973). Continuous positive airway pressure after open-heart operations in infancy. *Lancet*, **2**, 470.
53. Reynolds, E. O. R. (1975). Management of hyaline membrane disease. *Brit. Med. Bull.*, **31**, 18.
54. Swyer, P. R. and Levison, H. (1965). The current status of the respiratory distress syndrome of the newly born. *Canad. Med. Assoc. J.*, **93**, 335.
55. Davies, P. A., Robinson, R. J., Scopes, J. W., Tizard, J. P. M. and Wigglesworth, J. S. (1972). In *Medical Care of Newborn Babies*. London: Spastics International Medical Publications.
56. Reynolds, E. O. R. and Taghizadeh, A. (1974). Improved prognosis of infants mechanically ventilated for hyaline membrane disease. *Arch. Dis. Childh.*, **49**, 505.
57. Manginello, F. P. Grassi, A. E., Schechner, S., Krauss, A. N. and Auld, P. A. M. (1978). Evaluation of methods of assisted ventilation in hyaline membrane disease. *Arch. Dis. Childh.*, **53**, 878.
58. Fujiwara, T., Maeta, H., Morita, T., Watabe, Y., Chida, S. and Abe, T. (1980). Artificial surfactant therapy in hyaline membrane disease. *Lancet*, **1**, 55.
59. Harries, J. T. (1978). Aspects of intravenous feeding in childhood. In *Advances in Parenteral Nutrition*. Ed. by Ivan Johnston. Lancaster: MTP Press.
60. Harries, J. T. (1971). Intravenous feeding in infants. *Arch. Dis. Child.*, **46**, 855.

## SUGGESTED FURTHER READING

Bennett, E. J. (1975). *Fluids for Anesthesia and Surgery in the Newborn and Infant*. Springfield. Ill: Thomas.

Brown, T. C. K. and Fisk, G. C. (1979). *Anaesthesia for Children*. Oxford: Blackwell Scientific.

Bush, G. H. (1971). Intravenous fluid therapy in paediatrics. *Ann. Roy. Coll. Surg. Engl.*, **49**, 92.

Davies, J., Dobbing, J. eds. (1981). *Scientific Foundation of Paediatrics*. 2nd edit. London: Heinemann.

Godfrey, S. and Baum, J. D. (1979). *Clinical Paediatric Physiology*. Oxford: Blackwell Scientific.

Hatch, D. J. and Sumner, E. (1981). *Neonatal Anaesthesia*. London: Edward Arnold.

Jackson Rees, G. and Gray, T. C. (1981). *Paediatric Anaesthesia—Trends in current practice*. London: Butterworths.

Rickham, P. P., Lister, J. and Irving, I. M. (1978). *Neonatal Surgery*, 2nd edit. London: Butterworths.

Schaffer, A. J. and Avery, M. E. (1977). *Diseases of the Newborn*. 4th edit. Philadelphia: Saunders.

Smith, R. M. (1980). *Anesthesia for Infants and Children*. 4th edit. St. Louis: C. V. Mosby Co.

Stehling L. C. and Zander, H. L. (1979). *Anesthetic Implications of Congenital Anomalies in Children*. New York: Appleton-Century-Crofts.

Swyer, P. R. (1975). The intensive care of the newly born: physiological principles and practice. *Monographs in Paediatrics*, volume 6. Basel: Karger.

*Section Seven*

# SPECIAL SITUATIONS

**CHAPTER 43**

# Anaesthesia for Dental and Oral Surgery

---



---

## INTRODUCTION

Dental anaesthesia has a unique place in the range of general anaesthesia for several reasons. The first recorded administration of general anaesthesia was when Gardner Quincy Colton gave nitrous oxide to Horace Wells for the extraction of a tooth in 1844. Thomas Evans, an American dental surgeon first demonstrated this technique in London in 1868. Dental anaesthesia is the commonest single branch of anaesthesia. In the United Kingdom, about 1·5 million general anaesthetics are given for dental patients each year, equivalent to half the total given for all branches of surgery. In the United States of America the number is about 5 million, equivalent to one quarter of the total every year. Finally, the majority of dental anaesthetics are given by non-specialist anaesthetists, usually dental surgeons, in surgeries outside a hospital setting. The problems of dental anaesthesia are often very different from those of conventional general anaesthesia, and demand specialist training in this discipline for all would-be practitioners.

## MORTALITY AND MORBIDITY

The number of deaths associated with dental anaesthesia is about 1 in 100,000 in both the United Kingdom and United States of America. Although small in statistical terms, these cases represent personal tragedies, as the patients are usually young, fit people undergoing anaesthesia for relatively trivial procedures. It also seems likely that most of these deaths are due to preventable causes. Although the total number of general anaesthetics given for dental surgery is falling steadily, due to the increased use of sedation and local anaesthesia, the mortality rate is increasing. This has led to a number of publications examining the cause of deaths during dental anaesthesia.[1–3]

Bourne tried to show that most of the sudden deaths in the dental chair have followed unrecognised fainting in the sitting position. Tomlin, however, felt that hypoxia was the most common cause of death, and that posture was seldom causally related. Coplans and Curson's detailed analysis of mortality statistics confirm Tomlin's view that posture is not related to anaesthetic deaths in the dental chair. They showed that as the supine position has become more popular so deaths in that position have increased.

Minor morbidity such as pain, headache, nausea and vomiting is common after dental extractions. Surprisingly, the incidence is similar following local or general anaesthesia.[4] There is a very high incidence of side-effects following minor oral surgery in the intubated outpatient.[5,6] Adequate home conditions are essential for the intubated day-stay patient. If these are not available, overnight stay in hospital is advisable.

Most morbidity surveys only record minor symptoms. There is no data available on major complications such as mental changes following anaesthesia. Alterations in personality or memory are not known, due to the problems of neurological testing and collection of information. This leads to erroneous statements about safety of certain techniques. For example, hypoxic methods using nitrous oxide have been quoted as safe when analysing death rates and minor morbidity. Hypoxia with a normal cerebral circulation quickly leads to destruction of cerebral neurones, which cannot regenerate. It is quite likely that fine neurological testing could demonstrate changes in intellect, memory and personality following hypoxic dental anaesthesia. It cannot be stated too strongly that the use of oxygen lack to produce unconsciousness has no place in modern dental anaesthesia.

## ANAESTHESIA FOR DENTAL EXTRACTIONS

The great majority of extractions are performed in dental surgeries. A smaller proportion are done in outpatient clinics. The patients often present as emergencies, and therefore arrive poorly assessed in comparison to a normal hospital population. Extractions take place in the dental chair, most commonly in the sitting position. The operation rarely lasts longer than a few minutes. Recovery facilities are often limited, requiring an early return to street fitness. All these factors combine to make local anaesthesia the method of choice for simple dental extractions. General anaesthesia should only be used if there is a strong positive indication.

### Indications for General Anaesthesia

#### Definite

There are certain situations where general anaesthesia is definitely indicated:

*Young children with multiple extractions.*—Surgery in several quadrants of the mouth will need many injections, and more than one visit. This can be very upsetting for a small child. General anaesthesia is probably kinder, and less likely to cause fear of dentistry.

*Acute infections.*—Local anaesthesia is often unsuccessful in patients with dental abscesses due to the altered pH of the tissues. Local injections may also spread the infection. General anaesthesia overcomes these problems, allowing immediate extraction of the tooth and drainage of the abscess. Caution must be used if there is associated tissue oedema causing trismus, or potential airway problems.

*Previous radiotherapy to the jaw.*—It is probably unwise to use local injections in the jaw which has been irradiated, as this may lead to necrosis, especially in the mandible.

*Allergy to local anaesthetic drugs.*—True allergy to lignocaine is rare but does occur. Most patients with a history of so-called allergy, are usually describing fainting reactions or unpleasant sequelae to absorbed vasoconstrictors, particularly adrenaline.

Reactions to vasoconstrictors can be prevented by using plain solutions. Persistent fainters should be treated in the supine position. However, patients with a genuine history of lignocaine allergy, such as skin reactions or angioneurotic oedema, should be given general anaesthesia.

Patients who are severely *mentally or physically handicapped* may not be able to co-operate sufficiently to allow dental treatment under local anaesthesia.

### Relative Indications

General anaesthesia is often advocated in other situations where careful patient management will, in fact, allow local anaesthesia to be successfully used.

*Extremely nervous patients* who request general anaesthesia. Most of these patients can be treated successfully under local anaesthesia, by sympathetic and experienced dentists, with the use of anxiolytics such as diazepam if necessary. A few have severe dental phobia and will need general anaesthesia.

*Previous faint reactions* under local anaesthesia. This is often due to poor patient management and inexperienced operators. Treatment in the supine position by a sympathetic and experienced operator will often overcome these problems.

Patients who require *surgery in all four quadrants of the mouth* are often offered general anaesthesia to facilitate treatment in a single session. This practice underestimates the dangers of general anaesthesia, and should be discouraged.

*Epileptic patients* are often treated under general anaesthesia, as local anaesthesia may precipitate seizures. Although possible, this reason represents an inaccurate conclusion on the relative dangers of local and general anaesthesia in the epileptic patient. In the well-controlled epileptic the overall risks of general anaesthesia still outweigh those of local anaesthesia. Diazepam can always be used to protect patients with seizure disorders being treated under local anaesthesia. If general anaesthesia is used in these patients, thiopentone is the intravenous induction agent of choice. All the other commonly used induction agents can produce epileptiform reactions.

### Contra-indications

There are certain absolute contra-indications to outpatient general anaesthesia in the dental chair. Firstly, serious medical disease. Only ASA 1 or 2 class patients should be anaesthetised in the dental chair. Patients with serious cardiovascular, respiratory, or other medical disorders should be admitted to hospital. Similarly, patients with oral infection leading to severe trismus, or oedema of the floor of the mouth and pharynx, must be admitted to hospital. There may be life-threatening airway problems if general anaesthesia is administered to this group of patients.

## Equipment

### The Dental Chair and Posture

Traditionally, dental anaesthesia has been given with the patient in the erect position sitting in the dental chair. In 1957, Bourne[7] drew attention to the possibility of unrecognised fainting occurring during general anaesthesia in the sitting position. He postulated that many unexplained deaths during dental anaesthesia were due to fainting and could be prevented by using the supine position. This has led to increasing use of the supine position during the last two decades. However, Tomlin[2] concluded that posture was seldom causally related to deaths in dental anaesthesia. This view was supported by a detailed analysis of mortality statistics carried out by Coplans and Curson.[3] Comparative studies carried out by Forsyth and colleagues[8] and McCormick[9] failed to show significant cardiovascular differences between the supine and erect positions during dental anaesthesia. Thus, it would seem unwise to abandon the sitting position purely on cardiovascular criteria. The respiratory problems of airway control and pulmonary inhalation must also be evaluated when selecting an ideal posture. McCormick showed that pharyngeal soiling with blood was increased in the supine position.[9] Vital capacity is reduced and airway obstruction is more common in the supine position. Thus, although the debate on posture is still not settled, available evidence would support Forsyth's[8] view that the semi-recumbent position with legs elevated gives the ideal combination of respiratory and cardiovascular conditions (Fig. 1). It provides the airway advantages of an erect head and neck, with the cardiovascular advantages of a semi-reclining position and elevated legs. It is therefore important to use a dental chair with an adjustable head-rest, allowing manipulation of the head and neck on the trunk. The fully contoured chair with integral head-rest, used for conservative dentistry, is not satisfactory in this respect. The chair must also be capable of being placed in the horizontal position rapidly for the purposes of cardiopulmonary resuscitation, even if there is a power failure.

If the supine position is adopted, a tilting trolley can be used instead of the dental chair. This is more stable and provides easier recovery facilities, but lack of height adjustment with this system may create problems. Available evidence would suggest that fully supine patients should be intubated for complete airway protection.

### Anaesthetic Machines

Historically, the isolation of dental anaesthesia has led to the development of an anaesthetic machine not used in other branches of general anaesthesia. This is the intermittent- or demand-flow machine; the most popular models being the B.O.C. "Walton" series and the McKesson. The distinctive features of this type of apparatus are firstly, the ability to change rapidly the relative concentrations of oxygen and nitrous oxide, using a single calibrated control, and secondly, the ability of gas flow to follow the patients inspiratory effort or function on demand. It is also necessary for high gas-flows to be delivered, thus overcoming the problems of high resistance to inspiration caused by the twin narrow-bore delivery tubes traditionally used. However, modern dental anaesthesia does not require several of these facilities. Hypoxic mixtures should no longer be used, and it is therefore unnecessary constantly to change the inspired oxygen concentration. The development of the Goldman nose-piece with its single wide-bore tubing overcomes the problem of high resistance to inspiration. This allows the use of low inspired gas flows. Surveys have shown that old intermittent-flow machines are inaccurate and dangerous.[10,11] These machines should be phased out and replaced by machines of the standard Boyles type. Many companies now manufacture smaller versions of conventional anaesthetic machines suitable for dental anaesthesia. Alternatively, a wall- or cabinet-mounted Quantiflex Monitored Dial Mixer can be used. This machine is suitable for both relative analgesia and general anaesthesia. It is necessary to ensure that reliable vaporisers are included, which will deliver accurate concentrations of the volatile agents such as halothane or enflurane.

Atmospheric pollution with anaesthetic gases is particularly high in dental surgeries. This is

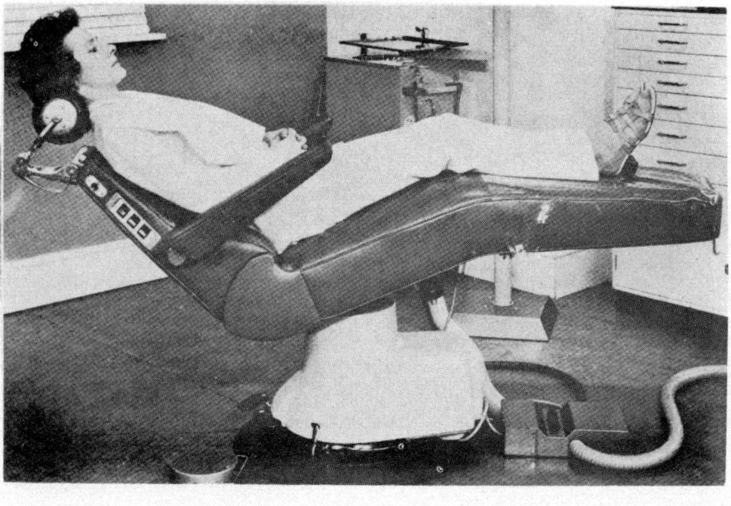

43/FIG. 1.—Reclining posture. (Courtesy of Dr. R. A. Green and Dr. M. P. Coplans, and H. K. Lewis and Co. Ltd., 1973.[57])

due to the problems of scavenging and lack of good air-conditioning. Work is still in progress on an ideal scavenging system.[12]

### Mouth Props, Gags, Packs and Airways

A variety of equipment is available in this area and final choice is a matter of personal preference. However, certain important points need to be kept in mind. Mouth props must be large enough to allow access for packing and surgery without restricting the available space for the dental surgeon. The McKesson prop is ideal for adults, whereas the Devonshire prop is more suitable for children. The mouth pack is the single most important item in the prevention of airway complications during dental anaesthesia. Incorrect packing may lead to respiratory obstruction, or inhalation of blood and debris. The best type of pack is a 3-in (7·5 cm) wide gauze, using the method recommended by Coplans and Barton.[13] This consists in placing layers of gauze in such a way as to isolate the operation site without unduly depressing the tongue (Fig. 2).

A mouth gag may be necessary if trismus is present or an emergency occurs. Nasopharyngeal airways can be invaluable in patients where it is difficult to maintain a good nasal airway. It is absolutely essential to have a reliable and efficient form of suction apparatus.

### Resuscitation Equipment

It is mandatory to have a full range of oral and nasal endotracheal tubes, together with laryngoscopes and any accessories necessary for intubation. Perks[14] has drawn attention to the serious emergencies that can arise in a dental surgery. Thus, it is becoming increasingly important for dental surgeries to be fully equipped for cardiopulmonary resuscitation. This includes provision of an electrocardiogram, defibrillator, and a set of resuscitation drugs. Delay in starting definitive treatment, whilst awaiting transfer to hospital, greatly reduces any chance for successful resuscitation from cardiac arrest. Practising dental anaesthetists must be able to insert an endotracheal tube and set up an intravenous infusion.

## Anaesthetic Management

### Pre-operative Preparation and Premedication

As with all patients presenting for general anaesthesia, pre-operative assessment can be subdivided into history, physical examination, and investigations.

The most efficient way to record a history from dental patients is to use a printed questionnaire. This will save time and prevent omissions, which is important in a busy dental clinic where several patients are presenting as emergencies. In elective cases the questionnaire can be filled in at the initial visit. Only generally fit patients in the ASA 1 or 2 classes are suitable for general anaesthesia in the dental chair.

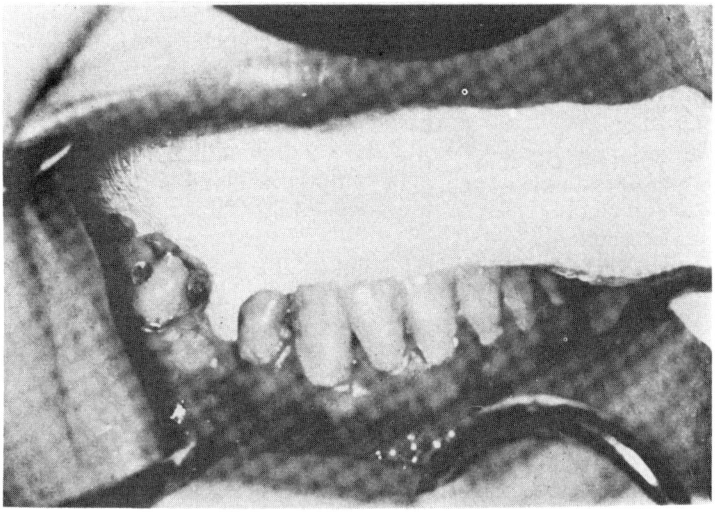

43/Fig. 2.—Pack in position for extraction of lower posterior teeth. Gap demonstrates that the pack has been tucked deeply into the lingual sulcus. (Courtesy of Dr. R. A. Green and Dr. M. P. Coplans, and H. K. Lewis and Co. Ltd., 1973.[57])

When the history is unremarkable it has often been standard practise to omit physical examination in dental clinics. It is difficult to defend the administration of general anaesthesia without prior examination of the patient. Auscultation of the chest together with recording of the pulse, blood pressure and weight should become a minimum acceptable practice. At the same time it is possible to evaluate the nasal airway and condition of the teeth.

Laboratory investigations have usually been omitted in patients with a clear history. However, Meyer[15] showed that 11 per cent of patients passed fit for out-patient general anaesthesia had abnormalities in blood and urine tests. In 2 per cent of patients, these abnormalities constituted a contra-indication to general anaesthesia. Thus, it is now becoming accepted that a haemoglobin estimation and urine analysis are a minimum work up in any patient presenting for general anaesthesia. It is absolutely essential to perform a haemoglobin estimation and sickle test in any black patient presenting for general anaesthesia. Patients with sickle-cell trait should be treated in hospital clinics, whilst those with sickle-cell disease must be admitted and given in-patient treatment.

Final preparation consists of ensuring that the consent form has been signed, an escort is available to accompany the patient home, and clear written postoperative instructions have been given. Prior to induction, it is essential for the patient to empty bladder and bowels. Dentures and contact lenses must be removed.

Premedication is best avoided in out-patient dental anaesthesia. Sedative and anxiolytic drugs will delay recovery, whilst anticholinergic drugs are not necessary and are also unpleasant for the patient. The majority of these patients are children, and good rapport established before anaesthesia commences together with kind and confident management of the child during induction, obviate the need for premedication.

Occasionally an uncontrollable child, commonly in the five- to ten-years age group, will need sedation prior to anaesthesia. Heavy premedication with drugs such as trimeprazine elixir 4 mg/kg is probably more reliable than the use of anxiolytics in these children.

### Induction

Position of the patient, as previously discussed, is still controversial. The semi-recumbent position with legs elevated in the dental chair, would seem the best posture on current evidence (Fig. 1, p. 1126). The head-rest must be adjusted to keep the head and neck in an erect position, thus making the airway easier to control. Small children will need a special seat to raise their head to the level of the head-rest.

**Inhalational induction.**—This is most commonly used in young children although older children, and adults with a fear of needles, will occasionally request gaseous induction. Young children may benefit from having a parent in the room holding their hand during induction. In a child under five years, it may prove easier to induce anaesthesia with it seated on its parent's lap in the dental chair.

Gaseous induction should commence with a nitrous oxide and oxygen mixture, using high gas-flows, and not less than 25 per cent inspired oxygen concentration. Initially, it is better to cup ones hand around the nose-piece, holding a high concentration of anaesthetic gases near the child's mouth and nose, rather than placing the nose-piece directly on the child's face. The most commonly used volatile supplement is halothane, and this can be introduced at a 0·5 per cent concentration. Every few breaths the concentration is increased by 0·5 per cent, until a concentration of between 3–4 per cent is reached. During this stage, the child may struggle slightly but the parent's reassuring presence, and restraint if necessary, coupled with firm but kind management by the anaesthetist, soon results in loss of consciousness. The nose-piece can now be placed firmly on the child's face, and halothane concentration reduced to 2–3 per cent until surgical anaesthesia is achieved. It is often helpful to tell the child a story during the induction stage, thus distracting its attention. Older children and adults will usually accept a mask placed directly on the face from the beginning of induction.

The most reliable signs of surgical anaesthesia are regular respiration and loss of muscle tone. The pupils will eventually become central, but it is often unnecessary to reach this plane of anaesthesia for one or two simple extractions. Older children and adults will accept a mouth prop before induction starts, but this is not advisable with younger children. In the latter group, it is better to insert the prop just prior to surgery.

**Intravenous induction.**—Intravenous induction is being increasingly used in out-patient dental anaesthesia, and is the method of choice for older children and adults. It is quick, causes less salivation, reduces the incidence of cardiac dysrhythmias, and results in less atmospheric pollution from anaesthetic gases. The main disadvantages, especially in the hands of part-time anaesthetists, are a higher incidence of associated fainting due to venepuncture, and the potential dangers of rapid injection into the circulation of potent drugs. Transition from intravenous induction to gaseous maintenance, can also prove more difficult than a purely inhalational technique.

Methohexitone is the most common agent for intravenous induction in out-patient dental anaesthesia. Normal induction doses are about 1·5 mg/kg for adults and 2 mg/kg for children. It has proved a safe and reliable drug with good, early recovery, free from nausea and vomiting, and a low incidence of anaphylactoid reactions. Disadvantages are pain on injection, especially when used in small veins on the dorsum of the hand, occasional hiccups, and abnormal muscle movements. Injection pain is a real problem in young children, but can be reduced by the addition of a small amount of intravenous lignocaine to the syringe of methohexitone just before injection. Methohexitone is contra-indicated in epileptic patients.

Thiopentone is less satisfactory in out-patients due to slower initial recovery. However, it is the drug of choice in epileptics, does not produce pain on injection, and may be used if desired.

Other intravenous induction drugs sometimes used are propanidid, Althesin and etomidate. Propanidid produces excellent recovery with little "hangover" but is associated with frequent anaphylactoid reactions; reported frequency varies between 1 in 540 to 1 in 1700 administrations. Althesin may also produce anaphylactoid reactions in 1 in 1000 administrations, but has only been associated with one death, and is probably the best non-barbiturate induction agent for dental anaesthesia. Etomidate causes severe pain on injection, frequent abnormal muscle movements, and is not suitable for out-patient dental anaesthesia.

It is wise to insert the mouth prop before induction, as this may be difficult if there is inadequate relaxation at the end of the injection.

**Maintenance**

Once a plane of surgical anaesthesia is achieved, the mouth pack can be inserted and surgery commenced. Anaesthesia is maintained, via the nose-piece at a light plane which normally requires about 1 per cent halothane.

Airway obstruction is prevented by pulling the mandible upwards and forwards, thus keeping the tongue from occluding the pharynx. Control of mandibular position is best achieved by a hand placed behind the angle. In difficult airways it may be necessary to use both hands.

At the end of surgery the prop is removed, and the pack placed over the sockets leaving the airway clear. The head should be held well forward to prevent blood and debris soiling the pharynx.

Halothane has become the most popular volatile agent for dental anaesthesia. It is non-explosive, non-irritant and produces rapid induction and recovery times with a low incidence of postoperative nausea and vomiting. Recently, enflurane has been suggested as a better volatile agent for outpatient dental anaesthesia as it produces less cardiac dysrhythmias.[16] Its lower blood/gas solubility coefficient should also produce faster induction and recovery times. In practice, enflurane has proved a less satisfactory agent than halothane for out-patient dental anaesthesia. Inhalational induction and satisfactory maintenance has proved difficult to achieve in young children, even using the maximum 5 per cent concentration available on British Enfluratec vaporisers.[17,18] A higher concentration in the 5–10 per cent range may be needed in this age group. This will increase the risks of EEG spiking and neuromuscular excitatory phenomena, especially as hypocarbia due to overventilation may also be present during induction. Recovery times are very similar after such brief anaesthetics, although the faster recovery seen with enflurane may be relevant in longer operations. In summary, halothane, remains the best volatile agent for brief out-patient dental anaesthesia, a view supported by Ryder and Wright.[19]

**Recovery**

Tomlin's[2] investigation of deaths in dental anaesthesia, showed that 30 per cent of all sudden deaths occurred in the recovery period. It is essential to observe the patient closely during recovery until they are awake. Patients anaesthetised on a trolley in the supine position should be turned on their sides with the trolley tipped 15 degrees head-down for recovery. Patients anaesthetised in the dental chair can also be placed on a trolley for recovery, or allowed to wake up in the chair.

A return to street fitness usually takes at least 30 minutes. Patients should be examined to ensure they can stand unsupported, and that all bleeding has stopped. It is imperative that they are escorted home, preferably in a car. They should be given a supply of oral analgesics and written postoperative instructions. These must explain that driving or operating machinery is forbidden for the remainder of the day, and that the consumption of alcohol is unwise. Clear instructions must also be given as to what to do and who to contact if a complication occurs.

There is some evidence to suggest that recovery of skilled movement is better following anaesthesia with inhalational rather than intravenous agents.[20]

### Monitoring

Monitoring of the patient in such brief procedures is difficult and usually kept to a minimum. Observation of the reservoir bag and colour of the patient may be all that is possible in the respiratory system. The high incidence of cardiac dysrhythmias seen with dental anaesthesia make some form of cardiovascular monitoring essential. Muir[21] showed that pulse monitors were unsatisfactory due to vasoconstriction and occasional patient movement. An ECG is the only reliable method to monitor cardiac rhythm and diagnose dysrhythmias. This should be used routinely in dental anaesthesia. The electrodes may be placed after induction in young children, when pre-operative connection may cause undue apprehension.

In longer procedures, a mono-aural precordial stethoscope may be used to monitor breath and heart sounds. Blood pressure can be measured by an oscillotometer or an automated blood-pressure monitor.

### Complications

**Respiratory.**—Airway complications are the most common source of problems during dental anaesthesia. *Airway obstruction* is usually due to the tongue, and can be corrected by manipulation of the mandible upwards and forwards. Incorrect positioning of the mouth prop and pack is a common cause of obstruction. It is important for the dentist and anaesthetist to work as a team and pay particular attention to technique in this area. The use of a second prop placed in position before the first is removed, when moving from one side of the mouth to the other, may be helpful in bilateral extractions. A soft, nasopharyngeal airway may be useful in persistent airway obstruction.

*Mouth breathing* is another common problem which will make it difficult to keep the patient asleep. This may be caused by incorrect positioning of the mouth prop and pack. If adjustment does not improve the situation, a nasopharyngeal airway should be inserted. In persistent cases it may be necessary to deepen anaesthesia intermittently, using a full face mask.

*Apnoea* is either due to breath-holding when anaesthesia is too light, or true respiratory depression when it is too deep. Diagnosis should be obvious and appropriate treatment instituted. In breath-holding it is only necessary to wait, as the patient will usually recommence breathing; however, apnoea due to excessive anaesthetic is a serious complication, and the patient must be ventilated with 100 per cent oxygen using a full face mask until breathing restarts.

*Laryngospasm* is a dangerous complication. It usually presents as crowing or inspiratory stridor. It is due either to surgical stimulation under too light an anaesthetic, or to the presence of secretions or foreign matter such as blood in the larynx. If the anaesthesia is excessively light, it must be deepened before surgical stimulation is re-applied. Large amounts of secretions or blood in the pharynx may need to be cleared by suction. When laryngospasm is present it is important to increase the inspired oxygen concentration, as hypoxia will increase the degree of laryngeal closure. In severe laryngospasm it may be necessary to administer oxygen under positive pressure using a full face mask, or to intubate the larynx. *Bronchospasm* is less common but may be seen in asthmatics or occasionally in normal patients under dental anaesthesia.

*Pulmonary aspiration* may be caused by vomiting or regurgitation of the stomach contents entering the trachea from below, or blood and tooth debris entering it from above. Correct packing should prevent blood and tooth debris entering the pharynx but the challenge to the mouth pack is much greater in the supine position. McCormick[9] found that pharyngeal soiling was more common with the patient flat. Regurgitation is also more likely to occur when the patient is supine, especially if a hiatus hernia is present. Thus, for absolute safety, tracheal intubation is necessary to protect the lungs and ensure a perfect airway when the supine position is used for dental anaesthesia.

**Cardiovascular.** — Although respiratory problems are more common, cardiovascular complications may be lethal, and could explain the sudden deaths that occur in the dental chair. There is marked lability of the cardiovascular system, resulting from autonomic overactivity, in patients who present for dental treatment with a combination of fear and pain. Sympathetic hyperactivity associated with raised plasma adrenaline levels will result in hypertension and tachycardia with pulse rates up to 200 beats per minute.[22] There may also be associated parasympathetic hyperactivity, partially explaining the high incidence of fainting seen in dental patients.[23] Against this background, anaesthesia may cause dramatic changes in the cardiovascular system, with serious consequences.

*Fainting* results from emotional factors, such as fear and anxiety, stimulating areas in the cingulate gyrus of the limbic cortex. This activates anterior hypothalamic centres, which stimulate sympathetic vasodilator fibres, mainly in muscle, causing profound vasodilatation. There is also increased parasympathetic activity originating from the hypothalamus and resulting in bradycardia due to vagal stimulation of the heart. Fainting is therefore an active reflex, resulting in severe hypotension, which may cause unconsciousness due to cerebral ischaemia. In critical situations, the blood supply to the brain is normally improved by the patient falling to a horizontal position, thereby restoring an adequate cerebral circulation. However, under anaesthesia the sitting dental patient may remain erect, with a consequent danger of brain damage and death.

Fainting may occur suddenly, but is often preceded by sweating, pallor, and sometimes complaints of nausea. Treatment consists of placing the patient flat, and giving intravenous atropine if there is associated bradycardia. It is wise to administer oxygen by mask in these circumstances. Adoption of the supine position usually results in a rapid return to consciousness, but Forsyth and associates[8] showed that fainting produces cardiovascular depression, prolonged sometimes in excess of one hour. It is therefore wise to abandon the procedure once fainting has occurred. Although less common, fainting can occur in the supine position, where it may be severe and prolonged.[24]

Fainting is common under local anaesthesia. Hannington-Kiff[25] found that 2 per cent of 3000 consecutive patients presenting for dental treatment had fainting reactions. It is more common in young patients, and likely fainters can be predicted using personality testing.[26] Pre-operative starvation and inexperienced operators will increase the incidence, whilst a tranquil environment, an experienced operator, and the supine position will reduce it.

During general anaesthesia, emotional fainting can only occur during the induction phase, especially in association with venepuncture. Although rare, this must always be anticipated. If fainting occurs on venepuncture, no further induction agent must be given, as this will increase cardiovascular depression with potentially lethal consequences. The patient must be laid flat, treated as necessary, and the procedure abandoned. By definition, fainting cannot occur when the patient is unconscious, and the use of this word to describe all severe hypotension seen during dental anaesthesia has resulted in much confusion. Hypotension and bradycardia occurring under general anaesthesia are due to different mechanisms and should be considered separately.

*Cardiac dysrhythmias*.—There is a high incidence of cardiac dysrhythmias during general anaesthesia for dental surgery.[27,28] When anaesthesia with halothane is used the incidence is about 25 per cent. Of these, three-quarters will show ectopic beats, nodal rhythm accounting for most of the remainder. Bradycardia is rare, occurring in less than 1 per cent of patients.

The final common pathway appears to be the beta effect of catecholamines on the myocardium. Afferent reflexes which elevate myocardial catecholamine levels are trigeminal-nerve stimulation due to extraction,[29] and possibly cervical sympathetic discharge following pharyngeal stimulation. Volatile agents such as halothane will increase the incidence in direct proportion to their ability to sensitise the myocardium to the action of catecholamines.[30,19] These dysrhythmias can be prevented by the prophylactic use of beta blockers.[31–34]

Local anaesthesia, and general anaesthesia using solely intravenous agents, are associated with a very low incidence of dysrhythmias. Intravenous induction will reduce both the incidence and severity of dysrhythmia seen, even if followed by maintenance with halothane. Dental anaesthesia with enflurane produces significantly fewer dysrhythmias than halothane, but is less satisfactory in other respects.[19] The use of atropine doubles the incidence, presumably due to a reduction in parasympathetic tone on the heart.[35] The presence of airway obstruction markedly increases cardiac dysrhythmias, whilst position of the patient makes no difference.

Ectopic rhythms seen in young, fit patients presenting for dental extractions in the chair have not been shown to cause any fall in cardiac output or blood pressure.[36,16] The potential danger is more likely to result from an irritable myocardium developing ventricular fibrillation. It remains possible that these ectopic rhythms are essentially benign in normal patients, but in any patient with unsuspected myocardial disease may prove to be lethal. Tomlin[2] reports two deaths in patients with unsuspected viral myocarditis. Cardiac arrest has also occurred in a patient with undiagnosed cardiomyopathy during dental anaesthesia.

Although significance of these cardiac dysrhythmias is still debatable, the ECG should be monitored. If an ectopic rhythm develops, surgical stimulation should be stopped, and the airway checked to ensure that no obstruction or hypoxia is present. This often results in spontaneous resolution of the ectopic rhythm. However, if the ectopic beats persist, an intravenous dose of lignocaine 1–2 mg/kg, or a small dose of an appropriate beta blocker will restore normal rhythm and prevent a recurrence. Although effective, prophylactic beta blockade is not recommended for routine use.

*Hypotension*.—The normal cardiovascular response to general anaesthesia for dental extractions is a small fall in blood pressure after induction, followed by a rise in blood pressure and heart rate during surgery.[36,37] This hypertensive response is seen in both supine and erect positions. Indeed, Forsyth and colleagues[8] and McCormick[9] could not show any significant differences in heart rate and blood pressure during dental anaesthesia in four different postures, ranging from the erect to fully supine.

In a few patients hypotension may occur. This is often accompanied by bradycardia and has been loosely termed as "fainting". Bradycardia occurring during surgery is not due to fainting, and probably results from direct trigeminal stimulation following extraction. Pain pathways in the trigeminal nerve travel in a long descending and ascending tract through the medulla. Painful stimuli may activate vagal neurones through radiating fibres, causing bradycardia. Severe bradycardia may cause hypotension, especially if nodal rhythm develops. The effects of hypotension will be more marked in the erect position. However, ECG monitoring can quickly diagnose this abnormality, which is easily reversed by intravenous atropine.

The whole subject of cardiovascular changes occurring during dental anaesthesia has recently been comprehensively reviewed by Thurlow.[38]

## ANALGESIA AND SEDATION FOR CONSERVATIVE DENTISTRY

It has been estimated that up to 50 per cent of patients in Western countries do not attend for regular dental treatment due to fear. This has led to a proliferation of techniques aimed at producing sedation and analgesia, thus making dentistry more acceptable to these patients.

### General Principles

It is important to understand the pharmacology of the drugs used and to choose an appropriate drug for a desired effect. Drugs used can be classified into three main groups: anxiolytics, sedatives and analgesics. Drugs should not be used to produce effects they do not possess. For example, subanaesthetic doses of barbiturates are not analgesic; in fact they probably *lower* pain threshold. The use of incremental methohexitone to obtain analgesia will only succeed when the drug is given in sufficient amount to produce full general anaesthesia.

When selecting a technique for controlled sedation, certain criteria should be fulfilled. The drug should produce reliable sedation without loss of consciousness. Verbal contact must be maintained at all times between dentist and patient. The surgical conditions must be satisfactory without gagging or involuntary muscle movements. There must be minimal cardiovascular and respiratory depression, with a rapid recovery to street fitness. Amnesia is helpful, but the drug must cause no serious side-effects. It should have a wide safety margin, making unintended loss of consciousness unlikely.

Other factors are important in the practical management of these patients. A supportive and sympathetic patient manner combined with expert technique in local blockade are essential. Drugs cannot compensate for poor patient management and inadequate local analgesia. The fitness of the patient must be assessed, as for general anaesthesia, especially when powerful intravenous drugs will be used. Prolonged preoperative starvation will make hypoglycaemia and fainting more common. Patients should be allowed food up to three hours, and fluids up to two hours, before the procedure. An escort should be available to accompany the patient home, especially when intravenous sedation is used. Controlled sedation, properly given, should not compromise the patient's airway, and treatment is best performed in the reclining position using the modern contoured dental chair.

### Oral Sedation

Anxiolytics, such as diazepam, may be used orally, commencing on the day before treatment. A dose of 2–5 mg three times a day is sufficient. Occasionally, this proves adequate to overcome the patient's fear, and allow dental treatment without further supplementation.

### Intramuscular Sedation

This route is not recommended as it is impossible to titrate the dosage of drugs used and produce reliable sedation. Subsequently, this route of administration will produce prolonged recovery. Occasionally it is the only alternative in difficult young children and mentally handicapped patients. However, these two groups will often require full general anaesthesia for dental treatment. Drugs used intramuscularly are ketamine and the normal range of premedication agents.

### Intravenous Sedation

This is the preferred route for controlled sedation as it is possible to titrate the drug precisely against effect.

**Jorgensen technique.**—This is one of the original and best known methods of intravenous sedation, introduced by Jorgensen at Loma Linda University, California in 1945. Pentobarbitone in 10 mg doses is injected every 30 seconds until the patient is relaxed and lightly sedated. This is then supplemented by a mixture of pethidine 25 mg and hyoscine 0·32 mg diluted in 5 ml, to obtain optimum conditions. Local blockade is performed, and dental treatment carried out.

This technique, although relatively safe, requires long induction and recovery times. Patients are very drowsy and have prolonged "hangover" effects. Since its introduction, variations on the original Jorgensen technique have been tried, using a wide variety of sedative and analgesic drugs. Many of these combinations can be dangerous in inexperienced hands and generally their use should be discouraged.

**Diazepam.**—This drug was first used in 1968. It is a very effective anxiolytic, and produces good amnesia for about 30 minutes. It is a mild sedative and is the most popular and effective drug for intravenous controlled sedation at the present time.

A suggested method of administration is to inject 2·5–5 mg every 30 seconds until satisfactory sedation is achieved. Drooping of the upper eyelid over the pupil, sometimes known as Verrill's sign, is a useful end-point. Average intravenous dose is 0·2 mg/kg, with a normal range of 10–20 mg in adults. Total dose should not exceed 0·3 mg/kg due to the dangers of respiratory depression. Failure to achieve adequate conditions at this dose may require alternative techniques in a small minority of patients. Diazepam has no analgesic effect and local blockade should be given as soon as sedation is achieved.

Diazepam in a dose of 0·2 mg/kg produces minimal effects on the cardiovascular system, apart from a transient tachycardia.[39,40] It is a potent respiratory depressant when given intravenously, and must be injected slowly, titrating dose against effect. Protective laryngeal reflexes may be impaired for the first few minutes after intravenous administration, and surgery should not commence for at least five minutes.[39]

The least satisfactory aspect of diazepam sedation is slow recovery. Return to street fitness will take at least one hour. There may also be a recurrence of drowsiness 6–8 hours postoperatively, due to the reappearance of diazepam and its active metabolite desmethyl-diazepine in the bloodstream.[41,42] It is therefore essential that the patient is accompanied home, and does not drive a car or operate machinery for at least 12–24 hours.[43]

Care must be taken not to inject the drug into an artery, where it may produce thrombosis and gangrene. Standard diazepam also causes frequent pain on injection, and subsequent thrombophlebitis, due to the propylene glycol solvent used. Several suggestions have been made to avoid this problem including using large veins, diluting the drug with saline or the patient's own blood prior to injection, and the addition of Cremophor. Current work suggests that the solution of diazepam in oil (Diazemuls) avoids the problem of pain and thrombophlebitis, and is the preparation of choice for dentistry.[44]

Although diazepam is an excellent drug for controlled sedation, adequate conditions cannot be achieved in a few patients. Some operators supplement diazepam with analgesics, such as pentazocine and fentanyl, in this group. This may result in severe respiratory depression, and should only be used if the operator has the skills and equipment to ventilate an apnoeic patient.

Prolonged recovery remains the main problem with diazepam sedation. Newer benzodiazepines with shorter recovery times, such as midazolam, are at present under investigation. Specific benzodiazepine antagonists may also be available in the near future.

**Incremental methohexitone.**—This technique introduced by Drummond-Jackson in 1962, claimed to produce a state of "ultralight" anaesthesia, with a lack of response to painful stimuli, and amnesia, but stopping short of full surgical anaesthesia with its attendant dangers. This supposition would seem unlikely, knowing barbiturate pharmacology.

Thorough investigation by two research teams showed that adequate conditions were only achieved by producing full surgical anaesthesia.[45,46] This caused respiratory problems such as airway obstruction and loss of protective laryngeal reflexes. During long procedures the circulatory system was compromised and could not respond to further insults such as hypoxia. Patients were placed at risk from hypotension and hypertension.

The use of this drug to produce controlled sedation is dangerous, especially when given by the single-handed operator-anaesthetist and should be discouraged.

### Inhalational

Klock in the United States of America and Tom in the United Kingdom originally suggested the use of nitrous oxide to provide "amnalgesia" 30 years ago. More recently, Langa[47] has popularised the use of nitrous oxide to produce sedation, analgesia and amnesia, a state commonly termed "relative analgesia". Nitrous oxide is given via a nose-piece in increasing concentrations starting at 10 per cent and working up to a maximum of 50 per cent to achieve the desired effects. In most patients it is unnecessary to exceed 30 per cent. This technique is safe, produces quick recovery, and is becoming increasingly popular. The subject has been well reviewed recently by Roberts.[48]

### Other Techniques

Hypnosis and acupuncture are sometimes used in dentistry. They certainly have a place in the control of pain and anxiety, but need specialised training to use, and are only effective in a limited proportion of patients.

Occasionally, it is impossible to produce adequate surgical conditions with controlled sedation. This may occur in very young children, the mentally or physically handicapped, and a small proportion of phobic adults. In these cases, general anaesthesia will be necessary. It is probably safest to intubate these patients, although in shorter procedures it may be possible to use a nasopharyngeal airway and careful packing.

## ANAESTHESIA FOR MINOR ORAL SURGERY

Minor oral surgery consists of complicated dental extractions such as impacted wisdom teeth, simple cysts, and other small procedures in the mouth. These are short operations taking

20–40 minutes on average, and rarely exceeding 60 minutes. It has been estimated that 25 per cent of medical costs could be saved by performing minor oral surgery on a day-stay out-patient basis. Many patients, especially children, prefer not to be admitted to hospital. These two facts suggest that minor oral surgery is best performed on a day-stay basis whenever possible.

### Day-Stay Surgery

Strict criteria must be used when selecting patients for day-stay surgery. Patients should be between the ages of 2 and 60 years, the extremes of age being avoided. They must be essentially fit, and free from serious cardiovascular or respiratory disease, falling into ASA 1 or 2 categories. The surgery must by straightforward and should not exceed one hour. Social conditions at home must be adequate for postoperative care. Ideally, the patient should not have to travel too far, and should be driven home. A responsible escort must accompany him, and be able to look after him at home for at least 24 hours.

Ideally, day-stay surgery is best performed in custom-built day-stay units or "surgicenters". These provide proper admission and assessment areas, together with good facilities for immediate and long-term recovery. Patients can fill in an anaesthetic questionnaire, and certain basic investigations such as haemoglobin estimation and urine analysis can be performed at the initial booking visit. This acts as a screening procedure and provided it is satisfactory, physical examination can be deferred until the patient arrives for surgery. It is best to operate in the morning, as this allows full time for recovery and reduces the period of pre-operative starvation for the patient. Premedication is best avoided as sedative drugs will delay recovery.

Anaesthetic technique is extremely important in day-stay surgery, as it is vital that postoperative morbidity is reduced to a minimum in ambulant patients returning home. Most of these patients will require tracheal intubation, although a few can sometimes be managed with nasopharyngeal airways and careful packing. Nasal endotracheal tubes are used. Bevel design makes introduction through the right nostril easier in most patients. Tubes may be plain uncuffed, or with a streamlined cuff. Choice will depend on the amount of bleeding expected and whether spontaneous or controlled ventilation is used. Tubes should be well lubricated before insertion. Plastic tubes are harder than rubber, and more likely to traumatise the nasal mucosa, causing excessive bleeding. Red rubber tubes also have a better preformed curve, allowing for easier insertion. It is usually necessary to select a nasal tube about 1·0 mm smaller in diameter than the appropriate oral tube for any particular patient.

If the trachea is intubated, the patient can be placed either fully supine or semi-reclining in the dental chair, depending on surgical preference. The semi-reclining position allows good visualisation of the larynx and presents no problems for intubation. When the supine position is adopted a trolley can be used, thus allowing the patient to recover without being moved.

After positioning the patient, the blood pressure should be checked, and an indwelling needle or cannula inserted. Induction is usually with intravenous agents except in young children. Methohexitone is a safe and popular induction agent for out-patients. Although Althesin and propanidid produce less "hangover" and better long-term recovery, the higher incidence of anaphylactoid reactions with these drugs makes them more dangerous in day-stay units. Intubation can be most easily performed following muscle relaxation with suxamethonium. However, the frequency of postoperative muscle pains in ambulant patients and the occasional prolonged apnoea following this drug make it a less than ideal agent for day-stay units. Alternatives to suxamethonium are intubation under deep spontaneous breathing often using the "blind nasal" technique, or intubation with non-depolarising muscle relaxants if a controlled ventilation technique is to be used. When suxamethonium is given, the severity of muscle pains can be reduced by prior administration of a small dose of a non-depolarising muscle relaxant. Following intubation, it is essential to pack the pharynx, using either moistened gauze or a preformed throat pack. The eyes must be protected and all connections secured, as the face is firmly wrapped in sterile drapes.

Anaesthesia is usually maintained by a volatile agent such as halothane or enflurane with the patient breathing spontaneously. Alternatively, a short-acting narcotic such as fentanyl may be given, or volatile agents given with controlled ventilation. Thomas and associates[49] compared spontaneous ventilation using nitrous oxide, oxygen and halothane with a controlled ventilation technique using nitrous oxide, oxygen, tubocurarine and fentanyl. They recommended the controlled-ventilation technique as providing more rapid recovery, avoidance of suxamethonium and halothane, and abolition of cardiac dysrhythmias. Subsequent work showed that although initial recovery was better following controlled ventilation with fentanyl, this group of patients felt less well on discharge and at home.[6] It is possible that narcotics and muscle relaxants produce more postoperative morbidity in ambulant patients than do volatile agents which are more rapidly eliminated. Other studies have shown a surprisingly high incidence of postoperative minor morbidity in day-stay patients undergoing minor oral surgery.[5] In an attempt to investigate anaesthetic causes of minor morbidity following out-patient anaesthesia, Fahy and Marshall[50] showed that length of operation was the only factor which significantly affected the occurrence and severity of symptoms. Thus, choice of anaesthetic agents remains a personal preference, and an ideal technique has yet to be evolved.

The cardiovascular system is very labile during minor oral surgery, and the ECG and blood pressure should be monitored. A precordial stethoscope is a useful, non-invasive monitor.

When surgery has finished, the throat pack should be removed under direct vision, and the pharynx suctioned. The endotracheal tube is best removed with the patient turned on his side. Due to the possibility of blood in the mouth and a compromised airway, it is safest to allow the patient to wake up before extubating the larynx.

Following immediate recovery the patient should remain for at least 2 to 3 hours to ensure that all bleeding has stopped, and that he is fit to return home. Several tests of street fitness have been devised. One of the easiest and most reliable is the ability of the patient to walk along a straight line without staggering or swaying.[51] On discharge, it is essential to give the patient a written set of postoperative instructions, a plentiful supply of analgesics, and to ensure they are escorted home, preferably in a car.

### In-Patient Surgery

When more extensive surgery is required, or the patient's medical or social condition contraindicates out-patient treatment, he should be admitted to hospital.

Pre-operative assessment and premedication are similar to any routine general anaesthetic. Likewise, anaesthetic technique will follow the principles already discussed for day-stay surgery. However, drugs do not have to be selected with immediate recovery and early ambulation as a necessity.

Special problems include patients presenting for dental clearance prior to cardiac surgery, and also haemophiliacs. Cardiac patients for dental clearance may have poor cardiovascular function and should be anaesthetised by doctors skilled in cardiac anaesthesia, with full antibiotic cover. Patients with haemophilia or other bleeding diatheses will need full pre-operative preparation by a haematologist. Intramuscular injections should be avoided, and it is safer to use oral endotracheal tubes, as the nasal route can produce severe haemorrhage.

## ANAESTHESIA FOR MAJOR ORAL AND MAXILLO-FACIAL SURGERY

Operations can be divided into elective and emergency procedures. Moore[52] divided elective operations into three main categories.

*Corrective operations* of the jaws such as mandibular and maxillary osteotomies, and building up procedures which may include the use of bone grafts.

*Removal of tumours* of the mandible and maxilla, ranging from the enucleation of the simple cysts to the removal of extensive jaw carcinoma which may involve excision of adjacent soft tissues.

*Operations on the tongue* and floor of the mouth.

Emergency operations follow trauma to the facial skeleton, and vary from simple fractures of the nasal bones to complicated bony injuries with associated soft-tissue damage.

### Elective Surgery

### Normal Airway

Anaesthetic management in patients with a

normal airway causing no intubation problems is similar to that for routine general anaesthesia, with specific attention to a few important points.

Normal premedication may be given after a full pre-operative assessment. Endotracheal intubation is essential and the choice between oral and nasal tubes depends upon the site of surgical intervention. In general a nasal tube provides better surgical access for all intra-oral procedures whereas an oral tube is more suitable for surgery on the remainder of the face. Nasal tubes should have a streamlined cuff. Oral tubes must be non-kinkable and armoured as they may be considerably distorted. Although cuffed endotracheal tubes are always used, it is important to insert a pharyngeal pack in addition. This prevents blood and foreign material from entering the stomach, where it may cause postoperative vomiting. It also prevents blood and debris settling above the cuff in the larynx, and possibly entering the lungs on cuff deflation at the end of operation.

Maintenance of anaesthesia can be with volatile agents or narcotics, using either controlled or spontaneous ventilation. Final choice depends upon length of operation and personal preference, but it is essential to select a technique which allows smooth and rapid recovery with an absence of vomiting. Neuroleptanalgesia using droperidol and fentanyl or controlled ventilation with a volatile supplement have both proved satisfactory. Blood loss may be heavy, and induced hypotension is often used in these cases. Patients undergoing reconstructive surgery may have several operations requiring multiple anaesthetics. Both these factors will affect final choice of anaesthetic technique.

Extubation, especially if airway problems are anticipated, is best performed with the patient awake in the lateral position. A nasopharyngeal airway may be left in place for easy suctioning of the pharynx. Patients are best nursed in an intensive therapy unit for the first 24 to 48 hours, especially if the jaws are wired together, and wire cutters should be immediately available.

### The Difficult Intubation

Many patients will have abnormal anatomy and present considerable problems for intubation. Certain crucial points must be borne in mind with these patients.

The majority of difficult intubations are predictable. Factors which will make visualisation of the larynx difficult include limited mouth opening, prominent upper teeth, a high arched palate, a receding mandible and a short immobile neck. Careful pre-operative assessment, with radiographs if necessary, is vital in predicting potential problems.[53]

A previous easy intubation does not guarantee an absence of problems. For example, following hemimandibulectomy and radiotherapy, intubation may become increasingly difficult.[54]

Certain tumours, especially of the larynx, do not compromise the airway when the patient is awake, but may cause obstruction when muscle tone is lost under anaesthesia.

The patient must never be paralysed before it has been established that controlled ventilation is possible with a face mask.

Where difficulty is anticipated, a variety of laryngoscopes, endotracheal tubes, bougies and bronchoscopes should be available.

Facilities for emergency tracheostomy or cricothyrotomy must be present.

**Awake intubation with local anaesthesia.**—This is the safest technique, and is the method of choice in serious airway problems. Premedication consists of an antisialogogue, with an anxiolytic if necessary. Opiates and respiratory depressants should be avoided in patients with potential airway problems. The nasal route is preferable whenever surgically possible. The nasal mucosa is first anaesthetised using cocaine. The nose may be prepacked with ribbon gauze, sprayed or, alternatively, cotton buds dipped in 10 per cent cocaine solution, or 25 per cent cocaine paste can be directly inserted into the nasal cavity. When it is necessary to use the oral route, the tongue and oral cavity are anaesthetised using a lignocaine spray, viscous gel or lozenge. This allows a laryngoscope blade to be gently introduced, following which the remainder of the larynx and glottis can be sprayed. Alternatively, the larynx above the vocal cords can be anaesthetised by bilateral superior laryngeal nerve blocks. If desired, the area below the vocal cords can be anaesthetised by direct instillation of 2 ml of lignocaine through a cricothyroid membrane puncture.

Good topical anaesthesia will allow a well-lubricated nasal endotracheal tube to be passed blindly into the larnyx, the patients virtually inhaling their own tube. The oral route is more difficult and requires laryngoscopy with some manipulation of the oral armoured tube.

The introduction of the fibre-optic bronchoscope has greatly simplified awake intubation. It is easier to visualise the larynx with this instrument when the patient is awake, as normal muscle tone prevents the tongue falling backwards and obscuring the view. The patient should be positioned sitting up at 45°, which also helps to keep the tongue away from the pharynx. After anaesthetising the nasal mucosa, a well-lubricated nasal tube is passed gently into the pharynx. The tube must have an internal diameter of at least 7 mm to accept introduction of the fibre-optic bronchoscope. The bronchoscope is then passed through the nasal tube into the pharynx. The bronchoscope can now be advanced under direct vision into the larynx, anaesthetising the airway in advance by instillation of lignocaine through the side arm. The nasal endotracheal tube can now be advanced over the bronchoscope, which is used as a bougie. The bronchoscope is withdrawn and, immediately correct endotracheal tube placement is confirmed, general anaesthesia can be induced with an intravenous agent.

The oral route is more difficult as the anterior angulation, sometimes necessary to enter the larynx, can be difficult to achieve with the fibre-optic instrument. However, if surgically necessary, this route is adopted, using an oral armoured tube in the same manner as previously described.

**General anaesthesia.**—Children will not co-operate sufficiently for awake intubation, and present-day fibre-optic bronchoscopes can only pass through endotracheal tubes of at least 7 mm internal diameter. General anaesthesia is therefore used in children, and is often employed when airway problems are mild in adults.

Premedication should again consist of an antisialogogue. An anxiolytic may be given if necessary, but opiates and powerful respiratory depressants must be avoided.

*Nasal intubation.*—Intubation is often only possible using a blind technique in these patients. The head should be placed on one pillow producing mild flexion of the cervical spine. Slight extension of the atlanto-occipital joint results in a "sniffing the morning air" position. It is advisable to use a cocaine nasal pack pre-operatively, which will shrink the nasal mucosa and make passage of the tube easier. When severe airway problems exist it is safer to use an inhalational induction. The addition of 5–10 per cent carbon dioxide will produce overbreathing and aid the procedure.

A well-lubricated nasal endotracheal tube can now be passed, rotating the tube as necessary to enter the pharynx. An immediate attempt can be made to pass the tube into the larynx. Alternatively, the endotracheal tube may be reconnected to the breathing circuit, allowing anaesthesia to be maintained or deepened. The tube can then be manipulated directly above the glottal opening by watching the respiratory excursion in the reservoir bag. Elevation of the lower jaw will lift the epiglottis away from the posterior pharyngeal wall. By listening to breath sounds the tube can then be guided towards the larynx and inserted with a final quick movement. In difficult cases the position of the larynx can be manipulated by external pressure, and it may also be necessary to increase flexion or laterally rotate the head.

*Oral intubation.*—Again a purely inhalational technique is safest using spontaneous ventilation to produce deep anaesthesia. Laryngoscopy is then carried out and the problem assessed. If the larynx is visible, intubation can proceed either under deep spontaneous ventilation or following a short-acting muscle relaxant. If only the posterior portions of the arytenoid cartilages are visible, intubation may be possible using a gum elastic bougie or stilette threaded through the endotracheal tube.

When no portion of the glottal opening is visible, it may still be possible to intubate by probing blindly behind the epiglottis with a stiff gum elastic bougie threaded through the endotracheal tube. If this is unsuccessful, visualisation of the larynx may be achieved by a rigid or fibre-optic bronchoscope, or the Huffman prism.[55] A new blade has been described which will allow blind oral passage of an endotracheal tube into the larynx.[56] If none of these techniques is successful, the nasal route should be tried.

In severe cases, or when attempts at intubation have failed, it will be necessary to perform a pre-operative tracheostomy under local anaesthesia. In emergencies it is possible to maintain oxygenation by cricothyroid puncture with a

14 gauge cannula. Ventilation can also be achieved through this cannula using a high-frequency positive pressure ventilator.

## Emergency Surgery

Major trauma may cause multiple injuries. First priority must be given to the establishment of a clear airway and restoration of an adequate circulation. Associated injuries to the head, chest and abdomen may require treatment before correction of maxillofacial damage.

In severe cases an obstructed airway is frequently present due to blood, teeth and bone fragments lying in the pharynx. There may be active bleeding in the pharynx, and the stomach will contain blood and food. The pharynx may be cleared gently using a finger, but pre-operative passage of a wide-bore stomach tube is often impossible.

If the mouth can be opened sufficiently, intubation is best achieved by a "crash induction" technique, using pre-oxygenation, followed by an intravenous induction agent and suxamethonium with cricoid pressure. Topical anaesthesia is not usually effective, due to active bleeding. Inhalation induction is difficult to achieve as a face mask cannot readily be applied. In extreme cases, where the mouth cannot be opened, preliminary tracheostomy under local anaesthesia may have to be performed.

Once a cuffed endotracheal tube is in place and the airway has been secured, all blood and debris can be removed from the pharynx. A wide-bore oesophageal tube can now be passed to empty the stomach. In most cases an oral endotracheal tube will be used, but occasionally, the nature of the injuries makes a nasal tube the better choice. When a cerebrospinal fluid leak is present, or there is a fracture at the base of the skull, it is thought advisable to avoid nasal tubes as they may cause meningitis. Maintenance of anaesthesia is similar to that described for elective operations, with a rapid and smooth recovery mandatory.

Postoperative management should be in an intensive therapy unit. Patients with immobilised jaws will need special attention. Sedation must be kept to a minimum and analgesic drugs only given on demand.

## REFERENCES


1. Bourne, J. G. (1970). Deaths with dental anaesthetics. *Anaesthesia*, **25**, 473.
2. Tomlin, P. J. (1974). Death in outpatient dental practice. *Anaesthesia*, **29**, 551.
3. Coplans, M.P. and Curson, I. (1982). Deaths associated with dentistry. *Brit. dent. J.*, **153**, 357.
4. Muir, V. M. J., Leonard, M. and Haddaway, E. (1976). Morbidity after dental extraction: a comparative survey. *Anesthesia*, **31**, 171.
5. Smith, B. L. and Young, P. N. (1976). Day stay anaesthesia. A follow up of day patients undergoing dental operations under general anaesthesia with endotracheal intubation. *Anaesthesia*, **31**, 181.
6. Heneghan, C., MacAuliffe, R., Thomas, D. and Radford, P. (1981). Morbidity after outpatient anaesthesia. A comparison of two techniques of endotracheal anaesthesia for dental surgery. *Anaesthesia*, **36**, 4.
7. Bourne, J. G. (1957). Fainting and cerebral damage. *Lancet*, **2**, 499.
8. Forsyth, W. D., Allen, G. D. and Everett, G. B. (1972). An evaluation of cardiorespiratory effects of posture in the dental outpatient. *Oral Surg.*, **34**, 77.
9. McCormick. *see* Thurlow, A. C. (1981). The postural evolution. *Anaesthesia*, **36**, 565.
10. Nainby-Luxmore, R. C. (1967). Some hazards of dental gas machines. *Anaesthesia*, **22**, 545.
11. Hutchinson, R. I. (1975). The accuracy and efficiency of general anaesthetic machines in dental practice. *Brit. dent. J.*, **138**, 187.
12. Whitcher, C. E., Zimmerman, D. C., Tonn, E. M. and Piziali, R. L. (1977). Control of occupational exposure to nitrous oxide in the dental operatory. *J. Amer. dent. Assoc.*, **95**, 763.
13. Coplans, M. P. and Barton, P. R. (1964). Nasal breathing and the dental pack. *Brit. dent. J.*, **116**, 209.
14. Perks, E. R. (1977). The diagnosis and management of sudden collapse in dental practice. *Brit. dent. J.*, **143**, 196.
15. Meyer, R. (1970). Pre-operative laboratory screening before administration of general anaesthesia in the office. *J. Oral Surg.*, **28**, 332.
16. Wright, C. J. (1980). Dysrhythmias during oral surgery. A comparison of halothane and enflurane anaesthesia. *Anaesthesia*, **35**, 775.
17. Black, G. W., Johnston, M. M. L. and Scott, M. G. (1977). Clinical impressions of Enflurane. *Brit. J. Anaesth.*, **49**, 975.
18. Farnsworth, G. (1981). Dysrhythmias during oral surgery. *Anaesthesia*, **36**, 77.
19. Ryder, W. and Wright, P. A. (1981). Halothane and enflurane in dental anaesthesia. *Anaesthesia*, **36**, 492.
20. Korttila, K., Tammisto, T., Ertama, P., Pfaffli, P., Blomgren, E. and Hakkinen, S. (1977). Recovery, psy-

chomotor skills, and simulated driving after brief inhalational anesthesia with halothane or enflurane combined with nitrous oxide and oxygen. *Anesthesiology*, **46**, 20.
21. Muir, V. M. J. (1973). Pulse monitors in outpatient dental anaesthesia. *Anaesthesia*, **28**, 312.
22. Edmondson, H. D., Roscoe, B. and Vickers, M. D. (1972). Biochemical evidence of anxiety in dental patients. *Brit. med. J.*, **4**, 7.
23. Taggart, P., Hedworth-Whitty, R., Carruthers, M. and Gordon, P. D. (1976). Observations on electrocardiogram and plasma catecholamines during dental procedures: the forgotten vagus. *Brit. med. J.*, **2**, 787.
24. Verrill, P. J. and Aellig, W. H. (1970). Vasovagal faint in the supine position. *Brit. med, J.*, **4**, 348.
25. Hannington-Kiff, J. G. (1969). Fainting and collapse in dental practice. *Dent. Practit. (dent. Rec.)*, **20**, 2.
26. Ruetz, P. P., Johnson, S. A., Callahan, R., Meade, R. C. and Smith, J. J. (1967). Fainting. A review of its mechanisms and a study in blood donors. *Medicine (Baltimore)*, **46**, 363.
27. Ryder, W. and Townsend, D. (1974). Cardiac rhythm in dental anaesthesia: a comparison of five anaesthetic techniques. *Brit. J. Anaesth.*, **46**, 760.
28. Gotta, A. W., Sullivan, C. A., Pelkofski, J., Kangwalklai, S. R. and Kozam, R. (1976). Aberrant conduction as a precursor to cardiac arrhythmias during anaesthesia for oral surgery. *J. Oral Surg.*, **34**, 421.
29. Plowman, P. E., Thomas, W. J. W. and Thurlow, A. C. (1974). Cardiac dysrhythmias during anaesthesia for oral surgery. The effect of local blockade. *Anaesthesia*, **29**, 571.
30. Reisner, L. S. and Lippmann, M. (1975). Ventricular arrhythmias after epinephrine injection in enflurane and in halothane anesthesia. *Anesth. Analg. Curr. Res.*, **54**, 468.
31. Tolas, A. G. and Allen, G. D. (1970). Propranolol in prevention of cardiac arrhythmias. *J. Oral Surg.*, **28**, 181.
32. Rollason, W. N. and Hall, D. J. (1973). Dysrhythmias during inhalational anaesthesia for oral surgery: incidence and prevention and treatment with practolol. *Anaesthesia*, **28**, 139.
33. Ryder, W., Charlton, J. E. and Gorman, P. B. W. (1973). Oral atropine and practolol premedication in dental anaesthesia. *Brit. J. Anaesth.*, **45**, 745.
34. Whitehead, M. H., Whitmarsh, V. B. and Horton, J. N. (1980). Metoprolol in anaesthesia for oral surgery. The effect of pre-treatment on incidence in cardiac dysrhythmias. *Anaesthesia*, **35**, 779.
35. Thurlow, A. C. (1972). Cardiac dysrhythmias in outpatient dental anaesthesia in children. The effect of prophylactic intravenous atropine. *Anaesthesia*, **27**, 429.
36. Allen, G. D., Ward, R. J., Tolas, A. and Danziger, F. (1965). Cardiovascular responses during general anaesthesia on dental outpatients. *J. Oral Therap. Pharmacol.*, **1**, 602.
37. Al-Khishali, T., Padfield, A., Perks, E. R. and Thornton, J. A. (1978). Cardiorespiratory effects of nitrous oxide, oxygen halothane anaesthesia administered to dental patients in the upright posture. *Anaesthesia*, **33**, 184.
38. Thurlow, A. C. (1983). Cardiovascular effects. In *Anaesthesia and Sedation in Dentistry*. Edited by M. P. Coplans and R. A. Green. Amsterdam: Elsevier/North Holland Biomedical Press.
39. Healy, T. E. J., Robinson, J. S. and Vickers, M. D. (1970). Physiological responses to intravenous diazepam as a sedative for conservative dentistry. *Brit. med. J.*, **3**, 10.
40. Allen, G. D., Everett, G. B. and Butler, L. A. (1976). Human cardiorespiratory and analgesic effects of intravenous diazepam and local anaesthesia. *J. Amer. dent. Assoc.*, **92**, 744.
41. Baird, E. S. and Hailey, D. M. (1972). Delayed recovery from a sedative: correlation of the plasma levels of diazepam with clinical effects after oral and intravenous administration. *Brit. J. Anaesth.*, **44**, 803.
42. Ghonheim, M. M., Mewlad, T. S. P. and Ambre, J. (1975). Plasma levels of diazepam and mood ratings. *Anesth. Analg. Curr. Res.*, **54**, 173.
43. Dixon, R. A. and Thornton, J. A. (1973). Tests of recovery from anaesthesia and sedation; intravenous diazepam in dentistry. *Brit. J. Anaesth.*, **45**, 207.
44. Jensen, S., Huttel, M. S. and Olesen, A. S. (1981). Venous complications after i.v. administration of Diazemuls (diazepam) and Dormicum (midazolam). *Brit. J. Anaesth.*, **53**, 1083.
45. Wise, C. C., Robinson, J. S., Heath, M. J. and Tomlin, P. J. (1969). Physiological responses to intermittent methohexitone for conservative dentistry. *Brit. med. J.*, **2**, 540.
46. Mann, P. E., Hatt, S. D., Dixon, R., Griffin, K. D. Perks, E. R. and Thornton, J. A. (1971). A minimal increment methohexitone technique in conservative dentistry. *Anaesthesia*, **26**, 3.
47. Langa, J. (1976). *Relative Analgesia in Dental Practice*. 2nd edit. Philadelphia: W. B. Saunders Co.
48. Roberts, G. J. R. (1983). Relative analgesia in clinical practice. In *Anaesthesia and Sedation in Dentistry*. Edited by M. P. Coplans and R. A. Green. Amsterdam: Elsevier/North Holland Biomedical Press.
49. Thomas, V. J. E., Thomas, W. J. W. and Thurlow, A. C. (1976). Cardiac arrhythmia during outpatient dental anaesthesia. A comparison of controlled ventilation with and without halothane. *Brit. J. Anaesth.*, **48**, 919.
50. Fahy, A. and Marshall, M. (1969). Postanaesthetic morbidity in outpatients. *Brit. J. Anaesth.*, **41**, 433.
51. Korttila, K. (1976). Recovery after intravenous sedation. *Anaesthesia*, **31**, 724.
52. Moore, P. (1973). Anaesthesia in maxillo-facial surgery. In *Anaesthesia and Analgesia in Dentistry*. Edited by R. A. Green and M. P. Coplans, London: H. K. Lewis.
53. White, A. and Kander, P. L. (1975). Anatomical factors in difficult direct laryngoscopy. *Brit. J. Anaesth.*, **47**, 468.
54. Berwick, E. P. (1983). Anaesthesia for facio-maxillary surgery. In *Anaesthesia and Sedation in Dentistry*. Edited by M. P. Coplans and R. A. Green, Amsterdam: Elsevier/North Holland Biomedical Press.
55. Huffman, J. P. and Elam, J. O. (1971). Prisms and fibreoptics for laryngoscopy. *Anesth. Analg. Curr. Res.*, **50**, 64.
56. Liban, J. B. and Liban, S. R. (1977). A new blade for blind endotracheal intubation. *Brit. J. Anaesth.*, **49**, 1279.
57. Green, R. A. and Coplans, M. P. (1973). (Eds.) *Anaesthesia and Analgesia in Dentistry*. London: H. K. Lewis.

## FURTHER READING

*Anaesthesia and Analgesia in Dentistry*. (1973). Edited by R. A. Green and M. P. Coplans. London: H. K. Lewis.

*Dental Anesthesia and Analgesia (Local and General)* (1979). 2nd edit. G. D. Allen. Baltimore: Williams and Wilkins.

*Anaesthesia and Sedation in Dentistry*. (1983). Edited by M. P. Coplans and R. A. Green. Amsterdam: Elsevier/North Holland Biomedical Press.

*General Anaesthesia for Dental Surgery*. (1971). Edited by A. R. Hunter and G. H. Bush. Altrincham: J. S. Sherratt.

Thurlow, A. C. (1983). Outpatient anaesthesia; Current concepts. In: *Inhalation Anaesthesiology* (Clinics in Anaesthesiology Vol. 1, No. 2), Ed. R. I. Mazze. London: W. B. Saunders.

CHAPTER 44

# Anaesthesia for Special Situations



## PRE-OPERATIVE PREPARATION AND PREMEDICATION

This account is not intended as a guide to pre-existing conditions which interfere with the conduct of anaesthesia but rather as an outline of the aims of a pre-operative visit.

Since patients are often presented for surgery with a condition that is also the cause for surgery, it is difficult or impossible to be dogmatic regarding the suitability of patients for anaesthesia. For instance, patients in renal failure are frequently presented with circulatory haemoglobin levels of 7 g per cent or less, whereas a patient for hysterectomy with such a low haemoglobin level would give rise to a more emotive but certainly no less practical problem.

However, a thorough knowledge of a patient's clinical state enables the anaesthetist to provide a complete service. This concept may be ideal in theory, but in practical terms an anaesthetist's time is limited and a systematic approach has to be adopted with a history that is succinct and pertinent:

1. Cardiorespiratory: exercise tolerance
2. Intercurrent disease and therapy:
   e.g. Hypertension—$\beta$-blocking drugs
   Diabetes—insulin
3. Dental state: Diseased teeth
   Prostheses, e.g. crowns, bridge
4. Smoking habits: cough, sputum
5. Drugs: sensitivities
   allergies
   steroids
6. Alcohol: tolerance
   barbiturates

The physical examination of the patient often consists of a brief auscultation of lung and heart sounds, although these signs are no more or less important than a glance at the patient's weight, or his ability to perform a forced vital capacity. Skeletal disabilities associated with arthritic diseases can cause practical difficulties such as restricted neck mobility or arthritis of the temporomandibular joint.

The matter of routine pre-operative investigations is a much more contentious issue, as many investigations are performed which are quite valueless and can be disregarded. Routine chest radiographs involve considerable use of radiological services and consequent expense. Kerr[1] rationalises its use to all smokers, those with evidence of respiratory disorder, and all patients over the age of 50. An ECG is also frequently performed on patients over the age of 50, but this will rarely reveal an abnormality unless it is performed during exercise.

Routine blood tests are considered prudent by most anaesthetists. Certainly all patients of African extraction should be screened for the presence of the sickle-cell condition. Again, it should be stressed that once it is decided that the operation is imperative, the outcome of the sickle test is of interest but not vital, as the patient will not be treated in any more or less hazardous manner, whatever the result of the test. It should be noted that occasionally acute abdominal conditions are the result of intra-abdominal manifestations of the sickle-cell disease, e.g. splenic infarct.

The estimation of haemoglobin levels as a routine is not difficult, any may be contributory in respect of sustainable blood losses or the detection of anaemia. However, children admitted for minor surgery do not often relish the process of a blood test whether by venepuncture or fingerprick and the result is the alienation of the patient. Only very occasionally is an unsuspected blood disorder detected.

## Premedication

In an account of the place of premedication in anaesthetic practice by far the most important question is "What is the objective?" The answer is divided into those aspects that affect the patient and those that assist the anaesthetist, and the two criteria are not always in agreement.

Firstly, from the patient's point of view, some will argue that a person who is apprehensive of the outcome of the operation desires to be rid of this anxiety. Sedative drugs do not necessarily fulfill this objective. On the contrary, sedation of an anxious patient can merely add to the problems. Sound advice and reassurance are obviously of great value here, and mere lip-service to this approach is inadequate. However, there are still some patients with a morbid fear of anaesthesia and operations, and anxiolytic tranquillising drugs can assist greatly. It should be obvious that such therapy cannot be of great benefit to the patient if it is only administered in the hour preceding the operation. Here, tranquillity is provided mostly for the anaesthetist and only partly for the patient.

### Anxiolytic Drugs

The benzodiazepine group of drugs have been widely employed for this purpose in a pre-operative capacity. Diazepam or lorazepam are examples and can be administered either orally or parenterally.

The opiate drugs have euphoric side-effects, and when the analgesic action is not primarily the reason for their administration the drug is given for its euphoriant effect, which will allay many of the patient's fears.

The phenothiazine drugs used in premedication vary from an hypnotic action to major tranquillising effects. Promethazine is largely hypnotic, whereas chlorpromazine is a potent transquilliser with many side-effects that may profoundly influence the conduct of subsequent anaesthesia.

The second objective of premedicant therapy is to provide an integral part of the anaesthetic technique. In this respect, three actions need to be considered.

1. To provide a basal narcotic state in a patient who is to receive light general anaesthesia combined with muscle relaxants. Many unfortunate reports of awareness during general anaesthesia occur as a result of inadequate regard for this aspect.

2. To counter the adverse effects of certain general anaesthetic agents. As an example, atropine is given as a premedicant drug to obviate the cholinergic action of suxamethonium or the bradycardia that occasionally accompanies the use of halothane.

3. To dry the secretions produced by the respiratory mucous membrane. Whilst this action may have been necessary when ether anaesthesia was common, it is rarely imperative during current anaesthetic practice, except with small children. Many anaesthetists feel that to deprive patients of food and fluid and then finally to inhibit their ability to salivate with atropine or hyoscine merely adds to their distress.

## Antisialogogues

*Atropine and hyoscine.*—Both atropine sulphate and hyoscine hydrobromide are used extensively as antisialogogues in pre-operative premedication. As both are tertiary ammonium compounds they readily cross the blood-brain barrier. Hyoscine also has a CNS-depressant action which often combines well with the opiates to provide good sedation. The amnesic or euphoric effect are often much appreciated by patients. However, in the elderly with cerebral arteriosclerosis it is contra-indicated as it can lead to confusional states. Atropine sulphate does not produce a similar depression and is therefore the drug of choice in these circumstances. The combination of hyoscine for premedication with large doses of atropine (with neostigmine) to reverse paresis at the end of the operation has been thought to give rise to the cholinergic syndrome sometimes seen in the recovery period. An alternative antisialogogue which does not cross the blood-brain barrier is glycopyrronium (glycopyrrolate).

*Glycopyrronium.*—This is a long-acting[2] anticholinergic agent with a potency between two and five times that of atropine.[3] Selectivity of action has been claimed with relatively more antisialogogue activity and less effect on heart rate.[4] For this reason, the use of glycopyrronium has been advocated in the elderly and those with cardiovascular problems; however, further studies have shown that the onset of action of glycopyrronium is slower than that of atropine, and that when glycopyrronium is used with neostigmine to reverse neuromuscular paralysis, the simultaneous onset of action of the two drugs masks any tachycardia that might be produced by glycopyrronium alone.[5] Intravenous administration of glycopyrronium during anaesthesia has been shown to be effective in increasing heart rate at doses of 5–15 $\mu$g/kg.[5] Glycopyrronium has no anti-emetic activity, due to its poor penetration of the blood-brain barrier,[6] and this lack of central action also means that the transient bradycardias possible with intravenous atropine administration do not occur. The quaternary ammonium structure of glycopyrronium is responsible for its poor oral absorption.

One action of anaesthesia that is most undesirable is the occurrence of emetic side-effects. Not infrequently this is initiated by the opiate drugs given pre-operatively, but a great deal may be done to prevent this by judicious use of drugs or combination of drugs. Hyoscine, whilst adding to the sedation of papaveretum will tend to limit the emetic effects of the opiate by virtue of its anti-emetic action.

Various combinations of drugs, such as the above example of papaveretum and hyoscine, have been evolved to cover the desired objectives outlined in the preceding paragraphs. A few other examples are:

morphine/atropine
promethazine/pethidine
promethazine/pethidine/hyoscine

## Adverse Reactions to Hyoscine

Certain agents, principally belladonna alkaloids, phenothiazines, butyrophenones and tricyclic antidepressants, can cause partial or complete block of central cholinergic transmission. This produces a syndrome known as central anticholinergic syndrome (CAS). The main features of the condition are drowsiness or coma, occasionally excitation and agitation, hallucinations, motor inco-ordination and a pyrexia. This condition can be encountered in the elderly or susceptible following premedication with hyoscine, although the other agents mentioned may also trigger the response.

CAS is treated by elevating the circulatory level of acetylcholine within the central nervous system, and this may be achieved by administration of physostigmine. This is available as physostigmine salicylate. The dosage is 0·5–1·0 mg i.v., given cautiously to avoid excessive muscarinic effects on the heart.

## Oculogyric Crises Caused by Phenothiazine

Although this subject is slightly out of context in this section, the phenothiazines are frequently administered as premedicant drugs. The phenothiazine which causes extrapyramidal side-actions with regularity is perphenazine (Fentazin). This is associated with the piperazine side-chain. Perphenazine is usually used as an anti-emetic, but is occasionally given as a premedicant drug. Other phenothiazines may also cause extrapyramidal side-effects.

The condition is frequently confined to the musculature of the tongue, face and eyes. The action of the tongue is unco-ordinated and it is moved in and out of the mouth, the facial muscles may twitch and the eyes are rolled about. This has become known as an oculogyric crisis.

Treatment consists of cessation of the offending drug and the administration of an anti-parkinsonism agent such as procyclidine (Kemadrin), which is most effective in this type of drug-induced parkinsonism. The dose of procyclidine is 5–10 mg i.v., and this may be repeated if ineffective.

## SPECIAL SITUATIONS

This section is not intended to be a complete account of the interaction of specialised anaesthesia for specialised surgical applications, but rather to discuss certain specific aspects of each subject.

### Ear Nose and Throat Surgery

#### The Ear

Much of the surgery performed on the ear is microsurgery of the middle ear. From the anaesthetists point of view, this entails utilising an anaesthetic technique which provides optimal conditions for the surgery. As quite small quantities of blood can obscure the entire operating field, the problem is not quite the same as is encountered when attempting to limit bleeding over larger operating fields. Attention to details of technique ensuring clear airways, avoidance of hypercarbia and careful posturing of the patient, will be as rewarding as any sophisticated technique of hypotensive anaesthesia. In many cases, the prudent application of small quantities of a local vasoconstrictor are indicated.

It is well to remember that the gas contained within the middle ear cavity is likely to increase in volume by ingress of *nitrous oxide* as a gas, and could "lift off" a delicate graft such as in a myringoplasty operation.

#### The Nose

Operations on the nose have one common feature—that they involve surgery on a particularly vascular structure. For the anaesthetist who is anxious to assist in reducing the vascularity of the nose many methods exist and are described elsewhere in the book. One technique is worth mentioning here, and that is the method described by Moffett[7] and still widely used. A solution is prepared as follows:

Cocaine 8 per—2 ml
Sodium bicarbonate 1 per cent—2 ml
Adrenaline 1:1000—1 ml

Macintosh and Ostlere[8] describe a modification of the technique where the Moffett solution is deposited in the spheno-ethmoidal recess to block the anterior ethmoidal nerve and the sphenopalatine ganglion. The same technique may be employed in providing topical analgesia for fibre-optic bronchoscopy when combined with pharyngeal topical analgesia.

#### Tonsillectomy/Adenoidectomy

In the infant, anaesthesia for adeno-tonsillectomy is generally administered via an orotracheal tube. The oral tube is held in a slot in the tongue-blade of the Doughty modification of the Boyle-Davis gag. Adult tonsillectomy is performed with nasotracheal control of the airway by the anaesthetist. A cuffed tube adds an extra element of safety. Pharyngeal packing is not necessary as it tends to obscure and intrude on the operative field. As the surgeon is working with direct vision, he must aspirate any blood to prevent inhalation around the endotracheal tube.

#### The Larynx

Operations on the larynx often present some of the most difficult problems for the anaesthetist, as surgical access and maintenance of an unobstructed airway form two irreconcilable objectives. However, with close co-operation between anaesthetist and surgeon, most procedures become feasible.

#### Laryngoscopy and Microlaryngoscopy

In order to perform laryngoscopy under general anaesthesia, a moderate degree of muscular relaxation is necessary, and it is also necessary to obtund the gagging reflex. This may be achieved using inhalational anaesthesia to a sufficient depth that all anaesthetic gases may be withdrawn and the laryngoscopy performed whilst the patient continues to ventilate spontaneously. This necessarily limits the effective anaesthesia time.

Increasingly, laryngoscopy is performed through a microscope. The laryngoscope is held in a steady position by a support, called a laryngostat, which rests on the subject's sternum.

The procedure tends to be more protracted

than a simple hand-held laryngsocopy and several anaesthetic techniques have been described to deal with this special circumstance.

(a) General anaesthesia. Spontaneous breathing is maintained with intravenous supplements and topical analgesia. Drawback: muscle relaxation is minimal.
(b) General anaesthesia is maintained with insufflated anaesthetic gases and spontaneous breathing. Drawback: minimal relaxation; considerable atmospheric pollution.
(c) General anaesthesia with muscle relaxants and maintained with intravenous supplements. Ventilation using jet venturi principle, either with a rigid catheter through the larynx or with an injector attached to the laryngoscope blade. Drawbacks: exhaled vapour causes movement of vocal cords; paralysed patient; lack of airway control.
(d) General anaesthesia with muscle relaxants, controlled ventilation with anaesthetic gases administered via a small specialised endotracheal tube. Drawback: the endotracheal tube, however small or transparent, may intrude upon or obscure the operating area.

A further complication has been introduced to microlaryngeal surgery in the form of the *carbon dioxide laser*. This device is used to thermocoagulate tumours of the larynx. It is a very precise tool but will damage any tissue it lands upon. Consequently, if the cords abduct as the beam is directed upon them, damage will be caused to the trachea. It is prudent, therefore, to place a wet swab in the larynx to prevent accidental tracheal damage.

It follows that the anaesthetic technique requires an endotracheal tube. However, there have been several reports of PVC endotracheal tubes being damaged by the laser beam, and actually igniting in the presence of oxygen. Some authors have advocated wrapping the endotracheal tube in aluminium foil, or having a flexible metal tube specially constructed (see Chapter 8).

### Total Laryngectomy

Fortunately this operation is becoming less common as a result of more effective radiotherapy for laryngeal neoplasms. However, it is occasionally performed and demands a special anaesthetic technique. The patient may have laryngeal obstruction and once paralysed with suxamethonium the obstruction may become complete and prevent the lungs being inflated (i.e. ball-valving). Therefore, *spontaneous* respiration should always be retained until it has been established that *controlled* respiration can be achieved with ease. When the trachea has been intubated, the operation can proceed, but it may be necessary to perform a tracheostomy initially, merely to re-establish an airway. Towards the end of the procedure, the endotracheal tube is removed, the trachea divided and anaesthesia continued by means of a special endotracheal tube (Montando). Clearly, a delay in performing the tracheostomy from the time of removal of the endotracheal tube will lead to ventilatory problems should the patient be paralysed. It is prudent, therefore, to have the patient breathing spontaneously at this time.

## Anaesthesia for Radiological Examinations

Many radiological examinations, particularly angiographic procedures, are unpleasant, and general anaesthesia is often preferred. When patients with arterial disease require angiography, the same precautions are necessary as for the definitive correction. It should be noted that many patients with arterial disease also suffer from hypertension and may be in borderline or frank left ventricular failure. The sudden administration of large quantities of contrast medium containing a considerable amount of sodium may be sufficient to tip the balance and precipitate the patient into pulmonary oedema. Iopamidol (Niopam) is one of a new generation of water-soluble, non-ionic contrast media with a considerably reduced general toxicity. For the same concentration of iodine it has a much lower osmolarity, and is isosmolar with plasma. Therefore there is less risk of circulatory complications. It can be given intravenously without pain, and when combined with Digital Subtraction Angiography (DSA) general anaesthesia is often unnecessary.

**Translumbar aortography** is performed with the patient lying prone, and the needle is introduced into the aorta percutaneously. The patient should be positioned and supported so that adequate respiratory exchange and chest movement can take place, and controlled ventilation is preferred.

**Peripheral angiography** can, and is, frequently performed without general anaesthesia. Carotid and cerebral angiography require carefully controlled physiological states and are dealt with elsewhere.

**Specialised neuroradiological procedures.**— The use of intrathecal air studies has declined dramatically since the introduction of Computerised Axial Tomography (CAT scans). The former is extremely demanding on anaesthetic techniques as the patient is often moved through 360° in either plane, with consequent effects on cardiovascular stability.

## Vascular Surgery

This is a vast topic and naturally involves many other specialised areas of anaesthesia. It is intended, therefore, to consider cerebral and carotid vascular surgery as part of neurosurgical anaesthesia, and confine the following remarks to vascular surgery, other than in the head and neck (see also Chapter 28).

The necessity for surgical intervention in vascular disorders is usually due to the pathological consequences of atherosclerosis. Thus the disease is widespread and rarely confined to one part of the vascular system. It is wise, therefore, to assess the adequacy of the patient's cerebral and coronary vessels before embarking upon anaesthesia, and to remember that atherosclerosis is frequently associated with diabetes mellitus.

## Aortic Surgery

Surgery of the arch of the aorta and the thoracic aorta is dealt with in the section on cardiac surgery but here consideration is given to the abdominal aorta.

The surgical procedures involve

1. Bypass of a discrete aortic blockage with a straight prosthesis
2. Bypass of a bifurcation blockage with a "trouser" graft from aorta to both iliac arteries, or occasionally to one iliac artery
3. Bypassing a completely occluded aorta with a prosthesis from one or other axillary artery to one or both femoral arteries.

The aorta may become occluded by atherosclerosis or may become aneurysmal. An aortic aneurysm may present as an acute episode with dissection of the layers of the aneurysm wall, or may present as a pulsatile swelling in the abdomen.

An acute dissecting aneurysm presents a very different clinical picture from that of the uncomplicated aneurysm. The patient will have lost a considerable quantity of blood, either into the aortic wall or into the surrounding retroperitoneal space. The abdomen is usually distended and a measurement of the girth will give some indication of the progressive nature of the condition. The patient will be in great pain and generally will exhibit the features of oligaemic shock. The femoral pulses will be lost and urinary output may be severely curtailed. If the upwards extension of the dissection involves the renal arteries, a very grave situation exists.

Thus, before embarking upon general anaesthesia for the surgical repair of a dissecting abdominal aneurysm, the prudent anaesthetist will have a reliable infusion running, a urinary catheter in position, a cannula in a central vein to assess the right atrial filling pressure and, if the means of measuring the arterial pressure by the intravascular technique with a transducer is readily available, this would be appropriate. Conventional methods of measuring blood pressure become difficult in such situations if there is severe vasoconstrictive compensation taking place.

The following anaesthetic technique has much to commend it:

Surgeons are ready, gowned and gloved, and the patient is on the table suitably resuscitated, with a blood transfusion in place and fully prepared and draped. The various intravenous and arterial lines have already been positioned under local anaesthesia. Anaesthesia is induced either by gaseous inhalation or intravenous agent, whilst an infusion of blood is running. Particular care must be exercised if an intravenous agent is used, especially a barbiturate, as the loss of vasomotor tone may be sufficient to cause a critical loss of coronary or cerebral blood flow, and for the patient to collapse. Ketamine has been used as an induction agent because of its property of enhancing vasomotor tone during induction. As soon as anaesthesia is induced, the surgeon may start. The primary surgical objective should be to acquire proximal control of the aorta to prevent further dissection or blood loss. The advantage of this technique is that it minimises the delay that will inevitably occur from the time anaesthesia is commenced. Anaesthesia will cause a loss of vasoconstrictive tone, but also the loss of abdominal muscle tone will allow a change in the intra-abdominal pressure to occur which may be sufficient to restart aortic bleeding which had stopped due to the balance of pressure inside and outside the aorta.

The subsequent management of the anaesthetic will be to maintain or restore an adequate right atrial pressure by transfusion and to monitor the urinary output. Once the aneurysm has been resected and the circulation restored, the acid-base balance can alter dramatically and accumulated acid metabolites may overwhelm the buffering capacity of the patient, causing a metabolic acidosis. This can be anticipated by the judicious administration of sodium bicarbonate 8·5 per cent just prior to the release of the proximal aortic clamp.

Many other complications can arise, as the quantity of transfused blood can be very great, and this is dealt with in Chapter 17.

**Peripheral Vascular Surgery**

This generally involves bypassing occluded, diseased vessels, usually from the iliac arteries downwards, depending upon the site of the major occlusion. Anaesthetic management is fairly straightforward but it should be stressed again that localised arterial occlusion is often part of a generalised disease process and the blood supply to vital organs may be critical. Such patients are often heavy smokers and their respiratory reserve may be very limited. The success of a surgical manoeuvre can be jeopardised if the blood flow to the operating area is diminished. This will lead to blood-clotting, particularly in prosthetic vessels. As diseased vessels are fairly unreactive to vasomotor tone, flow is very dependent upon pressure, and the anaesthetic technique should be aimed at producing as little fall as possible in arterial pressure during the procedure and, very importantly, in the postoperative period.

## Ophthalmic Anaesthesia

Ophthalmic operations can be divided into intra-ocular and extra-ocular procedures.

Examples of intra-ocular operations are:

1. Cataract extraction
2. Peripheral iridectomy
3. Trabeculectomy.

From the technical aspect, corneal grafting can be included in this category, whilst not exactly intra-ocular surgery.

The conditions required for intra-ocular operations are:

1. No change in intra-ocular pressure
2. No straining or elevation of venous pressure.

When surgery is proposed in a case of penetrating eye injury, it is important to prevent even a transient rise in intra-ocular pressure as this may result in vitreous loss.

To achieve these conditions, one is often faced with a dilemma. For instance, an elderly patient is to have cataract surgery and in other circumstances a fairly light anaesthetic would be indicated. The risk of the patient straining during cataract extraction under injudiciously light anaesthesia leads the anaesthetist to err on the side of caution and employ an anaesthetic technique which will ensure a still, relaxed patient. Occasionally, this conflict of interest is not easily resolved, and it is necessary to administer a local anaesthetic. Furthermore, cataracts can occur in younger people who have generalised debilities such as myotonia dystrophica or diabetes. Endotracheal intubation is always indicated with adequate topical anaesthesia of the trachea. Suxamethonium has been shown to increase intra-ocular pressure and this increase may not totally be prevented by pre-treatment with tubocurarine or gallamine.

There are considerable differences of opinion regarding the maintenance of anaesthesia, and particularly whether it is necessary to paralyse the patient with non-depolarising muscle relaxants and provide intermittent positive-pressure ventilation. Undoubtedly paralysis of the external ocular muscles removes any likelihood of their activity and thereby decreases the intra-ocular pressure. IPPV may lead to hypocarbia, and that will lower the intra-ocular pressure. The administration of acetazolamide 500 mg intravenously will inhibit aqueous humour secretion and thus restrict any rise in the intra-ocular pressure. Similarly, the use of an osmotic diuretic such as mannitol will also control the intra-ocular pressure. However, many anaesthetists prefer to use spontaneous respiration in order to avoid the difficult transition back from controlled ventilation to spontaneous breathing with its accompanying dangers of straining and coughing. The technique is not as important as a close adherence to the principles required to produce satisfactory conditions.

One problem frequently associated with cataract surgery is the short interval which commonly exists between two operations on bilaterally affected eyes. Until recently, halothane was the only acceptable inhalational agent for this procedure. However, with the advent of enflurane it is now no longer necessary to use halothane on two closely-linked occasions, as the former has been proved a most acceptable alternative in intra-ocular surgery.

It is very undesirable that a patient having had intra-ocular surgery should suffer from postoperative nausea and vomiting, with concomitant strain being put upon the eye. All effort should be made to minimise the possibility of causing emetic sequelae. Firstly the premedicant drugs should be considered, as opiates can affect the chemo-emetic trigger-zone in the medulla. Drugs with anti-emetic actions, such as droperidol and haloperidol, or phenothiazines such as promethazine, are to be preferred. The administration of intravenous opiates during the anaesthetic should also be avoided for the same reason. Anti-emetic drugs should be administered at the first complaint of any such symptoms in the postoperative period.

**Extra-ocular procedures** include all other operations associated with the eye:

1. Operations for retinal detachment
2. Strabismus (squint) correction
3. Orbital surgery.

The principle involved in the correction of retinal detachment is that of indenting the sclera from outside the eye thus reapproximating the retina to the choroid. It will attach as a result of the reaction caused by a cryotherapy probe applied around the area of retinal detachment. The indentation of the sclera will reduce the volume of the eye and the intra-ocular pressure will increase. If the anaesthetist attempts to obviate this increase in pressure by lowering the intra-ocular pressure, the result will tend to prevent the surgical reapproximation of the retina, choroid and sclera. Another consequence of increasing the intra-ocular pressure will be to counter the pressure within the central retinal artery. If the increased intra-ocular pressure exceeds the pressure within the artery, flow will cease, the eye will be in danger of becoming ischaemic, and blindness may ensue.

The anaesthetist must therefore ensure that the arterial pressure is at a level which will provide adequate retinal perfusion throughout the indentation procedure, and also that the blood pressure does not fall much below that level postoperatively.

**Vitrectomy** is a procedure during which the vitreous humour is aspirated with a specialised probe and replaced with a crystalloid fluid such as Hartmann's solution. Clearly, the intra-ocular pressure is largely in the surgeons control during this procedure and the anaesthetist need not be over-concerned by that particular aspect of the anaesthetic technique. It should be noted that occasionally a gas bubble is left in the eye which consists of a mixture of air and sulphur hexafluoride. As with other gas-filled cavities within a body which is receiving nitrous oxide, the latter gas tends to leave the solution and enter the bubble, increasing its volume. The anaesthetist may therefore be asked to stop using nitrous oxide during the bubble formation.

**Strabismus.**—It should be noted that occasionally a squint may be the presenting sign of a neurological disorder such as a IV or VI nerve palsy or of myasthenia gravis. During surgery for squint correction, traction on the external ocular muscles can cause cardiac irregularities which should be anticipated.

## Plastic, Reconstructive, Cosmetic and Microvascular Surgery

As the title suggests, this discipline covers a wide span of surgical technique. The correction of cutaneous deformities, whether congenital or due to trauma or burns, often involves a protracted series of procedures. This aspect immediately presents an anaesthetic problem of repeated anaesthetics at relatively brief intervals. It is desirable, therefore, that the anaesthetist should consider the surgical plan when considering a course of treatment, so that the technique may be appropriate to the stage of the procedure.

In addition, reconstructive surgery can involve the face and neck and thus may cause difficulties with intubation or the maintenance of an airway. The introduction of ketamine as a general anaesthetic agent has enabled the anaesthetist to provide safe conditions for short procedures without the hazard of attempting a difficult intubation. However, ketamine has other side-effects which may be sufficient to prevent its use.

The treatment of burns is a vast subject in itself, and it is not intended to attempt to deal with it here. However, the anaesthetist should be aware of the particular hazards which may arise. Suxamethonium has been reported frequently to cause cardiac arrest following burn injury, especially in children, and this disposition may persist for many months following the original injury.

### Cosmetic Surgery

This is surgery designed to improve the aesthetic appearance of a patient. Operations include mammoplasty, face-lift, rhinoplasty and others. The success of the operation often depends on carefully avoiding such complications as bleeding and haematoma formation which can cause fibrotic scarring. Such a result would rather nullify any aesthetic improvement. As the anaesthetist is often required to provide operative conditions with little or no bleeding, careful consideration must be given to balancing this with the patient's safety, and this can be a matter that is not easily resolved.

### Microvascular Surgery

Fresh challenges are presented to the anaesthetist in this relatively new field. The operations involve transplanting grafts of skin, or skin and bone, together with the nutrient blood vessels. The graft viability is dependent upon restoration of the blood supply and the vessels are anastomosed under the microscope. The procedure tends to be prolonged and peripheral blood flow becomes a critical factor. Under most circumstances, heat loss by the patient is not so great as to jeopardise the outcome of the surgery, but with microvascular techniques this becomes a very pertinent factor. Furthermore, compensatory vasoconstriction in response to positive-pressure respiration is undesirable.

A technique which provides very satisfactory conditions consists of positive-pressure ventilation, with sodium nitroprusside infusion to prevent peripheral vasoconstriction, and warming blankets and space-blankets for insulation. Considerable heat conservation can be achieved by using an efficient humidifier and maintaining right atrial filling pressures to a generous level to ensure maximal cardiac output in a vasodilated patient.

Other methods have been described, including continuous extradural anaesthesia, with the common objective of providing peripheral vasodilatation, but heat conservation is of paramount importance in any such technique.

## Orthopaedic Surgery

Orthopaedic surgery is frequently concerned with the correction of deformities or with acute trauma. In the former it may be due to a congenital condition such as talipes, or it may be the result of a generalised disease such as rheumatoid arthritis. The widespread nature of such a disease may well confront the anaesthetist with other problems, particularly as the temporomandibular and cervical joints may be affected, causing difficulties with intubation.

Occasionally, severely kyphoscoliotic patients present for surgical correction of the spinal deformity, and added to this they can have thoracic deformities and may not be ventilated adequately when anaesthetised. Great care should be exercised in the use of muscle relaxants in such patients as their ability to fully aerate their lungs and expectorate postoperatively may be restricted.

Some orthopaedic operations such as total hip replacement, may involve extensive exposure of vascular areas of bone. As this is rarely performed in the younger age group, methods of limiting operative blood loss demand prudent consideration. In one series Keith[9] compared the operative, postoperative and total blood loss in three groups of patients undergoing total hip replacement. He compared the blood losses associated with the anaesthetic techniques of epidural anaesthesia, halothane and spontaneous respiration anaesthesia, and neuroleptanaesthesia combined with controlled ventilation. The operative blood loss associated with epidural anaesthesia was significantly less than that of either of the other two groups; but the epidural group had a higher postoperative loss and there was no difference when total blood loss (operative and postoperative) was compared in the epidural and halothane groups.

Other workers have advocated deliberate hypotension with ganglion-blocking agents or sodium nitroprusside infusion. These agents may only be safely employed when the general condition of the patient will allow and the cardiovascular reserve will feature predominantly. Both an ECG and chest x-ray will be required routinely and will enable the anaesthetist to assess the presence or absence of respiratory disease, and measure the size of cardiac shadow. An ECG will not exclude coronary ischaemia, but may reveal evidence of previous myocardial infarction.

If the patient is postured laterally, or if the operating table is tilted laterally for the operation, a beneficial degree of postural hypotension can be created without marked alteration of the systemic blood pressure. This may be achieved by producing vasodilatation in the area of the hip joint, using spinal or epidural anaesthesia and, if the operated hip is tilted so that it is then uppermost, a great deal of blood loss can be averted. Similarly, if systemic ganglion blockade or sodium nitroprusside is used to diminish vasomotor tone, this may be titrated so that significant postural hypotension is present at the level of the operated hip whilst the systemic blood pressure remains virtually unchanged.

A danger which is always present following surgery, particularly hip surgery, which renders the patient immobile postoperatively, is that of deep-vein thrombosis and pulmonary embolism. As it is thought that deep-vein thrombosis is initiated during the operation, the anaesthetist should be aware of the danger and take whatever steps are considered desirable by the surgical team, whether it be the administration of Dextran 70, low-dose heparin, calf-muscle stimuli, or the use of pneumatic pumps.

In the early development of prosthetic joint replacement there were frequent reports of systemic effects being noted during the phase of acrylic-cement implantation. This danger has now been virtually eliminated by the careful preparation of the cement, the amounts of polymer and co-polymer being exactly correct, thus averting the possibility of excess co-polymer being absorbed and giving rise to vascular effects such as hypotension and even cardiac arrest.

**Fat Embolism**

By its very nature, orthopaedic surgery involves manipulation of marrow cavities which are highly vascular but which also contain much fat. Occasionally during surgery, but more frequently following trauma, some of this medullary fat is embolised into the blood stream. This is usually filtered off by the pulmonary capillary bed, causing a syndrome not unlike pulmonary embolism, with arterial hypoxaemia, and chest pain of a pleuritic nature. However, some fat globules are sufficiently small to traverse the pulmonary circulation and may end up in the skin as petechial haemorrhages or, in the glomeruli of the kidney as urinary fat globules and/or haematuria. They may prove fatal if they occlude vital vessels such as the coronaries or those of the brain stem.

**Use of Tourniquets**

Many orthopaedic operations on the limbs are performed with ischaemic conditions provided by the application of a tourniquet around the limb. This is a safe procedure provided certain rules are adhered to, and only a pneumatic tourniquet is used—other devices being regarded as dangerous. For instance, winding elastic bandages around a limb can apply a very great deal of pressure to that point. Nerve injury (or tourniquet paralysis, as the condition has been known) has virtually disappeared following the widespread adoption of the pneumatic tourniquet. However, the danger of excessive pressure still exists if regular checks are not made on the accuracy of the aneroid manometers. The tourniquet cuff should be applied to a part of the limb where nerves will not be directly compressed against a bony protuberance. Therefore, the cuff is most readily applied to the thigh or upper arm, but it may be used on the lower calf above the ankle. It should not be applied over a joint as nerves are vulnerable directly around the knee, elbow and ankle joints. It must also be remembered that the cuff should not be directly applied to the skin, as small folds of skin may be trapped under the cuff; to avoid this, 2 or 3 layers of orthopaedic wool should be wound around the limb initially.

Obviously the pressure applied to the cuff must be sufficient to occlude the arterial input. In a large limb the pressure formed within is a function of the pressure within the cuff, the width of the cuff, the size of the limb and the arterial pressure of the patient.

Generally speaking the following cuff pressures are sufficient and safe:

| | *Adult* | *Child* |
|---|---|---|
| Leg | 500 mm Hg | 250 mm Hg |
| Arm | 300 mm Hg | 150 mm Hg |

The limb should be exsanguinated by winding an Esmarch (elastic) bandage around the limb, starting distally until the level of the pneumatic cuff is reached, which is then inflated and the time noted. If it is impossible to apply the

Esmarch bandage, the limb should be elevated as nearly vertical as possible for about 5 minutes. Inflow occlusion by pressure on the major limb artery will help lessen the inflow and aid the venous drainage.

Tourniquets should not be applied to ischaemic limbs in the presence of sepsis, or to limbs where there is a deep-vein thrombosis for fear of pulmonary embolism. It may be argued that the tourniquet lessens the chance of embolisation, but it must be released at some point and the application may have dislodged a thrombus. Patients with sickle-cell disease are said to be unsuitable for tourniquet application, but patients with sickle-cell trait may be considered provided complete exsanguination is achieved.

Considerable differences exist regarding the safe duration for the application of a tourniquet. Two hours is considered as long as is prudent in a lower limb, but an upper limb may be longer. Safety may be increased for a prolonged tourniquet application if the limb is kept cool, i.e. with frequent bathing in ice-cold saline. Operating lights will tend to warm the operative site and thus increase the danger of prolonged ischaemia.

Following release of the tourniquet, there will be a period of reactive hyperaemia, the extent and severity of which is related to the duration of ischaemia. If the cuff has to be released before the completion of a procedure, it should be noted that tissue oxygenation takes a little time to become re-equilibrated with that of the arterial inflow.

## Gynaecological Anaesthesia

There are only a few anaesthetic problems associated with gynaecological operations that are not applicable to general surgery. It should be noted that frequently patients requiring hysterectomy do so as a result of excessive menstrual loss, and may be quite severely anaemic. This equally applies to the preliminary curettage examination which may be necessary. In younger patients where a hysterectomy is not indicated and the surgical excision of a fibroid (myomectomy) is necessary, the anaesthetist should be prepared for a greater than average blood loss as the uterus tends to be a very vascular structure.

### Laparoscopy

Laparoscopic examination of the pelvis is a most satisfactory procedure. The patient can be positioned head-down to empty the pelvis of intestines and enable the surgeon to examine the pelvic organs in detail.

Laparoscopy is frequently performed under general anaesthesia, although this need not be so. As 2–3 litres of gas are introduced into the peritoneum, the degree of respiratory embarrassment is considerable and the danger of gastric reflux great. The patient should therefore be intubated and given intermittent positive-pressure ventilation at a rate sufficient to discharge the absorbed carbon dioxide.

### Termination of Pregnancy

Vacuum aspiration of uterine contents is not a particularly stimulating procedure, and an anaesthetic technique consisting of barbiturate induction with intravenous supplement, nitrous oxide and oxygen, usually suffices. The intravenous supplement can be a further barbiturate (for example methohexitone) with intravenous diazepam, or a short-acting opiate such as fentanyl. It is generally considered inadvisable to use halothane in the inhaled mixture as this can cause relaxation of the uterine muscle and postoperative blood loss.[10]

## Anaesthesia in Remote Situations

Occasionally an anaesthetist may be required to administer anaesthesia in remote or difficult situations when medical gases are not readily available. The choice of agent is then either intravenous or inhalational. *Intravenous agents* are available which will provide total anaesthesia for emergency surgery, with greater or lesser degrees of protection against the potential aspiration of stomach contents.

Ketamine is a most suitable agent in this respect, with the added advantage of being able to be administered intramuscularly should an intravenous route not be readily available. The dose when given intravenously is 2–4 mg/kg body weight, or 5–10 mg/kg for intramuscular use.

The intravenous induction agents in current use may be given by incremental injection or continuous infusion, but will not provide anaesthesia without loss of protective glottic reflexes.

**Inhalational technique.**—If medical gases are not available, then inhalational general anaesthesia must be administered by a draw-over system where the patient inspires to draw air over a volatile liquid anaesthetic, such as ether.

**The EMO vaporiser** is a well-proven piece of anaesthetic apparatus and is a most suitable source of ether vapour in air. It can be used as a draw-over system for spontaneous respiration, or for controlled ventilation using the bellows attachment.

**The Triservice anaesthetic apparatus.**—This is another draw-over system which utilises atmospheric air as the carrier gas, but the vaporiser is designed to use either halothane or trichloroethylene as the volatile anaesthetic. The vaporiser will also produce vapour from other volatile anaesthetic agents. The apparatus incorporates the facility to enrich atmospheric air with oxygen.[11]

## REFERENCES


1. Kerr, I. H. (1974). The preoperative chest x-ray. *Brit. J. Anaesth.*, **46**, 558.
2. Mirakhur, R. K., Dundee, J. W. and Jones, C. J. (1978). Evaluation of the anticholinergic actions of glycopyrronium bromide. *Brit. J. Clin. Pharmacol.*, **5**, 77.
3. Mirakhur, R. K. (1979). Anticholinergic drugs. *Brit. J. Anaesth.*, **51**, 671.
4. Mirakhur, R. K., Dundee, J. W. and Clarke, R. S. J. (1977). Glycopyrrolate-neostigmine mixture for the antagonism of neuromuscular block: comparison with atropine-neostigmine mixture. *Brit. J. Anaesth.*, **49**, 825.
5. Mirakhur, R. K., Jones, C. J. and Dundee, J. W. (1981). Effects of intravenous administration of glycopyrrolate and atropine in anaesthetised patients. *Anaesthesia*, **36**, 277.
6. Mirakhur, R. K. and Dundee, J. W. (1981). Lack of anti-emetic effect of glycopyrrolate. *Anaesthesia*, **36**, 819.
7. Moffett, A. J. (1947). Nasal analgesia by postural instillation. *Anaesthesia*, **2**, 31.
8. Macintosh, Sir R. and Ostlere, M. (1955). *Local Analgesia: Head and Neck*. Edinburgh: Livingstone.
9. Keith, I. (1977). Anaesthesia and blood loss in total hip replacement. *Anaesthesia*, **32**, 444.
10. Grant, I. S. (1980). Anaesthesia for termination of pregnancy. *Brit. J. Anaesth.*, **8**, 711.
11. Houghton, I. T. (1981). The Triservice anaesthetic apparatus. *Anaesthesia*, **36**, 1094.

*Section Eight*

# HISTORY

CHAPTER 45

# Anaesthetic Equipment—A Historical Perspective

'And now I see with eye serene,
The very pulse of the machine;
A being breathing thoughtful breath,
A traveller betwixt life and death.
She was a Phantom of Delight.'
*William Wordsworth.*

THE development of anaesthetic apparatus cannot be taken as an isolated subject. It is inextricably linked with the development of the speciality as a whole. Each refinement in the design of apparatus in the early years reflected either the introduction of a new anaesthetic agent or a desire to improve the quality of anaesthesia administered, usually in terms of safety. These still are the fundamental considerations in the development of new equipment.

This chapter will therefore review both subjects together so that the one can be seen as part of the other.

The practice of anaesthesia as we know it today has evolved from the first public demonstration of ether anaesthesia at the Massachusetts General Hospital, Boston on October 16th, 1846. This first demonstration was not a sudden spontaneous event but the result of a number of independent observations combined with a change in attitudes in medicine in general. Mankind has always been torn between two spectra—one which holds that the toleration of pain shows great physical and spiritual fortitude and the other more compassionate view that suffering should be minimised. All through the early civilisations we find attempts to decrease pain, often by altering conscious level, together with painful rituals to prove maturity and strength of character.

The Egyptian culture described many medical treatments which were said to alleviate pain, some even contained poppy seeds but to relieve headache these were applied as a poultice rather than given orally.[1] However all operations depicted by paintings or on mosaics show the patients with their eyes open which has lead to the assumption that surgical anaesthesia as we know it was unknown in this culture.

The Mesopotamian civilisation of the same era had its medical practice based firmly on magic, they believed that all disease was due to demons and thus described few therapeutic agents; depending rather on rituals and incantations to cure symptoms.

It was to be the Greek and Roman civilisations that were to make medicine into a science, although there are few indications that there was any reversible anaesthesia. Homer's references to "nepenthes", drugs which had the power "to rob grief and anger of their sting" and induce amnesia are often quoted but do not appear to be references to anaesthesia as we know it.[2]

There are many similar references to agents like carbon dioxide and hemp fumes inducing sleep which are often quoted in anaesthetic histories,[3] but despite the lack of evidence to show that they were used in operations, it seems a reasonable assumption that some forms of analgesia during surgical manoeuvres were attempted by these early cultures.

One of the most interesting agents to appear in the early literature is Mandragora (Fig. 1). Used by every civilisation after the Egyptians and remaining popular into the late Middle Ages, this extraordinary plant could be inhaled, eaten, drunk or rubbed into the body to induce analgesia. It is even said to have been used by the Romans to minimise the pain of crucifixion.[3] One of the earliest references to its use is by Dioscordes who used mandragora in wine to decrease the agony of operations. He was also to use the term anaesthesia for the first time in relation to the local application of "Memphitic stone" to relieve pain.[4] Mandragora or mandrake as it was also known contains alkaloids such as scopolamine which presumably were the basis for its use.

There is some evidence that cannabis was utilised by early civilisations, especially the Chinese, to produce painless operations as early as 200 AD. The concept of inhalation of drugs was certainly known to many early cultures.

From the second to the fifteenth centuries there seem to have been few attempts to alleviate any pain. Many cultures believed that to do so was sacrilegious or unnatural, so most therapeutic manoeuvres were based on the use of herbs. Mandragora used with wine and opium extracts occur intermittently in the medical literature of the era.

There were numerous occasions when physical as opposed to pharmacological anaesthesia was used. Occlusion of the carotid arteries is said to have been practised by the Assyrians prior to circumcision, and the use of cold water to allow abscesses to be lanced painlessly is recorded in an early Saxon leechbook of 1050, the *Lacnunga*.[5]

The Renaissance was a time when great advances were made in science as well as in the arts and the concept of painless surgery became more acceptable. Paré was to describe local anaesthesia produced by nerve compression in 1562 and refrigeration anaesthesia was to be used on several occasions in the seventeenth century only to be forgotten again.

Sir Christopher Wren was to make a notable contribution to anaesthetic history when he gave the first recorded injection of a drug intravenously. He used a bladder and quill for the apparatus, opium as the drug and the subject was a dog.[6]

The hundred years prior to 1846 could be termed the pre-anaesthetic era and were a time when several notable physicians introduced ideas that were to have profound effects later in anaesthetic practice. Joseph Priestley discovered oxygen in 1771, although most of his research on the gas was to take place after 1774. His next discovery was that of nitrous oxide during 1772 after some original work by Stephen Hales in 1731.[7]

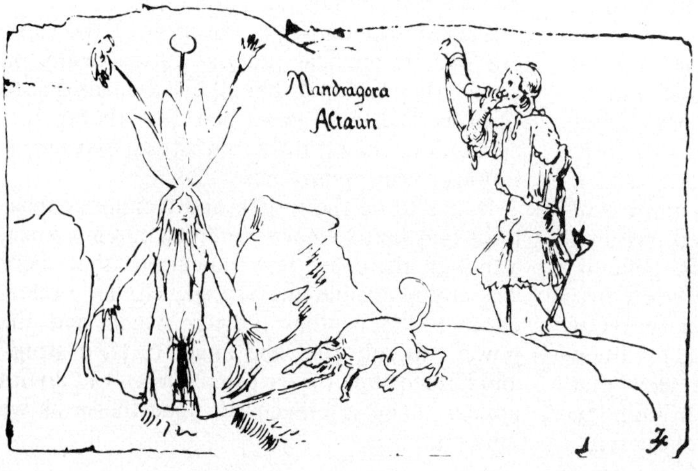


45/FIG. 1.—MANDRAGORA.

The evil spirit that was said to live amongst the roots would utter hideous cries if the plant was disturbed. These cries were fatal if heard and so a complex method of collection was necessary: having tied one's faithful dog to the plant, one retreated to a distance and called the dog to follow. The cries from the uprooted plant would kill the unfortunate animal but by blowing the horn the physician was protected and obtained the rare plant. (From *Anaesthetics Antient and Modern*, 75th Annual Meeting of the British Medical Association, Exeter, 1907. Courtesy of the Wellcome Trustees.)

Humphry Davy was to become interested in nitrous oxide as he started to study chemistry early in 1798 and was to continue this study when he moved to Bristol from his native Penzance to join Beddoes at the Pneumatic Medical Institution as its Superintendent. In April 1799 Davy inhaled nitrous oxide and in his book *Researches* (published the following year) he described the action of the gas in relieving his painful toothache and even suggested its use in relieving the pain of surgical procedures.[8] Davy was only twenty years old at the time and did not continue his researches in this field for long, he was soon to be promoted and take charge of the Chemistry department of the Royal Institution in London. It is incredible that no-one utilised his idea in medicine but perhaps this is related to the scarcity of his book which had only a limited edition published and to the fact that the medical profession do not often read books on chemical research! It is interesting to see that his work was repeated in America within a few years[9] and yet there was still no surgical application considered.

Advances were being made in other fields as well. Serturner isolated morphine from crude opium in 1806 thus allowing measured doses of the drug to be administered for the first time.[10] The following year Larrey who was Napoleon's surgeon observed that amputation of limbs could be performed painlessly during the battle of Eylau when the temperature on the battlefield was $-19°$ F.[11]

Henry Hickman started his medical practice in Shropshire in the 1820's and was the first to advocate and search for a means of producing surgical anaesthesia by inhalational means.[12] He chose to use carbon dioxide as his anaesthetic agent and experimented on animals with great success. He was unable to convince his colleagues that his ideas were worthwhile and he never tried the method on any patients. He even appealed to the French king, Charles X, in an attempt to influence the Royal Academy of Medicine in Paris to take up his work, but the medical profession in France were not impressed either and Hickman was to die at the age of twenty-nine a disappointed man seemingly unable to apply either his research clinically or even try alternative agents.[13]

A different approach to the problem was that of Friedrich Mesmer whose demonstrations of hypnotism suggested to others the possibilities of its use in surgery.[14–16] The technique was extremely effective in certain susceptible patients and is still in use today.

It was not to be an English physician who was to initiate anaesthesia even though Davy and Hickman had paved the way. In America in the 1830s and 40s ether and nitrous oxide were both very popular, especially among students who used them to produce intoxication at parties otherwise known as "ether frolics". There was also a vogue for travelling lecture tours on various scientific subjects which were aimed at and attended by the general public and which were very popular. It was to be a combination of these events that would lead to surgical anaesthesia.

In 1842 Crawford Williamson Long (Fig. 2) had just set up his general practice in Jefferson, Georgia, and remembering his medical student parties decided to try ether as an anaesthetic agent. He removed a lump in the neck from a Mr. James Venable on March 30th, 1842 and was so successful he performed a further eight cases up to 1846. His only equipment was a towel onto which the ether was slowly poured. He was a retiring man however and did not publish his results until many years later.[17] He thus is not recognised as the founder of modern anaesthesia; this accolade is given to Morton for his work in convincing the world of the use of ether.[18]

Before Morton was to succeed in demonstrating surgical anaesthesia there was to be one other major attempt. In 1844 a dentist called Horace Wells (Fig. 3) was to attend a travelling show where the actions of inhaling nitrous oxide gas were demonstrated by one Gardner Quincy Colton, a medical student who did not complete his studies. During the performance, which involved various people from the audience coming up on stage and breathing the gas, one of the people fell from the stage and badly gashed his leg. Wells questioned him and discovered that he had felt no pain. The potential of this was not lost on Wells and he immediately arranged to have one of his own healthy teeth removed by a colleague while Colton gave him nitrous oxide. The operation on the following day (the 11th December, 1844) was a great success and Wells continued to utilise the agent on several people over the next few weeks (making his own gas and administering it from

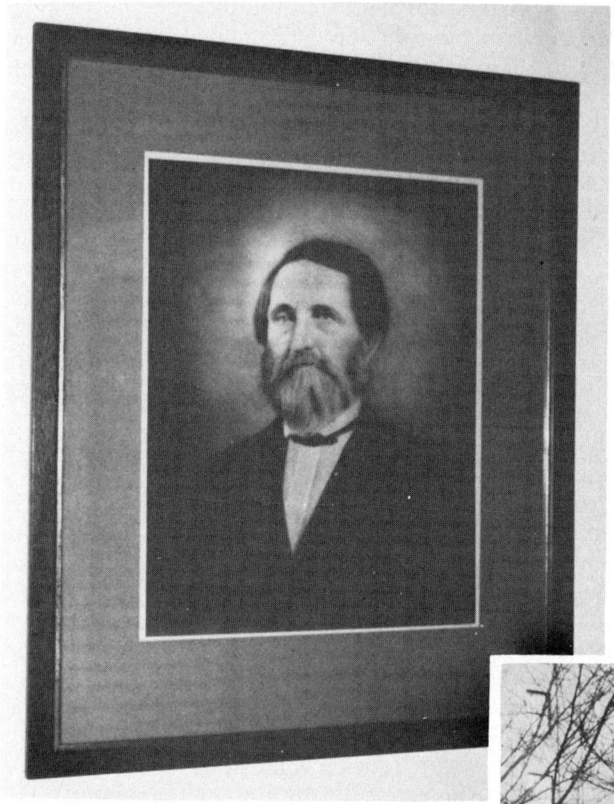

45/FIG. 2.—WILLIAM CRAWFORD LONG. (Courtesy of Dr. Charles Moore.)

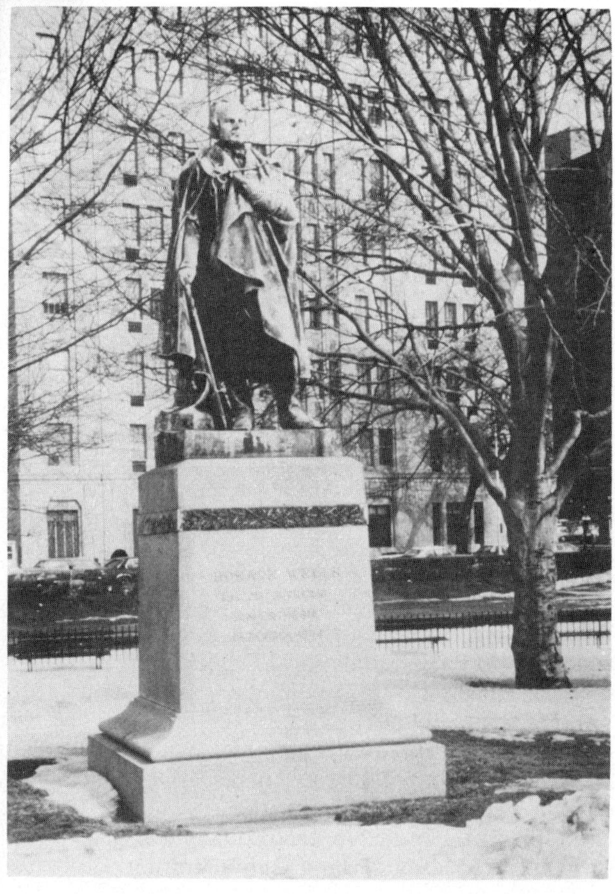

45/FIG. 3.—HORACE WELLS. (Courtesy of Dr. R. Calverley.)

an animal bladder) delivering it to the patient via a wooden tube.

In January of 1845 he arranged to give a demonstration at the Massachusetts General Hospital to the Harvard Medical College. Wells removed the tooth of a young man after an assistant had given nitrous oxide, the man cried out as the tooth was extracted and Wells left in disgrace to cries of "Humbug". He never recovered from this humiliation which was probably due to an inadequate volume of nitrous oxide being administered.[19] He was later to commit suicide in 1848 while in jail on an assault charge.

One of the people who helped to arrange this abortive demonstration was William Morton (Fig. 4) who had been a former partner of Wells. He continued to experiment with different drugs in an attempt to produce anaesthesia. He probably considered the effects of the "frolics" he had attended when he picked ether for his experiments. He tried the drug on his own household pets and even various insects before inhaling the agent himself. He undoubtedly received some advice from Charles Jackson, a physician and chemist, who was later to claim Morton stole his idea. It was probably Jackson who suggested the use of the glass vaporiser that Morton was to use. The first patient that Morton anaesthetised was one Eben Frost who presented with toothache on September 30th, 1846. Encouraged by his obvious success Morton arranged a public demonstration at the Massachusetts General Hospital, Boston, on October 16th, 1846. The patient, Gilbert Abbott, almost had no anaesthesia at all, as Morton was late arriving and the surgeon John Warren was about to start to remove a jaw tumour without him. Morton gave a successful anaesthetic and Warren remarked to the audience "gentlemen this is no humbug", a reference to the unlucky Wells.[20] The apparatus that Morton used was a glass inhaler containing liquid ether and a sponge wick (Fig. 5). It was a simple draw-over vaporiser which did not have to be particularly efficient as the surgeons of that time worked at speeds which are hardly believable today.[21]

A member of Morton's audience was Henry Bigelow, a surgeon of the hospital, and it was he who formally announced the discovery to the medical profession at a meeting of the American Academy of Arts and Sciences on November 3rd, 1846. He spoke also on November 9th

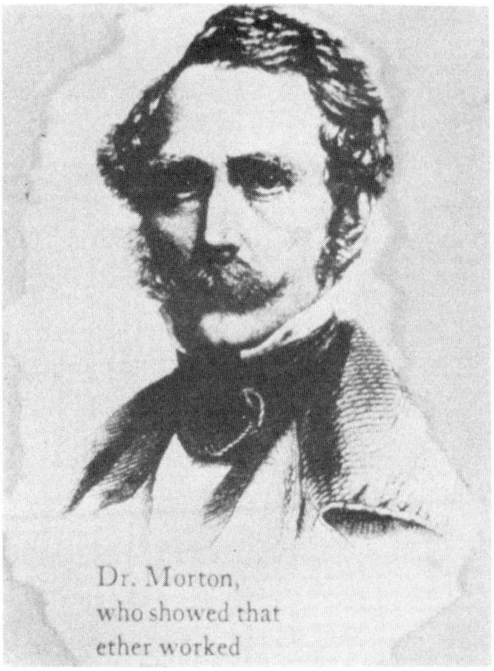


45/FIG. 4.—WILLIAM MORTON. (Courtesy of Bristol Laboratories, New York.)

to the Boston Society of Medical Improvement[22] and published a full account on November 18th, in a medical journal.[23] This was reprinted in part by a local newspaper in Boston. It is Bigelow who is credited with the quotation at Morton's original demonstration that, "he had seen something today that will go round the world".

The news spread quickly to Europe. Henry Bigelow's father, Jacob, wrote to a friend, Francis Boott, a dentist in Gower Street, London, of the efficacy of ether anaesthesia and on December 19th, 1846, Boott extracted a tooth under ether.[24] The anaesthetist was a Dr. Robinson who was to produce the first textbook on anaesthesia in Great Britain by April 1847. Boott's operation was followed on the 21st December 1846 by the amputation of a leg by Liston at University College Hospital, the anaesthetist being William Squires. Squires was to use as his inhaler a modified Nooth's apparatus which was originally designed for carbonating water.[25] Liston was most impressed and is quoted as saying "this Yankee dodge beats mesmerism hollow". The other popular inhaler

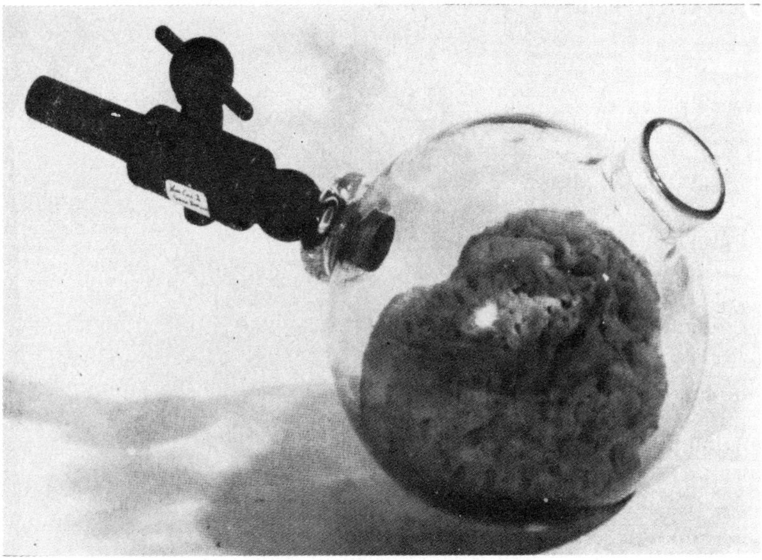

45/Fig. 5.—Morton Ether Inhaler (1846)

This is a photograph of a replica of the device used by Morton on 16th October, 1846. By the following day he had incorporated valves into a brass mouthpiece inserted into the globe. (Courtesy of the late Dr. K. Bryn Thomas and Blackwell Scientific Publications.[19])

at this time was the Hooper inhaler as used by Robinson. It was a glass vaporiser similar to the Squires apparatus utilising Morton's draw-over principle, again sponge pieces acted as wicks.[26]

James Simpson (Fig. 6) who was professor of midwifery at Edinburgh was always interested in any method to alleviate the pain of childbirth. He tried ether in his practice in January 1847 and was impressed with the results. The drug was not ideal for use in obstetrics, however, as it took some time to induce the patients, they often vomited and, because a large part of Simpson's practice was domiciliary, there were often open fires in the same room as the patient. Simpson then experimented with other drugs. He would often have dinner parties at the end of which the latest agent would be inhaled by those present. David Waldie a chemist and friend of Simpson suggested he tried chloroform but Simpson was not enthusiastic and waited several months before doing so. There was an historic dinner party on 4th November, 1847 when the company found themselves waking up under the dinner table after inhaling this new agent. Simpson was not slow to introduce it into clinical practice where he found it fast and effective in producing anaesthesia. He was to publish his first paper on the subject within a fortnight.[27]

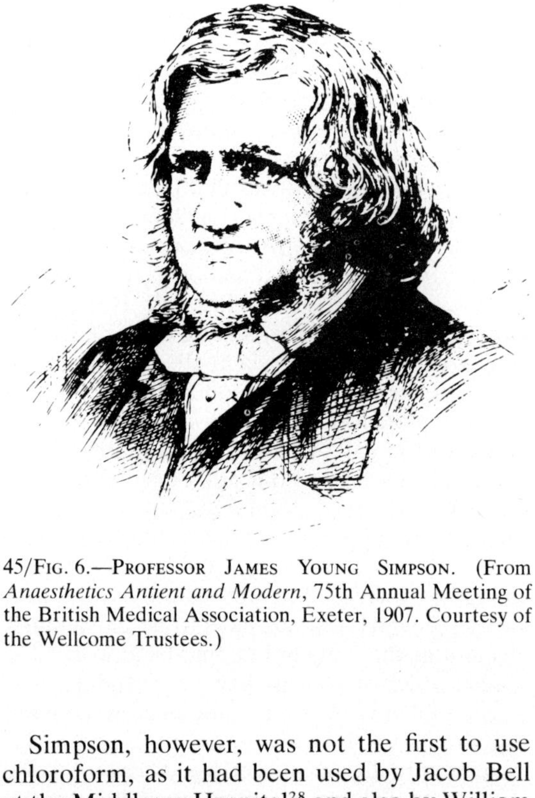

45/Fig. 6.—Professor James Young Simpson. (From *Anaesthetics Antient and Modern*, 75th Annual Meeting of the British Medical Association, Exeter, 1907. Courtesy of the Wellcome Trustees.)

Simpson, however, was not the first to use chloroform, as it had been used by Jacob Bell at the Middlesex Hospital[28] and also by William Lawrence at St. Bartholomew's Hospital[29] earlier in the year, but it is to Simpson that most of the accolades go. Simpson was to face enormous opposition to the use of anaesthesia in obstetrics from various powerful Churchmen in Great Britain and was to spend many years trying to persuade not only the clergy but also the general public that chloroform was beneficial. He advocated the use of a folded handkerchief or hollow sponge held over the patient's face onto which the chloroform was slowly dripped. Simpson felt one of the great advantages of the drug was that it needed no special apparatus for its administration and suggested folding the handkerchief into a cup-like shape for use in surgery.[27] The first deaths under ether anaesthesia were reported that year, one at Grantham and one at Colchester. Despite the fact that neither patient died during the anaesthetic or during the first few postoperative hours, ether was blamed and people began to talk again of the "usefulness of pain" in the disease process and the danger of its abolition. These cases were widely publicised and the medical profession in this country started to turn to chloroform as the agent of choice mainly because of the ease and speed of induction, but partly because of these deaths.

Chloroform was by no means safer and the first death reported using the drug was on 28th January, 1848 when Hannah Greener died during the removal of a toe nail.[30] Her anaesthetist noted her extreme anxiety pre-operatively[31] and described his resuscitation attempts. Hannah had already undergone uneventful surgery using ether[32] and yet despite this death chloroform continued to grow in popularity in the United Kingdom. More deaths were to occur and gradually two schools of thought developed, one in Edinburgh based on the work of Simpson and Syme, and the other in London where John Snow was the leading anaesthetist of his time.

John Snow (Fig. 7) was the first specialist anaesthetist in Great Britain and published a textbook on ether anaesthesia in September, 1847[33] less than one year after its introduction. In this book he described the signs and stages of anaesthesia so succinctly they were to remain unchallenged for eighty years. He was not impressed by the glass inhalers of Morton, Hooper and Squires that were available, and designed his own inhaler based on the Jeffrey's Spiral Steam Inhaler[34] which incorporated temperature compensation in the form of a water bath, a large surface area for the vaporisation of the ether and wide-bore tubing to decrease the resistance to respiration, quite advanced ideas for that era. Snow was not fully satisfied with ether and experimented with many other agents, eventually settling for chloroform. Much of this research work was carried out on animal models including mice, frogs and guinea-pigs. He was determined to explain the sudden deaths that were occurring with the drug and was sure that these were due to overdosage. He was convinced that the pulse should be palpated during induction as well as observing the respiration, and that an apparatus should be used which gave a controlled low concentration of chloroform in air. His research work and methods of administration were published together posthumously in 1858[35] but prior to this he had a long debate with Simpson, Syme and others in Scotland who believed that no specialised equipment was needed for chloroform anaesthesia and that one need only monitor the respiration which would fail before the pulse changed.

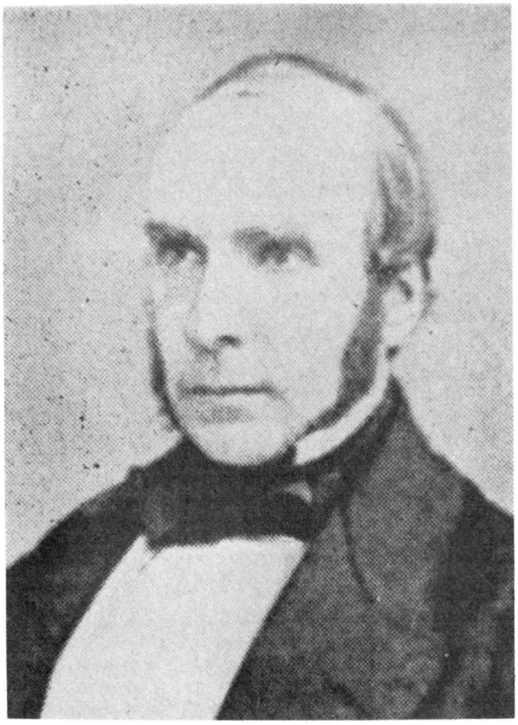

45/FIG. 7.—JOHN SNOW. (Courtesy of the Nuffield Department of Anaesthetics, Oxford, The Association of Anaesthetists of Great Britain and Ireland and the publishers, Blackwell Scientific Publications.[19])

Snow was also the anaesthetist who was invited to administer chloroform to Queen Victoria at the birth of Prince Leopold in 1853. This he was able to do utilising the analgesic phase of chloroform anaesthesia without inducing unconsciousness; this method of dropping chloroform onto a handkerchief was to be known as chloroform à la reine.

American anaesthesia had meanwhile been undergoing a turbulent period. Morton had petitioned Congress for some reward for his invention which he and his chemist friend Jackson had initially tried to patent under the name "Letheon". His claim to Congress was bitterly opposed by Jackson and friends of Wells (who had by now died) who claimed the invention as their own. Various testimonies were sought by the three main protagonists and the debate lasted from 1849 to 1854. The reward would have been $100,000 but in 1854 Crawford Long proved he had given ether some four years before the three rival claimants, who subsequently abandoned their fight. Long, a rather shy man, did not pursue the matter further and gained no financial rewards either.[36]

Chloroform never really achieved the popularity in America that it did in Europe and for the most part the American anaesthetists continued to use ether.

Following the death of Snow in 1858, Thomas Clover who was on the staff at University College and Westminster Hospitals in London took over the mantle of the leading researcher and practical anaesthetist in England. He initially worked on chloroform and being a supporter of Snow developed a fixed concentration apparatus which delivered 2½ per cent chloroform in air from a large reservoir bag which was carried on the anaesthetist's back (Fig. 8).[37]

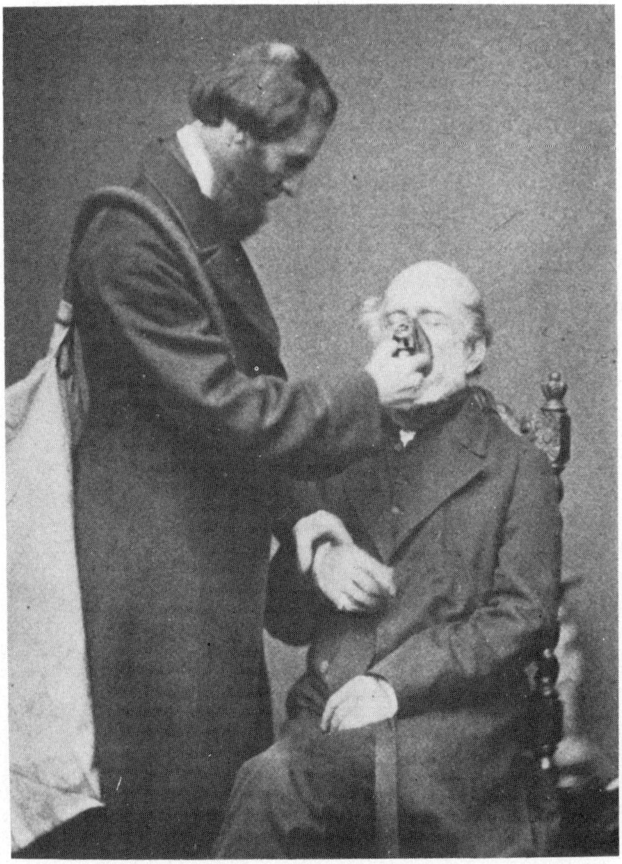

45/Fig. 8.—Thomas Clover.
This historic photograph not only demonstrates the use of Clover's chloroform bag but also shows Clover monitoring the patient's pulse. The induction and maintenance of anaesthesia in an upright position are also noteworthy! (Courtesy of the Nuffield Department of Anaesthetics, Oxford, The Association of Anaesthetists of Great Britain and Ireland and the publishers, Blackwell Scientific Publications.[19])

The same year saw the introduction of ACE by George Harley; this mixture of one part alcohol, two parts chloroform and three parts ether was advocated by many people to replace the toxic chloroform altogether but never achieved universal popularity, although similar mixtures were used in America extensively.[38]

1862 was also the year when the first wire frame mask was introduced.[39] Thomas Skinner was a Liverpool obstetrician who developed this apparatus to keep the cold lint off the patient's face; the whole mask could be folded flat and carried around inside one's top hat!! This mask antedated the better known Schimmelbusch mask by thirty years (Fig. 9).

Nitrous oxide was then to make a dramatic resurgence in America. The same Gardner Quincy Colton who had demonstrated nitrous oxide to Wells gave up his travelling show and formed a dental association in New Haven, Connecticut in which he provided anaesthetics for various dentists in the town.[40] He was to travel to Paris in 1867 and there met a Dr. Evans from London who proceeded to manufacture $N_2O$ in his rooms at the Langham Hotel, on his return to the capital. Evans then persuaded Barth to manufacture cylinders of the gas (1869) and Coxeter and Sons soon followed. The following year liquified $N_2O$ was manufactured in cast-iron cylinders by Coxeter and by 1873 they were available in New York produced by Johnson Brothers.[41]

It was to be from Europe that the next innovation was to come. Junker's chloroform bottle was the first "blow-over" apparatus designed (developed while Junker was resident in England) in which air was blown by means of a hand-held bellows through a glass bottle containing chloroform.[42] The apparatus was originally designed to give bichloride of methylene and soon became the most popular anaesthetic apparatus of its day. The design of the equipment was not ideal, however, and faulty connection of the bellows to the bottle resulted in liquid chloroform being blown into the patient! Almost every anaesthetist of that age brought out a "safe" modification of the Junker bottle (Fig. 10 *a* and *b*), much in the same way that everyone started to design wire frame masks.

The eighteen seventies was a period when ether began to regain its popularity from chloroform. This was largely the result of a visit by B. Joy Jeffries, an eye surgeon from Boston, who read a paper to the International Ophthalmological Conference in London and gave many personal demonstrations in London hospitals of the American technique of ether anaesthesia which involved the forcible physical restraint of the patient when the need arose during the second stage of a gaseous induction.[43]

Thomas Clover in the same year introduced his concept of sequential anaesthesia, starting with nitrous oxide and then switching to ether

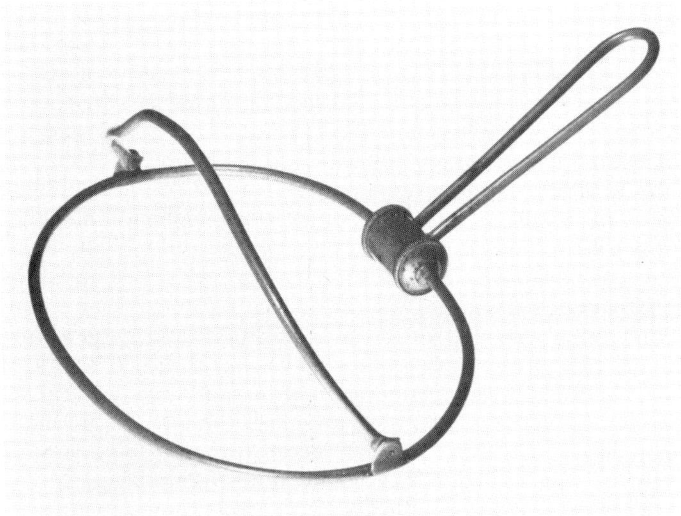

45/Fig. 9.—Skinner's wire frame mask.

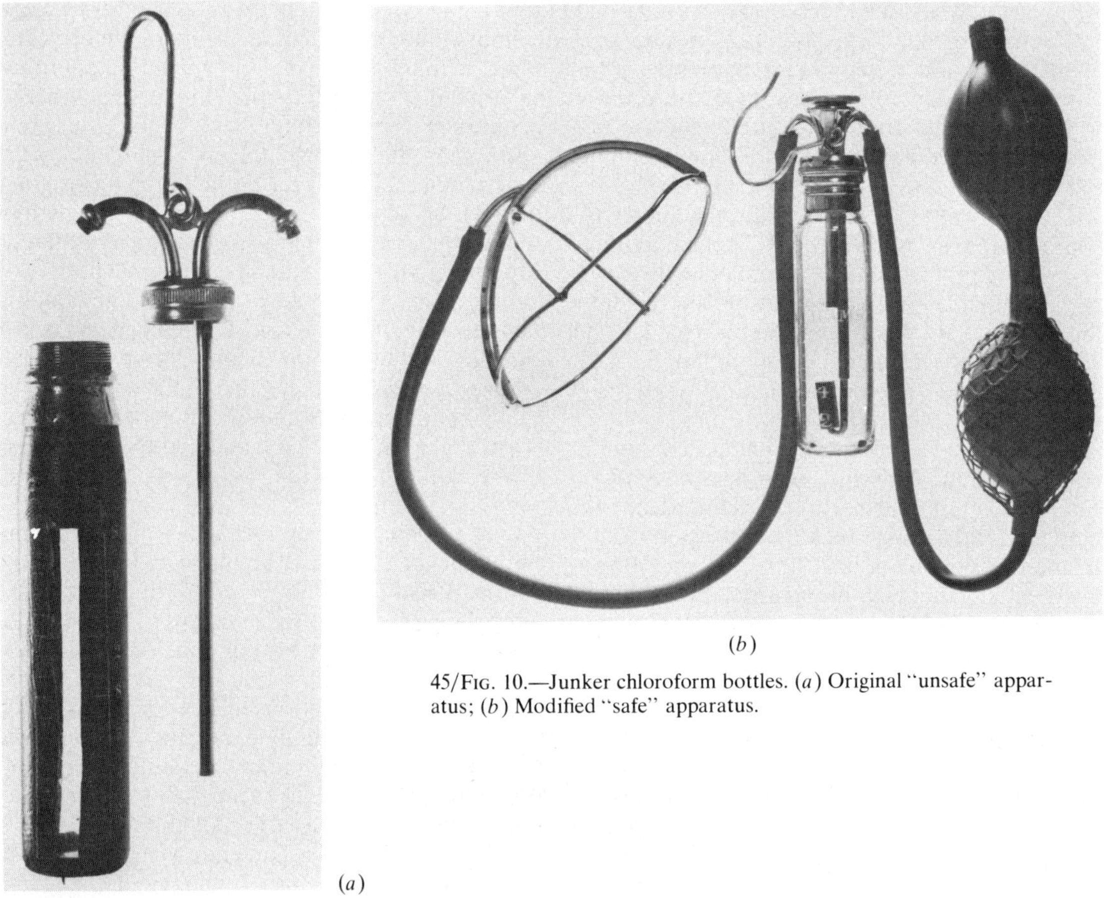

(*b*)

(*a*)

45/FIG. 10.—Junker chloroform bottles. (*a*) Original "unsafe" apparatus; (*b*) Modified "safe" apparatus.

when the patient was asleep.[44] The technique gained only limited popularity although Clover designed a specific apparatus for this purpose[45] and was replaced five years later when Clover introduced his portable regulating ether inhaler (Fig. 11). For the first time the amount of ether delivered to the patient could be regulated and the apparatus became very popular. It consisted of a metal sphere containing ether, onto which was soldered a water jacket; this sphere could be rotated round a central tube through which the patient breathed. By altering this rotation a variable amount of both inspiration and expiration passed through the vaporising chamber of the inhaler. Although graduated, the markings on the inhaler bore no relationship to percentage of vapour inhaled. When turned to the "F" mark, all of the tidal volume of the patient was diverted through the vaporising chamber. The apparatus was a fully closed circuit with no provision for carbon dioxide elimination or absorption, nor for the addition of air or oxygen. A reservoir bag was attached to the apparatus and often prefilled with nitrous oxide to facilitate the induction. When cyanosis occurred, the apparatus was removed from the patient's face and several breaths of room air allowed before replacing the inhaler back on the face. Clover deliberately designed the apparatus to exclude fresh air and felt that observation of the pulse, colour and respiratory pattern gave clear indication when air should be given to the patient. Clover claimed the equipment was economical, smooth and rapid in inducing patients and the majority of anaesthetists concurred.[46]

Soon everyone was producing modified Clover's Inhalers (in the same way as the wire

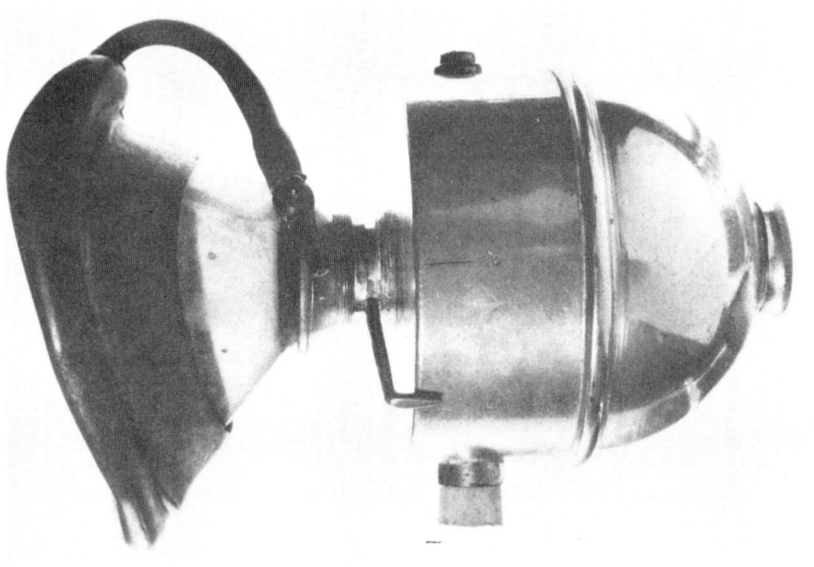

45/Fig. 11.—(*a*) Clover's portable regulating ether inhaler. (*b*) Cross-sectional diagram with valve fully closed. (*c*) Cross-sectional diagram with valve fully open. ((*b*) and (*c*) From *Anaesthetics and their Administration* by Sir Frederick W. Hewitt. Courtesy of Macmillan Publishers.)

frame masks and Junker's bottles) the most notable of which were the Ombredanne from France[47] and that of T. Wilson Smith.[48]

Barth, one of the main instrument makers in London at this time, were to introduce a simple valve apparatus, initially used to provide simple anaesthetics with nitrous oxide, but it quickly became associated with Clover's ether inhaler (Fig. 12).

The valve, with its attached mask and bag, permitted the anaesthetist to administer nitrous oxide with a complete rebreathing technique initially, and then by turning the control lever, allowed expired gas to escape to the atmosphere. Finally, the third control position permitted inspiration from room air instead of the reservoir bag.

The anaesthetist could thus vary the depth of his anaesthetic by turning a lever and without removing the apparatus from the patient's face. This valve arrangement, when used in conjunction with the Clover inhaler, made it a much simpler apparatus to use (Fig. 13).

One of the most far-reaching innovations in clinical anaesthesia to date was about to occur. At the Ophthalmological Conference in Heidelburg in 1884 Koller described the effects of a two per cent solution of cocaine instilled into the eye.[49] The following year Halstead and Hall in New York performed a mandibular nerve

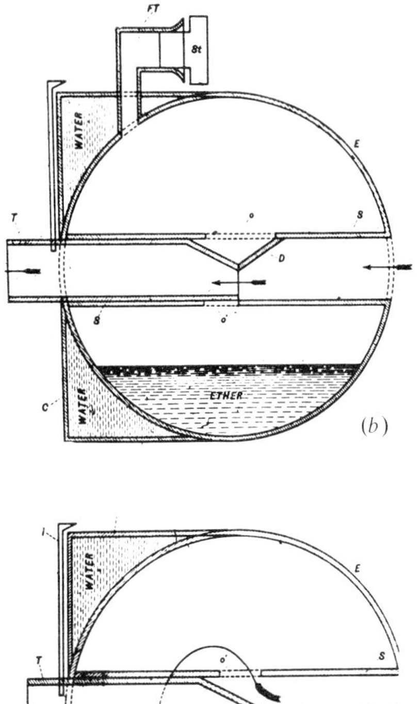


(*b*)

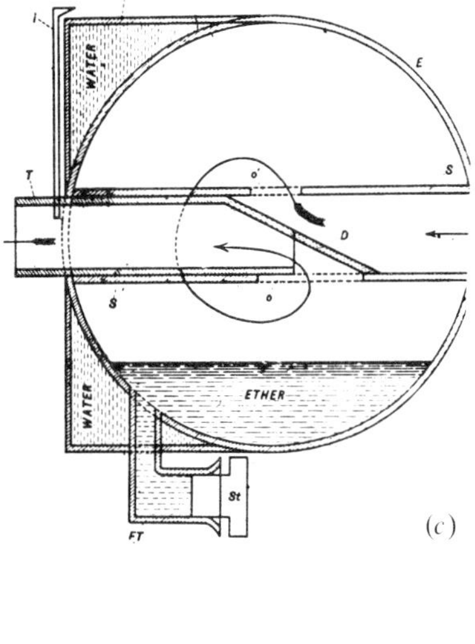


(*c*)

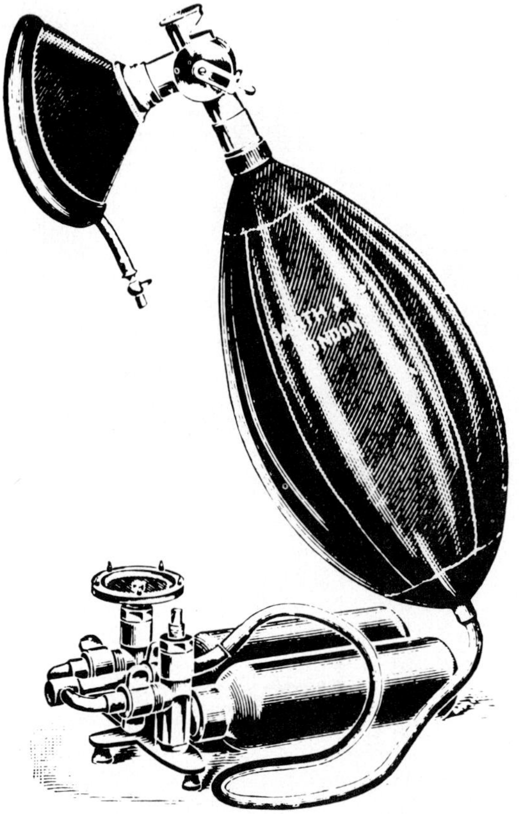

45/Fig. 12.—Barth valve and nitrous oxide cylinders. (Courtesy of Oxford University Press, in *Practical Anaesthetics*, by H. E. G. Boyle, Oxford Medical Manuals, 1911.)

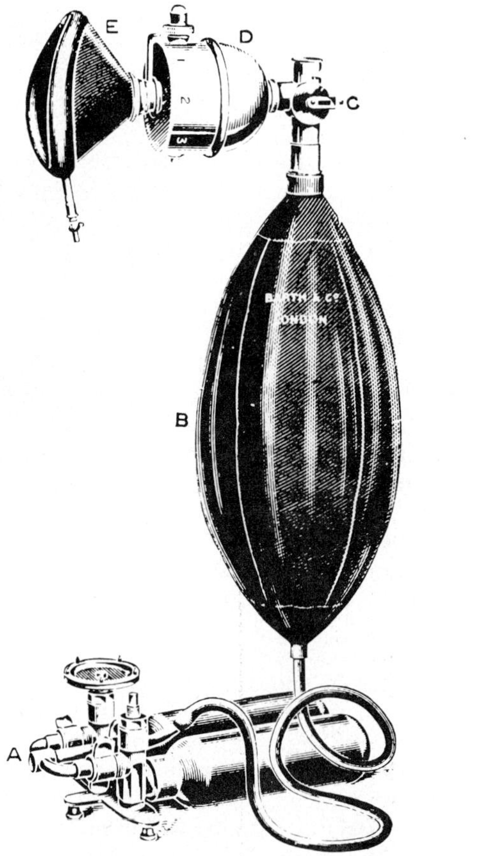


45/Fig. 13.—Clover's ether inhaler with Barth valve and nitrous oxide cylinders. (From *Anaesthetics Antient and Modern*, 75th Annual Meeting of the British Medical Association, Exeter, 1907. Courtesy of the Wellcome Trustees.)

block.[50] The medical profession were quick to take up the idea and cocaine was soon in use for all branches of operative surgery.[51] As with all new drugs, such a wide usage produced a series of reports of poisonings and caution was advocated with the agent.[52] Corning in New York, however, quickly demonstrated that by using tourniquets and thus arresting the circulation to an area, the duration of cocaine could be indefinitely prolonged and its side-effects minimised.[53] News of this research did not seemingly become known in Europe until much later.

Those who did not utilise this new concept still had the various volatile agents available. Gradually more and more concern was felt about the deaths occurring from chloroform. These could be divided into those that occurred on induction and those occurring later as a result of hepatic damage. Soon the anaesthetic world was divided into the chloroformers and the etherists both claiming that their particular agent was the safest and most effective. Most agreed that nitrous oxide was the safest of all but realised they could not prolong anaesthesia with this agent without incurring problems with hypoxia.

The debate on chloroform was to last some fifty years as society, after committee, after commission, investigated the toxic properties of the agent, each one producing clear evidence that chloroform had no effect on the heart when used in low concentrations and each one missing the point entirely.[54] Snow had pointed out the work of Glover in 1842 showing the effect of chloroform on the frog's heart and had repeated a great deal of the research himself[35] but despite this and the regular mortality, chloroform was to remain in everyday use for years to come (Fig. 14).

Many other anaesthetic agents were available for those who were tired of chloroform or ether; these included bromoform, amylene, methylene and bichloride of methylene. Each one had its protagonists and antagonists but none was to remain in clinical use for very long.

The eighteen nineties was a period when again much original work occurred with local anaesthetic techniques. Schleich was to introduce the concept of infiltration anaesthesia where isotonic saline solutions were injected subdermally and the oedematous tissue was found to be anaesthetised. This was later modified to use dilute cocaine solutions.[53] Within a few years Bier was to undergo spinal anaesthesia using 1 per cent cocaine based on the observations of Corning on dogs in 1885 and man in 1888[55] and the successful demonstration of lumbar puncture by Quincke in 1891.[56] Bier found, apart from a headache, that the technique produced excellent anaesthesia.[57] The process was rapidly popularised notably by Tuffier.[58]

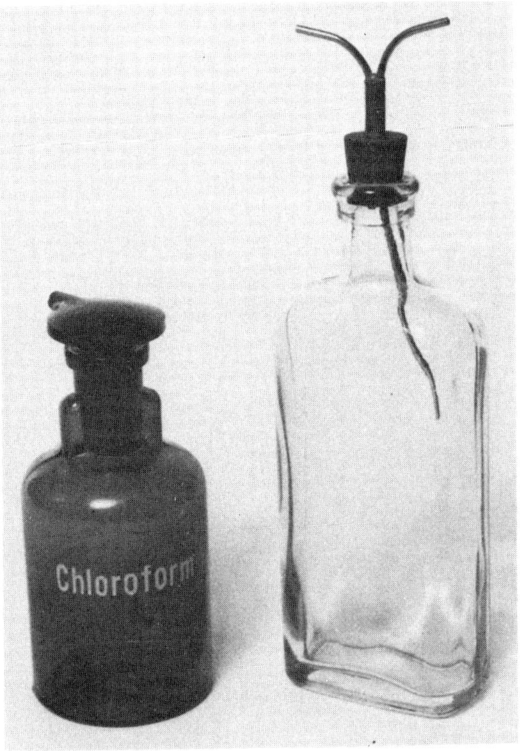


45/FIG. 14.—Chloroform and ether drop bottles. Note the difference in the size of the bottles. Essentially, ether drop bottles were larger than the chloroform bottles, reflecting the potency of chloroform.

There were other events occurring at this time that were to have far reaching effects later. Kirstein produced his direct vision laryngoscope in 1895 and Cushing had introduced anaesthetic record charts in the previous year. It was to be another American and inventor who would have perhaps the most far reaching effect on anaesthesia in the future.

Joseph O'Dwyer was appointed physician to the New York Foundling Hospital and was appalled by the death rate from croup or laryngeal diphtheria. The only treatment available was tracheostomy, a barbarous affair undertaken usually without anaesthesia in the end stages of asphyxiation. O'Dwyer developed a method of blind intubation of the larynx and despite much early criticism he persevered with his techniques. He published his results regularly and undertook extensive lecture tours to popularise the method (Fig. 15).[59,60] O'Dwyer manufactured adult tubes for the treatment of chronic laryngeal stenosis[61] and eventually collaborated with George Fell of Chicago to make the Fell-O'Dwyer apparatus. This early ventilator was made up of a bellows linked to an endotracheal tube by rubber tubing[62] and was eventually utilised in a modified form for thoracic anaesthesia by Matas and Madyl.[63] O'Dwyer was not the first to practise intubation but he, unlike his predecessors, notably MacEwen, was not discouraged by failure or criticism and persevered to popularise the technique.

The London Society of Anaesthetists was founded in 1893 by Silk and Dudley Buxton; this Society then became the notable Anaesthetic section of the Royal Society of Medicine in 1908. The Americans had by then founded the Long Island Society of Anesthetists under Erdmann which later evolved to a national body—the American Society of Anesthesiologists by 1945.

From the 1900's the speciality of anaesthetics began to develop even more rapidly in all fields. In local anaesthetic practice Sicard and Cathelin introduced caudal anaesthesia[64,65] while Braun

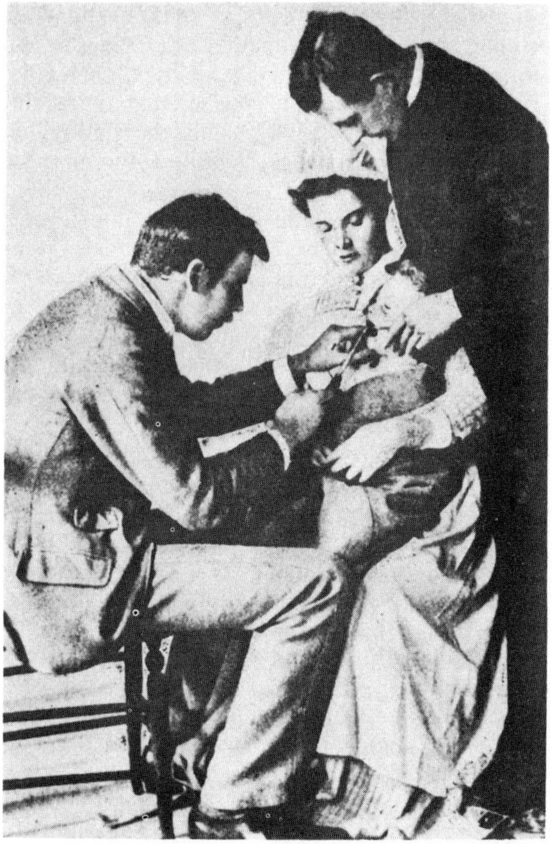

45/FIG. 15(*a*).—Method of intubation with O'Dwyer's apparatus.

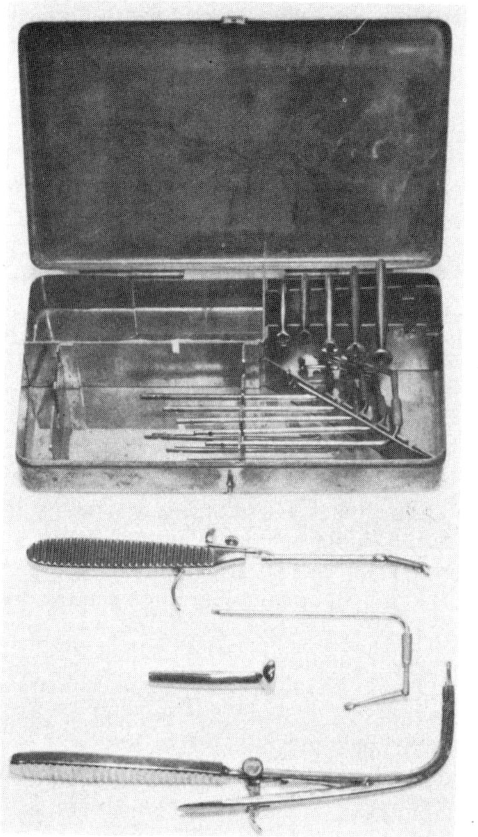

45/FIG. 15(*b*).—O'Dwyer's intubation set in case.

(*a*) and (*d*) Courtesy of British Medical Association, publishers of *British Medical Journal*, 1888.

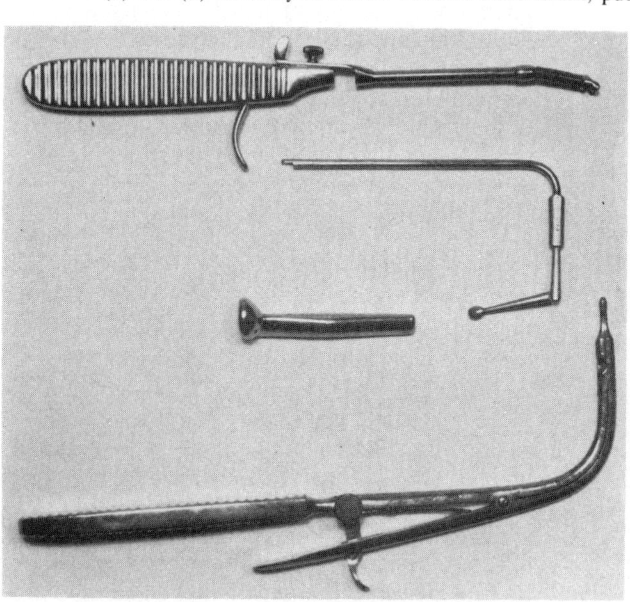

45/FIG. 15(*c*).—O'Dwyer's intubation apparatus.

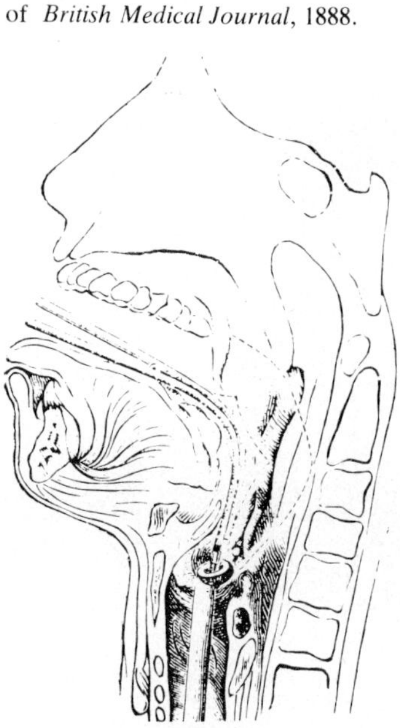

45/FIG. 15(*d*).—Intubation with O'Dwyer's apparatus.

firstly popularised the use of adrenaline combined with cocaine to achieve the same results as Corning some twenty years earlier and then did extensive clinical work on procaine in 1907, which had been suggested by Einhorn as a less toxic alternative to cocaine some two years earlier. At the same time Barker, a surgeon at University College Hospital, introduced "heavy" solutions of local anaesthetics for use in spinal blocks.[66] He was also to design a characteristic spinal needle (Fig. 16).

There were also developments taking place with inhalational anaesthesia. Hewitt produced a wide-bore modification of Clover's Inhaler in which, by increasing the internal diameter of the control tube, he felt that he had reduced the incidence of stertor and cyanosis occasioned by its use. He too advocated the use of a nitrous oxide induction and devised an ingenious stopcock to facilitate this process. The Hewitt inhaler also had the design advantage of the central tubes rotating within the fixed vaporising chamber, together with the ability to refill the apparatus during the anaesthetic. A smaller water reservoir was incorporated which meant the vaporiser had to be warmed before use.[67] Essentially the apparatus had the same failings as the original Clover (Fig. 17).

The chloroformists were busy developing vaporisers which limited the inspired concentration to below what they believed was the danger level of two per cent in air. One of the most popular of these was that designed by Vernon Harcourt. This apparatus was said to deliver not more than two per cent chloroform in air regardless of the respiratory volumes. It was calibrated as accurate over a specific temperature range and incorporated a form of thermometer in the vaporising chamber. This consisted of two special beads which floated or sank depending on the temperature of the liquid chloroform; the glass bottle containing the liquid could be heated on some models by the use of a candle to achieve the correct working temperature—this heating must have increased the levels of phosgene delivered considerably! However, the apparatus demonstrates many sophisticated design points that would be incorporated in later equipment notably its air bypass, temperature compensation, and compensation for the fall in chloroform levels by tapering the glass bottle in which it was held (Fig. 18).[68]

Research was taking place that was finally to prove the dangers of chloroform anaesthesia. Initially this was led by Dudley Buxton who

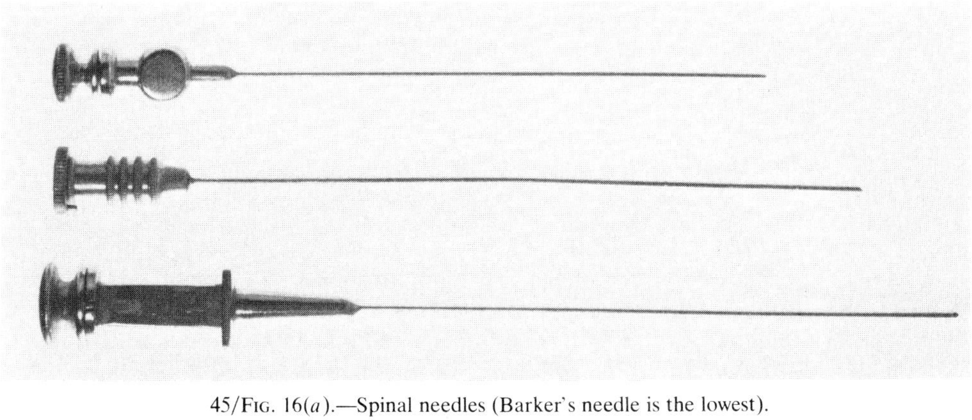

45/FIG. 16(*a*).—Spinal needles (Barker's needle is the lowest).

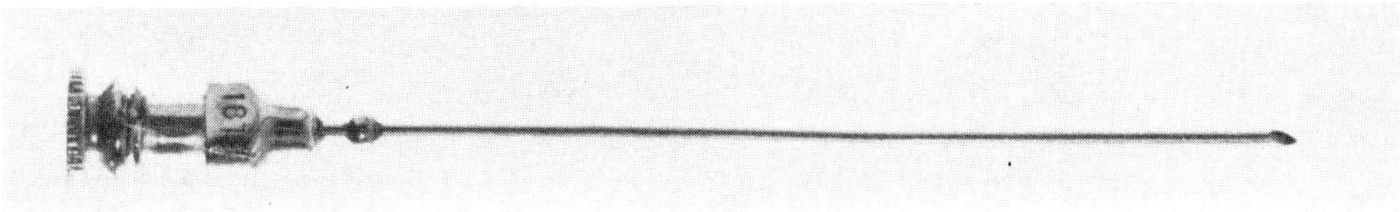

45/FIG. 16(*b*).—Caudal needle.

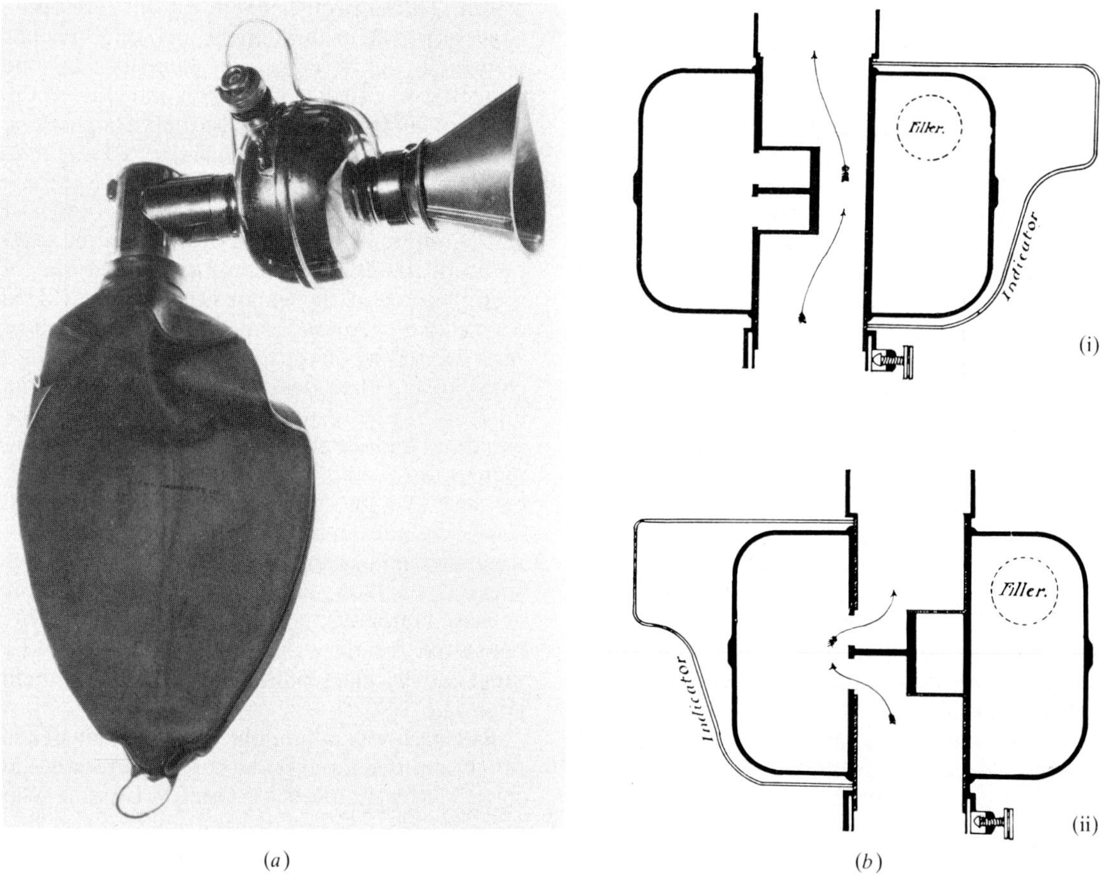


45/Fig. 17.—Hewitt's wide-bore modification of Clover's inhaler. (*a*) The inhaler; (*b*) Cross-section of apparatus: (i) Valve closed; (ii) valve open. ((*b*) From *Anaesthetics and Their Administration* by Sir Frederick W. Hewitt. Courtesy of Macmillan Publishers.)

campaigned constantly on the dangers of chloroform anaesthesia and was particularly scathing about the Hyderabad Commission reports. At a later date Embley working in Melbourne showed that chloroform produced vagal inhibition in morphinised dogs and stated that this was abolished by atropinisation.[69] He did not, however, advocate the use of atropine as a premedicant in man. It is interesting to note that routine premedication of patients was developing at this stage in Great Britain using morphine and hyoscine in an attempt to give a smoother ether anaesthetic, thus avoiding chloroform altogether.[70]

Following O'Dwyer's work, endotracheal anaesthesia was becoming more and more popular. Much of the early work was done in Europe and various endotracheal tubes were designed; one of the foremost exponents of this technique was Kuhn in Germany. This surgeon did extensive work on blind intubation with anaesthesia and produced some excellent apparatus for the purpose.[63]

America was to provide yet another innovation in this field with the development of intratracheal insufflation anaesthesia. Meltzer and Auer (1909)[71] working with dogs at the Rockefeller Institute, New York, showed that a continuous flow of air passing into the lungs via a tube placed in the trachea would keep the animal alive indefinitely, even when respiration was abolished with curare. With the addition of a bottle of ether to this circuit, anaesthesia could be induced and maintained. The tech-

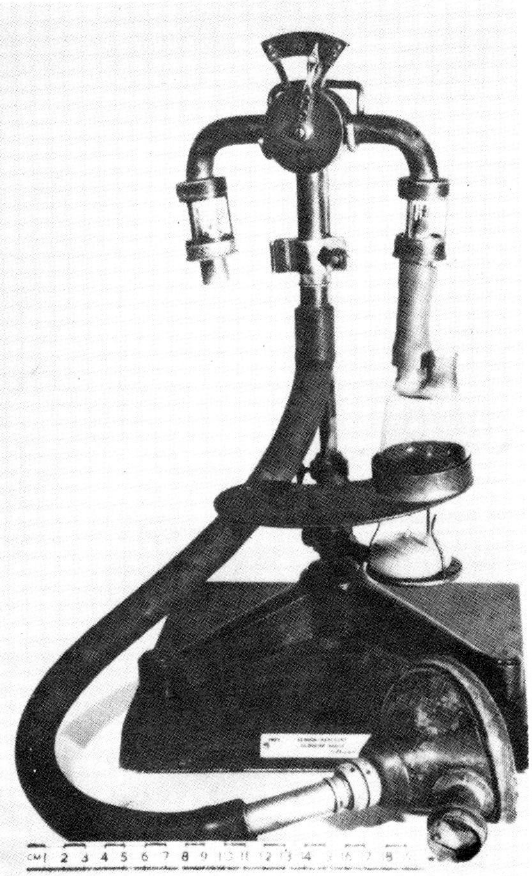

45/FIG. 18.—VERNON HARCOURT CHLOROFORM INHALER (1903)

Air is drawn through two unidirectional metal flap valves in glass cylinders on the side-arms, one connected to the chloroform-containing bottle. The two streams are controlled and mixed in the drum in the centre and then drawn by the patient down the centre tube to the face-mask. (Courtesy of the late Dr. K. Bryn Thomas and Blackwell Scientific Publications.[19])

nique was first adapted to human anaesthesia by Elsberg[72] and demonstrated in England by Kelly the following year. The equipment was highly complex and comprised a source of air (either an electric or a foot pump), a system of tubes linked to an ether reservoir and mercury manometer, a humidifier and a method of automatic blow-off should the pressure in the tube rise too high. This technique was especially valuable in thoracic and head and neck anaesthesia and also in those operations where it was necessary for the patient to be kept prone.

Intubation of these patients was facilitated by the laryngoscope recently developed by Chevalier Jackson. This had a straight blade and a light source which gave an excellent view of the larynx either under ether anaesthesia or after topical cocaine applications.

These insufflation techniques were largely to replace the need for the sedation provided by rectally administered ether in oil, which had until now been one of the few satisfactory techniques for head and neck surgery. Early work by Pirogoff in 1847 and Buxton in 1885 had been unsatisfactory owing to local tissue damage which often resulted in severe rectal bleeding. However Gwathmey's introduction of ether and olive oil per rectum in 1913 was very successful and many thousands of cases were performed using this method.[73]

It was at this time that McKesson of Toledo, Ohio, introduced his nitrous oxide and oxygen apparatus. This was a demand flow machine, the first of its kind and could generate any combination of oxygen and nitrous oxide required on a breath by breath basis.[74] McKesson believed that a degree of rebreathing and thus carbon dioxide retention was beneficial and this was an integral part of his equipment. The nitrous oxide or oxygen was fed via a reducing valve to a reservoir bag encased in two round discs. When the reservoir bag was filled the influx of fresh gas was stopped by means of a pinch valve. Inspiration by the patient triggered a demand valve which then allowed the patient to inhale a mixture of nitrous oxide and oxygen, as preset by a large dial on the top of the machine, from the two reservoirs. As soon as either gas was inhaled by the patient, fresh gas would refill the reservoir bags from the cylinders. The machine had a dial allowing the apparatus to be used in a continuous flow mode, instead of as a demand flow apparatus, and an oxygen bypass button. McKesson was to make regular modifications of this sophisticated apparatus over the next twenty years and even published textbooks on nitrous oxide and oxygen anaesthesia in dentistry (Fig. 19).[75]

McKesson was not the only person to develop apparatus for nitrous oxide and oxygen administration. Hewitt in England with his stopcock of 1893 and White of Philadelphia (1910) were both influenced by the writings of Paul Bert in

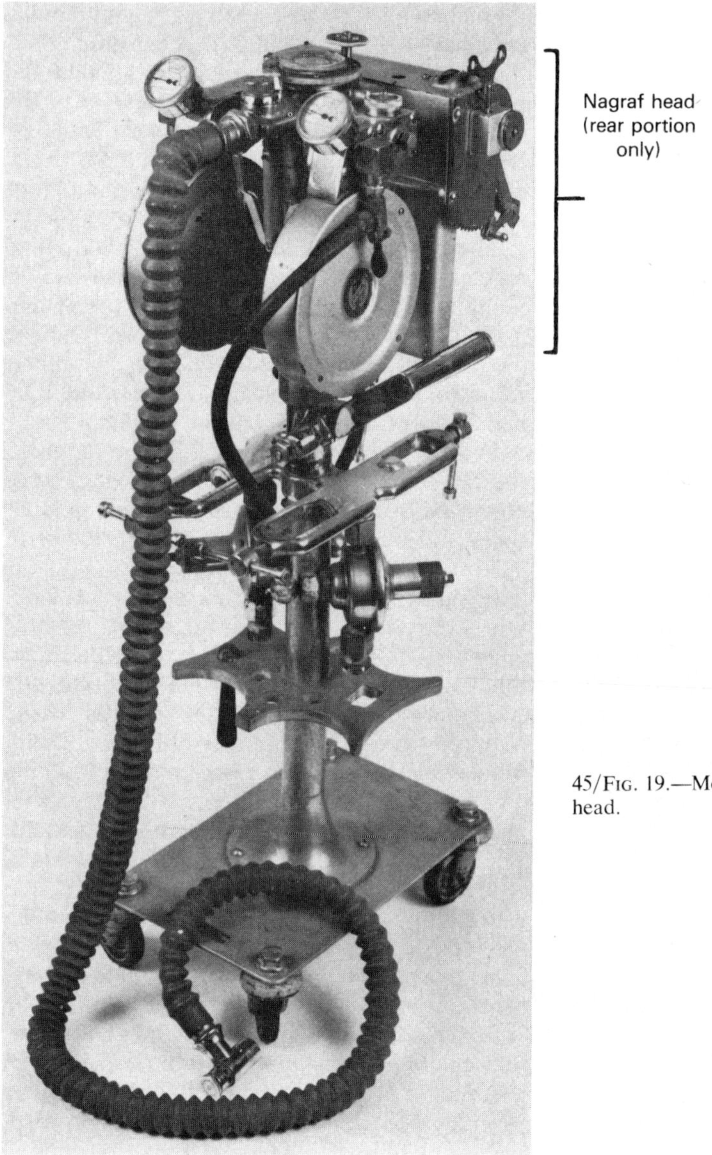


45/FIG. 19.—McKesson apparatus, with indicating Nagraf head.

the 1860's and Edmund Andrews of Chicago in 1868. All were convinced that nitrous oxide anaesthesia was improved by adding oxygen, but the idea was slow in coming to fruition. Following the introduction of McKesson's machine it was Gwathmey who was to make the next advances in this field. He developed his nitrous oxide and oxygen apparatus based on that of Cotton and Boothby (1912)[76] which he then persuaded Boyle to use. Their friendship, initially made in 1912 at the American Anesthetic Congress, was renewed when they met at the American Red Cross Hospital in France during the first world war. On returning to England in 1917 Boyle continued to use the Gwathmey apparatus bought by the Governors of St. Bartholomew's Hospital.[77] Being an American machine, there were a few drawbacks, especially in fitting British cylinders. To overcome this problem Boyle asked Coxeter to modify the Gwathmey, and they then developed the apparatus that was to become known as the Boyle's machine. Used for the first time at St. Bartholomew's Hospital in November 1917[78] it was then gradually modified by Boyle over the next twenty years, eventually evolving to the apparatus familiar to all anaesthetists today (Fig. 20).

An almost identical machine was designed by Geoffrey Marshall of Guy's Hospital at the same time whilst he too was working in France at the No. 17 Casualty Clearing Station, but Boyle was to publish his accounts before Marshall who waited until a clinical trial had been completed.[79] In a paper Boyle even pays tribute to Marshall's help in the use of this apparatus in France.[80]

The major modifications were the addition of a chloroform bottle, the development of plungers to facilitate ether vaporisation, the introduction of the dry bobbin flowmeters and finally the rotameters we are familiar with today. The early bubbling water-sight flowmeters were to solve some of the early respiratory problems encountered with ether anaesthesia related to the dry cylinder gases.

Sir Francis Shipway had attempted to overcome these problems in a different way in 1916 with his apparatus for delivering warmed ether and chloroform. The vapour was passed through a thermos flask filled with hot water but the ether, chloroform and air never directly came into contact with the warm water (Fig. 21).[81]

Most equipment designers, like Boyle and Shipway, continued to make minor changes in their apparatus throughout their clinical lives. Even the provision for chloroform anaesthesia was retained despite the work of Goodman Levy at this time. Levy showed the correlation between ventricular fibrillation and light chloroform anaesthesia in the presence of high circulating catecholamine levels.[82] This mechanism of myocardial sensitisation produced by chloroform explained the deaths on induction of anaesthesia that were so commonplace in the anxious unpremedicated patients at that time.

Gradually chloroform fell into disrepute and now few people in the Western World continue to use this agent. A good case can be made that with modern techniques of induction and well-designed vaporisers, chloroform and oxygen anaesthesia has much to recommend it.[83]

In America in the twenties, Guedel was to publish his observations made during and after the first world war on the clinical signs of ether anaesthesia.[84] These were to supplant the work of Snow and Plomley of 1847 and gave a simple guide to the depth of anaesthesia created.

In England, Magill and Rowbotham were providing anaesthesia for Gillies at the Plastics Unit in Sidcup. Starting with the techniques of intratracheal insufflation described by Elsberg and Kelly, they were firstly to develop a double-lumen insufflation catheter and, eventually, the concept of a wide-bore, soft rubber tube to allow the normal respiratory pattern (Fig. 22). This more physiological approach gained rapid widespread acceptance.[85] Magill was also to develop his simple delivery system for anaesthetic vapour as a means to keep out of the surgeons' way.[86] This circuit was soon to replace all previous methods of administration. Blind nasal intubation was another technique popularised by Magill, although it was Kuhn in Germany who was the first to write in detail on the technique some ten years previously.

Not all anaesthetists wished to have complex, unwieldy machines with heavy cylinders to carry round. Kenneth Pinson was to describe his "ether bomb" in 1921 as an alternative to these. A device which produced 100 per cent warmed ether vapour it was, like Shipway's apparatus, claimed to decrease postoperative respiratory problems[87] whilst needing no bellows or nitrous oxide delivery system.

The *British Journal of Anaesthesia* was published in 1923 and remained the sole specialist anaesthetic journal until 1940 when *Anesthesiology* appeared followed by *Anaesthesia* in 1947.

Inhalational anaesthesia was to receive yet another American innovation with the "to and fro" canister of Waters' closed-circuit system filled with soda-lime to absorb the carbon dioxide.[88] The use of carbon dioxide absorption in anaesthesia was first reported in 1868. Slaked lime was used by a dental surgeon in London called Alfred Coleman during nitrous oxide inhalations. This prolonged the use that could be made of the then expensive gas, as no metabolism of nitrous oxide took place during inhalation. This technique was used extensively at St. Bartholomew's and the London Dental Hospital for several years, but eventually Coleman gave up the method.[89] The Waters system was modified by Sword to the circle system[90]

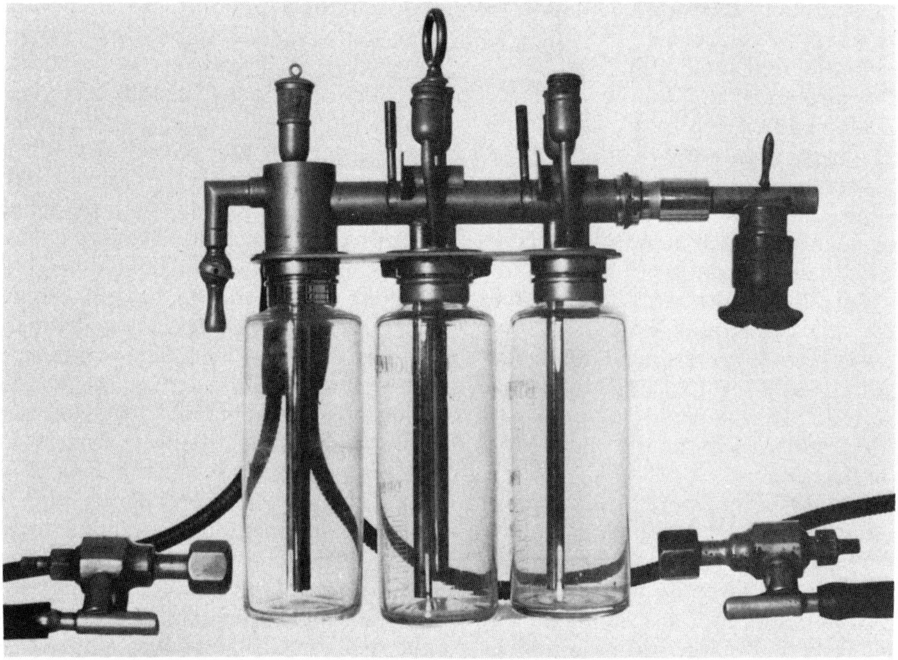

(*a*)

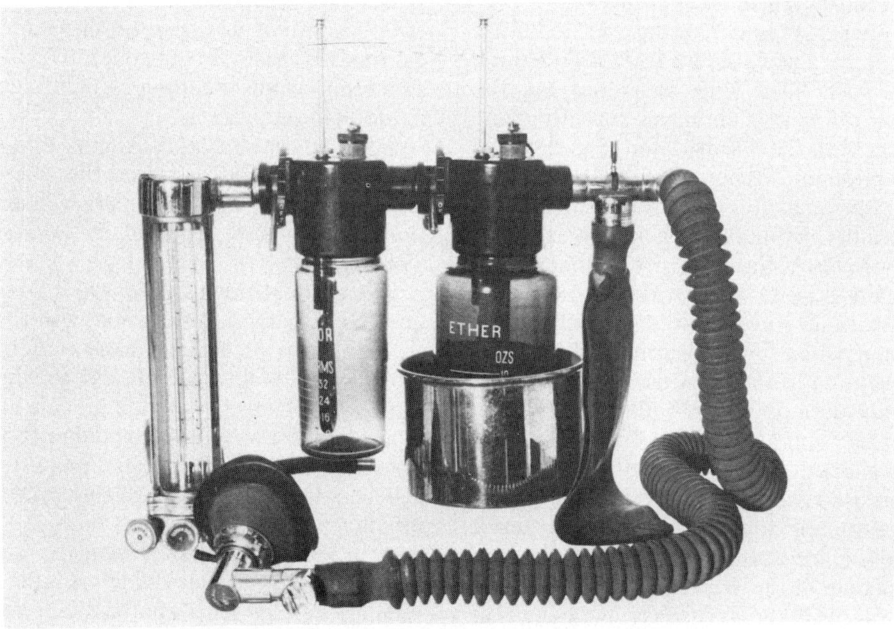


(*b*)

45/Fig. 20.—Boyle's machine.
(*a*) Early model showing water sight flowmeter; (*b*) Later model showing Coxeter dry bobbin flowmeter.

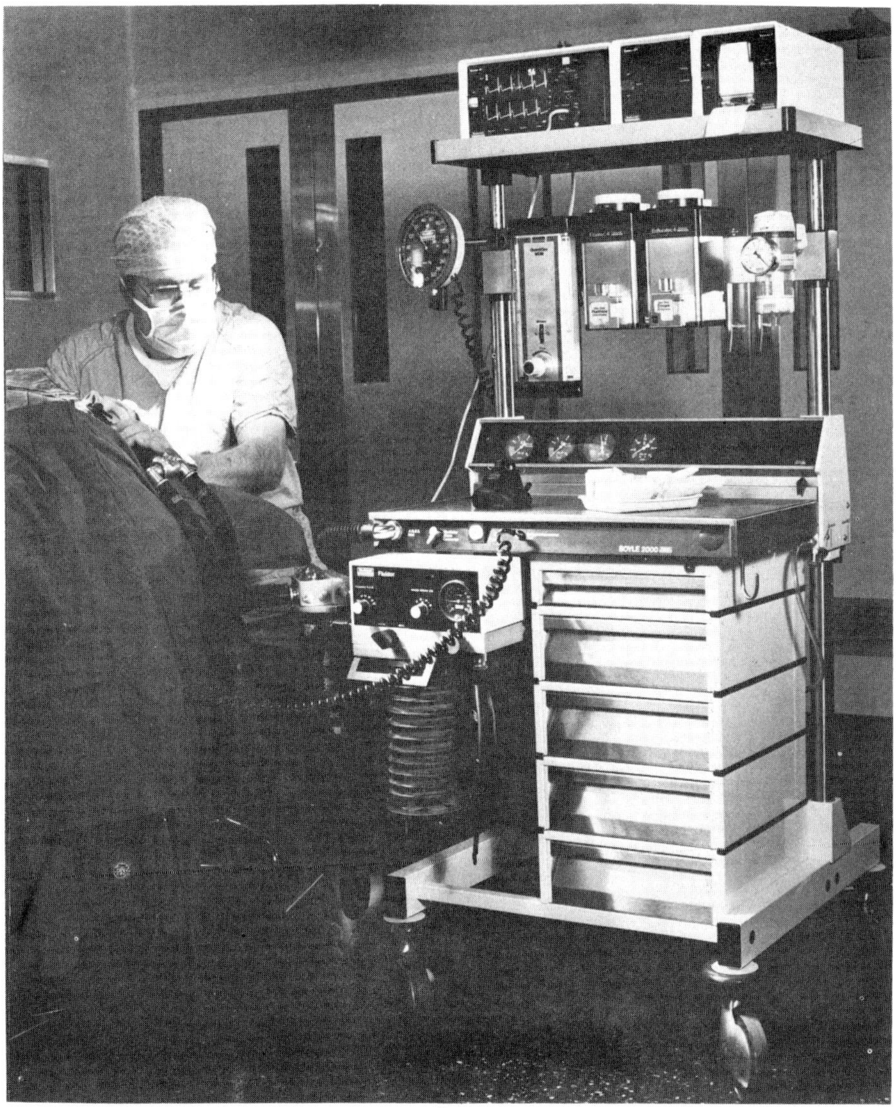

(*c*)

45/FIG. 20.—(*c*) Modern Boyle's machine. (Courtesy of Medishield.)

both circuits achieving world-wide popularity. Within a few years cuffed endotracheal tubes became available to "close" the circuit fully[91] and cyclopropane was then introduced for use primarily with the same circuit.[92]

The greatest development in the twenties and thirties was undoubtedly the introduction of intravenous barbiturates to induce anaesthesia. Chloral hydrate had been given by this route in 1872 in Lyons, France[93] and others had tried intravenous ether and chloroform.[94] Bardet used Somnifaine, a mixture of two barbiturates, with good results both on the Continent and in England[95] but it was the introduction of Per-

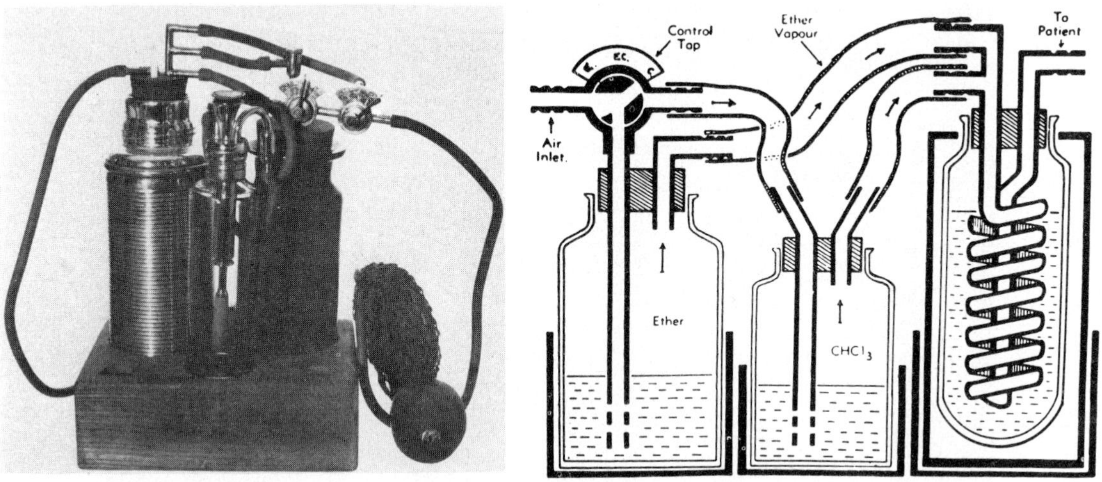


(*a*) (*b*)

45/FIG. 21.—(*a*) Shipway's insufflation apparatus; (*b*) Cross-section of apparatus. (From *Anaesthetic Methods*, 1946, by G. Kaye *et al.* Ramsay, Melbourne.[21])

nocton that was finally to assure the success of this technique.[96] The traumatic second stage of an inhalational anaesthetic sequence could now be bypassed and the search for newer agents continued. Amytal was the next to appear[97] while hexobarbitone was recorded as being used over twelve million times in its first twelve years.[98]

The introduction of thiopentone in America was to replace the majority of intravenous induction agents very quickly,[99] with the first use of the drug in England being recorded by Jarman.[100]

Local anaesthesia, too, was still evolving new techniques. Dogliotti in Italy popularised lumbar epidural anaesthesia[101] which had been described some ten years previously by the Spanish (Fig. 23).[102]

Obstetric anaesthetists were still searching for a method to provide safe analgesia for childbirth, preferably for use by unsupervised midwives. Chloroform was still in use for this purpose either from "brisettes", small ampoules of chloroform in gauze rolls[103] or from a Mennell chloroform inhaler, another modification of the Junker bottle.[104] The use of a drug, generally felt to be unsafe, by unsupervised midwives was not encouraged by the Royal College of Obstetricians and Minnitt was invited by the Liverpool Maternity Hospital to investigate the

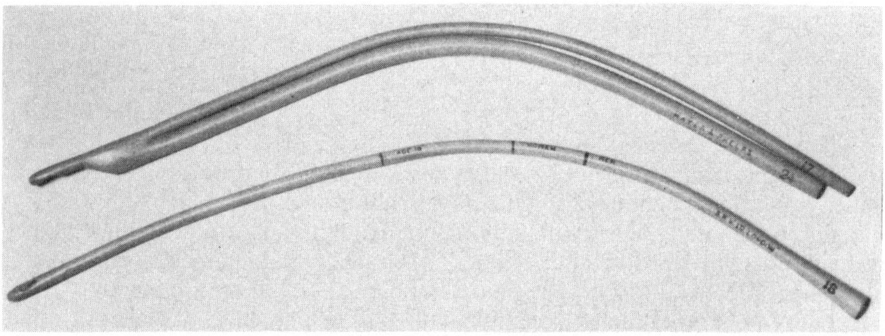

45/FIG. 22.—Magill's insufflation catheters.

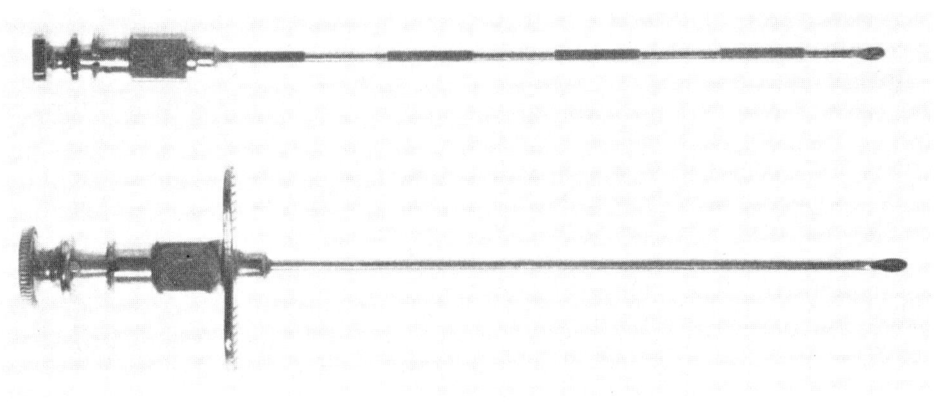

45/Fig. 23.—Epidural needles.

possibility of manufacturing a nitrous oxide apparatus for use in this field. He discussed the problem with Charles King, the instrument maker in London, and the first machine was used in Liverpool in October, 1933. It was a modified McKesson machine, utilising the nitrous oxide half of the apparatus and permitting air entrainment to dilute the nitrous oxide. Minnitt modified this machine several times and a whole series of so-called "gas and air" equipment was developed.[105] The apparatus was an instant success and was recognised by the Central Midwives Board for general use (Fig. 24).

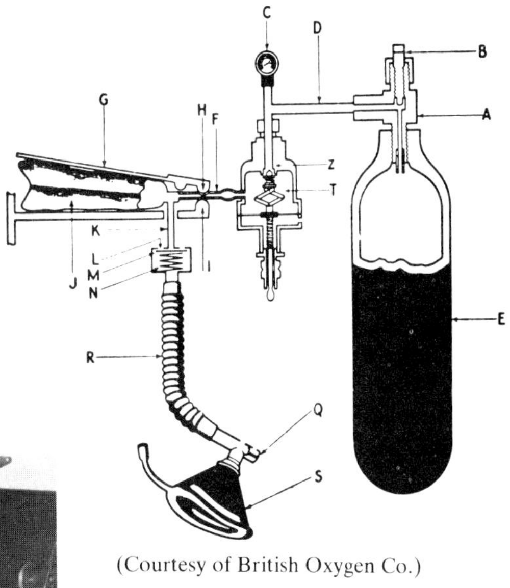


(Courtesy of British Oxygen Co.)

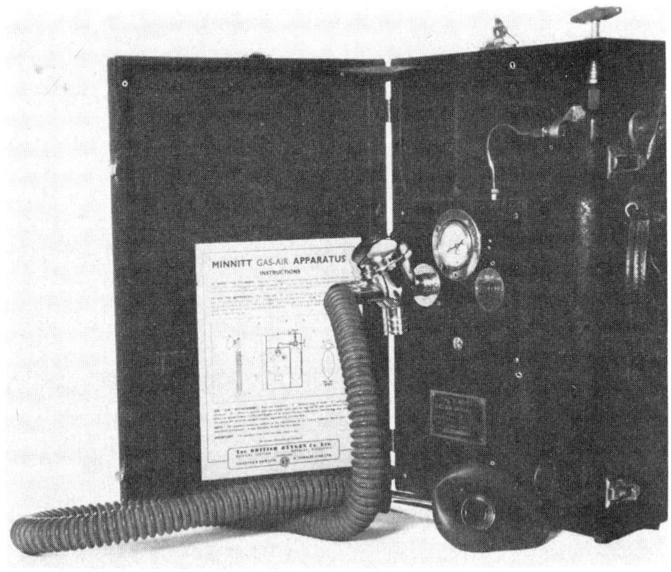


45/Fig. 24.—Minnitt's apparatus. (*left*) Minnitt's portable analgesia apparatus; (*above*) Cross-section of same apparatus.

It was to take thirty years for the medical profession to realise that hypoxic mixtures were inhaled with this machine.[106]

Like the first world war, the second was to provide further impetus for research. Pethidine was introduced in 1939 and trichloroethylene (Trilene) in 1941. Trilene had been used intermittently since 1911 but the need for a cheap, potent inhalational analgesic anaesthetic led the Medical Research Council to ask Hewer to investigate the agent. His favourable report led to its clinical introduction[107] its usefulness limited mainly by its slow induction when used as the sole agent. A plethora of Trilene and air machines were to follow in the next few years for self-administered analgesia. These included the Freedman inhaler, the Trilite inhaler, Burns Benson inhaler, Siebe Gorman-Hyatt inhaler, the Emotril and the Tecota Mark 6 inhalers. Only these latter two inhalers were passed as safe for use in obstetrics by the Central Midwives Board because of their temperature compensation, robust nature and accuracy at different flow rates (Fig. 25).

The war also demonstrated the need for portable anaesthetic machines for use in difficult circumstances or where cylinders of oxygen and nitrous oxide were not available. Such equipment had to be light, robust (perhaps to withstand a parachute drop) and yet accurate and reliable.

The machine that evolved to fill this need was

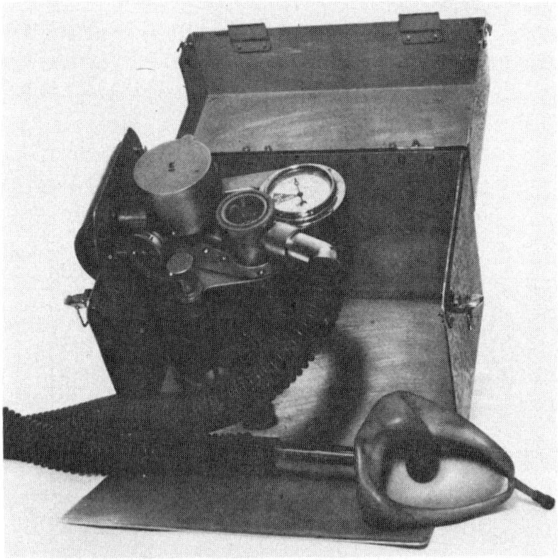

(*a*)

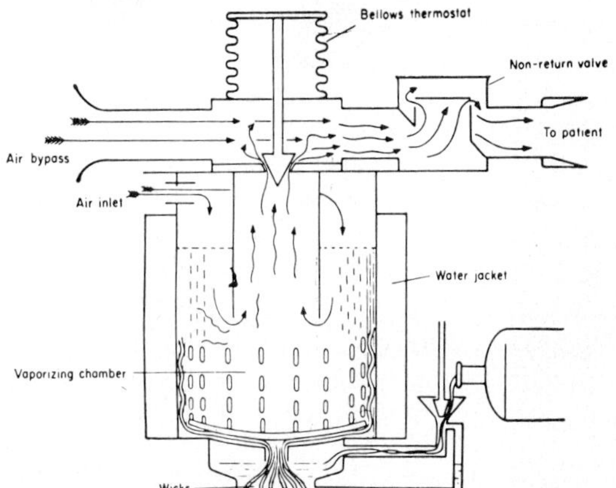


(*b*)

45/FIG. 25.—(*a*) Emotril inhaler; (*b*) Cross-sectional diagram of Emotril inhaler. ((*b*) Courtesy of Medical and Industrial Equipment Ltd.)

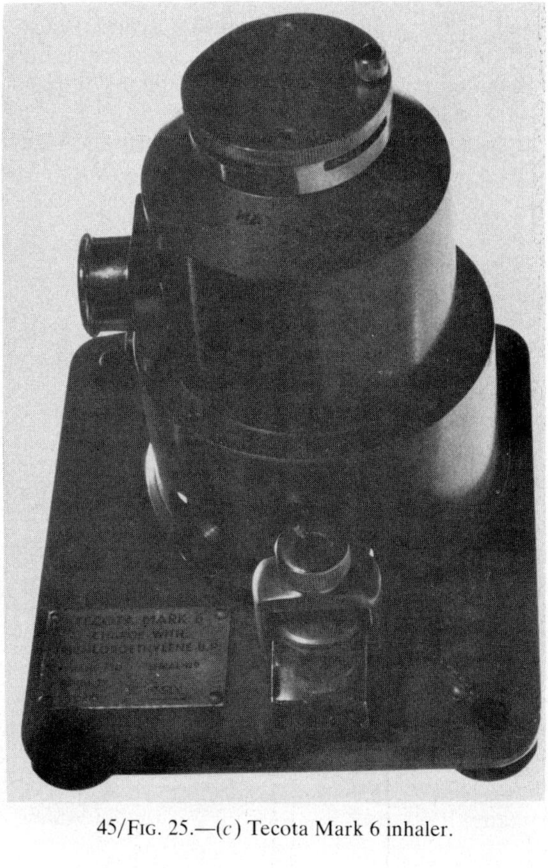

45/FIG. 25.—(*c*) Tecota Mark 6 inhaler.

the Oxford Vaporiser designed by Macintosh in 1941.[108] This apparatus had a calcium chloride heat-sink and was extremely popular. It was to be modified after the war to become the E.M.O. inhaler, possibly the most widely used anaesthetic machine in the world.[109]

Both machines were draw-over vaporisers which could be modified by the addition of bellows to become suitable for positive-pressure ventilation. The E.M.O. has a built in temperature compensation bellows system in addition to a water-bath heat reservoir (Fig. 26).

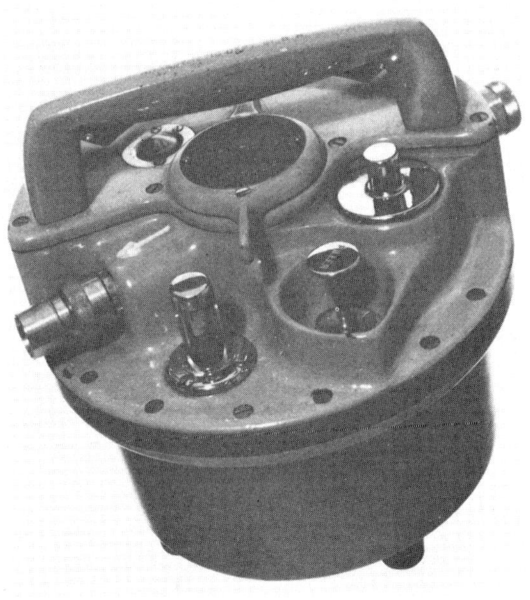

45/Fig. 26.—E.M.O. vaporiser.

The most dramatic innovation at this time, however, was the introduction of curare into clinical practice by Griffith and Johnson in Montreal, Canada. It seems incredible that it took 30 years after Meltzer and Auer had curarised dogs before others thought of the possibilities for clinical anaesthesia. Muscle relaxants were to make surgical procedures possible at a much lighter plane of anaesthesia and enhance postoperative recovery.[110] The short-acting muscle relaxants were to follow very quickly, decamethonium in 1949[111] and suxamethonium and gallamine in the same year.[112,113] Endotracheal intubation was to become a much simpler process using these drugs.

The next refinement in anaesthetic practice was the introduction of deliberate or controlled hypotension. The first technique was based on postural changes under total spinal block.[114] This was followed by arteriotomy pioneered by Hale[115] and refined in neurosurgical anaesthesia later.[116] Ganglion blocking agents, such as penta- and hexamethonium, were the next development.[117,118]

The 1950's saw the development of a large number of machines for intermittent positive-pressure ventilation. The Spiropulsator of Frenckner and Crafoord was received with little enthusiasm in England or America. The anaesthetists at that time had learnt to "feel" their way through an anaesthetic by the resistance of the reservoir bag of their closed circuit. This method had been popularised with cyclopropane anaesthesia[119] and the introduction of muscle relaxants had done little to change matters. Blease in 1945 developed a prototype pulmoflator designed to replace manual ventilation[120] but it took many years for the profession to adjust to the use of these machines. As curare became more and more widespread further ventilators followed, notably the Aintree[121] and the Fazakerley[122] in England. The Copenhagen poliomyelitis epidemic of 1952 provided yet further impetus for research and the Engström ventilator was developed in Sweden and the Beaver and Radcliffe ventilators in England.

In France in the 1950's Laborit was working on his lytic cocktail, a mixture of sparine, pethidine and chlorpromazine, which was to be a precursor of neuroleptanaesthesia and analgesia.[123] The term "neuroleptanalgesia" was used by Castro and Mundeleer to describe the state of neurovegetative block induced by the combination of powerful analgesics, such as fentanyl and phenoperidine, with sedatives of the butyrophenone type such as haloperidol and droperidol.[124]

Newer inhalational agents were then developed. Halothane was to provide a fast induction and recovery compared with its predecessors and quickly became the most popular anaesthetic agent in the world.[125] Initially administered from a Boyle's bottle, the development of the temperature compensated Fluotecs soon followed. The current Marks II III and IV have replaced the ill-fated Mark I which was introduced in 1957.[126] The Fluotecs utilise a bimetallic strip as a temperature compensation device and the later models are accurate at low flows and varying pressures (Fig. 27).

B.O.C. were to produce the Halox vaporiser as a variation of the copper kettle introduced by Lucien Morris in 1952.[127] This Halox apparatus was not universally popular owing to problems of rapid changes in temperature during use and has subsequently ceased to be manufactured (Fig. 28).

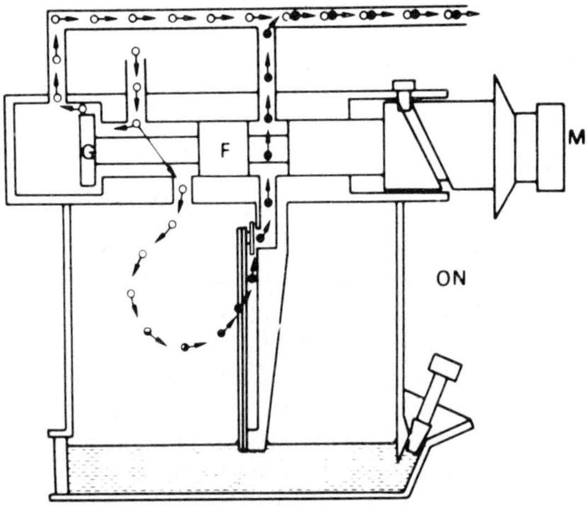


45/FIG. 27.—Fluotec Mark II vaporiser. (Courtesy of Dr. C. S. Ward and Baillière Tindall, publishers of *Anaesthetic Equipment: Physical Principles and Maintenance*.)

A simple vaporiser for use as draw-over or within closed circuit systems was designed by Goldman. It had no form of temperature compensation but has retained its popularity in its field.[128,129] A similar pattern vaporiser was used originally with a Minnitt's gas and air apparatus. This Rowbotham bottle is now used in a similar manner to the Goldman (Fig. 29).[130]

To speed the normally slow induction of ether with an EMO vaporiser the Bryce Smith induction unit using halothane was introduced (Fig. 30).[131]

It is still too early to say what the final outcome of the debate on halothane-induced jaundice will be but perhaps in the future this agent will be removed from clinical practice much the same as chloroform.[132] Other new inhalational agents followed halothane, methoxyflurane initially[133] then enflurane and isoflurane within a few years.[134]

Intravenous anaesthesia has seen many barbiturate drugs used in clinical practice but only methohexitone remains to challenge thiopentone.[135] There was a need for shorter-acting induction agents and many non-barbiturate drugs were investigated. Steroids were shown to have anaesthetic properties[136] and hydroxydione became available.[137] It was to be withdrawn quite quickly because of the high incidence of thrombophlebitis and its lack of potency. Althesin, a mixture of alphaxalone and alphadolone replaced this agent. It was found to be very potent, quickly metabolised and with a high safety margin.[138] The correlation between its use and a relatively high incidence of allergic responses have cast some doubt on the long-term future of this agent. The eugenol derivative propanidid seems to have suffered a similar fate after early enthusiasm.

Dissociative anaesthesia was introduced with the clinical use of phencyclidine.[139] This cataleptic state incorporating profound analgesia with amnesia also produced severe psychotic states on emergence with this drug. It was replaced by ketamine[140] whose emergence phenomena can be attenuated by the use of amnesic agents such as lorazepam.[141]

The introduction of ketamine anaesthesia has meant that complex surgical procedures can take place, if necessary, without any anaesthetic equipment at all except for a syringe and needle. This is a complete circle in a way from the days when all the anaesthetist needed was a dropper bottle and his handkerchief to continue his work.

As a speciality, anaesthesia appears to be in a relatively static state at present with the majority of research trying to improve and refine the various aspects of inhalational, intravenous and local anaesthesia and in the development of more efficient items of equipment. It seems likely that we are ready for a fundamental change in anaesthesia (such as came with the introduction of cocaine or curare) and perhaps that will come from the work on the endogenous opiates, endorphins and enkephalins.

Undoubtedly the anaesthetist of the future will be amused by the didactic statements of

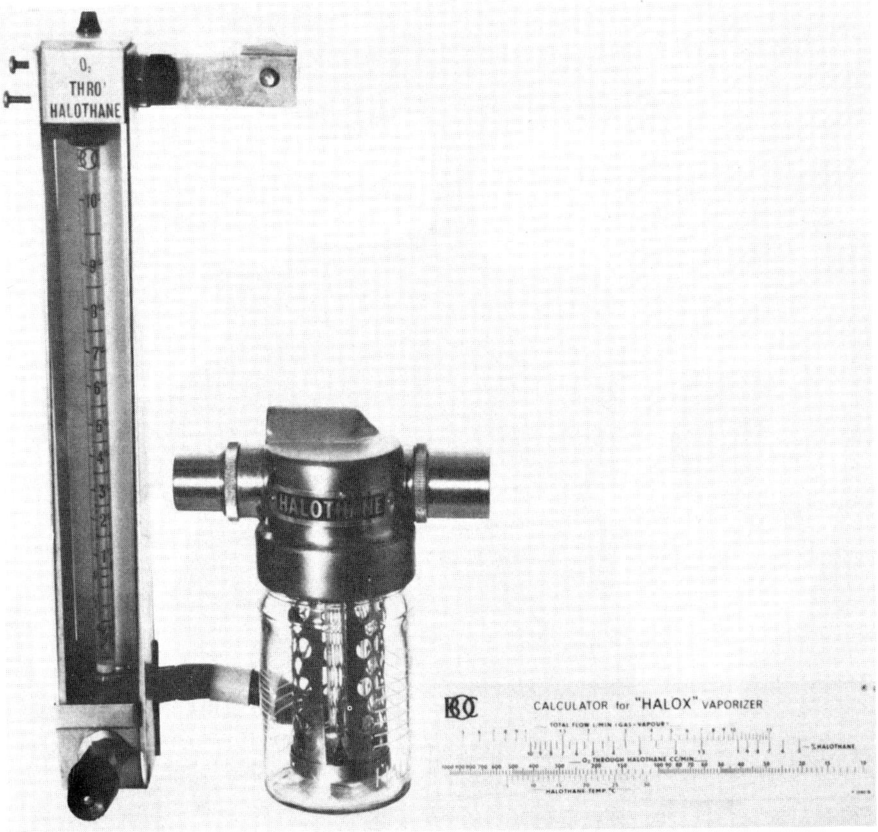


(a)

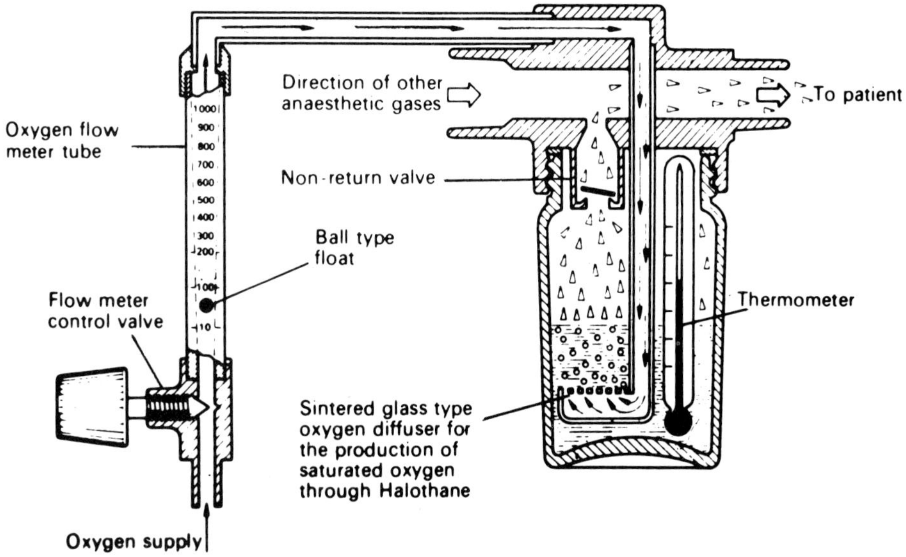


(b)

45/Fig. 28.—Halox vaporiser. (*a*) Rotameter, vaporiser and calculator. (*b*) Cross-sectional diagram of Halox vaporiser. ((*b*) Courtesy of Dr. C. S. Ward and Baillière Tindall, publishers of *Anaesthetic Equipment: Physical Principles and Maintenance.*)

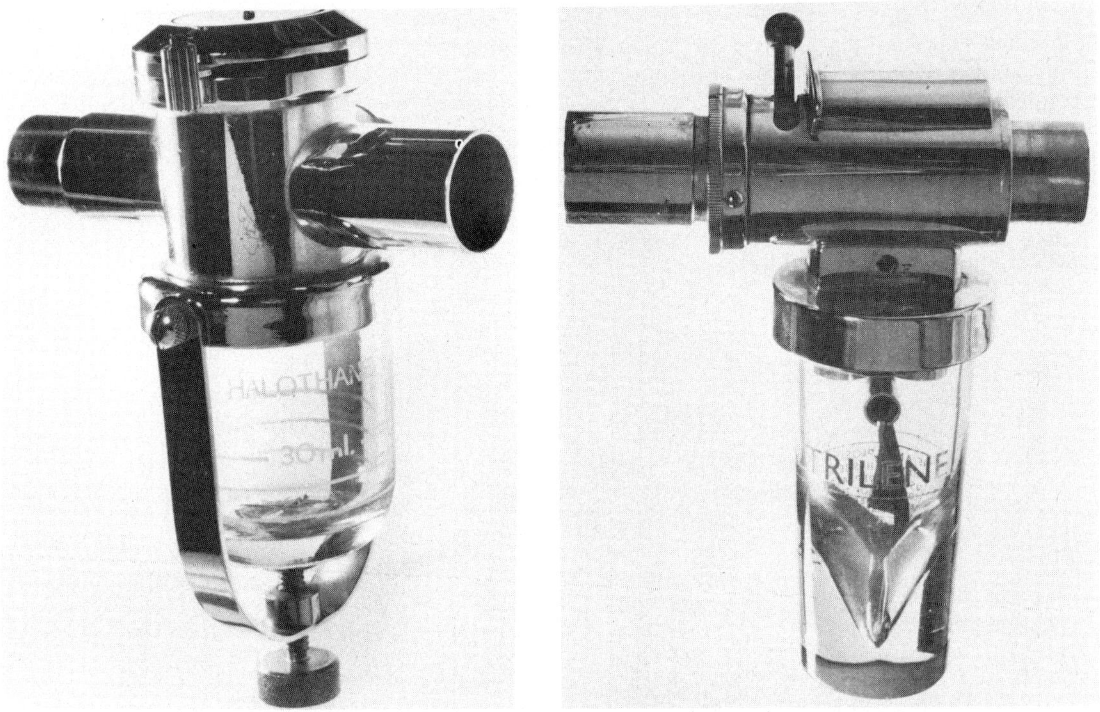


(*a*) (*b*)

45/Fig. 29.—Simple drawover vaporisers. (*a*) Goldman; (*b*) Rowbotham.

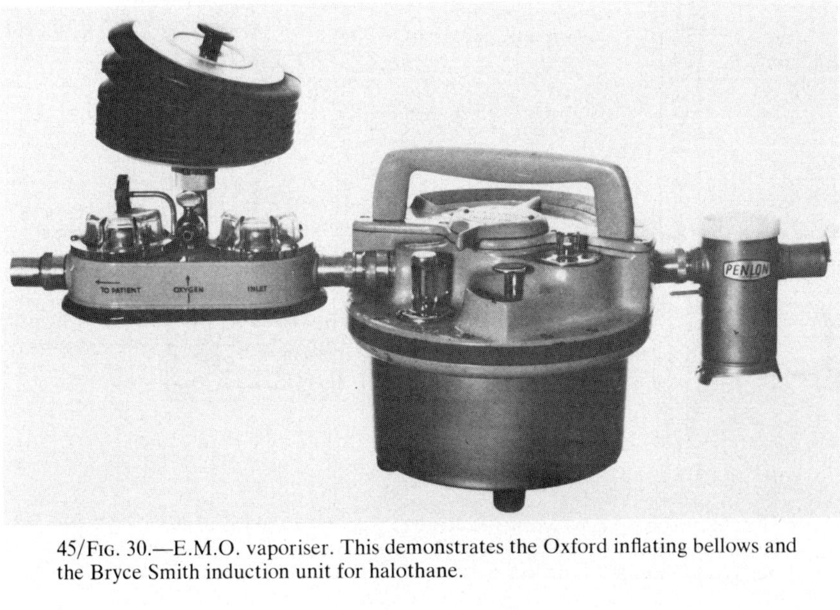


45/Fig. 30.—E.M.O. vaporiser. This demonstrates the Oxford inflating bellows and the Bryce Smith induction unit for halothane.

today, much as we may smile at quotations from the past such as "that it is doubtful if any agent will permanently replace chloroform for the general purposes of anaesthesia".[142] However, that same anaesthetist will be able to review the changes that have taken place in the development of anaesthetic apparatus by looking at one of the many anaesthetic museums present in Great Britain today (e.g. Leicester, Oxford, Cardiff, St. Bartholomew's Hospital, St. Thomas' Hospital and the Charles King collection). The preservation of our anaesthetic heritage to allow this review permits the reintroduction of ideas modified by current teaching that has dominated the development of anaesthesia as we know it today.

**REFERENCES**


1. Bryan C. P. (1930). *The Papyrus Ebers* p. 59–60. London: Geoffrey Bles.
2. Flagg, P. J. (1944). *The Art of Anesthesia*, p. 1. Philadelphia: J. B. Lippincott Co.
3. Gwathmey, J. T. (1914). *Anesthesia*, p. 2–3. New York: D. Appleton and Co.
4. Fulton, J. F. and Stanton, M. E. (1946). *The Centennial of Surgical Anesthesia*, p. 4–5. New York: Henry Schuman.
5. Armstrong-Davidson M. H. (1965). *The Evolution of Anaesthesia*, p. 46. Altrincham: John Sherratt and Son.
6. Dundee, J. W. and Wyant, G. M. (1974). *Intravenous Anaesthesia*, p. 1. Edinburgh: Churchill Livingstone.
7. Priestley, J. (1772). Observations on different kinds of air. *Phil. Trans. Roy. Soc.*, **62**, 210–211.
8. Davy, H. (1800). *Researches chemical and philosophical chiefly concerning nitrous oxide or dephlogisticated nitrous air and its respiration*, p. 556. London: Johnson.
9. Barton W. P. C. (1808). *A dissertation on the chymical properties and exhilarating effects of nitrous oxide gas.* Philadelphia: Lorenzo Press.
10. Serturner, F. W. A. (1806). Darstellung der reinen Mohnsaure (Opiumsaure) nebst einer chemischen untersuchung des opiums. Tromsdorff. *J. Pharm.*, **14**, 47–93.
11. Allen, C. W. (1914). *Local and Regional Anesthesia*, p. 19. Philadelphia: W. B. Saunders Co.
12. Hickman, H. H. (1824). A letter on suspended animation. Ironbridge: W. Smith.
13. Cartwright, F. F. (1952). *The English Pioneers of Anaesthesia.* Bristol: John Wright and Sons.
14. Elliotson, J. (1843). *Numerous cases of surgical operations without pain in the mermeric state.* London: H. Baillière.
15. Braid J. (1843). *Neurypnology.* London: John Churchill.
16. Esdaile J. (1846). *Mesmerism in India.* London: Longman Brown Green and Longman.
17. Long, C. W. (1849). An account of the first use of sulphuric ether by inhalation as an anesthetic in surgical operations. *Sth. Med. Surg.*, n.s. **5**, 705–713.
18. Ostler, W. (1918). The first printed documents relating to modern surgical anesthesia. *Proc. roy. Soc. Med.*, **11**, 65–69.
19. Thomas, K. B. (1975). *The Development of Anaesthetic Apparatus*, p. 117–118. Oxford: Blackwell.
20. Macintosh, R. R. and Bannister, F. B. (1943). *Essentials of General Anaesthesia*, 3rd edit., p. 5–7. Oxford: Blackwell.
21. Kaye, G., Orton, R. H. and Renton, D. G. (1946). *Anaesthetic Methods.* Melbourne: Ramsay Surgical Pty.
22. Fülöp-Miller, R. (1938). *Triumph Over Pain*, p. 189. Indianapolis: The Bobbs Merril Co.
23. Bigelow H. J. (1846). Insensibility during surgical operations produced by inhalation. *Boston med. Surg. J.*, **35**, 309–317.
24. Ellis, R. H. (1976). The introduction of ether anaesthesia to Great Britain. *Anaesthesia*, **31**, 766–777.
25. Zuck, D. (1978). Dr. Nooth and his apparatus. *Brit. J. Anaesth.*, **50**, 393–405.
26. Duncum, B. M. (1947). *The Devlopment of Inhalational Anaesthesia*, p. 131. London: Oxford Univ. Press.
27. Simpson, Y. J. (1847). *Account of a new anaesthetic agent as a substitute for sulphuric ether in surgery and midwifery.* Edinburgh: Sutherland and Knox.
28. Tomes, J. (1848). *Dental Physiology and Surgery*, p. 349. London: Parker.
29. Coote, H. (1847). Surgical operations performed by the inhalation of chloroform. *Lancet*, **2**, 571–572.
30. Medical Trials and Inquests (1848). Death from chloroform during a surgical operation. *Lond. Med. Gaz.*, **41**, n.s.6. 250–254.
31. Meggison, T. M. (1848). Letter on the Fatal Case of chloroform near Newcastle. *Lond. Med. Gaz.*, **41**, n.s.6. 254–255.
32. Potter, H. G. (1848). Letter on the effects produced by ether in the case of Hannah Greener. *Lond. med. Gaz.*, **41**, n.s.6, 255–256.
33. Snow, J. (1847). *On the Inhalation of the Vapour of Ether in Surgical Operations.* London: Churchill.
34. Slatter, E. M. (1960). The evolution of anaesthesia. 2. The first English ether inhalers. *Brit. J. Anaesth.*, **32**, 35–45.
35. Snow, J. (1858). *On Chloroform.* London: Churchill.
36. Gwathmey, J. T. (1914). *Anaesthesia*, p. 18. New York: D. Appleton and Co.
37. Traer, J. R. (1862). Surgical medical and obstetrical instruments in the International Exhibition of 1862. *Med. Tms. Gaz.*, **2**, 149.
38. Duncum, B. M. (1947). *The Development of Inhalational Anaesthesia*, p. 256. London: Oxford Univ. Press.
39. Skinner, T. (1862). Anaesthesia in midwifery with a new apparatus for its safer and more economical induction by chloroform. *Brit. med. J.*, **2**, 108–111.
40. Colton G. Q. (1873–4). Nitrous oxide. *Mth. Rev. dent. Surg.*, **2**, 26.
41. Galley, A. H. (1964). The debt of anaesthesia to pharmacy. *Ann. roy. Coll. Surg. Engl.*, **34**, 77–97.
42. Junker, F. A. (1867). Description of a new apparatus for administering narcotic vapours. *Med. Tms. Gaz.*, **2**, 590.

43. Jeffries, B. J. (1872). Ether in ophthalmic surgery. *Lancet*, **2**, 241–242.
44. Clover J. T. (1871). Discussion on ether and chloroform as anaesthetics. *Med. Tms. Gaz.*, **1**, 604.
45. Clover, J. T. (1876). On an apparatus for administering nitrous oxide gas and ether singly or combined. *Brit. med. J.*, **2**, 74–75.
46. Clover J. T. (1877). Portable regulating ether inhaler. *Brit. med. J.*, **1**, 69–70.
47. Ombredanne, L. (1908). Un appareil pour l'anesthesie par l'ether. *Gaz. Hop. (Paris)*, **81**, 1095–1100.
48. Smith, T. W. (1898). Improved ether inhaler. *Lancet*, **1**, 1005.
49. Koller, C. (1884). Ueber die verwendung des cocain zur anasthesitung am Auge. *Wien. med. Blatter*, **7**, 1352–1355.
50. Collins V. J. (1952). *Principles and Practice of Anesthesiology*, p. 211. London: Henry Kimpton.
51. *Medical Annual* (1885–6). London: Henry Kimpton. p. 26–27.
52. *Medical Annual* (1887). Bristol: John Wright and Co. p. 87–89.
53. Allen C. W. (1914). *Local and Regional Anaesthesia*, p. 150. Philadelphia: W. B. Saunders Co.
54. Thomas, K. B. (1975). *The Development of Anaesthetic Apparatus*, p. 60. Oxford: Blackwell.
55. Corning, J. L. (1888). Further contribution on local medication of the spinal cord with cases. *N.Y. med. Rec.*, **33**, 291–293.
56. Quincke, H. (1891). Die lumbalpunktur des hydrocephalis. *Berl. Klin. Wschr.*, **38**, 965–968.
57. Bier, A. (1899). Versuche uber cocainisirung des ruckenmarkes. *Dtsch. Z. Chir.*, **27**, 361–369.
58. Tuffier, T. (1901). *L'analgesie chirugicale par voie rachidienne (injections sous arachnoidiennes de cocaine) technique resultats indication*, 8th edit. Paris: Masson et Cie.
59. O'Dwyer, J. (1885). Intubation of the larynx. *N.Y. med. J.*, **42**, 145–147.
60. O'Dwyer, J. (1892). Intubation of the larynx. *Ann. Universal Med. Sci.*, **4**, G1–G10.
61. O'Dwyer, J. (1886). Chronic stenosis of the larynx. *N.Y. med. Rec.*, **29**, 641–642.
62. Northrup, W. P. (1896). Apparatus for artificial forcible respiration. *Med. Surg. Reps. Presbyterian Hosp.*, **1**, 127–136.
63. Mushin, W. W. and Rendell Baker, L. (1953). *Principles of Thoracic Anaesthesia*, p. 110–120. Oxford: Blackwell.
64. Sicard, A. (1901). Sur les injections epidurales sacrococcygiennes. *C. R. Soc. Biol. (Paris)*, **53**, 479–481.
65. Cathelin, F. (1901). Un mot d'histoire a propos des injections epidurales par le canal sacre et notes anatomique. *C. R. Soc. Biol. (Paris)*, **53**, 597–599.
66. Barker, A. E. (1907). A report on clinical experiences with spinal analgesia. *Brit. med. J.*, **1**, 665–674.
67. Hewitt F. W. (1901). *Anaesthetics*. London: Griffin.
68. Vernon-Harcourt, A. G. (1903). On a chloroform regulator. *Brit. med. J.*, **2**, Suppl., 143–4.
69. Embley, E. H. (1902). The causation of death during the administration of chloroform. *Brit. med. J.*, **1**, 817–821, 886–893 and 951–961.
70. Shearer, W. M. (1960). The evolution of premedication. *Brit. J. Anaesth.*, **32**, 554–562.
71. Meltzer and Auer (1909). Continuous respiration without respiratory movements. *J. exp. Med.*, **11**, 622–625.
72. Elsberg, C. A. (1911). Anaesthesia by the intratracheal insufflation of air and ether, a description of the technic of the method and of a portable apparatus for use in man. *Ann. Surg.* **53**, 161–168.
73. Evans, F. T. (1949). *Modern Practice in Anaesthesia*, p. 13. London: Butterworth and Co.
74. McKesson E. I. (1911). Nitrous oxide oxygen anesthesia with a description of a new apparatus. *Surg. Gynec. Obstet.*, **13**, 456–462.
75. McKesson, E. I. (1930). *Handbook of Nitrous Oxide and Oxygen Anesthesia in Dentistry*, 5th edit. Watford: McKesson Equipment Co.
76. Cotton F. J. and Boothby W. M. (1912). Nitrous oxide-oxygen, ether anaesthesia: notes on administration: a perfected apparatus. *Surg. Gynec. Obstet.*, **15**, 281–289.
77. Boyle, H. E. G. (1917). The use of nitrous oxide and oxygen with rebreathing in military surgery. *Lancet*, **2**, 667–669.
78. Hewer, C. L. (1978). Personal communication.
79. Marshall, G. (1920). Two types of portable gas oxygen apparatus. *Proc. roy. Soc. Med.*, **13**, 16–23.
80. Boyle, H. E. G. (1919). Recent developments in gas and oxygen anaesthesia. *St. Bart. Hosp. J.*, **27**, 22–23.
81. Shipway, F. E. (1916). The advantages of warm anaesthetic vapours and an apparatus for their adiministration. *Lancet*, **1**, 70–74.
82. Levy, G. A. (1912). The exciting causes of ventricular fibrillation in animals under chloroform anaesthesia. *Heart*, **4**, 319.
83. Payne, J. P. (1981). Chloroform in clinical anaesthesia. *Brit. J. Anaesth.*, **53**, Suppl. 1, 115.
84. Guedel, A. E. (1937). *Inhalational Anesthesia*. New York: MacMillan Co.
85. Gillespie, N. A. (1948). Endotracheal Anesthesia, 2nd edit., p. 22–23. Wisconsin: Univ. Wisconsin Press.
86. Magill, I. W. M. (1967). Discussion of fresh gas flow and rebreathing in the Magill circuit. *Proc. roy. Soc. Med.*, **60**, 750.
87. Wilson, S. R. and Pinson, K. B. (1921). A warm ether bomb. *Lancet*, **1**, 336.
88. Waters, R. M. (1924). Clinical scope and utility of carbon dioxide filtration in inhalation anaesthesia. *Curr. Res. Anesth.*, **3**, 20–22 and 26.
89. Foregger, R. (1961). Early use of the carbon dioxide absorption method in anaesthetic practice. *Brit. J. Anaesth.*, **33**, 470–475.
90. Sword, B. (1930). The closed circle method of administration of gas anaesthesia. *Curr. Res. Anesth.*, **9**, 198–202.
91. Guedel, A. E. and Waters, R. M. (1931). Endotracheal anesthesia a new technic. *Ann. Otol. Rhinol. Laryngol.*, **40**, 1139–1145.
92. Waters, R. M. and Schmidt, E. R. (1934). Cyclopropane anesthesia, *J. Amer. med. Ass.*, **103**, 975–983.
93. Oré, P. C. (1872). Des injection intraveineuses de chloral. *Bull. Soc. Chirurgie Paris*, **1**, 400–412.
94. Burkhardt, L. (1909). Die intravenose narkose mit Aether und Chloroform. *Münch. med. Wschr.*, **2**, 2365–2369.
95. Bardet D. (1921). Sur l'utilisation, comme anesthisique general d'un product nouveau le diethyl diallyl barbiturate de diethylamine. *Bull. gén. Ther. (Paris)*, **1**, 27–30.
96. Bumm, R. (1927). Intravenose Narkosen mit Barbitur-Saurederivaten. *Klin. Wschr.*, **6**, 725–6.
97. Zerfas, L. G. and Mcallum, J. T. C. (1929). The

analgesic and anesthetic properties of sodium isoamylethyl barbiturate. *J. Indiana med. Ass.*, **22**, 47–50.
98. Weese, H. and Scharpff, W. (1932). Evipan ein neuartiges einschlafmittel. *Dtsch. med. Wschr.*, **58**, 1205–1207.
99. Lundy, J. S. and Tovell, R. M. (1934). Some of the newer local and general anesthetic agents, methods of their administration. *Northw. Med. (Seattle)*, **33**, 308–311.
100. Jarman, R. and Abel, A. L. (1936). Intravenous anaesthesia with pentothal sodium. *Lancet*, **1**, 230 and 422–423.
101. Dogliotti, A. M. (1931). Eine neue methode der regionaren anesthesie 'Die peridurale segmentaire anesthesie'. *Zbl. Chir.*, **58**, 3141–3145.
102. Pages F. (1921). Anestesia metamerica. *Rev. Sanid. Milit. (Madrid)*, **3.5.11**, 351–385.
103. Rivett, L. C. (1933). Chloroform capsules during labour. *Brit. med. J.*, **2**, 778–779.
104. Mennell, Z. (1933). Modified Junker bottle for maternity analgesia. *Practitioner*, **130**, 519.
105. Minnitt, R. J. (1949). *Gas and Air Analgesia*, 4th edit. London: Baillière Tindall and Co.
106. Cole, P. V. and Nainby-Luxmore R. C. (1962). Respiratory volumes in labour. *Brit. med. J.*, **1**, 1118–1119.
107. Hadfield, C. F. and Hewer, C. L. (1941). Trichlorethylene as an inhalation anaesthetic. *Brit. med. J.*, **1**, 924–927.
108. Epstein, H. G., Macintosh, R. R. and Mendelsohn, K. (1941). The Oxford vaporiser no. 1. *Lancet*, **2**, 62–64.
109. Epstein, H. G. and Macintosh, R. R. (1956). An anaesthetic inhaler with automatic thermocompensation. *Anaesthesia*, **11**, 83–88.
110. Griffith, H. R. and Johnson, G. E. (1942). The use of curare in general anesthesia. *Anesthesiology*, **3**, 418–420.
111. Organe, G. S. W., Paton, W. D. M. and Zaimis, E. J. (1949). Preliminary trials of Bistrimethyl ammonium decane and pentane di iodide, $C_{10}$ and $C_5$, in man. *Lancet*, **1**, 21–23.
112. Bovet, D., Bovet-Nitti F., Guarino S., Longo, V. G. and Marotta, M. (1949). Proprieta farmacodinamiche di alcani derivati della succinilcolina dotati di azione curarica. *R. C. Ist. sup. Sanità*, **12**, 106–137.
113. Huguenard, P. (1949). Effets et applications d'un curarisant de synthese. *Brux.-méd.*, **27:2**, 2059–2065.
114. Griffiths, H. W. C. and Gillies, J. (1948). Thoracolumbar splanchnicectomy and sympathectomy. *Anaesthesia*, **3**, 134–146.
115. Hale, D. E. (1948). Controlled hypotension by arterial bleeding during operation and anesthesia. *Anesthesiology*, **9**, 498–505.
116. Jackson. I. (1954). Arteriotomy in neurosurgery. *Anaesthesia*, **9**, 13–16.
117. Paton, W. D. M. (1951). The paralysis of autonomic ganglia with special reference to the therapeutic effects of ganglion blocking drugs. *Brit. med. J.*, **1**, 773–778.
118. Enderby, G. E. H. and Pelmore, J. F. (1951). Controlled hypotension and postural ischaemia to reduce bleeding in surgery. *Lancet*, **1**, 663–666.
119. Nosworthy, M. D. (1941). Anaesthesia in chest surgery. *Proc. roy. Soc. Med.*, **34**, 479–506.
120. Musgrove, A. H. (1952). Controlled respiration in thoracic surgery. *Anaesthesia*, **7**, 77–85.
121. Esplen, J. R. (1952). A new apparatus for intermittent positive pressure inflation. *Brit. J. Anaesth.*, **24**, 303–311.
122. Esplen J. R. (1956). The Fazakerley respirator. *Brit. J. Anaesth.*, **28**, 176–186.
123. Laborit, H. and Huguenard, P. (1954). *Pratique de l'hibernotherapie en chirurgie et en medicine*. Paris: Masson.
124. De Castro, J. and Mundaleer, P. (1959). Anesthesie sans barbituriques: La neuroleptanalgesie. *Anesth. Analg. Réanimo*, **16**, 1022–1056.
125. Johnstone, M. (1956). The human cardiovascular response to fluothane anaesthesia. *Brit. J. Anaesth.*, **28**, 392–410.
126. Mackay I. M. (1957). Clinical evaluation of fluothane with special reference to a controlled percentage vaporiser. *Canad. Anaesth. Soc. J.*, **4**, 235–245.
127. Young, J. V. (1966). The practical use of the Halox vapouriser. *Anaesthesia*, **21**, 551–557.
128. Goldman, V. (1959). Fluothane in dental surgery. *Anesth. Analg. Curr. Res.*, **38**, 192–197.
129. Goldman, V. (1962). The Goldman vaporiser Mark II. *Anaesthesia*, **17**, 537–539.
130. Minnitt, R. J. and Gillies, J. (1948). *Textbook of Anaesthetics*, 7th edit., p. 320. Edinburgh: E. and S. Livingstone.
131. Bryce-Smith R. (1964). Halothane induction unit. *Anaesthesia*, **19**. 393–398.
132. Black G. W. (1979). Halothane related hepatitis. In: *Medical Annual 1979/80*, pp. 68–72. Bristol: John Wright.
133. Artusio J. F. (1960). A clinical evaluation of methoxyflurane in man. *Anesthesiology*, **21**, 512–517.
134. Dobkin, A. B., Heinrich, R. G., Israel, J. S., Levy, A. S., Neville, J. F. and Ounkasen, K. (1968). Clinical evaluation of a new inhalational agent. Compound 347. *Anesthesiology*, **29**, 275–287.
135. Stoelting, U. K. (1957). Use of a new intravenous oxygen barbiturate 25398 for intravenous anaesthesia. *Anesth. Analg. Curr. Res.*, **36**, 49–51.
136. Selye, H. (1941). Anaesthetic effects of steroid hormones. *Proc. Soc. exp. Biol. Med.*, **46**, 116–121.
137. Pan, S. Y., Gardocki, J. F., Hutcheon, D. E., Rudd, H., Kodet, M. J. and Laubach, G. D. (1955). General anaesthetic and other pharmacological properties of a soluble steroid 21—hydroxyprognanedione sodium succinate. *J. Pharmacol. exp. Ther.*, **115**, 432–441.
138. Campbell, D., Forrester, A. C., Miller, D. C., Hutton, I., Kennedy, J. A., Lawrie, T. D., Lorimer, A. R. and McCall D. (1971). A preliminary study of CT 1341. *Brit. J. Anaesth.*, **43**, 14–24.
139. Greifenstein, F. E. and De Vault, M. (1958). A study of l'aryl cyclohexaylamine for anaesthesia. *Anesth. Analg. Curr. Res.*, **37**, 283–294.
140. Corssen, G. and Domino, E. F. (1966). Dissociative Anesthesia: Further pharmacologic studies and first clinical experiences with the phencyclidine derivative CL—581. *Anesth. Analg. Curr. Res.*, **45**, 29–40.
141. Dundee, J. W. and Lilburn, J. K. (1978). Ketamine-lorazepam. *Anaesthesia*, **33**, 312–314.
142. *Medical Annual* (1887). Bristol: John Wright & Co. p. 16.

**APPENDIX I**

# Care and Sterilisation of Anaesthetic Equipment

Too little consideration is generally given to the cleanliness and sterility of apparatus used in anaesthesia, and particularly to those parts which indirectly or directly come into contact with the air passages. Absolute sterility is not always essential, since the upper air passages are in constant contact with the atmosphere, but there is evidence that infections have been spread from patient to patient through the use of contaminated anaesthetic or respiratory apparatus. This most clearly has been shown to occur with the use of ventilators (see Chapter 9). For this reason those parts of the anaesthetic system through which rebreathing takes place, and the apparatus such as an endotracheal tube, face-mask and laryngoscope which actually comes into direct contact with the patient, must be thoroughly washed after use and either sterilised, disinfected or at least kept clean until required again. If the equipment has been used for a patient suffering from a known infection then washing *must* be followed by sterilisation.

Constant washing and sterilisation of apparatus, particularly of rubber or plastic components, leads to some wear, but a more potent cause of deterioration is to be found in the use of lubricants containing Vaseline or greasy bases. The use of these, rather than repeated sterilisation, is the commonest cause of deterioration of cuffed tubes.[1] The lubricants should always be non-greasy and used either alone or incorporated with local anaesthetic; for example, K.Y. jelly and topical lignocaine 4 per cent jelly.

Lubricants can harbour organisms, so that they are best dispensed in small tubes which can be discarded daily before they become infected.

## DISINFECTION AND STERILISATION

A. *Disinfection* is the term used to signify the removal of most vegetative organisms which are easy to kill whilst spores may survive. There are four methods available for anaesthetic apparatus (where applicable):

(i) *Boiling water*—immersion for five minutes kills all vegetative bacteria and *some* spores.

(ii) *Low-temperature steam* (subatmospheric at 80° C)—kills all vegetative bacteria and *some* spores.

(iii) *Glutaraldehyde* (2·5 *per cent*; *Cidex*)—soaking for 30 minutes kills all vegetative bacteria and *many* spores. Automatic disinfecting machines using this agent are available.

(iv) *Chlorhexidine and spirit (70 per cent)*—soaking for 30 minutes kills all vegetative bacteria but *no* spores.

B. *Sterilisation* is the term used to signify the destruction of all organisms *including* spores. The principal methods available are:

(a) *Autoclaving*—the most commonly recommended routine is 134° C at 32 lb/sq in (221 kPa) for 3 minutes.

(b) *Gas Sterilisation*—two principal methods are available:

(i) Low-Temperature Steam (i.e. subatmospheric at 80° C) plus Formaldehyde is probably the most satisfactory method available to create sporicidal conditions and can be used for most anaesthetic equipment such as laryngoscopes, bronchoscopes, endotracheal tubes, etc. It is faster and cheaper than ethylene oxide and has the added advantage that it is devoid of toxic by-products that can be isolated from rubber and plastic materials after ethylene oxide.[2]

(ii) Ethylene Oxide—requires slightly longer exposure and is more toxic if either patients or attendants come into contact with the vapour. Sykes and his associates[3] recommend that ethylene oxide or liquid disinfectants should not be used for endotracheal tubes because they may leak out and cause tissue irritation.[4]

## Sterilisation of Anaesthetic Apparatus

**Airways.**—Ideally these are available in a disposable plastic. Expense may necessitate recycling in which case the rubber airway is more suitable. Great care must be taken to see that each airway is thoroughly washed in soap and water, both internally and externally, then dried and finally sterilised. Autoclaving is satisfactory for these items.

**Endotracheal tubes.**—Plastic disposable tubes are the most satisfactory (minimal irritation to laryngeal and tracheal mucosa) and are particularly important for those patients who may have to undergo prolonged ventilation. If recycling is essential then (as with airways) autoclaving is sufficient. Should ethylene oxide be used for sterilisation, particular care must be taken to ensure that none of the gas is retained in the rubber of endotracheal tubes which might later leak out *in situ*.

**Face-masks** are usually thoroughly washed in soap and water, dried and re-used. Unfortunately, they will not survive frequent autoclaving.

**Laryngeal sprays** are a potential source for the introduction of infection. Casewell and Dalton[5] report on six women who underwent general anaesthesia and later developed clinical evidence of respiratory tract infection. The common source was traced to a Forrester laryngeal spray which was found to be infected with *Pseudomonas aeruginosa*. All laryngeal sprays should be made of materials that can be *sterilised* frequently.

**Anaesthetic circuits.**—All corrugated tubing should be thoroughly washed and dried after every case. Ideally it should also be sterilised but frequent autoclaving causes damage to the material.

**Ventilators.**—See Chapter 9.

## Sterilisation of Plastic Materials

The introduction of plastic materials into clinical practice was largely brought about by the desire to control cross-infections in hospital by using disposable items. Also, many plastics are non-irritating to mucous membranes and therefore are to be preferred to red rubber when left in contact with the mucosa of the trachea or urethra for any prolonged period. In their disposable form, plastic items avoid all the problems of re-sterilisation, but rising costs have led some anaesthetists to reconsider the whole problem. It is essential to have some knowledge of the plastic materials available and their response to the various methods of sterilisation (see Table 1).

*Polyvinyl Chloride (PVC)* is the most widely used material, particularly for endotracheal and tracheostomy tubes. The great advantage of PVC is its flexibility so that with various additives (plasticisers) a wide range of hardness can be obtained.

### Methods of Sterilisation of PVC

**Gamma radiation.** (i) *Endotracheal tubes.*–Some degree of discolouration or yellowing will usually occur and this becomes more pronounced with prolonged storage. The colour change is due to the partial dechlorination of the PVC but the mechanical and functional properties of the material are not significantly affected. Repeated doses are not recommended as they lead to pronounced discolouration with undesirable changes in the pH of the aqueous extract and a perceptible stiffening of the material.

(ii) *Tracheostomy tubes.*—These are also made of PVC and therefore the same conditions apply as with endotracheal tubes. However, other parts (using different plastics) are often fitted to these tubes. For example, the Portex tracheostomy has a collar (made of acetyl polymer) attached to facilitate its use with swivel connectors. In these circumstances, the tracheostomy tube is not suitable for gamma radiation sterilisation.

**Steam sterilisation.**—This requires the high-speed vacuum process which is operated at

APPENDIX I/TABLE 1
THE EFFECT OF STERILISATION AND DISINFECTION PROCESSES ON MEDICAL AND SURGICAL PLASTICS

| *Material* | *Autoclaving* | *Dry heat* | *High-energy irradiation* | *Ethylene oxide* | *Boiling water* | *Liquid chemicals* | *Comments* |
|---|---|---|---|---|---|---|---|
| PVC (a) Flexible | Tubing satisfactory up to 136° C. Mouldings may distort. Avoid external loading while hot. | Unsuitable | Satisfactory up to 2·5 Mr. at higher doses discolours with liberation of hydrogen chloride. | Satisfactory | Satisfactory. Avoid external stress while hot. Mouldings may distort. | Not recommended. Attacked by some chemicals, in particular phenolic agents. | Flexible film and sheeting usually distorts on autoclaving. PVC tends to become opaque or cloudy in hot water or steam. Clarity restored on drying at R.T. more rapidly at 60° C. |
| (b) Rigid | Unsuitable because of deformation. Softens above 60° C. | Unsuitable | Medical grades usually unsatisfactory because of discolouration. | Satisfactory | Usually unsatisfactory because of dimensional changes. Thick sections less affected. Protect from external stresses. | Usually satisfactory. Phenolic agents should be avoided. | As for flexible PVC |
| Polyethylene Low density (L.D.) High density (H.D.) | Unsuitable L.D. softens at 80–100° C. H.D. softens at 120–130° C | Unsuitable | Satisfactory. Polyethylene becomes progressively harder and tougher above 2·5 Mr. and up to 25 Mr. | Satisfactory. Highly permeable to gases. Film may be used for packaging. | Usually satisfactory for H.D. polythene but L.D. polythene not satisfactory above 80° C. | Satisfactory | |
| Polypropylene | Satisfactory—mouldings may distort. | Unsuitable—softens at 145–150° C. | Not usually suitable. Some grades said to be more resistant. Oxidative degradation can occur especially on storage with subsequent embrittlement. | Satisfactory | Satisfactory | Satisfactory | |

(Reproduced with kind permission from *The Sterilisation of Plastics*, Portex Ltd.)

136° C. When autoclaving PVC it is particularly important to avoid any stress during the process (such as heavy weights from packing) because at autoclave temperatures PVC softens and can become permanently altered in shape.

Multiple autoclaving cycles can lead to a perceptible stiffening and discolouration of the material.

**Ethylene oxide.**—Sterilisation processes are usually operated at, or below, 55° C in order to avoid damage to heat-labile materials. Considered solely from the standpoint of possible damage to the product this is the best method available as it can be undertaken repeatedly without any perceptible effect on the PVC endotracheal and tracheostomy tubes. However, particular attention must be paid to adequate batch-by-batch biological monitoring of the efficacy of the sterilisation and also to the need for adequate post-sterilisation aeration of the product to avert hazards arising from ethylene oxide residues.

Other methods, such as the low-temperature steam/formalin process, are available but are considered less suitable because of the difficulty of ensuring the complete absence of any residual formalin. In conclusion, although re-sterilisation may be considered desirable on a cost basis, it must be remembered that with the unused sterilised manufactured product, provided the package is undamaged and if storage conditions are satisfactory, there is only one chance in one million of finding a product which is non-sterile.[6]

Further details of the effect of sterilisation and disinfection processes are shown in Table 1.

## REFERENCES

1. Buckley, R. W. (1952). Danger from endotracheal tubes. *Brit. med. J.*, **2**, 939.
2. Clinical Anaesthesia Conference (1969). Hazards associated with ethylene oxide sterilisation. *N.Y. St. J. Med.*, **69**, 1319.
3. Sykes, M. K., McNicol, M. W. and Campbell, E. J. M. (1976). *Respiratory Failure*, p. 172. Oxford: Blackwell Scientific Publications.
4. Rendell-Baker, L. (1972). Ethylene oxide. II aeration. In: Infections and Sterilisation Problems. Ed. R. B. Roberts. *Int. Anesthesiol. Clin.*, **10**, 101.
5. Casewell, M. W. and Dalton, M. T. (1977). Forrester laryngeal sprays as a source of pseudomonas respiratory tract infection. *Brit. med. J.*, **2**, 680.
6. Vincent, W. W. (1976). Portex Ltd. Personal communication.

## FURTHER READING

Cruikshank, R., Duguid, J. P., Marmion, B. P. and Swain, R. H. A. (1973). *Medical Microbiology*, Chap. 5. Edinburgh: Churchill Livingstone.

Lennette, E. H., Spaulding, E. H. and Truant, J. P. (1974). *Manual of Clinical Microbiology*, p. 852. Washington: Amer. Soc. Microbiol.

Lowbury, E. J. L., Ayliffe, G. A. J., Geddes, A. M. and Williams, J. D. (1981). *Control of Hospital Infection*, 2nd edit. London: Chapman and Hall.

APPENDIX II

# Useful Facts

## SI UNITS

THE SI system of units (Système International d'Unités) has been developed in an endeavour to reduce the enormous number of units in current use to a relatively small number of internationally acceptable units with standard symbols.

There are seven *base units* (Table 1), which may be combined by multiplication or division to produce *derived units* (Table 2).

APPENDIX II/TABLE 1
THE SI BASE UNITS

| *Physical quantity* | *Name of SI Unit* | *Symbol for SI Unit* |
|---|---|---|
| Length | metre | m |
| Mass | kilogram | kg |
| Time | second | s |
| Electric current | ampere | A |
| Thermodynamic temperature | kelvin | K |
| Amount of substance | mole | mol |
| Luminous intensity | candela | cd |

There are in addition *supplementary units* such as the radian and *special non-SI units* such as litre (l), day (d), hour (h), minute (min).

By attaching appropriate prefixes, decimal multiples and fractions of these units can be formed.

### The Mole

The quantity of a substance of known molecular weight is expressed in moles, where

$$\text{Number of moles (mol)} = \frac{\text{Weight in g}}{\text{Molecular Weight}}$$

and the units of concentration are therefore mol/l, mmol/l, μmol/l, etc. For univalent ions such as $Na^+$, $K^+$, $HCO^-{}_3$ $Cl^-$, millimoles and milliequivalents are numerically equal. In the case of a divalent ion such as $Ca^{++}$ the number of milliequivalents must be divided by 2 (the valency) to convert to millimoles. To convert results previously expressed as mg/100 ml to mmol/l the figure should be divided by the molecular weight of the substance concerned (to convert mg to mmol) and multiplied by 10 (to convert from 100 ml to 1 litre).

APPENDIX II/TABLE 2
SOME DERIVED SI UNITS

| *Physical quantity* | *Name of SI Unit* | *Symbol* | *Definition of SI Unit* |
|---|---|---|---|
| Volume | cubic metre | — | $m^3$ |
| Force | newton | N | $kg\ m\ s^{-2} = J\ m^{-1}$ |
| Pressure | pascal | Pa | $kg\ m^{-1}\ s^{-2} = N\ m^{-2}$ |
| Work | joule | J | $kg\ m^2\ s^{-2} = N\ m$ |
| Power | watt | W | $kg\ m^2\ s^{-3} = J\ s^{-1}$ |
| Surface tension | pascal metre | — | $Pa\ m = N\ m^{-1} = kg\ s^{-2}$ |
| Periodic frequency | hertz | Hz | $s^{-1}$ |

APPENDIX II/TABLE 3
SI PREFIXES AND THEIR SYMBOLS

| *Fraction* | *SI prefix* | *Symbol* | *Multiple* | *SI prefix* | *Symbol* |
|---|---|---|---|---|---|
| $10^{-1}$ | deci | d | 10 | deca | da |
| $10^{-2}$ | centi | c | $10^2$ | hecto | h |
| $10^{-3}$ | milli | m | $10^3$ | kilo | k |
| $10^{-6}$ | micro | μ | $10^6$ | mega | M |
| $10^{-9}$ | nano | n | $10^9$ | giga | G |
| $10^{-12}$ | pico | p | $10^{12}$ | tera | T |
| $10^{-15}$ | femto | f | | | |
| $10^{-18}$ | atto | a | | | |

| *Quantity* | *SI Unit or multiple* | | *Other Units* | *Conversion factors* Other Units to SI Units multiply by | *Conversion factors* SI Units to Other Units multiply by |
|---|---|---|---|---|---|
| Length | metre | (m) | inch | 0·0254 | 39·37 |
| | | | foot | 0·305 | 3·281 |
| Mass | kilogram | (kg) | ounce | 0·0284 | 35·27 |
| | | | pound | 0·454 | 2·205 |
| Force (mass×acceleration) | newton | (N) | dyne (cm g $s^{-2}$) | 0·00001 | 100,000 |
| | | | poundal (ft lb $s^{-2}$) | 0·138 | 7·233 |
| | | | [1]pound-force (lbf) | 4·448 | 0·225 |
| [2]Pressure (force÷area) | [3]kilopascal | (kPa) | mm Hg / Torr | 0·1333 | 7·501 |
| | | | kg f $cm^{-2}$ | 98·07 | 0·0102 |
| | | | cm $H_2O$ | 0·0981 | 10·19 |
| | | | Std atmosphere | 101·3 | 0·00987 |
| | | | lbf $in^{-2}$ | 6·895 | 0·145 |
| | | | bar | 100 | 0·01 |
| Work or Energy [4](force×distance or, pressure×volume) | [5]kilojoule | (kJ) | kilocalorie | 4·184 | 0·239 |
| Surface tension | pascal metre | (Pa m) | dynes/cm | 0·001 | 1,000 |
| Compliance | litres per kilopascal | (l $kPa^{-1}$) | l/cm $H_2O$ | 10·19 | 0·0981 |
| Resistance to flow | kilopascals×$litres^{-1}$ × seconds | (kPa $l^{-1}$ s) | cm $H_2O$ $l^{-1}$ sec | 0·0981 | 10·19 |
| Transfer factor | millimoles× $minutes^{-1}$× $kilopascals^{-1}$ | (mmol $min^{-1}$ $kPa^{-1}$) | ml $min^{-1}$ mm $Hg^{-1}$ | 0·335 | 2·986 |

1 This is a technical unit of force, where the mass (lb) is multiplied by the standard acceleration due to gravity (9·8 m $s^{-2}$).
2 Most pressure gauges read zero when the actual pressure = atmospheric pressure; so *gauge pressures* are pressures referred to atmospheric pressure, whereas *absolute pressures* are pressures referred to true zero pressure or vacuum.
3 The kilopascal has been given rather than the pascal, since in medical practice the kPa will be more commonly used.
4 Movement of gas in response to a pressure gradient.
5 The kilojoule has been given rather than the joule since in medical practice the kJ (and MJ) will be more commonly used.

Example: to convert 90 mg/100 ml glucose to mmol/l:

$$\frac{90 \times 10}{180 \text{ (molecular weight of glucose)}} = 5 \text{ mmol/l}$$

(when considering amount of substance, rather than concentration:

$$90 \text{ mg glucose} = \frac{90}{180} = 0{\cdot}5 \text{ mmol})$$

In the case of some substances the molecular weight is not known, for example the globulin fraction of plasma protein consists of a mixture of proteins of different molecular weights, so for these substances *mass concentration* is used (kg/l, g/l, mg/l, etc.). It has not yet been decided whether the molecular weight of haemoglobin will be calculated for the monomer (Hb) or tetramer ($Hb_4$), so haemoglobin concentration will continue to be reported in g/100 ml or g/dl.

### Volume

In 1964, the litre which had previously been defined in terms of the volume of 1 kg of pure water under standard conditions, was redefined as being equal to 1 cubic decimetre (1 l = 1 $dm^3$). The SI unit of volume is the cubic metre ($m^3$), but for medical purposes the litre will continue to be used.

1 pint = 0·568 l
1 litre = 1·760 pt
1 gallon (U.K.) = 1·201 gal (U.S.) = 4·546 l
1 gallon (U.S.) = 0·833 gal (U.K.) = 3·785 l

### Temperature

The SI unit is the kelvin (K), but for everyday use the degree Celsius (formerly called Centigrade) will be retained. The Fahrenheit scale is no longer used.

0° C = 273·15 K = 32·0°F
Celsius to Kelvin: K = °C + 273
Kelvin to Celsius: °C = K − 273
Celsius to Fahrenheit: °F = °C × $\frac{9}{5}$ + 32
Fahrenheit to Celsius: °C = (°F − 32) × $\frac{5}{9}$

## SPECIAL SYMBOLS*

### For Gases

| Primary Symbols (Large Capital Letters) | Examples |
|---|---|
| V = gas volume | VA = volume of alveolar gas |
| $\dot{V}$ = gas volume/unit time | $\dot{V}O_2$ = $O_2$ consumption/min. |
| P = gas pressure | $PAO_2$ = alveolar $O_2$ pressure |
| $\bar{P}$ = mean gas pressure | |
| F = fractional concentration in dry gas phase | $FIO_2$ = fractional concentration of $O_2$ in inspired gas |
| f = respiratory frequency (breaths/unit time) | |
| D = diffusing capacity | $DO_2$ = diffusing capacity for $O_2$ (ml $O_2$ min/mm/Hg) |
| R = respiratory exchange ratio | R = $\dot{V}CO_2/\dot{V}O_2$ |

| Secondary Symbols (Small Capital Letters) | Examples |
|---|---|
| I = inspired gas | $FICO_2$ = fractional concentration of $CO_2$ in inspired gas |
| E = expired gas | VE = volume of expired gas |
| A = alveolar gas | $\dot{V}A$ = alveolar ventilation/min |
| T = tidal gas | VT = tidal volume |
| D = dead space gas | VD = volume of dead space gas |
| B = barometric | PB = barometric pressure |

— Dash above any symbol indicates a *mean* value.
. Dot above any symbol indicates a *time derivative*.

* This list of special symbols with examples is reproduced from *The Lung* by the kindness of Professor Julius H. Comroe and the Year Book Medical Publishers, Incorporated.

## SPECIAL SYMBOLS—*contd.*

### For Blood

| Primary Symbols (Large Capital Letters) | Examples |
| --- | --- |
| Q = volume of blood | Qc = volume of blood in pulmonary capillaries |
| $\dot{Q}$ = volume flow of blood/unit time | $\dot{Q}c$ = blood flow through pulmonary capillaries/min. |
| C = content of gas in blood phase | $Ca_{O_2}$ = ml $O_2$ in 100 ml arterial blood |
| S = per cent saturation of Hb with $O_2$ or CO | $S\bar{v}O_2$ = saturation of Hb with $O_2$ in mixed venous blood |

| Secondary Symbols (Small Letters) | Examples |
| --- | --- |
| a = arterial blood | $Pa_{CO_2}$ = partial pressure of $CO_2$ in arterial blood |
| v = venous blood | |
| $\bar{v}$ = mixed venous blood | $P\bar{v}_{O_2}$ = partial pressure of $O_2$ in mixed venous blood |
| c = pulmonary capillary blood | $Pc_{CO}$ = partial pressure of CO in pulmonary capillary blood |

### For Lung Volumes

| | | |
| --- | --- | --- |
| VC | = Vital Capacity | = maximal volume that can be expired after maximal inspiration |
| IC | = Inspiratory Capacity | = maximal volume that can be inspired from resting expiratory level |
| IRV | = Inspiratory Reserve Volume | = maximal volume that can be inspired from end-tidal inspiration |
| ERV | = Expiratory Reserve Volume | = maximal volume that can be expired from resting expiratory level |
| FRC | = Functional Residual Capacity | = volume of gas in lungs at resting expiratory level |
| RV | = Residual Volume | = volume of gas in lungs at end of maximal expiration |
| TLC | = Total Lung Capacity | = volume of gas in lungs at end of maximal inspiration |

### Average Values for Adult Male at Rest

For further information about lung function tests see Cotes (1979).*

| | |
|---|---|
| Vital capacity | 4,800 ml |
| Functional residual capacity | 2,400 ml |
| Residual volume | 1,200 ml |
| Total lung capacity | 6,000 ml |
| Tidal volume | 600 ml |
| Respiratory frequency | 12/min |
| Minute volume | 8 l/min |
| Dead-space (Upright position) | |
| anatomical | 150 ml (2 ml/kg) |
| physiological | 190 ml (VD/VT $<0{\cdot}3$) |
| Alveolar ventilation | 5 l/min |
| Oxygen consumption (at rest) | 240 ml/min (10·7 mmol $min^{-1}$) |
| Carbon dioxide output (at rest) | 192 ml/min (8·6 mmol $min^{-1}$) |
| Respiratory exchange ratio (RQ) | 0·8 |
| Peak expiratory flow rate (PEFR) | 500 l/min |
| †($FEV_{1\cdot0}$/FVC)×100 | 85 per cent |
| Diffusing capacity (transfer factor) for carbon monoxide (Dco) | 30 ml $min^{-1}$ mm $Hg^{-1}$ (10 mmol $min^{-1}$ $kPa^{-1}$) |
| Compliance | |
| lungs | 0·2 l cm $H_2O^{-1}$ (2·04 l $kPa^{-1}$) |
| thorax | 0·2 l cm $H_2O^{-1}$ (2·04 l $kPa^{-1}$) |
| total | 0·1 l cm $H_2O^{-1}$ (1·02 l $kPa^{-1}$) |
| Airway resistance | 1·0 cm $H_2O$ $l^{-1}$ sec (0·1 kPa $l^{-1}$ s) |

* Cotes, J. E. (1979). *Lung Function*, 4th edit. Oxford: Blackwell Scientific Publications.

† This is the forced expiratory volume measured over 1 second (FEV 1·0) expressed as a percentage of the forced vital capacity (FVC).

## Composition of Dry Air (Vol per cent)[1]

| | |
|---|---|
| Nitrogen | 78·08 |
| Oxygen | 20·95 |
| Argon | 0·93 |
| Carbon dioxide | 0·03 |
| Other gases | trace amounts |

GAS TENSIONS IN INSPIRED AIR, ALVEOLAR GAS AND BLOOD

| | *Inspired air* | | *Alveolar gas* | | *Arterial blood* | | *Mixed venous blood* | |
|---|---|---|---|---|---|---|---|---|
| | mm Hg | (kPa) | mm Hg | (kPa) | mm Hg | (kPa) | mm Hg | (kPa) |
| Nitrogen | 590 | (78·6) | 564 | (75·2) | 567 | (75·6) | 567 | (75·6) |
| Oxygen | 158 | (21·1) | 102 | (13·6) | 99 | (13·2) | 40 | (5·3) |
| Carbon dioxide | [0·2 | (—)] | 40 | (5·3) | 40 | (5·3) | 46 | (6·1) |
| Water vapour | 5 | (0·7) | 47 | (6.3) | 47 | (6·3) | 47 | (6.3) |
| Total (excluding argon) | 753 | (100) | 753 | (100) | 753 | (100) | 700 | (93)[2] |

Note: 1. Partial pressure (kPa) and per cent composition of gas (at sea level) are numerically similar.
2. The sum of the partial pressures of gases in venous blood is considerably smaller than that in arterial blood.

## Conversion of Gas Volumes

1. To convert ml of gas/100 ml into mmol/l and vice versa:

$$\text{mmol/l} = \frac{\text{ml/100 ml}}{2{\cdot}24^*}$$

$$\text{ml/100 ml} = 2{\cdot}24 \times \text{mmol/l}$$

2. Temperature and pressure corrections
   ATPS = ambient temperature and pressure, saturated.
   BTPS = body temperature and ambient pressure, saturated.
   STPD = standard temperature (0° C) and pressure (760 mm Hg), dry.

Gas volumes may be measured under various conditions of temperature, pressure and saturation with water vapour. In the field of respiratory physiology, these volumes are usually corrected to BTPS. Conversions are made using the combined gas equation:

$$\frac{P_1V_1}{T_1} = \frac{P_2V_2}{T_2}$$

P = pressure minus the water vapour pressure
V = volume of gas
T = absolute temperature (K), = °C + 273

* (The molar volume of an *ideal* gas at 0° and 760 mm Hg is 22·414 l. In the case of $CO_2$, the molar volume is 22·257 l).

BIOCHEMICAL VALUES

For many of these values there is considerable variation in the "normal range" quoted by different laboratories.

| | *Old Units* | *SI Units* | *Conversion factors* Old Units to SI Units Multiply by: | *Conversion factors* SI Units to Old Units Multiply by: |
|---|---|---|---|---|
| Bicarbonate | 23–30 mEq/l | 23–30 mmol/l | — | — |
| Bilirubin | 0·3–1·2 mg/100 ml | 5–20 μmol/l | 17·1 | 0·0585 |
| Calcium (total) | 90–102 mg/l | 2·25–2·55 mmol/l | 0·025 | 40·1 |
| Calcium (ionised) | 46–50 mg/l | 1·15–1·25 mmol/l | 0·025 | 40·1 |
| Chloride | 95–110 mEq/l | 95–110 mmol/l | — | — |
| Cortisol | 8–26 μg/100 ml | 0·22–0·71 μmol/l | 0·0276 | 36·3 |
| Creatinine; | | | | |
| Men | 0·6–1·2 mg/100 ml | 53–106 μmol/l | 88·4 | 0·0113 |
| Women | 0·5–1·0 mg/100 ml | 44–88 μmol/l | | |
| Fasting Blood Glucose: | 75–105 mg/100 ml | 4·2–5·8 mmol/l | 0·056 | 18·0 |
| Iron | 67–150 μg/100 ml | 12–27 μmol/l | 0·179 | 5·59 |
| Iron Binding Capacity | 224–420 μg/100 ml | 40–75 μmol/l | 0·179 | 5·59 |
| Lead | 10–40 μg/100 ml | 0·5–1·9 μmol/l | 0·0483 | 20·7 |
| Magnesium | 1·5–2·4 mg/100 ml | 0·6–1·0 mmol/l | 0·411 | 2·43 |
| Phosphate | 2·4–4·3 mg/100 ml | 0·8–1·4 mmol/l | 0·323 | 3·10 |
| Potassium | 3·3–4·4 mEq/l | 3·3–4·4 mmol/l | | |
| Protein-bound Iodine | 4–8 μg/100 ml | 320–640 nmol/l | 78·8 | 0·0127 |
| Protein | | | | |
| Albumin | 4·0–5·5 g/100 ml | 40–55 g/l | 10 | 0·1 |
| Globulin | 1·5–3·0 g/100 ml | 15–30 g/l | | |
| Fibrinogen | 0·2–0·5 g/100 ml | 2–5 g/l | | |
| Total | 6·0–8·0 g/100 ml | 60–80 g/l | | |
| Sodium | 134–143 mEq/l | 134–143 mmol/l | — | — |
| Thyroxine (T4) | 4·8–10·3 μg/100 ml | 62–133 nmol/l | 12·9 | 0·078 |
| Triglycerides (fasting) | 60–160 mg/100 ml | 0·7–1·8 mmol/l | 0·0113 | 88·5 |
| Urate (Uric Acid) | | | | |
| Men | 3·6–8·0 mg/100 ml | 0·21–0·48 mmol/l | 0·0595 | 16·8 |
| Women | 2·1–6·0 mg/100 ml | 0·13–0·36 mmol/l | | |
| Urea | 18–41 mg/100 ml | 3·0–7·0 mmol/l | 0·167 | 6·01 |

(Enzymes have not been included because of the very different "normal ranges" quoted by various laboratories.)

## Haematological Values

| | *Old Units* | *SI Units* |
|---|---|---|
| B.12 (serum) | 180–1,000 pg/ml | 180–1,000 ng/l |
| Folate (serum) | 6–15 ng/ml | 14–34 nmol/l |
| Erythrocyte Sedimentation Rate (ESR)-Westergren | 2–12 mm in 1 hour | 2–12 mm in 1 hour |
| Haemoglobin: | | |
| Men | 14–18 g/100 ml | 14–18 g/dl |
| Women | 12–16 g/100 ml | 12–16 g/dl |
| At Birth | 17–20 g/100 ml | 17–20 g/dl |
| Haematocrit (PCV or packed cell volume) | | |
| Men | 42–52 per cent | 0·42–0·52 |
| Women | 37–47 per cent | 0·37–0·47 |
| Platelets | 150,000–400,000/$mm^3$ | 150–400 × $10^9$/l |
| Reticulocytes | 0·2–2·0 per cent | 0·2–2·0% |
| White Cells | 4,000–10,000/$mm^3$ | 4·0–10·0 × $10^9$/l |
| Neutrophils | 40–75 per cent | |
| Lymphocytes | 20–50 per cent | |
| Monocytes | 2–10 per cent | |
| Eosinophils | 1–6 per cent | |
| Basophils | 0–1 per cent | |

## Cerebrospinal Fluid

| | *Old Units* | *SI Units* |
|---|---|---|
| Cells | <5/$mm^3$ | <5 × $10^9$/l |
| Chloride | 120–130 mEq/l | 120–130 mmol/l |
| Glucose | 50–75 mg/100 ml | 2·8–4·2 mmol/l |
| Pressure | 70–180 mm $H_2O$ | 0·7–1·8 kPa |
| Protein, total | 15–45 mg/100 ml | 15–45 mg/100 ml |

## Urine

| | *Old Units* | *SI Units* |
|---|---|---|
| Calcium | 100–250 mg/24 hours | 2·5–6·2 mmol/24 hours |
| Creatinine | 0·8–1·8 g/24 hours | 7–16 mmol/24 hours |
| Inorganic phosphate | 0·5–1·5 g/24 hours | 16–48 mmol/24 hours |
| Potassium | 25–100 mEq/24 hours | 25–100 mmol/24 hours |
| Sodium | 130–260 mEq/24 hours | 130–260 mmol/24 hours |
| Urea | 10–30 g/24 hours | 170–500 mmol/24 hours |
| Vanillylmandelic acid (VMA) | 1–7 mg/24 hours | 5–35 μmol/24 hours |

## Body Water

Body water expressed as percentage of body weight:

| | *Adults* | | |
|---|---|---|---|
| | *Men* | *Women* | *Infants* |
| Total body water | 60 | 50 | 75 |
| Intracellular | 40 | 30 | 40 |
| Extracellular | 20 | 20 | 35 |
| a) Intravascular | 4 | 4 | 5 |
| b) Interstitial | 16 | 16 | 30 |

Water *intake* (Adult) per 24 hours

| | |
|---|---|
| As liquid........ | 1,500 ml |
| As food ......... | 1,000 ml (including 300 ml water of oxidation) |
| Total......... | 2,500 ml |

Water *elimination* (Adult) per 24 hours

| | |
|---|---|
| Skin.................. | 500 ml |
| Lungs................. | 400 ml |
| Faeces................. | 100 ml |
| Urine................. | 1,500 ml |
| Total............... | 2,500 ml |

## Gastric Secretion

Fasting juice

| | |
|---|---|
| Volume............. | 20–100 ml |
| pH................. | 0·9–1·5 |
| Emptying time....... | 3–6 hours |

# Index

# Index